TEXTBOOK OF AIDS MEDICINE

SECOND EDITION

TEXTBOOK OF AIDS MEDICINE

SECOND EDITION

Edited by

Thomas C. Merigan, Jr., MD
George E. and Lucy Becker Professor of Medicine
Director, Center for AIDS Research
Stanford University
Stanford, California

John G. Bartlett, MD
Professor of Medicine
Chief, Division of Infectious Diseases
Johns Hopkins University School of Medicine
Baltimore, Maryland

Dani Bolognesi, PhD
Director, Center for AIDS Research
James B. Duke Professor of Experimental Surgery
Vice-Chairman, Department of Surgery for Research and Development
Duke University Medical Center
Durham, North Carolina

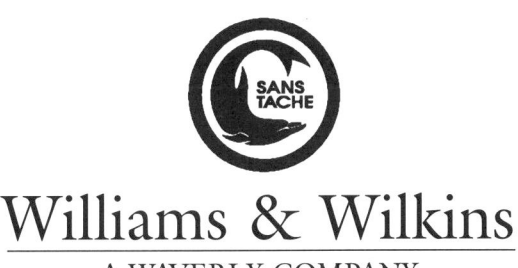

Williams & Wilkins
A WAVERLY COMPANY

BALTIMORE • PHILADELPHIA • LONDON • PARIS • BANGKOK
BUENOS AIRES • HONG KONG • MUNICH • SYDNEY • TOKYO • WROCLAW

Editor: Jonathan W. Pine, Jr.
Managing Editor: Molly L. Mullen
Marketing Manager: Peter Darcy
Project Editor: Peter J. Carley

Copyright © 1999 Williams & Wilkins

351 West Camden Street
Baltimore, Maryland 21201-2436 USA

Rose Tree Corporate Center
1400 North Providence Road
Building II, Suite 5025
Media, Pennsylvania 19063-2043 USA

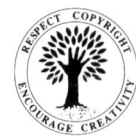

All rights reserved. This book is protected by copyright. No part of this book may be reproduced in any form or by any means, including photocopying, or utilized by any information storage and retrieval system without written permission from the copyright owner.

The publisher is not responsible (as a matter of product liability, negligence or otherwise) for any injury resulting from any material contained herein. This publication contains information relating to general principles of medical care which should not be construed as specific instructions for individual patients. Manufacturers' product information and package inserts should be reviewed for current information, including contraindications, dosages and precautions.

Printed in the United States of America

First Edition, 1994

Library of Congress Cataloging-in-Publication Data

Textbook of AIDS medicine.—2nd ed. / Thomas C. Merigan, Jr., John
  G. Bartlett, Dani Bolognesi. ome.
    p.   cm.
  Includes bibliographical references and index.
  ISBN 0-683-30216-7
  1. AIDS (Disease)   I. Merigan, Thomas C., 1934-   . II. Title:
Textbook of acquired immunodeficiency syndrome medicine.
  [DNLM: 1. Acquired Immunodeficiency Syndrome.   WC 503 T355 1999]
RC607.A26T48   1999
616.97′92—DC21
DNLM/DLC
for Library of Congress   97-42697
                                                                                                      CIP

The publishers have made every effort to trace the copyright holders for borrowed material. If they have inadvertently overlooked any, they will be pleased to make the necessary arrangements at the first opportunity.

To purchase additional copies of this book, call our customer service department at **(800) 638-0672** or fax orders to **(800) 447-8438**. For other book services, including chapter reprints and large quantity sales, ask for the Special Sales department.

Canadian customers should call **(800) 665-1148**, or fax **(800) 665-0103**. For all other calls originating outside of the United States, please call **(410) 528-4223** or fax us at **(410) 528-8550**.

Visit Williams & Wilkins on the Internet: **http://www.wwilkins.com** or contact our customer service department at **custserv@wwilkins.com**. Williams & Wilkins customer service representatives are available from 8:30 am to 6:00 pm, EST, Monday through Friday, for telephone access.

                                                                 99 00 01 02
                                             1 2 3 4 5 6 7 8 9 10

To our wives:

Joan Merigan
Jean Bartlett
Sarah Bolognesi

Preface to the Second Edition

This Second Edition of the *Textbook of AIDS Medicine* is now edited by Dani Bolognesi of Duke University, John Bartlett of Johns Hopkins University School of Medicine, and myself. We wish our former first edition colleague, Samuel Broder, the best in his new undertakings in industry.

This Second Edition of the book has changed with the continuing explosion of new information and insights in AIDS medicine. We have come to know much more about the virus and the way it affects the host, as well as how to control the infection in man and its complications, since 1994 when the First Edition premiered at the International AIDS Meeting in Berlin. Now we know more about this agent than any other pathogen infecting humans, including why some individuals seem to resist infection and why others have long periods without disease, as well as how to successfully combine drugs to control the infection and the disease that it causes.

It appears that, with proper albeit expensive treatment (hence, not available to most of the world's infected population), we can turn this infection into an arrested disease like hypertension or diabetes. Because the virus continues to be a moving target for drug therapy, continuing research on the mechanism underlying drug failure is also required. Experience with HIV infection has also allowed the development of new strategies for control of most of the opportunistic infections and, to some degree, for the cancers that complicate advanced HIV infection. Because of the diversity of viral strains, and the failure of candidate vaccines to achieve what we believe is protective immunity, we have not gone forward with attempts at large-scale vaccine programs to protect the "at risk" populations. However, we predict this will change in the next few years. Clearly, real successes have been achieved, but there is still a long way to go. We hope this volume will be the most comprehensive text available to provide a contemporary picture of where we are currently with this infection.

Thomas C. Merigan, Jr.

Preface to the First Edition

The acquired immunodeficiency disease (AIDS) and its related syndromes have changed (and in some cases shattered) virtually every aspect of medicine and society at large. AIDS has affected basic science, clinical practice, and societal perspectives.

First and foremost, we were required to accept the reality that even as the 20th century draws to a close, it is still possible for a previously unknown pathogen to initiate a pandemic that spares virtually no country. Second, we were made to realize that the distinction between those who perform basic research and those who engage in clinical care has become somewhat blurred. It is very difficult to engage in good science without being informed of the important epidemiological and clinical characteristics of the AIDS pandemic. By the same token, to be a good doctor responsible for the care of patients with AIDS, one must be informed as to the ever-changing developments in basic research and compartmentalization of medical disciplines. To "specialize" in AIDS requires a depth of knowledge in almost every field of medicine. For instance virtually every physician who sees large numbers of patients with AIDS must, in effect, develop some expertise in neoplastic diseases and the relationship between cancer and immune deficiency diseases. For those who view AIDS from a public health policy perspective, there must be a growing recognition that AIDS and poverty are strongly linked. And for those with a medicolegal orientation, any research or clinical agenda in AIDS will have multifaceted civil implications as to the rights and expectations of individuals who may already be facing oppression from society at large.

The purpose of this textbook is to provide the reader with an ability to survey the molecular, biological, immunological, epidemiological, clinical, psychosocial, and ethical issues that inform any discussion of AIDS, while at the same time permitting the reader to focus on any individual area of interest of an in-depth review. The book, in fact, has a special clinical orientation for physicians and physicians-in-training, but it is not intended for clinicians exclusively; and we believe it will have value from a basic research perspective as well.

AIDS, from any perspective, is not a simple disease; and this textbook makes no attempt to shield the reader artificially from this complexity. Moreover, in several arenas, there is no uniformity of opinion or consensus even on fundamental points. This book aims to draw together the views of leading figures in AIDS, and deliberately offers the viewpoints of different groups analyzing the same topic where we believe the reader can benefit from, or at least must know of, the diversity in thinking and analysis. Knowledge in AIDS, as perhaps in no other field of medicine, is in a constant state of flux; and several uncertainties as well as overt contradictions cannot be avoided. We believe it is better for the reader to have an opportunity to weigh and consider different points of view to better absorb new facts and ideas as they unfold in the future. Certain interrelated topics, such as the biochemical pharmacology of certain agents, therapeutic options, viral drug resistance, and so forth, are approached in multiple ways through the vehicle of several distinct chapters.

There is at this time no safe and effective vaccine against human immunodeficiency virus-1 (HIV-1), the causative agent of AIDS. Similarly, there is as yet no agent or combination of agents capable of curing the disease. Nevertheless, a substantial level of progress has been made; and there is no question that large numbers of patients can benefit from technologies already available, if such technologies are applied with skill and commitment. In one sense, we intend this textbook to serve as a source of optimism, albeit an optimism that must be tempered by the formidable characteristics of the disease. We have no illusions about how many challenges remain; but at the same time, our patients and the public at large are entitled to know the progress that has been made, so that the momentum for greater progress can be maintained.

Finally, progress against AIDS will certainly bring progress against many diseases not thought to be connected to AIDS. HIV-1 is one of the most complex retroviruses known. To illustrate, all retroviruses contain the gag, pol, and env genes, in addition to the *cis*-acting sequences acted on by the Gag and Pol proteins, plus important sequences affecting the control of transcription, splicing, and polyadenylation. In the cases of the known simpler animal retroviruses (e.g., murine leukemia virus), viral transcription, splicing, and polyadenylation are regulated by cell-encoded proteins. The additional genes found in complex retroviruses such as HIV-1 encode proteins that act in concert with cellular proteins to control transcription, splicing, and polyadenylation. Our ability to understand these steps is likely to enhance profoundly our ability to understand cellular differentiation and proliferation in normal and disease states particularly within the immune network where HIV-1 establishes residence and brings about dramatic dysfunction and dysregulation. Providing this message is a major goal of this book. We anticipate that this will be a long-term responsibility.

Samuel Broder
Thomas C. Merigan, Jr.
Dani Bolognesi

Contributors

Gordon L. Ada, DSc
Professor
John Curtin School of Medical Research
Australian National University
Canberra, Australia

Richard F. Ambinder, MD
Associate Professor
Departments of Oncology, Pathology, and Pharmacology
Johns Hopkins University School of Medicine
Baltimore, Maryland

Sam Avrett, MPH
Associate Scientific Director
International AIDS Vaccine Initiative
Washington, D.C.

Jan Balzarini, PhD
Professor
Department of Microbiology and Immunology
Faculty of Medicine
Katholieke Universiteit Leuven
Leuven, Belgium

John G. Bartlett, MD
Professor of Medicine
Chief, Division of Infectious Diseases
Johns Hopkins University School of Medicine
Baltimore, Maryland

Robert E. Baughn, MD
Associate Career Scientist
Research Service
Veterans Affairs Medical Center
Associate Professor
Microbiology and Immunology
Baylor College of Medicine
Houston, Texas

Joseph R. Berger, MD
Professor and Chairman
Department of Neurology and Internal Medicine
University of Kentucky School of Medicine
Lexington, Kentucky

William A. Blattner, MD
Professor of Medicine
Associate Director
Institute of Human Virology
University of Maryland
Baltimore, Maryland

Robert C. Bollinger MD, MPH
Associate Professor of Medicine and International Health
Division of Infectious Diseases
Johns Hopkins University School of Medicine
Department of International Health
Johns Hopkins University School of Hygiene and Public Health
Baltimore, Maryland

Dani Bolognesi, PhD
James B. Duke Professor of Experimental Surgery
Vice-Chairman, Department of Surgery for Research and Development
Duke University Medical Center
Durham, North Carolina

Jacques J. Bourgoignie, MD
Professor of Medicine
Director, Division of Nephrology and Hypertension
Department of Medicine
University of Miami School of Medicine
Miami, Florida

Mitchell S. Cappell, MD, PhD
Director, Gastrointestinal Motility and Laser Endoscopy Unit
Division of Gastroenterology
Department of Medicine
Robert Wood Johnson (Rutgers) Medical School
New Brunswick, New Jersey

Melvin D. Cheitlin, MD
Former Chief of Radiology
San Francisco General Hospital
Emeritus Professor of Medicine
University of California, San Francisco
San Francisco, California

Paul R. Clapham, PhD
Senior Virologist
Institute of Cancer Research
Chester Beatty Laboratories
London, United Kingdom

Clay J. Cockerell, MD
Director, Division of Dermatopathology
University of Texas Southwestern Medical Center
Associate Professor of Dermatology and Pathology
Dallas, Texas

Jon H. Condra, PhD
Senior Investigator
Antiviral Research
Merck Research Laboratories
West Point, Pennsylvania

Robert W. Coombs MD, PhD, FRCP(C)
Associate Professor
Departments of Laboratory Medicine and Medicine
University of Washington
Seattle, Washington

Deborah J. Cotton, MD, MPH
Assistant Professor of Medicine
Harvard Medical School
Infectious Disease Unit
Massachusetts General Hospital
Boston, Massachusetts

M. Patricia D'Souza, PhD
Scientist
Division of AIDS
National Institute of Allergy and Infectious Disease
National Institutes of Health
Bethesda, Maryland

Erik De Clerq, MD, PhD
Professor
Department of Microbiology and Immunology
Faculty of Medicine
Katholieke Universiteit Leuven
Leuven, Belgium

Don C. Des Jarlais, PhD
Director of Research
Chemical Dependency Institute
Beth Israel Medical Center
Professor of Community Medicine
Mt. Sinai School of Medicine
New York, New York

Elizabeth S. Didier, PhD
Research Scientist
Tulane Regional Primate Research Center
Adjunct Associate Professor
School of Public Health and Tropical Medicine
Tulane University
New Orleans, Louisiana

Jorge Diego, MD
Assistant Professor of Medicine
Division of Nephrology
Department of Medicine
University of Miami School of Medicine
Miami, Florida

Douglas T. Dieterich, MD, FACP
Associate Professor of Medicine
Department of Medicine
New York University School of Medicine
New York, New York

John P. Doweiko, MD
Staff Physician
Department of Medicine
Beth Israel Deaconess Medical Center
Division of Infectious Disease
Division of Hematology and Oncology
Harvard Medical School
Boston, Massachusetts

Michael P. Dubé, MD
Assistant Professor of Clinical Medicine
Division of Infectious Diseases
Department of Medicine
University of Southern California School of Medicine
Medical Director, Rand-Schrader 5P21 HIV Clinic
Los Angeles County–University of Southern California Medical Center
Cardinal Firm Director, Los Angeles County–University of Southern California Medical Service
Los Angeles, California

James P. Dunn, MD
Associate Professor
Department of Ophthalmology
Wilmer Eye Institute
Johns Hopkins Hospital
Baltimore, Maryland

Emelio A. Emini, PhD
Vice President
Department of Antiviral and Vaccine Research
Merck Research Laboratories
West Point, Pennsylvania

John W. Erickson, MD
Director, Structural Biochemistry Program
National Cancer Institute
Frederick Cancer Research and Development Center
Frederick, Maryland

Myron Essex, DVM, PhD
Chairman, Department of Cancer Biology
Harvard University School of Public Health
Chairman, Harvard AIDS Institute
Harvard University
Boston, Massachusetts

Anthony S. Fauci, MD
Director, National Institute of Allergy and Infectious Diseases
National Institutes of Health
Bethesda, Maryland

Margaret A. Fischl, MD
Director, Comprehensive AIDS Program
University of Miami School of Medicine
Miami, Florida

John C. Fletcher, PhD
Professor
Department of Biomedical Ethics and Religious Studies
University of Virginia
Charlottesville, Virginia

Ian W. Flinn
Assistant Professor
Department of Oncology
Division of Hematologic Medicine
Johns Hopkins University School of Medicine
Baltimore, Maryland

Samuel R. Friedman, PhD
Principal Investigator
National Development and Research Institutes, Inc.
New York, New York

Alvin E. Friedman-Kien, MD
Professor
Department of Dermatology and Microbiology
New York University Medical Center
New York, New York

Robert C. Gallo, MD
Professor and Director
Institute of Human Virology
University of Maryland
Baltimore, Maryland

Julie Louise Gerberding, MD, MPH
Associate Professor
Department of Medicine (Infectious Diseases) and Epidemiology and Biostatistics
University of California, San Francisco
Director, Epidemiology and Prevention Interventions Center
San Francisco General Hospital
San Francisco, California

Robert Goldin, MD, MRCPath
Senior Lecturer
Department of Histopathology
St. Mary's Hospital
London, United Kingdom

Michael S. Gottlieb, MD
Assistant Clinical Professor of Medicine
University of California, Los Angeles, School of Medicine
Los Angeles, California

Barney S. Graham, MD, PhD
Professor
Department of Medicine
Vanderbilt University School of Medicine
Nashville, Tennessee

John S. Greenspan, MD
Professor of Oral Biology and Oral Pathology
Chair, Department of Stomatology
Director, Oral AIDS Center, School of Dentistry
Professor of Pathology
Director, AIDS Clinical Research Center
School of Medicine, University of San Francisco
San Francisco, California

Deborah Greenspan, BSc, BDS, ScD
Clinical Professor
Department of Stomatology and Clinical Director
Oral AIDS Center, School of Dentistry
University of California, San Francisco
San Francisco, California

Tom Grothe, RN, ANP, MFCC
Charge Nurse
Coming Home Hospice
San Francisco, California

Carl Grunfeld, MD, PhD
Professor of Medicine
Department of Medicine
University of California, San Francisco
Co-Director, Special Diagnostic and Treatment Unit
Medical Service, Department of Veterans Affairs Medical Center
San Francisco, California

Holly Hagan, MPH
Seattle/King County Health Department
Seattle, Washington

Scott Hammer, MD
Associate Professor of Medicine
Beth Israel Deaconess Medical Center
Harvard Medical School
Boston, Massachusetts

David K. Henderson, MD
Associate Director for Quality Assurance and Hospital Epidemiology, Clinical Center
Office of the Director
Warren Grant Magnuson Clinical Center
National Institutes of Health
Bethesda, Maryland

Denis Henrard, PhD
V.I. Technologies, Inc.
New York, New York

Martin S. Hirsch, MD
Professor
Department of Medicine
Harvard Medical School
Director, Clinical AIDS Research
Massachusetts General Hospital
Boston, Massachusetts

Gary N. Holland, MD
Professor of Ophthalmology
University of California, Los Angeles, School of Medicine
Director, University of California, Los Angeles, Ocular Inflammatory Disease Center
Jules Stein Eye Institute
Los Angeles, California

Cecelia Hutto, MD
Associate Professor of Pediatrics
Division of Pediatric Infectious Diseases and Immunology
University of Miami School of Medicine
Miami, Florida

Margaret I. Johnston, PhD
Scientific Director, International AIDS Vaccine Initiative
Washington, D.C.

Phyllis J. Kanki, DVM, SD
Associate Professor of Pathobiology
Department of Cancer Biology
Harvard University School of Public Health
Boston, Massachusetts

Judith E. Karp, MD
Professor of Medicine
Department of Oncology
University of Maryland Cancer Center
Baltimore, Maryland

David T. Karzon, MD
Professor Emeritus of Pediatrics
Department of Pediatrics
Vanderbilt University Medical School
Nashville, Tennessee

Richard A. Kaslow, MD
Professor
Department of Epidemiology, Medicine, Microbiology
University of Alabama at Birmingham School of Public Health
Birmingham, Alabama

J. Michael Kilby, MD
Assistant Professor of Medicine
Division of Infectious Diseases
Medical Director
University of Alabama at Birmingham AIDS Outpatient Clinic
University of Alabama at Birmingham
Birmingham, Alabama

Marie Laga, MD, MSC
Epidemiologist
Institute of Tropical Medicine
Antwerp, Belgium

Stephen W. Lagakos, PhD
Professor
Department of Biostatistics
Scientific Director, Center for Biostatistics and AIDS Research
Harvard University School of Public Health
Boston, Massachusetts

Edward A. Lew, MD
Gastroenterology Fellow
Division of Digestive Diseases
University of California, Los Angeles
Los Angeles, California

xiv Contributors

Oliver Liesenfeld, MD
Department of Medical Microbiology
 and Infectious Diseases Immunology
Freie Universitat Berlin
Berlin, Germany

Jeffrey S. Loutit, MBCHB
Staff Physician
Department of Medicine
Palo Alto Veterans Administration
 Medical Center
Palo Alto, California

Janice Main, FRCP
Senior Lecturer
Department of Medicine
Imperial College of Medicine
St. Mary's Hospital
London, United Kingdom

Eugene O. Major, PhD
Chief, Laboratory of Molecular
 Medicine and Neuroscience
National Institute of Neurological
 Disorders and Stroke
National Institutes of Health
Bethesda, Maryland

Douglas J. Manion, MD
Research Fellow
Department of Medicine
Massachusetts General Hospital
Boston, Massachusetts

Henry Masur, MD
Chief, Critical Care Medicine
 Department
Warren Grant Magnuson Clinical
 Center
National Institutes of Health
Bethesda, Maryland

J. Allen McCutchan, MD, MSc
Professor of Medicine
Department of Medicine
University of California, San Diego
San Diego, California

Alastair McNair, MA, MRCP
Department of Medicine
St. Mary's Hospital Medical School
London, United Kingdom

Delinda E. Mercer, PhD
Counseling Psychologist
Department of Psychiatry
University of Pennsylvania
Philadelphia, Pennsylvania

Thomas C. Merigan, Jr., MD
George E. and Lucy Becker Professor
 of Medicine
Director, Center for AIDS Research
Stanford University Medical Center
Stanford, California

David S. Metzger, PhD
Director, Opiate/AIDS Research
Center for Studies of Addiction
Department of Psychiatry
University of Pennsylvania
Philadelphia, Pennsylvania

Michelle N. Meyer, MA
Doctoral Candidate, Religious Ethics
University of Virginia
Charlottesville, Virginia

Steven A. Miles, MD
Associate Professor of Medicine
Division of Hematology and Oncology
University of California, Los Angeles,
 School of Medicine
Clinic Director, University of
 California, Los Angeles, Center for
 Clinical AIDS Research and
 Education
Los Angeles, California

Hiroaki Mitsuya, MD, PhD
Chief, Experimental Retroviral Section
Department of Medicine Branch
National Institutes of Health National
 Cancer Institute
Bethesda, Maryland

José G. Montoya, MD
Assistant Professor of Medicine
Division of Infectious Diseases and
 Geographic Medicine
Stanford University Medical Center
Stanford, California

Daniel M. Musher, MD
Chief, Infectious Disease Section
Veterans Affairs Medical Center
Professor of Medicine
Professor of Microbiology/
 Immunology
Acting Chief, Infectious Disease
 Division
Baylor College of Medicine
Houston, Texas

Michelle Onorato, MD
Assistant Professor
Department of Internal Medicine
University of Texas Medical Branch
Galveston, Texas

Carmen Ortiz-Butcher, MD
Assistant Professor of Clinical Medicine
Division of Nephrology
University of Miami School of
 Medicine
Miami, Florida

June E. Osborn, MD
President, Josiah Macy, Jr. Foundation
New York, New York

Michael A. Poles, MD
Department of Internal Medicine
New York University Medical Center
New York, New York

Michael A. Polis, MD, MPH
Senior Investigator
Laboratory of Immunoregulation
Intramural AIDS Program
National Institutes of Health National
 Institute of Allergy and Infectious
 Diseases
Bethesda, Maryland

Richard B. Pollard, MD
Professor
Department of Internal Medicine,
 Microbiology, Immunology, and
 Pathology
University of Texas Medical Branch
Galveston, Texas

Maria S. Pombo de Oliveira, MD, PhD
Onco-Hematology-Immunology
Instituto Nacional de Cancer
Rio de Janeiro, Brazil

William G. Powderly, MD, FRCPI
Associate Professor of Medicine
Co-Director, Division of Infectious
 Diseases
Washington University
St. Louis, Missouri

Richard W. Price, MD
Professor
Department of Neurology
University of California, San Francisco
Chief, Neurology Service
San Francisco General Hospital
San Francisco, California

Thomas C. Quinn, MD, MSc
Professor of Medicine
Department of Medicine
Johns Hopkins University School of Medicine
Baltimore, Maryland

Robert R. Redfield, MD
Professor or Medicine
Profesor of Immunology and Microbiology
Associate Director
Institute of Human Virology
University of Maryland
Baltimore, Maryland

Patricia Reichelderfer, PhD
Program Virologist
Division of AIDS
National Institute of Allergy and Infectious Disease
National Institutes of Health
Rockville, Maryland

Jack S. Remington, MD
Professor of Medicine
Division of Infectious Diseases and Geographic Medicine
Stanford University School of Medicine
Marcus A. Krupp Research Chair and Chairman
Department of Immunology and Infectious Disease
Research Institute, Palo Alto Med. Foundation
Palo Alto, California

Douglas D. Richman, MD
Professor
Department of Pathology and Medicine
University of California, San Diego
La Jolla, California
Director, Virology Laboratory and Research Center for AIDS and HIV Infection
San Diego Veterans Affairs Medical Center
San Diego, California

Michael S. Saag, MD
Professor of Medicine
Division of Infectious Diseases
University of Alabama at Birmingham
Birmingham, Alabama

Sharon Safrin, MD, FACP
Director, Clinical Research
Gilead Sciences, Inc
Foster City, California
Associate Clinical Professor, Department of Medicine, and Epidemiology and Biostatistics
University of California, San Francisco
San Francisco, California

Fred R. Sattler, MD
Associate Professor of Medicine
Department of Medicine
University of Southern California School of Medicine
Los Angeles County–University of Southern California Medical Center
Los Angeles, California

Morris Schambelan, MD
Chief, Division of Endocrinology
San Francisco General Hospital
San Francisco, California

Dr. Bernhard Schwartländer, MD, PhD
Senior Epidemiologist
Team Leader Epidemiology, Monitoring and Evaluation
UNAIDS—The Joint United Nations Programme on HIV/AIDS
Geneva, Switzerland

Gwendolyn B. Scott, MD
Professor of Pediatrics
Director Division of Pediatric Infectious Disease and Immunology
Department of Pediatrics
University of Miami School of Medicine
Miami, Florida

Deborah E. Sellmeyer, MD
University of California, San Francisco
Postdoctoral Fellow
Division of Endocrinology
San Francisco, California

Mark S. Senak, JD
Senior Vice President
National Director, Health Policy
Manning, Selvage, and Lee
New York, New York

Leslie K. Serchuck, MD
Senior Clinical Investigator
HIV and AIDS Malignancy Branch
National Institutes of Health
Bethesda, Maryland

Robert W. Shafer, MD
Assistant Professor of Medicine
Division of Infectious Diseases and Geographic Medicine
Stanford University School of Medicine
Stanford, California

Rosemary Soave, MD
Associate Professor of Medicine and Public Health
Cornell University Medical College
Attending Physician
New York Hospital–Cornell Medical Center
New York, New York

Kenneth Stanley, PhD
Executive Director, Center for Biostatistics in AIDS Research
Harvard University School of Public Health
Boston, Massachusetts

Mario Stevenson, PhD
Professor
Program in Molecular Medicine
Department of Molecular Genetics and Microbiology
University of Massachusetts
Worcester, Massachusetts

Paul B. Tabereaux, MPH
Epidemiologic Staff Assistant
University of Alabama School of Medicine
University of Alabama at Birmingham School of Public Health
Birmingham, Alabama

Howard C. Thomas, BSc, MBBS, PhD, FRCPath
Professor
Department of Medicine
St. Mary's Hospital
London, United Kingdom

Sten H. Vermund, MD, PhD
Professor and Chair
Department of Epidemiology
University of Alabama at Birmingham School of Public Health
Director, Division of Geographic Medicine
Department of Medicine
University of Alabama School of Medicine
Birmingham, Alabama

Paul A. Volberding, MD
Professor of Medicine
University of California, San Francisco
Director, AIDS Program
San Francisco General Hospital
San Francisco, California

Robin A. Weiss, PhD
Professor of Viral Oncology
Institute of Cancer Research
Chester Beatty Laboratories
London, United Kingdom

Lauri Welles, MD
Clinical Associate
HIV and AIDS Malignancies Branch
National Institutes of Health National Cancer Institute
Bethesda, Maryland

Brian Wispelwey, MD
Associate Professor
Department of Medicine
Director, Division of Infectious Diseases Clinic
University of Virginia Health Science Center
Charlottesville, Virginia

Sin-Yew Wang, MD
Tan Tock Seng Hospital
Communicable Disease Center
Singapore

George E. Woody, MD
Chief, Substance Abuse Treatment Unit
Department of Psychiatry
Philadelphia Veterans Affairs Medical Center
Clinical Professor
Department of Psychiatry
University of Pennsylvania School of Medicine
Philadelphia, Pennsylvania

Robert Yarchoan, MD
Head, Retroviral Diseases Section
Department of Medicine Branch
National Institutes of Health National Cancer Institute
Bethesda, Maryland

Lowell S. Young, MD
Director, Kuzell Institute for Arthritis and Infectious Diseases
Medical Research Institute of San Francisco at California Pacific Medical Center
San Francisco, California

Contents

Preface to the First Edition   vii
Preface to the Second Edition   ix
Contributors   xi

Section I. Introduction

1/ **HIV/AIDS at the Millennium**
Robert R. Redfield, William A. Blattner, Robert C. Gallo   3

Section II. Basic Sciences

2/ **The Virus and Its Target Cells**
Paul R. Clapham, Robin A. Weiss   13

3/ **Viral Genes and Their Products**
Mario Stevenson   23

4/ **Natural History of HIV-1 Disease**
J. Michael Kilby, Michael S. Saag   49

5/ **Immunopathogenesis**
M. Patricia D'Souza, Anthony S. Fauci   59

6/ **An Immunologist's View of HIV Infection**
Gordon L. Ada   87

Section III. Epidemiology

7/ **Epidemiology of HIV Sexual Transmission**
Sten H. Vermund, Paul B. Tabereaux, Richard A. Kaslow   101

8/ **Epidemiology of AIDS in the Developing World**
Marie Laga, Bernhard Schwartländer   111

9/ **Public Health, HIV, and AIDS**
June E. Osborn   123

Section IV. Clinical

10/ INTRODUCTION TO THE CLINICAL SPECTRUM OF AIDS
Margaret A. Fischl — 139

11/ AIDS IN WOMEN
Deborah J. Cotton — 151

12/ SPECIAL CONSIDERATIONS IN CHILDREN
Cecelia Hutto, Gwendolyn B. Scott — 163

13/ HIV AMONG INJECTING DRUG USERS: EPIDEMIOLOGY AND EMERGING PUBLIC HEALTH PERSPECTIVES
Don C. Des Jarlais, Holly Hagan, Samuel R. Friedman — 179

14/ *PNEUMOCYSTIS CARINII* PNEUMONIA
Michael P. Dubé, Fred R. Sattler — 191

15/ TOXOPLASMOSIS IN THE SETTING OF AIDS
Oliver Liesenfeld, Sin-Yew Wang, Jack S. Remington — 225

16/ TUBERCULOSIS
Robert W. Shafer, José G. Montoya — 261

17/ NONTUBERCULOUS (ATYPICAL) MYCOBACTERIA
Lowell S. Young — 285

18/ SYPHILIS
Daniel M. Musher, Robert E. Baughn — 297

19/ BACILLARY ANGIOMATOSIS
Jeffrey S. Loutit — 303

20/ TROPICAL DISEASES IN THE HIV-INFECTED TRAVELER
Robert C. Bollinger, Thomas C. Quinn — 315

21/ INTESTINAL PARASITIC INFECTIONS: CRYPTOSPORIDIOSIS AND MICROSPORIDIOSIS
Rosemary Soave, Elizabeth S. Didier — 327

22/ FUNGI
William G. Powderly — 357

23/	**CYTOMEGALOVIRUS INFECTION IN PATIENTS WITH HIV INFECTION** *Michael A. Polis, Henry Masur*	373
24/	**HERPES SIMPLEX AND VARICELLA-ZOSTER VIRUS INFECTIONS IN HIV-INFECTED INDIVIDUALS** *Sharon Safrin*	391
25/	**PROGRESSIVE MULTIFOCAL LEUKOENCEPHALOPATHY** *Joseph R. Berger, Eugene O. Major*	403
26/	**KAPOSI'S SARCOMA AND CLOACOGENIC CARCINOMA: VIRUS-INITIATED MALIGNANCIES** *Steven A. Miles*	421
27/	**OVERVIEW OF AIDS-RELATED LYMPHOMAS: A PARADIGM OF AIDS MALIGNANCIES** *Judith E. Karp*	437
28/	**CLINICAL ASPECTS OF AIDS-RELATED LYMPHOMA** *Richard F. Ambinder, Ian W. Flinn*	451
29/	**OCULAR SEQUELAE** *James P. Dunn, Gary N. Holland*	457
30/	**NEUROLOGIC COMPLICATIONS OF HIV-1 INFECTION AND AIDS** *Richard W. Price*	477
31/	**CUTANEOUS MANIFESTATIONS OF HIV INFECTION** *Clay J. Cockerell, Alvin E. Friedman-Kien*	499
32/	**ORAL MANIFESTATIONS OF HIV INFECTION AND AIDS** *John S. Greenspan, Deborah Greenspan*	521
33/	**GASTROINTESTINAL MANIFESTATIONS OF HIV DISEASE, INCLUDING THE PERITONEUM AND MESENTERY** *Douglas T. Dieterich, Michael A. Poles, Mitchell S. Cappell, Edward A. Lew*	537
34/	**LIVER DISEASE AND AIDS** *Janice Main, Alastair McNair, Robert Goldin, Howard C. Thomas*	567
35/	**RENAL DISEASE AND AIDS** *Jacques J. Bourgoignie, Jorge Diego, Carmen Ortiz-Butcher*	585

36/ CARDIAC INVOLVEMENT IN THE PATIENT WITH AIDS
Melvin D. Cheitlin 601

37/ HEMATOLOGIC MANIFESTATIONS OF HIV INFECTION
John P. Doweiko 611

38/ ENDOCRINE ABNORMALITIES ASSOCIATED WITH HIV INFECTION AND AIDS
Deborah E. Sellmeyer, Carl Grunfeld, Morris Schambelan 629

39/ THE WASTING SYNDROME: PATHOPHYSIOLOGY AND TREATMENT
Carl Grunfeld, Morris Schambelan 643

40/ ASSAYS FOR THE DIAGNOSIS OF HIV INFECTION
Denis Henrard, Patricia Reichelderfer 661

41/ USE OF PLASMA HIV-1 RNA TO ASSESS PROGNOSIS AND MONITOR THERAPY IN HIV-1 INFECTION
Robert W. Coombs, Patricia Reichelderfer 673

Section V. Control and Prevention

42/ AIDS VACCINE DEVELOPMENT
Barney S. Graham, David T. Karzon 689

43/ DEVELOPING HIV VACCINES AND OTHER INTERVENTIONS TO PREVENT AIDS WORLDWIDE
Margaret I. Johnston, Sam Avrett 725

44/ IMMUNE-BASED THERAPIES FOR HIV INFECTION
Michelle Onorato, Richard B. Pollard 743

45/ DRUG DEVELOPMENT

45A/ DISCOVERY AND DEVELOPMENT OF ANTIRETROVIRAL THERAPEUTICS FOR HIV INFECTION
Hiroaki Mitsuya, John Erickson 751

45B/ ANTIRETROVIRAL TREATMENT FOR HIV INFECTION
Leslie K. Serchuck, Lauri Welles, Robert Yarchoan 780

46/ BIOSTATISTICAL CONSIDERATIONS IN THE DESIGN AND ANALYSIS OF AIDS CLINICAL TRIALS
Kenneth Stanley, Stephen W. Lagakos 807

47/ Biochemical Pharmacology

47A/ Nucleoside and Nonnucleoside Reverse Transcriptase Inhibitors Active against HIV
Jan Balzarini, Erik De Clerq   815

47B/ Protease Inhibitors
Emelio A. Emini, Jon H. Condra   848

48/ Strategies for Antiretroviral Therapy in Adult HIV Disease

48A/ Starting and Shifting of Antiretroviral Therapy
Paul A. Volberding   861

48B/ Strategy and Use of Antiretroviral Agents in Combination
Scott Hammer   872

48C/ Mechanisms Underlying Combination Antiretroviral Therapies
Douglas J. Manion, Martin S. Hirsch   885

49/ Viral Resistance to Antiviral Drugs
Douglas D. Richman   891

50/ Alternative, Unconventional, and Unproven Therapies
J. Allen McCutchan   903

51/ Psychotherapy and Counseling for HIV-Positive Individuals
George E. Woody, Delinda E. Mercer, David S. Metzger   911

52/ Hospice Care and Symptom Management
Tom Grothe, Michael Gottlieb   923

53/ HIV Transmission in the Health Care Environment
David K. Henderson   935

54/ Managing Occupational Exposures to HIV
Julie Louise Gerberding   947

55/ AIDS and Ethics: Clinical, Social, and Global
John C. Fletcher, Michelle N. Meyer, Brian Wispelwey   951

56/ LEGAL MANIFESTATIONS OF AIDS
Mark S. Senak 979

Section VI. Diseases Associated with Other Retroviruses

57/ HUMAN IMMUNODEFICIENCY VIRUS TYPE 2 (HIV-2)
Myron Essex, Phyllis J. Kanki 985

58/ HUMAN T-LYMPHOTROPIC VIRUSES: HTLV-I AND HTLV-II
William A. Blattner, Maria S. Pombo de Oliveira 1003

Index 1031

Color Plates

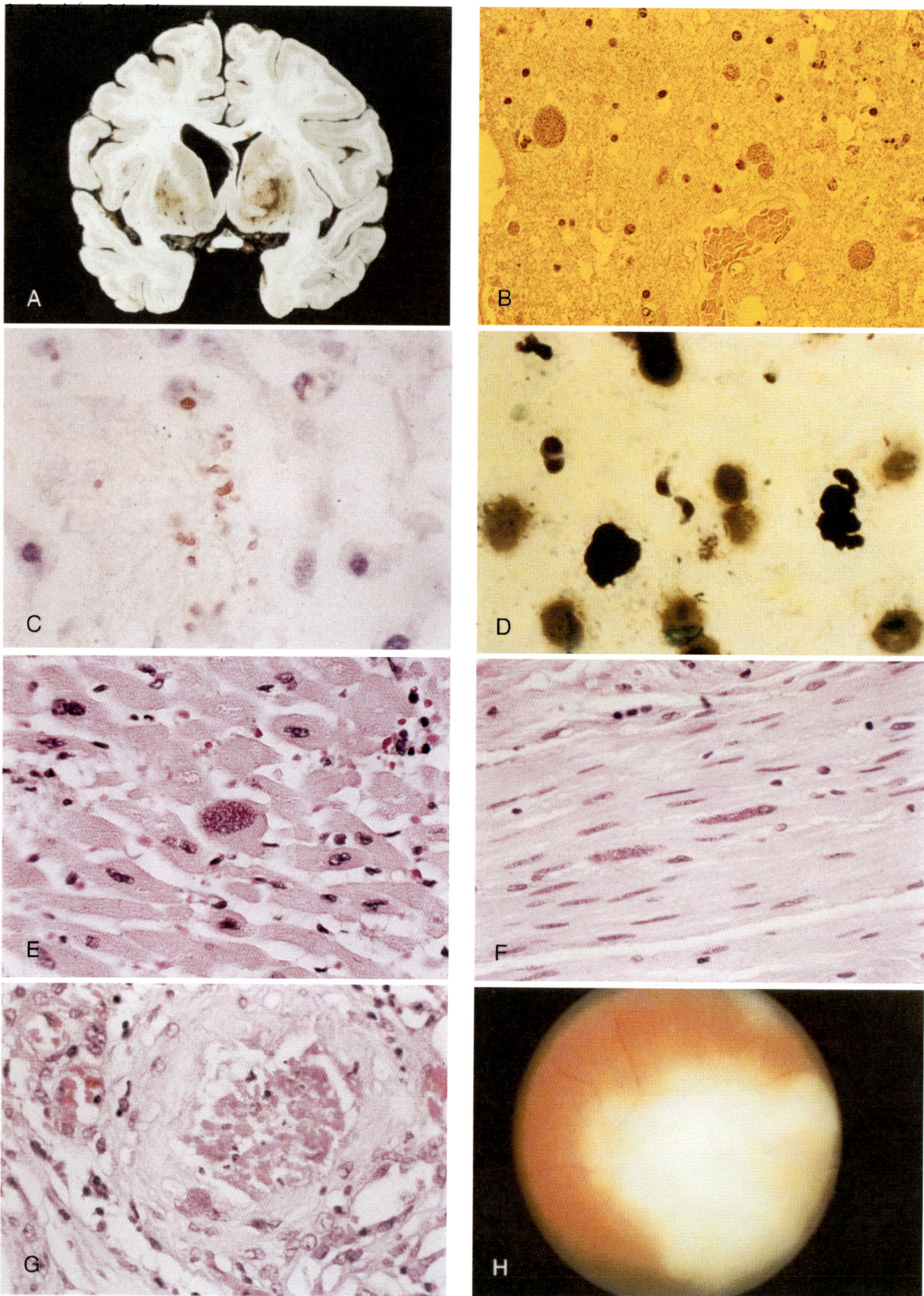

Color Plates

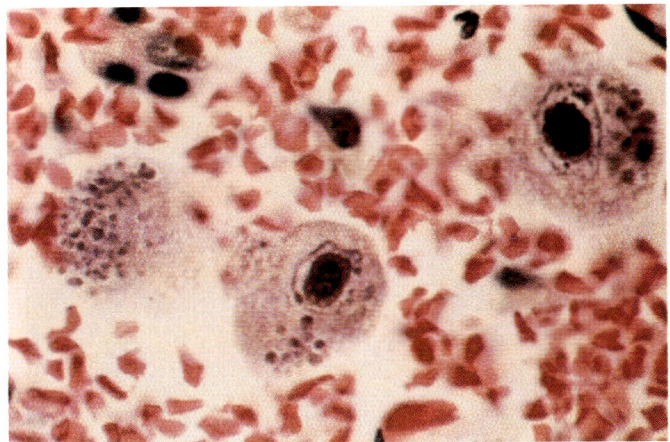

23.1

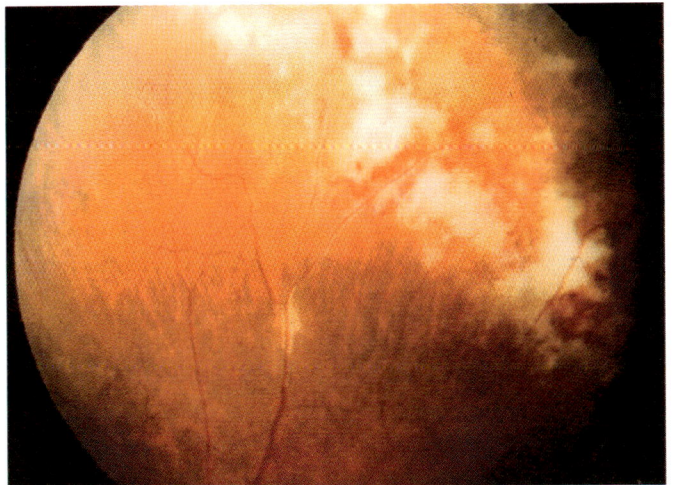

23.2

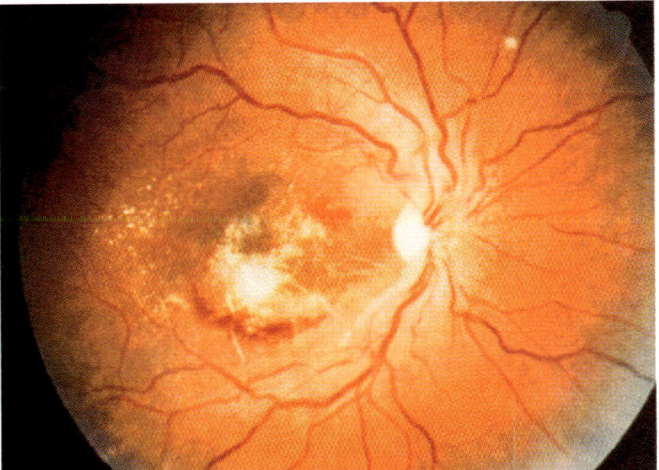

23.3

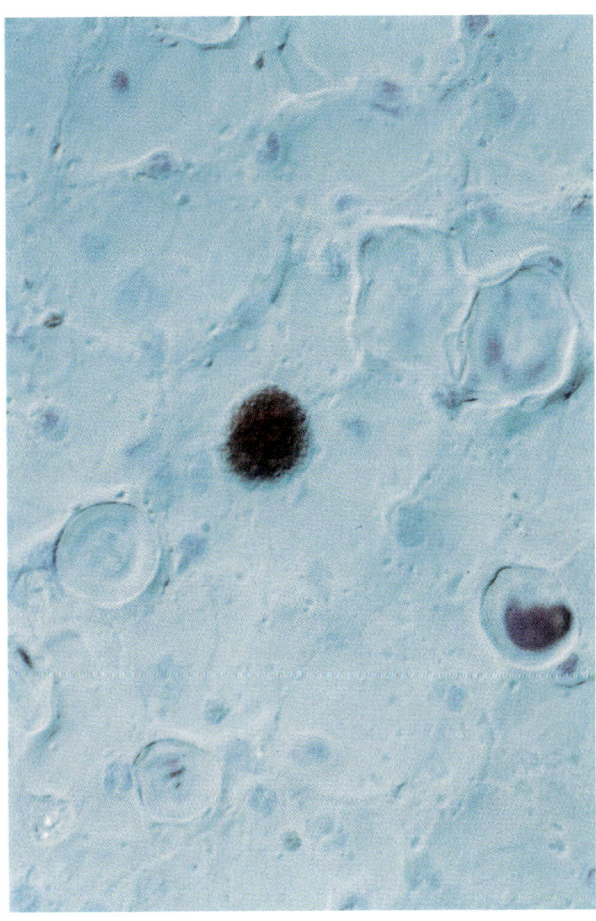

25.8

Color Plates

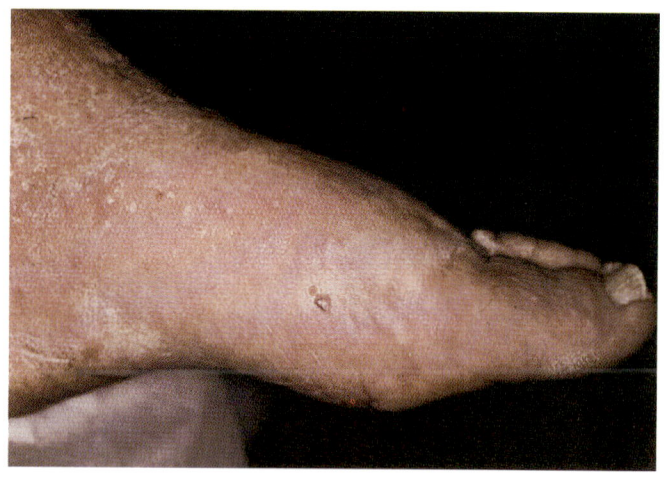
26.1

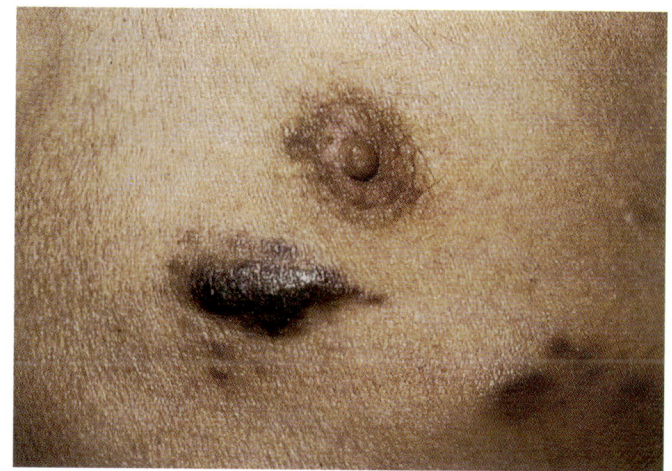
26.2

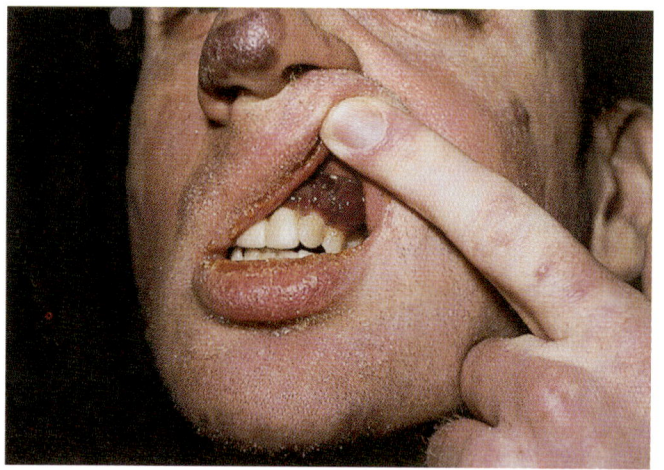
26.3

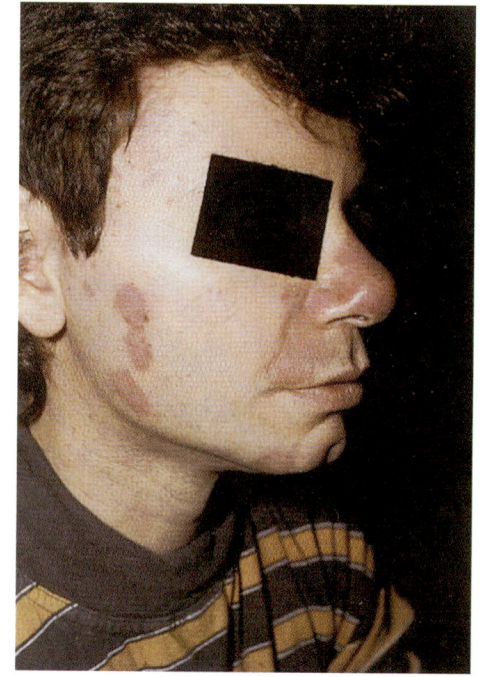
26.4

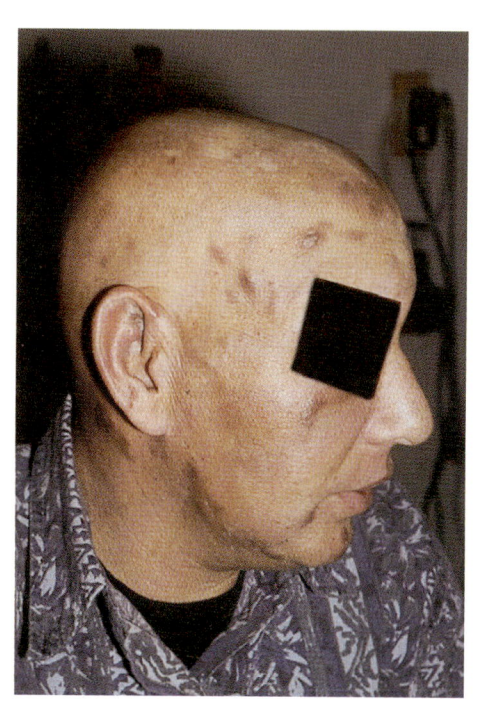
26.5

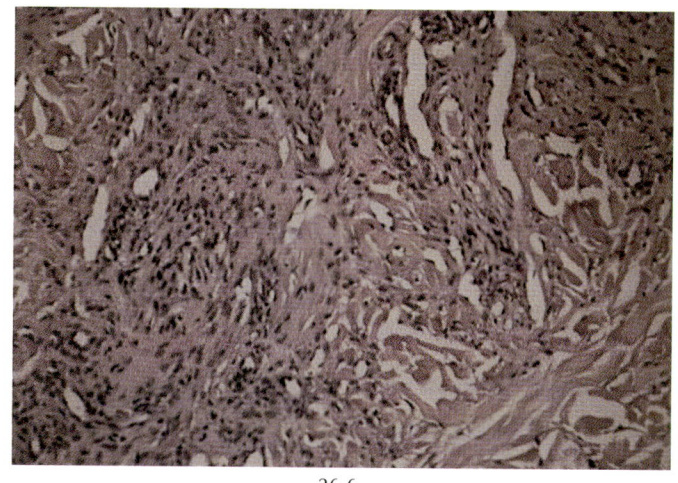
26.6

Color Plates

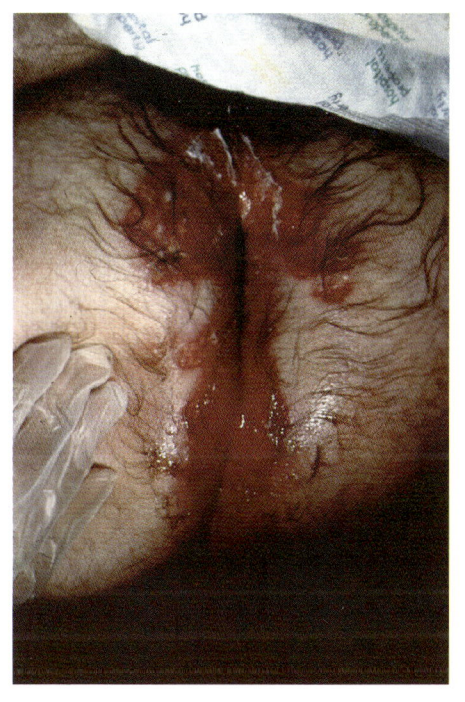

31.1

31.2

31.3

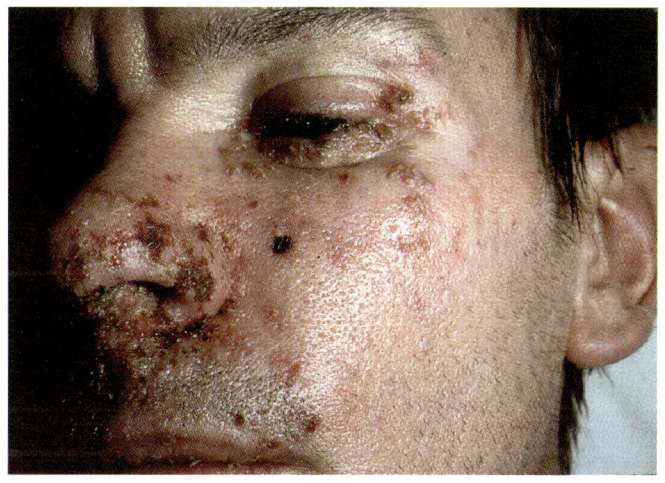

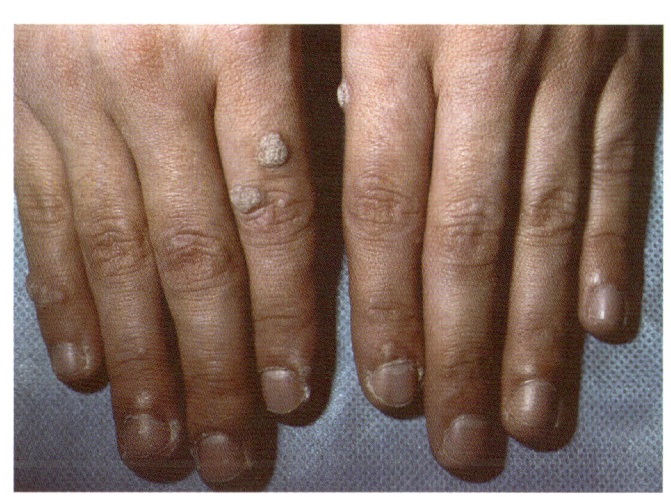

31.4

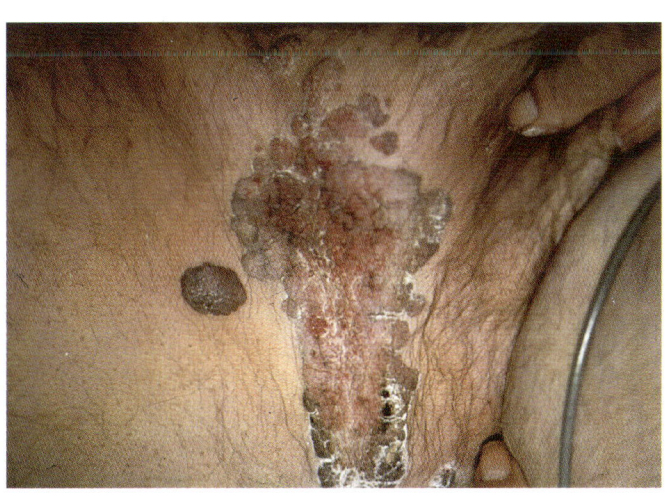

31.5

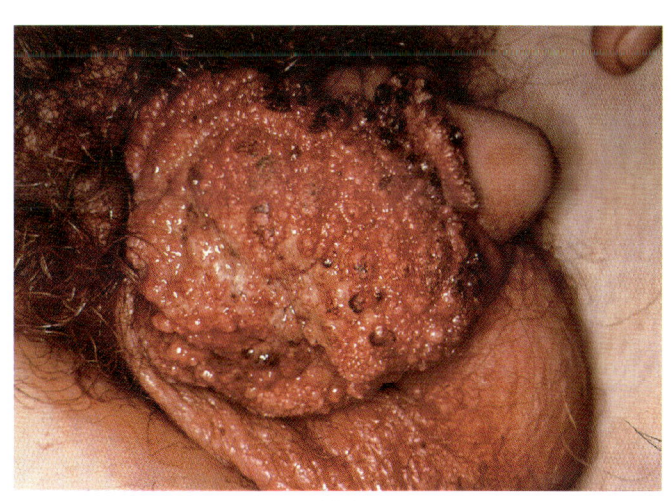

31.6

Color Plates

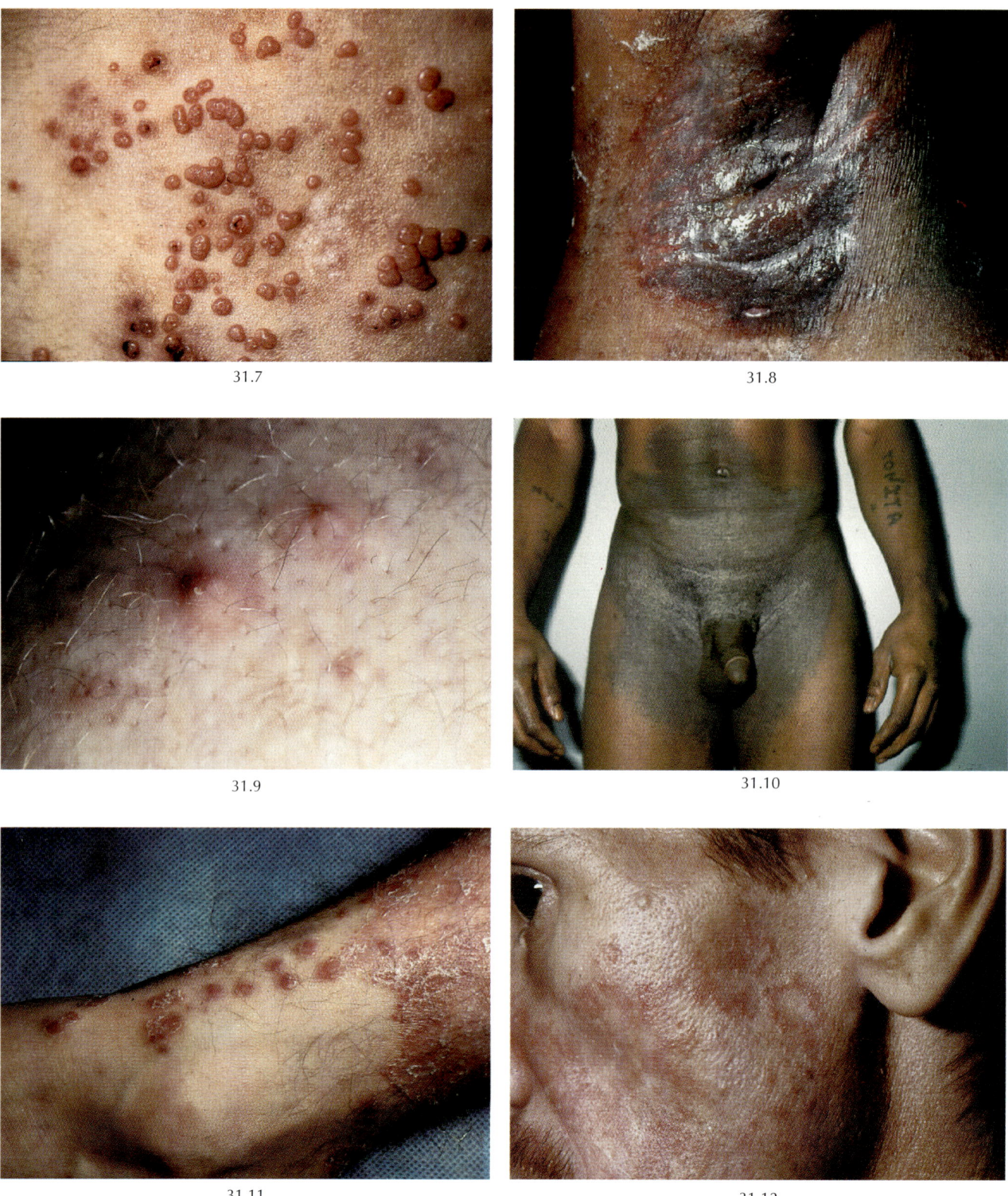

31.7

31.8

31.9

31.10

31.11

31.12

Color Plates

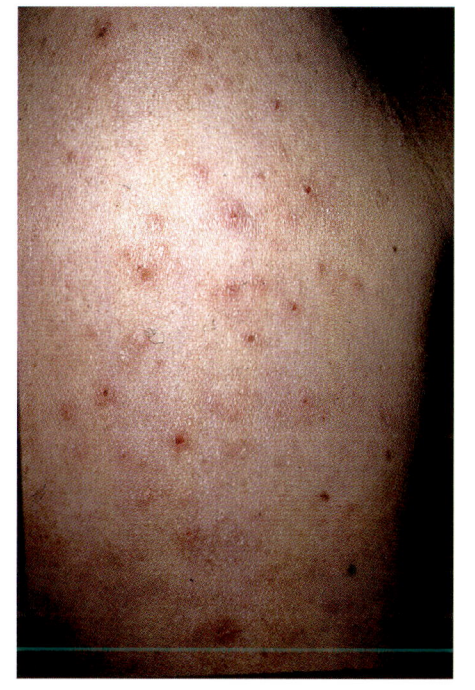
31.13

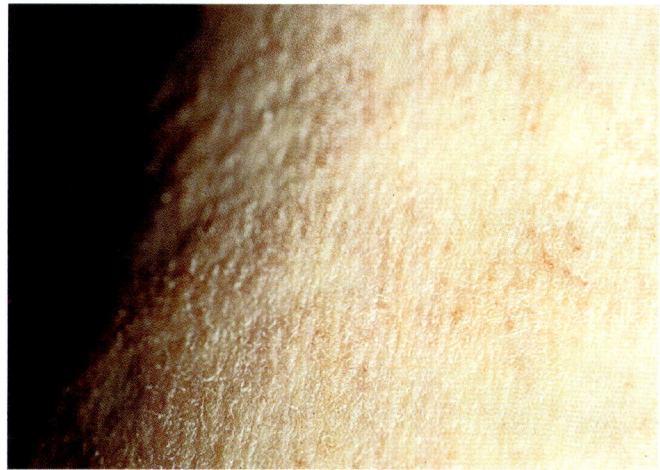
31.14

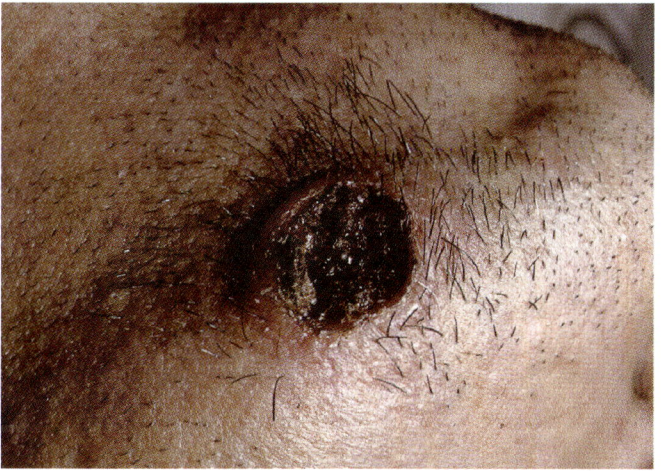
31.15

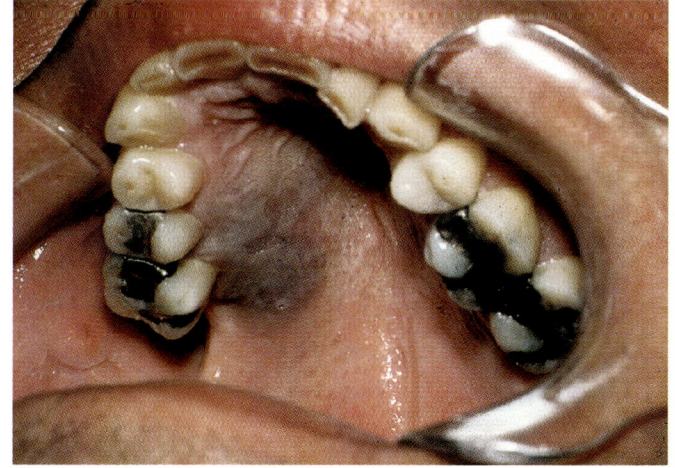
32.1

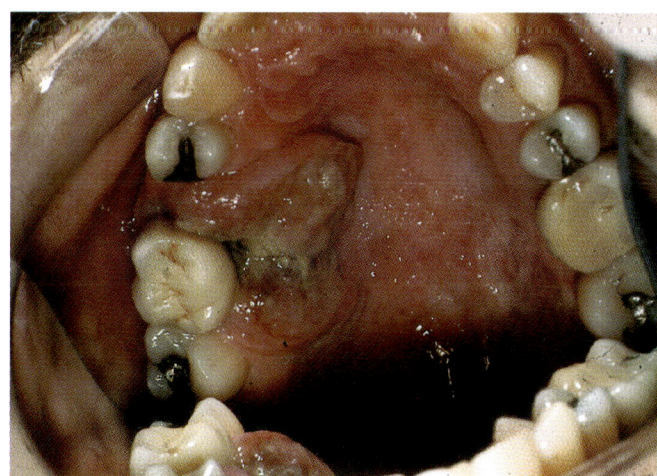
32.2

Color Plates

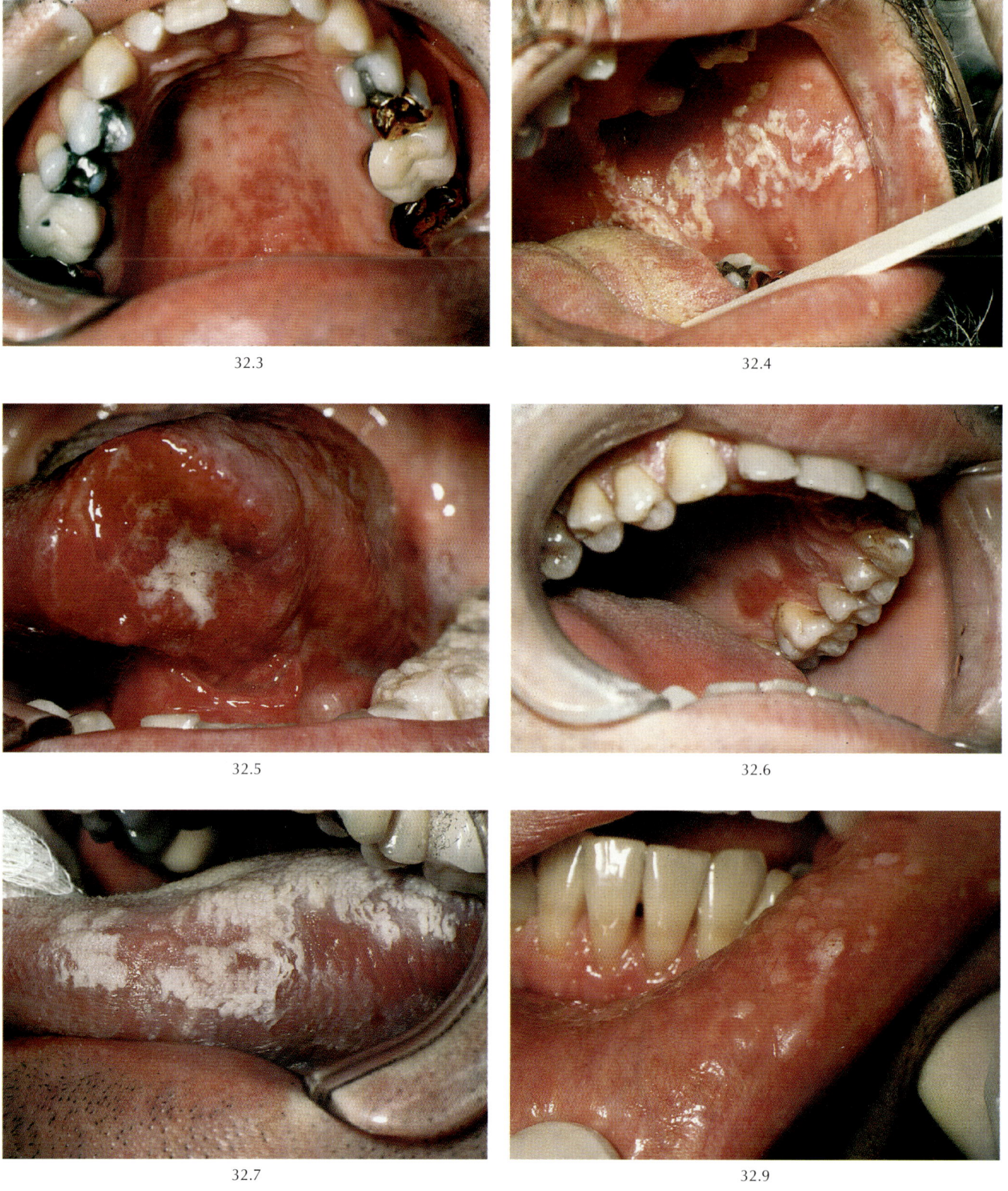

32.3

32.4

32.5

32.6

32.7

32.9

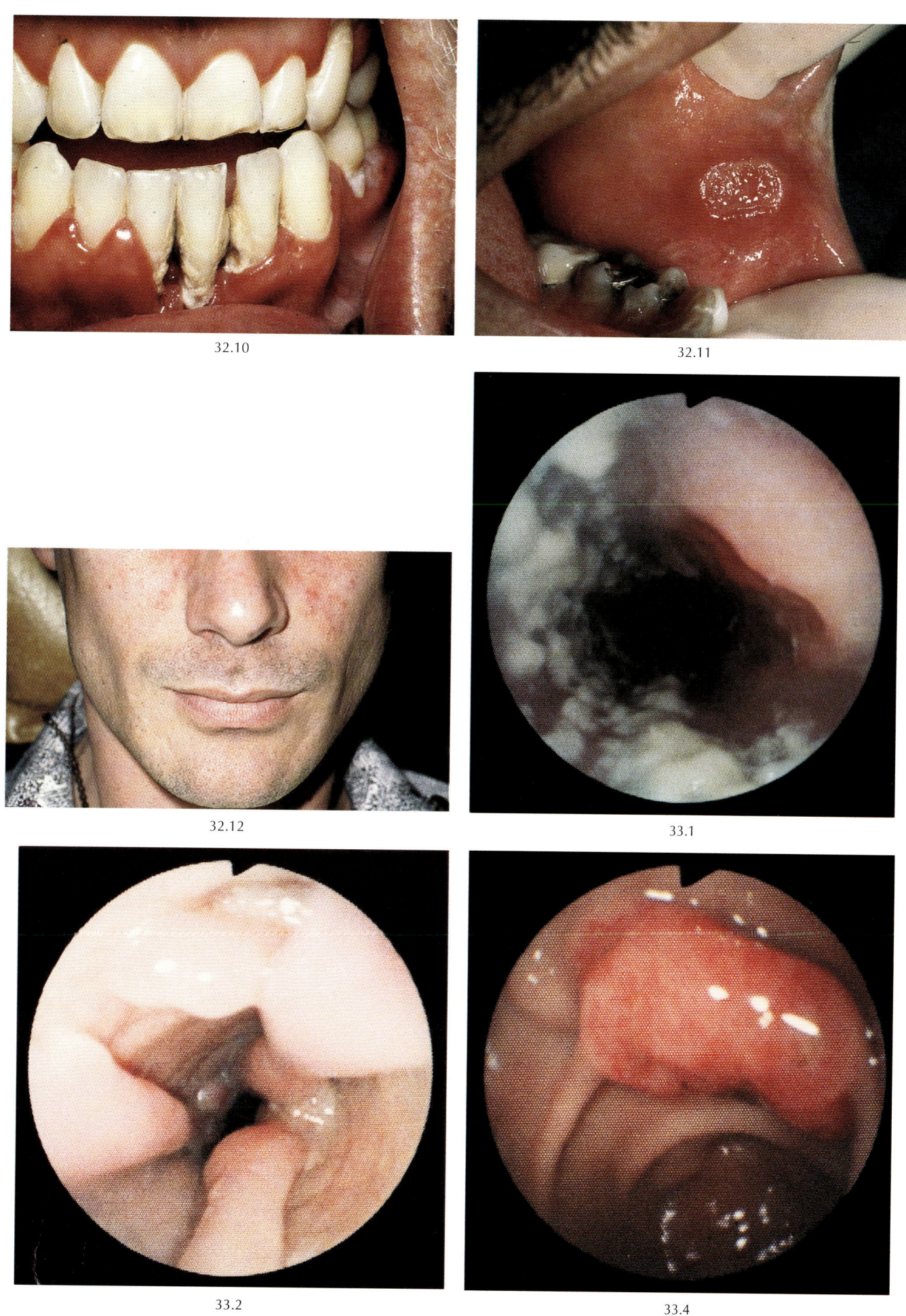

32.10

32.11

32.12

33.1

33.2

33.4

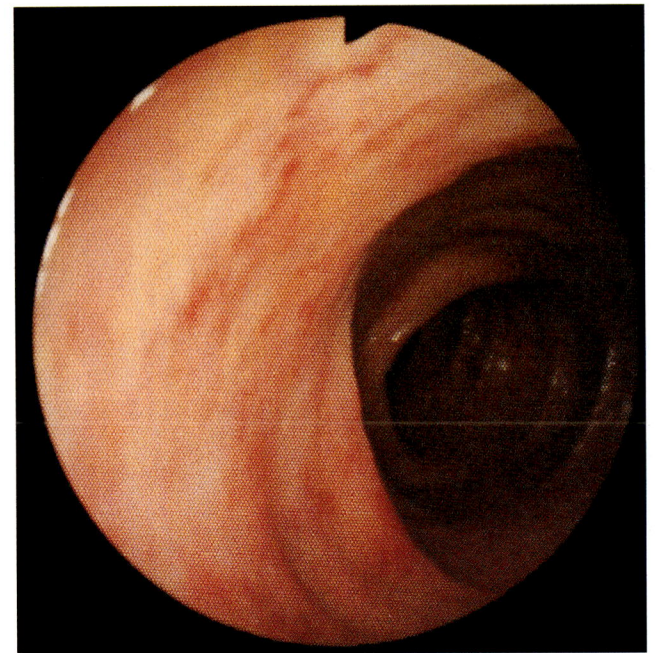

33.6

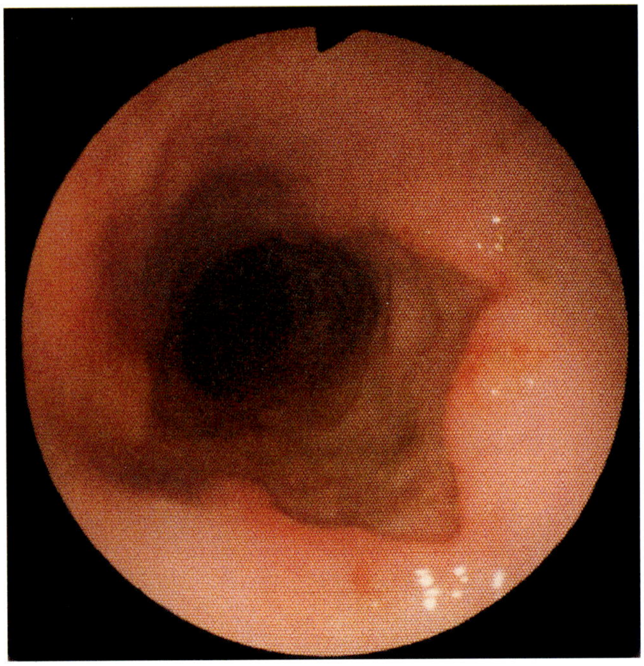

33.7

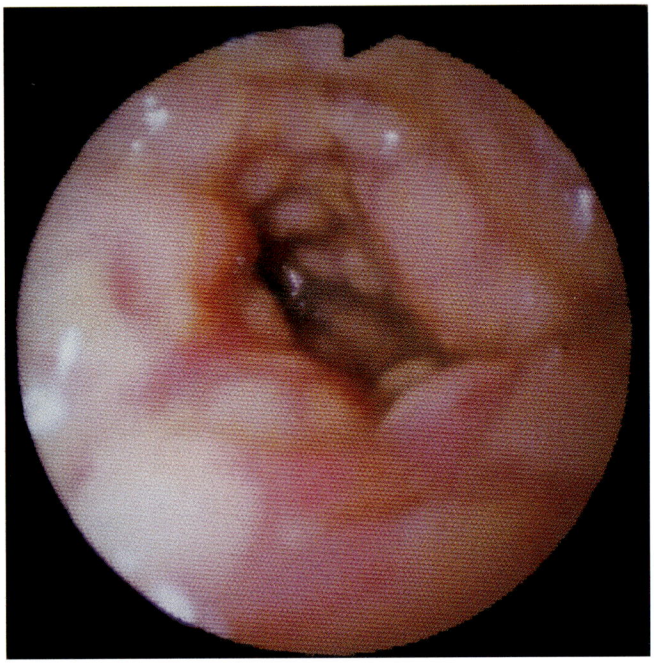

33.8

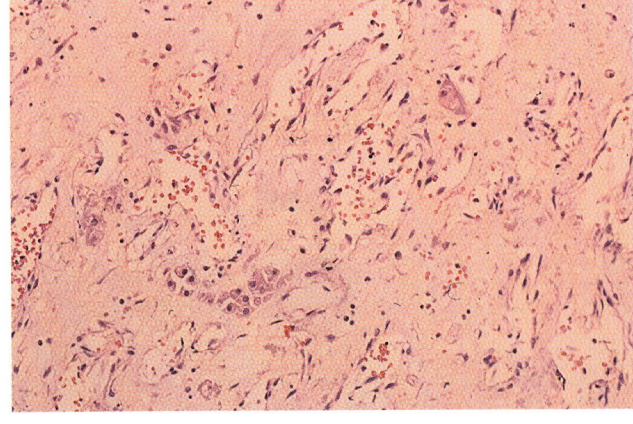

33.9

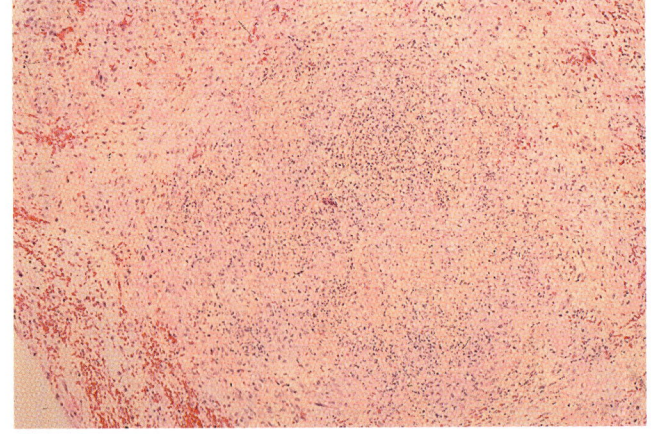

33.10

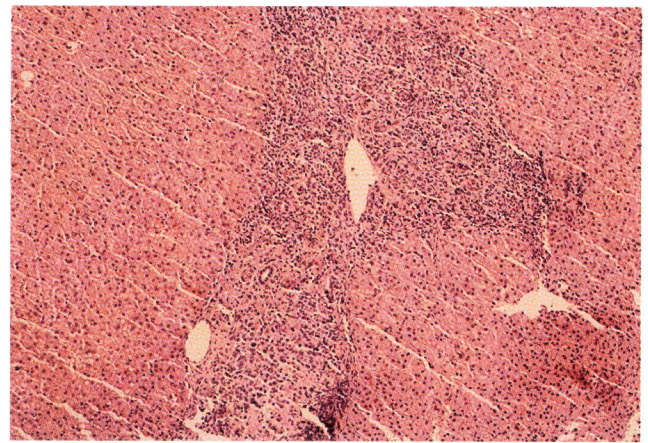

33.11

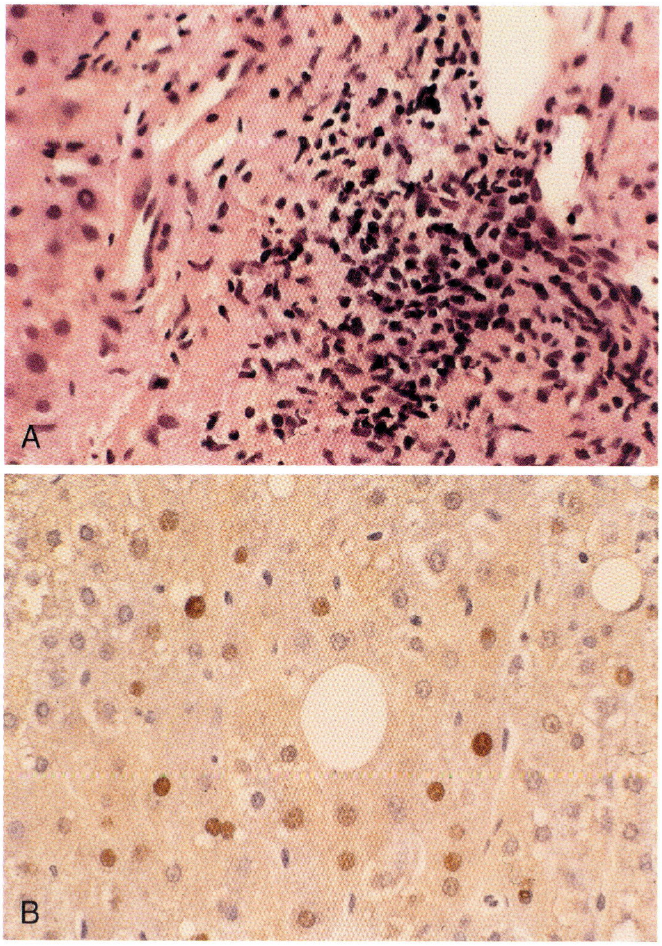

34.1A & B

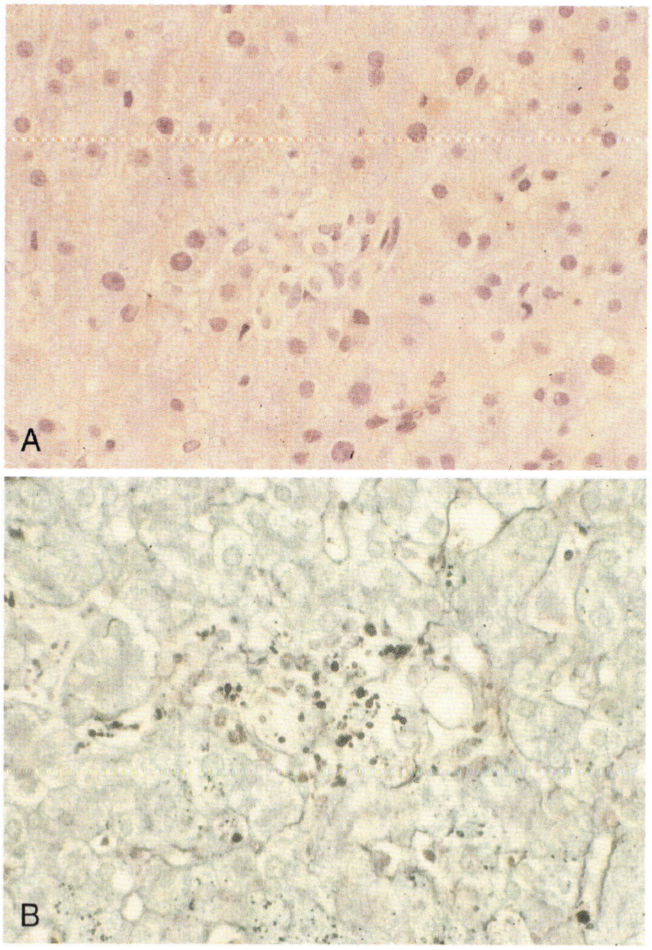

34.2A & B

Color Plates

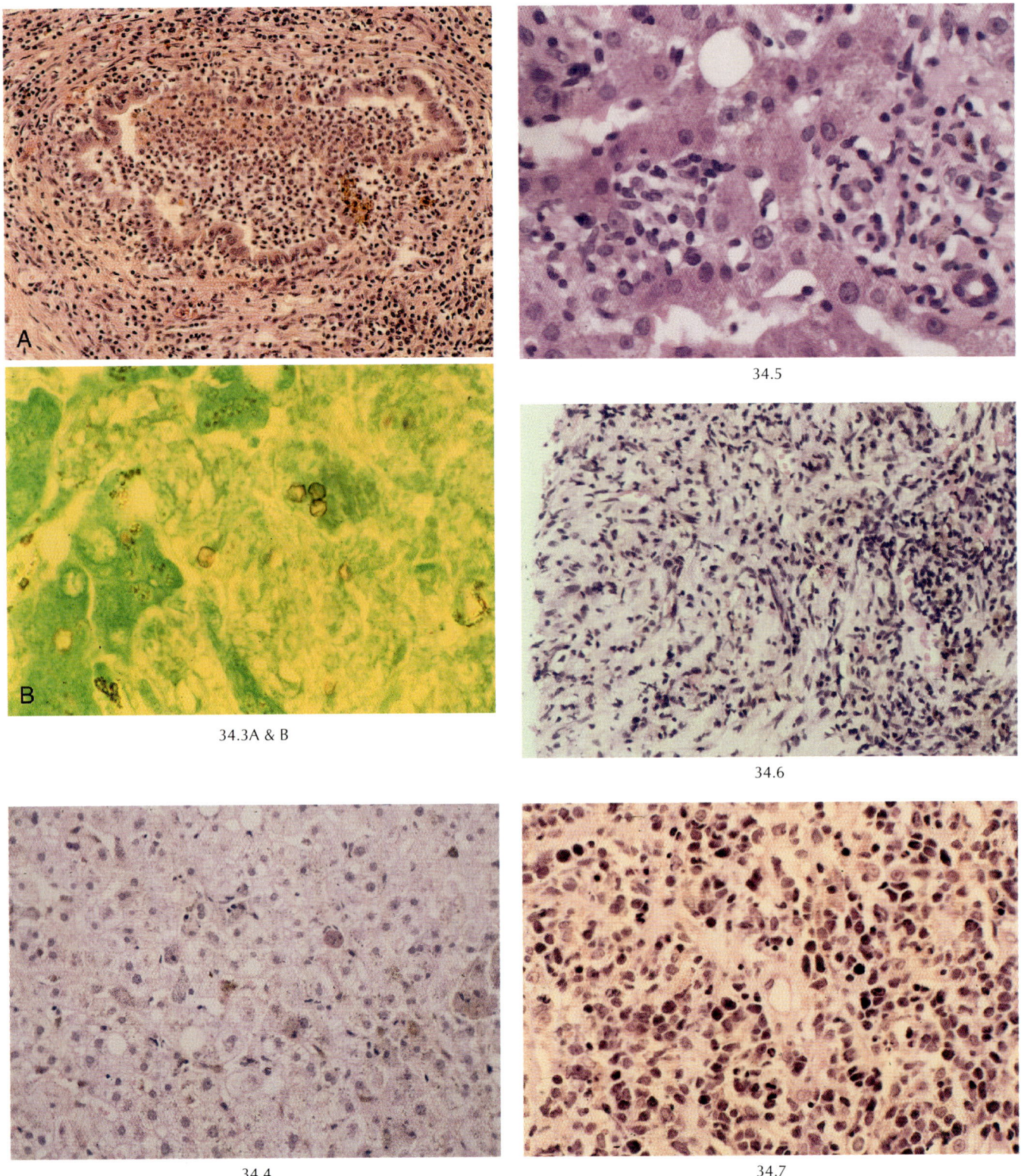

34.3A & B

34.5

34.6

34.4

34.7

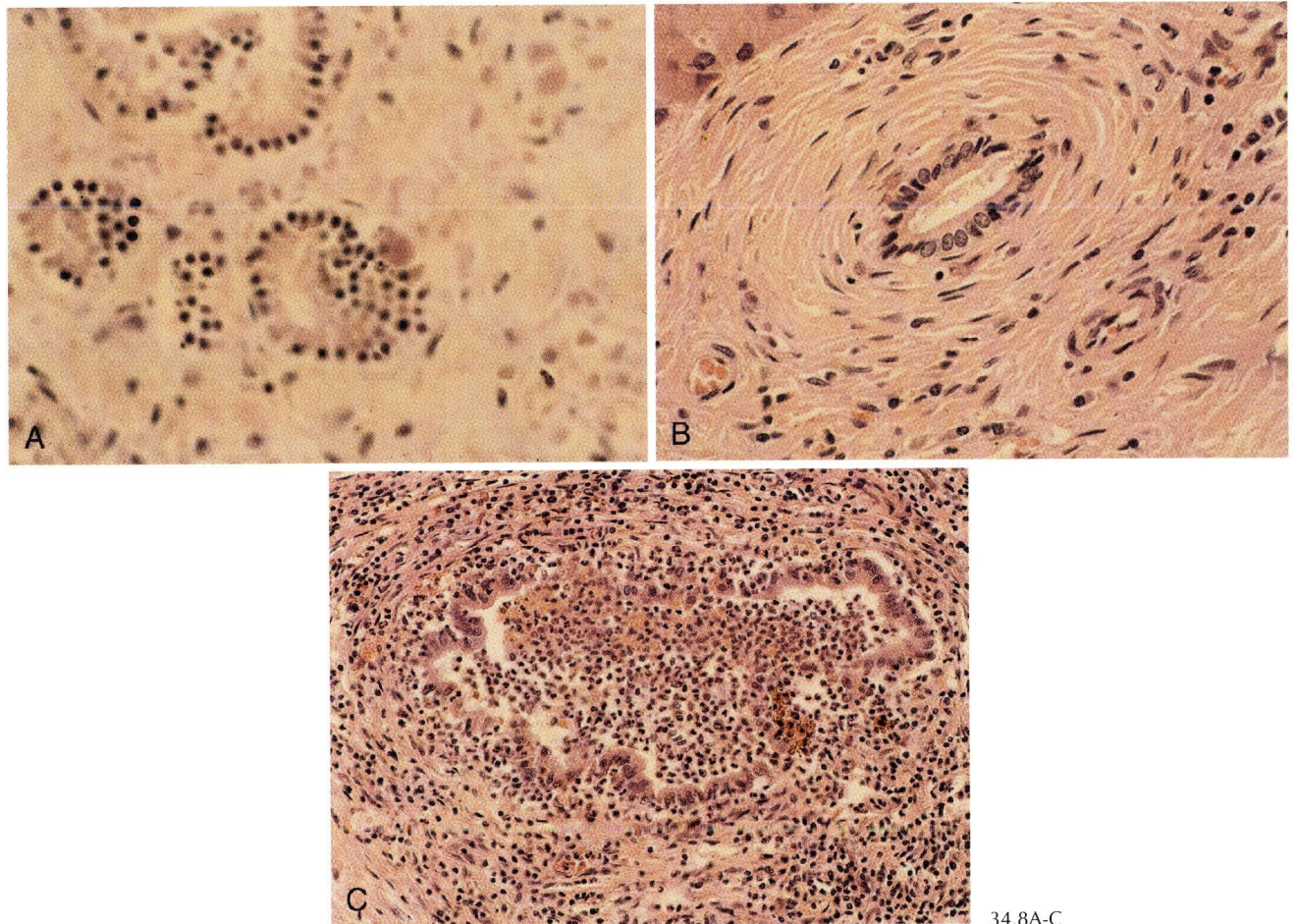

34.8A-C

Color Plates

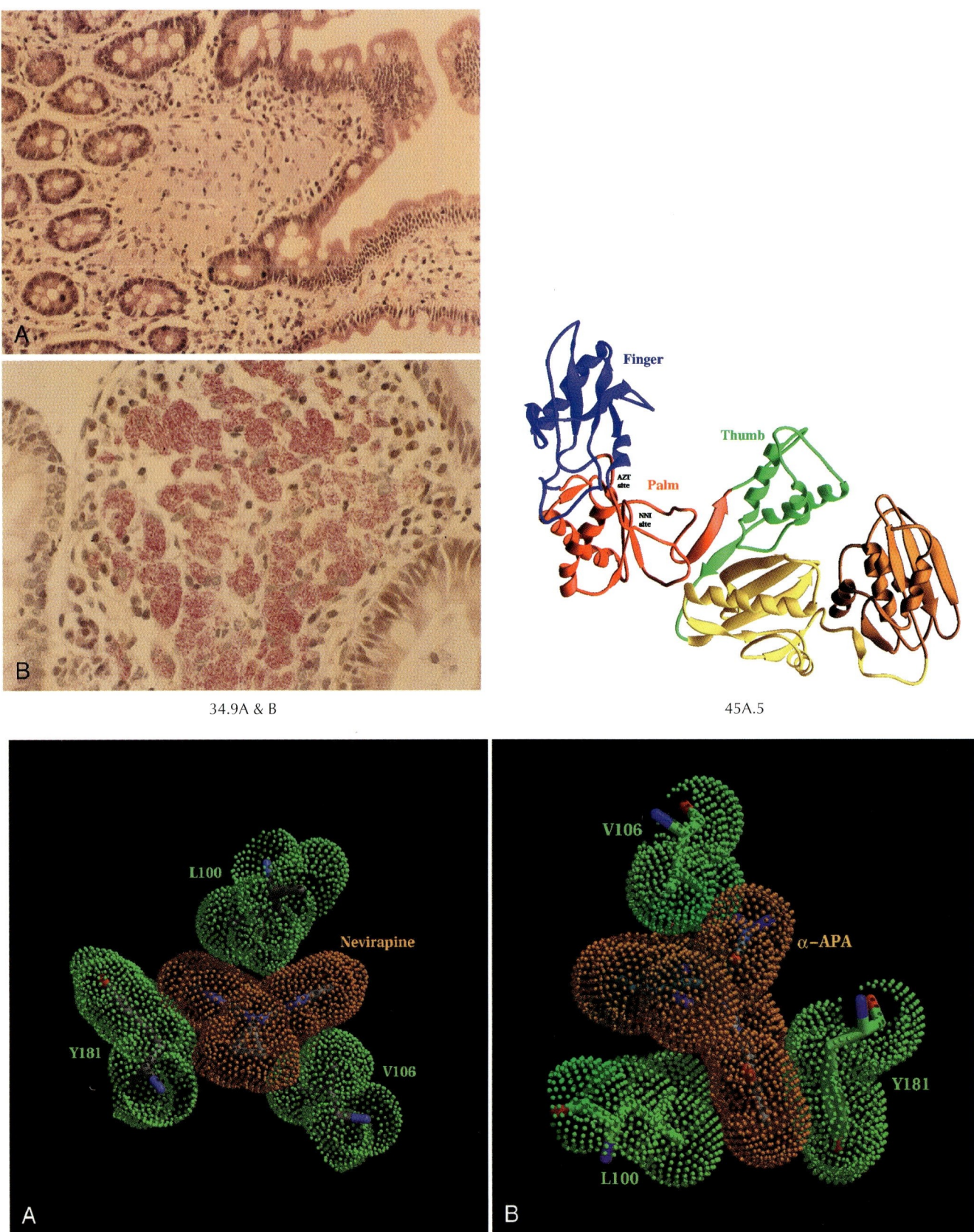

34.9A & B

45A.5

45A.6A & B

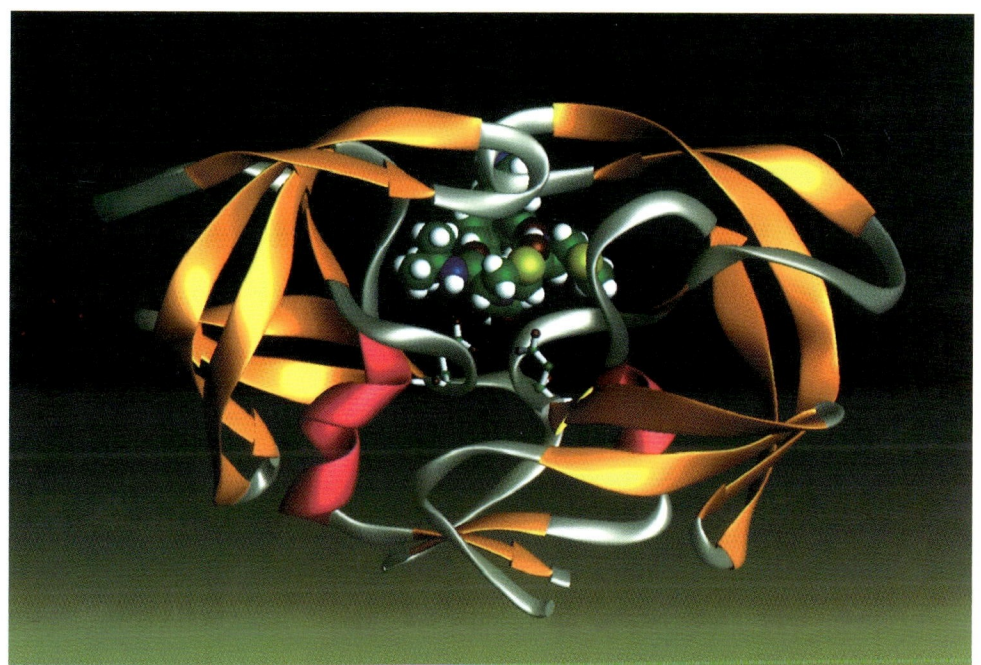

45A.7

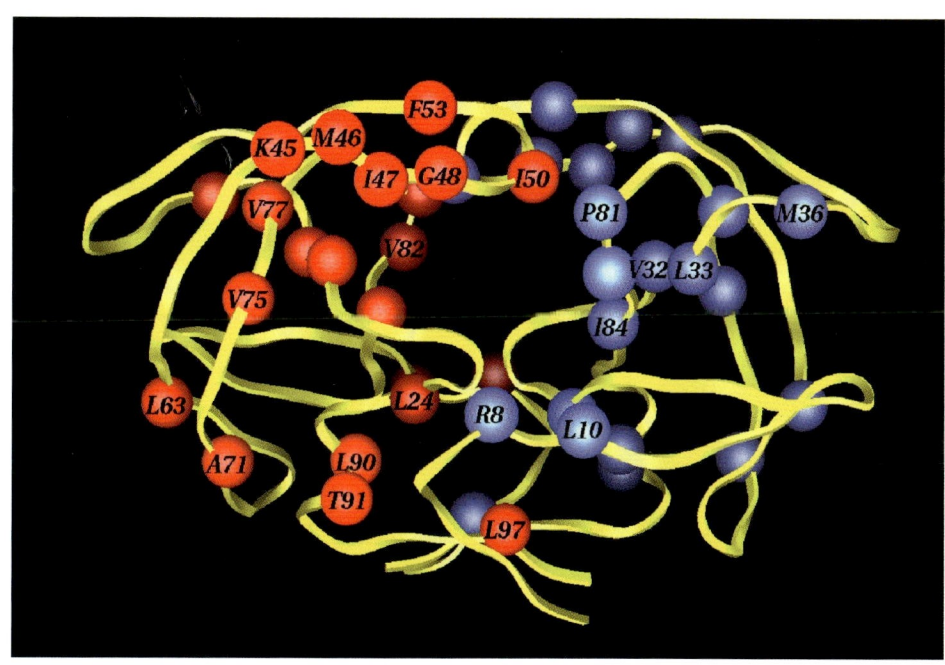

45A.8

Color Plates

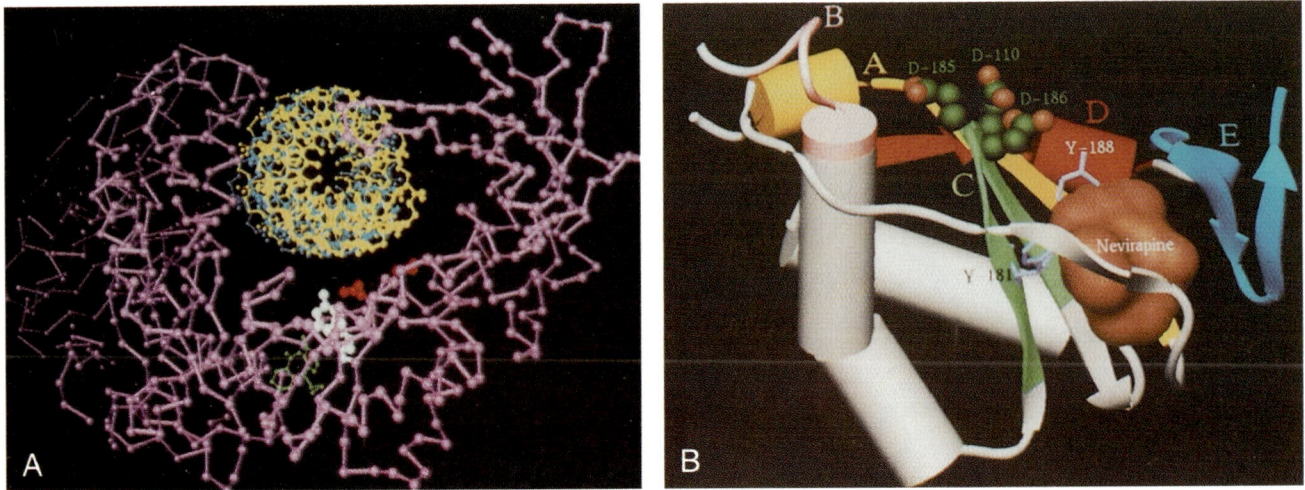

49.5A & B

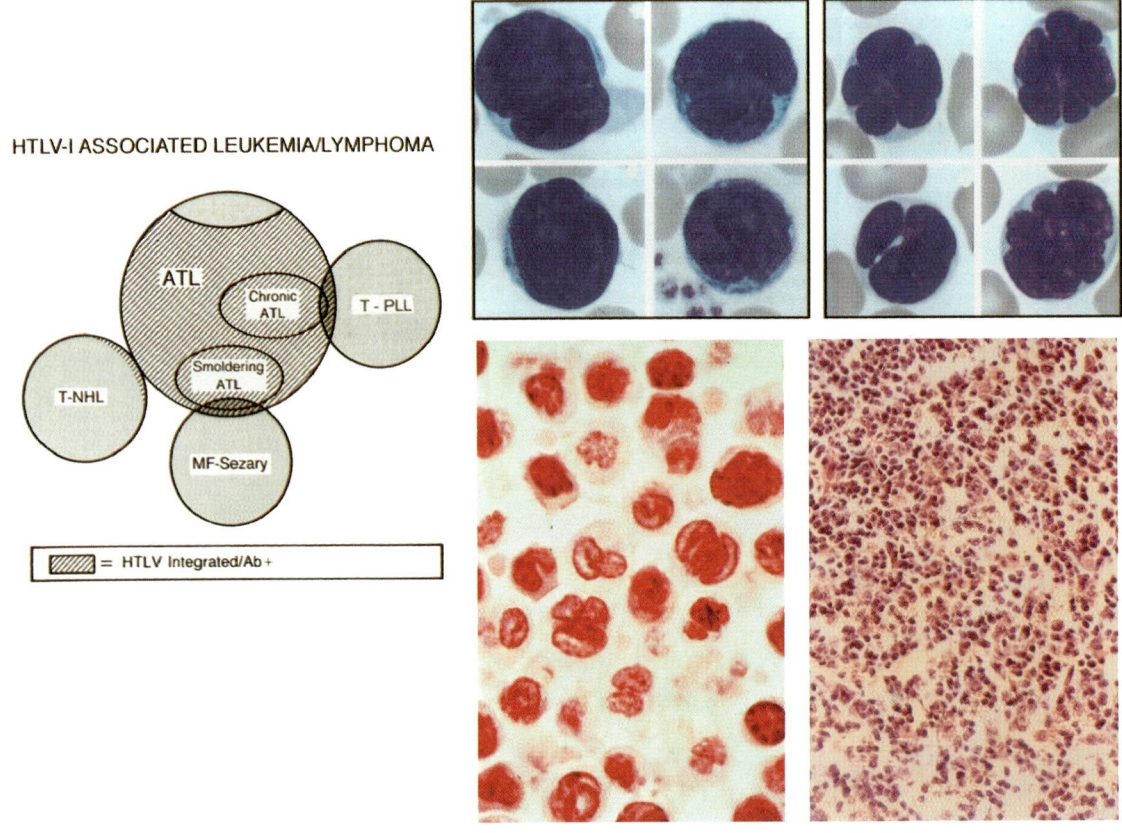

58.6

Section I
Introduction

1
HIV/AIDS AT THE MILLENNIUM

Robert R. Redfield, William A. Blattner, and Robert C. Gallo

The end of the twentieth century, the beginning of the third millennium, will see an epidemic of human immunodeficiency virus (HIV)/acquired immunodeficiency syndrome (AIDS) that is, despite impressive progress in basic and clinical science, grudgingly affected by these discoveries. Although mortality and morbidity have been favorably affected in affluent venues such as the United States and Europe by combinations of highly active antiretroviral therapy (HAART), these therapies are not universally effective, either as a result of intolerance because of side effects or as a result of drug resistance, and they are not affordable to the 95% of HIV-infected persons who reside in the developing world. Behavioral research has affected the rate of new infections in some locales, but these impacts are not durable, and infections remain at a rate at which new infections continue in epidemic proportions, save for the United States and Europe, where these parameters have reverted to a tenuous endemic pattern. A long-awaited preventive vaccine remains an elusive target, seemingly in sight but just over the horizon. Thus, the current edition of *Textbook of AIDS Medicine* is an important anchor of relevant and up-to-date information in a rapidly changing and sometimes confusing landscape of information.

In the few years since the first edition of this textbook, remarkable progress has been made in refining insights about HIV/AIDS based on the discoveries of the first decade of the epidemic. In this chapter, we highlight certain themes of discovery today that are likely to affect the field over the near-horizon interval between the second and third editions of this text.

ADVANCES IN BASIC SCIENCE

Characterization of the HIV genome is important in understanding the structure and function of the genes of HIV. Incremental progress has led to a refined understanding of the function of the genes of HIV-1 and their role in HIV pathogenesis. Understanding of the function of HIV's regulatory genes also opens new avenues for innovative therapy. For example, the further definition of the viral *vpr* gene and of its effects in promoting viral replication through impacts on cell-cycle kinetics not only provides a tool for studying viral host cell interaction, but also provides a target for attenuating viral replication. Studies of the *nef* gene have been more disappointing because investigators previously hypothesized that attenuation of this regulatory gene could severely affect the pathogenicity of HIV. Such attenuation is the focus of attempts to develop a live attenuated HIV vaccine. However, studies of *nef*-deleted viruses in human subjects have provided inconclusive results, and infection with *nef*-deleted simian viruses has yielded contradictory results, with some investigators reporting no adverse impacts on the host and others finding such viruses to be pathogenic, particularly in young animals whose immune systems are not fully developed. Studies of HIV *tat* have identified its critical role in immune pathogenesis of T-cell anergy and have defined its important function as a critical factor in the development of AIDS-associated Kaposi's sarcoma (KS).

The identification of the crystal structure of certain other genes has facilitated the rational development of antiviral therapies. Such information was critical in the development of the potent anti-HIV protease inhibitors. Identification of the zinc finger motif of the p17 gene has also provided a rational basis for identifying new potential targets, and certain domains of the envelope involved in cell fusion have provided the impetus to develop new approaches to therapy. Recent studies of the fusion domain of the HIV envelope have also proved a useful tool for targeting molecules that alter the kinetics of this process. Prototype therapeutics based on small, biologically active molecules blocking this mechanism have shown encouraging results in early phase studies.

An expanded understanding of the worldwide diversity of HIV-1 has documented two major groups of HIV-1: group M and group O. Group M subgroups, termed clades A to H, have been defined based on molecular sequencing. Most clades are represented in sub–Saharan Africa, a finding that lends credence to the concept that HIV originated on the African continent. The various subtypes have been disseminated throughout the world, and their diversity challenges the development of a universal HIV vaccine. A major controversy in HIV virology is the question whether subtypes vary in transmissibility and pathogenicity. Investigators have hypothesized that the explosive epidemics of heterosexually transmitted HIV, recognized in Asia and recently in Southern Africa, may relate to intrinsic characteristics of the virus. Thus, certain clades such as clade E in Thailand and clade C in South Africa have been linked to explosive heterosexual epidemics, whereas clade B viruses are associated with largely homosexual and injection drug use epidemics. In vitro studies have suggested differences in tropism from dendritic cells derived from penile foreskin, but this finding is controversial. Pathogenicity in some measure is determined by the growth phenotype of the virus with syncytium-inducing viruses associated with advanced HIV progression. Recently, recombination has been regularly identified among different clades of HIV where multiple clades of virus coexist in the same region. The pathogenic implications of this recombination are the focus of ongoing HIV research.

A major recent advance has been the discovery of the second receptor for HIV. The search for such a receptor dates back to the mid–1980s, when the first receptor, CD4, was identified. A critical step in the discovery of this second receptor was the recognition that a factor secreted by CD8 cells could block HIV infection. Laboratories had searched for this CD8 factor since the 1980s, when the removal of CD8 cells from coculture experiments aimed at propagating HIV-1 was found to enhance such propagation. Recent experiments identified at least one of these CD8 factors to be members of the C-C chemokine family. In particular, the chemokines termed macrophage inflammatory protein-1α and 1β (MIP-1α and MIP-1β) and regulated-on-activation normal T-expressed and secreted (RANTES), which bind to a seven-transmembrane receptor termed CCR5, have the capacity to block infection of monocyte tropic viruses but not T-cell tropic syncytium-inducing strains. This observation opened the door to the recognition that the second receptor for HIV is the chemokine receptor. Subsequently, a related receptor, CXCR4, was identified for the T-tropic viruses. Further studies have identified additional chemokines, termed macrophage-derived chemokines (MDCs), which block both classes of HIV and use additional receptors. One of the important insights gained from this research was the recognition that genetic polymorphisms of these receptors for the virus affect host susceptibility to HIV infection. Those with homozygous deletions of the receptor are largely resistant to HIV infection, by mechanisms thought to involve blocking of binding of HIV to the host cell. In other instances, heterozygotes for these polymorphisms appear resistant to infection and disease progression through mechanisms thought to involve increased production of the chemokine ligand itself, findings suggesting that these molecules may play a role in viral pathogenesis and perhaps in modulating infection and disease progression.

Major advances in understanding the dynamics of HIV infection have emerged from the convergence of therapeutic innovation and molecular and immunologic tools that have allowed studies of HIV viral dynamics and compartmentalization of virus in the immune system. The availability of potent combination chemotherapy has allowed careful quantification of viral production and clearance. In situ tools for detecting HIV virus in lymphatic tissues and precise quantitative tools for measuring virions in blood have coupled to provide an increasingly clear picture of a virus with broad tissue distribution and substantial capacity to replicate to maintain itself and to persist in the face of potent antiviral therapies. Some attempts to model the capacity of current HAART to eliminate HIV infection have proved wanting because of recent studies that document the capacity of HIV to persist productively in lymphocytes. A substantial reservoir of infectious virions is trapped in the follicular dendritic cells of the lymph node, but in the face of effective antiviral therapy, this reservoir is also cleared of virions. Such detailed studies provide a useful basis for developing strategies for eliminating HIV from the human host, a goal likely to be pursued with increasing sophistication in the coming years.

An infectious cause of KS has been postulated based on epidemiologic studies that demonstrated a disproportionate incidence of KS in homosexual men compared with other HIV-infected patients. The discovery of human herpesvirus type 8 (HHV-8) used new molecular approaches called differential representation analysis to identify novel genes present in KS tissue. These genes were identified as having homology to Herpes saimiri, a primate herpesvirus. Subsequently, the complete sequence of HHV-8 was achieved, and the virus was identified as being a γ herpesvirus with unique characteristics. In particular, certain novel genes were identified with homology to cellular genes, including regulatory and lymphokine and chemokine gene homologs. Study of these genes in disease pathogenesis is a major focus of ongoing research. In addition to a strong epidemiologic relationship of HHV-8 with all forms of KS, HHV-8 is also linked to body cavity lymphoma and Castleman's disease. An indirect relationship has also been suggested in the pathogenesis of multiple myeloma, although this link is controversial. Whether HHV-8 is not only necessary, but also sufficient to cause KS is a point of controversy. Clearly, the large excess of KS among HIV-infected persons compared with rates in other immunosuppressed populations has raised questions concerning the role for other factors in pathogenesis. For example, the HIV *tat* has the capacity to stimulate certain pathways that affect the immunologic milieu to favor proliferation of the target spindle cell, and whether some of the abundance of HHV-8 in KS tumor tissue could also reflect cell tropism is unclear. Understanding the pathogenic basis of KS formation and the role of HHV-8 in KS pathogenesis has substantial implications for understanding the cause of an important AIDS-associated malignancy.

Advancement has continued in the understanding of the human immune system and its interaction with HIV infection. Whereas the hallmark of HIV infection remains the development of a progressive quantitative and qualitative deficiency of the T-helper cell population, both endogenous and exogenous factors can contribute to the disease outcome of viral host interaction. Laboratory-based research continues to demonstrate multiple potential mechanisms of CD4 T-lymphocyte destruction and dysfunction. Mechanisms of CD4 cell destruction include viral lytic cytopathic infection, CD4 cell death as consequence of HIV-mediated syncytia formation, and host-directed immune response–mediated T-cell death as a consequence of HIV-specific cytotoxic T-cell responses, antibody-dependent cellular cytotoxicity, and natural killer cell activity. Clinically relevant immune dysfunction may be induced by cytokine dysregulation, HIV protein–induced T-cell anergy, and T-cell dysfunction resulting from terminal differentiation and apoptosis. The interaction among specific cytokines and the induction and the suppression of HIV transcription have also been characterized in understanding HIV pathogenesis. Yet despite these advances, the in vivo relevance of these potential mechanisms remains to be determined, for example, through proof of concept phase I intervention studies that target specific immunologic pathways and targets of HIV-1 infection.

Characterization of the human immune response to HIV continues to be elucidated. Investigators now recognize that after acute HIV infection, the human host mounts a vigorous multifaceted immune response. Innate immunoregulatory mechanisms, cytokine and chemokine production coupled with natural killer cell activity, previously underappreciated as important HIV defenses, are now areas of intense research. A reevaluation of the role of both humoral and cellular immune responses in in vivo viral control and viral diversity will likely yield important insights and an understanding of the complexities of HIV-specific immunity and viral control. New observations related to antibodies directed against regulatory proteins such as tat, nef, and vpr will likely lead to additional therapeutic concepts to be tested.

Before AIDS, most of the principles of human viral immunology were developed based on acute, self-limited pathogens such as influenza virus and poliovirus. Viral clearance and subsequent protection were associated with the production of a high-affinity antibody directed against immunodominant viral epitopes. A sine qua non of chronic viral infection is the lack of viral clearance by the host. Improved understanding of specific cytokine patterns (TH-1 and TH-2) has provided new insights concerning the relationship of the cytokine milieu and the maturation of the host-directed immune response. For acute viral pathogens, clearance frequently depends on a vigorous B-cell response; yet for chronic viral pathogens, this evolution may be but a viral defense mechanism for persistence. With further understanding of the interrelationship between the cytokine network and host-directed antiviral effector mechanisms, the possibility of altering the persistence of chronic viral pathogen may be on the horizon. Additionally, HIV-preventive vaccines that induce a predominant TH-1 or TH-2 immune response, or a balanced TH-1 and TH-2 response, afford an opportunity for enlightening the relevant correlates of effective anti-HIV immunity.

ADVANCES IN TREATMENT AND CLINICAL CARE

Since the first edition of the *Textbook of AIDS Medicine,* significant therapeutic advances have occurred. The first decade of AIDS research was highlighted with notable advancement in the field of molecular virology and viral pathogenesis. New diagnostic technology such as polymerase chain reaction methods and human immunologic reagents were developed and applied to the study of AIDS, and they provided important tools for the study of human disease in general. We have seen HIV medicine advance at a rapid pace, yielding to an evolving awareness of the need for the integration of primary and subspecialty care into one. This change has led to the emergence of a new care structure involving highly subspecialized HIV clinical care experts who provide primary care in a chronic care disease management model.

Physicians of the later half of the twentieth century have experienced the successes of scientific discovery over many of the diseases of humankind. AIDS treatment in the 1980s was a stark reminder of the limits of medicine without science. During that period, clinicians experienced what their predecessors had endured for infectious diseases in the preantibiotic era: to diagnose, to counsel, and to care for patients they served, fully understanding that medicine was but an art form whose limits were set by the state of science of the time. Treatment consisted of the use of interventions of limited temporal benefit and measurable toxicity. Physicians looked forward to more practical advances that could be translated into clinical benefits and could enhance clinical decision making. In this regard, the first edition of *Textbook of AIDS Medicine* served as a foundation for the evolving clinical practice of the 1990s, and the current edition provides the scientific basis as well as the clinical standard for care now and into the next millennium.

The development and application of combination antiretroviral chemotherapy, predicted in the first edition of *Textbook of AIDS Medicine,* are true advances in the treatment and control of HIV disease and its consequences. After nearly 15 years of increasing mortality rates throughout the world, combination antiretroviral chemotherapy and prophylactic use of antibiotics to prevent opportunistic infections have had an impact on population-based mortality rates in the United States and have reduced morbidity of countless HIV-1–infected persons. Rational drug development based on understanding the structure of the virus and its function have targeted critical enzymes of the viral life cycle. To date, seven reverse transcriptase inhibitors (five nucleoside analogs—zidovudine, didanosine, zalcitabine, lamivudine, and stavudine—and two nonnucleoside agents—nevirapine and delvaridine) are in clinical practice. This class of drugs targets the viral reverse transcriptase, a viral enzyme critical to the early life cycle of the virus. Two additional agents of this class, BW 1592 and MD 266, soon to be approved, are currently available in expanded access programs. To date, five protease inhibitors (saquinavir, ritonavir, indinavir, nelfinavir, and fortovase) targeting posttranslation viral assembly late in viral life cycle are in routine clinical practice. Additional reverse transcriptase inhibitors (both nucleoside and nonnucleoside) and protease drugs are at various stages of clinical evaluations. Prototype drugs targeting the viral enzyme integrase are also in clinical trials. New drug development is likely to continue at an accelerated pace fueled by the continued emergence of viral resistance, the pharmocokinetics of current agents (twice-daily and thrice-daily dosing regimens), and the limitations of current formulations requiring two to six tablets per dose.

Consensus reports, developed by various expert panels, outline recommendations related to important day-to-day clinical practice, such as when to institute antiviral therapy, what combinations of agents to use, and when to change treatment regimens. These documents have a major impact on current practice standards in the United States and abroad. These recommendations are based largely on expert opinion, but they lack evidence-based outcome data to validate optimal approaches. Prior recommendations by similar groups influenced many physicians to adopt treatment recommendations with sequential monotherapy, a recommendation that, in retrospect, was a suboptimal strategy because of frequent drug resistance When to start treatment is a particularly important issue. "Treat early, treat hard" has been advocated by some experts as a means of abrogating the destructive effects of ongoing HIV replication. Unanswered are questions of drug toxicity, drug resistance, and compliance and whether such approaches have lasting, long-term benefits. Additionally, suppressive chemotherapy instituted too early in treatment may adversely effect the full development of host-directed anti-HIV immunoregulatory mechanisms. Emerging data reinforce the importance of the host-directed adaptive immune response.

Although referred to as HAART, the current application of combination chemotherapy has significant limitations. These are complex drug regimens requiring patients to take multiple pills frequently, to endure recurrent gastrointestinal side effects such as nausea or chronic diarrhea, and to approach these treatment regimens with a commitment to strict adherence.

Current treatment algorithms follow a strategy of a multiagent regimen with sequential changes in treatment based on evidence of in vivo virologic failure. Frequently, this treatment failure is a direct consequence of the development of viral resistance. Characterization of molecular resistance secondary to point mutations of viral gene products continues to be appreciated. Cross-resistance is a major limitation of the nonnucleotide reverse transcriptase inhibitors and an increasing problem noted with protease inhibitors. Nonadherence to complex chemotherpeutic regimens continues to result in the emergence of drug resistance. In addition, novel biologic mechanisms of resistance (such as the induction of multidrug-resistant cellular gene products by protease inhibitor use) continue to be defined.

Drugs with improved pharmocokinetic profiles to enable once-daily dosing will continue to improve adherence and will potentially affect the emergence of viral resistance. However, primary viral resistance to pharmacologic agents with target viral enzymes will continue to represent a major limitation to drug therapy. Addition limitations of the current chemotherapeutic approach include end-organ toxicity, side effects with significant impact on quality of life, and cost. Another significant limitation of multiagent chemotherapy is its high cost, which restricts its availability to most the people living with HIV infection worldwide. This problem is unlikely to be solved in the future. Alternative approaches to treatment that are feasible for worldwide application must continue to be a focus of scientific exploration.

Additionally, chemotherapeutic strategies have been developed that exploit interactions between the virus and the host cell. A notable example is the use of hydroxyurea in combination with didanosine, initially proposed by Gallo and colleagues, to reduce the cellular nucleoside pool and thereby to enhance the antiviral activity of nucleoside analog agents. Combination antiretroviral therapy results in a 2- to 3-log decrease in measurements of viral expression, with the majority of treated patients demonstrating virologic responses below threshold detection levels. Despite this drug-induced response, when treatment is discontinued, viral rebound occurs. These observations underscored the important of resting cells as specific viral reservoirs of infection. In vivo studies also demonstrate that the unique combination of didanosine and hydroxyurea inhibited the establishment of persistent infection in peripheral blood mononuclear cells infected under nonactivating conditions. Despite limited clinical experience, many practicing clinicians are routinely using this combination as part of ongoing treatment regimens.

The implementation of treatment strategies to minimize the emergence of drug resistance is an ongoing focus. Advances in diagnostic technology that will improve viral detection from current thresholds of hundreds of copies to tens of copies are likely in the near future. Systematic studies of the impact of maintaining plasma viral loads at undetectable versus low- or high-level viral persistence will prove informative. The degree of persistent viral replication probably will predict treatment failure. However, recent clinical observation have noted a persistence of higher levels of CD4 cells in some patients with clinical responses to HAART but rising viral load. These data emphasize the importance of identifying relevant immunologic markers of clinical response.

Combination chemotherapy needs to be evaluated in terms of body compartment (i.e., blood, tissue, central nervous system); cell type (T-cell macrophage), and cell cycle (resting or activated). Different chemotherapeutic combinations will have antiviral activity in different biologic environments. To date, few patients have been treated with multiple drug regimens that are active in all biologic environments.

Regimens designed to induce viral suppression, followed by regimens to maintain viral suppression in resting compartments, are being clinically evaluated. Such approaches involving induction and maintenance regimens may prolong the utility of current drugs by limiting drug resistance. Unfortunately, increasing numbers of patients are presenting for salvage therapy, with few choices of agents available.

The capacity of current chemotherapy to facilitate immunologic reconstitution is not established. Patients receiving HAART therapy experience substantial increases in CD4 cells, but often these cells are immunologically naive. Longer-term study is needed to understand the immunologic impacts of such therapy. Further, we need to understand which drugs are directly immunotoxic and which have intrinsic immune-enhancing properties. Optimal use will require more careful clinical characterization of specific chemotherapeutic regimens in terms of immunologic impact.

Immune-based therapy is in development. The heightened awareness of the lack of immune reconstitution, coupled with the growing number of patients in whom combination antiretroviral therapy fails, has increased attention to the development of immune-based therapy. Strategies to modify immune response that are under development include the following: replacement cytokine therapy, such as therapeutic cytokines (interleukin-2) currently in phase III evaluation; modification of the cytokine milieu, such as ongoing studies of interferon-α as an active immunogen to regulate the interferon pathway; and active vaccination (vaccine therapy) with viral components to alter or augment specific anti-HIV immune responses. Direct immune reconstitution is also under intense investigation, including reinfusion of ex vivo expanded gene-modified T cells, human thymic and stem cell transplantation, and xenotropic transplantation. The pace of these efforts will depend on further advances in research related to basic human immunology, in vivo immune reeducation, and immune organ transplantation.

New research efforts continue to explore novel approaches to treatment. Recent discoveries by Gallo and colleagues related to chemokines and chemokine receptors will likely yield the development of biologically active molecules that will mimic the antiviral activity of natural chemokines and also will facilitate understanding of pathways to upregulate in vivo chemokine production. The potential of ex vivo gene modification of T cells to express altered chemokine receptors with poor HIV-binding capacity may serve as an additional approach to treatment, especially for patients with advanced disease.

Another area that holds great promise is related to the recent discovery of small, biologically active molecules excreted in the urine during early pregnancy that demonstrate various biologic activities including potential antiviral and proimmunologic effects. The potential of the endocrine immune interaction warrants additional investigation, particularly as related to gestational development, cell growth, and differentiation factors, which may yield a source of novel approaches to inhibit HIV replication and induce immune reconstitution.

Progress in the prevention of opportunistic infection has had significant impacts on patients over the past 10 years. *Pneumocystis carinii* pneumonia, candidiasis, and infections with *Mycobacterium avium intracellulare,* herpes simpex virus, and cytomegalovirus are now frequently preventable with current prophylactic regimens. Other diseases such as cryptosporidiosis and KS seem to be disappearing without a clear explanation, perhaps related to antiviral therapy, whereas others are more refractory, such as wasting and nutritional failure, lymphoma, and degenerative neurologic disease, although effective antiviral therapy has positively benefited therapy-responsive patients with these diseases.

ADVANCES IN PREVENTION AND VACCINE DEVELOPMENT

Developing an effective HIV vaccine has proved to be a daunting task. Similar to the quest for a malaria vaccine, which has eluded development, HIV presents many of the same challenges, an organism with potent means for eluding immunologic control. In particular, HIV's tropism for the very cells whose role it is to eliminate foreign invaders provides a difficult target. Certain issues have framed the debate about which path to follow in vaccine development. The stigma of HIV antibody positivity and the difficulty of distinguishing those who are infected from those who are immunized directed vaccine developers toward approaches that used subunits rather than whole viral vaccines. Moreover, successes in developing subunit vaccines using modern vaccinology approaches such as recombinant hepatitis B vaccines pointed toward a plethora of alternative approaches. Further, the debate has been affected by an ongoing discussion between those in the scientific community who favor full understanding of host–virus interactions to tailor a suitable vaccine and those with a more empiric approach who would rather implement trials with available candidates and study the successes and failures. Considerable effort has been expended in defining immunologic markers associated with protection against HIV-1 infection, so-called correlates of immunity. This debate has focused on defining the role of antibody-mediated versus cell-mediated responses and mucosal versus systemic immunity. Initial efforts focused on inducing strong humoral responses, and considerable effort was expended on defining neutralizing antibodies and means of enhancing such responses through the use of various adjuvants. In the early 1990s, the scientific community was poised to embark on the first trials of subunit candidate HIV vaccines, but the lack of conviction that these candidates promoted sufficient relevant immunity put a hold on going forward and redirected scientific efforts to define correlates of immunity and strategies for inducing a broader array of immune responses. The current scientific focus is on better understanding the role of cellular immunity in the process of controlling HIV, largely driven by emerging evidence that cellular responses temporally correlate with the abrogation of high-level HIV viremia early in HIV infection. Studies of highly exposed and uninfected individuals have suggested that cell-mediated immunity may correlate with protection because, for example, cytotoxic lymphocyte responses are reported by some investigators in such individuals, and other cell-mediated detection systems such as induction of interferon responses are observed in such individuals. However, controversy continues, and the scientific community is still divided on the validity of these claims. The vaccine trials design debate focuses on whether sterilizing immunity is achievable or whether the vaccine will protect against disease, but not infection. If the latter is the case, trials of much larger size and long duration will be required to define vaccine efficacy fully.

Despite these debates, substantial progress, albeit incremental, is ongoing. Various approaches are in preclinical and clinical development. The broad strategies being developed include several vaccine approaches. Synthetic peptides or recombinant antigens using a variety of adjuvants induce largely humoral immune responses. Live vector systems such as canarypox or bacteria such as *Salmonella* prove a means of packaging subunits of the HIV virus in a short-lived, live vector to expose the cellular arm of the immune system. Naked DNA vaccine candidates, delivering portions of the HIV genome attached to colloidal gold, also provide a means for stimulating cellular immunity. Based on controversial studies of *nef*-deleted variants of HIV, some members of the scientific community are promoting the concept of a live attenuated HIV vaccine. However, substantial safety concerns have been raised because, in some experiments on young animals, the so-called attenuated strain proved pathogenic.

To date, many individuals have participated in phase I and II trials, and participants have received various candidate vaccines. Most participants have received HIV subunit vaccines, primarily components of the viral envelope, usually gp120 or gp160, which have been developed for their ability to induce antibody responses. In the early 1990s, trials with these vaccines were considered for implementation in phase III efficacy trials, but the relative inefficiency of these candidates for inducing high titer antibodies and several instances of HIV-1 "breakthrough" infection during the course of phase II trials, which included some high-risk participants, led to the decision not to implement efficacy trials with these candidates in the United States. In retrospect, some of those who became infected did so early in the course of vaccination and before a full complement of booster injections was completed. Currently, trials with modified versions of these subunits tailored to the prevailing strains in Thailand and including a clade B construct derived from a field, nonlaboratory isolate have received approval for phase II testing, with the goal of proceeding to phase III efficacy testing by the year 2000 in Thailand. The induction of cytotoxic T-cell responses in persons receiving some canarypox-vectored products provided impetus to proposed vaccine trials involving the "prime boost" regimen. In the original proposal, priming with the canarypox-vectored HIV construct would be followed by a boost with subunit vaccine. Current approaches give the vectored product and subunit material at each visit over several months. A phase III efficacy trial involving this approach is proposed to begin by the year 2001 or before. Other candidates, including naked DNA, *Salmonella*-vectored HIV subunits, are in earlier phase development. Live attenuated candidates are under development with a much longer time frame because of unresolved safety issues and the lack of a precise animal model for safety testing. Current candidates are limited to a few clades. Unresolved is the question whether current candidates will provide sufficient cross-protection or whether a polyvalent vaccine will be required, and, if so, what the implications of emerging recombinant viruses will have on future vaccine design.

FUTURE SCOPE OF THE EPIDEMIC

Although the modes of spread of HIV are well understood, and preventive campaigns have been organized in virtually every country, the spread of HIV continues. Investigators currently estimate that, worldwide, 16,000 new infections take place daily. In early 1998, 30.6 million people worldwide are estimated to be living with HIV/AIDS. By the year 2000, this number will exceed 40 million. More than 1.1 million children younger than 15 years are HIV positive, largely through maternal–infant transmission, which is now potentially preventable through the use of antiviral drugs in the peripartum period. Of new infections worldwide, most are occurring in developing countries. Through 1997, the cumulative total of AIDS-associated deaths worldwide numbered 11.7 million, with 9 million deaths among adults and 2.7 million among children. In 1998, annual deaths from HIV will surpass those attributed to malaria. The social implications of the epidemic are vast, with reversal of favorable mortality trends in many developing countries and the emergence of approximately 8.2 million children younger than 15 years of age orphaned because of the premature deaths of their parents from HIV/AIDS.

In the United States, more than 640,000 cases of AIDS were reported as of January, 1998. The total number of persons living with HIV infection in the United States is estimated to range between 650,000 and 900,000, of whom 235,470 are living with AIDS. A cumulative total of 379,258 deaths due to AIDS has now been reported, making AIDS the second leading cause of death in the United States among persons 25 to 44 years old.

The future of the HIV epidemic in the United States is predicted by recent trends. First, the impact of HAART has reversed AIDS incidence trends, with declines of 10 to 15% attributed to the impact of therapy. Second, AIDS-related mortality has declined by 40 to 50% in some locales, again a reflection of the impact of therapy on HIV natural history. A less dramatic, but detectable, therapeutic effect was reported on AIDS incidence in 1987, the result of the introduction of zidovudine into therapy. However, that effect was short-lived as drug resistance developed with monotherapy. An important future question will be the sustainability of the HAART therapeutic effect, especially given emerging clinical reports of multidrug resistance and poor compliance with complex drug regimens among some populations.

The incidence of new infections is increasingly the result of heterosexual transmission, a trend reflected in the shift of cases to people of color and the rising number of women with

HIV/AIDS. Injection drug use is another major source of new infections. The incidence of infection among young gay men continues to be substantial in some locales, despite intensive educational campaigns. However, in the United States, unlike in many parts of the world, the number of new HIV infections is currently in a tenuous equilibrium with the number of persons dying of AIDS.

Recent reports have also documented the detection of new clades of HIV into locales with prevalent HIV infection. In some places, such as the Philippines and South Africa, viruses adapted to more efficient heterosexual transmission seem to be driving more robust epidemics. Whether this pattern is a harbinger of the future of the epidemic in other locales is not yet apparent. Similarly, the implications of viral recombination on HIV growth characteristics and spread remain to be established.

Critical to assessing the future of the epidemic worldwide will be the capacity to extend effective therapy to broader segments of the world population. This will require the successful development of alternative strategies to treatment other than sequential combination chemotherapy. Therapeutic vaccination, if feasible, would be more accessible worldwide. Perinatal intervention, in which relatively low-cost therapy such as short-term zidovudine treatment can prevent a substantial number of perinatal infections, is feasible for worldwide deployment. With international leadership and a multinational commitment, this program could prevent numerous children from dying of AIDS and could lay the groundwork for future international prevention programs. However, the main hope for dealing with the worldwide epidemic is the development of an effective and affordable preventive vaccine. Unfortunately, the results of the first phase III efficacy trials, which are currently in planning stages, will not be available when the next edition of this textbook is published, and thus prevention of HIV infection and of clinical AIDS will depend on measures currently available and detailed in the chapters of this textbook.

Section II
Basic Sciences

2
THE VIRUS AND ITS TARGET CELLS

Paul R. Clapham and Robin A. Weiss

The human immunodeficiency viruses (HIV-1, HIV-2) belong to the lentivirus subfamily of retroviruses. As with all retroviruses, the genome in the virus particle is diploid, comprising two single-stranded RNA molecules. On infection, the viral enzyme, reverse transcriptase, catalyzes the synthesis of a haploid, double-stranded DNA provirus, which becomes inserted into chromosomal DNA of the host cell (Fig. 2.1). This integrated provirus may remain latent in an inexpressed form, particularly in resting lymphocytes; in actively infected cells, however, RNA transcripts and proteins are produced, leading to the synthesis of new virions. Even during the asymptomatic period of infection, HIV replication and turnover of infected cells are remarkably dynamic (see Chap. 3). The replication of HIV depends on an intimate interplay between host transcriptional activators, such as NFkB, and viral regulatory genes, such as *tat* and *rev*. Immune-activated T-lymphocytes and macrophages are most permissive to HIV replication.

The molecular biology of HIV replication is reviewed elsewhere (see Chap. 3). In this chapter, the early steps in virus infection are depicted, and the cell-surface receptors exploited by HIV are described with reference to cellular tropism. The cellular targets for HIV infection are surveyed with regard to viral pathogenesis, therapeutic intervention, and vaccination. Table 2.1 shows the main cell types that become infected in vivo. Further cell types may physically adsorb virus without necessarily becoming infected. A long list of cells of nonhematopoietic origin can be infected in vitro with varying degrees of sensitivity by laboratory strains of HIV-1 and HIV-2. With some cell lines, entry is independent of CD4 but inefficient; the relevance, if any, of these culture phenomena to HIV in vivo and to disease remains obscure.

CD4–gp120 INTERACTIONS

The major cell-surface receptor for adsorption of HIV-1, HIV-2, and simian immunodeficiency virus (SIV) is the CD4 differentiation antigen. The natural function of CD4 on T lymphocytes is to interact with class II major histocompatibility (MHC-II) molecules presenting peptides on the surface of antigen-presenting cells. Thus, CD4 is an invariant accessory molecule in the T-cell receptor complex that determines restriction to MHC-II interaction. CD4 is expressed on T-helper lymphocytes and less densely on macrophages and microglial cells, as well as on dendritic cells and Langerhans cells. Because these are the major target cells for HIV infection in vivo, the determination of the cellular tropism of the virus at the first step of infection by binding to a specific receptor already goes a long way to explain the pathogenesis of HIV. The depletion or malfunctioning of CD4+ cells eventually leads to immune deficiency.

The highly glycosylated outer surface (SU) glycoprotein of HIV, gp120, specifically binds to CD4. The outer envelope of HIV is studded with knobs, probably as trimers of the transmembrane protein, gp41, to which gp120 is attached. These oligomeric knobs represent the machinery by which the virus attaches to and enters CD4+ cells. The gp120–CD4 interaction has been thoroughly analyzed with the use of site-specific mutagenesis, with monoclonal antibodies, and, since the crystallization of soluble CD4 molecules, in structural studies. The tertiary structure for the gp120, however, has not yet been fully resolved. Conformational changes both in gp120/gp41 oligomer and in CD4 appear to take place during the events leading to fusion. The viral fusion effector is thought to be a hydrophobic domain at the N-terminal part of gp41, which is held within the glycoprotein spike until receptor activation occurs.

The CD4 antigen belongs to the immunoglobulin (Ig) superfamily, with four extracellular domains (D1 to D4) resembling Ig light-chain variable domains. Crystallography data indicate that CD4 can form dimers by interactions among D4s, the membrane proximal domains. A CDR2-like region in the D1 domain is essential for gp120 binding. Conservative changes in this region (amino acid residues 43–50) from human to mouse sequences abrogate binding, and, conversely, substitution of human sequences in rat CD4 is sufficient to bind gp120. After gp120 binding by CDR2, the CD4 molecules engage in subsequent interaction with gp120 in which an induced fit effect is seen at physiologic temperature; some monoclonal antibodies to regions such as CDR3 on D1 and to D2 and D3 can block events leading to HIV envelope–cell membrane fusion even though they do not interfere with the primary binding of HIV to CD4.

CORECEPTORS

Biologic evidence accumulated for over a decade implied that a coreceptor was needed in addition to CD4 for HIV

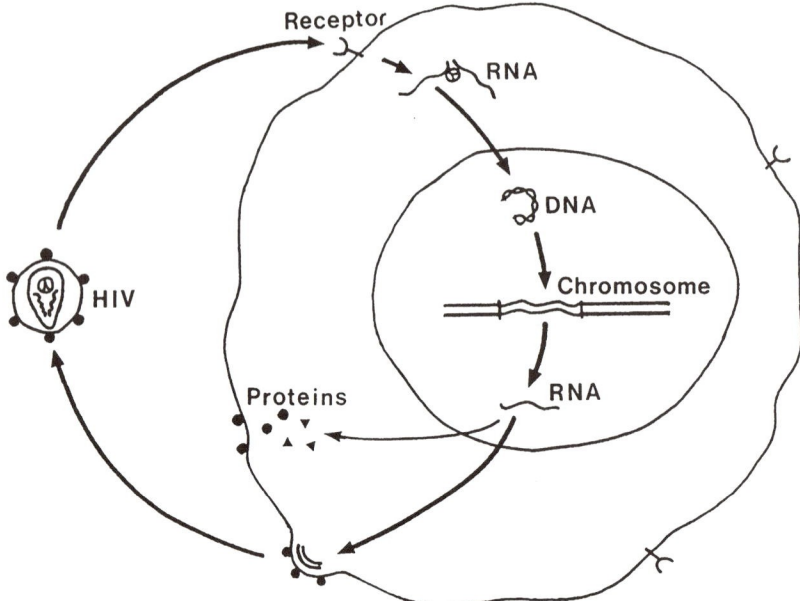

Figure 2.1. Simplified replication cycle of HIV.

Table 2.1. Cellular Targets for HIV

Infection	CD4+ T lymphocytes
	CD4+ monocytes and macrophages, including microglia
	CD4+ dendritic cells, including Langerhans cells
Attachment or presentation	Follicular dendritic cells in lymph nodes
	M cells on Peyer's patches
	Galactosylcerebroside+ cells in brain and gut

entry. When CD4 was expressed on the surface of many nonhuman cell types, gp120 and virus particles attached, but HIV entry and infection were not triggered. Even some human cell lines restricted CD4-induced entry by HIV at this postadsorption step. Moreover, evidence suggested that several coreceptors were exploited by different HIV and SIV strains that have distinct tropisms for different cell types. Different coreceptors were also thought likely to explain the different biologic phenotypes of primary HIV-1 isolates. Primary strains can generally be categorized into two groups, those that infect cell lines and induce syncytia in infected cultures of blood lymphocytes or particular CD4+ T-cell lines and those that do not. These two groups were given various names: 1) slow/low and rapid/high, 2) syncytium inducing (SI) and nonsyncytium inducing (NSI), and 3) T-cell line tropic or macrophage tropic.

An indicator to the identification of coreceptors came in 1995 when it was shown that the β-chemokines, known as macrophage inflammatory proteins (MIPs) (MIP-1α, MIP-1β, and RANTES), inhibited NSI, but not SI viruses, replicating in primary blood lymphocytes. In early 1996, a G-protein–coupled receptor with seven transmembrane (7TM) domains was shown to act as a coreceptor for HIV-1 T-cell line–adapted SI viruses. This receptor (initially called fusin) was related to the family of receptors for chemokines such as MIP-1α, MIP-1β, and RANTES. Thus, the coreceptor for NSI strains seemed likely to be the receptor for MIP-1α, MIP-1β, and RANTES. This receptor, CCR5 (newly identified at the time), was shown by several groups to function as a coreceptor for NSI strains but not T-cell line–adapted SI viruses.

Fusin had been previously cloned by several groups and variously designated L5, D2S201E, hFB22, HM89, and LESTR. A ligand for fusin was identified later in 1996 as stroma-derived factor (SDF-1). Because SDF-1 is a CXC α-chemokine, the term fusin was superceded by CXCR4.

All HIV-1 strains so far tested use CCR5, CXCR4, or both as coreceptors, although investigators now know that many HIV-1 viruses can use several coreceptors including CCR2b, CCR3, CCR8, and the orphan receptors termed BOB/GPR-15 and BONZO/STRL-33 (Table 2.2). The cross-reactivity with non-CCR5 coreceptors is thought to broaden as disease progresses, and many primary SI isolates use both CXCR4 and CCR5 as well as other coreceptors. Some primary SI strains are specific for CXCR4, however, and whether they evolve from strains using a broad range of coreceptors or switch directly from CCR5 is unclear.

What are chemokines and chemokine receptors? Chemokines are small, soluble, 8- to 10-kd proteins that act as chemoattractants, directing cells to appropriate sites in the body. β-Chemokines potently attract cells into sites of inflammation. Chemokines are divided mainly into two groups, depending on the arrangement of the first two cysteine residues nearest the N-terminus. Thus, α-chemokines have a –CXC– arrangement, and β-chemokines have a –CC– sequence. Chemokine receptor terminology depends on their respective chemokine ligands. Thus, CCRs,

Table 2.2. Immunodeficiency Virus Receptors[a]

	CD4	CCR5	CXCR4	CCR3	CCR2b	CCR8	BONZO STRL33	BOB GPR15	GPR1	US28
HIV-1 NSI	+	+	–	+	–	+	+	+	–	+
SI	+	+	+	+	+	+	+	+	–	+
SIV$_{MAC}$	+	+	–	–	–	?	+	+	+	?
Natural ligands	MHC class II	MIP-1α MIP-1β RANTES	SDF-1	Eotaxin RANTES MCP-3 MCP-4	MCP-1 MCP-2 MCP-3	I-309	?	?	?	?

[a]All HIV and SIVs bind to CD4. Nine coreceptors are shown that bind different HIV and SIV strains.
+, the appropriate coreceptor is active for at least one virus strain;
–, no viruses have yet been shown to use that coreceptor;
?, not yet tested or unknown;
MCP, monocyte chemoattractant protein; MHC, major histocompatibility complex; MIP, macrophage inflammatory protein; SDF, stroma-derived factor; SI and NSI, syncytium inducing and nonsyncytium inducing.

such as CCR5, are receptors for –CC– or β-chemokines, whereas CXCRs, such as CXCR4, are receptors for –CXC– or α-chemokines. This terminology runs into difficulties when a receptor binds both α- and β-chemokines, such as Duffy antigen. Chemokine specificity is complex. Some chemokines are specific for a single receptor, as are MIP-1β for CCR5 and SDF-1 for CXCR4, whereas others are promiscuous, such as RANTES, which binds to CCR1, CCR3, and CCR5. Such complexity presumably results in subtle networks of cell–cell signaling and cell trafficking at different sites throughout the body.

HOW DO CORECEPTORS TRIGGER HIV ENTRY?

HIV enters cells by inducing fusion of its lipid envelope with the membrane of the cell (Figs. 2.2 and 2.3). This fusion event is driven by structural changes in the spike glycoproteins, so a hydrophobic fusion domain at the N-terminus of gp41 is exposed and penetrates the cell membrane. These changes in envelope structure are driven by their interaction with CD4 and coreceptors on the cell surface. When gp120 docks with CD4, conformational changes in gp120 itself and probably also in CD4 are induced. These structural alterations are thought to form a site on gp120 that binds to the coreceptor, so a heterotrimolecular complex of gp120, CD4, and coreceptor is formed. The gp120–coreceptor interaction presumably triggers the remaining molecular rearrangements in gp41 needed for fusion. These structural changes are thought to be similar to those described for influenza virus fusion, as described elsewhere (1).

The variable loops, V1/V2, are not needed for gp120 to bind to the coreceptor, consistent with the observation that an HIV mutant deleted for V1/V2 is viable for replication. Inhibition of gp120–coreceptor binding by specific monoclonal antibodies indicates that the V3 loop and gp120 epitopes exposed on binding to CD4 are important. The precise gp120 site that interfaces with the coreceptor is still not clear; however, a broad conformational site that contacts two regions of the coreceptor is envisaged (see later).

The site on the coreceptor that is recognized by gp120 is also complex. Sequences at the N-terminus and in the second

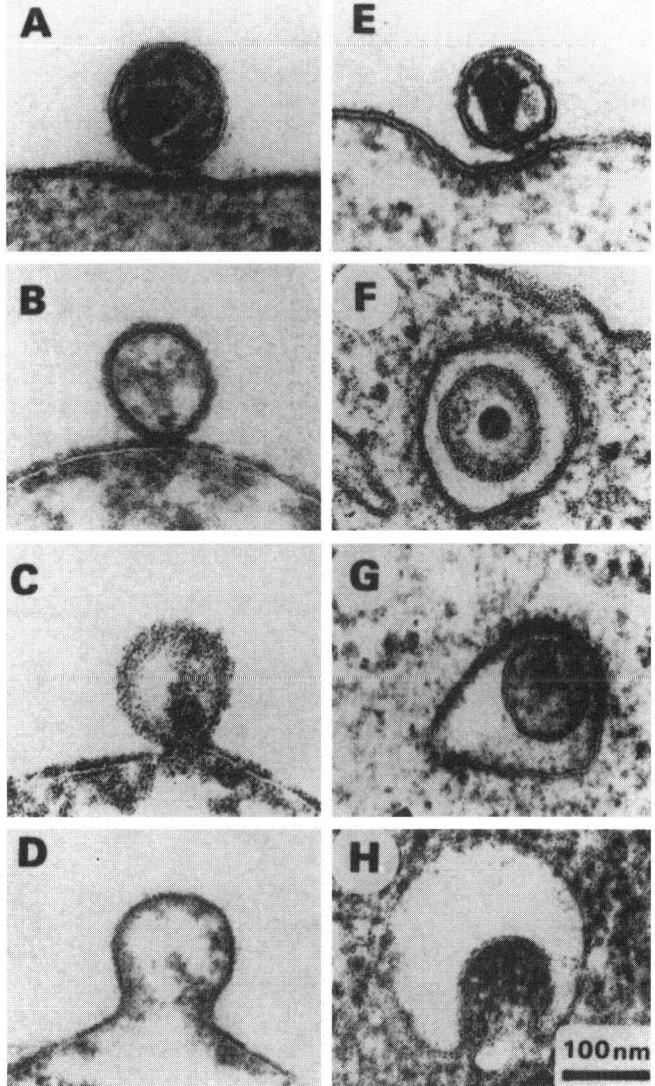

Figure 2.2. Electron micrographs showing stages of fusion of HIV-1 with cell membranes. **A–D.** Cell-surface fusion. **E–H.** Endocytic fusion. (Adapted from Grewe C, Beck A, Gelderblom HR. Early virus-cell interactions. J Acquir Immune Defic Syndr 1990;3:965–974.)

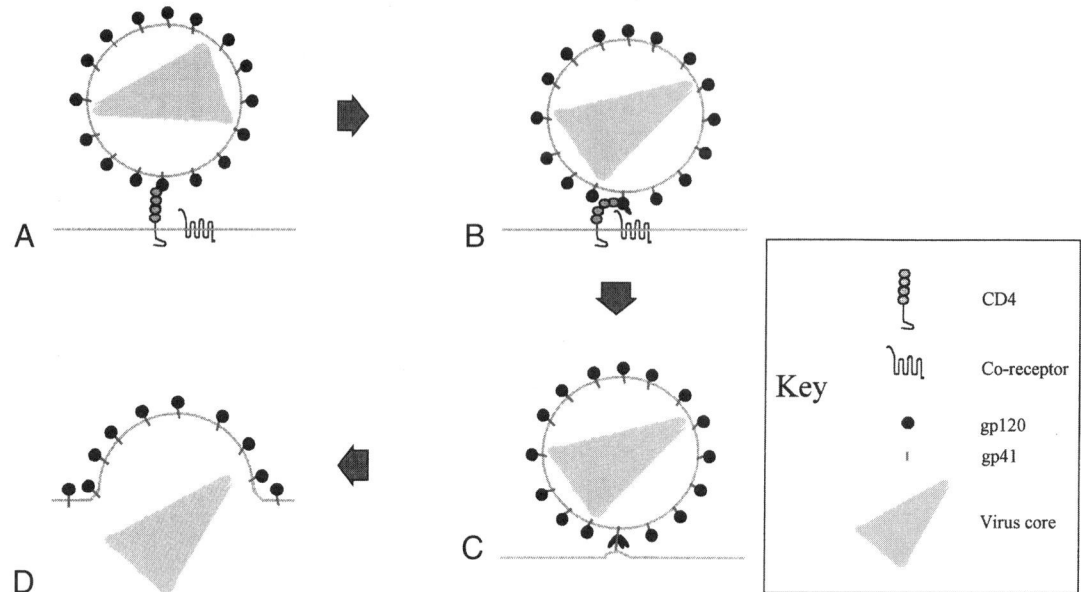

Figure 2.3. Attachment and fusion model for HIV-1 entry. *A,* attachment to CD4; gp120 interacts with CD4; *B,* the gp120–CD4 interaction results in conformational changes in gp120 and probably also in CD4; these structural alterations result in formation of a binding site for the 7TM coreceptor; *C,* further conformational changes are induced; gp41 is likely to extend so the hydrophobic fusion domain inserts into the cell membrane; two distal regions of gp41 interact together (not shown) allowing the cell and virion membranes to become closer; the exact process of cell and virion membrane fusion is poorly understood; the fate of gp120, CD4 and coreceptors is not known; *D,* an initial narrow fusion pore connects the cell cytoplasm and virion, this widens to allow the virus core to enter the cell cytoplasm.

extracellular loop (E2) seem most important. Remarkably, on CXCR4, E2 sequences are critical for recognition by HIV, whereas on CCR5, the N-terminal sequences are most important. This point was emphasized by a chimeric coreceptor that contained the N-terminus of CCR5 and E2 of CXCR4 and functioned as a coreceptor for a broad range of both NSI and SI strains of HIV. The reciprocal chimeric receptor exhibited only weak coreceptor activity for the same strains. It is unlikely that the mechanisms leading to fusion would be different for NSI and SI strains. Thus, both N-terminal and E2 sequences are likely to be involved in the gp120–coreceptor interaction, even though different sites on these coreceptors have been selected for gp120 recognition. Furthermore, different HIV strains react differently with coreceptors. Short deletions at the N-terminus of CXCR4 have no effect on the infection of some strains, whereas others are completely compromised. Moreover, as NSI strains adapt to use other coreceptors such as CXCR4, their interaction with CCR5 is altered, becoming exquisitely sensitive to amino acid substitutions in the extracellular loops of CCR5. In contrast to NSI strains, these dual tropic viruses are particularly sensitive to inhibition by CCR5 ligands such as RANTES on cell lines expressing only CCR5.

OTHER HIV RECEPTORS

CD4 may not be the only cell-surface molecule that functions as an adsorption receptor for HIV. Table 2.3 lists some of the molecules that have been studied as alternative receptors. Some of these receptors seem to function weakly as

Table 2.3. Cell-Surface Receptors Involved in HIV Attachment, Entry, and Fusion

CD4 differentiation antigen
Seven-transmembrane receptors
Galactosylcerebroside glycolipid
Placental membrane binding protein
LFA-1 adhesion receptor
Fc receptors
Complement receptors

receptors for HIV entry, whereas others may simply aid HIV attachment to cells when CD4 expression is low, such as on macrophages.

One possible alternative receptor is a membrane glycolipid with terminal galactose–ceramide residues called galactosylcerebroside. This is expressed on neuronal cells, oligodendrocytes, and possibly astrocytes, as well as on certain colorectal carcinoma cell lines. HIV gp120 binds to galactosylcerebroside with almost as high affinity as to CD4, but the efficiency of infection of cell lines after binding to this receptor is much lower. Little indication exists that neuronal cells become infected by HIV in vivo, although the evidence for infection of astrocytes is stronger. Galactosylcerebroside may present a route for infection.

A gene encoding another receptor (placental membrane binding protein, PMBP) that bound gp120 was cloned from human placenta. This receptor contained a lectin-like domain and bound gp120 with an affinity similar to the gp120/CD4 interaction. Expression of PMBP on HeLa cells efficiently captured HIV virions, which were internalized into endosomes but did not initiate new infections or replication.

Antibodies to the cell adhesion molecule, LFA-1, inhibit syncytium induction by HIV-1. T cells from patients genetically deficient in LFA-1 are also refractory to HIV-1-induced cell fusion, yet cell-free infection by virus is less dependent on LFA-1. The role of LFA-1, therefore, may be largely an artifact of the syncytium induction assay; anti-LFA-1 prevents cells from clumping together, a prerequisite for subsequent cell–cell fusion.

Fc and complement receptors also play a role in the infection of cells by HIV particles coated with antibody molecules. Such opsonized virions can attach to the FcR and CR2 receptors, and this engenders a slight enhancement of infection of CD4+ lymphocytes in vitro. Because most plasma virions in seropositive HIV-infected individuals are opsonized, it will be important to determine whether this phenomenon is relevant to HIV spread in vivo. Thus far, data are lacking.

NATURAL RESISTANCE TO HIV ENTRY

Many uninfected individuals have encountered HIV-1 on multiple occasions yet remain uninfected. Moreover, many HIV-1–positive individuals have been infected for many years but show no symptoms or progress slowly to acquired immunodeficiency syndrome (AIDS). Both these groups are under intense investigation in an attempt to understand their natural resistance to infection or disease progression, respectively. Knowledge of natural protective mechanisms may allow development of novel antiviral strategies.

We now know that up to 20% of the white population carries a defective CCR5 gene (Δ32), which has a 32-nucleotide deletion. This mutated gene therefore contains a premature stop codon, and the resulting truncated CCR5 protein does not reach the cell surface. Individuals who are homozygous for Δ32 CCR5 (about 0.1%) are substantially protected against infection by HIV-1, and this genotype is overrepresented among individuals who have been exposed to virus on many occasions yet remain uninfected. The protection given by Δ32 homozygosity is not complete, however, and several such individuals who are infected with HIV-1 have been reported. These reports do not contain a thorough examination of the virus phenotype harbored, although V3 sequences are consistent with the idea that the infecting virus is SI and uses CXCR4. These observations therefore show that, on some occasions, coreceptors other than CCR5 are exploited for transmission into the new host. Infected individuals who are heterozygous for Δ32 (Δ32 CCR5/CCR5) seem to progress more slowly to AIDS compared with those with normal CCR5/CCR5, although not all studies support this conclusion. The reasons for this slower disease course are unclear.

The Δ32 genotype has not been found outside the white population. Moreover, the frequency of Δ32 varies across Europe, with the highest levels found in the north and the lowest in the south around the Mediterranean. The exclusive presence of Δ32 in whites suggests that the mutation arose relatively recently and after the separation of this human population. The high frequency of Δ32 suggests that it must have been strongly selected for at some time in the past. One theory suggested that a catastrophic epidemic occurred in which individuals bearing Δ32 had a massive survival advantage. It is tempting to imagine that a CCR5-using, HIV-like virus may have been the cause. Such speculation is appealing, yet other unknown reasons could also explain the high frequency of Δ32 in the white population.

A point mutation in the CCR2 gene (CCR2-V64I) has been identified in all ethnic groups with a frequency of 15 to 25%. This modification results in a valine-to-isoleucine switch in the first transmembrane region of CCR2. For infected individuals who are homozygous or heterozygous for this mutation, progression to AIDS and death is slowed. Thus, in total, about one-fourth of long-term nonprogressors are heterozygous either for CCR2-V64I or for Δ32. The reason that CCR2-V64I protects is less clear even than Δ32. Although CCR2 does act as a coreceptor, it is used only by a few HIV-1 isolates. The V64I mutation has no effect on a range of CCR2 activities including its capacity to function as a coreceptor. Moreover, a second study failed to show a protective role for CCR2-V64I. The CCR2 gene is adjacent to CCR5, and this mutation may be a marker genetically linked to a determinant of CCR5 expression.

We do not know currently whether other polymorphisms in the genes of coreceptors will be discovered. Several groups are studying coreceptor promoters because defects in expression may also confer protection and long-term survival in infected individuals. Most long-term progressors and multiply exposed but uninfected individuals, however, do not contain the mutations described previously. Their condition must be explained by other mechanisms, some of which may not act to block HIV interaction with receptors and entry into cells.

EVOLUTION

Why does HIV need two receptors to trigger fusion? Several observations suggest that CD4 was acquired as a "second" receptor recently in lentivirus evolution. First, several HIV-2 variants that efficiently infect CD4– cell types were identified. Subsequently, these viruses were shown to be able to exploit CXCR4 without CD4 to trigger fusion of virion and cell membranes and therefore cell entry. Second, several SIV isolates from macrophages infect CCR5+ cells without CD4. Furthermore, strains of another lentivirus, feline immunodeficiency virus (FIV), adapted for replication in cell lines, use CXCR4. Neither CD4 nor any other receptor is currently implicated in FIV infection. FIV envelope sequences that are equivalent to HIV sequences implicated in CD4 binding (V4-C5) are considerably shorter, whereas the V3 loop is longer compared with the HIV SU glycoprotein. What is the advantage of the "second" receptor, CD4? The need for an interaction with CD4, before engaging the "fusion" receptor, may enable HIV to "hide" the coreceptor determinants away from the immune system and neutralizing antibodies before and during entry. The sensitivity of CD4-independent infection by HIV-2 variants to neutralization by immune serum compared with CD4-dependent entry supports this possibility.

VIRAL TROPISM

Expression of CD4 and coreceptors determine the sensitivity of HIV for different cell types. Table 2.1 lists the cells that are the main targets for HIV in vivo. Controversy has existed, however, over the tropism of HIV for macrophages and T cells; the terms macrophage tropism and T-cell tropism are frequently used imprecisely. Most HIV strains replicate in peripheral blood mononuclear cells (PBMCs) stimulated by phytohemagglutinin and interleukin-2. These cultures contain CD4+ T lymphocytes. Nearly all NSI viruses also infect macrophage cultures. SI strains are often termed T-cell tropic, a term implying that they do not infect macrophages, and this is usually the case for most T-cell line–passaged, laboratory strains of SI HIV that infect macrophages inefficiently at best. However, these strains have often accrued mutations in accessory genes, such as *vpr*, that are essential for replication in primary macrophages, and they probably do not truly reflect HIV strains in vivo. In contrast, several groups have reported efficient replication of primary SI isolates in macrophages. Moreover, different procedures for preparing macrophages can affect coreceptor expression and sensitivity to infection. Some cultured macrophages express both CCR5 and CXCR4 consistent with a wide range of macrophage-tropic HIV strains. Taking these factors into account, there is a broad spectrum of the relative efficiency of HIV replication between primary T lymphocytes and macrophages for both NSI and SI strains, as illustrated in Figure 2.4.

Apart from CXCR4 and CCR5, at least five other 7TM receptors have been shown to function as coreceptors for HIV in vitro. Currently, investigators have little precise knowledge of the cell types on which these coreceptors are expressed, but much work is underway to establish the roles of each of these coreceptors in HIV infection of distinct cell types in different tissues and organs in vivo. For example, in the brain, microglial cells derived from the monocyte/macrophage lineage are the main target for HIV infection. Ligands to CCR3 and CCR5 block infection of microglia by NSI strains of HIV-1, thus indicating that these coreceptors are expressed.

Blood dendritic cells and the related Langerhans cells of the skin and mucous membranes also appear to be permissive to the replication of most HIV tropisms. Whether these cells genuinely propagate the virus or whether they physically present bound virus to lymphocytes is controversial, because the purity of cell preparations is debated. In vivo, electron microscopic evidence indicates replicating, budding virions in Langerhans cells. As discussed later, cultured Langerhans

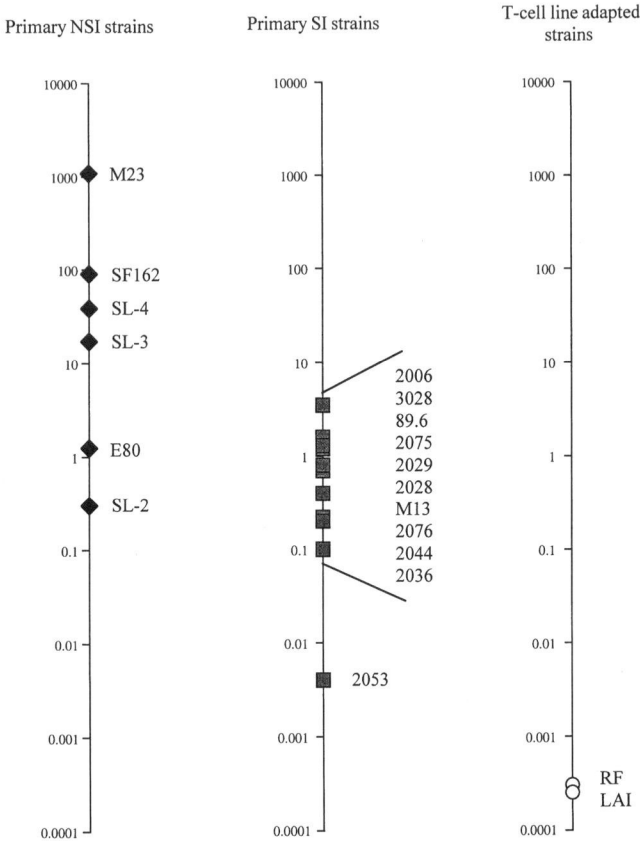

Figure 2.4. Macrophage median tissue culture infective dose (TCID$_{50}$)/peripheral blood mononuclear cell (PBMC) TCID$_{50}$. Relative efficiency of infection of HIV-1 isolates for cultured macrophages to primary PBMCs. (From Simmons et al. J Virol 1997;70:8355–8360.)

cells support replication by both NSI and SI virus. Inhibition of HIV infection by appropriate chemokines indicates that both CXCR4 and CCR5 are expressed, although uncultured Langerhans cells may not express CXCR4. Another distinct cell type is the follicular dendritic cell of the lymph node, which presents antigen to B lymphocytes in the lymphoid follicle. These cells may simply adsorb HIV to their surface without becoming infected, much like human U87 glioblastoma and rodent cell lines expressing human CD4.

The major viral determinant of tropism at the level of virus entry is the SU protein, gp120. The variable loops of gp120, V1/V2, and particularly V3 affect whether the virus is NSI or SI and which coreceptors are used for infection. These are regions of gp120 that are not directly connected with CD4 recognition but contain epitopes for neutralizing antibodies that act equally well before and after virus adsorption to cells. The genetic variation of the variable loops may be driven by escape from immune attack. Although this undoubtedly occurs, variation may also be driven by adaptation to infect different cell types as infection spreads within the individual.

HIV TROPISM AND TRANSMISSION

CCR5 is crucial for transmission of HIV to a new host because individuals homozygous for the 32-base pair deletion are largely resistant to infection (see earlier). CCR5-using NSI viruses are predominantly transmitted, but the reasons for this selectivity are not obvious. Isolates with an SI phenotype are readily isolated from semen of SI-virus carriers, a finding indicating no intrinsic barrier to SI transport and replication in seminal fluid lymphocytes. One opinion was that the first cells infected by HIV after transmission may selectively express CCR5, but not CXCR4. Cell types that are the main candidates for primary infection include dendritic cells, Langerhans cells present in mucosa and submucosal macrophages. Macrophages used for in vitro HIV infectivity studies are derived from blood monocytes. At first, these macrophages were not thought to express CXCR4 because they are relatively resistant to CXCR4-using T-cell line–passaged HIV-1 viruses. Yet the emerging consensus from fluoresence-activated cell sorter analysis using CXCR4 specific monoclonal antibodies is that these cultured macrophages do express CXCR4. Moreover, many primary SI viruses infect macrophages and are inhibited by CXCR4-specific ligands. However, whether these cultured macrophages are truly representative of tissue macrophages situated below the mucosal membranes of the vagina and rectum is unclear.

As with blood-derived macrophages, Langerhans cells isolated and cultured from human skin biopsies can be infected by HIV-1 strains that use either CCR5 or CXCR4. Moreover, ligands specific for these coreceptors block infection, a finding indicating the presence of both coreceptors on Langerhans cells. Uncultured Langerhans cells have been shown to express CCR5 but not CXCR4, although CXCR4 is rapidly upregulated on culture. If Langerhans cells at sites of transmission express CCR5 but not CXCR4, then the selective transmission of NSI viruses may be partly explained. Many SI isolates, however, use a broad range of coreceptors including CCR5 as well as CXCR4. The restrictions to these strains at transmission are therefore still obscure.

Investigators have reported that clade E HIV-1, which is spreading heterosexually in Thailand, readily infects Langerhans cells, whereas clade B virus, which has colonized Western homosexuals, does not. Investigators postulated that rectal infection, like parenteral infection, could bypass Langerhans cells in the mucosa and would favor T-cell tropic viruses. However, subsequent studies by other laboratories have not been able to confirm clade-specific tropisms, so it no longer appears likely that Langerhans cell tropism accounts for HIV variation between heterosexually and homosexually transmitted virus.

HIV TROPISM AND PATHOGENESIS

During the early phase of HIV infection before seroconversion, the virus propagates to appreciable plasma titers with little genetic variation. Primary infection may cause a temporary depletion of CD4+ PBMCs. HIV infection usually elicits strong cell-mediated immune responses (CD8+ cytotoxic T cells), which probably clear the high virus load, but fail to eradicate HIV infection altogether. During the long, so-called asymptomatic period, the virus is not latent but remains active in lymphoid tissue, as shown many years ago by immunofluorescence and electron microscopy. More sensitive in situ and polymerase chain reaction genome detection methods reveal high virus loads in affected lymph nodes and higher plasma and PBMC viremia than previously appreciated. In the early days of studying AIDS and HIV infection, physicians called the inflammatory signs of infection in the lymph nodes lymphadenopathy syndrome or persistent generalized lymphadenopathy. Indeed, the first HIV-1 isolate was called LAV, an abbreviation for lymphadenopathy virus, because it was derived by culture from an asymptomatic patient with swollen lymph glands.

The viruses most prevalent during the asymptomatic phase tend to be slow/low NSI variants that infect PBMCs and macrophages. Variants found in cerebrospinal fluid and the brain are similar and often have a greater propensity for macrophage tropism. However, the type of cell used for the propagation of these primary isolates affects their tropism. Possibly, HIV variants with different tropisms and coreceptor use account for different attributes of the overall syndrome of AIDS. Clearly, the T-helper cell depletion is associated with T-cell–tropic viruses, although indirect effects can also account in part for the decline in CD4+ cells. The SI variants that readily adapt in culture to propagation in T-cell lines usually appear late in disease and may emerge as a result of developing immune deficiency, although they presage the steepest decline of CD4+ lymphocytes in end-stage disease.

Other lentivirus infections may help to illuminate aspects of AIDS pathogenesis. For instance, direct inoculation of T-cell–tropic SI variants of SIV into the brain of macaque monkeys does not result in infection, whereas blood infection followed by a period of adaptation to macrophage tropism allows encephalopathic variants to emerge that then cause brain disease on direct inoculation into naive hosts. Visna/Maedi virus of sheep, the prototype lentivirus, resembles macrophage-tropic HIV without the appearance of T-cell–tropic variants. Infected susceptible sheep develop the wasting syndrome and central nervous system disease also characteristic of human AIDS in the absence of severe T-helper cell immune deficiency.

In understanding the virology of HIV pathogenesis, investigators must elucidate which parameters of infection are genuinely relevant to the development of disease. Is it total virus load, virus and infected cell turnover, antigenic diversity, or host immune responses resembling graft-versus-host disease? We still do not yet know the full significance of long-term survivors of HIV infection, and perhaps a related unknown issue is why some primate hosts infected with SIV or HIV manage to hold off disease manifestations indefinitely. A better understanding of these attributes of pathogenesis may point the way to therapeutic modalities aimed at postponing disease and to vaccines that prevent AIDS even if sterilizing prophylactic vaccination against HIV infection proved to be unattainable.

VIRUS NEUTRALIZATION

Neutralizing antibodies in seropositive patients can be divided into two types, those that broadly neutralize many HIV strains and those that are specific to particular variants. The latter, type-specific neutralizing antibodies, are usually directed to the V3 and sometimes to the V2 variable epitopes on gp120. The broadly cross-neutralizing antibodies recognize epitopes on gp120 and gp41, including complex, conformation-dependent regions of gp120 that interact with the CD4 receptor. Such antibodies compete weakly with CD4 for binding HIV virions. If stronger humoral immunity of this type could be developed, perhaps it would provide the basis for vaccine immunogens, because binding to CD4 is a conserved feature of all strains of HIV-1 and is generally shared with HIV-2. In addition, some V3 antibodies, particularly those to the crown of the epitope, show cross-neutralizing properties.

Most early experimental neutralization studies were conducted with virulent, T-cell line–passaged SI strains of HIV. Subsequent experiments revealed that primary isolates are substantially more resistant to a range of neutralizing antibodies of different specificities. These results suggest that a vaccine based solely on induction of neutralizing antibodies is unlikely to be effective.

Therefore, virus neutralization by antibodies is only one aspect of humoral immune defenses. Antibody-dependent cellular cytoxocity and antibody-dependent complement-mediated lysis of virions and of infected cells are other attributes that may be more important in vivo. Cytotoxic T-cell destruction of virus-infected cells is likely to be the major factor in clearing primary viremia. Nevertheless, as is the general experience with other viruses such as influenza or polio, the serum-neutralizing titers of vaccinated or recovered individuals correlate with protection to infection. Passive transfer of neutralizing antibody has been shown in a few cases to protect chimpanzees from challenge with HIV-1 and macaques from challenge with SIVmac. Thus, humoral immune responses may protect from de novo infection, although the extent of their role in delaying the progress of HIV pathogenesis in the persistently infected seropositive individual is controversial. Investigators are also interested in the possible role of neutralizing antibodies in protecting the fetus or newborn infant from maternal HIV infection.

Neutralizing antibodies that bind to domains of gp120 involved in CD4 recognition block the first step of infection, namely, adsorption to target cells. The most potently neutralizing monoclonal antibodies, however, are those to the V2 and V3 loops of gp120, and these also neutralize after adsorption to target cells, provided the virions have not yet become internalized. Probably, the neutralizing antibodies directed to gp41 can also act after attachment; indeed, one neutralizing monoclonal antibody that recognizes an epitope close to the virion membrane is a potent neutralizer of a broad range of primary HIV-1 strains.

THERAPEUTIC STRATEGIES

The therapeutic strategies based on blocking virus entry and hence spread to new cells have thus far been targeted to three processes: 1) blocking correct maturation of viral glycoproteins in the cells, producing HIV to render the virus noninfectious; 2) blocking HIV binding to CD4; and 3) blocking HIV interaction with coreceptors.

The first process blocks correct maturation of viral glycoproteins in the cells, producing noninfectious HIV. Compounds such as deoxynojirimycin and castanospermine interfere with proper glycosylation of HIV gp120 to reduce the infectivity of the virions. Because they are targeted to cellular enzymes, they are likely to have toxic side effects, but these drugs are worth pursuing experimentally, because, conversely, HIV should not develop resistance to them.

In the second process (blocking HIV binding to CD4), the major compounds targeted to inhibit the docking of the virus to its receptor are soluble recombinant proteins based on the CD4 receptor itself. Because the N-terminal domain alone binds to and neutralizes HIV, and it does not appear to be toxic or immunosuppressive, it can be tested as a pharmaceutical agent. Second-generation recombinant proteins comprising the N-terminal domains of CD4 linked with the Fc portion of IgG or IgM molecules have a much longer plasma half-life without loss of neutralizing properties. Clinical trials with such recombinant proteins have not shown significant benefit to date. One reason is that primary HIV isolates are much less sensitive to soluble CD4 (sCD4) inactivation than are T-cell line–adapted SI strains. New constructs, however, could lead to a renaissance of this approach.

Why does such a large discrepancy exist between the sensitivity of laboratory and clinical isolates of HIV-1? The primary affinity of sCD4 for gp120 is similar between the two types of HIV-1. However, the laboratory-adapted strains after in vitro passage in the absence of immunity and neutralizing antibodies are highly sensitive to uncoupling of gp120 from gp41 by sCD4, whereas clinical isolates retain sCD4 to form a tertiary complex of sCD4/gp120/gp41. In other words, sCD4 inactivates laboratory strains of HIV-1 by inducing the irreversible shedding of gp120, whereas sCD4 merely binds to the clinical isolates to compete with cell-anchored CD4 for infection. sCD4 has also been shown to enhance infection by some primary strains, presumably by inducing extra sites for binding to coreceptors. Another approach to exploiting our knowledge of CD4 as the HIV receptor has been to generate recombinant sCD4 coupled to toxic proteins such as bacterial exotoxin or the ricin A-chain. Such receptor toxin molecules bind with high affinity to cells expressing gp120/gp41 at the cell surface. Experiments with HIV-expressing cells in vitro show that the sCD4 toxins are efficacious in killing HIV-infected cells, but they are likely to be toxic and immunogenic in vivo. CD4, however, remains the only cell-surface receptor that binds all HIV strains and is essential for infection of the major cell types targeted by HIV in vivo. New approaches to block this interaction would therefore be worthwhile. For instance, small-molecular-weight compounds should be screened for inhibition of HIV attachment to CD4.

Gene therapy approaches that deliver genes encoding toxic proteins are also envisaged. These avenues may exploit the novel observation that CD4 and coreceptors can be assembled onto budding virus particles. These pseudotype viruses will specifically infect cells expressing HIV envelope glycoproteins by a "reverse fusion" event.

Strong interest has been expressed in developing novel drugs that target the coreceptors. Agents aimed at CCR5 could be used in contraceptives or as part of postexposure treatment. If infected individuals are treated early enough with drugs targeted to CCR5, then replication and variation of HIV could be slowed or halted, thus preventing the occurrence of cytopathic strains that use other coreceptors such as CXCR4. Drugs aimed at CXCR4 could be useful in the later stages of disease when SI strains that use this coreceptor have emerged or are likely to emerge.

CCR5 is an attractive target for therapeutics because individuals homozygous for the 32-base pair deletion seem to suffer no ill effects. Therefore, drugs that specifically block the natural function of CCR5 should not be overly toxic or immunosuppressive. Moreover, investigators must ensure that drugs do not activate CCR5 or other coreceptors because hyperallergic responses could result.

Currently, two main types of candidate exist for drug development. Chemokines themselves are candidates because they inhibit HIV infection in vitro. Chemokines interact with two sites on the receptor, first with the receptor's N-terminus. Then the N-terminus of the chemokine "hits" a second site within the receptor. This second site is thought to be crucial for signaling to ensue. Modification of a chemokine at the N-terminus can therefore abrogate its capacity to signal without affecting recognition and binding to its receptor. Such modified chemokines are potentially ideal for therapy because they should be incapable of activating inflammation while maintaining the capacity to interfere with HIV entry. Modification of RANTES at the N-terminus by chemical addition of several hydrocarbon residues, to form aminooxypentane (AOP)–RANTES, renders it inactive for chemotaxis and antagonistic for other CCR5 ligands. Remarkably, AOP–RANTES was more efficient for HIV inhibition by CCR5 than RANTES itself. The efficient inhibition seems to result from the capacity of AOP–RANTES to bind CCR5 with high affinity, to occupy all CCR5 molecules at the cell surface, and to induce rapid, mainly irreversible internalization of CCR5 into endosomes. Because RANTES interacts with other chemokine receptors as well as CCR5, it may not be the ideal starting point for drug development; however, the striking properties of AOP–RANTES suggest a future role for chemokine derivatives in therapy.

The second approach is to screen libraries of small organic molecules for their capacity to interact specifically with appropriate coreceptors. Modification of molecules identified in this way could then improve the potency of HIV inhibition and receptor specificity. A bicyclam derivative (AMD3100) has been reported that binds CXCR4 and potently inhibits HIV infection by this coreceptor. Drugs based on small organic molecules may be administered orally and may be efficiently absorbed and dispersed throughout the body. The cost of production could be substantially lower than that of protein-based reagents.

At this stage, it is difficult to assess how quickly HIV variants that evade coreceptor drugs will appear. Agents such as AOP–RANTES that strip CCR5 from the cell surface may help to prevent such escape mutants from emerging.

Reference

1. Stuart D. Virus structure: docking mission accomplished. Nature 1994;371:19–20.

Suggested Readings

Berger EA. HIV entry and tropism: the chemokine receptor connection. AIDS 1997;11(Suppl A):S3–S16.

Clapham PR, Weiss RA. Immunodeficiency viruses: spoilt for choice of co-receptors. Nature 1997;388:230–231.

Dimitrov DS, Broder CC. HIV and membrane receptors. New York: Landes Bioscience. Chapman & Hall, 1997.

Levy JA. HIV pathogenesis of AIDS. Washington, DC: ASM Press, 1998.

O'Brien SJ, Dean M. In search of AIDS-resistance genes. Sci Am 1997; September:28–35.

3
VIRAL GENES AND THEIR PRODUCTS

Mario Stevenson

The primate lentiviruses, human immunodeficiency virus-1 (HIV-1), HIV-2, and simian immunodeficiency virus (SIV), contain 10 open-reading frames. These open-reading frames encode viral gene products that provide structural integrity to the virion, provide enzymatic functions for virus replication, or regulate viral gene expression. In addition to the extensively characterized viral gene products are a potentially greater number of cellular proteins that interact with the viral gene products and mediate their function. Ultimately, perpetuation of the virus life cycle and dissemination of the virus in the host requires both viral proteins and their cellular intermediaries. The interaction between viral gene products and their cellular ligands represents a relatively unexplored area for therapeutic intervention of primate lentivirus replication. An essential prerequisite in any strategy aimed at blocking the action of viral proteins is a thorough understanding of the function of that viral gene product. Much of what is known regarding structural and enzymatic proteins of the primate lentiviruses has been modeled on studies with animal oncoretroviruses and, in particular, with murine leukemia virus, Rous sarcoma virus, and avian leukosis virus. As a consequence, a better understanding of the action of the viral enzymes has been gained, and agents that block the action of these enzymes have been developed and are used clinically. On the other hand, a deeper understanding of the functions of the regulatory and the accessory gene products has not been so readily forthcoming. Counterparts for most of the accessory gene products have not been identified outside the primate lentivirus lineages, nor to date have any cellular homologues of primate lentivirus accessory gene products been characterized.

Although little imagination is required to understand the requirement for the structural and enzymatic proteins, the role of the accessory gene products in the lentivirus life cycle is far from obvious. Whereas certain properties have been assigned to some of the accessory gene products, which of these properties, if any, relate to the actual functions of the protein in virus replication is by no means clear. In addition, a general theme emerging from the study of the regulatory and accessory gene products is that more than one property can be attributed to each protein, perhaps not surprising for a virus expected to carry out diverse biochemical actions with only a handful of virus-encoded proteins. In this chapter, I review the current status of research efforts into the molecular biology of HIV, its genomic organization, replication cycle, and properties associated with viral gene products, as well as a discussion of cellular proteins identified to date that interact with these viral gene products. I attempt to put viral gene products into perspective by discussing possible functions for the viral proteins and, in particular, the accessory viral proteins.

GENOMIC ORGANIZATION OF PRIMATE LENTIVIRUSES

The primate lentiviruses include HIV-1 and HIV-2 and the nonhuman primate lentiviruses, collectively referred to as SIVs. SIVs have been identified in various Old World monkey species (1) including mandrills (SIV_{MND}; subscript denotes species of origin) sooty mangabey (SIV_{SM}), African green monkey (SIV_{AGM}), macaque (SIV_{MAC}), and Sykes' monkey (SIV_{SYK}). An SIV variant that is more closely related to HIV-1 than the other nonhuman primate lentiviruses, SIV_{CPZ}, has been isolated from chimpanzees (2). The known primate lentiviruses form five main groups (3). Phylogenetic relationships among primate lentiviruses, as derived from pol protein sequences, are illustrated on Figure 3.1. Primate lentiviruses appear to be generally nonpathogenic in the natural host. HIV-1 and HIV-2 infection of humans and SIV_{MAC} infection of macaques are a result of cross-species transmission. Evidence of cross-species transmission is provided by phylogenetic relationships between SIV_{CPZ} and SIV_{SM}, which are of the same lineage as HIV-1 and HIV-2, respectively, and which, based on the divergence of the five major lineages, appear to have arisen from their respective simian counterparts recently. In a nonnatural host, selective pressure drives evolution of viral variants that better exist within the new environment but that, as a consequence, may acquire virulence. A fuller understanding of how primate lentiviruses are virulent in nonnatural hosts may be provided through an understanding of how primate lentivirus replication in a natural host can be supported without any pathogenic effects.

The genomic organization of the primate and animal lentiviruses is outlined in Figure 3.2. The genome of the simple animal oncoretrovirus, murine leukemia virus, is shown for comparison. The structural *gag* and *envelope (env)*

24 Section II. Basic Sciences

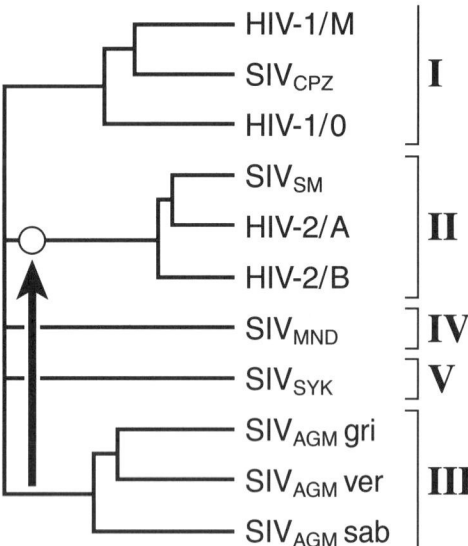

Figure 3.1. **Phylogenetic relationships among primate lentiviruses derived from pol protein sequences.** The five major and roughly equidistant lineages are indicated by Roman numerals. The diversity of HIV-1 is indicated by samples of groups M and O; diversity of HIV-2 is indicated by subtypes A and B. SIV subscripts denote species of origin (see text). Horizontal branch lengths are drawn to scale: the *scale bar* represents 0.05 amino acid replacements per site, that is, 5% difference, after correction for multiple hits; vertical separation is for clarity only. (Adapted from Sharp PM, Bailes E, Stevenson M, et al. Gene acquisition in HIV and SIV. Nature 1996;383:586–587.)

genes and the pol open-reading frame encoding the enzymatic proteins are common to all retroviruses. The 5′ long terminal repeat (LTR) contains the site for initiation of viral transcription (4). Distinct functional domains within the LTR are known as U3, R, and U5. Cellular factors that modulate viral transcription interact primarily with sequences in U3. Some of these sequences connect the transcriptional activity of the provirus to the activation state of the host cell. For example, T-cell mitogens and cytokines increase NF-κB levels in the nucleus that, in turn, act on sequences within the enhancer region of U3, thereby promoting transcription from the LTR (5–10). A *cis*-acting sequence designated the Tat-response element (TAR) located in R mediates the action of the viral transactivator, Tat (4). The *gag* and *env* genes encode multiple structural proteins that give the virion its integrity and promote its entry into cells. Many of the functions of the *gag* gene products can be thought of as simply protecting viral nucleic acids, because they are in transit from producer to target cell. However, it is becoming apparent that structural virion proteins and, in particular, the gag matrix (MA) and gag capsid (CA) proteins, serve important roles during virus entry into the new host cell. The regulatory proteins, Tat and Rev, act in *trans* on *cis*-acting signals within the provirus to control its transcriptional activity and the relative abundance of genomic and subgenomic viral RNAs, respectively.

Figure 3.2. **Preintegration events in lentivirus replication:** 1) The mature virion contains processed proteins derived from gag and gag pol polyproteins. Gag MA has been assigned mainly to the inner phospholipid leaflet of the host cell-derived virion membrane. Capsid constitutes the virion core. Viral enzymes involved in cDNA synthesis and integration are contained within the core, likely in association with genomic viral RNA. The accessory gene products, Vpr/Vpx, are specifically packaged within virions through their interaction with gag p6. Vpx and likely Vpr are contained within the viral core. Cyclophilin A is encapsidated within virions through its association with CA. In addition, the accessory gene products, Nef and Vif, are contained within virions, although their mechanism of virion incorporation and their location within the virion are unknown. 2) Infection of the cell is initiated on formation of a trimolecular complex between envelope on the virion and CD4/coreceptor molecules on the target cell. 3) Fusion of viral and target cell membranes is initiated on exposure of the fusogenic domains in the viral envelope. Two virion proteins (cyclophilin and Vif) are implicated in the uncoating process in which viral nucleic acids, in association with virion proteins, are deposited in the host cell cytoplasm. 4) The uncoating process results in deposition of a high-molecular-weight reverse transcription complex (also referred to as the preintegration complex) in the host cell cytoplasm. In addition to the enzymes RT and IN, the virion proteins MA and Vpr/Vpx remain associated with the reverse transcription complex as it translocates to the host cell nucleus. The mechanism through which the Vpr/Vpx and MA proteins associate with the complex is not well understood but may be mediated through interaction with gag p6. However, whether gag p6 is associated with the complex is unknown. Because the NC protein is implicated in synthesis of viral cDNA and in integration, by inference, it may also be a component of the reverse transcription complex. Although gag CA is excluded from the complex during uncoating, MA is retained. MA molecules that remain associated with the reverse transcription complex probably were originally located in the virion core, whereas the bulk of MA is on the exterior of the virion core. Phosphorylation of gag MA by a virion-associated kinase may promote dissociation of the reverse transcription complex from the membrane at the point of virus entry. Although reverse transcription in some cases may be initiated in the virion, most early and intermediate strand synthesis likely occurs in the cytosol. The reverse transcription process may be influenced by the activation state of the host cell such that in quiescent cells, low dNTP pools may impair the extent of reverse transcription. 5) Nuclear translocation of the reverse transcription complex occurs rapidly after infection of the cell. Components of the reverse transcription complex can be detected in the host cell nucleus within 15 to 30 minutes of infection. By comparison, complete synthesis of viral cDNA in vivo requires approximately 3 hours. As a consequence, most plus-strand cDNA synthesis may take place in the nucleus. In a nondividing target cell, translocation of the reverse transcription complex across the nuclear envelope is a saturable receptor-mediated and active process. Nucleophilic proteins within the reverse transcription complex interact with cellular importins, which direct the complex to the nuclear pore. Gag MA and Vpr/Vpx proteins have so far been implicated in the nuclear translocation process. The complex enters the nucleus through pores in the nuclear envelope because translocation of the complex is impaired by inhibitors of nuclear pore-mediated transport. In quiescent T cells, nuclear translocation of the reverse transcription complex is inefficient, likely because of the limited availability of active nuclear pores through which large nucleoprotein complexes can translocate. 6) After translocation of the reverse transcription complex to the nucleus and completion of viral cDNA synthesis, the cellular protein HMG I(Y) associates with the complex, and this association is necessary for integration of viral with host cell DNA 7). Integration of viral DNA appears to occur randomly and does not appear to be influenced by the transcriptional state of the integration site. However, the reported role of INI 1 in the integration process suggests that this cellular factor may remodel chromatin and thus may promote the ability of cellular DNA to act as a substrate for integration.

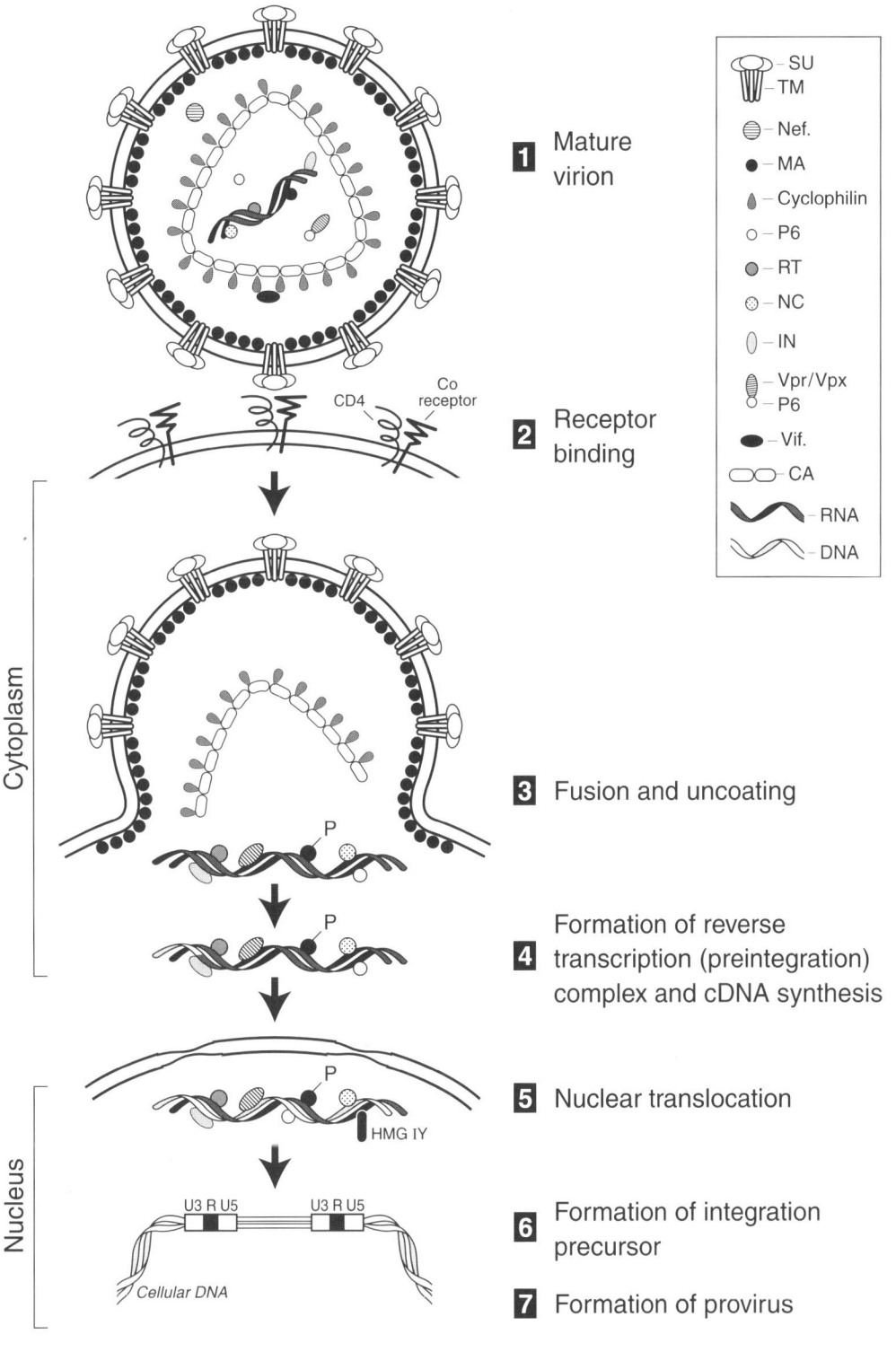

Tat and Rev are not unique to the primate lentiviruses, and homologous functions exist in the human T-cell leukemia viruses types 1 and 2 (4), human spuma retrovirus, otherwise known as human foamy virus (11), and feline and ungulate lentiviruses, including feline immunodeficiency virus (FIV), bovine immunodeficiency virus (BIV), caprine arthritis/encephalitis virus (CAEV), and equine infectious anemia virus (EIAV) (12) (see Fig 3.2). The remaining primate lentiviral genes are collectively referred to as the accessory genes, and with the exception of *vif*, which has been identified in FIV, BIV, and CAEV, they have no counterparts in any other retrovirus (see Fig 3.2). The primate lentiviruses differ in their relative composition of accessory genes, a difference that likely reflects the divergent evolution and adaptation to the respective primate host. However, although a particular accessory gene product may be absent from a primate lentivirus variant, its property is retained and exhibited by another viral protein. The differences among the primate lentiviral genomes involve genes of the so-called "middle region" located between *vif* and *env* genes. In this region, HIV-1 and SIV_{CPZ} encode *vpr* and *vpu* genes. In contrast, HIV-2/SIV_{SM}/SIV_{MAC} viruses lack *vpu* and, in its place, contain a gene termed *vpx* (see Fig 3.2). Nevertheless, a *vpu*-like property contained within envelope genes of HIV-2 otherwise lacks a *vpu* open-reading frame (13). In addition, properties ascribed to *vpx* are exhibited by HIV-1 vpr (14). The SIV_{MND}, SIV_{SYK}, and SIV_{AGM} viruses contain a single open-reading frame, namely, vpr in the "middle region," and it is likely that the functions exhibited by the missing *vpu* and *vpx* genes are provided by *envelope* and *vpr* genes, respectively. This conservation of function provides a strong argument that certain ascribed properties of these accessory gene products are essential for some certain aspects of primate lentivirus replication. These properties are discussed in detail in this chapter.

VIRION COMPOSITION

Primate lentiviruses have a spherical diameter of approximately 110 nm. The virion core spans almost the entire diameter of the virion, being approximately 100 nm in length (15). A distinguishing feature of primate lentiviruses is the presence of a structure designated the core or capsid–envelope link through which the virion core and the lipid bilayer are linked (16). Although the composition of the capsid–envelope link is unknown, this structure possibly provides a basis for the association of MA protein with components of the viral core, thus allowing this protein to be retained within the reverse transcription complex after host cell infection (17). Genomic RNA is present within viral particles as a dimer linked through hydrogen bonding (18). Dimerization of genomic viral RNA may also be promoted by the nucleocapsid protein (19, 20). A small fraction of viral particles isolated from infected tissue culture cells and from body fluids of infected individuals contain products of reverse transcription and predominantly minus-strand strong-stop DNA (21–23). These incomplete DNA forms may facilitate infection of cells in which low deoxynucleotide pools would otherwise restrict efficient infection and initiation of reverse transcription (24, 25).

Some viral and cellular proteins that do not appear to be involved in virion integrity or in receptor interaction have been identified in association with the virion. In many cases, the actual roles played by these proteins are not obvious, although a virion association argues for their involvement in an early step in the viral life cycle at a point preceding de novo expression of viral proteins. An important consideration regarding virion-associated proteins is whether those proteins are packaged, that is, whether their concentration in the virion exceeds their relative concentration in the cell. Several structural enzymatic and accessory gene products are packaged within the virion (Fig 3.3). Many other proteins, both viral and cellular, identified in association with the virion, do not appear to be specifically packaged (with the exception of cyclophilin). Their presence within the virion may be dictated by their association with cellular components that are virion incorporated (for example, plasma membrane). Nevertheless, many of these virion-associated proteins appear to be important for virus replication even though they may not be specifically "packaged" in the virus particle.

VIRAL GENE PRODUCTS

Envelope Glycoproteins

Envelope glycoprotein comprises two subunits cleaved from a gp160 precursor molecule. Synthesis and processing of envelope glycoproteins proceed in the cellular secretory pathway. Glycosylation and formation of disulfide bonds proceed in the endoplasmic reticulum (ER), resulting in the formation of a folded gp160 monomer (26). At this point, the envelope precursor acquires the capacity to bind CD4 and, as a consequence, rapidly binds nascent CD4 molecules as they too are synthesized and processed through the secretory pathway. The intracellular complex between gp160 and CD4 accounts, to a large degree, for the eventual depletion of surface CD4 expression after HIV infection of the host cell (27–31). On transport from the ER to the Golgi apparatus, additional processing leads to viral glycoproteins with both complex and hybrid carbohydrate side chains (32). Glycosylation greatly influences envelope glycoprotein function. N-linked glycosylation sites primarily in the N-terminal half of gp120 appear critical for viral infectivity (33). Envelope glycosylation also modulates immunogenicity of the envelope glycoprotein, for example, by occluding peptide epitopes and providing a means to avoid surveyance by immune responses (34). Most of the neutralizing antibody present in HIV-1 infected individuals recognizes sequences in the envelope glycoprotein. Most of these antibodies recognize the V3 loop, although sequences in V2 and C4 domains are also targets for neutralizing antibody (35, 36). The envelope precursor (gp160) is cleaved by a cellular endopeptidase to yield the extracellular portion (gp120 or SU) and the membrane-spanning portion (gp41 or TM). Precursor processing is essential for virion infectivity and for syncytium formation (37). Because the external glycoprotein subunit is noncovalently linked to the transmembrane portion, it easily dissociates from the virion. Routine purification procedures in which viral particles are sedimented through sucrose lead to marked reductions in particle infectivity. Soluble CD4 and neutralizing antibodies to HIV-1 gp120 inhibit viral infectivity by promoting dissociation of the external subunit from the virion (38, 39). It is also likely that shearing forces exerted on virions as they circulate in body fluids and between tissue spaces cause dissociation of the external envelope glycoprotein subunit. For this and other reasons, investigators have estimated that approximately 1 in 60,000 plasma virions is infectious (40).

Although biochemical studies have suggested dimeric, trimeric and tetrameric organization for SU (41–44), high-resolution electron microscopy suggests a trimeric structure (15). Because the envelope glycoprotein contains domains for the recognition of neutralizing antibody and for the

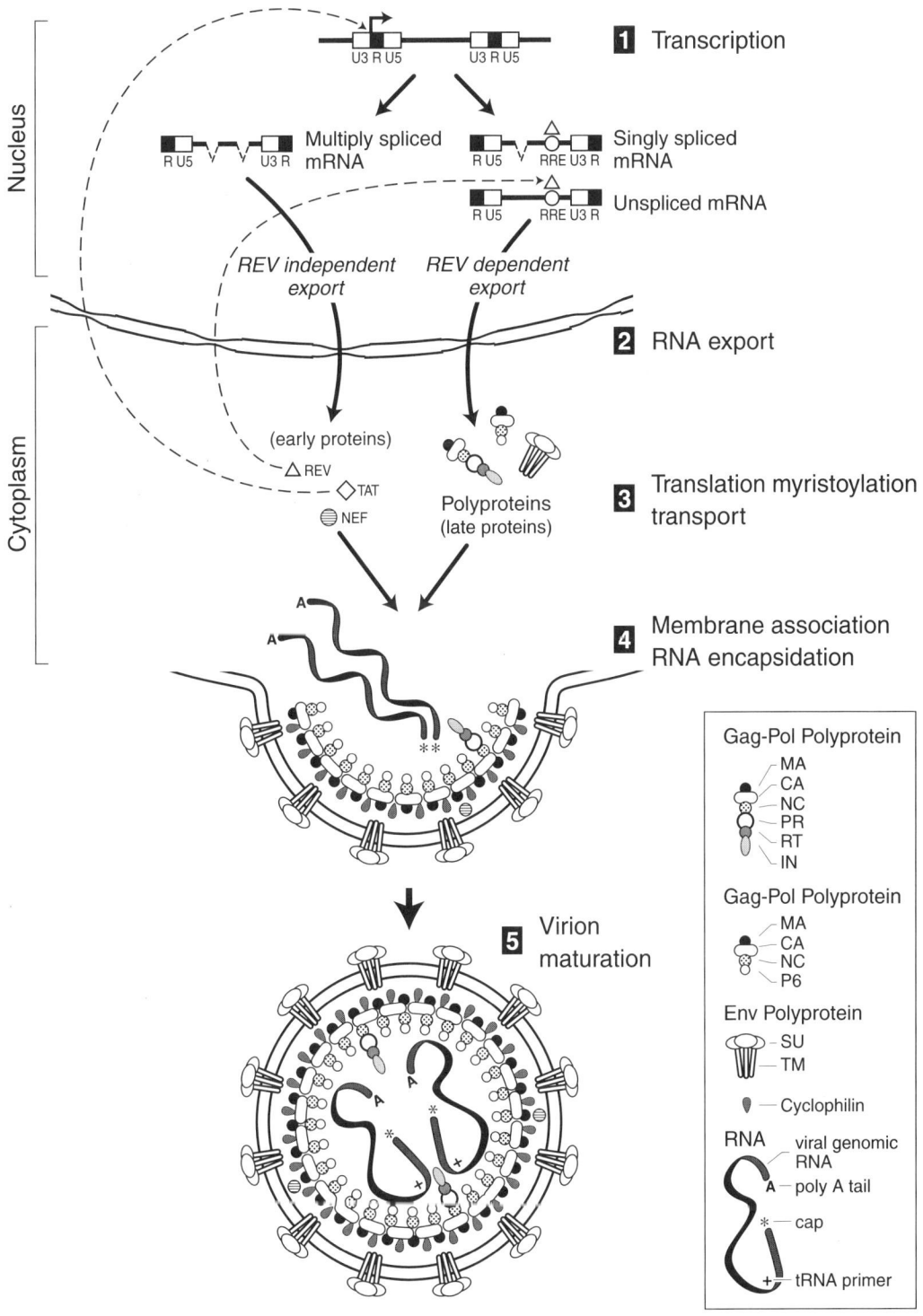

Figure 3.3. Postintegration events in lentivirus replication: 1) Proviral DNA serves as a template for the production of both genomic (unspliced) viral RNA that is destined for incorporation into progeny virions as well as spliced mRNAs for viral protein synthesis. Two major classes of spliced messages are produced. Small (less than 2 kb) multiply spliced messages are produced early after activation of the provirus and encode the Tat, Rev, and Nef proteins. Rev is translocated to the nucleus, where it interacts with the Rev-responsive element, which is only present in unspliced and singly-spliced transcripts. 2) The binding of Rev to the RRE promotes stability, nuclear export, and translation of RRE-containing transcripts (Rev-dependent pathway). This leads to the expression of gag, gag/pol, and env polyproteins, as well as the accessory gene products, Vif, Vpu, and Vpr/Vpx. 3) Nascent viral proteins are cotranslationally and posttranslationally modified through phosphorylation, myristoylation, and glycosylation. Whether viral precursor proteins associate initially in the cell cytosol to produce an assembly intermediate or whether the association occurs after precursor molecules localize to the plasma membrane is unclear. Interaction with gag and gag/pol polyproteins with the cell membrane is mediated by a basic domain at the N-terminus of the MA domain of $Pr^{55\ gag}$. The MA domain of $Pr^{55\ gag}$ is also important for the inclusion of envelope glycoproteins during virion assembly. 4) Selective packaging of full-length viral RNA is mediated by interaction between a *cis*-acting packaging element or "psi" located near the 5' end of full-length viral transcripts and the NC domain of $Pr^{55\ gag}$. As a consequence, unspliced RNAs are packaged from a large excess of spliced messages. 5) Virion maturation involves proteolytic processing of gag, gag/pol, and env precursor proteins by the PR domain of $Pr^{160\ gag/pol}$. Proteolytic processing is likely initiated during formation of electron-dense nucleoprotein complexes at the cell membrane and continues after detachment of the immature virion.

engagement of primary and secondary cell-surface receptors, escape from neutralizing antibody and adaptation to infection of different cell types provides the driving forces for sequence heterogeneity in the SU portion of the envelope glycoprotein. SU contains five variable regions interspersed with conserved regions. Selection pressure placed on viral populations (e.g., immunologic suppression by the host and competition between viruses for available target cells) results in the generation of a population of microvariants (quasispecies) (45, 46), and envelope variation within virus populations of an infected individual (intrapatient or intrastrain variation) ranges from 1 to 6%. By comparison, envelope sequences of viruses from distinct geographic locations (interpatient variation) can vary up to 25%. Intrapatient and interpatient genetic variability is the direct consequence of the infidelity of reverse transcription. As a consequence, one nucleotide sequence change is generated for each viral genome synthesized. Although mutations introduced during reverse transcription are predicted to be distributed randomly across the entire genome, only nonlethal mutations emerge in the virus population. The expansion of viruses of a particular genotype ultimately depends on the relative "fitness" of that virus, that is, whether it can compete with other viral genotypes for available host cells and whether it can exist in the face of environmental challenge (e.g., immunologic clearance and drug pressure). An immediate consequence of the extensive heterogeneity within SU regards the affinity with which envelope glycoproteins of different viruses bind to CD4. The increased binding of envelope molecules from primary isolates to CD4 likely accounts for the higher concentrations of soluble CD4 that are required to neutralize primary HIV-1 isolates (47–49).

The interaction between SU and CD4 initiates infection of the cell. This interaction likely leads to conformational rearrangement in both SU and CD4 (50) that ultimately leads to the generation of a binding site for interaction with coreceptor molecules including CXCR4 and CCR5 (51–53). The binding site for coreceptor molecules likely lies in gp120 in the region known as the variable V3 loop. Antibodies that block the V3/gp120 interaction also prevent the interaction of CCR5 with gp120 (52, 53). This is consistent with previous studies demonstrating that V3 loop sequences from monocytotropic HIV-1 variants conferred monocytotropism when inserted within the envelope of T-lymphotropic virus variants (54–57). Although processes that lead to activation of fusion between virion and cell membranes are not well understood, a likely situation is that formation of a heterotrimeric complex of gp120, CD4, and coreceptor leads to a conformational rearrangement in the transmembrane envelope subunit, exposing an N-terminal hydrophobic fusion peptide. This domain then initiates fusion after it is inserted into the target cell membrane. The fusogenic properties of the transmembrane domain may represent a major mechanism for virus-mediated cytopathicity (58).

Envelope and Virus-Mediated Cytopathicity

The fusogenic activity of gp41 is required for fusion of viral with host cell plasma membranes during virus entry (59–61). A fusogenic peptide is defined by a 20–amino acid hydrophobic domain at the N terminus of gp41 (amino acids 512 to 527). Expression of viral envelope glycoprotein in CD4+ cells leads to the formation of large multinucleated giant cells or syncytia and death of cells within the syncytia. Whether rapid T-cell turnover reported in vivo is mediated by the fusion of infected and uninfected cells through syncytium formation (58) or whether single cell killing proceeds in the absence of syncytium induction (28, 62) is unclear. Nevertheless, the fusogenic properties of envelope glycoprotein are likely to be critical determinants for both syncytium-dependent and independent cell killing. In this regard, individual HIV isolates exhibit a differential potential to induce fusion (63, 64). The terms syncytium-inducing (SI) and nonsyncytium-inducing (NSI) are used to describe the capacity of a particular HIV isolate to induce syncytia in MT-2 cultures. In actual terms, the distinction is not absolute because NSI isolates induce syncytia in primary macrophage cultures and in T-cell lines transfected with 7-transmembrane coreceptors (65). Most SI viruses replicate faster and to higher levels in peripheral blood mononuclear cell (PBMC) cultures (66). Although NSI variants exhibit variable replication rates in vitro, some of these exhibit replication profiles similar to those of SI strains.

Another distinction between SI and NSI strains regards their tropism. SI viruses are usually T-cell tropic in that they replicate within immortalized T-cell lines and infect macrophages inefficiently, whereas NSI strains infect primary monocyte-derived macrophages in vitro and PBMCs, but only a few T-cell lines. Again, however, this distinction is not absolute. Most SI viruses have been lab-adapted through in vitro passage in T-cell lines. This has been proposed to result in an increased viral affinity for CD4 that, as a consequence, allows infection of T-cell lines with low amounts of CD4 (67, 68). Thus, changes in CD4 affinity, rather than altered coreceptor usage, may explain the efficient infection of T-cell lines by SI strains. Similarly, primary SI viruses that have not been extensively passaged in T-cell lines infect macrophages as efficiently as NSI viruses (69, 70). A good but not absolute correlation exists between coreceptor usage and cell tropism. Monocyte-derived macrophages express CCR5 and low levels of CXCR4 (71) and can be infected by most CCR5 using NSI viruses. Because macrophages derived from individuals containing a homozygous deletion in CCR5 are resistant to infection by NSI viruses (72, 73), these results support the notion that CCR5 is the main coreceptor on macrophages for infection by NSI isolates. Lab-adapted strains that are CXCR4 specific infect macrophages inefficiently, a finding suggesting that CXCR4 is not in an appropriate confirmation to trigger fusion by such viruses (69). That primary SI viruses that can use either CCR5 and CXCR4 or exclusively CXCR4 can infect macrophages as well as T cells suggests that CXCR4 may, in some circumstances, be functional in macrophage lineage cells, or alternatively, that an unidentified coreceptor is mediating macrophage infection by these viruses. CCR5 usage does not automatically confer ability to infect primary macrophages, because strains that use CCR5 yet are unable to infect CCR5+ macrophages have been described (74). Although these results illustrate that the capacity of coreceptors to induce virus fusion may depend on cell type and that additional coreceptors await identification, additional virus-encoded factors dictate the ability to replicate in macrophages and may account for the differential ability of CCR5-using viruses to infect monocyte-derived macrophages in vitro (see the following section).

Gag Gene Products

Gag protein products primarily promote virion integrity and additionally direct the virion encapsidation of genomic viral RNA. The mature capsid proteins MA (p17), CA (p24), p2, NC (p7), p1, and p6 (75, 76) are derived from the gag polyprotein (Pr55^{gag}) through proteolytic processing by the virus-encoded protease. Proteolytic processing of gag polyprotein is activated during virion assembly and continues within the budded virus particle, but it can proceed entirely within the budded virion. Virus particles prepared in the presence of reversible protease inhibitors are released into the extracellular medium and contain uncleaved gag polyprotein. On removal of the inhibitor, gag processing leads to formation of infectious virions (77). The HIV-1 MA protein is the first retroviral matrix protein to be structurally characterized. The solution structure of gag MA has been determined by magnetic resonance imaging (MRI) (78, 79), and, additionally, the crystal structure of HIV-1 MA has been determined at 2.3-Å resolution (80). The protein is composed of four to five α helices and a three-strand mixed β sheet that provides a positively charged surface for interaction with the inner phospholipid leaflet of the viral membrane. In crystal lattices, MA protein forms trimers and associates with the viral membrane as a trimer (81). Trimerization creates a bipartite membrane-binding surface in which exposed basic amino acid residues likely cooperate with the N-terminal myristoyl group to mediate anchoring of the protein on the inner phospholipid leaflet of the virus membrane (80). Comparison of the MA proteins of HTLV-2 and HIV-1 indicates that the topologic structures of the exposed cationic membrane-binding surface are conserved features of retroviral MA proteins (82). Furthermore, the structure of HIV-1 MA suggests that membrane and nuclear localization properties of the protein are mediated by complex tertiary structures, rather than by simple linear motifs (78).

According to current models of virion structure (15), most MA within the virion lies on the inner phospholipid leaflet of the host cell-derived virion plasma membrane. Shortly after translation, the initiating methionine at the N-terminus is removed, and myristic acid is attached to the N-terminal glycine residue by the host cell enzyme, N-myristyl transferase (83). Gag MA facilitates virion association of envelope glycoprotein (84). The first 31 amino acids of MA contain a high proportion of basic amino acids, which appear to be important for membrane association (85). The action of this domain and the myristoylation modification are important for targeting the gag polyprotein to the cell plasma membrane. Mutations that abrogate myristoylation impair virion assembly and infectivity (85–87). MA is also posttranslationally modified by phosphorylation on serine and tyrosine residues (88, 89).

After infection of the cell, HIV-1 nucleic acids are reverse transcribed in a high-molecular-weight nucleoprotein reverse transcription complex or preintegration complex (17). The reverse transcription complexes of HIV-1 contain gag MA as well as the viral enzymes, reverse transcriptase (RT), and integrase (IN) (17, 90–92) (see also the section of this chapter on Vpr/Vpx proteins) but lack gag capsid proteins (CA; see Fig 3.2). The process through which CA is excluded from viral reverse transcription complexes, yet MA is retained, is not well understood. However, the binding of MA to viral reverse transcription complexes is maintained even in the presence of 600 mM postassium chloride (93, 94), a finding suggesting a high-affinity interaction between MA and a component of the viral reverse transcription complex. Phosphorylation of gag MA on a C-terminal tyrosine has been proposed to mediate the interaction of MA with IN, a mechanism implicated in tethering MA protein to the viral reverse transcription complex (95). However, binding of MA to the reverse transcription complex is maintained at salt concentrations that promote dissociation of IN from the complex (94), a finding suggesting that MA is bound to the complex by an IN-independent mechanism. Because of its association with the reverse transcription complex, MA has a potential to influence early stages in the virus life cycle (see Fig 3.3). Mutations within the C-terminus of MA that have no effect on virus particle production are nevertheless noninfectious (90). Similar phenotypes have been described for MA mutants of Rous sarcoma virus (91). Additional investigations should determine whether these phenotypes are related to the proposed role of MA in promoting membrane dissociation and nuclear translocation of the reverse transcription complex.

The tight association of MA with viral reverse transcription complexes has important consequences for virus infectivity. Because gag MA is myristoylated on infection of the cell, viral reverse transcription complexes would be predicted to remain associated with the host cell membrane at the point of virus entry. Investigators have demonstrated that phosphorylation of gag MA on serine residues promotes dissociation of gag MA (and its tethered reverse transcription complex) from the cell membrane, thus allowing subsequent nuclear translocation of the complex (89). In the newly infected cell, between 1 and 10% of the MA molecules are phosphorylated and localized to the nucleus (88, 89). Rapid nuclear localization of gag MA within the newly infected cell and the presence of a basic domain highly reminiscent of nuclear targeting signals of nuclear proteins (96) are consistent with a model in which gag MA of HIV-1 facilitates nuclear translocation of the reverse transcription complex. Thus, phosphorylation of gag MA likely provides a mechanism through which the opposing membrane targeting and nuclear targeting properties of gag MA are regulated (97) (see the section later in this chapter on the Vpr protein). Whether gag MA is directly involved in facilitating nuclear translocation of the viral reverse transcription complex remains to be determined. Gag MA appears to contain a nuclear targeting signal (NLS) (96). This sequence mediates binding of gag MA with α and β importins (98), consistent with the ability of this protein to act as a nuclear targeting factor. Recently, Fouchier and associates demonstrated that, when expressed in mammalian cells, gag MA does not undergo nuclear localization (99), a finding that suggests that MA is "piggy-backed" to the nucleus through the nuclear import properties of another reverse transcription complex component (for example, Vpr). However, the stoichiometry of MA within the reverse transcription complex and its phosphorylation probably are both necessary for the rapid nuclear translocation of MA and its tethered complex.

Capsid protein (CA) is a major component of the virion core. The three-dimensional structure of the amino terminal core domain of HIV-1 CA has been shown by MRI (100). In addition, the crystal structures of dimeric HIV-1 CA protein (101) and of the amino terminal domain of HIV-1 CA bound to human cyclophilin A, a peptidyl prolyl isomerase (102), have been described. The protein consists of seven α helices, five of which are arranged in a coiled structure. Cyclophilin A is incorporated into HIV-1 virions through its association with HIV-1 CA (103, 104). The interaction of cyclophilin with gag was first identified using the GAL4 two-hybrid system (105). The interaction of cyclophilin with HIV-1 gag CA is disrupted by cyclosporine (105), a fungal metabolite widely used as an immunosuppressive drug. Production of virus particles in the presence of cyclosporine prevents association of capsid protein with cyclophilin and prevents its incorporation into virions, and, as a result, virions are rendered noninfectious (103, 104).

The requirement of cyclophilin A for HIV-1 infectivity is unique among retroviruses and is differentially required for infectivity of primate lentiviruses. For example, cyclophilin A is required for the replication of group M HIV-1 and SIV_{CPZ}, but it is not required for group O HIV-1 variants or other primate immunodeficiency viruses (106, 107). The region of gag CA involved in binding cyclophilin A has been identified through mutagenesis studies (103, 104, 108, 109). In addition, the cocrystal structure of the CA–cyclophilin A complex indicates that binding is mediated exclusively by an exposed capsid loop that spans residues PRO 85 to PRO 93 (102, 110). Passage of HIV-1 in the presence of cyclosporine selects for variants that contain mutations in this exposed capsid loop (107). At present, the mechanism through which cyclophilin A modifies capsid function and promotes viral infectivity is not well understood. Modeling based on the crystal lattice indicates that gag CA molecules assemble into continuous planar strips (102). These strips may associate side by side to allow CA to form the surface of the viral core, and investigators have proposed that cyclophilin A may promote a weakening of the association between the capsid strips (102). Cyclophilin A may facilitate uncoating of the viral core immediately after fusion of the viral with the host cell membrane. Thus, mutations in capsid that impair cyclophilin A binding may lead to viruses that uncoat inefficiently. As a consequence, proper assembly of a functional reverse transcription complex is prevented. Gag CA is phosphorylated, although a role for this modification has not been identified (75). Recombinant CA has been shown to bind genomic viral RNA with high specificity (111). Although CA is a major structural component of the virion core, it does not appear to remain associated with the viral reverse transcription complex after infection of the host cell (17). Thus, the processes of uncoating and virus entry likely involve an orchestrated series of events that allow MA to associate with viral reverse transcription complexes yet exclude CA from these structures.

The NC protein appears dispensable for virus production, but it facilitates encapsidation of genomic viral RNA. A general model for the packaging of genomic viral RNA involves interaction between NC protein (as part of the gag polyprotein) and an ordered stem loop structure in the 5′ nontranslated region of the genome (otherwise known as the Psi or packaging signal) (19, 20, 112, 113). Consistent with this is the reported affinity of NC for genomic viral RNA (114). The presence of two copies of a cysteine–histidine (cys–his) motif reminiscent of metal-binding domains of nucleic acid–binding proteins additionally supports a role for NC in mediating packaging or facilitating condensation of viral RNA during the packaging reaction. Mutations within the cys–his motifs of NC protein or the presence of zinc ejector drugs impair viral replication (115, 116). NC remains associated with viral reverse transcription complexes after infection of the host cell (17, 117), a finding consistent with the reported role of NC protein in reverse transcription and integration (118–120). For example, nucleocapsid promotes specific initiation of minus-strand DNA synthesis in vitro (118), whereas Guo and colleagues demonstrated that HIV-1 nucleocapsid promotes efficient strand transfer during reverse transcription by inhibiting self-priming from minus-strand strong-stop DNA in the presence of TAR (119). In this case, nucleocapsid appears to be destabilizing secondary structures that otherwise promote self-priming. HIV-1 NC also stimulates magnesium-dependent IN-mediated strand transfer in vitro (120), a finding suggesting that NC may promote provirus establishment during virus infection. By comparison, the zinc finger motif of the Friend murine leukemia virus NC protein has been shown to be critical for viral cDNA synthesis in vitro and in vivo (121).

The C-terminal cleavage product of the gag polyprotein (p6) is important for late stages in virus replication, and HIV-1 variants with mutations in p6 show an aberrant pattern of particle release (122). The virion protein p6 mediates the packaging of HIV-1 Vpr (123, 124) and Vpx of HIV-2/SIV (125). This association between p6 and Vpr/Vpx proteins likely provides a basis through which these proteins are retained within the reverse transcription complex after host cell infection (14, 92, 126)

Pol Gene Products

Three distinct enzymatic functions are encoded by the pol open-reading frame. High-resolution crystal structures have been obtained for each viral enzyme including RT (127, 128), protease (129) and RNase H (130). A translational frameshift between overlapping *gag* and *pol* genes (131) leads to generation of a gag/pol polyprotein (Pr160$^{gag/pol}$). A short homopolymeric sequence at the junction between gag and pol open-reading frames promotes a frameshifting of the ribosome into the minus 1 position (131). Because frameshifting occurs at a frequency of around 10%, nine gag precursor molecules are produced for every gag/pol precursor (131–133). This balance is necessary to permit sufficient production of structural gag proteins for incorporation into the next generation of progeny virions. Processing of the gag/pol polyprotein by the viral protease requires autocatalytic activation in *cis* and in *trans* by protease homodimers (134, 135). Processing is tightly regulated, and autocatalytic activation of protease probably does not occur until initiation of virus budding from the host cell. Lentiviral proteases are related to other aspartyl proteases that contain an N-T/S-G motif in their active site (134). Protease remains a critical antiviral target through the use of peptidomimetic and nonpeptidomimetic inhibitors.

Synthesis of viral DNA from genomic viral RNA and DNA templates is catalyzed by RT, which is an RNA-dependent DNA polymerase. Cleavage of the p160 precursor by protease releases a p66 domain that contains polymerase and RNase H activities. After formation of a p66 homodimer, the RNase H domain is released on one subunit to yield a p66/p51 heterodimer (130, 136, 137) (Figs. 3.4 and 3.5). The structure of this heterodimer complexed with the nonnucleoside analog inhibitor nevirapine (127, 138, 139) and with double-stranded DNA (140) has been determined. Major functional domains of RT include the deoxyribonucleoside triphosphate (dNTP) binding site (residue 63 to 84 and 120 to 150 [140]), polymerization active site (residues 151 to 244 [141]), primer binding domain (residues 195 to 244 [142, 143]), and dimerization motif (residues 283 to 310 and 398 to 414 [144]) (see Fig 3.5).

The heterodimer and the p66 homodimers exhibit RT and RNase H activities; however, the p51 subunit alone is not active (145, 146). Reverse transcription itself proceeds through a highly ordered series of events that involve both genomic virion RNAs (147) (Fig 3.6). The reverse transcription process proceeds within the context of a high-molecular-weight nucleoprotein reverse transcription complex (see the section later in this chapter on Vpr/Vpx proteins). The infidelity of reverse transcription provides the basis for the genetic diversity of retroviruses (148). Based on in vitro experiments with recombinant enzyme and synthetic templates, the mutation rate of HIV-1 RT has been estimated at between 5 and 10 misincorporations generated per genome (149, 150). The actual mutation rate during virus replication in vivo is less well-understood and is likely to be influenced by host cell differences in activation state that lead to differences in dNTP levels in the cell. Reverse transcription, which has been reported to occur within virions, may promote the initiation of DNA synthesis in cellular environments with restricted dNTP levels (21–25).

Despite detailed structural information available for HIV-1 RT, many aspects of the process of reverse transcription in the infected cell are less well understood. After fusion of viral and host cell membranes, viral nucleic acids are deposited in the cytosol of the target cell in the form of a high-molecular-weight nucleoprotein reverse transcription complex, also referred to as the preintegration complex. The exact point at which reverse transcription is initiated after virus infection is not well understood. Current models of retroviral reverse transcription indicate that the process is initiated on entry of the reverse transcription complex into the target cell (151). However, products of reverse transcription can be detected within virions (21, 22), and reverse transcription was demonstrated to occur within virus particles (so-called endogenous reverse transcription) (24, 25). This endogenous reverse transcription (24, 25) can be augmented by polyamines and high dNTP concentrations (23). Investigators have proposed that endogenous reverse transcription facilitates infection of cells containing low dNTP pools (such as quiescent T cells and macrophage-lineage cells) in which reverse transcription otherwise may be inefficient (24, 25). Current models of retroviral reverse transcription indicate that viral cDNA synthesis is completed within the cytoplasm of the acutely infected cell (147). However, reverse transcription complexes of HIV-1 rapidly undergo nuclear translocation and can be detected within the nucleus within 15 to 30 minutes of infection (89). Because reverse transcription in vivo proceeds at approximately one to three nucleotides incorporated per second (152), complete synthesis of minus- and plus-strand DNA takes on the order of 3 hours. Thus, reverse transcription and nuclear transport of viral nucleic acids likely proceed concurrently, and completion of viral DNA synthesis probably occurs in the host cell nucleus (17).

The interaction of nascent viral cDNA comprising full-length plus- and minus-strand DNA with host cell DNA is catalyzed by the viral IN. The crystal structure of the catalytically active core domain of IN has been determined t 2.5 Å (153). The integration of viral into host cell DNA is essential for completion of subsequent events in the virus life cycle (154). IN is released from the 3′ end of the p160$^{gag/pol}$ precursor by the action of the viral protease. Integration involves three distinct processes. IN first trims two nucleotides from the 3′ ends of the plus and minus strands to create a staggered end. IN then cleaves host cell DNA and links the recessed 3′ end of the viral cDNA to the 5′ ends of the host cell DNA. Ligation of the remaining unjoined ends is

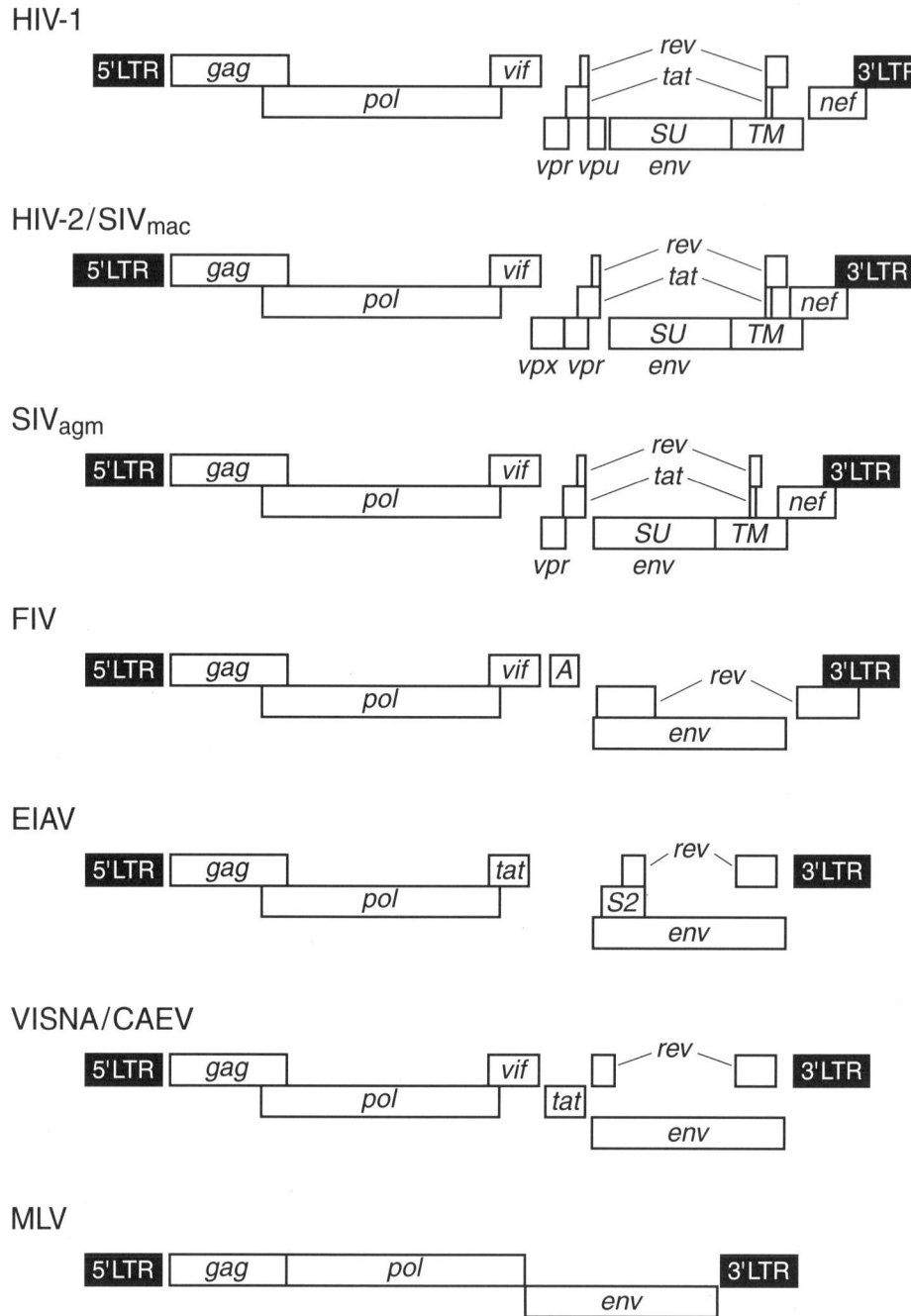

Figure 3.4. **Genomic organization of primate and nonprimate lentiviruses.** *Vpr* is encoded by HIV-1 and HIV-2 and some strains of SIV. *Vpx* is encoded by members of the HIV-2/SIV$_{SM}$ lineage. *Vpu* is encoded only by HIV-1. With the exception of EIAV, *Vif* is common to primate and nonprimate lentiviruses. The genome of the simple animal oncoretrovirus, murine leukemia virus, is shown for comparison.

effected by the host cell DNA repair system. The resulting integrated viral genome is called the provirus. Major functional domains in IN include a zinc-binding domain containing a highly conserved zinc finger motif that may be required for DNA binding (residues 1 to 50 [155]), an enzyme active site involved in dimerization and DNA binding (residues 50 to 212 [156–159]), and a third region (residues 212 to 288) implicated in DNA binding and dimerization. Homodimers of IN mediate integration by a single active site (156).

Integration in vitro can be reconstituted with recombinant IN and substrate DNA (160–162). Concerted integration in which both ends of the viral DNA are modified and coupled to substrate DNA can only be achieved when reverse transcription complexes from acutely infected cells or extracts from purified virions are used as sources of integration activity (163–165). Thus, other viral and cellular functions are probably required to promote concerted integration. Using a yeast genetic screen, HIV-1 IN has been shown to interact with Ini-1, which is a human homolog of the yeast transcription factor Snf-5 (166). Possibly, highly condensed regions of genomic DNA are poor substrates for integration, and Ini-1 affects target site selection by influencing the topology of substrate DNA. The presence of such a mechanism may be more important during provirus establishment in nondividing macrophage-lineage cells in which genomic DNA is highly condensed, but less important in cycling cells in which DNA replication during the cell cycle reduces DNA topology constraints.

Recently, a second host protein required for integration has been identified (93). Purification of preintegration complexes from acutely infected cells in the presence of 600-mM potassium chloride strips these complexes of a factor required for integration activity. Integration activity is restored on addition of an uninfected cell extract. The complementing factor was identified as HMG I(Y), a nonhistone chromosomal protein involved in chromosomal architecture and transcriptional control. HMG I(Y) does not appear to be incorporated into virions or associated with the preintegration complex, but rather, it is acquired from the infected cell during translocation of the preintegration complex to the host cell nucleus. The mechanism through which HMG I(Y) promotes integration by viral preintegration complexes is not well understood. Investigators have proposed that HMG I(Y) may position the two ends of the viral cDNA before integration. Alternatively, HMG I(Y) may prevent the preintegration complex from using its own cDNA as an integration target (93).

In addition to the role of IN in integration, several studies implicate IN in additional steps in viral entry. IN mutants that retain in vitro integration activity yet are incapable of provirus establishment have been described (167–169). Possibly, in vitro integration activity does not faithfully predict the capacity to promote integration in vivo. Alternatively, IN serves an additional, unidentified function in virus entry. The development of inhibitors that block integration function in vivo has been hampered by the inability of in vitro integration assays to represent all aspects of integration faithfully in vivo, and compounds that block in vitro integration activity have poor antiviral activity (170). HIV-1 IN contains a nuclear localization signal, and IN is localized to the host cell nucleus (171). By comparison, Kukolj and colleagues demonstrated that IN of avian sarcoma virus, but not that of HIV-1, underwent nuclear localization (172). The nuclear localization properties of HIV-1 IN have been suggested to promote nuclear targeting of the viral preintegration complex (171). This property of IN is additive with the roles of gag MA and Vpr in promoting nuclear translocation of HIV-1 preintegration complexes in nondividing target cells. Mutations in

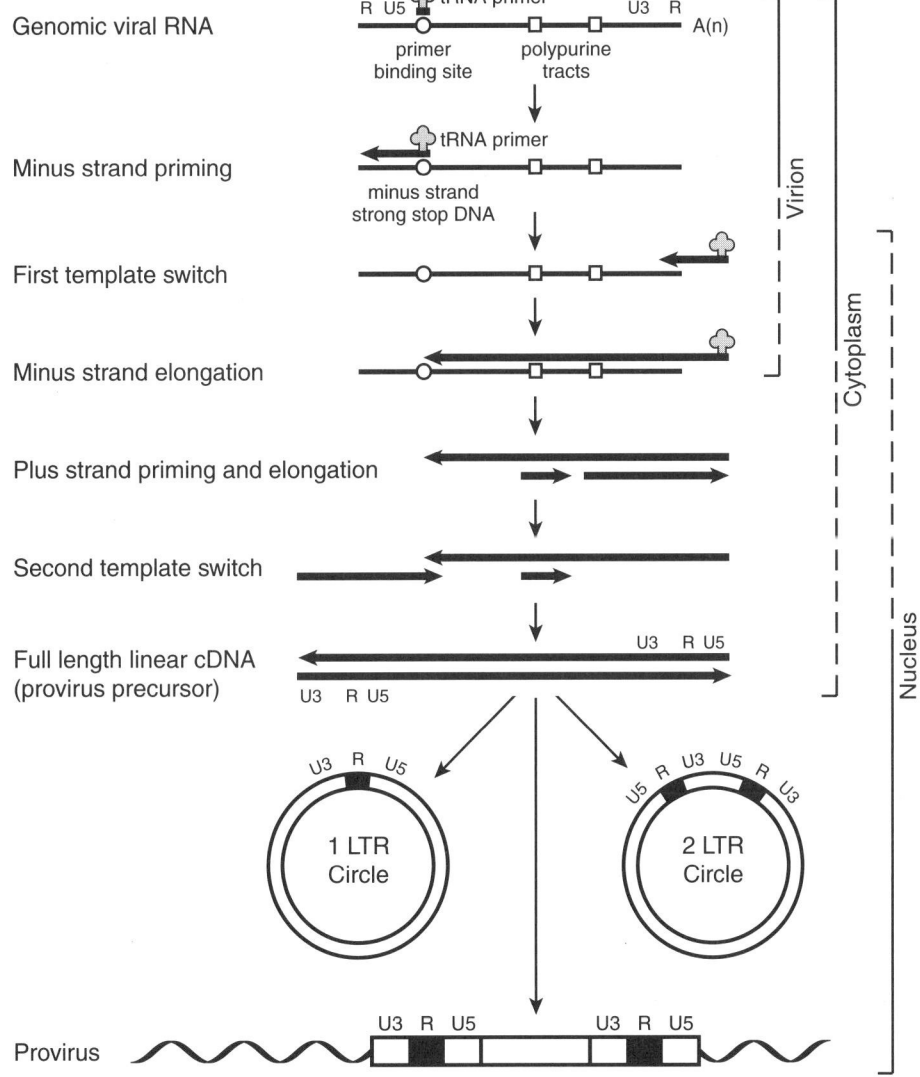

Figure 3.5. Schematic of the RT domain of HIV-1 polymerase. Boundaries of RT and RNase H domains of HIV polymerase are outlined. The action of protease yields a p66 homodimer and cleavage on one p66 subunit leads to the active p66/p51 heterodimer. The three-dimensional structure of p66 has been likened to that of a hand in which the thumb and fingers form the active site for the polymerase; the palm provides the location for positioning of the RNA template and the tRNA primer. Active residues in the polymerase domain include ASP 110 and ASP 185, 186. (Adapted from Kohlstaedt LA, Wang J, Friedman JM, et al. Crystal structure at 3.5 Å resolution of HIV-1 reverse transcriptase complexed with an inhibitor. Science 1992;256:1783–1790.)

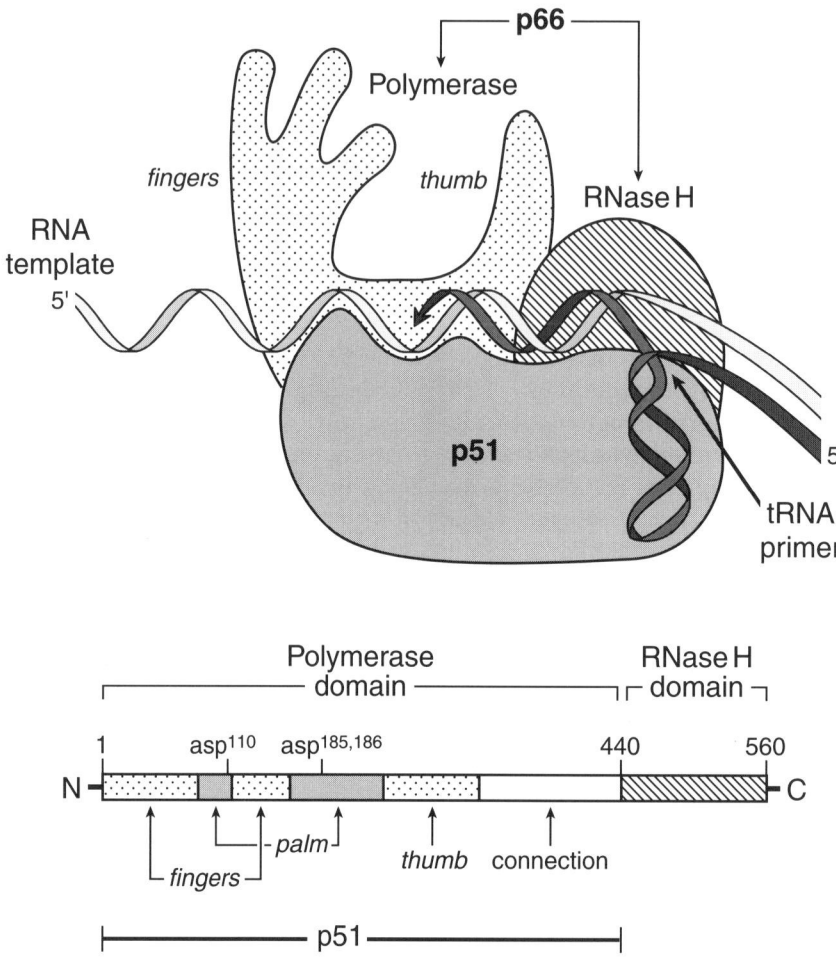

Figure 3.6. Genetic throughput of retroviruses. Reverse transcription is initiated on binding of a tRNA^{LYS} primer to the primer binding site, resulting in the formation of an 18-bp duplex. DNA synthesis proceeds to the 5' end of the viral genome, resulting in the formation of a minus-strand strong-stop cDNA, which is the first detectable cDNA product in infected cells. Minus-strand strong-stop products can also be detected in a small percentage of intact cell-free virions. After degradation of viral RNA, minus-strand strong-stop DNA recognizes redundant sequences in the 3' end of the second RNA template (first template switch), thus allowing minus-strand cDNA synthesis to continue (minus-strand elongation). As elongation occurs, the action of RNase H generates a series of staggered primers located within polypurine tracks near the boundary of the 3' LTR, allowing plus-strand cDNA synthesis to proceed (plus-strand priming and elongation). A second template switch facilitated by base complementarity at the primer binding site leaves the formation of a circular molecule, which allows completion of plus-strand synthesis. The final product contains full-length plus and minus strands in a linear configuration by an incompletely characterized process. Some linear cDNA molecules undergo recombination and end–end ligation to form 1 and 2 LTR circles, respectively. These circular products are detectable only in the nucleus of the infected cell and appear to be dead-end products in virus replication. The linear cDNA serves as the direct precursor to the integrated provirus. Thin lines denote RNA; thick lines denote cDNA. Primer binding sites and polypurine tracks are indicated by circles and squares, respectively. Poly A of the viral genomic RNA is represented as A(n). Subcellular location for distinct steps in reverse transcription are indicated. Hatched lines denote uncertainty in the boundaries of the cellular compartment in which that cDNA product is generated. Because cDNA synthesis and nuclear import are concurrent processes, a discrete stage in reverse transcription confined exclusively to either compartment is unlikely.

HIV-1 IN appear to perturb nuclear translocation of the viral preintegration complex only in viruses that lack functional gag MA and Vpr proteins.

Previous studies (173) indicated that nuclear targeting of large particles requires the participation of multiple NLS motifs and increasing the valency of NLS motifs on a particle increased rate and extent of its nuclear import (173). The presence of multiple import proteins in preintegration complexes of primate lentiviruses supports a model in which the presence of multiple NLS-containing proteins within the preintegration complex is necessary to drive efficient nuclear translocation of the ribosome-sized preintegration complex. Perhaps the nuclear targeting properties of HIV-1 IN are not directly involved in promoting nuclear targeting of the viral preintegration complex in nondividing cells. Avian sarcoma virus IN possesses a functional nuclear localization signal (172), yet this virus does not infect nondividing cells. This finding suggests that nuclear transport of IN may be involved in other aspects of retrovirus entry such as nuclear retention of the preintegration complex. Such a mechanism would be necessary to prevent exclusion of the viral preintegration complex from the nuclear compartment during reassembly of the nuclear envelope during host cell mitosis.

After infection of the target cell, nuclear translocation of the viral preintegration complex and establishment of the provirus are profoundly influenced by the activation state of the host cell (174–177). Quiescent lymphocytes support entry of viral nucleic acids, but virus replication is blocked at a stage preceding proviral integration (174–177). Previous studies suggested that low dNTP levels in quiescent T lymphocytes hamper efficient reverse transcription (174, 178). Other groups indicated that nuclear translocation of viral reverse transcription complexes is severely impaired in quiescent T lymphocytes (175, 176). In some studies, viral nucleic acids synthesized within infected quiescent cells underwent complete reverse transcription, nuclear translocation, and provirus establishment on subsequent activation of the infected cell (174–176). More recent studies have determined that the prevalent form of HIV-1 DNA in resting T cells is a full-length, linear cDNA in which ends of the linear cDNA have failed to undergo processing by viral IN (177). Whether the lack of end processing by HIV-1 IN is due to suboptimal levels of cellular integration cofactors (Ini-1; HMG I(Y)) in quiescent T cells (179) remains to be determined.

Long Terminal Repeat

After establishment of the provirus, the activity of the LTR depends on *cis*- and *trans*-acting regulatory factors, and the activity of these factors itself depends on the activation state of the host cell (4). The viral LTRs are divided into three domains that have distinct roles in transcription. Basal promoter elements, including the TATAA box for initiation of transcription by RNA pol 2 and SP1 binding sites, are contained within the U3 domain. The U3 region itself can be further subdivided into core–basal, enhancer, and modulatory domains (4). The enhancer of HIV-1 comprises a duplicated NF-κB site (between −104 and −81). NF-κB controls the activity of several cellular genes such as interleukin-2 (IL-2)/IL-2 receptor, tumor necrosis factor-α, class I/II major histocompatibility complex (MHC), and immunoglobulin-k light chain. The requirement of NF-κB for replication of primate lentiviruses is poorly understood, given that SIV variants lacking functional NF-κB (and SP-1) binding sites replicate efficiently in primary lymphocyte cultures in vitro and induce AIDS in (180, 181). The action of NF-κB may be more pronounced when the host cell is quiescent. In nonstimulated cells, NF-κB is inactive through its complexing with the inhibitor I-κB. Dissociation of the complex occurs during cell activation, thus allowing NF-κB to translocate to the nucleus and activate transcription. For this reason, cytokines and mitogens augment LTR activity by changing levels of NF-κB (5–10). Although NF-κB minus SIV can induce AIDS, in the host infected with multiple virus variants or quasispecies (46), competition among different virus variants is likely to favor the emergence of viruses with advantageous phenotypes. The conservation of NF-κB elements argues for a selective pressure to maintain such motifs. The core domain of U3 contains the TATAA box, which mediates binding of TFIID, a complex of cellular factors comprising TATAA-binding protein and RNA pol-II (4). The modulatory region of the U3 domain contains *cis*-acting transcriptional or regulatory elements that do not appear to contribute to promoter activity in vitro but appear to be important for virus replication (182). The LTR R domain contains a *cis*-acting sequence (TAR) that mediates Tat function as well as sites for binding of cellular transcription factors. The TAR element is located at the 5′ end of all HIV-1 transcripts. The structure itself comprises a 3 base pair (bp) bulge, a 4-bp stem, and a 6-bp loop. The Tat protein binds to the bulge, and cellular factors that cooperate with Tat in activating gene expression interact with loop sequences. Viruses that lack a functional TAR element or are unable to encode Tat protein are noninfectious. Signals in the U5 region of the 3′ LTR only are recognized by cellular polyadenylation machinery (183, 184), which adds poly-A tails to the 3′ end of viral transcripts.

Tat and Rev Proteins

Primate lentivirus gene expression is regulated by Tat and Rev proteins at the transcriptional and posttranscriptional levels, respectively (4). Tat protein is derived from two exons, the second of which is largely dispensable for transactivation (185). Functional domains that have been identified within Tat protein include the N-terminal, cysteine-rich, and basic domains. Binding of Tat to the *cis*-acting TAR is mediated by sequences in the basic and C-terminal domains. Current models of Tat transactivation have implicated a cellular coactivator protein that interacts with the activation domain, which, in turn, recruits RNA pol-II (186–190). Although the general consensus is that Tat transactivation increases the number of transcripts through increasing the rate of viral transcription (191, 192), possibly Tat may also be required for processive transcription. Thus, in the presence of Tat, long transcripts in the LTR are produced, whereas in the absence of Tat, only short, nonfunctioning transcripts are produced. Prematurely terminated transcripts have been identified in infected cells in vitro and in lymphocytes from HIV-1–infected individuals (193, 194). Presumably, in nonactivated host cells, Tat is rate-limiting; conditions that do not favor processive transcription. Consequently, activation of the infected cell leads to increases in basal transcription and to increases in levels of Tat, thus favoring processive transcription of viral RNA (194). Although Tat is critical for virus replication, Tat remains elusive as a target for antiviral therapy.

Rev is derived from two exons, the second of which contains functional domains that include an RNA-binding domain (residues 35 to 51) flanked by two oligomerization domains (195) and an activation domain (residues 73 to 84). Nuclear translocation of Rev is effected by sequences in the RNA binding domain (196, 197). Rev interacts with a *cis*-acting Rev-responsive element (RRE) located in the central portion of the viral *envelope* gene (198). Rev acts at the posttranscriptional level to increase the half-life of RRE containing HIV-1 mRNAs, to facilitate transport of HIV-1 mRNAs from the nucleus to the cytoplasm, and additionally to promote efficient translation of viral mRNAs. Rev binds to a high-affinity site within the RRE as a monomer. Additional Rev monomers then assemble onto the RRE, and this multimerization is necessary for Rev function (199).

Several models have been suggested to explain the mechanism through which Rev acts. For example, Rev may influence the splicing efficiency of transcripts containing an RRE by binding transcripts in the nucleus, thus increasing their half-life (198, 200–202). As a consequence, Rev may divert precursor viral transcripts from the splicing apparatus of the cell (203, 204). In a second model, viral transcripts contain *cis*-acting repressive sequences, also known as instability elements (201, 205), that promote degradation of viral transcripts (206–208). The effects of these instability elements are counterbalanced on Rev binding the RRE. In a third model, Rev may facilitate transport of RRE containing transcripts from the nucleus to the cytoplasm (198, 200). Consistent with this mechanism are demonstrations that the activation domain of Rev interacts with a cellular protein (hRab/Rip) that has homology with nucleoporins, a class of proteins mediating nucleocytoplasmic transport. This protein that binds the Rev activation domain when Rev is assembled onto its RNA target (209, 210) may play a role in mediating nucleoporin interaction during the nuclear export of viral RNA. Transdominant mutants of Rev that are nonfunctional yet otherwise bind the RRE prevent the activity of wild-type Rev. A transdominant Rev mutant termed M-10 (211) is currently undergoing clinical trials.

ACCESSORY GENE PRODUCTS

Nef Protein

The Nef protein represents the first accessory gene product for which structural information is available. The Nef binding surface for the SH3 domain of the tyrosine protein kinase Hck has been mapped by MRI (212). Furthermore, the crystal structure of the conserved core of HIV-1 Nef has been determined in complex with the SH3 domain of a point mutant of the tyrosine kinase, Fyn (213). Nef is myristoylated and localized on the plasma membrane of the infected cell (214). In addition, Nef is phosphorylated, but no function has been attributed to this modification (215, 216). Nef is one of the earliest detectable gene products after transcriptional activation of the provirus (217). In infected cells, Nef is found as a homodimer because of intermolecular disulfide bonds between highly conserved cysteine residues (218). Nef contains conserved acidic region at the N-terminus, followed by conserved PXX repeats characteristic of SH3 recognition motifs of protein tyrosine kinases (219). This region mediates interaction with Hck in vitro (213, 220) and in vivo (221). Nef can be detected in virus particles, where it is proteolytically processed by the viral protease (222–225). Although Nef associates with viral particles, whether Nef is specifically packaged or whether virion localization of Nef is important for Nef function is unclear.

PROPERTIES OF Nef

Nef mutants of HIV-1 are attenuated for replication and lymphocyte depletion in severe combined immunodeficiency mouse models of HIV in which human lymphocytes are reconstituted in the mouse by implantation of human thymic tissue (226). In addition, *nef* mutants of SIV are attenuated in macaque models of lentivirus pathogenesis (227). A few HIV-1 infected individuals with a long-term nonprogressor phenotype contain viruses with mutated *nef* genes (228, 229), enforcing the view that Nef is critical for primate lentivirus pathogenicity. These in vivo observations are in stark contrast to the minor requirement for Nef during HIV and SIV replication in primary lymphocytes and macrophages and in established T-cell lines in vitro. Properties of *nef* genes and identification of cellular ligands that interact with Nef are beginning to throw some light on how Nef may be influencing virus replication and pathogenicity in vivo.

Nef AND CD4 DOWNREGULATION

Nef induces rapid endocytosis and lysosomal degradation of CD4 that results in downregulation of CD4 expression on the surface of the infected host cell (215, 230, 231). This mechanism of Nef-mediated CD4 downregulation is additive with the effects of Vpu and envelope, which, by distinct mechanisms, also downregulate CD4 expression on the cell surface (28, 30, 232). Cell-surface receptor downregulation by animal oncoretroviruses (233) and by HIV-1 (28) protects the cell from reinfection by progeny virions. This process of superinfection has been implicated in viral cytopathicity. However, no evidence indicates that the requirements of Nef for primate lentiviral pathogenicity (227) are related to the effect of Nef on CD4 downregulation. Reduction of CD4 expression on the cell surface may also lead to an increase in the amount of intracellular CD4–p56 lck complexing (234) that, in turn, could affect the activation status of the infected host cell.

Nef AND CELLULAR KINASES

Studies of several groups suggest that Nef associates with cellular serine–threonine (235–242) and tyrosine protein kinases (220, 221, 239, 240, 243–245). Some groups have turned their attention to characterizing the kinase or kinases that associate with HIV and SIV Nef proteins. Nef has been shown to associate with a serine–threonine kinase that is structurally and functionally related to the p21-activated kinase PAK (235) through a double arginine motif in the C-terminus of Nef. In a subsequent study (235, 236), replications of SIV variants containing mutations in this motif were impaired in rhesus macaques (237), and resumption in high virus loads correlated with the reversion of point mutations and restoration of serine–threonine kinase interaction. In a more recent study, Lang and associates identified residues in Nef that abrogate serine–threonine kinase association and concluded that this association was dispensable for efficient replication and pathogenicity of SIV$_{MAC}$ in rhesus macaques (246). Several groups have also demonstrated association of Nef with the Src family tyrosine kinase Lck, which is expressed predominantly in T cells (239, 240, 245). Using Nef as an affinity reagent to probe cytoplasmic extracts of T cells, Greenway and colleagues identified that the Src family tyrosine kinase lck and the serine–threonine kinase MAPK/ERK could bind to Nef (239). Nef was further shown to bind Src homology 2 (SH2) and SH3 domains of lck, and Nef was phosphorylated on tyrosine as a consequence of this interaction (240, 245).

Nef also forms an extremely high-affinity interaction with the Src family tyrosine kinase Hck, which is expressed predominantly in myeloid cells (220, 221, 243, 244). These studies demonstrated that the SH3 domain of HIV-1 Nef was necessary and sufficient to induce full activation of Hck. The interaction of Nef with Hck has been difficult to reconcile with the myeloid-restricted expression of this kinase. Nevertheless, this observation and with the presence of conserved motifs within HIV that facilitate infection of macrophages (see the section of this chapter on Vpr and Vpx) support the notion that macrophage lineage cells may be critical for certain aspects of primate lentivirus pathogenicity.

The interaction of Nef with cellular kinases has several implications. Nef-associated serine–threonine kinase activity enhances the phosphorylation of the viral gag matrix protein on serine (247), and phosphorylation of matrix on serine has been implicated in facilitating membrane dissociation of the viral reverse transcription complex during virus entry (89). As a virion protein, Nef may promote virion incorporation of its associated kinase, which, in turn, leads to phosphorylation of virion proteins.

Nef AND VIRAL INFECTIVITY

Nef enhances virion infectivity (248, 249). Infection of quiescent lymphocytes by HIV leads to a nonproductive infection characterized by a labile intracellular replication intermediate (154, 174, 176). Virus replication can be renewed on subsequent activation of the host cell (154, 174). In this setting, Nef significantly promotes the extent of virus replication induced from this nonproductive state (248, 249). This enhancement of virus infectivity may be mediated at an early step in the virus life cycle, that is, before integration of viral with host cell DNA (Fig 3.7) (250–252). Enhancement of virus infectivity by Nef appears to be functionally and genetically separable from its effects on CD4 expression (253, 254), although it has been related to the association of Nef with cellular serine–threonine kinases (238). Whether the enhancement of HIV infectivity by the Nef-associated serine–threonine kinase is related to the mechanism through which cellular kinases promote gag MA phosphorylation and membrane dissociation of viral reverse transcription complexes during HIV entry is unclear (89, 247).

Nef AND LYMPHOCYTE ACTIVATION

Activation of the host cell is an essential prerequisite for productive infection of PBMCs by primate lentiviruses (154, 174). The interaction of Nef with cellular tyrosine kinases provides a basis for the modulation of host cell activation pathways on HIV infection. An acutely lethal variant of SIV (SIV$_{SM}$ PBj) replicates within nonactivated cultures, and this property is determined by the *Nef* gene, and specifically by an SH2 domain within Nef that binds Src (255). However, all other infectious HIV and SIV isolates identified to date require exogenous activation of T cells for their productive infection. Although replication within quiescent cells is not a representative property of primate lentiviruses, the highly conserved nature of SH2 recognition domains in SIV Nef and of SH3 recognition domains in HIV Nef supports the notion that, through Nef, the virus is tapped into activation pathways of the host cell. Thus, there exists the possibility that *Nef* genes of HIV and SIV promote virus replication by augmenting host cell activation status. In support of this concept, *Nef* genes of SIV and HIV have been shown to promote production of IL-2 in an IL-2–dependent rhesus T-cell line (256). However, investigators subsequently demonstrated that replacement of Nef with IL-2 was not sufficient to restore the pathogenic phenotype of SIV Δnef in rhesus macaques (257). Although earlier reports indicate that Nef inhibits lymphocyte activation (214, 245, 258–260), proteins that regulate signaling pathways in the cell probably can both stimulate and inhibit signaling pathways, depending on host cell type, level of expression, and the state of cell cycle during which expression is induced. The interaction of Nef with Lck may explain the inhibitory effects of Nef on activation pathways in T cells (239, 245, 261). More recently, however, expression of Nef in antigen-dependent T-cell clones did not influence any gross defects in T-cell antigen responsiveness (262). These differences may be explained by differences in viral strain used because the association of Nef with cellular serine–threonine kinases is viral isolate dependent (242).

Nef AND MHC CLASS I DOWNREGULATION

The recent demonstration that HIV-1 Nef induces MHC class I endocytosis (263) raises the intriguing possibility that HIV-1 Nef may be involved in protecting the infected host cell from recognition by CD8+ cytotoxic T cells (CTLs). However, investigators have demonstrated that the presence of a high CTL precursor frequency directed against an epitope in HIV-1 envelope resulted in a rapid and complete replacement of the CTL-sensitive virus population with a CTL-resistant population (264). The rate with which the CTL-sensitive population was replaced by a CTL-resistant population paralleled that observed when a drug-sensitive virus population is replaced by a drug-resistant population during antiretroviral drug therapy (265, 266). The study of Borrow and colleagues provides direct evidence that CTLs exhibit strong selective pressure on virus populations in vivo (264). In addition, long-term nonprogressors lacking a

Figure 3.7. Effects of HIV accessory gene products on the virus life cycle. 1) Vif is absolutely required for infection of primary cells. In the absence of Vif, virions may be noninfectious because of defects in gag/pol processing. 2) The effects of Vif may be manifest at the level of fusion and uncoating, and Vif may be necessary for promoting uncoating of the virus core. 3) Vif mutants of HIV show impaired viral DNA synthesis, and, in addition, reverse transcription complexes containing full-length cDNA appear to be unstable when Vif is absent. However, Vif does not appear to be a component of the reverse transcription complex; therefore, the defects are likely introduced earlier in the virus life cycle. In some cell lines, Nef mutants also show impaired cDNA synthesis. 4) Vpr/Vpx proteins promote nuclear translocation of the reverse transcription complex, a process that is necessary when the nuclear envelope is intact, as is the case after infection of nondividing macrophages. Vpr has also been suggested to contain weak transcriptional activating properties. 5) Translation of env and CD4 proteins occur in the same subcellular compartment, and subsequent interaction between CD4 and env in the ER interferes with appropriate transport of env. Vpu causes dissociation of env from CD4 and directs CD4 for lysosomal degradation, thus freeing envelope to resume transport to the cell surface. Nef causes downregulation of CD4, which likely also minimizes premature engagement of CD4 and env in the cell interior. 6) Vpu is important in virus maturation. Mutants of Vpu show defects in virus release. Vif may ensure appropriate maturation of gag and gag/pol polyproteins. 7) As virion proteins, Vif and Nef may be involved in virion maturation after the virus buds from the host cell. Defects at these steps may be manifest by impairment of viral DNA synthesis in the target cell.

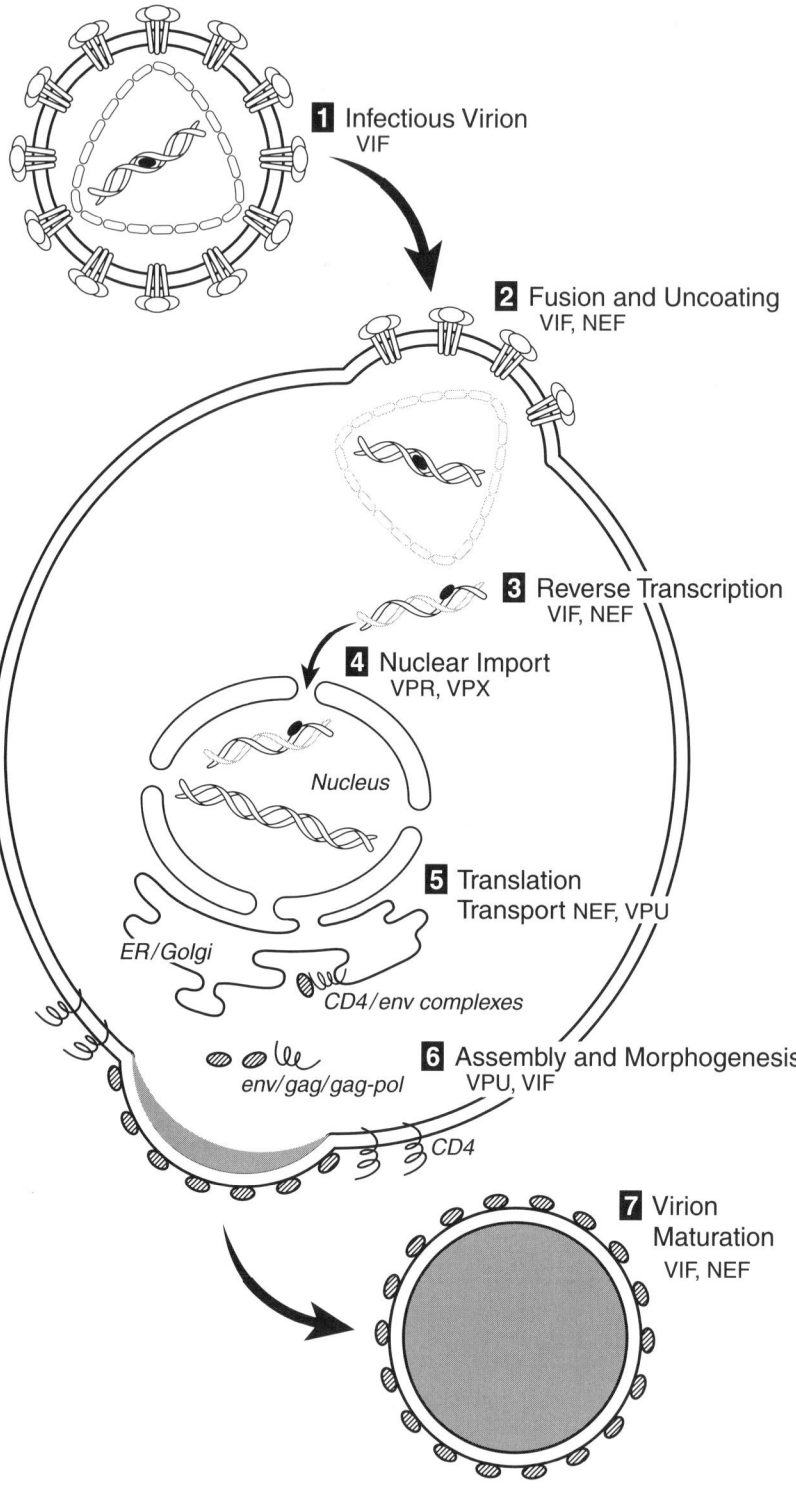

functional *nef* gene (228, 229) exhibit low but sustained levels of virus replication. Presumably, the absence of a functional nef gene in these virus populations would be expected to prevent the recognition and control by CTLs if indeed HIV-1 Nef is affording some protection from CTL surveillance.

Vif Protein

With the exception of EIAV, all lentiviruses encode a *vif* gene (see Fig 3.2). Vif is a phosphoprotein (267). The subcellular localization of the Vif protein is not fully understood. Initially, Vif was demonstrated to associate with the Golgi complex in infected cells (268). Subsequently, investigators demonstrated that Vif is a cytoplasmic protein existing in both a soluble cytosolic form and a membrane-associated form (269), and more recently, association of Vif with the cytoskeleton was reported in HeLa cells expressing Vif protein (270). In contrast, in T cells expressing Vif protein, 90% of Vif was associated with the plasma membrane (271).

Recent studies have demonstrated that Vif is incorporated into virus particles (270, 272); however, this does not appear to involve a specific packaging mechanism because Vif abundance in the virion does not exceed its relative concentration in the infected cell. Vif appears dispensable for virus production but is essential for virus replication in primary T cells and macrophages and certain cell lines. For example, "permissive" cells, such as H-9 and CEM, are Vif independent in that they support efficient replication of Vif-minus viruses. These T-cell lines may express a Vif-like factor that is absent from the primary cells and compensates for the absence of Vif. Another possibility is that primary cells contain a factor that restricts HIV replication and is counteracted by Vif, but the Vif-independent T-cell lines lack this inhibitory factor and, therefore, do not require Vif. Vif is required in the virus-producing cell.

Vif mutant viruses produced from nonpermissive cells do not establish infection in either permissive or nonpermissive target cells under single-cycle conditions (273–276). Single-cycle infectivity is restored if Vif is expressed in *trans* in the producer cell (275, 277). Electron microscopy analysis has suggested that Vif may be involved in maturation of the virion core and that virions lacking Vif do not exhibit the characteristic conic core structure (278, 279). Vif is implicated in proteolytic processing of the gag p55 precursor (278, 280). In contrast, Fouchier and associates did not observe any effects of Vif on processing or incorporation of structural viral proteins (281). In CAEV, the *vif* gene does not appear to be necessary for virus infectivity, but it is required for efficient virus production (282). Whether the effects of Vif on processing of structural viral proteins is related to the reported effects of Vif on reverse transcription after infection of the target cell is unclear (273, 276–278, 283). Some reports have demonstrated that *vif* mutant viruses are incapable of initiating reverse transcription after entry into the target cell (276, 278), whereas other reports have suggested that reverse transcription is initiated but does not go to completion (284, 285) (see Fig 3.7). More recently, investigators have demonstrated, however, that reverse transcription appears to go to completion after infection by *vif*-defective viruses, but these reverse transcripts are unstable and rapidly degraded (273). This finding suggests that proper functioning of the viral reverse transcription complex may require the action of the Vif protein (see Fig 3.7). Until biochemical assays that reconstitute Vif function in vitro are available, the identification of agents that block Vif function will not readily be forthcoming.

Vpu Protein

Vpu is encoded by HIV-1 and the related SIV_{CPZ} but is absent from the genomes of HIV-2 and all other SIV isolates characterized to date (see Fig 3.2) (286). Vpu is an amphipathic membrane protein that exhibits a perinuclear localization in infected cells (287). Although Vpu is a membrane protein, it does not appear to be incorporated into virus particles (287). Vpu is phosphorylated on serine by casein kinase 2 (288). Vpu appears to be relatively dispensable for virus replication in vitro. Two independent properties have been assigned to the Vpu protein. The first involves rapid degradation of CD4 in the endoplasmic reticulum of virus-infected cells or of cells expressing Vpu and CD4 (see Fig 3.7) (232). By reducing the intracellular half-life of CD4, Vpu likely reduces the formation of intracellular envelope–CD4 complexes reported by other groups (28, 31, 232, 234). Possibly, envelope–CD4 complexing interferes with efficient membrane transport of envelope glycoproteins and thus could impair virus production (see Fig 3.7). In the presence of Vpu, interference from CD4 during viral envelope transport would be less. Intriguingly, at least three different viral proteins are involved in the downregulation of CD4, namely, Vpu, Nef (215, 230, 231), and envelope (28, 289). The presence of three functionally distinct mechanisms for CD4 downregulation supports the notion that this process is necessary for some aspect of viral replication. Vpu has also been shown to facilitate virus budding. HIV-1 variants lacking an intact vpu gene are less efficient at releasing virions (290, 291), with the result that virions accumulate in intracytoplasmic vesicles. Although Vpu is not encoded by HIV-2, a Vpu-like function has been demonstrated in this virus (13), and it appears also to be involved in facilitating release of virus particles from the infected cell. The two properties of Vpu appear to be independent in that enhancement of virion release by Vpu does not require CD4 (292) but does appear to depend on phosphorylation (293).

Vpr/Vpx Proteins

Within the so-called "central viral region" (the region overlapping the vif and tat open-reading frames), primate lentiviruses encode either one or two small open-reading frames. HIV-1, SIV_{CPZ}, SIV_{AGM}, SIV_{SYK}, and SIV_{MND} each contain a single gene, usually termed *vpr* (see Fig 3.2). HIV-2 and several other SIV strains (SIV_{SM}, SIV_{MAC}) encode an additional gene in this region that has been termed *Vpx*. Based on the sequence similarity between *Vpx* and *Vpr* genes and their juxtaposition in the HIV-2/SIV_{SM}/SIV_{MAC} genome, investigators suggested that these genes had arisen from a gene duplication event (294). More recently, based on analysis of a more comprehensive database of Vpr and Vpx sequences (see Fig 3.1), investigators have proposed that the presence of an additional *vpx* gene in HIV-2/SIV_{SM} viruses is due to an ancestral nonhomologous recombination event (295). In infected cells, Vpr exists as an oligomer (296) and is localized mainly in the nucleus when expressed in the absence of other HIV-1 proteins (123). Because no classic nuclear localization signal in the Vpr protein has been identified, the possibility exists that Vpr directly interacts with the nuclear import apparatus of the cell or, alternatively, is "piggy-backed" through its affinity with another nuclear import protein. An α-helical structure at the N-terminus of Vpr has been implicated in both nuclear localization and virion incorporation (297–299). Both Vpr and Vpx are virion-associated proteins packaged primarily through their interaction with the C-terminal p6 protein of gag, most likely within the context of gag polyprotein (see Fig 3.5) (123–

125, 300–303). A conserved LXXLF motif in p6 appears important in governing virion association of Vpr (304) The Vpx protein has been identified in association with cores of HIV-2 (305). Because Vpr and p6 interact with a 1:1 stoichiometry, these proteins are packaged in virions in equimolar concentrations relative to gag (approximately 2000 to 3000 molecules per virion).

Most information regarding properties of primate lentiviral Vpr and Vpx proteins in vitro has been derived from studies on HIV-1 Vpr. Both Vpr and Vpx proteins appear to be largely dispensable for replication within established T-cell lines and primary PBMC cultures (14, 126, 306–309). However, Vpr of HIV-1 (126, 308, 310) and of SIV$_{AGM}$ (311) and Vpx of HIV-2/SIVS$_M$ (14, 306) are necessary for efficient replication in primary macrophages. Although some groups have suggested defects in replication of Vpr and Vpx mutants in primary lymphocytes (307, 311, 312), these effects appear to be donor dependent and to manifest only in PBMC cultures that inefficiently replicate virus. In animal studies, Vpr and Vpx mutants appear to be the least attenuated when compared with other accessory gene mutants. In the SCID-Hu PBL model, HIV-1 Vpr mutants exhibit replication and infectivity properties similar to those of wildtype viruses (313). In addition, mutants of SIV$_{MAC}$ that lack functional *vpx* or *vpr* genes appear to retain their in vivo pathogenicity (314–316).

Vpr AND CELL-CYCLE ARREST

Long-term passage of viruses with intact *vpr* genes leads to the outgrowth of viruses with mutations in *vpr* that truncate the Vpr reading frame. This is a direct consequence of the effect of Vpr on the cell cycle in which expression of Vpr within CD4+ T-cell lines leads to an accumulation of cells in the G$_2$ stage of the cell cycle (317–320). The mechanism through which Vpr arrests cell cycle is not known. For example, investigators have suggested that Vpr inhibits the activation of p34^{CDC2}-cyclin B, which controls the entry of the cell into mitosis (317, 319). Investigators have demonstrated that arrest of cell cycle by Vpr leads to the induction of apoptosis in the target cell (321). The effect of Vpr on cell-cycle arrest is not restricted to mammalian cells and has also been exhibited in the fission yeast, *Schizosaccharomyces pombe* (322). Because the effects of Vpr are phenotypically similar to those of the DNA alkalating agent nitrogen mustard, investigators have suggested that the Vpr mitotic block is similar to that of G$_2$ DNA damage checkpoint control (323). In contrast, Bartz and colleagues have demonstrated that the effects of Vpr are cytostatic, rather than cytotoxic, and the effect is upstream of activation of the mitotic cyclin-dependent kinase and is qualitatively different from that of G$_2$ DNA damage checkpoint control (324). Cell-cycle arrest is exhibited by Vpr alleles of all primate lentiviruses (325), and the conservation of this property across lentiviral lineages suggests that cell-cycle arrest by Vpr is important for some aspect of primate lentiviral pathogenicity. However, as yet, researchers have no clear understanding of the mechanism through which Vpr-mediated G$_2$ arrest supports primate lentiviral replication.

Vpr INTERACTION WITH URACIL DNA GLYCOSYLASE

Vpr of HIV-1 (326) and of HIV-2/SIV$_{SM}$ (327) interact with uracil DNA glycosylase (UDG), a DNA repair enzyme. The function of UDG is specifically to remove the RNA base uracil from DNA. The binding of Vpr to UDG does not impair the enzymatic activity of UDG (326). Intriguingly, the pol genes of EIAV (328), FIV, and CAEV (329) contain a deoxyuridine triphosphatase (dUTPase) domain responsible for preventing dUTP incorporation into viral cDNA during reverse transcription. Although the mechanisms of action of UDG and dUTPase are distinct, both ultimately minimize incorporation of uracil into cDNA (330). dUTPase mutants of FIV (331) and EIAV (328, 332) and of caprine and ovine lentiviruses (333) exhibit wild-type replication kinetics in dividing cells but are attenuated in primary macrophages. One explanation for the selective attenuation of dUTPase mutants in macrophages may relate to the low dNTP pools in these nondividing cells when compared with proliferating cells (334). Under such noncycling conditions, when the ratio of dUTP to thymidine triphosphate (TTP) in the cell is likely to be high, action of the viral encoded dUTPase would reduce the dUTP levels (by conversion to dUMP), thus minimizing incorporation of dUTP into viral cDNA. Such a property may be less important in dividing cells, in which high concentrations of TTP would make misincorporation of dUTP into viral cDNA less likely. The association of Vpr with UDG therefore raises the possibility that the attenuated replication of Vpr mutants of HIV-1 and of HIV-2/SIV (14, 126, 308, 310, 311) may be a consequence of the removal of UDG activity from the virus. However, in SIV$_{SM}$ PBj, Vpx is necessary for replication in macrophages, whereas Vpr is dispensable (14). Recent studies have demonstrated that SIV$_{SM}$ PBj Vpr, but not Vpx, interacts with UDG (327). This finding suggests that the role of HIV-1 Vpr and HIV-2/SIV$_{SM}$ Vpx in macrophage infection is not related to the association of these accessory gene products with the DNA repair enzyme UDG. Similarly, the interaction of Vpr with UDG is not necessary for induction of cell-cycle arrest by Vpr (327). Nevertheless, the interaction of HIV-1 *Vpr* and HIV-2/SIV$_{SM}$ *Vpr* genes with UDG argues that this association is important for primate lentivirus replication.

Vpr/Vpx PROTEINS AND NUCLEAR TRANSPORT

Immediately after fusion of viral with host cell membranes, viral nucleic acids are synthesized within a high-molecular-weight nucleoprotein reverse transcription complex (17, 164, 335, 336). This complex is subsequently transported to the host cell nucleus, where integration of viral with host cell DNA occurs (see Fig 3.3). After infection of target cells, virion-associated HIV-1 Vpr and virion-associated SIV$_{SM}$ Vpr and Vpx proteins remain associated with the viral reverse transcription complex (14, 92, 126). In nondividing primary macrophages, nuclear translocation of the viral reverse transcription complex appears dependent on Vpr and Vpx proteins. Thus, Vpr mutants of HIV-1 (126) and SIV$_{AGM}$ (311) and Vpx mutants of HIV-2/SIV$_{SM}$ (14) inefficiently translocate to the host cell nucleus of nondividing macrophages. Based on these observations, investigagtors have suggested that Vpr/Vpx proteins of primate lentiviruses facilitate nuclear translocation of the reverse transcription complex (219), and this property provides the mechanism by which these proteins facilitate macrophage infection. This model is consistent with the observation that Vpr proteins of HIV-1 exhibit a nuclear localization; however, no direct evidence indicates that Vpr/Vpx proteins of primate lentiviruses exhibit a classic NLS or bind to importins that mediate nuclear translocation of nuclear proteins. Thus, whether Vpr/Vpx proteins of primate lentiviruses are classic nuclear import proteins or whether they promote nuclear translocation of the reverse transcription complex by a novel or "piggy-back" mechanism remains to be determined. The presence of highly conserved mechanisms that facilitate infection of nondividing macrophages supports the notion that macrophage lineage cells are important for certain aspects of primate lentivirus pathogenicity.

References

1. Gardner MB, Endres M, Barry P. The simian retroviruses. In: Levy JA, ed. The retroviridae. vol. 3. New York: Plenum Press, 1994.
2. Huet T, Cheynier R, Meyerhans A, et al. Genetic organization of a chimpanzee lentivirus related to HIV-1. Nature 1990;345:356–359.
3. Sharp PM, Robertson DL, Hahn BH. Cross-species transmission and recombination of "AIDS" viruses. Philos Trans R Soc Lond B Biol Sci 1995;349:41–47.
4. Ou IS-H, Gaynor RB. Intracellular factors involved in gene expression of human retroviruses. In: Levy JA, ed. The retroviridae. vol. 4. New York: Plenum Press, 1995.
5. Biswas DK, Ahlers CM, Dezube BJ, et al. Pentoxifylline and other protein kinase C inhibitors down-regulate HIV-1 LTR NF-κB induced gene expression. Mol Med 1994;1:31–43.
6. Kaufman JD, Valandra G, Rodriquez G, et al. Phorbol ester enhances human immunodeficiency virus-promoted gene expression and acts on a repeated 10-base-pair functional enhancer element. Mol Cell Biol 1987;7:3759–3766.
7. Gabel G, Baltimore D. An inducible transcription factor activates expression of human immunodeficiency virus in T cells. Nature 1987;326:711–713.
8. Renjifo B, Speck NA, Winandy S, et al. *Cis*-acting elements in the U3 region of a simian immunodeficiency virus. J Virol 1990;64:3130–3134.
9. Siekevitz M, Josephs SF, Dukovich M, et al. Activation of the HIV-1 LTR by T cell mitogens and the *trans*-activator protein of HTLV-1. Science 1987;238:1575–1578.
10. Tong-Starksen S, Luciw PA, Peterlin BM. Human immunodeficiency virus long terminal repeat responds to T-cell activation signals. Proc Natl Acad Sci U S A 1987;84:6845–6849.
11. Löchelt M, Flügel RM. The molecular biology of human and primate spuma retroviruses. In: Levy JA, ed. The retroviridae. vol. 4. New York: Plenum Press, 1995.
12. Joag SV, Stephens EB, Narayan O. Lentiviruses. In: Fields BN, Knipe DM, Howley PM, et al, eds. Field's virology. 3rd ed. Philadelphia: Lippincott–Raven, 1996.
13. Bour S, Schubert U, Peden K, et al. The envelope glcoprotein of human immunodeficiency virus type 2 enhances viral particle release: a Vpu-like factor? J Virol 1996;70:820–829.
14. Fletcher TMI, Brichacek B, Sharova N, et al. Nuclear import and cell cycle arrest functions of the HIV-1 Vpr protein are encoded by two separate genes in HIV-2/SIM$_{SM}$. EMBO J 1996;15:6155–6165.
15. Gelderblom HR. Assembly and morphology of HIV: potential effects of structure on viral function. AIDS 1991;5:617–638.
16. Hoglund S, Ofverstedt L-G, Nilsson A, et al. Spatial visualization of the maturing HIV-1 core and its linkage to the envelope. AIDS Res Hum Retroviruses 1992;8:1–7.
17. Bukrinsky MI, Sharova N, McDonald TL, et al. Association of integrase, matrix, and reverse transcriptase antigens of human immunodeficiency virus type 1 with viral nucleic acids following acute infection. Proc Natl Acad Sci U S A 1993;90:6125–6129.
18. Marquet R, Baudin F, Gabus C, et al. Dimerization of human immunodeficiency virus (type 1) RNA: stimulation by cations and possible mechanism. Nucleic Acids Res 1991;19:2349–2357.
19. Sakaguchi K, Zambrano N, Baldwin ET, et al. Identification of a binding site for the human immunodeficiency virus type 1 nucleocapsid protein. Proc Natl Acad Sci U S A 1993;90:5219–5223.
20. Darlix JL, Lapadat-Tapolsky M, de Rocquigny H, et al. First glimpses as structure-function relationships of the nucleocapsid protein of retroviruses. J Mol Biol 1995;254:523–537.
21. Trono D. Partial reverse transcripts in virions from human immunodeficiency and murine leukemia viruses. J Virol 1992;66:4893–4900.
22. Lori F, Veronese FD, DeVico AL, et al. Viral DNA carried by human immunodeficiency virus type 1 virions. J Virol 1992;66:5067–5074.
23. Zhang H, Zhang Y, Spicer TP, et al. Reverse transcription takes place within extracellular HIV-1 virions: potential biological significance. AIDS Res Hum Retroviruses 1993;9:1287–1295.
24. Zhang H, Dornadula G, Pomerantz RJ. Endogenous reverse transcription of human immunodefciency virus type 1 in physiological microenvironments: an important stage for viral infection of nondividing cells. J Virol 1996;70:2809–2824.
25. Zhang H, Dornadula G, Yong W, et al. Kinetic analysis of intravirion reverse transcription in the blood plasma of human immunodeficiency virus type 1-infected individuals: direct assessment of resistance to reverse transcriptase inhibitors in vivo. J Virol 1996;70:628–634.
26. Fennie C, Laksy L. Model for intracellular folding of the human immunodeficiency virus type 1 gp120. J Virol 1989;63:639–646.
27. Stevenson M, Zhang XH, Volsky DJ. Downregulation of cell surface molecules during noncytopathic infection of T cells with human immunodeficiency virus. J Virol 1987;61:3741–3748.
28. Stevenson M, Meier C, Mann AM, et al. Envelope glycoprotein of HIV induces interference and cytolysis resistance in CD4+ cells: mechanism for persistence in AIDS. Cell 1988;53:483–496.
29. Crise B, Buonocore L, Rose JK. CD4 is retained in the endoplasmic reticulum by the human immunodeficiency virus type 1 glycoprotein precursor. J Virol 1990;64:5585–5593.
30. Hoxie JA, Alpers JD, Rackowski JL, et al. Alterations in T4 (CD4) protein and mRNA synthesis in cells infected with HIV. Science 1986;234:1123–1127.
31. Jabbar MA, Nayak DP. Intracellular interaction of human immunodeficiency virus type 1 (ARV-2) envelope glycoprotein gp160 with CD4 blocks the movement and maturation of CD4 to the plasma membrane. J Virol 1990;64:6297–6304.
32. Ratner L. Glucosidase inhibitors for treatment of HIV-1 infection. AIDS Res Hum Retroviruses 1992;8:165–173.
33. Lee W-R, Syu W-J, Du B, et al. Nonrandom distribution of gp 120 N-linked glycosylation site important for infectivity of human immunodeficiency virus type 1. Proc Natl Acad Sci U S A 1993;89:2213–2217.
34. Bosch ML, Andeweg AC, Schipper R, et al. Insertion of N-linked glycosylation sites in the variable regions of the human immunodeficiency virus type 1 surface glycoprotein through AAT triplet reiteration. J Virol 1994;68:7566-7569.
35. Chanh T, Dreesman GR, Kanda P, et al. Induction of anti-HIV neutralizing antibodies by synthetic peptides. EMBO J 1986;5:3065–3071.

36. Connick E, Schooley RT. HIV-1 specific immune responses. In: Morrow WJW, Haigwood N, eds. HIV-molecular organization, pathogenicity and treatment. Amsterdam: Elsevier, 1993.
37. McCune JM, Rabon LB, Feinberg MB, et al. Endoproteolytic cleavage of gp160 is required for the activation of human immunodeficiency virus. Cell 1988;53:55–67.
38. Moore JP, McKeating JA, Weiss RA, et al. Dissociation of gp120 from HIV-1 virions induced by soluble CD4. Science 1990;250:1139–1142.
39. Poignard P, Fouts T, Naniche D, et al. Neutralizing antibodies to human immunodeficiency virus type-1 gp120 induce envelope glycoprotein subunit dissociation. J Exp Med 1996;183:473–484.
40. Piatak Jr. M, Saag MS, Yang LC, et al. High levels of HIV-1 in plasma during all stages of infection determined by competitive PCR. Science 1993;259:1749-1754.
41. Earl PL, Doms RW, Moss B. Oligomeric structure of the human immunodeficiency virus type 1 envelope glycoprotein. Proc Natl Acad Sci U S A 1990;87:648–652.
42. Earl PL, Moss B, Doms RW. Folding, interaction with GRP78-BiP, assembly, and transport of the human immunodeficiency virus type 1 envelope protein. J Virol 1991;65:2047–2055.
43. Rey M-A, Krust B, Laurent AG, et al. Characterization of human immunodeficiency virus type 2 envelope glycoproteins: dimerization of the glycoprotein precursor during processing. J Virol 1989;63:647–658.
44. Weiss CD, Levy JA, White JM. Oligomeric structure of gp120 on infectious human immunodeficiency virus type 1 particles. J Virol 1990;64:5674–5677.
45. Burns DPW, Desrosiers RC. Envelope sequence variation, neutralizing antibodies, and primate lentivirus persistence. Curr Top Microbiol Immunol 1994;188:185–219.
46. Wain-Hobson S. Human immunodeficiency virus type 1 quasispecies in vivo and ex vivo. Curr Top Microbiol Immunol 1992;176:181.
47. Ashkenazi A, Smith DH, Marsters SA, et al. Resistance of primary isolates of human immunodeficiency virus type 1 to soluble CD4 is independent of CD4-gp120 binding affinity. Proc Natl Acad Sci U S A 1991;88:7056–7060.
48. Brightly DW, Rosenberg M, Chen ISY, et al. Envelope proteins from clinical isolates of human immunodeficiency virus type 1 that are refractory to neutralization by soluble CD4 possess high affinity for the CD4 receptor. Proc Natl Acad Sci U S A 1991;88:7802–7806.
49. Fantini J, Cook DG, Nathanson N, et al. Infection of colonic epithelial cell lines by type 1 human immunodeficiency virus is associated with cell surface expression of galactosylceramide, a potential alternative gp120 receptor. Proc Natl Acad Sci U S A 1993;90:2700–2704.
50. Clapham PR, Weiss RA. Immunodeficiency viruses: spoilt for choice of coreceptors. Nature 1997;388:230–231.
51. Lapham CK, Ouyang J, Chandrasekhar B, et al. Evidence for cell-surface association between fusin and the CD4-gp120 complex in human cell lines. Science 1996;274:602–605.
52. Trkola A, Dragic T, Arthos J, et al. CD4-dependent, antibody-sensitive interactions betwen HIV-1 and its coreceptor CCR-5. Nature 1996;384:184–187.
53. Wu L, Gerard NP, Wyatt R, et al. CD4-induced interaction of primary HIV-1 gp120 glycoproteins with the chemokine receptor CCR-5. Nature 1996;384:179–183.
54. Westervelt P, Gendelman HE, Ratner L. Identification of a determinant within the human immunodeficiency virus 1 surface envelope glycoprotein critical for productive infection of primary monocytes. Proc Natl Acad Sci U S A 1991;88:3097–3101.
55. O'Brien WA, Koyanagi Y, Namazie A, et al. HIV-1 tropism for mononuclear phagocytes can be determined by regions of gp120 outside the CD4-binding domain. Nature 1990;348:69–73.
56. Cheng-Mayer C, Quiroga M, Tung JW, et al. Viral determinants of human immunodeficiency virus type 1 T-cell or macrophage tropism, cytopathogenicity, and CD4 antigen modulation. J Virol 1990;64:4390–4398.
57. Hwang SS, Boyle TJ, Lyerly HK, et al. Identification of the envelope V3 loop as the primary determinant of cell tropism in HIV-1. Science 1991;253:71–74.
58. Sodroski J, Haseltine W, Kowalski M. Role of the human immunodeficiency virus type I envelope glycoprotein in cytopathic effect. Adv Exp Med Biol 1991;300:193–199.
59. Freed EO, Myers DJ, Risser R. Characterization of the fusion domain of the human immunodeficiency virus type 1 envelope glycoprotein gp41. Proc Natl Acad Sci U S A 1990;87:4650–4654.
60. Horth M, Lambrecht B, Khim MC, et al. Theoretical and functional analysis of the SIV fusion peptide. EMBO J 1991;10:2747–2755.
61. Kowalski M, Potz J, Basiripour L, et al. Functional regions of the envelope glycoprotein of human immunodeficiency virus type 1. Science 1987;237:1351–1355.
62. Somasundaran M, Robinson HL. A major mechanism of human immunodeficiency virus-induced cell killing does not involve cell fusion. J Virol 1987;61:3114–3119.
63. Tersmette M, de Goede RE, Al BJ, et al. Differential syncytium-inducing capacity of human immunodeficiency virus isolates: frequent detection of syncytium-inducing isolates in patients with acquired immunodeficiency syndrome (AIDS) and AIDS-related complex. J Virol 1988;62:2026–2032.
64. Schuitemaker H, Koot M, Kootstra NA, et al. Biological phenotype of human immunodeficiency virus type 1 clones at different stages of infection: progression of disease is associated with a shift from monocytotropic to T-cell-tropic virus populations. J Virol 1992;66:1354–1360.
65. Deng H, Liu R, Ellemeier W, et al. Identification of a major coreceptor for primary isolates of HIV-1. Nature 1996;381:661.
66. Asjo B, Morfeldt-Manson L, Albert J, et al. Replicative capacity of human immunodeficiency virus from patients with varying severity of HIV infection. Lancet 1986;2:660–662.
67. Kozak SL, Platt EJ, Madani N, et al. CD4, CXCR-4, and CCR-5 dependencies for infections by primary patient and laboratory-adapted isolates of human immunodeficiency virus type 1. J Virol 1997;71:873–882.
68. Platt EJ, Madani N, Kozak SL, et al. Infectious properties of human immunodeficiency virus type 1 mutants with distinct affinities for the CD4 receptor. J Virol 1997;71:883–890.
69. Simmons G, Wilkinson D, Reeves JD, et al. Primary, syncytium-inducing human immunodeficiency virus type 1 isolates are dual-tropic and most can use either Lestr or CCR5 as coreceptors for virus entry. J Virol 1996;70:8355–8360.
70. Valentin A, Albert J, Fenyö EM, et al. Dual tropism for macrophages and lymphocytes is a common feature of primary human immunodeficiency virus type 1 and 2 isolates. J Virol 1994;68:6684–6689.
71. McKnight A, Wilkinson D, Simmons G, et al. Inhibition of human immunodeficiency virus fusion by a monoclonal antibody to a coreceptor (CXCR-4) is both cell type and virus strain dependent. J Virol 1997;71:1692–1696.
72. Connor RI, Paxton WA, Sheridan KE, et al. Macrophages and CD4+ T lymphocytes from two multiply exposed, uninfected individuals resist infection with primary nonsyncytium-inducing isolates of human immunodeficiency virus type 1. J Virol 1996;70:8758–8764.
73. Rana S, Besson G, Cook DG, et al. Role of CCR5 in infection of primary macrophages and lymphocytes by macrophage-tropic strains of human immunodeficiency virus: resistance to patient-derived and prototype isolates resulting from the $\triangle ccr5$ mutation. J Virol 1997;71:3219–3227.
74. Dittmar MT, McKnight A, Simmons G, et al. HIV-1 tropism and coreceptor use. Nature 1997;385:495–496.
75. Henderson LE, Bowers MA, Sowder II RC, et al. Gag proteins of the highly replicative MN strain of human immunodeficieincy virus type 1: posttranslational modifications, proteolytic processings, and complete amino acid sequences. J Virol 1992;66:1856–1865.
76. Sanchez-Pescador R, Power MD, Barr PJ, et al. Nucleotide sequence and expression of an AIDS-associated retrovirus (ARV-2). Science 1985;227:484–492.

77. McQuade TJ, Tomasselli AG, Liu L, et al. A synthetic HIV-1 protease inhibitor with antiviral activity arrests HIV-like particle maturation. Science 1990;247:454–456.
78. Massiah MA, Starich MR, Paschall C, et al. Three-dimensional structure of the human immunodeficiency virus type 1 matrix protein. J Mol Biol 1994;244:198–223.
79. Matthews S, Barlow P, Boyd J, et al. Structural similarity between the p17 matrix protein of HIV-1 and interferon-τ. Nature 1994;370:666–668.
80. Hill CP, Worthylake D, Bancroft DP, et al. Crystal structures of the trimeric human immunodeficiency virus type 1 matrix protein: implications for membrane association and assembly. Proc Natl Acad Sci U S A 1996;93:3099–3104.
81. Massiah MA, Worthylake D, Christensen AM, et al. Comparison of the NMR and X-ray structures of the HIV-1 matrix protein: evidence for conformational changes during viral assembly. Protein Sci 1996;5:2391–2398.
82. Christensen AM, Massiah MA, Turner BG, et al. Three-dimensional structure of the HTLV-II matrix protein and comparative analysis of matrix proteins from the different classes of pathogenic human retroviruses. J Mol Biol 1996;264:1117–1131.
83. Schultz AM, Henderson LE, Oroszlan S. Fatty acylation of proteins. Annu Rev Cell Biol 1988;4:611.
84. Dorfman T, Mammano F, Haseltine WA, et al. Role of the matrix protein in the virion association of the human immunodeficiency virus type 1 envelope glycoprotein. J Virol 1994;68:1689–1696.
85. Zhou W, Parents LJ, Wills JW, et al. Identification of a membrane-binding domain within the amino-terminal region of human immunodeficiency virus type 1 gag protein which interacts with acidic phospholipids. J Virol 1994;68:2556–2569.
86. Bryant M, Ratner L. Myristoylation-dependent replication and assembly of human immunodeficiency virus 1. Proc Natl Acad Sci U S A 1990;87:523–527.
87. Gottlinger HG, Sodroski JG, Haseltine WA. Role of capsid precursor processing and myristoylation in morphogenesis and infectivity of human immunodeficiency virus type 1. Proc Natl Acad Sci U S A 1989;86:5781–5785.
88. Gallay P, Swingler S, Aiken C, et al. HIV-1 infection of nondividing cells: C-terminal tyrosine phosphorylation of the virla matrix protein is a key regulator. Cell 1995;80:379–388.
89. Bukrinskaya AG, Ghorpade A, Heinzinger NK, et al. Phosphorylation-dependent human immunodeficiency virus type 1 infection and nuclear targeting of viral DNA. Proc Natl Acad Sci U S A 1996;93:367–371.
90. Yu XF, Yuan X, Matsuda Z, Lee TH, et al. The matrix protein of human immunodeficiency virus type 1 is required for incorporation of viral envelope protein into mature virions. J Virol 1992;66:4966–4971.
91. Parent LJ, Wilson CB, Resh MD, et al. Evidence for a second function of the MA sequence in the rous sarcoma virus gag protein. J Virol 1996;70:1016–1026.
92. Hansen MST, Bushman FD. Human immunodeficiency virus type 2 preintegration complexes: activities in vitro and response to inhibitors. J Virol 1997;71:3351–3356.
93. Farnet CM, Bushman FD. HIV-1 cDNA integration: requirement of HMG I(Y) protein for function of preintegration complexes in vitro. Cell 1997;88:483–492.
94. Miller MD, Farnet CM, Bushman FD. Human immunodeficiency virus type 1 preintegration complexes: studies of organization and composition. J Virol 1997;71:5382–5390.
95. Gallay P, Swingler S, Song J, et al. HIV nuclear import is governed by the phosphotyrosine-mediated binding of matrix to the core domain of integrase. Cell 1995;83:569–576.
96. Bukrinsky M, Haggerty S, Dempsey MP, et al. A nuclear localization signal within HIV-1 matrix protein that governs infection of non-dividing cells. Nature 1993;365:666–669.
97. Stevenson M. Portals of entry: uncovering HIV nuclear transport pathways. Trends Cell Biol 1996;6:9–15.
98. Gallay P, Stitt V, Mundy C, et al. Role of the karyopherin pathway in human immunodeficiency virus type 1 nuclear import. J Virol 1996;70:1027–1032.
99. Fouchier RA, Meyer BE, Simon JH, et al. HIV-1 infection of non-dividing cells: evidence that the amino-terminal basic region of the viral matrix protein is important for Gag processing but not for post-entry nuclear import. EMBO J 1997;16:4531–4539.
100. Gitti RK, Lee BM, Walker J, et al. Structure of the amino-terminal core domain of the HIV-1 capsid protein. Science 1996;273:231.
101. Momany C, Kovari LC, Prongay AJ, et al. Crystal structure of dimeric HIV-1 capsid protein. Nature Structur Biol 1996;3:763–770.
102. Gamble TR, Vajdos FF, Yoo S, et al. Crystal structure of human cyclophilin A bound to the amino-terminal domain of HIV-1 capsid. Cell 1996;87:1285–1294.
103. Franke EK, Yuan HEH, Luban J. Specific incorporation of cyclophilin A into HIV-1 virions. Nature 1994;372:359–362.
104. Thali M, Bukovsky A, Kondo E, et al. Functional association of cyclophilin A with HIV-1 virions. Nature 1994;372:363–365.
105. Luban J, Bossolt KL, Franke EK, et al. Human immunodeficiency virus type 1 gag protein binds to cyclophilins A and B. Cell 1993;73:1067–1078.
106. Braaten D, Franke EK, Luban J. Cyclophilin A is required for the replication of group M human immunodeficiency virus type 1 (HIV-1) and simian immunodeficiency virus $SIV_{CPZ}GAB$ but not group O HIV-1 or other primate immunodeficiency virus. J Virol 1996;70:4220–4227.
107. Braaten D, Aberham C, Franke EK, et al. Cyclosporin A–resistant human immunodeficiency virus type 1 mutants demonstrate that gag encodes functional target of cyclophilin A. J Virol 1996;70:5170–5176.
108. Colgan J, Yuan HEH, Franke EK, et al. Binding of the human immunodeficiency virus type 1 gag polyprotein to cyclophilin A is mediated by the central region of capsid and requires gag dimerization. J Virol 1996;70:4299–4310.
109. Dorfman T, Göttlinger HG. The human immunodeficiency virus type 1 capsid p2 domain confers sensitivity to the cyclopholin-binding drug SDZ NIM 811. J Virol 1996;70:5751–5757.
110. Yoo S, Myszka DG, Yeh C, et al. Molecular recognition in the HIV-1 capsid/cyclophilin A complex. J Mol Biol 1997;269:780–795.
111. Luban J, Goff SP. Binding of human immunodeficiency virus type 1 (HIV-1) RNA to recombinant HIV-1 gag polyprotein. J Virol 1991;65:3203–3212.
112. Berkowitz RD, Luban J, Goff SP. Specific binding of human immunodeficiency virus type 1 gag polyprotein and nucleocapsid protein to viral DNAs detected by RNA mobility shift assays. J Virol 1993;67:7190–7199.
113. Berkowitz RD, Goff SP. Analysis of binding elements in the human immunodeficiency virus type 1 genomic RNA and nucleocapsid protein. Virology 1994;202:233–246.
114. Karpel RL, Henderson LE, Oroszlan S. Interactions of retroviral structural proteins with single-stranded nucleic acids. J Biol Chem 1987;262:4961–4967.
115. Aldovini A, Young RA. Mutations of RNA and protein sequences involved in human immunodeficiency virus type 1 packaging result in production of noninfectious virus. J Virol 1990;64:1920–1926.
116. Turpin JA, Terpening SJ, Schaeffer CA, et al. Inhibitors of human immunodeficiency virus type 1 zinc fingers prevent normal processing of gag precursors and result in the release of noninfectious virus particles. J Virol 1996;70:6180–6189.
117. Tanchou V, Gabus C, Rogemond V, et al. Formation of stable and functional HIV-1 nucleoprotein complexes in vitro. J Mol Biol 1995;252:563–571.
118. Li X, Quan Y, Arts EJ, Li Z, et al. Human immunodeficiency virus type 1 nucleocapsid protein (NCp7) directs specific initiation of minus-strand DNA synthesis primed by human $tRNA_3Lys$ in vitro: studies of viral RNA molecules mutated in regions that flank the primer binding site. J Virol 1996;70:4996–5004.

119. Guo J, Henderson LE, Bess J, et al. Human immunodeficiency virus type 1 nucleocapsid protein promotes efficient strand transfer and specific viral DNA synthesis by inhibiting TAR-dependent self-priming from minus-strand strong-stop DNA. J Virol 1997;71:5178–5188.
120. Carteau S, Batson SC, Poljak L, et al. Human immunodeficiency virus type 1 nucleocapsid protein specifically stimulates Mg2+-dependent DNA integration in vitro. J Virol 1997;71:6225–6229.
121. Yu Q, Darlix JL. The zinc finger of nucleocapsid protein of friend murine leukemia virus is critical for proviral DNA synthesis in vivo. J Virol 1996;70:5791–5798.
122. Gottlinger HG, Dorfman T, Sodroski JG, et al. Effect of mutations affecting the p6 gag protein on human immunodeficiency virus particle release. Proc Natl Acad Sci U S A 1991;88:3195–3199.
123. Lu Y-L, Spearman P, Ratner L. Human immunodeficiency virus type 1 viral protein R localization in infected cells and virions. J Virol 1993;67:6542–6550.
124. Paxton W, Connor RI, Landau NR. Incorporation of Vpr into human immunodeficiency virus type 1 virions: requirement for the p6 region of *gag* and mutational analysis. J Virol 1993;67:7229–7237.
125. Wu X, Conway JA, Kim J, et al. Localization of the Vpx packaging signal within the C terminus of the human immunodeficiency virus type 2 gag precursor protein. J Virol 1994;68:6161–6169.
126. Heinzinger N, Bukrinsky M, Haggerty S, et al. The Vpr protein of human immunodeficiency virus type 1 influences nuclear localization of viral nucleic acids in nondividing host cells. Proc Natl Acad Sci U S A 1994;91:7311–7315.
127. Kohlstaedt LA, Wang J, Friedman JM, et al. Crystal structure at 3.5 Å resolution of HIV-1 reverse transcriptase complexed with an inhibitor. Science 1992;256:1783–1790.
128. Arnold E, Jacobo-Molina A, Nanni RG, et al. Structure of HIV-1 reverse transcriptase/DNA complex at 7 A resolution showing active site locations. Nature 1992;357:85.
129. Navia MA, Fitzgerald PMD, McKeever B, et al. Three-dimensional structure of aspartyl protease from human immunodeficiency virus HIV-1. Nature 1989;337:615–620.
130. Davies JF, Hostomska Z, Hostomsky Z, et al. Crystal structure of the ribonuclease H domain of HIV-1 reverse transcriptase. Science 1991;252:88.
131. Jacks T, Power MD, Masiarz FR, et al. Characterization of ribosomal frameshifting in HIV-1 *gag-pol* expression. Nature 1988;331:280–283.
132. Parkin NT, Chamorro M, Varmus HE. Human immunodeficiency virus 1 *gag-pol* frameshifting is dependent on downstream mRNA secondary structure: demonstration by expression in vivo. J Virol 1992;66:5147–5151.
133. Wilson W, Braddock M, Adams SE, et al. HIV expression strategies: ribosomal frameshifting is directed by a short sequence in both mammalian and yeast systems. Cell 1988;55:1159–1169.
134. Skalka AM. Retroviral proteases: First glimpses at the anatomy of a processing machine. Cell 1989;56:911.
135. Debouck C. The HIV-1 protease as a therapeutic target for AIDS. AIDS Res Hum Retroviruses 1992;8:153.
136. Sharma SK, Fan N, Evans DB. Human immunodeficiency virus type 1 (HIV-1) recombinant reverse transcriptase: asymmetry in p66 subunits of the p66/p66 homodimer. FEBS Lett 1994;343:125–130.
137. Wang J, Smerdon SJ, Jager J, et al. Structural basis of asymmetry in the human immunodeficiency virus type 1 reverse transcriptase heterodimer. Proc Natl Acad Sci U S A 1994;91:7242–7246.
138. Smerdon SJ, Jager J, Wang J, et al. Structure of the binding site for nonnucleoside inhibitors of the reverse transcriptase of human immunodeficiency virus type 1. Proc Natl Acad Sci U S A 1994;91:3911–3915.
139. Jacobo-Molina A, Ding J, Nanni RG, et al. Crystal structure of human immunodeficiency virus type 1 reverse transcriptase complexed with double-stranded DNA at 3.0 A resolution shows bent DNA. Proc Natl Acad Sci U S A 1993;90:6320.
140. Cheng N, Merrill BM, Dainter GR, et al. Identification of the nucleotide binding site of HIV-1 reverse transcriptase using dTTP as a photoaffinity label. Biochemistry 1993;32:7630–7634.
141. Larder BA, Purifoy DJM, Powell KL, et al. Site-specific mutagenesis of AIDS virus reverse transcriptase. Nature 1987;327:716–717.
142. Basu A, Tirumalai RS, Modak MJ. Substrate binding in human immunodeficiency virus reverse transcriptase: an analysis of pyridoxal 5′-phosphate sensitivity and identification of lysine 263 in the substrate-binding domain. J Biol Chem 1989;264:8746–8752.
143. Sobol RW, Suhadolnik RJ, Kumar A, et al. Localization of a polynucleotide binding region in the HIV-1 reverse transcriptase: Implications for primer binding. Biochemistry 1991;30:10623–10631.
144. Becerra SP, Kumar A, Lewis MS, et al. Protein-protein interactions of HIV-1 reverse transcriptase: implication of central and C-terminal regions in subunit binding. Biochemistry 1991;30:11707–11719.
145. Hostomsky Z, Hostomska Z, Hudson GO, et al. Reconstitution in vitro of RNase H activity by using purified N-terminal and C-terminal domains of human immunodeficiency virus type 1 reverse transcriptase. Proc Natl Acad Sci U S A 1991;88:1148–1152.
146. Le Grice SFJ, Naas T, Wohlgensingerr B, et al. Subunit-selection mutagenesis indicates minimal polymerase activity in heterodimer-associated p51 HIV-1 reverse transcriptase. EMBO J 1991;10:3905–3939.
147. Arts EJ, Wainberg MA. Human immunodeficiency virus type 1 reverse transcriptase and early events in reverse transcription. Adv Virus Res 1996;46:97–155.
148. Coffin JM. Genetic diversity and evolution of retroviruses. Curr Top Microbiol Immunol 1992;176:143–164.
149. Preston BD, Poiesz BJ, Loeb LA. Fidelity of HIV-1 reverse transcriptase. Science 1988;242:1168–1171.
150. Roberts JD, Bebenek K, Kunkel TA. The accuracy of reverse transcriptase from HIV-1. Science 1988;242:1171–1173.
151. Weiss R, Teich N, Varmus H, et al. RNA tumor viruses. Cold Spring Harbor, NY: Cold Spring Harbor Laboratory, 1982.
152. Klarmann GJ, Schauber CA, Preston BD. Template-directed pausing of DNA synthesis by HIV-1 reverse transcriptase during polymerization of HIV-1 sequences in vitro. J Biol Chem 1993;268:9793–9802.
153. Dyda F, Hickman AB, Jenkins TM, et al. Crystal structure of the catalytic domain of HIV-1 integrase: similarity to other polynucleotidyl transferases. Science 1994;266:1981–1985.
154. Stevenson M, Haggerty S, Lamonica CA, et al. Integration is not necessary for expression of human immunodeficiency virus type 1 protein products. J Virol 1990;64:2421–2425.
155. Burke CJ, Sanyal G, Bruner MW, et al. Structural implications of spectroscopic characterization of a putative zinc-finger peptide from HIV-1 integrase. J Biol Chem 1992;267:9639.
156. Vincent KA, Ellison V, Chow SA, et al. Characterization of human immunodeficiency virus type 1 integrase expressed in *Escherichia coli* and analysis of variants with amino-terminal mutations. J Virol 1993;67:425–437.
157. Sherman PA, Fyfe JA. Human immunodeficiency virus integration protein expressed in *Escherichia coli* possesses selective DNA cleaving activity. Proc Natl Acad Sci U S A 1990;87:5119–5123.
158. Vink C, Oude AAM, Plasterk RHA. Identification of the catalytic and DNA-binding region of the human immunodeficiency virus type 1 integrase protein. Nucleic Acids Res 1993;21:1419–1425.
159. Bushman FD, Engelman A, Palmer I, et al. Domains of the integrase protein of human immunodeficiency virus type 1 responsible for polynucleotidyl transfer and zinc binding. Proc Natl Acad Sci U S A 1993;90:3428–3432.
160. Fujiwara T, Craigie R. Integration of mini-retroviral DNA: a cell-free reaction for biochemical analysis of retroviral integration. Proc Natl Acad Sci U S A 1989;86:3065–3069.
161. Brown PO, Bowerman B, Varmus HE, et al. Retroviral integration: structure of the initial covalent product and its precursor, and a role for the viral IN protein. Proc Natl Acad Sci U S A 1989;86:2525–2529.
162. Ellison V, Abrams H, Roe T, et al. Human immunodeficiency virus integration in a cell-free system. J Virol 1990;64:2711–2715.

163. Farnet CM, Haseltine WA. Integration of human immunodeficiency virus type 1 DNA in vitro. Proc Natl Acad Sci U S A 1990;87:4164–4168.
164. Bukrinsky MI, Sharova N, Dempsey MP, et al. Active nuclear import of human immunodeficiency virus type 1 preintegration complexes. Proc Natl Acad Sci U S A 1992;89:6580–6584.
165. Goodarzi G, Im GJ, Brackman K, et al. Concerted integration of retrovirus-like DNA by human immunodeficiency virus type 1 integrase. J Virol 1995;69:6090–6097.
166. Kalpana GV, Marmon S, Wang W, et al. Binding and stimulation of HIV-1 integrase by a human homolog of yeast transcription factor SNF5. Science 1994;266:2002–2006.
167. Leavitt AD, Robles G, Alesandro N, et al. Human immunodeficiency virus Type 1 integrase mutants retain in vitro integrase activity yet fail to integrate viral DNA efficiently during infection. J Virol 1996;70:721–728.
168. Cannon PM, Wilson W, Byles E, et al. Human immunodeficiency virus type 1 integrase: effect on viral replication of mutations at highly conserved residues. J Virol 1994;68(8):4768–4775
169. Engelman A, Englund G, Orenstein JM, et al. Multiple effects of mutations in human immunodeficiency virus type 1 integrase on viral replication. J Virol 1995;69:2729–2736.
170. Hazuda D, Felock P, Hastings J, et al. Equivalent inhibition of half-site and full-site retroviral strand transfer reactions by structurally diverse compounds. J Virol 1997;71:807–811.
171. Gallay P, Hope T, Chin D, et al. HIV-1 infection of nondividing cells through the recognition of integrase by the importin/karyopherin pathway. Proc Natl Acad Sci U S A 1997;94:9825–9830.
172. Kukolj G, Jones KS, Skalka AM. Subcellular localization of avian sarcoma virus and human immunodeficiency virus type 1 integrases. J Virol 1997;71:843–847.
173. Dworetzky SI, Lanford RE, Feldherr CM. The effects of variations in the number and sequence of targeting signals on nuclear uptake. J Cell Biol 1988;107:1279–1287.
174. Zack JA, Arrigo SJ, Weitsman SR, et al. HIV-1 entry into quiescent primary lymphocytes: molecular analysis reveals a labile, latent viral structure. Cell 1990;61:213–222.
175. Stevenson M, Stanwick TL, Dempsey MP, et al. HIV-1 replication is controlled at the level of T cell activation and proviral integration. EMBO J 1990;9:1551–1560.
176. Bukrinsky MI, Stanwick TL, Dempsey MP, et al. Quiescent T lymphocytes as an inducible virus reservoir in HIV-1 infection. Science 1991;254:423–427.
177. Chun TW, Carruth L, Finzi D, et al. Quantification of latent tissue reservoirs and total body viral load in HIV-1 infection. Nature 1997;387:183–188.
178. Gao W, Cara A, Gallo RC, et al. Low levels of deoxynucleotides in peripheral blood lymphocytes: a strategy to inhibit human immunodeficiency virus type 1 replication. Proc Natl Acad Sci U S A 1993;90:8925–8928.
179. Stevenson M. Molecular mechanisms for the regulation of HIV replication, persistence and latency. AIDS 1997;11:S25–S33.
180. Ilyinskii PO, Desrosiers RC. Efficient transcription and replication of simian immunodefciency virus in the absence of NFκB and Sp1 binding elements. J Virol 1996;70:3118–3126.
181. Ilyinskii PO, Simon MA, Czajak SC, et al. Induction of AIDS by simian immunodeficiency virus lacking NF-κB and SP1 binding elements. J Virol 1997;1997:1880–1887.
182. Kim JY, Gonzalez-Scarano F, Zeichner SL, et al. Replication of type 1 human immunodeficiency viruses containing linker scanning mutations in the -201 to -130 region of the long terminal repeat. J Virol 1993;67:1658–1662.
183. Cherrington J, Ganem D. Regulation of polyadenylation in human immunodeficiency virus (HIV): contributions of promoter proximity and upstream sequences. EMBO J 1992;11:1513–1524.
184. DeZazzo JD, Scott JM, Imperiale MJ. Relative roles of signals upstream of AAUAAA and promoter proximity in regulation of human immunodeficiency virus type 1 mRNA 3′ end formation. Mol Cell Biol 1992;12:5555–5562.
185. Peterlin BM. Molecular biology of HIV. In: Levy JA, ed. The retroviridae. vol. 4. New York: Plenum Press, 1995.
186. Nelbock P, Dillon PJ, Perkins A, et al. A cDNA for a protein that interacts with the human immunodeficiency virus tat transactivator. Science 1990;248:1650–1653.
187. Desai K, Loewenstein PM, Green M. Isolation of a cellular protein that binds to the human immunodeficiency virus Tat protein and can potentiate transactivation of the viral promoter. Proc Natl Acad Sci U S A 1991;88:8875.
188. Jeang KT, Chun R, Lin NH, et al. In vitro and in vivo binding of human immunodeficiency virus type 1 Tat protein and Sp1 transcription factor. J Virol 1993;67:6224.
189. Herrmann CH, Rice AP. Specific interaction of the human immunodeficiency virus Tat proteins with a cellular protein kinase. Virology 1993;197:601.
190. Kashanchi F, Piras G, Radnonovich MF, et al. Direct interaction of human TFIID with the HIV-1 transactivator Tat. Nature 1994;367:295–299.
191. Cullen BR. Mechanism of action of regulatory proteins encoded by complex retroviruses. Microbiol Rev 1992;56:375.
192. Frankel AD. Activation of HIV transcription by Tat. Curr Opin Genet Dev 1992;2:293.
193. Kao S-Y, Calmen AF, Luciw AP, Peterlin BM. Anti-termination of transcription within the long terminal repeat of HIV-1 by *tat* gene product. Nature 1987;330:489–493.
194. Adams M, Sharmeen L, Kimpton J, et al. Cellular latency in human immunodeficiency virus-infected individuals with high CD4 levels can be detected by the presence of promoter-proximal transcripts. Proc Natl Acad Sci U S A 1994;91:3862–3866.
195. Gait MJ, Karn J. RNA recognition by the human immunodeficiency virus Tat and Rev proteins. Trends Biochem Sci 1993;18:255.
196. Cochrane AW, Perkins A, Rosen CA. Identification of sequences important in the nucleolar localization of human immunodeficiency virus rev: relevance of nucleolar localization to function. J Virol 1990;64:881–885.
197. Olsen HS, Beidas S, Dillon P, et al. Mutational analysis of the HIV-1 Rev protein and its target sequence, the Rev response element. J Acquir Immune Defic Syndr 1991;4:558.
198. Malim MH, Hauber J, Le S-Y, et al. The HIV-1 rev *trans*-activator acts through a structured target sequence to activate nuclear export of unspliced viral mRNA. Nature 1989;338:254–257.
199. Malim MH, Cullen BR. HIV-1 structural gene expression requires the binding of multiple Rev monomers to the viral RRE: implications for HIV-1 latency. Cell 1991;65:241–248.
200. Emerman M, Vazeux R, Peden K. The *rev* gene product of the human immunodeficiency virus affects envelope-specific RNA localization. Cell 1989;57:1155–1165.
201. Felber BK, Hadzopoulou-Claradas M, Claradas C, et al. Rev protein of HIV-1 affects the stability and transport of viral mRNA. Proc Natl Acad Sci U S A 1989;86:1495–1499.
202. Hammarskjold M-L, Heimer J, Hammarskjold B, et al. Regulation of human immunodeficiency virus *env* expression by the *rev* gene product. J Virol 1989;63:1959–1966.
203. Chang DD, Sharp PA. Regulation by HIV rev depends upon recognition of splice sites. Cell 1989;59:789–795.
204. Lu X, Heimer J, Rekosh D, Hammarskjold M-L. U1 small nuclear RNA plays a direct role in the formation of a rev-regulated human immunodeficiency virus env mRNA that remains unspliced. Proc Natl Acad Sci U S A 1990;87:7598–7602.
205. Rosen CA, Terwilliger E, Dayton A, et al. Intragenic *cis*-acting *art* gene-responsive sequences of the human immunodeficiency virus. Proc Natl Acad Sci U S A 1988;85:2071–2075.
206. Cochrane AW, Jones KS, Beidas S, et al. Identification and characterization of intragenic sequences which repress human immunodeficiency virus structural gene expression. J Virol 1991;65:5305–5313.

207. Schwartz S, Campbell M, Nasioulas G, et al. Mutational inactivation of an inhibitory sequence in human immunodeficiency virus type 1 results in rev-independent gag expression. J Virol 1992;66:7176–7182.
208. Schwartz S, Felber BK, Pavlakis GN. Distinct RNA sequences in the gag region of human immunodeficiency virus type 1 decrease RNA stability and inhibit expression in the absence of rev protein. J Virol 1992;66:150–159.
209. Bogerd HP, Fridell RA, Madore S, et al. Identification of a novel cellular cofactor for the Rev/Rex class of retroviral regulatory proteins. Cell 1995;82:485–494.
210. Fritz CC, Zapp ML, Green MR. A human nucleoporin-like protein that specifically interacts with HIV Rev. Nature 1995;376:530–533.
211. Malim MH, Freimuth WW, Liu J, et al. Stable expression of trans-dominant rev protein in human T cells inhibits human immunodeficiency virus replication. J Exp Med 1992;176:1197–1201.
212. Grzesiek S, Bax A, Clore GM, et al. The solution structure of HIV-1 Nef reveals an unexpected fold and permits delineation of the binding surface for the SH3 domain of Hck tyrosine protein kinase. Nat Struct Biol 1996;3:340–345.
213. Lee CH, Saksela K, Mirza UA, et al. Crystal structure of the conserved core of HIV-1 nef complexed with a Src family SH3 domain. Cell 1996;85:931–942.
214. Niederman TM, Hastings WR, Ratner L. Myristoylation-enhanced binding of the HIV-1 nef protein to T cell skeletal matrix. Virology 1993;197:420–425.
215. Guy B, Kieny MP, Riviere Y, et al. HIV F/3′ orf encodes a phosphorylated GTP-binding protein resembling an oncogene product. Nature 1987;330:266–269.
216. Yu G, Felsted RL. Effect of myristoylation on p27 nef subcellular distribution and suppression of HIV-LTR transcription. Virology 1992;187:46–55.
217. Robert-Guroff M, Popovic M, Gartner S, et al. Structure and expression of tat-, rev-, and nef-specific transcripts of human immunodeficiency virus type 1 in infected lymphocytes and macrophages. J Virol 1990;64:3391–3398.
218. Kienzle N, Freund J, Kalbitzer HR, et al. Oligomerization of the Nef protein from human immunodeficiency virus (HIV) type 1. Eur J Biochem 1993;214:451.
219. Stevenson M. Pathway to understanding AIDS. Nat Struct Biol 1996;3:303–306.
220. Saksela K, Cheng G, Baltimore D. Proline-rich (PxxP) motifs in HIV-1 Nef bind to SH3 domains of a subset of Src kinases and are required for the enhanced growth of Nef+ viruses but not for down-regulation of CD4. EMBO J 1995;14:484–491.
221. Briggs SD, Sharkey M, Stevenson M, et al. SH3-mediated Hck tyrosine kinase activation and fibroblast transformation by the Nef protein of HIV-1. J Biol Chem 1997;272:17899–17902.
222. Schorr J, Kellner R, Fackler O, et al. Specific cleavage sites of Nef proteins from human immunodeficiency virus types 1 and 2 for the viral proteases. J Virol 1996;70:9051–9054.
223. Welker R, Kottler H, Kalbitzer HR, et al. Human immunodeficiency virus type 1 Nef protein is incorporation into virus particles and specifically cleaved by the viral proteinase. Virology 1996;219:228–236.
224. Pandori M, Fitch NJS, Craig HM, et al. Producer-cell modification of human immunodeficiency virus type 1: Nef is a virion protein. J Virol 1996;70:4283–4290.
225. Bukovsky AA, Dorfman T, Weimann A, et al. Nef association with human immunodeficiency virus type 1 virions and cleavage by the viral protease. J Virol 1997;71:1013–1018.
226. Jamieson BD, Aldrovandi GM, Planelles V, et al. Requirement of human immunodeficiency virus type 1 nef for in vivo replication and pathogenicity. J Virol 1994;68:3478–3485.
227. Kestler III HW, Ringler DJ, Mori K, et al. Importance of the nef gene for maintenance of high virus loads and for development of AIDS. Cell 1991;65:651–662.
228. Kirchhoff F, Greenough TC, Brettler DB, et al. Brief report: absence of intact nef sequences in a long-term survivor with nonprogressive HIV-1 infection. N Engl J Med 1995;332:228–232.
229. Deacon NJ, Tsykin A, Solomon A, et al. Genomic structure of an attenuated quasi species of HIV-1 from a blood transfusion donor and recipients. Science 1995;270:988–991.
230. Garcia JV, Miller AD. Serine phosphorylation independent downregulation of cell-surface CD4 by Nef. Nature 1991;350:508.
231. Aiken C, Konner J, Landau NR, et al. Nef induces CD4 endocytosis: requirement for a critical dileucine motif in the membrane-proximal CD4 cytoplasmic domain. Cell 1994;76:853–864.
232. Willey RL, Maldarelli F, Martin MA, et al. Human immunodeficiency virus type 1 Vpu protein regulates the formation of intracellular gp160- CD4 complexes. J Virol 1992;66:226–234.
233. Weiss R. Tissue-specific transformation by human T-cell leukemia virus. Nature 1984;310:273–274.
234. Crise B, Rose JK. Human immunodeficiency virus type 1 glycoprotein precursor retains a CD4-p56lck complex in the endoplasmic reticulum. J Virol 1992;66:2296–2301.
235. Sawai ET, Baur A, Struble H, et al. Human immunodeficiency virus type 1 Nef associates with a cellular serine kinase in T lymphocytes. Proc Natl Acad Sci U S A 1994;91:1539–1543.
236. Sawai ET, Baur AS, Peterlin BM, et al. A conserved domain and membrane targeting of Nef from HIV and SIV are required for association with a cellular serine kinase activity. J Biol Chem 1995;270:15307–15314.
237. Sawai ET, Khan IH, Montbriand PM, et al. Activation of PAK by HIV and SIV Nef: importance for AIDS in rhesus macaques. Curr Biol 1996;6:1519–1527.
238. Wiskerchen M, Cheng-Mayer C. HIV-1 Nef association with cellular serine kinase correlates with enhanced virion infectivity and efficient proviral DNA synthesis. Virology 1996;224:292–301.
239. Greenway A, Azad A, McPhee D. Human immunodeficiency virus type 1 nef protein inhibits activation pathways in peripheral blood mononuclear cells and T cell lines. J Virol 1995;69:1842–1850.
240. Baur AS, Sass G, Laffert B, et al. The N-terminus of Nef from HIV-1/SIV associates with a protein complex containing Lck and a serine kinase. Immunity 1997;6:283–291.
241. Nunn MF, Marsh JW. Human immunodeficiency virus type 1 Nef associates with a member of the p21-activated kinase family. J Virol 1996;70:6157–6161.
242. Luo T, Garcia JV. The association of Nef with a cellular serine/threonine kinase and its enhancement of infectivity are viral isolate dependent. J Virol 1996;70:6493–6496.
243. Lee C, Leung B, Lemmon MA, Z et al. A single amino acid in the SH# domain of Hck determines its high affinity and specificity in binding to HIV-1 Jef protein. EMBO J 1995;14:5006–5015.
244. Moarefi I, LaFevre-Bernt M, Sicheri F, et al. Activation of the Src-family tyrosine kinase Hck by SH3 domain displacement. Nature 1997;385:650–653.
245. Collette Y, Dutartre H, Benziane A, et al. Physical and functional Interaction of Nef with Lck. J Biol Chem 1996;271:6333–6341.
246. Lang SM, Iafrate AJ, Stahl-Hennig C, et al. Association of simian immunodeficiency virus Nef with cellular serine/threonine kinases is dispensable for the development of AIDS in rhesus macaques. Nat Med 1997;3:860–865.
247. Swingler S, Gallay P, Camaur D, et al. The Nef protein of human immunodeficiency virus type 1 enhances serine phosphorylation of the viral matrix. J Virol 1997;71:4372–4377.
248. Miller MD, Warmerdam MT, Gaston I, et al. The human immunodeficiency virus-1 nef gene product: a positive factor for viral infection and replication in primary lymphocytes and macrophages. J Exp Med 1994;179:101–113.
249. Spina CA, Kwoh TJ, Chowers MY, et al. The importance of nef in the induction of human immunodeficiency virus type 1 replication from primary quiescent CD4 lymphocytes. J Exp Med 1994;179:115–123.

250. Chowers MY, Spina CA, Kwoh TJ, et al. Optimal infectivity in vitro of human immunodeficiency virus type 1 requires an intact *nef* gene. J Virol 1994;68:2906–2914.
251. Aiken C, Trono D. Nef stimulates human immunodeficiency virus type 1 proviral DNA synthesis. J Virol 1995;69:5048–5056.
252. Schwartz O, Dautry-Varsat A, Goud B, et al. Human immunodeficiency virus type 1 nef induces accumulation of CD4 in early endosomes. J Virol 1995;69:528–533.
253. Chowers MY, Pandori CA, Spina CA, et al. The growth advantage conferred by HIV-1 nef is determined at the level of viral DNA formation and is independent of CD4 downregulation. Virology 1995;212:451–457.
254. Goldsmith MA, Warmerdam MT, Atchison RE, et al. Dissociation of the CD4 downregulation and viral infectivity enhancement functions of human immunodeficiency virus type 1 nef. J Virol 1995;69:4112–4121.
255. Du Z, Lang SM, Sasseville VG, et al. Identification of a *nef* allele that causes lymphocyte activation and acute disease in macaque monkeys. Cell 1995;82:655–674.
256. Alexander L, Du Z, Rosenweig M, et al. A role for natural simian immunodeficiency virus and human immunodeficiency virus type 1 *nef* alleles in lymphocyte activation. J Virol 1997;71:6094–6099.
257. Gundlach BR, Linhart H, Dittmer U, et al. Construction, replication, and immunogenic properties of a simian immunodeficiency virus expressing interleukin-2. J Virol 1997;71:2225–2232.
258. Baur AS, Sawai ET, Dazin P, et al. HIV-1 Nef leads to inhibition or activation of T cells depending on its intracellular localization. Immunity 1994;1:373–384.
259. Graziani A, Galimi F, Medico E, et al. The HIV-1 nef protein interferes with phosphatidylinositol 3-kinase activation 1. J Biol Chem 1996; 271:6590–6593.
260. Luria S, Chambers I, Berg P. Expression of the type 1 human immunodeficiency virus Nef protein in T cells prevents antigen receptor-mediated induction of interleukin 2 mRNA. Proc Natl Acad Sci U S A 1991;88:5326–5330.
261. Skowronski J, Parks D, Mariani R. Altered T cell activation and development in transgenic mice expressing the HIV-1 *nef* gene. EMBO J 1993;12:703–713.
262. Page KA, van Schooten WCA, Feinberg MB. Human immunodeficiency virus type 1 does not alter T-cell sensitivity to antigen-specific stimulation. J Virol 1997;71:3776–3787.
263. Schwartz O, Marechal V, Le Gall S, et al. Endocytosis of major histocompatibility complex class I molecules is induced by the HIV-1 Nef protein. Nat Med 1996;2:338–342.
264. Borrow P, Lewicki H, Wei X, et al. Antiviral pressure exerted by HIV-1-specific cytotoxic T lymphocytes (CTLs) during primary infection demonstrated by rapid selection of CTL escape virus. Nat Med 1997;3:205–211.
265. Wei X, Ghosh SK, Taylor ME, et al. Viral dynamics in human immunodeficiency virus type 1 infection. Nature 1995;373:117–122.
266. Ho DD, Neumann AU, Perelson AS, et al. Rapid turnover of plasma virions and CD4 lymphocytes in HIV-1 infection. Nature 1995;373: 123–126.
267. Yang X, Goncalves J, Gabuzda D. Phosphorylation of Vif and its role in HIV-1 replication. J Biol Chem 1996;271:10121–10129.
268. Guy B, Geist M, Dott K, et al. A specific inhibitior of cysteine proteases impairs a vif–dependent modification of human immunodeficiency virus type 1 env protein. J Virol 1991;65:1325–1331.
269. Goncalves J, Jallepalli P, Gabuzda DH. Subcellular localization of the Vif protein of human immunodeficiency virus type1. J Virol 1994;68: 704–712.
270. Karczewski MK, Strebel K. Cytoskeleton association and virion incorporation of the human immunodeficiency virus type 1 Vif protein. J Virol 1996;70:494–507.
271. Simon JHM, Fouchier RAM, Southerling TE, et al. The Vif and Gag proteins of human immunodeficiency virus type 1 colocalize in infected human T cells. J Virol 1997;71:5259–5267.
272. Liu H, Wu X, Newman M, et al. The Vif protein of human and simian immunodeficiency viruses is packaged into virions and associates with viral core structures. J Virol 1995;69:7630–7638.
273. Simon JHM, Malim MH. The human immunodeficiency virus type 1 Vif protein modulates the postpenetration stability of viral nucleoprotein complexes. J Virol 1996;70:5297–5305.
274. Chowdhury IH, Chao W, Potash MJ, et al. *vif*-negative human immunodeficiency virus type 1 persistently replicates in primary macrophages, producing attenuated progeny virus. J Virol 1996;70: 5336–5345.
275. Simon JHM, Southerling TE, Peterson JC, et al. Complementation of *vif*-defective human immunodeficiency virus type 1 by primate, but not nonprimate, lentivirus *vif* genes. J Virol 1995;69:4166–4172.
276. Courcoul M, Patience C, Rey F, et al. Peripheral blood mononuclear cells produce normal amounts of defective vif– human immunodeficiency virus type 1 particles which are restricted for the prererotranscription steps. J Virol 1995;69:2068–2074.
277. Reddy TR, Kraus G, Yamada O, et al. Comparative analyses of human immunodeficiency virus type 1 (HIV-1) and HIV-2 vif mutants. J Virol 1995;69:3549–3553.
278. Borman AM, Quillent C, Charneau P, et al. Human immunodeficiency virus type 1 Vif- mutant particles from restrictive cells: role of Vif in correct particle assembly and infectivity. J Virol 1995;69:2058–2067.
279. Hoglund S, Ohagen A, Lawrence K, et al. Role of vif during packing of the core of HIV-1. Virology 1994;201:349–355.
280. Simm M, Shahabuddin M, Chao W, et al. Aberrant gag protein composition of a human immunodeficiency virus type 1 *vif* mutant produced in primary lymphocytes. J Virol 1995;69:4582–4586.
281. Fouchier RAM, Simon JHM, Jaffe AB, et al. Human immunodeficiency virus type 1 Vif does not influence expression or virion incorporation of *gag*-, *pol*-, and *env*-encoded proteins. J Virol 1996; 70:8263–8269.
282. Harmache A, Bouyac M, Audoly G, et al. The *vif* gene is essential for efficient replication of caprine arthritis encephalitis virus in goat synovial membrane cells and affects the late steps of the virus replication cycle. J Virol 1995;69:3247–3257.
283. Goncalves J, Korin Y, Zack J, et al. Role of Vif in human immunodeficiency virus type 1 reverse transcription. J Virol 1996;70:8701–8709.
284. Sova P, Volsky DJ. Efficiency of viral DNA synthesis during infection of permissive and nonpermissive cells with *vif*-negative human immunodeficiency virus type 1. J Virol 1993;67:6322–6326.
285. von Schwedler U, Song J, Aiken C, et al. *vif* is crucial for human immunodeficiency virus type 1 proviral DNA synthesis in infected cells. J Virol 1993;4945–4955.
286. Myers G, Korber B, Wain-Hobson S, et al. Human retroviruses and AIDS: a compilation and analysis of nucleic acid and amino acid sequences. Los Alamos, NM: Los Alamos National Laboratory, 1994.
287. Strebel KTK, Maldarelli F, Martin MA. Molecular and biochemical analyses of human immunodeficiency virus type 1 *vpu* protein. J Virol 1989;63:3784–3791.
288. Schubert U, Strebel K. Differential activities of the human immunodeficiency virus type 1-encoded Vpu protein are regulated by phosphorylation and occur in different cellular compartments. J Virol 1994;68:2260–2271.
289. Hoxie JA, Alpers JD, Rackowski JL, et al. Alterations in T4 (CD4) protein and mRNA synthesis in cells infected with HIV. Science 1986;234:1123–1127.
290. Klimkait T, Strebel K, Hoggan MD, et al. The human immunodeficiency virus type 1-specific protein *Vpu* is required for efficient virus maturation and release. J Virol 1990;64:621–629.
291. Terwilliger EF, Cohen EA, Lu Y, et al. Functional role of human immunodeficiency virus type 1 *vpu*. Proc Natl Acad Sci U S A 1989;86:5163–5167.
292. Yao XJ, Göttlinger H, Haseltine WA, et al. Envelope glycoprotein and CD4 independence of *vpu*-facilitated human immunodeficiency virus type 1 capsid export. J Virol 1992;66:5119–5126.

293. Schubert U, Bour S, Ferrer-Montiel AV, et al. The two biological activities of human immunodeficiency virus type 1 Vpu protein involve two separable structural domains. J Virol 1996;70:809–819.
294. Tristem M, Marshall C, Karpas A, et al. Origin of *vpx* in lentiviruses. Nature 1990;347:341–342.
295. Sharp PM, Bailes E, Stevenson M, et al. Gene acquisition in HIV and SIV. Nature 1996;383:586–587.
296. Zhao LJ, Wang L, Mukherjee S, et al. Biochemical mechanism of HIV-1 Vpr function: oligomerization mediated by the N-terminal domain. J Biol Chem 1994;269:32131–32137.
297. Yao XJ, Subbramanian RA, Rougeau N, et al. Mutagenic analysis of human immunodeficiency virus type 1 Vpr: role of a predicted N-terminal alpha-helical structure in Vpr nuclear localization and virion incorporation. J Virol 1995;69:7032–7044.
298. Di Marzio P, Choe S, Ebright M, et al. Mutational analysis of cell cycle arrest, nuclear localization, and virion packaging of human immunodeficiency virus type 1 Vpr. J Virol 1995;69:7909–7916.
299. Mahalingam S, Collman RG, Patel M, et al. Functional analysis of HIV-1 Vpr: identification of determinants essential for subcellular localization. Virology 1995;212:331–339.
300. Yu X-F, Ito S, Essex M, et al. A naturally immunogenic virion-associated protein specific for HIV-2 and SIV. Nature 1988;335:262–265.
301. Cohen EA, Dehni G, Sodroski JG, et al. Human immunodeficiency virus *vpr* product is a virion-associated regulatory protein. J Virol 1990;64:3097–3099.
302. Lavallée C, Ladha Z, Göttlinger H, et al. Requirement of the Pr55^{gag} precusor for incorporation of the Vpr product into human immunodeficiency virus type 1 viral particles. J Virol 1994;68:1926–1934.
303. Kondo E, Mammano F, Cohen EA, et al. The p6^{gag} domain of human immunodeficiency virus type 1 is sufficient for the incorporation of vpr into heterologous viral particles. J Virol 1995;69:2759–2764.
304. Kondo E, Gottlinger HG. A conserved LXXLF sequence is the major determinant in p6^{gag} required for the incorporation of human immunodeficiency virus type 1 vpr. J Virol 1996;70:159–164.
305. Kewalramani VN, Emerman M. Vpx association with mature core structures of HIV-2. Virology 1996;218:159–168.
306. Yu X-F, Yu Q-C, Essex M, et al. The *vpx* gene of simian immunodeficiency virus facilitates efficient viral replication in fresh lymphocytes and macrophages. J Virol 1991;65:5088–5091.
307. Guyader M, Emerman M, Montagnier L, et al. VPX Mutants of HIV-2 are infectious in established cell lines but display a severe defect in peripheral blood lymphocytes. EMBO J 1989;8:1169–1175.
308. Bailliet JW, Kolson DL, Eiger G, et al. Distinct effects in primary macrophages and lymphocytes of the human immunodeficiency virus type I accessory genes *vpr*, *vpu* and *nef*: mutational analysis of a primary HIV-1 isolate. Virology 1994;200:623–631.
309. Gibbs JS, Regier DA, Desrosiers RC. Construction and in vitro properties of HIV-1 mutants with deletions in "nonessential" genes. AIDS Res Hum Retroviruses 1994;10:343–350.
310. Connor RI, Chen BK, Choe S, et al. Vpr is required for efficient replication of human immunodeficiency virus type-1 in mono-nuclear phagocytes. Virology 1995;206:935–944.
311. Campbell BJ, Hirsch VM. Vpr of simian immunodeficiency virus of African green monkeys is required for replication in macaque macrophages and lymphocytes. J Virol 1997;71:5593–5602.
312. Kappes JC, Conway JA, Lee S-W, et al. Human immunodeficiency virus type 2 vpx protein augments viral infectivity. Virology 1991;184:197–209.
313. Aldrovandi GM, Zack JA. Replication and pathogenicity of human immunodeficiency virus type 1 accessory gene mutants in SCID-hu mice. J Virol 1996;70:1505–1511.
314. Gibbs JS, Lackner AA, Lang SM, et al. Progression to AIDS in the absence of a gene vor *vpr* and *vpx*. J Virol 1995;69:2378–2383.
315. Hoch J, Lang SM, Weeger M, et al. *vpr* deletion mutant of simian immunodeficiency virus induces AIDS in rhesus monkeys. J Virol 1995;69:4807–4813.
316. Lang SM, Weeger M, Stahl-Hennig C, et al. Importance of *vpr* for infection of rhesus monkeys with simian immunodeficiency virus. J Virol 1993;67:902–912.
317. He J, Choe S, Walker R, DiMarzio P, et al. Human immunodeficiency virus type 1 viral protein R (Vpr) arrests cells in the G$_2$ phase of the cell cycle by inhibiting p34^{cdc2} activity. J Virol 1995;69:6705–6711.
318. Jowett JBM, Planelles V, Poon B, et al. The human immunodeficiency virus type 1 *vpr* gene arrests infected T cells in the G$_2$ + se of the cell cycle. J Virol 1995;69:6304–6313.
319. Re F, Braaten D, Franke EK, et al. Human immunodefciency virus type 1 Vpr arrests the cell cycle in G$_2$ by inhibiting the activation of p34^{cdc2}-cyclin B. J Virol 1995;69:6859–6864.
320. Rogel ME, Wu LI, Emerman M. The human immunodeficiency virus type 1 *vpr* gene prevents cell proliferation during chronic infection. J Virol 1995;69:882–888.
321. Stewart SA, Poon B, Jowett JBM, et al. Human immunodeficiency virus type 1 Vpr induces apoptosis following cell cycle arrest. J Virol 1997;71:5579–5592.
322. Zhao Y, Cao J, O'Gorman MRG, et al. Effect of human immunodeficiency virus type 1 protein R (*vpr*) gene expression on basic cellular function of fission yeast *Schizosaccharomyces pombe*. J Virol 1996;70:5821–5826.
323. Poon B, Jowett JBM, Stewart SA, et al. Human immunodeficiency virus type 1 *vpr* gene induces phenotypic effects similar to those of the DNA alkylating agent, nitrogen mustard. J Virol 1997;71:3961–3971.
324. Bartz SR, Rogel ME, Emerman M. Human immunodefciency virus type 1 cell cycle control: Vpr is cytostatic and mediates G$_2$ accumulation by a mechanism which differs from DNA damage checkpoint control. J Virol 1996;70:2324–2331.
325. Stivahtis GL, Soares MA, Vodicka MA, et al. Conservation and host specificity of Vpr-mediated cell cycle arrest suggest a fundamental role in primate lentivirus evolution and biology. J Virol 1997;71:4331–4338.
326. Bouhamdan M, Benichou S, Rey F, et al. Human immunodeficiency virus type 1 Vpr protein binds to the uracil DNA glycosylase DNA repair enzyme. J Virol 1996;70:697–704.
327. Selig L, Benichou B, Rogel ME, et al. Uracil DNA glycosylase specifically interacts with Vpr of both human immunodeficiency virus type 1 and simian immunodeficiency virus of sooty mangabeys, but binding does not correlate with cell cycle arrest. J Virol 1997;71:4842–4846.
328. Threadgill DS, Steagall WK, Flaherty MT, et al. Characterization of equine infectious anemia virus dUTPase: growth properties of a dUTPase-deficient mutant. J Virol 1993;67:2592–2600.
329. Elder JH, Lerner DL, Hasselkus-Light CS, et al. Distinct subsets of retroviruses encode dUTPase. J Virol 1992;66:1791–1794.
330. Myers LC, Vardine GL. DNA repair proteins. Curr Opin Struct Biol 1994;4:51–59.
331. Wagaman PC, Hasselkus-Light CS, Henson M, et al. Molecular cloning and characterization of deoxyuridine triphosphatase from feline immunodeficiency virus (FIV). Virology 1993;196:451–457.
332. Lichtenstein DL, Rushlow KE, Cook RF, et al. Replication in vitro and in vivo of an equine infectious anemia virus mutant deficient in dUTPase activity. J Virol 1995;69:2881–2888.
333. Turelli P, Petursson G, Guiguen F, et al. Replication properties of dUTPase-deficient mutants of caprine and ovine lentiviruses. J Virol 1996;70:1213–1217.
334. Terai C, Carson DA. Pyrimidine nucleotide and nucleic acid synthesis in human monocytes and macrophages. Exp Cell Res 1991;193:375–381.
335. Bowerman B, Brown PO, Bishop JM, et al. A nucleoprotein complex mediates the integration of retroviral DNA. Genes Dev 1989;3:469–478.
336. Farnet CM, Haseltine WA. Determination of viral proteins present in the human immunodeficiency virus type 1 preintegration complex. J Virol 1991;65:1910–1915.

4
NATURAL HISTORY OF HIV-1 DISEASE

J. Michael Kilby and Michael S. Saag

Infection with human immunodeficiency virus type 1 (HIV-1) results in a progressive loss of immune system function, ultimately leading to the opportunistic infections and malignancies of the acquired immunodeficiency syndrome (AIDS). The variability of disease expression depends on both host and viral factors. Recent discoveries point particularly to the influence of host genetic determinants on the risk of acquiring HIV-1 infection or of progression of disease once HIV infection has been established. Although the rate of disease progression has been shown to vary substantially among patients not treated with antiretroviral therapy, the median time from initial infection to the development of AIDS has been approximately 10 years.

Important advances in treatment have significantly altered the natural history of HIV-1 infection, especially when highly active antiretroviral therapy (HAART) regimens are administered to previously untreated patients. At the same time, development and standardization of new methods to quantitate HIV-1 viremia (viral load) have introduced clinically available assays to estimate prognosis for infected individuals as well as to monitor responses to antiretroviral interventions rapidly. Although the relative risk of developing certain opportunistic diseases is still estimated based on CD4 cell count values, the best overall predictions for progression to AIDS or death can be made based on the combined use of absolute CD4 counts and viral load measurements. This chapter reviews the natural history at each stage of HIV-1 infection with special emphasis on the relation of viral and cellular dynamics to the progression of disease.

VIRAL LOAD, CD4 COUNTS, AND CLINICAL STAGING

Before the identification of HIV as the cause of AIDS and the ability to quantify plasma viremia reliably, patients were identified strictly on the basis of the presence of an AIDS-defining opportunistic infection or malignant disease (1, 2). After the discovery of HIV, patients with HIV infection were categorized as having AIDS, AIDS-related complex (ARC), or asymptomatic disease. As more information has been gathered regarding the natural history of HIV disease, these terms have become outdated. Indeed, the term "AIDS" has little, if any, clinical utility. Its use is confined to an epidemiologic role in tracking the number of cases in a consistent fashion.

Shortly after the discovery of HIV, Walter Reed staging (3) and similar systems based on measurements of immune system function were proposed, but these approaches have generally become outmoded in the era of viral load and CD4 quantitation. Several studies demonstrated the value of the CD4 cell count as the best predictive marker of relative risk for the development of HIV-related opportunistic diseases (4). The current Centers for Disease Control and Prevention (CDC) case definition of AIDS is based on 1) the development of one of the AIDS-defining conditions (including one of the more recent additions to this list: tuberculosis, recurrent bacterial pneumonia, or invasive cervical carcinoma) or 2) an absolute CD4 count of less than 200 cells/mm^3 (5) (Table 4.1).

Although CD4 quantitation remains clinically useful to predict the risk of opportunistic infections and other HIV-related complications (4, 6–8), this test has several limitations as a marker of disease progression. Diurnal variation may account for shifts of as much as 50 to 150 cells/mm^3 in normal adults, although the degree of this change is less in patients with lower CD4 counts (9). Substantial laboratory-to-laboratory variability has been reported, and entities that do not perform this procedure frequently or do not have quality assurance programs may produce inaccurate test results. Compounding this problem, extended delay (more than 48 hours) between the time of sampling and actual specimen processing results in inaccurate values. The dependence of the CD4 count measurement on the total white cell count, which may change substantially from day to day and is influenced by several factors, is also a potential source of variability. Although some investigators advocated the use of the CD4 percentage as a more stable marker than the use of absolute values (10), most clinicians now follow the absolute CD4 count or a combination of absolute count and CD4 percentage values. Patients who have undergone splenectomy may have a deceptive elevation in the absolute CD4 count after this procedure, and the CD4 percentage may provide a more accurate indicator of the degree of immune dysfunction in this special population (11).

A strong correlation exists between the slope of CD4

Table 4.1 Revised Classification System of HIV Disease Centers for Disease Control and Prevention (January 1993)

CD4 Count	A	B	C
>500	A1	B1	C1
200–500	A2	B2	C2
<200	A3	B3	C3

Category A
- Asymptomatic HIV infection
- Persistent generalized lymphadenopathy
- Acute retroviral syndrome

Category B (formerly "ARC")
- Bacillary angiomatosis
- Candidiasis
  Oral
  Recurrent vaginal
- Cervical dysplasia
- Constitutional symptoms (e.g., fever or diarrhea) >1 month
- Hairy leukoplakia, oral
- Herpes zoster
- Idiopathic thrombocytopenia purpura
- Listeriosis
- Pelvic inflammatory disease
- Peripheral neuropathy

Category C (AIDS-defining conditions)
- CD4 count less than 200 cells/mm^3
- Candidiasis
  Pulmonary
  Esophageal
- Cervical cancer
- Coccidioidomycosis
- Cryptococcosis, extrapulmonary
- Cryptosporidiosis
- Cytomegalovirus
- Encephalopathy, HIV
- Herpes simplex Chronic (>1 month) Esophageal
- Histoplasmosis
- Isosporiasis
- Kaposi's sarcoma
- Lymphoma
- *Mycobacterium avium*
- *Mycobacterium kansasii*
- *Mycobacterium tuberculosis*
- *Pneumocystis carinii*
- Pneumonia, recurrent
- Progressive multifocal leukemia
- Salmonellosis

cell count decline and the rate of clinical disease progression (4, 12, 13). Individuals who have a decreased CD4 percentage value of 7% or more over a 1-year period have a relative risk of developing AIDS that is 35 times higher than the risk in persons with stable CD4 cell percentages over the same period (10). To use these data, patients should have serial CD4 counts obtained at frequent intervals (every 4 to 6 months at a minimum). Frequent serial measurements of CD4 cell values also help to compensate for intrinsic variability of CD4 cell measurements. Although the CD4 count remains a useful assessment of the stage of HIV disease, and increases in absolute CD4 counts indicate beneficial effects of changes in therapy, using the CD4 count alone provides an incomplete surrogate marker for clinical progression (14, 15). Thus, a need has existed for a more direct measurement of the disease process to determine prognosis, risk of disease progression, and responses to therapeutic interventions.

Various clinical and laboratory "surrogate markers" have been shown to have at least a weak relationship with clinical outcomes. Oral candidiasis, oral hairy leukoplakia, and, to a lesser degree, dermatomal varicella-zoster virus reactivation were identified in several cohort studies to be associated with varying degrees of disease progression (6, 16, 17). In the San Francisco General Hospital cohort, for example, men with lymphadenopathy, shingles, thrush, hairy leukoplakia, and constitutional symptoms were 22%, 25%, 39%, 42%, and 100% likely to progress to AIDS over a 2-year period compared with 16% of individuals who had none of these symptoms (6).

Laboratory markers of cellular activation, such as serum β_2-microglobulin and neopterin, were shown to correlate significantly with disease progression in several cohort studies (18, 19). Studies have also attempted to characterize patterns in the expression of proinflammatory cytokines (such as tumor necrosis factor-α, interferon-γ, and several of the interleukins) that predict progression of HIV disease (20–22). Thus far, these assays have been difficult to standardize and highly variable based on the techniques used, the individuals studied, and the clinical situations involved. A more specific virologic test, the p24 antigen assay, was developed as a marker of the degree of viral replication (19, 23). This assay was used in various clinical trials to demonstrate the effects of interventions; however, many HIV-infected patients have undetectable levels of this antigen, and the assay has a restricted dynamic range that limits the ability to stratify patients into distinct groups at risk for progression. None of these surrogate markers achieved consistent, widespread use in the clinical care of HIV-infected patients.

Important early studies using HIV-1 cultures and p24 antigen levels revealed that the level of viral burden increases with advancing disease (24–26). The development of polymerase chain reaction (PCR)–based assays for the quantitation of HIV genetic material (RNA) revealed that significant amounts of plasma HIV were present at all stages of HIV-1 infection (27). Investigations of the rapid decay of plasma HIV RNA (or viral load) in patients treated with potent combinations of antiretroviral drugs reveal persistent, ongoing viral replication even when the infected host is asymptomatic and has a relatively stable CD4 count (28, 29) (Fig. 4.1).

Monitoring changes in viral load on therapy has been shown to provide important prognostic information that is independent from, and complementary to, changes in abso-

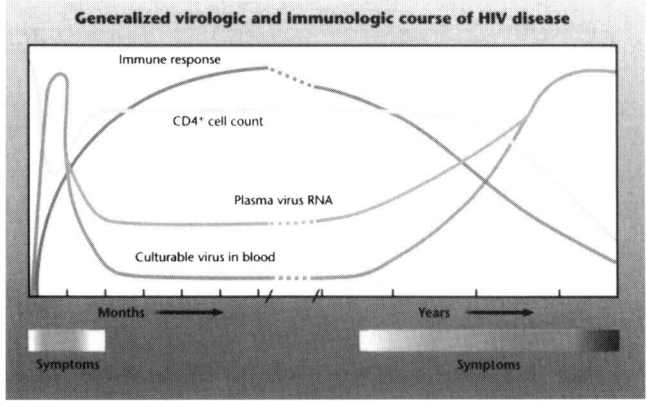

Figure 4.1. Schematic representation of the natural history of HIV disease. (Modified from Saag MS, Holodniy M, Kuritzkes DR, et al. HIV viral load markers in clinical practice. Nature Med 1996;2:625–629.)

lute CD4 count (30, 31). Viral load has been demonstrated in several cohorts to be the strongest known predictor of progression to AIDS and death (32–34). For example, HIV-infected men in the Multicenter AIDS Cohort Study were divided into four quartiles based on baseline viral load levels: the proportion of subjects who progressed to AIDS within 5 years among those with baseline viral loads (copies/mL) of less than 4530, 4531 to 13,020, 13,021 to 36,270, and more than 36,270 were 8%, 26%, 49%, and 62%, respectively (Fig. 4.2) (33). Because most of these men did not receive antiretroviral therapy in the course of the study, this prognostic information largely reflects the untreated natural history of HIV progression. The combination of viral load and absolute CD4 count provides better discrimination of outcome than either measurement alone. Mellors and associates used both variables to stratify patients into discrete groups with risks for progression to AIDS or death within 6 years that ranged from less than 2 to 98% (Fig. 4.3) (35).

Viral load monitoring has been available clinically for a relatively short period, and current data are insufficient to allow prospectively validated guidelines for its clinical use. However, many clinicians have rapidly accepted HIV RNA monitoring as a routine part of clinical practice. A panel of investigators and clinicians provided interim recommendations (36) regarding the clinical use of viral load testing, whereas large studies are in progress to develop standardized testing and treatment strategies further. HIV RNA levels can guide decision-making about the initiation of antiretroviral therapy. Based on prognostic considerations (33–35) (see Fig. 4.2), most clinicians would strongly recommend therapy if the viral load exceeds approximately 10,000 copies/mL or if viral load is more than 5000 copies/mL and the clinical status suggests disease progression. Many physicians agree that the potential benefits of combination antiretroviral therapy should be discussed with all HIV-infected individuals, regardless of disease stage. Two measurements taken several weeks before therapy may be helpful to establish a "baseline" viral load.

A repeat viral load determination should be obtained 3 to 4 weeks after initiation of therapy or after a change in therapy. The minimum change in viral load that is indicative of a true biologic difference (rather than random variation) such as a response to antiviral therapy is in the range of 0.4 to 0.5 log (more than 2.5-fold change) (30, 36). A target level of HIV RNA should be selected by the patient and clinician before the administration of therapy. This target range may vary in different clinical situations. A newly diagnosed patient with early disease may reasonably have the expectation for combination therapy to result in sustained "undetectable" HIV RNA by currently available PCR-based assays (less than 25 to 500 copies/mL depending on the assay). Many patients and caregivers may be content to maintain the viral load within the range of the most favorable prognostic quartile (less than about 5000 copies/mL), although this higher threshold may be associated with more antiretroviral resistance. In the case of a patient with extremely advanced disease in whom all available therapies have failed, a 10-fold reduction in viral

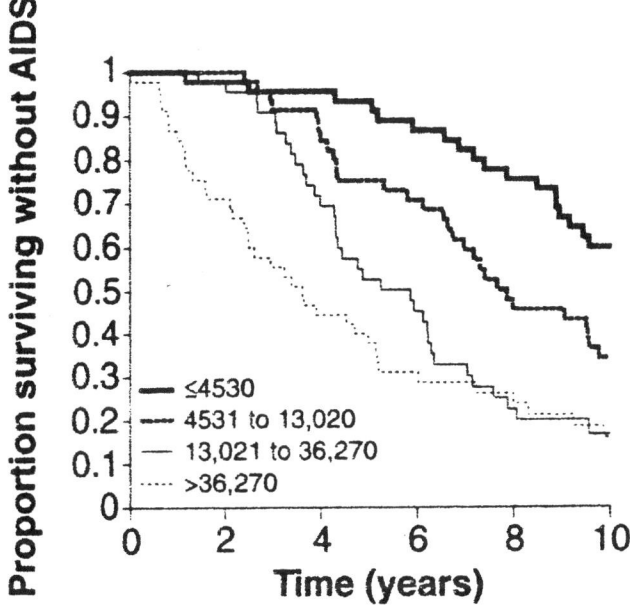

Figure 4.2. Relation between baseline markers and prognosis: Kaplan–Meier curves for AIDS-free survival. (From Mellors JW, Rinaldo CR Jr, Gupta P, et al. Prognosis in HIV-1 infection predicted by the quantity of virus in plasma. Science 1996;272:1167–1170.)

load could be interpreted as a favorable response to a new intervention regardless of the absolute nadir achieved. Further experience will be necessary to clarify whether a clinically significant "threshold" of viral load would constitute the appropriate target range, although treatment strategies will continue to be individualized.

Because procedures in HIV RNA determinations require meticulous, reproducible techniques, samples should be sent to a laboratory with expertise and experience in these methods. The currently available PCR and branched-chain DNA methods correlate relatively well with one another, but ideally a patient should be monitored longitudinally using the same assay. Although the proper processing and transport of blood samples vary based on the specific assay used, in general the most accurate results will be obtained if the plasma is separated from whole blood and frozen within 6 hours of acquisition. The within-assay variation for most available tests is in the range of 0.15 to 0.2 log. Relatively larger (approximately 0.3 log) is the biologic variation encountered in the measurement of plasma HIV RNA levels. In particular, clinical events or interventions that modulate the activation state of the cellular immune system can influence the viral load. Immunoactivation may at least transiently increase plasma viral load, for example, during an opportunistic infection (37), after routine vaccinations (38), or when intravenous interleukin-2 is administered (39). On the other hand, patients with advanced AIDS with paradoxic immunoactivation and wasting syndrome may demonstrate temporary declines in viral load when immunosuppressive corticosteroid therapy is given (40). Thus, investigators are interested in the potential influence of more sustained alterations in immunoactivation status on the natural history of HIV infection.

LESSONS FROM THE EXTREMES OF DISEASE PROGRESSION

Although the combination of viral load and CD4 count provides the most reliable predictor of outcomes based on the typical natural history of HIV infection, much scientific interest has been expressed in characterizing atypical cases of HIV progression (very rapid or very slow) to gain insights into viral pathogenesis and the determinants of disease progression. Previous investigations of "long-term nonprogressors," individuals documented to have been infected with HIV for many years without any signs of progressive immunosuppression, suggested that these rare individuals constituted a heterogenous group characterized by combinations of (less virulent) viral and (more effective) host immune response factors (41, 42). Several discoveries have pointed to the potential influence of host genetic determinants on susceptibility to HIV acquisition and the subsequent development of disease.

Studies involving persons who have been exposed repeatedly to HIV infection without becoming infected were critical for understanding the importance of CCR5, a coreceptor for HIV entry into host cells. Individuals who remain uninfected with HIV despite risk factors for infection are statistically more likely to have an uncommon homozygous deletion of the CCR5 coreceptor, rendering their cells less susceptible to HIV entry (43, 44). Heterozygotes for this coreceptor defect, relatively common among the general population (e.g., up to 20% of whites in the United States), are overrepresented among patients with long-term nonprogressive HIV infection as compared with HIV-infected patients with more usual disease progression (43, 45). CCR5 tends to be the primary coreceptor for the nonsyncytium-inducing (NSI) isolates of HIV, whereas isolates that induce syncytial cell formation (SI) in the laboratory primarily use a different coreceptor, designated CXCR4 (46). Patients with early asymptomatic HIV infection have a predominance of NSI viral variants. In contrast, patients with advanced HIV infection have more aggressive SI viruses that predominate. The conversion from NSI to SI phenotype has been associated with precipitous falls in CD4 counts (47). Evidence demonstrates an analogous evolution of HIV-1 coreceptor usage as disease progresses (48). The clinical utility of NSI/SI and CCR5 coreceptor phenotype determinations remains to be established. Further study of CCR5 and other HIV coreceptors will likely better define the host determinants for HIV progression.

Further support for the importance of host immunologic factors in determining the natural history of disease comes

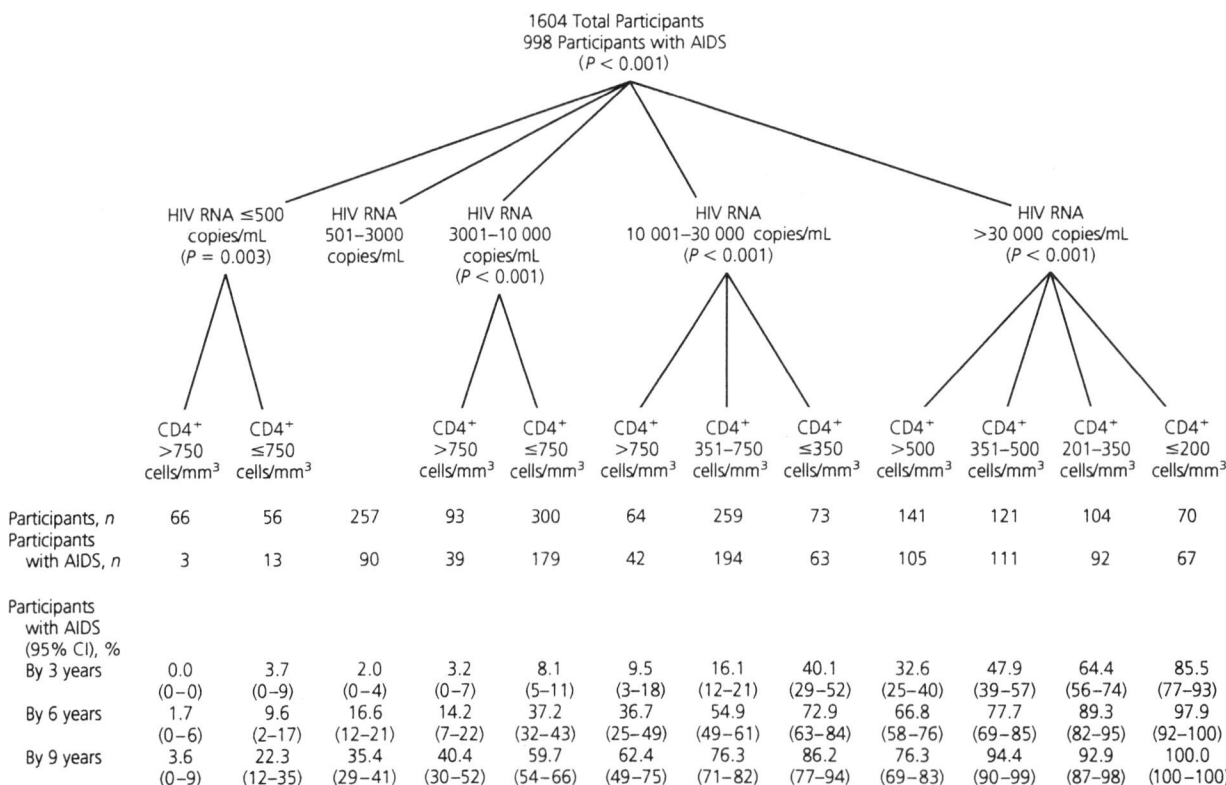

Figure 4.3. Probability of developing AIDS according to HIV-1 concentration and CD4+ lymphocyte count. The *P* values are derived from the likelihood ratio test using Cox regression. Mean 95% confidence intervals were derived from 500 bootstrap samples using the percentile method. (From Mellors JW, Muñoz A, Giorgi JV, et al. Plasma viral load and CD4+ lymphocytes as prognostic markers of HIV-1 infection. Ann Intern Med 1997;126:946–954.)

from studies correlating major histocompatibility complex gene products with the course of HIV infection; certain HLA haplotype combinations are associated with more rapid HIV disease progression (49). Rare patients with unfavorable HLA haplotypes have been described who fail to develop diagnostic HIV antibodies (seroconvert) and who die of rapidly progressive AIDS (50, 51).

DISEASE STAGING

A reasonable way to categorize the natural history of HIV disease clinically is to divide the stages of illness into five categories based on CD4 count, as follows: acute infection (seroconversion); early disease (CD4 count greater than 500 cells/mm^3); middle stage disease (CD4 count between 200 and 500 cells/mm^3); late disease (CD4 count between 50 and 200 cells/mm^3); and advanced disease (CD4 count less than 50 cells/mm^3). The remainder of this chapter is based on this format.

Acute Retroviral Seroconversion Syndrome

A schematic representation of the time course of HIV infection is presented in Figure 4.1. Within 2 to 4 weeks after initial infection, high levels of circulating free virus can be cultured from the plasma (52, 53). This period of high-titer plasma viremia is associated with high levels of p24 antigen, and the viral load by PCR-based techniques is often in the range of 1 million copies/mL. Peak levels of plasma viremia are generally associated with the development of clinical symptoms of acute seroconversion. Within 10 to 21 days of the onset of symptoms, a detectable antibody response is noted. Anti-gp160 and p24 antibodies are detected first, followed by antibodies to gp120 and gp41. Antibodies to the envelope portion of the virus (e.g., gp120 and gp41) persist for life, whereas the anti-p24 antibody response may diminish to nondetectable levels in late disease. As discussed earlier, rare individuals with delayed or inadequate HIV antibody production may have a less favorable prognosis. Evidence suggests that the quality and quantity of the HIV-specific cellular immune response during acute infection, particularly cytotoxic CD8+ T cells, are other host factors that affect the natural history of HIV infection (54–56).

Previously, investigators were uncertain whether treatment of acute retroviral syndrome would be of any benefit to the patient. Because more recent data demonstrate that the amount of plasma HIV RNA early after infection is the single strongest predictor for the rate of disease progression, several trials have investigated the effects of early intervention. A European study suggested that administering zidovudine alone to acutely infected patients altered the clinical course of HIV disease and helped to preserve immune function compared with acutely infected patients given placebo (57). More recently, much more dramatic effects have been demonstrated when acutely infected patients were given HAART (typically a protease inhibitor and two reverse transcriptase inhibitors, although various drug combinations are being evaluated). These individuals have had sustained suppression of viral load below the level of detectability in both blood and tissue assays for more than 1 year in several cases (58). Although prolonged viral suppression does not appear to be synonymous with viral eradication (59), the sustained suppression of HIV replication will likely significantly alter the natural history of HIV infection for these patients. Intervening as early as possible in the disease process, while the virus population is homogenous and the immune system remains intact, has theoretic advantages, and studies are underway to evaluate the benefits of very early therapy further. For example, one report indicates that aggressive, very early antiretroviral treatment (before seroconversion) can result in maintenance of HIV-specific CD4-cell proliferative responses that are similar to the responses seen in long-term nonprogressors (60).

The diagnosis of the acute retroviral syndrome can be established by a demonstration of p24 antigen positivity or HIV RNA levels concurrent with negative antibody tests (enzyme-linked immunosorbent assay [ELISA] and Western blot) in the appropriate clinical setting. Although the syndrome is straightforward to diagnose, the challenge is to improve the ability to identify these patients as rapidly and efficiently as possible.

Initial primary infection with HIV often is unrecognized clinically, but investigators have known for over a decade that many of these individuals develop symptoms of a "viral illness" (61). Because these symptoms are nonspecific and temporary, only an estimated 20 to 30% of symptomatic individuals actually seek medical attention, and the possibility of acute HIV infection is frequently not explored even when a health care worker is involved.

The onset of symptoms usually occurs within 2 to 6 weeks after exposure (52, 53, 62). Among those patients presenting for medical evaluation, the most common symptom reported is fever, followed by adenopathy, pharyngitis, or skin rash, characterized as a transient morbilliform eruption. The type and relative frequency of symptoms are summarized in Table 4.2 (52, 62). Signs of immune deficiency can be seen even in this early stage of infection. Oral candidiasis, esophageal candidiasis, and even *Pneumocystis* pneumonia have been reported during the acute seroconversion syndrome. This is understandable because some acutely infected patients have abnormally low absolute CD4+ counts (15% less than 399, 7% less than 300 cells/mm^3) (62). Certain oropharyngeal signs and symptoms including pharyngitis, odynophagia, oral and tonsillar ulcers, and idiopathic esophageal ulcers have been well described in this setting (52, 62, 63). Although uncommon, neurologic manifestations such as meningismus (with or without cerebrospinal fluid pleocytosis and positive cerebrospinal fluid cultures), peripheral neuropathy, myelopathy, brachial neuritis, Bell's palsy, or, rarely, self-limited encephalitis or Guillain-Barré syndrome have been reported.

The usual duration of symptoms varies, but nonspecific symptoms that are prolonged provide additional incentive to rule out acute HIV infection in the right setting; the mean duration of fever and headache among acutely infected patients with these complaints in one study, for example, was

Table 4.2 Signs and Symptoms of Acute HIV-1 Infection

Sign or Symptom	Frequency (%)
Fever	97
Adenopathy	77
Pharyngitis	73
Rash	70
Myalgia or arthralgia	58
Thrombocytopenia	51
Leukopenia	38
Diarrhea	33
Headache	30
Elevated serum aminotransferase levels	23
Nausea or vomiting	20
Hepatosplenomegaly	17
Oral thrush	10
Encephalopathy	8
Neuropathy	8

16.9 and 25.8 days, respectively (64). Longer duration of symptoms of acute seroconversion syndrome has been associated with more rapid progression to AIDS (65). Unfortunately, combining these symptoms into a well-defined syndrome (such as the "mononucleosis-like" symptoms of fever, sore throat, and cervical adenopathy) is not a sensitive screening strategy (64).

The laboratory findings during acute seroconversion are characterized by marked lymphopenia with depletion of both CD4 and CD8 lymphocytes. Atypical lymphocytes are commonly seen in the peripheral blood and may be seen at levels of 20 to 30%. Anemia and thrombocytopenia are sometimes seen as well. The initial lymphopenia is followed by a period of relative lymphocytosis, predominantly of CD8+ T cells. After clinical symptoms of the acute seroconversion syndrome resolve, the CD8+ lymphocytosis normalizes; however, the CD4 cell count, although increasing, does not return to baseline values (4). In a few cases, the CD4 lymphocyte count remains suppressed, with no rebound effect. Patients who experience more severe lymphopenia generally have a more accelerated course of progressive HIV disease.

Early Disease (CD4 Count Higher Than 500 Cells/mm^3)

Most individuals with high CD4 counts generally have no symptoms related to HIV infection, with the exception of mild-to-moderate lymphadenopathy. Early in the epidemic, the presence of lymphadenopathy was considered a poor prognostic sign; more likely, however, the loss of lymphadenopathy is a sign of impending disease progression (66). When symptoms are present, the most common HIV-associated findings in patients with early disease are dermatologic, although most of the skin manifestations mentioned here actually increase in frequency as the CD4 count declines. Seborrheic dermatitis, especially in the nasolabial folds or along the hairline, is common. Patients with psoriasis may have more difficulty controlling their disease, and some who never had psoriasis before may develop this disorder. Pruritic folliculitis ("itchy red bumps"), onychomycosis, and extremely dry skin can be chronic problems. Eosinophilic folliculitis, sometimes associated with mild peripheral eosinophilia, is of unclear origin; some patients respond to topical corticosteroids. Perifollicular skin disorders most often represent insect bites (some HIV-infected patients appear to have a heightened and prolonged reaction to insect bites) or molluscum contagiosum. Scabies is an especially pruritic cause of perifollicular dermatitis and should be considered in all patients with itchy red bump disorders.

Although more common later in the disease, oral hairy leukoplakia may be identified at this stage of disease along the lateral margins of the tongue. When present, this entity is virtually diagnostic of underlying HIV infection. Aphthous ulcerations may be present in up to 2 to 5% of patients with early HIV infection. These lesions are thought to be immune mediated rather than infectious; this theory is supported by the favorable responses to immunomodulation with corticosteroids or thalidomide therapy. Herpes simplex labialis may be seen in early disease, but it is a more common complication of later stage HIV infection. A listing of common complications associated with each stage of disease is given in Table 4.3.

Because of 1) the demonstration that high levels of viral replication are present even among stable, asymptomatic patients and 2) the ability of HAART to suppress this viral load to extremely low levels in most treatment-naive patients,

Table 4.3 Common Complications (Pathogens or Diseases) Associated with Stages of HIV Disease[a]

Early	Middle	Late
Acute seroconversion	Bacterial disease	Bacterial disease
Varicella-zoster virus	*Mycobacterium tuberculosis*	*Mycobacterium avium* complex
Herpes simplex virus	*Bartonella*	*Mycobacterium tuberculosis*
Epstein–Barr virus	*Salmonella*	*Rhodococcus equi*
	Syphilis	*Bartonella*
	Clostridium difficile	*Salmonella*
	Neisseria gonorrhoeae	*Clostridium difficile*
	Herpes simplex virus	*Nocardia*
	Epstein–Barr virus	*Cryptococcus*
		Histoplasmosis
	Pneumocystis carinii pneumonia	*Aspergillus*
	Lymphoma	Coccidioidomycosis (*Candida* sp.)
	(Kaposi's sarcoma or human herpes virus type 8)	(Herpes simplex virus/varicella-zoster virus)
		Cytomegalovirus
		Toxoplasmosis
		Pneumocystis carinii pneumonia
		Lymphoma
		(Kaposi's sarcoma)

[a]Complications in parentheses indicate disease processes that commonly occur in more than one stage of disease.

many clinicians are offering antiretroviral therapy to patients regardless of stage of disease. Even without therapy, the likelihood of patients with early HIV infection will develop an AIDS-defining condition and die within 18 to 24 months is less than 5% (23). Instead, a slow, progressive decline in CD4+ cells is typically seen during this time. Although the rate of decline may vary and is difficult to predict, a decrease of 40 to 80 cells/mm^3 per year on average is generally expected in patients who do not receive antiretroviral therapeutic intervention. With therapeutic intervention, CD4 counts often increase considerably, and this increase can lead to uncertainty about characterizing the relative stage of immunosuppression and the need for continued opportunistic infection prophylaxis.

Middle Stage Disease (CD4 Counts Between 200 and 500 Cells/mm^3)

Even though the CD4 counts are lower in this group of patients, most individuals at the middle stage of disease remain asymptomatic or have only mild disease manifestations. Many of the skin and oral lesions described in the discussion of the early period persist or perhaps worsen through the middle stage. In addition, other disorders, previously referred to as ARC, begin to appear. These symptoms consist of recurrent herpes simplex disease, varicella-zoster virus disease (shingles), mild oropharyngeal or vaginal candidiasis, oral hairy leukoplakia, recurrent seborrheic dermatitis, pruritic folliculitis, recurrent diarrhea, intermittent fever, and unexplained weight loss (more than 10 lb over 6 to 8 weeks). Other "constitutional symptoms," such as myalgias, arthralgias, headache, and fatigue, can also be seen in patients at this stage and anecdotally appear to correlate with higher levels of HIV viremia in some patients.

Mycobacterium tuberculosis infection tends to result in typical cavitating apical lung lesions among patients in this CD4 range, whereas patients with AIDS are more likely to have atypical pulmonary disease or extrapulmonary disease including dissemination and mycobacteremia. Routine bacterial infections, most frequently presenting as sinusitis, bronchitis, or pneumonia, are also common. These infections are generally caused by community-acquired organisms such as *Streptococcus pneumoniae* and *Haemophilus influenzae*. However, pathogens generally associated with nosocomial infections such as *Staphylococcus aureus* and *Pseudomonas aeruginosa* are encountered more commonly in these patients than in the routine outpatient care of adults without HIV infection. HIV-infected persons are more likely to have positive blood cultures than individuals without HIV infection when common bacterial infections are diagnosed (e.g., *S. pneumoniae*, *H. influenzae*, and *Salmonella enteritidis*).

When left untreated, patients with middle stage HIV disease have a 20 to 30% chance of developing an AIDS-defining condition or dying within the next 18 to 24 months; with zidovudine therapy, the risk is reduced two- to threefold (23, 67). As stated earlier, most clinicians now recommend combination antiretroviral therapy for patients in the early or middle stage of HIV disease, based on the encouraging results of clinical trials. Interim recommendations regarding specific drug regimen options and broad treatment strategies have been published (68), but the details are likely to evolve substantially as studies in progress provide new information and novel therapies become available.

Late Disease (CD4 Counts Between 50 and 200 Cells/mm^3)

By the CDC definition, all patients with fewer than 200 CD4+ cells/mm^3 have AIDS. A large clinical trial has demonstrated a clear clinical benefit when patients with AIDS are given a protease inhibitor–containing HAART regimen as compared with those patients receiving two reverse transcriptase inhibitors (69). Because many patients with earlier stage HIV infection are also now receiving this more aggressive form of therapy, the "AIDS" designation has little practical impact on decisions regarding the initiation of antiretroviral therapy. However, decisions regarding prophylaxis and empiric treatment of possible opportunistic conditions are critically affected, because the risk of developing AIDS-defining conditions rises substantially when CD4 counts drop below 200 cells/mm^3 (23).

Patients with late stage disease are at high risk of developing certain opportunistic infections including *Pneumocystis carinii* pneumonia, *Toxoplasma gondii* encephalitis, cryptosporidiosis, isosporiasis, tuberculosis, lymphoma, Kaposi's sarcoma, and esophageal candidiasis. *P. carinii* prophylaxis is indicated for all patients in this category, and trimethroprim–sulfamethoxazole can provide dual prophylaxis for patients with positive serologic tests for *Toxoplasma*.

Previously described symptoms of ARC also become more prevalent and frequently more severe. Fundoscopic examination may reveal the well-circumscribed cotton-wool spots of HIV retinopathy. Mononeuritis, myelitis, cranial nerve palsies (e.g., Bell's palsy), and idiopathic peripheral neuropathies may be noted. On rare occasion, unexplained transient ischemic attacks may occur. In such instances, underlying neurologic processes (e.g., neurosyphilis or cytomegalovirus [CMV] encephalitis) should be excluded. Human papillomavirus–associated malignancies, such as cervical cancer in women and carcinoma of the rectum in men, are reported with increased frequency at this stage of disease. HIV-associated idiopathic thrombocytopenia, anemia, neutropenia, and isolated elevation in lactose dehydrogenase occur with increased frequency. Hypogonadism and menstrual irregularities begin to appear. On occasion, patients develop idiopathic adrenal insufficiency. A subgroup of patients may develop progressive azotemia in association with high-grade proteinuria, constituting the syndrome of HIV-associated nephropathy. Such patients have rapidly progressive glomerulonephritis that leads to end-stage renal disease within 4 to 6 months, although prednisone therapy appears to slow this progression in many patients (70).

Advanced HIV Disease (CD4 Counts Less Than 50 Cells/mm^3)

Before the HAART era, all patients with advanced disease had a considerable likelihood of developing a new AIDS-defining illness or dying within 2 years. In addition, many patients have an inadequate response to combination antiretroviral therapy, especially those who have had an extensive prior treatment history or who are unable to afford or to comply with multidrug regimens. Certain opportunistic infections are associated with the most advanced stages of immunosuppression. Disseminated *Mycobacterium avium* complex disease, cryptococcal meningitis, progressive multifocal leukoencephalopathy, invasive aspergillosis, disseminated coccidioidomycosis, disseminated histoplasmosis, and invasive *Penicillium marneffei* disease are much more likely to occur during this stage of disease. CMV retinitis is the leading cause of blindness in these patients, and this virus also causes various other end-organ diseases including esophagitis, colitis, and polyradiculopathy characterized by ascending paralysis and cauda equina enhancement on magnetic resonance scans. Typically, these advanced patients develop coexisting opportunistic processes. Once a specific disease is identified and treatment is initiated, relapsing disease is the rule in most patients, although successful antiretroviral treatment may alter the presentation and frequency of recurrences.

Neurologic disease processes become especially prevalent at this stage of infection. Primary central nervous system lymphoma and progressive multifocal leukoencephalopathy, caused by the JC virus, create difficult management issues. Some patients develop so-called "HIV-associated dementia" during this period. This entity is characterized by cerebral atrophy and diminished cognitive function. The incidence of HIV-associated dementia has decreased substantially since the routine administration of antiretroviral therapy.

HIV wasting syndrome is seen with increased frequency in patients with advanced HIV infection, although it appears to be less common when effective antiretroviral intervention is possible. Defined as involuntary loss of more than 10 lb of usual body weight, the diagnosis of wasting syndrome implies that a thorough search for underlying opportunistic infections and malignant diseases has been undertaken and is negative. The cause of wasting can be characterized as decreased oral intake, gastrointestinal malabsorption, increased catabolism, or a combination of any of these factors. Patients with advanced HIV disease frequently have poor appetites, often as a result of underlying opportunistic diseases or as a side effect of medications. Some patients with advanced disease may have fat malabsorption. Increased catabolism is believed to be mediated, at least in part, by HIV-induced production of certain cytokines including tumor necrosis factor-α and interleukin-6. Occult Addison's disease may also be the cause of wasting in occasional patients.

Prophylaxis for disseminated *Mycobacterium avium* complex is recommended for patients when the CD4 count has dropped below the range of 50 to 75 cells/mm^3. Systemic antifungal therapy does diminish the incidence of disseminated fungal infections such as cryptococcosis or histoplasmosis, but generally the cost-to-benefit ratio is unfavorable for preventing these less common conditions. Although it is much more prevalent, mucosal candidiasis is generally benign if treated early, such that prophylaxis is unnecessary and expensive; however, patients with multiple recurrences or severe manifestations (such as refractory vaginal candidiasis or esophagitis) may require long-term therapy with an antifungal such as fluconazole. Concerns about the development of multiresistant pathogens are also an issue if widespread prophylaxis for mycobacterial and fungal infections becomes routine. Although oral ganciclovir appears to reduce the risk of CMV disease in patients with advanced disease, no broad consensus exists on the use of this expensive therapy for primary prophylaxis. It is conceivable that, in the future, prophylaxis for CMV and other infections will be provided to a more targeted population with a particularly high risk of disease based on virologic, genetic, or immunologic factors.

With more aggressive antiretroviral regimens, earlier identification of opportunistic processes, and more effective treatments of specific opportunistic infections, patients with advanced disease are living substantially longer than they did earlier in the epidemic (71). Recently, the incidence of AIDS-related deaths among all AIDS cases declined for the first time in the history of the epidemic, thus suggesting that advancements in the treatment of HIV and its complications are extending the lives of the most immunosuppressed HIV-infected patients (72).

Staging HIV Infection in the HAART Era

Studies have concluded that HAART regimens favorably alter the natural history of HIV infection and decrease the development of clinical end points in patients with AIDS. However, evidence indicates that the "immune reconstitution" associated with successful viral suppression is not complete. A patient, for example, whose CD4 count rises from 40 to 250 cells/mm^3 may not have achieved cellular immune responses synonymous with those this same individual had when he or she had a "natural complement" of 250 cells/mm^3 years before. The mean absolute CD4 count for patients initially diagnosed with CMV retinitis has shifted upward over the last several years according to a recent multicenter study (73); this finding suggests that CMV disease may be occurring among patients receiving HAART at CD4 count ranges that are higher than usual for this opportunistic infection. Investigators have proposed that, although the increases seen in CD4+ cells in patients receiving combination therapy are associated with functional benefits, the overall repertoire of memory and naive T cells may be altered, so the risk of infection with a certain opportunistic pathogen remains. Preliminary reports have also suggested that patients who have recently initiated HAART may have atypical manifestations when they develop infections associated with advanced AIDS; for example, patients who have *Mycobacterium avium* complex infection diagnosed after a rise in CD4 cells (from less than 50 to more than 200 cells/mm^3) may have tender, localized adenopathy rather than disseminated mycobacteremia (74). Some clinicians have noted that opportunistic infections sometimes are diagnosed immediately after the initiation of HAART, a finding suggesting that the partial return of cellular immune responses may contribute to signs and symptoms such as fever, local inflammation, or pain.

Until these observations are confirmed or refuted in larger clinical trials, most experts are recommending that patients continue prophylaxis or maintenance therapies that reflect the lowest CD4 counts they had before starting antiretroviral therapy. Further studies are necessary to develop staging systems that take into account the effects of significant viral suppression on the risk of infectious complications and on the long-term prognosis of HIV infection. Advances in understanding HIV immunopathogenesis will continue to provide insights into predicting disease progression and providing the most effective treatment strategy for each HIV-infected individual.

References

1. Centers for Disease Control. Classification system for human T-lymphotropic virus type III/lymphadenopathy-associated virus infections. MMWR Morb Mortal Wkly Rep 1986;35:334–339.
2. Centers for Disease Control. Revision of the CDC surveillance case definition for acquired immunodeficiency syndrome. MMWR CDC Surveill Summ 1987;36(Suppl 1S):1S–5S.
3. Redfield RR, Wright DC, Tramont EC. The Walter Reed staging classification for HTLV-III/LAV infection. N Engl J Med 1986;314:131–132.
4. Stein DS, Korvick JA, Vermund SH. CD4+ lymphocyte cell enumeration for prediction of clinical course of human immunodeficiency virus disease: a review. J Infect Dis 1992;165:352–363.
5. Centers for Disease Control and Prevention. 1993 Revised classification system for HIV infection and expanded surveillance of definition for AIDS among adolescents and adults. MMWR Morb Mortal Wkly Rep 1992;41:1–19.
6. Moss AR, Bacchetti P, Osmond D, et al. Seropositivity for HIV and the development of AIDS or AIDS-related condition: three year follow up of the San Francisco General Hospital Cohort. Br Med J 1988;296:745–750.
7. Jacobson MA, Bacchetti P, Kolokathis A, et al. Surrogate markers for survival in patients with AIDS and AIDS related complex treated with zidovudine. Br Med J 1991;302:73–78.
8. Selwyn PA, Alcabes P, Hartel D, et al. Clinical manifestations and predictors of disease progression in drug users with human immunodeficiency virus infection. N Engl J Med 1992;327:1697–1703.
9. Malone JL, Simms TE, Gray GC, et al. Sources of variability in repeated T-helper lymphocyte counts from human immunodeficiency virus type 1-infected patients: total lymphocyte count fluctuations and diurnal cycle are important. J Acquir Immune Defic Syndr 1990;3:144–151.
10. Burcham J, Marmor M, Dubin N, et al. CD4% is the best predictor of development of AIDS in a cohort of HIV-infected homosexual men. AIDS 1991;5:365–372.
11. Zurlo JJ, Wood L, Gaglione MM, et al. Effect of splenectomy on T lymphocyte subsets in patients infected with HIV. Clin Infect Dis 1995;20:768–771.
12. Phillips AN, Lee CA, Elford J, et al. Serial CD4 lymphocyte counts and development of AIDS. Lancet 1991;337:389–392.
13. Saah AJ, Munoz A, Kuo V, et al. Predictors of the risk of development of acquired immunodeficiency syndrome within 24 months among gay men seropositive for human immunodeficiency virus type 1: a report from the multicenter AIDS cohort study. Am J Epidemiol 1992;135:1147–1155.
14. Choi S, Lagakos SW, Schooley RT, et al. CD4+ lymphocytes are an incomplete surrogate marker for clinical progression in persons with asymptomatic HIV infection taking zidovudine. Ann Intern Med 1993;118:674–680.
15. DeGruttola V, Wulfsohn M, Fischl M, et al. Modeling the relationship between survival and CD4+-lymphocytes in patients with AIDS and AIDS-related complex. J Acquir Immune Defic Syndr 1993;6(4):359–365.
16. Melbye M, Goeddert JJ, Grossman RJ, et al. Risk of AIDS after herpes zoster. Lancet 1987;1:728–730.
17. Greenspan D, Greenspan JS, Hearst NG, et al. Relation of oral hairy leukoplakia to infection with human immunodeficiency virus and the risk of developing AIDS. J Infect Dis 1987;155:475–481.
18. Moss AR, Bacchetti P. Natural history of HIV infection. AIDS 1989;3:55–61.
19. Fahey JL, Taylor JMG, Detels R, et al. The prognostic value of cellular and serologic markers in infection with human immunodeficiency virus type 1. N Engl J Med 1990;322:166–172.
20. Mosmann TR. Cytokine patterns during the progression to AIDS. Science 1994;265:193–194.
21. Thea DM, Porat R, Nagimbi K, et al. Plasma cytokines, cytokine antagonists, and disease progression in African women infected with HIV-1. Ann Intern Med 1996;124:757–762.
22. Than S, Hu R, Oyaizu N, et al. Cytokine pattern in HIV-infection progression in HIV-infected children. J Infect Dis 1997;175:47–56.
23. MacDonell KB, Chimiel JS, Poggensee L, et al. Predicting progression to AIDS: combined usefulness of CD4 lymphocyte counts and p24 antigenemia. Am J Med 1990;89:706–712.
24. Ho DD, Moudgil T, Alam M. Quantitation of human immunodeficiency virus type 1 in the blood of infected persons. N Engl J Med 1989;321:1618–1625.
25. Coombs RW, Collier AC, Allain J-P, et al. Plasma viremia in human immunodeficiency virus infection. N Engl J Med 1989;321:1626–1631.
26. Saag MS, Crain MJ, Decker WD, et al. High level viremia in adults and children infected with human immunodeficiency virus: relation to disease stage and CD4+ lymphocyte levels. J Infect Dis 1991;164:72–80.
27. Piatak M, Saag MS, Yang LC, et al. High levels of HIV-1 plasma during all stages of infection determined by competitive PCR. Science 1993;259:1749–1754.
28. Wei X, Ghosh SK, Taylor ME, et al. Viral dynamics in HIV-1 infection. Nature 1995;373:117–122.
29. Ho DD, Neumann AU, Perelson AS, et al. Rapid turnover of plasma virions and CD4 lymphocytes in HIV-1 infection. Nature 1995;373:123–126.
30. Hughes MD, Johnson VA, Hirsch MS, et al. Monitoring plasma HIV-1 RNA levels in addition to CD4+ lymphocyte count improves assessment of antiretroviral therapeutic response. Ann Intern Med 1997;126:929–938.
31. O'Brien WA, Hartigan PA, Daar ES, et al. Changes in plasma HIV RNA levels and CD4+ lymphocyte counts predict both response to antiretroviral therapy and therapeutic failure. Ann Intern Med 1997;126:939–945.
32. Mellors JW, Kingsley LA, Rinaldo CR, et al. Quantitation of HIV-1 RNA in plasma predicts outcome after seroconversion. Ann Intern Med 1995;122:573–579.
33. Mellors JW, Rinaldo CR, Gupta P, et al. Prognosis in HIV-1 infection predicted by the quantity of virus in plasma. Science 1996;272:1167–1170.
34. Obrien TR, Blattner WA, Waters D, et al. Serum HIV-1 RNA levels and time to development of AIDS in the multicenter hemophilia cohort study. JAMA 1996;276:105–110.

35. Mellors JW, Munoz A, Giorgi JV, et al. Plasma viral load and CD4+ lymphocytes as prognostic markers of HIV-1 infection. Ann Intern Med 1997;126:946–954.
36. Saag MS, Holodniy M, Kuritzkes DR, et al. HIV viral load markers in clinical practice. Nature Med 1996;2:625–629.
37. Donovan RM, Bush CE, Markowitz NP, et al. Changes in virus load markers during AIDS-associated opportunistic diseases in HIV-infected persons. J Infect Dis 1996;174:401–403.
38. O'Brien WA, Grovit-Ferbas K, Namazi A, et al. HIV-1 replication can be increased in peripheral blood of seropositive patients after influenza vaccination. Blood 1995;86:1082–1089.
39. Kovacs JA, Baseler M, Dewar RJ, et al. Increases in CD4 T lymphocytes with intermittent courses of interleukin-2 in patients with HIV infection. N Engl J Med 1995;332:567–575.
40. Kilby JM, Tabereaux PB, Mulanovich V, et al. Effects of tapering doses of oral prednisone on viral load among HIV-infected patients with unexplained weight loss. AIDS Res Hum Retroviruses 1997;13:1533–1537.
41. Cao Y, Qin L, Zhang L, et al. Virologic and immunologic characterization of long-term survivors of HIV-1 infection. N Engl J Med 1995;332:201–208.
42. Pantaleo G, Menzo S, Vaccarezza M, et al. Studies in subjects with long-term nonprogressive HIV infection. N Engl J Med 1995;332:209–216.
43. Dean M, Carrington M, Winkler C, et al. Genetic restriction of HIV-1 infection and progression to AIDS by a deletion allele of the CKR5 structural gene. Science 1996;273:1856–1862.
44. Liu R, Paxton WA, Choe S, et al. Homozygous defect in HIV-1 coreceptor accounts for resistance of some multiply-exposed individuals to HIV-1 infection. Cell 1996;86:367–377.
45. Michael NL, Chang G, Louie LG, et al. The role of viral phenotype and CCR-5 gene defects in HIV-1 transmission and disease progression. Nature Med 1997;3:338–340.
46. Feng Y, Broder CC, Kennedy PE, et al. HIV-1 entry cofactor: functional cDNA cloning of a seven-transmembrane G protein-coupled receptor. Science 1996;272:872–877.
47. Koot M, Keet IPM, Vos AHV, et al. Prognostic value of HIV-1 syncytium-inducing phenotype for rate of CD4+ cell depletion and progression to AIDS. Ann Intern Med 1993;118:681–688.
48. Scarlatti G Tresoldi E, Bjorndal A, et al. In vivo evolution of HIV-1 co-receptor usage and sensitivity to chemokine-mediated suppression. Nature Med 1997;3:1259–1265.
49. Kaslow RA, Carrington M, Apple R, et al. Influence of combinations of human major histocompatibility complex genes on the course of HIV-1 infection. Nature Med 1996;2:405–411.
50. Montagnier L, Brenner C, Chameret S, et al. HIV infection and AIDS in a person with negative serology. J Infect Dis 1997;175:955–959.
51. Michael NL, Brown AE, Volgt RF, et al. Rapid disease progression without seroconversion following primary HIV-1 infection: evidence for highly susceptible human hosts. J Infect Dis 1997;175:1352–1359.
52. Clark SJ, Saag MS, Decker WD, et al. High titers of cytopathic virus in plasma of patients with symptomatic primary HIV-1 infection. N Engl J Med 1991;324:954–960.
53. Daar ES, Moudgio T, Meyer RD, et al. Transient high levels of viremia in patients with primary human immunodeficiency virus type 1 infection. N Engl J Med 1991;324:961–964.
54. Pantaleo G, Demarest JF, Soudeyns H, et al. Major expansion of CD8+ T cells with a predominant Vβ usage during the primary immune response to HIV. Nature 1994;370:463–467.
55. Borrow P, Lewicki H, Wei X, et al. Antiviral pressure exerted by HIV-1-specific cytotoxic T lymphocytes (CTLs) during primary infection demonstrated by rapid selection of CTL escape virus. Nature Med 1997;3:205–211.
56. Musey L, Hughes J, Schacker T, et al. Cytotoxic T-cell responses, viral load, and disease progression in early HIV-1 infection. N Engl J Med 1997;337:1267–1274.
57. Kinloch-De Loes S, Hirschel BJ, Hoen B, et al. A controlled trial of zidovudine in primary HIV infection. N Engl J Med 1995;333:408–413.
58. Markowitz M, Cao Y, Vesanen M, et al. Recent HIV infection treated with AZT, 3TC, and a potent protease inhibitor [abstract LB8]. Presented at the 4th Conference on Retroviruses and Opportunistic Infections, Washington, DC, 1997.
59. Wong JK, Hezareh M, Gunthard HF, et al. Recovery of replication-competent HIV despite prolonged suppression of plasma viremia. Science 1997;278:1291–1295.
60. Rosenberg ES, Billingsley JM, Caliendo AM, et al. Vigorous HIV-1-specific CD4+ T cell responses associated with control of viremia. Science 1997;278:1447–1450.
61. Cooper DA, Gold JA, MacLean P, et al. Acute retrovirus infection: definition of a clinical illness associated with seroconversion. Lancet 1985;1:137–140.
62. Schacker T, Collier AC, Hughes J, et al. Clinical and epidemiologic features of primary HIV infection. Ann Intern Med 1996;125:257–264.
63. Rabeneck L, Popovic M, Garner S, et al. Acute HIV infection presenting with painful swallowing and esophageal ulcers. JAMA 1990;263:2318–2322.
64. Vanhems P, Allard R, Cooper DA, et al. Acute HIV-1 disease as a mononucleosis-like illness: is the diagnosis too restrictive? Clin Infect Dis 1997;24:965–970.
65. Pedersen C, Lindhardt BO, Jensen BL, et al. Clinical course of primary HIV infection: consequences for subsequent course of infection. Br Med J 1989;299:154–157.
66. Osmond D, Chaisson RE, Moss AR, et al. Lymphadenopathy in asymptomatic patients seropositive for HIV. N Engl J Med 1987;317:246.
67. Volberding PA, Lagakos SW, Koch MA, et al. Zidovudine in asymptomatic human immunodeficiency virus infection: a controlled trial in persons with fewer than 500 CD4-positive cells per cubic millimeter. N Engl J Med 1990;322:941–949.
68. Carpenter CCJ, Fischl MA, Hammer SM, et al. Antiretroviral therapy for HIV infection in 1997: updated recommendations of the International AIDS Society–USA Panel. JAMA 1997;277:1962–1969.
69. Hammer SM, Squires KE, Hughes MD, et al. A controlled trial of two nucleoside analogues plus indinavir in persons with HIV infection and CD4 cell counts of 200 per cubic millimeter or less. N Engl J Med 1997;337:725–739.
70. Smith MC, Austen JL, Carey JT, et al. Prednisone improves renal function and proteinuria in HIV-associated nephropathy. Am J Med 1996;101:41–48.
71. Moore RD, Hidalgo J, Sugland BW, et al. Zidovudine and the natural history of the acquired immunodeficiency syndrome. N Engl J Med 1991;324:1412–1416.
72. Centers for Disease Control and Prevention. Update: trends in AIDS incidence, deaths, and prevalence—United States, 1996. MMWR Morb Mortal Wkly Rep 1997;46:165–173.
73. Jacobson MA, Zegans M, Pavan PR, et al. Cytomegalovirus retinitis after initiation of highly active antiretroviral therapy. Lancet 1997;399:1443–1445.
74. Race EM, Adelson-Mitty J, Kriegel GR, et al. Focal mycobacterial lymphadenitis following initiation of protease inhibitor therapy in patients with advanced HIV-1 disease. Lancet 1998;351:252–255.

5
IMMUNOPATHOGENESIS

M. Patricia D'Souza and Anthony S. Fauci

The human immunodeficiency virus (HIV) was first identified in 1983 and was shown to be the cause of acquired immunodeficiency syndrome (AIDS) in 1984 (1–3). Since that time, extraordinary progress has been made in our understanding of this pathogen. Studies on the pathogenesis of AIDS have unraveled many, but not all, of the mysteries of how HIV causes disease. The principal cells targeted by HIV in vivo are helper T lymphocytes and cells of the monocyte–macrophage lineage. HIV entry and infection are typically initiated by the binding of the HIV envelope glycoprotein to its primary cellular receptor, the CD4 antigen (4–6). However, the high-affinity binding between envelope and CD4 is insufficient to activate the membrane fusion process; investigators have shown recently that HIV also requires the presence of a fusion cofactor (7–12). Once infection is established, active viral replication and high levels of circulating plasma viremia result in seeding of the lymphoid organs, which subsequently function as the primary site of virus replication and serve as a reservoir of infectious virus (13). A consequence of the persistent viral replication is a vicious cycle of immune activation, cytokine secretion, and virus spread, all of which contribute to a complex array of pathogenic mechanisms ultimately resulting in the depletion of CD4+ T cells, destruction of lymphoid tissue, and the onset of life-threatening opportunistic infections and neoplasms (13).

In this chapter, we focus on the pathogenic mechanisms of HIV disease, particularly immunopathogenic mechanisms. The complex process of viral–host interactions at the cellular and molecular level that lead paradoxically to both immune responses and disease progression is discussed.

HOST CELL RECEPTORS

CD4

The most predominant cellular target for HIV infection is a subset of T cells characterized by the expression of the CD4 molecule—the CD4+ T cell. CD4 serves as a ligand for the major histocompatibility complex (MHC) II molecules during antigen presentation (14, 15). HIV attaches to the CD4+ T cell by virtue of a high-affinity interaction between CD4 and the viral surface glycoprotein, gp120, a product of the *env* gene.

The envelope glycoproteins are synthesized as a polyprotein precursor, gp160, that is subsequently cleaved by host cell proteases into the gp120 and gp41 subunits, which remain noncovalently associated in an oligomeric complex (16–18). The association of CD4 with gp120 initiates a complex cascade of conformational changes in the envelope protein and in the CD4 molecule, and this culminates in a pH-independent fusion of the virion and host membranes (19). However, the ability of HIV to enter and infect a host cell through the CD4 receptor depends on additional features of the target cell. For example, expression of human CD4 on murine cells permitted binding of the HIV gp120 molecule, indicating that the human CD4 was functionally intact (6), but viral entry did not occur. This block in viral entry is manifested at the level of membrane fusion because it could be overcome by fusing nonhuman cells expressing human CD4 to human cells to form transient or stable hybrids (20, 21). These and other findings suggest that critical human components required for the fusion process reside in the plasma membrane of human cells and not in most nonhuman cells.

Coreceptors for HIV Entry

The previously unrecognized component of the fusion and entry process was recently identified when investigators demonstrated that the seven-transmembrane (7TM) domain, G-protein–coupled glycoprotein named fusin, now redesignated CXCR4, was the fusion coreceptor for T-lymphocytotropic (T-tropic) HIV strains (7). T-tropic HIV strains, also known as syncytium-inducing (SI) viruses, can replicate in primary CD4+ T cells as well as in established CD4+ T-cell lines; however, they replicate poorly in monocyte/macrophages. The major physiologic function of the family of 7TM receptors is to activate intracellular calcium fluxes or cyclic adenosine monophosphate increases in response to extracellular ligands; these receptors are widely expressed in different tissues (22–26). Among known ligands for the 7TM family of receptors are various neuropeptides, chemokines, and peptide hormones; members of this superfamily are also involved in smell, taste, and vision transduction tissues (22–26). CXCR4 is most homologous to members of the α or C-X-C chemokine receptor family, and its natural ligand has been recently identified as the α-chemokine, stromal cell–derived growth factor-1 (SDF-1) (27, 28). Shortly after fusin was identified as the coreceptor for T-tropic strains of HIV, the β-chemokine receptor 5 (CCR5) was shown to be its counterpart for envelope-mediated fusion and entry of monocytotropic (M-tropic) isolates (8–12). M-tropic HIV strains, sometimes called nonsyncytium-inducing (NSI) viruses, can replicate in primary CD4+ T cells and macrophages; however, they replicate poorly in T-cell lines. CCR5 is a member of the β or C-C chemokine receptor superfamily of the 7TM receptors; its ligands are RANTES (regulated-on-activation, normal T expressed and secreted), macrophage inflammatory protein-1α (MIP-1α) and macrophage inflammatory protein-1β (MIP-1β) (Fig 5.1). A subset of M-tropic viral isolates can also use two additional β-chemokine receptors, CCR3 and CCR2b, as fusion cofactors (9, 10).

The in vivo importance of the CCR5 receptor was recently demonstrated when investigators found that individuals homozygous for a 32 base-pair deletion in the CCR5 coding sequence do not express the protein at the cell surface, and, consequently, their CD4+ T cells resist in vitro infection with M-tropic isolates of HIV (29–31). Individuals homozygous for this defect are highly, but not completely, resistant to HIV infection on in vivo exposure (32). This new information highlights the importance of the chemokine receptors in HIV transmission and provides an example of a defined genetic resistance to infection with HIV. A more thorough discussion of second-receptor biology can be found elsewhere (33, 34).

INFECTION OF LYMPHOID CELLS

CD4+ T Lymphocytes

Several important pieces of evidence led to the recognition that the primary target for infection with HIV was the helper subset of T lymphocytes expressing the CD4 antigen (4, 5, 35). These include the dramatic loss of CD4+ T cells during progressive HIV infection, the ability of monoclonal antibodies against CD4 to block HIV replication in culture (5, 36), the demonstration that gp120 forms an immunoprecipitable complex with CD4 (36), and, finally, the demonstration that transfection of the human CD4 gene into otherwise noninfectable human cells rendered them susceptible to HIV infection (6). In infected individuals, the absolute loss of CD4+ T cells or their functional impairment is central to the pathogenesis of HIV disease, and it contributes significantly to the profound immunosuppression characteristic of AIDS. These topics are addressed in detail in the following sections.

Hematopoietic Cells

A central immunologic feature of HIV disease is the loss of CD4+ T cells. Accelerated destruction of these cells by certain direct and indirect mechanisms (discussed later) is likely the major cause of cell loss. However, impaired regeneration of mature CD4+ T cells from the precursor cell pool is also likely to contribute to the ultimate depletion of these cells. In this regard, HIV infection of bone marrow, thymic precursor

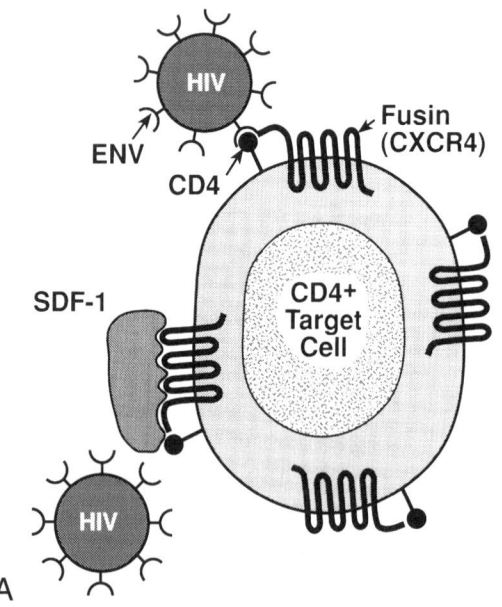
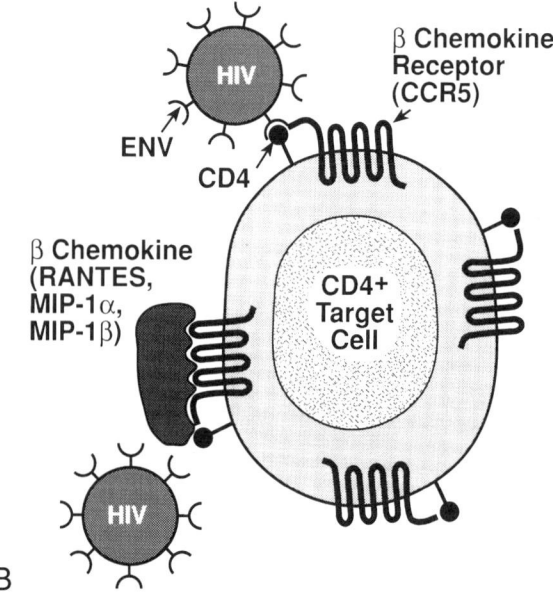

Figure 5.1. Coreceptors for M- and T-tropic strains of HIV-1 on CD4+ T cells. CXCR4 is the major coreceptor for T-tropic strains, entry of which is inhibited by its ligand SDF-1. CCR5 is the major coreceptor for M-tropic strains, and their entry is inhibited by its natural ligands RANTES, MIP-1α, and MIP-1β. (Adapted from Fauci AS. Host factors and the pathogenesis of HIV-induced disease. Nature 1996;384:529–534.)

cells, or the thymic and lymphoid tissue stromal environment could impair the regenerative process. Furthermore, HIV-infected individuals experience various cytopenias and other hematologic abnormalities, some of which are believed to arise from depressed hematopoiesis (37).

The thymus is the principal site where pluripotent hematopoietic stem cells mature into T lymphocytes (38, 39). Successful T-cell development within the thymic environment is a dynamic process requiring specific cellular and soluble factors (40, 41). Many of the stromal and lymphoid cells of the thymus and lymph node express CD4 and are thus susceptible to HIV infection. The most immature subset of thymocytes expresses the CD34 antigen, but not the CD3/T-cell receptor (TCR) complex or CD8 antigen, and little or no CD4 antigen. These cells expand and proliferate to express both CD4 and CD8 and are referred to as double-positive (DP) thymocytes. The final stage of intrathymic T-cell development involves the selective loss of either CD4 or CD8 antigen on DP thymocytes, resulting in single-positive CD4+ or CD8+ thymocytes that also express high levels of TCR (42).

Results of in vitro experiments demonstrated that HIV can infect CD34+ progenitor cells in human bone marrow (43), as well as the DP thymocytes and the single-positive CD4+ thymocytes (44). Ex vivo studies using DNA polymerase chain reaction (PCR) demonstrated that variable numbers of CD34+ cells in the bone marrow of HIV-infected individuals were infected. This finding was almost exclusively confined to individuals with advanced stage disease (45). Other studies could not demonstrate infection of CD34+ (46–48). The reasons for these discrepancies are unclear and may relate to differences in cellular tropisms of the infecting viruses. The mechanism by which HIV affects hematopoiesis is likely multifactorial. HIV may directly infect and destroy hematopoietic cells. Alternatively, HIV infection of cells in the bone marrow could affect hematopoiesis by causing abnormal cytokine secretion and disruption of the microenvironment required for hematopoietic regulation (46, 47, 49–53).

Although compelling evidence indicates that thymocytes are permissive for HIV infection in vitro, the in vivo relevance of these observations, particularly in HIV-infected adults, is unclear. To delineate the effects of HIV on the human thymus further, the severe combined immunodeficient (SCID)-hu animal mouse model was used. In this model, human thymus development could be recapitulated by transplantation of human fetal, liver, and thymus tissue under the renal capsule. Using SCID-hu mice, HIV-infection of the human thymus was demonstrated (54–56), and DP thymocytes were eliminated or significantly decreased (55). Further studies demonstrated that injection of virus directly into the thymic tissue of these mice resulted in a spreading cytopathic infection, depletion of both DP thymoctyes and single-positive CD4+ and CD8+ populations, and disruption of the thymic stromal network (54). Another important finding from the SCID-hu mouse studies was that different viral isolates exhibited varying effects on the thymus; certain viral strains were more cytopathic to thymocytes, whereas other strains were more destructive to the thymic stroma (54–56). An analogous situation may exist in HIV-infected individuals in whom viral isolates of different cellular tropisms may differentially affect the thymus and the thymic microenvironment.

INFECTION OF NONLYMPHOID CELLS
Monocyte/Macrophages

Whereas CD4+ T lymphocytes are the primary targets for HIV infection in vitro as well as in vivo, other cells that express the CD4 molecule are also susceptible to infection with HIV. Peripheral blood monocytes and tissue macrophages both express surface CD4 and are susceptible to HIV infection (57–59). Virus present within cells of the macrophage lineage may play a unique role in HIV pathogenesis. First, monocyte/macrophages are relatively resistant to the cytopathic effects of HIV, and thus they may serve as tissue reservoirs for HIV (60). Second, most of the HIV in infected monocytes/macrophages is sequestered in intracellular vacuoles, with few, if any, viral particles associated with the plasma membrane (61). Consequently, the virus can escape detection by the immune system. Third, infection of monocyte/macrophages is associated with the release of proinflammatory cytokines, some of which are potent inducers of HIV expression in CD4+ T cells, as well as in other infected monocyte/macrophages (57). In addition, infection of microglial cells (which are of monocytic lineage) in the central nervous system is also associated with the release of cytokines and neurotoxins that may contribute to HIV-related encephalopathy (62–64).

Although peripheral blood monocytes express greater numbers of CD4 molecules than tissue macrophages, they appear less susceptible to HIV infection than monocytes that have been propagated in culture (65, 66). The differing susceptibility of monocytes and macrophages to HIV infection may not merely be a reflection of the level of CD4 antigen expression but may reflect different coreceptor expression and usage, as well as different patterns of chemokine/cytokine expression as cells differentiate or activate. Recently, investigators have shown that the CCR3 and CCR5 molecules serve as major receptors with CD4 on brain microglial cells for HIV-1 infection of the central nervous system (67). The natural ligands for CCR3 and CCR5 could inhibit entry of selective HIV isolates that use these receptors (67). The surface expression of CCR3 and CCR5 on lymphocytes, and possibly nonlymphoid lineages as well, in culture is increased on phytohemagglutinin stimulation and interleukin (IL)-2 priming (68), perhaps explaining the increasing susceptibility of peripheral blood monocytes to HIV infection on culturing in vitro.

Studies on peripheral blood monocytes from HIV-infected individuals have identified a low proportion of infected cells (35, 69), compared with the higher frequency of infected macrophages isolated from lung and brain tissue of HIV-infected patients (70–72). These findings indicate that tissue maturation or immune activation may be critical for the susceptibility of these cells to HIV infection. In this regard, the level of HIV replication in peripheral blood monocytes and peritoneal macrophages from two HIV-infected individuals was shown to increase in the presence of opportunistic pathogens (73). These findings are consistent with recent observations that immune stimulation resulting from infection (74–76) or immunization (77–80) can result in a transient increase in plasma viral load.

Dendritic Cells

Dendritic cells (DCs) are important cells of the immune system that arise from CD34+ progenitors in the bone marrow. DCs include Langerhans cells (LCs) or epidermal DCs, dermal DCs, circulating blood DCs, interdigitating cells and tissue DCs (81). The two major portals for DC trafficking are the blood and the afferent lymphoid system, where DCs home to the T-cell regions of the spleen and lymph nodes, respectively (82, 83). DCs exhibit three primary functions: 1) they effectively take up antigens from the periphery and at mucosal surfaces; 2) when activated, they migrate to sites with a high probability of interaction with naive and memory T cells (84); and 3) they efficiently present processed peptides in the context of MHC class II and MHC class I products and activate T cells that recognize the presented peptides (85, 86). DCs are capable of eliciting a primary immune response, whereas other antigen-presenting cells induce predominantly secondary responses.

DCs can express the CD4 receptor (87), but authors of published studies disagree about the infectability of DCs and their ability to replicate virus (88). The contradictory findings about HIV infection of DCs may be explained at least in part by the existence of three or more populations of CD4+ cells with dendritic morphology that are present in blood, of which only one is susceptible to infection with HIV in vitro (88).

Two major hypotheses exist concerning the role of HIV-infectable DCs in HIV pathogenesis. The first suggests that blood DCs are prime targets for HIV infection in vitro and in vivo (89, 90). Supporting this hypothesis is evidence suggesting that viral infection leads to destruction of these cells and a decline in their ability to stimulate T-cell immunity. The other view is that DCs are infected at a low level (91), and their ability to bind and activate T cells remains uncompromised. However, if these cells are mixed with either activated or quiescent memory T cells, they can efficiently transmit virus to CD4+ T cells and can promote extensive viral replication (91–94). Overall, DCs appear to play an important role in pathogenesis, and, together with CD4+ cells, they support extensive virus replication and transmission in vitro and in vivo.

Other cell types that express little or no CD4 or only CD4 mRNA and yet are susceptible to HIV infection in vitro are discussed in Chapter 1. The HIV genome and its products are covered in Chapter 2, viral tropism is considered in Chapter 1, and the dynamics of HIV infection is discussed in Chapter 3.

CLINICAL COURSE OF HIV INFECTION: IMPLICATIONS FOR UNDERSTANDING MECHANISMS OF PATHOGENESIS

The median time course of HIV infection and progression to AIDS is approximately 8 to 10 years. Although this continuum varies from patient to patient, it is convenient to conceptualize the progression of HIV infection in three stages: the first phase of primary infection, a second clinically latent period when viral replication continues, and a third phase of advanced disease (13) (Fig 5.2). Each phase has its own distinguishing but overlapping immunologic and virologic events, which are discussed separately in the following sections.

Primary HIV Infection

Primary infection generally refers to the period from initial infection until the immune response to HIV gains some measure of control over viral replication, usually a few weeks to months. Approximately 30 to 70% of newly infected individuals experience signs and symptoms during acute HIV-1 infection that may include fever, malaise, rash, lymphadenopathy, pharyngitis, headache, diarrhea, and occasionally neurologic manifestations (95–97). This complex is referred to as the "acute retroviral syndrome."

Primary HIV infection is characterized by active viral replication and extremely high levels of plasma viremia (97–99). During this period, the virus disseminates throughout the body and seeds lymphoid organs, where its replication is incompletely suppressed (100). Concomitant with the high level of viremia is the frequent observation of a precipitous decline in CD4+ T-cell counts. With the development of an immune response to HIV and a reduction in levels of plasma viremia, the CD4+ T-cell counts generally rebound, but rarely to preinfection levels.

The initially high levels of HIV replication and plasma viremia generally decrease with the appearance of an HIV-specific immune response. The decreasing viral levels gradually stabilize within 6 months to 1 year at a virologic "set-point." Investigators have demonstrated that the virologic set-point directly correlates with the rate of HIV-mediated disease progression (101, 102). In this regard, plasma HIV RNA levels are the single most important predictor of disease progression. The viral and host factors that mediate the virologic set-point in an infected individual are unknown and constitute a topic of intense investigation.

Observations on the diversity and dynamics of the interaction between HIV and the immune system in early HIV infection suggest that the quality of the immune response is one factor influencing the set-point of the viral load. During primary HIV infection, subsets of CD8+ T cells that manifest cytolytic function are mobilized and expand to variable degrees. These subsets are composed of 24 families desig-

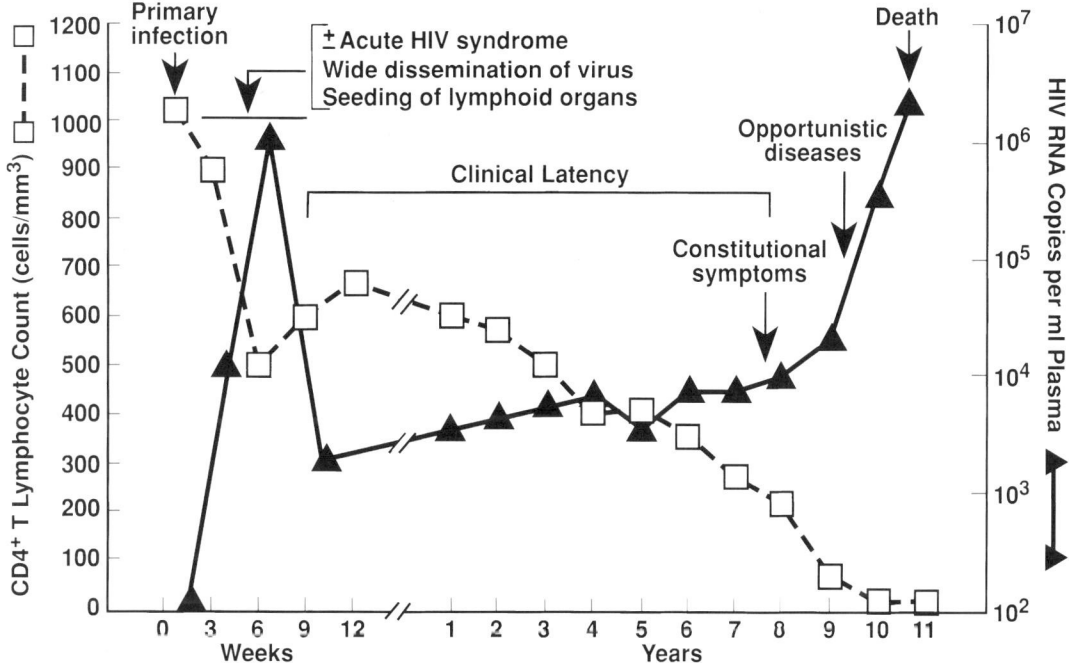

Figure 5.2. Typical course of HIV infection. After primary infection is widespread dissemination of virus and a plummeting of CD4+ T cells in peripheral blood. An immune response to HIV ensues, with a decrease in detectable viremia *(triangles)*, followed by a prolonged period of clinical latency. The CD4+ T-cell count declines *(squares)* during the following years, until it reaches a critical level below which the risk of opportunistic diseases is substantial. (Adapted from Pantaleo G, Graziosi C, Fauci AS. The immunopathogenesis of human immunodeficiency virus infection. N Engl J Med 1993;328:327–335.)

nated on the basis of the variable (V) region of the β chain of the TCR and are referred to as Vβ families. By examining the response of the CD8+ T-cell Vβ repertoire during primary HIV infection, investigators demonstrated that those individuals who mount a restricted response manifested by a major expansion of a single Vβ family generally exhibit a rapidly progressive clinical course. By comparison, individuals who mount a more heterogeneous or diffuse response characterized by no major expansions or minor expansions of multiple Vβ subsets experience an attenuated disease course (103). Major expansions of Vβ subsets in primary HIV infection are thought to result in depletion of the high-affinity HIV-specific cytotoxic T lymphocyte (CTL) clonotypes within those subsets leading to a compromise of the HIV-specific CTL response and viral escape from immune system control (104).

During primary infection, the number of CTL precursors directed against the viral Gag, Pol, and envelope proteins correlates with a decrease in the burst of plasma viremia, suggesting that CTLs play a fundamental role in the control of HIV infection (105, 106). In fact, CTL clones specific for the HIV envelope protein have been expanded from the blood of patients as early as 2 days after the onset of acute symptoms, well before antibody seroconversion. These clones specifically recognize sequences expressed by the transmitted expanded virus (107). In rhesus monkeys acutely infected with simian immunodeficiency virus (SIV), the CTL response also develops early and is temporally associated with clearance of viral antigenemia (108, 109). Evidence of the importance of CTLs in viral containment was provided in a recent study of a patient whose early CTL response was focused on a highly immunodominant epitope in gp160. This patient had rapid elimination of the transmitted virus strain and selection for a virus population bearing amino acid changes at a single residue within this epitope. This mutation conferred escape from recognition by primary CTLs by 136 days after the onset of the acute syndrome (110).

The cellular immune response appears to be more important than the humoral response in controlling HIV replication during acute infection, because neutralizing antibodies against HIV are not detected for at least 30 to 60 days after the resolution of the peak viremia (111). Neutralizing antibodies are more effective at blocking the infectivity of free HIV virions, rather than cell-to-cell transmission. Nonneutralizing antigen-binding antibodies to envelope and p24 (viral capsid protein) develop much earlier than neutralizing antibodies (112). Their appearance coincides with seroconversion, or the first detection of an antibody response to HIV, and they may be important in mediating antibody-dependent cellular cytotoxicity (ADCC) (see later). Antibodies may play a role in reducing the rate of infection of new cells beyond the acute phase (111).

CD8+ T-cell–mediated soluble, suppressorlike activity has been reported in some patients during primary HIV infection. This nonlytic activity also appears to be temporally associated with a decrease in plasma viremia, a finding suggesting that it, too, may play an important role in controlling viral replication (113).

Clinical Latency

The relative stabilization of the level of plasma viremia at a set-point generally signifies the beginning of a clinically latent period that may last for years. This phase is characterized by chronic immune activation and persistent viral replication despite a lack of consistent signs or symptoms of disease. Typically, this is the longest lasting of the three stages of HIV-infection, representing approximately 80% of the total course (114). During this phase, the number of circulating CD4+ T cells slowly declines by about 50 to 70 cells/μL per year, signaling the onset of progressive immune deficiency. The declining CD4+ T-cell numbers are likely due to ongoing viral replication with accompanying direct cytotoxicity, immune-mediated elimination of infected cells, and the failure to replace adequately the dying CD4+ T cells. The inability to regenerate CD4+ T cells may be a direct consequence of infection of progenitor cells, or it may be due to an indirect effect of the virus on the lymphoid microenvironment (see earlier). During this asymptomatic stage of infection, the numbers of infected cells in the peripheral blood, the plasma viral RNA levels, and the number of cells expressing virus in lymphoid tissue are generally low, although detectable. In contrast, one often sees a large quantity of virus trapped on the follicular DCs (FDCs) in the germinal centers of the lymph nodes. Recent data quantitating the viral burden in lymphoid tissue indicate that large pools of virus are present on FDCs; these levels are 100 to 10,000 times greater than the amount found in association with CD4+ T cells, monocytes, and macrophages. Even when virus was below the level of 5000 copies/mL as measured by the branched-chain DNA assay in peripheral blood (115), more than 1 million copies of viral RNA per gram of lymphoid tissue were found in the FDC pool (116). However, high levels of plasma viremia may occur during the clinically latent period and almost invariably lead to the transition to advanced stage disease.

The pivotal role of CTLs in controlling virus replication continues throughout the chronic phase of infection. However, the specificity of the CTLs, as well as the magnitude of the response, varies among infected individuals (117, 118). In patients who adequately control their viral load, CTLs to Env, Gag-Pol, as well as Nef, and Tat are continuously detected. Eventually, the effective CTL response declines and plasma viremia escalates. The factors that lead to the decline of an effective CTL response are not entirely clear and remain an important issue to resolve. One compelling hypothesis for the decline of the CTLs is the development of viral escape mutants that evade recognition by CTLs both early and late in disease (110, 119–121). In support of this hypothesis, a recent study of two HIV-infected individuals has identified a single mutation in an immunodominant CTL epitope late in HIV infection. This resulted in a provirus population capable of evading immune recognition and contributing to the collapse of the immune response (122).

Neutralizing antibodies are also present throughout the asymptomatic phase of disease, albeit at relatively low levels (123, 124). In addition to neutralizing antibodies, binding antibodies to Env, Nef, Rev, Vpr, Vpu, and Tat are also detected, but they tend to decline as disease progresses (117). Antibodies to p24 rise to their highest levels during this phase and then fall, usually to undetectable levels, before the onset of AIDS (97, 98).

Advanced Disease

Advanced disease is characterized by an AIDS-defining illness or a decline in the levels of circulating CD4+ T cells to below 200 cells/μL (125). Plasma viremia usually increases during this stage of disease (114) and is correlated with a sharp decrease in CD4+ T-cell counts.

Immune function is diminished, as evidenced by the loss of CD4+ T cells, the destruction of lymphoid tissue architecture, and the loss of CD8+ CTLs and noncytolytic viral suppression (114). The reasons for the faster CD4+ T-cell decline at this time are not fully appreciated. One possibility is that the increased plasma viremia accelerates the CD4+ T-cell destruction; a second is the failure to repopulate dying cells. The reasons for the decline of the CD8+ T-cell population are also not clear; however, as with CD4+ T cells, the decline may be due in part to a block in the regeneration of CD8+ T cells from progenitors. Another possibility is that high levels of viremia or viral proteins contribute to the sequestration of CD4+ and CD8+ T cells out of the circulation.

Levels of neutralizing antibodies are generally low or undetectable at this stage of disease, and titers of nonneutralizing antibodies to viral proteins are diminished (118). In addition, aberrant production of immunoregulatory or proinflammatory cytokines occurs (114). Thus, as a direct consequence of the loss of the regulatory function of the CD4+ T lymphocytes, and the impaired CD8+ T-cell populations, immune activation and cytokine secretion may ultimately become inappropriate and may lead to a compounding of detrimental effects.

Finally, the late stage of disease is also characterized by destruction of lymphoid tissue and collapse of the FDC network. Because the FDCs play an important role in maintaining the integrity of the immune system, dissolution of this network is likely to be a prime component of the severe immune deficiency observed at this stage of disease, leaving individuals at high risk for developing life-threatening opportunistic infections and malignant diseases. In addition, the loss of virus-trapping capability of the FDCs contributes to the "spillover" of virus into the circulation (see later).

LYMPHOID ORGANS AND HIV

HIV directly interacts with many of the cells of the lymphoid system. The immune response to invading pathogens is generated in lymphoid tissue, where foreign antigens are trapped and presented to T and B cells. Within lymphoid tissue, two types of DCs predominate: bone marrow–derived DCs, which are involved in all aspects of T-cell development, including stimulation of naive cells, and expansion of the memory and effector T-cell populations; and FDCs, a distinct cell type found only within the lymphoid follicles, which interact primarily with B cells (126). DCs and FDCs are key components in the acquisition and presentation of antigens and in the development of cellular and humoral immunity.

DCs and FDCs play a prominent role in different stages of HIV infection. DCs are among the first cells that interact with HIV at the sites of viral entry; they can form complexes with T cells and migrate to the draining lymph node or splenic white pulp (127). Support for the role of DCs in the early establishment of infection is found in the SIV-infected macaque model; DCs in the cervicovaginal mucosa were the first cells infected after experimental vaginal inoculation of SIV (127).

In contrast, FDCs in the lymph nodes trap and retain virus particles that are coated with antibody or complement (128, 129). These trapped complexes are localized within specialized regions of lymphoid tissue, called germinal centers (129–131). Germinal centers are characterized by foci of rapidly proliferating antigen-specific B cells and antigen-bearing FDCs; antigen-specific T cells, which are usually found in the paracortical regions of lymph nodes, infiltrate the germinal centers to provide help to B cells during an immune response (132, 133). Within the germinal center, these cells respond by production of cytokines needed for germinal center development, the differentiation of B cells and antibody production, and the development of a memory response. The germinal center thus represents an environment in which HIV or its antigens can be trapped and retained, allowing for the generation and maintenance of a memory response to the virus.

HIV-infected individuals often develop significant lymphadenopathy, an indication of the cellular activation and immune response to the virus within the lymphoid tissue microenvironment (96–98). Germinal center hyperplasia is a prominent histologic finding (100). Early in primary infection, numerous virus-expressing cells are detected in lymph nodes; the largest number of virus-expressing cells in these organs is found preceding or coinciding with the peak titer of plasma viremia, a finding suggesting that the lymphoid tissue is the source of circulating virus (Fig 5.3). Peak plasma viremia and tissue dissemination of virus occur in association with the abrupt decrease in circulating CD4+ T cells observed during primary infection. At the same time, CD4+ T cells accumulate in the nodes, either because of in situ proliferation or as a result of their migration from the periphery to the lymph nodes (96–98, 134).

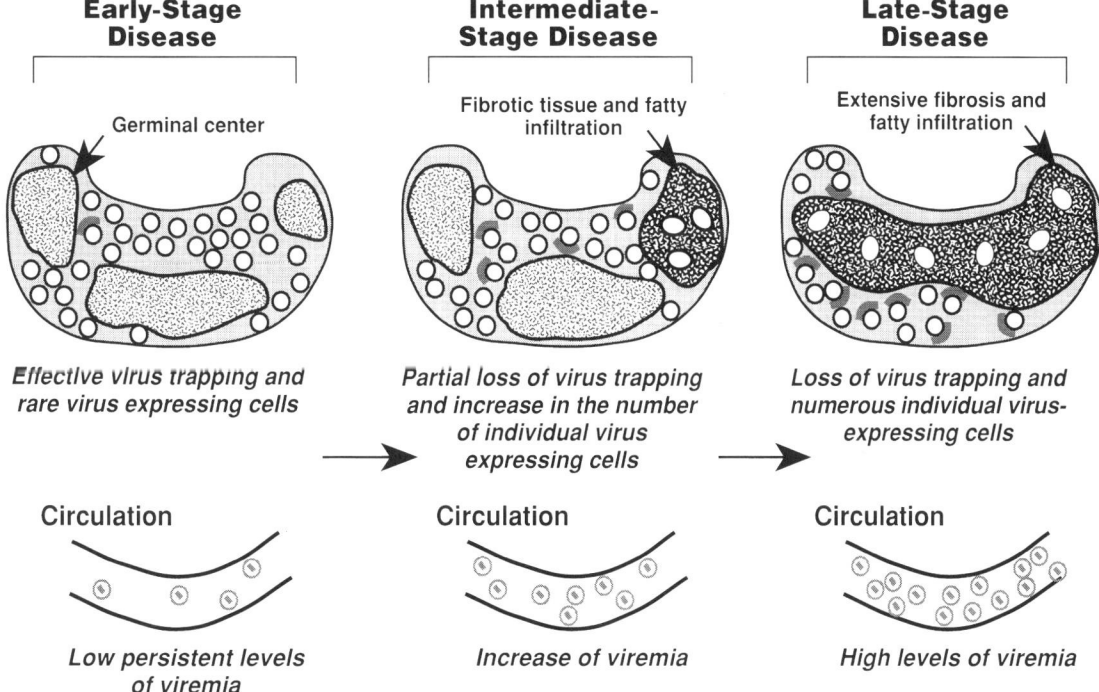

Figure 5.3. Schematic representation of virus distribution, histopathology, and viremia associated with the progression of HIV disease. In primary stage disease, one sees extensive germinal center formation in lymph node, effective virus trapping into the FDC network (gray area), few virus-expressing cells, and low levels of viremia. In clinical stage disease, large areas of the lymphoid tissue undergo involution (i.e., fibrosis and fatty infiltration), and both the number of virus-expressing cells in lymph node and the levels of viremia increase. In advanced stage disease, most of the lymphoid tissue is replaced by fibrosis and fatty infiltration; virus trapping is generally lost; numerous virus-expressing cells and high levels of viremia are noted. (Adapted from Pantaleo G, Fauci AS. New concepts in the immunopathogenesis of HIV infection. Annu Rev Microbiol 1996; 50:825–854.)

With the development of an immune response to HIV, one sees a rapid downregulation of virus-expressing cells in the lymphoid organs and plasma and an increase in virus trapping in the FDC network in the germinal center. These trapped virus particles are coated with anti-HIV antibodies and complement, and this permits their attachment to the FDCs, likely by virtue of the complement receptors on these cells. These trapped virions or viral antigens are the dominant form of virus present in the lymphoid tissue during the clinically latent period. Although the FDCs themselves are not usually infected (135), the trapped HIV virions remain infectious for CD4+ T cells (136), even when coated with neutralizing antibodies (137).

The microenvironment of the lymphoid tissue is ideal for establishing and propagating HIV infection, either by stimulating secretion of cytokines such as tumor necrosis factor-α (TNF-α), IL-6, IL-10, and interferon-γ (IFN-γ) or by maintaining a pool of activated target cells that may support virus replication (138). Supporting this notion is the observation that a substantial proportion of CD4+ T cells (25 to 50%) are activated in the lymph nodes of patients with HIV infection, compared with a smaller percentage (5 to 10%) in the blood (139); these cells are susceptible to infection and contribute to the propagation of viral replication (95). Thus, the microenvironment of the lymphoid organs is ideal for both the initiation and the maintenance of HIV infection.

Because of prolonged virus replication during the course of HIV disease, the lymphoid architecture deteriorates, and involution of germinal centers becomes apparent (95) (see Fig. 5.3). Gradually, disruption of the lymphoid tissue microenvironment directly affects the function of germinal center B cells, which are critical for maintaining a humoral immune response against a new antigenic challenge. This may contribute to the general immune system failure observed in the late stage of HIV infection.

During the advanced stage of disease, the destruction of the FDC network is severe, resulting in the loss of HIV-trapping ability. This is coincident with the marked increase in plasma viremia (95, 100, 130, 140). Dissolution of the FDC network with release of previously trapped virus contributes at least in part to the increased viral burden in peripheral blood (128). Lymph node architecture is destroyed, and lymphoid tissue is replaced by fibrotic tissue or fatty infiltration (see Fig. 5.3). The earlier sequence of events is reversed in that one sees an increase in mononuclear cells expressing viral RNA in the paracortical area; the proportion of these cells increases as disease progresses (130). The loss of lymphoid architecture at this stage of HIV disease is an important component of the severe immune deficiency and increased susceptibility to opportunistic infections. In addition, the capacity of the immune system to control virus spreading and replication is diminished (see Fig. 5.3).

LONG-TERM NONPROGRESSION

The natural history and pathogenic processes of HIV infection are complex and variable and are influenced by genetic factors, virulence of HIV variants, and host immunologic response to the virus (104, 114, 118). Projections based on models of survival from cohort studies suggest that between 10 and 17% of infected individuals will remain free of clinical AIDS 20 years after the initial infection (141, 142); these individuals are termed long-term survivors. Within this group exist a subset of persons (less than 5% of HIV-infected people) called long-term nonprogressors (LTNPs) (143–145); these are individuals whose CD4+ T counts are stable and have not declined over several years (8 to 10 years at least) of HIV infection and whose disease has not progressed even though they have not received antiretroviral therapy. What proportion of LTNPs will continue to remain stable and healthy is unclear. Some individuals who were originally termed LTNPs have experienced disease progression. Further, longitudinal observations in these populations should clarify this issue.

LTNPs are a topic of intense investigation because an understanding of their immune system may delineate the biologic and virologic factors that prevent progression of their disease. The benign course of disease in these individuals likely is due to both viral and host factors. To date, research has focused on three areas: 1) viral strain and phenotype; 2) immune response; and 3) genetic factors.

LTNPs from different cohorts have significantly lower plasma viremia (124, 144, 146–150), when compared with HIV-infected individuals with progressive disease. The level of viral replication in LTNPs is significantly lower than in progressors, even though virus could be identified by PCR techniques in virtually all LTNPs. Isolation of HIV from the blood of LTNPs is difficult, although the virus is sometimes culturable from lymph node mononuclear cells (146). LTNPs typically harbor HIV variants exhibiting the NSI phenotype that use CCR5 as a fusion cofactor (123, 151). In addition, HIV variants isolated from LTNPs are diverse rather than homogeneous, and investigators have suggested that this viral heterogeneity may reflect an effective immune response to HIV (119, 152).

Some studies have focused on the viral strain present in LTNPs in the hope of discovering virologic parameters that may modulate nonprogression. One focus of activity has been the *nef* gene because previous studies showed that it is a major determinant of pathogenicity in vivo; it is required for the maintenance of high levels of viral replication and the development of AIDS in SIV-infected adult rhesus monkeys (153). A recently published study from the Sydney Bloodbank cohort describes a single blood donor infected with a defective strain of HIV and a cohort of 6 blood or blood-product recipients infected by this donor. These individuals have remained free of disease 10 to 14 years after infection (154). The authors speculated that the deletion in the *nef* gene and in the region of overlap of *nef* and the U3 region of the long terminal repeat (LTR) in the transmitted virus is responsible for the lack of progression to disease in both the donor and the recipients. In a different study, 1 of 5 LTNPs infected with HIV had a deletion in the *nef*-LTR region as well as additional deletions in the *nef*-

LTR over a period of 10 years (147). Defects in viral proteins in addition to Nef may also be responsible for viral attenuation. For example, no deletions in *nef* were found in a single LTNP hemophiliac (155) and in another group of 10 LTNPs (156); 2 of the individuals had undefined defects in the NF-κB and Sp1 sites (157).

Studies of the immune response in LTNPs have not revealed any single immune response uniformly associated with nonprogression. One study reported that few cells expressing virus were found in lymphoid tissue by in situ hybridization, and the structure of the lymph node architecture and the FDC were preserved (146). These investigators noted a high frequency of anti-HIV–specific memory CTLs against envelope (146); and memory CTLs against Gag, Pol, and envelope were also present at high levels compared with levels in patients with intermediate and advanced stage disease (150, 158). Activated, circulating CTLs to p17, p24, RT, envelope, and Nef that are broadly cross-reactive against multiple HIV variants in LTNPs have also been reported in patients with low viral loads who had been infected for up to 17 years (159). In contrast, another study found no activated CTLs in LTNPs with CD4+ T-cell counts higher than 1000/μL (160). The demonstration of strong CTL responses and low viral load is consistent with a potential role of CTL as a protective host defense. However, LTNPs appear to be a heterogeneous group of individuals in which multiple factors may contribute to the state of nonprogression.

Studies on the level of antibodies in LTNPs have also proved inconsistent. In some studies, LTNPs exhibit potent and broad neutralizing antibody responses against laboratory-adapted isolates as well as a diverse panel of primary HIV isolates (123, 124, 146); however, a study of LTNPs from the San Francisco City Clinic revealed weak to undetectable titers against a panel of 10 primary isolates (159). Other studies have described high titers of antibodies to the core proteins, p24 and p17 (149, 161). These antibody responses may be a sign of a complex immune response, because loss of anti-p24 is a surrogate marker of a deteriorating immune system and the onset of AIDS.

Supporting the concept that the chronic state of immune activation in individuals who progress to disease is due to persistent viral replication is the observation that LTNPs exhibited little CD8+ T-cell activation and little expression of the HLA-DR+ CD38+ phenotype (162). HLA-DR and CD38 are two unique cellular markers present on subsets of cytotoxic CD8+ T cells that become activated at seroconversion and predict disease progression (163).

The CD8+ T cells of LTNPs demonstrate elevated levels of soluble suppressor activity when compared with rapid progressors (124). Although RANTES, MIP-1α, and MIP-1β have been identified as responsible for some of the soluble suppressor activity that blocks viral entry of M-tropic virus in CD4+ T cells (164) (see the section of this chapter on inhibition of HIV entry by chemokines), these three β-chemokines do not appear to be entirely responsible for the elevated suppressor activity in LTNPs. Thus, other as yet unidentified factors may be responsible for the CD8+ T-cell–mediated suppression in LTNPs (165–168).

Certain genes are associated with rates of disease progression. Genes of the MHC region are directly involved in the generation of the immune response to pathogens. These genes encode various polymorphic proteins that display antigens on the cell surface. Antigen recognition varies at the level of MHC type, so not all individuals recognize all viral antigens equally (169). In fact, some MHC genes have been associated with protection against HIV disease progression (170). The most compelling evidence of a gene that protects against disease progression has been the observation that individuals who express one normal and one mutant allele for CCR5 have significantly lower viral loads and slower rates of CD4+ T-cell decline when compared with individuals with two normal alleles; thus, the presence of the heterozygous CCR5 state modestly impedes disease progression (31, 171, 172). Other forms of genetically mediated resistance to HIV infection will likely be identified with further study.

RAPID DISEASE PROGRESSION

Survival analyses have demonstrated that approximately 6% of HIV-infected individuals experience a rapid decline in CD4+ T-cell levels within 2 to 3 years and develop full-blown AIDS within 3 years after primary HIV infection (141, 173). Rapid progressors uniformly exhibit higher HIV RNA levels in the plasma as well as higher HIV DNA load in peripheral blood mononuclear cells (PBMCs) when compared with nonprogressors. This higher viral load is usually noted soon after seroconversion and persists throughout the course of disease (101, 174). A recent study has confirmed and extended these observations, demonstrating that, in a cohort of infected homosexual and bisexual men, 50% of the men with more than 10,900 HIV RNA copies/mL died within 6 years of study entry (102).

Rapid progressors exhibit more homogeneity among HIV isolates compared with nonprogressors, a finding implying that the immune response to HIV is less effective and is less capable of driving HIV variant diversification in the former group (119, 152). Some rapid progressors harbor viruses with a more virulent SI phenotype (175) that use CXCR4 as a fusion cofactor (7). The tissue distribution of CXCR4 is broader than that of CCR5, perhaps allowing the virus access to a wider range of potential target cells and thereby facilitating HIV replication and spread (176).

The breadth and diversity of the immune responses in rapid progressors are variable, suggesting that the state of rapid progression is not attributable to a single immunologic parameter. Some rapid progressors exhibit high frequencies of precursor Gag-specific CTLs early in infection that wane with time and coincide with the loss of CD4+ T cells (158). Other studies have reported the presence of circulating anti-HIV CTL activity against multiple viral proteins (150). Soluble suppressors of HIV replication are present in rapid progressors, but levels diminish with disease progression (177, 178). Again, this noncytolytic suppressor activity is not attributable entirely to RANTES, MIP-1α, and MIP-1β (165–168).

Rapid progressors exhibit low levels or no detectable antienvelope-neutralizing antibodies to the autologous virus (179, 180). They either do not develop or have lower levels of anti-p24 and anti-p17 antibodies (149, 181). Individuals who experience a more rapid course of disease progression also manifest an unusual degree of immune activation, a likely consequence of persistent virus replication, as monitored by the level of expression of the CD38 antigen, which is an indicator of poor prognosis (163). Elevated levels of serum markers of immunologic activation, such as neopterin and β-2 microglobulin, have also been reported to correlate with more rapid disease progression and HIV-mediated immune system destruction (182, 183). Overall, increased plasma RNA levels, together with diminishing anti-HIV immune responses and elevated levels of CD8+ CD38+ T cells, have been correlated with rapid disease progression.

CELLULAR ACTIVATION AND ENDOGENOUS CYTOKINES IN THE PATHOGENESIS OF HIV DISEASE

Although HIV disease ultimately results in severe immune deficiency, a major factor in the immunopathogenesis of HIV infection is aberrant immune activation (13). The ongoing replication of HIV and new infection of target cells result in the constant processing and presentation of HIV antigen, thus generating a robust immune response that partially suppresses HIV but provides a stimulus for persistent immune activation. This activation is intimately linked to a change in the profile of detectable cytokines in the blood and lymph nodes of HIV-infected individuals (138, 184).

Effects of HIV on Cytokine Production

Cytokines are key components in the regulation of inflammation, as well as in the differentiation and activation of immune effector cells. They have complex effects on the replication of HIV that, in turn, directly affect cytokine production. In this regard, in vitro infection of cells with HIV results in increased production of TNF-α, IL-6, IL-1β, and other cytokines (184). However, productive infection with HIV does not appear to be a requirement for these effects. For instance, the binding of HIV envelope protein to the CD4 receptor on monocytes enhances the secretion of granulocyte-macrophage (GM)–colony-stimulating factor (CSF), TNF-α, IL-6, and IL-1β (184–188). Similarly, soluble viral proteins such as Tat and gp120 can mimic productive viral infection and can induce the secretion of TGF-β (185, 189). In vivo, these cytokines may play a role in regulating HIV expression; for example, elevated levels of TGF-β have been found in brain tissue of HIV-infected individuals and in the circulation (190–192).

IL-2 is a cytokine that regulates the proliferation and differentiation of lymphocytes, including CD4+ T cells. IL-2 levels are decreased in both blood and lymph nodes of HIV-infected individuals, and in vitro, production of IL-2 from PBMCs obtained from HIV-infected individuals is decreased compared with uninfected individuals (193). Administration of exogenous IL-2 in HIV infection was tested to determine its immunotherapeutic benefit on the expansion of CD4+ T cells, despite cell culture data showing that IL-2 activated lymphocytes and enhanced HIV growth. IL-2 was administered to HIV-infected patients with CD4+ T-cell counts greater than 200/μL (mean approximately 400 μL), on an intermittent schedule of 5 days of IL-2, followed by an 8-week rest period. Over the course of several cycles of IL-2, a significant boost in the CD4+ T-cell number to normal levels (between 800 and 1200/μL) was achieved (194, 195). Transient increases in plasma viremia were directly associated with the infusion of IL-2 and occurred in most patients, in association with the reported stimulatory effects of IL-2 on HIV replication (196). However, the total viral load did not change, and increases in plasma virus returned to baseline after the treatment (194, 195). Investigation into the mechanism of IL-2 induced CD4+ T-cell expansion supports the hypothesis that the new cells are of extrathymic origin and therefore represent an amplification of the existing CD4+ T-cell repertoire. In patients with CD4+ T-cell counts below 200/μL, IL-2 was not effective. This may result from the irreversible loss of such a large proportion of the T-cell repertoire. The combination of protease inhibitors to suppress viral replication and IL-2 therapy to sustain CD4+ T-cell counts may be a promising therapeutic approach for treating HIV-infected individuals. However, its ultimate clinical benefit awaits the results of larger efficacy trials.

Cytokine Induction of HIV Expression

Cytokines that increase the growth and expression of HIV in different cell culture systems include IL-1β, IL-2, IL-3, IL-6, IL-12, TNF-α, TNF-β, M-CSF, and GM-CSF (184). The original finding that crude supernatants from PBMC cultures induce viral expression in chronically infected cell lines (197) led to the discovery that numerous individual cytokines induce HIV expression either by endogenous manipulation or when added exogenously to acutely or chronically infected cell cultures (184). Of the inductive cytokines, TNF-α, IL-6, and IL-1β are the most investigated, and they are discussed in this section.

Both in vitro and in vivo studies have demonstrated that TNF-α plays a critical role in HIV pathogenesis. Endogenous TNF-α was observed to drive HIV replication in vitro in monocytic and T-cell lines and in primary macrophages and PBMCs (33, 198). In vivo studies have shown that PBMCs isolated from HIV-infected patients spontaneously, as well as in response to exogenous stimulants, secrete higher levels of TNF-α than do PBMCs isolated from uninfected individuals (186, 199–202). Elevated levels of TNF-α have been demonstrated in plasma, and increased expression of TNF-α has been demonstrated in the lymph nodes of HIV-infected individuals (138, 193). In addition, TNF-α secretion by pulmonary alveolar macrophages obtained from HIV-infected individuals is higher than that observed in cells from uninfected individuals, and this is independent of opportunistic infections (203, 204).

The upregulation of TNF-α expression by HIV infection is only one facet of the TNF-α autocrine–paracrine loop. TNF-α also potently upregulates HIV production from chronically infected monocyte and T-cell lines as well as from PBMCs derived from HIV-infected individuals (184, 198, 205–207). TNF-α appears to upregulate HIV expression by activating the important cellular transcription factor, NF-κB (207, 208). NK-κB proteins bind to NK-κB-specific consensus sequences within the LTR of the HIV genome and induce transcription from the proviral DNA.

Investigators have demonstrated that IL-6 can induce HIV replication in chronically infected monocyte cultures and can synergize with TNF-α (208–210). Elevated levels of IL-6 in serum, plasma, cerebrospinal fluid, and lymphoid tissue have been reported in HIV-infected individuals, and PBMCs from these individuals produce higher levels of IL-6 when compared with cells from healthy controls (199, 211, 212). The mechanism of IL-6–mediated HIV induction is not fully understood, but it is likely a posttranscriptional effect (208, 213). When IL-6 and TNF-α interact synergistically to induce HIV expression, both transcriptional and posttranscriptional pathways are involved. Furthermore, interaction of gp120 with a cell-surface component of B cells, that is not CD4, resulted in increased production of TNF-α and IL-6 (200). This gp120-dependent upregulation of cytokine expression was observed exclusively in B cells from HIV-infected individuals and did not occur in activated B cells obtained from uninfected controls (200). The identity of the B-cell receptor for the gp120 is unknown; however, it is likely to be a cell-surface immunoglobulin specific for gp120, based on previous observations that a substantial proportion of B-cell response in HIV-infected individuals are directed at HIV proteins (214).

IL-1β directly induces expression of HIV in monocytic cell lines and synergizes with IL-6 to upregulate virus expression (213). This inductive effect is blocked by TGF-β and antibodies to IL-1. IL-1β is thought to induce HIV expression at the viral transcription level in an NF-κB–independent manner, predominantly by posttranscriptional mechanisms (184). IL-1β can also directly induce expression of HIV in PBMCs activated with IL-2, and an anticytokine antibody or a natural cytokine antagonist to IL-1β could abrogate this effect (198, 213).

GM-CSF and liposaccharide (LPS) can also upregulate HIV expression in primary cells and chronically infected cell lines, both independently (215) and in synergy with TNF-α (210). Virus production independent of TNF-α was demonstrated to depend on the secretion of endogenous IL-1β (215). This cytokine is believed to act at a posttranscriptional step in the HIV life cycle.

Cytokine Suppression of HIV Expression

The steady state of virus replication in HIV-infected individuals is influenced, at least in part, by a balance between the inductive effects of the proinflammatory cytokines, discussed earlier, and the suppressive effects of various other cytokines, discussed later. In contrast to the cytokines that induce HIV replication, IFN-α and IFN-β exert a predominantly suppressive effect. In vitro, studies have demonstrated that IFN-α can affect multiple steps of the HIV replication cycle in vitro; in acutely infected T cells and monocytes, the major block occurs at the preintegration level, before formation of the provirus (216), whereas in chronically infected cells, the block is at the level of viral assembly (217). Investigators have also reported that IFN-α inhibits the activation of HIV provirus by indirectly interfering with the NF-κB–specific interaction (216). In cell culture, HIV infection of monocytes blocked production of IFN-α, but not TNF-α, IL-6, or IL-1 after stimulation (218, 219). Monocytes infected in vivo and tested in cell culture also do not secrete IFN-α. In vitro studies of virus isolates from patients in early disease demonstrate that HIV replication is sensitive to IFN-α mediated inhibition. However, late in disease, in some patients, high levels of IFN-α are detectable in serum simultaneous with high levels of viral replication (220–222). These patients progress to death more quickly when compared with IFN-α negative patients matched for CD4+ T-cell counts. This paradox is resolved with the observation that HIV isolates display a broad range of sensitivities to IFN-α in vitro, and prevalence of IFN-α–resistant variants increases during progression to AIDS (223). The emergence of resistance to IFN-α during HIV disease is an indicator that this cytokine is critical to the overall balance between viral activation and host response; however, whether resistance to IFN-α antecedes or results from disease progression is unclear.

A third category of cytokines can induce or suppress HIV, depending on the ex vivo culture conditions. These include TGF-β, IL-4, IL-10, IL-13, and IFN-γ. The HIV-inductive effect of these cytokines depends on certain factors, including the type of infected cell, whether the cells are primary or in established cultures, and the timing of cytokine treatment relative to HIV infection. For example, IFN-γ upregulates virus expression in T cells in an autocrine manner (224), in primary monocyte/macrophage cultures treated before HIV infection (209), and in chronically infected monocytoid cell lines (225). In contrast, HIV expression was downregulated by IFN-γ when the monocyte/macrophage cultures were pretreated with IFN-γ before HIV infection (209). Likewise, IL-4 can either upregulate or downregulate HIV expression from monocytes, depending on the time of treatment of the cells with the cytokine (226). IL-10 is a pleiotropic cytokine that exhibits both inhibitory and stimulatory activities on mononuclear cells, depending on the concentration of cytokine used. At high concentrations (10 ng/mL) IL-10 blocks HIV replication in vitro by inhibiting the production of the HIV-inducing cytokines TNF-α and IL-6 (227); at lower

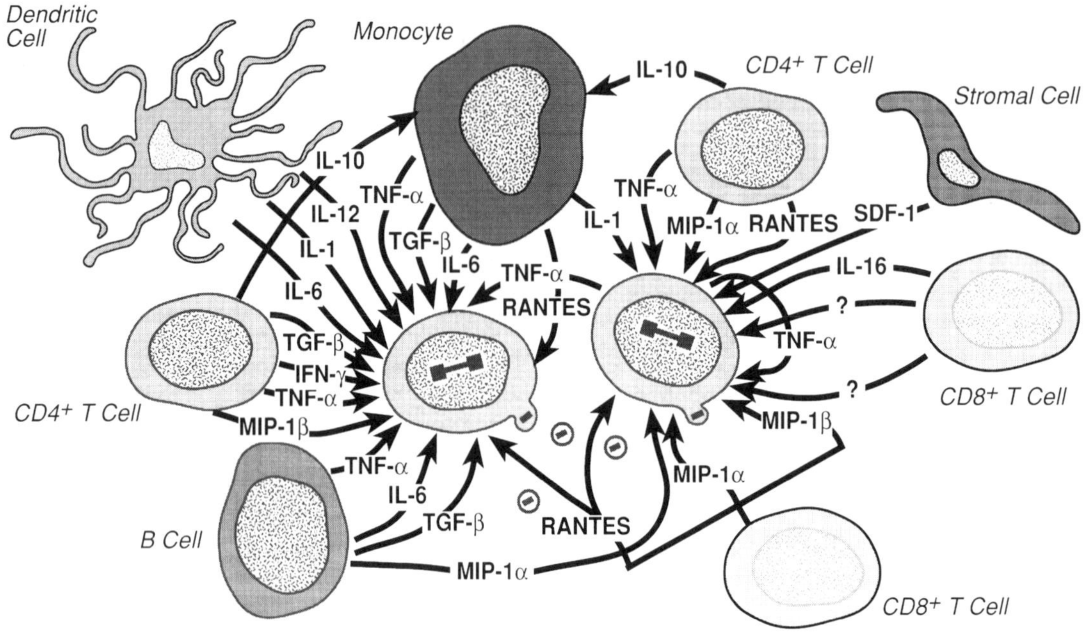

Figure 5.4. Endogenous cytokines regulating viral replication in CD4+ T cells. Numerous cytokines, particularly the proinflammatory cytokines TNF-α, IL-1β, and IL-6, strongly upregulate replication. TGF-β and IL-10 downregulate it. The β-chemokines, which are secreted by various cell types including CD8+ and CD8− mononuclear cells, strongly inhibit infection by M-tropic strains of HIV-1, whereas SDF-1 inhibits infection with T-tropic strains. (Adapted from Fauci AS. Host factors and the pathogenesis of HIV-induced disease. Nature 1996;384:529–534.)

concentrations, IL-10 acts synergistically to enhance HIV-replication induced by other cytokines (228). In vivo administration of a single dose of IL-10 to HIV-infected individuals rendered their PBMCs refractory to LPS-induced cytokine secretion in vitro. In addition, it resulted in a transient decrease (measured in hours) in the levels of plasma viremia that was believed to be due to a transient inhibition of the endogeneous cytokine network that maintains the steady state of virus replication in vivo. IL-10 induced inhibition of cellular activation likely also contributed to this effect (229).

Another cytokine with pleiotropic effects on HIV is TGF-β. This cytokine has been shown to inhibit HIV expression in a chronically infected monocytic cell line stimulated with either phorbol myristate acetate or IL-6 (218). TGF-β has also been reported to have dichotomous effects on HIV replication in primary monocyte/macrophage cultures and can either enhance or inhibit virus production, depending on the conditions (230–232).

In addition to the compelling in vitro data mentioned earlier, a considerable amount of evidence indicates that the delicate balance between HIV-inducing and HIV-suppressing cytokines plays a major role in regulating the net replication of HIV in vivo and thus in affecting the steady-state level of plasma viremia (33) (Fig 5.4). This is clearly seen in studies with IL-2 and IL-10, as well as in studies in which immunization (77–80) and ongoing infections (74–76), which are associated with enhanced expression of HIV-inducing cytokines, profoundly, but transiently, increase the levels of plasma viremia.

Cytokines and Hematopoietic Cells

Endogenous cytokines that are produced by cells within the hematopoietic microenvironment not only affect HIV replication, but also affect the proliferation and differentiation of hematopoietic cells in the bone marrow and thymus by acting locally through close cell-to-cell contact (233). Cytokines have positive or negative regulatory influences on early T-cell development. Cytokines with positive regulatory effects include stem cell factor, also known as c-kit ligand, leukemia inhibitory factor, IL-1, IL-13, IL-6, GM-CSF, erythropoietin, and thrombopoietin. Those with negative regulatory effects include TGF-β, TNF-α, MIP-1α, IFN-α, IFN-β, IFN-γ, and IL-4. In the human thymus, IL-4 and stem cell factor have been implicated as positive regulators of thymopoiesis and lymphoiesis, and some (234), but not all (235), studies indicate that the TGF-β family may negatively regulate the division of intrathymic progenitor T cells. Consequently, HIV infection of the hematolymphoid microenvironment such as bone marrow, fetal liver, or thymus can induce or suppress the expression of these cytokines and can impair hematopoiesis.

In long-term bone marrow cultures, HIV-induced suppressive effects on erythropoiesis and myelopoiesis have been associated with the expression of TNF-α, IL-4, and IFN-α (53, 236). Hematopoietic progenitor cells from HIV-infected patients are more sensitive to the inhibitory effects of these cytokines. (237). Although these events have not been studied within the microenvironment of the bone marrow or thymus, HIV infection of these organs could potentially lead to enhanced secretion of cytokines that are both hematosuppressive and stimulatory to viral replication.

Th1/Th2 Cytokine Patterns

A paradigm involving differential activation of two subsets of CD4+ T-helper (Th) cell clones, Th1 and Th2, with different patterns of cytokine production has been proposed to explain, at least in part, the T-cell dysfunction observed in progressive HIV-related disease (238). In the mouse, Th1-type responses favor strong cellular immunity with normal or increased levels of IL-2, IL-12, and IFN-γ production. Th2 responses result in increased IL-4, IL-5, IL-6, and IL-10 cytokines and promote B-cell differentiation and expansion (238). In the absence of a prominent differentiation to Th1 or Th2 cells, most CD4+ T cells produce both Th1- and Th2-type cytokines and are referred to as Th0 cells (239). This strict Th1/Th2 dichotomy is not observed in humans because other cell types secrete these cytokines, further complicating the issue. The major cytokine facilitator of a Th1 response is IL-12, whereas that of a Th2 response is IL-4. The major cytokine suppressor of a Th1 response is IL-10; the major suppressor of a Th2 response is IFN-γ (240–242). Previous studies have suggested that a "switch" from a Th1 cytokine phenotype to a Th2 phenotype is a critical step in the progression of HIV disease (243, 244). In addition, investigators have observed that Th2 T-cell clones are much more susceptible to HIV infection than are Th1 T-cell clones (245). However, careful analyses of cytokine expression in unfractionated and purified cell populations from peripheral blood and lymph nodes of HIV-infected individuals at different stages of disease have revealed no selective increase in levels of IL-4 and IL-10 gene expression associated with advanced disease (193, 245); IL-10 secretion from macrophages derived from patients at different stages of disease was not increased, as would have been expected in this model (246). Rather, the data demonstrated that HIV can favor a shift to the Th0 phenotype in response to recall antigens and preferentially replicate in CD4+ T cells producing Th2- and Th0-type cytokines (245). The dominant in vivo cytokine responses to HIV infection appear to be an increase in levels of TNF-α, IFN-γ, and IL-6 concomitant with reduced levels of IL-2 as determined by plasma levels and lymph node cytokine patterns (193, 245, 247, 248). Therefore, other than the increased IL-10 gene expression in lymph nodes that has been demonstrated to be sustained from the onset of infection, the specific role of Th2 cytokines in the progression of HIV disease remains unclear (193).

Inhibition of HIV Entry by Chemokines

In addition to the endogenous cytokines that suppress replication of HIV (see earlier), the ability of soluble factors secreted by CD8+ T cells to suppress HIV replication in a noncytolytic manner has been known since the mid-1980s (177, 249, 250); however, the precise identity of these factors remained obscure (251, 252). An important advance in this regard was the observation in 1995 that β-chemokines suppress the binding and entry of M-tropic isolates of HIV into CD4+T cells. β-Chemokines are structurally related peptides that exhibit potent leukocyte activation and chemotactic activity. They are characterized by two linked cysteine residues without an intervening amino acid (C-C). Three β-chemokines, RANTES, MIP-1α, and MIP-1β, inhibited the replication of M-tropic isolates in lymphocytes from uninfected donors or T-cell lines (164). Similarly, SDF-1, inhibited binding and fusion with T-tropic isolates of HIV (27, 28). SDF-1 is an α-chemokine characterized by an intervening amino acid between the two cysteine residues (C-X-C).

The suppressor activity of β-chemokines is mostly restricted to HIV entry in CD4+ T cells. A cocktail of neutralizing antibodies against the three chemokines abrogated the inhibitory activity of the three chemokines in cultures of PBMCs, but not macrophages that were infected with M-tropic HIV. In contrast, a soluble CD8+ T-cell supernatant suppressed infection of M-tropic and T-tropic HIV in PBMCs and M-tropic HIV in macrophages (253). Furthermore, antibodies to the β-chemokines could not abrogate completely the inhibitory effects of a CD8+ T-cell supernatant on infection of PBMCs with an M-tropic virus (254). In summary, these data indicate that CD8+ T cells produce factors that are capable of suppressing HIV. Some of these factors, as yet unidentified, inhibit the replication of M-tropic as well as T-tropic viruses in both macrophage and T cells, and they appear to inhibit HIV-replication after viral integration (253). In contrast, β-chemokines, which are secreted by both CD4+ and CD8+ T cells, suppress replication of M-tropic viruses only in CD4+ T cells by inhibiting the viral entry process.

DEPLETION AND DYSFUNCTION OF CD4+ T CELLS

The loss of CD4+ T cells is the central immunologic abnormality of HIV infection and is largely responsible for the profound immunodeficiency characteristic of late stages of the disease. In infected individuals, the rate of CD4+ T-cell loss reflects the balance between ongoing cell destruction and an inadequate repopulation from progenitor cells.

CD4+ T cells may be lost through several potential mechanisms, both direct and indirect. Infected cells may be depleted through direct cytopathic effects of the virus, by virus-specific CTLs, or by antibody-dependent cell mediated cytotoxicity (ADCC) (255, 256). CTL lysis of infected cells is mediated by both CD8+ or CD4+ lymphocytes and is directed at processed viral antigens expressed on the cell surface in the context of MHC class I or class II molecules. ADCC is mediated by natural killer (NK) cells through Fc receptor binding of specific antiviral antibodies. In ADCC, the viral antigen does not have to be endogenously produced or processed, but merely expressed on the surface of the cell. The specificity is at the level of the antibody, not at the level of the cytolytic effector cell. In this regard, several recent studies have provided compelling evidence for the destruction of uninfected CD4+ T cells that have bound free circulating HIV antigens (257, 258). In addition, uninfected cells may be destroyed as a result of cell-to-cell fusion and the formation of syncytia (259, 260). Binding of gp120 to CD4 also interferes with the function of these cells and renders them susceptible to apoptosis induced by cross-linking of CD4 by gp120 (Table 5.1). Although all these mechanisms operate in vitro, their precise pathogenic significance in vivo is unclear. The prominent mechanisms for CD4+ T-cell loss are discussed in the following sections.

HIV-Mediated Direct Cytopathicity

Some virally induced cytopathic effects operate on single infected cells and directly induce their death (261, 262). One explanation for direct cytopathicity of the virus is an accumulation of unintegrated viral DNA in the cell. However, recent data show no association between the accumulation of unintegrated HIV DNA and single cell killing (263, 264). This has led to increased speculation that HIV-induced single cell killing involves interactions between the envelope protein and the CD4 molecule. In productively infected CD4+ lymphoblasts, both gp160 and CD4 are synthesized in the rough endoplasmic reticulum, where an opportunity for intracellular interaction of newly synthesized gp160 and CD4 molecules exists (265). This interaction can have two effects: cellular toxicity as a consequence of the gp160–CD4 binding (266); and intracellular sequestration of CD4 molecules resulting in a decreased surface expression of CD4 (267, 268). The resulting absence of CD4 on the cell membrane could impair MHC class II–CD4 interactions, a requisite step in antigen-specific responses (see later).

In other studies, the envelope protein has been directly implicated in HIV-induced cytopathic effects by initiating autofusion events that disrupt cell membrane integrity, leading to single cell death (266, 269, 270). In one study, serial passage of an HIV isolate in a cell line led to isolation of an HIV variant with a reduced ability to mediate single cell killing (271). A detailed molecular analysis of envelope has localized cytopathic determinants to both gp120 and gp41 subunits (256, 271, 272). Amino acid mutagenesis of this region led to a loss of syncytium formation and single cell killing without affecting viral replication.

HIV-Mediated Syncytia Formation

The interaction of noninfected CD4+ T cells with HIV-expressing cells in syncytia also provides a mechanism for depletion of uninfected cells. In some experimental systems, cell-to-cell fusion occurs between infected cells expressing HIV envelope protein and uninfected cells expressing CD4, leading to the formation of giant multinucleated cells or syncytia (259, 260, 273). Cell adhesion molecules such as leukocyte functional antigen 1 (LFA-1) also appear to play a role in facilitating syncytium formation; anti–LFA-1 antibodies block syncytium formation (274, 275).

A direct relation between the presence of syncytia and the cytopathicity of the virus in individual cells has been demonstrated in vitro (276–278), and HIV isolated from patients during advanced disease has a greater capacity to induce syncytia in vitro (278–280). Although abundant in vitro data support syncytia formation as a mechanism of CD4+ T-cell loss, in studies of lymph nodes and spleen from infected individuals, giant cells are observed only rarely (281). Thus, the pathogenic relevance of this mechanism in vivo remains unclear.

HIV-Specific Cytotoxic T Lymphocytes

HIV-specific CTLs that are both MHC class I (CD8+ CTLs) and MHC class II (CD4+ CTLs) restricted have been identified. Although CD8+ CTLs play an important role in the early control of HIV replication and spread (105, 106), their levels wane with the onset of AIDS (282). HIV-specific CD8+ CTLs may also play a role in the immunopathogenesis of HIV infection by contributing to the depletion of HIV-infected antigen-presenting cells and infected CD4+ T cells, as well as through immunopathologic damage to lymphoid tissue as a result of the secretion of proinflammatory cytokines (283). In addition to CD8+ CTLs, precursors of CD4+ CTLs have also been identified in peripheral blood of HIV-infected individuals (284) and in noninfected persons who have been immunized with recombinant gp160 (285). The in vivo relevance of CD4+ CTLs for the control of HIV infection is unclear.

Antibody-Dependent Cellular Cytotoxicity

Noninfected CD4+ T cells in the vicinity of productively infected cells may absorb sufficient amounts of soluble gp120, which is or becomes bound to anti-gp120 antibodies and become susceptible to destruction by an ADCC mechanism mediated by NK cells (286). Previous studies have demonstrated that uninfected CD4+ T cells incubated with purified gp120 could be destroyed by ADCC in the presence of anti-gp120 antibodies (287). The extent to which this mechanism contributes to CD4+ T-cell depletion in vivo is unknown. In addition, the quantity of free, circulating gp120

Table 5.1. Potential Mechanisms of CD4+ T-Lymphocyte Dysfunction/Depletion in HIV Infection

HIV-mediated direct cytopathicity (single-cell killing)
HIV-mediated syncytia formation
Virus-specific immune responses:
    HIV-specific cytolytic T lymphocytes
    Antibody-dependent cellular cytotoxicity
    Natural killer cells
Autoimmune mechanisms
Superantigen-mediated pertubation of T-cell subsets
Apoptosis

(Adapted from Pantaleo G, Graziosi C, Fauci AS. The immunopathogenesis of human immunodeficiency virus infection. N Engl J Med 1993; 328:327–335.)

and anti-gp120 antibodies that block monomer gp120 binding to CD4 and the potential impairment of the CD16+-expressing, NK population during disease progression are factors that would affect the role of this pathway.

Autoimmune Mechanisms

Envelope glycoprotein subunits (gp120 and gp41) and MHC class II molecules share some degree of antigenic homology and can bind to the CD4 molecule. Investigators have postulated that antibodies to envelope could potentially cross-react with common determinants on MHC class II antigens, thus impairing antigen processing, presentation, and helper CD4+ T-cell functions (288). The sera of HIV-infected individuals have been shown to contain various anti-lymphocyte antibodies that can cross-react with viral proteins. For example, antibodies that cross-react with both gp41 and MHC class II molecules (289), as well as antibodies that recognize common determinants on IL-2 and HIV envelope protein (290), have been observed. Autoantibodies have also been reported against antigens on platelets and neutrophils (291, 292) and the partially sialylated form of CD43 on normal human thymocytes (293). A sequence homology between the MHC class I determinants and envelope protein has also been observed (294). Thus, antigenic homology between viral and host cell proteins could result in the immunologic destruction of uninfected CD4+ T cells by the HIV-induced immune response (295, 296).

Superantigen-Mediated Perturbation of T-Cell Subsets

Superantigens are proteins that activate entire subsets of T cells by binding to a specific variable (V) region of the β chain (β) of the TCR (297). The TCR is composed of an α and β chain, each of which is divided into variable and constant region gene segments encoded by different exons (298, 299). The variable gene segments of the TCR α and β chains are divided into families; these are 29 Vα and 24 Vβ families (300). Superantigens can stimulate and activate large numbers of T cells by binding only to the V region of the β chain in association with binding to the β chain of the MHC class II molecule. In addition, superantigens do not require processing for T-cell stimulation; they bind as intact molecules to a site on the MHC class II molecule that is outside the peptide binding groove, thus circumventing the antigen processing pathway for T-cell recognition (301). Because of this less restricted specificity of superantigens, they can induce massive stimulation and expansion of all those T cells bearing specific β-chain regions potentially leading to anergy and deletion. By contrast, conventional antigens specifically interact with particular components of the V, diversity (D) and joining (J) regions of the TCR α and β chains. This restricted specificity permits stimulation of only a small fraction of T cells.

In one published study of AIDS patients, a specific deletion in certain Vβ subsets was demonstrated, whereas asymptomatic HIV-infected patients showed no differences in the pattern of expression of their TCR Vβ regions (302). However, these results have not been corroborated (303). A different study in monozygotic twins discordant for HIV infection provided direct evidence for specific perturbation in the Vβ13 and Vβ21 families expressed in CD4+ T cells in the HIV-infected twin. This latter study is of particular relevance because the observed perturbations in the Vβ families cannot be attributed to the effects of HLA or other loci on the expressed TCR (304). Yet another study has shown HIV to replicate more efficiently in Vβ12 cells (305). This same subset specifically proliferated in response to cells from HIV-positive patients, suggesting the presence of a Vβ12-directed superantigen.

No convincing evidence indicates that the HIV genome encodes a superantigen that may be responsible for the induction of T-cell anergy or deletion. More likely, the virus exerts a superantigen-like effect by activating T-cell subsets, rendering them susceptible to viral infection (see earlier). Superantigens present in other opportunistic organisms possibly also could play a role in HIV disease pathogenesis; for example, a gene product of cytomegalovirus enhanced replication of HIV in the Vβ12 subset (306).

Apoptosis

Apoptosis is a regulated mechanism of cell death that is critical to organogenesis as well as to various physiologic processes (307). It is important in the development of the immune system and in the maintenance of normal immune function (307). It is characterized by activation of a family of proteolytic enzymes, nuclear condensation, and DNA fragmentation. Apoptosis does not require direct infection of the cell; rather, cross-linking of the CD4 molecule by gp120 or gp120 immunocomplexes, followed by conventional antigen or superantigen activation of the TCR, can initiate this process. Activation signals are inherent to the process of apoptosis. Besides priming a cell for apoptosis, other immunologic repercussions of the gp120–CD4 interaction include aberrant immune activation resulting in cytokine secretion and lymphocyte anergy or resistance to subsequent stimulation by the TCR (308, 309).

Early studies demonstrated that activated or immortalized CD4+ T cells infected with HIV in culture undergo apoptosis (310, 311). CD4+ T cells from HIV-seronegative individuals undergo apoptosis in vitro if the CD4 antigen is bound by gp120 immune complexes and the cells are subsequently activated (310). Apoptosis is also an important mechanism in the loss of progenitor cells in vitro. When purified uninfected CD34+ cells are exposed to HIV or to recombinant gp120, apoptosis is induced, and a reduction in the number of colony-forming cells is observed in the absence of viral infection (49, 312, 313). In addition, the presence of viral peptides that can be presented to developing T cells through MHC molecules may lead to tolerance or anergy in the developing cells and may contribute further to the immune dysfunction associated with HIV infection. Additional in vitro studies have demonstrated that apoptosis also occurs in CD4+ and CD8+ T cells in HIV-infected adults (314–319), and the level of apoptosis measured in vitro is apparently related to the general state of immune activation and does not correlate with the clinical stage of disease progression or with viral burden (314, 320).

In vivo, apoptosis has been demonstrated in lymphoid tissue of infected individuals (314), in human neonates, and in SIV-infected macaques (257), as well as in models of HIV pathogenesis such as human thymic transplants in SCID-hu mice (54–56). Studies in lymph node tissues from children and macaques infected perinatally with HIV or SIV, respectively (257), have demonstrated that productively infected cells are resistant to apoptosis, and the uninfected or bystander CD4+ and CD8+ T cells are killed in HIV and SIV infection. Supporting the notion that HIV-infected cells are resistant to apoptosis is the observation that, in cocultures of DCs and memory T cells, apoptosis occurs in noninfected CD4+ T cells (321).

Examination of the molecular mechanisms in apoptosis has revealed the importance of Fas antigen in the induction of apoptosis (322–325). Fas antigen is a cell-surface molecule designated CD95. When CD95 interacts with Fas ligand, it induces apoptosis without affecting viral replication. Recent experiments have shown that the Fas antigen is upregulated (309) in peripheral blood CD4+ T cells in which the CD4 molecules are cross-linked and induced to apoptosis in the absence of a secondary TCR activation signal (319).

Lymphocyte Regeneration

As discussed earlier, HIV infection of progenitor cells and the disruption of the hematopoietic microenvironment may diminish the regenerative capacity of the CD4+ T-cell pool (54). Another possibility is that the rapid proliferation of mature lymphocytes may also exhaust their renewal ability (326). Measurement of telomere length has been used to monitor turnover of CD4+ naive and memory lymphocytes; this technique has been demonstrated to provide an indication of the extent of replication of the cell population (326). Telomeres consist of long hexameric repeats at the ends of chromosomes; they serve a role in in chromosome protection, positioning, and replication (327). In normal somatic cells, the chromosomes lose approximately 100 nucleotides per cell division because of the inability of DNA polymerase to replicate the ends of linear DNA (328–330). By measuring the mean terminal restriction fragment length of the telomere, investigators have shown that telomeres in both naive and memory lymphocytes shorten with age, a finding suggesting that both populations are turning over. New data show that the mean terminal restriction fragment length of CD8+ T cells is shorter in HIV-infected individuals than noninfected individuals, indicating that these cells have undergone increased cell divisions (331, 332). However, no significant changes were noted in the CD4+ cells; this unexpected result requires further study, given the assumptions of the high rate of CD4+ T-cell turnover in HIV infection (333–336).

Investigators have demonstrated that naive CD4+ and CD8+ lymphocytes exhibiting the CD45RA+CD62L+ phenotype are preferentially lost during the course of HIV infection in adults and children (337, 338). The depletion of this population of cells could progressively impair the ability of the infected host to mount immune responses to new antigens. In examining the lymphocyte changes in vivo in individuals followed longitudinally in the Multicenter AIDS Cohort Study (MACS), investigators observed that whereas CD4+ T cells are lost, CD8+ lymphocytes increase in a seemingly compensatory fashion, resulting in a constant level of total T cells without regard to whether the cells express a CD4+ or CD8+ phenotype; this compensation persists until the advanced stage of disease (339). This phenomenon has been termed T-cell homeostasis (340). Investigators have hypothesized that lymphocyte numbers are maintained through the regulation of total CD3+ T-cell number; as CD4+ cells are destroyed by HIV, they are replenished with both CD4+ and CD8+ T cells (339). Such a process would lead to the more pronounced depletion of CD4+ T cells and loss of the biologic functions associated with that subset.

Nature of T-Cell Dysfunctions in HIV Infection

Infection of CD4+ T cells leads to numeric depletion of this population as well as to impaired immune function of surviving cells. HIV infection of hematopoietic cells alters the function of these cells and leads to impaired differentiation and proliferation and to reduced colony-forming capacity (341–343). By analyzing the in vitro proliferative capacities of infected CD4+ memory T cells, a diminished response to recall antigens (i.e., tetanus toxoid and influenza virus peptides), mitogens, anti-CD3 antibodies, and HLA self-restricted alloantigens was observed (233, 344). In addition, defective IL-2 and IL-2 receptor production (345), defective T-cell colony formation, and impairment of the autologous mixed lymphocyte reaction were observed (346) (Table 5.2). These dysfunctions are not due to an impairment of antigen-presenting cells because identical results were obtained in the absence of monocytes (347) or when using cells from identical twins who were discordant for HIV-infection (348). HIV-infection of CD4+ T cells has also been reported to decrease expression of CD4 as a result of intracellular complexing of CD4 with gp120 or by direct inhibition of CD4 biosynthesis (267, 268). A reduction in CD4 expression on the cell surface may, in turn, impair the MHC class II–CD4 interactions that are necessary for antigen-specific responses.

Quantitative and functional defects in CD8+ T cells have also been observed as disease progresses (349, 350). The reasons for these abnormalities are unknown and are likely to be multifactorial, including diminished CD4+ T-helper cell functions and IL-2 production and a failure to regenerate from progenitor cells. The broad cytolytic effector mechanisms of CD8+ CTLs in AIDS patients are intact (349), but a defect is noted in the clonal expansion of precursor anti-HIV CTLs into mature populations (351). CD8+ T cells also exhibit elevated levels of certain activation markers that

Table 5.2. Lymphocyte Dysfunctions in HIV-Infected Individuals

CD4+ T cells
  Defects in:
    T-cell colony formation
    Autologous mixed lymphocyte reactions
    IL-2 receptor production
    IL-2 receptor expression
    Diminished proliferation to recall antigens, anti-CD3 antibodies, alloantigens, mitogens
CD8+ cells
  Deficiency in MHC-restricted CTL function
  Impaired clonogenic ability
B cells
  Aberrant polyclonal and oligoclonal activation

are prognostic for disease progression (163). In addition to the defective anti-HIV CTLs, functional defects in other CD8+ CTLs directed at influenza and CMV antigens have also been demonstrated (352, 353).

B-CELL DYSFUNCTIONS

B cells from HIV-infected individuals are polyclonally activated even early in disease (354); antigen-specific and nonspecific B-cell responses are impaired in HIV-infected patients probably as a result of this spontaneous hyperactivity. The generalized B-cell hyperactivity is thought to contribute to lymph node hyperplasia in HIV infection (355). Some of the features of B-cell hyperactivity include elevated serum immunoglobulin levels, increased spontaneous overproduction of immunoglobulins, decreased production of immunoglobulin in response to pokeweed in the presence of adequate T-helper activity (356), and increased secretion of the proinflammatory cyotokines TNF-α and IL-6, as well as increased spontaneous transformation of B cells by Epstein–Barr virus and a higher incidence of non–Hodgkin's lymphoma (357). A decrease in the level of circulating B cells early in the course of infection that becomes more pronounced as disease progresses has also been reported (358) (see Table 5.2). One potential explanation for this depletion is the observation that a subset of B cells expresses the heavy-chain variable region, VH3, that functions as a cellular receptor for gp120 resulting in viral binding, cellular proliferation, and subsequent depletion of B cells bearing VH3 (359).

Although HIV does not appear to infect normal, untransformed B cells, some of the functional abnormalities of B cells in HIV-infected individuals can be mimicked in vitro by exposing B cells to intact virus or viral proteins. For example, the carboxyl terminal end of gp41 was capable of polyclonally activating B cells, achieving levels of proliferation and immunoglobulin production comparable to those of other B-cell mitogens (360). Significant numbers of circulating B cells from HIV-infected individuals at all stages of infection spontaneously secrete antibodies against HIV antigens, principally envelope, but also Gag and Pol proteins (361–364). Thus, abnormal B-cell function in HIV infection may in part result from HIV-induced spontaneous activation of these cells and subsequent failure of these chronically stimulated cells to respond to specific activation signals (365, 366).

NATURAL KILLER CELL DYSFUNCTIONS

NK cells bear surface receptors for the FcR portion of IgG. They lyse certain tumor cell lines or virally infected cells. One mechanism of NK-mediated cytolysis is ADCC. Some HIV-infected individuals express a defect in NK cell function early in the course of disease that is magnified as disease progresses (367). Investigators have reported a selective depletion of a CD16+ CD56+ CD8+ subset of NK cells during HIV infection (368) and a reciprocal elevation of a subset of NK cells expressing the CD16+ CD56– phenotype with low lytic activity in infected individuals when compared with uninfected individuals (369). Some reports have suggested that NK cells in HIV-infected patients exhibit reduced non–MHC-restricted cytotoxicity to various target cells because of the presence of autoantibodies complexed with the surface receptors on these cells; the presence of these autoantibodies can disrupt the normal function of NK cells (370) (Table 5.3). However, most reports indicate that NK cells mediate cytolysis normally in HIV infection (371, 372).

Incubation with IL-2 (373), IL-12 (374), or mitogens enhances NK cell function in cells from HIV-infected individuals, a finding suggesting that NK cells from these subjects are not intrinsically defective but lack the appropriate inductive signals. Probably, both a numeric depletion of this population and the absence of appropriate signals from CD4+ T cells contribute to the observed NK abnormalities in vivo. A consequence of reduced NK cell function may be a reduced capacity to provide protection of the host against viral pathogens.

MONOCYTE/MACROPHAGE DYSFUNCTIONS

HIV infection of macrophages in vitro significantly impairs several aspects of their function. Phagocytic ability against certain opportunistic pathogens is diminished, as are chemotactic and antigen presentation functions. Fc receptor function, oxidative burst responses, and tumor surveillance

Table 5.3. Dysfunctions in Other Immune-Competent Cells in HIV-Infected Individuals

Monocyte/macrophages
  Defects in:
    Chemotaxis
    Fc-receptor function
    C3-receptor–mediated clearance
    Oxidative burst responses
Dendritic cells
  Defects in:
    Antigen presentation
    T-cell proliferation
Natural killer cells
  Defects in:
    Release of NK cytotoxic factors

are also decreased (73, 375). HIV-infected macrophages exhibit an altered profile of cytokine secretion with higher levels of IL-1β, IL-6, IL-8, and TNF-α and lower amounts of IL-12 (376). The decreased antigen-presenting function may be a result of interference with expression of accessory molecules (377) (see Table 5.3). In the early stages of HIV infection, monocytic functions are preserved (378); however, monocytes isolated from symptomatic and long-term asymptomatic HIV-infected persons appear to be defective in monocyte-dependent systems of T-cell proliferation (379). Mounting evidence indicates that HIV-infected macrophages and microglia play a role in the pathogenesis of HIV-related encephalopathy and AIDS–dementia complex (ADC). HIV-infected macrophages can be readily visualized in the brain and spinal cord of patients with ADC and vacuolar myelopathy, a finding linking productive viral replication within macrophages and tissue disorders.

DENDRITIC CELL DYSFUNCTIONS

Considerable disagreement exists concerning the degree of infectability of DCs by HIV (81, 88), nonetheless, DCs appear to play a significant role in HIV pathogenesis. Several studies performed on DCs derived from peripheral blood of infected individuals show up to 20% of cells expressing the HIV provirus (380), with depletion of a subpopulation of DCs (380, 381). Certain studies suggest that antigen-presenting abilities of DCs are also deficient and are attributable to HIV infection of the DCs (380). Other studies, however, show only rare infection of DCs and have observed neither a selective depletion of DCs nor a decrease in antigen-presenting function (382). Tissue-derived LCs isolated from cadaveric skins of AIDS patients show approximately 1% infectivity (383). LCs were also deficient in their capacity to stimulate T-cell proliferation (384) (see Table 5.3).

Although the central role of DCs in AIDS pathogenesis is apparent, the extent of DC-associated viral burden and the levels of productive infection remain controversial. The discrepancies among various published studies may reflect the existence of different populations of cells with dendritic morphology, only some of which are infectable with HIV (88), different methods of purifying and culturing DCs, and the possibility of laboratory contamination by T cells.

CONCLUSION

The pathogenic mechanisms of HIV disease are multifaceted and multifactorial; they involve both virologic and host factors. Paramount among host factors are the HIV-specific immune responses that play a major role in the containment of HIV replication. However, certain immunologic responses paradoxically contribute to the propagation of HIV replication. For example, although HIV-induced activation of the immune system is essential for triggering HIV-specific immune responses, it also leads to a favorable milieu for virus replication. In this regard, the complex network of immunoregulatory and proinflammatory cytokines, which are closely linked to the state of immune activation, are critical in modulating the steady state of HIV replication. Nonspecific host factors, several of which are genetically determined, also play a major role in the pathogenesis of HIV disease. Delineation of these complex mechanisms is important for the design of therapeutic and vaccine strategies.

References

1. Barre-Sinoussi F, Chermann JC, Rey F, et al. Isolation of a T-lymphotropic retrovirus from a patient at risk for acquired immune deficiency syndrome (AIDS). Science 1983;220:868–871.
2. Gallo RC, Salahuddin SZ, Popovic M, et al. Frequent detection and isolation of cytopathic retroviruses (HTLV-III) from patients with AIDS and at risk for AIDS. Science 1984;224:500–503.
3. Neumann M, Harrison J, Saltarelli M, et al. Splicing variability in HIV type 1 revealed by quantitative RNA polymerase chain reaction. AIDS Res Hum Retroviruses 1994;10:1531–1542.
4. Dalgleish AG, Beverley PC, Clapham PR, et al. The CD4 (T4) antigen is an essential component of the receptor for the AIDS retrovirus. Nature 1984;312:763–767.
5. Klatzmann D, Champagne E, Chamaret S, et al. T-lymphocyte T4 molecule behaves as the receptor for human retrovirus LAV. Nature 1984;312:767–768.
6. Maddon PJ, Dalgleish AG, McDougal JS, et al. The T4 gene encodes the AIDS virus receptor and is expressed in the immune system and the brain. Cell 1986;47:333–348.
7. Feng Y, Broder CC, Kennedy PE, et al. HIV-1 entry cofactor: functional cDNA cloning of a seven-transmembrane, G protein-coupled receptor. Science 1996;272:872–877.
8. Dragic T, Litwin V, Allaway GP, et al. HIV-1 entry into CD4+ cells is mediated by the chemokine receptor CC-CKR-5. Nature 1996;381:667–673.
9. Doranz BJ, Rucker J, Yi Y, et al. A dual-tropic primary HIV-1 isolate that uses fusin and the beta-chemokine receptors CKR-5, CKR-3, and CKR-2b as fusion cofactors. Cell 1996;85:1149–1158.
10. Choe H, Farzan M, Sun Y, et al. The beta-chemokine receptors CCR3 and CCR5 facilitate infection by primary HIV-1 isolates. Cell 1996; 85:1135–1148.
11. Alkhatib G, Combadiere C, Broder CC, et al. CC CKR5: a RANTES, MIP-1alpha, MIP-1beta receptor as a fusion cofactor for macrophage-tropic HIV-1. Science 1996;272:1955–278.
12. Deng H, Liu R, Ellmeier W, et al. Identification of a major co-receptor for primary isolates of HIV-1. Nature 1996;381:661–666.
13. Fauci AS. Multifactorial nature of human immunodeficiency virus disease: implications for therapy. Science 1993;262:1011–1018.
14. Gay D, Maddon P, Sekaly R, et al. Functional interaction between human T-cell protein CD4 and the major histocompatibility complex HLA-DR antigen. Nature 1987;328:626–629.
15. Doyle C, Strominger JL. Interaction between CD4 and class II MHC molecules mediates cell adhesion. Nature 1987;330:256–259.
16. Allan JS, Coligan JE, Barin F, et al. Major glycoprotein antigens that induce antibodies in AIDS patients are encoded by HTLV-III. Science 1985;228:1091–1094.
17. Veronese FD, DeVico AL, Copeland TD, et al. Characterization of gp41 as the transmembrane protein coded by the HTLV-III/LAV envelope gene. Science 1985;229:1402–1405.
18. Willey RL, Bonifacino JS, Potts BJ, et al. Biosynthesis, cleavage, and degradation of the human immunodeficiency virus 1 envelope glycoprotein gp160. Proc Natl Acad Sci U S A 1988;85:9580–9584.
19. Sattentau QJ, Moore JP. The role of CD4 in HIV binding and entry. Philos Trans R Soc Lond Biol 1993;342:59–66.
20. Broder CC, Dimitrov DS, Blumenthal R, et al. The block to HIV-1 envelope glycoprotein-mediated membrane fusion in animal cells expressing human CD4 can be overcome by a human cell component(s). Virology 1993;193:483–491.

21. Dragic T, Charneau P, Clavel F, et al. Complementation of murine cells for human immunodeficiency virus envelope/CD4–mediated fusion in human/murine heterokaryons. J Virol 1992;66:4794–4802.
22. Neote K, DiGregorio D, Mak JY, et al. Molecular cloning, functional expression, and signaling characteristics of a C-C chemokine receptor. Cell 1993;72:415–425.
23. Gao JL, Kuhns DB, Tiffany HL, et al. Structure and functional expression of the human macrophage inflammatory protein 1 alpha/RANTES receptor. J Exp Med 1993;177:1421–1427.
24. Bacon KB, Premack BA, Gardner P, et al. Activation of dual T cell signaling pathways by the chemokine RANTES. Science 1995;269:1727–1730.
25. Raport CJ, Schweickart VL, Chantry D, et al. New members of the chemokine receptor gene family. J Leukoc Biol 1996;59:18–23.
26. Wells TN, Power CA, Lusti-Narasimhan M, et al. Selectivity and antagonism of chemokine receptors. J Leukoc Biol 1996;59:53–60.
27. Bleul CC, Farzan M, Choe H, et al. The lymphocyte chemoattractant SDF-1 is a ligand for LESTR/fusin and blocks HIV-1 entry. Nature 1996;382:829–833.
28. Oberlin E, Amara A, Bachelerie F, et al. The CXC chemokine SDF-1 is the ligand for LESTR/fusin and prevents infection by T cell line-adapted HIV-1. Nature 1996;382:833–835.
29. Liu R, Paxton WA, Choe S, et al. Homozygous defect in HIV-1 coreceptor accounts for resistance of some multiply-exposed individuals to HIV-1 infection. Cell 1996;86:367–377.
30. Samson M, Libert F, Doranz BJ, et al. Resistance to HIV-1 infection in caucasian individuals bearing mutant alleles of the CCR-5 chemokine receptor gene. Nature 1996;382:722–725.
31. Dean M, Carrington M, Winkler C, et al. Genetic restriction of HIV-1 infection and progression to AIDS by a deletion allele of the CKR5 structural gene: Hemophilia Growth and Development Study, Multicenter AIDS Cohort Study, Multicenter Hemophilia Cohort Study, San Francisco City Cohort, ALIVE Study. Science 1996;273:1856–1862.
32. Biti R, Ffrench R, Young J, et al. HIV-1 Infection in an individual homozygous for the CCR5 deletion allelle. Nat Med 1997;3:252–253.
33. Fauci AS. Host factors and the pathogenesis of HIV-induced disease. Nature 1996;384:529–534.
34. D'Souza MP, Harden VA. Chemokines and HIV-1 second receptors. Confluence of two fields generates optimism in AIDS research. Nat Med 1996;2:1293–1300.
35. Schnittman SM, Psallidopoulos MC, Lane HC, et al. The reservoir for HIV-1 in human peripheral blood is a T cell that maintains expression of CD4 [published erratum appears in Science 1989;245:preceding 694]. Science 1989;245:305–308.
36. McDougal JS, Kennedy MS, Sligh JM, et al. Binding of HTLV-III/LAV to T4+ T cells by a complex of the 110K viral protein and the T4 molecule. Science 1986;231:382–385.
37. Zon LI, Arkin C, Groopman JE. Haematologic manifestations of the human immune deficiency virus (HIV). Br J Haematol 1987;66:251–256.
38. Terstappen LW, Loken MR. Myeloid cell differentiation in normal bone marrow and acute myeloid leukemia assessed by multidimensional flow cytometry. Anal Cell Pathol 1990;2:229–240.
39. Haynes BF, Heinly CS. Early human T cell development: analysis of the human thymus at the time of initial entry of hematopoietic stem cells into the fetal thymic microenvironment. J Exp Med 1995;181:1445–1458.
40. Owen JJ, Jenkinson EJ. Early events in T lymphocyte genesis in the fetal thymus. Am J Anat 1984;170:301–310.
41. Tjonnfjord GE, Veiby OP, Steen R, et al. T lymphocyte differentiation in vitro from adult human prethymic CD34+ bone marrow cells. J Exp Med 1993;177:1531–1539.
42. Patel DD, Hale LP, Haynes BF. HIV in lymph node and thymus. In: Gupta S, ed. Immunology of HIV infection. New York: Plenum, 1996:95–121.
43. Folks TM, Kessler SW, Orenstein JM, et al. Infection and replication of HIV-1 in purified progenitor cells of normal human bone marrow. Science 1988;242:919–922.
44. Schnittman SM, Denning SM, Greenhouse JJ, et al. Evidence for susceptibility of intrathymic T-cell precursors and their progeny carrying T-cell antigen receptor phenotypes TCR alpha beta + and TCR gamma delta + to human immunodeficiency virus infection: a mechanism for CD4+ (T4) lymphocyte depletion. Proc Natl Acad Sci U S A 1990;87:7727–7731.
45. Stanley SK, Kessler SW, Justement JS, et al. CD34+ bone marrow cells are infected with HIV in a subset of seropositive individuals. J Immunol 1992;149:689–697.
46. Molina JM, Scadden DT, Sakaguchi M, et al. Lack of evidence for infection of or effect on growth of hematopoietic progenitor cells after in vivo or in vitro exposure to human immunodeficiency virus. Blood 1990;76:2476–2482.
47. Davis BR, Schwartz DH, Marx JC, et al. Absent or rare human immunodeficiency virus infection of bone marrow stem/progenitor cells in vivo. J Virol 1991;65:1985–1990.
48. De Luca A, Teofili L, Antinori A, et al. Haemopoietic CD34+ progenitor cells are not infected by HIV-1 in vivo but show impaired clonogenesis. Br J Haematol 1993;85:20–24.
49. Louache F, Henri A, Bettaieb A, et al. Role of human immunodeficiency virus replication in defective in vitro growth of hematopoietic progenitors. Blood 1992;80:2991–2999.
50. von Laer D, Hufert FT, Fenner TE, et al. CD34+ hematopoietic progenitor cells are not a major reservoir of the human immunodeficiency virus. Blood 1990;76:1281–1286.
51. Scadden DT, Zeira M, Woon A, et al. Human immunodeficiency virus infection of human bone marrow stromal fibroblasts. Blood 1990;76:317–322.
52. Zauli G, Re MC, Davis B, et al. Impaired in vitro growth of purified (CD34+) hematopoietic progenitors in human immunodeficiency virus-1 seropositive thrombocytopenic individuals. Blood 1992;79:2680–2687.
53. Schwartz GN, Kessler SW, Rothwell SW, et al. Inhibitory effects of HIV-1–infected stromal cell layers on the production of myeloid progenitor cells in human long-term bone marrow cultures [published erratum appears in Exp Hematol 1995;23:181]. Exp Hematol 1994;22:1288–1296.
54. Stanley SK, McCune JM, Kaneshima H, et al. Human immunodeficiency virus infection of the human thymus and disruption of the thymic microenvironment in the SCID-hu mouse. J Exp Med 1993;178:1151–1163.
55. Bonyhadi ML, Rabin L, Salimi S, et al. HIV induces thymus depletion in vivo. Nature 1993;363:728–732.
56. Aldrovandi GM, Feuer G, Gao L, et al. The SCID-hu mouse as a model for HIV-1 infection. Nature 1993;363:732–736.
57. Poli G, Fauci AS. The role of monocyte/macrophages and cytokines in the pathogenesis of HIV infection. Pathobiology 1992;60:246–251.
58. Crowe S, Mills J, McGrath MS. Quantitative immunocytofluorographic analysis of CD4 surface antigen expression and HIV infection of human peripheral blood monocyte/macrophages. AIDS Res Hum Retroviruses 1987;3:135–145.
59. Gartner S, Markovits P, Markovitz DM, et al. The role of mononuclear phagocytes in HTLV-III/LAV infection. Science 1986;233:215–219.
60. Meltzer MS, Nakamura M, Hansen BD, et al. Macrophages as susceptible targets for HIV infection, persistent viral reservoirs in tissue, and key immunoregulatory cells that control levels of virus replication and extent of disease. AIDS Res Hum Retroviruses 1990;6:967–971.
61. Orenstein JM, Meltzer MS, Phipps T, et al. Cytoplasmic assembly and accumulation of human immunodeficiency virus types 1 and 2 in recombinant human colony-stimulating factor-1–treated human monocytes: an ultrastructural study. J Virol 1988;62:2578–2586.
62. Genis P, Jett M, Bernton EW, et al. Cytokines and arachidonic metabolites produced during human immunodeficiency virus (HIV)-

infected macrophage-astroglia interactions: implications for the neuropathogenesis of HIV disease. J Exp Med 1992;176:1703–1718.
63. Giulian D, Vaca K, Noonan CA. Secretion of neurotoxins by mononuclear phagocytes infected with HIV-1. Science 1990;250:1593–1596.
64. Gendelman HE, Lipton SA, Tardieu M, et al. The neuropathogenesis of HIV-1 infection. J Leukoc Biol 1994;56:389–398.
65. Schuitemaker H, Kootstra NA, Koppelman MH, et al. Proliferation-dependent HIV-1 infection of monocytes occurs during differentiation into macrophages. J Clin Invest 1992;89:1154–1160.
66. Rich EA, Chen IS, Zack JA, et al. Increased susceptibility of differentiated mononuclear phagocytes to productive infection with human immunodeficiency virus-1 (HIV-1). J Clin Invest 1992;89:176–183.
67. He J, Chen Y, Farzan M, et al. CCR3 and CCR5 are co-receptors for HIV-1 Infection of microglia. Nature 1997;385:645–649.
68. Bleul CC, Wu L, Hoxie JA, et al. The HIV coreceptors CXCR4 and CCR5 are differentially expressed and regulated on human T lymphocytes. Proc Natl Acad Sci U S A 1997;94:1925–1930.
69. Simmonds P, Balfe P, Peutherer JF, et al. Human immunodeficiency virus-infected individuals contain provirus in small numbers of peripheral mononuclear cells and at low copy numbers. J Virol 1990;64:864–872.
70. Koenig S, Gendelman HE, Orenstein JM, et al. Detection of AIDS virus in macrophages in brain tissue from AIDS patients with encephalopathy. Science 1986;233:1089–1093.
71. Plata F, Autran B, Martins LP, et al. AIDS virus-specific cytotoxic T lymphocytes in lung disorders. Nature 1987;328:348–351.
72. Shaw GM, Harper ME, Hahn BH, et al. HTLV-III infection in brains of children and adults with AIDS encephalopathy. Science 1985;227:177–182.
73. Crowe SM. Role of macrophages in the pathogenesis of human immunodeficiency virus (HIV) infection. Aust N Z J Med 1995;25:777–783.
74. Goletti D, Weissman D, Jackson RW, et al. Effect of *Mycobacterium tuberculosis* on HIV replication: role of immune activation. J Immunol 1996;157:1271–1278.
75. Claydon EJ, Bennett J, Gor D, Forster SM. Transient elevation of serum HIV antigen levels associated with intercurrent infection. AIDS 1991;5:113–114.
76. Ho DD. HIV-1 viraemia and influenza. Lancet 1992;33:1549.
77. Stanley Sk, Ostrowski MA, Justement JS, et al. Effect of immunization with a common recall antigen on viral expression in patients infected with human immunodeficiency virus type 1. N Engl J Med 1996;334:1222–1230.
78. O'Brien WA, Grovit-Ferbas K, Namazi A, et al. Human immunodeficiency virus-type 1 replication can be increased in peripheral blood of seropositive patients after influenza vaccination. Blood 1995;86:1082–1089.
79. Staprans SI, Hamilton BL, Follansbee SE, et al. Activation of virus replication after vaccination of HIV-1–infected individuals. J Exp Med 1995;182:1727–1737.
80. Brichacek B, Swindells S, Janoff EN, et al. Increased plasma human immunodeficiency virus type 1 burden following antigenic challenge with pneumococcal vaccine. J Infect Dis 1996;174:1191–1199.
81. Cameron P, Pope M, Granelli-Piperno A, et al. Dendritic cells and the replication of HIV-1. J Leukoc Biol 1996;59:158–171.
82. Austyn JM, Kupiec-Weglinski JW, Hankins DF, et al. Migration patterns of dendritic cells in the mouse: homing to T cell-dependent areas of spleen, and binding within marginal zone. J Exp Med 1988;167:646–651.
83. Fossum S. Dendritic leukocytes: features of their in vivo physiology. Res Immunol 1989;140:883–891; discussion 918–912.
84. Bujdoso R, Hopkins J, Dutia BM, et al. Characterization of sheep afferent lymph dendritic cells and their role in antigen carriage. J Exp Med 1989;170:1285–1301.
85. Bhardwaj N, Friedman SM, Cole BC, et al. Dendritic cells are potent antigen-presenting cells for microbial superantigens. J Exp Med 1992;175:267–273.
86. Pancholi P, Steinman RM, Bhardwaj N. Dendritic cells efficiently immunoselect mycobacterial-reactive T cells in human blood, including clonable antigen-reactive precursors. Immunology 1992;76:217–224.
87. O'Doherty U, Steinman RM, Peng M, et al. Dendritic cells freshly isolated from human blood express CD4 and mature into typical immunostimulatory dendritic cells after culture in monocyte-conditioned medium. J Exp Med 1993;178:1067–1076.
88. Weissman D, Li Y, Ananworanich J, et al. Three populations of cells with dendritic morphology exist in peripheral blood, only one of which is infectable with human immunodeficiency virus type 1. Proc Natl Acad Sci U S A 1995;92:826–830.
89. Patterson S, Knight SC. Susceptibility of human peripheral blood dendritic cells to infection by human immunodeficiency virus. J Gen Virol 1987;68:1177–1181.
90. Langhoff E, Terwilliger EF, Bos HJ, et al. Replication of human immunodeficiency virus type 1 in primary dendritic cell cultures. Proc Natl Acad Sci U S A 1991;88:7998–8002.
91. Pope M, Betjes MG, Romani N, et al. Conjugates of dendritic cells and memory T lymphocytes from skin facilitate productive infection with HIV-1. Cell 1994;78:389–398.
92. Weissman D, Li Y, Orenstein JM, Fauci AS. Both a precursor and a mature population of dendritic cells can bind HIV: however, only the mature population that expresses CD80 can pass infection to unstimulated CD4+ T cells. J Immunol 1995;155:4111–4117.
93. Fauci AS, Pantaleo G, Stanley S, et al. Immunopathogenic mechanisms of HIV infection. Ann Intern Med 1996;124:654–663.
94. Cameron PU, Freudenthal PS, Barker JM, et al. Dendritic cells exposed to human immunodeficiency virus type-1 transmit a vigorous cytopathic infection to CD4+ T cells [published erratum appears in Science 1992;257:1848]. Science 1992;257:383–387.
95. Pantaleo G, Graziosi C, Fauci AS. The immunopathogenesis of human immunodeficiency virus infection. N Engl J Med 1993;328:327–335.
96. Tindall B, Cooper DA. Primary HIV infection: host responses and intervention strategies [editorial]. AIDS 1991;5:1–14.
97. Clark SJ, Saag MS, Decker WD, et al. High titers of cytopathic virus in plasma of patients with symptomatic primary HIV-1 infection. N Engl J Med 1991;324:954–960.
98. Daar ES, Moudgil T, Meyer RD, et al. Transient high levels of viremia in patients with primary human immunodeficiency virus type 1 infection. N Engl J Med 1991;324:961–964.
99. Piatak M Jr, Saag MS, Yang LC, et al. High levels of HIV-1 in plasma during all stages of infection determined by competitive PCR. Science 1993;259:1749–1754.
100. Pantaleo G, Graziosi C, Demarest JF, et al. Role of lymphoid organs in the pathogenesis of human immunodeficiency virus (HIV) infection. Immunol Rev 1994;140:105–130.
101. Mellors JW, Kingsley LA, Rinaldo CR Jr, et al. Quantitation of HIV-1 RNA in plasma predicts outcome after seroconversion. Ann Intern Med 1995;122:573–579.
102. Mellors JW, Rinaldo CR Jr, Gupta P, et al. Prognosis in HIV-1 infection predicted by the quantity of virus in plasma. Science 1996;272:1167–1170.
103. Pantaleo G, Demarest JF, Soudeyns H, et al. Major expansion of CD8+ T cells with a predominant V beta usage during the primary immune response to HIV. Nature 1994;370:463–467.
104. Pantaleo G, Demarest JF, Schacker T, et al. The qualitative nature of the primary immune response is a prognosticator of disease progression independent of the initial level of plasma viremia. Proc Natl Acad Sci U S A 1997;94:254–258.
105. Koup RA, Safrit JT, Cao Y, et al. Temporal association of cellular immune responses with the initial control of viremia in primary human immunodeficiency virus type 1 syndrome. J Virol 1994;68:4650–4655.
106. Borrow P, Lewicki H, Hahn BH, et al. Virus-specific CD8+ cytotoxic T-lymphocyte activity associated with control of viremia in primary human immunodeficiency virus type 1 infection. J Virol 1994;68:6103–6110.

107. Safrit JT, Andrews CA, Zhu T, et al. Characterization of human immunodeficiency virus type 1–specific cytotoxic T lymphocyte clones isolated during acute seroconversion: recognition of autologous virus sequences within a conserved immunodominant epitope. J Exp Med 1994;179:463–472.
108. Yasutomi Y, Reimann KA, Lord CI, et al. Simian immunodeficiency virus–specific CD8+ lymphocyte response in acutely infected rhesus monkeys. J Virol 1993;67:1707–1711.
109. Reimann KA, Tenner-Racz K, Racz P, et al. Immunopathogenic events in acute infection of rhesus monkeys with simian immunodeficiency virus of macaques. J Virol 1994;68:2362–2370.
110. Borrow P, Lewicki H, Wei X, et al. Antiviral pressure exerted by HIV-1–specific cytotoxic T lymphocytes (CTLs) during primary infection demonstrated by rapid selection of CTL escape virus. Nat Med 1997;3:205–211.
111. Moore JP, Cao Y, Ho DD, et al. Development of the anti-gp120 antibody response during seroconversion to human immunodeficiency virus type 1. J Virol 1994;68:5142–5155.
112. Moore JP, Ho DD. Antibodies to discontinuous or conformationally sensitive epitopes on the gp120 glycoprotein of human immunodeficiency virus type 1 are highly prevalent in sera of infected humans. J Virol 1993;67:863–875.
113. Mackewicz CE, Yang LC, Lifson JD, et al. Non-cytolytic CD8 T-cell anti-HIV responses in primary HIV-1 infection. Lancet 1994;344:16/1–16/3.
114. Pantaleo G, Fauci AS. New concepts in the immunopathogenesis of HIV infection. Annu Rev Microbiol 1996;50:825–854.
115. Pachl C, Todd JA, Kern DG, et al. Rapid and precise quantification of HIV-1 RNA in plasma using a branched DNA signal amplification assay. J Acquir Immune Defic Syndr Hum Retrovirol 1995;8:446–454.
116. Haase AT, Henry K, Zupancic M, et al. Quantitative image analysis of HIV-1 infection in lymphoid tissue. Science 1996;274:985–989.
117. Haynes BF. Immune responses to HIV infection. In: De Vita VT, Hellman S, Rosenberg SA, eds. AIDS: etiology, diagnosis, treatment and prevention. 3rd ed. Philadelphia: JB Lippincott, 1992:77–86.
118. Haynes BF, Pantaleo G, Fauci AS. Toward an understanding of the correlates of protective immunity to HIV infection. Science 1996;271:324–328.
119. Wolinsky SM, Korber BT, Neumann AU, et al. Adaptive evolution of human immunodeficiency virus-type 1 during the natural course of infection. Science 1996;272:537–542.
120. Phillips RE, Rowland-Jones S, Nixon DF, et al. Human immunodeficiency virus genetic variation that can escape cytotoxic T cell recognition. Nature 1991;354:453–459.
121. Carmichael A, Jin X, Sissons P, et al. Quantitative analysis of the human immunodeficiency virus type 1 (HIV-1)–specific cytotoxic T lymphocyte (CTL) response at different stages of HIV-1 infection: differential CTL responses to HIV-1 and Epstein–Barr virus in late disease. J Exp Med 1993;177:249–256.
122. Goulder PJ, Phillips RE, Colbert RA, et al. Late escape from an immunodominant cytotoxic T-lymphocyte response associated with progression to AIDS. Nat Med 1997;3:212–217.
123. Montefiori DC, Pantaleo G, Fink LM, et al. Neutralizing and infection-enhancing antibody responses to human immunodeficiency virus type 1 in long-term nonprogressors. J Infect Dis 1996;173:60–67.
124. Cao Y, Qin L, Zhang L, et al. Virologic and immunologic characterization of long-term survivors of human immunodeficiency virus type 1 infection. N Engl J Med 1995;332:201–208.
125. Centers for Disease Control. HIV/AIDS surveillance. Atlanta: Centers for Disease Control, 1992:1–18.
126. Tew JG, Kosco MH, Burton GF, et al. Follicular dendritic cells as accessory cells. Immunol Rev 1990;117:185–211.
127. Spira AI, Marx PA, Patterson BK, et al. Cellular targets of infection and route of viral dissemination after an intravaginal inoculation of simian immunodeficiency virus into rhesus macaques. J Exp Med 1996;183:215–225.
128. Fox CH, Tenner-Racz K, Racz P, et al. Lymphoid germinal centers are reservoirs of human immunodeficiency virus type 1 RNA [published erratum appears in J Infect Dis 1992;165:1161]. J Infect Dis 1991;164:1051–1057.
129. Tenner-Racz K, Racz P, Dietrich M, et al. Altered follicular dendritic cells and virus-like particles in AIDS and AIDS-related lymphadenopathy [letter]. Lancet 1985;1:105–106.
130. Pantaleo G, Graziosi C, Demarest JF, et al. HIV infection is active and progressive in lymphoid tissue during the clinically latent stage of disease. Nature 1993;362:355–358.
131. Embretson J, Zupancic M, Ribas JL, et al. Massive covert infection of helper T lymphocytes and macrophages by HIV during the incubation period of AIDS. Nature 1993;362:359–362.
132. Tew JG, DiLosa RM, Burton GF, et al. Germinal centers and antibody production in bone marrow. Immunol Rev 1992;126:99–112.
133. Szakal AK, Kosco MH, Tew JG. Microanatomy of lymphoid tissue during humoral immune responses: structure function relationships. Annu Rev Immunol 1989;7:91–109.
134. Gaines H, von Sydow MA, von Stedingk LV, et al. Immunological changes in primary HIV-1 infection. AIDS 1990;4:995–9.
135. Reinhart TA, Rogan MJ, Viglianti GA, et al. A new approach to investigating the relationship between productive infection and cyopathicity in vivo. Nat Med 1997;3:218–221.
136. Schrager LK, Fauci AS. Human immunodeficiency virus: trapped but still dangerous. Nature 1995;377:680–681.
137. Heath SL, Tew JG, Szakal AK, et al. Follicular dendritic cells and human immunodeficiency virus infectivity. Nature 1995;377:740–744.
138. Graziosi C, Pantaleo G, Fauci AS. Comparative analysis of constitutive cytokine expression in peripheral blood and lymph nodes of HIV-infected individuals. Res Immunol 1994;145:602–605; discussion 605–607.
139. Pantaleo G, Fauci AS. New concepts in the immunopathogenesis of HIV infection. Annu Rev Immunol 1995;13:487–512.
140. Pantaleo G, Graziosi C, Fauci AS. The role of lymphoid organs in the immunopathogenesis of HIV infection. AIDS 1993;7(Suppl 1):S19–S23.
141. Munoz A, Kirby AJ, He YD, et al. Long-term survivors with HIV-1 infection: incubation period and longitudinal patterns of CD4+ lymphocytes. J Acquir Immune Defic Syndr Hum Retrovirol 1995;8:496–505.
142. Phillips AN, Sabin CA, Elford J, et al. Use of CD4 lymphocyte count to predict long-term survival free of AIDS after HIV infection. BMJ 1994;309:309–313.
143. Schrager LK, Young JM, Fowler MG, et al. Long-term survivors of HIV-1 infection: definitions and research challenges. AIDS 1994;8(Suppl 1):S95–S108.
144. Buchbinder SP, Katz MH, Hessol NA, et al. Long term HIV 1 infection without immunologic progression. AIDS 1994;8:1123–1128.
145. Easterbrook PJ. Non-progression in HIV infection [published erratum appears in AIDS 1994;8:1514]. AIDS 1994;8:1179–1182.
146. Pantaleo G, Menzo S, Vaccarezza M, et al. Studies in subjects with long-term nonprogressive human immunodeficiency virus infection. N Engl J Med 1995;332:209–216.
147. Kirchhoff F, Greenough TC, Brettler DB, et al. Brief report: absence of intact nef sequences in a long-term survivor with nonprogressive HIV-1 infection. N Engl J Med 1995;332:228–232.
148. Harrer T, Harrer E, Kalams SA, et al. Cytotoxic T lymphocytes in asymptomatic long-term nonprogressing HIV-1 infection: breadth and specificity of the response and relation to in vivo viral quasispecies in a person with prolonged infection and low viral load. J Immunol 1996;156:2616–2623.
149. Hogervorst E, Jurriaans S, de Wolf F, et al. Predictors for non- and slow progression in human immunodeficiency virus (HIV) type 1 infection: low viral RNA copy numbers in serum and maintenance of high HIV-1 p24-specific but not V3-specific antibody levels. J Infect Dis 1995;171:811–821.

150. Rinaldo C, Huang XL, Fan ZF, et al. High levels of anti-human immunodeficiency virus type 1 (HIV-1) memory cytotoxic T-lymphocyte activity and low viral load are associated with lack of disease in HIV-1–infected long-term nonprogressors. J Virol 1995; 69:5838–5842.
151. Michael NL, Chang G, Louie LG, et al. The role of viral phenotype and CCR-5 gene defects in HIV-1 transmission and disease progression. Nat Med 1997;3:338–340.
152. Delwart EL, Sheppard HW, Walker BD, et al. Human immunodeficiency virus type 1 evolution in vivo tracked by DNA heteroduplex mobility assays. J Virol 1994;68:6672–6683.
153. Kestler HW III, Ringler DJ, Mori K, et al. Importance of the nef gene for maintenance of high virus loads and for development of AIDS. Cell 1991;65:651–662.
154. Deacon NJ, Tsykin A, Solomon A, et al. Genomic structure of an attenuated quasispecies of HIV-1 from a blood transfusion donor and recipients. Science 1995;270:988–991.
155. Greenough TC, Somasundaran M, Brettler DB, et al. Normal immune function and inability to isolate virus in culture in an individual with long-term human immunodeficiency virus type 1 infection. AIDS Res Hum Retroviruses 1994;10:395–403.
156. Huang Y, Zhang L, Ho DD. Biological characterization of nef in long-term survivors of human immunodeficiency virus type 1 infection. J Virol 1995;69:8142–8146.
157. Huang Y, Zhang L, Ho DD. Characterization of nef sequences in long-term survivors of human immunodeficiency virus type 1 infection. J Virol 1995;69:93–100.
158. Klein MR, van Baalen CA, Holwerda AM, et al. Kinetics of Gag-specific cytotoxic T lymphocyte responses during the clinical course of HIV-1 infection: a longitudinal analysis of rapid progressors and long-term asymptomatics. J Exp Med 1995;181:1365–1372.
159. Harrer T, Harrer E, Kalams SA, et al. Strong cytotoxic T cell and weak neutralizing antibody responses in a subset of persons with stable nonprogressing HIV type 1 infection. AIDS Res Hum Retroviruses 1996;12:585–592.
160. Ferbas J, Kaplan AH, Hausner MA, et al. Virus burden in long-term survivors of human immunodeficiency virus (HIV) infection is a determinant of anti-HIV CD8+ lymphocyte activity. J Infect Dis 1995;172:329–339.
161. Keet IP, Krol A, Klein MR, et al. Characteristics of long-term asymptomatic infection with human immunodeficiency virus type 1 in men with normal and low CD4+ cell counts. J Infect Dis 1994;169: 1236–1243.
162. Giorgi JV, Ho HN, Hirji K, et al. CD8+ lymphocyte activation at human immunodeficiency virus type 1 seroconversion: development of HLA-DR+ CD38ms CD8+ cells is associated with subsequent stable CD4+ cell levels. The Multicenter AIDS Cohort Study Group. J Infect Dis 1994;170:775–781.
163. Giorgi JV, Liu Z, Hultin LE, et al. Elevated levels of CD38+ CD8+ T cells in HIV infection add to the prognostic value of low CD4+ T cell levels: results of 6 years of follow-up. The Los Angeles Center, Multicenter AIDS Cohort Study. J Acquir Immune Defic Syndr Hum Retrovirol 1993;6:904–912.
164. Cocchi F, DeVico AL, Garzino-Demo A, et al. Identification of RANTES, MIP-1 alpha, and MIP-1 beta as the major HIV-suppressive factors produced by CD8+ T cells. Science 1995;270:1811–1815.
165. Clerici M, Balotta C, Trabattoni D, et al. Chemokine production in HIV-seropositive long-term asymptomatic individuals. AIDS 1996; 10:1432–1433.
166. Zanussi S, D'Andrea A, Simonelli C, et al. Serum levels of RANTES and MIP-1α in HIV-positive long-term survivors and progressor patients. AIDS 1996;10:1431–1432.
167. Chen Y, Gupta P. CD8+ T-cell–mediated suppression of HIV-1 infection may not be due to chemokines RANTES, MIP-1α and MIP-1β. AIDS 1996;10:1434–1435.
168. Blazevic V, Heino M, Ranki A, et al. RANTES, MIP and interleukin-16 in HIV infection. AIDS 1996;10:1435–1436.
169. Rammensee HG, Falk K, Rotzschke O. Peptides naturally presented by MHC class I molecules. Annu Rev Immunol 1993;11:213–244.
170. Kaslow RA, Carrington M, Apple R, et al. Influence of combinations of human major histocompatibility complex genes on the course of HIV-1 infection. Nat Med 1996;2:405–411.
171. Huang Y, Paxton WA, Wolinsky SM, et al. The role of a mutant CCR5 allele in HIV-1 transmission and disease progression. Nat Med 1996;2:1240–1243.
172. Zimmerman PA, Buckler-White A, Alkhatib G, et al. Inherited resistance to HIV-1 conferred by an inactivating mutation in CC chemokine receptor 5: studies in populations with contrasting clinical phenotypes, defined racial background and quantified risk. Mol Med 1997;3:22–35.
173. Munoz A, Wang MC, Bass S, et al. Acquired immunodeficiency syndrome (AIDS)-free time after human immunodeficiency virus type 1 (HIV-1) seroconversion in homosexual men. Multicenter AIDS Cohort Study Group. Am J Epidemiol 1989;130:530–539.
174. Saksela K. HIV-1 RNA in blood and pathogenesis of HIV infection. Ann Med 1995;27:625–628.
175. Schuitemaker H, Koot M, Kootstra NA, et al. Biological phenotype of human immunodeficiency virus type 1 clones at different stages of infection: progression of disease is associated with a shift from monocytotropic to T-cell–tropic virus population. J Virol 1992;66: 1354–1360.
176. Bleul CC, Fuhlbrigge RC, Casasnovas JM, et al. A highly efficacious lymphocyte chemoattractant, stromal cell-derived factor 1 (SDF-1). J Exp Med 1996;184:1101–1110.
177. Walker CM, Moody DJ, Stites DP, et al. CD8+ lymphocytes can control HIV infection in vitro by suppressing virus replication. Science 1986;234:1563–1566.
178. Mackewicz CE, Ortega HW, Levy JA. CD8+ cell anti-HIV activity correlates with the clinical state of the infected individual. J Clin Invest 1991;87:1462–1466.
179. Pincus SH, Messer KG, Nara PL, et al. Temporal analysis of the antibody response to HIV envelope protein in HIV-infected laboratory workers. J Clin Invest 1994;93:2505–2513.
180. Cavacini LA, Emes CL, Power J, et al. Loss of serum antibodies to a conformational epitope of HIV-1/gp120 identified by a human monoclonal antibody is associated with disease progression. J Acquir Immune Defic Syndr Hum Retrovirol 1993;6:1093–1102.
181. Janvier B, Mallet F, Cheynet V, et al. Prevalence and persistence of antibody titers to recombinant HIV-1 core and matrix proteins in HIV-1 infection. J Acquir Immune Defic Syndr Hum Retrovirol 1993;6:898–903.
182. Sheppard HW, Lang W, Ascher MS, et al. The characterization of non-progressors: long-term HIV-1 infection with stable CD4+ T-cell levels. AIDS 1993;7:1159–1166.
183. Phair J, Jacobson L, Detels R, et al. Acquired immune deficiency syndrome occurring within 5 years of infection with human immunodeficiency virus type-1: the Multicenter AIDS Cohort Study. J Acquir Immune Defic Syndr Hum Retrovirol 1992;5:490–496.
184. Poli G, Fauci AS. Cytokine cascades in HIV infection. In: Gupta S, ed. Immunology of HIV infection. New York: Plenum, 1996:285–301.
185. Clouse KA, Cosentino LM, Weih KA, et al. The HIV-1 gp120 envelope protein has the intrinsic capacity to stimulate monokine secretion. J Immunol 1991;147:2892–2901.
186. Merrill JE, Koyanagi Y, Chen IS. Interleukin-1 and tumor necrosis factor alpha can be induced from mononuclear phagocytes by human immunodeficiency virus type 1 binding to the CD4 receptor. J Virol 1989;63:4404–4408.
187. Oyaizu N, Chirmule N, Ohnishi Y, et al. Human immunodeficiency virus type 1 envelope glycoproteins gp120 and gp160 induce interleukin-6 production in CD4+ T-cell clones. J Virol 1991;65: 6277–6282.
188. Poli G, Fauci AS. The effect of cytokines and pharmacologic agents on chronic HIV infection. AIDS Res Hum Retroviruses 1992; 8:191–197.

189. Zauli G, Davis BR, Re MC, et al. Tat protein stimulates production of transforming growth factor-beta 1 by marrow macrophages: a potential mechanism for human immunodeficiency virus-1–induced hematopoietic suppression. Blood 1992;80:3036–3043.
190. Allen JB, Wong HL, Guyre PM, et al. Association of circulating receptor Fc gamma RIII-positive monocytes in AIDS patients with elevated levels of transforming growth factor-beta. J Clin Invest 1991;87:1773–1779.
191. Kekow J, Wachsman W, McCutchan JA, et al. Transforming growth factor beta and noncytopathic mechanisms of immunodeficiency in human immunodeficiency virus infection. Proc Natl Acad Sci U S A 1990;87:8321–8325.
192. Wahl SM, Allen JB, McCartney-Francis N, et al. Macrophage- and astrocyte-derived transforming growth factor beta as a mediator of central nervous system dysfunction in acquired immune deficiency syndrome. J Exp Med 1991;173:981–991.
193. Graziosi C, Pantaleo G, Gantt KR, et al. Lack of evidence for the dichotomy of TH1 and TH2 predominance in HIV-infected individuals. Science 1994;265:248–252.
194. Kovacs JA, Vogel S, Albert JM, et al. Controlled trial of interleukin-2 infusions in patients infected with the human immunodeficiency virus. N Engl J Med 1996;335:1350–1356.
195. Kovacs JA, Baseler M, Dewar RJ, et al. Increases in CD4 T lymphocytes with intermittent courses of interleukin-2 in patients with human immunodeficiency virus infection: a preliminary study. N Engl J Med 1995;332:567–575.
196. Kinter A, Fauci AS. Interleukin-2 and human immunodeficiency virus infection: pathogenic mechanisms and potential for immunologic enhancement. Immunol Res 1996;15:1–15.
197. Folks TM, Justement J, Kinter A, et al. Cytokine-induced expression of HIV-1 in a chronically infected promonocyte cell line. Science 1987;238:800–802.
198. Kinter AL, Poli G, Fox L, et al. HIV replication in IL-2–stimulated peripheral blood mononuclear cells is driven in an autocrine/paracrine manner by endogenous cytokines. J Immunol 1995;154:2448–2459.
199. Rautonen J, Rautonen N, Martin NL, et al. Serum interleukin-6 concentrations are elevated and associated with elevated tumor necrosis factor-alpha and immunoglobulin G and A concentrations in children with HIV infection. AIDS 1991;5:1319–1325.
200. Rieckmann P, Poli G, Fox CH, et al. Recombinant gp120 specifically enhances tumor necrosis factor-alpha production and Ig secretion in B lymphocytes from HIV-infected individuals but not from seronegative donors. J Immunol 1991;147:2922–2927.
201. von Sydow M, Sonnerborg A, Gaines H, et al. Interferon-alpha and tumor necrosis factor-alpha in serum of patients in various stages of HIV-1 infection. AIDS Res Hum Retroviruses 1991;7:375–380.
202. Vyakarnam A, Matear P, Meager A, et al. Altered production of tumour necrosis factors alpha and beta and interferon gamma by HIV-infected individuals. Clin Exp Immunol 1991;84:109–115.
203. Israel-Biet D, Cadranel J, Beldjord K, et al. Tumor necrosis factor production in HIV-seropositive subjects: relationship with lung opportunistic infections and HIV expression in alveolar macrophages. J Immunol 1991;147:490–494.
204. Millar AB, Miller RF, Foley NM, et al. Production of tumor necrosis factor-alpha by blood and lung mononuclear phagocytes from patients with human immunodeficiency virus-related lung disease. Am J Respir Cell Mol Biol 1991;5:144–148.
205. Clouse KA, Powell D, Washington I, et al. Monokine regulation of human immunodeficiency virus-1 expression in a chronically infected human T cell clone. J Immunol 1989;142:431–438.
206. Folks TM, Clouse KA, Justement J, et al. Tumor necrosis factor alpha induces expression of human immunodeficiency virus in a chronically infected T-cell clone. Proc Natl Acad Sci U S A 1989;86:2365–2368.
207. Duh EJ, Maury WJ, Folks TM, et al. Tumor necrosis factor alpha activates human immunodeficiency virus type 1 through induction of nuclear factor binding to the NF-kappa B sites in the long terminal repeat. Proc Natl Acad Sci U S A 1989;86:5974–5978.
208. Poli G, Bressler P, Kinter A, et al. Interleukin 6 induces human immunodeficiency virus expression in infected monocytic cells alone and in synergy with tumor necrosis factor alpha by transcriptional and post-transcriptional mechanisms. J Exp Med 1990;172:151–158.
209. Koyanagi Y, O'Brien WA, Zhao JQ, et al. Cytokines alter production of HIV-1 from primary mononuclear phagocytes. Science 1988;241:1673–1675.
210. Latham PS, Lewis AM, Varesio L, et al. Expression of human immunodeficiency virus long terminal repeat in the human promonocyte cell line U937: effect of endotoxin and cytokines. Cell Immunol 1990;129:513–518.
211. Birx DL, Redfield RR, Tencer K, et al. Induction of interleukin-6 during human immunodeficiency virus infection. Blood 1990;76:2303–2310.
212. Breen EC, Rezai AR, Nakajima K, et al. Infection with HIV is associated with elevated IL-6 levels and production. J Immunol 1990;144:480–484.
213. Poli G, Kinter AL, Fauci AS. Interleukin 1 induces expression of the human immunodeficiency virus alone and in synergy with interleukin 6 in chronically infected U1 cells: inhibition of inductive effects by the interleukin 1 receptor antagonist. Proc Natl Acad Sci U S A 1994;91:108–112.
214. Amadori A, Zamarchi R, Veronese ML, et al. B cell activation during HIV-1 infection. II. Cell-to-cell interactions and cytokine requirement. J Immunol 1991;146:57–62.
215. Goletti D, Kinter AL, Hardy EC, et al. Modulation of endogenous IL-1 beta and IL-1 receptor antagonist results in opposing effects on HIV expression in chronically infected monocytic cells. J Immunol 1996;156:3501–3508.
216. Shirazi Y, Pitha PM. Interferon alpha-mediated inhibition of human immunodeficiency virus type 1 provirus synthesis in T-cells. Virology 1993;193:303–312.
217. Shirazi Y, Pitha PM. Alpha interferon inhibits early stages of the human immunodeficiency virus type 1 replication cycle. J Virol 1992;66:1321–1328.
218. Poli G, Fauci AS. The role of monocyte/macrophages and cytokines in the pathogenesis of HIV infection. Pathobiology 1992;60:246–251.
219. Poli G, Fauci AS. Cytokine modulation of HIV expression. Semin Immunol 1993;5:165–173.
220. Francis ML, Meltzer MS. Induction of IFN-alpha by HIV-1 in monocyte-enriched PBMC requires gp120–CD4 interaction but not virus replication. J Immunol 1993;151:2208–2216.
221. Eyster ME, Goedert JJ, Poon MC, et al. Acid-labile alpha interferon: a possible preclinical marker for the acquired immunodeficiency syndrome in hemophilia. N Engl J Med 1983;309:583–586.
222. Edlin BR, St.Clair MH, Pitha PM, et al. In-vitro resistance to zidovudine and alpha-interferon in HIV-1 isolates from patients: correlations with treatment duration and response [published erratum appears in Ann Intern Med 1992;117:879]. Ann Intern Med 1992;117:457–460.
223. Kunzi MS, Farzadegan H, Margolick JB, et al. Identification of human immunodeficiency virus primary isolates resistant to interferon-alpha and correlation of prevalence to disease progression. J Infect Dis 1995;171:822–828.
224. Vyakarnam A, McKeating J, Meager A, et al. Tumour necrosis factors (alpha, beta) induced by HIV-1 in peripheral blood mononuclear cells potentiate virus replication. AIDS 1990;4:21–27.
225. Biswas P, Poli G, Kinter AL, et al. Interferon gamma induces the expression of human immunodeficiency virus in persistently infected promonocytic cells (U1) and redirects the production of virions to intracytoplasmic vacuoles in phorbol myristate acetate-differentiated U1 cells. J Exp Med 1992;176:739–750.
226. Kazazi F, Mathijs JM, Chang J, et al. Recombinant interleukin 4 stimulates human immunodeficiency virus production by infected monocytes and macrophages. J Gen Virol 1992;73:941–949.

227. Weissman D, Poli G, Fauci AS. Interleukin 10 blocks HIV replication in macrophages by inhibiting the autocrine loop of tumor necrosis factor alpha and interleukin 6 induction of virus. AIDS Res Hum Retroviruses 1994;10:1199–1206.
228. Weissman D, Poli G, Fauci AS. IL-10 synergizes with multiple cytokines in enhancing HIV production in cells of monocytic lineage. J Acquir Immune Defic Syndr Hum Retrovirol 1995;9:442–449.
229. Weissman D, Ostrowski M, Daucher JA, et al. Interleukin-10 decreases HIV plasma viral load: results of a phase 1 clinical trial. In: 4th Conference on Retroviruses and Opportunistic Infections. Washington, DC: IDSA Foundation for Retrovirology and Human Health, 1997;37:71.
230. Poli G, Kinter AL, Justement JS, et al. Transforming growth factor beta suppresses human immunodeficiency virus expression and replication in infected cells of the monocyte/macrophage lineage. J Exp Med 1991;173:589–597.
231. Lazdins JK, Klimkait T, Woods-Cook K, et al. In vitro effect of transforming growth factor-beta on progression of HIV-1 infection in primary mononuclear phagocytes. J Immunol 1991;147:1201–1207.
232. Novak RM, Holzer TJ, Kennedy MM, et al. The effect of interleukin 4 (BSF-1) on infection of peripheral blood monocyte-derived macrophages with HIV-1. AIDS Res Hum Retroviruses 1990; 6:973–976.
233. Williams DA. Ex vivo expansion of hematopoietic stem and progenitor cells: robbing Peter to pay Paul? [editorial]. Blood 1993;81:3169–3172.
234. Plum J, De Smedt M, Leclercq G, et al. Influence of TGF-beta on murine thymocyte development in fetal thymus organ culture. J Immunol 1995;154:5789–5798.
235. d'Angeac AD, Dornand J, Emonds-Alt X, et al. Transforming growth factor type beta 1 (TGF-beta 1) down-regulates interleukin-2 production and up-regulates interleukin-2 receptor expression in a thymoma cell line. J Cell Physiol 1991;147:460–469.
236. Schwartz GN, Kessler SW, Szabo JM, et al. Negative regulators may mediate some of the inhibitory effects of HIV-1 infected stromal cell layers on erythropoiesis and myelopoiesis in human bone marrow long term cultures. J Leukoc Biol 1995;57:948–955.
237. Geissler RG, Ottmann OG, Kojouharoff G, et al. Influence of human recombinant interferon-alpha and interferon-gamma on bone marrow progenitor cells of HIV-positive individuals. AIDS Res Hum Retroviruses 1992;8:521–525.
238. Romagnani S. Biology of human TH1 and TH2 cells. J Clin Immunol 1995;15:121–129.
239. del Prete G, de Carli M, Almerigogna F, et al. Human IL-10 is produced by both type 1 helper (Th1) and type 2 helper (Th2) T cell clones and inhibits their antigen-specific proliferation and cytokine production. J Immunol 1993;150:353–360.
240. Chehimi J, Trinchieri G. Interleukin-12: a bridge between innate resistance and adaptive immunity with a role in infection and acquired immunodeficiency. J Clin Immunol 1994;14:149–161.
241. Mosmann TR, Moore KW. The role of IL-10 in crossregulation of TH1 and TH2 responses. Immunol Today 1991;12:A49–A53.
242. Abehsira-Amar O, Gibert M, Joliy M, et al. IL-4 plays a dominant role in the differential development of Tho into Th1 and Th2 cells. J Immunol 1992;148:3820–3829.
243. Clerici M, Shearer GM. The Th1–Th2 hypothesis of HIV infection: new insights. Immunol Today 1994;15:575–581.
244. Clerici M, Shearer GM. A TH1→TH2 switch is a critical step in the etiology of HIV infection. Immunol Today 1993;14:107–111.
245. Maggi E, Mazzetti M, Ravina A, et al. Ability of HIV to promote a TH1 to TH0 shift and to replicate preferentially in TH2 and TH0 cells. Science 1994;265:244–248.
246. Chehimi J, Starr SE, Frank I, et al. Impaired interleukin 12 production in human immunodeficiency virus-infected patients. J Exp Med 1994;179:1361–1366.
247. Fan J, Bass HZ, Fahey JL. Elevated IFN-gamma and decreased IL-2 gene expression are associated with HIV infection. J Immunol 1993;151:5031–5040.
248. Mosmann TR. Cytokine patterns during the progression to AIDS. Science 1994;265:193–194.
249. Walker CM, Levy JA. A diffusible lymphokine produced by CD8+ T lymphocytes suppresses HIV replication. Immunology 1989;66:628–630.
250. Brinchmann JE, Gaudernack G, Vartdal F. CD8+ T cells inhibit HIV replication in naturally infected CD4+ T cells: evidence for a soluble inhibitor. J Immunol 1990;144:2961–2966.
251. Brinchmann JE, Gaudernack G, Vartdal F. In vitro replication of HIV-1 in naturally infected CD4+ T cells is inhibited by rIFN alpha 2 and by a soluble factor secreted by activated CD8+ T cells, but not by rIFN beta, rIFN gamma, or recombinant tumor necrosis factor-alpha. J Acquir Immune Defic Syndr Hum Retrovirol 1991;4:480–488.
252. Mackewicz CE, Ortega H, Levy JA. Effect of cytokines on HIV replication in CD4+ lymphocytes: lack of identity with the CD8+ cell antiviral factor. Cell Immunol 1994;153:329–343.
253. Moriuchi H, Moriuchi M, Combadiere C, et al. CD8+ T-cell-derived soluble factor(s), but not beta-chemokines RANTES, MIP-1 alpha, and MIP-1 beta, suppress HIV-1 replication in monocyte/macrophages. Proc Natl Acad Sci U S A 1996;93:15341–15345.
254. Kinter AL, Ostrowski M, Goletti D, et al. HIV replication in CD4+ T cells of HIV-infected individuals is regulated by a balance between the viral suppressive effects of endogenous beta-chemokines and the viral inductive effects of other endogenous cytokines. Proc Natl Acad Sci U S A 1996;93:14076–14081.
255. Fauci AS. The human immunodeficiency virus: infectivity and mechanisms of pathogenesis. Science 1988;239:617–622.
256. Siliciano RF. The role of CD4 in HIV envelope-mediated pathogenesis. Curr Top Microbiol Immunol 1996;205:159–179.
257. Finkel TH, Tudor-Williams G, Banda NK, et al. Apoptosis occurs predominantly in bystander cells and not in productively infected cells of HIV- and SIV-infected lymph nodes. Nat Med 1995;1:129–134.
258. Su L, Kaneshima H, Bonyhadi M, et al. HIV-1–induced thymocyte depletion is associated with indirect cytopathogenicity and infection of progenitor cells in vivo. Immunity 1995;2:25–36.
259. Sodroski J, Goh WC, Rosen C, et al. Role of the HTLV-III/LAV envelope in syncytium formation and cytopathicity. Nature 1986;322:470–474.
260. Lifson JD, Reyes GR, McGrath MS, et al. AIDS retrovirus induced cytopathology: giant cell formation and involvement of CD4 antigen. Science 1986;232:1123–1127.
261. Stevenson M, Meier C, Mann AM, et al. Envelope glycoprotein of HIV induces interference and cytolysis resistance in CD4+ cells: mechanism for persistence in AIDS. Cell 1988;53:483–496.
262. Somasundaran M, Robinson HL. A major mechanism of human immunodeficiency virus-induced cell killing does not involve cell fusion. J Virol 1987;61:3114–3119.
263. Bergeron L, Sodroski J. Dissociation of unintegrated viral DNA accumulation from single-cell lysis induced by human immunodeficiency virus type 1. J Virol 1992;66:5777–5787.
264. Laurent-Crawford AG, Hovanessian AG. The cytopathic effect of human immunodeficiency virus is independent of high levels of unintegrated viral DNA accumulated in response to superinfection of cells. J Gen Virol 1993;74:2619–2628.
265. Crise B, Buonocore L, Rose JK. CD4 is retained in the endoplasmic reticulum by the human immunodeficiency virus type 1 glycoprotein precursor. J Virol 1990;64:5585–5593.
266. Koga Y, Sasaki M, Yoshida H, et al. Cytopathic effect determined by the amount of CD4 molecules in human cell lines expressing envelope glycoprotein of HIV. J Immunol 1990;144:94–102.
267. Agy MB, Wambach M, Foy K, et al. Expression of cellular genes in CD4 positive lymphoid cells infected by the human immunodeficiency virus, HIV-1: evidence for a host protein synthesis shut-off induced by cellular mRNA degradation. Virology 1990;177:251–258.
268. Kawamura I, Koga Y, Oh-Hori N, et al. Depletion of the surface CD4 molecule by the envelope protein of human immunodeficiency virus expressed in a human CD4+ monocytoid cell line. J Virol 1989;63:3748–3754.

269. Cao J, Park IW, Cooper A, et al. Molecular determinants of acute single-cell lysis by human immunodeficiency virus type 1. J Virol 1996;70:1340–1354.
270. Koga Y, Tanaka K, Lu YY, et al. Priming of immature thymocytes to CD3-mediated apoptosis by infection with murine cytomegalovirus. J Virol 1994;68:4322–4328.
271. Stevenson M, Haggerty S, Lamonica C, et al. Cloning and characterization of human immunodeficiency virus type 1 variants diminished in the ability to induce syncytium-independent cytolysis. J Virol 1990;64:3792–3803.
272. Kowalski M, Bergeron L, Dorfman T, et al. Attenuation of human immunodeficiency virus type 1 cytopathic effect by a mutation affecting the transmembrane envelope glycoprotein. J Virol 1991;65:281–291.
273. Lifson JD, Feinberg MB, Reyes GR, et al. Induction of CD4–dependent cell fusion by the HTLV-III/LAV envelope glycoprotein. Nature 1986;323:725–728.
274. Pantaleo G, Butini L, Graziosi C, et al. Human immunodeficiency virus (HIV) infection in CD4+ T lymphocytes genetically deficient in LFA-1: LFA-1 is required for HIV-mediated cell fusion but not for viral transmission. J Exp Med 1991;173:511–514.
275. Hildreth JE, Orentas RJ. Involvement of a leukocyte adhesion receptor (LFA-1) in HIV-induced syncytium formation. Science 1989;244:1075–1078.
276. Fisher AG, Ensoli B, Looney D, et al. Biologically diverse molecular variants within a single HIV-1 isolate. Nature 1988;334:444–447.
277. Cheng-Mayer C, Seto D, Tateno M, et al. Biologic features of HIV-1 that correlate with virulence in the host. Science 1988;240:80–82.
278. Fenyo EM, Morfeldt-Manson L, Chiodi F, et al. Distinct replicative and cytopathic characteristics of human immunodeficiency virus isolates. J Virol 1988;62:4414–4419.
279. Tersmette M, Gruters RA, de Wolf F, et al. Evidence for a role of virulent human immunodeficiency virus (HIV) variants in the pathogenesis of acquired immunodeficiency syndrome: studies on sequential HIV isolates. J Virol 1989;63:2118–2125.
280. Tersmette M, Lange JM, de Goede RE, et al. Association between biological properties of human immunodeficiency virus variants and risk for AIDS and AIDS mortality. Lancet 1989;1:983–985.
281. Macher AM. The pathology of AIDS. Public Health Rep 1988;103:246–254.
282. Hoffenbach A, Langlade-Demoyen P, Dadaglio G, et al. Unusually high frequencies of HIV-specific cytotoxic T lymphocytes in humans. J Immunol 1989;142:452–462.
283. Zinkernagel RM, Hengartner H. T-cell-mediated immunopathology versus direct cytolysis by virus: implications for HIV and AIDS. Immunol Today 1994;15:262–268.
284. Sethi KK, Naher H, Stroehmann I. Phenotypic heterogeneity of cerebrospinal fluid-derived HIV-specific and HLA-restricted cytotoxic T-cell clones. Nature 1988;335:178–181.
285. Stanhope PE, Liu AY, Pavlat W, et al. An HIV-1 envelope protein vaccine elicits a functionally complex human CD4+ T cell response that includes cytolytic T lymphocytes. J Immunol 1993;150:4672–4686.
286. Weinhold KJ, Lyerly HK, Stanley SD, et al. HIV-1 GP120-mediated immune suppression and lymphocyte destruction in the absence of viral infection. J Immunol 1989;142:3091–3097.
287. Lyerly HK, Matthews TJ, Langlois AJ, et al. Human T-cell lymphotropic virus IIIB glycoprotein (gp120) bound to CD4 determinants on normal lymphocytes and expressed by infected cells serves as target for immune attack. Proc Natl Acad Sci U S A 1987;84:4601–4605.
288. Ziegler JL, Stites DP. Hypothesis: AIDS is an autoimmune disease directed at the immune system and triggered by a lymphotropic retrovirus. Clin Immunol Immunopathol 1986;41:305–313.
289. Golding H, Shearer GM, Hillman K, et al. Common epitope in human immunodeficiency virus (HIV) I-GP41 and HLA class II elicits immunosuppressive autoantibodies capable of contributing to immune dysfunction in HIV I-infected individuals. J Clin Invest 1989;83:1430–1435.
290. Bost KL, Hahn BH, Saag MS, et al. Individuals infected with HIV possess antibodies against IL-2. Immunology 1988;65:611–615.
291. Klaassen RJ, Mulder JW, Vlekke AB, et al. Autoantibodies against peripheral blood cells appear early in HIV infection and their prevalence increases with disease progression. Clin Exp Immunol 1990;81:11–17.
292. Klaassen RJ, Goldschmeding R, Dolman KM, et al. Anti-neutrophil cytoplasmic autoantibodies in patients with symptomatic HIV infection. Clin Exp Immunol 1992;87:24–30.
293. Ardman B, Sikorski MA, Settles M, et al. Human immunodeficiency virus type 1–infected individuals make autoantibodies that bind to CD43 on normal thymic lymphocytes. J Exp Med 1990;172:1151–1158.
294. Grassi F, Meneveri R, Gullberg M, et al. Human immunodeficiency virus type 1 gp120 mimics a hidden monomorphic epitope borne by class I major histocompatibility complex heavy chains. J Exp Med 1991;174:53–62.
295. Ardman B, Kowalski M, Bristol J, et al. Effects on CD4 binding of anti-peptide sera to the fourth and fifth conserved domains of HIV-1 gp120. J Acquir Immune Defic Syndr Hum Retrovirol 1990;3:206–214.
296. Gurley RJ, Ikeuchi K, Byrn RA, et al. CD4+ lymphocyte function with early human immunodeficiency virus infection. Proc Natl Acad Sci U S A 1989;86:1993–1997.
297. Mew D, Balza F, Towers GH, et al. Anti-tumour effects of the sesquiterpene lactone parthenin. Planta Med 1982;45:23–27.
298. Toyonaga B, Mak TW. Genes of the T-cell antigen receptor in normal and malignant T cells. Annu Rev Immunol 1987;5:585–620.
299. Davis MM, Bjorkman PJ. T-cell antigen receptor genes and T-cell recognition [published erratum appears in Nature 1988;335:744]. Nature 1988;334:395–402.
300. Wilson RK, Lai E, Concannon P, et al. Structure, organization and polymorphism of murine and human T-cell receptor alpha and beta chain gene families. Immunol Rev 1988;101:149–172.
301. Dellabona P, Peccoud J, Kappler J, et al. Superantigens interact with MHC class II molecules outside of the antigen groove. Cell 1990;62:1115–1121.
302. Imberti L, Sottini A, Bettinardi A, et al. Selective depletion in HIV infection of T cells that bear specific T cell receptor V beta sequences. Science 1991;254:860–862.
303. Soudeyns H, Rebai N, Pantaleo GP, et al. The T cell receptor V beta repertoire in HIV-1 infection and disease. Semin Immunol 1993;5:175–185.
304. Rebai N, Pantaleo G, Demarest JF, et al. Analysis of the T-cell receptor beta-chain variable-region (V beta) repertoire in monozygotic twins discordant for human immunodeficiency virus: evidence for perturbations of specific V beta segments in CD4+ T cells of the virus-positive twins. Proc Natl Acad Sci U S A 1994;91:1529–1533.
305. Laurence J, Hodtsev AS, Posnett DN. Superantigen implicated in dependence of HIV-1 replication in T cells on TCR V beta expression. Nature 1992;358:255–259.
306. Dobrescu D, Ursea B, Pope M, et al. Enhanced HIV-1 replication in V beta 12 T cells due to human cytomegalovirus in monocytes: evidence for a putative herpesvirus superantigen. Cell 1995;82:753–763.
307. Cohen JJ. Apoptosis: the physiologic pathway of cell death. Hosp Pract 1993;28:35–43.
308. Chirmule N, Kalyanaraman VS, Oyaizu N, et al. Inhibition of functional properties of tetanus antigen-specific T-cell clones by envelope glycoprotein GP120 of human immunodeficiency virus. Blood 1990;75:152–159.
309. Oyaizu N, McCloskey TW, Than S, et al. Cross-linking of CD4 molecules upregulates Fas antigen expression in lymphocytes by inducing interferon-gamma and tumor necrosis factor-alpha secretion. Blood 1994;84:2622–2631.
310. Banda NK, Bernier J, Kurahara DK, et al. Crosslinking CD4 by human immunodeficiency virus gp120 primes T cells for activation-induced apoptosis. J Exp Med 1992;176:1099–1106.

311. Laurent-Crawford AG, Krust B, Muller S, et al. The cytopathic effect of HIV is associated with apoptosis. Virology 1991;185:829–839.
312. Zauli G, Re MC, Visani G, et al. Evidence for a human immunodeficiency virus type 1–mediated suppression of uninfected hematopoietic (CD34+) cells in AIDS patients. J Infect Dis 1992;166:710–716.
313. Zauli G, Re MC, Furlini G, et al. Human immunodeficiency virus type 1 envelope glycoprotein gp120-mediated killing of human haematopoietic progenitors (CD34+ cells). J Gen Virol 1992;73:417–421.
314. Muro-Cacho CA, Pantaleo G, Fauci AS. Analysis of apoptosis in lymph nodes of HIV-infected persons: intensity of apoptosis correlates with the general state of activation of the lymphoid tissue and not with stage of disease or viral burden. J Immunol 1995;154:5555–5566.
315. Lewis DE, Tang DS, Adu-Oppong A, et al. Anergy and apoptosis in CD8+ T cells from HIV-infected persons. J Immunol 1994;153:412–420.
316. Gougeon ML, Garcia S, Heeney J, et al. Programmed cell death in AIDS-related HIV and SIV infections. AIDS Res Hum Retroviruses 1993;9:553–563.
317. Groux H, Torpier G, Monte D, et al. Activation-induced death by apoptosis in CD4+ T cells from human immunodeficiency virus-infected asymptomatic individuals. J Exp Med 1992;175:331–340.
318. Meyaard L, Otto SA, Jonker RR, et al. Programmed death of T cells in HIV-1 infection. Science 1992;257:217–219.
319. Oyaizu N, McCloskey TW, Coronesi M, et al. Accelerated apoptosis in peripheral blood mononuclear cells (PBMCs) from human immunodeficiency virus type-1 infected patients and in CD4 cross-linked PBMCs from normal individuals. Blood 1993;82:3392–3400.
320. Katsikis PD, Wunderlich ES, Smith CA, et al. Fas antigen stimulation induces marked apoptosis of T lymphocytes in human immunodeficiency virus-infected individuals. J Exp Med 1995;181:2029–2036.
321. Cameron PU, Pope M, Gezelter S, et al. Infection and apoptotic cell death of CD4+ T cells during an immune response to HIV-1–pulsed dendritic cells. AIDS Res Hum Retroviruses 1994;10:61–71.
322. Newell MK, Haughn LJ, Maroun CR, et al. Death of mature T cells by separate ligation of CD4 and the T-cell receptor for antigen. Nature 1990;347:286–289.
323. Suda T, Takahashi T, Golstein P, et al. Molecular cloning and expression of the Fas ligand, a novel member of the tumor necrosis factor family. Cell 1993;75:1169–1178.
324. Takahashi T, Tanaka M, Brannan CI, et al. Generalized lymphoproliferative disease in mice, caused by a point mutation in the Fas ligand. Cell 1994;76:969–976.
325. Lynch DH, Watson ML, Alderson MR, et al. The mouse Fas-ligand gene is mutated in gld mice and is part of a TNF family gene cluster. Immunity 1994;1:131–136.
326. Weng NP, Levine BL, June CH, et al. Human naive and memory T lymphocytes differ in telomeric length and replicative potential. Proc Natl Acad Sci U S A 1995;92:11091–11094.
327. Zakian VA. Telomeres: beginning to understand the end. Science 1995;270:1601–1607.
328. Hastie ND, Dempster M, Dunlop MG, et al. Telomere reduction in human colorectal carcinoma and with ageing. Nature 1990;346:866–868.
329. Vaziri H, Dragowska W, Allsopp RC, et al. Evidence for a mitotic clock in human hematopoietic stem cells: loss of telomeric DNA with age. Proc Natl Acad Sci U S A 1994;91:9857–9860.
330. Watson JD. Origin of concatemeric T7 DNA. Nat New Biol 1972;239:197–201.
331. Wolthers KC, Bea G, Wisman A, et al. T cell telomere length in HIV-1 infection: no evidence for increased CD4+ T cell turnover. Science 1996;274:1543–1547.
332. Effros RB, Allsopp R, Chiu CP, et al. Shortened telomeres in the expanded CD28 − CD8+ cell subset in HIV disease implicate replicative senescence in HIV pathogenesis. AIDS 1996;10:F17–F22.
333. Wei X, Ghosh SK, Taylor ME, et al. Viral dynamics in human immunodeficiency virus type 1 infection. Nature 1995;373:117–122.
334. Ho DD, Neumann AU, Perelson AS, et al. Rapid turnover of plasma virions and CD4 lymphocytes in HIV-1 infection. Nature 1995;373:123–126.
335. Coffin JM. HIV population dynamics in vivo: implications for genetic variation, pathogenesis, and therapy. Science 1995;267:483–489.
336. Perelson AS, Neumann AU, Markowitz M, et al. HIV-1 dynamics in vivo: virion clearance rate, infected cell life-span, and viral generation time. Science 1996;271:1582–1586.
337. Rabin RL, Roederer M, Maldonado Y, et al. Altered representation of naive and memory CD8 T cell subsets in HIV-infected children. J Clin Invest 1995;95:2054–2060.
338. Roederer M, Dubs JG, Anderson MT, et al. CD8 naive T cell counts decrease progressively in HIV-infected adults. J Clin Invest 1995;95:2061–2066.
339. Margolick JB, Munoz A, Donnenberg AD, et al. Failure of T-cell homeostasis preceding AIDS in HIV-1 infection: the Multicenter AIDS Cohort Study. Nat Med 1995;1:674–680.
340. Stanley SK, Fauci AS. T cell homeostasis in HIV infection: part of the solution, or part of the problem? J Acquir Immune Defic Syndr Hum Retrovirol 1993;6:142–143.
341. Steinberg HN, Crumpacker CS, Chatis PA. In vitro suppression of normal human bone marrow progenitor cells by human immunodeficiency virus. J Virol 1991;65:1765–1769.
342. Watanabe M, Ringler DJ, Nakamura M, et al. Simian immunodeficiency virus inhibits bone marrow hematopoietic progenitor cell growth. J Virol 1990;64:656–663.
343. Potts BJ, Hoggan MD, Lamperth L, et al. Replication of HIV-1 and HIV-2 in human bone marrow cultures. Virology 1992;188:840–849.
344. Lane HC, Depper JM, Greene WC, et al. Qualitative analysis of immune function in patients with the acquired immunodeficiency syndrome: evidence for a selective defect in soluble antigen recognition. N Engl J Med 1985;313:79–84.
345. Noronha IL, Daniel V, Schimpf K, et al. Soluble IL-2 receptor and tumour necrosis factor-alpha in plasma of haemophilia patients infected with HIV. Clin Exp Immunol 1992;87:287–292.
346. Mallet F, Hebrard C, Livrozet JM, et al. Quantitation of human immunodeficiency virus type 1 DNA by two PCR procedures coupled with enzyme-linked oligosorbent assay. J Clin Microbiol 1995;33:3201–3208.
347. Bentin J, Tsoukas CD, McCutchan JA, et al. Impairment in T-lymphocyte responses during early infection with the human immunodeficiency virus. J Clin Immunol 1989;9:159–168.
348. Fauci AS. AIDS: immunopathogenic mechanisms and research strategies. Clin Res 1987;35:503–510.
349. Pantaleo G, De Maria A, Koenig S, et al. CD8+ T lymphocytes of patients with AIDS maintain normal broad cytolytic function despite the loss of human immunodeficiency virus–specific cytotoxicity. Proc Natl Acad Sci U S A 1990;87:4818–4822.
350. Walker BD, Plata F. Cytotoxic T lymphocytes against HIV. AIDS 1990;4:177–184.
351. Margolick JB, Volkman DJ, Lane HC, et al. Clonal analysis of T lymphocytes in the acquired immunodeficiency syndrome: evidence for an abnormality affecting individual helper and suppressor T cells. J Clin Invest 1985;76:709–715.
352. Shearer GM, Salahuddin SZ, Markham PD, et al. Prospective study of cytotoxic T lymphocyte responses to influenza and antibodies to human T lymphotropic virus-III in homosexual men: selective loss of an influenza-specific, human leukocyte antigen–restricted cytotoxic T lymphocyte response in human T lymphotropic virus-III positive individuals with symptoms of acquired immunodeficiency syndrome and in a patient with acquired immunodeficiency syndrome. J Clin Invest 1985;76:1699–1704.
353. Rook AH, Manischewitz JF, Frederick WR, et al. Deficient, HLA-restricted, cytomegalovirus-specific cytotoxic T cells and natural killer cells in patients with the acquired immunodeficiency syndrome. J Infect Dis 1985;152:627–630.

354. Lane HC, Masur H, Edgar LC, et al. Abnormalities of B-cell activation and immunoregulation in patients with the acquired immunodeficiency syndrome. N Engl J Med 1983;309:453–458.
355. Jacobson DL, McCutchan JA, Spechko PL, et al. The evolution of lymphadenopathy and hypergammaglobulinemia are evidence for early and sustained polyclonal B lymphocyte activation during human immunodeficiency virus infection. J Infect Dis 1991;163:240–246.
356. Miedema F, Petit AJ, Terpstra FG, et al. Immunological abnormalities in human immunodeficiency virus (HIV)–infected asymptomatic homosexual men: HIV affects the immune system before CD4+ T helper cell depletion occurs. J Clin Invest 1988;82:1908–1914.
357. Birx DL, Redfield RR, Tosato G. Defective regulation of Epstein–Barr virus infection in patients with acquired immunodeficiency syndrome (AIDS) or AIDS-related disorders. N Engl J Med 1986;314:874–879.
358. Reddy MM, Goetz RR, Gorman JM, et al. Human immunodeficiency virus type-1 infection of homosexual men is accompanied by a decrease in circulating B cells. J Acquir Immune Defic Syndr Hum Retrovirol 1991;4:428–434.
359. Berberian L, Goodglick L, Kipps TJ, et al. Immunoglobulin VH3 gene products: natural ligands for HIV gp120. Science 1993;261:1588–1591.
360. Chirmule N, Kalyanaraman VS, Saxinger C, et al. Localization of B-cell stimulatory activity of HIV-1 to the carboxyl terminus of gp41. AIDS Res Hum Retroviruses 1990;6:299–305.
361. Amadori A, Zamarchi R, Ciminale V, et al. HIV-1–specific B cell activation: a major constituent of spontaneous B cell activation during HIV-1 infection. J Immunol 1989;143:2146–2152.
362. Amadori A, Gallo P, Zamarchi R, et al. IgG oligoclonal bands in sera of HIV-1 infected patients are mainly directed against HIV-1 determinants. AIDS Res Hum Retroviruses 1990;6:581–586.
363. Vendrell JP, Segondy M, Ducos J, et al. Analysis of the spontaneous in vitro anti-HIV-1 antibody secretion by peripheral blood mononuclear cells in HIV-1 infection. Clin Exp Immunol 1991;83:197–202.
364. Shirai A, Cosentino M, Leitman-Klinman SF, et al. Human immunodeficiency virus infection induces both polyclonal and virus-specific B cell activation. J Clin Invest 1992;89:561–566.
365. Katz IR, Krown SE, Safai B, et al. Antigen-specific and polyclonal B-cell responses in patients with acquired immunodeficiency disease syndrome. Clin Immunol Immunopathol 1986;39:359–367.
366. Amadori A, Chieco-Bianchi L. B-cell activation and HIV-1 infection: deeds and misdeeds. Immunol Today 1990;11:374–379.
367. Rinaldo CR Jr, Beltz LA, Huang XL, et al. Anti-HIV type 1 cytotoxic T lymphocyte effector activity and disease progression in the first 8 years of HIV type 1 infection of homosexual men. AIDS Res Hum Retroviruses 1995;11:481–489.
368. Lucia B, Jennings C, Cauda R, et al. Evidence of a selective depletion of a CD16+ CD56+ CD8+ natural killer cell subset during HIV infection. Cytometry 1995;22:10–15.
369. Hu PF, Hultin LE, Hultin P, et al. Natural killer cell immunodeficiency in HIV disease is manifest by profoundly decreased numbers of CD16+CD56+ cells and expansion of a population of CD16dimCD56– cells with low lytic activity. J Acquir Immune Defic Syndr Hum Retrovirol 1995;10:331–340.
370. Muller C, Szangolies M, Kukel S, et al. Characterization of autoantibodies to natural killer cells in HIV-infected patients. Scand J Immunol 1996;43:583–592.
371. Katz JD, Mitsuyasu R, Gottlieb MS, et al. Mechanism of defective NK cell activity in patients with acquired immunodeficiency syndrome (AIDS) and AIDS-related complex. II. Normal antibody-dependent cellular cytotoxicity (ADCC) mediated by effector cells defective in natural killer (NK) cytotoxicity. J Immunol 1987;139:55–60.
372. Ojo-Amaize E, Nishanian PG, Heitjan DF, et al. Serum and effector-cell antibody-dependent cellular cytotoxicity (ADCC) activity remains high during human immunodeficiency virus (HIV) disease progression. J Clin Immunol 1989;9:454–461.
373. Rook AH, Masur H, Lane HC, et al. Interleukin-2 enhances the depressed natural killer and cytomegalovirus-specific cytotoxic activities of lymphocytes from patients with the acquired immune deficiency syndrome. J Clin Invest 1983;72:398–403.
374. Sirianni MC, Ansotegui IJ, Aiuti F, et al. Natural killer cell stimulatory factor (NKSF)/IL-12 and cytolytic activities of PBL/NK cells from human immunodeficiency virus type-1 infected patients. Scand J Immunol 1994;40:83–86.
375. Wahl SM, Orenstein JM, Smith PD. Macrophage functions in HIV-1 Infection. In: Gupta S, ed. Immunology of HIV infection. New York: Plenum, 1996:303–336.
376. Merrill JE. Cytokines and retroviruses. Clin Immunol Immunopathol 1992;64:23–27.
377. Knight SC, Macatonia SE. Effect of HIV on antigen presentation by dendritic cells and macrophages. Res Virol 1991;142:123–128.
378. Clerici M, Stocks NI, Zajac RA, et al. Accessory cell function in asymptomatic human immunodeficiency virus-infected patients. Clin Immunol Immunopathol 1990;54:168–173.
379. Prince HE, Moody DJ, Shubin BI, et al. Defective monocyte function in acquired immune deficiency syndrome (AIDS): evidence from a monocyte-dependent T-cell proliferative system. J Clin Immunol 1985;5:21–25.
380. Macatonia SE, Lau R, Patterson S, et al. Dendritic cell infection, depletion and dysfunction in HIV-infected individuals. Immunology 1990;71:38–45.
381. Eales LJ, Farrant J, Helbert M, et al. Peripheral blood dendritic cells in persons with AIDS and AIDS related complex: loss of high intensity class II antigen expression and function. Clin Exp Immunol 1988;71:423–427.
382. Cameron PU, Forsum U, Teppler H, et al. During HIV-1 infection most blood dendritic cells are not productively infected and can induce allogeneic CD4+ T cells clonal expansion. Clin Exp Immunol 1992;88:226–236.
383. Cimarelli A, Zambruno G, Marconi A, et al. Quantitation by competitive PCR of HIV-1 proviral DNA in epidermal Langerhans cells of HIV-infected patients. J Acquir Immune Defic Syndr Hum Retrovirol 1994;7:230–235.
384. Blauvelt A, Clerici M, Lucey DR, et al. Functional studies of epidermal Langerhans cells and blood monocytes in HIV-infected persons. J Immunol 1995;154:3506–3515.

6

AN IMMUNOLOGIST'S VIEW OF HIV INFECTION

Gordon L. Ada

It is convenient to divide infections into two groups—acute infections, and chronic, persisting infections. In acute infections, the host is either overwhelmed by the infection and dies within a few days or a week, or the immune response of the host is sufficiently rapid and comprehensive so the infection is cleared, and the host recovers. After this initial infection, the host usually resists a further exposure to the same infectious agent; the host has become immune. This memory may last for the lifetime of the host. This is the experience of most people exposed to infections such as smallpox, polio, yellow fever, measles, mumps, and rubella, to name a few. Sometimes, the host experiences a series of similar acute infections by the same organism because the development of broadly protective immunity takes some time. The classic case is influenza. The virus, by one of two general types of genetic mechanisms (antigenic drift or antigenic shift), undergoes changes in the amino acid sequence and hence the antigenicity of the surface antigens, the hemagglutinin and neuraminidase. In this way, a later isolate of influenza virus is able to "bypass" or "evade" the antibody present as a result of an earlier infection, and reinfection occurs. A study of viruses causing acute infections, particularly in an animal model such as the mouse, has led to an understanding of: 1) the different immune responses that occur after infection, and the role of each in preventing, limiting and finally clearing the infection; and 2) the nature of immunologic memory induced as part of the immune response.

Persisting infections, many also inducing chronic disease, occur either because the host fails to generate protective immune responses or because these responses, although generated, fail to control the infection for one or more of several possible reasons. Many important infectious diseases, including the major parasitic infections such as malaria, are in this category. Because of its public health importance, particularly the early indication that the mortality rate may come close to 100%, infection by the human immunodeficiency virus (HIV) early became the target for detailed immunologic examination. Furthermore, because of the lack of a suitable and readily available animal model, most attention has necessarily focused on human infection. The pattern that has emerged is that, over a variable period but averaging about 10 years for most of those infected, critical cells of the immune system are either directly infected by the virus or are affected by the resulting immunopathology. This leads to a state of immune deficiency that allows chronic infection by opportunistic infectious agents and leads finally to death. The fascination for immunologists is threefold:

1. To understand the nature of the infectious process, the immune responses that occur after infection, the reasons they are generally ineffective, allowing a slow but progressive decrease in immune capability, and the immunopathology that results
2. To judge or predict the chances of success of immunologic prophylaxis to prevent or to limit and then clear the infection in those at risk of infection, that is, to convert what is normally a persisting infection into an acute infection
3. If item number 2 is not possible, to prevent or delay immunodeficiency in most cases so individuals survive for a significantly longer period and become noninfectious or much less infectious to others

In this chapter, the nature of the adaptive immune system and the role of the immune responses that occur in an acute infection are first briefly described, followed by a description of the different patterns seen during HIV infections. The combined information forms the basis for a discussion of the requirements of a vaccine for HIV prophylaxis.

IMMUNE RESPONSES THAT OCCUR DURING AN ACUTE VIRAL INFECTION

Two classes of immune responses are seen during an infection. They are the innate (or nonadaptive, nonspecific) and the adaptive (or specific) responses.

Innate Immunity

Various different cell types, cytokines, and other soluble factors mediate the response that occurs generally within minutes or hours after an infection is initiated. The cell types include neutrophils, natural killer (NK) cells, macrophages/monocytes, eosinophils, and mast cells. Cytokines include the interferons (IFNs) α, β, and γ, which can be induced early in the response. Proteins include those of the complement cascade and the C-reactive protein. Investigators now realize that components of the innate and adaptive systems interact and overlap. For example, IFN-γ used to be called immune interferon because it is produced by T lymphocytes, but it is now known to be produced also by NK cells. Although some responses, such as NK cells, may show a degree of selectivity in their action, none is specific; furthermore, no evidence to date indicates that any component of the innate system has a memory effect.

Adaptive Immunity

The adaptive responses are characterized by two features—specificity and memory. The only cell type that displays both these characteristics is the lymphocyte, of which two classes are known. B cells make antibodies, a humoral effector response, which once secreted, become widely distributed around the body. T cells not only have regulatory roles through helper (Th) and suppressor (Ts) activities, but also they may have effector activity, mediating delayed-type hypersensitivity (DTH) or cytotoxicity (cytotoxic T lymphocytes or CTLs), that is, lysis of infected cells. These responses are adaptive because, after specific stimulation by antigen, activation, replication, and differentiation of B and T cells occur. The receptors for antigen on both T and B cells show great specificity. In the case of B cells, affinity maturation of the antibody produced over time is seen. Although T-cell responses are largely mediated by short-range factors (cytokines, interleukins), they are generally referred to as cell-mediated immune (CMI) responses.

Antibody, or the immunoglobulin (Ig) receptor on B cells (mainly IgM), may recognize amino acid (or sugar) sequences (called epitopes) on virus or individual antigens either free in solution or present on the surface of infected cells. Such sequences may be "continuous" or discontinuous (e.g., formed by adjacent molecules), but in each case, they may have a preferred conformation. In contrast, the T-cell receptor (TCR) recognizes peptides derived either from degraded antigens or from newly synthesized foreign or self-proteins, complexed with major histocompatibility complex (MHC) antigens. In this case, parts of the peptide and the MHC molecule form the epitope, so the peptide component is sometimes simply called a determinant. Two main classes of such complexes are recognized. Peptides derived from the processing in lysosomes of exogenous antigens associate with class II MHC antigens and are recognized by Th cells; hence these responses are called class II MHC restricted, and the responding T cell is characterized by a membrane marker, the CD4 molecule. In contrast, peptides derived from endogenous proteins (self-proteins or viral proteins synthesized in the cytoplasm) associate with class I MHC antigens and are recognized by the TCR on CTLs; hence these responses are called class I MHC restricted, and the membrane marker on these cells is the CD8 molecule. In the latter case, the peptide is 8 to 10 amino acids long (usually 9) and has a "motif," that is, must have certain amino acids in particular positions to complex with a given molecule.

The peptide–MHC complex is presented to T cells by antigen-presenting cells (APCs). The most effective APCs, sometimes called "professional" APCs, include macrophages and especially dendritic cells. Such cells clearly must express MHC molecules, as well as a "costimulator" molecule for which the T cells express a receptor, and must secrete certain cytokines. T cells are both major producers of and responders to cytokines. Two types of Th cells—Th1 and Th2—have now been described both in mice and in humans, and investigators have proposed the existence of a precursor population, Th0. These cells are distinguished by the profiles of secreted cytokines (Table 6.1). The profile for Th1 cells is similar to that of CTLs, so the tendency is to group Th1 and CTLs as type 1 T cells and Th2 cells as type 2 T cells. Of all the cytokines now recognized, two, at least in the mouse, play a dominant role in directing the immune response. Interleukin (IL)-4 strongly favors a type 2 T-cell response, and IL-12 a type 1 T-cell response. In addition, investigators have found, at least in vitro, that on exposure to IL-4, CTLs can convert to a population that secretes a profile of cytokines similar to that of type 2 cells; these two populations have been called Tc1 and Tc2, to correspond to Th1 and Th2 (see Table 6.1).

The foregoing is a simplified version of our current knowledge of the immune system. More detailed accounts can be found elsewhere (1, 2).

Table 6.1. Characteristics of T-Lymphocyte Subsets

	CD4+ T cells		CD8+ T cells	
	Th1	Th2	Tc1	Tc2
Secreted factors				
IL-2	+	−	+	−
IL-3	+	−	−	−
IL-4	−	+	−	+
IL-5	−	+	−	+
IL-6	−	+	−	?
IL-10	−	+	−	?
IL-13	−	+	−	?
TNF-α	+	+	−	−
TNF-β	+	−	+	−
IFN-γ	+	−	+	−
Chemokines[a]	−	−	+	−
CD8+ T-cell suppressor factors			+	
Effector activities				
Cytotoxicity	−	−	+	+
DTH	+	−	+/−	−
B-cell help	IgG2a[b], IgG1[c]	IgG1[b], IgA[b], IgE[b]	−	+

DTH, delayed-type hypersensitivity; IFN, interferon; IL, interleukin; TNF, tumor necrosis factor.
[a]MIP-1α, MIP-1β, RANTES.
[b]In mice.
[c]In humans.

IMMUNOLOGIC MEMORY

A major feature of the adaptive system is immunologic memory. After interaction with activated Th cells, rapidly dividing B cells (the centrocytes) in the germinal centers (GCs) of lymphoid tissue undergo somatic hypermutation. B cells with Ig receptors of higher affinity are selected for further differentiation by antigen that, in the form of aggregates of antigen and antibody, has attached to the *surface* of follicular dendritic cells (FDCs) in the GC. Especially if they are resistant to proteases, antigens are known to persist on FDCs for many months, and some are thought to do so for years (1). After differentiation, some cells become antibody-secreting cells, and others become memory cells that may have Ig receptors of different isotypes (G, A, and E). B memory cells continually recirculate, and on further contact with antigen, the foregoing cycle may be repeated. A second dose of antigen may amplify this sequence of events and may boost the recruitment of memory cells.

Little is known about the development of T-cell memory, except their induction does not seem to be restricted to any special site, the TCR does not undergo affinity maturation, and the cells survive for long periods in the absence of specific antigen. The requirements for their stimulation are much less stringent than those for naive T cells. They can be stimulated by APCs that do not express costimulator molecules (3), and the kinetics of activation is short (4)—two critical properties of an effective vaccine. This field has been reviewed (5).

One of the specific contributions of HIV vaccine development was the demonstration (6) that volunteers immunized first with a gp160 recombinant vaccinia virus and later boosted with a recombinant gp160 prepared in baculovirus-transfected cells developed anti-gp160 antibody titers substantially higher than volunteers receiving only doses of the same product. This finding suggests that some forms of immunogen may be better at inducing a memory response than others, and it has opened up a new aspect of vaccination strategies.

ROLE OF DIFFERENT IMMUNE RESPONSES, PARTICULARLY DURING AN INFECTION

Prevention of Infection

Specific antibody is the only mechanism for completely or largely preventing a viral infection. Infants, particularly in countries where many viral diseases are endemic, are protected from virally induced disease by antibody that is maternally derived at birth and is supplemented by breast-feeding. Numerous examples have shown that transfer of specific immune sera has protected a susceptible host from disease. In the development of many vaccines, a primary aim has been to induce a strong antibody response with the aim of preventing a challenge infection. Whether complete prevention—"sterilizing immunity"—ever occurs is unclear, but it is unlikely, as shown by the experiments of Parker Small and colleagues in mice. Transfer of specific IgG limited subsequent influenza viral replication in the lung but did not prevent tracheitis, that is, infection of epithelial cells at the mucosal surface (7). However, transfer of a hybridoma expressing anti-influenza poly-IgA prevented infection in most, but not all, mice; in this case, the poly-IgA was converted to secretory IgA (sIgA) in passage through the epithelial cells to the lumen (8). Treatment of mice convalescing from a respiratory influenza infection with anti-α but not anti-μ or anti-γ sera destroyed their resistance to a second infection of mucosal cells with the homologous virus (9). The natural route of infection by many viruses, including HIV, is through a mucosal surface. That secretory IgA (sIgA) can neutralize viral infectivity extracellularly is well established. Substantial evidence indicates that IgA antibodies can neutralize viruses intracellularly if the virus is infecting an epithelial cell through which the IgA is passing en route to the lumen (10).

Limitation of Viral Replication

Many innate immune responses, such as the production of the IFNs and enhanced NK cell activity, usually occur shortly after infection and may limit the extent of viral replication before components of the adaptive immune response are activated and become effector cells. In an outbred population such as humans, assessing the extent of the contribution of such responses to controlling an infection is difficult. If a virus has a rapid replication cycle, such as less than 10 hours, the absence of such responses could mean the difference between life or death. The absence of a neutrophil response could be devastating in the case of infection by rapidly replicating bacteria. No evidence from any model viral system indicates that, in the absence of a specific immune response, activated innate responses can clear an infection.

Recovery from an Infection

In an acute viral infection, such as murine influenza virus, specific lymphocyte responses are detected in the following sequence: regulatory T cells (Th2), effector T cells (such as CTLs), and finally, antibody. The role of antibody and effector T cells in controlling or clearing a viral infection has been elucidated mainly by transfer experiments. Antibody of the correct specificity can contribute to the recovery from infection, by neutralizing the infectivity of cell-free viral progeny (e.g., preventing or minimizing viremia), by lysing infected cells expressing viral antigens (by antibody-dependent cellular cytotoxicity [ADCC] or by complement-dependent lysis). After immunization with inactivated polio vaccine, systemic antibody prevents spread of polio virus from the mucosa to the nervous system, and antibody of the correct specificity should prevent the viremia seen after HIV infection.

In several examples in mice lacking effector CTLs, a viral infection has been cleared. The list includes egg-grown influenza (11, 12) and vaccinia virus (13, 14). Antibody may have been responsible for some of these results. High-titer antibody has cleared virus from cells infected either with

Table 6.2. Evidence Supporting a Dominant Role for Cytotoxic T Lymphocytes (CTLs) in the Control and Clearance of Viral Infections

General arguments
1. Clearance of many viral infections is associated with the induction of a CTL response before the appearance of neutralizing antibody.
2. Nearly all mammalian cell types express class I MHC antigens. Exceptions include gametes, neurons, red blood cells, and cells of the trophoblast.
3. CTLs secrete potent cytokines with antiviral and macrophage-activating properties, such as interferon γ and tumor necrosis factor α as well as a range of chemokines.
4. Infected cells become susceptible to lysis by CTLs long before viral progeny is made.

More direct evidence
1. Transfer of specific effector CTLs into an MHC-compatible host clears established infections in a specific organ or protects from death following an otherwise lethal infection (1). In humans, CTLs reconstitute specific cytomegalovirus (19, 20) and Epstein–Barr virus (21) immunity after allogeneic bone marrow transplants.
2. Using lymphocytic choriomeningitis virus (LCMV, a noncytopathic virus) infections of mice, CTLs have been shown to lyse infected cells in vivo (22) as well as in vitro. Similarly, virus-specific CTLs transferred to transgenic mice expressing the hepatitis B surface antigen caused apoptosis of the hepatocytes (23). The cytotoxicity of LCMV-specific CTLs is greatly impaired in perforin -ve mice (24).

respiratory syncytial virus (RSV) (15) or Sindbis virus (16). In contrast, CTLs are necessary for the clearing of murine lymphocytic choriomeningitis (LCM) virus, ectromelia, and Theiler's virus infections (17). One difference is that the latter three are mouse pathogens, whereas influenza, vaccinia, and Sindbis viruses and RSV are not.

Starting with the discovery of MHC restriction in 1974 (18), increasing evidence has suggested that CTLs are the major mechanism for controlling and clearing an acute viral infection, and this subject has been reviewed (17). Some aspects are listed in Table 6.2 (19–24).

STRUCTURE AND ANTIGENIC PROPERTIES OF HIV-1

Structure

For relatively small viruses, HIV-1 and HIV-2 have an extraordinarily complex composition, possessing both structural and regulatory proteins. The HIV-1 proviral genome is 9.7 kb in length and includes regulatory sequences at either end, long terminal repeats, and genes coding for proteins that have structural (env, gag) or enzymatic (pol) properties. The env consists of two glycosylated proteins, linked noncovalently: gp41, which spans the viral envelope; and gp120, which is entirely external. The latter has five "loops" that are held in that conformation by disulfide bonds.

All other proteins are inside the viral envelope. The gag (group-specific) protein is translated as a polyprotein precursor molecule, p55, which is cleaved to form four products: p7, p9, p17, and p24. The products of the *pol* gene have enzymatic activities—a reverse transcriptase, an endonuclease, a protease, and an integrase. An elaborate collection of regulatory genes determines whether and how much infectious virus is produced. They include *vpr, rev, vif, tat, vpu,* and *nef*; the last is required for the prolific replication of the virus in vivo, as has been well shown for simian immunodeficiency virus (SIV) (25). Their function has become better understood in recent years, but in this chapter, their main interest is as a source of T-cell determinants early in the cycle of viral replication. Peptides from these molecules, in association with MHC molecules, provide not only an early stimulus by infected cells for the induction of T-cell responses, but also an early recognition of an infected cell by effector CTLs.

Antigenic Properties of the Viral Proteins

EPITOPES RECOGNIZED BY B CELLS

The two classes are those composed of linear sequences of amino acids or sugars, called continuous epitopes, and those composed of spatially adjacent sequences, either on the same molecule or contributed by adjacent molecules and called discontinuous sequences. Both can have a particular conformation. Examples of the different epitopes are illustrated in Figure 6.1.

The five types of epitopes of particular interest are those recognized by antibody that 1) neutralizes viral infectivity; 2) takes part in ADCC; 3) can enhance viral infectivity; 4) may share some homology with sequences in host proteins (molecular mimicry), and hence if used for immunization, may lead to the development of autoimmunity; and 5) those present on host antigens that may be incorporated into the structure of the agent. This last case became important when investigators found that SIV could contain antigens derived from the human cellular substrate, and this led to a misleading interpretation about the immunogenicity of inactivated SIV in monkeys (26).

All these types of epitopes are present in HIV, but the first was initially and has remained of the greatest interest and relevance for vaccine development, and is mainly discussed in this article; gp120 contains 5 conserved (C1 to C5) and 5 variable (V1 to V5) regions. The V3 loop has long been regarded as the principal neutralizing domain, meaning that it is sufficiently immunogenic during an infection or when env preparations are used for vaccination to be recognized by most infected or vaccinated individuals. Apart from a partly conserved 4-amino acid sequence at the tip of the loop, as many as 12 different amino acids may occupy some of the other residue positions (27). Thus, antibodies to this region tend to be strain specific. Some neutralizing antibodies were found to recognize sequences in the V2 loop as well as a discontinuous sequence in a region near the binding site of gp120 to the primary cellular receptor for HIV, the CD4 molecule. The evidence suggested that antibody to the latter site may be more antigenically cross-reactive, but it required a prolonged immunization schedule to obtain adequate titers, a finding suggesting that this site may be poorly immunogenic (28).

Strong evidence supports the existence of coreceptors for the virus. The receptors for certain chemokines on susceptible cells act as coreceptors for syncytium-inducing (SI) (fusin, 29) and nonsyncytium-inducing (NSI) (CC-CKR-5, 30, 31) variants. The b-chemokines RANTES (regulated-on-activation, normal T expressed and secreted), the macrophage inflammatory proteins (MIP-1a and MIP-1b), which bind to CC-CKR-5, inhibit HIV-1 (32) in a manner similar to that observed by soluble factors from CD8+ T cells (33). This area has been reviewed (34), but it is worthwhile stressing that the CC chemokines blocked infection by some primary HIV isolates (32), and the ability of the CD4+ T cells of some individuals to resist infection by HIV (35) correlated with the presence of these factors (32).

NEUTRALIZATION OF FIELD STRAINS OF HIV-1 BY ANTIBODY

The setback to HIV vaccine development seemed substantial when the two most advanced candidate vaccines for HIV, produced by the Genentech and Biocine companies, were not approved by the National Institute of Allergy and Infectious Diseases (NIAID) to proceed to phase III clinical trials. Both candidates were the env antigen prepared in mammalian cell culture and would have been expected to have an appropriate conformation. Although many reasons were given for the decision, an important one was that the antibody induced by these preparations neutralized laboratory-adapted strains, but not field strains of the virus. This finding was formally confirmed in a later publication (36). There seemed to be two possible explanations: 1) that some modification of the neutralization assay would "correct" this anomaly; or 2) because investigators generally agree that the only epitopes recognized by neutralizing antibody occur in the env, then the conformation of this antigen in a newly isolated field strain virus must differ in some subtle way from that on the surface of laboratory-adapted virus, which is usually grown in cultured CD4+ T cells. In contrast, chimpanzees immunized with rpg160 and boosted with a V3 peptide (MN strain) were protected from challenge with a heterologous strain that was passaged in blood mononuclear cells and hence was considered equivalent to a primary isolate (37). In a second case, DNA coding for a Japanese V3 loop sequence and a mycobacterial protein was transfected into bacille Calmette-Guérin (BCG), which, after administration to and replication in hu-PBL-SCID mice, secreted the chimeric protein. The antibody induced by this construct neutralized the infectivity of a primary HIV isolate that possessed the same V3 motif sequence (38).

Investigators have since proposed that antibody recognizing epitopes on gp120 oligomers, probably trimers, is critical for the neutralization of the infectivity of primary strains HIV (39), a view consistent with the finding that primary isolates of HIV-1 are relatively resistant to neutralization by monoclonal antibodies to monomeric gp120 (40). Studies (41, 42) including other findings in a review article (43), support this interpretation. In the infected cell, some of the monomeric precursor gp160 oligomerizes probably to a trimer for transport to the plasma membrane; gp41, the transmembrane component, remains as a trimer in the membrane, whereas the secreted gp120 may be more unstable. In addition, large amounts of monomeric gp160 may be shed into the medium when the infected cell dies. One human antibody, 2F5, specific for the external sequence 662-667 near the plasma membrane, neutralizes clade B primary HIV-1 strains, and in trials with chimpanzees, considerably delayed seroconversion after challenge (44). Two antibodies that bind to oligomeric gp120 have been shown to neutralize primary isolates. One

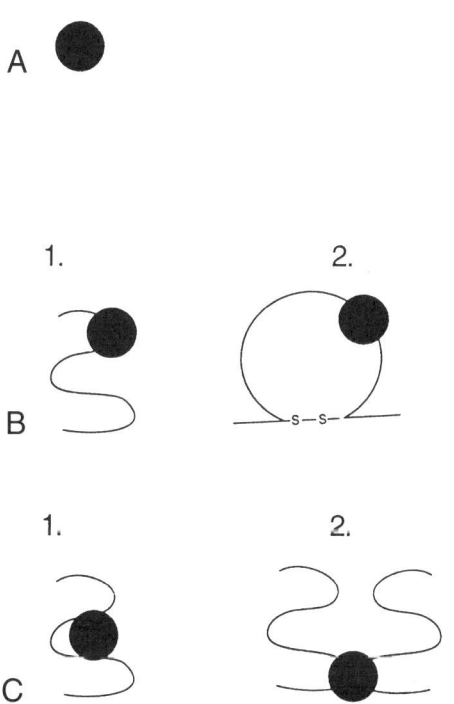

Figure 6.1. Examples of different typews of epitopes seen by the binding site of an antibody. A. The shape (epitope) seen by a binding site. The total surface area of contact and interaction may be as high as 800 A^2, although much of the specificity is primarily determined by a central area of 250 to 400 A^2 (1). **B.** Continuous (linear) sequences. **B1.** Linear sequence in a protein. **B2.** Linear sequence in a peptide loop, linked by a disulfide bond. This occurs in the V3 loop of gp120. **C.** Discontinuous (nonlinear) sequences. **C1.** Formed by sequences within a molecule adn adjacent because of the overall conformation of a protein. **C2.** Formed by adjacent sequences on proteins in close proximity; such epitopes occur in the surface antigens of influenza and polio viruses (1) and have been postulated (39) to occur in HIV-1 env, and more recent findings support this conclusion (40–43).

epitope, CD4bd, is close to the CD4 binding site. One recombinant antibody recognizing this site, IgGb12, at relatively high concentrations neutralized all 35 primary isolates, including some nonclade B isolates (JA Kessler, PM McKenna, EA Emini, et al, quoted in 43), and protected hu-SCID mice from infection with a primary isolate (M-C Gauduin, RA Koup, quoted in 43). This antibody is sensitive to mutations occurring in the V2 loop. The other, 2G12, recognizes an epitope that appears to contain residues from the base of the V3 loop and the V4 region (45). This epitope is also expressed on monomeric gp120. Other antibodies are in the process of being defined (43).

To date, preparations of defined antibodies that neutralize primary strains are mainly either monoclonal antibodies or are made from phage combinatorial libraries. If antibodies of this specificity are formed during an infection, they may represent only a tiny proportion of the total antibody made to env. In fact, investigators have proposed that nearly all the antibody response during an infection is to unprocessed gp160 liberated especially when infected cells die, in effect "infected cellular debris" (45). The critical epitopes recognized by antibodies that can neutralize a primary isolate are most likely poorly immunogenic, so the question arises, will it be possible to devise an immunization protocol that would result in the generation of high-titer antibody of these specificities? An inactivated whole virion (free of "cellular debris") has been suggested (46). Moss and colleagues (41) have constructed a recombinant vector that leads to the formation in cells of an oligomeric gp140 containing the entire gp120 and the ectoderm of gp41; the gp41 is truncated just prior to the transmembrane domain. It is secreted from the vector-infected cells and so can be purified to homogeneity with relative ease.

DETERMINANTS RECOGNIZED BY T CELLS

Virtually all HIV antigens have been screened for determinants that bind to class I or II MHC antigens of different haplotypes, and many of these were published in an earlier review (47). In the case of class I MHC peptide determinants, most are nonapeptides with particular motifs at certain residue positions for different HLA haplotypes. This has made it straightforward to screen HIV antigens for nonapeptides, which, in association with the particular HLA molecule, should be recognized by CTLs. The role of CTLs in the control and recovery of many infections is summarized earlier. Before reviewing the evidence consistent with a similar role for CTLs in HIV infections, the different patterns of HIV infection now seen are briefly reviewed.

DIFFERENT PATTERNS OF HIV INFECTION

For the first decade after the discovery of HIV, essentially only one pattern was seen (Fig. 6.2B). The first sign of infection, usually a few weeks after exposure, was the occurrence of a brief viremia that, in severe cases, necessitated hospitalization. This was accompanied by a temporary de-

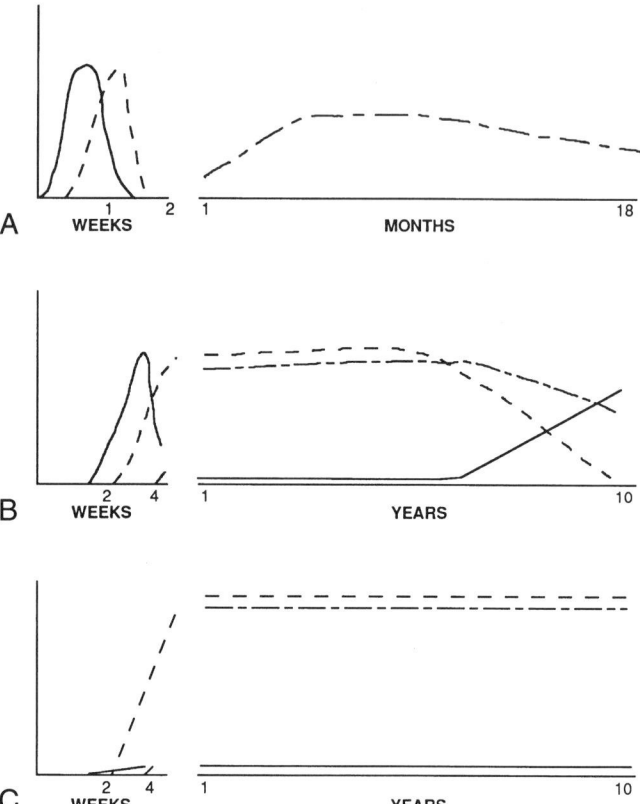

Figure 6.2. Presence of infectious virus and immune responses in an acute versus a chronic persisting infection. Ordinates: *LHS*, log infectious virus titer; *RHS*, increase in CTL effector activity and neutralizing antibody titers. Abcissa: time after infection. **A.** Levels of infectious influenza virus in the mouse lung after intranasal inoculation. The virus undergoes cycles of replication *(solid line)*, but the prevention of further replication and clearance of virus coincides with the appearance of CTLs *(line comprising dashes of equal size)*. Neutralizing antibody appears later and persists *(line comprising long and short dashes)*. **B.** Levels of infectious virus in the circulation of an individual infected with HIV *(solid line)* who progresses to AIDS in 10 years or less. The decrease in early viremia coincides with the appearance of CTLs, and this activity may persist for some years *(equal dashes)*. The later decrease in CTL activity approximately coincides with the decrease in CD4+ T cells in the circulation. Neutralizing antibodies *(long and short dashes)* are detected later than CTL activity. **C.** Levels of infectious HIV *(solid line)*, CTL activity *(equal dashes)*, and neutralizing antibody *(long and short dashes)* in the circulation of a long-term nonprogressor *(LTNP)* HIV-infected individual.

crease of CD4+ T-cell levels. These returned to near-normal levels and, in most cases, remained high for up to 6 to 8 years. During this time, the viral levels in the blood remained low, but as the CD4+ T-cell levels began to fall, blood viral levels increased, and an individual became the target for different opportunistic infections. After infection, the average time until death was about 10 years, although in some cases it was shorter. The clinically asymptomatic period was initially called a latent period, but subsequent studies (48, 49) showed that during this period, the battle between the virus and the immune system was intense, especially in lymphoid tissues. For example, up to 10^9 viral particles and 2×10^9 CD4+ T cells were produced daily, to replace losses of cells that had become infected. Investigators inferred (50) that much higher levels of virus would have been detected were it not for strong CTL activity during this period. The presence in the blood of effector CTLs (not requiring in vitro stimulation) after the viremic period and persisting for several years is one of the unique features of a human infection. A close association between the control of viremia and the detection of CTL activity was found (51, 52), a result reminiscent of findings in tissues of experimental animals infected with other viruses (1). Seroconversion occurred at about the time of viremia, but neutralizing antibody was usually not detected until later (53), sometimes much later (43). On the other hand, the presence of ADCC was also said to correlate well with the initial decline in viremia (54, 55), so this response could also contribute.

The last few years have seen the emergence of a subset of infected individuals who have survived for considerably more than 10 years with high CD4+ T-cell levels and little if any immunodeficiency (56–58). They are called long-term nonprogressors (LTNPs). Although some may have been infected with defective virus (59, and see later), robust immune responses are generally thought to be important contributory factors. This interpretation has been strengthened by a publication (60) in which the antibody response, especially early neutralizing activity against primary isolates, was compared between LTNPs and short-term nonprogressors or progressors. The findings indicated that generally, neutralizing antibody responses were slow to develop during a primary infection, a finding confirming that their presence did not correlate with the control of viremia. An important point was that, over time, they became uniquely broad in their activity against heterologous primary isolates in LTNPs. A comparison of infectious virus levels, CTL, and neutralizing activities of progressors versus LTNPs is shown in Figure 6.1. In comparison with the responses in an acute infection (influenza virus in the mouse lung; see Fig. 6.1A), high CTL effector activity and neutralizing antibody levels persist in LTNPs.

In one report (61), several recipients of blood from an HIV-1–infected individual (who has remained free of AIDS) did not result in immunodeficiency in the infected recipients. The transmitted virus was a naturally occurring attenuated form, with deletions in the *nef* gene and in the U3 region of the long terminal repeat (62). One case has also been reported of the disappearance of HIV in a child born to an infected mother (63). Unfortunately, no immunologic studies were conducted.

CTL RESPONSES TO AND CONTROL OF HIV INFECTIONS

Although the evidence that CTL responses play an important part in controlling HIV-1 infections is indirect, mainly by association with a favorable outcome of the infection, the case is becoming more persuasive. Transfer experiments could give a clear answer. Under conditions in which high concentrations of specific antibody could protect hu-PBL-SCID mice from a challenge HIV-1 infection, transfer of CTLs either 1 day before or on the day of challenge gave only partial protection in two of five mice (64). The cells transferred were cloned human cells with a specificity against a single determinant in nef. Two points can be made. Although the protection was HLA restricted, cells specific for several determinants restricted by the same MHC haplotype could have given more impressive results; and cultured T cells have abnormal migration patterns in mice (Ada GL, unpublished data). Repeated transfer of much larger numbers of cells resulted in complete protection, but this was not HLA restricted (64), a finding suggesting a role also for secreted suppressor factors.

Activated CD8+ T cells may secrete chemokines, and this may explain a recent finding. In a novel approach to stimulate protective immunity in the genitorectal tracts of female monkeys, they were immunized through iliac lymph nodes, which drain the genitorectal mucosa. They and control monkeys, which had not been immunized, were then challenged with SIV by the rectal route. Complete or partial protection was achieved by this vaccination Although protection did not correlate with the level of sIgA produced at the mucosa by the immunized monkeys, a correlation existed between protection and with IgA secreting cells, with CD8 suppressor factor, and with levels of RANTES and MIP-1b in the draining lymph nodes (65). Although the form of the immunogen used should not have generated specific CTLs, others pointed out (66) that memory CD8+ T cells specific for other antigens can be converted to effector cells by interaction with APCs expressing costimulator molecules and antigens of unrelated specificities. In other words, such cells may have been the source of the protective factors.

The possible association between different immune responses and rapid, slow, or lack of progression to AIDS is reviewed elsewhere (67). Increasing evidence indicates that nonprogressors have high blood levels of CD8+ class I–restricted CTLs that do not decrease over time and of CD8+ non–MHC-restricted suppressor activity. Different HLA alleles are associated with rapid progression to AIDS compared with long-term survival (67), as could be expected if CTLs were an important contributor to protection. In the case of the restriction element HLA-B57, which is common in ethnic groups in Africa where HIV is prevalent, five new conserved peptide determinants have been detected in slow progressors and may represent the dominant HIV-specific CTL response (68). Investigators have proposed that CTLs targeted at a major immunodominant rather than several less dominant determinants of HIV may lead to effective control (69), and a trial peptide-based therapy to test this concept is in progress (67). The internal antigen gag is particularly rich in CTL determinants, and an association between such responses and a decreased risk of progression to AIDS-related complex or to AIDS has been reported (70).

Four recently described "experiments of nature" are particularly fascinating. Investigators are seeing small but increasing numbers of individuals who have been exposed to HIV but who are seronegative, in whom HIV has not been detected or isolated, but who have mounted a CTL response to peptide determinants considered specific for HIV. These are:

1. Long-term partners of infected men or women (71)
2. Babies born of infected mothers (72, 73)
3. In a small proportion of long-term female prostitutes in Africa. In one set, viral peptide determinants recognized by the CTLs were identified in 5 of 6 cases (74 and McMichael A, unpublished data).
4. In 7 of 20 health care workers knowingly exposed once to HIV-infected blood (75). Only CTLs recognizing determinants in the env protein were sought.

That four such separate situations have now been described must add more credence to the generality of the findings. Several comments can be made:

1. According to immunologic dogma, a CD8+ CTL response is consistent with the interpretation that HIV infection occurred in all these situations, at least to the extent that viral protein synthesis took place.
2. The findings do not prove that the CTL responses protected the individuals from a continuing HIV infection, but together with the previously discussed findings, they send a clear message to vaccine developers—take note!
3. One could argue that in the first three cases in the foregoing list, the initial exposure was to an attenuated or defective strain of HIV, but this seems unlikely in the case of randomly selected health care workers exposed to HIV.
4. The findings with health care workers, especially if extended in further studies with other viral antigens such as gag and nef, suggests that the original estimate in the United States of only 1% or less of exposures to HIV result in infection, as judged by seroconversion (76), may be a considerable underestimate. Possibly, in the four groups of infections described previously, the recipients received only a small dose of virus. It is encouraging that macaque monkeys inoculated with a "subinfectious dose" of SIV made a cellular but no antibody response; yet they resisted a later challenge with a high dose of SIV (77). The concept that a low dose of antigen preferentially stimulates a type 1 T-cell response has been advocated by Bretscher (78).

Why do CTLs not clear nearly all HIV infections, as they do in several murine viral model infectious systems? Several explanations have been proposed (79), but I still argue in favor of an early proposal (80) that virus hides and may persist in sites (sanctuaries) where, for one reason or another, it is "unavailable" to the immune system (Fig 6.3). A recent finding illustrates one example. Intact HIV can localize, presumably complexed with antibody, on the *surface* of follicular dendritic cells (FDCs) in lymphoid tissues and can remain infectious, even in the presence of neutralizing antibody (81); that is, a "sanctuary" can exist in the very organ that is the site of the intense struggle between the virus and the immune system. It is also a potentially efficient method for the virus to contact and infect passing CD4+ T

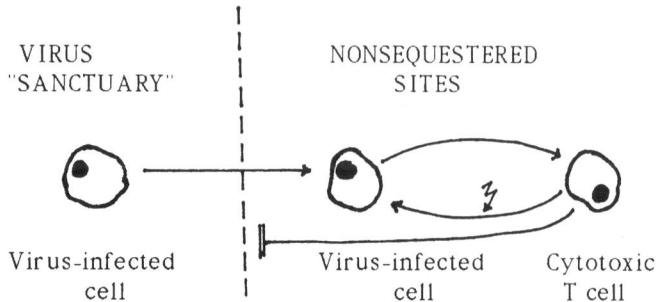

Figure 6.3. Possible interpretation of the finding that, despite a strong CTL response in many infected people, infectious virus persists. On the RHS (see Fig. 6.2), an HIV-infected cell acts as an antigen-presenting cell, inducing the formation of CTLs, which can then lyse or inhibit the growth of virus in infected cells. In contrast to an acute viral infection (see Fig. 6.2A), the virus is not cleared (see Fig. 6.2B and C). This suggests the presence in the body of other infected cells (LHS; see Fig. 6.2) that are not accessible to CTLs (hence the idea of a barrier), but continually feed infectious virus into the system. Examples of such a viral "sanctuary" include immunoprivileged sites, an infected cell not processing viral proteins correctly or not expressing sufficient peptide–MHC complexes at the cell surface.

cells. As more rapid progression to AIDS-related complex and AIDS occurs, the structure of infected lymphoid tissue disintegrates, including the integrity of FDCs.

ROUTES OF INFECTION BY HIV

Five routes are known: 1) intravenous, by transfer of infected blood or blood products, either by transfusion or by the sharing of needles by drug users; 2) receptive anal intercourse; 3) receptive vaginal intercourse; 4) from infected mother to fetus or baby at or before parturition; and 5) breast-feeding by infected mothers. The first two are common in many developed countries, but worldwide, infection by vaginal intercourse is by far the most common. Sixty percent of infections occur in sub–Saharan Africa, where transmission between adults is mainly heterosexual.

The ability to analyze the properties of the infecting virus present during viremia (82), that is, within a few weeks after infection, has shown that the latter is largely due to the replication of virus of a single antigenic specificity (83), even though the viral population in the donor is usually antigenically heterogeneous. Mutants (quasispecies) begin to predominate after viremia has occurred (84).

To follow the fate of virus after intravenous inoculation would be difficult. One has a greater opportunity to do so after a vaginal infection and to study the localized immune response. Such studies are now being reported. One report suggests that dendritic cells and macrophages in the monkey vaginal mucosa become infected by SIV, and these cells act as vectors of the virus to the draining lymph nodes, where other cells, including CD4+ T cells, become infected. India ink, inoculated into the vaginal submucosa of macaques, localized in the draining lymph nodes within 72 hours (85).

Investigators have shown that antiviral CTLs are present in the vaginal epithelium of SIV-infected monkeys (86).

Similarly, virus-specific CD8+ CTLs have been found in cytobrush specimens from the genital mucosa of HIV-infected women (87). The CTL clones obtained after in vitro stimulation lysed pol or gag-expressing target cells, as did clones isolated from blood specimens. All eight subjects with CD4+ T-cell counts above 500 cells/mL were positive, whereas only 4 of 11 with lower T-cell counts were positive.

PROSPECTS FOR PROPHYLACTIC HIV VACCINES

When the decision not to proceed with phase III trials of the two leading candidate HIV vaccines was made by the NIAID, it slowed down HIV vaccine development by some companies. "The pipeline is almost shut down" is a comment attributed to Bolognesi (88). A major reason was the failure of antibody induced by these vaccines to neutralize field isolates. This had one beneficial effect—a push to identify the reasons for this failure, as discussed earlier. Even though HIV showed such marked antigenic variation (much greater than influenza), a second reason was that the leading vaccine candidates were primarily designed to stimulate an antibody response, with the desirability or need for the vaccine to induce as well a strong CTL response something of an afterthought. This message has also now got through. The opening sentence of the abstract of a recent article reads (89): "A *fundamental goal* [my italics] of current strategies to develop an efficacious vaccine for AIDS is the elicitation of broadly reactive cytotoxic T lymphocyte (CTL) reactivities capable of destroying virally infected targets." The article is notable for several reasons: 1) the histocompatible cells used as targets for CTLs were not pulsed with peptides or infected with recombinant viruses, but were infected with HIV field isolates of different clade specificities; 2) the candidate vaccines used were recombinant canarypox constructs expressing gp160 (MN) or the *env, gag,* and protease genes; 3) particularly in the last case, the vaccine elicited broad CTL activities capable of recognizing viruses belonging to genetically diverse HIV-1 clades; that is, the vaccine achieved the goal for which it was designed, although it required a daunting series of immunizations. The findings are completely consistent with the much earlier work with influenza virus: immunizing mice with the nucleoprotein of one viral subtype induced CTLs that lysed target cells infected with any influenza A virus subtype (90). "I think chemokines and CTLs are going to be the answer for (HIV) vaccines" is a comment attributed to Gallo (91).

In conclusion, once a reproducible technique is found for inducing antibody responses that strongly neutralize the infectivity of field isolates, it should be possible to devise a protocol for immunization that will induce the major protective responses. Particularly for the control of heterosexual infection, the aim (92) is to:

1. Neutralize the infectivity of incoming virus to as high a level as possible, by generating persisting high levels of sIgA, as well as IgG
2. Generate as large a pool of memory CTL as possible against conserved peptide sequences that are common to different viral clades, and, where possible, are immunodominant
3. Maximize the production of CD8 T-cell–suppressor factors and the appropriate chemokines

    Regarding 2 and 3, HIV-1 CTLs mediate antiviral suppression by both cytolytic and noncytolytic mechanisms. Both mechanisms are triggered in an antigen-specific and HLA-restricted fashion, but the latter acts without HLA restriction (93).
4. Within the first few days to a week after initiation of infection, to
    a. Have memory CTLs converted to effector cells, which would then destroy or inhibit viral replication in infected cells in the regional lymph nodes and associated vessels draining the infected mucosal site, thus limiting production of progeny virus;
    b. Prevent viremia, through CTLs and preformed IgG, so the spread of HIV to other sites in the body is prevented or severely limited

The primary aim of such a vaccination protocol is the conversion of what is normally a chronic persisting infection by HIV into an acute infection. The transfer of infected cells, even latently infected cells, by a donor is not regarded as especially serious because, in most cases, they should be rapidly destroyed by a host-versus-graft reaction (94).

We still have some way to go to achieve this objective, but more tools are available now than previously. The most successful vaccination protocol used to date is a live, attenuated (*nef*—) SIV preparation, but the balance between efficacy and safety is so fine (95) that it is unlikely that similar HIV preparations would be acceptable as vaccines. However, a study of the SIV preparation shows that this immunization protects against a challenge with virulent SIV, whether the latter is administered by a systemic (96) or a rectal route (97). In the latter case, the immunization resulted in the presence of neutralizing antibodies and CTLs in the circulation and SIV-binding antibodies in rectal fluids. Virus-specific CTLs were also found in gut-associated lymph nodes, and investigators proposed that these could have had a role in limiting the subsequent superinfection.

Investigators are exploring new approaches to achieving more comprehensive and enhanced immune responses, such as DNA immunization or mixed regimens, for example, priming with DNA and boosting with a chimeric live vector (98), or selectively inducing desired immune responses by the incorporation into plasmids or live vectors of DNA coding for certain cytokines, such as GM-CSF, IFN-γ, IL-12, and IL-6. Progress is being made with inducing improved immune responses at mucosal surfaces by immunizing adjacent to the draining lymph nodes (65), but obtaining persisting mucosal responses is still a challenge. Building a closer relationship between academia and pharmaceutical and biotechnology companies involved in HIV vaccine research and development is desirable, and this is a goal of the NIAID Division of AIDS and of the International AIDS

Vaccine Initiative, a program sponsored by the Rockefeller Foundation.

Acknowledgments

I wish to express my appreciation to Drs. Richard Burton and David Montefiori for supplying preprints of manuscripts accepted for publication.

References

1. Ada G, Ramsay A. Vaccines, vaccination and the immune response. Philadelphia: Lippincott–Raven, 1997:1–247.
2. Paul WE, ed. Fundamental immunology. 3rd ed. New York: Raven Press, 1993.
3. Mullbacher A, Flynn K. Aspects of cytotoxic T cell memory. Immunol Rev 1996;150:113–128.
4. Flynn K, Mullbacher A. The generation of memory antigen-specific cytotoxic T cell responses by CD28/CD80 interactions in the absence of antigen. Eur J Immunol 1997;27:456–462.
5. Doherty PD, Ahmed R. Immune responses to viral infections. In: Nathanson N, ed. Viral pathogenesis. Philadelphia: Lippincott–Raven, 1996:143–162.
6. Graham BS, Matthews TJ, Belshe RB, et al. Augmentation of human immunodeficiency virus type 1 neutralizing antibody by priming with gp160 recombinant vaccinia and boosting with rgp160 in vaccinia naive adults. J Infect Dis 1993;167:533–537.
7. Ramphal R, Cogliano RB, Shands JW, et al. Serum antibody prevents lethal murine influenza pneumonitis but not tracheitis. Infect Immun 1979;29:992–996.
8. Renegar KB, Small PA. Passive transfer of local immunity to influenza virus infection by IgA antibody. J Immunol 1991;146:1972–1978.
9. Renegar KB, Small P. Immunoglobulin A mediates murine anti-influenza virus immunity. J Virol 1992;65:2146–2148.
10. Lamm ME. Interaction of antigens and antibodies at mucosal surfaces. Annu Rev Microbiol 1997;51.
11. Scherle PA, Palladino G, Gerhardt W. Mice can recover from pulmonary influenza virus infection in the absence of class I MHC–restricted cytotoxic T cells. J Immunol 1992;148:212–221.
12. Eichelberger M, Allan W, Zijlstra M, et al. Clearance of influenza virus respiratory infection in mice lacking class I major histocompatibility complex–restricted CD8+ T cells. J Exp Med 1991;174:875–880.
13. Ramshaw IA, Ramsay A, Ruby J, et al. Expression of cytokines by recombinant vaccinia viruses: a model for studying cytokines in viral infections in vivo. Immunol Rev 1992;127:157–182.
14. Spriggs MK, Koller BH, Sato T, et al. β_2–Microglobulin, CD8+ T cell–deficient mice survive inoculation with high doses of vaccinia virus and exhibit altered IgG responses. Proc Natl Acad Sci U S A 1992;89:6070–6074.
15. Taylor G. The role of antibody in controlling and/or clearing virus infections. In: Ada GL, ed. Strategies in vaccine design. Austin, TX: RG Landes, 1994:17–34.
16. Griffin DE, Levine B, Tyor WB, et al. The immune response in viral encephalitis. Semin Immunol 1992;4:111–119.
17. Ada GL, McElrath MJ. HIV–vaccine induced cytotoxic T cell response: potential role in vaccine efficacy. AIDS Res Hum Retroviruses 1996;13:243–246.
18. Zinkernagel RM, Doherty PC. Restriction of in vitro cell-mediated cytotoxicity in lymphocytic choriomeningitis with a syngeneic or semi-allogeneic system. Nature 1974;248:701–702.
19. Riddell SR, Watanabe KS, Goodrich JM, et al. Restoration of viral immunity in immunodeficient humans by the adoptive transfer of T cell clones. Science 1992;257:238–241.
20. Walter EA, Greenberg PD, Gilbert MJ, et al. Reconstitution of cellular immunity against cytomegalovirus in recipients of allogeneic bone marrow by transfer of T cell clones from the donor. N Engl J Med 1995;33:1038–1044.
21. Rooney CM, Smith CA, Ng CY, et al. Use of gene-modified virus-specific lymphocytes to control Epstein-Barr virus–related lymphoproliferation. Lancet 1995;345:9–13.
22. Kyburz D, Speiser DE, Battegay M, et al. Lysis of infected cells in vivo by anti-viral cytotoxic T cells demonstrated by release of cell internal viral proteins. Eur J Immunol 1993;23:1540–1545.
23. Ando K, Guidotti LC, Wirth S, et al. Class I–restricted cytotoxic T lynmphocytes are directly cytopathic for their target cells in vivo. J Immunol 1994;152:3245–3253.
24. Kagi D, Ledermann B, Burki K, et al. Cytotoxicity mediated by T cells and natural killer cells is greatly impaired in perforin-deficient mice. Nature 369;31–36:1994.
25. Desrosier RC. HIV with multiple gene deletions as a live attenuated vaccine for AIDS. AIDS Res Hum Retroviruses 1992;8:411–418.
26. Stott EJ. Anti-cell antibody in macaques. Nature 1991;353:393.
27. LaRosa GJ, Davide JP, Weinhold K, et al. Conserved sequence and structural elements in the HIV-1 principal neutralizing determinant. Science 1990;249:932–935.
28. Haigwood NL, Nara PL, Brooks E, et al. Native but not denatured recombinant human immunodeficiency virus type-1 gp120 generates broad spectrum neutralizing antibodies in baboons. J Virol 1992;66:172–182.
29. Feng Y, Broder C, Kennedy P, et al. HIV-1 entry cofactor:functional cDNA cloning of a seven-transmembrane, G protein–coupled receptor. Science 1996;272:872–877.
30. Deng HK, Liu R, Ellmeier W, et al. Identification of a major coreceptor for primary isolates of HIV-1. Nature 1996;381:661–666.
31. Dragic T, Litwin V, Allaway GP, et al. HIV-1 entry into CD4+ cells is mediated by the chemokine receptor CC-CKR-5. Nature 1996;381:667–673.
32. Cocchi F, DeVico AL, Garzino-Demon A, et al. Identification of RANTES, MIP-1a and MIP-1b as the major HIV suppressive factors produced by CD8+ T cells. Science 1995;270:1811–1815.
33. Walker CM, Moody DJ, Stites DP, et al. CD8+ lymphocytes can control HIV infection in vitro by suppressing virus replication. Science 1998;234:1563–1566.
34. Heeney JL, Bruck C, Goudsmit J, et al. Immune correlates of protection from HIV infection and AIDS. Immunol Today 1997;18:4–8.
35. Paxton WA, Martin SR, Tse D, et al. Relative resistance to HIV-1 infection of CD4 lymphocytes by persons who remain uninfected despite multiple high-risk sexual exposure. Nat Med 1996;2:412–417.
36. Mascloa JR, Snyder SW, Weislow OS, et al. Immunization with envelope subunit vaccine products elicits neutralizing antibodies against laboratory-adapted but not primary isolates of human immunodeficiency virus type-1. J Infect Dis 1996;173:340–348.
37. Girard M, Meigner B, Barre-Sinoussi F, et al. Vaccine-induced protection of chimpanzees against infection by a heterologous human immunodeficiency virus type 1. J Virol 1995;69:6239–6248.
38. Honda M, Matsuo K, Nakasone T, et al. Protective immune response induced by secretion of a chimeric soluble protein from a recombinant *Mycobacterium bovis* bacillus. Proc Natl Acad Sci U S A 1995;92:10693–10696.
39. Sattentau QJ, Moore JP. Human immunodeficiency virus type 1 neutralization is determined by epitope exposure on the gp120 oligomer. J Exp Med 1995;182:185–196.
40. Moore JP, Cao Y, Qing L, et al. Primary isolates of human immunodeficiency virus type 1 are relatively resistant to neutralization to monoclonal antibodies to gp120, and their neutralization is not predicted by studies to monomeric gp120. J Virol 1995;69:101–109.
41. Earl PL, Broder CC, Doms RW, et al. Epitope map of human immunodeficiency virus type 1 gp41 derived from 47 monoclonal antibodies produced by immunization with oligomeric envelope protein. J Virol 1997;71:2674–2684.
42. Fouts TR, Binley JM, Trkola A, et al. Neutralization of the human immunodeficiency virus type 1 primary isolate JR–FL by human monoclonal antibodies correlates with antibody binding to the oligomeric form of the envelope glycoprotein complex. J Virol 1997;71:2779–2785.

43. Burton DR. A vaccine for HIV type-1: the antibody response. Proc Natl Acad Sci U S A 1997;94:10018–10023.
44. Conley ASJ, Kessler AJ II, Boots IJ, et al. The consequence of passive administration of an anti-human immunodeficiency virus type 1 neutralizing monoclonal antibody before challenge of chimpanzees with a primary virus isolate. J Virol 1996;70:6571–6578.
45. Trieola A, Punscher M, Muster T, et al. Human monoclonal antibody 2G12 defines a distinctive neutralization epitope on the gp120 glycoprotein of human immunodeficiency virus type 1. J Virol 1996;70: 1100–1108.
46. Parren PWHI, Burton DR. Antibody response to HIV-1: debris or virion? Nat Med 1997;3:366–367.
47. Nixon DF, Broliden K, Ogg G, et al. Cellular and humoral antigenic epitopes in HIV and SIV. Immunology 1992;76:515–534.
48. Ho DD, Neumann AU, Perelson AS, et al. Rapid turnover of plasma virions and CD4+ lymphocytes in HIV-1 infection. Nature 1995;373: 123–127.
49. Wei X, Ghosh SK, Taylor ME, et al. Viral dynamics in human immunodeficiency virus type-1 infection. Nature 1995;373:117–122.
50. Wain-Hobson S. Virological mayhem. Nature 1995;373:102.
51. Koup RA, Safrit JT, Cao Y, et al. Temporal association of cellular immune responses with the initial control of viremia in primary human immunodeficiency virus type-1 infection. J Virol 1994;68:4650–4655.
52. Borrow P, Lewcki H, Hahn B, et al. Virus-specific CD8+ cytotoxic T lymphocyte activity associated with control of viremia in primary human immunodeficiency virus type-1 infection. J Virol 1994;68: 6103–6110.
53. Ariyoshi K, Harwood E, Chiongsong-Popov R, et al. Is clearance of HIV-1 viremia at seroconversion mediated mediated by neutralizing antibodies? Lancet 1992;340:1257–1258.
54. Connick E, Marr DG, Zhang X–Q, et al. HIV-specific cellular and humoral immune responses in primary HIV infection. AIDS Res Hum Retroviruses 1996;12:1129–1140.
55. D'Souza MP, Mathieson B. Early phases of HIV infection. AIDS Res Hum Retroviruses 1996;12:1–9.
56. Buchbinder SP, Katz MH, Hussal NA, et al. Long-term HIV-1 infection without immunologic progression. AIDS 1994;8:1123–1128.
57. Sheppard HW, Lang W, Ascher MS, et al. The characterization of non-progressors: long-term HIV-1 infection with stable CD4+ T cell levels. AIDS 1993;7:1159–1166.
58. Munoz A, Kirby AJ, He YD, et al. Long-term survivors with HIV-1 infection: incubation period and longitudinal patterns of CD4+ lymphocytes. N Engl J Med 1995;332:209–216.
59. Kirchoff F, Greenough TC, Bruttler DB, et al. Absence of intact nef sequences in a long-term survivor with non-progressive HIV-1 infection. N Engl J Med 1995;332:228–232.
60. Pilgrim AK, Pantaleo G, Cohen OJ, et al. Neutralizing antibody responses to human immunodeficiency virus type 1 in primary infection and long-term non-progressive infection. J Infect Dis 1997;176: 924–932.
61. Learmont J, Tindall LJ, Evans L, et al. Long-term symptomless HIV-1 infection in recipients of blood products from a single donor. Lancet 1992;340:863–867.
62. Deacon NJ, Tsykin A, Solomon A, et al. Genomic structure of an attenuated quasi species of HIV-1 from a blood transfusion donor and recipients. Science 1995;270:988–992.
63. Bryson Y, Pang S, Wei L, et al. Clearance of HIV infection in a perinatally infected infant. N Engl J Med 1995;332:833–838.
64. Mosier DE. Human immunodeficiency virus infection of human cells transplanted to severe combined immunodeficient mice. Adv Immunol 1996;63:79–126.
65. Lehner T, Wang Y, Cranage M, et al. Protective mucosal immunity elicited by targeted iliac lymph node immunization with a subunit SIV envelope and core vaccine in macaques. Nat Med 1996;2:767–776.
66. Ada GL, Mullbacher A. SIV and HIV prophylaxis. Nat Med 1996;2: 1054–1055.
67. Haynes BF, Pantaleo G, Fauci AS. Towards an understanding of the correlates of protectoive immunity to HIV infection. Science 1996; 271:324–328.
68. Goulder PJR, Bunce M, Krausa P, et al. Novel, cross-restricted, conserved and immunodominant cytotoxic T lymphocyte epitopes in slow progressors in HIV-1 type infection. AIDS Res Hum Retroviruses 1996;12:1691–1698.
69. Nowak M, May RM, Phillips RE, et al. Antigenic oscillations and shifting immunodominance in HIV-1 infections. Nature 1995;375: 606–611.
70. Riviere Y, McChesney MB, Porrot F, et al. Gag-specific cytotoxic responses of HIV type 1 are associated with a decreased risk of progression to AIDS-related complex or AIDS. AIDS Res Hum Retroviruses 1995;11:903–907.
71. Langlade-Demoyen P, Ngo-Giang-Huong N, Ferchat F, et al. Human immunodeficiency virus (HIV) nef-specific cytotoxic T lymphocytes in noninfected heterosexual contacts of HIV-infected patients. J Clin Invest 1994;93:1293–1297.
72. Chenynier R, Langlade-Demoyen P, Marescot M, et al. CTL response in the PBMC of children born to HIV-infected mothers. Eur J Immunol 1992;22:2211–2217.
73. Rowland-Jones S, Sutton J, Ariyoshi K, et al. HIV-specific CTL activity in an HIV-exposed but uninfected infant. Lancet 1993;341:860–861.
74. Rowland-Jones S, Sutton J, Ariyoshi K, et al. HIV-specific cytotoxic T cells in HIV-exposed but uninfected Gambian women. Nat Med 1995;1:59–64.
75. Pinto LA, Sullivan J, Berzofsky JA. Env-specific cytotoxic T lymphocytes in HIV-seronegative health care workers occupationally exposed to HIV-contaminated body fluids. J Clin Invest 1995;96:867–876.
76. Blattner WA. HIV epidemiology: past, present and future. FASEB J 1991;5:2340–2349.
77. Clerici M, Clark E, Polacino P, et al. T cell proliferation to subinfectious SIV correlates with a lack of infection after challenge of macaques. AIDS 1994;8:1391–1395.
78. Bretscher P. Requirements and basis for efficacious vaccination by a low antigen dose regimen against intracellular pathogens uniquely susceptible to a cell-mediated attack. In: Ada GL, ed. Strategies in vaccine design. Austin, TX: RG Landes, 1994:99–112.
79. Bevan MJ, Braciale TJ. Why can't cytotoxic T cells handle HIV? Proc Natl Acad Sci U S A 1995;92:5765–5767.
80. Ada GL. Prospects for HIV vaccines. J Acquir Immune Defic Syndr Hum Retrovirol 1988;1:295–303.
81. Heath SL, Tew J Grant, Tew JF et al. Follicular dendritic cells and human immunodeficiency virus infectivity. Nature 1995;377: 740–744.
82. Daar ES, Moudgil T, Myer RD, et al. Transient high levels of viremia in patients with primary human immunodeficiency virus type-1 infection. N Engl J Med 1991;324:961–964.
83. Wolf TWF, Zwart G, Bakker M, et al. Naturally occuring mutations within HIV-1 V3 genomic RNA lead to antigenic variation dependent upon a single amino acid substitution. Virology 1991;185:195–205.
84. Wain-Hobson S. Human immunodeficiency virus type-1 quasispecies in vivo and ex vivo. Curr Top Microbiol Immunol 1992;176: 181–193.
85. Miller CJ. Mucosal transmission of simian immunodeficiency virus. Curr Top Microbiol Immunol 1994;188:107–123.
86. Lohman BL, Miller CJ, McChesney MB. Antiviral cytotoxic T lymphocytes in vaginal mucosa of simian immunodeficiency virus–infected rhesus macaques. J Immunol 1995;155:5855–5860.
87. Musey L, Hu Y, Eckert L, et al. HIV-1 induces cytotoxic T lymphocytes in the cervix of infected women. J Exp Med 1997;185:293–303.
88. Cohen J. Vaccine drought spurs NIAID plan to improve industry ties. Science 1996;271:1227–1228.
89. Ferrari G, Humphrey W, McElrath MJ, et al. Clade B–based HIV-1 vaccines elicit cross-clade cytotoxic T lymphocyte reactivities in uninfected volunteers. Proc Natl Acad Sci U S A 1997;94:1396–1401.

90. Ada GL, Jones PD. The immune response to influenza infection. Curr Top Microbiol Immunol 1986;128:1–54.
91. Cohen J. Exploiting the HIV–chemokine nexus. Science 1997; 275:1261–1264.
92. Kent SJ, Clancy, RL, Ada GL. Prospects for a prophylactic HIV vaccine. Med J Aust 1996;165:211–215.
93. Yang OO, Kalams SA, Trocha A, et al. Suppression of human immunodeficiency virus type 1 replication by CD8+ cells:evidence for HLA class 1–restricted triggering of cytolytic and noncytolytic mechanisms. J Virol 1997;71:3120–3128.
94. Ada GL, Blanden, RV, Mullbacher A. HIV: To vaccinate or not to vaccinate. Nature 1992;359:572.
95. Baba TW, Jeong YS, Penninck D, et al. Pathogenicity of live, attenuated SIV after mucosal infection of neonatal macaques. Science 1995;267: 1820–1826.
96. Marthas ML, Sujipto S, Higgins J, et al. Immunization with a live attenuated simian immunodeficiency virus (SIV) prevents early disease but not infection in rhesus macaques challenged with pathogenic SIV. J Virol 1990;64:3694–3700.
97. Cranage MP, Whatmore AM, Sharpe SA, et al. Macaques infected with live attenuated SIVmac are protected against superinfection via the rectal mucosa. Virology 1997;229:143–154.
98. Leong KH, Ramsay AJ, Morin MJ, et al. Generation of enhanced immune responses by consecutive immunization with DNA and recombinant fowlpox virus. In: Brown F, Chanock R, Ginsberg H, et al, eds. Vaccines 95. Cold Spring Harbor, NY: Cold Spring Harbor Laboratory Press, 1998:327–331.

Section III
Epidemiology

Chapter 7
EPIDEMIOLOGY OF HIV SEXUAL TRANSMISSION

Sten H. Vermund, Paul B. Tabereaux, and Richard A. Kaslow

The epidemiology of human immunodeficiency virus (HIV) disease includes the population distribution of infection and disease, risk exposure characteristics that help to determine who is infected and who is not, access to care issues that help to determine who is diseased and who is not, and those factors that alter the pathogenic processes or natural history of disease. This chapter emphasizes the principal problem in worldwide HIV control: sexual transmission and its prevention.

A human being is infected with HIV every 10 seconds on average, as estimated conservatively by demographers and epidemiologists at the World Health Organization and the Joint United Nations Programme on HIV/AIDS (UNAIDS). Sexual transmission may account for 90% of new HIV cases worldwide (1). In the most heavily affected countries, nearly 40% of young adults are infected with HIV, as is well documented in Malawi, Zambia, Uganda, and elsewhere (1–6). The magnitude of the epidemic in two of Africa's most populous nations, Nigeria and South Africa, has risen in the mid-1990s; other countries such as India are now experiencing continued rapid spread of the infection (1, 7–11). Transmission of HIV in Latin America has resulted in about twice as many infections as in North America, although the latter epidemic is far more familiar to the world press (12). In Asia, the numbers of infected are growing so rapidly that more new HIV infections may now be occurring per year there than in Africa. Revised estimates in 1997 suggest that more than 30 million persons globally are infected with HIV and more than 10 million additional persons have died of HIV disease (7).

The number of sexual partners, the risk characteristics of partners, failure to use condoms, anal exposure, and uninhibited behavior associated with drug or alcohol use are among the best documented *behavioral* risk factors for sexual transmission. Among the most compelling *biologic* risk factors are the presence of other sexually transmitted infections, high HIV viral load, and low CD4+ lymphocyte count in the infectious contact (9, 13). Other likely but less well-documented cofactors include the lack of male circumcision, cervical ectopy, genetic characteristics of human leukocyte antigens (HLAs) and chemokine receptors, coinfections with nonsexually transmitted agents and immune activation, and viral virulence and tropism. Even less certain is the importance of factors such as vitamin A deficiency, oral contraceptive use, failure to use other barriers such as spermicides to prevent transmission, vaginal douching, abnormal anatomic features, immune modulation from drug or alcohol use, or personal hygiene factors. Epidemiology has contributed much to the early clarification of HIV risk factors, but other, more subtle confounded factors such as those listed in this paragraph have proved elusive.

Preventive guidelines focused on condom use and sexual risk reduction based on insights from epidemiologic and behavioral research were promulgated in the first few years of the epidemic, even before the cause of acquired immunodeficiency syndrome (AIDS) was apparent. More recently, control of ulcerogenic and inflammatory sexually transmitted infections has been shown to prevent HIV transmission. Multiple points of vulnerability in the HIV transmission cycle can be attacked both in industrialized and developing countries if cultural and political taboos can be overcome and prevention programs can be mounted. Yet our prevention approaches using tools such as condoms, risk reduction education, and control of sexually transmitted disease (STD) are few in number and are difficult to implement. Given the high cost of treatment, worldwide HIV prevention would seem to be logically the compelling paradigm for research and intervention. It is not (Table 7.1). Without conventional economic incentives inherent in the development of pharmaceutical products for Western markets, prevention research takes a distant second place to the therapeutics component of worldwide investment in research and development. For example, the AIDS budget of the National Institutes of Health (NIH) in the 1997 fiscal year was approximately $1.4 billion, of which $450 million was classified as therapy oriented and $89 million as behavior and vaccine oriented. Beyond these maldistributed public research monies in the United States are the vast corporate funds infused into research and development for chemotherapy or immunotherapy, compared with the minute

Table 7.1. National Priorities for Public Funds: Contrasts for Prevention and Therapy

Prevention Research	Therapy Research
Prevention is the abstract achievement of a nonexistent event.	Therapy is needed, is real, is life-giving.
Prevention costs money, but makes no money—vaccines, education, condoms.	Therapy represents huge, long-term pharmaceutical and health care income for companies and health care providers.
Market forces do not drive prevention research and development.	Major companies have large HIV drug research and development programs.

private sector expenditures for developing and testing new barrier contraceptives, STD control strategies, or novel behavior change approaches.

Key cofactors for the sexual transmission of HIV have been identified largely through field epidemiologic research, complemented by experiments using simian immunodeficiency virus (SIV) in rhesus macaques or HIV in chimpanzees. The identification of risk factors has allowed innovative public sector–sponsored HIV prevention research to be conducted in many parts of the world, but this research is hindered by resource constraints and market forces less favorable for investments in prevention than in therapeutic research (14).

VIRAL FACTORS IN INFECTIOUSNESS

HIV binds avidly to immunologic cells expressing the CD4 molecule and the CCR5 (for macrophages) or CXCR4 (for lymphocytes) molecular coreceptors; any physical or physiologic facilitator of this contact may be expected to enhance this binding reaction and thereby to increase the risk of transmission (15–21). The complex relationships that may exist among sexual risk factors and the difficulties in measuring these factors make it difficult to identify the same significant factors consistently in all populations. Risk of sexual transmission is greatest when the infected partner has a high circulating virus load, which correlates with a high genital tract virus load. A coincident STD in an HIV-infected individual may be associated with increased genital tract inflammation and HIV load in the semen (22). When an HIV-infected individual is in the so-called "window period" between infection and seroconversion, virus load is extremely high (23, 24). Seroconversion represents the onset of a vigorous host immune response, with cell-mediated activity recognizable weeks before host humoral immunity is evident. Viral clearance from the peripheral circulation probably correlates with a substantial decline in infectiousness.

Viral phenotype and viral tropism (e.g., macrophages versus lymphocytes) are highly relevant to infectiousness (15). An assay using a living cell line (MT-2) indicates whether an HIV-1 strain results in the clumping of cells. The syncytium-inducing (SI) strains are associated with rapid disease progression and are thought to be more pathogenic (25, 26). However, SI strains are much less often transmitted than non-SI (NSI) forms that do not clump cells in the MT-2 assay. In vitro studies and HIV-1 transmission experiments in chimpanzees suggest enormous heterogeneity in infectiousness by viral strain, although whether one genetic subtype of HIV-1 may be more or less infectious than another is not known (27). These observations are helpful in prevention efforts insofar as they highlight priorities for vaccine and drug development.

In addition to the transient period of early infection, a more prolonged time period of high infectiousness occurs late in the course of infection as immunodeficiency supervenes. High plasma viremia and increased quantities of free and cell-associated virus particles in cervicovaginal secretions, rectal fluids, and seminal fluid correlate with the decline in CD4+ and CD8+ lymphocytes and the deterioration of lymph node architecture. The lymph nodes trap circulating virus for presentation to local humoral and cellular defenses; overwhelming viral reproduction occurs when these defense sentinels are destroyed (28–30).

Although increased transmission rates are likely associated with depleted CD4+ cells among HIV-infected sexual partners, causality is difficult to establish with epidemiologic methods because higher transmission rates in late stage disease may also reflect longer duration of exposure to an infected partner. Longitudinal studies that simultaneously monitor sexual behavior along with clinical and immunologic status of HIV-discordant sexual partners have not resolved these issues. Nor will the answer come easily in North American and European settings, where relatively low seroconversion rates are a likely and desirable "study effect" of enrollment within a cohort that offers education and counseling, STD screening and treatment, and condom distribution (31). The relatively high seroconversion rates still observed in African cohorts of discordant couples, despite the impact of intervention, make such research more feasible in those settings (32–36).

GENETICS AND RISK

Viral attachment and penetration as well as cellular susceptibility to infection depend on the "lock-and-key" fit of viral envelope glycoproteins with target cellular molecules. The primary CD4+ receptor appears to be uniformly expressed in all human populations studied. However, host genes encoding HLA molecules, transporters associated with antigen processing (TAP), and chemokine receptors are highly variable (16). In turn, some persons may be more infectious as a consequence of their greater genetic susceptibility to rapid progression because they manifest their viral loads in a shorter time period than slow progressors. Genetically determined variability in the integrity of the CCR5 and CXCR4 chemokine-binding secondary receptors for HIV may 1) promote HIV passage from infected to uninfected cells (wild-type homozygous form), 2) retard progression of disease (heterozygous for wild-type and mutant forms), or 3) protect against HIV infection after heavy exposure (homozygous mutant form) (19).

Variability in HLA and TAP gene products influences long-term progression and may even protect against viral infection (37, 38). Among homosexual men and commercial sex workers with multiple, unprotected sexual encounters with known HIV-infected individuals, genetic profiles suggesting inherent resistance to infection or to disease progression have been discovered (37–42). Prior exposure to HIV or cellular antigens without infection can theoretically result in vaccine-like protection (43–47). Whether this phenomenon occurs to any great extent in human populations and whether its occurrence would imply that strong mucosal immunity can be established through vaccination is not yet clear.

COINFECTION AND GENITAL ECOLOGY

Inflammation and ulcers lead to disruption of the normal integrity of genital epithelial surfaces. Ulcers and inflammation increase the likelihood that HIV will contact a CD4+ cell, both by thinning the usual protective squamous epithelium and by recruiting more CD4+ cells, follicular dendritic cells, or macrophages that are targets for HIV. Sexually transmitted infections that produce frank genital ulcers include herpes, syphilis, and chancroid. Urethritis and cervicitis are more diffuse inflammatory and exudative processes caused by chlamydia, gonorrhea, trichomoniasis, bacterial vaginosis, vaginal candidiasis, and others. Women and men with any of these reproductive infections are likely to be more susceptible to infection than persons with normal genital anatomy and microbial flora.

Among HIV-infected persons, recruitment of infectious lymphocytes, macrophages, or other cells into seminal or vaginal secretions may increase transmissibility of HIV. Hence, sexually transmitted infections accompanied by urethral, prostatic, cervical, vaginal, and anal inflammatory responses increase HIV infectiousness (22). Mucosal ulceration, inflammation, exudation, or trauma to protective epithelial surfaces, as occurs with genital infection or "dry sex" (women in some cultures use vaginal drying agents), is likely to increase the efficiency of viral release as well as viral entry. In addition, patients with STDs commonly report other high-risk activities and multiple partners, combining increased biologic risk with behavioral risk.

Colonization by normal vaginal flora produces a dynamic ecosystem containing a limited variety of salutary bacterial species. The presence of these commensal species may interfere with acquisition of nonendogenous, harmful organisms. Therefore, trauma to the vaginal environment by antibiotic use, vaginal douching, or physical or mechanical damage may disrupt vaginal ecology, may alter susceptibility of women to STDs, and may increase the risk of HIV infection. Hydrogen peroxide–producing lactobacilli occupy an ecologic niche and guard against infection by various pathogens including *Escherichia coli*, *Enterococcus*, and *Gardnerella* species (48–54). Loss of these lactobacilli correlates with the occurrence of bacterial vaginosis and increased inflammatory change.

It is hypothesized but not known whether systemic coinfections in the HIV-infected person increase infectiousness. Cytomegalovirus, Epstein–Barr virus, human T-cell lymphotropic virus (HTLV) types 1 or 2, human herpesviruses types 6 or 7, *Mycobacterum tuberculosis*, *Mycoplasma fermentans*, and others have been suggested as promoters of HIV expression in vitro and could increase in vivo viremia and infectiousness. Immune cells activated by some of these agents are more easily infected than resting cells in vitro; and an in vivo correlate remains plausible. In cross-sectional studies, coinfection in HIV-1 (with HTLV-1, for example) may be more common among persons whose lower CD4+ cell counts are the consequence of longer duration of infection or higher-risk behavior (55–57). Epidemiologic studies have not confirmed these hypothesized relationships, although negative data do not disprove the hypotheses (58).

An uncircumcised man may have a higher intraurethral and subpreputial load of potentially infectious cells than a circumcised man, a finding suggesting a mechanism by which lack of circumcision serves as a risk factor for transmission to a sexual partner (59). The effects may be low or nil in industrialized countries in temperate climates where opportunities for personal hygiene are greater (60). Whether differences in clothing and dressing patterns (i.e. tighter clothing) may alter the genital fluid contact time through postcoital genital friction in men is not known; a habit of dress could be a risk factor for HIV.

Genital anatomic variations may account for longer or shorter contact time with infectious genital secretions after sexual intercourse. Female genital mutilation, for example, could be expected to increase the risk of acquiring HIV from contaminated cutting instruments, infundibulectomy, increased trauma and bleeding during coitus, and increased anal sexual exposure. An HIV-infected African woman who has experienced genital mutilation may be more infectious as a consequence of coital trauma associated with her unnatural postsurgical genital anatomy (61).

INFECTIOUSNESS AND ANTIRETROVIRAL CHEMOTHERAPY

Use of highly active antiretroviral therapy with three or more different agents may substantially reduce the infectiousness of the recipient. Whether cumulative infectiousness after initiation of effective treatment is increased through the patient's extended life span or decreased as viral load diminishes is not known. Although transmissibility may be lower early in the course of chemotherapy, prolonged survival with good health may promote high-risk sexual activity if educational messages and *personal experience* do not establish and maintain safe sexual practices. The drug-naive, HIV-infected recipient of an optimal antiretroviral regimen nearly always experiences a decline in viral load and a rise in CD4+ cell count. However, nonadherence to the complex and expensive treatment regimen is common, and with suboptimal therapy, this benefit is likely to be transient because of the development of drug resistance. The issue of resistance highlights the urgency of maintaining safe sexual practices along with optimal chemotherapy in HIV-infected persons.

RISK FOR HIGH SUSCEPTIBILITY

Biologic or behavioral factors are likely to increase susceptibility among infected persons in several ways. First, increased contact with blood and infectious genital secretions during sexual acts probably increases transmission probability. Second, STDs or other mucosal disruptions increase the number and vulnerability of target cells in the mucosal epithelia of the rectum, cervix, vagina, or oral cavity. Third, increased volume of or contact time with infectious secretions increases risk. This last phenomenon is a likely reason why male-to-female transmission is more efficient than female-to-male transmission and why uncircumcised men may be at higher risk for heterosexual transmission from vaginal sex than circumcised men.

Susceptibility to infection is related to specific sexual behaviors rather than to sexual orientation or preference. Behavioral risk for seroconversion is associated with increasing numbers of sexual partners, nonsteady or casual partners, and partners who have HIV or are themselves at high behavioral risk of HIV infection. Among heterosexuals, the men at highest risk had multiple exposures to women in risk categories defined by the United States Centers for Disease Control and Prevention (CDC) (e.g., injection drug users, women with HIV-infected sexual partners) (62). Multiple homosexual encounters were shown in the Multicenter AIDS Cohort Study to be one of the strongest predictors in increasing prevalence of disease (63). The number of exposures to an infected index case increases the risk of HIV transmission (64, 65), as does behavioral synergy of psychoactive drug use during sexual activity (66, 67).

Disruption of the integrity of the epithelial mucosa of the exposed sexual, oral, or rectoanal orifice facilitates access to the circulation and to specific immunologic cells (68, 69). Genital trauma increases susceptibility. Among gay men in the Multicenter AIDS Cohort Study, HIV seropositivity was 7.7-fold more common at the highest level of rectal trauma and more than 3-fold more common with receptive anal intercourse (50).

Receptive anal intercourse is likely to be an efficient mode of HIV transmission for either men or women. Trauma with penile insertion beyond the epithelialized areas can infect rectal mucosal cells directly. Because high levels of virus are detectable in preejaculate, whether withdrawal before ejaculation provides highly effective risk reduction is uncertain (70–73).

Mechanical barriers, primarily latex condoms, for blocking HIV infection have been shown to decrease the risk of transmission dramatically. Many studies have now concluded that consistent use of condoms is highly effective in preventing the transmission of HIV. Through an increase in condom use in men alone from 14 to 94% during a 5-year period, Thailand's HIV-control program achieved a reduction in annual incidence from 2.6 to 1.6% as well as a 79% reduction in STDs (74–78). Studies of the efficacy of a currently marketed spermicide, nonoxynol-9, have not shown benefit (79, 80). Female condoms are being studied for both efficiency and effectiveness.

Cervical ectopy is the exocervical exposure of the columnar epithelium along the exposed junction known as the transformation zone; this zone is normally found within the relatively protected endocervical region. Ectopic endocervical cells are exposed to both trauma and infection, thus enhancing their susceptibility to STDs, including HIV (relative risks ranging from 1.7 to 5.0 in published studies). Adolescents who are at increased risk because of a larger number of sexual partners or higher incidence of STDs run even higher risks of transmission of infection because of cervical ectopy covering as much as half the cervix as a normal developmental variation (39, 49, 78, 81).

Cervical ectopy accompanying oral contraceptive use may increase HIV risk. Studies of oral contraceptive use remain equivocal about the role of these agents in increasing or decreasing susceptibility to HIV infection. Altered risk of transmission with oral contraceptive use may be attributable to salutary or harmful hormonal influences. The issue is complicated by the finding that studies thus far have failed to report the duration of use. Moreover, studies have not always taken into account that women protected from pregnancy may not take additional precautions (i.e. latex condoms) to prevent spread of STDs (39, 82, 83). Studies in Kenya implicate oral hormonal contraceptives in the production of higher genital HIV load among infected women (39). A woman's need to prevent HIV may conflict with her desire to control her fertility, introducing a complex moral dilemma for public health practice.

Nutritional status, particularly vitamin A deficiency, has emerged as a likely cofactor for perinatal transmission (84–90). It will be important to assess whether sexual transmis-

Table 7.2. Selected Challenges in Prevention Research: Behavior

Early recognition and intervention
    Women recognizing risk: among men, for themselves, for their fetus
    Health care providers recognizing risk among **women and men**
    Facilitating treatment of drug addiction, interim risk reduction
    Improving access and adherence to prophylaxis and antiretroviral therapies
    Assisting in tuberculosis diagnosis and prevention
    Screening for preventable cancers
Male factors
    Behavioral and cultural antecedents for promiscuity and lying
    Prevention of violence and sexual abuse toward women and children
    Understanding of destructive preferences for "dry sex" and sex with girls
Early prevention interventions for later high-risk behavior
    Prevention and identification of child sexual abuse
    Building of women's negotiating skills
    Self-esteem and independent judgment
    Delay of coital debut
    Widespread acceptance of use of barriers in coitus

sion occurs more easily in vitamin A–deficient adults, because administration of vitamin A represents a practical and affordable opportunity for intervention in developing countries (91). In addition, observations on vitamin A provide an incentive to investigate many other nutritional variables such as folic acid, zinc, selenium, and others that may affect immune activation, mucosal integrity, or cellular function (92).

PREVENTION OF SEXUAL TRANSMISSION

Although interest in ascertaining additional cofactors that facilitate or inhibit HIV transmission is considerable, from the earliest days of the epidemic investigators knew enough to declare that unprotected sex with a high-risk partner is the principal risk factor for sexual acquisition of HIV (Table 7.2). However, the difficulty inherent in changing human sexual behavior has necessitated further efforts to delineate possible points of intervention through a more detailed appreciation of the biologic cofactors for transmission (Table 7.3). Careful evaluations will help to determine the ultimate effectiveness of the programs judged most successful at behavioral and community-based education and cofactor reduction throughout the world. Although condoms can substantially reduce the risk of HIV transmission, their use depends on acceptance by both partners during sexual activity. In heterosexual or homosexual encounters, the inability of some women or men to negotiate use of a condom barrier emphasizes the need for development of barriers that can be controlled independent of the partner's preference (93–95).

Studies have evaluated the female condom, a device that may be effective in helping women to negotiate safer sex and to protect themselves from HIV infection. Although the female condom is now available, its relatively high cost and the difficulty of obtaining the device have hindered its acceptance. Although studies have begun to demonstrate acceptance among female condom users, efficacy is still unknown. It is encouraging that populations as diverse as low-income African–American women and men and women in developing countries have reported favorable experiences with the female condom (96–98).

Spermicides are currently recommended by many health departments or agencies for protection against sexually transmitted infections, including HIV. The first trial in Kenya used high doses in a potentially excoriative vaginal sponge. Lower doses of nonoxynol-9–based spermicides showed early promise, but a major efficacy trial in Cameroon in 1997 using only 70 mg nonoxynol-9 in a benign film vehicle to block HIV did not suggest protection (80). Hence, attention is now drawn to experiments with other compounds and to less frequent use of nonoxynol-9 (99).

Microbicides may have the potential to reduce HIV transmission in formulations such as gels, creams, films, foams, tablets, and suppositories that are applied topically to genital mucosal surfaces. Mechanisms of action of these potent compounds may include the following: 1) nonspecific antimicrobial effects of surfactants, acid pH buffers, and natural products; 2) inhibition of binding of HIV or other STD pathogens to mucosal target cells; 3) inhibition of replication of HIV or other STD pathogens after initial infection; and 4) combinations of these. Evaluations of available microbicides must be conducted in rigorous clinical trial environments to ensure proper safety precautions and surveillance for side effects as well as proper measurement of intended outcomes. Additionally, researchers should strive to develop microbicides for infection control without sperm-killing properties for women whose religious or personal preferences prevent them from using contraception (100). A vaginal suppository containing *Lactobacillus crispatus* is an example of a natural microbial product used to maintain healthy vaginal ecology and perhaps to decrease the acquisition of STD and HIV infections among women (52–52, 54).

Treatment of symptomatic STDs has been demonstrated to reduce HIV transmission 42% in 2 years in a controlled trial in Tanzania (101). Thus, low-technology syndromic management of STDs can be an important tool in HIV prevention. A more appealing theoretic strategy is for health care workers to screen persons at highest risk and HIV-infected persons to provide early curative therapy for all sexually transmitted infections they detect, whether or not these are symptomatic. In poor countries, however, investments in diagnosis may detract from resources for therapy. Mass periodic chemotherapy of persons with recurrent infections may be more cost-efficient than screening and treatment in areas with the highest prevalence; this hypothesis is being tested in the Rakai region of Uganda (102, 103).

Future testing of improved barriers, including female condoms and cervical caps or diaphragms, is essential in providing options for women. The impact of latex barriers with or without spermicides on STDs is being studied in

Table 7.3. Selected Challenges in Prevention Research: Biology

Maintenance and restoration of natural barriers
   Normal vaginal ecology
      Avoidance of douching
      Avoidance of unnecessary antibiotic use
      Renewal of H_2O_2–producing lactobacilli
   STD detection and treatment
      Consumer-friendly settings for diagnosis and treatment
      Provision of resources and leadership
      Facilitation of screening in high-risk settings
      Resolution of civil liberties issues in contact tracing
Maintenance and restoration of artificial barriers
   Use of technologies that women and men like and use
      Female condoms
      Cervical caps and diaphragms
      Microbicides and spermicides
      Erotic social marketing of condoms
      Social change to permit widely available condoms
   Development of new products and methods
   Economic incentives for prevention development
Anatomic risks for women
      Importance of cervical ectopy: adolescents, oral contraceptive users
      Anal sex risk, bleeding risk, coital trauma
      Role of female genital mutilation

Alabama and elsewhere, as are female condom slippage and breakage (104).

In the absence of effective vaccine strategies, reliance on HIV prevention behaviors is the only, and therefore crucial, option for averting further escalation of new infections, particularly among women of lower socioeconomic status who are at high risk of HIV infection. Women's research in HIV/AIDS has taken a more prominent position of priority in recent years (Table 7.4).

ASSESSING THE IMPACT OF HIV CHEMOTHERAPY ON HIV TRANSMISSION

Numerous HIV prevention approaches combining control efforts from the STD epidemic are available worldwide and are clearly not being exploited, even within the United States. STD control efforts in the northwestern United States have proved successful in chlamydia, gonorrhea, and syphilis control. However, this success has not been translated adequately into major regional prevention programs, as needed in areas such as the southeastern United States, where STD rates are the highest in the country and the occurrence of HIV/AIDS has the fastest growth trajectory (104–110). Contact tracing and other classically successful approaches to STD control make more sense than ever for HIV because early chemotherapeutic intervention is indicated for any HIV-infected individual with a high viral load (111). The impact of HIV chemotherapy on HIV transmission is likely to be substantial (112). The use of barrier methods to prevent HIV transmission is currently problematic. Social marketing and education about use of condoms are heavily controlled by media interests worried about unpopular reactions from certain groups of subscribers. Condoms are not readily obtained in public places in the United States; availability is largely restricted to pharmacies and a few automotive service station rest rooms. Among the highest prevention research priorities are developing and assessing barriers that women (and men who have sex with men) can use even without their partner's knowledge or consent. The female condom, cervical caps and diaphragms, microbicides and spermicides, and effective male condoms useful for latex-sensitive persons represent current products in research on physical barriers to genital infection. The drug abuse epidemic and sexual transmission of HIV are closely related. Sexual activity in exchange for drugs and sex with intravenous drug users are risk factors for HIV acquisition. Proved to be effective, yet socially controversial, are risk-reduction strategies such as needle exchange, readily accessible methadone programs, and street outreach, all of which are not currently widespread but could be implemented in the United States within a relatively short time.

Obviously, an effective HIV vaccine is the ideal tool for preventing HIV infection. However, HIV vaccine development is in a state of controversy at present. Despite protection afforded to chimpanzees using recombinant envelope subunit products and their availability for use since 1992, no efficacy trial has been conducted. This delay in the vaccine evaluation process is due to the judgment of some influential scientists that the human immune system generates responses to these products that are inadequate to neutralize circulating wild virus. However, that judgment has effectively precluded efforts to determine whether the immune response to these vaccine constructs blocks transmission, even imperfectly. The most promising approaches to vaccine development are also the most worrisome from the point of view of safety: use of live attenuated HIV and DNA vaccines (112–117). Even more disturbing is the modest industrial investment into HIV vaccine research and development. The slow pace and meager support of HIV vaccine research have been direct consequences of the distorted investment in therapy from both private and government funding sources. Whether the 1997 statement of the Clinton Administration in the United States highlighting the need for HIV vaccine development will be reflected in increased funding for this endeavor as part of the larger effort to sustain a partnership among government, academia, and industry, including empiric approaches toward efficacy trials, is uncertain (118).

In conclusion, given the rapid recognition of the principal modes of transmission of HIV more than a decade ago, the failure of subsequent control activities to stem the pandemic (e.g., Asia) is a discouraging reminder of the difficulties of translating knowledge into practice. Bold policy has been rare in confronting separate local and regional HIV epidemics. In the realm of public policy and behavior change in socially sensitive areas, the AIDS epidemic requires political and community leaders to take risks with their leadership positions to advocate effective, albeit controversial, strategies for control of HIV transmission. Similarly, in the scientific arena, renewed commitment to the development of an HIV vaccine is needed. Vaccines represent a vital technologic tool to complement behavioral change and barriers such as condoms and microbicides. Only a long-term sustained partnership of all nations will succeed in developing and applying an HIV vaccine. Despite the impediments, researchers are currently conducting HIV vaccine trials. Although hope is great that the scientific community will be able to develop an efficacious

Table 7.4. Women's Research in 1987 and in 1997

1987	1997
Poor clinical trial representation	Better clinical trial accrual, but not meeting proportion within the epidemic
Lack of specific women-focused working groups in clinical trials network	Established women-focused clinical trials research agenda
Virtual absence of women living with HIV in clinical trials planning	Presence of major women's cohorts, results now forthcoming
Absence of women in prospective cohorts, except pregnant women	Explosion of interest in women's prevention modalities with important new discoveries
Small size of women-focused studies	Suboptimal services and disease recognition
Emphasis on pregnancy	
Poor clinical and social services and slow disease recognition	

and universally acceptable vaccine, this vaccine will take years to formulate and to test. Meanwhile, more immediate efforts to reduce sexual transmission must focus on available technologies and strategies of behavioral intervention, STD control, condom social marketing, optimal prenatal care, and risk reduction for drug abusers.

References

1. Quinn TC. Global burden of the HIV pandemic. Lancet 1996;348: 99–106.
2. Fylkesnes K, Musonda RM, Kasumba K, et al. The HIV epidemic in Zambia: socio-demographic prevalence patterns and indications of trends among childbearing women. AIDS 1997;11:339–345.
3. Needham D. The reality of despair: AIDS in Malawi. Can Med Assoc J 1996;155:91–92.
4. Nunn AJ, Wagner H-U, Kamali A, et al. Migration and HIV-1 seroprevalence in a rural Ugandan population. AIDS 1995;9:503–506.
5. Mulder DW, Nunn AJ, Kamali A, et al. Two-year HIV-1–associated mortality in a Ugandan rural population. Lancet 1994;343:1021–1023.
6. Wawer MJ, Sewankambo NK, Berkley S, et al. Incidence of HIV-1 infection in a rural region of Uganda. BMJ 1994;308:171–173.
7. Global Programme on AIDS. The current global situation of the HIV–AIDS pandemic [http://www.unaids.org/highband/document/epidemio/report97.html]. Geneva: World Health Organization, 1997.
8. Weniger BG, Takebe Y, Ou C-Y, et al. The molecular epidemiology of HIV in Asia. AIDS 1994;8(Suppl 2):S13–S28.
9. Bollinger RC, Tripathy SP, Quinn TC. The human immunodeficiency virus epidemic in India. Medicine (Baltimore) 1995;74:97–106.
10. Rodrigues JJ, Mehendale SM, Shepherd ME, et al. The biological and behavioural risk factors for prevalent HIV infection in sexually transmitted disease clinics in India. BMJ 1995;311:283–286.
11. Mehendale SM, Rodrigues JJ, Brookmeyer RS, et al. HIV–1 incidence and predictors of seroconversion in patients attending sexually transmitted diseases clinics in India. J Infect Dis 1995;172:1486–1491.
12. Quinn TC, Narain JP, Zacarias FR. AIDS in the Americas: a public health priority for the region. AIDS 1990;4:709–724.
13. Haverkos HW, Quinn TC. The third wave: HIV infection among heterosexuals in the United States and Europe. Int J STD AIDS 1995;6:227–232.
14. Vermund SH. The role of prevention research in HIV vaccine trials. AIDS Res Hum Retroviruses 1994;10:S303–S305.
15. Moore JP. Coreceptors: implications for HIV pathogenesis and therapy. Science 1997;276:51–52.
16. Paxton WA, Martin SR, Tse D, et al. Relative resistance to HIV-1 infection of CD4 lymphocytes from persons who remain uninfected despite multiple high-risk sexual exposure. Nature Med 1996;2: 412–417.
17. Huang Y, Paxton WA, Wolinsky SM, et al. The role of a mutant CCR5 allele in HIV-1 transmission and disease progression. Nature Med 1996;2:1240–1243.
18. Liu R, Paxton WA, Choe S, et al. Homozygous defect in HIV-1 coreceptor accounts for resistance of some multiply exposed individuals to HIV-1 infection. Cell 1996;86:367–377.
19. Dean M, Carrington M, Winkler C, et al. Genetic restriction of HIV-1 infection and progression to AIDS by a deletion allele of the CKR5 structural gene: Hemophilia Growth and Development Study, Multicenter AIDS Cohort Study, Multicenter Hemophilia Cohort Study, San Francisco City Cohort, ALIVE Study. Science 1996; 273:1856–1862.
20. Trkola A, Dragic T, Arthos J, et al. CD4-dependent, antibody-sensitive interactions between HIV-1 and its co-receptor CCR-5. Nature 1996;384:184–187.
21. Bleul CC, Wu L, Hoxie JA, et al. The HIV coreceptors CXCR4 and CCR5 are differentially expressed and regulated on human T lymphocytes. Proc Natl Acad Sci U S A 1997;94:1925–1930.
22. Cohen MS, Hoffman IF, Royce RA, et al. Reduction of concentration of HIV-1 in semen after treatment of urethritis: implications for prevention of sexual transmission of HIV-1. AIDSCAP Malawi Research Group. Lancet 1997;349:1868–1873.
23. Koopman JS, Longini IMJ, Jacquez JA, et al. Assessing risk factors for transmission of infection. Am J Epidemiol 1991;133:1199–1209.
24. Daar ES, Moudgil T, Meyer RD, et al. Transient high levels of viremia in patients with primary human immunodeficiency virus type 1 infection. N Engl J Med 1991;324:961–964.
25. Roos MTL, Koot M, Tersmette M, et al. T cell function and HIV SI phenotype are prognostic markers for development of AIDS in HIV-1 infected homosexual men [abstract WS-BO1-1]. In: 9th International Conference on AIDS, Berlin, 1993:44.
26. Koot M, Keet IPM, Vos AH, et al. Prognostic value of HIV-1 syncytium-inducing phenotype for rate of CD4+ cell depletion and progression to AIDS. Ann Intern Med 1993;118:681–688.
27. Soto–Ramirez LE, Renjifo B, McLane MF, et al. HIV-1 Langerhans' cell tropism associated with heterosexual transmission of HIV. Science 1996;271:1291–1293.
28. Embretson J, Zupancic M, Ribas JL, et al. Massive covert infection of helper T lymphocytes and macrophages by HIV during the incubation period of AIDS. Nature 1993;362:359–362.
29. Pantaleo G, Graziosi C, Demarest JF, et al. HIV infection is active and progressive in lymphoid tissue during the clinically latent stage of disease. Nature 1993;362:355–358.
30. Reinhart TA, Rogan MJ, Viglianti GA, et al. A new approach to investigating the relationship between productive infection and cytopathicity in vivo. Nature Med 1997;3:218–221.
31. DeHovitz JA, Kelly P, Feldman J, et al. Sexually transmitted diseases, sexual behavior, and cocaine use in inner city women. Am J Epidemiol 1994;140:1125–1134.
32. Allen S, Serufilira A, Gruber V, et al. Pregnancy and contraception use among urban Rwandan women after HIV testing and counseling. Am J Public Health 1993;83:705–710.
33. Allen S, Tice J, Van De Perre P, et al. Effect of serotesting with counseling on condom use and seroconversion among HIV discordant couples in Africa. BMJ 1992;304:1605–1609.
34. Tice J, Allen S, Serufilira A, et al. Impact of HIV testing on condoms/spermicide use among HIV discordant couples in Africa [abstract]. In: 6th International Conference on AIDS, San Francisco, 1990:262.
35. Lindan C, Allen S, Nsengumuremyi F, et al. HIV testing and education promote safer sex among urban women in Rwanda [abstract]. In: 6th International Conference on AIDS, San Francisco, 1990:256.
36. Allen S, Serufilira A, Van De Perre P, et al. HIV seroconversion in urban Rwandan women before and after a prevention program [abstract]. In: 6th International Conference on AIDS, San Francisco, 1990:104.
37. Kaslow RA, Carrington M, Apple R, et al. Influence of combinations of human major histocompatibility complex genes on the course of HIV-1 infection. Nature Med 1996;2:405–411.
38. Plummer FA, Simonsen JN, Cameron DW, et al. Cofactors in male–female sexual transmission of human immunodeficiency virus type 1. J Infect Dis 1991;163:233–239.
39. Plourde PJ, Plummer FA, Pepin J, et al. Human immunodeficiency virus type 1 infection in women attending a sexually transmitted diseases clinic in Kenya. J Infect Dis 1992;166:86–92.
40. Greggio NA, Cameran M, Giaquinto C, et al. DNA HLA-DRB1 analysis in children of positive mothers and estimated risk of vertical HIV transmission. Dis Markers 1993;11:29–35.
41. Itescu S, Mathur–Wagh U, Skovron ML, et al. HLA-B35 is associated with accelerated progression to AIDS. J Acquir Immune Defic Syndr Hum Retrovirol 1992;5:37–45.

42. Kroner BL, Goedert JJ, Blattner WA, et al. Concordance of human leukocyte antigen haplotype-sharing, CD4 decline and AIDS in hemophilic siblings: Multicenter Hemophilia Cohort and Hemophilia Growth and Development Studies. AIDS 1995;9:275–280.
43. Arthur LO, Bess JW Jr, Urban RG, et al. Macaques immunized with HLA-DR are protected from challenge with simian immunodeficiency virus. J Virol 1995;69:3117–3124.
44. Chan WL, Rodgers A, Grief C, et al. Immunization with class I human histocompatibility leukocyte antigen can protect macaques against challenge infection with SIVmac-32H. AIDS 1995;9:223–228.
45. Gallimore A, Cranage M, Cook N, et al. Early suppression of SIV replication by CD8+ nef-specific cytotoxic T cells in vaccinated macaques. Nature Med 1995;1:1167–1173.
46. Arthur LO, Bess JW Jr, Sowder RC, et al. Cellular proteins bound to immunodeficiency viruses: implications for pathogenesis and vaccines. Science 1992;258:1935–1938.
47. Eddy GA, Lewis MG, McCutchan FE, et al. Animal models: active and passive immunization induced by envelope peptides protects rhesus macaques from SIV AIDS. AIDS Res Hum Retroviruses 1993; 9(Suppl 1):S105–S110.
48. Bouvet E, de Vincenzi I, Ancelle-Park RA, et al. Defloration as risk factor for heterosexual HIV transmission. Lancet 1989;1:615.
49. Clemetson DB, Moss GB, Willerford DM, et al. Detection of HIV DNA in cervical and vaginal secretions: prevalence and correlates among women in Nairobi, Kenya. JAMA 1993;269:2860–2864.
50. Hillier SL. A healthy vaginal ecosystem is important for prevention of HIV transmission: why and how? In: Conference on Advances in AIDS Vaccine Development. Bethesda, MD: National Institutes of Health, 1996:56.
51. Martin HL, Nyange PM, Richardson BA, et al. Association between presence of vaginal lactobacilli and acquisition of HIV and STDs [abstract Tu-12]. In: 11th International Conference on AIDS, Vancouver, 1997:383.
52. Hawes SE, Hillier SL, Benedetti J, et al. Hydrogen peroxide–producing lactobacilli and acquisition of vaginal infections. J Infect Dis 1996;174:1058–1063.
53. Agnew KJ, Hillier SL. The effect of treatment regimens for vaginitis and cervicitis on vaginal colonization by lactobacilli. Sex Transm Dis 1995;22:269–273.
54. Hillier SL, Krohn MA, Rabe LK, et al. The normal vaginal flora, H_2O_2-producing lactobacilli, and bacterial vaginosis in pregnant women. Clin Infect Dis 1993;16(Suppl 4):S273–S281.
55. Figueroa JP, Morris J, Brathwaite A, et al. Risk factors for HTLV-I among heterosexual STD clinic attenders. J Acquir Immune Defic Syndr Hum Retrovirol 1995;9:81–88.
56. Schechter M, Harrison LH, Halsey NA, et al. Coinfection with human T-cell lymphotropic virus type I and HIV in Brazil: impact on markers of HIV disease progression. JAMA 1994;271:353–357.
57. Dada AJ, Oyewole F, Onofowokan R, et al. Demographic characteristics of retroviral infections (HIV-1, HIV-2, and HTLV-I) among female professional sex workers in Lagos, Nigeria. J Acquir Immune Defic Syndr Hum Retrovirol 1993;6:1358–1363.
58. Hawkins RE, Rickman LS, Vermund SH, et al. Association of *Mycoplasma* and HIV infections: detection of amplified *Mycoplasma fermentans* DNA in blood. J Infect Dis 1992;581–585.
59. Seidlin M, Vogler M, Lee E, et al. Heterosexual transmission of HIV in a cohort of couples in New York City [published erratum appears in AIDS 1993;7:following 1541]. AIDS 1993;7:1247–1254.
60. Laumann EO, Masi CM, Zuckerman EW. Circumcision in the United States. JAMA 1997;277:1052–1058.
61. Caldararo N. The HIV/AIDS epidemic: its evolutionary implications for human ecology with special reference to the immune system. Sci Total Environ 1996;191:245–269.
62. Levin LI, Peterman TA, Renzullo PO, et al. Risk behaviors associated with recent HIV-1 seroconversion among young men in the United States Army. Am J Public Health 1995;85:1500–1506.
63. Chmiel JS, Detels R, Kaslow RA, et al. Factors associated with prevalent human immunodeficiency virus (HIV) infection in the Multicenter AIDS Cohort Study. Am J Epidemiol 1987;126:568–577.
64. Blower SM, Boe C. Sex acts, sex partners, and sex budgets: implications for risk factor analysis and estimation of HIV transmission probabilities. J Acquir Immune Defic Syndr 1993;6:1347–1352.
65. Padian NS, Shiboski SC, Jewell NP. The effect of number of exposures on the risk of heterosexual HIV transmission. J Infect Dis 1990;161:883–887.
66. Rubinstein A, Sicklick M, Gupta A, et al. Acquired immunodeficiency with reversed T4/T8 ratios in infants born to promiscuous and drug-addicted mothers. JAMA 1983;249:2350–2356.
67. Blower SM, Hartel D, Dowlatabadi H, et al. Drugs, sex and HIV: a mathematical model for New York City. Philos Trans R Soc Lond Biol Sci 1991;331:171–187.
68. Wasserheit JN. Epidemiological synergy: interrelationships between human immunodeficiency virus infection and other sexually transmitted diseases. Sex Transm Dis 1992;19:61–77.
69. Stamm WE, Handsfield HH, Rompalo AM, et al. The association between genital ulcer disease and acquisition of HIV infection in homosexual men. JAMA 1988;260:1429–1433.
70. Agnew J. Some anatomical and physiological aspects of anal sexual practices. J Homosex 1985;12:75–96.
71. Padian N. The heterosexual transmission of acquired immunodeficiency syndrome (AIDS): international perspectives and national projections. Rev Infect Dis 1987;9:947–960.
72. Mastro TD, Satten GA, Nopkesorn T, et al. Probability of female-to-male transmission of HIV-1 in Thailand [comments]. Lancet 1994;343:204–207.
73. Anderson DJ, Wolff H, Pudney J, et al. Presence of HIV in semen. In: Alexander NJ, Gabelnick HL, Spieler JM, eds. Heterosexual transmission of AIDS. New York: Wiley–Liss; 1990:167–180.
74. Hanenberg RS, Rojanapithayakorn W, Kunasol P, et al. Impact of Thailand's HIV-control programme as indicated by the decline of sexually transmitted diseases. Lancet 1994;344:243–245.
75. Stratton P, Alexander NJ. Prevention of sexually transmitted infections: physical and chemical barrier methods. Infect Dis Clin North Am 1993;7:841–859.
76. de Vincenzi I. A longitudinal study of human immunodeficiency virus transmission by heterosexual partners: European Study Group on Heterosexual Transmission of HIV [comments]. N Engl J Med 1994;331:341–346.
77. Laga M, Alary M, Nzila N, et al. Condom promotion, sexually transmitted diseases treatment, and declining incidence of HIV-1 infection in female sex workers. Lancet 1994;344:246–248.
78. Saracco A, Musicco M, Nicolosi A, et al. Man-to-woman sexual transmission of HIV: longitudinal study of 343 steady partners of infected men. J Acquir Immune Defic Syndr Hum Retrovirol 1993;6:497–502.
79. Kreiss J, Ngugi E, Holmes K, et al. Efficacy of nonoxynol 9 contraceptive sponge use in preventing heterosexual acquisition of HIV in Nairobi prostitutes. JAMA 1992;268:477–482.
80. Roddy RE, Leopold Z, Kelly RA, et al. A randomized controlled trial of the effect of nonoxynol-9 film use on male-to-female transmission of HIV-1. In: National Conference on Women and HIV, Los Angeles, 1997:215.3.
81. Moss GB, Clemetson D, d'Costa L, et al. Association of cervical ectopy with heterosexual transmission of human immunodeficiency virus: results of a study of couples in Nairobi, Kenya. J Infect Dis 1991;164:588–591.
82. Morrison CS, Schwingl PJ. Oral contraceptive use and infectivity of HIV-seropositive women. JAMA 1993;270:2298.
83. Simonsen JN, Plummer FA, Ngugi EN, et al. HIV infection among lower socioeconomic strata prostitutes in Nairobi. AIDS 1990;4:139–144.
84. Semba RD, Miotti P, Chiphangwi JD, et al. Maternal vitamin A deficiency and child growth failure during human immunodeficiency virus infection. J Acquir Immune Defic Syndr Hum Retrovirol 1997;14:219–222.

85. Semba RD, Farzadegan H, Vlahov D. Vitamin A levels and human immunodeficiency virus load in injection drug users. Clin Diagn Lab Immunol 1997;4:93–95.
86. Rahman MM, Mahalanabis D, Alvarez JO, et al. Effect of early vitamin A supplementation on cell-mediated immunity in infants younger than 6 mo. Am J Clin Nutr 1997;65:144–148.
87. Rassekh CH, Johnson JT, Myers EN. Accuracy of intraoperative staging of the N0 neck in squamous cell carcinoma. Laryngoscope 1995;105:1334–1336.
88. Schriefer A, Barral A, Carvalho EM, et al. Serum soluble markers in the evaluation of treatment in human visceral leishmaniasis. Clin Exp Immunol 1995;102:535–540.
89. Sproston AR, Roberts SA, Davidson SE, et al. Serum tumour markers in carcinoma of the uterine cervix and outcome following radiotherapy. Br J Cancer 1995;72:1536–1540.
90. Stancovski I, Gonen H, Orian A, et al. Degradation of the proto-oncogene product c-Fos by the ubiquitin proteolytic system in vivo and in vitro: identification and characterization of the conjugating enzymes. Mol Cell Biol 1995;15:7106–7116.
91. Camp WL, Allen S, Alvarez JO, et al. Serum retinol and HIV-1 RNA viral load among rapid and slow progressors. J Acquir Immune Defic Syndr Hum Retrovirol (in press).
92. Baum MK, Shor-Posner G, Lu Y, et al. Micronutrients and HIV-1 disease progression. AIDS 1995; 9:1051–1056.
93. Johnson AM. Condoms and HIV transmission. N Engl J Med 1994;331:391–392.
94. Vermund SH. Transmission of HIV-1 among adolescents and adults. In: DeVita VT Jr, Hellman S, Rosenberg SA, et al., eds. AIDS. Philadelphia: JB Lippincott, 1996:147–165.
95. Stigum H, Magnus P, Veierod M, et al. Impact on sexually transmitted disease spread of increased condom use by young females, 1987–1992. Int J Epidemiol 1995;24:813–820.
96. Elias C. Female-controlled methods to prevent sexual transmission of HIV [abstract Tu-12]. In: 11th International Conference on AIDS, Vancouver, 1997:214.
97. Musaba E, Morrison CS, Sunkutu MR, et al. Long-term use and acceptability of the female condom among couples at high risk of HIV in Zambia [abstract Th-12]. In: 11th International Conference on AIDS, Vancouver, 1997:238.
98. Purohit A, Tamashiro H, Steinberg J, et al. Prevention issues of male and female condoms [abstract Th-12]. In: 11th International Conference on AIDS, Vancouver, 1997:329.
99. Rosenberg ZF. Topical microbicides:the pathway to female-controlled HIV prevention strategies. National Conference on Women and HIV, Los Angeles, 1997:101.1.
100. Elias C, Heise L. The development of microbicides : a new method of HIV prevention for women. New York (1 Dag Hammarskjold Plaza, New York, NY 10017): Population Council, 1993–1997;6:105.
101. Grosskurth H, Mosha F, Todd J, et al. Impact of improved treatment of sexually transmitted diseases on HIV infection in rural Tanzania: randomised controlled trial. Lancet 1995;346:530–536.
102. Wawer MJ, Sewankambo NK, Gray RH, et al. Community-based trial of mass STD treatment for HIV control, Rakai, Uganda: preliminary data on STD declines [abstract Mo-12]. In: 11th International Conference on AIDS, Vancouver, 1997:39.
103. Scarlett M, Macaluso M, Duerr A. Acceptability of microbicides among women attending a sexually transmitted disease clinic in Alabama. National Conference on Women and HIV, Los Angeles, 1997:1.15.
104. Wasserheit JN, Aral SO. The dynamic topology of sexually transmitted disease epidemics: implications for prevention strategies. J Infect Dis 1996;174(Suppl 2):S201–S213.
105. Aral SO, Holmes KK, Padian NS, et al. Overview: individual and population approaches to the epidemiology and prevention of sexually transmitted diseases and human immunodeficiency virus infection. J Infect Dis 1996;174(Suppl 2):S127–S133.
106. Hillis SD, Wasserheit JN. Screening for chlamydia: a key to the prevention of pelvic inflammatory disease [editorial; comment]. N Engl J Med 1996;334:1399–1401.
107. Holmes KK. Human ecology and behavior and sexually transmitted bacterial infections. Proc Natl Acad Sci U S A 1994;91:2448–2455.
108. Wasserheit JN. Effect of changes in human ecology and behavior on patterns of sexually transmitted diseases, including human immunodeficiency virus infection. Proc Natl Acad Sci U S A 1994;91:2430–2435.
109. McCormack WM, Mogabgab WJ, Jones RB, et al. Multicenter, comparative study of cefotaxime and ceftriaxone for treatment of uncomplicated gonorrhea. Sex Transm Dis 1993;20:269–273.
110. Anonymous. Update: trends in AIDS incidence, deaths, and prevalence—United States, 1996. MMWR Morb Mortal Wkly Rep 1997;46:165–173.
111. Landis SE, Schoenbach VJ, Weber DJ, et al. Results of a randomized trial of partner notification in cases of HIV infection in North Carolina [comments]. N Engl J Med 1992;326:101–106.
112. Anderson DJ, O'Brien TR, Politch JA, et al. Effects of disease stage and zidovudine therapy on the detection of human immunodeficiency virus type 1 in semen. JAMA 1992;267:2769–2774.
113. Cohen J. Naked DNA points way to vaccines [news; comment]. Science 1993;259:1691–1692.
114. McDonnell WM, Askari FK. DNA vaccines [review]. N Engl J Med 1996;334:42–45.
115. Boyer JD, Ugen KE, Wang B, et al. Protection of chimpanzees from high-dose heterologous HIV-1 challenge by DNA vaccination. Nature Med 1997;3:526–532.
116. Hoth DF, Bolognesi D, Corey L, et al. HIV vaccine development: a progress report. Ann Intern Med 1994;121:603–611.
117. Vermund SH, Fischer RD, Hoff R, et al. Preparing for HIV vaccine efficacy trials: partnerships and challenges. AIDS Res Hum Retroviruses 1993;9(Suppl 1):S27–S33.
118. Mitchell A. Clinton calls for AIDS vaccine as goal [abstract]. New York Times, May 19, 1997:A11.

8

EPIDEMIOLOGY OF AIDS IN THE DEVELOPING WORLD

Marie Laga and Bernhard Schwartländer

During the first years after the original description of the acquired immunodeficiency syndrome (AIDS), the disease appeared largely confined to middle-class homosexual men, intravenous drug users, and recipients of blood products in the Western world. The epidemic is now evolving into a mainly heterosexually transmitted disease of the developing world and of poor and marginalized populations in the industrialized world, as is the case for many other infectious diseases. This chapter discusses specific features of the epidemiology of human immunodeficiency virus (HIV) infection and AIDS in the developing world, as well as the impact of the epidemic on individuals and society, particularly in Africa.

SIZE OF THE PROBLEM: GLOBAL INCIDENCE AND PREVALENCE OF AIDS AND HIV INFECTION

As of December 1997, the number of people living with HIV/AIDS globally was estimated at 30.6 million (1). Of those, 12.1 million were women and 1.1 million were children (younger than 15 years old). Since the beginning of the epidemic, about 11.7 million people have died of AIDS; of those, 2.3 million died during 1997 (Table 8.1). These data are obtained from estimations based on HIV prevalence data and ad hoc surveys.

Figure 8.1 exhibits the estimated regional distribution of cumulative HIV infections in adults in the world and shows that more than 70% of cases occurred in Africa. These incidence figures reveal little about the actual spread of the disease, except they continue to increase at a staggering rate. Thus, in 1997 alone, nearly 5.8 million people became infected (1). Most of these new infections occurred in sub–Saharan Africa, India, and Southeast Asia. Much controversy and uncertainty exist about the future spread of HIV and about the ultimate global dimensions of the epidemic. Whereas short-term (less than 3 years) projections can be made with a reasonable degree of accuracy, long-term forecasting is, at best, unreliable and should always be interpreted with caution.

A plausible, although conservative, estimate is that, by the year 2000, one will see a minimal cumulative total of 40 million cases of HIV infection and of 10 million adult AIDS cases, approximately 90% of which will have occurred in the developing world. The regional comparison of the current situation with regard to the epidemiology of HIV/AIDS is summarized in Table 8.2. The following sections examine more closely the spread of HIV infection in various parts of the developing world.

AFRICA

Sub–Saharan Africa is undoubtedly still the worst affected area in the world. With about 10% of the world's population, it is now thought to harbor two-thirds of the total number of people living with HIV worldwide (2, 3). Although the epidemic spread of HIV in Africa began silently in the late 1970s, recognition of the severe implications of HIV/AIDS for the continent occurred a decade later. Today, with 20 million adults and children infected, AIDS is the most serious of Africa's many public health problems.

The levels of HIV and the epidemic patterns within Africa still vary across regions, with wide variety among and even within countries (Fig. 8.2). This mosaic of different HIV epidemics is clearly a result of a heterogeneous distribution of individual and societal risk factors, such as sexual networks or population mobility and migration (2). Although more than 90% of adults in sub–Saharan Africa become infected through heterosexual contact, most children acquire their infection from their mothers. Africa can be schematically divided into five areas, each with roughly similar epidemiologic features of the HIV epidemic: west, central, east, south, and north.

In East Africa, HIV began already to spread rapidly and widely in the late 1970s and early 1980s, resulting in prevalence rates among pregnant women in urban areas ranging from 15 to 30% (see Fig. 8.2). An estimated 36% of all persons with HIV live in East Africa, and HIV prevalence rates continue to increase in some countries such as Kenya. In other countries, the rates have reached a plateau at high levels in some areas, and for the first time, prevalence rates appear to be declining in some urban areas in Uganda (4, 5). Although these trends are open to many interpretations, impressive prevention efforts resulting in a reduced rate of new infections probably are partly responsible (5). The movement of people along the trans–African highway is a major drive of the epidemic in East Africa.

Southern Africa has witnessed both well-established severe epidemics in Zambia, Zimbabwe, and Malawi for a long time and more recent, explosive epidemics such as those in Botswana, Lesotho, and South Africa (2). In urban areas of Zambia and Zimbabwe, prevalence rates among adults now range from 20 to 45% in the 20- to 30-year age groups (Fig. 8.3) (6). In Botswana, where HIV was rare in the mid-1980s 43% of pregnant women in Francistown were HIV positive in 1997 (see Fig. 8.3). By 1997, the South African government estimated that 2.4 million people (or 6% of the population), including 1.4 million women, were living with HIV in the country, a rise of one-third over 1995.

In West Africa, the epidemic started later than in East Africa and is mainly dominated by the epidemiologic situation of Côte d'Ivoire, which acts as an economic magnet,

Table 8.1 Global Summary of the HIV/AIDS Epidemic as of December 1997

People newly infected with HIV in 1997	Total	5.8 million
	Adults	5.2 million
	Women	2.1 million
	Children <15 y	590 000
No. of people living with HIV/AIDS	Total	30.6 million
	Adults	29.5 million
	Women	12.1 million
	Children <15 y	1.1 million
AIDS deaths in 1997	Total	2.3 million
	Adults	1.8 million
	Women	820 000
	Children <15 y	460 000
Total no. of AIDS deaths since the beginning of the epidemic	Total	11.7 million
	Adults	9.0 million
	Women	4.0 million
	Children <15 y	2.7 million
Total no. of AIDS orphans[a] since the beginning of the epidemic		8.2 million

[a]Defined as HIV-negative children who lost their mother or both parents to AIDS when they were under the age of 15 y.
(From Joint United Nations Programme on HIV/AIDS (UNAIDS)/World Health Organization (WHO). Report on the global HIV/AIDS epidemic: fact sheet. Geneva: UNAIDS/WHO, 1997.)

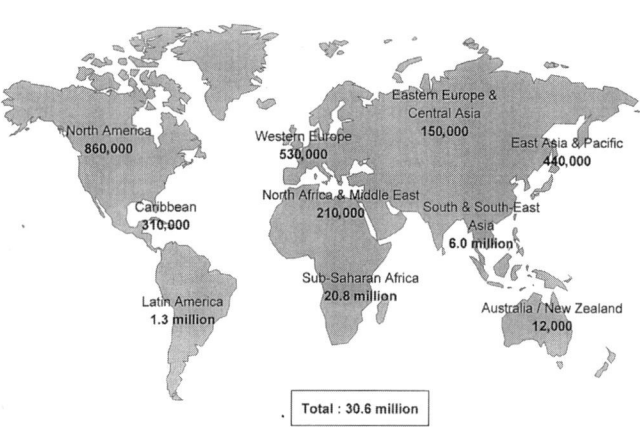

Figure 8.1. Adults and children estimated to be living with HIV/AIDS as of end 1996. (From Joint United Nations Programme on HIV/AIDS (UNAIDS)/World Health Organization (WHO). Report on the global HIV/AIDS epidemic: fact sheet. Geneva: UNAIDS/WHO, 1997.)

Table 8.2 Regional HIV/AIDS Statistics and Features as of December 1997

Region	Epidemic Started	Adults and Children Living with HIV/AIDS	Adult Prevalence Rate[a] (%)	Cumulative No. of Orphans[b]	Percentage of HIV-Positive Adults Who are Women (%)	Main Mode(s) of Transmission for Adults Living with HIV/AIDS
Sub–Saharan Africa	late 1970s–early 1980s	20.8 million	7.4	7.8 million	50	Heterosexual
North Africa and Middle East	late 1980s	210 000	0.13	14 200	20	IDU, Heterosexual
South and Southeast Asia	late 1980s	6.0 million	0.6	220 000	25	Heterosexual
East Asia and Pacific	late 1980s	440 000	0.05	1 900	11	IDU, Heterosexual, MSM
Latin America	late 1970s–early 1980s	1.3 million	0.5	91 000	19	MSM, IDU, Heterosexual
Caribbean	late 1970s–early 1980s	310 000	1.9	48 000	33	Heterosexual, MSM
Eastern Europe and Central Asia	early 1990s	150 000	0.07	30	25	IDU, MSM
Western Europe	late 1970s–early 1980s	530 000	0.3	8 700	20	MSM, IDU
North America	late 1970s–early 1980s	860 000	0.6	70 000	20	MSM, IDU, Heterosexual
Australia and New Zealand	late 1970s–early 1980s	12 000	0.1	300	5	MSM, IDU
Total		30.6 million	1.0	8.2 million	41	

MSM, men who have sex with men; IDU, injecting drug users.
[a]The proportion of adults living with HIV/AIDS in the adult population (15 to 49 years of age)
[b]Orphans are defined as HIV-negative children who lost their mother or both parents to AIDS when they were under age 15
(From Joint United Nations Programme on HIV/AIDS (UNAIDS)/World Health Organization (WHO). Report on the global HIV/AIDS epidemic: fact sheet. Geneva: UNAIDS/WHO, 1997.)

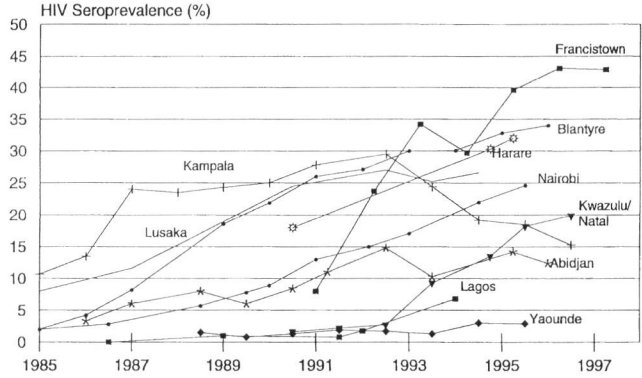

Figure 8.2. HIV seroprevalence for pregnant women in selected urban areas of Africa from 1985 to 1997. (From United States Bureau of the Census, HIV/AIDS Surveillance Data Base, 1998.)

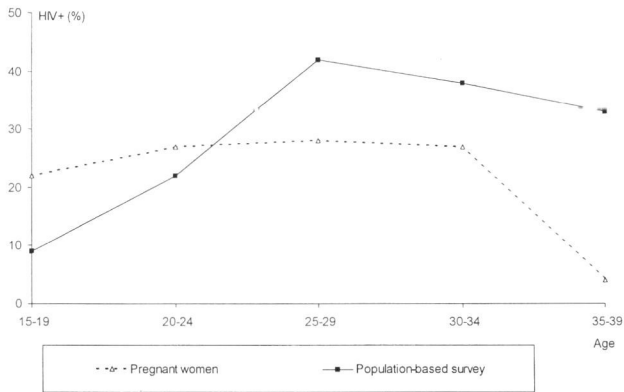

Figure 8.3. HIV prevalence in Lusaka, Zambia estimated by a population-based survey and by screening of antenatal women in 1996. (From Fylkesnes K, Musonda RM, Kasumba K, et al. The HIV epidemic in Zambia: socio-demographic prevalence patterns and indications of trends among childbearing women. AIDS 1997;11:339–345.)

drawing intense migration from neighboring countries (2, 4, 7). Although prevalence rates among pregnant women in Abidjan, the capital city, reached 10 to 15% in 1996, similar rates have been found in smaller towns and rural areas in Côte d'Ivoire, as well as in some neighboring countries such as Burkina Faso. In other countries in these regions, HIV has remained or has stabilized at much lower levels, such as in Senegal, where HIV rates among antenatal attendees have not exceeded 2 to 3%. West Africa is also characterized by the occurrence and spread of HIV-2. Although HIV-2 is found in population samples in nearly all West African countries, with the epicenter in Guinea-Bissau (more than 7% prevalence in pregnant women), HIV-2 is less transmissible as well as less pathogenic than HIV-1 (8–10). In most countries, increasing HIV-1 infection rates now far exceed those of HIV-2 or rates of dual reactivity, both of which tended to remain stable or to decline over the past several years. With the improvement of diagnostic methods to detect HIV-2, it is likely that most, if not all, dually reactive individuals are actively infected with both HIV-1 and HIV-2 (11).

Central Africa has been less severely affected than the other regions, despite the evidence that HIV was present there for a long time. HIV infection rates typically vary around 5% among pregnant women. An interesting and intriguing observation has been the relatively low and stable prevalence from 1985 to 1995 in Kinshasa, Democratic Republic of Congo (around 5%), as well as in Congo, Gabon, and, until recently, Cameroon (see Fig. 8.2) (2).

In North African countries, the rates of HIV among the general population still remain low (less than 1%), and the modes of transmission involve a mix of heterosexual and homosexual contact and injecting drug use (2, 4).

LATIN AMERICA

Monitoring the HIV/AIDS epidemics in Latin America and the Caribbean has been done mostly through AIDS case reporting and analysis. The region has only a few functioning HIV sentinel surveillance programs, so it is difficult to assess the current status of HIV epidemics. Even more difficult to predict is the future of these epidemics.

In general, epidemic spread of HIV began about the same time as in North America (late 1970s). At the end of 1997, investigators estimated that about 1.6 million people were living with HIV/AIDS in Latin America and the Caribbean, and about 580,000 had died of AIDS since the beginning of the epidemic (see Table 8.2).

From scattered studies of HIV prevalence in various countries, the HIV epidemics seem to be just starting or are concentrated in marginalized or neglected populations, and these features make surveillance especially difficult. Whereas homosexual transmission in men was the major mode of spread in the beginning of the epidemic in many countries, transmission by heterosexual contact and among injecting drug users has become increasingly important since the mid-1980s (12–14). Thus, in Brazil, although the absolute numbers of AIDS cases attributed to male homosexual contacts have been stable, the relative proportion of cases in men who have sex with men (MSM) declined from approximately 70% in 1980 to 1986 to about 30% of all cases with information on the transmission category at the end of 1997, as a result of steady increases of heterosexual cases and cases in intravenous drug users. Accounting for more than 40% of cases, heterosexual transmission was the most frequently reported category at the end of 1997 (Fig. 8.4). This ongoing dynamic of the HIV epidemics in Latin America is also illustrated by a changing sex ratio among the reported AIDS cases, with overall increases in the proportion of female cases (Fig. 8.5).

However, rates of HIV infection in MSM are still high, ranging from 5% in Costa Rica to more than 30% in Mexico City in 1993 and 1994 (Fig. 8.6) (4). Rates in injecting drug users range from 5 to 11% in Mexico to close to 50% in Argentina and Brazil (1, 4).

The situation in the Caribbean shows diverse epidemic patterns. Although in some countries, such as Barbados, Trinidad and Tobago, and Martinique, sex between men still

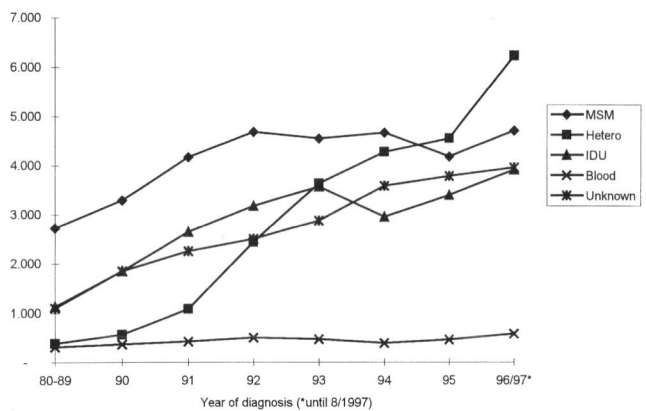

Figure 8.4. AIDS cases by transmission category and year of diagnosis in Brazil. MSM, men who have sex with men.

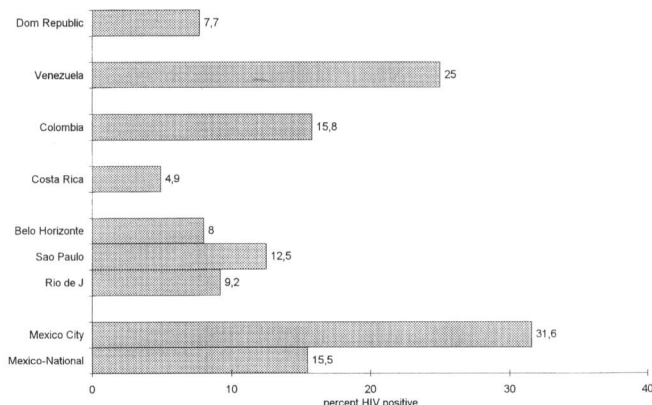

Figure 8.6. Prevalence rates in men who have sex with men (MSM) in Latin America.

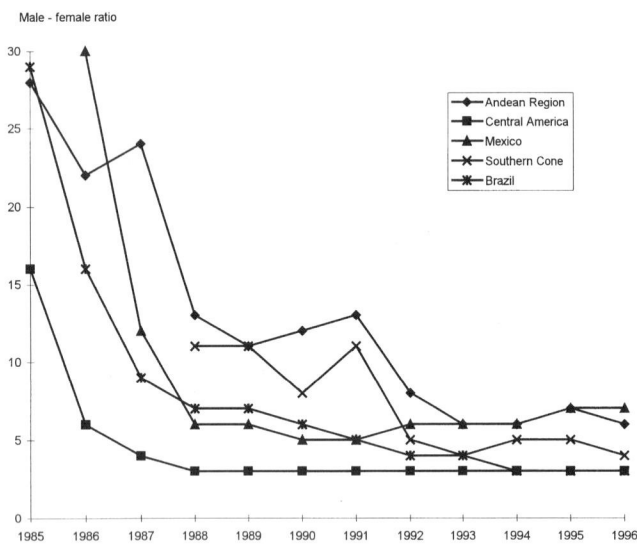

Figure 8.5. Male-to-female ratio in reported AIDS cases in Latin America from 1985 to 1996.

seems to be the predominant mode of transmission, in other countries, such as the Bahamas and Guyana, heterosexual transmission is more frequent, with prevalence rates of 4 and 7% in pregnant women in 1992, respectively (15).

In the Latin Caribbean, high rates of infection have been seen in the general population, with prevalence of HIV in pregnant women as high as 8.4% in Haiti in 1993 and similar rates in the Dominican Republic in 1996, where HIV levels were low in the early stages of the epidemic (4). In male patients with sexually transmitted diseases (STDs) in Haiti, the rate was 25% in 1992, and in sex workers, it was 42% in 1989. In the Dominican Republic, where HIV levels were low in the early years of the epidemic, 2% of pregnant women were HIV positive in 1995 (15–18).

ASIA

With more than half the world's population, Asia, like Latin America, has diverse patterns of HIV spread. In general, the spread of HIV started in the late 1980s. Because the epidemics in this part of the world are still at an early stage, surveillance systems are limited, and it is difficult to apply results from limited studies to the large populations in most of these countries. At the end of 1997, investigators estimated that about 6 million people were living with HIV/AIDS in South and Southeast Asia, and about 440,000 were infected in East Asia and the Pacific, excluding Australia and New Zealand (see Fig. 8.1 and Table 8.2). Because of the early stage of the epidemics, the number of people who had already died of AIDS by the end of 1997, 750,000, is low when compared with the total number of people living with HIV in the region. The full impact of the epidemic will be seen at the beginning of the next century, when currently infected people will develop AIDS and—in the absence of affordable treatment—subsequently will die.

Although overall rates are still low when compared with those in sub–Saharan Africa, the numbers are high because of the region's large populations. As of late 1997, India already had an estimated 3 to 5 million people living with HIV/AIDS. It is the country with by far the greatest number of HIV infections in the world, and, given current trends, a doubling of these numbers until the year 2000 does not seem unrealistic (1). This statistic shows that the future course of the global HIV epidemic will be heavily influenced by the spread of HIV in this region.

HIV initially spread in explosive epidemics in populations of intravenous drug users in South and Southeast Asia (19), that is, in various areas of Thailand, Myanmar, India, Malaysia, Cambodia, China, and Vietnam, to reach seroprevalence levels in the tested populations as high as 50% within a short period (20–25). However, heterosexual transmission has been rapidly increasing and is now the predominant mode of HIV transmission in Asia. This first became obvious from rapidly increasing infection rates among female prostitutes in Thailand and in Bombay, India. In Bombay, prevalence rates exploded from 0% in 1987 to more than 20% in 1991 (4, 26, 27). In Thailand, HIV levels reached from 15% in the northeastern part of the country to up to 40% in the northern provinces in 1991 in this population (4, 21, 28, 29).

Subsequently, the rates of infection, especially in young Thai men, increased to reach nationwide levels of 4% in 1993, with highest rates, up to 20%, in the northern provinces (30). However, after recognizing these dramatic developments, the Thai government started one of the most effective public health programs, the so-called 100% Condom Use Program (31). As a consequence of the excellent collaborations between the government and the well-established Thai sex industry, condom use, especially in sexual encounters between sex workers and their clients, increased dramatically, resulting in decreasing trends in young Thai men since 1993 (Fig. 8.7) (32–34). This decrease has not yet been seen in pregnant women, in whom levels have seemed to stabilize around 2%. This success story may serve as a useful example for other countries in the region (29).

At the end of 1996, the Chinese government estimated the number of people living with HIV/AIDS in China to be around 200,000. Current estimates show that this number may have doubled by the end of 1997 in the country, where two major epidemics are under way. One is in injecting drug users in the mountainous southwest of the country. The other, newer epidemic is now surfacing among heterosexuals, especially along the prosperous eastern seaboard, where prostitution is reemerging as the gap grows between rich and poor (35). The warning signs of high-risk behavior are worryingly clear: the incidence of STDs has shot up in recent years, and no evidence suggests that the upward trend will be broken.

Despite well-documented commercial sex industries, several Southeast Asian nations have low rates of HIV infection. In Indonesia, Malaysia, the Philippines, and Singapore, for instance, infection rates are well under 0.5%. Other countries in the region, however, show much higher levels of HIV spread (36).

In Indochina, the picture is mixed. It is bleakest in Cambodia, where 1 in 20 pregnant women, 1 in 16 soldiers and policeman, and 1 in 2 sex workers tested positive in sentinel HIV surveillance (37). Although condom use has grown rapidly (condom sales have risen from virtually nothing to around a million units a month in the space of under 3 years), commercial sex remains common: in a recent survey, three-fourths of respondents in the military and the police force and two-fifths of students said they had visited a sex worker in the last year. In neighboring Vietnam and in Myanmar, the incidence of HIV infection is also rising rapidly. In Myanmar, HIV infection among sex workers rose from 4% in 1992 to more than 20% in 1996, whereas 2 of 3 injecting drug users are infected. Among pregnant women in the general population, a relatively constant 2% are infected (4, 38).

MODES OF TRANSMISSION

Sexual Transmission

In a global sense, HIV infection is primarily an STD. In contrast to the epidemic in industrialized countries, heterosexual intercourse accounts for most cases of HIV infection acquired sexually in developing countries. Overall estimates are that 75% of cases worldwide are acquired by sexual contact (1).

Unprotected receptive anal intercourse is the most effective mode of sexual transmission of HIV (39). It is practiced not only by homosexual and bisexual men, but also by heterosexual couples. Whereas this practice seems to be unusual in sub–Saharan Africa, it may play a significant role in the spread of HIV in Latin America in selected Caribbean countries and in some Asian cities (40, 41). Expression of a homosexual lifestyle is severely repressed in most developing countries. Although data on sexual behavior in men underestimate homosexual activity for this reason, indicators such as the declining male-to-female ratio among AIDS cases suggest that heterosexual intercourse has become the driving force of the epidemic worldwide.

Vaginal–penile heterosexual intercourse is an inefficient mode of transmission of HIV, particularly from an infected woman to a man (42, 43). However, the efficiency of heterosexual transmission can be enhanced in the presence of well-defined biologic risk factors, including more advanced immunodeficiency in the infecting partner, the presence of conventional STDs in either partner, lack of circumcision, anal intercourse, and sex during menses or use of vaginal products (Table 8.3) (44, 45). Solid evidence now indicates that the presence of ulcerative and nonulcerative STDs facilitate sexual transmission of HIV, and, more important, STD control does have an impact on the rate of HIV infection (46–48). Probably, a rampant and sustained heterosexual epidemic in developing countries is only possible because of a common occurrence of such amplifying factors, in addition to high-risk sexual behavior patterns. At a population level, the overall efficiency of heterosexual transmission may increase as the epidemic progresses, as more infected people become immunodeficient. This may be a relevant factor currently in Africa.

Investigators have also come to realize over the years that HIV acquisition is not only a result of individual risk behavior, but also is determined by "societal" vulnerability such as urbanization, single-sex migration, or low status of women, factors that increase individuals' vulnerability to HIV. This realization has important implications on the design of prevention programs (3, 49).

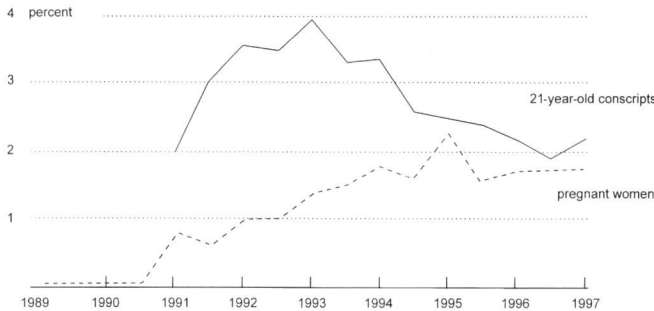

Figure 8.7. HIV prevalence in pregnant women and in 21-year-old conscripts in Thailand.

Table 8.3 Variables Influencing the Sexual Spread of HIV Infection in a Population

Biologic variables
    Level of viremia
    Prevalence of other sexually transmitted diseases
    Lack of male circumcision
    Use of certain vaginal products
    Infectivity and virulence of HIV strains(?)
Behavioral variables
    Rate of partner change
    Sexual mixing patterns
    Size of and rate of contact with core groups
    Type of sexual intercourse (anal intercourse, intercourse during menses)
    Level of condom use
    Behavior and infection rate of partners
    Prevalence of injecting drug use
Demographic variables
    Proportion of sexually most active age groups
    Male-to-female ratio
    Rate and growth or urbanization
    Migration patterns
Economic and political factors
    Performance of the health care system
    Response to the epidemic
    Poverty, deprivation, lack of education
    War and social disturbance
    Women's status
    Attitudes toward sex

(Adapted from Piot P, Laga M, Ryder RW, et al. The global epidemiology of HIV infection: continuity, heterogeneity and change. J Acquir Immune Defic Syndr 1990;3:403–412.)

Mother-to-Child Transmission

On a worldwide scale, transmission of HIV from mother to child during or after pregnancy is the second most common mode of spread of HIV. It is the major source of HIV infection in children. It has become a true public health problem in much of Africa, where, as of December 1997, 2.7 million children had died of AIDS, and 1.1 million children were living with HIV/AIDS (see Table 8.1 and Fig. 8.1).

In general, higher frequencies of mother-to-child transmission have been observed in Africa (30 to 40%), compared with the Western world (50). The reasons for this apparently higher transmission rate in Africa may be more advanced immunodeficiency in the mother, which increases the risk for transmission (51). Probably, the higher viral load associated with immune depletion and with early infection is a major determinant of the degree of infectiousness, whether for sexual or vertical transmission.

Another, and undoubtedly the most important, factor contributing to this difference in mother-to-child transmission is breast-feeding (50, 52). This risk factor is particularly important in mothers who become infected during late pregnancy or lactation. In this situation, the risk of transmission through breast milk may be as high as 50% (52). However, the rate of postnatal transmission of HIV-1 from mothers who were already infected during pregnancy is lower, estimated at between 5 and 15% (53).

Although the rates, timing, and risk factors for mother-to-child transmission of HIV have been better described, the greatest challenge for developing countries will be to find ways of benefiting from the advances made in prevention mother-to-child transmission in industrialized countries. In view of the ongoing trials in Africa and Asia with short-course antiretroviral agents, vitamin A, vaginal cleansing, and breast milk alternatives, investigators should know in the next few years whether any of these interventions can significantly lower the perinatal transmission rate of HIV. If efficacy is shown, public health authorities will be faced with major challenges to implement these strategies on a large scale. Although mother-to-child transmission of HIV-2 undoubtedly can occur, it seems unusual, with a much lower rate of transmission than for HIV-1 (54).

Transmission by Blood Products

Sharing of injection equipment among drug users is the most common route of HIV transmission by blood in Asia, Latin America, and the Caribbean. Illicit injecting drug use is mainly associated with the major routes of drug trafficking, and several populations have had a recent shift from smoking or inhaling drugs to injection (55). The fulminant spread of HIV-1 among injecting drug users in Bangkok in the late 1980s paralleled closely the patterns of spread of HIV-1 among injecting drug users in several cities in the industrialized world. Imprisonment and injecting with equipment previously used by multiple other drug users were the two strongest predictors of HIV-1 infection (56). Whereas intravenous drug use in Thailand began mainly in urban slum areas, it is now spreading in rural areas as well (57).

Blood transfusion is the most efficient mode of HIV transmission; nearly all recipients of HIV-seropositive blood become infected (58). Whereas transmission by contaminated blood transfusion and blood products has become unusual in most Asian and Latin American countries, blood transfusion remains the third most common route of HIV infection in Africa, after heterosexual and perinatal transmission, especially among children. This is largely because of an inability to implement screening of blood donors and other measures to ensure a safe blood supply, as a result of a failing health care system (59). The continuing transmission of HIV through contaminated blood is particularly tragic because the technology to prevent it is available.

The role of injections administered for medical reasons in the spread of HIV in the developing world is not well documented, but it is probably low (59). However, outbreaks in Eastern Europe demonstrate that injection-associated nosocomial HIV transmission is possible, and it may be a source of HIV infection in the community (60).

DYNAMICS OF HIV SPREAD

Over the past decade, investigators have come to realize not only that the epidemiology of HIV-1 is not homogeneous throughout the world, but also that it is in continuous evolution (1–4, 44). Monitoring this heterogeneity in the epidemic is essential for ensuring an adequate public health response. Table 8.3 lists major variables that influence the spread of HIV infection in a population. They can be grouped in biologic, demographic, behavioral, and economic/political determinants.

As a rule, the spread of a sexually transmitted agent such as HIV is defined by the equation $R_o = BcD$, where R_o is the reproductive rate, B is the average probability that infection is transmitted from an infected person to a susceptible individual, c is the average rate at which new partners are acquired, and D is the average duration of infection (61). The mix and interaction of risk determinants directly (biologic or behavioral variables) or indirectly (demographic and economic/political variables) influencing these three factors determine how HIV-1 infection spreads in a population. Conversely, interventions affecting any of these factors decrease the reproductive rate.

Biologic Variables

African HIV-1 isolates exhibit an unusually high degree of genetic variability, and evidence also indicates the occurrence of distinct subtypes of HIV-1 in Southeast Asia. The epidemiologic and clinical significance of these different HIV-1 subtypes is unclear, except for HIV-1 versus HIV-2 (62). Whether some subtypes are more closely associated with heterosexual spread and others with transmission among injecting drug users may simply reflect differences in geographic distribution or among social and sexual networks.

Several other conditions amplify the efficiency of sexual transmission of HIV by increasing both the infectiousness of an individual and the susceptibility of a noninfected sex partner to HIV-1 (46). The prevalence of various STD is high in many parts of the world, particularly in urban populations (63, 64). STD prevalence and incidence are even higher in so-called "core" groups for HIV infection, such as prostitutes and their clients, long-distance truck drivers, and military personnel (47). High levels of STD are linked not only with unsafe sexual behavior, but also with inadequate clinical services for patients with an STD.

Behavioral Variables

Sexual behavior is the most important determinant of the spread of HIV. The heterogeneity of sexual behavior among and within populations is high and probably influences the heterogeneity of the AIDS epidemic in the developing world (65). Table 8.4 summarizes the rates of casual and commercial sex reported in three surveys in Africa. These surveys show that men have more sexual partners than women and that, in some societies, higher socioeconomic status is associated with higher rates of partner change.

High rates of partner change increase the risk of HIV-1 infection, but the infection status of one's partner is equally important. In general, sexual behavior patterns that involve contacts with a highly infected core group are associated with the most rapid spread of HIV-1. Such behavior is determined not only by cultural values, but also by economic and demographic factors (see later).

In addition, the sexual mixing patterns largely define how rapidly HIV-1 spreads in a population, particularly in the early stages of the epidemic (66, 67). Thus, in cities with a high male-to-female ratio, such as Harare, Nairobi, or Bombay, the rate of casual and commercial sex is increased, resulting in high HIV-1 prevalence rates in prostitutes and their clients and in rapid spread in the general population. In contrast, sexual patterns involving roughly equal numbers of men and women in the general population may imply a slower spread of HIV. However, as the prevalence of HIV infection increases in the general population, a higher number of people (particularly women) become infected without practicing high-risk sexual behavior themselves. This phenomenon is illustrated by data from Rwanda showing that an increasing proportion of women with HIV-1 have their regular partner or husband as their only sexual contact (68).

Sexual practices such as intercourse during menses and particularly anal intercourse also vary among and within societies, and they may influence the rate of spread of HIV-1. Anal intercourse is thought to be more frequent in some Latin American populations, in whom bisexual behavior seems also to be more common (41).

Condoms are increasingly popular in the developing world, mainly as a result of intensive social marketing programs (69). The reduction in HIV-1 incidence after condom use has been well documented in prostitutes and discordant couples in Zaire (47). Probably, massive condom use will further slow the spread of HIV.

Demographic Variables

The most active age groups represent a much larger proportion of the population in the developing world. This finding in itself is associated with higher incidence rates of STDs, including HIV infection. Because of high birth rates, this population of young adults will become even larger in the near future.

Large urban concentrations and migratory populations have also been linked with above-average rates of STDs. Whereas significant rural-to-urban migration is occurring throughout the developing world, some regions also experience extensive international and transnational migrations, such as within Brazil and to Côte d'Ivoire from its neighbor-

Table 8.4 Urban Men and Women Reporting Commercial or Casual Sex in the Last 12 Months by Level of Education

Country	Education Level			
	No School (%)	Primary (%)	Secondary (%)	Higher (%)
Central African Republic				
Male	15	20	25	35
Female	7	10	6	
Côte d'Ivoire				
Male	16	24	43	44
Female	5	12	12	9
Kenya				
Male	21	25	25	32
Female		9	8	7

(From Caraël M. Sexual behaviour. In: Cleland J, Ferry B, eds. Sexual behaviour and AIDS in the developing world. London: Taylor and Francis, 1995: 75–123.)

ing countries. The system of migrant labor causes long absences and predisposes to increased family breakdown and larger numbers of sexual partners (70).

The balance between supply and demand of sexual contact between the sexes is an important determinant of HIV-1 epidemiology. Cities with such an imbalance may experience a more rapid spread of HIV-1. This situation may result from an unusually high number of men, usually from migration of male laborers into cities, but it may also be due to social constraints on sexuality, such as a tendency of men to marry late and the social stance against premarital and extramarital sex among women. An extreme example of this imbalance is that of the migrant miners under apartheid in South Africa (71). Such urban demographic patterns may have a marked influence on sexual behavior by favoring prostitution and high rates of STDs.

Economic and Political Factors

The efficacy of the response of society to the AIDS epidemic will ultimately determine the extent of HIV spread. This response is uniformly insufficient, although Thailand has demonstrated that an energetic and adequate national reaction to an emerging AIDS epidemic is possible. A major problem is a lack of international funds for AIDS control programs in the developing world, programs that need about 20 times more resources than are currently available. As a result of poor management, low political priority given to health and social services (as compared with military expenditure), and structural readjustment plans, the health care system has severely deteriorated, particularly in many African countries (72). This problem has been accompanied by declining access to health services and less control of STDs, as well as fewer opportunities for preventive activities.

Poverty is one of the most powerful driving forces of epidemics and is the most difficult factor to change. It engenders prostitution, homelessness in adults and the presence of street children, poorly educated citizens, migration, and separated families, all fertile ground for the spread of HIV.

Finally, the sexual norms of society undoubtedly influence both the spread of HIV and the response to an STD epidemic. Indicators of poor status of women correlate well with high and rapid spread of HIV, a finding suggesting that women's status plays some role in this epidemic (63).

IMPACT OF THE AIDS/HIV EPIDEMIC

The impact of AIDS on the individual and on society has not become fully visible as yet and goes beyond the suffering of infected individuals and their relatives and friends. More than any disease of our time, AIDS will have a long-term impact on the demography, economy, social system, and health sector in seriously affected countries.

Demographic Impact

The ultimate demographic impact of the AIDS epidemic is controversial, but it will vary among countries in proportion to the level reached by the epidemic. A conservative estimate is that, in sub–Saharan Africa, the population growth rate will decline from an average of 3% to less than 2% per year around the year 2000 (73). However, in the most severely affected countries of eastern and southern Africa, a greater effect on population growth is anticipated. In countries with a slower population growth, such as in Asia or Latin America, a severe AIDS epidemic may even lead to negative population growth.

Such reductions in population growth will be due to increased mortality, mainly among young adults, who are the driving force of a nation. In Thailand, investigators estimate that, by the year 2000, 30% of all deaths will be from AIDS, and in Abidjan, Côte d'Ivoire, AIDS is now the leading cause of death in adults (74, 75). Instead of benefiting the population by reducing its growth rate, the consequent doubling or quadrupling of the mortality rate in persons aged 15 to 44 years would have tragic effects on the economy, the social structure, and the fabric of society (63).

Not only are adult mortality rates increasing significantly as a result of the AIDS epidemic, but also mortality in children under 5 years old is increasing. AIDS is now reversing the gains of child survival initiatives in a growing number of developing countries (Fig. 8.8). Finally, the historic trend of a gradual increase of the life expectancy at birth has been reversed in several sub–Saharan African countries, as illustrated in Figure 8.9.

Impact on the Health Sector

Among the most visible aspects of the burden of HIV infection are the large numbers of emaciated men and women with AIDS in many African hospitals. In many cities, these people constitute up to half of all patients, and AIDS is the major cause of death among hospitalized patients (75).

As an increasing number of people with HIV develop AIDS, the demand for health care will rise rapidly, and hospitals in some Asian and American cities will probably face situations similar to those encountered in Africa today. AIDS patients not only will occupy beds that could be used for patients with treatable diseases, but also they will account for both absolute and relative increases in health care expendi-

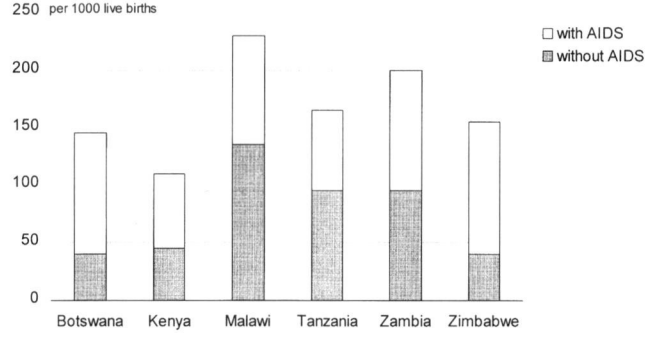

Figure 8.8. Estimated impact of AIDS on mortality rates in children younger than 5 years of age in selected African countries in 2010. (From United States Bureau of the Census.)

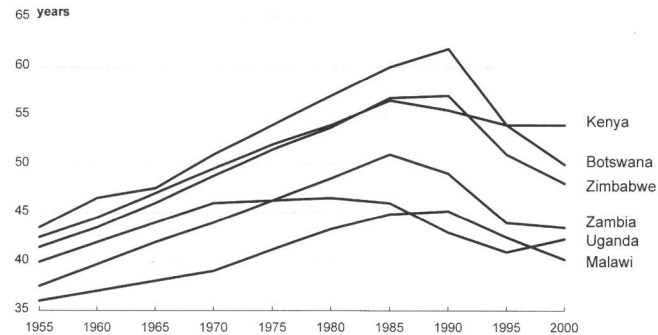

Figure 8.9. Projected life expectancy at birth in selected sub–Saharan countries. (From United Nations Population Division. World Population Prospects. rev. ed. New York: United Nations Population Division, 1996.)

ture. Planning for absorbing this enormous burden of patients is a top priority for health care systems in the developing world, in addition to the challenging issue of making antiviral drugs available (76).

Accompanying Epidemic of Tuberculosis

Each year, nearly 3 million people die of tuberculosis, which is the leading cause of death from infectious diseases in the world (77). Most of these cases occur in the developing world, mainly in Asia (more than 50% of the fatal cases in the world) and in Africa (approximately 25%), where between 50 and 80% of adults are infected with *Mycobacterium tuberculosis*.

This disease of major public health significance has been affected by the HIV epidemic, with rising incidence rates wherever HIV has become endemic (78). This rise in incidence is entirely attributable to HIV infection. HIV-induced immunodeficiency is thought to lead to reactivation of latent infection with *Mycobacterium tuberculosis*, and it is the driving force behind a new tuberculosis epidemic accompanying the AIDS epidemic. HIV seroprevalence rates among tuberculosis patients in Africa and Haiti are from 30 to 80% (78).

Additional problems for tuberculosis control programs include a high mortality rate among tuberculosis patients with HIV infection (mostly because of HIV-related diseases), a growing problem of multidrug resistance by *Mycobacterium tuberculosis*, and a 5- to 10-fold increase in severe skin rashes during antituberculosis therapy in HIV-positive patients (78).

Economic and Social Impact

AIDS has become one of the five leading causes of lost health in sub–Saharan cities, and it accounts for 15% of the total disease burden (63). AIDS affects mainly young adults in the most productive years of their lives and has an impact on various economic and social sectors. Whereas the direct medical costs to society are large, the magnitude of the far more important indirect costs is enormous (79).

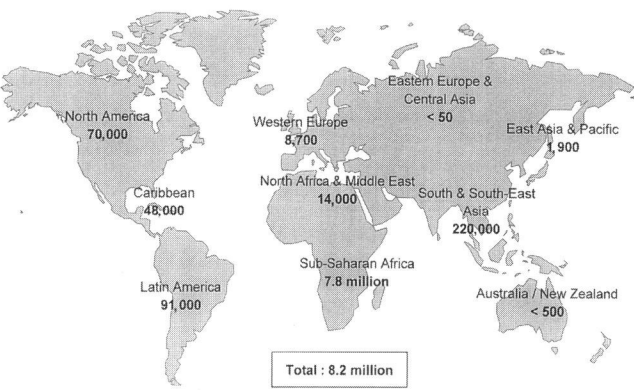

Figure 8.10. Cumulative number of children estimated to have been orphaned by AIDS at age 14 years or younger. Orphans are defined as HIV-negative children who lost their mother or both parents to AIDS.

The loss of productivity in industry, agriculture, and services will affect the gross domestic product (GDP) in severely affected countries. Thus, in Tanzania, experts have estimated that the real GDP growth rate in the period 1985 to 2010 will decline by 15 and 28%, from 4% per annum to 2.9 to 3.4% per annum, as a result of AIDS (79).

Finally, AIDS has a profound impact on the household and basic community as a result of illness, death of breadwinners, a growing number of orphans, increased expenses for health care, and loss of purchasing power (80). Figure 8.10 summarizes the number of children estimated to have been orphaned by AIDS at the age of 14 years or younger, by region. AIDS truly may become a destabilizing factor in society as a whole.

References

1. Joint United Nations Programme on HIV/AIDS (UNAIDS)/World Health Organization (WHO). Report on the global HIV/AIDS epidemic: fact sheet. Geneva: UNAIDS/WHO, 1997.
2. Tarantola D, Schwartländer B. HIV/AIDS epidemics in sub–Saharan Africa: dynamism, diversity and discrete declines? In: Laga M, De Cock K, Kaleeba N, eds. AIDS in Africa. 2nd ed. London: Rapid Science, 1997:S5–S21.
3. Tarantola D, Mann J. Global overview: a powerful HIV/AIDS pandemic. In: Mann J, Tarantola D, eds. AIDS in the world II. New York: Oxford University Press, 1996:5–40.
4. United States Bureau of the Census. Recent HIV seroprevalence levels by country: January 1997. Washington, DC: Population Division, US Bureau of the Census, 1997.
5. Asiimwe-Okiror G, Opio AA, Musinguzi J, et al. Change in sexual behaviour and decline in HIV infection among young pregnant women in urban Uganda. AIDS 1997;11:1757–1763.
6. Fylkesnes K, Musonda RM, Kasumba K, et al. The HIV epidemic in Zambia: socio-demographic prevalence patterns and indications of trends among childbearing women. AIDS 1997;11:339–345.
7. Djomand G, Greenberg A, Sassan-Morokro M, et al. The epidemic of HIV/AIDS in Abidjan, Côte d'Ivoire: a review of data collected by project RETRO-CI from 1987 to 1993. J Acquir Immune Defic Syndr Hum Retrovirol 1995;10:358–365.
8. De Cock KM, Adjorlolo G, Ekpini E, et al. Epidemiology and transmission of HIV-2: why there is no HIV-2 pandemic. JAMA 1993;270:2083–2086.
9. Kanki PJ, Peeters M, Guéye-Ndiaye A. Virology of HIV-1 and HIV-2: implications for Africa. AIDS 1997;11(Suppl B):S33–S42.

10. Anderson S, Albert J, Norrgen H, et al. Trends of incidence and prevalence of HIV-1 in Guinea-Bissau, West Africa, and preliminary data on subtypes [abstract Mo.C.1480]. Presented at the 11th International Conference on AIDS, Vancouver, 1996.
11. Ghys PD, Diallo MO, Ettiègne-Traore V, et al. Dual seroreactivity to HIV-1 and HIV-2 in female sex workers in Abidjan, Côte d'Ivoire. AIDS 1995;9:955–958.
12. Quinn TC, Narrain JP, Zacarias FRK. AIDS in the Americas: a public health priority for the region. AIDS 1990;4:709–724.
13. Hospedales J, White F, Gayle C, et al. Epidemiology of HIV/AIDS in the Caribbean. In: Lamptey P, White F, Figueroa FP, et al., eds. The handbook for AIDS prevention in the Caribbean. Research Triangle Park, NC: Family Health International, 1992:1–23.
14. Basset D, Narain J. Changing pattern of HIV transmission in the Caribbean. In: AIDS: profile of an epidemic. Scientific publication no. 514. Pan American Health Organization, 1988:200–204.
15. Joint United Nations Programme on HIV/AIDS (UNAIDS)/World Health Organization (WHO). HIV/AIDS/STD epi fact sheet: Caribbean. Geneva: UNAIDS/WHO, 1997.
16. Bouloa R, Halsey N, Kissinger P, et al. Stable HIV-1 seroprevalence rates in pregnant women residing in an Haitian urban slum [abstract MC 3015]. Presented at the 7th International Conference on AIDS, Florence, Italy, 1991.
17. Liautaud B, Mellon LR, Denize-Vieux J, et al. Preliminary data on STDs in Haiti [abstract PoC 4302]. Presented at the 7th International Conference on AIDS, Amsterdam, 1992.
18. Giordano M, Pape J, Blattner W, et al. The seroprevalence of HTLV-1 and HIV-1 co-infection in Haiti [abratct M.G.P. 3]. Presented at the 5th International Conference on AIDS, Montreal, 1989.
19. Li PCK, Yeoh EK. Current epidemiological trends of HIV infection in Asia. AIDS Clin Rev 1992;1–24.
20. Des Jarlais DC, Friedman SR, Chooanya K, et al. International epidemiology of HIV and AIDS among injecting drug users. AIDS 1992;6:1053–1068.
21. Weniger BG, Limpakarnjanarat K, Ungchusok K, et al. The epidemiology of HIV infection and AIDS in Thailand. AIDS 1991;5(Suppl 2):S71–S85.
22. Ford N, Koetsawang S. The socio-cultural context of the transmission of HIV in Thailand. Soc Sci Med 1991;33:405–414.
23. Naik TN, Sarkar S, Singh HL, et al. Intravenous drug users: a new high risk group for HIV infection in India. AIDS 1991;5:117–118.
24. Sarkat S, Mokerjee P, Roy A, et al. Descriptive epidemiology of intravenous heroin users: a new risk group for transmission of HIV in India. J Infect Dis 1991;23:201–207.
25. Zhang JP. An epidemiological study on HIV infection in Ruili County, Yennan Province. Chung Hua Liu Hsing Ping Hsueh Tsa Chih 1991;12:9–12.
26. Bhave GG, Wagle UD, Tripathy SP. HIV sero-surveillance in promiscuous females of Bombay, India [abstract FC 612]. Presented at the 6th International Conference on AIDS, San Francisco, 1991.
27. Boonchalaksi W, Guest P. Prostitution in Thailand. Institute for Population and Social Research publication no. 171. Bangkok: Mahidol University, 1994.
28. Siraprapasiri T, Thanprasertsuk S, Rodklay A, et al. Risk factors for HIV among prostitutes in Chiangmai, Thailand. AIDS 1991;5:579–582.
29. Ministry of Heath, Thailand. Surveillance report. Bangkok: Ministry of Health, 1997.
30. Jugsudee A, Tanormklom S, Junlananto P, et al. HIV-1 seroprevalence among young adult populations in Thailand, 1990–1995 [abstract Mo.C.1519]. Presented at the 11th International Conference on AIDS, Vancouver, 1996.
31. Rojanapithayakorn W, Hanenberg R. The 100% Condom Program in Thailand: editorial review. AIDS 1996;10:1–7.
32. Nelson K, Celentano D, Eiumtrakol S, et al. Changes in sexual behavior and a decline in HIV infection among young men in Thailand. N Engl J Med 1996;335:297–303.
33. Brody S. Decline in HIV infections in Thailand. N Engl J Med 1996;335:1998–1999.
34. Brown T, Sittitrai W, Vanichseni S, et al. The recent epidemiology of HIV and AIDS in Thailand. AIDS 1994;8(Suppl 2):S131–S141.
35. Chinese Academy for Preventive Medicine. Sexually transmitted diseases in China. Beijing: Chinese Academy for Preventive Medicine, 1997.
36. World Health Organization (WHO), Regional Office for the Western Pacific. STD, HIV and AIDS surveillance report, issue 10; and Report on the global epidemic. Geneva: UNAIDS, 1997.
37. National AIDS Programme. Report of the National AIDS Programme, Cambodia. Phnom Penh: National AIDS Programme, 1997.
38. National AIDS Prevention and Control Programme. Report of the National AIDS Prevention and Control Programme, Myanmar. Rangoon: National AIDS Prevention and Control Programme, 1997.
39. Detels R, English P, Visscher BR, et al. Seroconversion, sexual activity, and condom use among 2915 HIV seronegative men followed for up to 2 years. J Acquir Immune Defic Syndr 1989;2:77–83.
40. Quinn TC, Mann JM, Curran JW, et al. AIDS in Africa: an epidemiological paradigm. Science 1986;16:516–519.
41. Parker RG, Tawil O. Bisexual behavior and HIV transmission in Latin America. In: Tielman R, Carballo M, Hendriks A, eds. Bisexuality and HIV/AIDS. New York: Prometheus Press, 1991.
42. Johnson AM, Laga M. Heterosexual transmission of HIV. AIDS 1988;2(Suppl 1):S49–S56.
43. Holmberg SD, Horsburgh CR Jr, Ward JW, et al. Biological factors in the sexual transmission of human immunodeficiency virus. J Infect Dis 1989;160:116–125.
44. Piot P, Laga M, Ryder RW, et al. The global epidemiology of HIV infection: continuity, heterogeneity and change. J Acquir Immune Defic Syndr 1990;3:403–412.
45. Moses S, Plummer FA, Bradley JE, et al. Male circumcision and the AIDS epidemic in Africa. Health Trans Rev 1995;5:100–103.
46. Ghys PD, Fransen K, Diallo MO, et al. The associations between cervicovaginal HIV shedding, sexually transmitted diseases and immunosuppression in female sex workers in Abidjan, Côte d'Ivoire. AIDS 1997;11:F85–F93.
47. Laga M, Alary M, Nzila N, et al. Condom promotion, STD treatment leading to a declining incidence of HIV-1 infection in female Zairean sex workers. Lancet 1994;344:246–248.
48. Grosskurth H, Mosha F, Todd J, et al. Impact of improved treatment of sexually transmitted diseases on HIV infection in rural Tanzania: randomised controlled trial. Lancet 1995;346:530–536.
49. Caraël M, Buvé A, Awusabo-Asare K. The making of HIV epidemics: what are the driving forces? AIDS 1997;11(Suppl B):S23–S31.
50. Working Group on Mother-to-Child Transmission of HIV. Rates of mother-to-child transmission of HIV-1 in Africa, America and Europe: results from 13 perinatal studies. J Acquir Immune Defic Syndr 1995;8:506–510.
51. Ryder RW, Temmerman M. The effect of HIV-1 infection during pregnancy and the perinatal period on maternal and child health in Africa. AIDS 1991;5(Suppl 1):S75–S85.
52. Van de Perre P, Simonon A, Msellati P, et al. Postnatal transmission of human immunodeficiency virus in infants born to seropositive mothers. N Engl J Med 1991;325:593–599.
53. Wiktor SZ, Ekpini E, Nduati RW. Prevention of mother-to-child transmission of HIV-1 in Africa. AIDS 1997;11(Suppl B):S79–S87.
54. Adjorlolo G, De Cock KM, Ekpini E, et al. Prospective comparison of HIV-1 and HIV-2 perinatal transmission in Abidjan, Côte d'Ivoire. JAMA 1994;272:462–466.
55. Des Jarlais DC, Friedman SR, Choopanya K, et al. International epidemiology of HIV and AIDS among injecting drug users. AIDS 1992;6:1053–1068.
56. Choopanya K, Vanichseni S, Des Jarlais DC, et al. Risk factors and HIV seropositivity among injecting drug users in Bangkok. AIDS 1991;5:1509–1513.
57. Ford N, Koetsawang S. The socio-cultural context of the transmission of HIV in Thailand. Soc Sci Med 1991;33:405–414.
58. Colebunders R, Ryder R, Francis H, et al. Seroconversion rate, mortality and clinical manifestations associated with the receipt of a

human immunodeficiency virus infected blood transfusion. J Infect Dis 1991;164:450–456.
59. Van de Perre P, Diakhate L, Watson-Williams J. Prevention of blood-borne transmission of HIV. AIDS 1997;11(Suppl B):S89–S98.
60. Hersh BS, Popovici F, Apetrei RC, et al. Acquired immunodeficiency syndrome in Romania. Lancet 1991;338:645–649.
61. Anderson RM, May RM. Transmission dynamics of HIV infection. Nature 1987;26:137–142.
62. Workshop report from the European Commission (DG XII, INCO-DC) and Joint United Nations Programme on HIV/AIDS. HIV-1 subtypes: implications for epidemiology, pathogenicity, vaccines and diagnostics. AIDS 1997;11:UNAIDS 17–UNAIDS 36.
63. Over M, Piot P. HIV infection and sexually transmitted diseases. In: Jamison DT, Mosley WH, eds. Disease control priorities in developing countries. Washington, DC: World Bank, 1993.
64. Hira SR. Sexually transmitted diseases: a menace to mothers and children. World Health Forum 1986;7:243–247.
65. Caraël M. Sexual behaviour. In: Cleland J, Ferry B, eds. Sexual behaviour and AIDS in the developing world. London: Taylor and Francis, 1995:75–123.
66. Larson A. Social context of HIV transmission in Africa: historical and cultural bases of east and central African sexual relations. Rev Infect Dis 1989;11:71–73.
67. Boily MC, Anderson RM. Sexual contact patterns between men and women and the spread of HIV-1 in urban centres in Africa. IMA J Math Appl Med Biol 1991;8:221–247.
68. Allen S, Lindan C, Serufila A, et al. Human immunodeficiency virus infection in urban Rwanda: demographic and behavioural correlates in a representative sample of childbearing women. JAMA 1991;226:1657–1663.
69. Lamptey P, Goodridge GAW. Condom issues in AIDS prevention in Africa. AIDS 1991;5(Suppl 1):S183–S191.
70. Hunt CW. Migrant labor and sexually transmitted disease: AIDS in Africa. J Health Soc Behav 1989;30:353–373.
71. Stein Z, Zwi A, eds. Action on AIDS in southern Africa: Maputo Conference on Health in Transition in Southern Africa (CHISA), April 1990. New York: CHISA, 1991.
72. Sanders D, Sambo A. AIDS in Africa: the implications of economic recession and structural adjustment. Health Pol Planning 1991;6:157–165.
73. Whiteside A, Stover J. The demographic and economic impact of AIDS in Africa. AIDS 1997;11(Suppl B):S55–S61.
74. Armstrong J, Bos E. The demographic, economic, and social impact of AIDS. In: Mann J, Tarantola DJM, Netter TW, eds. AIDS in the world. Cambridge, MA: Harvard University Press, 1992:195–226.
75. De Cock KM, Barrere B, Diaby L, et al. AIDS: the leading cause of adult death in the west African city of Abidjan, Ivory Coast. Science 1990;249:793–796.
76. Gilks CF, Katabira E, De Cock KM. The challenge of providing effective care for HIV/AIDS in Africa. AIDS 1997;11(Suppl B):S99–S106.
77. Murray CJL, Styblo K, Rocillon A. Tuberculosis in developing countries: burden, intervention and cost. Bull Int Union Tuberc Lung Dis 1990;65:6–24.
78. Perriëns JH, Mukadi Y, Nunn P. Tuberculosis and HIV infection: implications for Africa. AIDS 1991;5(Suppl 1):S127–S134.
79. Bertozzi SM. Combating HIV in Africa: a role for economic research. AIDS 1991;5(Suppl 1):S45–S54.
80. Barnett T, Blaikie P. AIDS in Africa: its present and future impact. London: Bellhaven Press, 1992.

9
PUBLIC HEALTH, HIV, AND AIDS

June E. Osborn

The epidemiology of the acquired immunodeficiency syndrome/human immunodeficiency virus (AIDS/HIV) epidemic is described in detail in the preceding chapters. However, for purposes of developing the themes of appropriate public health response, certain facets of the patterns of transmission and dissemination of HIV deserve emphasis.

DEFINITIONS

Initial Patterns of Epidemic Expression

DEFINITION OF AIDS

The first recognition of AIDS cases in 1981 heralded a worldwide pandemic, as became clear over the next few years. Initially, however, a major problem was definition of the new illness, inasmuch as it presented as a syndrome or constellation of disease manifestations rather than as one precise entity. For purposes of careful surveillance, therefore, the United States Centers for Disease Control (CDC) deliberately adopted a conservative case definition, requiring underlying CD4+ T-cell depletion accompanied by one or more specific opportunistic infections or tumors. The diseases on that list became known as AIDS-defining conditions (1).

As experience with the syndrome broadened, additional disorders including primary neurologic disease were added to the list, which currently has at least 30 entries. As international reports linked the epidemic to systemic phenomena such as profound tissue wasting (so-called "slim disease" in East Africa), an international definition was adopted that was different from that of CDC.

Of particular significance to the surveillance definition thus created was the relative absence of women among recognized AIDS cases in the first few years. This meant that experience with HIV disease in women was limited, and it had the unintended result of omission of gender-specific entities such as chronic *Candida* vaginitis or distinctively aggressive cervical neoplasia from the AIDS-defining list.

The AIDS case definition and its evolution are relevant to descriptions of the early years of the AIDS pandemic, because each change was designed to be more inclusive of the range of manifestations of advanced HIV disease, once it became possible to test for infection with HIV (2, 3). The most recent broadening by the CDC of the AIDS definition occurred in 1993 (4), when several manifestations that occurred strikingly in women or in injection drug users (IDUs) were added. These manifestations included rapidly invasive cervical carcinoma, pulmonary tuberculosis (extrapulmonary tuberculosis was already a defining condition), and recurrent bacterial pneumonias in an HIV-seropositive person. Furthermore, as of 1993, the confirmed finding of a CD4+ T-cell count below 200 cells/mm^3 in an HIV-positive person became a sufficient criterion to warrant an AIDS diagnosis, even in the absence of defining opportunistic infections or tumors.

The artificiality of the surveillance definition of AIDS became clear once the HIVs were discovered and characterized and their causal link to the emerging syndrome of immune suppression and its consequences was established. Most clinicians concluded that the defined syndromes of AIDS were, in fact, the end stage of progressive HIV-mediated damage, including depletion of CD4+ T cells or other facets of HIV replication resulting in tissue wasting or in central or peripheral neurologic damage. Thus, many observers argued that it would make sense to refer to the overall entity as HIV disease, with individual cases progressing along a continuum from asymptomatic to gradually increasing clinical manifestations of illness resulting from the underlying pathogenetic process. In such a construct, what is currently called AIDS would be the usual (but not invariable) end stage of progression of HIV disease. The cogency of the argument, in terms of assessing epidemic impact, is evident when one notes that, before the 1993 change, many people died of HIV-related illness without ever "qualifying" for the AIDS definition. However, the term AIDS (and thus the definition of the syndrome) had acquired socioeconomic meaning quite apart from diagnostic or epidemiologic concerns. Complicating factors such as qualification for reimbursement for care as well as mandatory case reporting of AIDS-defined cases created a circumstance in which sudden transition to "HIV disease" would have had disruptive effects (5–7). Thus, the broadening of the definition of AIDS in 1993 was important and went far toward rectifying the earlier problems of measuring disease impact among women and IDUs.

EARLY FEATURES OF THE EPIDEMIC AS A DETERMINANT OF SUBSEQUENT PUBLIC PERCEPTION

Several accidents of history served initially to obscure the broad threat presented by the emergence of HIV as a pandemic pathogen. In particular, that the first cases in the developed world were recognized in marginalized communities of gay men or IDUs led to a false reassurance that "risk groups" existed. That, in turn, allowed for widespread denial that the new syndrome could present any threat to people who did not perceive themselves as belonging to those groups. Much distortion of public health discussions has resulted from such perceptions, and it is critical to development of sound policy that the issue of HIV transmission be clearly addressed.

The first recognition of AIDS cases, reported in the summer of 1981 in the United States, was followed quickly by both prospective and retrospective reporting of similar cases nationally and worldwide. Although most cases early in the epidemic in the United States were recognized either in gay men with many sexual partners or in IDUs, other patterns of epidemic expression were seen elsewhere. In particular, in large areas of the world where neither openly gay sexuality nor injecting drug use prevailed, HIV was spread predominately by heterosexual sex (8). In those areas, women were at least as frequently involved as were men, in a pattern that mimicked that of familiar sexually transmitted diseases (STDs); for example, women tended to be younger than men at time of disease expression.

To describe these early variations in epidemic pattern, the Global Programme on AIDS of the World Health Organization (WHO) initially proposed that the former constellation (i.e., AIDS appearing primarily in gay men and IDUs) be referred to as type I and the latter (suggestive of heterosexual spread) as type II. Even as the construct was proposed, it was evident that in some countries and cultures the two patterns appeared simultaneously, so a third designation of "mixed types I/II" was suggested. Finally, a type III designation was applied to those countries that were spared (by a few years) the arrival of overt AIDS, which throughout the 1980s included much of Asia and Eastern Europe.

Using that nomenclature for descriptive convenience, one can summarize that, in the early epidemic in the industrialized Western world, the type I pattern predominated, as did (in general) the associated stigmatization and denial. In sub-Saharan Africa, type II initially spread in central and eastern African countries, but it soon spread both south and west. North African countries have reported little AIDS, although whether that finding reflects a true exception to an otherwise global spread or simply a deficit in surveillance or reporting is not clear.

Many Caribbean countries were involved from the onset, but their pattern of disease expression was mixed, with evidence of both type I and type II spread. The same was true of Brazil and subsequently of Mexico and other nations in Latin America.

As another accident of history, much of Asia and Eastern Europe experienced overt AIDS cases a few years later than their recognition in the West, thus earning the early designation of type III countries. The pause was brief, however, and dramatic spread in Thailand, India, and southern China has occurred recently, leading to knowledgeable predictions that Asia may account for over 40% of HIV infections by the turn of the century (9).

Thus, the sense of invulnerability that characterized many cultures and countries in the first years of the epidemic has given way to an awareness that the pandemic is indeed universal. With time, it became clear that every continent (with the possible exception of Antarctica) and every country had at least some HIV if not overt cases of AIDS, that only a few modes of transmission were operant, and that the artificial distinctions suggested by type I, II, and III "patterning" had not only lost their utility, but were indeed fostering a denial of involvement on the part of people and (in particular) of their governmental leadership. The phenomenon of denial until overt AIDS cases appeared was a regular occurrence in countries around the globe, the consequences of which were particularly dire inasmuch as the long, silent asymptomatic stage of HIV disease in infected individuals meant that years of preventive activities were lost thereby. What was vividly clear by the end of the first decade was that HIV/AIDS was a new, deadly disease to which the whole human race was approximately equally susceptible, and that no corner of the earth would escape (10).

Modes of Transmission

As noted previously, even in the earliest years of AIDS recognition, the primary routes of virus spread—by sexual intercourse or by injection—were evident. As case numbers climbed and diagnostic acumen sharpened, it became clear that transmission through blood and blood products was a matter of urgent concern. Pediatric cases presented a more challenging diagnostic problem because their clinical expression varied widely both in timing and manifestation; however, it became evident that birth to an infected mother constituted a risk for 15 to 30% of infants born in that circumstance (11).

Thus, by 1984, the major routes of transmission of the newly isolated HIV had been delineated, and cumulative experience suggested that virus spread by any other means was rare, if it occurred at all. With the advent of the diagnostic capability provided by serologic tests for HIV antibody (enzyme-linked immunosorbent assay or ELISA) and Western blot in 1985, and with the capacity for HIV cultivation developed in many clinical laboratories, assessing virus routes of transmission in both prospective and retrospective studies became possible. On the basis of the accumulating data, in turn, the sharply restricted capacity of HIV to transfer from host to host was confirmed. With effective measures to protect the blood supply, strategies could be devised that allowed public health officials and health care professionals to warn of risk behaviors, avoidance of which could then place people out of the range of HIV.

TRANSMISSION: WHAT *DOES NOT* WORK

The complete inefficacy of so-called casual contact to transmit HIV has been demonstrated repeatedly in careful epidemiologic studies. Even tears and saliva, which occasionally have been shown in the laboratory to contain small amounts of virus, have not been implicated in HIV spread from one person to another.

Friedland and colleagues followed 206 members of families in which a person with diagnosed AIDS had been cared for at home for weeks or months without precautions. Without exception, when no sexual contact occurred, no family member was infected secondarily despite the sharing of utensils, razors, cups, toilet facilities, and affectionate kisses, not to mention the unprotected handling of secretions (12, 13).

In similar studies, now involving many thousands of people, casual contagion has consistently failed to be implicated. This conforms well to the finding that, even as the epidemic widened, the "no identified risk" category of AIDS occurrence at CDC gradually decreased as a percentage of the whole (14). Most of the individuals on that list had either died before follow-up was possible or had been unwilling to cooperate fully with epidemiologic investigation. Now, with millions of infected people, the occasional rare exception to the rule of transmission only by sex, blood, or birth to an infected mother emphasizes just how restricted HIV is in its modes of spread.

TRANSMISSION: WHAT *DOES* WORK

Sex

By contrast with the resoundingly negative findings noted previously for "casual" contact, all forms of sexual intercourse carry at least some risk of HIV transfer from infected to uninfected partner, although the efficiency of transmission varies, depending on the type of intercourse. Anal receptive intercourse is severalfold more efficient than other sexual modes; the high level of risk has been shown most clearly in prospective studies of male–male couples (15), but investigators have suggested that a similarly high risk may pertain to women who engage in receptive anal intercourse with infected male partners (16). Unfortunately, the prevalence of heterosexual anal intercourse is poorly documented; efforts to study its frequency have suggested that it is more widespread and frequent than commonly believed. Insertive anal intercourse and vaginal intercourse appear to carry lower levels of risk. Investigators have suggested that male-to-female transmission is more efficient than the reverse (17), although data on this issue are inconsistent. Some of the variations in findings may reflect the enhanced efficiency of transmission of HIV in the presence of other STDs, which often was a moot factor in studies of heterosexual transmission.

However, in considering relative efficiencies of sexual transmission, several caveats are important. First, that each of these modes of intercourse can effectively spread the virus to a sexual partner is not disputed; what is at issue is relative efficiency. Second, the matter of whether the likelihood of transfer is greater from male to female than the reverse is still unresolved: longitudinal studies of monogamous couples in which only one partner was infected initially have suggested nearly equal efficiency of transmission in either direction (18). Third, as yet unknown factors influence transmission, because in any sexual partnership setting in which one partner was infected and the other susceptible, clear instances of failure to transmit the virus over sustained intervals have been reported (19), just as in other studies there seem to be "high-efficiency transmitters" (20). When repeated unprotected sexual exposure fails to result in infection, a recent finding suggests that a specific genotype, found only in the white population thus far, with about a 1% frequency (21), may render those individuals insusceptible to HIV because they lack necessary coreceptors. The latter case may be explained in part by the fact that highest concentrations of HIV are present in patients extremely early and extremely late in their HIV infection; however, that fact alone is insufficient to explain variability of transmission. Finally, instances of HIV transmission during a single act of intercourse are well documented; efforts to estimate "risk-per-sex-act" (22, 23) are rendered perilous by these several caveats.

Two final issues concerning sexual spread require brief comment. The riskiness of oral sex has been difficult to assess in the context of HIV transmission inasmuch as it usually is not the sole mode of sexual intercourse; however, several reports establish firmly that HIV can be transmitted by this means, albeit infrequently (24–26). Similarly, the low level of risk from female–female sex has led some investigators to assert that lesbians are not at risk; that conclusion is unwarranted (27). In fact, awareness of HIV risk is important in all contexts of sexuality, and it underlies the strategies of prevention and public health intervention discussed later in this chapter.

Blood

The transmission of HIV is at its most efficient through injection of infected blood or blood products.

1. *Transfusion and infusion.* Transfusion of whole blood or blood components such as platelets or red blood cells carries a great likelihood of HIV transfer when the donor is infected, although the risk is not 100% (28). The contamination of the blood supply by HIV was recognized in the United States in 1983, followed quickly by institution of policies of self-exclusion, unit-exclusion, and (as of May 1985, when blood screening became possible through ELISA and Western blot assays for HIV antibodies) direct testing for evidence of HIV infection. Further refinements of testing allow detection of HIV (antibody, antigen, or RNA) early in infection, leaving only a brief "window period." The result has been a virtual elimination of HIV transmission through transfused blood: currently, the estimated risk is less than 1 in 500,000 per unit, relating directly to the likelihood of donors' being in the early or "window" period of infection

(29, 30). That finding underscores the value of self-exclusion and unit-exclusion, in addition to screening, as important elements of the blood safety policy. Despite the advance in technology, discussion of risk behavior with potential donors (especially first-time donors) remains central to the strategy in place to protect the blood supply.

Fractionation of blood into plasma components reduces HIV infectivity to a variable extent. γ-Globulin preparations have been shown repeatedly to be free of HIV under standard conditions of fractionation (31, 32), whereas both factor VIII and IX concentrates were found to be contaminated early in the epidemic (33). The addition of a heat-treatment step in preparation of these clotting factors greatly reduced the likelihood of HIV transmission even before systemic screening of blood and blood products for HIV antibodies (34), which began in 1985 in the United States. However, the disastrous consequence of the prescreening contamination of large pools of factor VIII concentrate was that as many as 70% of severely hemophiliac patients became HIV infected before recognition of their special risk in 1983 (35).

Since the advent of screening, efforts have been devoted to creating blood product substitutes that could free hemophiliac populations from such unknown risks. Chief among these are the development of recombinant factor VIII and IX (36) products that could eliminate blood contamination as a hazard for people with those congenital clotting disorders.

HIV-2 was recognized shortly after its identification in West Africa to share the transmission properties of HIV-1 and as such raised the issue of screening for that agent as well (37). Initial screening tests for HIV-1 had only marginal ability to recognize the cross-reacting antibodies present in HIV-2–infected sera. However, newer ELISA tests directed at HIV-1 were able to pick up 90% of HIV-2 infections as well, and since 1991, blood screening tests in the United States have been able to identify both sets of antibodies inclusively (38).

2. *Injection: licit and illicit*. Reuse of injection apparatus also carries a high risk of HIV transmission. Dramatic outbreaks of HIV in nurseries in both the (former) Soviet Union and Romania (9) have underscored the hazard of reuse of unsterilized equipment in the health care setting, whereas IDUs who share needles and syringes have been infected thereby in great numbers in cities in many parts of the world. The east coast of the United States experienced that type of mass HIV infection phenomenon in the early years of the epidemic such that, by 1986, more than 50% of new AIDS cases in New York City occurred in IDUs or their sexual partners (39).

The potential for rapid spread within a drug-injecting population has been demonstrated repeatedly since then. Edinburgh, Bangkok, and numerous cities in Spain and Italy have sustained dramatic increases in numbers of HIV infections in drug-using populations within a few months, usually associated with addicts' difficulty in obtaining injection apparatus. Conversely, needle-exchange programs designed to make it possible for users to avoid contaminated needles have correlated closely with leveling off of HIV spread or actual decline of surrogate markers of blood-borne infection such as hepatitis B among addicted populations (40).

In recent years, the use of needle exchange as one facet of overall "harm-reduction" programs has gained wide acceptance (41). That access to sterile injection apparatus does not increase drug use is well established, and it also significantly decreases HIV transmission. Drug treatment programs, of course, are effective: even though addiction is a chronic, relapsing condition with the difficulty of "cure" characteristic of other chronic diseases, there is benefit to be gained during treatment intervals themselves. Clearly, much needs to be done to take full advantage of the harm-reduction interventions now documented to be effective in diminishing the potential scale of the HIV epidemic (42, 43).

Uninjected illicit drugs can also facilitate HIV spread: "crack" cocaine has been implicated as the vehicle whereby STDs in general and HIV in particular have been disseminated rapidly, particularly in adolescent populations through multiple sexual partners and use of sex as currency for drugs (44).

Injections of "licit" materials have also been suggested as a vehicle for HIV transmission. Early in the epidemic, international health workers noted that "injectionism" (the frequent use of needles as therapeutic interventions per se) or scarification rituals could play an important role in places where such activities were prevalent, inasmuch as sterilization was rarely part of such practices. Despite those early concerns, such customs have been only slightly implicated in actual HIV epidemic spread, in contrast to the more dominant modes of sexual transmission, blood infusion, and needle sharing during injecting drug use, which usually involves actual drawing of blood into the syringe before injection. Nevertheless, investigators strongly advise that such practices, including tattooing and ear-piercing procedures, be viewed as risky and conducted only in the context of careful sterilization procedures.

Birth to an Infected Mother

Early uncertainty about whether pediatric AIDS occurred was largely a consequence of the diagnostic difficulty that resulted from variability of HIV disease expression in children. Not until 1983 was severe illness from HIV fully accepted as a pediatric condition, and even then it was evident that manifestations were more various than in adults and required a different pediatric AIDS definition (45).

The situation was further confused by the finding that not all children born to HIV-infected mothers were themselves infected, even though all would test HIV positive for the first several months of life by prevalent antibody tests, because of transplacental transfer of maternal IgG antibody. With time, a clearer picture of maternal HIV transmission and of pediatric AIDS has emerged. The frequency of maternal-to-fetal transmission of HIV appears to be between 15 and 30%

of live births, with most infections occurring in the puerperium. In well-documented instances, the first, but not the second, of a pair of twins has been infected (46, 47). Earlier infection in utero seems to occur with a lesser frequency, and breast-feeding by an infected mother adds to cumulative risk for an infant.

As discussed elsewhere (see Chap. 12), a major advance in pediatric AIDS was the finding, in a study dubbed "076," that administration of oral zidovudine in the fourth quartile of pregnancy, intravenously during the puerperium, and then orally for 6 weeks to the newborn dropped the rate of HIV transmission from 25 to 8% of recipient infants. Studies continue to reinforce the findings of that initial trial (48–50), and some investigations are exploring variations on the 076 protocol, including different dosage strategies and possible use of combination therapies.

Breast-Feeding

The finding that breast-feeding by an HIV-infected mother enhances her offspring's risk of HIV infection is troubling, but it has been supported by numerous studies. The likelihood of HIV transmission appears to increase incrementally to nearly double the rate of perinatal infection, if the infant breast-feeds over a period of months (51). Those findings are sufficiently firm to justify the recommendation that HIV-infected mothers should not breast-feed their infants, under conditions of clean water and adequate alternative nutrition. However, unsafe water supplies and inanition can pose a much more likely and immediate hazard to an infant's life in many parts of the world, and where that is the case, breast-feeding should still be advised (52, 53).

SPECIAL ISSUES: PATIENTS AND HEALTH CARE WORKERS

The possibility that HIV could be transmitted in the health care setting has been a focus of intense concern since the onset of the epidemic. Although health care workers have been found to be infected, investigators have not suggested that different modes of transmission were involved. Indeed, the prevalence of HIV positivity among health care workers has regularly reflected that in the general population, and recognized risk behaviors (discussed earlier) have been associated with most of those infections. Indeed, despite the enormity of the pandemic of HIV spread, only about four dozen instances of patient-to-caregiver transmission were documented in the first decade (54); most of these resulted from substantial accidents involving significant parenteral exposure to HIV-infected bloody fluids.

Several approaches have been taken to assess the risk of health care workers' acquiring HIV from infected patients. Some of the most compelling approaches have taken advantage of the fact that hepatitis B, although spread by the same routes as HIV, is 30- to 100-fold more readily transmitted. Kuhls and associates (55) undertook studies in Los Angeles in which significant injury occurred to female health care workers caring for patients dually infected with HIV and either hepatitis B or herpes simplex. Among 246 such instances, hepatitis B seroconversion followed in 1 case and herpes simplex in 1 case, whereas no instance of HIV infection resulted (55).

Prospective studies have been carried out in the context of needlestick injuries involving patients known to be HIV infected. Such injured health care workers have been followed by the CDC, and the estimated likelihood of HIV infection resulting from such direct injury is 3 per 1000 (56).

The context of such injuries has also been analyzed, and recommendations have emerged that substantially lessen the likelihood of "sharps" accidents. These include double gloving in surgery, elimination of such risky procedures as needle capping, and careful provision for disposal of sharp instruments in health care settings (57). When serious needlestick accidents or other HIV exposures do occur in the health care workplace, policies and procedures have been developed to deal with them, as detailed elsewhere in this text (see Chap. 54).

The reverse issue, that of HIV transmission from infected health care worker to patient, was quiescent until 1990, although it was still a focus of ongoing attention. During the first several years of the epidemic, some retrospective studies had been conducted on patients who had been cared for by HIV-positive physicians after the possibility of HIV exposure came to light. In no instance was medical or surgical care implicated in HIV transmission. Then, in 1990, five patients in one dental practice in Florida were shown to be HIV infected with isolates that shared virtual molecular identity of the HIV strain infecting that dentist, who had already died of AIDS and whose records were incomplete. The initial presumption, that the dentist had bled into wounds during invasive oral procedures, led to intense concern and debate about HIV-infected health care workers (58, 59).

Subsequent analysis of the events in that practice, coupled with further extensive CDC retrospective studies of thousands of patients cared for by HIV-infected health care professionals (60), resulted in findings that underscore the singularity of the Florida cases. No other instance of transmission from health care worker to patient has been found or even suspected. That several patients (rather than just one) were so infected has suggested breaks in infection control procedures that seem to have characterized that unique dental practice; and analysis of experience with hepatitis B in health care settings since 1987 (when the CDC advised universal precautions as the appropriate safeguard against blood-borne pathogens in the health care workplace) has confirmed the efficacy of the universal precautions policy as an appropriate means of ensuring safety for both patient and provider in the context of health care (61).

PUBLIC HEALTH ROLES IN THE EPIDEMIC IN THE UNITED STATES

Prevention

The definitive knowledge that HIV transmission occurs solely through sex, blood injection, or birth to an infected mother has made it possible, from the earliest years of the epidemic, to intervene with strategies of prevention. Securing the safety of blood supplies, of paramount importance; was effectively accomplished in the United States by mid-1985. That success opened the way for reliance on education as a primary weapon of prevention, inasmuch as avoidance of risky behavior could ensure safety from HIV.

The importance of that fact cannot be overemphasized because avoidance of risk behaviors can ensure complete protection, whereas even the best vaccines we have against other microbial pathogens are only 98% (or less) protective. The tendency has been to "wait until the vaccine comes," especially when available educational strategies require open discussion of sensitive topics such as sex and illicit drug use; but vaccines will not supplant strategies that are currently available and whose efficacy is already demonstrable.

EDUCATION

Education of the population at every level is central to the future containment and control of the HIV pandemic. That educational effort must convey, first and foremost, what does and does not transmit HIV. In that context, programs to date have only been partially successful: American populations are generally aware that sex and drug use carry risk, but they continue to worry, distractingly, about more casual modes of transmission. Such misplaced concern not only diffuses the focus on behaviors that do convey risk, but it also fuels ongoing fear and resultant discrimination against people with HIV and AIDS. That discriminatory effect has a negative impact on public health strategies because it diminishes the likelihood that people will seek to know their HIV status.

Furthermore, even risk behaviors such as sex and drug use have been misperceived: the reiterative to homosexual sex and drug addiction conveys inadvertent reassurance that heterosexual intercourse or "recreational" drug use is not risky. Additionally, a common misperception is that, because education (as opposed, for instance, to vaccine) is simple and "low tech," it cannot be effective as a primary preventive strategy.

In fact, much has been learned during the first years of AIDS about health education that is broadly useful. First, the validity of the approach has been affirmed for HIV prevention in communities at special risk, where uncensored and explicit messages have been delivered repeatedly and by multiple means. Most dramatically, in longitudinal studies of several hundred men in San Francisco who were at high risk from homosexual sex, the annual incidence of new HIV infections dropped from 18% in 1982 to 0% 2 years later (62). Similar dramatic decreases in new HIV infections were observed in comparable communities in New York and other cities where defined communities of gay men could be reached. However, such success cannot be extrapolated directly to all men with same-sex orientation, inasmuch as many live "closeted" lives and are not reached by such openly formulated programs of education about "safer sex."

Subsequently, in those same populations where dramatic initial successes were achieved, the completeness of the prevention victory has been eroded; more recently, new infections have occurred at a rate of 1 to 3% per year. That number still represents an impressive decrement in HIV spread, but analysis of the "failures" is also enlightening. Some represent genuine "relapse," with a return to unsafe sexual practices (see later), whereas many—perhaps most—result from young men entering the homosexual population and rejecting warnings from older, established members of the community (63, 64), a vivid illustration of a generation gap.

Despite setbacks, however, considerable data attest to the potential efficacy of education as a major weapon against HIV spread. To be effective, however, prevention messages must be delivered clearly, reiteratively, and in the language of their intended listeners. Innovations such as teenage peer education, dramatic portrayal of AIDS messages, and popularization of AIDS issues (e.g., in "rap" songs and media portrayals) have shown considerable promise and deserve extensive pursuit as the epidemic moves relentlessly toward younger populations of people at risk, especially adolescents. In addition, focus on relationships, rather than on stark facts about transmission, adds to the effectiveness of intervention.

The central messages of AIDS educational programs need to include the facts that sex and injection drug use are risky behaviors and that abstinence is the only guarantee of safety, but thoughtful approaches to sexuality are of enormous importance and can reduce risk substantially for those who do not choose to be abstinent. In the latter context, reduction of numbers of sexual partners and avoidance of high-risk sexual practices (unprotected sex, anal intercourse) need to be emphasized, as does enhancement of HIV transmission in the presence of other STDs (65, 66).

The issue of concomitant HIV and other sexually transmitted infections has taken on increasing importance, not only because similar risk behavior sets the stage for both, but also because the likelihood of HIV transmission is enhanced as much as severalfold when common STDs are present as well. This finding has, in fact, led to promising efforts to achieve some degree of containment of HIV through vigorous (more affordable) treatment regimens aimed at eliminating treatable STDs, in areas of the world where antiviral therapy is economically infeasible.

CONDOMS AND BARRIER TECHNIQUES

The foregoing discussion delineates the broad fundamentals of a message designed to decrease risk of sexual transmission of HIV. "Unprotected sex" refers to the occurrence of sexual intercourse without prevention of "exchange of bodily fluids," that is, preejaculation or vaginal fluids or semen, or exposure to other sexually transmitted pathogens that can enhance the likelihood of HIV spread. The recommended mode of protection against such exchange or exposure is the use of condoms, specifically, latex condoms, with a nonoil-based lubricant. So-called "natural" condoms do not provide an effective barrier against HIV, and oil-based lubricants destroy the integrity of latex condoms.

The efficacy of condom usage in this context has been repeatedly questioned, inasmuch as their relative inefficiency as a means of pregnancy prevention is accepted by many as a truism. However, results of studies have shown that properly applied condoms used invariably during sexual intercourse have decreased HIV spread by at least ninefold, a major success in the face of such a threatening pathogen (68, 69). The earlier apparent failures of condoms may well be explained by lack of instruction in their proper usage throughout the act of intercourse or by inconstancy in their use over time. In any event, condom usage clearly plays a central role in so-called safer sex for those individuals who are not mutually monogamous.

A major drawback to this easily articulated public health recommendation has been that, in many cultures and circumstances, the proposal that condoms be used during intercourse is received with hostility by a sexual partner. In particular, women who have nondominant roles in a sexual relationship may invoke actual corporal, social, or economic punishment at such a suggestion; for this reason, many have urged that priority be given to finding barrier methods of HIV prevention that lend themselves to female control (70). The so-called "female condom" is an early version of such a device, but its relative expense and reported awkwardness argue for further intensive effort in this regard. Similarly, efforts are intensifying to expand the repertoire of vaginal microbicides, which would further empower women in sexual situations (71).

DRUG TREATMENT AND NEEDLE ISSUES

The remarkable efficiency of HIV spread through needle sharing has been demonstrated repeatedly around the world in the context of illicit drug use (see Chap. 13). Although even recreational injecting drug use carries that risk, those who are addicted are clearly at enormous, repeated risk of infection; and with them, their sexual partners and offspring become exposed to HIV, with further amplification of the virus pool in the population. Thus, it is a matter of urgent public health priority that such spread be aborted.

The most obvious means to accomplish that end is to remove IDUs from the path of the virus, preferably by effective treatment for their addiction, which, in turn, eliminates the risk of exposure through sharing of injection apparatus. Treatment for addiction, although clearly suboptimal in its success rate, can be accomplished effectively for a substantial plurality of IDUs; for heroin addicts, methadone maintenance can effectively eliminate HIV from the clinical picture. Thus, the availability of drug treatment on demand for addicted IDUs has been the highest-priority recommendation of virtually every public healthy advisory group that has made recommendations concerning HIV policy (72–74). Unfortunately, in the United States, as of this writing, long waiting lists for treatment exist in every major city for poor, addicted people.

Even if national policies were revised to accommodate for drug treatment programs on a much broader scale, such changes would take time to put in place. Although such treatment options and resources are being contemplated or deployed, the HIV threat is ever present. For that reason, strategies of needle exchange have been devised and implemented in other parts of the world and in a growing number of cities in the United States. In such programs, addicted people can be assured of exchanging used for sterile injection apparatus at convenient locales and without fear of immediate reprisal. In no instance has such a civic policy led to increased drug use, as was warned by opponents (75), and HIV spread has been diminished thereby in some places (76). When needle exchange cannot be implemented, investigators have suggested that careful instruction on the use of bleach to clean injection apparatus can be moderately effective and well received by IDUs, although the "harm-reduction" effect is far less certain that that of needle-exchange interventions.

Such interventions in the difficult context of intravenous drug use and addiction must be given the highest priority in any public health program to contain HIV. However, their implementation is likely to have several predictable effects besides HIV containment, effects that should be planned for in an overall prevention program targeted to IDUs. First, many addicted people have no access to health care of any kind, and simple intervention concerning HIV quickly invokes a latent need for primary health care. Second, investigators have observed almost routinely that changes in injection risk taking are much easier to accomplish than are changes in sexual risk taking in IDU populations. Well-designed public health interventions must encompass both categories of risk behavior to achieve an optimal effect (77).

TESTING AND SCREENING AS METHODS OF PREVENTION

Since the advent of the capacity to identify HIV-infected persons by laboratory testing techniques in 1985, the call to use the HIV test as a primary means of HIV prevention has been persistent. There is nothing inherently wrong with that suggestion, except it usually refers solely or predominately to the *testing*, whereas counseling is omitted or undervalued.

In the absence of counseling, serious distortions can occur in the overall usefulness of this approach to prevention. First, those who test positive may fail to appreciate the significance of that fact or to know how to protect others from their HIV infection (see later). In most public health programs, those pitfalls have been recognized and dealt with, so persons with a positive test result are indeed counseled and followed.

Negative tests may not be dealt with so intelligently, however. An underinformed person who has sought testing because of self-perceived risk behavior may interpret a negative test as a sign that he or she is some way immune to HIV and thus may resume risky practices with a false sense of impugnity.

One of the major impediments to the effective deployment of counseling and testing in the context of HIV control is the logistics of its availability. In the context of public care, scant resources have sometimes made access difficult: testing centers are often located in worrisome areas of cities, waiting lists are long, and obtaining results can involve daunting difficulties. All these features of the public health response to the epidemic are susceptible to improvement (77).

Responding to the apparent opportunity to increase testing by easing access, pharmaceutical companies have created home test kits that enable a concerned person to send a dried blood sample by mail for HIV antibody testing. In the initial versions of such kits, care was given to providing results in the context of telephone counseling. Versions now under development propose to substitute saliva for blood and even to omit the obligatory counseling step. Such shortcuts are worrisome for the same reason noted earlier: counseling is central to the effective use of HIV testing in a clinical or public health program of epidemic control.

More problematic still is the perceived use of test results. Mandatory testing has been rejected by every major public health advisory group that has considered it, on the grounds that the coercion in the testing policy would drive people at greatest risk "underground" and thus would be counterproductive. That dynamic pertains as well to test results, however. In the continuing, discriminatory climate that surrounds the HIV/AIDS epidemic in the United States, even the perception that one could be at risk of HIV infection has resulted in loss of life and health insurance, jobs, apartment leases, and even friendships and family support. Thus, the importance of access to confidential or anonymous counseling and testing resources remains critically important in this facet of prevention (78).

One special instance of testing that threatens to become mandatory is that of pregnant women. With the advent of the encouraging findings from the 076 study of zidovudine use in late pregnancy, legislative calls for mandating HIV testing during pregnancy became louder. Some states that had already mandated blinded cord blood screening of newborns proposed to "unblind" the results and mandate notification of seropositive women concerning their HIV status. These issues are evolving, but clearly they must be guided at least in part by access to treatment and care, which is often problematic for such women.

BLOOD SUPPLY ISSUES

The urgency of blood supply protection is addressed earlier. In brief, present policies have established greater safety in the blood supply of the United States from all known blood-borne pathogens than has ever been the case before, and the risk from HIV-1 and HIV-2 has been reduced close to zero. Although over 12,000,000 units of blood and blood products are administered each year in the United States, the range of risk from HIV is estimated to be about 2 per million units transfused (29, 79). Because transfusion is a procedure used when its absence would be life threatening, those risks are extremely low compared with the risks inherent in the medical conditions necessitating the use of blood.

This point is important, because the principle of avoidance of risk pertains equally to this context as it does to the behavioral risks of sex and injection. All efforts to reduce the use of blood in clinical therapeutics are desirable, as is the practice of autoinfusion—donation of one's own blood for future use when possible. Blood donation carries no risk at all, inasmuch as careful sterilization procedures pervade the blood banking protocols. However, that fact is still lost on a worrisomely high number of potential donors who shun blood centers for fear of HIV. With these points in mind, achievement of the present level of safety of the blood supply in the United States and other developed nations so quickly after the recognition of AIDS and (subsequently) HIV represents an impressive scientific and public health accomplishment.

Early Intervention and Care

The capacity of health professionals to intervene in the context of established HIV infection was limited in the early years of the epidemic. However, as discussed elsewhere in this text (see Chap. 48), systemic studies have established the efficacy of several clinical interventions in delaying the onset of disabling HIV disease and AIDS, especially if these interventions are instituted before the onset of overt, diagnostic illness. This general set of approaches is referred to as early intervention, and because early recognition of HIV infection is prerequisite to such intervention, several issues of public health policy arise.

With the advent of combination antiviral therapy, the rationale for early initiation of treatment to diminish viral load has gained new support. The timing of such active intervention is discussed elsewhere (see Chap. 48), but other facets of care and prevention of further spread remain as central as before to the concept of early intervention.

SCREENING, COUNSELING, AND TESTING

Many issues involved in counseling and testing are discussed earlier in this chapter. They provide part of the substance of the ongoing screening debate in public health: how widely and how routinely should screening for HIV be done, in what populations, and with what goals in mind? Such discussions are often carried out as if cost were not an issue. However, the dynamic nature of the epidemic means that any one effort at widespread screening of large populations would become dated quickly (in the absence of other effective public health measures such as education), and the costs are far from trivial. For instance, the call for testing health care workers in 1991, in the wake of the singular dentist transmission events, prompted an analysis by Gerberding, who found that HIV testing of health care workers and their patients in the context of seriously invasive procedures at one 350-bed hospital in San Francisco would cost an estimated $860,000 in the first year alone (80).

In the context of a private practice or managed-care setting, these issues can be resolved readily; and a good case can be made for offering HIV testing regularly, as part of overall health assessment, to sexually active adults and others who perceive themselves to be at special risk. Physicians who undertake such a policy of preventive care should, of course, be in a position to provide counseling about risk avoidance as well. However, to view HIV testing as routine even in such favorable circumstances is unwise. The law requires that a person's consent be obtained before HIV testing (exceptions in hospitals generally involve unusual life-or-death circumstances), and failure to gain that consent in advance and to provide pretest counseling sets the stage for great clinical difficulties if results of an unannounced test are positive.

In the context of such private care, a person who tests HIV positive can be the beneficiary of the many facets of early intervention: good maintenance of general health and nutrition, intermittent assessment of immunologic status through CD4+ testing, and institution of antiinfective therapies to prevent *Pneumocystis carinii* pneumonia and to treat aggressively those early manifestations of HIV disease such as candidiasis or herpes simplex that could otherwise progress to debilitating levels before recognition. Institution of antiretroviral therapies directed at HIV can be guided by careful follow-up, and, of course, ongoing counseling can be implemented to help such a person adjust to the facts of living with HIV and to protect loved ones from risk.

In the context of public care, at least in the United States at present, many of these positive outcomes of HIV diagnosis are unavailable. Even mandated access to such HIV-specific programs as CD4+ testing or zidovudine availability may be of limited or no value to an HIV-infected person if the programs are discontinuous or if primary care is not available as well.

The reemergence of tuberculosis in the United States in the late 1980s reflects the importance of many of these points. Tuberculosis gained much of its amplified territory from the undue susceptibility of HIV-infected people (81), including prisoners, whose numbers had increased dramatically over the preceding decade by mandatory drug-sentencing laws in many states, resulting in crowding far beyond initial prison design. The spread of tuberculosis in such circumstances was an obvious threat, but the failure to provide care in the prisons in many places, or continuity of care after release in others, helped to escalate the tuberculosis epidemic. Furthermore, failure to provide for follow-up of such prisoners after release, to ensure compliance with antitubercular regimens, accelerated the development of multidrug-resistant tuberculosis with its frightening potential for further dissemination (81, 82).

In summary, early intervention is a major opportunity in the HIV epidemic, both for individual care and for public health strategies of curtailment of further viral spread. However, failure to implement it through lack of access or discontinuity of intervention strategies often makes it worse than irrelevant for those whose social and medical circumstances put them outside the private health care system (83).

PARTNER NOTIFICATION

In addition to identification of persons who are themselves infected, the traditional public health approach to STDs has included contact tracing or, in more recent parlance, partner notification. This practice evolved in the context of syphilis and gonorrhea, wherein the interval between infection and illness on the part of the identified, infected person was short and wherein the likelihood of real infectious risk to the exposed sexual partners after even a single sexual contact was high. In the aggregate, neither of these conditions pertains in the HIV epidemic: the interval between infection and disease can be many years, and the likelihood of transmission per infectious act has been estimated to be as low as 1/1000 acts of sexual intercourse (84). Thus the cost-effectiveness of extensive efforts at partner notification deserves careful assessment in the context of competing public health needs.

In considering partner notification as a public health strategy, a clear distinction between public and individual health must be drawn. Little or no question exists that partner notification is an important goal in complete medical and health care of an individual known to be infected with HIV. Whether that pursuit of potentially infected sexual (or drug-using) contacts should be conducted by the index case, the private physician, or other health care workers is often best determined in the context of individual personal and social circumstances. Such pursuit should be done in the context of accessible counseling and testing for those contacted, inasmuch as the likelihood of actual HIV transmission is so widely variable and the induced fear inherent in such a pursuit is sure to be disruptive. Thus, in the context of individual medical practice, maximal flexibility must be available to those deciding how to contact past partners.

The public health practice of contact tracing raises issues beyond those involved in individual health care. In particular, it is personnel intensive and therefore expensive, and so its role in the present epidemic is problematic when evaluated in competition with other public health budget categories such as making the voluntary counseling and testing options discussed earlier more accessible. Indeed, in assessing the overall role of partner notification as a public health strategy for HIV control, the WHO concluded (in part) as follows:

Partner notification programmes should be considered, but within the context of a comprehensive AIDS prevention and control programme.... Partner notification has potential benefits and risks, including the potential to help prevent HIV transmission and reduce the morbidity and mortality of HIV infection but also the potential to produce individual and social harm and detract from other AIDS prevention and control activities.... (85)

To illustrate the point, it may be a prudent use of public health budgeted funds to support partner notification activities in a state where only a few dozen instances of known HIV infection existed. By contrast, it would be a poor diversion of resources in a community in which HIV seroprevalence rates were already at or higher than 20%. The point is (for circumstances between those two extremes) that partner notification must be weighed and evaluated as one of many possible public health strategies.

In making such a choice, the positive factors are obvious: persons so notified, who had been unaware that they had been placed at risk of HIV, can seek to know their status and can respond accordingly. This allows them to learn about HIV with the goal of avoidance of further risk, if the test result is negative, or early intervention and care, if indeed they prove to be infected. The negatives must be kept in mind, however; the "underground effect," referred to earlier, it is a regular force in the HIV/AIDS epidemic, and coercive partner notification is clearly a threat that enhances it. Furthermore, anonymity of sexual partners was a contributor to the initial HIV explosion in some high-risk communities, and enforced partner notification could readily result in the resumption of such grossly unsafe practices.

CONTINUUM OF CARE OPTIONS

Although health care policy and management are considered to comprise a separate and complex field, they are often subsumed in discussions of public health aspects of the epidemic, and brief comments are therefore warranted here. Specifically, the cost of caring for persons with HIV/AIDS has been an alarming aspect of the epidemic from the onset. Early estimates set the lifetime price (before the advent of antiviral drugs) of care for an individual patient with AIDS at well over $100,000 (86); and initial pricing of pharmaceuticals developed for people with HIV/AIDS threatened to escalate that exorbitant cost still further. Recent success with combination therapies, including at least one protease inhibitor among three antivirals administered together, has had included promising effects on the viral load and immunologic status of many patients. However, the cost of such therapy is estimated to be at least $10,000 per year in antiretroviral drugs alone, and some clinicians propose that this treatment be initiated when CD4+ cells drop below $500/mm^3$, if not earlier still. Thus, major shifts in overall cost of care can be expected. Whether the decline in hospitalizations is sufficient to make up for the cost of maintenance therapy in the outpatient setting remains to be seen. What would constitute a duration of treatment sufficient to result in permanent HIV suppression is unclear.

Issues Arising from Demographic Features of the Epidemic

The preponderance of the HIV epidemic's impact has been leveled against young adult populations, and increasingly it is moving to younger and younger age groups. Certain particularly difficult facets of the overall disruption reflect these demographic facts, associated as they are with insecure employment status, paucity or lack of health insurance protection, and other facets of juniority in society in the United States. These trends have significant impact on both public health and medical responses to the epidemic and are therefore be addressed briefly here.

HOUSING

Experts who study issues of housing and homelessness in the United States caution, as a guidepost, that when 50% or more of personal income is devoted to housing cost, homelessness is imminent. This dynamic has been played out relentlessly in the AIDS epidemic. Illness or lack of stamina progressively interferes with employment, part-time or lower-paying substitute employment follows, and in due course the ability to maintain a mortgage payment or lease is compromised. The result has been homelessness for many people living with AIDS. Estimates suggest that the ranks of the homeless have been increased by 10 to 20% in many large American cities, and the same pressures toward loss of domicile pertain in smaller communities and rural areas as well. This consideration is not peripheral to the issues of health, because even minor illness in a homeless and therefore dependent person may lead to hospitalization; and many municipalities have instituted well-meaning regulations that persons with AIDS may not be discharged without a domicile. Thus, efforts to create communal or supportive housing are intergral and important aspects of an HIV care strategy; and government supports for maintenance of housing of people with HIV/AIDS can have a cost-effective result in terms of health care as well as quality of life (87–89).

DISCRIMINATION

The unreasoning fear of people with HIV/AIDS among the undereducated public has led to discriminatory phenomena that have intensified the problems of caring for and coping with large numbers of seriously ill young adults. This dynamic has contributed to eviction and therefore the homelessness cited earlier, but more broadly, it has involved almost all facets of life including employment, insurance, and health care (both giving and receiving). The discriminatory dynamic was intense in 1990 when the Americans with Disabilities Act was considered and ultimately was passed by Congress and signed into law by the president, effective the summer of 1992. That act makes it a violation of federal law to discriminate against, among others, persons with disabilities resulting from either HIV infection or *perception of their risk of HIV infection*. The latter provision was necessitated by the serious discriminatory effects encountered even by loved ones, family members, and friends of people caught in the path of the HIV epidemic.

It is important to realize that such a federal law exists, but it is even more important to understand that discrimination will continue to play a significant, and sometimes determinant, role in health care and public health policies until the federal intent is enforced at the community level and is empowered by state and local legislation. Reliance on federal legal protection per se is a time-consuming and costly recourse available almost solely to sophisticated and knowledgeable members of society who are not the most likely to experience the effects of discrimination.

In the health care setting, the threat of discrimination has menaced even the availability of health care. In the wake of the revelations of the Florida dentist case (90) (see earlier), widespread anxiety prompted the demand that all HIV-infected health care workers reveal their status to persons potentially under their care. For a while, such a current of popular opinion held sway despite the total lack of evidence of HIV transmission from health care worker to patient in hospitals, clinics, or any other setting except for that unique cluster of cases in a single dental practice.

Happily, as in an earlier analog in which parents demanded separation of their offspring from HIV-infected children in schools, panic eased, and the CDC ultimately published guidelines that created expert advisory panels (locally based) to judge whether a rare risk of HIV transmission could exist in a given circumstance, considering not only kinds of procedures but skills of the professional in question. Thus, the nation, and much of the world that tends to follow the lead of the United States in such matters, was saved the needless and discriminatory exile of talented health care professionals from their vitally needed practice of skills (91). Such discriminatory tides of public opinion are remarkably strong and are likely to arise in other contexts before they recede entirely in the face of well-informed reason.

PRISONS

Throughout the world, the health care of incarcerated people is marginal or problematic. In the United States, that was strikingly the case even before the AIDS epidemic. Unhappily, the advent of HIV and AIDS coincided with a national war on drugs that was fought primarily through interdiction efforts at the borders coupled with mandatory sentencing laws for persons convicted of drug-related offenses. Because drug users were at special risk of HIV infection, those combined policies had the effect of focusing a crucial part of the HIV epidemic in prisons.

That result could have brought to potential intervention the gain of access to the most difficult part of the population. Concentration of people at risk is so dramatic that, in the early 1990s, as many as 14% of men and women in New York State prisons, for instance, were found to be seropositive for HIV (92). With mandatory sentencing for drug-related crimes crowding the prisons with people at high HIV risk, that figure may be even higher.

However, this major public health opportunity for intervention has thus far been lost, because most prison health care has remained rudimentary for lack of funding. As discussed earlier, the result has been failure to take advantage of the potential access to such difficult populations to initiate care for and to educate large numbers of people with HIV, to protect their sexual partners and offspring, and to establish continuity of care with community health centers and other agencies on their release from prison. Worse, the crowding, discontinuity of interventions, and HIV prevalence combined synergistically to create conditions conducive to a fresh tuberculosis epidemic that, in its worst dimension, includes multidrug-resistant tuberculosis. The issue of prison health, long viewed as eccentric or at least peripheral to issues of public health, should occupy a central place in discussions of containment of three threatening epidemics: HIV/AIDS, drugs, and tuberculosis (93).

RURAL HEALTH CARE

In close analogy to the discussions of prison health care, simmering issues of inadequate rural health care have been intensified by HIV/AIDS. Two key factors have contributed to that effect: first, the misperception on the part of rural populations that HIV/AIDS was a phenomenon of large urban centers and therefore of no relevance to them; and second (as a direct result), the belief that no planning need take place concerning their strategies to care for people with HIV disease. The result has been that small, rural hospitals have often been caught by surprise by a single AIDS case and have reacted unknowledgeably with unnecessarily prolonged hospitalization or excessive isolation procedures that have exhausted contingency funds and have threatened their very survival as health care institutions. Much unnecessary hospitalization can be avoided by planning and constructing options that offer a continuum of care. Nowhere has the failure to do so exacted a higher cost than in rural hospitals.

HIV/AIDS as a Sexually Transmitted Disease

The point is made repeatedly in this chapter that much HIV transmission follows the pattern of an STD, and indeed much of the cumulative experience of STD control in public health is pertinent to problems posed by AIDS. However, that generalization has its limitations in guiding public health response, because STD control programs have been of variable quality and suboptimal efficacy in many areas. Briefly, two points are worth noting about using the STD model as the dominant approach to HIV. First, many of the features of HIV infection, notably its extremely long asymptomatic interval and relative inefficiency of transmission, raise serious issues about the cost-effectiveness of traditional STD approaches, notably contact tracing. Second, HIV is now so widely disseminated in populations that do not identify with STD patterns of risk that the awareness of the universality of HIV as a threat to young people could be lost if the standard approach is pursued predominately through STD clinics. From STD programs that have been administered particularly well and effectively much can be learned and joint public health initiatives can be undertaken. Indeed, the synergistic effect of other STDs on HIV transmission dictates that STDs be given a high level of attention in their own right. However, subsuming of HIV/AIDS under the rubric of STD programs has hazards that should be weighed carefully.

IMMIGRATION AND TRAVEL

One issue that has proved difficult and distracting in the HIV epidemic has been that of proposed restrictions on travel and immigration for people with HIV/AIDS. That matter was addressed carefully in 1987 by the Global Programme on AIDS of the World Health Organization, as summarized by von Reyn and colleagues (94). In general, travel restrictions are costly in both human and economic terms, and they discriminate without justification. Issues of immigration relate sufficiently closely to broader economic and health care issues that they are not addressed here, except to note that AIDS presents approximately the same problem as do other chronic diseases such as severe diabetes or heart disease and thus should be considered equitably in a broader context. On the other hand, the issue of international travel is much more important to understand, given that the restriction of free movement across international borders of individuals because they are HIV infected not only infringes on their human rights without justification, but it also sends a false message to the public, by suggesting that these people pose a threat. The appropriate protection of a national population is education for avoidance of risk behavior. Limitation of travel contributes nothing to such protection and may lead to public misapprehension of the source of risk.

AIDS IN THE DEVELOPING WORLD: SIMILARITIES AND DIFFERENCES

This chapter focuses on the HIV/AIDS epidemic as it relates to public health in the United States. Much of the commentary pertains also to other developed nations, where resource constraints are not (or need not be) necessarily determinants of policy. The special problems presented by difficulties of health care access and financing in the United States are less generally applicable. Space does not permit a broad discussion of public health issues raised by HIV and AIDS in the developing world. Those topics are explored thoroughly in *AIDS in the World II* (9). Nonetheless, a few comments are needed to alert the reader to sharp differences arising from extreme resource limitations in many countries hard hit by HIV.

First, most of the discussion of public health programs and priorities has been predicated on the assumption that bloodborne dissemination of HIV is under control. That is still not true in many places; even though screening test costs have been sharply reduced, they may still approximate the annual per capita investment in total health care in many developing nations. The securement of the blood supply must occupy the highest priority everywhere; and where resources are limited, efforts to curtail the conditions that lead to blood usage must be intensified (e.g., prevention of iron deficiency anemia of pregnancy, which could otherwise make transfusion mandatory in the peripartum period).

Second, those familiar with the general underfunding of public health programs and the burden of other "competing" diseases in many countries recognize that AIDS could overwhelm existing systems. It is an important point of caution; AIDS and HIV threaten many populations so severely that a net negative impact on population growth is forecast, so a response must be undertaken to curtail further HIV spread. Nonetheless, this can be done in ways that support or even build the infrastructure of overall public health if careful attention is given to the modes of response. For this reason, among many, resorting to extensive general screening of populations can be particularly destructive, because it is time and disease specific and tends to divert health personnel from more broadly applicable initiatives such as health education.

Third, it is important to recognize the global nature of the HIV/AIDS epidemic, including the need for the development of drugs and vaccines that are accessible to rich and poor nations alike. In the past, little thought was given to making technologic and scientific developments available to all, but with the worldwide dynamics of this pandemic, that issue must be readdressed. Countries in sub-Sarahan Africa or Asia may well prove suitable venues for vaccine trials, but they must then be in a position to share in the products of such trials, and their people must have access to current standards of care to justify ethically the interposition of vaccine protocols.

References

1. United States Congress, Office of Technology Assessment. The CDC's case definition of AIDS: implications of the proposed revisions-background paper, OTA-BP-H-89. Washington, DC: US Government Printing Office, 1992.
2. Centers for Disease Control. Revision of the case definition of acquired immunodeficiency syndrome for national reporting: United States. Ann Intern Med 1985;103:402–403.
3. Centers for Disease Control. Revision of the CDC surveillance case definition for acquired immunodeficiency syndrome. MMWR Morb Mortal Wkly Rep 1987;36:1–15.
4. Centers for Disease Control. 1993 revised classification system for HIV infection and expanded surveillance case definition for AIDS among adolescents and adults. MMWR Morb Mortal Wkly Rep 1992;41:961–962.
5. Osborn JE. The changing definition of AIDS. What's in a name? J Am Health Pol 1991;1:19–22.
6. Buehler JW. The surveillance definition of AIDS. Am J Public Health 1992;82:1462–1464.
7. Des Jarlais DC, Wenston J, Friedman SR, et al. Implications of the revised surveillance definition: AIDS among New York City drug users. Am J Public Health 1992;82:1531–1533.
8. Mann JM. The global picture of AIDS. J Acquir Immune Defic Syndr 1988;1:209–216.
9. Mann JM, Tarantola D, eds. AIDS in the world. II. The Global AIDS Policy Coalition. Oxford: Oxford University Press, 1996.
10. Mann JM. AIDS—the second decade: a global perspective. J Infect Dis 1992;165:245–250.
11. Caldwell MB, Rogers MF. Epidemiology of pediatric HIV infection. Pediatr Clin North Am 1991;38:1–16.
12. Friedland GH, Saltzman BR, Rogers MF, et al. Lack of transmission of HTLV-III/LAV infection to household contacts of patients with AIDS or AIDS-related complex with oral candidiasis. N Engl J Med 1986;314:344–349.
13. Friedland G, Kahl P, Saltzman B, et al. Additional evidence for lack of transmission of HIV infection by close interpersonal (casual) contact. AIDS 1990;4:639–644.
14. Castro KG, Lifson AR, White CR, et al. Investigations of AIDS patients with no previously identified risk factors. JAMA 1988;259:1338–1342.
15. Ginzberg HM, Fleming PL, Miller KD. Selected public health observations derived from the multicenter AIDS cohort study. J Acquir Immune Defic Syndr 1988;1:2–7.
16. Royce RA, Sena A, Cates W Jr, et al. Sexual transmission of HIV. N Engl J Med 1977;336:1072–1078.
17. Neal JJ, Fleming PL, Green TA, et al. Trends in heterosexually acquired AIDS in the United States, 1988 through 1995. J Acquir Immune Defic Syndr Hum Retrovirol 1997;14:465–474.
18. Padian NS, Shiboski SC, Jewell NP. Female-to-male transmission of human immunodeficiency virus. JAMA 1991;266:1664–1667.

19. Redfield RR, Burke DS Shadow on the land: the epidemiology of HIV infection. Viral Immunol 1987;1:69–81.
20. Palenicek J, Fox R, Margolick J, et al. Longitudinal study of homosexual couples discordant for HIV-1 antibodies in the Baltimore MACS study. J Acquir Immune Def Syndr 1992;5:1204–1211.
21. Huang Y, Paxton WA, Wolinsky SM, et al. The role of a mutant CCR5 allele in HIV-1 transmission and disease progression. Nat Med 1996; 2:1240–1243.
22. Clumeck N, Taelma H, Hermans P, et al. A cluster of HIV infection among heterosexual people without apparent risk factors. N Engl J Med 1989;321:1460–1462.
23. Padian NS, Shiboski SC, Jewell NP. The effect of number of exposures on the risk of heterosexual HIV transmission. J Infect Dis 1990;161: 883–887.
24. Keet IPM, van Lent NA, Sandfort TGM, et al. Orogenital sex and the transmission of HIV among homosexual men. AIDS 1992;6:223–226.
25. Lifson AR, O'Malley PM, Hessol NA, et al. HIV seroconversion in two homosexual men after receptive oral intercourse with ejaculation: implications for counseling concerning safe sex practices. Am J Public Health 1990;80:1509–1511.
26. Mayor KH, DeGruttola V. Human immunodeficiency virus and oral intercourse. Ann Intern Med 1987;107:428–429.
27. Dicker BG. Risk of AIDS among lesbians. Am J Public Health 1989;79:1569.
28. Centers for Disease Control. Human immunodeficiency virus infection in transfusion recipients and their family members. MMWR Morb Mortal Wkly Rep 1987;36:137–140.
29. Williams AE, Thomson RA, Schreiber GB, et al. Estimates of infectious disease risk factors in U.S. blood donors. JAMA 1997;277:967–972.
30. Sloand EM, Pitt E, Chiarello RJ, et al. HIV testing: state of the art. JAMA 1991;266:2861–2866.
31. Cuthbertson B, Perry RJ, Foster PR, et al. The viral safety of intravenous immunoglobulin. J Infect Dis 1987;15:125–133.
32. Centers for Disease Control. Safety of therapeutic immune globulin preparations with respect to transmission of human T-lymphotrophic virus type III/lymphadenopathy–associated virus infection. MMWR Morb Mortal Wkly Rep 1986;5:231–233.
33. Johnson RE, Lawrence DN, Evatt BL, et al. Acquired immunodeficiency syndrome among patients attending hemophilia treatment centers and mortality experience of hemophiliacs in the United States. Am J Epidemiol 1985;121:797–810.
34. Schimpf K, Brackmann HH, Kreuz W, et al. I. Absence of anti-human immunodeficiency virus types 1 and 2 seroconversion after the treatment of hemophilia A or Von Willebrand's disease with pasteurized factor VIII concentrate. N Engl J Med 1989;321:1148–1152.
35. Hilgartner MW. AIDS and hemophilia. N Engl J Med 1987;317:1153–1154.
36. Schwartz RS, Abildgaard CF, Aleadort LM, et al. Human recombinant DNA–derived antihemophilic factor (factor VIII) in the treatment of hemophilia A. N Engl J Med 1990;323:1800–1805.
37. O'Brien TR, George JR, Holmberg SD. Human immunodeficiency virus type 2 infection in the United States: epidemiology, diagnosis, and public health implications. JAMA 1992;267:2775–2779.
38. Centers for Disease Control. Testing for antibodies to human immunodeficiency virus type 2 in the United States. MMWR Morb Mortal Wkly Rep 1992;41:1–9.
39. Des Jarlais DC, Friedman SR. AIDS and IV drug use. Science 1989;245:578.
40. Hagan H, Reid T, Des Jarlais DC, et al. The incidence of HBV infection and syringe exchange programs. JAMA 1991;266:1646–1647.
41. Gostin LO, Lazzarini Z, Jones TS, et al. Prevention of HIV/AIDS and other blood-borne diseases among injection drug users: a national survey on the regulation of syringes and needles. JAMA 1997;277:53–62.
42. Des Jarlais DC, Friedman P, Hagan H, et al. The protective effect of AIDS-related behavioral change among injection drug users: a cross-national study. Am J Public Health 1996;86:1780–1785.
43. Osborn JE. Editorial:drug use and behavior change. Am J Public Health 1996;86:1698–1699.
44. Chiasson MA, Stoneburner RL, Hilderandt DS, et al. Heterosexual transmission of HIV-1 associated with the use of smokable freebase cocaine (crack). AIDS 1991;5:1121–1126.
45. Pitt J, Brambilla D, Reichelderfer P, et al. Maternal immunologic and virologic risk factors for infant human immunodeficiency virus type 1 infection: findings from the Women and Infants Transmission Study. J Infect Dis 1997;175:567–575.
46. Palca J. HIV risk higher for first-born twins. Science 1991;254:1729.
47. Task Force on Pediatric AIDS. Perinatal human immunodeficiency virus (HIV) testing. Pediatrics 1992;89:791–794.
48. Condor EM, Sperling RS, Gelber R, et al. Reduction of maternal–infant transmission of human immunodeficiency virus type 1 with zidovudine treatment. N Engl J Med 1994;331:1173–1180.
49. Cooper ER, Nugent RP, Diaz C, et al. After AIDS Clinical Trial 076: the changing pattern of zidovudine use during pregnancy, and the subsequent reduction in the vertical transmission of human immunodeficiency virus in a cohort of infected women and their infants. J Infect Dis 1996;174:1207–1211.
50. Sperling RS, Shapiro DE, Coombs RW, et al. Maternal viral load, zidovudine treatment, and the risk of transmission of human immunodeficiency virus type 1 from mother to infant. N Engl J Med 1996:335: 1621–1629.
51. Guay LA, Hom DL, Mmiro F, et al. Detection of human immunodeficiency virus type 1 (HIV-1) DNA and p24 antigen in breast milk of HIV-1 infected Ugandan women and vertical transmission. Pediatrics 1996;98:438–444.
52. Martino M, Tovo P-A, Tozzi AE, et al. HIV-1 transmission through breast-milk: appraisal of risk according to duration of feeding. AIDS 1992;6:991–997.
53. Dunn DT, Newell ML, Ades AE, et al. Risk of human immunodeficiency virus type 1 transmission through breastfeeding. Lancet 1992; 340:585–588.
54. Chamberland ME, Conley LJ, Bush TJ, et al. Health care workers with AIDS: national surveillance update. JAMA 1991;266:3459–3462.
55. Kuhls TL, Viker S, Parris NB, et al. Occupational risk of HIV, HBV, and HSV-2 infections in health care personnel caring for AIDS patients. Am J Public Health 1987;77:1306–1309.
56. Miike L, Ostrowsky J. HIV in the health care workplace. Background paper 7. Washington, DC: Office of Technology Assessment, 1991.
57. Gerberding JL. Surgery and AIDS: reducing the risk. JAMA 1991;265: 1572–1573.
58. Ciesielski C, Marianos D, Ou C-Y, et al. Transmission of human immunodeficiency virus in a dental practice. Ann Intern Med 1992; 116:798–805.
59. Ou C-Y, Ciesielski CA, Myers G, et al. Molecular epidemiology of HIV transmission in a dental practice. Science 1992;256:1165–1171.
60. Centers for Disease Control. Update: investigations of patients who have been treated by HIV-infected health-care workers. MMWR Morb Mortal Wkly Rep 1992;41:345–346.
61. Rogers DE, Gellin BG. The bright spot about AIDS: it is very tough to catch. AIDS 1990;4:695–696.
62. Winkelstein W, Samuel M, Padian NS, et al. The San Francisco Men's Health Study. III. Reduction in human immunodeficiency virus transmission among homosexual/bisexual men, 1982–86. Am J Public Health 1987;76:685–689.
63. Stall R, Barrett D, Bye L, et al. A comparison of younger and older gay men's HIV risk-taking behaviors: the communication technologies 1989 cross-sectional survey. J Acquir Immune Defic Syndr 1992;5: 682–687.
64. Stall R, Ekstrand M, Pollack L, et al. Relapse from safer sex: the next challenge for AIDS prevention efforts. J Acquir Immune Defic Syndr 1990:3:1181–1187.
65. Cates W, Hinman AR. Sexually transmitted diseases in the 1990s. N Engl J Med 1991;325:1368–1370.

66. Quinn TC, Groseclose SL, Spence M, et al. Evolution of the human immunodeficiency virus epidemic among patients attending sexually transmitted disease clinics: a decade of experience. J Infect Dis 1992; 165:541–544.
67. Reference deleted.
68. Kamenga M, Ryder RW, Jingu M, et al. Evidence of marked sexual behavior change associated with low HIV-1 seroconversion in 149 married couples with discordant HIV-1 serostatus: experience at an HIV counseling center in Zaire. AIDS 1991;5:61–67.
69. Cates W, Stewart FH, Trussell J. Commentary:the quest for women's prophylactic methods: hopes vs science. Am J Public Health 1992;82: 1479–1482.
70. Rosenberg MJ, Davidson AJ, Chen J-H, et al. Barrier contraceptives and sexually transmitted diseases in women:a comparison of female-dependent methods and condoms. Am J Public Health 1992;82:669–674.
71. Pauwels R, De Clercq E. Development of vaginal microbicides for the prevention of heterosexual transmission of HIV. J Acquir Immune Defic Syndr Hum Retrovirol 1996;11:211–221.
72. National Commission on AIDS. America living with AIDS. Washington, DC: US Government Printing Office, 1991.
73. Report of the Presidential Commission on the Human Immunodeficiency Virus Epidemic. Washington, DC: US Government Printing Office, 1988.
74. Committee on a National Strategy for AIDS of the Institute of Medicine. Confronting AIDS: directions for public health, health care, and research. Washington, DC: National Academy Press, 1986.
75. Des Jarlais DC, Stepherson B. History, ethics, and politics in AIDS prevention research. Am J Public Health 1991;81:1393–1394.
76. Ljungberg B, Christensson B, Tunving K, et al. HIV prevention among injecting drug users:three years of experience from a syringe exchange program in Sweden. J Acquir Immune Defic Syndr 1991;4:890–895.
77. Osborn JE. AIDS:politics and science. N Engl J Med 1988;318:444–447.
78. Kegeles SM, Catania JA, Coates TJ, et al. Many people who seek anonymous HIV-antibody testing would avoid it under other circumstances. AIDS 1990;4:585–588.
79. Dodd RY. The risk of transfusion-transmitted infection. N Engl J Med 1992;327:419–421.
80. Gerberding JL. Expected costs of implementing a mandatory human immunodeficiency virus and hepatitis B virus testing and restriction program for health care workers performing invasive procedures. Infect Control Hosp Epidemiol 1991;12:443–447.
81. Dooley SW, Jarvis WR, Martone WK, et al. Multidrug-resistant tuberculosis. Ann Intern Med 1992;117:257–259.
82. National Commission on AIDS Report. HIV disease in correctional facilities. Washington, DC: National Commission on AIDS, 1991.
83. Brewer TF, Derrickson J. AIDS in prison: a review of epidemiology and preventative policy. AIDS 1992;6:623–628.
84. Padian NS, Shiboski SC, Jewell NP. Female-to-male transmission of human immunodeficiency virus. JAMA 1991;266:1664–1667.
85. Global Programme on AIDS and Programme of STD. Report of the consultation on partner notification for preventing HIV transmission. Geneva: World Health Organization, 1989.
86. Scitovsky AA, Rice DP. Estimates of the direct and indirect costs of acquired immunodeficiency syndrome in the United States:1985, 1986, and 1991. Public Health Rep 1987;102:5–17.
87. Weisfeld VD, ed. AIDS health services at the crossroads: lessons for community care. Princeton, NJ: Robert Wood Johnson Foundation, 1991.
88. Makadon HJ, Seage GR, Thorpe KE, et al. Paying the medical cost of the HIV epidemic: a review of policy options. J Acquir Immune Defic Syndr 1990;3:123–133.
89. National Commission on AIDS. Housing and the HIV/AIDS epidemic: recommendations for action. Washington, DC, National Commission on AIDS, 1992.
90. Ciesielski C, Marianos D, Ou C-Y, et al. Transmission of human immunodeficiency virus in a dental practice. Ann Intern Med 1992; 116:798–805.
91. United States Congress, Office of Technology Assessment. HIV in the health care workplace: a background paper. AIDS Patient Care 1992; 6:169–185.
92. Moini S, Hammett TM. 1989 Update: AIDS in correctional facilities. Washington, DC: National Institute of Justice, 1990.
93. National Commission on AIDS. HIV disease in correctional facilities. Washington, DC: National Commission on AIDS, 1991.
94. von Reyn CF, Mann JM, Chin J. International travel and HIV infection. Bull World Health Organ 1990;68:251–259.

Section IV
Clinical

10

Introduction to the Clinical Spectrum of AIDS

Margaret A. Fischl

The purpose of this chapter is to provide an overview and introduction to other chapters in this book that deal with specific pathogens or organ-system damage linked to the acquired immunodeficiency syndrome (AIDS). Since AIDS was first recognized in the early 1980s, the manifestations and natural history of human immunodeficiency virus (HIV) disease have slowly emerged. Investigators now recognize that HIV infection induces a chronic and progressive process with a broad spectrum of manifestations and complications from primary infection to life-threatening opportunistic infections, malignancies, and wasting. The course of the infection is marked by increasing viral replication, emergence of a more virulent viral strain, and progressive destruction of the immune system with dysfunction and depletion of CD4 cells, if left untreated.

After primary infection, HIV disease represents a spectrum from asymptomatic infection to symptomatic disease with intermittent and chronic manifestations and the potential for life-threatening processes. The availability of increasingly more effective treatments not only has improved overall outcome, but also has dramatically decreased the incidence of life-threatening opportunistic infections, malignancies, and wasting (1). Based on the chronicity and broad scope of the disease, HIV infection is currently staged by CD4 cell counts, HIV symptoms, and complications, as outlined in Table 10.1. However, with an increasing understanding of the pathogenesis of HIV infection, HIV disease may more accurately be staged by CD4 cell counts and HIV RNA levels (Table 10.2). Caution should be used in the use of any staging system because the boundaries between stages are not necessarily discrete, and patients do not always make the transition directly from one stage to the next.

ACUTE PRIMARY HIV INFECTION

Primary infection with HIV is typically asymptomatic; however, 50 to 80% of patients may have symptoms. Because of patients' and clinicians' lack of consideration of HIV, acute primary HIV infection frequently goes unrecognized (2).

Acute primary infection (also known as acute retroviral syndrome) is characterized by fever, headache, malaise, myalgia, arthralgia, pharyngitis, nausea, and a diffuse erythematous rash (3). Symmetric lymphadenopathy is common. Hepatitis and meningitis are seen less frequently, as well as pneumonitis. Mucocutaneous ulcers and rare cases of oral candidiasis and *Candida* esophagitis have been reported (4, 5).

Laboratory abnormalities are nonspecific and suggest an acute viral illness. Leukopenia and lymphopenia are common, and occasionally leukocytosis is seen. Atypical lymphocytes may be noted as patients' symptoms resolve. An increase in CD8 cell counts with a resultant inversion in the CD4:CD8 ratio is frequently noted. A decrease in CD4 cell count is common, and this count typically increases with resolution of symptoms.

The incubation period is normally 2 to 4 weeks, and symptoms generally resolve within days to weeks. Persistent symptoms beyond several weeks and suppression of CD4 cells suggest rapidly progressive HIV infection.

Infection with HIV occurs with a single genotype that evolves over time into genetically distinct viral variants, HIV-1 quasispecies. Virologic evaluation initially shows a large number of infected cells in the peripheral blood and high titers of infectious virions in the plasma (6). Viral titers rapidly decline with the development of a cellular immune response (Fig 10.1). However, HIV RNA levels in the plasma may still remain detectable. HIV p24 antigenemia may be detectable before HIV Gag and Env protein antibodies appear. HIV p24 antigen levels subsequently decline with the development of anti-HIV antibodies, and only a few patients with asymptomatic HIV infection have detectable levels of serum HIV p24 antigen early in the course of HIV disease. Current studies suggest that cellular immunity plays a major role in controlling viral replication, because antibody-dependent cellular cytotoxicity (ADCC) activity and HIV-specific cytotoxic T lymphocytes (CTLs) are detected before the appearance of neutralizing antibodies (7).

HIV-1 antibodies become detectable several weeks after the onset of symptoms. The initial humoral response consists of IgM antibodies followed by IgG antibodies. The determination of serum p24 HIV antigen levels or proviral DNA

Table 10.1. Stages of HIV Disease

Stage and Clinical Features	Typical Duration	CD4+ Cell Count Range (cells/mm^3)
Acute primary HIV infection	1–2 wk	1,000–500
Asymptomatic (no symptoms or signs other than lymphadenopathy)	10+ y	750–500
Early symptomatic (non–life-threatening infections, or chronic or intermittent symptoms)	0–5 y	500–100
Late symptomatic (increasingly severe symptoms, life-threatening infections, or cancers)	0–3 y	200–50
Advanced (increasing hazard of death and serious "opportunistic" infections)	1–2 y	50–0

Adapted from Volberding P. Clinical spectrum of HIV disease. In: DeVita VT, Hellman S, Rosenberg SA, eds. AIDS: etiology, diagnosis, treatment, and prevention. 3rd ed. Philadelphia: JB Lippincott, 1992:123–140.)

Table 10.2. HIV RNA/CD4 and HIV Disease Risks

Stage of Disease	HIV RNA titer (copies/mL)	CD4 cell count (cells/mm^3)	Percentage with AIDS over 6 years (%)
Early	< 3,000	—	1.7–9.6
	< 10,000	> 750	14.2
Intermediate	< 10,000	< 750	37.2
	< 30,000	> 350	36.7–54
Advanced	10,000–30,000	< 350	72.9
	> 30,000	> 350	68.8–77
Late	> 30,000	< 350	89.3–97

(Adapted from Mellors JW, Muñoz A, Giorgi JV, et al. Plasma viral load and CD4+ lymphocytes as prognostic markers of HIV-1 infection. Ann Intern Med 1997; 126:946–954.)

sequence by polymerase chain reaction (PCR) is more sensitive for the detection of HIV during primary infection. Although circulating HIV RNA can be detected through quantitative PCR or branched-chain DNA (bDNA), these assays are not currently quality controlled as diagnostic tests and should be used cautiously. False-positive test results may occur in up to 3% of cases, especially at the lower range of quantitation of the current assay (less than 1000 copies/mL). If acute primary HIV infection is suspected, serum p24 HIV antigen levels or proviral DNA sequences by PCR should be obtained. Testing for the presence of HIV-1 antibody should also be done. Detection of HIV-1 antibody by enzyme-linked immunosorbent assay (ELISA) is widely used and initially may be negative or indeterminate. The Western blot assay is used for the confirmation of positive ELISA test results and may demonstrate no or select antibody bands. HIV-1 antibody testing should be repeated to document conversion from negative to positive results. Monitoring plasma HIV RNA levels is not unreasonable, because levels are typically high and decrease to a stable level.

Initial treatment of acute primary infection is supportive. Antiretroviral therapy in symptomatic patients may afford an early opportunity to control and potentially to eliminate viral infection and minimize immune dysfunction. However, the long-term benefits of antiretroviral therapy in this setting are unknown. Based on our current understanding of HIV pathogenesis and viral dynamics (8), if therapy is chosen, combination regimens with three or more antiretroviral drugs should be used. Regimens that include nucleoside reverse transcriptase inhibitors, nonnucleoside reverse transcriptase inhibitors, and HIV-1 protease inhibitors should be considered (9). The transmission of resistant virus between sexual partners has been described and may affect response to initial treatment regimens (10).

ASYMPTOMATIC HIV INFECTION

Although diffuse lymphadenopathy and headache may be present, generally no chronic signs or symptoms are attributable to HIV during the early or asymptomatic phases of infection. However, many laboratory abnormalities are seen, including anemia, leukopenia, neutropenia, lymphopenia, thrombocytopenia, and elevation in transaminases. Hematologic abnormalities are typically mild, although thrombocytopenia may be severe and require therapy. Thrombocytopenia is likely a result of decreased platelet survival resulting from platelet-directed antibodies and circulating immune complexes and decreased platelet production resulting from HIV infection of megakaryocytes (11). Elevations in serum transaminases may be associated with an acute or chronic hepatitis or the reactivation of viral hepatitis with progressive immunosuppression (12). Increases in total serum globulin levels and decreases in albumin and cholesterol levels may also be seen.

HIV infection is characterized by a high level of viral turnover and CD4 cell destruction and replacement (13).

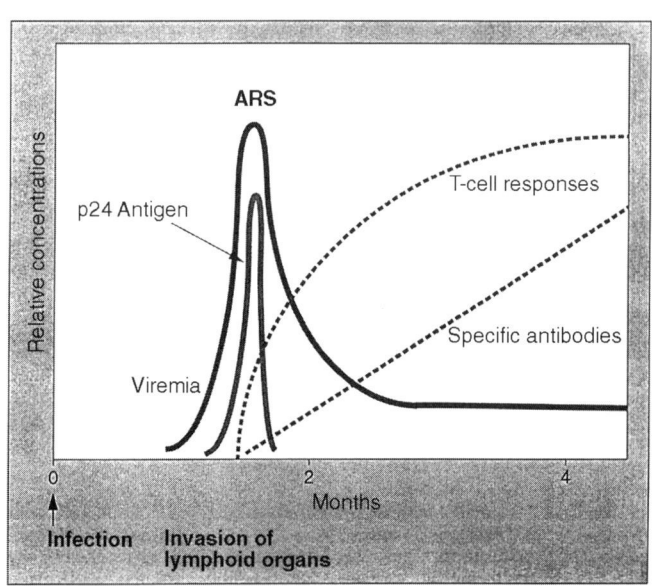

Figure 10.1. Rapid decline of viral titers with development of cellular immune response.

Table 10.3. Laboratory Test Evaluation of Asymptomatic and Symptomatic HIV Disease

Test	Indications
HIV RNA level	Consideration for antiretroviral therapy and changes in antiretroviral therapy
CD4 cell count	Consideration for antiretroviral therapy and chemoprophylaxis for opportunistic infections
Complete blood count	Assessment of hematologic complications of HIV disease
PPD	Assessment of coinfection with *Mycobacterium tuberculosis*
Syphilis serology	Assessment of coinfection with *Treponema pallidum*
Hepatitis serology	Assessment for acute and chronic hepatitis and future risk of reactivation of latent infection
Toxoplasma IgG antibody	Assessment of prior exposure to *Toxoplasma* and future risk for reactivation of latent infection
Papanicolaou smear	Detection of cervical cytologic abnormalities in women

Table 10.4. Chemoprophylaxis for Opportunistic Infection

PPD ≥ 5 mm:	
Mycobacterium tuberculosis	Isoniazid, 300 mg daily, and pyridoxine, 50 mg daily, for 12 months (isoniazid-sensitive organism)
	Rifampin, 600 mg daily, for 12 months (isoniazid-resistant organism)
CD4 cell count < 200 cells/mm^3:	
Pneumocystis carinii pneumonia	Trimethoprim–sulfamethoxazole, once daily or three times per week
	Dapsone, 50 mg twice per day or 100 mg daily
	Dapsone, 50 mg once daily, plus pyrimethamine, 50 mg once weekly (leucovorin, 25 mg, once weekly)
	Dapsone, 200 mg once weekly, plus pyrimethamine, 75 mg once weekly (leucovorin, 25 mg, once weekly)
	Atovaquone, 750 mg, twice per day
	Inhaled pentamidine, 300 mg via a Respigard II nebulizer every 3 or 4 weeks
CD4 cell count < 100 cells/mm^3:	
Toxoplasma gondii	Trimethoprim–sulfamethoxazole, once daily vs three times per week
	Dapsone, 50 mg once daily, plus pyrimethamine, 50 mg once weekly (leucovorin, 25 mg, once weekly)
CD4 cell count < 50 cells/mm^3:	
Mycobacterium avium	Clarithromycin, 500 mg, twice a day
	Azithromycin, 1200 mg, once weekly
	Rifabutin, 300 mg daily

CD4 cell count, CD8 cell count, and plasma HIV-1 RNA level are direct measures of HIV disease. Circulating levels of HIV-1 RNA correlate with HIV disease stage and are strong predictors of disease outcome, including CD4 cell decline, AIDS events, and mortality (14). The absolute number of circulating CD4 cells is also predictive of disease progression and death, particularly among patients with lower CD4 cell counts (15).

Over time, laboratory evidence of progressive immunodeficiency is noted, with a decline in the absolute number of circulating CD4 cells, if left untreated. Although variation in CD4 cell counts can be seen, a decline of 40 to 80 cells/mm^3 per year can be seen in the untreated patient. This decline varies from patient to patient; some patients may have a more rapid decline in CD4 cells, whereas others may have more stable counts over long periods (16, 17).

Once HIV infection is adequately documented, CD4 cell counts and plasma HIV-1 RNA levels should be monitored in a reliable laboratory. CD4 cell counts and plasma HIV-1 RNA levels should be obtained approximately every 6 months (Table 10.3). A complete blood count should be monitored every 6 months to identify hematologic complications of HIV infection. Liver function tests should also be considered to monitor for other infections, such as hepatitis.

Because of the increased incidence of coinfection with *Mycobacterium tuberculosis* and the risk for reactivation of latent infection, skin testing for tuberculous infection should be done at the earliest assessment. The Mantoux test (5 units of purified protein derivative, PPD) is preferred, and an induration of 5 mm or more is considered a positive test in patients with HIV disease (18). As the CD4 cell count declines, skin test anergy is common and interferes with the detection of prior tuberculous infection. Patients with a positive PPD should receive isoniazid therapy to prevent tuberculosis (Table 10.4). The use of other skin tests to document anergy is not useful and is no longer recommended.

Serologic evaluation for syphilis is warranted as a result of the increased incidence of coinfection with *Treponema pallidum* in this patient population. Because the natural history of syphilis differs among patients with HIV disease, careful attention must be given to the diagnosis and treatment of syphilis (19). Patients with HIV infection are at an increased risk for acute and chronic hepatitis and reactivation of hepatitis with progressive immunosuppression. Screening for hepatitis B and C virus infection is recommended. Reactivation of latent infection with *Toxoplasma gondii* is common and typically occurs among patients with preexisting anti-

Table 10.5. Clinical Syndromes and Pathogens Associated with HIV Disease by Organ System

Respiratory tract
  Pneumonia
    Pneumocystis carinii
    Streptococcus pneumoniae
    Haemophilus influenzae
    Staphylococcus aureus
    Rhodococeus equi
    Nocardia asteroides
    Histoplasma capsulatum
    Coccidioides immitis
    Candida species
    Aspergillus species
    Mycobacterium avium-complex
    Toxoplasma gondii
    Strongyloides stercoralis
    Cytomegalovirus
    Herpes simplex virus
    Lymphoid interstitial pneumonitis
Gastrointestinal tract
  Mouth and esophagus
    Pain and odynophagia
      Candida species
      Cytomegalovirus
      Herpes simplex virus
    Other
      Hairy leukoplakia
      Erosive gingivitis
      Aphthous ulcers
  Intestine and colon
    Gastrointestinal/colitis
      Salmonella species
      Shigella species
      Campylobacter jejuni
      Mycobacterium avium-complex
      Cryptosporidium species
      Isospora belli
      Blastocystis hominis
      Entamoeba histolytica
      Giardia lamblia
      Microsporida
      Strongyloides stercoralis
      Cytomegalovirus
      Adenovirus
    Other
      Nonspecific enteropathy with diarrhea and malabsorption
  Rectum and Anus
    Proctitis
      Herpes simplex virus
      Cytomegalovirus
      Chlamydia trachomatis
      Neisseria gonorrhoeae
      Treponema pallidum
  Biliary tract and gallbladder
    Infection
      Cytomegalovirus
      Cryptosporidium
      Microsporida
    Other
      Cholecystitis
      Extrahepatic obstruction and sclerosing cholangitis
Liver
  Bacillary peliosis hepatitiis
  Adenovirus (fatal hepatic necrosis)

Nervous system
  Central nervous system
    Encephalitis or dementia
      Subacute encephalopathy
      Herpes simplex virus
      Cytomegalovirus
      Progressive multifocal leukoencephalopathy
      Varicella-zoster virus
      Treponema pallidum
      Mycobacterium avium-complex
    Discrete mass lesion/abscess
      Toxoplasma gondii
      Neoplasm
      Kaposi's sarcoma
      Primary or metastatic lymphoma
      Cryptococcus neoformans
      Coccidioides immitis
      Candida albicans
      Mycobacterium tuberculosis
      Nocardia asteroides
    Meningitis
      Listeria monocytogenes
      Aseptic
        HIV
        Herpes simplex virus
        Varicella-zoster virus
        Cytomegalovirus
        Cryptococcus neoformans
        Coccidioides immitis
        Mycobacterium tuberculosis
        Treponema pallidum
      Lymphomatous meningitis
  Spinal cord or peripheral nerves
    Myelitis or neuropathy
      Vacuolar myelopathy
      Chronic inflammatory polyneuropathy
      Distal symmetric sensory motor neuropathy
      Varicella-zoster virus radiculitis
      Cytomegalovirus myelitis
Eye
  Retinitis
    Cytomegalovirus
    Varicella-zoster virus
    Candida albicans
    Histoplasma capsulatum
    Toxoplasma gondii
  Keratoconjunctivitis
    Microsporida
Disseminated
  Infection processes
    Mycobacterium avium-complex
    Mycobacterium tuberculosis
    Cryptococcus neoformans
    Coccidioides immitis
    Histoplasma capsulatum
    Cytomegalovirus
    Pneumocystis carinii
    Cat-scratch disease
    Kaposi's sarcoma
    Non–Hodgkin's lymphoma

Table 10.6. Skin Conditions Commonly Associated with HIV Disease

Condition	Findings	Location
Staphylococcal folliculitis	Erythematous pustules or papules; possibly pruritic	Face, trunk, groin
Eosinophilic folliculitis	Urticaria or papules	Face, trunk
Bacillary angiomatosis	Friable, vascul papules, plaques, or subcutaneous nodules	Skin, bone, liver, spleen, lymph node
Herpes simplex	Grouped vesicles, ulcers, fissures	Orolabial, anogenital
Herpes zoster (shingles)	Clustered vesicles on erythematous bases	Dermatomal distribution; possible spillage onto adjacent dermatoses
Molluscum contagiosum	Small pearly papules, with central umbilication	Face, anogenital area
Insect bite reactions	Erythematous, urticarial papules	Axillae, groin, finger webs (scabies), lower legs (flea bites), upper and lower extremities, and exposed areas (mosquitoes)
Photosensitivity	Eczematous eruption	Face (tip of nose), extensor forearms, neck
Drug eruption	Erythemalous macules and papules, urticaria, erythema multiforme, Stevens–Johnson syndrome	Face, trunk, lower extremities, palms, soles of feet
Kaposi's sarcoma	Pigmented macules, violaceous or nodules	All surfaces (face, tip of nose, ears, trunk, extremities, groin, anogenital area)
Seborrheic dermatitis	White scaling without erythema, patches and plaques of erythema with indistinct margins and yellowish, greasy scales	Scalp, cheeks, eyebrows, nasolabial folds, chest, upper back, axillae, groin
Psoriasis and Reiter's syndrome	Sharply marginated plaques with a silvery scale	Elbows, knees, lumbosacral area

bodies to *Toxoplasma*. Determination of serum immunoglobulin (IgG) *Toxoplasma* antibodies is therefore recommended for patients who are at increased risk of *Toxoplasma* infection.

The incidence of cervical intraepithelial neoplasia is two- to threefold higher among women with HIV infection (20). Therefore, routine screening of HIV-infected women by Papanicolaou smear is recommended for the detection of cervical cytologic abnormalities. A Papanicolaou smear should be performed every 6 months after the initial diagnosis of HIV infection and then once per year.

Streptococcal pneumonia is a common community-acquired pneumonia. Patients with HIV infection who have a CD4 cell count of at least 200 cells/mm^3 should receive a single dose of 23-valent polysaccharide pneumococcal vaccine, if they have not been vaccinated in the past 5 years. For patients with CD4 cell counts lower than 200 cells/mm^3, the clinical utility of pneumococcal vaccination is likely to be diminished because of a blunted humoral response, but it still should be offered.

Table 10.7. Oral Manifestations of HIV Disease

Fungal	Malignant
Candidiasis	Kaposi's sarcoma
Histoplasmosis	Non–Hodgkin's lymphoma
Cryptococcosis	Squamous cell carcinoma
Viral	Other
Herpes simplex	Gingivitis
Varicella zoster	Aphthous ulcers
Cytomegalovirus	
Hairy leukoplakia	

increased risk for disease progression, and enlargement of lymph nodes may indicate non–Hodgkin's lymphoma or tuberculosis. Enlargement of the liver and spleen can also be seen and is typically nonspecific early in the disease. Many different mucocutaneous conditions can occur and should alert the physician to the possible presence of HIV infection (Tables 10.5 to 10.7).

EARLY SYMPTOMATIC HIV DISEASE

Early clinical manifestations of HIV disease include constitutional symptoms such as headache, fatigue, malaise, myalgia, fever, night sweats, anorexia, diarrhea, and weight loss. Symptoms may be present alone or in combination. Generalized lymphadenopathy involving extrainguinal sites may persist during both the asymptomatic and symptomatic phases of the disease. Persistent generalized lymphadenopathy may be present with or without other manifestations of HIV disease and is not predictive of disease progression. However, regression of lymphadenopathy may indicate an

Headache

Headache is a common complication of HIV disease and can be seen at all stages of the illness. At early stages, no specific cause may be found for recurring headaches, and treatment is symptomatic. Headache can indicate the presence of an opportunistic infection or malignancy, especially as the CD4 cell count declines. Patients who have persistent headaches should be evaluated for a central nervous system (CNS) infection or malignancy (see Table 10.5). Computed tomographic (CT) scan or, preferably, magnetic resonance imaging (MRI) of the brain should be done. If meningitis is suspected, a lumbar puncture should be performed. Headache can accompany systemic infections and typically resolves with the treatment of the systemic infection. Adverse reaction to medications, particularly antiretroviral drugs, and acute hypersensitivity reactions may also cause headache.

Fatigue

Fatigue is an early manifestation of HIV disease and may be worse in the evening and after strenuous activity. Progressive or debilitating fatigue should alert the physician to the presence of an opportunistic infection or progressive HIV disease. Fatigue may also occur as an adverse reaction to several antiretroviral drugs.

Fever and Night Sweats

Fever can be a manifestation of HIV disease and may also herald complications of HIV disease, including opportunistic infections and malignancies (21). The latter is especially true for temperatures higher than 102°F and for those patients with declining CD4 cell counts. For patients with a CD4 cell count of 100 to 200 cells/mm^3, fever should prompt an evaluation for tuberculosis, *Pneumocystis carinii* pneumonia, bacterial infections, and HIV-related non–Hodgkin's lymphoma. For patients with a CD4 cell count lower than 100 cells/mm^3, disseminated infection with *Mycobacterium avium* should also be considered. Fever may also reflect other less serious infections such as sinusitis or an adverse reaction to a medication. If no cause is found, fever can be managed with anti-inflammatory agents.

Night sweats are typically nonspecific. They may be recurrent and drenching, and they may or may not be accompanied by fever. When night sweats are associated with fever, the presence of an opportunistic infection, particularly tuberculosis, should be considered.

Diarrhea

Diarrhea is a manifestation of HIV disease and may reflect direct consequences of HIV or various enteric, parasitic, and opportunistic infections (see Table 10.5). Determining the cause of diarrhea may be difficult, and careful examination of the stool for specific pathogens is required (22). Early in HIV disease, enteric pathogens (*Salmonella* sp., *Shigella* sp., *Campylobacter* sp.) and parasitic organisms (*Giardia lamblia, Entamoeba histolytica*) should be suspected. In advanced disease, *Cryptosporidium, Isospora belli, Mycobacteria, Candida* sp., and cytomegalovirus infection are more common.

Mucocutaneous Conditions

Several dermatologic conditions are seen with increased frequency among patients with early symptomatic HIV disease and should raise the suspicion of the presence of HIV infection (23). Common skin disorders are outlined in Table 10.6. The diagnosis of these disorders is typically based on clinical appearance. Biopsy or culture should be considered for atypical findings, persistent findings that are unresponsive to initial therapy, and in cases of possible bacillary angiomatosis or Kaposi's sarcoma. Kaposi's sarcoma may be seen early in HIV disease, and careful examination of the skin and oral cavity should be done routinely.

Herpes simplex virus and varicella zoster virus infection should raise the suspicion of HIV infection. In early HIV disease, herpes simplex infection is typically manifested by limited, often recurrent orolabial and anogenital infection. With more advanced HIV disease, chronic mucocutaneous herpes simplex virus disease may be seen. In late stage HIV disease, ulcers may coalesce and form large denuded areas. Acyclovir should be administered for acute disease persisting for more than 5 to 7 days, and suppressive therapy with acyclovir is indicated for recurring disease.

Oral complications during the course of HIV disease are common (see Table 10.7) (24). Candidiasis is a prominent feature of HIV disease and is typically mild during early symptomatic HIV disease and more severe in later stages. Oral candidiasis can first appear with isolated findings in the mouth or with more extensive disease involving the esophagus, gastrointestinal tract, anogenital areas, vaginal mucosa, and cervix. Skin involvement is uncommon. Oral candidiasis typically causes white plaques or patches and smooth, erythematous patches. Less commonly, *Candida* causes hyperkeratosis and angular cheilitis. Hyphae and budding yeast forms are easily seen on microscopic examinations.

Hairy leukoplakia (Epstein–Barr virus infection) results in white, painless, oral changes on the lateral aspects of the tongue and less commonly the buccal mucosa. Oral hairy leukoplakia can be seen in earlier stages of HIV disease and may be an early indication of HIV infection. Oral aphthous ulcers occur in patients with HIV disease, especially as the CD4 cell count declines. Painful lesions of unknown origin in the mouth suggest aphthous ulcers and should be distinguished from herpes virus infections including herpes simplex and cytomegalovirus. Topical solutions with corticosteroids are useful for the treatment of aphthous ulcers. For patients with severe or refractory disease, systemic corticosteroids or thalidomide should be tried. Herpes virus infection secondary to either herpes simplex or cytomegalovirus can involve the lips, palate, and gingiva. Oral ulcers from cytomegalovirus are typically associated with disseminated disease.

Anogenital complications include venereal warts, herpes simplex infection, candidiasis, and Kaposi's sarcoma. Several other sexually transmitted diseases including syphilis, gonorrhea, and chlamydia can be seen. The diagnosis of mucosal disorders is frequently based on clinical findings. However, atypical or persistent findings and lesions suggestive of a malignancy or sexually transmitted disease should prompt biopsy, culture, or serologic testing.

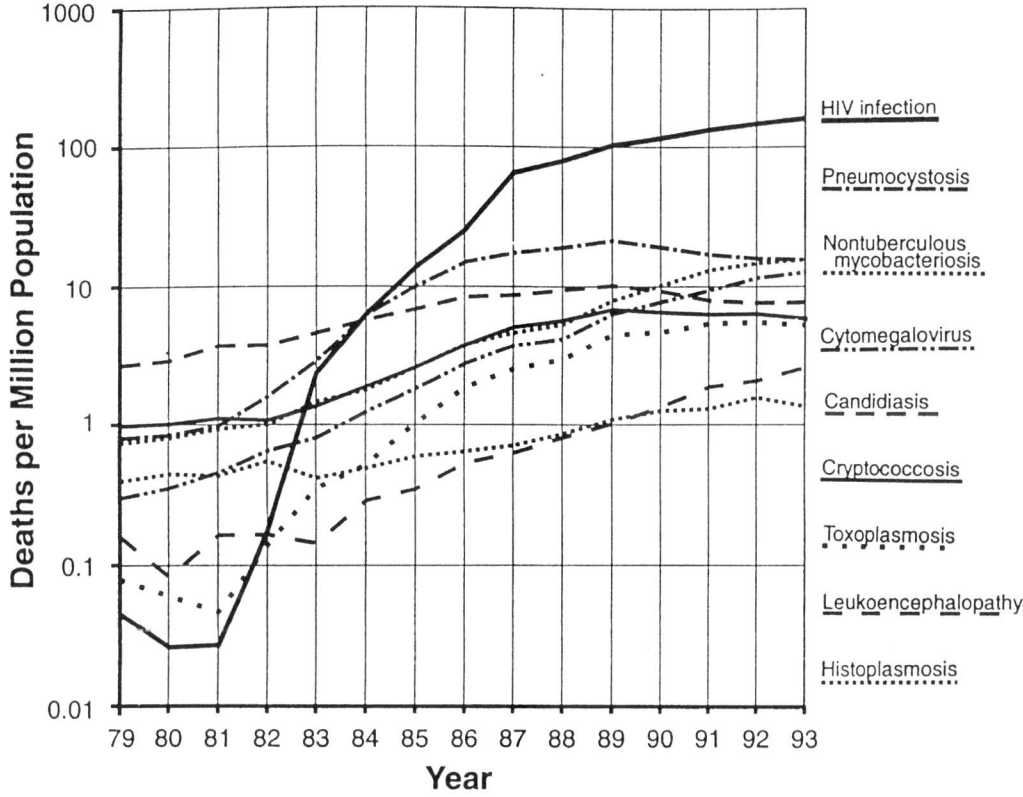

Figure 10.2. Increased risk of death from various opportunistic infections in patients with HIV disease.

Laboratory Abnormalities

Anemia, leukopenia, lymphopenia, and thrombocytopenia may be noted. Proteinuria, hypoalbuminemia, and elevation in serum blood urea nitrogen or creatinine levels may indicate HIV nephropathy. Mild elevations in serum transaminase are common and typically are nonspecific. More modest elevations in serum transaminase should suggest the presence of an opportunistic infection or malignancy, hepatitis, or possible adverse reaction to a medication. Decreases in serum cholesterol and increases in serum globulins may also be seen.

Progressive declines in CD4 cell counts are commonly noted without treatment. A decline in the CD4 cell count to fewer than 200 cells/mm^3 represents an increased risk of disease progression and warrants administration of chemoprophylaxis (see Table 10.4). The risk of disease progression is approximately 20 to 30% over a 24-month period without treatment.

Management

Plasma HIV RNA levels, CD4 cell counts, complete blood counts, and liver function studies should be repeated every 3 to 6 months to identify the need for antiretroviral therapy or chemoprophylaxis for opportunistic infections and to identify potential complications of HIV disease. As with asymptomatic HIV disease, patients should be evaluated for coinfection with *Mycobacterium tuberculosis*, syphilis, hepatitis, and *Toxoplasma*, if these tests have not already been completed (see Table 10.3). With CD4 cell count declines, chemoprophylaxis for *Pneumocystis carinii* pneumonia, *Toxoplasma*, and *M. avium* infection should be instituted as outlined in Table 10.4 (25). In addition, patients who have a positive PPD and who have received chemoprophylaxis should receive isoniazid for the prevention of tuberculosis.

Prevention of Opportunistic Infections

Plasma HIV RNA levels strongly predict decreases in CD4 cell counts and progression to AIDS and death. In addition, the number of circulating CD4 cells is closely correlated with the risk of developing several opportunistic infections associated with HIV disease. Opportunistic infections are the most common cause of death in patients with HIV infection (26), and HIV disease has increased the risk of death from several opportunistic infections (Fig 10.2). Improvements in clinical outcome and survival are associated with the use of appropriate chemoprophylaxis for opportunistic infections (see Table 10.4). As the CD4 cell count declines to fewer than 200 cells/mm^3, chemoprophylaxis for *Pneumocystis carinii* pneumonia should be given. Chemoprophylaxis should also be considered for patients with thrush and those with unexplained fevers (higher than 100°F) for more than 2 weeks. Trimethoprim–sulfamethoxazole given once daily is the preferred regimen. Three times weekly trimethoprim–sulfamethoxazole, dapsone, dapsone plus pyrimethamine, atovaquone, and aerosolized pentamidine have been successfully used for the prevention of *P. carinii* pneumonia.

Patients who have CD4 cell counts lower than 100 cells/mm^3 and who have detectable IgG antibody to *Toxoplasma* should receive chemoprophylaxis for toxoplasmosis. Trimethoprim–sulfamethoxazole and dapsone in combination with pyrimethamine appear affective in the prevention of toxoplasmosis (27). Chemoprophylaxis for *Mycobacterium avium* infection has been associated with both prevention of *M. avium* disease and improved survival. Chemoprophylaxis is therefore recommended when the CD4 cell count declines to fewer than 50 cells/mm^3. Either clarithromycin or azithromycin are recommended (28, 29). Rifabutin can be used as an alternative for those who are unable to tolerate or take clarithromycin or azithromycin. Patients who have been recently exposed to tuberculosis or those with a tuberculin skin test reaction of 5 mm or more of induration should receive chemoprophylaxis for tuberculosis. In addition, patients with a previous history of a positive tuberculin skin test who have not received chemoprophylaxis in the past should receive chemoprophylaxis. Currently, chemoprophylaxis for cytomegalovirus is optional and can be considered for patients with a CD4 cell count below 50 cells/mm^3 who has detectable antibodies to cytomegalovirus.

LATE SYMPTOMATIC DISEASE

Late symptomatic HIV disease may be characterized by declining CD4 cell count (50–200 cells/mm^3), persistent or progressive constitutional symptoms, opportunistic infections, malignancies, wasting, and dementia. Common constitutional symptoms include fatigue, fever, anorexia, nausea, vomiting, diarrhea, and weight loss. Fatigue may be profound and signal the presence of an opportunistic infection. Fever should prompt an evaluation for opportunistic infections (see Table 10.5). Typically, fever is accompanied by symptoms that should direct the initial evaluation. Anorexia, nausea, and vomiting may suggest a gastric process secondary to *Candida, Mycobacterium avium* infection, cytomegalovirus infection, Kaposi's sarcoma, lymphoma, or an adverse reaction to any number of medications. Vomiting may also reflect a CNS process. Diarrhea may be debilitating and result in progressive weight loss and wasting. Large volumes of watery diarrhea with abdominal pain and weight loss suggest enteropathy. In addition to enteric pathogens, *Cryptosporidium, Isospora belli, Microsporida*, and *M. avium* infection should be suspected (see Table 10.5). Frequent small volumes of diarrhea with lower abdominal pain suggest colitis. The most frequent pathogen is cytomegalovirus.

The broad spectrum of complications associated with HIV disease is outlined in Table 10.5. Physicians still must be cognizant of the Centers for Disease Control and Prevention (CDC) case definition for AIDS for reporting purposes (30).

The revised definition issued in January, 1993 now includes patients who have CD4 cell counts lower than 200 cells/mm^3 or a CD4 percentage lower than 14% and the addition of pulmonary tuberculosis, recurrent bacterial infection, and invasive cervical cancer.

With the advent of potent antiretroviral therapy and the ability to suppress viral replication to low levels in the circulation, the incidence of opportunistic complications has decreased. In addition, overall survival for HIV disease has improved, and patients with HIV disease are increasingly ambulatory with less need for hospitalization. Emerging data suggest a direct relationship between the suppression of viral replication and the decreasing incidence of opportunistic infections. Although CD4 cell counts may dramatically increase during potent antiretroviral therapy, currently no recommendations exist to stop chemoprophylaxis for opportunistic infections, until further data are available about the safety of such a practice.

Pulmonary Disease

Respiratory tract infections and malignancies are frequent complications of HIV disease. *Streptococcus pneumoniae, Haemophilus influenzae, Staphylococcus aureus, Klebsiella pneumoniae*, and other common pathogens can cause bacterial pneumonitis. Bacterial pnuemonias are more commonly seen among patients with CD4 cell counts lower than 200 cells/mm^3, injection drug users, and smokers. Presentation typically includes cough, fever, and shortness of breath. A more abrupt onset of symptoms and the presence of pleuritic chest pain may help to distinguish bacterial pneumonia from other processes. In addition, the chest radiograph is more likely to show lobar or segmental consolidation (Table 10.8).

Tuberculosis has been a frequent complication of HIV disease (31). Reactivation of latent infection may be seen at earlier stages of the disease (CD4 cell count is at least 200 cells/mm^3). However, tuberculosis can occur in patients with late symptomatic HIV disease, and there is an increased

Table 10.8. Chest Radiograph Findings in HIV Disease

Condition	Findings
Bacterial pneumonia	Lobar consolidation, pleural effusion; rare cavitation
Pneumocystis carinii pneumonia	Diffuse, bilateral infiltrates; rare focal nodules with or without cavitation
Mycobacterium tuberculosis	Coarse diffuse interstitial infiltrates; hilar or mediastinal adenopathy; pleural effusions
Fungal infection	Poorly defined nodular infiltrates; adenopathy; cavitations, consolidation, pleural infiltrates less frequent
Cytomegalovirus infection	Diffuse find reticular interstitial infiltrates
Kaposi's sarcoma	Scattered nodular infiltrates; pleural effusions frequent
Lymphoma	Enlarging mass; hilar adenopathy; interstitial infiltrates

risk of active tuberculosis after primary exposure. Pulmonary tuberculosis may mimic *Pneumocystis carinii* pneumonia and may be difficult to distinguish from other opportunistic infections. The findings of more coarse interstitial changes and hilar or mediastinal adenopathy on the chest radiograph should suggest the presence of tuberculosis. Pleural effusions can be seen in 10 to 20% of the cases (see Table 10.8).

The most common pulmonary complication of HIV disease is *Pneumocystis carinii* pneumonia, which is seen with increasing frequency among patients who have a CD4 cell count lower than 200 CD4 cells/mm^3. Presentation includes dry cough, shortness of breath, and fever. The chest radiograph typically shows diffuse interstitial infiltrates. On rare occasions, focal nodules with or without cavitation may be seen. A decrease in oxygen saturation or an increase in the arterial–alveolar gradient is common on arterial blood gas assessment. Elevation in serum lactic dehydrogenase, although nonspecific, is typically seen in patients with *P. carinii* pneumonia. Diagnosis can be made by examination of sputum, bronchial lavage material, or lung tissue obtained from a transbronchial biopsy. Prompt recognition and treatment of *P. carinii* pneumonia are important in improving outcome and survival. The use of chemoprophylaxis for *P. carinii* pneumonia has decreased the occurrence of this pulmonary complication and should be considered for any patients with a prior diagnosis of *P. carinii* pneumonia or patients with a CD4 cell count less than or equal to 200 cells/mm^3 or symptoms.

Systemic fungal infections may result in pulmonary disease. Hilar adenopathy, pulmonary nodules, and interstitial, reticulonodular, or cavitary infiltrates can be seen in cryptococcosis, histoplasmosis, blastomycosis, and coccidioidomycosis.

Gastrointestinal Disease

The entire gastrointestinal tract can be involved sometime during the course of HIV disease. Esophageal and diarrheal diseases are more frequently seen (32, 33). The presence of dysphagia or odynophagia suggests the presence of esophageal disease. Esophageal disease may also present with anorexia, nausea, and epigastric pain. The most frequent cause of esophageal disease is infection with *Candida*, and approximately 70 to 80% of patients with *Candida esophagitis* also have oral candidiasis. Patients who present with dysphagia or odynophagia should be treated with oral antifungal agents. If symptoms persist or worsen, then other causes of esophageal disease, such as herpes simplex infection, cytomegalovirus infection, or aphthous ulceration, must be considered. Extrinsic compression from mediastinal lymphadenopathy related to tuberculosis, fungal infections, or lymphoma may also present with dysphagia. The diagnosis of esophageal disease is best made by endoscopy with biopsy and brushings of affected areas.

Diarrhea is the most common manifestation of intestinal complications of HIV disease. Small intestinal disease typically presents with midepigastric cramping, bloating, and nausea in association with a secretory-type diarrhea. This can result in dehydration and volume depletion. Infections secondary to *Cryptosporidium, Microspora, Isospora belli,* and *Mycobacterium avium* are more common in late symptomatic HIV disease. In contrast, colitis more typically presents with fever, lower abdominal pain, and smaller volumes of diarrhea frequently associated with mucus. Infection secondary to cytomegalovirus is most frequent. However, *Cryptosporidium, M. avium,* and *Clostridium difficile* toxin can also be seen. Anorectal disease can also be seen. The presence of anorectal ulcers is most consistent with herpes simplex infection and, less commonly, cytomegalovirus infection.

Neurologic Disease

Several CNS infections and lymphoma can be seen in late symptomatic HIV disease (see Table 10.5) (34). Lymphoma may occur as a primary malignancy of the brain or as metastatic disease from extraneural sites. The most common presentation of primary CNS lymphoma is focal or multifocal neurologic deficits. CNS infections typically present with focal neurologic deficits, seizures, headache, and fever. General debilitation, confusion, altered mental status, lethargy, and coma can also be seen. The diagnosis of CNS lymphoma or infections is based on neuroimaging procedures, identification of the etiologic agent by lumbar puncture or brain biopsy, and response to therapy. MRI is generally superior to CT. If a CT scan is done, a contrast-enhanced CT with a double dose of contrast to increase the detection of lesions should be done. For patients who have atypical findings or those who do not respond to therapy, a brain biopsy may be needed (35). A lumbar puncture should be done if meningitis or neurosyphilis is suspected.

HIV dementia is a less frequent complication of late symptomatic HIV disease because of the increasing use of antiretroviral drugs. Vacuolar myelopathy is the most common cause of spinal cord complications. Infectious pathogens and malignancies, including lymphoma, *Mycobacteria, Toxoplasma,* and cytomegalovirus infection, can cause myelopathy.

Peripheral neuropathy is a common complication of HIV disease and can occur at any stage of the disease. In late HIV disease, sensory axonal neuropathy typically occurs. Treatment is symptomatic and includes tricyclic antidepressants and narcotic analgesics, if needed. Several of the nucleoside analogs used to treat HIV disease, including zalcitabine, didanosine, and stavudine, can cause toxic peripheral neuropathy.

Malignancies

Several malignancies are associated with HIV infection and typically have a more aggressive course, especially late in HIV disease. Malignancies reported among patients with HIV infection include Kaposi's sarcoma, non–Hodgkin's lymphoma, system high-grade lymphoma, primary CNS lymphoma, Hodgkin's disease, anogenital squamous cell carcinoma, anal carcinoma, and cervical carcinoma. Kaposi's sarcoma, non–Hodgkin's lymphoma, and invasive cervical carcinoma are also considered AIDS-defining illnesses, according to the CDC guidelines.

Management

The management of late symptomatic HIV disease is directed toward the recognition, treatment, and prevention of opportunistic processes (see Tables 10.4 and 10.5). Symptomatic treatment of constitutional symptoms and complications of infections such as diarrhea may be needed. Careful examination of the skin, oral cavity, anorectal area, groin, genitalia, vaginal mucosa, and cervix is essential for the early recognition of infections, Kaposi's sarcoma, and cervical cancer.

Plasma HIV RNA levels and CD4 cell counts should be monitored at least every 3 months, and complete blood counts, blood chemistry studies, and renal and liver function studies should be repeated as clinically indicated. Based on the availability of potent antiretroviral therapy, every effort should be made to maximally suppress viral replication.

ADVANCED (END-STAGE) HIV DISEASE

Patients with advanced HIV disease have an increased likelihood of disseminated infection with *Mycobacterium avium* and cytomegalovirus, severe wasting, dementia, and death (36). Wasting syndrome is characterized by unexplained progressive weight loss with or without diarrhea and severe debilitation (37). Because several infections can lead to diarrhea and cachexia, a careful evaluation for *Cryptosporidium,* cytomegalovirus, and *M. avium* should be done. Appetite stimulants such as megesterol acetate, cannabinoids, anabolic steroids, testosterone, and human growth hormone may be useful (38). Fat malabsorption is common in advanced HIV disease, and diets containing medium-chain triglycerides may be helpful. The precise mechanism for wasting is unknown but may be related to several cytokines, including tumor necrosis factor.

Patients with persistent fever of unknown origin should be evaluated for *Pneumocystis carinii* pneumonia, mycobacterial infections, and disseminated cytomegalovirus infection. Evaluation should include a chest radiograph, blood cultures (including isolator tubes for intracellular organisms), bone marrow aspirate and biopsy, and liver biopsy if abnormalities in liver function are noted. Symptomatic treatment of fever with nonsteroidal anti-inflammatory agents may be helpful. Patients with advanced HIV disease may have severe and debilitating myalgias and pain; adequate analgesics should be used.

AIDS–dementia complex is characterized by cognitive, behavioral, and motor dysfunction and is most common in late HIV disease after the development of HIV-related opportunistic infections or malignancies (39). Impaired concentration, forgetfulness, and slowed cognitive function are early symptoms. Changes in personality and behavior characterized by apathy and withdrawal may also be noted. In rare cases, agitation, irritability, confusion, and psychosis may be seen. Motor symptoms, including gait disturbances, loss of coordination, and leg weakness, can occur. With progressive complaints, confusion, psychosis, impaired rapid movements, hyperreflexia, release reflexes (snout, glabella, and grasp), weakness, ataxia, spasticity, bladder and bowel incontinence, and myoclonus can be found. Ataxia is a late feature and can be disabling in the face of progressive leg weakness. Cerebral atrophy and patchy or diffusely increased signal intensity in the white matter and less frequently the basal ganglia or thalamus are typical neuroimaging findings. Cerebrospinal fluid examination can show a mild elevation in protein and mild pleocytosis with a predominance of mononuclear cells and can assist in the exclusion of a diagnosis of meningitis or neurosyphilis.

Progressive multifocal leukoencephalopathy can be seen in advanced HIV disease and is characterized by multiple areas of white matter demyelination. Hypodense, nonenhancing lesions are prominent on MRI evaluation.

Management

Treatment of advanced HIV disease should focus on the recognition, treatment, and prevention of opportunistic infections and maximizing antiretroviral therapy. Management of symptoms during this phase of the disease is important. The prevalence of pain increases with advancing HIV disease and needs careful evaluation and treatment, when appropriate. Dyspnea, nausea, vomiting, diarrhea, and asthenia can be prominent features of advanced disease and need careful attention. Psychosocial support may be necessary throughout the course of HIV disease, but it is particularly important to dying patients.

ANTIRETROVIRAL TREATMENT OF HIV DISEASE

HIV replication takes place predominantly in productively infected T cells and macrophages. Limited amounts of virus are derived from latently infected cells that are activated. The major reservoir for the virus is lymphoid tissues. Circulating levels of HIV RNA correlate with HIV disease stage and are strong predictors of HIV disease outcome after seroconversion. In addition, HIV RNA levels discriminate disease risk at all levels of CD4 cell counts and predict declines in CD4 cells. From the lowest to the highest HIV RNA category, the percentages of patients progressing to AIDS by 6 years were 5.4% (fewer than 500 copies/mL), 16.6% (more than 500 to 3000 copies/mL), 31.7% (more than 3000 to 10,000 copies/mL), 55.2% (more than 10,000 to 30,000) and 80.0% (more than 30,000 copies/mL).

The most effective therapies for HIV infection include the HIV-1 reverse transcriptase and protease inhibitors. Without the proven ability to eradicate HIV infection and the emergence of viral resistance with partial suppression of viral replication, therapeutic approaches must be optimized through the use of combination regimens. Based on current knowledge of HIV dynamics, therapeutic interventions must be used to maximize the suppression of viral replication overtime, to avoid viral resistance, and to prevent immunologic dysfunction. To achieve these goals, early treatment intervention and the most potent of regimens are needed. Eleven antiretroviral drugs are approved for the treatment of HIV disease, including five reverse transcriptase inhibitors (zidovudine, didanosine, zalcitabine, stavudine, and lamivudine), two nonnucleoside reverse transcriptase inhibitor (nevirapine and delavirdine), and four protease inhibitors (saquinavir, ritonavir, indinavir, and nelfinavir). Several agents including 1592U89, DMP-266, and 141W94 are under evaluation.

Initiating Antiretroviral Therapy

Patients with HIV infection should consider antiretroviral therapy if they have symptoms, a CD4 cell count lower than 500 cells/mm^3, or an HIV RNA level of 5000 to 10,000 copies/mL regardless of CD4 cell count or symptoms. Judging the adequacy of therapy is more feasible with the use of HIV RNA and CD4 cell determinations. Ideally, the HIV RNA level should fall to low levels (lower than 500 to 5000 copies/mL) during therapy. How tightly HIV replication should be controlled within this range is unknown. Emerging data with protease inhibitors suggest the need for maximal suppression HIV replication (fewer than 200 to 500 RNA copies/mL) to improve long-term durability and to decrease the risk of viral resistance (9).

Antiretroviral Treatment Regimens

NUCLEOSIDE ANALOGS

Studies have shown that combination regimens are superior to zidovudine monotherapy at all stages of disease (40, 41). Several combination regimens, including zidovudine with either didanosine, zalcitabine, or lamivudine, are associated with clinical and survival benefits (12). Combination regimens with didanosine and stavudine or lamivudine and either didanosine or stavudine show promise and are reasonable additional options.

NONNUCLEOSIDE REVERSE TRANSCRIPTASE INHIBITORS

Nonnucleosides are a potent class of compounds that inhibit HIV-1 reverse transcriptase and differ from nucleosides that mimic the normal deoxynucleotide triphosphate and act as chain terminators. These drugs bind to a common region in the reverse transcriptase and are susceptible to several amino acid substitutions, which confer high-level resistance. Although combinations with nonnucleoside analogs are associated with enhanced effectiveness, resistance is still a long-term problem. At least one study has shown that the combination of zidovudine, didanosine, and nevirapine is associated with greater viral suppression and decreased drug resistance (43). Thus, three-drug regimens that include nonnucleoside analogs are reasonable alternatives, especially for patients with earlier stages of HIV disease.

HIV-1 PROTEASE INHIBITORS

The HIV-1 protease enzyme is responsible for mediating the maturation of newly formed viral particles in infected cells. Protease inhibition results in immature HIV particles that cannot perpetuate new cycles of infection. Four HIV-1 protease inhibitors are approved for the treatment of HIV infection: saquinavir, ritonavir, indinavir, and nelfinavir.

Clinical benefits had been seen with ritonavir in a large study that included patients with advanced HIV disease and the concurrent use of up to two approved nucleosides. Clinical benefits have also been noted with saquinavir when given with zalcitabine to patients with 50 to 300 CD4 cells/mm^3 and at least 16 weeks of prior zidovudine or zidovudine intolerance. The direct comparison of a three-drug regimen (zidovudine or stavudine, lamivudine, and indinavir) versus a two-drug regimen (zidovudine or stavudine and lamivudine) in patients with nucleoside experience who had a CD4 cell count less than or equal to 200 cells/mm^3 demonstrated that the three-drug regimen provided superior clinical and survival benefits (44). These finding support the routine use of three-drug regimens, particularly those containing an HIV-1 protease inhibitors for the treatment of patients with HIV infection and low CD4 cell counts or high RNA levels. Profound suppression of viral replication as measured by HIV RNA levels occurs with triple-drug therapy that contains an HIV-1 protease inhibitors in patients with earlier stages of HIV disease (45) and would warrant the consideration of three-drug regimens for patient at all stages of HIV disease.

Treatment Failure and Changing Antiretroviral Therapy

Changes in current antiretroviral therapy should be considered when one is faced with unacceptable toxicities, failure to attain an adequate antiviral response (HIV RNA levels lower than 500 to 5000 copies/mL), and relapse (HIV RNA levels that rise above 5000 to 35,000 copies/mL). In the face of treatment failures, at least two new drugs should be considered. Sequential therapy or adding a single new drug to a failing regimen increases the likelihood of drug resistance and circumvents the goals of combination therapy. When considering alternative drugs, one must consider potency, tolerance, and resistance patterns; using drugs with overlapping resistance patterns is unlikely to be successful.

References

1. Centers for Disease Control and Prevention. Update: trends in AIDS incidence—United States, 1996. MMWR Morb Mortal Wkly Rep 1996;46:861–867.

2. Schacker T, Collier AC, Hughes J, et al. Clinical and epidemiologic features of primary HIV infection. Ann Intern Med 1996; 125:257–264.
3. Kinloch-de Loës S, de Saussure P, Saurat JH, et al. Symptomatic primary infection due to human immunodeficiency virus type 1: review of 31 cases. Clin Infect Dis 1993;17:59–65.
4. Rabeneck L, Popvic M, Gartner S, et al. Acute HIV infection presenting with painful swallowing and esophageal ulcers. JAMA 1990;263:2318.
5. Peña JM, Martínez-López MA, Arnalich F, et al. Esophageal candidiasis and immunodeficiency associated with acute HIV infection. AIDS 1988;13:872.
6. Piatak M, Saag MS, Yang LC, et al. High levels of HIV-1 in plasma during all stages of infection determined by competitive PCR. Science 1993;259:1749–1754.
7. Connick E Marr DG, Zhang XQ, et al. HIV-specific cellular and humoral immune responses in primary HIV infection. AIDS Res Hum Retroviruses 1996:12:1129–1140.
8. Perelson AS, Neumann AU, Markowitz M, et al. HIV-1 dynamics in vivo: virion clearance rate, infected cell life-span, and viral generation time. Science 1996;271:1582–1586.
9. Carpenter CC, Fischl MA, Hammer SH, et al. Antiretroviral therapy for HIV infection in 1997: updated recommendations of the International AIDS Society-USA Panel. JAMA 1997;277:1962–1969.
10. Erice A, Mayers DL, Strike DG, et al. Primary infection with zidovudine-resistant human immunodeficiency virus type 1. N Engl J Med 1993;328:1163–1165.
11. Dominquez A, Gamallo G, Garcia R, et al. Pathophysiology of HIV related thrombocytopenia: an analysis of 41 patients. J Clin Pathol 1994;47:999.
12. Hadler SC, Judson FN, O'Malley PM, et al. Outcome of hepatitis B virus infection in homosexual men and its relation to prior human immunodeficiency virus infection. J Infect Dis 1991;163:454.
13. Perelson AS, Essunger P, Cao Y, et al. Decay characteristics of HIV-1-infected compartments during combination therapy. Nature 1997;387:188–191.
14. Mellors JW, Muñoz A, Giorgi JV, et al. Plasma viral load and CD4+ lymphocytes as prognostic markers of HIV-1 infection. Ann Intern Med 1997;126:946–954.
15. Philips AN, Lee CA, Elford J, et al. Serial CD4 lymphocyte counts and development of AIDS. Lancet 1991;337:389.
16. Cao Y, Qin L, Zhang L, et al. Virologic and immunologic characteristics of long-term survivors of human immunodeficiency virus type 1 infection. N Engl J Med 1995;332:201–208.
17. Pantaleo G, Menzo S, Vaccarezza M, et al. Studies in subjects with long-term nonprogressive human immunodeficiency virus infection. N Engl J Med 1995;332:209–216.
18. Markowitz N, Hansen NI, Hopewell PC, et al. Incidence of tuberculosis in the United States among HIV-infected persons. Ann Intern Med 1997;126:123–132.
19. Rolfs RT, Joesoef MR, Hendershot EF, et al. A randomized trial of enhanced therapy for early syphilis in patients with and without human immunodeficiency virus infection. N Engl J Med 1997;337:307–314.
20. Wright TC Jr, Ellerbrook TV, Chiasson MA, et al. Cervical intraepithelial neoplasia in women infected with human immunodeficiency virus: prevalence, risk factors, and validity of Papanicolaou smears. Obstet Gynecol 1994;84:591–597.
21. Septowitz KA, Telzak EE, Carrow M, et al. Fever among outpatients with advanced human immunodeficiency virus infection. Arch Intern Med 1993;153:1909–1912.
22. Johnson JF, Sonnenberg A. Efficient management of diarrhea in the acquired immunodeficiency syndrome (AIDS): a medical decision analysis. Ann Intern Med 1990;112:942–948.
23. Valle S-L. Dermatologic findings related to human immunodeficiency virus infection in high-risk individuals. J Am Acad Dermatol 1987; 17:951.
24. Feigal DW, Katz MH, Greenspan D, et al. The prevalence of oral lesions in HIV-infected homosexual and bisexual men: three San Francisco epidemiology cohorts. AIDS 1991;5:519.
25. CDC. 1997 USPHS/IDSA guidelines for the prevention of opportunistic infections in person infected with human immunodeficiency virus. MMWR Morb Mortal Wkly Rep 1997;46:1–47.
26. Selik RM, Karon JM, Ward JW. Effect of the human immunodeficiency virus epidemic on mortality from opportunistic infections in the United States in 1993. J Infect Dis 1997;176:632–636.
27. Podazamezer D, Salazar A, Jiménez J, et al. Intermittent trimethoprim-sulfamethoxazole compared with dapsone-pyrimethamine for the simultaneous primary prophylaxis of Pneumocystis carinii pneumonia and toxoplasmosis in patients infected with HIV. Ann Intern Med 1995; 122:755–761.
28. Havlir DV, Dubé MP, Sattler FR, et al. Prophylaxis against disseminated Mycobacterium avium complex with weekly azithromycin, daily rifabutin, or both. N Engl J Med 1996; 335:392–398.
29. Pierce M, Crampton S, Henry D, et al. A randomized trial of clarithromycin as prophylaxis against disseminated Mycobacterium avium complex infection in patients with advanced acquired immunodeficiency syndrome. N Engl J Med 1996:335:384–391.
30. Centers for Disease Control and Prevention. 1993 revised classification system for HIV infection and expanded surveillance case definition for AIDS among adolescents and adults. MMWR Morb Mortal Wkly Rep 1992;41:RR-17.
31. Sepkowitz KA, Raffalli J, Riley L, et al Tuberculosis in the AIDS era. Clin Microbiol Rev 1995;8:180–199.
32. Pantongrag-Brown L, Nelson AM, Brown AE, et al. Gastrointestinal manifestations of acquired immunodeficiency syndrome: radiologic–pathologic correlation. Radiographics 1995;15:1155–1178.
33. Wicox CM. Serious gastrointestinal disorders associated with human immunodeficiency virus infection. Crit Care Clin 1993;9:73–88.
34. Simpson DM, Tagliati M. Neurologic manifestations of HIV infection. Ann Intern Med 1994;121:769–785.
35. Holloway RG, Mushlin AI. Intracranial mass lesions in acquired immunodeficiency syndrome: using decision analysis to determine the effectiveness of stereotactic brain biopsy. Neurology 1996;46: 1010–1015.
36. Drew LJ. Cytomegalovirus infection in patients with AIDS. Clin Infect Dis 1992;14:608–615.
37. Grunfield C, Geingold KR. Seminars in medicine of the Beth Israel Hospital, Boston: metabolic disturbances and wasting in the acquired immunodeficiency syndrome. N Engl J Med 1992;327:329–337.
38. Coodley GO, Loveless MO, Merrill TM. The HIV wasting syndrome: a review. J Acquir Immune Defic Syndr 1994;7:681–694.
39. Portgies P, Enting RH, De Gans J, et al. Presentation and course of AIDS dementia complex: 10 years of follow-up in Amsterdam, The Netherlands. AIDS 1993;7:669–675.
40. Hammer SM, Katzenstein DA, Hughes MD, et al. A trial comparing nucleoside monotherapy with combination therapy in HIV-infected adults with CD4 cell counts from 200 to 500 per cubic millimeter: AIDS Clinical Trials Groups Study 175 study team. N Engl J Med 1996;335: 1081–1090.
41. Delta Coordinating Committee. Delta: a randomized double-blind controlled trial comparing combinations with zidovudine plus didanosine or zalcitabine with zidovudine alone in HIV infected individuals. Lancet 1996;348:283–291.
42. Staszewski K, Hill AM, Barlett J, et al. Reductions in HIV-1 disease progression for zidovudine/lamivudine relative to control treatments: a meta-analysis. AIDS 1997;11:577–83.
43. D'Aquila ART, Hughes MD, Johnson VA, et al. Nevirapine, zidovudine, and didanosine compared with zidovudine and didanosine in patients with HIV-1 infection: a randomized, double-blind, placebo-controlled trials. Ann Intern Med 1996;1019–1030.
44. Hammer SM, Squires KE, Hughes MD, et al. A controlled trials of two nucleoside analogues plus indinavir in persons with human immunodeficiency virus infection and CD4 cell counts of 200 per cubic millimeter or less. N Engl J Med 1997;337:725–733.
45. Gulick RM, Mellors JW, Havlir D, et al. Treatment with indinavir, zidovudine, and lamivudine in adults with human immunodeficiency virus infection and prior antiretroviral therapy. N Engl J Med 1997; 337:734–739.

11
AIDS IN WOMEN

Deborah J. Cotton

Acquired immunodeficiency syndrome (AIDS) is now the fourth leading cause of death in American women of childbearing age, and an estimated 107,000 to 160,000 women in the United States are currently living with human immunodeficiency virus (HIV) infection (1). Most these women are young, indigent, and faced with social challenges that often pose more of an immediate threat to their well-being and that of their families than HIV.

Worldwide, estimates are that, by the year 2000, new infections in women will equal those in men (2). The rising global burden of AIDS in women can ultimately be attributed in large measure to the disadvantaged social position of women throughout most of the world. Countless women are not able to determine their sexual experiences or partners. Moreover, they are prevented from learning about or using safer sex techniques. Thus, both here and abroad, one can argue that AIDS in women is a separate epidemic, and approaches to its control need to be gender specific.

EPIDEMIOLOGY AND TRANSMISSION OF HIV INFECTION IN WOMEN

Globally, most women have acquired HIV infection through vaginal intercourse. The efficiency of HIV transmission during vaginal intercourse is greater from man to woman than vice versa (3, 4). Genital ulceration, caused by sexually transmitted diseases (STDs), increases the risk of heterosexual transmission of HIV (5, 6). Nonulcerating STDs may increase the number of inflammatory cells in the genital tract that can serve as target cells for the virus (7). A recent study suggests that bacterial vaginosis may also predispose to HIV transmission (8). Factors that disrupt the lower genital tract epithelium such as tampon use or reaction to intravaginal spermicides may also increase the risk of acquisition of HIV by women (9, 10). HIV has been isolated from menstrual blood (11), and sexual intercourse during menses has been shown to increase the risk of HIV transmission to men (12).

Data on whether oral contraceptives increase the risk of infection are conflicting. Progesterone implants have been shown to increase the risk of infection from inoculation of simiam immunodeficiency virus (SIV) in rhesus macaques, an increase that is believed to be due to thinning of vaginal epithelium (13). Cervical ectopy, which is associated with oral contraceptive use as well as with pregnancy, may also increase the risk of HIV transmission to women (14).

Anal intercourse appears significantly more likely to result in HIV transmission to women than vaginal intercourse, probably because of increased fragility of the anal mucosa (15, 16). Anecdotal cases of female-to-female transmission have been reported, although this mode of transmission appears uncommon (17).

In some industrialized countries such as the United States and many countries of Western Europe, transmission of HIV through intravenous drug use is a major contributor to infection in women (18). Roughly half of all cumulative cases of HIV in women in the United States are in current or past intravenous drug users. Moreover, women who use intravenous drugs are also at risk of HIV infection from sexual partners who have acquired their own infection from intravenous drug use. Attributing all AIDS in women who use intravenous drugs to their drug use may thus underestimate the risk of heterosexual transmission. Use by women of nonintravenous drugs, including alcohol, also contributes to infection through the disinhibiting effects of these agents and through exchange of sex for drugs (19).

In the United States, AIDS cases in women that are caused by heterosexual transmission are now increasing dramatically; in most parts of the country, heterosexual transmission has surpasssed intravenous drug use as the dominant mode of transmission to women (20). Geographically, HIV infection in women has been concentrated in low-income inner-city neighborhoods of major urban areas of the Atlantic seaboard. In these areas, HIV infection is only one of many threats to family health and safety. Drug abuse, domestic and street violence, and lack of availability of basic educational, medical, and social services are major problems. Besides the rising incidence of HIV infection in urban cities, rural areas in the southeastern United States are also showing a rapid increase in the incidence of AIDS in women, largely from heterosexual transmission (21).

Blood transfusion, including that administered for obstetric indications, represented a significant risk factor among women before widespread HIV screening of the blood supply was introduced in industrialized countries in the mid-1980s, and it remains a risk in some parts of the world today. In addition, in many countries, use of unsterilized medical equipment has amplified the epidemic. Finally, most health care workers are women, and although the risk of occupational transmission is low, the number of women at risk through such exposure is large.

NATURAL HISTORY OF HIV INFECTION IN WOMEN

Until recently, few prospective cohort studies were conducted that could assess gender differences in survival or clinical manifestations of HIV. As a result, conclusions regarding the natural history of HIV infection in women have often been based on small case series and anecdotal reports, and they have yielded conflicting data. Although early studies reported significantly shorter survival in women with AIDS compared with men (22, 23), several more recent studies have demonstrated that women have had less access to routine HIV care and to the best current therapies for HIV infection than have men, a finding that confounds assessment of possible biologic differences in survival (24–27). Two large, federally sponsored cohort studies of women in the United States have been established, the Women's Interagency Cohort Study and the HIV Epidemiology Research Study. These studies should provide more detailed data on gender differences in the natural history of HIV infection in the next few years. A third study, the Womens and Infants Transmission Study, was established in 1989 and follows pregnant women and their infants.

The pattern of opportunistic infection and other complications associated with HIV infection differs minimally between women and men (28, 29). Esophageal candidiasis, cytomegalovirus (CMV) disease, and herpes simplex virus disease appear more common in women. Pronounced risk-group differences in the occurrence of HIV-related Kaposi's sarcoma have long been known, with few cases reported in women (30). A recent study suggests that when Kaposi's sarcoma does occur in women, it is more likely to be noncutaneous, to have lymph node involvement, and to be diagnosed later (31). Kaposi's sarcoma is now believed to be due to a novel herpes virus (32).

Gynecologic Disease in Women

Cervical dysplasia and invasive cervical cancer are more prevalent in HIV-infected than in HIV-negative women and are directly correlated with the degree of immunosuppression (33–35). Cervical dysplasia and cancer are believed to be caused by the human papillomaviruses (HPVs); four of these viruses (HPV 16, 18, 31, and 45) account for more than 80% of all such cancers (36, 37).

A recently published prospective study showed that the cumulative presence and persistence of HPV DNA shedding were higher in HIV-seropositive than in HIV-seronegative women, and this was true for all types of HPV including HPV-16 and 18 (38). Persistence was strongly associated with lower CD4 cell counts. Persistent shedding of HPV has been associated with the development of squamous epithelial lesions, and thus it likely accounts for the increased incidence of cervical dysplasia seen in HIV-infected women. Although a direct causal role of HIV in the development of cervical dysplasia has been postulated, present evidence best supports an indirect role of HIV in pathogenesis through its immunosuppressive effects. No evidence has indicated a dramatic increase in the overall incidence of cervical cancer coincident with the HIV epidemic in women to date.

Although pelvic inflammatory disease (PID) is frequent in HIV-infected women, determination of a causal role of HIV in its occurrence or course is even more difficult than with cervical dysplasia and cancer (39–41), because of the known association of PID with a history of early and multiple sex partners (39–41) and with a history of sexually transmitted diseases. Many different menstrual abnormalities have been reported among women with AIDS. However, a recent large, well-controlled study showed no differences in intermenstrual or irregular bleeding or in amenorrhea in HIV-positive compared with HIV-negative women (42). A second study only showed some increase in delayed cycles and amenorrhea and fewer premenstrual symptoms in HIV-positive women (43). Finally, vaginal candidiasis may occur earlier than oral candidiasis and may serve as an early marker of HIV infection in women (44).

In 1993, the United States Centers for Disease Control and Prevention (CDC) added cervical cancer to the list of AIDS-defining conditions (45). Vulvovaginal candidiasis, cervical dysplasia, cervical carcinoma in situ, and PID were also added to the revised classification system of HIV infection, under category B. Category B includes conditions that, although not considered to meet the definition of CDC-defined AIDS, are considered attributable to HIV infection or indicative of a defect in cell-mediated immunity. In addition, category B includes conditions considered by physicians to have a clinical course or to require management that is complicated by HIV infection.

HIV Infection in Pregnancy

Early report of deaths during pregnancy in HIV-infected women led to concerns that HIV could have a significant negative public health impact on maternal morbidity and mortality (46). However, most experts now believe that the risk of pregnancy-accelerated HIV disease progression is low, at least in women who are not in advanced stages of disease. The frequency of bacterial infections in HIV-infected women does appear to be higher during pregnancy and the peripartum period (47–49).

Increasingly effective prophylaxis and therapy for HIV-related opportunistic infections, as well as antiviral therapy, may improve the chances for maternal survival sufficiently to preclude any immediate deleterious effect of intercurrent pregnancy even in women with advanced disease. The greatest maternal danger occurs when HIV infection is not detected or when inadequate prenatal or routine HIV care is received.

VERTICAL TRANSMISSION OF HIV

HIV is vertically transmitted, and estimates of such transmission have varied from 14 to 40% in the absence of antiretroviral therapy (50–52). Women with low CD4 cell counts, high viral load, or symptomatic disease are more likely to transmit infection (50–54). Vitamin A deficiency, smoking, illicit drug use, and coinfection with hepatitis C are also associated with increased risk of vertical transmission (55–58). Evidence to support a major role of intrapartum transmission of HIV includes absence of circulating virus at birth in most infants ultimately found to be infected (59). An increased risk of infection in the firstborn twin and in infants delivered after prolonged rupture of membranes supports the importance of direct contact with virus in the maternal genital tract in vertical transmission (55, 60–63). The association of chorioamnionitis with vertical transmission suggests that placental transmission may also be important (64). Virus has been isolated from fetuses early in gestation; a role of HIV in fetal loss has been suggested (65). Invasive techniques such as amniocentesis, vacuum extraction, fetal monitoring, and use of forceps appear to increase the risk of transmission (63). A role of cesarean section in reducing HIV transmission has been suggested by results of several studies, but it remains controversial (66–69); a meta-analysis did not show a protective effect (70). Breast-feeding is believed to transmit HIV to a previously uninfected infant about 15% of the time, and the risk of transmission appears directly related to the duration of breast-feeding (71, 72).

IMPACT OF AIDS ON WOMEN'S HEALTH CARE

The woman with HIV infection often is a member of an infected family. She may have acquired her infection from her husband or other sexual partner recently or in the distant past. One or more of her children may have been infected vertically. She is often the primary caregiver for other ill family members, despite her own disease, and experience suggests that when women are responsible for others, their own needs are often ignored (73, 74). Even though HIV infection is often a disease of a whole family, care is often fragmented.

Women with HIV infection often have inadequate access to appropriate medical care, either because they live in countries with few services overall or because they are members of socioeconomic groups that rely on clinics or emergency rooms with resultant poor continuity of care. When pregnant, these women may receive late or even no prenatal care. Older women with HIV infection may have one or more significant comorbid medical conditions, complicating overall management.

In addition, because in some countries AIDS is commonly perceived as a disease of men, practitioners may neglect to consider a diagnosis of HIV infection even in the face of symptoms or signs that would prompt HIV testing in a male patient. Because women are often unaware of risk factors in their sexual partners, they may not identify risk even if directly asked.

Additional issues are raised when attempting to provide women with access to clinical trials of promising drugs. In the past, women were often excluded from such protocols, as has traditionally been the case in other diseases, because of concerns over possible teratogenic effects of experimental drugs. Although most HIV trials permit the enrollment of nonpregnant women, participation has lagged when compared with the proportion of AIDS cases in women (75). Enrollment of pregnant women in trials other than those concerning prevention of perinatal transmission remains controversial. Experimental sites often do not provide the types of support services, such as transportation and child care, that are needed by women to participate successfully in drug trials.

MANAGEMENT OF NONPREGNANT WOMEN WITH HIV INFECTION

Initial Assessment

The initial evaluation of the nonpregnant woman with HIV infection should consist of the same elements as for men; that is, a careful medical history and physical examination should be conducted for symptoms and signs indicative of immune dysfunction. Immunizations should be given according to recently published guidelines for the use of vaccines in HIV infection. Serologic testing for syphilis, CMV, and toxoplasmosis should be performed; screening for prior infection with these organisms is especially important for women, given their ramifications for possible future pregnancies. Women who are CMV seronegative who require blood products should receive CMV-negative or leukocyte-filtered preparations. To prevent infection with CMV from young children, careful handwashing should be stressed. Women who are seronegative for *Toxoplasma gondii* should be carefully instructed in measures to avoid acquisition of this organism. Skin testing for tuberculosis should be performed.

In addition to standard evaluations, a detailed sexual and gynecologic history should be obtained, and a full pelvic examination should be performed. Contraceptive advice should be given, and safer sex techniques should be explained. The need for use of both condoms and additional effective birth control should be stressed; women should not rely on condoms alone for pregnancy prevention.

Laboratory Testing and Monitoring

Because some enzyme-linked immunosorbent assays (ELISAs) and all Western blots use whole viral lysates as the source of HIV antigens that can contain human lymphocyte antigens (HLAs), multiparous women may have a higher frequency of false-positive ELISA tests and indeterminate Western blot results because of presence of (HLA) antibodies formed as a consequence of immunization through pregnancy (76). In questionable cases, such as routine pregnancy screening in the absence of known epidemiologic risks, antibody testing should be repeated and viral load and CD4 testing performed to ascertain true infection.

Few data are available on any gender differences in CD4 cell or HIV viral load dynamics. A recent small study showed that women matched for CD4 count and duration of infection had significantly lower serum viral loads than men (77). However, current guidelines for use of these tests for initiation and assessment of antiretroviral treatment and as thresholds for initiation of opportunistic infection prophylaxis should be used for women.

Antiviral Therapy

Concerns have been raised that women may respond differently to antiviral therapies than men; however, only a few clinical trials have enrolled sufficient numbers of women to permit statistically valid subgroup analysis. In addition, few pharmacokinetic studies of drugs used for HIV infection have been performed in women. In a case series of fulminant hepatic necrosis (hepatic steatosis) secondary to zidovudine, most patients were obese women (78). Studies of possible gender differences in drug efficacy and toxicity in women are being conducted in the AIDS Clinical Trials Group (ACTG); analysis of one large trial suggested that women had more didanosine discontinuation and had a more sustained increase in CD4 cells during zidovudine monotherapy compared with men (79). Several other recent antiviral trials showed no gender differences in drug efficacy (80, 81). Protease inhibitors may alter blood levels of oral contraceptives; an alternate form of pregnancy prevention should be used (82, 83).

Prevention and Treatment of Opportunistic Infection

As with antiviral therapy, at present few data are available on the development, detection, or course of opportunistic infection in women compared with men. As previously noted, women may develop esophageal candidiasis more frequently than men, and clinicians should carefully question women about dysphagia or chest pain. Whether women with recurrent vaginal candidiasis are more likely to develop esophageal disease is unknown. Current guidelines for opportunistic infection prophylaxis and treatment should be applied to women. The dangers of inadvertent pregnancy while taking drugs used for treatment of HIV and its complications should be stressed.

MANAGEMENT OF GYNECOLOGIC COMPLICATIONS OF HIV INFECTION

As previously discussed, cervical dysplasia is common in HIV-infected women. Papanicolaou (PAP) testing should be performed every 6 months initially, then yearly if results are normal, given concern that cervical dysplasia may progress more quickly in HIV-infected women. Although a small study suggested that routine PAP smears may be insufficiently sensitive to detect a high proportion of abnormalities subsequently found on colposcopy (84), more recent, larger studies concluded that HIV positivity was not associated with any increased risk of cytologic or histologic discrepancy (34, 85). Thus, most experts continue to recommend PAP smears as the initial screen for cervical dysplasia in HIV-infected women, but with prompt referral of patients with any abnormalities (or with uninterpretable PAP smear results) for consideration of colposcopic evaluation or other follow-up.

Women with asymptomatic HIV infection often have recurrent vaginal yeast infection that may be refractory to treatment. Topical therapy is insufficient in many cases, and repeated courses or long-term suppressive therapy with oral fluconazole may be necessary. When systemic therapy is used, the smallest possible dose and frequency should be prescribed, to prevent emergence of resistance. A recent study in HIV-infected women demonstrated the efficacy of weekly fluconazole at a dose of 200 mg per week in preventing both oropharyngeal and vaginal candidiasis, but not esophageal candidiasis, with in vitro or clinical resistance occurring in less than 5% of isolates (86).

PID is widely believed to be more common and more aggressive in HIV-infected women, although data from formal epidemiologic studies are inconclusive (39–41). Antibiotics should be used that cover the wide range of organisms implicated in PID. In a recent cross-sectional study, women with HIV infection and PID were found to have delayed defervescence and a more frequent need to change antibiotics (87). No differences were noted in the frequency of tuboovarian absess or need for surgery. However, clinicians should have a low threshold for hospitalizing women and initiating aggressive intravenous therapy when the possibility of abscess or peritonitis exists or when the patient fails to respond to outpatient management. Menstrual abnormalities are common in HIV-infected women, but they are not specific; workup and treatment should proceed in the same manner as for HIV-negative women (42, 43).

MANAGEMENT OF HIV INFECTION IN PREGNANCY

Women often learn of their pregnancy and HIV diagnosis at nearly the same time, and they must be educated rapidly to make decisions regarding pregnancy termination, antiretroviral therapy, or prenatal care. Clinics or programs geared to the unique needs of pregnant HIV-infected women are ideal. Wherever care is delivered, attention should be paid to non–HIV-related issues that can have a major impact on maternal and fetal well-being such as nutrition, smoking cessation, immunization, and psychosocial needs. Addicted women are often motivated by pregnancy to seek sobriety, and this decision needs to be supported actively. Recommendations regarding specific management of complications of HIV infection in pregnant women are hampered by a lack of data on the efficacy, toxicity, and teratogenicity of drugs when used in pregnancy.

CD4 Cell Count and Viral Load Monitoring

In a large cohort study of HIV-infected women, CD4 and CD8 percentages remained stable throughout pregnancy. CD4 counts increased modestly; trends of all measurements varied widely (88). At present, the use of standard CD4 cell count thresholds for initiation of antiviral therapy and of opportunistic infection prophylaxis appears warranted. Viral load appears stable during pregnancy in the absence of antiretroviral therapy (53, 89).

The clinician should obtain any known prepregnancy values of CD4 count and viral load, and these values should be measured at the first prenatal visit and tests repeated at least once during the second and third trimesters and at the postpartum visit. Women receiving combination antiretroviral therapy require more frequent testing to assess treatment response.

Immunizations

Updated recommendations on immunization in HIV-infected persons have recently been published (90). Pneumococcal, *Haemophilus influenzae* B, and hepatitis B vaccines are killed preparations that can be given during pregnancy according to standard recommendations. Although some concern has been raised that HIV viral load may increase after immunization, such increases appear to be transient, and their clinical significance is unknown (91, 92). Some experts advise delaying immunization until antiretroviral therapy has maximally suppressed viral load. Influenza vaccine should be given yearly to HIV-positive women regardless of pregnancy status. For pregnant women traveling to areas where polio is endemic, the enhanced, inactivated (Salk) vaccine should be given. Despite the possibility of vaccine-induced maternal and congenital infection, pregnant women who have CD4 cell counts higher than 200 cells/mm^3 can receive measles, mumps, and rubella vaccines when the risk of native disease is considered greater than the theoretic risks of vaccine-induced illness such as for example during an ongoing measles epidemic. Women with more advanced disease should not receive these vaccines because of reports of vaccine-induced disease such as measles pneumonitis (93). Instead, for travel or during an epidemic, they should receive intravenous immunoglobulin.

Antiviral Therapy

The demonstration, in 1994, that zidovudine monotherapy could dramatically reduce the risk of vertical transmission of HIV was a landmark event. More recently, a rapid evolution in understanding of HIV pathogenesis has led to increasingly aggressive management of HIV infection with potent combinations of antiretroviral drugs. These developments have made current care of the pregnant woman with HIV infection extraordinarily complex. In addition, the patient's prior therapy, stage of gestation, and severity of HIV infection need to be taken into account. *The reader is urged to consult primary references and to obtain expert opinion in the management of pregnant women on a case-by-case basis; recommendations that appear here may become quickly outdated.*

ACTG 076

ACTG 076 was a placebo-controlled trial comparing the ability of zidovudine monotherapy versus placebo to decrease vertical transmission of HIV (94). Pregnant women with more than 200 CD4 cells/mm^3 between 14 and 34 weeks' gestation were eligible. The trial was stopped early because of a significant decrease in perinatal transmission rate in women treated with zidovudine (8.3%) versus those who received placebo (25.5%). No maternal side effects were associated with treatment. Neonates who received zidovudine had decreased hemoglobin that reverted to normal levels spontaneously after treatment ended.

Further studies and clinical experience have demonstrated that zidovudine confers a similar benefit in reducing vertical transmission in women with fewer than 200 CD4 cells and in those with prior zidovudine exposure. Only about one-third of the reduction in vertical transmission can be explained by a reduction in maternal HIV plasma viral load (52). There is no viral load threshold below which perinatal transmission has not occurred. Similarly, there is no threshold above which transmission always occurs. Part of the efficacy of zidovudine in preventing vertical transmission may be due to inhibition of reverse transcriptase in the infant; thus, not all currently available antiretroviral agents may be as effective as zidovudine in interrupting vertical transmission.

On the basis of ACTG 076, investigators now recommend that all HIV-infected pregnant women be treated with the 076 regimen. However, in practice, modifications have been made; the current recommendations for zidovudine use as monotherapy in pregnancy are as follows (95):

During pregnancy, at any time after 14 weeks' gestation: zidouvudine 100 mg orally five times daily *or* 200 mg orally three times daily (the latter is now more commonly used)

During labor and delivery: zidovudine, 2-mg/kg intravenous loading dose followed by 1 mg/kg per hour intravenously intrapartum until the umbilical cord is clamped; the regimen should be started 4 hours before scheduled cesarean section.

For the neonate: zidovudine elixir, 2 mg/kg orally four times daily starting at 6 hours of life and continued until 6 weeks of age.

Limitations of ACTG 076 include the inability to determine the relative contribution of each component of therapy (antepartem, intrapartum, or neonatal) to transmission reduction and the lack of data on long-term effects of therapy on women, infected children, and uninfected children. However, to date, no negative long-term outcomes in children in the study have been observed. Small studies and clinical experience have suggested that each component of therapy may be beneficial (96); thus, investigators recommend that pregnant women presenting for care at any time after 14 weeks' gestation be treated, as well as neonates up to 1 week of life born to untreated mothers who are known to be infected with HIV or who are at high risk of HIV infection.

CURRENT PRINCIPLES OF ANTIRETROVIRAL THERAPY IN PREGNANCY

In the last 2 years, new insights into viral pathogenesis have led to increasing use of combination antiretroviral therapy at all stages of HIV infection, and zidovudine monotherapy has been abandoned as a treatment modality for nonpregnant adults. Thus, an increasing number of women are likely to become pregnant while taking combination antiviral therapy. In addition, controversy exists on treatment of pregnant women who present with untreated HIV infection. Several evolving principles may help to guide management:

1. Whenever possible, antiretroviral therapy that maximizes maternal health should be chosen.
2. Pregnant women should be fully informed about what is known of the safety and efficacy of antiretroviral treatments when used in pregnancy, and they should be involved as fully as possible in therapeutic decision-making.
3. In previously untreated women, antiretroviral therapy generally should be deferred until 14 weeks' gestation.
4. Women who present in the first trimester of pregnancy who are already receiving antiretroviral therapy generally should have that therapy continued. Although the risk of teratogenicity of antiretroviral therapies other than zidovudine is currently unknown, cessation of therapy is believed likely to lead to increased levels of circulating virus and viral resistance, potentially both increasing the risk of vertical transmission and adversely affecting maternal prognosis.
5. Because only some of the benefit of zidovudine could be explained through its reduction of plasma viral load, zidovudine should be included as a part of any combination therapy used during pregnancy, except when significant adverse treatment-related effects have occurred or when use would preclude optimal management of the mother's illness.
6. Pregnant women must be informed that no combination of drugs has been shown to be equally or more effective than zidovudine monotherapy in decreasing vertical transmission, although one hopes that combined regimens, through reduction of viral load or other mechanisms, may further reduce the vertical transmission rate below that seen with zidovudine alone in ACTG 076.
7. When a woman has previously not received zidovudine is asymptomatic, has relatively high CD4 counts and low viral load, and is reluctant to assume the risk of newer drugs to her fetus, zidovudine monotherapy may continue to be a reasonable therapeutic modality during pregnancy. Frequent viral load testing should be performed, and a more potent regimen should be given to the mother after delivery.

USE OF COMBINATION ANTIRETROVIRAL THERAPY IN PREGNANCY

At present, no single approach to combination antiretroviral therapy in pregnancy is favored, and clinical trials of pharmacokinetics of antiviral agents in pregnancy are ongoing. Didanosine crosses the placenta, where it is extensively metabolized (97). Nevirapine, a nonnucleoside reverse transcriptase inhibitor, crosses both the blood–brain and placental barriers in rats (98). A recent phase I study of nevirapine in pregnant women demonstrated a long half-life, no maternal or fetal toxicities, and good placental transfer, findings suggesting that this agent may be highly active when given during the intrapartum period (99). A recent trial of intravenous immunoglobulin (IVIG) in combination with zidovudine compared with zidovudine alone in preventing vertical transmission was stopped because of low rates in each arm of the trial, precluding the ability detect significant differences in efficacy between treatments (100). An overview of use of antiretroviral therapy in pregnancy has recently been published (101), and a pregnancy registry sponsored by Glaxo-Wellcome, Inc., has been established. The reader is urged to report confidentially each patient treated with antiviral therapy during pregnancy to that registry: 1-800-722-9292. Information on specific antiviral agents in pregnancy is presented in Table 11.1.

Management of Labor and Delivery

A possible benefit of cesarean delivery in reducing vertical transmission of HIV remains controversial (63, 66–69), and most data are from studies conducted before use of antiviral therapy in pregnancy became widespread. A clinical trial of cesarean section to decrease perinatal transmission has begun in Europe (68). At present, cesarean section should be used for the same indications as in non–HIV-infected women.

Interventions that could either introduce maternal blood into the fetus or increase exposure to maternal secretions should be avoided, such as the use of scalp electrodes, forceps, and vacuum extraction. Fetal membranes should be left intact for as long as possible because transmission has been associated with prolonged membrane rupture; delivery should be completed within 4 hours of membrane rupture (55, 62).

CARCINOGENICITY OF ZIDOVUDINE

Zidovudine has been reported to cause malignant genitourinary tumors in the offspring of rats and mice treated with high doses of the drug for prolonged periods (102). The relevance of these findings to human use is currently unknown; no such tumors have been seen in the offspring of women who received zidovudine as part of ACTG 076 (103). At present, the clear benefit of zidovudine in interrupting vertical transmission is believed to outweigh these possible risks (104).

Table 11.1. Antiretrovirals in Pregnant Women, Neonates, and Children

| | FDA Approved | | | | | |
	For Prevention of Transmission	In Neonates	In Children	FDA Pregnancy Category[a]	Placental Passage	Liquid Form Available
Antiretroviral Agent						
Nucleoside analog reverse transcriptase inhibitors						
Didanosine (ddI, Videx)	No	Yes	Yes	B	Yes (human)	Yes
Lamivudine (3TC, Epivir)	No	No	Yes (>4 mo)	C	Yes (human)	Yes
Stavudine (d4t, Zerit)	No	No	Yes (>1 mo)	C	Yes (rhesus)	Yes
Zalcitabine (ddC, Hivid)	No	No	No	C	Yes (rhesus)	Yes, investigational
Zidovudine (AZT, Retrovir)	Yes	Yes	Yes	C	Yes (human)	Yes
Nonnucleoside reverse transcriptase inhibitors						
Delaviridine (Rescriptor)	No	No	No	C	Unknown	No
Nevirapine (Viramune)	No (phase II study underway)	No	No	C	Yes (human)	Yes, investigational
Protease inhibitors						
Indinavir (Crixivan)	No[b]	No[b]	No	C	Yes (rats)	No
Nelfinavir (Viracept)	No[b]	No[b]	Yes (>2 yr)	B	Unknown	Yes
Ritonavir (Norvir)	No[b]	No[b]	Yes (>2 yr)	B	Yes (rats)	Yes
Saquinavir (Invirase)	No[b]	No[b]	No	B	Unknown	No

[a]US Food and Drug Administration pregnancy categories are:
A. Adequate and well-controlled studies of pregnant women fail to demonstrate a risk to the fetus during the first trimester of pregnancy (with no evidence of risk during later trimesters).
B. Animal reproduction studies fail to demonstrate a risk to the fetus, and adequate, but well-controlled, studies of pregnant women have not been conducted.
C. Safety in human pregnancy has not been determined; animal studies are either positive for fetal risk or have not been conducted, and the drug should not be used unless the potential benefit outweighs the potential risk to the fetus.
D. Positive evidence of human fetal risk is based on adverse reaction data from investigational or marketing experiences, but the potential benefits from the use of the drug in pregnant women may be acceptable despite its potential risks.
X. Studies in animals or reports of adverse reactions have indicated that the risk associated with the use of the drug for pregnant women clearly outweighs any possible benefit.
[b]Phase 1 perinatal protocols underway in the AIDS Clinical Trials Group.
(Data from Federal Register July 9 and October 30, 1997; Perinatal and pediatric HIV guidelines drafts; and Pitts J, Cotton D. Treating the HIV-infected pregnant woman and her child. *AIDS Clin Care* 1997; 9[12].)

PROPHYLAXIS AND THERAPY OF OPPORTUNISTIC INFECTIONS

Almost all opportunistic infections in pregnancy are life-threatening, and thus the benefit to the mother of treatment generally far outweighs any risk to the fetus. Detailed information concerning the use of specific drugs in pregnancy is limited. Standard references, on which most of the following recommendations are based, should be consulted in individual cases (90, 105–107).

Pneumocystis Pneumonia

Although theoretic concern exists that trimethoprim-sulfamethoxazole (TMP–SMX) could cause neonatal kernicterus when given to women at term, most authorities consider TMP–SMX the first-line agent for prevention and therapy of *Pneumocystis carinii* pneumonia (PCP) in pregnant women at all stages of gestation, given its excellent efficacy in the treatment and prophylaxis of PCP (108). A few experts recommend deferring PCP prophylaxis with TMP–SMX until after the first trimester of pregnancy, to avoid any teratogenic risk.

In cases of serious TMP–SMX allergy or intolerance, few data are available to guide choice of agents for prophylaxis or therapy during pregnancy. Intravenous pentamidine is effective for therapy of PCP; however, data on teratogenicity of this agent are limited. Dapsone–trimethoprim or primaquine–clindamycin are reasonable alternatives to TMP–SMX for therapy. Dapsone has been used for many years for treatment of leprosy during pregnancy without evidence of teratogenicity; however, the drug interferes with the glucose-6-phosphate dehydrogenase system. Experience using primaquine during pregnancy in the treatment of malaria is extensive, without reported teratogenicity (109). Primaquine can, however, cause fetal hemolysis. No data are available on the efficacy or safety of aerosolized pentamidine during pregnancy; however, absorption is minimal. Atovaquone is a new oral therapy for PCP; use in pregnant women has been only anecdotal thus far. Trimetrexate should be used only if one has no other alternatives because it is a folate antagonist, and the closely related drug, methotrexate, is a known teratogen (106). Adjunctive steroid therapy should be used in PCP during pregnancy according to the usual guidelines.

Systemic Fungal Disease

Although animal studies have demonstrated possible antiestrogen effects of fluconazole, limited human data have shown no toxicity (110). Anecdotal clinical experience using amphotericin B in pregnancy is substantial, with no reported associated teratogenicity (111–113). Therefore, treating cases of acute cryptococcal meningitis (or other systemic mycosis) with amphotericin appears prudent because this agent has been shown in clinical trials to be more effective than fluconazole alone for acute treatment of cryptococcal meningitis. However, for maintenance therapy of cryptococcal meningitis, fluconazole has clearly been shown to be superior to amphotericin; one approach in pregnancy is to use maintenance therapy with weekly or biweekly amphotericin (1 mg/kg) in the first trimester and to switch to fluconazole beyond 12 to 14 weeks of gestation.

Viral Diseases

Acyclovir use during pregnancy has not revealed any significant teratogenic effects (114). Ganciclovir is a potent cytotoxic agent and has been reported to be both mutagenic and teratogenic in animals; it should be avoided at all stages of pregnancy unless no other alternative exists and disease is considered life-threatening. Foscarnet has been associated with some fetal abnormalities in animal studies; however, the risk appears lower than that associated with ganciclovir, and thus it is the agent of choice to treat life-threatening CMV disease in pregnancy (115). If asymptomatic CMV retinitis is picked up on routine examination, or if symptomatic disease is minimal, it may be possible to delay therapy until after 12 to 14 weeks' gestation. If disease is confined to one eye, ganciclovir or foscarnet implants may also be considered during the first trimester.

Cerebral Toxoplasmosis

Sulfa drugs including sulfadiazine are considered safe in pregnancy despite theoretic concerns regarding neonatal kernicterus when used at term. Similarly, clindamycin has been used widely in pregnant women without apparent adverse fetal outcomes. Pyrimethamine is a mainstay in the therapy of cerebral toxoplasmosis. Although it interferes with folic acid metabolism and is not recommended until after 12 to 14 weeks' gestation, anecdotal use in humans has not demonstrated teratogenicity. In the first trimester of pregnancy, sulfadiazine alone could be used, or, if it is possible to obtain, spiramycin can be added (116). Because pyrimethamine interferes with folic acid metabolism, when it is used, leucovorin should be given as adjunctive therapy. For prophylaxis of toxoplasmosis, nonpyrimethamine-containing regimens should be used.

Tuberculosis and *Mycobacterium avium intracellulare* Infection

Experience with antituberculosis drugs in pregnancy is significant, and, in general, the same indications for prophylaxis and treatment of tuberculosis should be used in pregnant women as in nonpregnant HIV-infected patients (117). Isoniazid, ethanbutol, and rifampin are all considered safe. Data on teratogenicity from pyrazinamide are limited; no teratogenicity has been demonstrated with widespread use. Isoniazid prophylaxis can be deferred in most cases until after the first trimester. Given the morbidity and mortality of *Mycobactrium avium intracellulare* complex and the high risk of occurrence in patients with fewer than 50 CD4 cells/mm^3, prophylaxis is warranted during pregnancy. Azithromycin is the prophylactic drug of choice during pregnancy, because clarithromycin has been shown to be a teratogen in animals (90).

PREVENTION OF HIV INFECTION IN WOMEN

Programs to prevent HIV infection for the most part have focused on the use of condoms and voluntary change of sexual behaviors. However, women face a more complex set of challenges in AIDS prevention. First, it is easier for them to become infected during vaginal intercourse than men, and thus, the use of a condom for each act of intercourse is essential. However, a woman often does not determine whether a condom is used and may suffer many negative consequences including physical violence if she demands condom use.

The development and recent licensure of the "female condom," a vaginal sheath designed to serve both as a contraceptive and safer sex device, as well as other female-controlled contraceptives, are promising developments (118). However, the female condom was given a conditional license without proof of efficacy for prevention of either pregnancy or STD transmission because of the urgency of the epidemic. Factors associated with the use of this device are currently under study (119, 120).

As discussed previously, some studies have suggested that although nonoxynol-9, the active ingredient in spermicides, can effectively kill HIV in vitro (121), it may actually increase the transmission of HIV to women during vaginal intercourse, through vaginal irritation, by altering the vaginal microbiologic flora, or by other means. Some studies suggest that oral contraceptives may also increase the risk of transmission. Trials of vaginal microbicides and gel spermicides are now underway (112, 123). At present, making recommendations to women at risk for HIV for both contraception and infection prevention is difficult; condom use must remain the mainstay of HIV prevention.

HIV TESTING OF WOMEN AT RISK

The detection of HIV infection in women is of the utmost importance to identify and treat affected women and to prevent infection to their sexual partners and offspring. The CDC now recommends that all pregnant women be offered counseling and voluntary HIV testing (124). States receiving HIV funding through the Ryan White Care Act may have to demonstrate either significant reduction in perinatal HIV infection rates or achievement of target goals for HIV testing of pregnant women by 1998 to continue to receive such funding. If goals are not met, states may be required to institute mandatory testing of all infants born of mothers who have refused prenatal HIV testing. Much controversy surrounds the issue of mandatory testing of pregnant women or their infants.

Virtually all experts in HIV infection recommend routine counseling regarding HIV infection for all pregnant women, and some recommend that women be routinely tested for HIV unless they explicitly refuse. At a minimum, physicians and other health care providers should incorporate HIV counseling and voluntary testing into their practices; they should educate themselves on state laws regarding consent and confidentiality of such tests, and they should have a plan in place for care or referral of those patients found to be HIV positive.

While vigorously promoting testing, health care providers must remain mindful of its possible negative consequences. Women who reveal positive serostatus to abusive partners may be harmed. In addition, the pregnant population in the United States is at overall low risk of HIV infection (125), and the issue of false-positive tests and their ramifications must be considered.

In conclusion, HIV infection in women differs in many respects from the disease in men. Women are younger, more impoverished, and more likely to belong to ethnic minorities than men with this disease. Although few clear-cut biologic differences are noted in the course and spectrum of HIV infection in women, less access to health care and HIV drug therapy by women has resulted in poorer survival. Female-specific manifestations of infection including gynecologic complications may lead to additional morbidity and mortality. Major advances in the prevention of vertical transmission create new challenges for the detection and treatment of pregnant women with HIV infection. Finally, methods of prevention of infection in women are currently inadequate, and therefore, the incidence of this disease likely will continue to increase dramatically in women in the United States and worldwide.

References

1. Centers for Disease Control and Prevention. Mortality attributable to HIV infection among persons ages 25–44 years: United States, 1994. MMWR Morb Mortal Wkly Rep 1995;45:121–125.
2. Quinn TC. Global burden of the HIV pandemic. Lancet 1996;348: 480–481.
3. Nicolosi A, Correa Leite ML, Musicco M, et al. The efficiency of male-to-female and female-to-male sexual transmission of the human immunodeficiency virus: a study of 730 stable couples. Italian Study Group on HIV Heterosexual Transmission. Epidemiology 1994; 5:570–575.
4. European Study of the Heterosexual Transmission of HIV. Comparison of female-to-male and male-to-female transmission of HIV in 563 stable couples. BMJ 1992;304:809–813.
5. Plummer FA, Simonsen JN, Cameron DW, et al. Cofactors in male-female sexual transmission of human immunodeficiency virus type 1. J Infect Dis 1991;163:233–239.
6. Rompalo AM, Shepherd M, Lawlor JP, et al. Definitions of genital ulcer disease and variation in risk for prevalent human immunodeficiency virus infection. Sex Transm Dis 1997;24:436–442.
7. Laga M, Manoka A, Kiuuvo M, et al. Nonulcerative sexually transmitted diseases as risk factors for HIV-1 transmission in women: results from a cohort study. AIDS 1993;7:95–102.
8. Sewankambo N, Gray RH, Wawer MJ, et al. HIV-1 infection is associated with abnormal vaginal flora morphology and bacteria vaginosis. Lancet 1997;350:546–550.
9. Raudront D, Frappart L, DeHaas P, et al. Study of the vaginal mucous membrane following tampon utilization: aspect on colposcopy, scanning electron microscopy and transmission electron microscopy. Eur J Obstet Gynecol Reprod Biol 1989;31:53–65.
10. International Working Group on Vaginal Microbicides. Recommendations for the development of vaginal microbicides. AIDS 1996;10:1–6.
11. Vogt MW, Witt DJ, Craven DE, et al. Isolation patterns of human immunodeficiency virus from cervical secretions during the menstrual cycle of women at risk for the acquired immunodeficiency syndrome. Ann Intern Med 1987;106:380–382.
12. Stratton P, Alexander NJ. Prevention of sexually transmitted infections: physical and chemical barrier methods. Infect Dis Clin North Am 1993;7:841–859.
13. Marx PA, Spira AI, Gettie A, et al. Progesterone implants enhance SIV vaginal transmission and early virus load. Nat Med 1996;10: 1084–1089.
14. Moss GB, Clemetson D, D'Costa L, et al. Association of cervical ectopy with heterosexual transmission of human immunodeficiency virus: results of a study of couples in Nairobi, Kenya. J Infect Dis 1991;164:588–591.
15. Lazzarin A, Saracco A, Musicco M, et al. Man-to-woman sexual transmission of the human immunodeficiency virus: risk factors related to sexual behavior, man's infectiousness, and woman's susceptibility. Italian Study Group on HIV Heterosexual Transmission. Arch Intern Med 1991;151:2411–2416.
16. Seidlin M, Vogler M, Lee E, et al. Heterosexual transmission of HIV in a cohort of couples in New York City. AIDS 1993;9:1247–1254.
17. Chu SY, Hammett TA, Buehler JW. Update: epidemiology of reported cases of AIDS in women who report sex only with other women, United States, 1980–1991. AIDS 1992;6:518–519.
18. Wortley PM, Chu SY, Berkelman RC. The epidemiology of HIV/AIDS in women and the impact of the expanded 1993 CDC surveillance definition of AIDS. In: Cotton D, Watts DH, eds. The medical management of AIDS in women. New York: Wiley–Liss, 1997:3–14.
19. Malow RM, Jager KB, Ireland SJ, et al. Alcohol and drug abuse: HIV infection and risky sexual behaviors among women in treatment for noninjection drug dependence. Psychiatr Serv 1996;47:1197–1199.
20. Wortley PM, Fleming PL. AIDS in women in the United States: recent trends. JAMA 1997;278:911–916.
21. Ellerbrock TV, Lieg S, Harrington PE, et al. Heterosexually transmitted human immunodeficiency virus infection among pregnant women in a rural Florida community. N Engl J Med 1992;327:1704–1709.
22. Rothenberg R, Woelfel M, Stoneburner R, et al. Survival with the acquired immunodeficiency syndrome. N Engl J Med 1987;317: 1297–1302.
23. Friedland GH, Saltzman B, Vileno J, et al. Survival differences in patients with AIDS. J Acquir Immun Defic Syndr 1991;4:144–153.
24. Stein M, Piette J, Mor V, et al. Differences on access to zidovudine among symptomatic HIV-infected persons. J Gen Intern Med 1991; 6:35–40.
25. Chaisson RE, Deruly JC, Moore RD. Race, sex, drug use, and progression of human immunodeficiency virus disease. N Engl J Med 1995;333:751–756.
26. Lemp G, Hirozawa A, Cohen J, et al. Survival for women and men with AIDS. J Infect Dis 1992;166:74–79.
27. Melnick SL, Sherer R, Louis TA, et al. Survival and disease progression according to gender of patients with HIV infection: the Terry Beirn Community Programs for Clinical Research on AIDS. JAMA 1994; 272:1915–1921.
28. Fleming PL, Ciesielski VA, Byers RH, et al. Gender differences in reported AIDS-indicative diagnoses. J Infect Dis 1993;168:61–67.
29. Clark RA, Brandon W, Dumestre J, et al. Clinical manifestations of infection with the human immunodeficiency virus in women in Louisiana. Clin Infect Dis 1993;17:173–177.
30. Rabkin CS, Biggar RJ, Horm JW. Increasing incidence of cancers associated with the human immunodeficiency virus epidemic. Int J Cancer 1991;47:692–696.
31. Cooley TP, Hirschhorn LR, O'Keane JC. Kaposi's sarcoma in women with AIDS. AIDS 1996;10:1221–1225.

32. Chang Y, Casarman E, Pessin MS, et al. Identification of herpesvirus-like DNA sequences in AIDS-associated Kaposi's sarcoma. Science 1994;266:1865–1869.
33. Vermund SH, Kelley KF, Klein RS, et al. High risk of human papillomavirus infection and cervical squamous intraepithelial lesions among women with symptomatic human immunodeficiency virus infection. Am J Obstet Gynecol 1991;165:392–400.
34. Wright TC Jr, Ellerbrock TV, Chiasson MA, et al. Cervical intraepithelial neoplasia in women infected with human immunodeficiency virus: prevalence, risk factors, and validity of Papanicolaou smears: New York Cervical Disease Study. Obstet Gynecol 1994;84:591–597.
35. Sun XW, Ellerbrock TW, Lungo O, et al. Human papillomavirus infection in human immunodeficiency virus-seropositive women. Obstet Gynecol 1995;85:680–686.
36. International Agency for Research on Cancer (IARC). Human papillomaviruses: IARC monograph on the evaluation of carcinogenic risks to humans. vol. 64. Lyon, France: IARC, 1995.
37. Shah KV. Human papillomaviruses and anogenital cancers. N Engl J Med 1997;1386–1388.
38. Sun XW, Kuhn L, Ellerbrock TV, et al. Human papillomavirus infection in women infected with the human immunodeficiency virus. N Engl J Med 1997;337:1343–1349.
39. Hoegsberg B, Abulafia O, Sedlis A, et al. Sexually transmitted diseases and human immunodeficiency virus infection among women with pelvic inflammatory disease. Am J Obstet Gynecol 1990;1135–1139.
40. Korn AP, Landers DV, Green JR, et al. Pelvic inflammatory disease in human immunodeficiency virus-infected women. Obstet Gynecol 1993;82:765–768.
41. Irwin KL, Rice RJ, Sperling RS, et al. Potential for bias in studies of the influence of human immunodeficiency virus infection on the recognition, incidence, clinical course, and microbiology of pelvic inflammatory disease. Obstet Gynecol 1994;84:463–469.
42. Ellerbrock TV, Wright TC, Bush TJ, et al. Characteristics of menstruation in women infected with human immunodeficiency virus. Obstet Gynecol 1996;87:1030–1034.
43. Chirgwin KD, Feldman J, Muneyyirci-Delale O, et al. Menstrual function in human immunodeficiency virus–infected women without acquired immunodeficiency syndrome. J Acquir Immune Defic Syndr Hum Retrovirol 1996;12:489–494.
44. Imam W, Carpenter C, Mayer K, et al. Hierarchical pattern of mucosal *Candida* infections in HIV seropositive women. Am J Med 89:142–146.
45. Centers for Disease Control and Prevention. 1993 revised classification system for HIV infection and expanded surveillance case definition for AIDS among adolescents and adults. MMWR Morb Mortal Wkly Rep 1992;41:1–19.
46. Koonin LM, Elklerbrock TV, Atrawsh HK, et al. Pregnancy-associated deaths due to AIDS in the United States. JAMA 1989;3:1306–1309.
47. Goedert JJ, Landesman SH. Serious infections during pregnancy among women with advanced human immunodeficiency virus infection. Am J Obstet Gynecol 1990;162:30–34.
48. Minkoff HL, Willoughby A, Mendes H, et al. Serious infections during pregnancy among women with advanced human immunodeficiency virus infection. Am J Obstet Gynecol 1990;162:30–34.
49. Vermund S, Galbraith M, Ebner SC, et al. Human immunodeficiency syndrome in pregnant women. Ann Epidemiol 1992;2:773–803.
50. Ryder RW, Nsa W, Hassig SE, et al. Perinatal transmission of the human immunodeficiency virus type 1 to infants of seropositive women in Zaire. N Engl J Med 320:1637–1642.
51. European Collaborative Study. Risk factors for mother-to-child transmission. Lancet 1992;339:1007–1012.
52. Sperling RS, Shapiro DE, Coombs RW, et al. Maternal viral load, zidovudine treatment, and the risk of transmission of human immunodeficiency virus type 1 from mother to infant: Pediatric AIDS Clinical Trials Group Protocol 076 Study Group. N Engl J Med 1996;335:1621–1629.
53. Mayaux MJ, Dussaix E, Isopet J, et al. Maternal virus load during pregnancy and mother-to-child transmission of human immunodeficiency virus type 1: the French perinatal cohort studies. SEROGEST Cohort Group. J Infect Dis 1997;175:172–175.
54. Mofenson LM. Mother-to-child HIV-1 transmission: timing and determinants. Obstet Gynecol Clin North Am 1997;24(4):759–784.
55. Burns DN, Landesman S, Meunz LR, et al. Cigarette smoking, premature rupture of membranes, and vertical transmission of HIV-1 among women with low CD4+ levels. J Acquir Immune Defic Syndr 1994;7:718–726.
56. Rodriquez EM, Mofenson LM, Chang BH, et al. Association of maternal drug use during pregnancy with maternal HIV culture positivity and perinatal HIV transmission. AIDS 1996;10:273–282.
57. Greenberg BL, Semba RD, Vink PE, et al. Vitamin A deficiency and maternal–infant transmissions of HIV in two metropolitan areas in the United States. AIDS 1997;11:325–332.
58. Hershow RC, Riestser KA, Lew J, et al. Increased vertical transmission of human immunodeficiency virus from hepatitis C virus-coinfected mothers. Women and infants transmission study. J Infect Dis 1997;176:414–420.
59. Kalish LA, Pitt J, Lew J, et al. Defining the time of fetal or perinatal acquisition of human immunodeficiency virus type 1 infection on the basis of age at first positive culture: Women and Infants Transmission Study (WITS). J Infect Dis 1997;175:712–715.
60. Goedert JJ. Duliege Am, Amos CT, et al. High risk of HIV-1 infection for first-born twins. Lancet 1991;1471–1475.
61. Duliege AM, Amos CI, Felton S, et al. Birth order, delivery route, and concordance in the transmission of human immunodeficiency virus type 1 from mothers to twins: International Registry of HIV-Exposed Twins. J Pediatr 1995;126:625–632.
62. Landesman SH, Kalish LA, Burns DN, et al. Obstetrical factors and the transmission of human immunodeficiency virus type 1 from mother to child. N Engl J Med 1996;334:1617–1623.
63. Mandelbrot L, Mayaux MJ, Bongain A, et al. Obstetric factors and mother-to-child transmission of human immunodeficiency virus type 1: the French perinatal cohorts. Am J Obstet Gynecol 1996;175:661–667.
64. Temmerman M, Nyong'o AO, Bwayo J, et al. Risk factors for mother-to-child transmission of human immunodeficiency virus-1 infection. Am J Obstet Gynecol 1995;172:700–705.
65. Langston C, Lewis DE, Hammill HA, et al. Excess intrauterine fetal demise associated with maternal human immunodeficiency virus infection. J Infect Dis 1995;172:1451–1460.
66. Newell ML, Dunn D, Peckham CS, et al. Caesarean section and risk of vertical transmission of HIV-1 infection: European Collaborative Study. Lancet 1994;343:1464–1467.
67. Tovo PA, de Martino M, Gabiano C, et al. Mode of delivery and gestational age influence perinatal HIV-1 transmission: Italian Register for HIV infection in Children. J Acquir Immune Defic Syndr Hum Retrovirol 1996;11:88–94.
68. Peckham C, Newell ML. Human immunodeficiency virus infection and mode of delivery. Acta Paediatr Suppl 1997;421:104–106.
69. Bobat R, Coovadia H, Coutsoudis A, et al. Determinants of mother-to-child transmission of human immunodeficiency virus type 1 infection in a cohort from Durban, South Africa. Pediatr Infect Dis J 1996;15:604–610.
70. Dunn DT, Newell ML, Mayaux C, et al. Mode of delivery and vertical transmission of HIV-1: a review of prospective studies. J Acquir Immune Defic Syndr Hum Retrovirol 1994;7:1064–1066.
71. Dunn DT, Newell ML, Ades AE, et al. Risk of human immunodeficiency virus type 1 transmission through breast-feeding. Lancet 1992;340:585–588.
72. Bertolli J, St. Louis ME, Simonds RJ, et al. Estimating the timing of mother-to-child transmission of human immunodeficiency virus in a breast-feeding population in Kinshasa, Zaire. J Infect Dis 1996;174:722–726.
73. Callaway CC, Brady MT, Crim LB, et al. Family-centered care provides women with a one-stop shopping approach [abstract P2.52]. In: National Conference on Women with HIV, Los Angeles, 1997:185.

74. Kloser P. Primary care of women with HIV disease. In Cotton D, Watts H, eds. The medical management of AIDS in women. New York: Wiley–Liss, 1997.
75. Cotton DJ, Finkelstein DM, He W, et al. Determinants of accrual of women to a large, multicenter clinical trials program of human immunodeficiency virus infection. J Acquir Immune Defic Syndr 1993;6:1322–1328.
76. Sayers MH, Beatty PG, Hansen JA. HLA antibodies as a cause of false-positive reactions in screening enzyme immunoassays for antibodies to human T-lymphotrophic virus type III. Transfusion 1986; 26:113–115.
77. Evans JS, Nims T, Cooley J, et al. Serum levels of virus burden in early-stage human immunodeficiency virus type 1 disease in women. J Infect Dis 1997;175:795.
78. Freiman SP, Helfert KE, Hamrell MR, et al. Hepatomegaly with severe steatosis in HIV-seropositive patients. AIDS 1993;7:379–385.
79. Currier JS, Spino CS, Grimes J, et al. Gender differences in toxicity rates and CD4 responses to nucleoside analogue therapy in ACTG 175 [abstract 290]. In: 11th International Conference on AIDS, Vancouver, 1996:224.
80. Bartlett JA, Benoit SL, Johnson VA, et al. Lamivudine plus zidovudine compared with zalcitabine plus zidovudine in trial: North American HIV Working Party. Ann Intern Med 1996;125:161–172.
81. Everson RE, Weidle PJ, Perdue BE, et al. Evaluation of drug interactions with indinavir [abstract 611]. In: 4th Conference on Retroviruses and Opportunistic Infection. Washington, DC: American Society for Microbiology, 1997:177.
82. Ouellet D, Hsu A, Qian J, et al. Effect of ritonavir on the pharmacokinetics of ethinyl estradiol in healthy female volunteers [abstract Mo.B.1198]. In: 11th International Conference on AIDS, Vancouver, 1996;88.
83. Saravolatz LD, Winslow DL, Collins G, et al. Zidovudine alone or in combination with didanosine or zalcitabine in HIV-infected patients with the acquired immunodeficiency syndrome or fewer than 200 CD4 cells per cubic millimeter. N Engl J Med 1996;335:1099–1106.
84. Maiman M, Tarricone N, Viera J, et al. Colposcopic evaluation of human immunodeficiency virus–seropositive women. Obstet Gynecol 1991;78:84–88.
85. Boardman LA, Peipert JF, Cooper AS, et al. Cytologic–histologic discrepancy in human immunodeficiency virus-positive women referred to a colposcopy clinic. Obstet Gynecol 1994;84:1016–1020.
86. Schuman P, Capps L, Peng G, et al. Weekly fluconazole for the prevention of mucosal candidiasis in women with HIV infection: a randomized, double-blind, placebo-controlled trial. Terry Beirn Community Programs for Clinical Research on AIDS. Ann Intern Med 1997;126:689–696.
87. Barbosa C, Macasaet M, Brockmann S, et al. Pelvic inflammatory disease and human immunodeficiency virus infection. Obstet Gynecol 1997;89:65–70.
88. Tuomala RE, Kalish LA, Zorilla C, et al. Changes in total, CD4+, and CD8+ lymphocytes during pregnancy and one year postpartum in human immunodeficiency virus–infected women: the Women and Infants Transmission Study. Obstet Gynecol 1997;89:967–974.
89. Melvin AJ, Burchett SK, Watts DH, et al. Effect of pregnancy and zidovudine therapy on viral load in HIV-1–infected women. J Acquir Immune Defic Syndr Hum Retrovirol 1997;14:232–236.
90. United States Public Health Service/Infectious Disease Society of America (USPHS/IDSA) Prevention of Opportunistic Infection Working Group. 1997 USPHS/IDSA guidelines for the prevention of opportunistic persons infected with the human immunodeficiency virus. Ann Intern Med 1997;127:922.
91. Jackson CR, Vavro CL, Valentine ME, et al. Effect of influenza immunization on immunologic and virologic characteristics of pediatric patients infected with human immunodeficiency virus. Pediatr Infect Dis J 1997;16:200–204.
92. Fowke KR, D'Amico R, Chernoff DN, et al. Immunologic and virologic evaluation after influenza vaccination of HIV-1–infected patients. AIDS 1997;11:1013–1021.
93. MMWR Morb Mortal Wkly Rep. Measles pneumonitis following measles–mumps–rubella vaccination of a patient with HIV infection, 1993. MMWR Morb Mortal Wkly Rep 1996;45:603–606.
94. Connor E, Sperling R, Gelber R, et al. Reduction of maternal–infant transmission of human immunodeficiency virus 1 with zidovudine treatment: results of AIDS Clinical Trials Group Protocol 076. N Engl J Med 1994;331:1173–1180.
95. United States Public Health Service. US Public Health Service recommendations for use of antiretroviral drugs during pregnancy for maternal health and reduction of perinatal transmission of human immunodeficiency virus type 1 in the United States. Federal Register July 3, 1997;62(131).
96. Simpson BJ, Shapiro ED, Andiman WA. Reduction in the risk of vertical transmission of HIV-1 associated with treatment of pregnant women with orally administered zidovudine alone. J Acquir Immune Defic Syndr Hum Retrovirol 1997;14:145–152.
97. Henderson GI, Perez AB, Yang Y, et al. Transfer of dideoxyinosine across the human isolated placenta. Br J Clin Pharmacol 1994;38:237–242.
98. Siverstein H, Riska P, Johnstone JN, et al. Nevirapine, a nonnucleoside reverse transcriptase inhibitor, freely enters the brain and crosses the placental barrier [abstract no. Tu.B.2325]. In: 11th International Conference on AIDS, Vancouver, 1996;321.
99. Mirochnick M, Sullivan J, Cort S, et al. Safety and pharmacokinetics (pk) of nevirapine (NVP) in HIV-1 infected pregnant women and their newborns: ACTG Protocl 250 Team. In: American Pediatric Association and Society for Pediatric Research annual meeting, May 6–10, 1996, Washington, DC. Pediatr AIDS HIV Infect 1996;7:280.
100. McKinney RE Jr. Ongoing and future trials of antiretroviral therapy in the pediatric AIDS clinical trials group (PACTG) [abstract 173]. In: 3rd Conference on Retroviruses and Opportunistic Infection. Washington, DC: American Society for Microbiology, 1996.
101. Minkoff H, Augenbraun M. Antiretroviral therapy for pregnant women. Am J Obstet Gynecol 1997;176:478–489.
102. Ayers KM, Torrey CE, Reynolds DJ. A transplancental carcinogenicity bioassay in CD-1 mice treated with zidovudine. Fundam Appl Toxicol 1997;38:195–198.
103. Hanson IC, Cooper E, Antonelli T, et al. Lack of tumors in infants with perinatal HIV exposure and fetal/neonatal exposure to zidovudine (AZT).
104. Rowe PM. US expert panel reaffirms benefit of perinatal zidovudine. Lancet 1997;349:258.
105. Rayburn WF. Chronic medical disorders during pregnancy: guidelines for prescribing drugs. J Reprod Med 1997,42:1–24.
106. Sorosky JI, Sood AK, Bueker TE. The use of chemotherapeutic agents during pregnancy. Obstet Gynecol Clin North Am 1997;24:591–599.
107. United States Pharmacopeia. DI: drug information for the health care professional. 17th ed. vol. 1. Rockville, MD: United States Pharmacopeial Convention, 1997.
108. Decker CF, Masur A. Management and prevention of *Pneumocystis carinii* pneumonia. In: Cotton D, Watts H, eds. The medical management of AIDS in women. New York: Wiley–Liss, 1997.
109. Phillips-Howard PA, Wood D. The safety of antimalarial drugs in pregnancy. Drug Saf 1996;14:131–145.
110. Inman W, Pearce G, Wilton L. Safety of fluconazole in the treatment of vaginal candidiasis: a prescription-event monitoring study, with special reference to the outcome of pregnancy. Eur J Clin Pharmacol 1994;46:115–118.
111. Ismail MA, Lerner SA. Disseminated blastomycosis in a pregnant woman: review of amphotericin B usage during pregnancy. Am Rev Respir Dis 1982;126:350–353.
112. Stafford CR, Fisher JF, Fadel HE, et al. Cryptococcal meningitis in pregnancy. Obstet Gynecol 1983;62:35–37.

113. Dean JL, Wolf JE, Ranzini AC, et al. Use of amphotericin B during pregnancy: case report and review. Clin Infect Dis 1994;18:364–368.
114. Andrews EB, Yankaskas BC, Cordero JF, et al. Acyclovir in pregnancy registry: six years' experience: the Acyclovir in Pregnancy Registry Advisory Committee. Obstet Gynecol 1992;79:7–13.
115. Hitti J, Watts H. Antiviral therapy in pregnancy. In: Cotton D, Watts H, eds. The medical management of AIDS in women. New York: Wiley–Liss, 1997:218–219.
116. Mariuz P, Bosler EM, Luft BJ. Toxoplasmosis in HIV-infected women. In: Cotton D, Watts H, eds. The medical management of AIDS in women. New York: Wiley–Liss, 1997:321–343.
117. Brost BC, Newman RB. The maternal and fetal effects of tuberculosis therapy. Obstet Gynecol Clin North Am 1997;24:659–673.
118. Elias CJ, Coggis C. Female-controlled methods to prevent sexual transmission of HIV. AIDS 1996;3:43–51.
119. McCabe E, Golub S, Lee AC. Making the female condom a "reality" for adolescents. J. Pediatr Adolesc Gynecol 1997;10:15–23.
120. Sly DF, Quadagno D, Harrison DF, et al. Factors associated with use of the female condom. Fam Plann Perspect 1997;29:181–184.
121. Jennings R, Clegg A. The inhibitory effect of spermicidal agents on replication of HSV-2 and HIV-1 in-vitro. J Antimicrob Chemother 1993;32:71–82.
122. Biggar RJ, Miotti PG, Taha TE, et al. Perinatal intervention trial in Africa: effect of birth canal cleansing intervention to prevent HIV transmission. Lancet 1996;347:1647–1650.
123. Martin HL Jr, Stevens CE, Richardson BA, et al. Safety of a nonoxynol-9 vaginal gel in Kenyan prostitutes: a randomized clinical study. Sex Transm Dis 1997;24:279–283.
124. Centers for Disease Control. US Public Health Service recommendations for human immunodeficiency virus counseling and voluntary testing for pregnant women. MMWR Morb Mortal Wkly Rep 1995;44:1–14.
125. Rogers MF. Epidemiology of HIV/AIDS in women and children in the USA. Acta Paediatr Suppl 1997;421:15–26.

12

SPECIAL CONSIDERATIONS IN CHILDREN

Cecelia Hutto and Gwendolyn B. Scott

Many aspects of human immunodeficiency virus type 1 (HIV-1) infection in children and adults are similar. The epidemiology of pediatric AIDS mirrors the epidemiology of HIV-1–infected women, and many of the opportunistic infections and other associated clinical diseases are not unlike those described for adults. However, certain characteristics of HIV-1 are unique to children. The most significant differences may be secondary to the route and timing of infection for the overwhelming majority of infected children, that is, perinatal acquisition. Perinatal transmission leads to diagnostic considerations that are different for young infants than for older children and adults, and it contributes to differences in both the natural history of infection and the spectrum of clinical disease. In this chapter, aspects of HIV-1 infection unique to children are emphasized.

EPIDEMIOLOGY

In the United States and in most areas of the world today, the primary route of HIV-1 infection in children is by intrauterine or perinatal transmission of virus from the mother to her child. Data from the Centers for Disease Control and Prevention (CDC) indicate that 7689 cases of AIDS had been reported in children younger than 13 years of age by December 1996 (1). Of these, 90% were associated with perinatal transmission, 8% with exposure to infected blood or blood products, and, in 2%, a route of transmission was not identified. Children may also become infected through sexual abuse, but the incidence of infection by this route in children is not known (2).

The magnitude of the HIV-1 epidemic in children in the United States is not known because reporting of HIV-1 infections is not required by all states. Using data from the National HIV-1 Surveillance of HIV-1 Seropositivity Among Childbearing Women Project and from a multicenter pediatric HIV-1 surveillance project, investigators from the CDC estimated that about 15,000 HIV-1–infected children were born in the United States between 1978 and 1983 (3). This estimation, although still underrepresenting the epidemic, provides a clearer picture than data that include only cases of AIDS.

States with large urban areas in the eastern United States including New York, New Jersey, and Florida have reported the largest number of pediatric cases. In 1996 alone, more than 40% of the 678 pediatric cases were reported from New York and Florida. However, almost all states and territories of the United States have reported cases of AIDS in children. Pediatric HIV-1 infections are seen increasingly in less populated states, smaller cities, and even rural areas.

Most cases of AIDS in children have been reported in minority populations. The proportion of all reported cases by race and ethnicity is as follows: white, not Hispanic 18%; black, not Hispanic 58%; Hispanic 23%; and others, less than 1%.

PEDIATRIC CASE DEFINITION AND CLASSIFICATION

Criteria for diagnosis of HIV-1 infection in infants and children younger than 13 years of age and for classification of infected children have been published by the CDC. Increasing experience and knowledge of the natural history of HIV-1 infection and its associated disease has led to revisions in these criteria over time. The most recent criteria were published in 1994 (Tables 12.1 to 12.4) (4). The definition of infection in infants and children is age dependent. Diagnosis of infection in infants requires laboratory assays that can detect the virus directly such as polymerase chain reaction (PCR) or antigen assays. In children older than 18 months of age, the demonstration of HIV-1 immunoglobulin G (IgG) antibody by a reactive enzyme immunoassay and secondary confirmatory assay may be used for diagnosis of infection.

The most recent classification system for HIV-1–infected children is based on both clinical and immunologic criteria (see Tables 12.2 to 12.4). The immunologic criteria use the absolute CD4+ lymphocyte number and the CD4+ lymphocyte percentage. Because the CD4+ lymphocyte numbers and CD4+ lymphocyte percentages vary by age, the criteria for classifying children according to the level of immunosuppression is based on age-adjusted norms. In addition to immunologic classification, children are also classified based on clinical criteria into one of four stages that include N, A, B, or C. Stage N is the most benign classification and includes only children who are asymptomatic. Children with the most serious disease manifestations, AIDS-defining illnesses, are classified as stage C. Lymphoid interstitial pneumonitis (LIP) is the only AIDS-defining illness not classified as stage C but is a stage B manifestation. The categories are mutually exclusive, and a child's clinical classification is based on the most severe manifestation of the infection.

PERINATAL TRANSMISSION

Transmission of HIV-1 from mother to fetus or infant is the route by which most children throughout the world acquire infection. For simplicity, this route of transmission is termed "perinatal transmission" despite the recognition that transmission may occur months before delivery as well as around the time of delivery. Many studies provide both direct and indirect evidence that transmission from mother to child can occur in utero by transplacental passage of virus, intrapartum through contact with infected maternal blood and cervical secretions, or in the postpartum period through breast-feeding.

The demonstration of HIV-1 in fetal tissues by in situ studies and PCR as early as the first trimester of pregnancy is the most direct evidence of intrauterine infection (5–7). Evidence of intrapartum transmission, which is presumed to occur by contact of the infant during labor and delivery with infected maternal blood or secretions in the birth canal, is less direct. Studies of twins born to infected mothers provide evidence for intrapartum transmission. Both twins may be infected, they may be uninfected, or they may have a discordant outcome. Studies of twins with discordant infection outcomes found that the firstborn twin of either a vaginal or cesarean delivery has a significantly greater risk of infection than the secondborn twin (8). Because the firstborn twin is the one most exposed to maternal blood and secretions during delivery, this finding suggests that intrapartum exposure is important for transmission of infection and helps to explain the greater risk of infection for the firstborn twin. In more than 50% of infants born to HIV-1 seropositive mothers who are subsequently determined to be infected, one cannot detect virus at birth by either culture or PCR (9, 10). Infection can be detected in most of these infants by 2 months of age. Although the presence of virus in lymph nodes or another privileged site at the time of delivery cannot be excluded, investigators assume that the failure to detect virus at birth results from intrapartum transmission of virus in quantities that cannot be detected at birth. The inability to detect virus in infected infants until a week or more after birth has been used as an empiric definition of intrapartum transmission (11). Other evidence supporting the occurrence of intrapartum transmission is provided by studies that report a higher risk of transmission in infants who are born after rupture of maternal amniotic membranes for more than

Table 12.1. Definition of HIV Infection in Children

1. A child < 18 months of age, who is known to be HIV seropositive or born to an HIV-infected mother and:
   - Has positive results on two separate determinations (excluding cord blood) using one or more of the following HIV detection tests:
     HIV virus culture
     HIV polymerase chain reaction
     HIV antigen (p24) OR
   - Meets diagnosis of AIDS based on the 1987 AIDS case definition
2. A child ≥ 18 months of age born to an HIV-infected mother or a child infected by blood, blood products, or other known mode of transmission such as sexual contact who
   - Is HIV antibody positive by repeatedly reactive enzyme immunoassay and a confirmatory test (e.g., Western blot, immunofluorescence assay) OR
   - Meets any of the criteria in (1) above

(From Centers for Disease Control and Prevention. 1994 revised classification system for human immunodeficiency virus infection in children under 13 years of age. MMWR Morb Mortal Wkly Rep 1994;43:1–9.)

Table 12.2. Pediatric HIV Classification

Immunologic Categories	Clinical Categories			
	N: No signs/symptoms	A: Mild signs/symptoms	B: Moderate signs/symptoms	C: Severe signs/symptoms
1: No evidence of suppression	N1	A1	B1	C1
2: Evidence of moderate suppression	N2	A2	B2	C2
3: Severe suppression	N3	A3	B3	C3

(From Centers for Disease Control and Prevention. 1994 revised classification system for human immunodeficiency virus infection in children under 13 years of age. MMWR Morb Mortal Wkly Rep 1994;43:1–9.)

Table 12.3. Immunologic Categories Based on Age-Specific CD4+ T-Lymphocyte Counts and Percentage of Total Lymphocytes

Immunologic Category	Age of Child					
	< 12 mo		1–5 y		6–12 y	
	Count	Percentage (%)	Count	Percentage (%)	Count	Percentage (%)
1: No evidence of suppression	≥ 1,500	(≥ 25)	≥ 1,000	(≥ 25)	≥ 500	(≥ 25)
2: Evidence of moderate suppression	750–1,499	(15–24)	500–999	(15–24)	200–499	(15–24)
3. Severe suppression	< 750	(< 15)	< 500	(< 15)	< 200	(< 15)

(From Centers for Disease Control and Prevention. 1994 revised classification system for human immunodeficiency virus infection in children under 13 years of age. MMWR Morb Mortal Wkly Rep 1994;43:1–9.)

Table 12.4. Clinical Categories for Children with HIV Infection

Category N: Not symptomatic
  Children who have no signs or symptoms considered to be the result of HIV infection or who have only one of the conditions listed in category A
Category A: Mildly symptomatic
  Children with two or more of the conditions listed below but none of the conditions listed in categories B and C
  - Lymphadenopathy (≥ 0.5 cm at more than two sites; bilateral indicates one site)
  - Hepatomegaly
  - Splenomegaly
  - Dermatitis
  - Parotitis
  - Recurrent or persistent upper respiratory infection, sinusitis, or otitis media
Category B: Moderately symptomatic
  Children who have symptomatic conditions other than those listed for category A or C that are attributed to HIV infection; examples of conditions in clinical category B include but are not limited to:
  - Anemia (< 8 g/dL), neutropenia (< 1000/mm^3), or thrombocytopenia (< 100,000/mm^3) persisting ≥ 30 d
  - Bacterial meningitis, pneumonia, or sepsis (single episode)
  - Candidiasis, oropharyngeal (thrush), persisting (> 2 months) in children > 6 mo of age
  - Cardiomyopathy
  - Cytomegalovirus infection, with onset before 1 mo of age
  - Diarrhea, recurrent or chronic
  - Hepatitis
  - Herpes simplex virus (HSV) stomatitis, recurrent (more than two episodes within 1 yr)
  - HSV bronchitis, pneumonitis, or esophagitis with onset before 1 mo of age
  - Herpes zoster (shingles) involving at least two distinct episodes or more than one dermatome
  - Leiomyosarcoma
  - Lymphoid interstitial pneumonia or pulmonary lymphoid hyperplasia complex
  - Nephropathy
  - Nocardiosis
  - Persistent fever (lasting > 1 mo)
  - Toxoplasmosis, onset before 1 mo of age
  - Varicella, disseminated (complicated chickenpox)
Category C: Severely symptomatic
- Serious bacterial infections, multiple or recurrent (i.e., any combination of at least two culture-confirmed infections within a 2-y period), of the following types: septicemia, pneumonia, meningitis, bone or joint infection, or abscess of an internal organ or body cavity (excluding otitis media, superficial skin or mucosal abscesses, and indwelling catheter–related infections)
- Candidiasis, esophageal or pulmonary (bronch, trachea, lungs)
- Coccidioidomycosis, disseminated (at site other than or in addition to lungs or cervical or hilar lymph nodes)
- Cryptococcosis, extrapulmonary
- Cryptosporidiosis or isosporiasis with diarrhea persisting > 1 mo
- Cytomegalovirus disease with onset of symptoms at age > 1 mo (at a site other than liver, spleen, or lymph nodes)
- Encephalopathy (at least one of the following progressive findings present for at least 2 mo in the absence of a concurrent illness other than HIV infection that could explain the findings): a) failure to attain or loss of developmental milestones or loss of intellectual ability, verified by standard developmental scale or neuropsychological tests; b) impaired brain growth or acquired microcephaly demonstrated by head circumference measurements or brain atrophy demonstrated by CT or MRI (series imaging is required for children < 2 y of age); c) acquired symmetric motor deficit manifested by two or more of the following: paresis, pathologic reflexes, ataxia, or gait disturbance
- Herpes simplex virus infection causing a mucocutaneous ulcer that persists for > 1 mo; or bronchitis, pneumonitis, or esophagitis for any duration affecting a child > 1 mo of age
- Histoplasmosis, disseminated (at a site other than or in addition to lungs or cervical or hilar lymph nodes)
- Kaposi's sarcoma
- Lymphoma, primary, in brain
- Lymphoma, small, noncleaved cell (Burkitt's), or immunoblastic or large cell lymphoma of B-cell or unknown immunologic phenotype
- *Mycobacterium tuberculosis,* disseminated or extrapulmonary

(From Centers for Disease Control and Prevention. 1994 revised classification system for human immunodeficiency virus infection in children under 13 years of age. MMWR Morb Mortal Wkly Rep 1994;43:1–9.)

4 hours (12). Finally, most infected infants are born at term and are asymptomatic, a finding that is consistent with transmission either in late gestation or at delivery.

Breast-feeding is another potential route of perinatal infection that has been established for infants. HIV-1 can be isolated from breast milk (13). Case reports of mothers who became infected in the postpartum period through blood transfusions they required because of peripartum complications and who subsequently breast-fed their infants, who were also later determined to be infected, provides strong indirect evidence of transmission through breast-feeding (14–18). Although breast-feeding is not as significant a route of transmission in the United States and other industrialized countries where infected women are counseled not to breast-feed, it is a major concern in developing countries where no safe alternatives for infant feeding exist. A meta-analysis of prospective studies that attempted to quantify the risk associated with breast-feeding reported risks that ranged from 7 to 22 % (19). A study in South Africa evaluated two groups of women for rate of perinatal transmission (20). The women were grouped according to whether they chose to formula-feed or breast-feed their infants. The rate of transmission for the two groups of mothers, who were not significantly different for mode of delivery or CD4+ lymphocyte number, was 46% for breast-fed infants and 18% for infants receiving formula; this finding suggests that the risk associated with breast-feeding is high in some populations. Why the risk is so variable is not clear, but factors such as stage of maternal infection, maternal viral load, and duration of feeding may be important.

The overall rate of perinatal infection among populations studied throughout the world has ranged from 13% to almost 40% (21–26). The lowest rates were reported from Europe and the highest from countries in Africa (23, 24, 26). The transmission rate among infants in a large prospective study in Miami, Florida was 30% (22). Determining why the majority of infants born to seropositive mothers are not infected has been the focus of intense study. Several maternal demographic, clinical, virologic, and immunologic factors, as well as obstetric practices and complications, have been investigated to understand their role in transmission (Table 12.5). The maternal factors that have been most consistently correlated with perinatal HIV-1 transmission are maternal clinical stage, CD4+ lymphocyte number, and viral load at delivery. The risk of transmission is greatest among mothers with AIDS during pregnancy (23, 25), and an inverse correlation exists between maternal CD4+ lymphocyte number during pregnancy and risk of perinatal transmission (27–31). Because clinical stage is closely correlated to CD4+ cell number, these two variables probably are interdependent. Maternal viral load has been shown to be directly correlated with risk of transmission. Studies using p24 antigenemia, quantitative cell culture, and quantitative DNA assays have shown a direct correlation between transmission and virus burden in the mother (24, 27, 30–33). More recently, RNA PCR studies that quantitate maternal plasma virus have also demonstrated a striking correlation between transmission risk and HIV-1 plasma RNA copy number (30, 34–36). A wide range in the plasma RNA copy number has been reported in infected pregnant women, and transmission has been reported in association with the entire spectrum of maternal RNA levels. Transmission rates were highest, however, in women with the highest levels of plasma RNA. Sperling and coinvestigators, using data from the AIDS Clinical Trials Group (ACTG) 076 trial, which studied the effect of zidovudine (ZDV) in reducing perinatal transmission, grouped mothers by quartiles in which their RNA copy numbers fell (34). Transmission was greater than 40% among women who were in the highest quartile for plasma RNA levels.

Perinatal transmission is clearly correlated with maternal disease stage, CD4+ lymphocyte number, and viral load, but transmission also occurs in women with low RNA levels, in those with normal CD4+ lymphocyte numbers, and in women who are asymptomatic. This finding suggests that other factors also play a role in transmission. Data from studies examining the role of antibodies in protecting against transmission have been conflicting. Many investigators have failed to find a difference between transmitting and nontransmitting mothers when they correlated antibodies to epitopes of the HIV-1 gp120 V3 region and transmission (37, 38). Several studies have reported a role for neutralizing antibody to HIV-1 in preventing transmission (39–42). Both Bryson and coworkers and Kliks and coworkers found that neutralizing antibody to autologous virus was present more frequently in mothers who were nontransmitters (40, 42). Khouri and colleagues used a competitive inhibition assay to demonstrate lower levels of antibody to the CD4 binding epitope in mothers who transmit virus to their infants when compared with those who do not (39). Another group of investigators, however, were unable to correlate neutralizing antibody with transmission (41).

The biologic characteristics of maternal viral isolates have also been studied to determine whether specific phenotypes can be identified that are more likely to result in infection. Syncytial-inducing isolates have been correlated with advanced disease stage, but in studies of isolates transmitted to infants, the nonsyncytial-inducing virus is found more frequently (42). A few studies have also reported that viruses with specific replication kinetics, termed "rapid, high" producers, are most likely to be transmitted, but these studies have been performed in only a limited number of infants (42, 43).

In addition to maternal factors, obstetric factors have been investigated for their influence on perinatal transmission. Despite data that support intrapartum transmission as the route of transmission in many infected infants, most studies from the United States have failed to show that the mode of delivery correlates with the risk of transmission (22, 28, 30). The French Collaborative Study also reported that transmission for infants in their study was not influenced by mode of delivery (44). The European Collaborative Study, however, reported an odds ratio of 0.56 for cesarean section compared with vaginal delivery when correlated with infection risk

Table 12.5. Factors that May Influence Perinatal Transmission

Maternal
   Stage of disease
   CD4+ lymphocyte number
   Virus load
   Neutralizing or other functional antibody
   Virus phenotype
Obstetric
   Route of delivery
   Prolonged rupture of amniotic membranes
   Events that increase exposure to maternal blood
   Chorioamnionitis

(24), and a study that combined data from both European and United States studies and included more than 3000 infants in the analysis reported an odds ratio for cesarean section versus vaginal delivery of 0.80 (95% confidence interval [CI] 0.63 to 1.00) (45). These data suggest that the question regarding the role of delivery in transmission remains in question. For route of delivery and other potential obstetric or maternal factors that may affect transmission, the timing of infection (intrauterine or intrapartum) is likely to be influential because factors that may affect intrapartum transmission may not be important in intrauterine transmission and vice versa. Duration of ruptured membranes before delivery may affect the role of mode of delivery in transmission. Duration of ruptured amniotic membranes has been reported to be directly correlated with transmission if rupture occurs more than 4 hours before delivery (28).

Diagnosis of HIV-1 Infection in Children

The definition of HIV-1 infection in children is age dependent (see Table 12.1). For children 18 months of age or older, diagnosis can be made using the enzyme-linked immunosorbent assay (ELISA) and Western blot or another confirmatory assay if the ELISA is positive. Diagnosis of infection in children younger than 18 months of age using antibody assays that detect IgG antibody to HIV-1 is complicated by the presence of maternal IgG antibody in infants. All infants born to HIV-1 seropositive mothers have IgG antibody to HIV-1 at birth because of passive transfer of maternal antibody across the placenta. The median time for disappearance of maternal antibody is 10 months in uninfected infants (46). Uninfected children who continue to have measurable antibody beyond 10 months of age will serorevert by 18 months of age. The presence of HIV-1 antibody beyond 18 months of age indicates infection. Tests that rely on detection of IgG antibody such as the ELISA and Western blot cannot be used for diagnosis of infection in most infants who are younger than 18 months of age.

Currently, the most commonly used assays for diagnosis of infection in infants for whom the ELISA and Western blot cannot be used are assays that detect virus directly. These assays include viral culture, PCR assays, and antigen assays. Commercial assays using PCR for detection of viral DNA are probably the most frequently used assays in the United States because of their sensitivity and availability. Studies comparing PCR with virus culture, the current standard for diagnosis of HIV-1 infection in children, have found that PCR assays are both sensitive and specific for early diagnosis in infants. Because of costs, biohazard concerns, and the complexity of performing cultures, virus cultures are generally available only in research facilities. Antigen assays that detect the HIV-1 core protein, p24, are also used for diagnosis. The antigen assay that uses acid or heat treatment of serum to dissociate antigen from immune complexes has greater sensitivity than the first-generation p24 antigen assay. Neither assay, however, is as sensitive as PCR for diagnosis.

Another approach to diagnosis in younger infants is the use of antibody assays that detect antibody isotypes to HIV-1 that cannot be transported across the placenta. Assays for detection of both HIV-1 IgA and IgM have been tested (47–50). The IgA assays are the most promising because of their greater sensitivity in infants. Although their sensitivity is less during the first 3 months of life, the sensitivity is significantly better by 6 months of age.

PERINATAL HIV-1 INFECTION

Many characteristics of the natural history of HIV-1 infection are unique to children. Not only are specific diseases common in children and rare or unknown in adults, but also the duration of the incubation period varies before the development of disease, particularly AIDS-defining illnesses, and, in many children, HIV-1 causes a much more aggressive infection than that seen in most adults.

Most HIV-1–infected neonates are asymptomatic at birth and cannot be distinguished from uninfected neonates. The time interval from birth to development of AIDS among perinatally infected infants varies widely. Data from the CDC that describe the age of children when AIDS-defining illnesses were first diagnosed provides some insight into the variable period between infection and the development of AIDS. The largest number of AIDS cases occurred in children who were younger than 24 months of age, but the remaining cases occurred evenly across the age spectrum from 2 to 12 years. Studies by Auger and coinvestigators used parametric and nonparametric statistics to estimate the incubation period for AIDS in children with data from perinatally infected pediatric patients in New York City (51). Their data identified two risk populations: the largest risk population had a median incubation time of 6.1 years, and the second, smaller population had a median incubation time of 4.1 months. These data suggest the presence of a subset of perinatally infected children who, like adults, do not have significant disease for years after their infection and the presence of a second subset of children who develop the most serious manifestations of infection during the first 2 years of age.

Clinical signs of infection are common in HIV-1 infection even in the absence of AIDS. Forsyth and coworkers described the occurrence of clinical findings as defined by the CDC 1987 Classification of Pediatric HIV Disease in a population of 75 infected children, all of whom had been examined in infancy by the investigators and for whom clinical information was available during the first year of life; in addition, all had follow-up until at least 18 months of age (52). In this study cohort, 64% had at least one abnormal clinical finding by 6 months of age, and 79% did by 12 months of age. These findings are similar to a report by the European Collaborative Study in which more than 90% of children followed prospectively had clinical signs of infection by 12 months of age (44). Immunologic abnormalities also develop early in many infected infants. Eighty-three percent of the infants followed by the European Collaborative Study had immunologic abnormalities by 6 months of age (46).

The diversity in the occurrence of clinical disease and degree of immunodeficiency as measured by absolute CD4+ lymphocyte number and percentage of CD4+ lymphocytes over time is reflected in the 1994 revised CDC Classification of Pediatric HIV Infection in which children are staged by age according to their clinical disease and their CD4+ lymphocyte number and percentage (4).

With the development of the HIV RNA PCR assay, which permits the quantitation of plasma virus levels, preliminary data about the relationship among viral burden, clinical disease, and prognosis and viral burden in relation to CD4+ cell number have been reported. Unlike adults, in whom high HIV-1 RNA levels usually occur soon after primary infection but then decline by as much as 1000-fold over the subsequent 2 to 3 months, perinatally infected infants develop and often maintain high levels of virus during the first 2 years of life. These high levels can occur in asymptomatic infants with normal CD4+ lymphocyte counts (53), as well as in symptomatic infants. Mofenson and coworkers reported a geometric mean RNA copy number at baseline of approximately 100,000 copies/mL in 92 children enrolled in the National Institute of Child Health and Human Development Intravenous Immunoglobulin Clinical Trial, a HIV-1 plasma RNA level much higher than that seen in adults whose duration of infection was similar (54). These data suggest that children may have high viral loads even beyond infancy. The data from this study also indicate that both the baseline RNA values and CD4+ lymphocyte percentages were independent predictors of mortality risk. Studies that correlate survival with RNA copy numbers in children by age have not been reported.

A retrospective analysis of 172 perinatally infected infants in Miami, Florida showed that the age at diagnosis of a serious HIV-1 related illness is a prognostic indicator of survival (55). In as many as one-third of perinatally infected infants, the onset of serious clinical disease occurs at a young age, often 6 months of age or younger (56). With its onset, one sees an exacerbated evolution of disease, and death occurs early. These infants have been termed "rapid progressors," and they have been the subject of intense study in an effort to understand the pathogenesis of HIV-1 infection. Children with rapid progression characteristically develop AIDS-defining illnesses by 2 years of age. Severe encephalopathy is a frequent clinical manifestation, and opportunistic infections such as *Pneumocystis carinii* pneumonia (PCP) and *Candida* esophagitis are also commonly diagnosed. Clinical disease in rapid progressors is accompanied by a rapid decline in CD4+ lymphocyte number. Blanche and coworkers reported a rate of survival of 48 ± 24% at 3 years of age in children with characteristics of rapid progressors in their population in comparison with 97 ± 3% in children without these characteristics (56).

To understand the pathogenesis of disease in rapid progressors, De Rossi and her coinvestigators investigated the disease outcome in 11 infected infants who were studied sequentially from birth in relation to their pattern of viral replication (57). In this small group of infants, three patterns were discerned. Infants who developed AIDS early had a rapid and sustained increase in both their plasma RNA levels and cell-associated proviral DNA during the first few weeks of life. RNA levels as high as more than 1,000,000 copies/mL of plasma and more than 1000 HIV-1 DNA copies/10^5 peripheral blood mononuclear cells were measured in these infants. The patterns observed in infants with slower disease evolution were described as either a rapid replication to a high titer of RNA or DNA levels that were not sustained, or replication to maximum RNA levels lower than those of the other two groups of infants. A similar difference in pattern of viral replication measured by plasma RNA levels between groups of infants who were divided on the basis of disease evolution was reported by Shearer and coworkers (53). Other investigators studying the pathogenesis of disease in rapid progressors have focused on the cause of the rapid loss of CD4+ lymphocytes (58). Kourtis and coworkers proposed that the loss of CD4+ lymphocytes in this group of infants could be due to defective generation of CD4+ cells by the thymus, as occurs in infants with DiGeorge syndrome, rather than destruction. These investigators found that 75% of 17 infants with immunophenotypes that resembled that of DiGeorge syndrome developed AIDS by 12 months of age in comparison with 14% of 42 children without this immunophenotype (58). Studies in other populations will be important to confirm these findings. Other investigators studying the pathogenesis of infection are examining virus phenotype, the role of antibodies and cell-mediated immunity, and genetic influences on disease progression.

In perinatally infected children who are not rapid progressors, the natural history of infection is more variable. These children are at risk for both acute and chronic infections. In addition, HIV-1–associated disease can involve virtually any organ system. Infected children may have a disease course primarily characterized by excessive infections, or their course may involve primarily organ system diseases such as pulmonary or renal disease. Some children have a combination of both infections and organ system involvement.

Until the early 1990s, the prognosis of survival beyond the first decade of life for perinatally infected children was considered to be extremely poor. This prognosis, however, has clearly changed. An increasing proportion of children are now surviving into the second decade of life. In Miami, 25% of the population of 266 children are older than 10 years of age. This improvement in prognosis is related in part to more potent antiretroviral drugs and to a better understanding of the risk of opportunistic infections and the use of prophylaxis to prevent these infections. Factors other than treatment are important, however, because some children are not diagnosed until the end of the first decade of life after being well clinically for years. A small subset of children followed for several years has maintained a normal CD4+ lymphocyte number and has no evidence of disease despite the absence of any therapy. This group is similar to the long-term nonprogressors described in the adult population (59). Studies of this group of long-term nonprogressors, as well as studies of rapid progressors, may provide important insights into the pathogenesis of HIV-1 infection in children and the variation in its natural history.

DISEASES OF THE ORGAN SYSTEMS

Organ system disease associated with HIV-1 infection is common in children. Some organ systems are more frequently affected than others, but any organ can be affected. Some diseases that are typical of infection among adults such as Kaposi's sarcoma and other malignancies are unusual in children, whereas diseases such as LIP and HIV-1–associated encephalopathy are more characteristic of pediatric infection.

LIP occurs in many infected children in the United States. It may be less common in children in other areas of the world, however. Studies from the United States reported that as many as 40% of children have LIP in comparison with a report from Italy, where LIP occurred in 14% of children in this population (60, 61). The occurrence of LIP in children younger than 1 year of age is unusual. In most children, the initial presentation of LIP is the development of an abnormal radiograph without accompanying clinical symptoms. The radiographic characteristics of LIP are bilateral reticulonodular infiltrates in which hilar lymphadenopathy may or may not be present (62). These radiographic changes, which persist for at least 2 months and are not responsive to antimicrobial therapy, is the definition of LIP as defined by the CDC (4). The clinical course associated with LIP is variable. Some children remain asymptomatic. If disease evolves, it is often an indolent process. Chronic lung disease associated with recurrent infection, hypoxemia, and eventually the development of bronchiectasis can ensue in many children. Steroid therapy may be efficacious in children who develop hypoxemia (63). The etiology and pathophysiology of this infection are not clear. Biopsy of the lung in children with LIP reveals a peribronchial infiltration of lymphocytes and plasma cells. Several studies have suggested an association with Epstein–Barr virus infection (64). LIP is an AIDS-defining disease in children. Because experience has suggested that the prognosis for survival in children with this disease is better than for other AIDS-defining conditions, children with LIP but no other AIDS-defining illnesses are classified as category B rather than category C.

Central nervous system abnormalities are common in children and include a spectrum of manifestations. The most severe manifestation is a progressive encephalopathy that may occur in as many as 10% of infected children. It typically develops in young children and is associated with a poor prognosis (55). The encephalopathy is manifested by changes in muscle tone that may result in severe hypertonia and spastic quadriparesis. Children may also have regression in their developmental milestones and develop microcephaly. Radiographic studies of the brain show cerebral atrophy, enlargement of the ventricles, and basal ganglia calcifications. HIV-1 has been cultured from the cerebrospinal fluid in some children (65), but whether the pathogenesis of this disease is related to direct or indirect effects of the virus is not clear. Antiretroviral therapy, particularly ZDV, may stabilize or reverse central nervous system abnormalities. Improvement in cognition, brain growth, and reversal of abnormalities on the CT scan of the brain have been reported (66–69).

Although the clinical manifestations and pathogenesis of HIV-1–associated disease affecting other organ systems such as the cardiac, renal, gastrointestinal, hematologic, and dermatologic may be different in adults and children, these diseases are common to both age groups. These diseases therefore are not discussed in this chapter.

INFECTIONS

Infections are a common manifestation of HIV-1 infection in children. Pediatric patients have an increased frequency of minor bacterial infections such as otitis media, sinusitis, impetigo, cellulitis, urinary tract infections, and pneumonia (70–72). Minor fungal infections such as oral candidiasis and *Candida* dermatitis are also common. Tinea capitis and tinea corporis infections may be recurrent or chronic.

Serious bacterial infections that include meningitis, osteomyelitis, septic arthritis, deep tissue abscesses, and bacteremia are frequent. The causative organisms are usually common childhood pathogens such as *Streptococcus pneumoniae* and *Salmonella* species. *Haemophilus influenzae* type b infections are rarely seen now, a change that most likely results from the use of *Haemophilus influenzae* vaccines. In children with the most advanced immunosuppression who have had frequent hospitalizations, *Staphylococcus aureus* and Gram-negative pathogens assume increased importance (73). In children, the occurrence of two or more serious bacterial infections within a 2-year period is an AIDS-defining condition. The increased susceptibility of bacterial infection occurs as a result of B-cell dysfunction induced by the virus that leads to a decreased or absent antibody response to specific antigens (74–76). This dysfunction is more important in children than in adults, presumably because HIV-1 infection occurs at a time when the immune response is immature and preexisting memory cells are not present. The ability to produce antibody to a vaccine antigen can be used to determine the individual child's ability to respond to other antigens in vivo and to assess B-cell function.

Children with HIV-1 infection and recurrent bacterial infections may benefit from intravenous γ-globulin given monthly or bimonthly (77–79). A multicenter, double-blind, placebo-controlled study comparing intravenous γ-globulin with albumin demonstrated that children with a CD4+ lymphocyte count higher than 200 had an increase in time to development of a serious infection, but no difference in survival was found between the groups of children (79). Some children in each group in this study received either ZDV or trimethoprim–sulfamethoxazole (TMP–SX). In contrast, the results of another multicenter, placebo-controlled trial in which all children received ZDV did not show enhanced protection from infection in children who were receiving TMP–SX (80). Present recommendations are that γ-globulin therapy be considered for use in HIV-

1–infected children with the following conditions: humoral immune dysfunction, as defined by a lack of antibody response to de novo antigens; hypogammaglobulinemia; recurrent serious bacterial infections occurring while receiving appropriate antibiotic prophylaxis; chronic lung disease with bronchiectasis; and lack of detectable antibody to measles in children who live in an area where measles is endemic (81).

The most common opportunistic infection in children and adults is PCP. PCP in children differs from the disease in adults in that it occurs most frequently in those who are the most recently infected, young infants, and it causes significant morbidity and mortality among this age group (82–85). Without prophylaxis, the mean age at which PCP is most likely to occur is between 3 and 6 months (86). TMP–SX is the drug of choice for initial therapy. Pentamidine and atovaquone are alternative therapies for children who do not respond to TMP–SX therapy or who are allergic to sulfa drugs. With increasing experience and understanding of the natural history of HIV-1 infection among children, prevention of PCP has become a primary focus of care for both infants at risk for infection and infected children. The United States Public Health Service published recommendations for PCP prophylaxis for both groups of children (Table 12.6) (86). Recommendations in infected children are based on CD4+ lymphocyte counts that are adjusted for age. Prophylaxis is also recommended beginning at 4 to 6 weeks of age for infants who are born to infected mothers and whose infection status is not yet determined. For children who are not infected with HIV and who serorevert, prophylaxis may be discontinued. In addition to these recommendations, any infected child who has had a prior episode of PCP or a CD4+ lymphocyte percentage equal to or less than 15% should receive prophylaxis. At this time, HIV-1–infected children who meet criteria for prophylaxis should continue therapy for life. The drug of choice for prophylaxis is TMP–SX. Pentamidine and dapsone are alternative drugs for prophylaxis.

Candida esophagitis is a common opportunistic infection among children and may occur without oral candidiasis. In infants and young children, its occurrence is suggested by the presence of fever, poor appetite, and vomiting. Older children may complain of substernal pain. Diagnosis can usually be made by barium swallow, but endoscopy and biopsy may be needed in some children. For early esophagitis, ketoconazole or oral fluconazole usually provides effective therapy, but, occasionally, amphotericin B is required, particularly in children who may have resistant fungi.

Disseminated infection with *Mycobacterium avium-intracellulare* occurs in severely immunocompromised children. Its presentation is similar to that described in adults. Therapeutic regimens used in adults have been adopted for therapy in children. Unlike in adults, studies in children to determine the efficacy of rifabutin, clarithromycin, or azithromycin for prophylaxis of this infection have not been done. Many physicians caring for children, however, have used the experience in adult trials to base decisions regarding prophylaxis for children. Despite the lack of studies to document the efficacy of this approach, prophylaxis is usually begun in children based on their CD4+ lymphocyte count: children younger than 12 months, less than 750 cells/mm^3; children 1 to 2 years old, less than 500/mm^3; children 2 to 6 years old, less than 75 cells/mm^3; and children 6 years or older, less than 50 cells/mm^3.

MANAGEMENT OF THE INFANT AT RISK FOR HIV INFECTION

Diagnosis of HIV-1 infection before or during pregnancy allows the woman to make informed decisions about her own care and interventions for reduction of perinatal transmission. Knowledge of maternal HIV-1 status facilitates early identification of infants at risk for HIV-1 and optimizes their medical management. Several compelling reasons exist for early identification of at risk infants. These include the prophylactic use of ZDV after birth to reduce transmission of HIV-1 infection, early diagnosis of HIV-1 infection, initiation of prophylaxis against PCP, monitoring for HIV-1–associated complications, and institution of combination

Table 12.6. Recommendations for *Pneumocystis carinii* Pneumonia (PCP) Prophylaxis and CD4+ Monitoring for HIV-Exposed Infants and HIV-Infected Children, by Age and HIV-Infection Status

Age/HIV-Infection Status	PCP Prophylaxis	CD4+ Monitoring
Birth to 4–6 wk; HIV exposed	No prophylaxis	1 mo
4–6 wk to 4 mo; HIV exposed	Prophylaxis	3 mo
4–12 mo		
HIV infected or indeterminate	Prophylaxis	6, 9, and 12 mo
HIV infection reasonably excluded	No prophylaxis	None
1–5 y; HIV infected	Prophylaxis if: CD4+ count is < 500 cells/µL or CD4+ percentage is < 15%[a]	Every 3–4 mo
6–12 y; HIV infected	Prophylaxis if: CD4+ count is < 200 cells/µL or CD4+ percentage is < 15%	Every 3–4 mo

[a]Children 1 to 2 years of age who were receiving PCP prophylaxis and had a CD4+ count of < 750 cells/µL or percentage of < 15% at < 12 months of age should continue prophylaxis.
(From Centers for Disease Control and Prevention: Guidelines for prophylaxis against *Pneumocystis carinii* pneumonia for children infected with human immunodeficiency virus. MMWR Morb Mortal Wkly Rep 1991;40:1–11.)

antiretroviral therapies in infants after diagnosis of HIV-1 infection. Recommendations for the evaluation and treatment of the HIV-1–exposed infant have been published by the American Academy of Pediatrics Committee on Pediatric AIDS (87).

The management of the child at risk for HIV-1 infection begins at birth. Medical visits should be scheduled at 2 weeks and at 2, 4, and 6 months of age, and they should include evaluation for HIV-1 as well as routine care and immunizations. Infants receiving ZDV for the first 6 weeks of life should be monitored at birth and at 2 weeks of age for hematologic toxicities (anemia, absolute neutropenia, or thrombocytopenia). Prophylaxis for PCP is begun between 4 and 6 weeks of age using TMP–SX given 3 days a week. Immune studies, including a CD4+ lymphocyte count and percentage should be monitored beginning at 2 to 3 months of age. A diagnostic test for HIV-1 should be done as soon after birth as possible, at 2 months of age, and again between 4 and 6 months of age. If the PCR tests for HIV-1 are negative and the clinical and immune parameters are normal at age 6 months, PCP prophylaxis can be discontinued, and the infant is followed with HIV-1 ELISA antibody tests to document disappearance of the antibody. In an infant who is not infected, the antibody disappears at a median age of 10 months; most infants have lost maternal HIV-1 antibody by 18 months of age (46). An algorithm for management of the HIV-1 exposed infant is presented in Figure 12.1. Using this schema, an infant is considered not infected if there are two negative DNA PCR assays for detection of HIV-1 (one of which was done after 4 months of age), two consecutive negative antibody tests for HIV-1 performed between 6 and 18 months of age, no other laboratory evidence of infection, and the absence of an AIDS-defining condition.

TREATMENT AND MANAGEMENT

Early diagnosis and improved therapies have changed pediatric HIV-1 infection from a rapidly progressive, fatal disease in many infants to a chronic disease with prolonged survival. Because HIV-1 infection is a family disease and other family members may be infected, the care system for HIV-1–infected children should be family centered, coordinated, and comprehensive. Case management services provide additional and needed support to families infected with HIV-1 to ensure access to medical care.

Medical evaluations and laboratory assessments should be performed at least every 3 months. Children with more advanced disease require more frequent medical evaluations. The child with fever should be evaluated promptly, undergo appropriate diagnostic tests, and be treated expectantly with antibiotics pending culture results. The frequency of laboratory assessments depends on the stage of disease and the medications prescribed. Children should be monitored for drug toxicities, changes in CD4+ lymphocyte percentage and absolute numbers, and changes in the viral load as measured by number of HIV-1 RNA copies/mL plasma (HIV RNA PCR) at 3-month intervals. If the lymphocyte count or

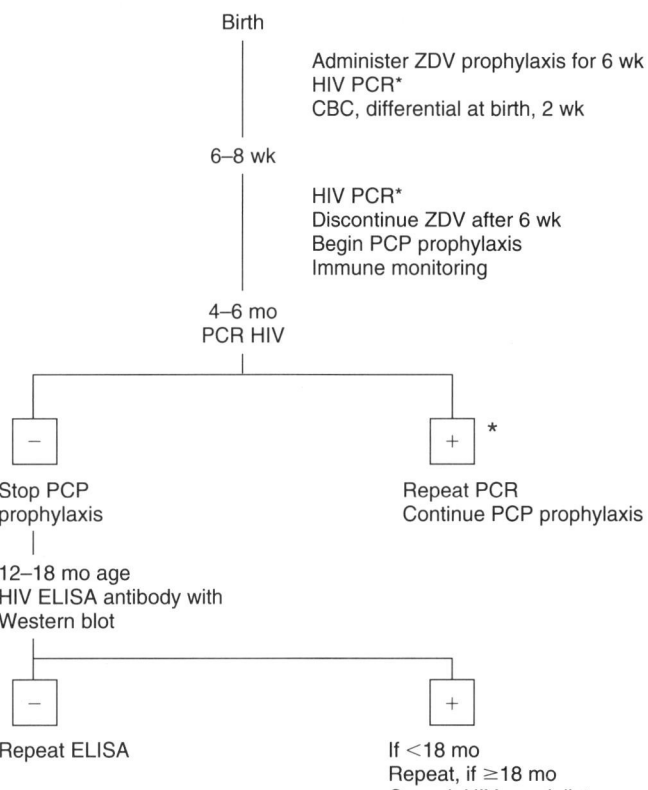

Figure 12.1. Management of the infant at risk for HIV. If HIV PCR is positive, repeat test. If it is positive again, the infant is infected with HIV, and an HIV specialist should be consulted regarding therapy.

percentage or the viral load is close to a threshold that would mandate beginning or changing therapy, the value should be repeated within 1 month.

Recommendations for immunization of children with HIV-1 infection have been issued by the American Academy of Pediatrics and the Advisory Committee on Immunization Practices (88, 89). Inactivated vaccines for protection against diphtheria, pertussis, tetanus, *Haemophilus influenzae* type b, and hepatitis B should be given according to the schedules for immunologically normal children. Live vaccines are usually contraindicated in the immunocompromised host; however, some exceptions are made in the case of HIV-1–infected children. Inactivated polio vaccine (IPV) is given in place of oral polio vaccine to prevent vaccine-related paralytic polio in the immunocompromised recipient as well as to avoid spread of the vaccine virus to other immunocompromised family members. Uninfected children residing in a household with HIV-1–infected adults or children should also receive IPV. Recommendations regarding the administration of measles, mumps, and rubella (MMR) vaccine have changed based on a case report of an adolescent with severe immune compromise who had received MMR vaccine and subsequently developed severe pneumonitis associated with the vaccine strain of the measles virus (90). Currently, measles vaccine is not recommended for use in severely immunocompromised children, adolescents, or adults with

Table 12.7. Recommendations for Routine Immunization of HIV-Infected Children in the United States

Vaccines	Known Asymptomatic HIV Infection	Symptomatic HIV Infection
Hepatitis B	Yes	Yes
Diphtheria-tetanus-acellular pertussis vaccine (or DPT)	Yes	Yes
Inactivated poliovaccine	Yes	Yes
Measles-mumps-rubella (MMR)	Yes	Yes[a]
Haemophilus influenzae type b vaccine	Yes	Yes
Pneumococcal	Yes	Yes
Influenza	Yes[b]	Yes
Varicella	No	No

[a] Severely immunocompromised children should *not* receive MMR vaccine.
[b] Influenza vaccine should be provided annually during the fall to HIV-exposed infants 6 months of age and older, to HIV-infected children and adolescents, and to household contacts of HIV-infected persons.

HIV-1 infection (Table 12.7). For children who are infected with HIV-1 and do not have severe immune compromise, the vaccine is recommended to be given between 12 and 15 months and again before school entry to prevent measles, which can be a life-threatening illness in children with HIV-1 infection (91). Influenza vaccine should be given yearly in the fall to infected children over 6 months of age, as well as to household contacts. The 23-valent pneumococcal vaccine is recommended for infected children over the age of 2 years because of the increased incidence of invasive pneumococcal infection. The American Academy of Pediatrics recommends a booster dose 3 to 5 years after the initial dose. A new protein-conjugated pneumococcal vaccine is being tested in clinical trials to determine its safety, tolerance, and immune response in young infants with HIV-1 infection. Varicella vaccine is currently not recommended for use in HIV-1–exposed or HIV-1–infected children. However, clinical trials of this vaccine are ongoing in this population to test its safety and potential use.

Some infected children, particularly those who are symptomatic, do not produce an adequate immune response despite immunization and remain susceptible to the disease (74, 76). Thus, for exposure to measles, prophylaxis with γ-globulin is recommended independent of vaccination status (92). If a child is receiving intravenous γ-globulin monthly, and exposure to measles occurred during the first 2 weeks after therapy, additional IgG is not necessary. Passive prophylaxis should also be given for tetanus-prone wounds and exposure to varicella, hepatitis A, and hepatitis B.

Antiretroviral Therapy

No cure exists for HIV-1 infection, but antiretroviral drugs can delay progression of disease in both adults and children and prolong survival. The most commonly used drugs in children are nucleoside analogs that inhibit the reverse transcriptase of the virus, ZDV (azidothymidine, AZT), didanosine (ddI, dideoxyinosine), lamivudine (3TC), stavudine (D4T), and zalcitabine (ddC, dideoxycytosine). With the exception of zalcitabine, all these drugs are available commercially as a pediatric formulation. A new reverse transcriptase inhibitor, 1592U89, is in clinical trials in children, and its use has been associated with a significant decrease in viral load when it is given to adults in combination with other drugs. The use of nonnucleoside reverse transcriptase inhibitors, particularly nevirapine, is increasing in children. No pediatric experience has been reported with delavirdine. A multicenter, randomized, double-blind clinical trial has evaluated various combinations of ZDV, ddI, and nevirapine in children, and the results of this trial are pending. Although published experience with use of protease inhibitors in children is limited, use is increasing as formulations appropriate for children become available. At present, ritonavir and nelfinavir are approved for use in children. Saquinavir and indinavir are not commercially available in pediatric formulations. Clinical trials performed by the National Cancer Institute Pediatric Branch and the Pediatric AIDS Clinical Trials Group (PACTG) are studying protease inhibitors in combination with nucleoside reverse transcriptase inhibitors. At present, no information is available regarding the pharmacokinetics of the protease inhibitors in neonates and young infants.

Treatment decisions have been based on clinical experience and results of clinical trials. Initial pediatric clinical trials with ZDV determined its pharmacokinetics, safety, and efficacy (93, 94). Pediatric clinical trials have shown no difference in clinical outcome using ZDV monotherapy at 90 mg/M^2 per dose as compared with the standard dose, 180 mg/M^2, given every 6 hours (95). The higher dose is often used in children with HIV-associated central nervous system involvement, because ZDV has been shown to cross the blood–brain barrier, and improvements in central nervous system function have been described (68, 94). In another multicenter, double-blind study, PACTG 152, drug-naive, symptomatic children between the ages of 3 months and 18 years were randomized to receive ZDV alone, ddI alone, or ZDV plus ddI. Results of this study showed a significantly higher risk of progression of HIV-1 infection or death after a median follow-up of 23 months in patients receiving ZDV monotherapy, and this arm of the study was discontinued. No significant differences in clinical end points were seen in the other two arms of the study after a median follow-up of 32 months. Thus, in this study of initial therapy in symptomatic HIV-1–infected children, ddI monotherapy or the combination of ZDV and ddI was superior to ZDV monotherapy (96). A subsequent clinical trial was designed to evaluate the efficacy of ZDV and lamivudine (3TC), ddI monotherapy, and ZDV and ddI combination therapy with regard to disease progression and death. This randomized trial was conducted in infants and children, 6 weeks to 18 years old, who had received more than 56 days of prior antiretroviral therapy. Results showed that patients receiving ddI monotherapy were more likely to experience disease progression or death. Thus, combination therapy was proven to be superior to ddI monotherapy and is recommended for initial treatment (97).

Data on the use of zalcitabine as initial treatment for children are limited, but the drug is well tolerated in pediatric patients with advanced HIV-1 disease (98).

Data are limited on the early treatment of children with perinatally acquired HIV infection before the development of advanced symptoms. A pediatric AIDS clinical trial evaluated the use of oral ZDV, ddI, and nevirapine in infants with perinatally acquired HIV-1 infection between 2 and 16 weeks of age. Seven of the eight children had reductions in viral load of at least 1.5 log within 4 weeks of initiating therapy. A pair of twins who began therapy at 10 weeks of age had clearance of detectable plasma HIV-1 RNA that persisted through 16 months of therapy (99). Thus, early, aggressive therapy of infants with perinatally acquired infection can result in significant and sustained reduction in viral load and maintenance of CD4 counts.

Guidelines for the use of antiretroviral agents in pediatric HIV infection have been developed by a working group convened by the National Pediatric and Family HIV Resource Center, the Health Resources and Services Administration, and the National Institutes of Health and will be published by early 1998. Treatment decisions are complex, taking into consideration the viral pathogenesis of disease, the interpretation of viral and immune markers of HIV-1 disease progression, and patterns of resistance. In making therapeutic decisions about pediatric patients, four areas need to be addressed: initiation of therapy in the infected newborn, initial therapy in the older infant or child, indications for a change of antiretroviral therapy, and the prevention of perinatal transmission.

INITIATION OF THERAPY: NEWBORNS AND INFANTS LESS THAN 1 YEAR OF AGE

Approximately 20% of all infants with perinatally acquired infection have a rapid onset and progression of disease with the development of an AIDS-defining illness by 1 year of age. Recent studies have indicated that the infected infant has a sustained high viral load over the first 2 years of life, and viral burden is associated with prognosis. Thus, pediatricians have a unique opportunity to treat infected newborns and infants early with reduction of the viral burden to low or undetectable levels that should ultimately influence outcome and survival. For the greatest success, this therapy should be aggressive and initiated early after diagnosis of infection. Aggressive combination therapy using three drugs is preferred for treatment of a newly diagnosed infant independent of clinical, virologic, or immunologic status. When three-drug combinations are used, usually two nucleoside reverse transcriptase inhibitors are used in combination with nevirapine or, as pharmacokinetic data become available in young children, a protease inhibitor. Infants who cannot tolerate or comply with a three-drug regimen should be given combination therapy with two nucleoside reverse transcriptase inhibitors.

INITIATION OF THERAPY: OLDER CHILD

The older child may present with asymptomatic or symptomatic HIV-1 infection. As outlined earlier, it is critical to evaluate clinical status, viral load, and immune parameters in the context of what is known about the pathogenesis of HIV-1. Immune values should be interpreted based on age-adjusted values (see Table 12.3). For older children and adolescents, until better information is obtained, the same CD4+ lymphocyte counts and percentages and viral load parameters recommended for initiation or change of therapy in adults are used (100). Thus, therapy is recommended if the viral load is higher than 5000 to 10,000 copies/mL of plasma. The preferred regimen for treatment includes three-drug therapy with two nucleoside reverse transcriptase inhibitors and a protease inhibitor or a nonnucleoside reverse transcriptase inhibitor, such as nevirapine, with the goal of maximum suppression of the virus. This, of course, requires education of both the child and the caregivers regarding the importance of compliance and adherence to the regimen for maximum drug benefit and delay in development of resistance. The asymptomatic older child who presents with a viral load lower than 5000 copies/mL plasma and a CD4+ lymphocyte count higher than 500/mm^3 has a low risk of disease progression, and some experts may elect not to treat such a patient with antiretroviral therapy, but to monitor clinical, viral, and immune parameters closely.

CHANGING THERAPY

The three major reasons for changing therapy are drug toxicity, intolerance to the medication, and drug treatment failure. Treatment failure can be defined in terms of clinical or laboratory parameters. A change of therapy should occur if one notes clinical deterioration as defined by weight loss or poor weight gain, progressive neurodevelopmental deterioration, or disease progression defined as a change in clinical classification. A significant change in viral load is defined by a return to baseline values or a threefold or greater increase and is an indication for change of therapy. Less well defined parameters for change in therapy are related to change in CD4+ lymphocyte status, but a progressive deterioration in counts or percentage is considered significant. When changing therapy, it is important to add at least two new drugs.

OTHER CONSIDERATIONS

Other considerations in drug therapy in children include the taste of the medications, the compliance of the child and the family in adhering to the drug regimen, and the potential benefits to the child. Education of the family and the child is essential, and older children should be aware of their diagnosis to increase drug compliance. In addition, particularly with the protease inhibitors, knowledge of potential drug interactions is critical, and patients should be counseled not to take new medications unless they have spoken with their physician to assess potential drug interactions. Based on clinical trial data, most HIV-1 specialists believe that early aggressive combination therapy decreases viral load, potentially preserves the immune system, provides a longer time to development of disease progression, and, ultimately, prolongs survival.

PREVENTION OF PERINATAL TRANSMISSION

Vertical transmission of HIV-1 accounts for most cases of HIV-1 infection in infants and children worldwide. Potential interventions for the reduction of perinatal transmission of HIV-1 are based on our knowledge of the timing of transmission and predisposing risk factors. A major breakthrough in HIV-1 prevention occurred when the results of a multicenter, double-blind, placebo-controlled study sponsored by the ACTG (Protocol 076) showed a decrease in HIV-1 transmission from 25.3% in the placebo group to 8.3% in the ZDV-treated group when ZDV was administered to HIV-1–infected women during the second and third trimesters of pregnancy, at delivery, and to their infants for the first 6 weeks of life (101). Women entering this trial had mild clinical HIV-1 disease and CD4+ lymphocyte counts higher than 200 cells/mm^3. Shortly after the results of this trial were announced, the United States Public Health Service issued guidelines for the use of ZDV in HIV-1–infected pregnant women (102). Although investigators do not know whether all parts of the regimen are equally important in reduction of transmission, it is recommended that ZDV be offered to HIV-1–infected pregnant women at delivery even if it was not received prenatally. Likewise, if the HIV-1–infected mother of an infant has not received ZDV, the infant should be offered ZDV therapy as soon as possible after birth. Frenkel and associates evaluated 188 HIV-1–infected pregnant women who received only prenatal ZDV and who were seen at five university centers before 1994. None of the infants received ZDV prophylaxis. The perinatal transmission rate was 12.5% in this group of women and suggests that prenatal therapy is important for reduction of perinatal transmission (103).

Another PACTG trial (Protocol 185), completed in April, 1997, evaluated the efficacy, safety, and tolerance of hyperimmune anti–HIV-1 Ig (HIVIG) compared with standard intravenous γ-globulin for the reduction of perinatal transmission in HIV-1–infected women receiving ZDV with CD4 counts lower than 500/mm^3. The results showed no difference in transmission in the two treatment arms, and the study was stopped because the perinatal transmission rate had dropped to 4.8% overall and a treatment effect could only be demonstrated by enrolling significantly larger numbers of women. This result confirms the efficacy of ZDV for prevention of perinatal transmission of HIV-1 not only in women with mild disease but also in women with more advanced disease and prior ZDV use (104).

Standards of care in pregnant women are evolving, and as more women are identified and offered early treatment, combination drug regimens will become standard therapy for pregnant women. The adult treatment guidelines indicate that appropriate antiretroviral therapy should not be withheld from a woman because of pregnancy. The woman and her physician must discuss potential risks and benefits for both the woman and her fetus of continued aggressive drug therapy during pregnancy. However, ZDV is the only drug with proven efficacy in the reduction of perinatal transmission, and it should be incorporated into the woman's drug regimen during pregnancy when possible. Phase I studies of newer nucleoside reverse transcriptase inhibitors (ddI, D4T, and 3TC), nonnucleoside reverse transcriptase inhibitors (nevirapine) and protease inhibitors (indinavir, ritonavir, and nelfinavir) in pregnant women and their neonates are in progress. Finally, an ongoing phase III, randomized, double-blind clinical trial (Protocol 316) will assess the efficacy of a nonnucleoside reverse transcriptase inhibitor, nevirapine, delivered in one dose to the mother during labor and one dose to the neonate between 48 and 72 hours of life. Women and their infants will also be offered the standard ZDV regimen for reduction of perinatal transmission. Nevirapine is rapidly absorbed, provides a rapid, high level of drug, and has a prolonged half-life, making this an ideal drug for prophylaxis of the infant.

The efficacy of ZDV in reduction of perinatal transmission has been a significant advance in prevention of HIV-1 infection. However, with increased use of ZDV in women, resistance to this drug will occur with a potential effect on transmission. Thus, it is important to have early access to new drugs and to continue to conduct clinical trials in pregnant women and their neonates. A better understanding of the timing and mechanism of transmission and of the pathogenesis of HIV-1 will allow us to design more effective therapeutic and preventive interventions. In addition, registries to document drugs used during pregnancy are important to determine the long-term side effects of antiretroviral drugs for both the women and their exposed children. Finally, prevention of perinatal transmission depends on the woman's knowing her HIV-1 infection status and on HIV counseling and offering of HIV-1 testing to all pregnant women as the standard of care (105).

In conclusion, pediatric HIV-1 infection has many unique aspects. This is a chronic, multisystemic disease, and much has been learned over the past 15 years about the natural history and prognosis of this infection in children. Investigators anticipate that new advances in management and aggressive therapy will prolong the time to development of disease and will increase survival in infected infants and children. Already, several perinatally infected children have survived into adolescence (106). Care should be directed to the family unit with attention to both medical and psychosocial needs. Care should be comprehensive and coordinated, and because of the complexity of the illness and decisions about treatment, care should be provided in consultation with a pediatric HIV-1 specialist. Numerous social issues need to be addressed including day care and school attendance, respite and foster care, legal guardianship, and confidentiality. Resources for care and treatment become increasingly important, and access to care and clinical drug trials needs to be ensured. An active research agenda to answer some of the important questions about the timing and mechanism of perinatal transmission, maternal factors associated with transmission, and determinants of progression of HIV-1 disease is critical. Clinical trials to determine optimal therapy are crucial. Pediatricians and obstetricians are working together to devise interventions that will reduce perinatal transmission to less than 2% and significantly reduce the number of infected infants and children. One of the major challenges will be to transfer knowledge and to develop practical approaches for prevention of HIV-1 infection and reduction of perinatal transmission worldwide. This is our hope as we approach the year 2000 and enter into the third decade of pediatric AIDS and HIV-1 infection.

Acknowledgment

We would like to acknowledge the support of National Institutes of Health grants U01 AI27560, R01 AI23524, and R01 HD34337.

References

1. Centers for Disease Control and Prevention. HIV-AIDS surveillance report. Atlanta, GA: Centers for Disease Control and Prevention, 1996;8:1–39.
2. Gutman LT, St Claire KK, Weedy C, et al. Human immunodeficiency virus transmission by child sexual abuse. Am J Dis Child 1991;145:137–141.
3. Davis SF, Byers RH, Lindesgren ML, et al. Prevalence and incidence of vertically acquired HIV infection in the United States. JAMA 274:952–955.
4. Centers for Disease Control and Prevention. 1994 revised classification system for human immunodeficiency virus infection in children under 13 years of age. MMWR Morb Mortal Wkly Rep 1994;43:1–9.
5. Soeiro R, Rubinstein A, Rashbabaum WK, et al. Maternal–fetal transmission of AIDS: frequency of HIV-1 nucleic acid sequences in human fetal DNA. J. Infect Dis 1992;166:699–703.
6. Lewis SH, Reynolds KC, Fox HI, et al. HIV-1 in trophoblastic and villous Hofbauer cells, and hematological precursors in 8 week old fetuses. Lancet 1990;335:565–568.
7. Langston C., Lewis DE, Hammil AH, et al. Excess intrauterine fetal demise associated with maternal human immunodeficiency virus infection. J. Infect Dis 1995;172:1451–1460.
8. Duliege AM, Amos CI, Biggar RJ, et al. Birth order, delivery route, and concordance in the transmission of human immunodeficiency virus type 1 from mothers to twins: International Registry of HIV-Exposed Twins. J Pediatr 1995;126:625–632.
9. Hutto C, Owens C, Dumond D, et al. Early detection of perinatal HIV-1 infection with polymerase chain reaction (PCR), virus culture, and p24 antigen: program issue APS/SPR. Pediatr Res 1992;31:164A.
10. Borkowsky W, Krasinski K, Pollack H, et al. Early diagnosis of human immunodeficiency virus infection in children 6 months of age: comparison of polymerase chain reaction, culture, and plasma antigen capture techniques. J Infect Dis 1992;166:616–619.
11. Bryson YJ, Luzuriago K, Sullivan JL, et al. Proposed definitions for in utero versus intrapartum transmission of HIV-1 [letter]. N Engl J Med 1992;327:1246–1247.
12. Minkoff H, Burns DN, Landesman S, et al. The relationship of the duration of ruptured membranes to vertical transmission of human immunodeficiency virus. Am J Obstet Gynecol 1995;173:585–589.
13. Thiry L, Sprecher-Goldberger S, Jonckheer T, et al. Isolation of AIDS virus from cell-free breast milk of three healthy virus carriers. Lancet 1985;2:891.
14. Ziegler JB, Cooper DA, Johnson RD, et al. Postnatal transmission of AIDS-associated retrovirus from mother to infant. Lancet 1985;1:896–897.
15. Lepage P, van de Perre P, Carael M, et al. Postnatal transmission of HIV from mother to child. Lancet 1987;2:400.
16. Weinbreck P, Loustaud V, Denis F, et al. Postnatal transmission of HIV infection. Lancet 1988;1:482.
17. Stiehm ER, Vink P. Transmission of human immunodeficiency virus infection by breast-feeding. J Pediatr 1991;118:410–412.
18. Van De Perre P, Simonon A, Msellati P, et al. Postnatal transmission of human immunodeficiency virus type 1 from mother to infant. N Engl J Med 1991;325:593–598.
19. Dunn DT, Newell ML, Ades AE, et al. Risk of human immunodeficiency virus type 1 transmission through breast feeding. Lancet 1992;340:585–588.
20. Gray G, McIntyre JA, Lyons SF. The effect of breast feeding on vertical transmission of HIV-1 in Soweto, South Africa. Presented at the 11th International Conference on AIDS, Vancouver, BC, Canada, 1996: abstract ThC415.
21. Blanche S, Rouzioux C, Moscato, MLSG, et al. A prospective study of infants born to women seropositive for human immunodeficiency virus type 1. N Engl J Med 1989;320:1643–1648.
22. Hutto C, Parks, WP, Lai S, et al. A hospital-based prospective study of perinatal infection with human immunodeficiency virus type 1. J Pediatr 1991;118:347–353.
23. Ryder RW, NSA W, Hassing S, et al. Perinatal transmission of HIV-1 to infants in seropositive women in Zaire. N Engl J Med 1989;320:1637–1642.
24. European Collaborative Study. Risk factors for mother-to-child transmission of HIV-1. Lancet 1992;339:1007–1012.
25. Gabiano C, Tovo P-A, deMartino M, et al. Mother-to-child transmission of human immunodeficiency virus type 1: risk of infection and correlates of transmission. Pediatrics 1992;90:369–374.
26. Hira SK, Kamamanga J, Bhat GL, et al. Perinatal transmission of HIV-1 in Zambia. BMJ 1989;299:1250–1252.
27. Mayaux MJ, Blanche S, Rouzioux C, et al. Maternal factors associated with perinatal HIV-1 transmission: the French Cohort Study: 7 years of follow-up observation. The French Pediatric HIV Infection Study Group. J Acquir Immune Defic Syndr Hum Retrovirol 1995;8:188–194.
28. Landesman SH. Kalish LA, Burns DN, et al. Obstetrical factors and the transmission of human immunodeficiency virus type 1 from mother to child. N Engl J Med 1996;334:1617–1623.
29. The European Collaborative Study. Vertical transmission of HIV-1: maternal immune status and obstetric factors. AIDS 1996;10:1675–1681.
30. Dickover RE, Garratty EM, Herman SA, et al. Identification of levels of maternal HIV-1 RNA associated with risk of perinatal transmission: effect of maternal zidovudine treatment on viral load. JAMA 1996;275:599–605.
31. Pitt J, Brambilla D, Reichelderfer P, et al. Maternal immunologic and virologic risk factors for infant human immunodeficiency virus type 1 infection: findings from the women and infants transmission study. J Infect Dis 1997;175:567–575.
32. Weiser B, Nachman S, Tropper P, et al. Quantitation of human immunodeficiency virus type 1 during pregnancy:relationship of viral titer to mother-to child transmission and stability of viral load. Proc Natl Acad Sci U S A 1994;91:8037–8041.
33. Borkowsky W., Krasinski K, Cao Y, et al. Correlation of perinatal transmission of human immunodeficiency virus type 1 with maternal viremia and lymphocyte phenotypes. J Pediatr 194;125:345–351.
34. Sperling RS, Shapiro DE, Coombs RW, et al. Maternal viral load, zidovudine treatment, and the risk of transmission of human immunodeficiency virus type 1 from mother to infant. N Engl J Med 1996;335:1621–1629.
35. Fang G, Burger H, Grimson R, et al. Maternal plasma human immunodeficiency virus type a RNA level: a determinant and projected threshold for mother-to-child transmission. Proc Natl Acad Sci U S A 1995;92:12100–12104.

36. Koup R, Yunzhen C, Ho D, et al. Lack of maternal viral threshold for vertical transmission of HIV-1. Presented at the 3rd International Conference on Retroviruses and Opportunistic Infections, Washington, DC, 1996: abstract LB2.
37. Parekh BS, Shaffer N, Paru CP, et al. Lack of correlation between maternal antibodies to V3 loop peptides of gp120 and perinatal HIV-1 transmission. AIDS 1991;5:1179–1184.
38. Goedert JJ, Dublin S. Perinatal transmission of HIV type 1: associations with maternal anti-HIV serological reactivity. Mothers and Infants Cohort Study and HIV-1 Perinatal Serology Working Group. AIDS Res Hum Retroviruses 1994;10:1125–1134.
39. Khouri YF, McIntosh K, Cavacini L, et al. Vertical transmission of HIV-1 correlation with maternal viral load and plasma levels of CD4 binding site anti-gp120 antibodies. J Clin Invest 1995;95:732–737.
40. Bryson YJ, Lehman D, Garratty E, et al. The role of maternal autologous neutralizing antibody in prevention of maternal fetal HIV-1 transmission. J Cell Biochem 1993;17E(Suppl):95.
41. Husson RN, Lan Y, Kojima E, et al. Vertical transmission of human immunodeficiency virus type: autologous neutralizing antibody, virus load, and virus phenotype. J Pediatr 1995;126:865–871.
42. Kliks SC, Wara DW, Landers DV, et al. Features of HIV-1 that could influence maternal-child transmission. JAMA 1994;272:467–474.
43. Scarlatti G, Hodara V, Rossi P, et al. Transmission of human immunodeficiency virus type 1 (HIV-1) from mother to child correlates with viral phenotype. Virology 1993;197:624–629.
44. Mandelbrot L, Mayaux MJ, Bongain A, et al. Obstetric factors and mother-to-child transmission of human immunodeficiency virus type 1: the French perinatal cohorts, Serogest French Pediatric HIV Infection Study Group. Am J Obstet Gynecol 1996;175:661–667.
45. Dunn DT, Newell ML, Mayaux MJ, et al. Mode of delivery and vertical transmission of HIV-1: a review of prospective studies. J Acquir Immune Defic Syndr 1994;7:1064–1066.
46. European Collaborative Study. Children born to women with HIV-1 infection: Natural history and risk of transmission. Lancet 1991;337: 253–260.
47. Weiblen BJ, Lee FK, Cooper ER, et al. Early diagnosis of HIV infection in infants by detection of IgA antibodies. Lancet 1990;335: 988–990.
48. Landesman S, Weiblen B, Mendez H, et al. Clinical utility of HIV-IgA immunoblot assay in the early diagnosis of perinatal infection. JAMA 1991;266:3443–3446.
49. Quinn TC, Kline RL, Halsey N, et al. Early diagnosis of perinatal HIV infection by detection of viral-specific IgA antibodies. JAMA 1991; 266:3439–3442.
50. Husson RN, Comeau AM, Hoff R. Diagnosis of human immunodeficiency virus infection in infants and children. Pediatrics 1990;86: 1–10.
51. Auger I, Thomas P, De Gruttola V, et al. Incubation periods for pediatric AIDS patients. Nature 1988;336:575–577.
52. Forsyth BWC, Andiman WA, O'Connor T. Development of a prognosis-based clinical staging system for infants infected with human immunodeficiency virus. J Pediatr 1996;129:648–655.
53. Shearer WT, Quinn TC, LaRussa P, et al. Viral load and disease progression in infants infected with HIV-1. N Engl J Med 1997;336: 1337–1342.
54. Mofenson LM, Korelitz J, Meyer WA, et al. The relationship between serum human immunodeficiency virus type 1 (HIV-1) RNA levels, CD4 lymphocyte percent, and long-term mortality risk in HIV-1-infected children. J Infect Dis 1997;175:1029–1038.
55. Scott G, Hutto C, Makuch R, et al. Survival in children with perinatally acquired human immunodeficiency virus type 1 infection. N Engl J Med 1989;321:1791–1796.
56. Blanche S, Tardieu M, Duliege AM, et al. Longitudinal study of 94 symptomatic infants with perinatally acquired human immunodeficiency virus infection: evidence for a bimodal expression of clinical and biological symptoms. Am J Dis Child 1990;144:1210–1215.
57. De Rossi A, Masiero S, Giaquinto C, et al. Dynamics of viral replication in infants with vertically acquired human immunodeficiency virus type 1 infection. J Clin Invest 1996;97:323–330.
58. Kourtis AP, Ibebu C, Nahmias AJ, et al. Early progression of disease in HIV-infected infants with thymus dysfunction. N Engl J Med 1996; 335:1431–1436.
59. Cao Y, Qin L, Zhang L, et al. Virologic and immunologic characterization of long-term survivors of human immunodeficiency virus type 1 infection. N Engl J Med 1995;332:201–208.
60. Rubinstein A, Morecki R, Silverman B, et al. Pulmonary disease in children with acquired immune deficiency syndrome and AIDS-related complex. J Pediatr 1986;108:498–503.
61. Tovo PA, De Martino M, Gabiano C, et al. Prognostic factors and survival in children with perinatal HIV-1 infection. Lancet 1992;339: 1249–1253.
62. Oldham SA, Castillo M, Jacobson FL, et al. HIV-associated lymphocytic interstitial pneumonia: Radiologic manifestations and pathologic correlation. Radiology 1989;170:83–87.
63. Rubinstein A, Bernstein LJ, Charytan M, et al. Corticosteroid treatment for pulmonary lymphoid hyperplasia children with the acquired immunodeficiency syndrome. Pediatr Pulmonol 1988;4: 13–17.
64. Andiman WA, Rubinstein MK, et al. Opportunistic lymphoproliferations associated with Epstein–Barr DNA in infants and children with AIDS. Lancet 1985;2:1390–1393.
65. Resnick L, Demarzo-Veronese F, Schupbach J, et al. Intrablood-brain barrier synthesis of HTLV-III-specific IgG in patients with neurologic symptoms associated with AIDS or AIDS-related complex N Engl J Med 1985;313:1498–1504.
66. McKinney RE, Maha MA, Connor EM, et al. A multicenter trial of oral zidovudine in children with advanced human immunodeficiency virus disease. N Engl J Med 324:1991;1018–1025.
67. Brouwers P, Moss H, Wolters P, et al. Effect of continuous-infusion zidovudine therapy on neuropsychologic functioning in children with symptomatic human immunodeficiency virus infection. J Pediatr 1990;117:980–985.
68. Decarli C, Fugate L, Faloon J, et al. Brain growth and cognitive improvement in children with human immunodeficiency virus-induced encephalopathy after 6 months of continuous infusion zidovudine therapy. J Acquir Immune Defic Syndr 1991;4:585–592.
69. Brivio L, Tornaghi R, Musetti L, et al. Improvement of auditory brainstem responses after treatment with zidovudine in a child with AIDS. Pediatr Neurol 1991;7:53–55.
70. Bernstein LJ, Kreiger BZ, Novick BZ, et al. Bacterial infection in the acquired immunodeficiency syndrome of children. Pediatr Infect Dis J 1985;4:472–475.
71. Krasinski K, Borkowsky W, Bonk S, et al. Bacterial infections in human immunodeficiency virus-infected children. Pediatr Infect Dis J 1988; 7:323–328.
72. Principi N, Marchisio P, Tornaght R, et al. Acute otitis media in human immunodeficiency virus-infected children. Pediatrics 1991;88: 566–571.
73. Vernon DD, Holzman BH, Lewis P, et al. Respiratory failure in children with acquired immunodeficiency syndrome and acquired immunodeficiency syndrome-related complex. Pediatrics 1988;82: 223–228.
74. Bernstein LJ, Ochs HD, Wedgwood RJ, et al. Defective humoral immunity in pediatric acquired immune deficiency syndrome. J Pediatr 1985;107:352–357.
75. Pahwa S, Fikrig S, Menez R, et al. Pediatric acquired immunodeficiency syndrome: demonstration of B lymphocyte defects in vitro. Diagn Immunol 1986;4:24–30.
76. Borkowsky W, Steele CJ, Grubman S, et al. Antibody responses to bacterial toxoids in children infected with human immunodeficiency virus. J Pediatr 1987;110:563–566.
77. Calvelli T, Rubinstein A. Intravenous gamma-globulin in infants with acquired immunodeficiency syndrome. Pediatr Infect Dis J 1989;5: S207–S210.
78. Pahwa S. Intravenous immune globulin in patients with acquired immune deficiency syndrome. J Allergy Clin Immunol 1989;84: 625-631.

79. National Institute of Child Health and Human Development Intravenous Immunoglobulin Study Group. Intravenous immune globulin for the prevention of bacterial infection in children with symptomatic human immunodeficiency virus infection. N Engl J Med 1991;325: 73–80.
80. Spector SA, Gelber RD, McGrath N, et al. A controlled trial of intravenous immune globulin for the prevention of serious bacterial infections in children receiving zidovudine for advanced human immunodeficiency virus infection. N Engl J Med 1994;331: 1181–1187.
81. Working Group on Antiretroviral Therapy, National Pediatric HIV Resource Center. Antiretroviral therapy and medical management of the HIV-infected child. Pediatr Infect Dis J 1993;12:513–522.
82. Kovacs A, Frederick T, Church J, et al. CD4 T-lymphocyte counts and *Pneumocystis carinii* pneumonia in pediatric HIV infection. JAMA 1991;265:1698–1702.
83. Connor E, Bagarazzi M, McSherry G, et al. Clinical and laboratory correlates of *Pneumocystis carinii* pneumonia in children infected with HIV. JAMA 1991;265:1693–1697.
84. Bye MR, Bernstein LJ, Glaser J, et al. *Pneumocystis carinii* pneumonia in young children with AIDS. Pediatr Pulmonol 1990;9:251–253.
85. Leibovitz E, Rigaud M. Pollack H, et al. *Pneumocystis carinii* pneumonia in infants infected with the human immunodeficiency virus with more than 450 CD4 T lymphocytes per cubic millimeter. N Engl J Med 1990;323:531–533.
86. Centers for Disease Control and Prevention: Guidelines for prophylaxis against *Pneumocystis carinii* pneumonia for children infected with human immunodeficiency virus. MMWR Morb Mortal Wkly Rep 1991;40:1–11.
87. American Academy of Pediatrics Committee on Pediatric AIDS. Evaluation and medical treatment of the HIV-exposed infant. Pediatrics 1997;99:909–917.
88. American Academy of Pediatrics. HIV infection. In: Peter G, ed. 1997 Red Book: Report of the Committee on Infectious Diseases. 24th ed. Elk Grove Village, IL: American Academy of Pediatrics, 1997: 279–304.
89. Centers for Disease Control and Prevention, General recommendations on immunization: recommendations of the Advisory Committee on Immunization Practices (ACIP) MMWR Morb Mortal Wkly Rep 1994;43:RR-1.
90. Centers for Disease Control and Prevention. Measles pneumonitis following measles-mumps-rubella vaccination of a patient with HIV infection, 1993. MMWR Morb Mortal Wkly Rep 1996;45:603–606.
91. Markowitz LE, Chandler FW, Roldan EO, et al. Fatal measles pneumonia without rash in a child with AIDS. J Infect Dis 1988;158: 480–483.
92. Centers for Disease Control and Prevention. Update: vaccine side effects, adverse reactions, contraindications, and precautions. Recommendations of the Advisory Committee on Immunization Practices (ACIP). MMWR Morb Mortal Wkly Rep 1996;45:1–33.
93. McKinney RE, Pizzo PA, Scott GB, et al. Safety and tolerance of intermittent intravenous and oral zidovudine therapy in human immunodeficiency virus–infected pediatric patients. J Pediatr 1990; 116:640–647.
94. McKinney RE, Maha MA, Connor EM, et al. A multicenter trial of oral zidovudine in children with advanced human immunodeficiency virus disease. N Engl J Med 1991;324:1018–1025.
95. Brady MT, McGrath N, Brouwers P, et al. Randomized study of the tolerance and efficacy of high-versus low-dose zidovudine in human immunodeficiency virus-infected children with mild to moderate symptoms (AIDS Clinical Trials Group 128). J Infect Dis 1996;173: 1097–1106.
96. Englund J, Baker C, Raskino C, et al, for the AIDS Clinical Trials Group (ACTG) Study 152 Team. Zidovudine, didanosine, or both as the initial treatment for symptomatic HIV-infected children. N Engl J Med 1997;336:1704–1712.
97. National Institute of Allergy and Infectious Disease Pediatric AIDS Clinical Trials Group ACTG Protocol 300 executive summary. Bethesda, MD: National Institutes of Health, 1997.
98. Spector S, Blanchard S, Wara D, et al. Comparative trial of two dosages of zalcitabine in zidovudine-experienced children with advanced human immunodeficiency virus disease. Pediatr Infect Dis J 1997;16: 623–626.
99. Luzuriaga K, Bryson Y, Krogstad P, et al. Combination treatment with zidovudine, didanosine, and nevirapine in infants with human immunodeficiency virus type I infection. N Engl J Med 1997; 336:1344–1349.
100. Carpenter C, Fischl M, Hammer, S, et al. Antiretroviral therapy for HIV infection in 1997: updated recommendations of the International AIDS Society-USA Panel. JAMA 1997;277:1962–1969.
101. Connor EM, Sperling RS, Gelber R, et al. Reduction of maternal–infant transmission of human immunodeficiency virus type 1 with zidovudine treatment. N Engl J Med 1994;331:1173–1180.
102. Centers for Disease Control and Prevention. Recommendations for the use of zidovudine to reduce perinatal transmission of human immunodeficiency virus. MMWR Morb Mortal Wkly Rep 1994;43: 1–20.
103. Frenkel LM, Cowles MK, Shapiro AJ, et al. Analysis of the maternal components of the AIDS Clinical Trials Group 076 zidovudine regimen in the prevention of mother-to-infant transmission of human immunodeficiency virus type 1. J Infect Dis 1997;174: 971–974.
104. National Institute of Child Health and Human Development. Pediatric AIDS Clinical Trials Group Protocol 185 executive summary. Bethesda, MD: National Institutes of Health, 1997.
105. Centers for Disease Control and Prevention. U.S. Public Health Service recommendations for human immunodeficiency virus counseling and voluntary testing for pregnant women. MMWR Morb Mortal Wkly Rep 1995;44:1–15.
106. Nielsen K, McSherry G, Petru A, et al. A descriptive survey of pediatric human immunodeficiency virus-infected long-term survivors. Pediatrics 1997;99:1–7.

# 13

HIV Among Injecting Drug Users: Epidemiology and Emerging Public Health Perspectives

Don C. Des Jarlais, Holly Hagan, and Samuel R. Friedman

INJECTION OF ILLICIT PSYCHOTROPIC DRUGS: POTENTIAL FOR TRANSMISSION OF INFECTIOUS PATHOGENS

A person who injects drugs intravenously inserts the needle into the skin, searches for a vein, and then typically pulls back on the plunger. Blood coming into the syringe is the indication that the needle has been successfully inserted into a vein and that the injected drug will rapidly travel to the brain. Completely pushing the plunger into the barrel of the syringe does not, however, lead to injection of all the blood–drug mixture; a small residue of blood and drug remains in the needle and syringe. If a second person then injects drugs with the same needle and syringe, the residue from the first user also will be injected into the vein of the second person. These microtransfusions provide an efficient method for transmitting blood-borne pathogens among persons who inject illicit drugs.

This simple "sharing" of needles and syringes is not the only method for transmitting blood-borne pathogens among injecting drug users (IDUs). Drug injectors often combine resources to purchase drugs. Because the drugs are sold through illicit markets, purchasers almost always obtain better prices if they combine finances and purchase in larger quantities. When two or more IDUs have purchased drugs together, they need to divide the jointly obtained drugs equitably. One of the simplest methods for dividing is to put all the drug into solution and then use a needle and syringe to divide this mixture. Because the syringes are finely calibrated with respect to volume of solution in the syringe, they are an excellent means for precise division of drugs. If the syringe used for dividing the drugs contains blood-borne pathogens, however, this division can lead to contamination of the drug solution and infection of the persons who inject the different parts of the drug solution. Syringe-mediated drug sharing has been associated with HIV infection (1).

In addition to needles and syringes, other equipment is used in the injection of psychoactive drugs. "Cookers" (containers such as bottle caps or spoons) are used to dissolve the drugs in water before injection, "cottons" (small pieces of cotton) or "filters" (usually cigarette filters) are often used to filter impurities out of the drug mixture before injecting, and "rinse water" (used to rinse blood out of used needles and syringes so the blood does not clot and render the needle or syringe inoperable) all may become contaminated with blood-borne pathogens, so multiperson use of these could also lead to transmission of the pathogens.

Persons who inject psychoactive drugs also participate in sexual relationships, so they can transmit infectious pathogens to sexual partners, or they can become infected from their sexual partners. Because persons who inject psychoactive drugs also have children, they can be the source of perinatal transmission of infectious pathogens.

GLOBAL EPIDEMIC OF ILLICIT DRUG INJECTION

The injection of illicit psychoactive drugs has been reported in 121 different countries (2). An estimated 5 million persons throughout the world inject illicit drugs (3), and this number probably is growing rapidly. Although much remains to be learned about the international diffusion of illicit drug injection, the following factors appear to be important:

1. Substantial international growth has occurred in the use of "licit" psychoactive drugs. Use of nicotine and alcohol has spread to many areas of the world where these psychoactive drugs are not part of the traditional culture (4–6). Nonmedical psychoactive drug use as a whole, and not simply illicit psychoactive drug use, has been increasing over the last several decades.
2. The globalization of the world economy is a factor. Improvements in communication and transportation and reductions in trade barriers have led to great increases in international trade. These same developments also facilitate international trade in illicit drugs.

3. Economies of scale in illicit drug production are factors. The large profit margins possible in the sale of illicit addicting substances also means that substantial profits can be made by selling these drugs, even to "poor" people. The large profit margins from selling illicit drugs in industrialized countries can be used to underwrite the development of new markets in developing countries. The economics of the international distribution of illicit drugs particularly facilitates the development of domestic drug markets in producing and transit countries.
4. Injecting produces a strong drug effect because of the rapid increase in the concentration of the drug in the brain. Injecting is also highly cost-efficient in that almost all the drug is actually delivered to the brain. On these grounds, intravenous injection can be considered a technologically superior method of psychoactive drug administration. Inexpensive technologic advances tend to disperse widely and are difficult (though not impossible) to reverse (7).

Although current efforts to reduce the supplies of illicit psychoactive drugs probably can be improved, the effectiveness of such efforts is likely to vary across time and place. Therefore, public health officials should plan in terms of further worldwide increases in illicit psychoactive drug injection, with the potential for severe public health consequences, including transmission of blood-borne pathogens such as HIV.

HIV INFECTION AMONG INJECTING DRUG USERS

HIV has been reported among IDUs in 80 countries (2). This is a substantial increase over the 59 countries with HIV infection among IDUs in 1989 (8). In some European countries, such as Spain and Italy, injecting drug use has long been the most common risk factor for HIV infection and AIDS (9). In the United States, injecting drug use has been associated with approximately one-third of the cumulative cases of AIDS (10). Over half the heterosexual transmission cases in the United States have involved transmission from an IDU, and over half the perinatal transmission cases have occurred in women who injected drugs themselves or who were the sexual partners of IDUs. In the most recent estimate of new HIV infections in the United States, approximately half of all new infections in the country are occurring among IDUs (11).

HIV may be introduced into a local population of IDUs through a "bridge population" such as men who have sex with men and who also inject drugs. This appears to be the way in which HIV was first introduced into the IDU population in New York City (12), which was also probably the introduction of HIV into the IDU population in the United States. Travel by IDUs may also introduce HIV into local populations. Contrary to popular stereotypes, many drug injectors do travel, including internationally (13). International "drug tourism" has been noted (14), although not yet well studied. Additionally, incarceration of IDUs from different geographic areas may also contribute to spread of blood-borne viruses among IDUs (15).

Outcomes of Infection

In sharp contrast to HIV infection among homosexual and bisexual men, HIV infection among IDUs leads to a wider variety of illnesses than the original opportunistic infections used to define AIDS. HIV infection has been associated with increased morbidity or increased mortality from tuberculosis, bacterial pneumonias, endocarditis (16), and cervical cancer (through a possible interaction with human papillomavirus) (17). The 1987 and 1993 revisions of the United States Centers for Disease Control (CDC) surveillance definition for AIDS were based in part on the studies of the wider spectrum of HIV-related illnesses among IDUs. Before these revisions, many IDUs were dying from HIV-related illnesses without ever being classified as having AIDS (16).

The mechanisms through which HIV infection leads to this wider spectrum of illnesses have not yet been identified. Tuberculosis infection is controlled primary through cell-mediated immunity, so one would expect HIV infection to lead to increased reactivation of latent tuberculosis infection and increased susceptibility to this infection. HIV infection can also affect humoral immune functioning (18), so resistance to many infectious agents may be compromised. The lifestyle of many IDUs may also put them at greater risk for exposure to many different pathogens and may reduce immune functioning through mechanisms such as poor nutrition.

Whether continued use of psychoactive drugs influences the course of HIV infection among IDUs has been an important question since AIDS was first noticed among IDUs. Many different psychoactive substances have at least some in vitro effects on components of the immune system. Studies comparing progression of HIV infection among IDUs and among men infected through male-with-male sex, however, have generally shown no differences in the rate of CD4 cell count loss or development of AIDS (19). At present, continued use of psychoactive drugs per se does not appear to have any strong effect on the course of HIV infection among IDUs. Immune system activation, however, may increase replication of HIV (20), so high frequencies of nonsterile injections, or that development of other infections such as bacterial pneumonias, may increase progression of HIV infection.

Rapid Transmission of HIV

In many areas, HIV has spread extremely rapidly among IDUs, with the HIV seroprevalence rate (the percentage of IDUs infected with HIV) increasing from less than 10 to 40% or more within 1 to 2 years (21). Several factors have been associated with extremely rapid transmission of HIV among IDUs: 1) lack of awareness of HIV/AIDS as a local threat; 2) restrictions on the availability and use of new injection equipment; and 3) mechanisms for rapid, efficient mixing within the local IDU population. Without an awareness of AIDS as a local threat, IDUs are likely to use each other's equipment frequently. Indeed, before awareness of HIV/AIDS is present, providing previously used equipment to another IDU is likely to be seen as an act of solidarity among IDUs or as a service for which one may legitimately charge a small fee.

Various types of legal restrictions can reduce the availability of sterile injection equipment and thus can lead to increased multiperson use (sharing) of drug injection equipment. In some jurisdictions, medical prescriptions are required for the purchase of needles and syringes. Possession of needles and syringes can also be criminalized as "drug paraphernalia," thereby putting users at risk of arrest if needles and syringes are found in their possession. In some jurisdictions, IDUs have also been prosecuted for possession of drugs based on the minute quantities of drugs that remain in a needle and syringe after it has been used to inject drugs. In addition to the possible legal restrictions on the availability of sterile injection equipment, the actual practices of pharmacists and police can create important limits. Even if laws permit sales of needles and syringes without prescriptions, pharmacists may choose not to sell without prescriptions or not to sell to anyone who "looks like a drug user." Similarly, police may harass IDUs found carrying injection equipment even if there are no laws criminalizing the possession of narcotics paraphernalia.

"Shooting galleries" (places where IDUs can rent injection equipment, which is then returned to the gallery owner for rental to other IDUs) and "dealer's works" (injection equipment kept by a drug seller, which can be lent to successive drug purchasers) are examples of situations that provide rapid, efficient mixing within an IDU population. The mixing is rapid in that many IDUs may use the gallery or the dealer's injection equipment within short periods of time. Several studies have indicated that the infectiousness of HIV is many times greater in 2 to 3 months after initial infection compared with the long "latency" period between initial infection and the development of severe immunosuppression (22). Thus, the concentration of new infections in these settings may synergistically interact with continued mixing and may lead to highly infectious IDUs' transmitting HIV to large numbers of other drug injectors. "Efficient" mixing refers to the sharing of drug injection equipment with few restrictions on who shares with whom. Thus, efficient mixing spreads HIV across potential social boundaries, such as friendship groups, which otherwise could have limited transmission.

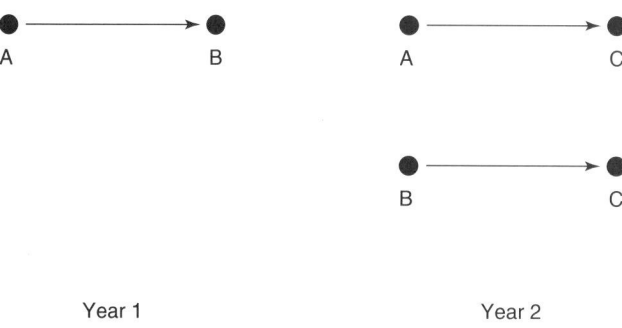

Figure 13.2. Serial monogamy sharing.

Some of the possible dynamics of transmission through rapid, efficient mixing is illustrated in Figure 13.1. In this hypothetic example, an HIV-infected IDU regularly uses shooting galleries and injects three times per day in galleries. This IDU was only recently infected with HIV and thus is in a highly infectious state. As a result of the three injections per day in shooting galleries, this IDU transmits HIV to two other IDUs per day. Each of these newly infected IDUs also uses shooting galleries three times per day, and each of them infects two other IDUs per day. The total number of HIV-infected IDUs thus *triples* every day.

One interesting aspect of the transmission through rapid, efficient mixing is that large-scale risk reduction can have only modest effects on transmission. In the example illustrated in Figure 13.1, consider what would happen if a syringe-exchange outreach worker started supplying the galleries with enough clean syringes so that, rather than having all injections administered with needles and syringes used by others, only half the injections were given with previously used equipment, and half were administered using clean equipment. Thus, the number of unsafe injections is reduced by half, and the number of new infections per infectious person is reduced from two per day to one per day. With this 50% reduction in unsafe injections, the number of infected persons now *doubles* every day instead of tripling every day. This reduction is meaningful, but, of course, it will not stop the ongoing epidemic of HIV transmission.

Figure 13.2 illustrates "serial monogamy" among IDUs, in which each person changes "sharing partners" once a year. Clearly, new HIV infections would occur in this situation, but at a low rate compared with the rapid mixing situation.

This example does contain several important simplifications: newly infected persons are not immediately infectious, the period of high infectiousness after initial HIV infection probably lasts only weeks to several months, and, as larger

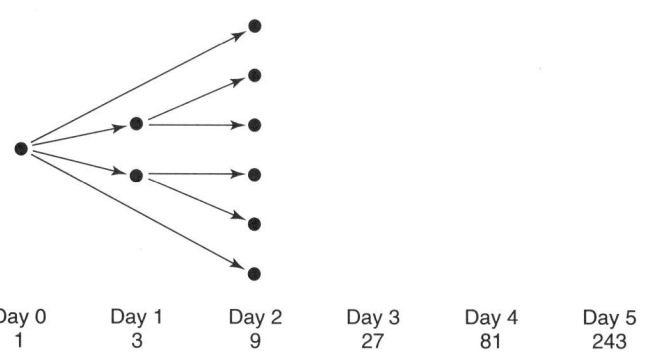

Figure 13.1. Rapid partner change sharing.

proportions of the population become infected, more sharing of needles and syringes in the shooting galleries is between persons who are already infected, and thus no new infections occur. Nevertheless, rapid, efficient mixing can be critical in HIV transmission among IDUs. Based on retrospective interviews we conducted with IDUs in New York City, approximately one-quarter of all injections occurred in shooting galleries, during the period of rapid HIV transmission (1978 to 1984) (23).

HIV/AIDS PREVENTION FOR INJECTING DRUG USERS

Early Studies

The common stereotype that IDUs are not at all concerned about health led to initial expectations that they would not change their behavior because of AIDS. In sharp contrast to these expectations, reductions in risk behavior were observed among IDU participants in many different early prevention programs, including outreach/bleach distribution (24, 25), "education only" (26, 27), drug abuse treatment (28), syringe exchange (29), increased over-the-counter sales of injection equipment (30, 31), and HIV counseling and testing (32, 33).

In addition, evidence indicates that IDUs reduce HIV risk behavior in the absence of any specific prevention program. IDUs in New York City reported risk reduction before the implementation of any formal HIV prevention programs (34, 35). IDUs had learned about AIDS through the mass media and the oral communication networks within the IDU community, and the illicit market in sterile injection equipment had expanded to provide additional equipment (36).

Rather than having to overcome indifference to AIDS among IDUs, the scientific problem became one of understanding and quantifying the change processes. The differences in research design and measurement instruments in these early studies have generally precluded any comparisons regarding the differential effectiveness of the different HIV prevention programs. It was also difficult to determine how a specific prevention program could be contributing to behavior change processes and the effects of the behavior change on the rate of new HIV infections among IDUs and their sexual partners.

Possible "social desirability" effects were also an important potential problem in interpreting the early behavior change studies. Subjects clearly were reporting reduced risk behavior, but this finding could have been a reflection that the subjects simply learned what the researchers wanted to hear and were providing socially desirable responses without any meaningful changes in risk behavior. Research conducted as part of the World Health Organization Multi-Centre Study showed significantly lower HIV infection rates among IDUs who reported changing their behavior in response to AIDS than the rates among IDUs who did not report changing their behavior in response to AIDS (37, 38). Although an important variation was noted across sites, the overall protective effect–adjusted odds ratio of self-reported behavior change against infection with HIV was 0.50. Social desirability effects still must be considered in any research on highly stigmatized behaviors such as injecting drug use and the sharing of drug injection equipment, but evidence indicates the construct validity of self-reported AIDS risk reduction among IDUs.

HIV Incidence Studies

Over the last 10 years, sufficient data have been accumulated to provide reasonable estimates of the likely HIV incidence after implementation of three types of prevention programs: street outreach, syringe exchange, and methadone maintenance treatment.

STREET OUTREACH

The National AIDS Demonstration Research/AIDS Targeted Outreach Model (NADR/ATOM) program was begun in the United States in 1987 and eventually included 41 projects in nearly 50 different cities (39). In all the cities, the NADR/ATOM project involved street outreach to IDUs not in treatment programs. The eligibility requirements for subjects to be enrolled in the research component of the NADR/ATOM projects required that the person must have injected illicit drugs in the previous 6 months and must not have been in drug abuse treatment in the preceding 1 month. Approximately 40% of the more than 30,000 subjects enrolled in the NADR/ATOM projects reported that they had never been in drug abuse treatment.

Many of the NADR/ATOM projects used experimental designs to test psychological theories of health behavior change. All subjects were provided with a "standard" intervention to reduce HIV risk behavior, which included information about HIV and AIDS, a baseline risk assessment, and the option of HIV counseling and testing. Some of these subjects were then randomly assigned to an "enhanced" condition, which typically involved several additional hours of counseling, education, and skill training incorporating components of the psychological theories of health behavior. Subjects were followed at 6-month intervals to assess changes in HIV risk behaviors and the incidence of new HIV infections.

The NADR/ATOM projects provided a wealth of data about HIV risk behaviors among IDUs not in drug treatment programs. With respect to changes in HIV risk behaviors, two strong and consistent findings were reported. First, almost all the NADR/ATOM projects showed substantial reductions in injection risk behavior from the baseline assessment to the follow-up interviews, with the percentage of IDUs reporting that they did not "always use a sterile needle" declining from 64 to 41%, whereas those reporting ever sharing needles declined from 54 to 23% (40).

The second general finding was that few of the different projects showed significant differences in risk reduction between the "standard" intervention and the "enhanced"

Table 13.1. HIV Seroprevalence and HIV Seroconversions per 100 Person-Years at Risk, Among Injecting Drug Users in 14 Localities,[a] by Legal Status of Over-the-Counter Syringe Sales

No. HIV−	No. HIV+	HIV+ (%)	Seroconversions	Person-Years at Risk[b]	Seroconversions per 100 Person-Years at Risk
Localities where over-the-counter sales are illegal:					
A. 288	311	51.9	4	49.3	8.11
B. 1,088	908	45.5	6	146.1	4.10
C. 855	589	40.8	3	81.9	3.66
D. 669	194	22.5	17	262.8	6.47
E. 1,222	76	5.9	2	956.1	0.21
F. 787	14	1.7	0	109.0	0.00
Localities where over-the-counter sales are legal:					
G. 1,760	138	7.3	7	184.0	3.80
H. 652	43	6.2	5	187.0	2.67
I. 1,968	61	3.0	8	732.5	1.09
J. 651	17	2.5	0	225.3	0.00
K. 2,099	31	1.5	2	765.1	0.26
L. 891	13	1.4	3	983.4	0.31
M. 372	4	1.1	0	18.0	0.00
N. 514	5	1.0	0	53.7	0.00

[a]The principal investigators of specific sites are preparing detailed analyses of their data on seroconversion rates; data are publicly available (with locality identifiers removed) through Nova Research Company, Bethesda, MD.
[b]Numbers presented for person-years at risk by locality do not add up to those for the summary table because of rounding error.

interview. The general lack of differences between the "standard" and the "enhanced" interventions should not be interpreted as meaning that the psychological theories of health behavior are not relevant to HIV risk reduction among IDUs. Rather, these results suggest two other possible explanations. First, after the provision of basic information about AIDS (as in the standard intervention), 2 to 6 hours of additional education and counseling do little to further "strengthen" anti-AIDS attitudes, perceptions, and intentions.

A second explanation is that risk reduction among IDUs—again, after basic HIV/AIDS education—is primarily a function of social processes rather than the characteristics of individual IDUs. Thus, information about HIV/AIDS, new attitudes toward risk behaviors, and skills in practicing new behaviors would have been transmitted among active IDUs, influencing persons who had not participated in the "enhanced" conditions.

The NADR/ATOM studies included follow-up of the participants with repeated HIV counseling and testing to detect new HIV infections. Table 13.1 presents data on new HIV infections among participants in the NADR/ATOM projects for which these outcome data are available (41). (The cities are not identified individually, because researchers in those cities are preparing individual research reports.)

Two findings from the NADR/ATOM HIV incidence (new infection) studies are clear. First, the new infection rates are substantially lower in the cities where the initial (background) HIV seroprevalence rates were low. Second, both background HIV seroprevalence and the new infection rates are generally much lower in areas that permit over-the-counter sales of sterile injection equipment (i.e., do not have prescription requirements for the sale of injection equipment).

The higher new infection rates in areas with higher HIV seroprevalence are easily understood in epidemiologic terms. An uninfected person who engages in high-risk behavior (sharing of drug injection equipment or unprotected sexual intercourse) is more likely to encounter an HIV-infected risk partner. Indeed, even within the low-seroprevalence cities, the NADR/ATOM seroincidence data showed was a direct relationship between higher background seroprevalence and higher incidence (41).

The overall incidence rate was also much lower in areas with legal over-the-counter sales of injection equipment (0.79 per hundred person-years at risk) than in areas with prescription requirements for sale of injection equipment (1.99 per hundred person-years at risk) (SR Friedman, et al, unpublished data). Current HIV seroprevalence is the product of past seroincidence (plus changes in the composition of the IDU population), and the presence of over-the-counter sales was also strongly linked with current seroprevalence (so strongly that multivariate analyses were not possible).

However, given the difficulties in establishing factors accounting for current HIV seroprevalence in United States cities where over-the-counter sales of injection equipment are legal, one must be cautious in drawing conclusions about causal relationships between such sales and lower rates of HIV incidence. The data in Table 13.1, however, strongly suggest that over-the-counter sales may be one factor in facilitating safer injection among IDUs. Studies from France (30, 42), Glasgow, Scotland (31), and Connecticut (43) all show HIV risk reduction associated with over-the-counter sales, supporting the interpretation of a causal role for over-the-counter sales in reducing HIV transmission among IDUs.

In addition to the NADR/ATOM outreach/bleach-distribution program data presented in Table 13.1, one such program deserves additional consideration. The NADR program in Chicago not only had one of the strongest theoretic bases, but the Chicago research group also was able to collect 4 years of HIV incidence data in the cohort of IDUs who participated in the program (44). The data showed a dramatic drop in injection risk behavior over the 4-year time period, from 95% of the subjects reporting recent injection risk behavior at the start of the project to only 15% reporting injection risk behavior in the fourth year. HIV incidence in the cohort fell from approximately 9 per 100 person-years at risk during the first year of the cohort follow-up to approximately 2 per 100 person-years at risk for the rest of the follow-up period. Most important was a strong relationship between self-reported injection risk behavior and actual HIV seroconversion: all the subjects who became infected with HIV were from among those who reported current injection risk behavior. All subjects who reported that they stopped injection risk behavior avoided HIV infection. The study did not include a comparison group, so caution is needed in making causal inferences. Nevertheless, the dramatic drop in reported injection risk behavior and the strong association between HIV incidence and reported injection risk behavior suggest that this project did lead to a substantial reduction in HIV transmission among IDUs in the study.

Many of the NADR/ATOM programs distributed small bottles of bleach to IDUs for disinfection of used injection equipment. Bleach is a strong viricide, but some investigators doubt whether the bleach disinfection as practiced by IDUs in the field actually protects against HIV infection. Studies from Baltimore (45) and New York City (46) failed to show any relationship between self-reported use of bleach to disinfect injection equipment and protection from infection with HIV. A third study from Miami, however, did find a significant protective effect against HIV incidence (C McCoy, unpublished data.) Of course, numerous difficulties arise in attempting to find such a relationship. Reporting on the frequency and circumstances of using bleach may not be accurate. IDUs may not now how to use bleach properly to disinfect injection equipment (the current recommendation is for 30 seconds of contact time of full-strength, not diluted bleach in the needle and syringe). Even if IDUs know how to use bleach properly, they may not be using it effectively under "field conditions" (47).

Thus, the effectiveness of the outreach/bleach-distribution programs in lowering rates of new HIV infections among IDUs may be a result of participants' obtaining more sterile injection equipment (from pharmacies or on the illicit market), rather than the result of the actual use of bleach to disinfect used injection equipment.

SYRINGE EXCHANGE

Table 13.2 presents HIV incidence data among participants in syringe-exchange programs. First, as with the outreach/bleach-distribution programs, HIV incidence is low in areas with low background HIV prevalence. HIV incidence is, among other factors, related to the probability of a seronegative IDU sharing equipment with a seropositive IDU. Therefore, perhaps almost any HIV prevention program will appear to be effective in a low-seroprevalence area. Conversely, the presence of syringe-exchange programs (or other easy access to sterile injection equipment) may itself be an important reason that HIV seroprevalence and HIV incidence have remained low in many populations of IDUs.

Table 13.2. Studies of HIV Incidence Among Syringe-Exchange Participants

City	HIV Prevalence[a]	Measured HIV Seroconversions[b]	Estimated HIV Seroconversions[c]	Reference
Lund, Sweden	Low	0	—	78
Glasgow	Low	—	0–1 (2)	13
Sydney	Low	—	0–1 (2)	13
Toronto	Low	—	102 (1)	13
England and Wales (except London)	Low	—	0–1 (1)	79
Kathmandu	Low	0	—	80
Tacoma, WA	Low	< 1	—	81
Portland, OR	Low	< 1	—	82
Montreal	Moderate	5–13	—	49
London	Moderate	—	1–2 (3)	79
Vancouver, BC	Moderate	18	—	50
Amsterdam	High	4	—	Van den Hoek, personal communication
Chicago, IL	High	3	—	Wiebel, personal communication
New York, NY	Very high	1.5	—	83
New Haven, CT	Very high	—	3 (4)	84

[a]Low, 0 to 5%; moderate, 6 to 20%; high, 21 to 40%; very high, 41+%.
[b]Cohort study or repeated testing of participants in per 100 person-years at risk.
[c]Estimated from: (1) stable, very low < 2% seroprevalence in area; (2) self-reports of previous seronegative test and a current HIV blood/saliva test; (3) stable or declining seroprevalence; (4) HIV testing of syringes collected at exchange per 100 person-years at risk.

IDUs from the Montreal and Vancouver exchange have an HIV incidence rate higher than that of the other cities in Table 13.2. The Montreal and Vancouver programs appear to attract a subgroup of IDUs with extremely high initial risk levels (48–50), including high rates of cocaine injection, high levels of unprotected commercial sex work, and homelessness (which may make it difficult to have clean needles available at the time of drug injection). Still, additional data are needed to explain the Montreal and Vancouver incidence rates fully, and new studies are being initiated in these cities.

The HIV incidence data from the three United States high-HIV seroprevalence cities (New Haven, Chicago, and New York) with syringe-exchange programs must be considered encouraging with respect to reducing HIV transmission in high-seroprevalence areas. The data from New Haven are generally consistent with the previously developed mathematical model to assess the effectiveness of the New Haven syringe-exchange program (51).

A major difficulty in interpreting the HIV incidence studies of syringe-exchange participants is the lack of meaningful comparison groups. In almost all areas, IDUs who do not use the syringe exchanges purchase sterile injection equipment from pharmacies, such as in the United Kingdom, Sydney, Australia, and Amsterdam. In the New York City study, however, only the IDUs who used the syringe exchanges had legal access to sterile injection equipment, because New York has a prescription law requirement. The New York City study did show a significantly higher HIV incidence rate among IDUs who did not use the syringe exchanges—5.3 per 100 person-years at risk (52). The New York City study is the first to show a difference in HIV incidence between IDUs who had full legal access to sterile injection equipment for injecting illicit drugs and IDUs who used illegal sources for obtaining their injection equipment.

A study of incident hepatitis B and hepatitis C infection among IDUs in Tacoma, Washington also provides support for the effectiveness of syringe-exchange programs on reducing transmission of blood-borne viruses (53). Tacoma/Pierce County is one of the four counties in the CDC Hepatitis Surveillance System, and thus it has among the best data on hepatitis incidence in the United States. A case-control design was used. Cases of hepatitis B and hepatitis C among IDUs were identified through the surveillance reporting system. Controls were identified among IDUs attending the drug treatment and HIV counseling clinics in the county. (Sera are collected at both clinics, and thus could be tested to identify IDUs who were seronegative for hepatitis.) Demographic data, drug-injection history data, and a determination of whether the subject had ever used the local syringe-exchange program were abstracted from the clinics' records.

Multiple logistic regression analyses were used to identify statistically independent factors differentiating the incident IDU hepatitis cases from the controls. Failure to use the local syringe exchange was strongly associated with both incident hepatitis B and incident hepatitis C. After statistical control for age, gender, race or ethnicity, and duration of injection,

Table 13.3. HIV Incidence among Methadone-Maintenance Patients

Location	Rate Per 100 Person-Years at Risk	Reference
Sweden	0	28
Los Angeles	0.07	57
New York City	0.88	58
Philadelphia	2.3	56
Amsterdam	4	59

the odds ratio for acute infection with hepatitis B among IDUs who had never used the exchange compared with any use of the exchange was over 5 for hepatitis C; the adjusted odds ratio also was over 5 for "never" versus "ever" using the exchange. One of the possible reasons for the strength of these associations is that the local syringe-exchange program is the primary HIV prevention program in the area. Although pharmacies in the area are legally permitted to sell injection equipment without a prescription, many pharmacists choose not to sell to persons suspected of being IDUs.

Of course, the HIV seroincidence data in Table 13.2 and the hepatitis data from the Tacoma study are far from constituting "experimental proof" of the effectiveness of syringe-exchange programs in reducing transmission of blood-borne viruses. Nevertheless, these data clearly indicate that IDUs will use syringe-exchange programs to protect themselves successfully against infection with blood-borne viruses.

METHADONE MAINTENANCE TREATMENT

Many different types of drug abuse treatment, including residential therapeutic communities, outpatient drug-free counseling, and methadone maintenance, have been shown to reduce the use of illicit drugs, including the injection of illicit drugs (54, 55). Thus, one can reasonably expect that participation in drug treatment would lead to reductions in unsafe drug injection and then to reductions in HIV incidence. Although this expectation should hold for all types of drug treatment that have been shown to be effective in reducing drug injection, data are sufficient to assess only methadone maintenance treatment with respect to rates of new HIV infection.

Various studies have shown that participation in methadone maintenance treatment is associated with low rates of HIV risk behavior and with lower HIV seroprevalence, compared with persons not in drug abuse treatment. Table 13.3 shows HIV incidence data among patients receiving methadone in selected cities. The rate among patients receiving methadone maintenance in the Swedish study (28) is particularly striking, given that HIV seroprevalence increased from 0% to approximately 50% over the same period among a group of heroin injectors who applied to the methadone program but could not be accepted because the program was already at capacity. The incidence rate among the Philadelphia methadone patients is not low, but in the same study, HIV incidence among a comparison group of IDUs who were not in methadone maintenance was six times as high (56).

The low rate seen in Los Angeles is undoubtedly a function of the low HIV seroprevalence among IDUs in the Los Angeles area (57). The incidence rate in the New York City program (58) also must be considered low given the high HIV seroprevalence in the city (between 40 and 50% at the time of data collection).

Amsterdam clearly has a high HIV incidence rate among its patients who receive methadone, and this rate is not different from the rate among IDUs in Amsterdam who did not participate in methadone maintenance programs (59). This finding may be due to several factors, including low methadone doses prescribed for the patients (in whom cross-tolerance to heroin and protection from heroin use occurs) and cocaine injection among the patients (methadone provides no pharmacologic protection against cocaine use). Since these data were collected, the Amsterdam program has increased the dosages of methadone that are prescribed.

Integrating Multiple Prevention Programs

Although assisting IDUs to practice safer injection and providing drug abuse treatment to reduce drug injection per se are often perceived as contradictory strategies, in practice they have been complementary strategies. One of the most important lessons of the early outreach programs was that the process of teaching IDUs how to practice safer injection uncovered a previously hidden demand for entry into drug abuse treatment. This unexpected demand for drug abuse treatment led to a program in which New Jersey outreach workers distributed vouchers that could be redeemed for no-cost detoxification treatment (26). Over 95% of the vouchers were redeemed by drug users entering treatment, many of whom had never before been in drug abuse treatment.

The NADR/ATOM projects also uncovered a previously hidden demand for treatment, and they were able successfully to refer many people for treatment (60). The limiting factor in the ability of these programs to place drug users into treatment was usually the lack of available treatment capacity in the different cities.

Syringe-exchange programs also have become important sources of referral to drug misuse treatment programs. For example, the New Haven program reported that 33% of the first 569 participants were referred to drug treatment (51). The Tacoma syringe-exchange program has become the leading source of referrals to the local drug treatment program (61). The capacity of outreach/bleach-distribution programs and syringe-exchange programs to make effective referrals to drug treatment programs may depend primarily on the availability of treatment in the local area and on whether the programs can afford the appropriate staff to make and follow through on referrals.

Although much progress has been made in providing referrals from outreach/bleach-distribution programs to drug abuse treatment programs, HIV prevention efforts in many countries, including the United States, are still hampered by a lack of "referrals" from drug abuse treatment programs to bleach-distribution and syringe-exchange programs. Whereas drug abuse treatment programs lead to substantial and well-documented reductions in illicit drug use (55), it would be unrealistic to expect that all IDUs who enter treatment programs will abstain from further illicit drug injection. Indeed, most are likely to fail to be treated completely, or they use illicit drugs while in treatment. Some drug treatment programs in the United States currently include information about the locations and hours of operation of local bleach-distribution and syringe-exchange programs as part of the "AIDS education" provided to all entrants into treatment. (Many European drug treatment programs actually provide syringe-exchange services on site.) In general, however, drug abuse treatment programs in the United States and in many developing counties have not yet developed strategies for reducing the likelihood that persons who relapse to drug injection will become infected with HIV through sharing of drug injection equipment.

Standards for Assessing Prevention Programs

Evaluation of HIV prevention programs is critical to reducing HIV transmission. The resources available for HIV prevention are limited—in many developing countries, these resources are severely limited. Thus, expending resources on ineffective programs involve great "opportunity lost" costs. Randomized clinical trials are the current standard for evaluating public health and medical interventions. However, many good reasons exist not to use randomized clinical trials for HIV prevention efforts. First, effective HIV prevention often occurs at a community level rather than at an individual level. This means that the community (or local population of IDUs) is the appropriate unit of analysis for evaluating prevention programs. Although community-level randomized clinic trials are possible, they are usually difficult and expensive to conduct. Second, HIV prevention may depend on the local context. As noted earlier, both street outreach programs and syringe-exchange programs are likely to be associated with low HIV incidence if they are implemented in populations with low seroprevalence. Local transportation systems may affect mixing patterns among IDUs and thus the potential for rapid-partner-change types of transmission. Thus, a large sample of communities may be needed to assess a particular type of HIV prevention program. Given the multiple difficulties in conducting randomized clinical trials for HIV prevention, we would suggest the following criteria for evaluating the public health effectiveness of HIV prevention programs:

1. A sound biologic, psychological or sociologic theory underlies the intervention. For example, at the biologic level, syringes obtained from pharmacies or exchanges do

not contain HIV, and HIV does not penetrate latex condoms. At a psychological level, persons with accurate information about how HIV is and is not transmitted are more likely to be able to reduce their risk behavior; persons who have options in selecting methods for reducing risk are more likely to change their risk behavior. At a social level, IDUs do influence each others' behavior and can thus act as influence agents to reduce the risk behavior or their peers. The underlying theory in the prevention program should be sufficiently well established that it would be unethical to conduct a randomized trial of that theory, although specific methods of operationalizing the theory may need to be tested empirically.

2. The prevention program is popular with the target audience. It attracts and retains large numbers of persons at risk for HIV transmission.
3. Participants in the program achieve a low HIV transmission rate. A "low" incidence rate must be determined with respect to HIV seroprevalence in the local population of IDUs. We would suggest that in areas where the seroprevalence is under 10%, a "low" incidence rate would be 1% per year or less. In areas with higher HIV seroprevalence rates, we would suggest that a "low" incidence rate would be 2% per year or less.

Randomized clinical trials may be the current standard for assessing HIV prevention programs, but conducting such studies is often resource intensive and logistically difficult. Additionally, for many aspects of HIV prevention, present knowledge would make a randomized clinical trial unethical, for example, providing access to condoms versus denying access to condoms or providing access to sterile injection equipment versus denying access to sterile injection equipment. Randomized clinical trial studies should thus be used when investigators are uncertain whether a specific type of prevention program will be effective and, if the program is effective, whether it is likely to have a large public health impact. In the absence of these two conditions, we would suggest that the foregoing three criteria should be used for assessing HIV prevention efforts.

Current Problematic Issues in Preventing Infection

Much has been learned in the last decade of research on prevention of HIV infection among IDUs. Most important, all studies to date have shown that the large majority of IDUs will modify their behavior to reduce the chances of becoming infected with HIV. The theoretic bases for HIV prevention efforts have expanded from "factual education" to psychological and social-change theories. Prevention programs are increasingly providing the means for behavior change (for safer injection and for reducing drug injection). Despite the progress in terms of research findings, increasing sophistication of prevention programs, and actual reduction in HIV transmission, some problem areas still exist with respect to prevention of new HIV infections among IDUs in some industrialized countries—the United States in particular—and in many developing countries.

HIV PREVENTION IN HIGH-SEROPREVALENCE AREAS

Current prevention programs for IDUs in low-seroprevalence areas appear capable of achieving control over HIV transmission (62). These programs cannot prevent all new HIV infections, but they appear to be able to maintain low seroprevalence indefinitely. In these areas of low HIV seroprevalence, almost all remaining risk behavior among IDUs occurs among persons who are HIV seronegative and therefore without transmission of the virus. In areas of high HIV seroprevalence, however, even moderate levels of injection risk behavior are likely to involve persons of different HIV serostatus and thus to lead to transmission of the virus. Recent analyses conducted by Holmberg of the CDC (11) suggest that transmission of HIV among IDUs in high-seroprevalence areas may account for the plurality of new HIV infections in the United States.

A new generation of HIV prevention programs may thus be needed for IDUs in high-HIV-seroprevalence areas. In addition to more intensive programs focusing on safer injection, programs are needed to reduce the numbers of persons injecting illicit drugs in high-seroprevelance areas. Massive expansion of drug abuse treatment could lead to large reductions in the numbers of persons who are injecting illicit drugs. Programs to reduce initiation into drug injection would also be useful for high-seroprevalence areas, because these would also lead to a reduction over time in the numbers of IDUs (63).

SEXUAL TRANSMISSION OF HIV

Although consistent evidence indicates that IDUs will make large changes in their injection risk behavior in response to concerns about AIDS, changes in sexual behavior appear to be much more modest. All studies that have compared changes in injection risk behavior with changes in sexual risk behavior found greater changes in injection risk behavior (64). In general, IDUs appear more likely to make risk-reduction efforts (reduced numbers of partners, increased use of condoms) in "casual" sexual relationships rather than in "primary" sexual relationships (64)

The reasons for the difficulties in changing the sexual behavior of IDUs have not been fully clarified, but the problem appears in many different cultural settings, including IDUs in Asia, Europe, and South America, as well as in the United States (13). To place the problem in perspective, however, IDUs have undoubtedly changed their sexual risk behavior more than noninjecting heterosexuals in the United States as a whole (65).

One factor that appears to be important in increasing condom use among IDUs is an altruistic desire to avoid transmitting HIV to a noninjecting sexual partner. In both Bangkok (66) and New York City (67), IDUs who know (or have reason to suspect) that they are HIV positive are particularly likely to use condoms in relationships with sexual partners who do not inject illicit drugs. Most programs that have urged IDUs to use condoms thus far have focused on the self-protective effects of condom usage. Appealing to altruistic feelings of protecting others from HIV infection may be an untapped source of motivation for increasing condom use.

Heterosexual transmission from IDUs to their sexual partners who do not inject drugs has occurred in the United States since the first heterosexual IDUs were infected with HIV. The use of crack cocaine is often associated with high frequencies of unsafe sexual behaviors. In cities such as New York and Miami, which have large numbers of HIV-infected IDUs who also use crack cocaine, the use of crack without injection drug use has itself become an important risk factor for infection with HIV (68). Although intervening in the nexus of injection drug use–crack use–unsafe sex will be difficult, one strategy that could be used is to provide prompt treatment for genital ulcerative sexually transmitted diseases such as syphilis. The presence of these ulcerative sexually transmitted diseases appears to increase the likelihood of HIV transmission (69).

Additional strategies are needed for increasing safer sex among IDUs who engage in male-with-male sexual activities. IDUs who also engage in male-with-male sex can act as a bridge population between nondrug-injecting men who engage in male-with-male sex and the larger IDU population. In many industrialized countries, HIV seroprevalence among men who engage in male-with-male sex is substantially higher than among exclusively heterosexual IDUs. Indications exist of "slippage" back to high-risk sexual behavior among men who have sex with men in San Francisco (70, 71) and Amsterdam (72). If slippage back to unsafe sex should occur among men who have sex with men in the United States as a whole, this could lead to more HIV infection among male IDUs who engage in male-with-male sex, followed by more transmission from these men to other IDUs.

"INSUFFICIENT" PROGRAMS

Considerable evidence indicates that outreach programs, programs to provide access to sterile injection equipment, and drug abuse treatment programs can substantially reduce HIV transmission among IDUs. Although most of these programs have been associated with low rates of new HIV infections, occasional examples of programs that were not sufficient in reducing HIV transmission have been reported. The methadone treatment program in Amsterdam and the syringe-exchange programs in Montreal and Vancouver are examples of insufficient programs discussed previously.

The "first generation" of HIV prevention studies demonstrated that prevention programs can be, and most are, effective in reducing HIV transmission. A "second generation" of research that identifies characteristics of effective and less than sufficient programs is now needed. This research will need to examine not only program characteristics and individual behavior change, but also the social contexts of drug use and the social networks, social influence, and mixing patterns among drug users.

PROVISION OF PREVENTION SERVICES

Although important questions still must answered with respect to the implementation of HIV prevention among IDUs, the biggest single problem may simply be the scarcity of HIV prevention services for IDUs in the world. For example, in the United States, the Presidential Commission on the HIV Epidemic recommended in 1988 that drug abuse treatment be provided to all persons who desire it. The United States National Commission on AIDS made the same recommendation in 1991 (73). The National Commission on AIDS also recommended the removal of "legal barriers to the purchase and possession" of sterile injection equipment. Although syringe-exchange services have expanded in the United States in the last several years, the Commission's recommendations would appear as valid today as when they were initially made. In many developing countries, drug addiction is not seen as a health problem, and scarce available resources are allocated only to law enforcement efforts at controlling illicit drug use.

HARM REDUCTION

The worldwide epidemic of HIV infection among IDUs has led to important conceptual developments on injecting drug use as a health problem. HIV and AIDS have dramatically increased the adverse health consequences of injecting drug use and thus have led to the perception of psychoactive drug use as more of a health problem and not just a criminal justice problem. At the same time, HIV infection can be prevented without requiring the cessation of injecting drug use. This potential separation of a severe adverse consequence of drug use from the drug use itself has encouraged analysis of other areas in which adverse consequences of drug use could be reduced without requiring cessation of drug use.

The ability of many IDUs to modify their behavior to reduce the chances of HIV infection has also led to consideration of drug addicts both as concerned about their health and as capable of acting on that concern (without denying the compulsive nature of drug dependence). These ideas have formed much of the basis for what has been termed the "harm reduction" perspective on psychoactive drug use (74–77). This perspective emphasizes the pragmatic need to reduce harmful consequences of psychoactive drug use while acknowledging that eliminating psychoactive drug use and misuse is not likely to be feasible in the foreseeable future. One of the major strengths of the harm reduction perspective is its applicability to both licit (alcohol, nicotine) and illicit psychoactive drugs.

Acknowledgments

Sections of this chapter were originally prepared as reports to the United Kingdom Department of Health and the United States Congress Office of Technology Assessment. Additional support was provided by grant DA R01 03574 from the National Institute on Drug Abuse.

References

1. Jose B, Friedman SR, Curtis R, et al. Syringe-mediated drug-sharing (backloading): a new risk factor for HIV among injecting drug users. AIDS 1993;7:1653–1660.
2. Des Jarlais DC, Stimson GV, Hagan H, et al. Emerging infectious diseases and the injection of illicit psychoactive drugs. Curr Issues Public Health 1996;2:102–137.
3. Mann J, Tarantola J, Netter T. AIDS in the world. Cambridge, MA: Harvard University Press, 1992:407–411.
4. Peto R. Smoking and death: the past 40 years and the next 40. BMJ 1994;309:937–939.
5. Mackay JL. The fight against tobacco in developing countries. Tuber Lung Dis 1994;75:8–24.
6. Ambler CH. Drunks, brewers and chiefs: alcohol regulation in colonial Kenya 1900–1939. In: Barrow S, Room R, eds. Drinking behaviour and belief in modern history. Berkeley, CA: University of California Press, 1991.
7. Rogers E. Diffusion of innovations. Vol 3. New York: Free Press, 1982.
8. Des Jarlais DC, Friedman SR. AIDS and IV drug use. Science 1989;245:578–579.
9. European Centre for the Epidemiological Monitoring of AIDS. Third quarterly report. Paris: European Centre for the Epidemiological Monitoring of AIDS, 1996.
10. Centers for Disease Control and Prevention. HIV/AIDS surveillance report. Atlanta, GA: Centers for Disease Control and Prevention, 1995.
11. Holmberg S. The estimated prevalence and incidence of HIV in 96 large US metropolitan areas. Am J Public Health 1996;86:642–654.
12. Des Jarlais DC, Friedman SR, Novick D, et al. HIV-1 infection among intravenous drug users in Manhattan, New York City, from 1977 through 1987. JAMA 1989;261:1008–1012.
13. Ball A, Des Jarlais DC, Donoghoe M, et al. Multi-Centre study on drug injecting and risk of HIV infection: Programme on Substance Abuse. Geneva: World Health Organization, 1994.
14. Simons M. Drug tourism in Europe. New York Times, April 20, 1994:A8.
15. Wright N, Vanichseni S, Akarasewi P, et al. Was the 1988 HIV epidemic among Bangkok's injecting drug users a common source outbreak? AIDS 1994;8:529–532.
16. Stoneburner R, Des Jarlais D, Benezra D, et al. A larger spectrum of severe HIV-1-related disease in intravenous drug users in New York City. Science 1988;242:916–919.
17. Vermund SH, Kelley KF, Klein RS, et al. High risk of human papillomavirus infection and cervical squamous intraepithelial lesions among women with symptomatic human immunodeficiency virus infection. Am J Obstet Gynecol 1991;165:392–400.
18. Zolla-Pazner S, Des Jarlais DC, Friedman SR, et al. Nonrandom development of immunologic abnormalities after infection with human immunodeficiency virus: implications for immunologic classification of the disease. Proc Natl Acad Sci U S A 1987;84:5404–5408.
19. Margolick JB, Munoz A, Vlahov D, et al. Direct comparison of the relationship between clinical outcome and change in CD4+ lymphocytes in human immunodeficiency virus–positive homosexual men and injecting drug users. Arch Intern Med 1994;154:868–875.
20. Zagury D, Bernard J, Leonard R, et al. Long-term cultures of HTLV-III–infected T cells: a model of cytopathology of T-cell depletion in AIDS. Science 1986;231:850–853.
21. Des Jarlais DC, Friedman SR, Choopanya K, et al. International epidemiology of HIV and AIDS among injecting drug users. AIDS 1992;6:1053–1068.
22. Jacquez J, Koopman J, Simon C, et al. Role of the primary infection in epidemic HIV infection of gay cohorts. J Acquir Immune Defic Syndr Hum Retrovirol 1994;7:1169–1184.
23. Des Jarlais DC, Friedman SR, Sotheran JL, et al. Continuity and change within an HIV epidemic: injecting drug users in New York City, 1984 through 1992. JAMA 1994;271:121–127.
24. Thompson PI, Jones TS, Cahill K, et al. Promoting HIV prevention outreach activities via community-based organizations. Presented at the 6th International Conference on AIDS, San Francisco, 1990.
25. Wiebel W, Chene D, Johnson W. Adoption of bleach use in a cohort of street intravenous drug users in Chicago. Presented at the 6th International Conference on AIDS, San Francisco, 1990.
26. Jackson J, Rotkiewicz L. A coupon program: AIDS education and drug treatment. Presented at the 3rd International Conference on AIDS, Washington, DC, 1987.
27. Ostrow DG. AIDS prevention through effective education. Daedalus 1989;118:29–254.
28. Blix O, Gronbladh L. AIDS and IV heroin addicts: the preventive effect of methadone maintenance in Sweden. Presented at the 4th International Conference on AIDS, Stockholm, 1988.
29. Buning EC, Hartgers C, Verster AD, et al. The evaluation of the needle/syringe exchange in Amsterdam. Presented at the 4th International Conference on AIDS, Stockholm, 1988.
30. Espinoza P, Bouchard I, Ballian P, et al. Has the open sale of syringes modified the syringe exchanging habits of drug addicts? Presented at the 4th International Conference on AIDS, Stockholm, 1988.
31. Goldberg D, Watson H, Stuart F, et al. Pharmacy supply of needles and syringes: the effect on spread of HIV in intravenous drug misusers. Presented at the 4th International Conference on AIDS, Stockholm, 1988.
32. Cartter ML, Petersen LR, Savage RB, et al. Providing HIV counseling and testing services in methadone maintenance programs. AIDS 1990;4:463–465.
33. Higgins DL, Galavotti C, O'Reilly KR, et al. Evidence for the effects of HIV antibody counseling and testing on risk behaviors. JAMA 1991;266:2419–2429.
34. Friedman SR, Des Jarlais DC, Sotheran JL, et al. AIDS and self-organization among intravenous drug users. Int J Addict 1987;22:201–219.
35. Selwyn P, Feiner C, Cox C, et al. Knowledge about AIDS and high-risk behavior among intravenous drug abusers in New York City. AIDS 1987;1:247–254.
36. Des Jarlais DC, Friedman SR, Hopkins W. Risk reduction for the acquired immunodeficiency syndrome among intravenous drug users. Ann Intern Med 1985;103:755–759.
37. Des Jarlais DC, Choopanya K, Vanichseni S, et al. AIDS risk reduction and reduced HIV seroconversion among injection drug users in Bangkok. Am J Public Health 1994;84:452–455.
38. Des Jarlais DC, Friedmann P, Hagan H, et al. The protective effect of AIDS-related behavioral change among injection drug users: a cross-national study. Am J Public Health 1996;86:1780–1785.
39. Brown BS, Beschner GM, eds. Handbook on risk of AIDS: injection drug users and sexual partners. Wesport, CT: Greenwood Press, 1993.
40. Stephens RC, Simpson DD, Coyle SL, et al. Comparative effectiveness of NADR interventions. In: Brown BS, Beschner GM, eds. Handbook on risk of AIDS. Westport, CT: Greenwood Press, 1993.
41. Friedman SR, Jose B, Deren S, et al. Risk factors for human immunodeficiency virus seroconversion amoung out-of-treatment drug injectors in high and low seroprevalance cities. Am J Epidemiol 1995;142:864–874.
42. Ingold FR, Ingold S. The effects of the liberalization of syringe sales on the behavior of intravenous drug users in France. Bull Narc 1989;41:67–81.
43. Groseclose SL, Weinstein B, Jones TS, et al. Impact of increased legal access to needles and syringes on practices of injecting-drug users and police officers: Connecticut, 1992–1993. J Acquir Immune Defic Syndr Hum Retrovirol 1995;10:82–89.
44. Wiebel W, Jimenez A, Johnson W, et al. Positive effect on HIV seroconversion of street outreach intervention with IDU in Chicago, 1988–1992. Presented at the 9th International Conference on AIDS, Berlin, 1993.
45. Vlahov D, Astemborski J, Solomon L, et al. Field effectiveness of needle disinfection among injecting drug users. J Acquir Immune Defic Syndr Hum Retrovirol 1994;7:760–766.
46. Titus S, Marmor M, Des Jarlais DC, et al. Bleach use and HIV seroconversion among New York City injection drug users. J Acquir Immune Defic Syndr Hum Retrovirol 1994;7:700–704.

47. Gleghorn AA, Jones TS, Doherty MC, et al. Acquisition and use of needles and syringes by injecting drug users in Baltimore, Maryland. J Acquir Immune Defic Syndr Hum Retrovirol 1995;10:97–103.
48. Lamothe F, Bruneau J, Soto J, et al. Risk factors for HIV seroconversion among injecting drug users in Montreal: the Saint-Luc Cohort experience. Presented at the 10th International Conference on AIDS, Yokohama, Japan, 1994.
49. Hankins C, Gendron S, Tran T. Montreal needle exchange attenders versus non-attenders: what's the difference? Presented at the 10th International Conference on AIDS, Yokohama, Japan, 1994.
50. Strathdee S, Patrick D, Currie S, et al. Needle exchange is not enough: Lessons from the Vancouver injection drug use study. AIDS 1997;11: F59–F65.
51. O'Keefe E, Kaplan E, Khoshnood K. Preliminary report: City of New Haven needle exchange program. New Haven, CT: Office of Mayor John C. Daniels, 1991.
52. Des Jarlais DC, Marmor M, Paone D, et al. HIV incidence among injecting drug users in New York City syringe-exchange programmes. Lancet 1996;348:987–991.
53. Hagan H, Des Jarlais DC, Friedman SR, et al. Reduced risk of hepatitis B and hepatitis C among injecting drug users participating in the Tacoma syringe exchange program. Am J Public Health 1995;85: 1531–1537.
54. Gerstein D, Harwood H, eds. Treating drug problems. Washington, DC: National Academy Press, 1990.
55. Hubbard RL, Marsden ME, Rachal JV, et al, eds. Drug Abuse Treatment: A National Study of Effectiveness. Chapel Hill, NC: University of North Carolina Press, 1989.
56. Metzger D, Woody G, McLellan AT, et al. Human immunodeficiency virus seroconversion among in- and out-of-treatment intravenous drug users: an 18 month prospective follow-up. J Acquir Immune Defic Syndr 1993;6:1049–1056.
57. Kerndt P, Weber M, Ford W. HIV incidence among injection drug users enrolled in a Los Angeles methadone program. JAMA 1995;278: 1831–1832.
58. Orr M, Friedmann P, Glebatis D, et al. Incidence of HIV infection among clients of a methadone maintenance program in New York City. JAMA 1996;276:99.
59. van Ameijden EJC, van den Hoek A, Coutinho RA. Risk factors for HIV seroconversion in injecting drug users in Amsterdam, the Netherlands. Presented at the 7th International Conference on AIDS, Florence: Italy, 1991.
60. Ashery RS, Davis H, Davis WH, et al. Entry into treatment of IDUs based on the association of outreach workers with treatment programs. In: Brown BS, Beschner GM, eds. Handbook on risk of AIDS. Westport, CT: Greenword Press, 1993:386–395.
61. Hagan H, Des Jarlais DC, Friedman SR, et al. Risk of human immunodeficiency virus and hepatitis B virus in users of the Tacoma syringe exchange program. In: Proceedings of the National Academy of Sciences Workshop on Needle Exchange and Bleach Distribution Programs. Washington: National Academy Press, 1994.
62. Des Jarlais DC, Hagan HH, Friedman SR, et al. Maintaining low HIV seroprevalence in populations of injecting drug users. JAMA 1995;274: 1226–1231.
63. Des Jarlais DC, Casriel C, Friedman SR, et al. AIDS and the transition to illicit drug injection: results of a randomized trial prevention program. Br J Addict 1992;87:493–498.
64. Friedman SR, Des Jarlais DC, Ward TP. Overview of the history of the HIV epidemic among drug injectors. In: Brown BS, Beschner GM, Consortium NAR, eds. Handbook on risk of AIDS: injection drug users and sexual partners. Westport, CT: Greenwood Press, 1993:3–15.
65. Laumann EO, Gagnon JH, Michael RT, et al. The social organization of sexuality: sexual practices in the United States. Chicago: University of Chicago Press, 1994.
66. Vanichseni S, Des Jarlais DC, Choopanya K, et al. Condom use with primary partners among injecting drug users in Bangkok, Thailand and New York City, United States. AIDS 1993;7:887–891.
67. Friedman SR, Jose B, Neaigus A, et al. Consistent condom use in relationships between seropositive injecting drug users and sex partners who do not inject drugs. AIDS 1994;8:357–361.
68. Edlin BR, Irwin KL, Faruque S, et al. Intersecting epidemics: crack cocaine use and HIV infection among inner-city young adults. N Engl J Med 1994;331:1422–1427.
69. Chiasson MA, Stoneburner RL, Hildebrandt DS, et al. Heterosexual transmission of HIV-1 associated with the use of smokable freebase cocaine (crack). AIDS 1991;5:1121–1126.
70. Ekstrand ML, Coates TJ. Maintenance of safer sexual behaviors and predictors of risky sex: the San Francisco Men's Health Study. Am J Public Health 1990;80:973–977.
71. Stall R, Ekstrand ML, Pollack L, et al. Relapse from safer sex: the next challenge for AIDS prevention efforts. J Acquir Immune Defic Syndr 1990;3:1181–1187.
72. de Wit JFB, de Vroome EMM, Sandfort TGM, et al. Safer sexual practices not reliably maintained by homosexual men. Am J Public Health 1992;82:615–616.
73. National Commission on AIDS. The twin epidemics of substance use and HIV. Washington, DC: National Commission on AIDS, 1991.
74. Brettle RP. HIV and harm reduction for injection drug users. AIDS 1991;5:125–36.
75. Des Jarlais DC, Friedman SR, Ward TP. Harm reduction: a public health response to the AIDS epidemic among injecting drug users. Annu Rev Public Health 1993;14:413–50.
76. Des Jarlais DC. Harm reduction: a framework for incorporating science into drug policy [editorial]. Am J Public Health 1995;85:10–12.
77. Heather N, Wodak A, Nadelmann E, et al, eds. Psychoactive drugs and harm reduction: from faith to science. London: Whurr Publishers, 1993.
78. Ljungberg B, Christensson B, Tunving K, et al. HIV prevention among injecting drug users: three years of experience from a syringe exchange program in Sweden. J Acquir Immune Defic Syndr Hum Retrovirol 1991;4:890–95.
79. Stimson GV. AIDS and injecting drug use in the United Kingdom, 1987–1993: the policy response and the prevention of the epidemic. Soc Science Med 1995;41:699–716.
80. Maharjan SH, Peak A, Rana S, et al. Declining risk for HIV among IDUs in Kathmandu: impact of a harm reduction programme. Presented at the 10th International Conference on AIDS, Yokohama, Japan, 1994.
81. Hagan H, Des Jarlais DC, Purchase D, et al. The Tacoma syringe exchange. J Addict Dis 1991;10:81–88.
82. Oliver K, Maynard H, Friedman SR, et al, eds. Behavioral and community impact of the Portland syringe exchange program. In: Proceedings: Workshop in Needle Exchange and Bleach Distribution Programs. Washington, DC: National Academy of Sciences, 1994: 35–39.
83. Des Jarlais DC, Marmor M, Paone D, et al. HIV incidence among syringe exchange participants in New York City. Lancet 1996;348: 987–991.
84. Kaplan EH, Heimer R. HIV incidence among needle exchange participants: estimates from syringe tracking and testing data. J Acquir Immune Defic Syndr Hum Retrovirol 1994;7:182–189.

14

PNEUMOCYSTIS CARINII PNEUMONIA

Michael P. Dubé and Fred R. Sattler

In the early years of the acquired immunodeficiency syndrome (AIDS) epidemic, *Pneumocystis* pneumonia was the initial case-defining event in nearly 60% of AIDS patients in North America (1), and almost 80% experienced at least one episode during their lifetime (2, 3). Most patients were treated in hospitals and experienced appreciable morbidity from cough, breathlessness, chest pressure, weight loss, and drug-induced toxicities. Mortality was high, and the cost for each hospital admission was estimated at $10,000 to $20,000. Some survivors required supplemental oxygen for months.

With the advent of effective prophylaxis, the relative incidence of *Pneumocystis* pneumonia has decreased (4–6). However, *Pneumocystis* is still a leading cause of death (4, 5) and in one survey the infection occurred in 22% of patients during the 6 months before death (7). Even with prophylaxis, *Pneumocystis* pneumonia still occurs, particularly among individuals with very low CD4 cell counts (8). *Pneumocystis* pneumonia therefore continues to be a major cause of human suffering and contributes greatly to health care costs for episodes requiring hospitalization.

For patients who are receiving regular medical care and who are monitored closely, diagnosis of *Pneumocystis* pneumonia is often difficult because the clinical presentation may be insidious or atypical, especially for those receiving prophylaxis (9–14). Careful vigilance and use of ancillary tests are often necessary for early detection and treatment while the infection is amenable to ambulatory care and oral therapy. Thus, *Pneumocystis* pneumonia will remain a major health care problem and challenge for clinicians and investigators into the next millennium.

ETIOLOGY AND INCIDENCE

Pneumocystis carinii was first described by Chagas, who misidentified the organism as the sexual state of *Trypanosoma cruzi* (15). The organism was identified as a unique microbe in Parisian sewer rats by the Delanoes in 1912 (16). *P. carinii* was not appreciated as a human pathogen until it was causally related to plasma cell pneumonia in 3- to 6-month-old premature, marasmic infants housed in post–World War II orphanages in Europe (17–19). After that time, approximately 100 cases of "*Pneumocystis* pneumonia" occurred each year in severely immunocompromised patients in the United States (20, 21). Not until the early years of the AIDS epidemic in North America, where *Pneumocystis* pneumonia occurred nearly 3 times more often than any other AIDS-defining event, did the infection receive widespread attention (1, 2).

Pneumocystis carinii is a eukaryotic microbe with a nuclear membrane and intracellular organelles. Its morphologic features, failure to grow on fungal culture media, and response to drugs used to treat protozoan infections suggested for years that it was a protozoan. However, the organism has an affinity for fungal stains, and detailed ultrastructural analysis suggested as early as 1970 that *P. carinii* had morphologic features more similar to those of fungi (22, 23). Molecular analysis of 16S ribosomal RNA and mitochondrial DNA from the organism revealed that it is a fungus and phylogenetically closely related to the *Ascomycetes* and *Basidiomycetes* yeasts (24–29). A 6785 base pair sequence of mitochondrial DNA from *P. carinii* contains the genes for the reduced nicotinamide adenine dinucleotide (NADH) dehydrogenase subunits 1, 2, 3, and 6, cytochrome oxidase subunit II and apocytochrome b (28). Analysis of these sequences showed a 60% similarity with fungi but only a 20% similarity with protozoa. Moreover, the dihydrofolate reductase (DHFR) of *P. carinii* is of lower molecular weight than protozoan DHFR because it lacks combined thymidylate synthetase–DHFR activity present in the corresponding protozoan protein function (30, 31). Finally, fungi possess an elongation factor for protein synthesis that is also present in *P. carinii* (32).

Pneumocystis carinii, however, has features that are atypical for a fungus. It is resistant to standard antifungal agents (e.g., amphotericin and azole drugs) that affect the outer sterol membranes of fungi. *P. carinii* lacks ergosterol and contains cholesterol instead, but so do some fungi (33–36). The cell wall of the trophozoite form of *P. carinii*, which is more abundant in infected lungs than the cyst form, is unusually fragile and contains β-glucan (37). Antifungal compounds (e.g., echinocandins and papulocandins) that inhibit β-glucan synthesis reduced both *P. carinii* cysts and trophozoites in immunosuppressed rats (38, 39). Finally, *P. carinii* contains only two copies of the ribosomal RNA gene, compared with most fungi, which contain hundreds of copies of the gene (40).

Considerable genotypic and antigenic variation exists among *Pneumocystis carinii* isolated from different host species as well as among *P. carinii* found in the same host species (41). Differences in various proteins have been described (42–47). Considerable genetic differences demonstrated by karyotyping (48) and sequencing analysis (49–61) definitively establish strain differences. However, whether these differences establish that multiple species of *P. carinii* exist remains controversial. At present, the different variants of *P. carinii* are referred to as "special forms." Using a trinomial nomenclature system, human *P. carinii* is known as *P. carinii* special form *hominis* (*P.c.* sp. f. *hominis*).

Genetic divergence also exists among isolates of *Pneumocystis carinii hominis* from different human sources. Variation in RNA (54, 62, 63) and in internal transcribed spacer (ITS) genes (64–66) has been demonstrated and suggests the existence of multiple human strains.

Better understanding of the molecular composition of the functional and structural constituents of *Pneumocystis carinii* will ultimately provide valuable insights into pathogenic mechanisms and targets for development of more effective therapies.

EPIDEMIOLOGY AND TRANSMISSION

Serologic testing with indirect fluorescent antibody (IFA) or enzyme-linked immunosorbent assay (ELISA) techniques and recent investigations to detect antibody to the major (40-kd) antigen of human *Pneumocystis carinii* indicate that 80 to 90% of children have been exposed to the organism during their first few years of life (67–72). The most generally accepted hypothesis for pathogenesis has been that organisms remain latent until persons become severely immune compromised when reactivation of *P. carinii* occurs. This theory provides the rationale for not isolating patients, but few data support the hypothesis.

In the laboratory, immune-suppressed rodents acquire infection through inhalation of *Pneumocystis carinii* (73–77). With electrophoretic karyotyping, *P. carinii* identified in the lungs of naive animals are the same as those in chronically infected animals and from which infections are acquired (78). Although humans are exposed to the organism at a young age (67, 68), little evidence supports the concept of colonization or a chronic carrier state. In fact, the organism has not been detected incidentally in lungs at autopsy of previously healthy adults (79–82) or in sputum or bronchoalveolar lavage (BAL) fluid by polymerase chain reaction (PCR) for mitochondrial rRNA sequences of human *P. carinii* (83–85). These studies suggest that *P. carinii* is not carried for any appreciable time in the lungs of normal individuals.

However, *Pneumocystis carinii* and increased lymphocyte subsets were found in the BAL of a 20-year-old bronchoscopy technician who had volunteered to be a control subject (86). She had no evidence of pneumonia, and a follow-up BAL 26 weeks later revealed no organisms and a normal BAL cell count. This individual may have had transient colonization or conversely subclinical infection that improved without therapy. Regardless, chronic carriage of *P. carinii* is probably infrequent in immune-competent humans.

Pneumocystis carinii has been found incidentally at autopsy in the lungs of up to 8% immunocompromised patients (81, 82). With PCR, genetic sequences of *P. carinii* have been detected in the absence of histologic evidence of infection (87) in patients receiving immunosuppressive therapies or those with human immunodeficiency virus (HIV) and low CD4 cells. Analysis of genetic variation at the ITS regions of the nuclear rRNA operon among isolates of *P. carinii* demonstrated different sequence types in four of seven recurrent episodes of pneumonia (66). These data suggest that both reactivation and exogenous reinfection may occur in immunocompromised patients (41).

The organism is probably not acquired from zoonotic sources because there are major genetic and antigenic differences among *Pneumocystis carinii* from different host species (42, 43, 88–90). In addition, there is host specificity for strains of *P. carinii* obtained from different host species (91). However, in one laboratory, PCR of certain specimens from human samples yielded DNA containing "patchwork" regions similar to sequences from *P. carinii* from rats (64, 65, 92). This finding suggests several possibilities: 1) coinfection with both human and rat forms of *P. carinii*; 2) sexual recombination of rat and human *P. carinii*; or 3) laboratory contamination with rat *P. carinii* (41). Further investigation will be necessary to clarify these issues.

Several reports involving clusters of cases or familial spread strongly support that infection can be spread by person-to-person contact or exposure to a common reservoir (93–98). In one of these studies, five recipients of renal transplants who shared outpatient facility waiting areas and treatment rooms with AIDS patients developed *Pneumocystis* pneumonia (97). In a natural history study of patients with HIV, upper respiratory infections peaked in winter months, followed by *Pneumocystis* pneumonia 4 months later, suggesting that *P. carinii* and respiratory viruses are transmitted concurrently (99). Antibody titers to *P. carinii* are elevated in health care workers frequently exposed to patients with *Pneumocystis* pneumonia (100), and *P. carinii* DNA has been detected in air samples taken from rooms of patients with pneumonia (101).

If person-to-person spread is a common mode of acquiring infection, this has implications for respiratory isolation of patients with *Pneumocystis* pneumonia from other compromised patients. *P. carinii* DNA has been detected in air samples from rooms of patients with *Pneumocystis* pneumonia (101), as well as in air from a rural outdoor location (62). Unfortunately, definitive data supporting airborne communicability among individuals have been hampered by the absence of epidemiologic markers. Future epidemiologic studies must therefore incorporate molecular technologies to determine the actual mode of transmission.

PATHOGENESIS AND PATHOPHYSIOLOGY

In vivo data show that *Pneumocystis carinii* is acquired by the airborne route (76). Once inhaled, the organism adheres to the type 1 alveolar cell of the lung and interacts with alveolar macrophages through the extracellular proteins fibronectin, vitronectin, and surfactant protein D, which bind the surface glycoprotein of *P. carinii* (102–111). After several weeks of cortisone treatment, small clusters of *P. carinii* can be detected in alveolar spaces throughout the lungs of rats. Later, air sacs are completely filled with organisms, a finding suggesting that replication is slow but proliferation in the lung is extensive.

Two distinct morphologic forms of the organism are detected during infection. One is a small, pleomorphic trophozoite that comprises most of the microorganisms in the lung, and the other is a more mature, larger, thick-walled cyst that contains up to eight intracystic bodies (112). In rats recovering from *Pneumocystis* pneumonia, tissue homogenates show an increase in the proportion of trophozoites compared with cysts (113). Examination of infected lung by light microscopy typically shows a foamy alveolar exudate consisting of degenerative cell membranes, surfactant, and host proteins (103). A few alveolar macrophages are present. As infection progresses, septal hypertrophy occurs, as well as an accumulation of interstitial edema and mononuclear cell infiltration. Similar abnormalities occur in humans. Pathophysiologic consequences have also been detected by electron microscopy and include subepithelial bleb formation resulting from increased alveolar–capillary permeability, degenerative changes in type I alveolar cells, and effacement of the basement membrane, the putative site of transport of serum, fibrin, and other proteins into alveoli (114).

Alterations in pulmonary surfactant appear intricately linked to the pathophysiology of *Pneumocystis*. During infection, one sees alterations in surfactant phospholipids (diminished phosphatidylcholine and increased sphingomyelin), and surfactant protein A, which regulates secretion and absorption of surfactant phospholipids, increases (115–120). The exact relation of these changes to lung injury is unknown (115, 117, 121), although deficiency of surfactant phospholipids likely results in abnormalities in alveolar surface tension, lung distensibility, and ventilation–perfusion. More is understood about surfactant protein A (119), which binds to the mannose residue of *P. carinii* gp120 (122), possibly enhancing attachment of organisms to type I pneumocytes and interfering with phagocytosis of *P. carinii* by alveolar macrophages (123). That surfactant is important in pathogenesis is supported by the observation that intratracheal instillation of surfactant improved oxygenation and pulmonary architecture in immune-suppressed laboratory animals with *Pneumocystis* pneumonia (118).

The physiologic consequences of these pathologic abnormalities include early impairment of gas exchange because of increased alveolar–capillary permeability (124), which is measured by decreased membrane diffusing capacity (125) and ultimately decreased compliance, total lung capacity, and vital capacity (126). Lung function is apparently further impaired by the host inflammatory response. In severe combined immunodeficiency (SCID) mice with *Pneumocystis* pneumonia, reconstitution of the immune system by bone marrow transplantation or infusion of CD4 cells resulted in early deaths from a hyperinflammatory pulmonary response, which cleared *P. carinii* from the lungs (127, 128). That the inflammatory response is deleterious in humans is supported by the deterioration in oxygenation that occurs soon after initiation of specific anti-*Pneumocystis* therapy and that is blunted by adjunctive corticosteroids (129), as well as the association of increased BAL neutrophils in patients destined for a poor outcome (130).

Multiple studies have supported an important role for inflammatory mediators in the pathogenesis of *Pneumocystis carinii* pneumonia. Local production of interleukin (IL)-1 (131), IL-6 (131, 132), IL-8 (133–135), granulocyte–macrophage colony-stimulating factor (GM-CSF) (136), tumor necrosis factor-α (TNF-α) (137), leukotriene B_4 (133, 135), and phospholipase A_2 are all increased in AIDS patients. In individuals with *Pneumocystis* pneumonia, IL-8 is elevated in BAL fluid and correlates with BAL fluid neutrophilia, arterioalveolar oxygen tension difference or (A-a)Do_2, and severity of illness; therapy with corticosteroids has resulted in a reduction in IL-8 levels (135). Conversely, although TNF-α expression by alveolar macrophages is also decreased by corticosteroid administration (138), TNF-α appears to be an essential component in the host defense against *P. carinii*. TNF-α production from alveolar macrophages is stimulated through a β-glucan–mediated mechanism (139). Antibody to TNF-α prevents the clearance of *P. carinii* that occurs after SCID mice are reconstituted with normal T cells (140). In humans, higher levels of TNF-α production by alveolar macrophages have correlated with lower organism numbers in BAL fluid (141) and higher arterial oxygen levels (142). The implication of these findings is that, with greater understanding of the immunopathogenesis of *Pneumocystis* pneumonia, adjunctive immunomodulator therapies may be tested to determine whether they could enhance the effects of specific antimicrobial therapies.

IMMUNORESPONSE AND RISK FOR INFECTION

Understanding the biology and pathogenesis of *Pneumocystis* has been hampered by difficulties propagating *P. carinii* in tissue culture. Thus, studies have relied heavily on animal models. Although *P. carinii* harvested from rats has different antigenic properties than human isolates of the organism (46), considerable insights into the pathogenesis of *Pneumocystis* pneumonia have been acquired from these models.

T-Cell–Mediated Response

In SCID mice, nude mice, laboratory rodents treated with corticosteroids or cytotoxic agents, and malnourished rodents receiving low-protein diets, the common immunologic deficit predisposing these animals to *Pneumocystis* pneumonia is severe depletion in T-cell function (75, 143–147). When the deficit is corrected by adoptive transfer of spleen T lymphocytes from phenotypically normal mice into *P. carinii*–infected, T-cell–deficient animals, lung cysts are cleared, and pneumonia resolves (148, 149). Other adoptive transfer experiments established that helper L3T4 (equivalent to human CD4 cells) lymphocytes were necessary to reconstitute delayed-type hypersensitivity to *Pneumocystis*, but suppressor lymphocytes were necessary for complete expression of resistance to *P. carinii* (150). Administration of monoclonal antibody to CD4 cells resulted in *Pneumocystis* pneumonia and inability to eradicate the infection, in conventional Balb/c mice and reconstituted SCID mice inoculated with *P. carinii*, respectively (151, 152). Finally, major surface glycoprotein (MSG) appears to be important to the development of host T-cell recognition and the immune response to *P. carinii* infection in rats (153). These experiments provide inferential evidence that depletion of CD4 cells is necessary for development of *Pneumocystis* pneumonia.

In humans without HIV infection, *Pneumocystis* pneumonia frequently occurs in association with lymphoreticular malignancies, certain congenital disorders, and chemotherapy with cyclosporine (154) or corticosteroids that have in common variable defects in T-cell function (154–156). By contrast, adults with pure hypogammaglobulinemia rarely develop *Pneumocystis* pneumonia. For HIV-positive persons, the risk of developing *Pneumocystis* pneumonia is related to deficiencies in their T-helper (CD4 surface phenotype) lymphocytes. Thus, impaired T-cell function is most likely the critical immune deficit necessary for this opportunistic infection to occur.

The degree of impaired T-cell function is also an important determinant of the risk of infection in humans. Most patients have CD4 lymphocyte counts in the range of 50 to 75 cells/mm^3 at the time of their first episode of *Pneumocystis* pneumonia (157), and more than 90% of episodes in fact occur when counts are lower than 200/mm^3 (158). Moreover, when individuals are receiving prophylaxis, failures of prophylaxis occur most commonly with very low CD4 cells counts (8). If patients with fewer than 200 CD4 cells are not given prophylaxis, the risk of developing *Pneumocystis* pneumonia was reported to be 8.4% at 6 months, 18.4% at 12 months, and 33.3% at 36 months (157). Some episodes do, however, occur in patients with higher CD4 counts when thrush and fever are present (158).

Humoral Response

Previous studies suggested that antibodies to *Pneumocystis carinii* had little effect on host defense against the organism. In one experiment, rats immunized with *P. carinii* responded with antibody titers of 1:64 to 1:256 but developed fatal *Pneumocystis* pneumonia when subjected to immunosuppression by corticosteroids (159). In another experiment, immune serum was ineffective in curing immune-suppressed mice that developed *Pneumocystis* (148). However, other studies suggest that antibodies to *P. carinii* may be important components of host defense to *P. carinii* (160, 161). In adoptive transfer of T cells and spleen cells from immunocompetent donors into SCID mice, B cells were necessary in addition to T cells for recipient mice to resolve preexisting *Pneumocystis* pneumonia (160). Moreover, immunoprophylaxis with monoclonal antibody or hyperimmune serum against major antigenic determinants of *P. carinii* provides protection and effective treatment of *Pneumocystis* pneumonia in several murine models (161, 162). In the latter experiments, a fatal hyperinflammatory response to *P. carinii* resulting from adoptive transfer of T cells to SCID mice was prevented by pretreatment with hyperimmune serum (162).

In humans, the most common antibody response is to the 40-kd antigen. In one study, AIDS patients with *Pneumocystis* pneumonia had more active immunoglobulin M (IgM) and IgG antibody response to the 40-kd antigen of *P. carinii* after a single episode, and the response was even greater with repeated episodes than for healthy persons (163). In another study, the frequency of IgG antibodies directed to purified surface antigen (gp95) was greater during *Pneumocystis* pneumonia than in HIV-infected patients without pneumonia (164). Perhaps the immune response augmented by recurrent episodes is directed against different epitopes.

The importance of the humoral response was inferred by the deficiency of anti-*Pneumocystis carinii* antibodies of at least one isotype in BAL from patients with *Pneumocystis* pneumonia compared with patients without HIV (165). Moreover, the presence of IgA antibody in BAL that binds to intraalveolar and extrapulmonary *P. carinii* but not to *P. carinii* in pulmonary granulomas suggests that the antibodies may also be related to the diversity of host response (165).

HISTOPATHOLOGY

Light microscopy of lung tissue from AIDS patients with *Pneumocystis* commonly shows prominent eosinophilic, foamy intraalveolar exudate accompanied by mild interstitial pneumonitis along with proliferation of type II pneumocytes (12, 166). The cysts are uniformly 5 to 7 μm and require special stains for identification. They appear as helmet, crescent, or banana shapes with darkly stained foci resulting from thickening of the capsule (167, 168).

Diffuse alveolar damage is commonly present in biopsy sections. Remarkably, the organizing phase is present more often than the acute exudative phase, and it has been detected as interstitial fibrosis in 63% and intraluminal fibrosis in 36% of biopsy specimens (12, 169). Because acute exudative alveolar damage is unusual, hyaline membranes have been detected in only 4% of biopsy samples, but they may be so prominent as to obscure the typical eosinophilic alveolar exudate (12, 169). In fact, eosinophilic alveolar exudate may be absent in up to 19% of cases because of artifact, biopsy-induced hemorrhage, atelectasis, or the presence of other processes such as alveolar damage of lymphocytic interstitial pneumonia (12).

Other histologic abnormalities that are uncommon in HIV-negative patients occur in patients with AIDS. These include pulmonary cysts and cavities, granulomatous inflammation, lymphocytic interstitial pneumonitis, microcalcifications, vascular permeation, vasculitis, and alveolar proteinosis. Pulmonary cysts and cavities are often associated with aerosol pentamidine and are usually located in upper lobes (12, 170–181). These cavities are usually multiple and bilateral and result from lung destruction and necrosis caused by *Pneumocystis carinii* (179, 182–184). Spontaneous pneumothorax may result from rupture of a cavity (185–188), and hemoptysis may occur if a blood vessel ruptures into a cavity (189). Rupture of subpleural lesions may cause pleural effusions (heretofore rare in *Pneumocystis* pneumonia) containing *P. carinii* (182, 190–192).

Other unusual findings include noncaseating granulomas with scattered giant cells (193–195) in up to 5% of lung biopsies (12). Cavitary granulomas (183) and granulomas with central calcifications (196) may also occur. Microcalcification is present in up to 2% of biopsies (12) and is bubbly, platelike, elongate, or conchoidal (197). Because calcifications can be detected without prior *Pneumocystis* pneumonia or anti-*Pneumocystis* therapy, calcifications may be a reaction to dying *P. carinii* (197). Vasculitis may also be detected and is associated with necrotizing or cavitary lesions (12, 177, 179, 182) and extrapulmonary dissemination (12, 170).

The most unusual histologic finding is pulmonary alveolar proteinosis (PAP) (198–200), which, unlike the typical foamy, alveolar exudates, is finely granular, with occasional clumps and cholesterol clefts. *Pneumocystis carinii* must be carefully sought in biopsy specimens with PAP inasmuch as *Pneumocystis* is far more common than idiopathic PAP. Both types of alveolar exudates stain with periodic acid–Schiff. Therefore, electron microscopic examinations for lipoproteinaceous material with myelinlike bodies (198) or specific immunochemical stains for apoprotein (198, 199) are necessary to diagnose alveolar proteinosis definitively.

CLINICAL MANIFESTATIONS

Symptoms

The onset of *Pneumocystis* pneumonia in AIDS patients is usually insidious, with symptoms present for at least 3 to 4 weeks (201, 202). Rarely, patients may be entirely asymptomatic, even with extensive involvement visible on a chest radiograph (14). The cardinal manifestation is chronic, nonproductive cough. Cough is occasionally associated with mucoid sputum (21, 201) or rarely hemoptysis (189, 203). Retrosternal chest tightness intensified with inspiration or coughing is a second, nearly global symptom (21, 201, 204). Fever occurs in 80 to 90% of cases, but it may be present for a shorter duration than cough or chest tightness. Dyspnea on exertion and breathlessness at rest occur late in the infection, when oxygenation is moderately to severely impaired.

Physical Findings

Abnormal physical findings are usually limited to the lung. Tachypnea is unusual with mild episodes, whereas respiratory distress and use of accessory respiratory muscles are often present in patients with severe episodes. Rales are detected in only 30 to 40% of cases and are usually present only in severe episodes (21, 205). Indeed, the absence of adventitial breath sounds should not be used to exclude the possibility of *Pneumocystis* pneumonia in persons at risk for AIDS.

Physical findings outside the lung are nonspecific but may assist the clinical assessment. In patients who have not been treated with topical or oral antifungal drugs, particularly those whose initial AIDS presentation is *Pneumocystis* pneumonia, oral thrush is frequent. Seborrheic dermatitis involving the face between the eyebrows, forehead, and upper cheeks is also common in patients with *Pneumocystis* pneumonia and is unusual in patients with other pulmonary complications of AIDS. However, generalized adenopathy with nodes larger than 1.0 cm is rare because patients with *Pneumocystis* pneumonia generally have severe immune deficiency and hypoplastic lymph nodes. Enlarged lymph nodes, particularly when found in a focal distribution, should suggest the presence of another opportunistic complication, although concurrent *Pneumocystis* pneumonia is possible.

Lung Cavitation and Spontaneous Pneumothorax

Spontaneous pneumothorax with resulting bronchopleural fistulas refractory to closure is increasingly frequent (184, 188, 203, 206–214). This complication appears related to lung cavitation (14, 180, 215, 216), which may occur in up to 10% of patients with *Pneumocystis* pneumonia and, manifested by solitary, thin-walled cavities or regional honeycombing, often precedes pneumothoraces (217). Such lesions may occur in nonsmokers, during first episodes of *Pneumocystis* pneumonia, and after bronchoscopy, aerosol therapy, and mechanical ventilation. These lesions may be due to chronic infection with *P. carinii*, which may result in activation of pulmonary macrophages that release elastase and thereby destroy lung tissue (218). The cavities of *P. carinii* pneumonia can mimic mycobacterial disease and may lead to diagnostic confusion (14).

Spontaneous pneumothorax without a precipitating cause was reported in 20 (2%) of 1030 patients with AIDS at one medical center (203). Use of aerosol pentamidine has been a major risk factor for pneumothorax, with odds ratios (ORs) of 3.9 to 17.6 (203, 219). In one study, prior *Pneumocystis* pneumonia was also a risk factor (OR = 14.5), and if both conditions existed, the incidence of spontaneous pneumothorax was 6.3% (203). Because deposition of pentamidine by aerosol in the periphery of the lung is less than in central regions (220), it may be that chronic subpleural *Pneumocystis* infection with lung destruction extends to involve the pleura (190, 192, 221). Regardless of the mechanism, 19 of 20 patients with pneumothoraces in the study described earlier had active *Pneumocystis* pneumonia requiring treatment (203). Thus, HIV-infected patients with spontaneous pneumothorax should undergo workup and treatment for *Pneumocystis* pneumonia along with management of the pneumothorax (184, 203).

Extrapulmonary Pneumocystosis

Pneumocystis carinii infection outside the lung (222–225) previously occurred in approximately 0.5 to 3.0% of patients with *Pneumocystis* pneumonia (222, 223, 226). Initial reports emphasized the relationship with aerosol pentamidine, but a review of cases shows that nearly half occurred without prior prophylaxis with pentamidine. Using nested PCR of the ITS of the rRNA genes (Pc-ITS-PCR), all 27 patients with proved *Pneumocystis* pneumonia were Pc-ITS-PCR positive in sera obtained at the time of bronchoscopy (227), a finding suggesting that dissemination occurs by hematogenous spread during acute pneumonia. In fact, 19 (55%) of 37 patients in one report had concurrent *Pneumocystis* pneumonia documented, and pulmonary involvement was suspected in others at the time disseminated lesions were detected (225).

Clinical presentations have included external auditory polyps (228), mastoiditis (229), choroiditis, cutaneous lesions (170, 230, 231) or digital necrosis secondary to vasculitis (170), obstruction of the small intestine (232), ascites with gross nodules in the stomach and duodenum, hepatitis (187, 233, 234), splenitis (233, 235), hilar or mediastinal lymphadenopathy (188, 233), thyroiditis, and hematologic cytopenias resulting from involvement of the bone marrow (233, 235–239). At autopsy, disseminated infection has been documented in other organs including abdominal lymph nodes (233, 235, 240), pancreas (233), brain (241), heart (233), kidneys (233), gastric mucosa (233, 240), and adrenal glands (233, 235). Lymph nodes, liver, spleen, and bone marrow appear to be the most commonly affected organs (223). Histologic examination of affected organs shows a striking resemblance to the pathologic features usually found in the lung. Typical foci of eosinophilic frothy exudates are present, and special staining reveals *Pneumocystis carinii* cysts. Unlike in the lung, these lesions are often calcified (punctate or rimlike), and one may see vasculitis with invasion of vessel walls by *P. carinii* organisms (188, 242, 243).

Signs and symptoms of extrapulmonary *Pneumocystis* infection are usually nonspecific (e.g., fever and sweats), although involvement of the choroid, thyroid, bone marrow, or liver results in organ-specific clinical manifestations. *P. carinii* involving the thyroid may present with neck pain and goiter, which may be multinodular or a solitary neck mass that is cold on iodine-125 scanning. Involvement of the thyroid may result in either hyperthyroidism or hypothyroidism (244–248). Diagnosis is usually established by fine-needle aspiration (245). Choroiditis is the other infection readily accessible to clinical diagnosis inasmuch as it has unique funduscopic features (249–258). Lesions consist of slightly elevated, yellow–white plaques, generally limited to the choroid without involvement of retinal vessels (unlike cytomegalovirus retinitis) and without evidence of intraocular inflammation (Fig 14.1). Identification of typical lesions may provide the first clue of *P. carinii* infection. In one series, the lung was also involved in 18 (86%) of 21 cases at the time of diagnosis (258), but in other cases, ocular involvement has been the only evidence of extrapulmonary infection.

Outcome is poor with extensive and widespread extrapulmonary involvement, which often results in organ failure and death (259, 260). By contrast, if only a single extrapulmonary site is involved and the patient has no concomitant pneumonia, chances for survival are good with specific therapy of *Pneumocystis carinii* infection (223). For prophylaxis, prevention of extrapulmonary *Pneumocystis* infection is one justification favoring systemic therapy. In fact, only one case of extrapulmonary *Pneumocystis* infection has been reported during prophylaxis with trimethoprim–sulfamethoxazole (TMP–SMX) (261). Prophylaxis with TMP–SMX likely prevents seeding of tissues outside the lung or provides early therapy of *P. carinii* at these distant sites.

LABORATORY ABNORMALITIES
Pulmonary Function Tests

The single most useful indirect marker of *Pneumocystis* pneumonia is the presence of hypoxemia (201, 262–266). A Pa_{O_2} lower than 80 mm Hg or an $(A\text{-}a)D_{O_2}$ higher than 15 mm Hg occurs in more than 80% of patients with *Pneumocystis* pneumonia (10, 267). Because patients with prior *Pneumocystis* pneumonia are often monitored closely, subsequent episodes may be associated with less severe hypoxemia because of early detection (263). The degree of hypoxemia at presentation is also of prognostic value. Room air Pa_{O_2} lower than 70 mm Hg and $(A\text{-}a)D_{O_2}$ higher than 35 mm Hg are associated with a sharp increase in risk for a fatal outcome (201, 263, 265, 266, 268). This finding has therapeutic importance because the United States Public Health Service has recommended adjunctive corticosteroids for patients with room air $(A\text{-}a)D_{O_2}$ higher than 35 mm Hg (268).

In documented cases in which blood gases and chest radiographs are normal or near normal, oxygen desaturation can be measured with pulse oximetry during exercise and the $(A\text{-}a)D_{O_2}$ generally widens (269–271).

The carbon monoxide diffusing capacity (D_{LCO}) is less than 70% of predicted values in nearly all patients with *Pneumocystis* pneumonia because the transmembrane diffusion of carbon monoxide is impaired (alveolar capillary block) by intraalveolar exudate (125, 272, 273). The test is not specific and may be abnormal in patients with pulmonary Kaposi's sarcoma, those with bacterial and mycobacterial infections of the lung, and intravenous drug users; however, in these conditions values are generally higher than 70% of normal (274). However, a normal or near-normal D_{LCO} makes *Pneumocystis* pneumonia unlikely. The test is also helpful in AIDS patients with asthma inasmuch as results should be normal in subjects whose hypoxemia is due solely to bronchospasm. Serial determinations of D_{LCO} in patients followed longitudinally were predictive of *Pneumocystis*

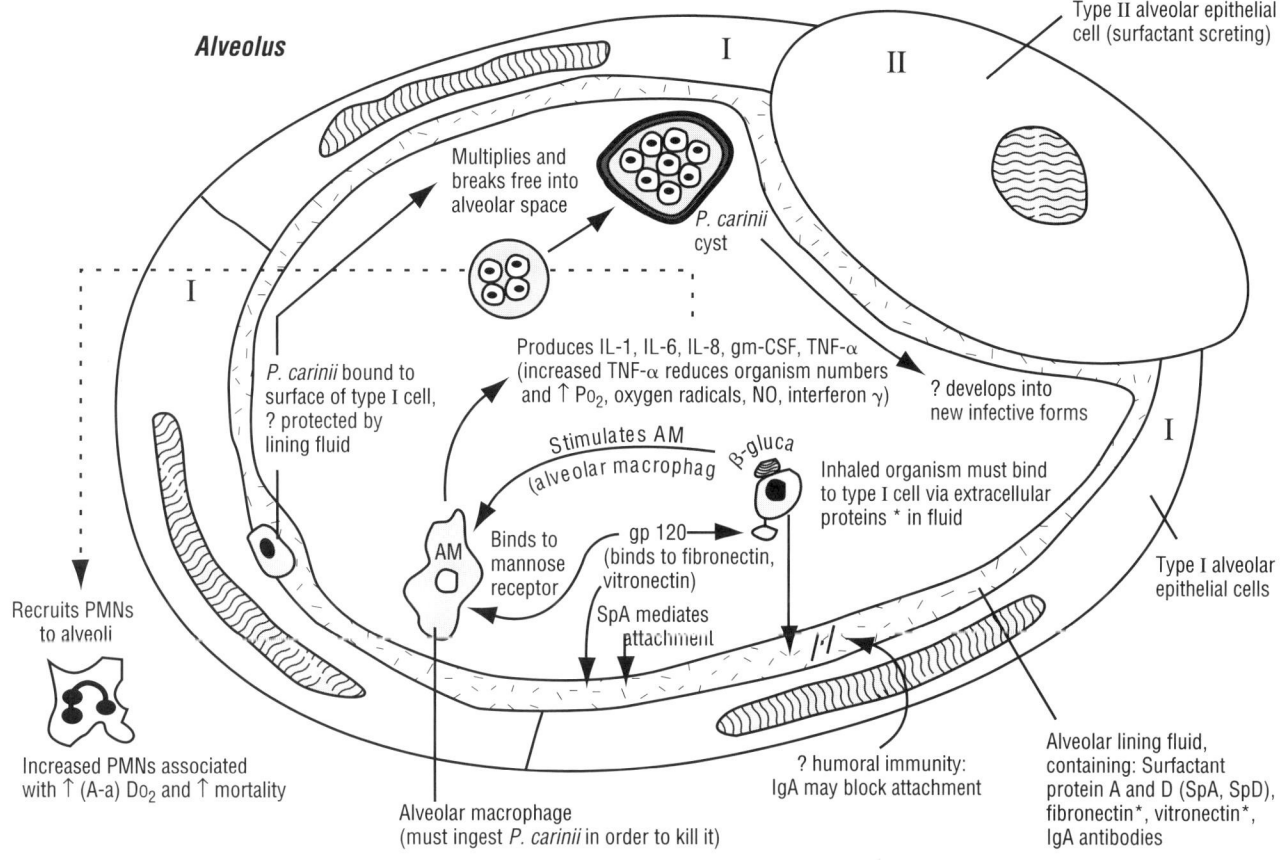

Figure 14.1. Pathogenesis of *Pneumocystis carinii* pneumonia.

pneumonia, but values tended to decrease over time even in the absence of pneumonia (275).

Lactate Dehydrogenase

Lactate dehydrogenase (LDH) has been studied extensively (10, 262, 265, 266, 276–279). Evaluation of BAL LDH isoenzymes suggests that LDH produced by the lung is selectively filtered by alveolar–capillary membranes before appearing in the serum (278). Serum LDH is a useful ancillary test because values are more highly elevated in patients with *Pneumocystis* pneumonia than matched patients without *P. carinii* (279, 280) and are usually elevated in more than 90% of hospitalized patients with *Pneumocystis* pneumonia (279). In one series of hospitalized patients, elevated LDH had diagnostic sensitivity of 78% and specificity of 74% for *Pneumocystis* pneumonia; the sensitivity rose to 94% for patients with dyspnea when the cutoff value was higher than 220 IU/L (280). Of equal import, serial tests gradually improve in survivors compared with nonsurvivors (279, 281). Moreover, survivors usually have lower values at outset, and values higher than 500 IU/L are associated with an increased risk of death (276, 279, 282).

CD4 Lymphocyte Counts

The absolute or relative number of CD4 lymphocytes is valuable in evaluating the risk for *Pneumocystis* pneumonia (157, 159, 283). The typical patient has a count in the range of 50 to 75 cells/mm^3, and more than 90% of individuals have values lower than 200 cells/mm^3 when first diagnosed with *Pneumocystis* pneumonia. However, in one natural history study of ambulatory subjects at risk for AIDS, 26% had CD4 counts higher than 200 cells/mm^3 (all but one had counts between 201 and 350 cells/mm^3) in the 6 months before the diagnosis of *Pneumocystis* pneumonia, but most of these patients had preceding fever and thrush.

Imaging Procedures

Typically, infiltrates on chest radiographs are interstitial; they begin in the perihilar areas and spread first to the lower and later to the upper lung fields, although the apices are usually spared (217, 219). As the disease progresses, an alveolar pattern with air bronchograms may be superimposed on the interstitial process and may be the initial presentation in up to 10% of cases (180, 217, 284). In 10 to 30% of cases, the radiographic presentation is atypical, with asymmetric or predominantly upper lobe infiltration, especially in patients who received prophylaxis with inhaled pentamidine (9–13, 207, 219, 285). Less frequent manifestations include nodules, cystic lesions with "honeycombing," overt cavitation, pneumatoceles, pneumothorax, hilar adenopathy with or without calcifications, pleural effusions, abscesses, lobar or segmental consolidation, solitary parenchymal nodules, and postobstructive infiltration secondary to endobronchial nodules of *Pneumocystis carinii* (190, 195, 203, 217, 219, 285–295). Upper lobe predominance with cystic or cavitary changes may mimic tuberculosis (Fig 14.2) (14, 195, 284, 292), whereas 10 to 20% of patients, generally those with mild episodes, have normal chest radiographs at presentation (219, 296–298).

Standard computed tomography (CT) and high-resolution CT (HRCT) have revealed fine diffuse alveolar consolidation with bronchial wall thickening even when chest radiographs are normal (173, 299–302). HRCT changes correlate well with histologic sections of lung (299). Unexpected changes have included regional consolidation, cystic airspaces, and subpleural sparing (173). Low-attenuation lesions and calcifications of lymph nodes, spleen, liver, and kidneys have been detected in patients with extrapulmonary involvement (242, 243, 301). The value of CT is probably limited to patients with normal chest radiographs or with unexpected extrapulmonary *Pneumocystis* infection.

Nuclear imaging has been of ancillary assistance in suspected cases. Gallium accumulates in activated macrophages through transferrin receptors in areas of lung inflammation, but pulmonary uptake is not specific for *Pneumocystis* infection (303–311). Sensitivity of the test has varied between 84 and 100% (309, 312). Specificity is reportedly improved if scans are designated as positive only when gallium uptake in the lungs equals or exceeds that of liver (311). However, patients with mild *Pneumocystis* pneumonia may have minimal or no lung uptake, and other pulmonary complications may produce positive scans. Gallium imaging is useful for patients with chronic lung disease who have worsening respiratory symptoms because blood gases and radiographs may be chronically abnormal in these individuals.

DIAGNOSIS

Diagnostic Procedures

SPUTUM INDUCTION

Unlike *Pneumocystis* pneumonia in other immunocompromised patients, enormous numbers of *P. carinii* may be present in deep respiratory secretions of patients with AIDS. Unfortunately, most patients with *Pneumocystis* pneumonia produce minimal or no sputum. Respiratory secretions can be obtained by ultrasonic nebulization of hypertonic saline (313, 314), although care must be taken because many patients experience arterial desaturation during the procedure (315). Concentrates of such specimens are difficult to examine unless treated with mucolytic agents to dissolve oral debris before staining (316). When the sediment is appropriately stained and slides are reviewed by experts, the procedure has a sensitivity of 15 to 94% (313, 314, 317–325), with corresponding negative predictive values that have also varied widely (39 to 96%). The procedure is laborious for respiratory therapists and laboratory technicians, but positive results often obviate the need for bronchoscopy. Fluorescent staining with monoclonal antibodies for *P. carinii* may increase the yield to more than 90% (318, 326). With the use of PCR techniques, the sensitivity of induced sputum may approach that of BAL (see the section of this chapter on molecular identification).

As for BAL, the yield of induced sputum may be lower for patients receiving aerosol pentamidine because the numbers of the organism may be reduced. In one study of 54 patients, the diagnosis was confirmed by induced sputum in 64.3% of those receiving aerosol pentamidine compared with 92.3% not receiving pentamidine ($P<.02$) (327). By contrast, the respective yields were 63% compared with 64% in another trial (328).

BRONCHOALVEOLAR LAVAGE

BAL is the standard for diagnosis (329). This procedure involves wedging the bronchoscope into a peripheral nondependent airway (usually the right middle lobe) and instilling 100 to 250 mL of nonbacteriostatic saline as 20- to 30-mL aliquots and aspirating fluid after each aliquot is instilled (330). When approximately 50 mL fluid has been recovered, the specimen is centrifuged, and the pellet is

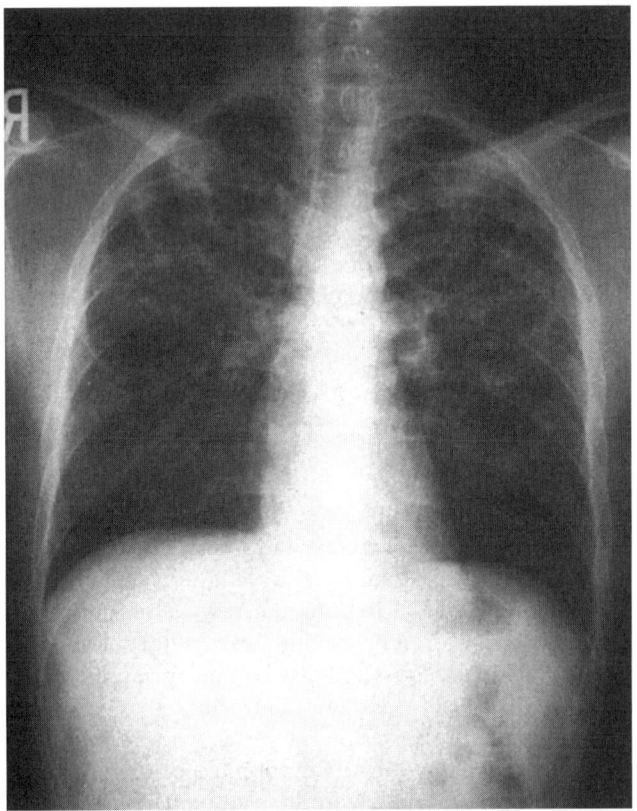

Figure 14.2. Chest radiograph of a 27-year-old AIDS patient who had received 13 months of aerosolized pentamidine as secondary prophylaxis for *Pneumocystis* pneumonia when recurrent infection was documented. Extensive cavitation in the upper lobes mimics tuberculosis.

stained for *Pneumocystis carinii*. In 86 to 97% of cases, *P. carinii* organisms are detected by this procedure (329, 331–338). Nonbronchoscopic techniques involving the blind placement of catheters into distal airways provide similar yields as BAL (335, 336, 339). These techniques require sedation and local anesthesia similar to BAL and therefore provide no advantage. Finally, for mechanically ventilated patients, lavage through the endotracheal tube resulted in a diagnosis of *P. carinii* in 19 of 20 patients in one study (340).

At one center, diagnostic yield of BAL declined to 62% for patients with acute *Pneumocystis* pneumonia who had been receiving inhaled pentamidine and who frequently had disease predominantly in upper lobes (284). Several approaches may improve yield. Bilateral BAL resulted in a diagnosis in 31 (94%) of 33 patients compared with 51 (84%) of 61 for historical patients previously undergoing BAL on one side (341). Similarly, the combination of multiple-lobe, site-directed BAL and monoclonal antibody staining increased the diagnostic yield from 80 to 98% (342). In patients with focal infiltrates, the combination of site-directed BAL and transbronchial biopsy led to a diagnosis in 90% of patients with a prior nondiagnostic BAL (343). That there may be a twofold increase in the number of *P. carinii* from upper lobes compared with lower lobes in these patients suggests that sampling from specific involved sites may increase the yield (344).

TRANSBRONCHIAL BIOPSY

When transbronchial biopsy specimens are obtained without crush artifact and contain at least 25 alveoli, the diagnostic yield is similar to that of BAL (329). If both BAL and transbronchial biopsy samples are obtained, the diagnostic sensitivity is additive and approaches 100% (329). However, pneumothoraces and bleeding may occur in up to 10% of subjects (331). Thus, many pulmonologists prefer to perform only BAL with the initial bronchoscopy. If the first procedure is nondiagnostic, BAL is repeated, and transbronchial biopsies are obtained. If specimens from both procedures are adequate and fail to show *Pneumocystis carinii* with standard histologic and cytologic stains, the diagnosis is considered to be excluded. Other investigators have suggested that biopsies do not increase the yield of BAL and only increase the chances for complications (345).

OPEN LUNG BIOPSY

Open lung biopsy is rarely needed in AIDS patients for diagnosis of *Pneumocystis* pneumonia because of the high yield with sputum induction and BAL. This technique is usually reserved for patients in whom bronchoscopy has been nondiagnostic (346, 347) because of technical problems with the procedure or in whom transbronchial biopsies are contraindicated because of bleeding disorders or concurrent management with mechanical ventilation. Open lung biopsy is safer than transbronchial biopsy for patients with abnormal coagulation because hemostasis is more reliably achieved intraoperatively than at bronchoscopy.

Laboratory Identification of *P. carinii*

CYST WALL STAINS

The standard means for identifying *Pneumocystis carinii* cysts has involved staining with Gomori's methenamine silver, because diagnostic sensitivity and specificity have both generally exceeded 95% (348–350). The procedure requires 4 to 6 hours, and up to 10% false-negative results may occur (351). Modifications have reduced processing time to 1 to 2 hours (351–353). Toluidine blue O also stains the cyst wall and is faster than standard silver stains (318, 354, 355). Calcofluor white, a chemifluorescent optical brightening agent that binds β-linked polysaccharides of fungi and *P. carinii* (356–359), had a sensitivity and specificity of 100 and 95%, respectively, in one study of 45 specimens (359).

NONCYST WALL STAINS

Wright–Giemsa and Diff–Quik have been used to stain trophozoites, nuclei of cysts, and intermediate forms and can be completed within 30 minutes (360–362). However, organisms may be missed in 10 to 15% of cases (360, 363). The method does allow polymorphonuclear neutrophils to be identified in BAL, a finding associated with greater impairment in pulmonary physiology and survival (130, 362, 364).

Papanicolaou stains the nonspecific foam surrounding large clusters of *Pneumocystis carinii*, but organisms are not readily identified (365). The method is quick and useful for screening. As with the Giemsa stain, sensitivity is only in the range of 80%. Fluorescent microscopy of Papanicolaou-stained BAL specimens detected *P. carinii* in 100% as brilliant yellow–green circular 5-μm structures with 1- to 3-μm fluorescent inclusions (366).

IMMUNOCHEMICAL STAINS

Direct and indirect immunofluorescent staining techniques using monoclonal antibodies are highly sensitive, with yields in excess of 90% for BAL specimens (326, 357, 367–370). These methods are more sensitive for sputum samples than silver or Wright–Giemsa stains (318, 357, 363, 368–371). Although false-positive results occasionally occur (367, 368), these techniques have become the primary diagnostic procedure in many clinical laboratories.

MOLECULAR IDENTIFICATION

PCR will likely increase diagnostic sensitivity, especially with induced sputum specimens (83, 372–382). In patients with *Pneumocystis* pneumonia documented by bronchoscopy, nested PCR detected *P. carinii* in all 17 (100%) of sputum samples compared with lesser sensitivity of immunofluorescent and toluidine blue O stains (38 to 53%) (83).

Similarly, in a study of 49 HIV-infected patients not receiving prophylaxis who were suspected of having *Pneumocystis* pneumonia, 6 had positive staining or immunofluorescence of induced sputum specimens, whereas patients with negative studies underwent bronchoscopy with BAL (381). Seven additional patients had positive standard staining of BAL specimens; all these were positive by PCR of induced sputum, yielding a sensitivity of 100% in this small clinical study. However, when PCR was applied to BAL fluid, it did not appear to increase sensitivity in most investigations (83, 227, 377, 379, 380, 382–384).

PCR has also been applied to blood specimens with varying degrees of sensitivity (83, 227, 380, 385). The most impressive results have been reported by Atzori and colleagues (227) using nested PCR of the *Pneumocystis carinii* ITS of the rRNA genes (Pc-ITS-PCR). All 27 patients with proved *Pneumocystis* pneumonia were Pc-ITS-PCR positive in sera obtained at the time of bronchoscopy, whereas all 18 AIDS patients without pneumocystosis and 25 control patients had negative Pc-ITS-PCR results on their sera.

Lack of a definitive standard makes it difficult to ascertain the true sensitivity and specificity of molecular techniques. At present, it appears reasonable to reserve PCR for sputum specimens that prove negative by immunofluorescence staining. Ultimately, the role of PCR for blood and respiratory specimens in the diagnosis of *Pneumocystis* pneumonia should be established by a clinical trial that analyzes patient outcomes and cost-effectiveness of a PCR-based diagnostic approach.

TREATMENT FOR ACUTE EPISODES

Initial Therapy

For mild episodes of *Pneumocystis* pneumonia in which oxygenation is minimally impaired, mortality rates have been below 5% in recent years (268, 386). However, the absence of hacking cough, fever, and typical radiographic infiltration and the presence of normal or near-normal LDH levels in many mild cases still challenge the diagnostic acumen of the most experienced AIDS practitioners. The importance of initiating treatment early in the course is emphasized by the finding that patients with initial Pao_2 lower than 70 mm Hg or $(A-a)Do_2$ higher than 35 mm Hg have a sharp increase in the risk of an unfavorable outcome (268, 387–389). In fact, fatality rates are in the range of 20 to 30% in patients with severe episodes even when corticosteroids are prescribed with conventional therapies. Mild to moderately severe episodes are thus defined by an $(A-a)Do_2$ lower than 35 mm Hg on room air and moderate-to-severe episodes as $(A-a)Do_2$ of at least 35 mm Hg.

Sputum induction and bronchoscopies are typically not available after hours or on weekends, and results of cytologic examination or stains may be delayed for 24 or more hours after specimens have been collected. Thus, most patients with typical clinical features of *Pneumocystis* infection should be treated empirically, especially if they have moderate-to-severe impairment in their arterial blood gases. This treatment does not impair the ability to establish a histologic or cytologic diagnosis because large numbers of *P. carinii* cysts and trophozoites remain in lung tissues and pulmonary secretions for weeks to months after therapy (126, 362, 390). Once treatment is initiated, every effort should be made to confirm the diagnosis, even if the patient appears to be responding to treatment.

Bacterial pneumonia may improve with several anti-*Pneumocystis* regimens. This is especially relevant for *Haemophilus influenzae*, which can cause diffuse interstitial infiltrates that mimic *Pneumocystis*. Similarly, nonspecific interstitial pneumonitis may improve spontaneously (391), and various conditions may transiently improve because of corticosteroid treatment. These situations can provide the false impression that improvement occurred as a result of anti-*Pneumocystis* therapy. Likewise, tuberculosis, fungal infection, Kaposi's sarcoma, and cytomegalovirus pneumonia may closely resemble *Pneumocystis* pneumonia. Each of these complications requires different therapies. Once patients fail to respond to empiric therapy for *Pneumocystis* pneumonia, they may be too ill for sputum induction, bronchoscopy, or open lung biopsy, thus denying them the opportunity to receive specific therapy.

Finally, standard therapies for *Pneumocystis* pneumonia are associated with high rates of adverse and often serious adverse reactions, which may prolong hospitalization (392–395). It is difficult to justify these toxic reactions for patients who do not have the infection. Thus, compelling reasons exist to establish a definitive diagnosis whenever possible. Empiric therapy may be justified when the clinical syndrome suggests *Pneumocystis* pneumonia and the patient refuses bronchoscopy or is too ill for invasive procedures. Table 14.1 summarizes standard therapies available for treatment of *Pneumocystis* pneumonia.

Severe Episodes

Initial therapy should be given parenterally for severe episodes. TMP and SMX, which have nearly complete bioavailability when administered orally (396), are erratically absorbed from the gut in subjects without AIDS but with severely impaired gas exchange (397). Patients in whom treatment has failed often have serum TMP concentrations lower than 5 µg/mL (397). In addition, AIDS patients may have achlorhydria and upper gut enteropathy with malabsorption, which could adversely affect bioavailability of therapies for *Pneumocystis* pneumonia.

TRIMETHOPRIM–SULFAMETHOXAZOLE

The antifolate combination of TMP–SMX was the first therapy licensed by the United States Food and Drug Administration for *Pneumocystis* pneumonia. Assessing the relative efficacy of TMP–SMX has been difficult because side effects are frequent with nearly all therapies used to treat patients with AIDS and thus many patients are unable to complete a full course of treatment with the initial therapy

Table 14.1. Therapies for Acute *Pneumocystis* Pneumonia

Mild-to-Moderate Episodes	
Low-dose oral TMP–SMX	12–15 mg/kg/d (TMP component)
Trimethoprim + dapsone	TMP, 12–15 mg/kg/d; dapsone, 100 mg/d
Primaquine + clindamycin	Primaquine, 15–30 mg base/d; clindamycin, 2400–2700 mg IV/d; 1350–1800 mg orally/d
Atovaquone	2250 mg/d (750 mg suspension TID)
Aerosolized pentamidine	600 mg once daily via the Respirgard II nebulizer
Moderate-to-Severe Episodes	
TMP–SMX IV	15–20 mg/kg/day (TMP component) IV, in 3–4 divided doses
Trimetrexate + leucovorin	45 mg/M^2/d[a] as a single IV infusion, plus leucovorin, 80 mg/M^2/d[a] (in four equal doses); consider adding dapsone 100 mg orally/d
Pentamidine IV	4 mg/kg/d as a single IV infusion
PLUS:	
Adjunctive corticosteroids (prednisone/methylprednisolone)	40/30 mg twice daily, days 1–5
	40/30 mg once daily, days 6–10
	20/15 mg once daily, day 11 to end of course

TMP–SMX, trimethoprim–sulfamethoxazole.
[a]Modified for hematologic toxicity (402).

(394, 398). In one study of patients with moderate-to-severe episodes in which median (A-a)Do$_2$ was 44 mm Hg, subjects were prospectively randomized to receive a full 3-week course of either TMP–SMX or pentamidine without being crossed over to the opposite therapy for apparent treatment failure or adverse drug reactions (399). Although the trial was not blinded, the noncrossover design allowed the relative efficacy and toxicities of these two therapies to be fully assessed. Of the patients treated with TMP–SMX, 86% survived, compared with 61% treated with pentamidine ($P<.05$). Moreover, room air Pao$_2$ in patients treated with TMP–SMX improved by at least 10 mm Hg 7 days earlier than for those receiving pentamidine. Differences in survival or Pao$_2$ were probably not affected by clinician–investigator bias.

All surviving patients completed the 3-week course of therapy. An average of 2.4 adverse reactions was ascribed to study therapy in 89% of individuals treated with TMP–SMX. Acetaminophen was prescribed for drug-induced fever, and antihistamines were administered for morbilliform rash. Generally, fever subsided and rashes coalesced and faded over several days to weeks. In addition, the dose of TMP–SMX was modified during therapy to maintain TMP serum concentrations of 5 to 8 μg/mL in attempt to prevent severe hematologic toxicities. With this approach, neutrophil counts remained higher than 500/mm^3 and platelet counts were higher than 25,000/mm^3. Efficacy was not compromised with the final average dose of 12 mg/kg per day, and thus 15 mg/kg per day should be adequate for even severe episodes and perhaps reduces toxicity (400). Moreover, the approach of "treating-through" toxicities allowed patients to be switched to oral TMP–SMX once they had improved and to complete therapy at home. The dosage of TMP–SMX does not need to be adjusted when therapy is changed from the intravenous to the oral route (396). Finally, therapeutic drug monitoring provided data to develop a nomogram to adjust dosage for impaired renal function (Table 14.2).

In prospective blind studies (Table 14.3), each involving more than 300 patients, TMP–SMX was more effective, albeit more toxic, than experimental therapies with atovaquone, aerosol pentamidine, and trimetrexate (386, 401, 402). Thus, sequential folate blockade with TMP–SMX appears to be the most effective therapy currently available.

Toxicities from TMP–SMX are more frequent in patients with AIDS and include leukopenia, anemia, thrombocytopenia, azotemia, rash, fever, gastrointestinal disturbances, and hepatitis. Recently, hyperkalemia has been recognized as a potentially serious toxic effect of TMP (403–410). Renal insufficiency increases the risk of hyperkalemia (406), and advanced age may also be a risk factor (411–413). The mechanism of hyperkalemia is thought to be an amiloride-like action that decreases potassium excretion at the distal tubule (405, 414).

PARENTERAL PENTAMIDINE

Parenteral pentamidine is often prescribed for severe episodes. In the aforementioned study (399), survival was inferior with pentamidine compared with TMP–SMX, but the dose of pentamidine was reduced for nephrotoxicity. Possibly, the final average dose of 3 mg/kg per day compromised outcome. In two small studies of individuals with less severe *Pneumocystis* pneumonia, 3 mg/kg per day resulted in a good outcome (415, 416). However, until the optimal dose is established, 4 mg/kg per day should be used for severe episodes.

Nephrotoxicity, hypoglycemia, and hypotension are the most frequent serious toxicities (394, 395, 399, 417). Impaired renal function is related to the cumulative dose and typically occurs after the initial week of therapy (418). The combination of pentamidine and amphotericin B is especially nephrotoxic (419). Hypotension usually lasts only several hours after an intravenous dose, although modestly low blood pressures may persist for several months. Acute hypotension can usually be corrected by hydration therapy and by placing patients in the reverse Trendelenburg position.

Hypoglycemia occurs in 10 to 50% of AIDS patients treated with pentamidine (399, 417, 418, 420–422) and is

Table 14.2. Dosing of Trimethoprim–Sulfamethoxazole (TMP–SMX) for Patients with Renal Impairment[a]

Serum Creatinine (mg/dL)	CL_{cr} (mL/min)	Loading Dose (mg)	Maintenance Dose (mg)	Dose Interval (h)	Maintenance Dose (mg/kg/d)	Peak Concentration (µg/mL)	Trough Concentration (µg/mL)
0.7	109	525	275	6	18.32	10.1	5.9
1.0	76	525	250	8	12.51	9.8	5.5
1.5	50	500	200	8	10.00	10.1	6.8
2.0	37	500	225	12	7.50	10.2	6.1
2.5	29	500	200	12	6.66	10.3	6.8
3.0	24	500	175	12	5.83	10.2	7.1
5.0	13	500	225	24	3.75	10.2	5.9
8.0	7	500	175	24	2.92	10.0	6.6
10.0	5	500	150	24	2.50	9.7	6.6

[a]This table was generated from an analysis of the time-concentration data from 179 serum TMP levels obtained from patients during therapeutic drug monitoring of patients receiving intravenous TMP–SMX. The analysis utilized a nonparametric EM population pharmacokinetic modeling program. The following population parameter values were obtained for TMP: The median V_d was 0.8016 ± 0.6415 L/kg and median K_{slope} was 0.0010067 ± 0.00136 (h [mL/min/1.73 M^2])$^{-1}$. The K_{int} was set and fixed at 0.01155 ± 0.01155 h^{-1}. The correlation between V_d and K_{slope}, analogous to the covariance between the parameters, was -0.36664.

For patients with renal failure defined by serum creatinine or serum clearance of creatinine, doses of intravenous TMP–SMX should be chosen to achieve true peak concentrations (level at the completion of the infusion) of 8–10 µg/mL and trough concentrations of 5–7 µg/mL. Dose values in the table were generated for a typical male AIDS patient who was 35 years old, 69 inches tall, weighed 60 kg, and whose muscle mass was 85% of normal.

potentially the most treacherous toxicity. This adverse effect results from sudden increases in serum insulin caused by lysis of pancreatic β cells (423–425). Pentamidine is bound tightly to tissues, and the risk of hypoglycemia is related to drug accumulation (417, 418, 422). Hypoglycemia is thus more likely in the second and third weeks of therapy. In fact, precipitous and fatal reactions have occurred up to 2 weeks after the last dose (418, 426). Thus, for any degree of hypoglycemia, pentamidine should be discontinued, and capillary glucose should be monitored for several weeks. Occasionally, patients must remain in the hospital to receive concentrated infusions of glucose to keep their serum concentrations higher than 40 mg/dL. Depletion of pancreatic insulin may lead to ketoacidosis, hyperosmolar coma, and the ultimate need for treatment with hypoglycemic agents (423, 427–429).

Intramuscular administration of the drug frequently causes painful sterile abscess and limits the usefulness of this route of administration. Other toxic effects occur less frequently and include hyperkalemia, pancreatitis, hypomagnesemia, hypocalcemia, bone marrow suppression, myositis and myoglobinuria, hematuria, ventricular tachycardia, and torsades de pointes.

TRIMETREXATE

Trimetrexate is a powerful antifolate drug that binds to the dihydrofolate reductase of *Pneumocystis carinii* nearly 1500 times more avidly than does TMP (3). Trimetrexate lacks the acidic carboxylic groups of methotrexate and is therefore concentrated in protozoan cells. Concurrent therapy with leucovorin (folinic acid) attenuates trimetrexate-induced hematologic toxicity. These features suggested that trimetrexate could be more effective than the combination of TMP–SMX and potentially less toxic as a single agent. In a dosage evaluation study, 36 patients with a median baseline (A-a)Do$_2$ higher than 30 mm Hg received 45 or 60 mg/M^2 of trimetrexate daily (430). Thirty four (94%) survived, and all completed a 21-day course of therapy. Hypersensitivity reactions were tolerable, and hematologic toxicities were reversed within several days by modifying doses of trimetrexate and leucovorin.

A phase III multicenter trial was initiated by the AIDS Clinical Trials Group (ACTG) to compare trimetrexate (45 mg/M^2 per day) and leucovorin with TMP–SMX (20 mg/kg TMP per day) (402). Three hundred three patients with *Pneumocystis* pneumonia and baseline room air (A-a)Do$_2$ higher than 30 mm Hg were enrolled. By day 10, 16% of patients assigned to TMP–SMX failed therapy compared with 27% receiving trimetrexate ($P=.064$). Failure rates were 20 and 38% by day 21 ($P=.008$). Estimated mortality during 3 weeks of study therapy was less striking, because the rate was 12±3% for patients assigned to TMP–SMX compared with 20±4% for trimetrexate ($P=.088$). By study day 49, the difference in mortality (16±4% versus 29±5%) was significant ($P=.028$), but the proportion dying of *Pneumocystis* was similar in both groups. The number of cumulative treatment-terminating adverse events including hematologic toxicities was less with trimetrexate ($P=.0002$). Thus, trimetrexate should be suitable for patients with severe episodes who cannot tolerate TMP–SMX or in whom treatment has failed.

The finding that treatment with this powerful DHFR inhibitor as a single agent resulted in a survival rate of 80% in patients with severe episodes suggests that combination with a sulfone or sulfonamide could improve outcome further. The combination of trimetrexate plus dapsone does not alter disposition of either drug and was safe in a small blinded comparison with TMP–SMX (431, 432). Larger trials will be needed to define the role of this combination for therapy of *Pneumocystis* pneumonia.

ADJUNCTIVE CORTICOSTEROIDS

Four controlled studies established that the addition of corticosteroids within 72 hours of beginning conventional therapy improves outcome and reduces mortality (129,

Table 14.3. Definitive Treatment Studies Comparing Trimethoprim–Sulfamethoxazole (TMP–SMX) with Other Therapies

Study Drug	Entry Criteria	Number (N)	Failure at End of Treatment	Outcome Variables	Survival at End of Treatment (%)	Comments
TMP-SMX[a] 15–20 mg/kg/d	No blood gas criteria[a]	36	Not available	Days for Pa_{O_2} to ↑ by ≥10 mm Hg:	86[c]	Doses altered
IV Pentamidine 4 mg/kg/d		33	—	day 7[c]	61	
				day 15		Survival day 49:
TMP-SMX[d] 20 mg/kg/d	$(A-a)D_{O_2} \geq 30$ mm Hg	109	20%[c]	$\Delta(A-a)D_{O_2}$ at day 10 of therapy:	88	84%[c]
Trimetrexate[e] 45 mg/m²/d		106	38%	−11 mm Hg	80	69%
				−5 mm Hg		Failure if $(A-a)D_{O_2}$ increased by >30:
TMP-SMX[f] 15 mg/kg/d	$Pa_{O_2} \leq 55$ mm Hg	144[b]	19.5%[c]	Pa_{O_2} day 9:	89	17%[c]
Aerosol pentamidine[g] 600 mg/d		143	28.9%	87.7 mm Hg	82.6	36%
				77.2 mm Hg		Death <28 d after treatment:
TMP-SMX[h] 15 mg/kg/d	$(A-a)D_{O_2} \leq 45$ mm Hg[i]	160	7%[c]	$\Delta(A-a)D_{O_2}$ or lactate dehydrogenase:	100	1[c]
Atovaquone 750 mg TID		162	20%	No data	100	11
				—		

[a]Sattler et al., 1988 (399)
[b]Median $(A-a)D_{O_2}$ at entry = 44 mm Hg
[c]$P < .05$
[d]Sattler et al., 1994 (402)
[e]Administered along with leucovorin at 80 mg/m² (20 mg/m² q6h)
[f]Montgomery et al., 1995 (401)
[g]Administered by Respirgard II jet nebulizer
[h]Hughes et al., 1993 (386)
[i]96 subjects with $(A-a)D_{O_2}$ 35–45 mm Hg received prednisone at 40 mg BID for days 1–5, 40 mg/d for days 6–10, and 20 mg/d for days 11–21

387–389), whereas a single study failed to demonstrate benefit (433). These studies are summarized in Table 14.4. In the largest trial, which evaluated 40 mg of prednisone twice daily for 5 days followed by tapering doses over 3 weeks, major clinical benefits were noted (387). Of 220 patients with proved and 31 with presumed *Pneumocystis* pneumonia, "oxygenation failure" (Pa_{O_2}/Fi_{O_2} lower than 75), the need for mechanical ventilation, and death were each reduced approximately 50% in patients randomized to receive corticosteroids compared with patients not receiving corticosteroids. There was no survival benefit for patients with mild episodes (baseline Pa_{O_2}/Fi_{O_2} higher than 350). The only adverse consequence of steroids was an increased incidence of mucocutaneous herpes infections (387). Subsequent, long-term studies have demonstrated no increased risk for late-occurring serious opportunistic infections (434–436).

The one trial that failed to demonstrate benefit (433) had several design limitations that are summarized by Bozzette and Morton (437). The primary end point in this study emphasized clinical recovery as opposed to clinical deterioration, whereas nonsignificant trends in favor of less deterioration in corticosteroid recipients were consistently observed. Finally, a metaanalysis (437) of five randomized controlled trials of early corticosteroids for confirmed *Pneumocystis* pneumonia, including the data from the study that failed to show benefit (433), showed a typical odds ratio for death in control subjects of 2.9 (exact 95% confidence interval [CI], 1.6, 5.3; $P<.001$). Taken together, these studies provide compelling evidence that adjunctive corticosteroids improve outcome and reduce mortality when prescribed early in the course of therapy for patients with initial room air Pa_{O_2} lower than 70 mm Hg or $(A-a)D_{O_2}$ higher than 35 mm Hg.

Adjunctive corticosteroids can have detrimental effects if prescribed empirically for pulmonary tuberculosis or fungal infection, which may mimic *Pneumocystis* pneumonia, if this treatment delays diagnosis and specific therapy. Such patients may initially improve in response to corticosteroids, thus providing the false impression that they had *Pneumocystis* pneumonia. Moreover, corticosteroids may aggravate and accelerate the progression of cutaneous and pulmonary Kaposi's sarcoma by stimulating a Kaposi's growth promotor or inhibiting a growth suppressor (438–445). Thus, every effort should be made to establish a definitive diagnosis of *Pneumocystis* pneumonia in patients treated with adjunctive corticosteroids. However, if *Pneumocystis* is present, concomitant tuberculosis or fungal infection should not be considered contraindications to corticosteroid therapy, if these other infections are also treated.

Salvage Therapy

Once patients have developed respiratory failure during treatment for *Pneumocystis* pneumonia, prognosis even with changing therapy is poor. Outcome may ultimately be determined more by the degree of lung injury from alveolar damage than by antimicrobial interventions. Although clinicians often change therapy when clinical deterioration occurs during an episode of *Pneumocystis* pneumonia, few data support such an approach, and criteria to guide when to switch therapy have not been established.

Possibly, decreased susceptibility to the administered antimicrobial agents may responsible for some therapeutic failures, but the lack of in vitro susceptibility testing applicable to clinical isolates of *Pneumocystis carinii* makes this a possibility that has not been evaluated. Mutations in the dihydropteroate synthase (DHPS) gene have been reported in four of six AIDS patients who developed *Pneumocystis* pneumonia while receiving sulfa-based prophylaxis (446). However, in this small study, these mutations were not associated with failure to respond to TMP–SMX therapy, and mutations were also detected in two of eight patients who did not receive sulfa drugs in the preceding year. The clinical importance of these observations is unknown. In a controlled trial of treatment of mild-to-moderate episodes of *Pneumocystis* pneumonia, antipneumocystis prophylaxis in the 30 days before treatment was not associated with subsequent failure to respond to treatment doses of the prophylactic agent (447).

TRIMETREXATE

Of 159 patients intolerant of both TMP–SMX and pentamidine and of 160 patients in who at least one conventional treatment had failed after 10 days or more, 84 (53%) and 48 (30%) of subjects in these respective groups were treated for at least 14 days with trimetrexate and were alive after 1 month of follow-up (448). Of 111 patients receiving mechanical ventilation at study entry, 18 (16%) were extubated and alive 1 month later. These results are similar to those obtained when patients with overt treatment failures with TMP–SMX or parenteral pentamidine are crossed over to the opposite therapy (398).

CLINDAMYCIN–PRIMAQUINE

In a study of 28 patients (11 were previously intolerant of, 13 were failing or intolerant of, and 4 had both failed and were intolerant of conventional therapies), patients received clindamycin intravenously (typically 900 mg every 8 hours) plus 30 mg of primaquine orally once daily until they had improved sufficiently to receive all oral therapy (449). Twenty-four (86%, 95% CI, 73 to 99%) were successfully treated with the regimen. Rash was the most common side effect. In a larger study of 109 patients with *Pneumocystis* pneumonia (70 proved and 39 probable), 35 patients had failed standard therapy, 15 were intolerant to conventional agents, and 59 were receiving the combination as initial therapy (450). Outcome was excellent with only 8 failures. This included 6 patients of 15 who had also failed to respond to standard therapies. Caution must be exercised with this regimen for severely hypoxemic patients. Because neither agent is highly effective alone against *P. carinii* in laboratory studies (451–454), outcome could be catastrophic if the

Table 14.4. Summary of Five Controlled Trials of Early Corticosteroids for *Pneumocystis* Pneumonia

Variable	Montaner et al., 1990 (129)	Bozzette et al., 1990 (387)	Gagnon et al., 1990 (388)	Nielsen et al., 1992 (389)	Walmsley et al., 1995 (433)
Number of subjects	38	251	23	59	78
Placebo-controlled	Yes	No	Yes	No	Yes
Entry criteria	O_2 saturation 85–90% on room air, or a 5% decrease with exercise	FiO_2 index > 75	PO_2 < 75 mm Hg on 35% inspired oxygen	PO_2 < 67.5 mm Hg on room air	PO_2 < 70 mm Hg on room air
Initial corticosteroid therapy	Oral prednisone 60 mg/d	Oral prednisone 40 mg every 12 h	IV methylprednisolone 40 mg every 6 h	IV methylprednisolone 0.5 mg/kg every 6 h	IV methylprednisolone 40 mg every 12 h
Mortality					
Corticosteroid	6%	14%	25%	11%	10%
Control	0%	29%	82%	45%	16%
P value	Not significant	.01	.008	.02	Not significant
Comments	Less deterioration in oxygenation	Less need for mechanical ventilation	Less need for mechanical ventilation	Less need for mechanical ventilation	Less discontinuation of TMP–SMX

TMP–SMX, trimethoprim–sulfamethoxazole.

primaquine or oral clindamycin is not absorbed by these patients.

ADJUNCTIVE CORTICOSTEROIDS

Anecdotal reports continue to suggest that adjunctive corticosteroids are beneficial when started well into the course of therapy for patients failing to respond to specific therapies for *Pneumocystis* pneumonia (455, 456). Unfortunately, no controlled studies have been done to support their clinical usage in this setting. To the contrary, in a trial in which 41 patients were randomized to receive 60 mg of methylprednisolone or placebo every 6 hours at any time when their $Pa o_2$ declined to less than 51 mm Hg, no advantage for corticosteroid treatment was noted (457). Most patients were randomized more than 3 days after initiation of anti-*Pneumocystis* treatment. However, the number of subjects studied may have been too small to demonstrate a small but significant benefit for corticosteroids (457). Moreover, perhaps higher dosages of corticosteroids or other anti-inflammatory therapies could improve outcome for patients in whom standard therapies fail.

Mild Episodes

For mild episodes, which are generally associated with an excellent outcome, treatments should be nontoxic, inexpensive, convenient, and suited for home therapy. TMP–SMX is inexpensive and conveniently administered orally, but it has a high frequency of side effects. Thus, other alternatives are needed.

TRIMETHOPRIM–DAPSONE

One modification of sequential folate blockade with TMP–SMX has been to replace SMX, which inhibits dihydropteroate synthetase, with diaminodiphenylsulfone (dapsone). Dapsone inhibits the same enzyme and alone is of comparable efficacy to TMP–SMX in the cortisone-treated rat model (458, 459). A randomized study of 60 patients with arterial Po_2 higher than 60 mm Hg treated with either dapsone plus TMP or TMP–SMX (460) showed similar efficacies (93 and 90%, respectively) but fewer serious toxicities occurred in the TMP–dapsone group (30% compared with 57% in the TMP–SMX group).

In a larger trial (ACTG 108) involving 181 patients with mild-to-moderate episodes, in which $(A-a)Do_2$ was lower than 45 mm Hg, TMP–dapsone was compared with TMP–SMX and clindamycin–primaquine (447). At baseline, the mean room air $(A-a)Do_2$ was 30.4 mm Hg; patients with $(A-a)Do_2$ of 35 to 45 mm Hg also received adjunctive corticosteroids. All 3 regimens had similar efficacy, with success rates of 88 to 93% (Table 14.5). However, the study had limited power to detect differences in therapeutic efficacy (447). Although adverse events were generally similar with the 3 regimens, severe rash and hepatotoxicity were less common with TMP–dapsone. These results further confirm that TMP–dapsone is an effective, well-tolerated alternative for treatment of mild episodes of *Pneumocystis* pneumonia. TMP–dapsone may be particularly useful in patients with underlying hepatic disease.

CLINDAMYCIN PLUS PRIMAQUINE

Clindamycin and the antimalarial drug primaquine together have excellent activity against *P. carinii* in a limited culture system and in cortisone-treated rats, although neither agent is highly effective alone (452–454). In the first clinical investigation of this combination, 23 (92%) of 25 patients treated with 600 mg of clindamycin intravenously every 6 hours and 15 mg of primaquine base by mouth once daily responded (454). However, 17 of the subjects had been treated previously with conventional therapies that may have contributed to the ultimate outcome.

In another study, 22 previously untreated patients with $(A-a)Do_2$ lower than 30 mm Hg received 900 mg clindamycin intravenously every 8 hours for 10 days and then 450 mg orally every 6 hours for 11 days along with 30 mg primaquine base orally once daily for 3 weeks (451). Of these patients 20 (91%) improved by day 7; in 2, therapy failed, and they were switched to other therapies; 4 patients were subsequently removed from the study because of rash; 16 patients (73%) successfully completed the 3-week course of therapy. Generalized rash was the most common toxicity and occurred in 15 cases but required treatment cessation in only 3 patients. Mild diarrhea occurred in 1 case. The trial was extended to

Table 14.5. Results of a Randomized Trial Comparing Three Regimens for Treatment of Mild-to-Moderate *Pneumocystis* Pneumonia

	Successful Treatment	Dose-limiting Toxicity	Dose-limiting Rash	Severe Rash	Severe Hematologic Toxicity	Hepatotoxicity
TMP–dapsone N = 35	88%	24%	10%	2%	12%	3%
TMP–SMX N = 32	91%	36%	19%	6%	11%	19%
Clindamycin–primaquine N = 30	93%	33%	21%	16%	28%	7%
P value	>.2	.2	.2	.07	.01	.003

TMP–SMX, trimethoprim–sulfamethoxazole.
(From Safrin S, Kinkelstein DM, Feinberg J, et al. Comparison of three regimens for treatment of mild to moderate *Pneumocystis carinii* pneumonia in patients with AIDS. Ann Intern Med 1996;124:792–802.)

assess all oral clindamycin (450 mg 3 times daily) and the same dose of primaquine in 46 patients who had baseline (A-a)Do$_2$ lower than 40 mm Hg. Of the first 14 patients, 13 (93%) responded. Rash occurred in 7 (54%) but was not treatment limiting.

In ACTG study 108 (described in the section on dapsone–TMP and in Table 14.5), patients with mild-to-moderate *Pneumocystis* pneumonia receiving clindamycin 600 mg orally every 8 hours plus primaquine 30 mg orally per day had outcomes similar to TMP–SMX and TMP–dapsone recipients (447). However, severe rash and hematologic toxicities were more frequent with clindamycin–primaquine. Thus, other regimens would be preferable in patients with severe myelosuppression at baseline.

ATOVAQUONE

Atovaquone is a hydroxynapthoquinone originally developed as an antimalarial compound. The drug inhibits mitochondrial electron transport necessary for the biosynthesis of pyrimidines in protozoa, but its actual mode of action against *Pneumocystis carinii* is unknown. In cortisone-treated rats, recurrences did not occur 1 month after therapy for *Pneumocystis* infection with atovaquone (461). It is the only clinical agent tested in the model that has shown this lethal effect. The drug has unique pharmacokinetic properties, including a terminal serum half-life of approximately 50 hours (462) and limited bioavailability that increases severalfold with food. This property has necessitated multiple daily dosing for maximal drug exposure.

Based on these features and on the results of early clinical trials (463, 464), a randomized, double-blind study of 322 patients with mild to moderately severe *Pneumocystis* pneumonia, characterized by (A-a)Do$_2$ lower than 45 mm Hg, compared oral atovaquone (750 mg) versus TMP (320 mg) plus SMX (1600 mg), with each regimen given 3 times daily (386). Failures from inadequate therapeutic response occurred in 31% of patients receiving atovaquone and 16% of those receiving TMP–SMX ($P=.002$). Therapeutic failures because of drug toxicity occurred in 7% of atovaquone-treated patients and in 20% of TMP–SMX-treated patients ($P=.001$). Although the proportion remaining on study therapy with either agent over the 21-day course of treatment was similar for both regimens, 11 patients randomized to receive atovaquone compared with only 1 receiving TMP–SMX died during the study.

Steady-state plasma levels of atovaquone were lower in patients failing to respond and were related to the occurrence of diarrhea (386). The unfavorable outcome was probably due to the inherently poor bioavailability of the tablet preparation used in that trial. The currently available suspension formulation of atovaquone is better absorbed, but unless greater efficacy is demonstrated, this drug should be reserved for patients with mild episodes of *Pneumocystis* pneumonia who have had severe intolerance to TMP–SMX.

AEROSOLIZED PENTAMIDINE

With aerosolized pentamidine, drug is delivered directly to alveoli in high concentration (416, 465). In a multicenter study (401), 364 patients with room air (A-a)Do$_2$ lower than 55 mm Hg were randomized to receive either 600 mg aerosolized pentamidine once daily with a jet nebulizer or TMP–SMX at 15 mg/kg per day (TMP component). Although no differences in survival were noted, Pao$_2$ improved significantly more quickly with TMP–SMX, and therapy in patients treated with TMP–SMX failed less often. In particular, for those with an initial (A-a)Do$_2$ of more than 30 mm Hg, 17% of TMP–SMX recipients had therapy discontinued by day 21, versus 36% for aerosolized pentamidine recipients ($P=.001$). As expected, toxicities occurred more often with TMP–SMX.

Aerosolized pentamidine has not been as effective as intravenous pentamidine. In one study, 45 patients with baseline room air Pao$_2$ higher than 55 mm Hg were randomized to aerosolized pentamidine at 600 mg once daily or intravenous pentamidine (416). Although initial failure rates were similar (12% versus 19%), recrudescence of symptoms (35% versus 0%) and relapse (24% versus 0%) were more common with aerosolized pentamidine ($P<.05$ for both). In the second study, only 6 of 11 patients randomized to receive inhaled pentamidine (8 mg/kg per day) responded, whereas all 10 assigned to the parenteral formulation responded ($P=.02$) (466). Nonresponders to inhaled pentamidine had lower mean baseline Pao$_2$ compared with responders (60 versus 81 mm Hg, $P=.005$). Aerosol treatment may not be as effective in areas of the lung with extensive airspace consolidation, which could predispose to early relapse. Moreover, in sicker patients with tachypnea and higher minute ventilation, peripheral alveolar deposition may be suboptimal, thereby predisposing these individuals to treatment failure. Thus, aerosolized pentamidine seems suited for patients who have mild *Pneumocystis* pneumonia and who are unable to tolerate other therapies.

DAPSONE (ALONE)

In an uncontrolled trial, 18 patients with mild-to-moderate episodes were treated with 100 mg per day of dapsone alone (467). The 39% failure rate was unacceptably high. A second study evaluated 200 mg dapsone daily for patients with initial room air Pao$_2$ higher than 60 mm Hg (468). This study was terminated after 7 patients had been enrolled because of 2 deaths and 5 failures. Treatment was terminated in 4 because of methemoglobinemia (9.5 to 17.4%) and respiratory distress, and none was able to complete a full course of therapy with dapsone successfully. These data indicate that dapsone should not be prescribed alone for treatment of *Pneumocystis* pneumonia.

ADJUNCTIVE CORTICOSTEROIDS

Corticosteroids resulted in more rapid improvement in exercise tolerance and less early deterioration compared with placebo in a small trial involving 23 subjects with mild episodes of *Pneumocystis* pneumonia (469). However, only 1 death occurred during the study, consistent with the expected low mortality rate among patients with mild *Pneumocystis* pneumonia. On balance, no compelling reason exists to use adjunctive corticosteroids in this population.

Experimental Agents

Several promising drugs are undergoing initial testing in humans, and other compounds have been identified with good activity against *Pneumocystis carinii* in vitro or in animal models.

PIRITREXIM

Piritrexim is an oral antifolate drug that binds the DHFR of *Pneumocystis carinii* approximately 1000 times more avidly than TMP (470). In a pilot study of 15 patients with a first episode of *Pneumocystis* pneumonia and a baseline Pao_2 Pao_2 higher than 60 mm Hg, 6 patients were treated with 150 mg/kg of piritrexim twice daily and 9 with 250 mg/kg twice daily for 3 weeks, along with 50 mg of leucovorin 4 times daily in both groups (471). All survived, and 4 of 6 patients responded favorably at the lower dose and 6 of 9 at the higher dose. None developed neutrophil counts lower than $750/mm^3$, but 9 (60%) patients relapsed within 3 months of completing therapy. If this drug proceeds further in clinical development, it could provide a companion drug for trimetrexate once patients with severe episodes are ready for oral therapy outside the hospital.

PENTAMIDINE ANALOGS AND 8-AMINOQUINOLINES

Analogs of pentamidine and the 8-aminoquinolines have been evaluated and used in developing countries for treatment of malaria and leishmaniasis. Several compounds from these two classes of drugs are at least as potent as pentamidine and primaquine against *Pneumocystis carinii* in the laboratory and demonstrate good bioavailability in animals (472, 473). WR-6026, an 8-aminoquinoline, was developed by the military and was used to treat *Leishmania* in Africa with a good safety profile. WR-6026 is the first of these agents to enter clinical trials for treatment of *Pneumocystis*.

OTHER AGENTS

Other experimental agents have been tested in animals with *Pneumocystis* and show promise. These include interferon-γ (IFN-γ) plus low-dose TMP–SMX (474, 475), eichinocandins and papulacandins (1,3-β-glucan synthesis inhibitors) (38, 476), urinary proteinase inhibitor (477), erythromycin plus sulfisoxazole (478), other macrolides plus sulfonamides (479), furazolidone and nitrofurantoin (480), and mycophenolate mofetil (481). Mycophenolate mofetil is unique in that not only does it have anti-*P. carinii* activity in rats with *Pneumocystis* pneumonia, but also the agent is immunosuppressive. IFN-γ warrants comment, inasmuch as it alone reduces lung cysts and, together with TMP–SMX, is synergistic in animals with *Pneumocystis* infection (389, 475). When aerosol IFN-γ was used as adjunctive therapy with TMP–SMX for patients with mild-to-moderate *Pneumocystis* pneumonia, all 19 recipients improved, and no toxicity was attributable to study therapy (482).

PROGNOSIS
Predictors of Outcome

The degree of alveolar damage as measured physiologically by $(A-a)Do_2$ higher than 35 mm Hg (268, 386), the histologic presence of interstitial edema (263), and indirectly by low triiodothyronine (T_3) and high reverse T_3 hormone concentrations (483, 484) or elevation of LDH to more than 500 IU/dL (265, 266, 276, 279, 282) have been predictors of increased risk for respiratory failure and death. Results of quantitative BAL for *Pneumocystis carinii* provide more evidence that the extent of infection and the corresponding inflammatory response are important determinants of outcome (130, 362, 485). In one study, the the number of *P. carinii* in clumps associated with 500 nucleated cells in BAL was determined in 56 patients after 21 days of therapy (362). For 24 of 25 responders who did not relapse within 6 months, a more than 50% decrease in clusters was seen. Responders with relapse and nonresponders had no change in the number of clusters.

Four studies have indicated that patients with more than 5% polymorphonuclear neutrophils in BAL cell counts are more likely to progress to respiratory failure or death (130, 362, 364, 486). Moreover, increased BAL neutrophils have been associated with the presence of α_2-globulins and high protein in BAL and with higher BAL protein to plasma protein, providing further evidence for increased capillary permeability during severe *Pneumocystis* pneumonia (486). At follow-up bronchoscopy in the trial discussed earlier, only 2 of 32 responders still had increased neutrophils compared with 17 of 24 nonresponders (362).

Supportive Care

Supportive care is an essential component for successful outcome of severely ill patients. Continuous positive airway pressure (CPAP) by face mask improves oxygenation in cases with tachypnea and desaturation refractory to standard masks, thereby mitigating the need for mechanical ventilation in some cases (487–490). In one report involving 36 episodes of respiratory failure, 23 of 25 patients were successfully managed with CPAP alone; in 11 others, intubation and mechanical ventilation were delayed (487).

Mechanical Ventilation and ICU Care

For patients receiving mechanical ventilation, mortality was in the range of 86 to 100% during the early years of the AIDS epidemic (272, 491–497). In the latter part of the 1980s, reports that 30 to 50% of patients in intensive care units (ICUs) receiving assisted ventilation were discharged from the hospital alive has supported the value of aggressive measures in some patients with severe episodes (264, 492, 498–503). More recently, however, increasing mortality rates have been reported from some centers (504). Ascertaining the reason for differing outcomes is difficult, but it may be related to patient selection. Low albumin, arterial pH lower than 7.35, the need for positive end-expiratory pressure higher than 10 cm H_2O after 96 hours in the ICU (492, 502), low CD4 cell count (504), the presence of pneumothorax (504), no prior use of prophylaxis (505), and prolonged ICU stay (506) portend a greater risk for a fatal outcome. Thus, patients with better nutritional status who are not acidotic or in respiratory failure with less severe alveolar damage may benefit most from ICU care.

PROPHYLAXIS

Patients with fewer than 200 CD4 cells but without prior *Pneumocystis* infection are at increased risk of *Pneumocystis* pneumonia. For patients experiencing an initial bout of *Pneumocystis* pneumonia, approximately 5% will relapse each month, or 60% by 12 months, if specific prophylaxis is not administered (507). Controlled studies have established that aerosol pentamidine, dapsone, and TMP–SMX are highly effective in preventing *Pneumocystis* pneumonia in these two groups of patients. Because it is not yet known whether CD4 cell increases induced by antiviral drug therapy restore immune competence to *P. carinii*, prophylaxis for *Pneumocystis* pneumonia should be based on an individual's lowest-ever CD4 cell count (508).

Aerosol Pentamidine

The pivotal study resulting in licensure of aerosol pentamidine involved 408 high-risk subjects at 14 community treatment centers in San Francisco (509). A dose of 300 mg given by jet nebulizer once monthly was more protective (P=.0008) than 2 other doses in patients with prior episodes (secondary prophylaxis). These results were confirmed in a second study of primary prophylaxis (no prior *Pneumocystis*) involving 223 patients with advanced AIDS-related complex or fewer than 200 CD4 cells (510). *Pneumocystis* pneumonia occurred in 8 patients receiving 300 mg monthly compared with 23 in a placebo group (P=.0021).

Results with an ultrasonic nebulizer have been equally compelling (511, 512). Induction therapy has consisted of 5 doses over 14 days followed by 1 dose on day 21 and then every 2 weeks. In one blinded study, 5 episodes of *Pneumocystis* pneumonia occurred among 84 patients receiving 60-mg doses compared with 27 episodes in 78 patients receiving placebo (P<.001) (511). Thus, despite differences in the efficiency of the 2 nebulizers (220), each produces sufficient respirable particles with mass median diameters 1 to 5 µm to be highly effective.

Toxicity has been limited to transient bad taste and cough. Prolonged coughing or bronchospasm occasionally occurs, usually in smokers or patients with asthma, but these complications can be prevented or attenuated by pretreatment with an aerosol bronchodilator (513, 514). In separate studies, 26%, 34%, and 100% of patients experienced 10%, 15%, and 21% average reductions in FEV_1, respectively, after a single treatment (513–515). However, no documented long-term deleterious effects of aerosol pentamidine on pulmonary function after more than 12 months of therapy have been reported (516–518).

Although little pentamidine is absorbed into the systemic circulation, generalized rash (519), pancreatitis (512, 520, 521), hypoglycemia (512, 522), renal insufficiency (523), and diabetes (524, 525), have occurred during aerosol therapy. Even in the absence of overt pancreatic insufficiency, aerosolized pentamidine can cause significant abnormalities in glucose homeostasis (526). Contact dermatitis and conjunctivitis may also occur (527). These systemic and cutaneous toxicities are uncommon. Disadvantages of inhaled pentamidine include the high cost of the drug, need for a compressed air source, lack of systemic prophylaxis for extrapulmonary *Pneumocystis carinii* infection, morbidity associated with spontaneous pneumothorax (203, 528), and incomplete protection provided for patients with prior *Pneumocystis* infection (10 to 30% recurrence after 1 to 2 years) (509, 511).

Trimethoprim–Sulfamethoxazole

By contrast, TMP–SMX is inexpensive, orally administered, and thus well suited for home therapy. Several controlled studies have established that TMP–SMX is more effective than aerosol pentamidine (506, 529–531) for both primary and secondary prophylaxis. For secondary prophylaxis, the most definitive study included 154 patients with a single prior episode of *Pneumocystis* pneumonia assigned to receive 1 double-strength tablet of TMP–SMX and 156 to receive 300 mg aerosol pentamidine monthly (529). By intent to treat, 14 and 36 of *Pneumocystis* pneumonia occurred in the 2 groups. The respective estimated 18-month recurrence rate was 11.4% versus 27.6% (P<.001). The frequency of severe hepatic and hematologic toxicities was similar in the two groups. Moreover, bacterial infections and cerebral toxoplasmosis occurred less often during therapy with TMP–SMX. In a study of 214 patients with fewer than 200 CD4 cells, TMP–SMX was also superior to monthly aerosol pentamidine for primary prophylaxis (530).

A large open-label trial involving 843 patients compared primary prophylaxis with TMP–SMX (1 double-strength tablet twice daily, which could be reduced to once daily if toxicity occurred), dapsone (50 mg twice daily, which could be reduced to once daily if toxicity occurred), and aerosolized pentamidine (300 mg per month) (506). No overall difference in *Pneumocystis* pneumonia incidence was seen among the 3 groups by intent-to-treat analysis, but for patients entering the study with fewer than 100 CD4 lymphocytes/ mm^3, the systemic therapies (dapsone and TMP–SMX) were superior to pentamidine. The 36-month cumulative risk of

Pneumocystis pneumonia for this subset of subjects was 33% with pentamidine, 19% with TMP–SMX, and 22% with dapsone ($P=.04$ favoring the 2 systemic therapies). The "on-treatment" analyses also favored TMP–SMX, but only 23% of patients were receiving full doses of their originally assigned treatment when they completed the study (506).

Intermittent TMP–SMX also appears effective (532–535). In 2 open-label studies testing 1 double-strength tablet given on Mondays, Wednesdays, and Fridays, only 4 cases of Pneumocystis pneumonia occurred (3 patients were noncompliant) in 220 high-risk patients after 12 to 18 months of observation (532, 533). Less than 10% of patients had treatment-terminating toxicities with the test regimens. In a comparative trial of secondary prophylaxis, 60 patients received 1 double-strength tablet of TMP–SMX twice daily on 2 days per week, and 73 received 300 mg aerosol pentamidine once monthly (534). One patient (1.7%) assigned to TMP–SMX and 31 (42.5%) assigned to pentamidine developed Pneumocystis pneumonia ($P<.0001$). Median disease-free intervals were 1153 and 496 days, respectively. Treatment-terminating toxicities occurred in 5% of patients in both groups. In a retrospective review of patients at risk for Pneumocystis pneumonia (38% with prior pneumocystis), 133 were treated with 1 double-strength tablet of TMP–SMX twice daily thrice weekly for a mean of 7 months, 77 received 50 mg dapsone daily for a mean of 5.7 months, and 125 received 300 mg aerosol pentamidine monthly for a mean of 9.3 months (535). No Pneumocystis pneumonia was seen with TMP–SMX after 981 patient-months, 5 cases occurred with dapsone after 437 patient-months, and 17 cases occurred with pentamidine after 1166 patient-months. These studies suggest that intermittent TMP–SMX may be effective, but they do not establish whether the regimens are as effective or better tolerated than daily TMP–SMX.

A randomized, open study comparing 480 mg to 960 mg of TMP–SMX daily as primary prophylaxis (median CD4 cell count 86 to 90) demonstrated no difference between the two doses, with no episodes of Pneumocystis pneumonia at a median follow-up of 376 days (536). Survival was similar in both treatment groups. However, the cumulative incidence of adverse events (not including death) was higher in patients in the group receiving 960 mg per day (31% versus 18% in the 480-mg group, $P=.007$). This study suggests that, for primary prophylaxis, lower doses of TMP–SMX may be sufficient. However, this study did not establish equal efficacy for the most severely immunocompromised patients (CD4 cell count less than 50).

Management of TMP–SMX Intolerance

Because studies have indicated that TMP–SMX is the most effective prophylactic therapy for Pneumocystis pneumonia in persons with fewer than 100 CD4 lymphocytes/mm^3, some reports have described different approaches to desensitize or rechallenge persons who have already experienced cutaneous hypersensitivity (537–546). This approach usually involves beginning with a low dose of diluted TMP–SMX elixir with gradual escalation to the doses used in the pill form. These protocols have resulted in variable success in desensitizing patients and thereby allowing them to take TMP–SMX without severe intolerance. Because comparisons among regimens have not been made, no compelling reason exists to recommend one regimen over another. Once desensitization is achieved, patients should be warned not to interrupt therapy for even as little as 1 or 2 days because desensitization may be lost, and reactions, often severe, may occur with subsequent doses.

ACTG 268 assessed whether "ramped" dosing with TMP–SMX should be done routinely during initiation of prophylaxis for Pneumocystis pneumonia (547). Subjects with median CD4 counts of 169 cells/mm^3 were randomized to standard prophylaxis with TMP–SMX versus ramped therapy at 3-day intervals beginning with 1 mL, followed by 2, 5, 10, and 20 mL. After 14 weeks, 84% patients who had their doses gradually escalated remained on study therapy compared with only 66% receiving standard therapy ($P=.0002$). The relative risk of discontinuing therapy was 2.2 for subjects receiving immediate standard therapy. Those with CD4 counts less than 100 cells/mm^3 were more likely not to tolerate prophylaxis regardless of the method of initiation, but assigned treatment was a greater predictive value. Use of gradual dose escalation of TMP–SMX should enable substantially more patients to tolerate this form of prophylaxis and ultimately should result in less Pneumocystis pneumonia.

Dapsone

Dapsone has been effective in open-label studies (548–550). In a controlled trial of primary prophylaxis, 47 patients were randomized to receive 100 mg dapsone daily and 39 to 1 double-strength tablet of TMP–SMX daily (550). After 862 and 776 patient-months in the respective groups, each therapy was associated with a single episode of Pneumocystis pneumonia, but the number of end points was too small to provide statistical confidence that the therapies were truly similar. The most serious toxicities associated with dapsone are hemolytic anemia and methemoglobinemia, but both are infrequent in HIV patients.

Several trials have compared dapsone, with or without pyrimethamine, to TMP–SMX or aerosolized pentamidine (506, 531, 551–554). In one study, aerosolized pentamidine recipients had a similar risk of Pneumocystis pneumonia compared with those assigned to dapsone, 50 mg per day, plus pyrimethamine, 50 mg per week (adjusted relative risk 1.13), but the risk of toxoplasmosis was higher with aerosolized pentamidine (relative risk 1.81, 95% CI, 1.12 to 2.94, $P=.02$) (552). More patients discontinued dapsone–pyrimethamine because of toxicity (42 versus 3 receiving pentamidine, $P<.001$) and no survival difference was seen. Bozzette and colleagues (506) showed no overall efficacy difference among TMP–SMX, dapsone, and aerosolized pentamidine, but dapsone at 50 mg twice daily appeared superior to dapsone at 50 mg daily. In the on-treatment analysis, the rate of Pneumocystis pneumonia per

100 patient-years was 2.6 for those receiving dapsone at the higher dose as compared with 11.3 for those receiving the reduced dose. These results suggest that trials that use doses of dapsone of 50 mg daily or less may underestimate the potential efficacy of dapsone because of suboptimal dosing.

Two trials have raised concerns about the possible association of increased mortality with dapsone use (531, 551). In one trial, the adjusted relative risk of death among those assigned to dapsone was 2.18 (95% CI, 1.27 to 3.74) compared with those assigned to pentamidine (551). However, this study used a formulation of dapsone available in France (Disulone; Specia, Paris) which also contained iron protoxalate that may have confounded the results. The other trial (531) used a low dose of dapsone (100 mg weekly, plus pyrimethamine) and had a strikingly higher rate of *Pneumocystis* pneumonia of 32.1 per 100 person-years compared with 10.2 for pentamidine and 2.0 for TMP–SMX. Although no survival difference was noted between patients assigned to dapsone compared with pentamidine, those assigned to dapsone were more likely to die compared with those assigned to TMP–SMX (adjusted relative risk 2.8, 95% CI, 1.1 to 7.3, $P=.037$). This difference probably relates to the dramatically lower prophylactic efficacy of the low dose of dapsone used. Multiple other studies have not documented decreased survival with dapsone (506, 553–555), and a meta-analysis failed to demonstrate decreased survival with dapsone-based regimens (556).

Other Agents

Pyrimethamine–sulfadoxine is an antifolate combination that can be administered once weekly and has shown protective efficacy in uncontrolled observations (557). Enthusiasm for this therapy was hampered by fatalities from Stevens–Johnson syndrome during prophylaxis for malaria and in one HIV-infected patient (558).

Atovaquone suspension is being compared, in a randomized open trial, to dapsone for patients intolerant of TMP–SMX. Results of this study are pending as of this writing, and no controlled data are available regarding the usefulness of this agent for prophylaxis.

Prophylaxis Recommendations

Based on the studies cited previously, TMP–SMX should be considered the agent of first choice, followed by dapsone and, finally, aerosolized pentamidine. The systemic therapies have the added advantage of providing some protection against toxoplasmosis and do not require specialized facilities for administration. The added protection of TMP–SMX and dapsone are probably limited to individuals with fewer than 100 CD4 cells/mm^3. For those with counts above 100 cells/mm^3, aerosolized pentamidine is of comparable protective efficacy. Present data are insufficient to recommend atovaquone or combinations of agents such as aerosolized pentamidine plus dapsone. For individuals with a prior history of intolerance to TMP–SMX and with fewer than 100 CD4 cells/mm^3, clinicians should strongly consider either rechallenge or desensitization with TMP–SMX.

References

1. Centers for Disease Control. Update: acquired immunodeficiency syndrome: United States. MMWR Morb Mortal Wkly Rep 1986;35:17–21.
2. Centers for Disease Control. Update: acquired immunodeficiency syndrome: United States. MMWR Morb Mortal Wkly Rep 1986;35:757–766.
3. Allegra CJ, Kovacs JA, Drake JC, et al. Activity of antifolates against *Pneumocystis carinii* dihydrofolate reductase and identification of a potent new agent. J Exp Med 1987;165:926–931.
4. Klatt EC, Nichols L, Noguchi NT. Evolving trends revealed by autopsies of patients with acquired immunodeficiency syndrome: 565 autopsies in adults with the acquired immunodeficiency syndrome, Los Angeles, Calif, 1992–93. Arch Pathol Lab Med 1994;118:884–890.
5. Selik RM, Chu SY, Word JW, et al. Trends on infectious diseases and cancers among persons dying of HIV infection in the United States from 1987 to 1992. Ann Intern Med 1995;123:933–936.
6. Moore RD, Chaisson RE. Natural history of opportunistic disease in an HIV infected urban clinical cohort. Ann Intern Med 1996;124:633–642.
7. Chan ISF, Neaton JD, Saravolatz LD, et al. Frequencies of opportunistic diseases prior to death among HIV-infected persons. AIDS 1995;9:1145–1151.
8. Saah AJ, Hoover DR, Peng Y, et al. Predictors for failure of *Pneumocystis carinii* pneumonia prophylaxis: Multicenter AIDS Cohort Study. JAMA 1995;273:1197–1202.
9. Quin JW, Baumgart KW, Garsia RJ. *Pneumocystis carinii* pneumonia: upper lobe recurrence following cotrimoxazole. Aust NZ J Med 1991;21:380–381.
10. Katz MH, Baron RB, Grady D. Risk stratification of ambulatory patients suspected of *Pneumocystis* pneumonia. Arch Intern Med 1991;151:105–110.
11. Edelstein H, McCabe RE. Atypical presentations of *Pneumocystis carinii* pneumonia in patients receiving inhaled pentamidine prophylaxis. Chest 1990;98:1366–1369.
12. Travis WD, Pittaluga S, Lipschik GY, et al. Atypical pathologic manifestations of *Pneumocystis carinii* pneumonia in the acquired immunodeficiency syndrome: review of 123 lung biopsies from 76 patients with emphasis on cysts, vascular invasion, vasculitis, and granulomas. Am J Surg Pathol 1990;14:615–625.
13. Shin MS, Veal CF, Jessup JG, et al. Apical *Pneumocystis carinii* pneumonia in AIDS patients not receiving inhaled pentamidine prophylaxis. Chest 1991;100:1462–1464.
14. Sarkar S, Dube MP, Jones BE, et al. *Pneumocystis* pneumonia masquerading as tuberculosis. Arch Intern Med 1997;157:351–355.
15. Chagas C. Nova tripanozomiaze humana. Mem Instit Oswlado Cruz 1909;1:159–218.
16. Delanoe P, Delanoe M. Sur les rapports des kystes de carinii du poumon des rats avec le trypanosoma lewisii: presenter par M. Laveran [note de Delanoe and Delanoe]. C R Acad Sci (Paris) 1912;155:658–660.
17. Dutz W. *Pneumocystis carinii* pneumonia. Pathol Annu 1970;5:309–341.
18. Dutz W. *Pneumocystis carinii* infection and interstitial pneumonia: what does history teach? Semin Diagn Pathol 1989;6:195–202.
19. Thomas SF, Dutz W, Khodadad EJ. *Pneumocystis carinii* pneumonia (plasma cell pneumonia); roentgenographic, pathologic and clinical correlation. Am J Roentgenol Radium Ther Nucl 1966;98:318–322.
20. Burke BA, Good RA. *Pneumocystis carinii* infection. Medicine (Baltimore) 1973;52:23–51.
21. Walzer PD, Perl DP, Krogstead DJ, et al. *Pneumocystis carinii* pneumonia in the United States: epidemiologic, diagnostic, and clinical features. Ann Intern Med 1974;80:83–93.

22. Vavra J, Kucera K. *Pneumocystis carinii* Delanoe: its ultrastructure and ultrastructural affinities. J Protozool 1970;17:463–483.
23. ul Haque A, Plattner SB, Cook RT, et al. *Pneumocystis carinii*: taxonomy as viewed by electron microscopy. Am J Clin Pathol 1987;87:504–510.
24. Fitch WM, Margoliash E. Construction of phylogenetic trees. Science 1967;155:279–284.
25. Sogin ML, Elwood HJ, Gunderson JH. Evolutionary diversity of eukaryotic small-subunit rRNA genes. Proc Natl Acad Sci U S A 1986;83:1383–1387.
26. Gunderson JH, Elwood HJ, Ingold A, et al. Phylogenetic relationships between chlorophytes, chrysophytes, and oomycetes. Proc Natl Acad Sci U S A 1987;84:5823–5827.
27. Edman JC, Kovacs JA, Masur H, et al. Ribosomal RNA sequence shows *Pneumocystis carinii* to be a member of the fungi. Nature 1988;334:519–522.
28. Pixley FJ, Wakefield AE, Banerji S, et al. Mitochondrial gene sequences show fungal homology for *Pneumocystis carinii*. Mol Microbiol 1991;5:1347–1351.
29. Van der Peer Y, Hendriks L, Goris A, et al. Evolution of basidiomycetous yeasts as deduced from small ribosomal subunit RNA sequences. Syst Appl Microbiol 1992;15:250–258.
30. Garrett CE, Coderre CE, Meek TD, et al. A bifunctional thymidilate synthetase-dihydrofolate reductase in protozoa. Mol Biochem Parasitol 1984;11:257–265.
31. Berverly SM, Ellenberger TE, Cordingley JS. Primary structure of the gene encoding the bifunctional dihydrofolate reductase-thymidilate synthetase of *Leishmania major*. Proc Natl Acad Sci U S A 1986;83:2584–2585.
32. Riis B, Rattan SIS, Clark BFC, et al. Eukaryotic protein elongation factors. Trends Biochem Sci 1990;15:420–424.
33. Chen YS, Haskins RH. Studies on the pigments of *Penicillium funiculsum*. I. Production of cholesterol. Canad J Chem 1963;41:1647–1649.
34. McCorkindale NJ, Hutchinison SA, Pursey BA, et al. A comparison of the types of sterol found in species of the Saprolenginales and Leptomitales with those found in other Phycomycetes. Phytochemistry 1969;8:861–867.
35. Ramgopal M, Bloch K. Sterol synergism in yeast. Proc Natl Acad Sci U S A 1983;80:712–715.
36. Rodriquez RJ, Taylor FR, Parks LW. A requirement for ergosterol to permit growth of yeast sterol auxotrophs on cholesterol. Biochem Biophys Res Commun 1982;106:435–441.
37. Matsumoto Y, Yamada M, Amagai T. Yeast glucan of *Pneumocystis carinii* cyst wall: an excellent target for chemotherapy. J Protozool 1991;38:6S–7S.
38. Schmatz DM, Romanchek MA, Pittarelli LA, et al. Treatment of *Pneumocystis carinii* pneumonia with 1,3-β-glucan synthesis inhibitors. Proc Natl Acad Sci U S A 1990;87:5950–5954.
39. Schmatz DM, Powles M, McFadden DC, et al. Treatment and prevention of *Pneumocystis carinii* pneumonia and further elucidation of the *P. carinii* life cycle with 1,3-β-glucan synthesis inhibitor L-671,329. J Protozool 1991;38:151S–153S.
40. Giuntoli D, Stringer SL, Stringer JR. Extraordinarily low number of ribosomal RNA genes in *P. carinii*. J Eukaryot Microbiol 1994;41:88S.
41. Stringer JR, Walzer PD. Molecular biology and epidemiology of *Pneumocystis carinii* infection in AIDS. AIDS 1996;10:561–571.
42. Kovacs JA, Halpern JL, Swann JC, et al. Identification of antigens and antibodies specific for *Pneumocystis carinii*. J Immunol 1988;140:2023–2031.
43. Walzer PD, Linke MJ. A comparison of the antigenic characteristics of rat and human *Pneumocystis carinii* by immunoblotting. J Immunol 1987;138:2257–2265.
44. Graves DC, McNabb SJ, Worley MA, et al. Analysis of rat *Pneumocystis carinii* antigens recognized by human and rat antibodies by using Western immunoblotting. Infect Immun 1986;54:96–103.
45. Linke MJ, Cushion MT, Walzer PD. Properties of the major antigens of rat and human *Pneumocystis carinii*. Infect Immun 1989;57:1547–1555.
46. Kovacs JA, Halpern JL, Lundgren B, et al. Monoclonal antibodies to *Pneumocystis carinii*: identification of specific antigens and characterization of antigenic differences between rat and human isolates. J Infect Dis 1989;159:60–70.
47. Bauer NL, Paulsrud JR, Bartlett MS, et al. *Pneumocystis carinii* organisms obtained from rats, ferrets, and mice are antigenically different. Infect Immun 1993;61:1315–1319.
48. Hong ST, Steele PE, Cushion MT, et al. *Pneumocystis carinii* karyotypes. J Clin Microbiol 1990;28:1785–1795.
49. Banerji S, Wakefield AE, Allen AG, et al. The cloning and characterization of the arom gene of *Pneumocystis carinii*. J Gen Microbiol 1993;139:2901–2914.
50. Cushion MT, Zhang J, Kaselis M, et al. Evidence for two genetic variants of *Pneumocystis carinii* coinfecting laboratory rats. J Clin Microbiol 1993;31:1217–1223.
51. Dyer M, Volpe F, Delves CJ, et al. Cloning and sequence of a beta-tubulin cDNA from *Pneumocystis carinii*. Mol Microbiol 1992;6:991–1011.
52. Edlind TD, Bartlett MS, Weinberg GA, et al. The beta-tubulin gene from rat and human isolates of *Pneumocystis carinii*. Mol Microbiol 1992;6:3365–3373.
53. Garbe TR, Stringer JR. Molecular characterization of clustered variants of genes encoding major surface antigens of human *Pneumocystis carinii*. Infect Immun 1994;62:3092–3101.
54. Keely SP, Stringer JR, Baughman RP, et al. Genetic variation among *Pneumocystis carinii* hominis isolates in recurrent pneumocystosis. J Infect Dis 1995;172:595–598.
55. Kovacs JA, Powell F, Edman JC, et al. Multiple genes encode the major surface glycoprotein of *Pneumocystis carinii*. J Biol Chem 1993;268:6034–6040.
56. Meade JC, Stringer JR. Cloning and characterization of an ATPase gene from *Pneumocystis carinii* which closely resembles fungal hydrogen ATPases. J Eukaryot Microbiol 1995;42:298–307.
57. Peters SE, Wakefield AE, Whitwell KE, et al. *Pneumocystis carinii* pneumonia in thoroughbred foals: identification of a genetically distinct organism by DNA amplification. J Clin Microbiol 1994;32:213–216.
58. Stringer JR, Stringer SL, Zhang J, et al. Molecular genetic distinction of *Pneumocystis carinii* from rats and humans. J Eukaryot Microbiol 1993;40:733–741.
59. Wada M, Kitada K, Saito M, et al. cDNA sequence diversity and genomic clusters of major surface glycoprotein genes of *Pneumocystis carinii*. J Infect Dis 1993;168:979–985.
60. Wright TW, Simpson Haidaris PJ, Gigliotti F, et al. Conserved sequence homology of cysteine-rich regions in genes encoding glycoprotein A in *Pneumocystis carinii* derived from different host species. Infect Immun 1994;62:1513–1519.
61. Zhang J, Stringer JR. Cloning and characterization of an alpha-tubulin-encoding gene from rat-derived *Pneumocystis carinii*. Gene 1993;123:137–141.
62. Wakefield AE, Fritscher CC, Malin AS, et al. Genetic diversity in human-derived *Pneumocystis carinii* isolates from four geographical locations shown by analysis of mitochondrial rRNA gene sequences. J Clin Microbiol 1994;32:2959–2961.
63. Latouche S, Roux P, Poirot JL, et al. Preliminary results of *Pneumocystis carinii* strain differentiation by using molecular biology. J Clin Microbiol 1994;32:3052–3053.
64. Lu J, Bartlett M, Shaw M, et al. Typing of *Pneumocystis carinii* strains that infect humans based on nucleotide sequence variation of internal transcribed spacers of rRNA genes. J Clin Microbiol 1994;32:2904–2912.
65. Lu J, Bartlett M, Smith J, et al. Typing of *Pneumocystis carinii* strains with type-specific oligonucleotide probes derived from nucleotide sequences of internal transcribed spacers of rRNA. J Clin Microbiol 1995;33:2973–2977.

66. Tsolaki AG, Miller RF, Underwood AP, et al. Genetic diversity at the internal transcribed spacer regions of the rRNA operon among isolates of *Pneumocystis carinii* from AIDS patients with recurrent pneumonia. J Infect Dis 1996;174:141–156.
67. Meuwissen JHE, Tauber I, Leeuwenber ADEM, et al. Parasitologic and serologic observations of infection with Pneumocystis in humans. J Infect Dis 1977;136:43–49.
68. Pfifer LL, Hughes WT, Stagno S, et al. *Pneumocystis carinii* infection: evidence for high prevalence in normal and immunosuppressed children. Pediatrics 1978;61:35–41.
69. Hofmann B, Odum N, Platz P, et al. Humoral responses to *Pneumocystis carinii* in patients with acquired immunodeficiency syndrome and in immunocompromised homosexual men. J Infect Dis 1985; 152:838–840.
70. Hofmann B, Nielsen PB, Odum N, et al. Humoral and cellular responses to *Pneumocystis carinii*, CMV, and herpes simplex in patients with AIDS and in controls. Scand J Infect Dis 1988;20:389–394.
71. Madison SE, Hayes GV, Slemenda SB, et al. Detection of specific antibody by enzyme-linked immunosorbent assay and antigenemia by counterimmunoelectrophoresis in humans infected with *Pneumocystis carinii*. J Clin Microbiol 1982;15:1036–1043.
72. Madison SE, Walls KW, Haverkos HW, et al. Evaluation of serologic tests for *Pneumocystis carinii* antibody and antigenemia in patients with acquired immunodeficiency syndrome. Diagn Microbiol Infect Dis 1984;2:69–75.
73. Hendley JO, Weller TH. Activation and transmission in rats of infection with Pneumocystis. Proc Soc Exp Biol Med 1971;137:1401–1404.
74. Walzer PD, Schnelle V, Armstrong D, Rosen PP. Nude mouse: a new experimental model for *Pneumocystis carinii* infection. Science 1977; 197:177–179.
75. Hughes WT, Smith B. Provocation of infection due to *Pneumocystis carinii* by cyclosporin A. J Infect Dis 1982;145:767.
76. Hughes WT, Bartley DL, Smith BM. A natural source of infection due to *Pneumocystis carinii*. J Infect Dis 1983;147:595.
77. Soulez B, Palluaalt F, Cesbron JY, et al. Introduction of *Pneumocystis carinii* in a colony of SCID mice. J Protozool 1991;38:123S–125S.
78. Cushion MT, Stringer JR, Walzer PD. Cellular and molecular biology of *Pneumocystis carinii*. Int Rev Cytol 1991;131:59–107.
79. Rodinson JJ. Two cases of pneumocystosis: observation in 203 adult autopsies. Arch Pathol 1961;50:156–159.
80. Easterly JA. *Pneumocystis carinii* in lungs of adults at autopsy. Am Rev Respir Dis 1968;97:935–937.
81. Sedaghation MR, Singer DB. *Pneumocystis carinii* in children with malignant disease. Cancer 1972;29:772–777.
82. Settnes OP, Genner J. *Pneumocystis carinii* in human lungs at autopsy. Scand J Infect Dis 1986;18:486–489.
83. Lipshcik GY, Gill VJ, Lundgren JD, et al. Improved diagnosis of *Pneumocystis carinii* infection by polymerase chain reaction on induced sputum and blood. Lancet 1992;340:203–206.
84. Wakefield AE, Pixley FJ, Banerji S, et al. Detection of *Pneumocystis carinii* with DNA amplification. Lancet 1990;336:451–453.
85. Peters SE, Wakefield AE, Sinclair K, et al. A search for *Pneumocystis carinii* in post mortem lungs by DNA amplification. J Pathol 1992; 166:195–198.
86. Stiller RA, Paradis IL, Dauber JH. Subclinical pneumonitis due to *Pneumocystis carinii* in a young adult with elevated antibody titers to Epstein–Barr virus. J Infect Dis 1992;166:926–930.
87. Leigh TR, Wakefield AE, Peter SE, et al. Comparison of DNA amplification and immunofluorescence for detecting *Pneumocystis carinii* in patients receiving immunosuppressive therapy. Transplantation 1992;54:3.
88. Graves DC, McNabb SJ, Ivey MH, et al. Development and characterization of monoclonal antibodies to *Pneumocystis carinii*. Infect Immun 1986;51:125–133.
89. Gigliotti F, Ballou LR, Hughes WT, et al. Purification and initial characterization of a ferret *Pneumocystis carinii* surface antigen. J Infect Dis 1988;158:848–854.
90. Sinclair K, Wakefield AE, Banerji S, et al. *Pneumocystis carinii* organisms derived from rat and human hosts are genetically distinct. Mol Biochem Parasitol 1991;45:183–184.
91. Gigliotti F, Harmsen AG, Haidaris CG, et al. *Pneumocystis carinii* is not universally transmissible between mammalian species. Infect Immun 1993;61:2886–2890.
92. Lee CH, Ju JJ, Bartlett MS, et al. Nucleotide sequence variation in *Pneumocystis carinii* strains that infect humans. J Clin Microbiol 1993;31:754–757.
93. Watanabe JM, Chinchinian H, Weitz C, et al. *Pneumocystis carinii* pneumonia in a family. JAMA 1965;193:685–686.
94. Goesch TR, Gotz G, Stellbrinck KH, et al. Possible transfer of *Pneumocystis carinii* between immunodeficient patients. Lancet 1990; 336:627.
95. Brazinsky JH, Phillips JE. *Pneumocystis carinii* transmission between patients with lymphoma. JAMA 1969;209:1527.
96. Benousan T, Garo B, Islam S, et al. Possible transfer of *Pneumocystis carinii* between kidney transplant recipients. Lancet 1990;336:1066–1067.
97. Chave JP, David S, Wauters JP, et al. Transmission of *Pneumocystis carinii* from AIDS patients to other immunosuppressed patients: a cluster of *Pneumocystis carinii* pneumonia in renal transplant recipients. AIDS 1991;5:927–932.
98. Jacobs JL, Libby DM, Winters RA, et al. A cluster of *Pneumocystis carinii* pneumonia in adults without predisposing illnesses. N Engl J Med 1991;324:246–250.
99. Hoover DR, Graham NMH, Bacellar H, et al. Epidemiologic patterns of upper respiratory illness and *Pneumocystis carinii* pneumonia in homosexual men. Am Rev Respir Dis 1991;144:756–759.
100. Leigh TR, Millet MJ, Jameson B, et al. Serum titres of *Pneumocystis carinii* antibody in health care workers caring for patients with AIDS. Thorax 1993;48:619–621.
101. Bartlett MS, Lee CH, Lu JJ, et al. *Pneumocystis carinii* detected in air. J Eukaryot Microbiol 1994;41:75S.
102. Lanken PN, Minda M, Pietra GG, et al. Alveolar response to experimental *Pneumocystis carinii* pneumonia in the rat. Am J Pathol 1980;99:561–578.
103. Yoneda K, Walzer PD. The interaction of *Pneumocystis carinii* with host cells: an ultrastructural study. Infect Immun 1980;29:692–703.
104. Yoneda K, Walzer PD. Attachment of *Pneumocystis carinii* to type I alveolar cells: study by freeze fracture electron microscopy. Infect Immun 1983;40:812–815.
105. Henshaw NG, Carson JL, Collier AM. Ultrastructural observations in *Pneumocystis carinii* attachment to rat lung. J Infect Dis 1985;151: 181–186.
106. Long EC, Smith JS, Meier JL. Attachment of *Pneumocystis carinii* to rat pneumocytes. Lab Invest 1986;54:609–614.
107. Pottratz ST, Martin WJ. Role of fibronectin in *Pneumocystis carinii* attachment to cultured lung cells. J Clin Invest 1990;85:351–356.
108. Pottratz ST, Paulsrud J, Smith JS, et al. *Pneumocystis carinii* attachment to cultured lung cells by pneumocystis gp 120, a fibrinonectin binding protein. J Clin Invest 1991;88:403–407.
109. Limper AH, Standing JE, Hoffman OA, et al. Vitronectin binds to *Pneumocystis carinii* and mediates organism attachment to cultured lung epithelial cells. Infect Immun 1993;61:4302–4309.
110. Neese LW, Standing JE, Olson EF, et al. Vitronectin, fibronectin, and antibody to gp120 enhance macrophage release of TNF-α in response to *Pneumocystis carinii*. J Immunol 1994;152:4549–4556.
111. O'Riordan DM, Standing JE, Kwon KY, et al. Surfactant protein D interacts with *Pneumocystis carinii* and mediates organism adherence to alveolar macrophages. J Clin Invest 1995;95:2699–2710.
112. Ruffolo JJ. *Pneumocystis carinii* cell structure. In: Walzer PD, Genta RM, eds. *Pneumocystis carinii* pneumonia. 2nd ed. New York: Marcel Dekker, 1993:25–43.
113. Sukura A. Trophozoite to cyst ratio increases during recovery from *Pneumocystis carinii* pneumonia in rats. APMIS 1995;103:300–306.

114. Yoneda K, Walzer PD. Mechanism of alveolar injury in experimental *Pneumocystis carinii* pneumonia in the rat. Br J Exp Pathol 1981;62:339–346.
115. Kernbaum S, Masliah J, Alcindor LG, et al. Phospholipase activities of bronchoalveolar lavage fluid in rat *Pneumocystis carinii* pneumonia. Br J Exp Pathol 1983;64:75–80.
116. Brun-Pascaud M, Pocidalo JJ, Kernbaum S. Respiratory alterations in experimental *Pneumocystis carinii* pneumonia in rats. Bull Eur Physiopathol Resp 1985;21:37–41.
117. Sheenan PM, Stokes DC, Yeh, Hughes WT. Surfactant phospholipids and lavage phospholipase A2 in experimental *Pneumocystis carinii* pneumonia. Am Rev Respir Dis 1986;134:526–531.
118. Eijking EP, van Daal GJ, Tenbrinck R, et al. Effect of surfactant replacement on *Pneumocystis carinii* pneumonia in rats. Intensive Care Med 1991;17:475–478.
119. Phelps DS, Fishman JA, Rose RM. Surfactant protein A levels in glucocorticoid-immunosuppressed rats infected with *Pneumocystis carinii*. Am Rev Respir Dis 1992;145:A246.
120. Su TH, Nararajan V, Martin WJ. Pulmonary surfactant in *Pneumocystis carinii* pneumonia is associated with a marked increase in sphingomyelin. Am Rev Respir Dis 1992;145:A246.
121. Pesanti EL. Phospholipid profile of *Pneumocystis carinii* and its interaction with alveolar type II epithelial cells. Infect Immun 1987;55:736–741.
122. Zimmersman PE, Voelker R, McCormack FX, et al. 120-kD surface glycoprotein of *Pneumocystis carinii* is a ligand for surfactant protein A. J Clin Invest 1992;89:143–149.
123. Koziel H, O'Riordan D, Phelps D, et al. Surfactant protein-a inhibits binding and internalization of *Pneumocystis carinii* by alveolar macrophages. Am Rev Respir Dis 1992;145:A247.
124. Mason GR, Duane GB, Mena I, et al. Accelerated solute clearance in *Pneumocystis carinii* pneumonia. Am Rev Respir Dis 1987;135:864–868.
125. Sankary RM, Turner J, Lipavsky A, et al. Alveolar-capillary block in patients with AIDS and *Pneumocystis carinii* pneumonia. Am Rev Respir Dis 1988;137:443–449.
126. Coleman DL, Dodek PM, Golden JA, et al. Correlation between serial pulmonary function tests and fiberoptic bronchoscopy in patients with *Pneumocystis carinii* pneumonia and the acquired immunodeficiency syndrome. Am Rev Respir Dis 1984;129:491–493.
127. Roths JB, Marshall JD, Allen RD, et al. Spontaneous *Pneumocystis carinii* pneumonia in immunodeficient mutant scid mice. Am J Pathol 1990;136:1173–1186.
128. Roths JB, Sidman CL. Both immunity and hyper-responsiveness to *Pneumocystis carinii* result from transfer of CD4+ but not CD8+ T cells into severe combined immunodeficiency mice. J Clin Invest 1992;90:673–678.
129. Montaner JSG, Lawson LM, Levitt N, et al. Corticosteroids prevent early deterioration in patients with moderately severe *Pneumocystis carinii* pneumonia and the acquired immunodeficiency syndrome (AIDS). Ann Intern Med 1990;113:14–20.
130. Mason GR, Hashimoto CH, Dickman PS, et al. Prognostic implications of bronchoalveolar lavage neutrophilia in patients with *Pneumocystis carinii* pneumonia and AIDS. Am Rev Respir Dis 1989;139:1336–1342.
131. Twigg HL, Iwamoto GK, Soliman DM. Role of cytokines in alveolar macrophage accessory cell function in HIV-infected individuals. J Immunol 1992;149:1462–1469.
132. Trentin L, Garbisa S, Zambello R, et al. Spontaneous production of IL-6 by alveolar macrophages of HIV-1 seropositive patients. J Infect Dis 1992;166:731–737.
133. Lipschik GY, Doerfler ME, Kovacs JA, et al. Leukotriene B4 and interleukin 8 in human immunodeficiency virus–related pulmonary disease. Chest 1993;104:763–769.
134. Denis M, Ghadirian E. Dysregulation of interleukin-8, interleukin-10, and interleukin-12 release by alveolar macrophages from HIV type 1-infected subjects. AIDS Res Hum Retroviruses 1994;10:1619–1627.
135. Benfield TL, Steenwuk RV, Nielsen TL, et al. Interleukin-8 amd eicosanoid production in the lung during moderate to severe *Pneumocystis carinii* pneumonia in AIDS: a role of interleukin-8 in the pathogenesis of P. carinii pneumonia. Respir Med 1995;89:285–290.
136. Agostini C, Trentin L, Zambello R, et al. Release of granulocyte-macrophage colony-stimulating factor by alveolar macrophages in the lung of HIV-1-infected patients. J Immunol 1992;149:3379–3385.
137. Agostini C, Zambello R, Trentin L, et al. Alveolar macrophages from patients with AIDS and AIDS-related complex constitutively synthesize and release tumor necrosis factor alpha. Am Rev Respir Dis 1991;144:195–201.
138. Huang ZB, Eden E. Effect of corticosteroids on IL1-beta and TNF-alpha release by alveolar macrophages from patients with AIDS and *Pneumocystis carinii* pneumonia. Chest 1993;104:751–755.
139. Hoffman OA, Standing JE, Limper AH. *Pneumocystis carinii* stimulates tumor necrosis factor-alpha release from alveolar macrophages through a beta-glucan-mediated mechanism. J Immun 1993;150:3932–3940.
140. Chen W, Havell EA, Harmsen AG. Importance of endogenous tumor necrosis factor alpha and gamma interferon in host resistance against *Pneumocystis carinii* infection. Infect Immun 1992;60:1279–1284.
141. Krishnan VL, Meager A, Mitchell DM, et al. Alveolar macrophages in AIDS patients: increased spontaneous tumour necrosis factor-alpha production in *Pneumocystis carinii* pneumonia. Clin Exp Immunol 1990;80:156–160.
142. Rayment N, Miller RF, Ali N, et al. Synthesis of tumor necrosis factor-alpha mRNA in bronchoalveolar lavage cells from human immunodeficiency virus–infected persons with *Pneumocystis carinii* pneumonia. J Infect Dis 1996;174:654–659.
143. Frenkel JK, Good JT, Schultz JA. Latent *Pneumocystis* infection in rats, relapse and chemotherapy. Lab Invest 1966;15:1559–1577.
144. Walzer PD, Powell RD, Yoneda K. *Pneumocystis carinii* pneumonia in different strains of cortisonized mice. Infect Immun 1979;24:939–947.
145. Walzer PD, Powell RD, Yoneda K, et al. Growth characteristics and pathogenesis of experimental *Pneumocystis* pneumonia. Infect Immun 1980;27:929–937.
146. Ruskin J, Hughes WT. *Pneumocystis carinii*. In: Remington JS, Klein J, eds. Infectious diseases of the fetus and newborn infant. Philadelphia: WB Saunders, 1983:507–543.
147. Hughes WT, Price RA, Sisko F, et al. Protein calorie malnutrition: a host determinant for *Pneumocystis carinii* infection. Am J Dis Child 1974;128:44–52.
148. Furuta T, Ueda K, Fujiwara K, et al. Cellular and humoral immune response of mice subclinically infected with *Pneumocystis carinii*. Infect Immun 1985;47:544–548.
149. Furuta T, Ueda K, Kyuwa S, et al. Effect of T-cell transfer on *Pneumocystis carinii* infection in nude mice. Jpn J Exp Med 1984;54:57–64.
150. Graves DC, Li X, Paiva W. Delayed-type hypersensitivity response in mice to *Pneumocystis carinii*. J Protozool 1991;38:49S–52S.
151. Harmsen AG, Stankiewicz M. Requirement for CD4+ cells in resistance to *Pneumocystis carinii* pneumonia in mice. J Exp Med 1990;1972:937–945.
152. Shellito J, Suzara VV, Blumenfeld W, et al. A new model of *Pneumocystis carinii* infection in mice selectively depleted of helper T lymphocytes. J Clin Invest 1990;85:1686–1693.
153. Theus SA, Andrews RP, Steele P, et al. Adoptive transfer of lymphocytes sensitized to the major surface glycoprotein of *Pneumocystis carinii* confers protection in the rat. J Clin Invest 1995;95:2587–2593.
154. Bunjes D, Hardt C, Rollinghoff M, et al. Cyclosporin A mediates immunosuppression of primary cytotoxic T cell responses by impairing the release of interleukin 1 and interleukin 2. Eur J Immunol 1981;11:657–661.
155. Gold E. Infection associated with immunologic deficiency disease. Med Clin North Am 1974;58:649–659.

156. Walzer PD, Schultz MG, Western KA, et al. *Pneumocystis carinii* pneumonia and primary immune deficiency disease. Natl Cancer Inst Monogr 1976;43:65–74.
157. Lidman C, Berglund O, Tynell E, et al. CD4+ cells and CD4+ percent as risk markers for *Pneumocystis carinii* pneumonia (PCP): implications for primary PCP prophylaxis. Scand J Infect Dis 1992; 24:157–160.
158. Phair J, Munoz A, Detels R, et al. The risk of *Pneumocystis carinii* pneumonia among men infected with human immunodeficiency virus type 1. N Engl J Med 1990;322:161–165.
159. Hughes WT, Ho-Kyun K, Price R, et al. Attempts at prophylaxis for murine *Pneumocystis carinii* pneumonitis. Curr Ther Res 1973;15: 581–587.
160. Harmsen AG, Stankiewicz M. T cells are not sufficient for resistance to *Pneumocystis carinii* pneumonia in mice. J Parasitol 1991;38: 44S–45S.
161. Gigliotti F, Hughes WT. Passive immunoprophylaxis with specific monoclonal antibody confers partial protection against *Pneumocystis carinii* pneumonitis in animal models. J Clin Invest 1988;81:1666–1668.
162. Graves DC, Smulian G, Walzer PD. Humoral and cellular immunity. In: Walzer PD, Genta RM, eds. *Pneumocystis carinii* pneumonia. 2nd ed. New York: Marcel Dekker, 1992:267–287.
163. Peglow SL, Smulian AG, Linke JM, et al. Serologic responses to *Pneumocystis carinii* antigens in health and disease. J Infect Dis 1990;161:296–306.
164. Lundgren B, Lundgren JD, Mathiesen L, et al. Antibody response to a major antigen in human immunodeficiency virus–infected patients with and without *P. carinii* pneumonia. J Infect Dis 1992;165:1151–1155.
165. Blumenfeld W, McCook O, Griffiss JM. Detection of antibodies to *Pneumocystis carinii* in bronchoalveolar lavage fluid by immunoreactivity to *Pneumocystis carinii* within alveoli, granulomas, and disseminated sites. Mod Pathol 1992;5:107–113.
166. Guamer J, Robey SS, Gupta PK. Cytologic detection of *Pneumocystis carinii*: a comparison of Papanicolaou and other histochemical stains. Diagn Cytopathol 1986;2:133–137.
167. Bedrossian CW. Ultrastructure of *Pneumocystis carinii*: a review of internal and surface characteristics. Semin Diagn Pathol 1989;6: 212–237.
168. Watts JC, Chandler FW. *Pneumocystis carinii* pneumonitis: the nature and diagnostic significance of the methenamine silver-positive intracystic bodies. Am J Surg Pathol 1985;9:744–751.
169. Askin FB, Katzenstein AL. *Pneumocystis* infection masquerading as diffuse alveolar damage: a potential source of diagnostic error. Chest 1981;79:420–422.
170. Davey RT Jr, Margolis D, Kleiner D, et al. Digital necrosis and disseminated *Pneumocystis carinii* infection after aerosolized pentamidine prophylaxis. Ann Intern Med 1989;111:681–682.
171. Praz JO, Lorenzi P, Chevrolet JC. *Pneumocystis carinii* pneumonia and acquired immunodeficiency syndrome: an atypical presentation with lung cavitations. Eur Respir J 1990;3:1221–1223.
172. Judson MA, Postic B, Weiman DS. *Pneumocystis carinii* pneumonia manifested as a hilar mass and cavitary lesion: an atypical presentation in a patient receiving aerosolized pentamidine prophylaxis. South Med J 1990;83:1309–1312.
173. Moskovic E, Miller R, Pearson M. High resolution computed tomography of *Pneumocystis carinii* pneumonia in AIDS. Clin Radiol 1990;42:239–243.
174. Summers QA, Helprin GA, Tarala RA, et al. Multiple pneumatoceles and bilateral tension pneumothoraces complicating pneumocystis pneumonia in AIDS. Aust NZ J Med 1990;20:257–260.
175. Gurney JW, Bates FT. Pulmonary cystic disease: comparison of *Pneumocystis carinii* pneumatocoeles and bullous emphysema due to intravenous drug abuse. Radiology 1989;173:27–31.
176. Rao NA, Zimmerman PL, Boyer D, et al. A clinical, histopathologic, and electron microscopic study of *Pneumocystis carinii* choroiditis. Am J Ophthalmol 1989;107:218–228.
177. Case records of the Massachusetts General Hospital. Weekly clinicopathological exercises. Case 9-1989: a 32-year-old man with AIDS and a cavitary pulmonary lesion. N Engl J Med 1989;320:582–587.
178. Pincus PS, Sandler MA, Naude GE, et al. Multiple pulmonary cavities-an unusual complication of *Pneumocystis carinii* pneumonia. S Afr Med J 1987;72:871–872.
179. Liu YC, Tomashefski JF Jr, Tomford JW, et al. Necrotizing *Pneumocystis carinii* vasculitis associated with lung necrosis. Arch Pathol Lab Med 1989;113:494–497.
180. Barrio JL, Suarez M, Rodriguez JL, et al. *Pneumocystis carinii* pneumonia presenting as cavitating and noncavitating solitary pulmonary nodules in patients with the acquired immunodeficiency syndrome. Am Rev Respir Dis 1986;134:1094–1096.
181. Gronbeck C. *Pneumocystis carinii* pneumonia presenting as cavitary lung disease. Milit Med 1988;153:314–316.
182. Balachandran I, Jones DB, Humphrey DM. A case of *Pneumocystis carinii* in pleural fluid with cytologic, histologic and ultrastructural documentation. Acta Cytol 1990;34:486–490.
183. Klein S, Warnock M, Webb WR, et al. Cavitating and noncavitating granulomas in AIDS patients with Pneumocystis pneumonitis. AJR Am J Roentgenol 1989;152:753–754.
184. Eng RHK, Bishburg E, Smith SM. Evidence for destruction of lung tissues during *Pneumocystis carinii* infection. Arch Intern Med 1987; 147:746–749.
185. McGarry TM. Pneumatoceles and pneumothorax in *Pneumocystis carinii*. N Y State J Med 1991;91:287–288.
186. Beers MF, Sohn M. Swartz M. Recurrent pneumothorax in AIDS patients with *Pneumocystis* pneumonia: a clinicopathologic report of three cases and review of the literature. Chest 1990;98:266–270.
187. Saldana MJ, Monew JM. Cavitation and other atypical manifestations of *Pneumocystis carinii* pneumonia. Semin Diagn Pathol 1989;6: 273–286.
188. Afessa B, Green WR, Williams WA, et al. *Pneumocystis carinii* pneumonia complicated by lymphadenopathy and pneumothorax. Arch Intern Med 1988;148:2651–2654.
189. Mascarenhas DAN, Vasudevan VP, Vaida KP. *Pneumocystis carinii* pneumonia: rare cause of hemoptysis. Chest 1991;99:251–253.
190. Mariuz P, Raviglione MC, Gould IA, et al. Pleural disease in *Pneumocystis carinii* infection. Chest 1991;99:774–776.
191. Elwood LJ, Dobrzanski D, Feuerstein IM, et al. *Pneumocystis carinii* in pleural fluid: the cytologic appearance. Acta Cytol 1991;35: 761–764.
192. Ewig S, von Kempis J, Rockstroh J, et al. *Pneumocystis carinii* pleuropneumonia after aerosolized pentamidine prophylaxis. Infection 1991;19:442–444.
193. Hartz JW, Geisinger KR, Scharyj M, et al. Granulomatous pneumocystosis presenting as a solitary pulmonary nodule. Arch Pathol Lab Med 1985;109:466–469.
194. Cupples JB, Blackie SP, Road JD. Granulomatous *Pneumocystis carinii* pneumonia mimicking tuberculosis. Arch Pathol Lab Med 1989;113: 1281–1284.
195. Blumenfeld W, Basgoz N, Owen WF Jr, et al. Granulomatous pulmonary lesions in patients with acquired immunodeficiency syndrome (AIDS) and *Pneumocystis carinii* infection. Ann Intern Med 1988;109:505–507.
196. Gal AA, Koss MN, Strigle S, et al. *Pneumocystis carinii* infection in the acquired immunodeficiency syndrome. Semin Diagn Pathol 1989;6: 287–299.
197. Lee MM, Schinella RA. Pulmonary calcification caused by *Pneumocystis carinii* pneumonia: a clinicopathological study of 13 cases in acquired immunodeficiency syndrome patients. Am J Surg Pathol 1991;15:376–380.
198. Tran Van Nhieu J, Vojtek AM, Bernaudin JF, et al. Pulmonary alveolar proteinosis associated with *Pneumocystis carinii*: ultrastructural identification in bronchoalveolar lavage in AIDS and immunocompromised non-AIDS patients. Chest 1990;98:801–805.

199. Ruben FL, Talamo TS. Secondary pulmonary alveolar proteinosis occurring in two patients with acquired immunodeficiency syndrome. Am J Med 1986;80:1187–1190.
200. Prakash UB, Barham SS, Carpenter HA, et al. Pulmonary alveolar phospholipoproteinosis: experience with 34 cases and a review. Mayo Clin Proc 1987;62:499–518.
201. Kovacs JA, Himenez JX, Macher AM. *Pneumocystis carinii* pneumonia: a comparison between patients with acquired immunodeficiency syndrome and patients with other immunodeficiencies. Ann Intern Med 1984;100:633–671.
202. Haverkos HW. Assessment of therapy for *Pneumocystis carinii* pneumonia. Am J Med 1984;76:501–508.
203. Sepkowitz KA, Telzak EE, Gold JWM, et al. Pneumothorax in AIDS. Ann Intern Med 1991;114:455–459.
204. Masur H, Michelis MA, Greene JB, et al. An outbreak of community-acquired *Pneumocystis carinii* pneumonia: initial manifestations of cellular immune dysfunction. N Engl J Med 1981;305:1431–1438.
205. Hopewell PC. *Pneumocystis carinii* pneumonia: diagnosis. J Infect Dis 1988;157:1115–1119.
206. Joe L, Gordon F, Parker RH. Spontaneous pneumothorax with *Pneumocystis carinii* infection: occurrence in patients with acquired immunodeficiency syndrome. Arch Intern Med 1986;146:1816–1817.
207. Sherman M, Levin D, Breidlbart D. *Pneumocystis carinii* pneumonia with spontaneous pneumothorax: a report of three cases. Chest 1986;90:609–610.
208. Goodman PC, Daley C, Minagi H. Spontaneous pneumothorax in AIDS patients with *Pneumocystis carinii* pneumonia. AJR Am J Roentgenol 1986;147:29–31.
209. Fleisher AG, McElvaney G, Lawson L, et al. Surgical management of spontaneous pneumothorax in patients with AIDS. Ann Thorac 1988;45:21–23.
210. Martinez CM, Romanelli A, Mullen MP, et al. Spontaneous pneumothoraces in AIDS patients receiving aerosolized pentamidine. Chest 1988;94:1317–1318.
211. Brynes TT, Brevig JK, Yeoh CB. Pneumothorax in patients with acquired immunodeficiency syndrome. J Thorac Cardiovasc Surg 1989;98:546–550.
212. Scannell KA. Pneumothoraces and *Pneumocystis carinii* pneumonia in two AIDS patients receiving aerosol pentamidine. Chest 1990;97:479–480.
213. Lee MJ. Aerosolized pentamidine and spontaneous pneumothoraces in AIDS patients. Chest 1990;97:510–511.
214. Metersky ML, Colt HG, Olson LK, et al. AIDS-related spontaneous pneumothorax: risk factors and treatment. Chest 1995;108:946–951.
215. Sandhu JS, Goodman PC. Pulmonary cysts associated with *Pneumocystis carinii* pneumonia in patients with AIDS. Radiology 1989;173:33–35.
216. Feuerstein IM, Archer A, Pluda JM, et al. Thin-walled cavities, cysts, and pneumothorax in *Pneumocystis carinii* pneumonia: further observations with histopathological correlation. Thorac Radiol 1990;174:697–702.
217. DeLorenzo LJ, Huang CT, Maguire GP, et al. Roentgenographic patterns of *Pneumocystis carinii* pneumonia in 104 patients with AIDS. Chest 1987;91:323–327.
218. Werb Z, Gordon S. Elastase secretion by stimulated macrophages: characterization and regulation. J Exp Med 1975;142:361–367.
219. Chaffey MH, Klein JS, Gamsu G, et al. Radiographic distribution of *Pneumocystis carinii* in patients with AIDS treated with prophylactic inhaled pentamidine. Radiology 1990;175:715–719.
220. Ilowite JS, Baskin MI, Sheetz MS, et al. Delivered dose and regional distribution of aerosolized pentamidine using different delivery systems. Chest 1991;99:1139–1144.
221. Dyner TS, Lang W, Busch DF, et al. Intravascular and pleural involvement by *Pneumocystis carinii* in a patient with AIDS. Ann Intern Med 1989;111:194.
222. Telzak EE, Cote RJ, Gold JWM, et al. Extrapulmonary *Pneumocystis carinii* infections. Rev Infect Dis 1990;12:380–386.
223. Raviglione MC. Extrapulmonary pneumocystosis: the first 50 cases. Rev Infect Dis 1990;12:1127–1138.
224. Northfelt DW, Clement MJ, Safrin S. Extrapulmonary pneumocystosis: clinical features in human immunodeficiency virus infection. Medicine (Baltimore) 1990;69:392–398.
225. Cohen OJ, Stoeckle MY. Extrapulmonary *Pneumocystis carinii* infections in the acquired immunodeficiency syndrome. Arch Intern Med 1991;151:1205–1214.
226. Witt K, Nielsen TN, Junge J. Dissemination of *Pneumocystis carinii* in patients with AIDS. Scand J Infect Dis 1991;23:691–695.
227. Atzori C, Lu JJ, Jiang B, et al. Diagnosis of *Pneumocystis carinii* pneumonia in AIDS patients by using polymerase chain reactions on serum specimens. J Infect Dis 1995;172:1623–1626.
228. Schinella RA, Breda SD, Hammerschlag PE. Otic infection due to *Pneumocystis carinii* in an apparently healthy man with antibody to the human immunodeficiency virus. Ann Intern Med 1987;106:399–400.
229. Gherman CR, Ward RR, Bassis ML. *Pneumocystis carinii* otitis media and mastoiditis as the initial manifestation of the acquired immunodeficiency syndrome. Am J Med 1988;85:250–252.
230. Hennessey NP, Parro EL, Cockerell CJ. Cutaneous *Pneumocystis carinii* infections in patients with acquired immunodeficiency syndrome. Arch Dermatol 1991;127:1699–1701.
231. Coulman CU, Greene I, Archibald WR. Cutaneous pneumocystosis. Ann Intern Med 1987;106:396–398.
232. Carter TR, Cooper PH, Petri WA Jr, et al. *Pneumocystis carinii* infection of the small intestine in a patient with acquired immunodeficiency syndrome. Am J Clin Pathol 1988;89:679–683.
233. Amin MB, Abrash MP, Mezger E, et al. Systemic dissemination of *Pneumocystis carinii* in a patient with acquired immunodeficiency syndrome. Henry Ford Hosp Med J 1990;38:68–71.
234. Poblete RB, Rodriquez K, Foust RT, et al. *Pneumocystis carinii* hepatitis in the acquired immunodeficiency syndrome (AIDS). Ann Intern Med 1989;110:737–740.
235. Unger PD, Rosenblum M, Krown SE. Disseminated *Pneumocystis carinii* infection in a patient with acquired immunodeficiency syndrome. Hum Pathol 1988;19:113–116.
236. Batra P, Wallace JM, Ovenfors CO, et al. Efficacy and complications of transthoracic needle biopsy of lung in patients with *Pneumocystis carinii* pneumonia and AIDS *Pneumocystis carinii* involvement of the bone marrow in the acquired immunodeficiency syndrome. Am J Med 1988;250–252.
237. Momose H, Lee S. *Pneumocystis carinii* as foamy exudate in bone marrow. JAMA 1991;265:1672.
238. Rossi JF, Eledjam JF, Delage A, et al. *Pneumocystis carinii* infection of bone marrow in patients with malignant lymphoma and acquired immunodeficiency syndrome: original report of three cases. Arch Intern Med 1990;150:450–452.
239. Raviglione MC, Garner GR, Mullen MP. *Pneumocystis carinii* in bone marrow. Ann Intern Med 1988;109:253.
240. Matsuda S, Urata Y, Shiota T, et al. Disseminated infection of *Pneumocystis carinii* in a patient with acquired immunodeficiency syndrome. Virchow Arch A Pathol Anat Histopathol 1989;414:523–527.
241. Mayayo E, Vidal F, Alvira R, et al. Cerebral *Pneumocystis carinii* in AIDS. Lancet 1990;336:1592.
242. Radin DR, Baker EL, Klatt EC, et al. Visceral and nodal calcification in patients with AIDS-related *Pneumocystis carinii* infection. AJR Am J Roentgenol 1990;154:27–31.
243. Lubat E, Megibow AJ, Balthazar EJ, et al. Extrapulmonary *Pneumocystis carinii* infection in AIDS. CT findings. Radiology 1990;174:157–160.
244. Ragni MV, Dekker A, DeRubertis FR, et al. *Pneumocystis carinii* infection as necrotizing thyroiditis and hypothyroidism. Am J Clin Pathol 1991;95:489–493.
245. Walts AE, Pitchon HE. *Pneumocystis carinii* in FNA of the thyroid. Diagn Cytopathol 1991;7:615–617.

246. Drucker DJ, Bailey D, Rotstein L. Thyroiditis as the presenting manifestation of disseminated extrapulmonary *Pneumocystis carinii* infection. J Clin Endocrinol Metab 1990;71:1663–1665.
247. Battan R, Mariuz P, Raviglione MC, et al. *Pneumocystis carinii* of the thyroid in a hypothyroid patient with AIDS: diagnosis by fine needle aspiration biopsy. J Clin Endocrinol Metab 1990;72:724–726.
248. Gallant JE, Enriquez RE, Cohen KL, et al. *Pneumocystis carinii* thyroiditis. Am J Med 1988;84:303–306.
249. Macher AM, Bardenstein DS, Zimmerman LE, et al. *Pneumocystis carinii* choroiditis in a male homosexual with AIDS and disseminated pulmonary and extrapulmonary P. carinii infection. N Engl J Med 1987;316:1092.
250. Roa NA, Zimmerman PL, Boyer D, et al. A clinical, histopathologic, and electron microscopic study of *Pneumocystis carinii* choroiditis. Am J Ophthalmol 1989;107:218–228.
251. Freeman WR, Gross JG, Labelle J, et al. *Pneumocystis carinii* choroidopathy: a new clinical entity. Arch Ophthalmol 1989;107:863–867.
252. Rosenblatt MA, Cunningham C, Teich S, et al. Choroidal lesions in patients with AIDS. Br J Ophthalmol 1990;74:610–614.
253. Dugel PU, Rao NA, Forster DJ, et al. *Pneumocystis carinii* choroiditis after long term aerosolized pentamidine therapy. Am J Ophthalmol 1990;110:13–17.
254. Sneed SR, Blodi CF, Berger BB, et al. *Pneumocystis carinii* choroiditis in patients receiving inhaled pentamidine. N Engl J Med 1990;322:936–937.
255. Friedberg DN, Brook DL. Asymptomatic disseminated *Pneumocystis carinii* infection detected by ophthalmoscopy. Lancet 1990;336:1256–1257.
256. Holland GN, MacArthur LJ, Foos RY. Choroidal pneumocystosis. Arch Ophthalmol 1991;109:1454–1455.
257. Foster RE, Lowder CY, Meisler DM, et al. Presumed *Pneumocystis carinii* choroiditis: unifocal presentation, regression with intravenous pentamidine, and choroiditis recurrence. Ophthalmology 1991;98:1360–1365.
258. Shami MJ, Freeman W, Friedberg D, et al. A multicenter study of pneumocystis choroidopathy. Am J Ophthalmol 1991;112:15–22.
259. Cote RJ, Rosenblum M, Telzak EE, et al. Disseminated *Pneumocystis carinii* infection causing extrapulmonary organ failure: clinical, pathologic, and immunohistochemical analysis. Mod Pathol 1990;3:25–30.
260. Telzak EE, Armstrong D. Extrapulmonary and other unusual manifestations of *Pneumocystis carinii*. In: Walzer PD, Genta RM, eds. *Pneumocystis carinii* pneumonia. 2nd ed. New York: Marcel Dekker, 1993:361–378.
261. Rockstroh J, Ewig S, Luster W, et al. Disseminated *Pneumocystis carinii* infection in an AIDS patient on trimethoprim/sulfamethoxazole prophylaxis after breakthrough PCP. Presented at the 7th International Conference on AIDS, Florence, Italy, 1991.
262. Kales CP, Murren JR, Torres RA, et al. Early predictors of inhospital mortality for *Pneumocystis carinii* pneumonia in the acquired immunodeficiency syndrome. Arch Intern Med 1987;147:1413–1417.
263. Brenner M, Ognibene FP, Lack EE, et al. Prognostic factors and life expectancy of patients with acquired immunodeficiency syndrome and *Pneumocystis carinii* pneumonia. Am Rev Respir Dis 1987;136:1199–1206.
264. El-Sadr W, Simberkoff MS. Survival and prognostic factors in severe *Pneumocystis carinii* pneumonia requiring mechanical ventilation. Am Rev Respir Dis 1988;137:1264–1267.
265. Garay SM, Greene J. Prognostic indicators in the initial presentation of *Pneumocystis carinii* pneumonia. Chest 1989;95:769–772.
266. Speich R, Weber R, Kronauer CHM, et al. Prognostic score for *Pneumocystis carinii* pneumonia. Respiration 1990;57:259–263.
267. Baughman RP, Frame PT. Predicting a positive result for immunocompromised patients undergoing BAL for fever and pulmonary symptoms. Chest 1989;95:192S–193S.
268. The National Institutes of Health-University of California Expert Panel for Corticosteroids as Adjunctive Therapy for Pneumocystis Pneumonia. Consensus statement on the use of corticosteroids as adjunctive therapy for *Pneumocystis* pneumonia in the acquired immunodeficiency syndrome. N Engl J Med 1990;323:1500–1504.
269. Smith DE, Wyatt J, Mcluckie A, et al. Severe exercise hypoxemia with normal or near normal X-rays: a feature of *Pneumocystis carinii* infection. Lancet 1982;2:1049–1052.
270. Balestra DJ, Hennigan SH, Ross GS. Clinical prediction of *Pneumocystis* pneumonia. Arch Intern Med 1992;152:623–624.
271. Stover DE, Greeno RA, Galgiardi AJ. The use of a simple exercise test for the diagnosis of *Pneumocystis carinii* pneumonia in patients with AIDS. Am Rev Respir Dis 1989;139:1343–1346.
272. Stover DE, White DA, Romano PA, et al. Spectrum of pulmonary diseases associated with the acquired immunodeficiency syndrome. Am J Med 1985;78:429–437.
273. Hopewell PC, Luce JM. Pulmonary involvement in the acquired immunodeficiency syndrome. Chest 1985;87:104–112.
274. Mitchell DM, Fleming J, Pinching AJ, et al. Pulmonary function in human immunodeficiency virus infection: a prospective 18-month study of serial lung function in 474 patients. Am Rev Respir Dis 1992;146:745–751.
275. Stansell JD, Osmond DH, Charlebois E, et al. Predictors of *Pneumocystis carinii* pneumonia in HIV-infected persons: Pulmonary Complications of HIV Infection Study Group. Am J Respir Crit Care Med 1997;155:60–66.
276. Benson CA, Spear J, Hines D, et al. Combined APACHE II score and serum lactate dehydrogenase as predictors of in-hospital mortality caused by first episode *Pneumocystis carinii* pneumonia in patients with acquired immunodeficiency syndrome. Am Rev Respir Dis 1991;144:319–323.
277. Kagawa FT, Kirsch CM, Yenokida GG, et al. Serum lactate dehydrogenase activity in patients with AIDS and *Pneumocystis carinii* pneumonia: an adjunct to diagnosis. Chest 1988;94:1031–1033.
278. Smith RL, Ripps CS, Lewis ML. Elevated lactate dehydrogenase values in patients with *Pneumocystis carinii* pneumonia. Chest 1988;93:987–992.
279. Zaman MK, White DA. Serum lactate dehydrogenase levels and *Pneumocystis carinii* pneumonia: diagnostic and prognostic significance. Am Rev Respir Dis 1988;137:796–800.
280. Grover SA, Coupal L, Suissa S, et al. The clinical utility of serum lactate dehydrogenase in diagnosing *Pneumocystis carinii* pneumonia among hospitalized AIDS patients. Clin Invest Med 1992;15:309–317.
281. Silverman BA, Rubinstein A. Serum lactate dehydrogenase levels in adults and children with acquired immunodeficiency syndrome (AIDS) and AIDS-related complex: possible indicator of B cell proliferation and disease activity: effect of intravenous gamma globulin on enzyme levels. Am J Med 1985;78:728–736.
282. Lipman ML, Goldstein E. Serum lactic dehydrogenase predicts mortality in patients with AIDS and *Pneumocystis* pneumonia. West J Med 1988;149:486?.
283. Masur H, Ognibene FP, Yarchoan R, et al. CD4 counts as predictors of opportunistic pneumonias in human immunodeficiency virus (HIV) infection. Ann Intern Med 1989;111:223–231.
284. Scott WW, Kuhlman JE. Focal pulmonary lesions in patients with AIDS: percutaneous transthoracic needle biopsy. Radiology 1991;180:419–421.
285. Jules-Elysee KM, Stover DM, Zaman MB, et al. Aerosolized pentamidine: effect on diagnosis and presentation *Pneumocystis carinii* pneumonia. Ann Intern Med 1990;112:750–757.
286. Kennedy CA, Goetz MB. Atypical roentgenographic manifestations of *Pneumocystis carinii* pneumonia. Arch Intern Med 1992;152:1390–1398.
287. Goodman PC. *Pneumocystis carinii* pneumonia. J Thorac Imaging 1991;6:16–21.
288. Naidich DP, McGuinness G. Pulmonary manifestations of AIDS: CT and radiographic correlations. Radiol Clin North Am 1991;29:999–1017.
289. Amorosa JK, Nahass RG, Nosher JL, et al. Radiologic distribution of pyogenic pulmonary infection from *Pneumocystis carinii* pneumonia in AIDS patients. Radiology 1990;175:721–724.

290. Groskin SA, Massi AF, Randall PA. Calcified hilar and mediastinal lymph nodes in an AIDS patient with *Pneumocystis carinii* pneumonia. Radiology 1990;175:345–346.
291. Gagliardi AJ, Stover DE, Zamman MK. Endobronchial *Pneumocystis carinii* infection in a patient with acquired immunodeficiency syndrome. Chest 1987;91:463–464.
292. Abd AG, Nierman DM, Ilowite JS, et al. Bilateral upper lobe *Pneumocystis carinii* pneumonia in a patient receiving inhaled pentamidine. Chest 1988;94:329–331.
293. de los Santos-Sastre S, Capote F, Pereira A. Atypical roentgenographic manifestations of *Pneumocystis carinii* pneumonia in AIDS. Chest 1988;94:219–220.
294. Scannell KA. Atypical presentation of *Pneumocystis carinii* pneumonia in a patient receiving inhalational pentamidine. Am J Med 1988;85:881–884.
295. Bleiweiss IJ, Jagirdar JS, Klein MJ, et al. Granulomatous *Pneumocystis carinii* pneumonia in three patients with the acquired immunodeficiency syndrome. Chest 1988;94:580–583.
296. Israel HI, Gottlieb JE, Schulman ES. Hypoxemia with normal chest roentgenogram due to *Pneumocystis carinii* pneumonia: diagnostic errors due to low suspicion of AIDS. Chest 1987;92:857–859.
297. Murray JF, Felton CP, Garay SM, et al. Pulmonary complications of the acquired immunodeficiency syndrome: report of a National Heart Lung and Blood Institute Workshop. N Engl J Med 1984;310:1682–1688.
298. Tow TWY, Rosen MJ, Tierswtein AS. Normal chest roentgenogram as a prognostic factor in *Pneumocystis carinii* pneumonia in patients with acquired immunodeficiency syndrome. Am Rev Respir Dis 1984;129:A54.
299. Bessis L, Callard P, Gotheil C, et al. High resolution CT of parenchymal lung disease: precise correlation with histologic findings. Radiographics 1992;12:45–58.
300. McFadden RG, Carr TJ, Mackie ID. Thoracic magnetic resonance imaging in the evaluation of HIV-1/AIDS pneumonitis. Chest 1992;101:371–374.
301. Feuerstein IM, Francis P, Raffeld M, et al. Widespread visceral calcifications in disseminated *Pneumocystis carinii* infection: CT characteristics. J Comput Asst Tomogr 1990;14:149–151.
302. Bergin CJ, Wirth RL, Berry GJ, et al. *Pneumocystis carinii* pneumonia: CT and HRCT observations. J Comput Asst Tomogr 1990;14:756–759.
303. Stevens DA, Allegra JC. Gallium accumulation in early pulmonary *Pneumocystis carinii* infection. South Med J 1986;79:1148–1151.
304. Kramer EL, Sanger JH, Garay SM, et al. Diagnostic implications of Ga-67 chest-scan patterns in human immunodeficiency virus–seropositive patients. Radiology 1989;170:671–676.
305. Charron M, Ackerman ES, Kolodny GM, et al. Focal lung uptake of gallium-67 in patients with acquired immunodeficiency syndrome secondary to *Pneumocystis carinii* pneumonia. Eur J Nucl Med 1988;14:424–426.
306. Kramer EL, Sanger JJ, Garay SM, et al. Gallium-67 scans of the chest in patients with acquired immunodeficiency syndrome. J Nucl Med 1987;28:1107–1114.
307. Bitran J, Bekerman C, Weinstein R, et al. Patterns of gallium-67 scintigraphy in patients with acquired immunodeficiency syndrome and the AIDS related complex. J Nucl Med 1987;28:1103–1106.
308. Picard C, Meignan M, Rosso J, et al. Technetium-99 DPTA aerosol and gallium scanning in acquired immunodeficiency syndrome. Clin Nucl Med 1987;12:501–506.
309. Woolfenden JM, Carrasquillo JA, Larson SM, et al. Acquired immunodeficiency syndrome: Ga-67 imaging. Radiology 1987;162:383–387.
310. Reiss TF, Golden J. Abnormal lung gallium-67 uptake preceding pulmonary physiologic impairment in an asymptomatic patient with *Pneumocystis carinii* pneumonia. Chest 1990;97:1261–1263.
311. Coleman DL, Hattner RS, Luce JM, et al. Correlation between gallium lung scans and fiberoptic bronchoscopy in patients with suspected *Pneumocystis carinii* pneumonia and the acquired immunodeficiency syndrome. Am Rev Respir Dis 1984;130:1166–1169.
312. Tumeh SS, Belville JS, Pugatch R, et al. Ga-67 scintigraphy and computed tomography in the diagnosis of *Pneumocystis carinii* pneumonia in patients with AIDS. A prospective comparison. Clin Nucl Med 1992;17:387–394.
313. Baughman RP, Dohn MN, Frame PT. Preference of *Pneumocystis carinii* for the upper lobes. Chest 1991;100:1275.
314. Johnson DL, Boylen CT, Barbers R, et al. A reevaluation of bronchoscopy in patients with possible *Pneumocystis carinii* pneumonia. Presented at the 3rd International Conference of Bronchoalveolar Lavage, Vienna, 1991.
315. Pitchenik AE, Ganjei P, Torres A, et al. Sputum examination for the diagnosis of *Pneumocystis carinii* pneumonia in the acquired immunodeficiency syndrome. Am Rev Respir Dis 1986;133:226–229.
316. Miller RF, Semple SJG, Kocjan G. Difficulties with sputum induction for diagnosis of *Pneumocystis carinii* pneumonia. Lancet 1990;1:112.
317. Miller RF, Buckland J, Semple SJ. Arterial desaturation in HIV positive patients undergoing sputum induction. Thorax 1991;46:449–451.
318. Zaman MK, Wooten OJ, Suprahmanya B, et al. Rapid noninvasive diagnosis of *Pneumocystis carinii* from induced liquified sputum. Ann Intern Med 1988;109:107–110.
319. Bigby TD, Margolskee D, Curtis JL, et al. The usefulness of induced sputum in the diagnosis of *Pneumocystis carinii* pneumonia in patients with the acquired immunodeficiency syndrome. Am Rev Respir Dis 1986;133:515–518.
320. Kovacs JA, Ng VL, Masur H, et al. Diagnosis of *Pneumocystis carinii* pneumonia: improved detection in sputum with use of monoclonal antibodies. N Engl J Med 1988;318:859–893.
321. Del Rio C, Guarner J, Honig EG, et al. Sputum examination in the diagnosis of *Pneumocystis carinii* pneumonia in the acquired immunodeficiency syndrome. Arch Pathol Lab Med 1988;112:1229–1232.
322. Masur H, Gill VJ, Ognibene FP, et al. Diagnosis of *Pneumocystis carinii* by induced sputum technique in patients without the acquired immunodeficiency syndrome. Ann Intern Med 1988;109:755–756.
323. Keigh TR, Hume C, Gazzard B, et al. Sputum induction for diagnosis of *Pneumocystis carinii* pneumonia. Lancet 1989;2:205–206.
324. O'Brien RF, Quinn JL, Miyahara BT, et al. Diagnosis of *Pneumocystis carinii* pneumonia by induced sputum in a city with moderate incidence of AIDS. Chest 1989;95:136–138.
325. Kirsch CM, Azzi RL, Yenokida GG, et al. Analysis of induced sputum in the diagnosis of *Pneumocystis carinii* pneumonia. Am J Med Sci 1990;299:386–391.
326. Willocks L, Burns S, Cossar R, et al. Diagnosis of *Pneumocystis carinii* in a population of HIV-positive drug users, with particular reference to sputum induction and fluorescent antibody techniques. J Infect 1993;26:257–264.
327. Miller RF, Kocjan G, Buckland J, et al. Sputum induction for the diagnosis of pulmonary disease in HIV positive patients. J Infect 1991;23:5–15.
328. Carmichael A, Bateman N, Nayagam M. Examination of induced sputum in the diagnosis of *Pneumocystis carinii* pneumonia. Cytopathology 1991;2:61–66.
329. Stover DE, Zaman MB, Hajdu SI, et al. Bronchoalveolar lavage in the diagnosis of diffuse pulmonary infiltrates in the immunosuppressed host. Ann Intern Med 1984;101:1–7.
330. Reynolds HY. Bronchoalveolar lavage. Am Rev Respir Dis 1987;135:250–263.
331. Broaddus C, Dake MD, Stulbarg MS, et al. Bronchoalveolar lavage and transbronchial biopsy for the diagnosis of pulmonary infections in the acquired immunodeficiency syndrome. Ann Intern Med 1985;102:747–752.
332. Gal AA, Klatt EC, Koss MN, et al. The effectiveness of bronchoscopy in the diagnosis of *Pneumocystis carinii* and cytomegalovirus pulmonary infections in acquired immunodeficiency syndrome. Arch Pathol Lab Med 1987;111:238–241.
333. Golden JA, Hollander H, Stulbarg MS, et al. Bronchoalveolar lavage as the exclusive diagnostic modality for *Pneumocystis carinii* pneumo-

nia: a prospective study among patients with acquired immunodeficiency syndrome. Chest 1986;90:18–22.
334. Orenstein M, Webber CA, Heurich AE. Cytologic diagnosis of *Pneumocystis carinii* infection by bronchoalveolar lavage in acquired immunodeficiency syndrome. Acta Cytol 1985;29:727–731.
335. Birriel JA, Adams JA, Saldana MA, et al. Role of flexible bronchoscopy and bronchoalveolar lavage in the diagnosis of pediatric acquired immunodeficiency syndrome-related pulmonary diseases. Pediatrics 1991;87:897–899.
336. Rutstein RM. Predicting risk of *Pneumocystis carinii* pneumonia in human immunodeficiency virus–infected children. Am J Dis Child 1991;145:922–924.
337. Bonfils-Roberts EA, Nickodem A, Nealon TF. Retrospective analysis of the efficacy of open lung biopsy in acquired immunodeficiency syndrome. Ann Thorac Surg 1990;49:115–117.
338. Define LA, Saleba KP, Gibson BB, et al. Cytologic evaluation of bronchoalveolar lavage specimens in immunosuppressed patients with suspected opportunistic infections. Acta Cytol 1987;31:235–242.
339. Martin WR, Ablertson TE, Siegel B. Tracheal catheters in patients with acquired immunodeficiency syndrome for the diagnosis of *Pneumocystis carinii* pneumonia. Chest 1990;98:29–32.
340. Caughey G, Wong H, Gamsu G, et al. Nonbronchoscopic bronchoalveolar lavage for the diagnosis for *Pneumocystis carinii* pneumonia in the acquired immunodeficiency syndrome. Chest 1985;88:659–662.
341. Tigg ME, Kohn DB, Sondel PM, et al. Tracheal aspirate examination for *Pneumocystis carinii* cysts as a guide to therapy of pneumocystis pneumonia. J Pediatr 1983;102:881–883.
342. Levine SJ, Kennedy D, Shelhame JH, et al. Diagnosis of *Pneumocystis carinii* pneumonia by multiple lobe, site-directed bronchoalveolar lavage with immunofluorescent monoclonal antibody staining in human immunodeficiency virus-infected patients receiving aerosolized pentamidine chemoprophylaxis. Am Rev Respir Dis 1992;146:838–843.
343. Cadranel J, Gillet-Juvin K, Antoine M, et al. Site-directed bronchoalveolar lavage and transbronchial biopsy in HIV-infected patients with pneumonia. Am J Respir Crit Care Med 1995;152:1103–1106.
344. Karpel JP, Prezant D, Appel D, et al. Endotracheal lavage for the diagnosis of *Pneumocystis carinii* pneumonia in intubated patients with acquired immunodeficiency syndrome. Crit Care Med 1986;14:741.
345. Meduri GU, Stover DE, Greeno RA, et al. Bilateral bronchoalveolar lavage in the diagnosis of opportunistic pulmonary infections. Chest 1991;100:1272–1276.
346. Levine SJ, Masur H, Gill VJ, et al. Effect of aerosolized pentamidine prophylaxis on the diagnosis of *Pneumocystis carinii* pneumonia by induced sputum examination in patients infected with human immunodeficiency virus. Am Rev Respir Dis 1991;144:760–764.
347. Metersky ML, Catanzaro A. Diagnostic approach to *Pneumocystis carinii* pneumonia in the setting of prophylactic aerosolized pentamidine. Chest 1991;100:1345–1349.
348. Fitzgerald W, Bevelaqua FA, Garay SM, et al. The role of open lung biopsy in patients with the acquired immunodeficiency syndrome. Chest 1987;91:659–661.
349. Grocott RG. A stain for fungi in tissue sections and smears using Gomori methenamine-silver nitrate technique. Am J Clin Pathol 1955;25:975–979.
350. Pintozzi RL, Blecka LJ, Nanos S. Morphologic identification of *Pneumocystis carinii*. Acta Cytol 1979;23:35–39.
351. Schumann GB, Swensen JJ. Comparison of Papanicolaou's stain with Gomori methenamine silver (GMS) stain for the cytodiagnosis of *Pneumocystis carinii* in bronchoalveolar lavage (BAL) fluid. Am J Clin Pathol 1991;95:583–586.
352. Mahan CT, Satle GE. Rapid methenamine silver stain for pneumocystis and fungi. Arch Pathol Lab Med 1978;102:351–352.
353. Limper AH, Offord KP, Smith TS, et al. *Pneumocystis carinii* pneumonia: differences in lung parasite number and inflammation in patients with and without AIDS. Am Rev Respir Dis 1989;140:1204–1209.

354. Gosey LL, Howard RM, Witzbsky FG, et al. Advantages of a modified toluidine blue O stain and bronchoalveolar lavage for the diagnosis of *Pneumocystis carinii* pneumonia. J Clin Microbiol 1985;22:803–807.
355. Paradis IL, Ross C, Dekker A, et al. A comparison of modified methenamine silver and toluidine blue stains for the detection of *Pneumocystis carinii* in bronchoalveolar lavage specimens from immunosuppressed patients. Acta Cytol 1990;34:511–516.
356. Walzer PD, Kim CK, Cushion MT. *Pneumocystis carinii*. In: Walzer PD, Genta RM, eds. Parasitic infections in the compromised host. New York: Marcel Dekker, 1989:83–178.
357. Stratton N, Hryniewicki J, Aarnaes SL, et al. Comparison of monoclonal antibody and calcofluor white stains for the detection of *Pneumocystis carinii* from respiratory specimens. J Clin Microbiol 1991;29:645–647.
358. Kim YK, Parulekar S, Yu PK, et al. Evaluation of Calcofluor white stain for detection of *Pneumocystis carinii*. Diagn Microbiol Infect Dis 1990;13:307–310.
359. Baselski VS, Robison MK, Pifer LW, et al. Rapid detection of *Pneumocystis carinii* in bronchoalveolar lavage samples by using Cellufluor staining. J Clin Microbiol 1990;28:393–394.
360. Tollerud RP, Strohofer SS, Weseler TA, et al. Use of a rapid differential stain for identifying *Pneumocystis carinii* in bronchoalveolar lavage fluid. Chest 1989;95:493–497.
361. Baughman RP, Strohofer S, Colangelo G, et al. Semiquantitative technique for estimating *Pneumocystis carinii* burden in the lung. J Clin Microbiol 1990;28:1425–1427.
362. Colangelo G, Baughman RP, Dohn MN, et al. Follow-up bronchoalveolar lavage in AIDS patients with *Pneumocystis carinii* pneumonia: *Pneumocystis carinii* burden predicts early relapse. Am Rev Respir Dis 1991;143:1067–1071.
363. Baughman RP, Strohofer SS, Clinton BA, et al. The use of an indirect fluorescent antibody test for detecting *Pneumocystis carinii*. Arch Pathol Lab Med 1989;113:1062–1066.
364. Smith RL, El-Sadr WM, Lewis ML. Correlation of bronchoalveolar lavage cell populations with clinical severity of *Pneumocystis carinii* pneumonia. Chest 1988;92:60–64.
365. Greaves TS, Strigle SM. The recognition of *Pneumocystis carinii* in routine Papanicolaou-stained smears. Acta Cytologica 1985;29:714–720.
366. Wehle K, Blanke M, Koenig G, et al. The cytological diagnosis of *Pneumocystis carinii* by fluorescence microscopy of Papanicolaou stained bronchoalveolar lavage specimens. Cytopathology 1991;2:113–120.
367. Wolfson JS, Waldron MA, Sierra LS. Blinded comparison of a direct immunofluorescent monoclonal antibody staining method and a Giemsa staining method for identification of *Pneumocystis carinii* in induced sputum and bronchoalveolar lavage specimens of patients infected with human immunodeficiency virus. J Clin Microbiol 1990;28:2136–2138.
368. Ng VL, Virani NA, Chaisson RE, et al. Rapid detection of *Pneumocystis carinii* using direct fluorescent monoclonal antibody stain. J Clin Microbiol 1990;28:2228–2233.
369. Midgley J, Parsons PA, Shanson DC, et al. Monoclonal immunofluorescence compared with silver stain for investigating *Pneumocystis carinii* pneumonia. J Clin Pathol 1991;44:75–76.
370. Ng VL, Yajko DM, McPhaul LW, et al. Evaluation of an indirect fluorescent-antibody stain for detection of *Pneumocystis carinii* in respiratory secretions. J Clin Microbiol 1990;28:975–979.
371. Cregan P, Yamamoto A, Lum A, et al. Comparison of four methods for rapid detection of *Pneumocystis carinii* in respiratory specimens. J Clin Microbiol 1990;28:2432–2436.
372. Hayashi Y, Watanabe J, Nakata K, et al. A novel diagnostic method of *Pneumocystis carinii*. In situ hybridization of ribosomal ribonucleic acid with biotinylated oligonucleotide probes. Lab Invest 1990;63:576–580.
373. Wakefield AE, Guiver L, Miller RF, et al. DNA amplification on induced sputum samples for diagnosis of *Pneumocystis carinii* pneumonia. Lancet 1991;1:337–338.

374. Blumenfeld W, McCook O, Holodniy M, et al. Correlation of morphologic diagnosis of *Pneumocystis carinii* with presence of pneumocystis DNA amplified by the polymerase chain reaction. Mod Pathol 1992;5:103–106.
375. Eisen D, Ross BC, Fairbairn J, et al. Comparison of *Pneumocystis carinii* detection by toluidine blue O staining, direct immunofluorescence and DNA amplification in sputum specimens from HIV positive patients. Pathology 1994;26:198–200.
376. Evans R, Joss WL, Pennington TH, et al. The use of a nested polymerase chain reaction for detecting *Pneumocystis carinii* from lung and blood in human infection. J Med Microbiol 1995;42:209–213.
377. Skøt J, Lerche AG, Kolmos HJ, et al. *Pneumocystis carinii* in bronchoalveolar lavage and induced sputum: detection with a nested polymerase chain reaction. Scand J Infect Dis 1995;27:363–367.
378. De Luca A, Tamburini E, Ortona E, et al. Variable efficiency of three primer pairs for the diagnosis of *Pneumocystis carinii* pneumonia by the polymerase chain reaction. Mol Cell Probes 1995;9:333–340.
379. Leibovitz E, Pollack H, Moore T, et al. Comparison of PCR and standard cytological staining for detection of *Pneumocystis carinii* from respiratory specimens from patients with or at high risk for infection by human immunodeficiency virus. J Clin Microbiol 1995; 33:3004–3007.
380. Roux P, Lavrard I, Poirot JL, et al. Usefulness of PCR for detection of *Pneumocystis carinii* DNA. J Clin Microbiol 1994;32:2324–2326.
381. Chouaid C, Roux P, Lavard I, et al. Use of the polymerase chain reaction technique on induced-sputum samples for the diagnosis of *Pneumocystis carinii* pneumonia in HIV-infected patients: a clinical and cost-analysis study. Am J Clin Pathol 1995;104:72–75.
382. Cartwright CP, Nelson NA, Gill VJ. Development and evaluation of a rapid and simple procedure for detection of *Pneumocystis carinii* by PCR. J Clin Microbiol 1994;32:1634–1638.
383. Leigh TR, Gazzard BG, Rowbottom A, et al. Quantitative and qualitative comparison of DNA amplification by PCR with immunofluorescence staining for diagnosis of *Pneumocystis carinii* pneumonia. J Clin Pathol 1993;46:140–144.
384. Armbruster C, Pokieser L, Hassl A. Diagnosis of *Pneumocystis carinii* pneumonia by bronchoalveolar lavage in AIDS patients: comparison of Diff-Quik, fungifluor stain, direct immunofluorescence test and polymerase chain reaction. Acta Cytol 1995;39:1089–1093.
385. Schluger N, Godwin T, Sepkowitz K, et al. Application of the polymerase chain reaction to pneumocystosis and frequent detection of *Pneumocystis carinii* in the serum of patients with pneumocystis pneumonia. J Exp Med 1992;176:1327–1333.
386. Hughes WT, Leoung G, Kramer F, et al. Comparison of atovaquone (566C80) with trimethoprim–sulfamethoxazole for the treatment of *Pneumocystis carinii* pneumonia in patients with acquired immunodeficiency syndrome (AIDS). N Engl J Med 1993;328:1521–1527.
387. Bozzette SA, Sattler FR, Chui J, et al. A controlled trial of early adjunctive treatment with corticosteroids for *Pneumocystis carinii* pneumonia in the acquired immunodeficiency syndrome. N Engl J Med 1990;323:1451–1457.
388. Gagnon S, Boota AM, Fischl MA, et al. Corticosteroids as adjunctive therapy for severe *Pneumocystis carinii* pneumonia in the acquired immunodeficiency syndrome: a double-blind, placebo controlled trial. N Engl J Med 1990;323:1444–1450.
389. Nielsen TL, Eeftinck-Schattenkerk JK, Jensen BN, et al. Adjunctive corticosteroid therapy for *Pneumocystis carinii* pneumonia in AIDS: a randomized European multicenter open label study. J Acquir Immune Defic Syndr Hum Retrovirol 1992;5:726–731.
390. Shelhamer JH, Ognibene FP, Macher AM, et al. Persistence of *Pneumocystis carinii* in lung tissue of acquired immunodeficiency syndrome patients treated for *Pneumocystis* pneumonia. Am Rev Respir Dis 1984;130:1161–1165.
391. Suffredini AF, Ognibene FP, Lack EE, et al. Nonspecific interstitial pneumonitis: a common cause of pulmonary disease in the acquired immunodeficiency syndrome. Ann Intern Med 1987;107:7–13.
392. Jaffe HS, Abrams DI, Ammann AJ, et al. Complications of co-trimoxazole in treatment of AIDS-associated *Pneumocystis carinii* pneumonia in homosexual men. Lancet 1983;2:1109–1111.
393. Gordin FM, Simon GL, Wofsy CB, et al. Adverse reactions to trimethoprim–sulfamethoxazole in patients with the acquired immunodeficiency syndrome. Ann Intern Med 1984;100:495–499.
394. Klein NC, Duncanson FP, Lenox TH, et al. Trimethoprim-sulfamethoxazole for *Pneumocystis carinii* in AIDS patients: results of a large prospective randomized treatment trial. AIDS 1992;6:301–305.
395. Sands FM, Kron MA, Brown RB. Pentamidine: a review. Rev Infect Dis 1985;7:625–634.
396. Chin TWF, Vandenbrouke A, Fong IW. Pharmacokinetics of trimethoprim–sulfamethoxazole in critically ill and non-critically ill AIDS patients. Antimicrob Agents Chemother 1995;39:28–33.
397. Miser JS, Savitch J, Bleyer WA. Management of *P. carinii* pneumonia. N Engl J Med 1977;296:47.
398. Wharton JM, Coleman DL, Wofsy CB, et al. Trimethoprim-sulfamethoxazole or pentamidine for *Pneumocystis carinii* pneumonia in the acquired immunodeficiency syndrome: a prospective randomized trial. Ann Intern Med 1986;105:37–44.
399. Sattler FR, Cowan R, Nielsen DM, et al. Trimethoprim-sulfamethoxazole compared with pentamidine for treatment of *Pneumocystis carinii* pneumonia in the acquired immunodeficiency syndrome: a prospective noncrossover study. Ann Intern Med 1988;109:280–287.
400. Fong IW, Chin T, Cheung A, et al. The toxicity of different doses of cotrimoxazole (TMP/SMX) in AIDS patients with *Pneumocystis carinii* pneumonia. In: Program and Abstracts of 17th International Congress on Chemotherapy. Munich: International Society of Chemotherapy, 1991: abstract 1706.
401. Montgomery AB, Edison RE, Sattler F, et al. Pentamidine aerosol versus trimethoprim–sulfamethoxazole for *Pneumocystis carinii* in acquired immune deficiency syndrome. Am J Respir Crit Care Med 1995;151:1068–1074.
402. Sattler FR, Frame P, Davis R, et al. Trimetrexate with leucovorin versus trimethoprim–sulfamethoxazole for moderate to severe episodes of *Pneumocystis carinii* pneumonia in patients with AIDS: a prospective, controlled multicenter investigation of the AIDS Clinical Trials Group Protocol 029/031. J Infect Dis 1994;170:165–172.
403. Perazella MA, Mahnensmith RL. Trimethoprim–sulfamethoxazole: hyperkalemia is an important complication regardless of dose. Clin Nephrol 1996;46:187–192.
404. Ougorets I, Asnis DS, Melchert A. Hyperkalemia and trimethoprim–sulfamethoxazole [letter]. Ann Intern Med 1996;125:779.
405. Eiam Ong S, Kurtzman NA, Sabatini S. Studies on the mechanism of trimethoprim-induced hyperkalemia. Kidney Int 1996;49:1372–1378.
406. Alappan R, Perazella MA, Buller GK. Hyperkalemia in hospitalized patients treated with trimethoprim–sulfamethoxazole. Ann Intern Med 1996;124:316–320.
407. Noto H, Kaneko Y, Takano T, et al. Severe hyponatremia and hyperkalemia induced by trimethoprim–sulfamethoxazole in patients with *Pneumocystis carinii* pneumonia. Intern Med 1995;34:96–99.
408. Greenberg S, Reiser IW, Chou SY. Hyperkalemia with high-dose trimethoprim–sulfamethoxazole therapy. Am J Kidney Dis 1993;22:603–606.
409. Choi MJ, Fernandez PC, Patnaik A, et al. Brief report: trimethoprim-induced hyperkalemia in a patient with AIDS. N Engl J Med 1993;328:703–706.
410. Greenberg S, Reiser IW, Chou SY, et al. Trimethoprim-sulfamethoxazole induces reversible hyperkalemia. Ann Intern Med 1993;119:291–295.
411. Modest GA, Price BP, Mascoli N. Hyperkalemia in elderly patients receiving standard doses of trimethoprim–sulfamethoxazole. Ann Intern Med 1994;120:437–438.
412. Pennypacker LC, Mintzer J, Pitner J. Hyperkalemia in elderly patients receiving standard doses of trimethoprim–sulfamethoxazole. Ann Intern Med 1994;120:437–438.

413. Canaday DH, Johnson JR. Hyperkalemia in elderly patients receiving standard doses of trimethoprim–sulfamethoxazole. Ann Intern Med 1994;120:437–438.
414. Velásquez H, Perazella MA, Ellison DH, et al. Renal mechanism of trimethoprim-induced hyperkalemia. Ann Intern Med 1993;119:296–301.
415. Conte JE, Hollander H, Golden JA. Inhaled or reduced-dose intravenous pentamidine for *Pneumocystis carinii* pneumonia. Ann Intern Med 1987;107:495–498.
416. Conte JE, Chernoff D, Feigal DW, et al. Intravenous or inhaled pentamidine for treating *Pneumocystis carinii* pneumonia in AIDS: a randomized trial. Ann Intern Med 1990;113:203–209.
417. Assan R, Perronne C, Assan D, et al. Pentamidine-induced derangements of glucose homeostasis: determinant roles of renal failure and drug accumulation. A study of 128 patients. Diabetes Care 1995;18:47–55.
418. Waskin H, Stehr-Green JK, Helmick CG, et al. Risk factors for hypoglycemia associated with pentamidine therapy for *Pneumocystis* pneumonia. JAMA 1988;269:345–347.
419. Antoniskis D, Larsen RA. Acute, rapidly progressive renal failure with simultaneous use of amphotericin B and pentamidine. Antimicrob Agents Chemother 1990;34:470–472.
420. Stahl-Bayliss C, Kalman CM, Laskin OL. Pentamidine-induced hypoglycemia in patients with acquired immunodeficiency syndrome. Clin Pharmacol Ther 1986;39:271–275.
421. Perrone C, Bricaire F, Leport C, et al. Hypoglycemia and diabetes mellitus following parenteral pentamidine mesylate treatment in AIDS patients. Diabet Med 1990;7:585–589.
422. Comtois R, Poutiot J, Vinet B, et al. Higher pentamidine levels in AIDS patients with hypoglycemia during treatment of *Pneumocystis carinii* pneumonia. Am Rev Respir Dis 1992;146:740–744.
423. Bouchard PH, Sai P, Reach G, et al. Diabetes mellitus following pentamidine-induced hypoglycemia in humans. Diabetes 1982;31:40–45.
424. Boillot D, Veld PI, Sai P, et al. Functional and morphological modifications induced in rat islets by pentamidine and other diamidines in vitro. Diabetologia 1985;28:359–364.
425. Sai P, Boillot D, Boitard C, et al. Pentamidine: a new diabetogenic drug in laboratory rodents. Diabetologia 1983;25:418–423.
426. Sattler FR, Waskin H. Pentamidine and fatal hypoglycemia. Ann Intern Med 1987;107:789–790.
427. Lambertus MW, Murphy AR, Nagami P, et al. Diabetic ketoacidosis following pentamidine therapy in a patient with acquired immunodeficiency syndrome. West J Med 1988;149:602–604.
428. Bryceson A. Pentamidine-induced diabetes mellitus. East Afr Med J 1969;46:170–173.
429. Osei K, Falka JM, Nelson KP, et al. Diabetogenic effect of pentamidine. Am J Med 1984;77:41–46.
430. Sattler FR, Allegra CJ, Verdegem TD, et al. Trimetrexate-leucovorin dosage evaluation study for treatment of *Pneumocystis carinii* pneumonia. J Infect Dis 1990;161:91–96.
431. Stansell JD, Dubé MP, Sharpe E, et al. Randomized phase I trial of trimetrexate glucuronate, leucovorin plus dapsone versus trimethoprim/sulfamethoxazole for treatment of moderate to severe *Pneumocystis carinii* pneumonia. In: Program and Abstracts of the 35th Interscience Conference on Antimicrobial Agents and Chemotherapy, San Francisco, 1995.
432. Koda RT, Stansell J, Li W, Chatterjee D, et al. Pharmacokinetics of trimetrexate, leucovorin and dapsone in AIDS patients with moderately severe *Pneumocystis carinii* pneumonia. In: Program and Abstracts of the 35th Interscience Conference on Antimicrobial Agents and Chemotherapy, San Francisco, 1995.
433. Walmsley S, Levinton C, Brunton J, et al. A multicenter randomized double-blind placebo-controlled trial of adjunctive corticosteroids in the treatment of *Pneumocystis carinii* pneumonia complicating the acquired immune deficiency syndrome. J Acquir Immune Defic Syndr Hum Retrovirol 1995;8:348–357.
434. Jones BE, Taikwel EK, Mercado AL, et al. Tuberculosis in patients with HIV infection who receive corticosteroids for presumed *Pneumocystis carinii* pneumonia. Am J Respir Crit Care Med 1994;149:1686–1688.
435. Gallant JE, Chaisson RE, Keruly JC, et al. The effect of adjunctive corticosteroids for the treatment of *Pneumocystis carinii* pneumonia (PCP) on mortality and subsequent complications. Presented at the 4th Conference on Retroviruses and Opportunistic Infections, Washington, DC, 1997.
436. Martos A, Podzamczer D, Martinez-Lacasa J, et al. Steroids do not enhance the risk of developing tuberculosis or other AIDS-related diseases treated for *Pneumocystis carinii* pneumonia. AIDS 1995;9:1037–1041.
437. Bozzette SA, Morton SC. Reconsidering the use of adjunctive corticosteroids in *Pneumocystis* pneumonia? J Acquir Immune Defic Syndr Hum Retrovirol 1995;8:345–347.
438. Gill P, Loureiro C, Berstein-Singer M, et al. Clinical effect of glucocorticoids on Kaposi's sarcoma related to the acquired immunodeficiency syndrome (AIDS). Ann Intern Med 1989;110:937–940.
439. Schulhafer EP, Grossman ME, Fagin G, et al. Steroid-induced Kaposi's sarcoma in a patient with pre-AIDS. Am J Med 1987;82:213–217.
440. Real FX, Krown SE, Koziner B. Steroid-related development of Kaposi's sarcoma in a homosexual man with Burkitt's lymphoma. Am J Med 1986;80:119–122.
441. Koop HO, Holodniy M, List A. Fulminant Kaposi's sarcoma complicating long term corticosteroid therapy. Am J Med 1987;83:787–789.
442. Nakamura S, Salahuddin SZ, Biberfeld P, et al. Kaposi's sarcoma cells: long-term culture with growth factor(s) from human retrovirus-infected CD4+ T cells. Science 1988;242:426–430.
443. Salahuddin SZ, Nakamura S, Biberfeld P, et al. Antigenic properties of Kaposi's sarcoma-derived cells after long-term culture in vitro. Science 1988;242:430–433.
444. Cai J, Zheng T, Lotz M, et al. Glucocorticoids induce Kaposi's sarcoma cell proliferation through the regulation of transforming growth factor-beta. Blood 1997;89:1491–1500.
445. Guo WX, Antakly T, Cadotte M, et al. Expression and cytokine regulation of glucocorticoid receptors in Kaposi's sarcoma. Am J Pathol 1996;148:1999–2008.
446. Locke A, Meshnick S, Lane B, et al. Mutations in *Pneumocystis carinii* associated with prophylaxis breakthroughs in AIDS patients. Presented at the 4th Conference on Retroviruses and Opportunistic Infections, Washington, DC, 1997.
447. Safrin S, Finklestein DM, Feinberg J, et al. Comparison of three regimens for treatment of mild to moderate *Pneumocystis carinii* pneumonia in patients with AIDS. Ann Intern Med 1996;124:792–802.
448. Feinberg JF, Katz D, McDermott C, et al. Trimetrexate (TMTX) salvage therapy of PCP in AIDS patients without therapeutic options: interim results of the 1st AIDS treatment IND protocol. In: Proceedings of the 5th International Conference on AIDS, Montreal, 1989.
449. Noskin GA, Murphy RL, Black JR, et al. Salvage therapy with clindamycin/primaquine for *Pneumocystis carinii* pneumonia. Clin Infect Dis 1992;14:183–188.
450. Toma E. Clindamycin/primaquine for treatment of *Pneumocystis carinii* in AIDS. Eur J Clin Microbiol Infect Dis 1991;10:210–213.
451. Black JR, Feinberg J, Murphy RL, et al. Clindamycin and primaquine as primary treatment for mild and moderately severe *Pneumocystis carinii* pneumonia in patients with AIDS. Eur J Clin Microbiol Infect Dis 1991;10:204–207.
452. Bartlett MS. Models for evaluating compounds for activity against *Pneumocystis carinii*. Eur J Clin Microbiol Infect Dis 1991;10:199–201.
453. Smith JW. Studies of the susceptibility of *Pneumocystis carinii* to clindamycin/primaquine in rats. Eur J Clin Microbiol Infect Dis 1991;10:201–203.
454. Queener SF, Bartlett MS, Richardson JD, et al. Activity of clindamycin and primaquine against *Pneumocystis carinii* in vitro and in vivo. Antimicrob Agents Chemother 1988;32:807–813.

455. LaRocco A Jr, Amundson DE, Wallace MR, et al. Corticosteroids for *Pneumocystis carinii* pneumonia with acute respiratory failure: experience with rescue therapy. Chest 1992;102:892–895.
456. Schiff MJ, Farber BF, Kaplan MH. Steroids for *Pneumocystis carinii* pneumonia in the acquired immunodeficiency syndrome: assessment. Arch Intern Med 1990;150:1819–1821.
457. Clement M, Edison R, Turner J, et al. Corticosteroids as adjunctive therapy in severe *Pneumocystis carinii* pneumonia: prospective placebo-controlled trial. Am Rev Respir Dis 1989;139(Suppl):A250.
458. Hughes WT, Smith BL. Efficacy of diaminodiphenylsulfone and other drugs in murine *Pneumocystis carinii* pneumonitis. Antimicrob Agents Chemother 1984;26:436–440.
459. Hughes WT. Comparison of dosages, intervals, and drugs in the prevention of *Pneumocystis carinii* pneumonia. Antimicrob Agents Chemother 1988;32:623–625.
460. Medina I, Mills J, Leoung G, et al. Oral therapy for *Pneumocystis carinii* pneumonia in the acquired immunodeficiency syndrome: a controlled trial of trimethoprim–sulfamethoxazole versus trimethoprim–dapsone. N Engl J Med 1990;323:776–782.
461. Hughes WT, Gray VL, Gutteridge WE, et al. Efficacy of a hydroxynaphthoquinone, 566C80, in experimental *Pneumocystis carinii* pneumonia. Antimicrob Agents Chemother 1990;34:225–228.
462. Hughes WT, Kennedy W, Shenep JL, et al. Safety and pharmacokinetics of 566C80, a hydroxynapthoquinone with anti-*Pneumocystis carinii* activity: a phase I study in HIV infected men. J Infect Dis 1991;163:943–948.
463. Falloon J, Kovacs J, Hughes W, et al. A preliminary evaluation of 566C80 for the treatment of *Pneumocystis carinii* pneumonia in patients with acquired immunodeficiency syndrome. N Engl J Med 1991;325:1534–1538.
464. Dohn MN, Frame PT, Baughman RP, et al. Open-label efficacy and safety trial of 42 days of 566C80 for *Pneumocystis carinii* pneumonia in AIDS patients. J Protozool 1991;38:220S–221S.
465. Debs RJ, Straubinger RM, Burnette EN, et al. Selective enhancement of pentamidine uptake in the lung by aerosolization and delivery in liposomes. Am Rev Respir Dis 1987;135:731–737.
466. Soo Hoo GW, Mohsenifar Z, Meyer RD. Inhaled or intravenous pentamidine therapy for *Pneumocystis carinii* pneumonia in AIDS: a randomized trial. Ann Intern Med 1990;113:195–202.
467. Mills J, Leoung G, Medina I, et al. Dapsone treatment of *Pneumocystis carinii* pneumonia in the acquired immunodeficiency syndrome. Antimicrob Agents Chemother 1988;32:1057–1060.
468. Safrin S, Sattler FR, Lee BL, et al. Dapsone as a single agent is suboptimal therapy for *Pneumocystis carinii* pneumonia. J Acquir Immune Defic Syndr Hum Retrovirol 1991;4:244–249.
469. Montaner JS, Guillemi S, Quieffin J, et al. Oral corticosteroids in patients with mild *Pneumocystis carinii* pneumonia and the acquired immune deficiency syndrome (AIDS). Tuber Lung Dis 1993;74:173–179.
470. Kovacs JA, Allegra CJ, Swan JC, et al. Potent antipneumocystis and antitoxoplasma activities of piritrexim, a lipid-soluble antifolate. Antimicrob Agents Chemother 1988;32:430–433.
471. Falloon J, Allegra C, Kovacs J, et al. Piritrexim with leucovorin for the treatment of *Pneumocystis* pneumonia (PCP) in AIDS patients. Clin Res 1990;38:361A.
472. Bartlett MS, Queener SF, Tidwell RR, et al. 8-Aminoquinolines from Walter Reed Army Institute for Research for treatment and prophylaxis of *Pneumocystis* pneumonia in rat models. Antimicrob Agents Chemother 1991;35:277–282.
473. Tidwell RR, Jones SK, Geratz JD, et al. Analogues of 1,5-bis(4-amidinophenoxy)pentane (pentamidine) in the treatment of experimental *Pneumocystis carinii* pneumonia. J Med Chem 1990;33:1252–1257.
474. Shear HL, Valladares G, Narachi MA. Enhanced treatment of *Pneumocystis carinii* in rats with trimethoprim/sulfamethoxazole. J Acquir Immune Defic Syndr Hum Retrovirol 1990;3:943–948.
475. Beck JM, Liggitt HD, Brunette EN, et al. Reduction in intensity of *Pneumocystis carinii* pneumonia in mice by aerosol administration of gamma interferon. Infect Immun 1991;59:3859–3862.
476. van Middlesworth F, Omstead MN, Schmatz D, et al. L-687,781, a new member of the papulacandin family of β-1,3-D-glucan synthesis inhibitors. I. Fermentation, isolation, and biological activity. J Antibiot 1991;44:45–51.
477. Akashi K, Ishimaru T, Shibuya T, et al. Human urinary proteinase inhibitor in the treatment of *Pneumocystis carinii* pneumonia. Chest 1991;99:1055–1056.
478. Hughes WT, Killer JT. Synergistic anti-*Pneumocystis carinii* effects of erythromycin and sulfisoxazole. J Acquir Immune Defic Syndr Hum Retrovirol 1991;4:532–537.
479. Hughes WT. Macrolide-antifol synergism in anti-*Pneumocystis carinii* therapeutics. J Protozool 1991;38:160S.
480. Walzer PD, Kim CK, Foy J, Zhang JL. Furazolidone and nitrofurantoin in the treatment of experimental *Pneumocystis carinii* pneumonia. Antimicrob Agents Chemother 1991;35:158–163.
481. Oz HS, Hughes WT. Novel anti-*Pneumocystis carinii* effects of the immunosuppressant mycophenolate mofetil in contrast to provocative effects of tacrolimus, sirolimus, and dexamethasone. J Infect Dis 1997;175:901–904.
482. Sattler F, Walser J, Golden J, et al. Recombinant interferon gamma (rIFNγ) aerosol for treatment of Pneumocystis pneumonia (PCP). In: Program and Abstracts of the 8th International Conference on AIDS, Amsterdam, 1993.
483. Lopresti JS, Fried JC, Spencer CA, Nicoloff JT. Unique alterations of thyroid hormone indices in the acquired immunodeficiency syndrome (AIDS). Ann Intern Med 1989;110:970–975.
484. Fried JC, LoPresti JS, Micon M, et al. Serum triiodothyronine values: prognostic indicators of acute mortality due to *Pneumocystis carinii* pneumonia associated with acquired immunodeficiency syndrome. Arch Intern Med 1990;150:406–409.
485. Blumenfeld W, Miller CN, Chew KL, et al. Correlation of *Pneumocystis carinii* cyst density with mortality in patients with acquired immunodeficiency syndrome and *Pneumocystis* pneumonia. Hum Pathol 1992;23:612–618.
486. Sadaghdar H, Huang ZB, Eden E. Correlation of bronchoalveolar lavage findings to severity of *Pneumocystis carinii* pneumonia in AIDS: evidence for the development of high permeability pulmonary edema. Chest 1992;102:63–69.
487. Gachot B, Clair B, Wolff M, et al. Continuous positive airway pressure by face mask or mechanical ventilation in patients with human immunodeficiency virus infection and severe *Pneumocystis carinii* pneumonia. Intensive Care Med 1992;18:155–159.
488. Prevedoros HP, Lee RP, Marriot D. CPAP, effective respiratory support in patients with AIDS-related *Pneumocystis carinii* pneumonia. Anesth Intensive Care 1991;19:561–566.
489. Miller RF, Semple SJ. Continuous positive airway pressure ventilation for respiratory failure with *Pneumocystis carinii* pneumonia. Respir Med 1991;85:133–138.
490. Gregg RW, Friedman BC, Williams JF, et al. Continuous positive airway pressure by face mask in *Pneumocystis carinii* pneumonia. Crit Care Med 1990;18:21–24.
491. Wachter RM, Luce JM, Turner J, et al. Intensive care of patients with the acquired immunodeficiency syndrome: outcome and changing patterns of utilization. Am Rev Respir Dis 1986;134:891–896.
492. Wachter RM, Russi MB, Bloch A, et al. *Pneumocystis carinii* pneumonia and respiratory failure in AIDS: improved outcomes and increased use of intensive care units. Am Rev Respir Dis 1991;143:251–256.
493. Murray JF, Garay SM, Hopewell PC, et al. NHLBI workshop summary: pulmonary complications of the acquired immunodeficiency syndrome: an update. Am Rev Respir Dis 1987;135:504–509.
494. Schein KRM, Fischl MA, Pitchenik AE, et al. ICU survival of patients with the acquired immunodeficiency syndrome. Crit Care Med 1986;14:1026–1027.

495. Rosen MJ, Cucco RA, Teirstein AS. Outcome of intensive care in patients with the acquired immunodeficiency syndrome. J Intensive Care Med 1986;1:55–60.
496. Garay S. Respiratory failure in AIDS. Am Rev Respir Dis 1986;133:A344.
497. Baggott LA, Boggott BB. *Pneumocystis carinii* pneumonia in AIDS patients in intensive care. Chest 1987;92:132S.
498. Montaner JSG, Russell JA, Ruedy J, et al. Acute respiratory failure secondary to *Pneumocystis carinii* pneumonia in the acquired immunodeficiency syndrome: a potential role for systemic corticosteroids. Chest 1989;95:881–884.
499. Friedman Y, Franklin LC, Rackow EC, et al. Improved survival in patients with acquired immunodeficiency syndrome, *Pneumocystis carinii* pneumonia, and severe respiratory failure. Chest 1989;96:862–866.
500. Efferen LS, Nadarajah D, Palat DS. Survival following mechanical ventilation for *Pneumocystis carinii* pneumonia in patients with the acquired immunodeficiency syndrome: a different perspective. Am J Med 1989;87:401–404.
501. Rogers PL, Lane HC, Henderson DK, et al. Admission of AIDS patients to a medical intensive care unit: causes and outcome. Crit Care Med 1989;17:113–117.
502. Peruzzi WT, Skoutelis A, Shapiro BA, et al. Intensive care unit patients with acquired immunodeficiency syndrome and *Pneumocystis carinii* pneumonia: suggested predictors of hospital outcome. Crit Care Med 1991;19:892–900.
503. Nielsen TL, Guldager H, Pedersen C, et al. The outcome of mechanical ventilation in patients with AIDS-associated primary episode *Pneumocystis carinii* pneumonia. Scand J Infect 1991;23:37–41.
504. Wachter RM, Luce JM, Safrin S, et al. Cost and outcome of intensive care for patients with AIDS, *Pneumocystis carinii* pneumonia, and severe respiratory failure. JAMA 1995;273:230–235.
505. Gallant JE, McAvinue SM, Moore RD, et al. The impact of prophylaxis on outcome and resource utilization in *Pneumocystis carinii* pneumonia. Chest 1995;107:1018–1022.
506. Bozzette SA, Finklestein DM, Spector SA, et al. A randomized trial of three antipneumocystis agents in patients with advanced human immunodeficiency virus infection. N Engl J Med 1995;332:693–699.
507. Fischl MA, Parker CB, Pettinelli C, et al. A randomized controlled trial of reduced daily dose of zidovudine in patients with the acquired immunodeficiency syndrome. N Engl J Med 1990;323:1010–1025.
508. Centers for Disease Control. 1997 USPHS/IDSA Guidelines for the Prevention of Opportunistic Infections in Persons Infected with Human Immunodeficiency Virus. MMWR Morb Mortal Wkly Rep 1997;46:1–46.
509. Leoung GS, Feigal DW, Montgomery AB, et al. Aerosolized pentamidine for prophylaxis against *Pneumocystis carinii*: the San Francisco Community Prophylaxis Trial. N Engl J Med 1990;323:769–775.
510. Hirschel B, Lazzarin A, Chopard P, et al. A controlled study of inhaled pentamidine for primary prevention of *Pneumocystis carinii* pneumonia. N Engl J Med 1991;324:1079–1083.
511. Montaner JS, Lawson LM, Gervais A, et al. Aerosolized pentamidine for secondary prophylaxis of AIDS-related *Pneumocystis carinii* pneumonia: a randomized, placebo-controlled study. N Engl J Med 1991;114:948–953.
512. Murphy RL, Lavelle JP, Allan JD, et al. Aerosol pentamidine prophylaxis following *Pneumocystis carinii* pneumonia in AIDS patients: results of a blinded dose-comparison study using an ultrasonic nebulizer. Am J Med 1991;90:418–426.
513. Leigh TR, Wiggins J, Gazzard BG, et al. Effect of terbutaline on bronchoconstriction induced by nebulized pentamidine. Thorax 1991;46:122–123.
514. Quiffin J, Hunter J, Schechter MT, et al. Aerosol pentamidine-induced bronchoconstriction: predictive factors and preventive therapy. Chest 1991;100:624–627.
515. Katzman M, Meade W, Iglar K, et al. High incidence of bronchospasm with regular administration of aerosolized pentamidine. Chest 1992;101:79–81.
516. Ong EL, Dunbar EM, Mandal BK. Efficacy and effects on pulmonary function tests of weekly 600 mg of aerosol pentamidine as prophylaxis against *Pneumocystis carinii* pneumonia. Infection 1992;20:136–139.
517. Camus F, de Picciotto C, Lepretre A, et al. Pulmonary tolerance of prophylactic aerosolized pentamidine in human immunodeficiency virus–infected patients. Chest 1991;99:609–612.
518. Tullis E, Yu DG, Rawji M, et al. The long-term effects of aerosol pentamidine on pulmonary function. Clin Invest Med 1992;15:42–48.
519. Berger TG, Tappero JW, Leoung GS, et al. Aerosolized pentamidine and cutaneous eruptions. Ann Intern Med 1989;110:1035–1036.
520. Murphy RL, Noskin GA, Ehrenpreis ED. Acute pancreatitis associated with aerosolized pentamidine. Am J Med 1990;88:53N–56N.
521. Hart CC. Aerosolized pentamidine and pancreatitis. Ann Intern Med 1989;111:691.
522. Karboski JA, Godley PJ. Inhaled pentamidine and hypoglycemia. Ann Intern Med 1988;108:490.
523. Chapelon C, Raguin G, De Gennes C. Renal insufficiency with nebulized pentamidine. Lancet 1989;2:1045–1046.
524. Chen JP, Braham RL, Squires KE. Diabetes after aerosolized pentamidine. Ann Intern Med 1991;114:913–914.
525. Fisch A, Prazuck T, Malkin JE, et al. Diabetes mellitus in a patient with AIDS after treatment with pentamidine aerosol. Br Med J 1990;301:875.
526. Uzzan B, Bentata M, Campos J, et al. Effects of aerosolized pentamidine on glucose homeostasis and insulin secretion in HIV-positive patients: a controlled study. AIDS 1995;9:901–907.
527. Lindley DA, Schleupner CJ. Aerosolized pentamidine and conjunctivitis. Ann Intern Med 1988;988.
528. Newsome GS, Ward DJ, Pierce PF. Spontaneous pneumothorax in patients with acquired immunodeficiency syndrome treated with prophylactic aerosolized pentamidine. Arch Intern Med 1990;150:2167–2168.
529. Hardy DW, Feinberg J, Finkelstein DM, et al. A controlled trial of trimethoprim–sulfamethoxazole or aerosolized pentamidine for secondary prophylaxis of *Pneumocystis carinii* pneumonia in patients with the acquired immunodeficiency syndrome. AIDS Clinical Trials Group Protocol 021. N Engl J Med 1992;327:1842–1848.
530. Schneider ME, Hopelman AIM, Eeftinck-Schattenkerk JKM, et al. A controlled trial of aerosolized pentamidine or trimethoprim–sulfamethoxazole as primary prophylaxis against *Pneumocystis carinii* pneumonia in patients with human immunodeficiency virus infection. N Engl J Med 1992;327:1836–1841.
531. Antinori A, Murri R, Ammassari A, et al. Aerosolized pentamidine, cotrimoxazole and dapsone–pyrimethamine for primary prophylaxis of *Pneumocystis carinii* pneumonia and toxoplasmic encephalitis. AIDS 1995;9:1343–1350.
532. Ruskin J, LaRiviere M. Low-dose co-trimoxazole for prevention of *Pneumocystis carinii* in human immunodeficiency virus disease. Lancet 1991;337:468–471.
533. Stein DS, Weems JJ, William CL. Use of low-dose trimethoprim–sulfamethoxazole thrice weekly for primary and secondary prophylaxis of *Pneumocystis carinii* in human immunodeficiency virus-infected patients. Antimicrob Agents Chemother 1991;35:1705–1709.
534. Carr A, Tindall B, Penny R, et al. Trimethoprim–sulfamethoxazole appears more effective than aerosolized pentamidine as secondary prophylaxis against *Pneumocystis carinii* pneumonia in patients with AIDS. AIDS 1992;6:165–171.
535. Martin MA, Cox PH, Beck K, et al. A comparison of the effectiveness of three regimens in the prevention of *Pneumocystis carinii* pneumonia human immunodeficiency virus-infected patients. Arch Intern Med 1992;152:523–528.
536. Schneider ME, Nielsoen TL, Nelsing S, et al. Efficacy and toxicity of two doses of trimethoprim–sulfamethoxazole as primary prophylaxis

against *Pneumocystis carinii* pneumonia in patients with human immunodeficiency virus. J Infect Dis 1995;171:1632–1636.

537. Caumes E, Guermonprez G, Lecomte C, et al. Efficacy and safety of desensitization with sulfamethoxazole and trimethoprim in 48 previously hypersensitive patients infected with human immunodeficiency virus. Arch Dermatol 1997;133:465–469.

538. Cortese LM, Soucy DM, Endy TP. Trimethoprim/sulfamethoxazole desensitization. Ann Pharmacother 1996;30:184–186.

539. Belchi Hernandez J, Espinosa Parra FJ. Management of adverse reactions to prophylactic trimethoprim–sulfamethoxazole in patients with human immunodeficiency virus infection. Ann Allergy Asthma Immunol 1996;76:355–358.

540. Nguyen MT, Weiss PJ, Wallace MR. Two-day oral desensitization to trimethoprim–sulfamethoxazole in HIV-infected patients. AIDS 1995;9:573–575.

541. Bissuel F, Cotte L, Crapanne JB, et al. Trimethoprim–sulphamethoxazole rechallenge in 20 previously allergic HIV-infected patients after homeopathic [letter]. AIDS 1995;9:407–408.

542. Gluckstein D, Ruskin J. Rapid oral desensitization to trimethoprim–sulfamethoxazole (TMP–SMZ): use in prophylaxis for *Pneumocystis carinii* pneumonia in patients with AIDS who were previously intolerant to TMP–SMZ. Clin Infect Dis 1995;20:849–853.

543. Absar N, Daneshvar H, Beall G. Desensitization to trimethoprim/sulfamethoxazole in HIV-infected patients. J Allergy Clin Immunol 1994;93:1001–1005.

544. Bachmeyer C, Salmon D, Guerin C, et al. Trimethoprim–sulphamethoxazole desensitization in HIV-infected patients: an open study [letter]. AIDS 1995;9:299–300.

545. Moreno JN, Poblete RB, Maggio C, et al. Rapid oral desensitization for sulfonamides in patients with the acquired immunodeficiency syndrome. Ann Allergy Asthma Immunol 1995;74:140–146.

546. Carr A, Penny R, Cooper DA. Efficacy and safety of rechallenge with low-dose trimethoprim–sulphamethoxazole in previously hypersensitive HIV-infected patients. AIDS 1993;7:65–71.

547. Para MF, Dohn M, Frame P, et al. ACTG 268 trial: gradual initiation of trimethoprim/sulfamethoxazole (T/S) as primary prophylaxis for *Pneumocystis carinii* pneumonia (PCP). Presented at the 4th Conference on Retroviruses and Opportunistic Infections, Washington, DC, 1997.

548. Hughes WT, Kennedy W, Dugdale M, et al. Prevention of *Pneumocystis carinii* pneumonia in AIDS patients with weekly dapsone. Lancet 1990;336:1066.

549. Kemper CA, Tucker RM, Lang OS, et al. Low-dose dapsone prophylaxis of *Pneumocystis carinii* pneumonia in AIDS and AIDS-related complex. AIDS 1990;4:1145–1148.

550. Blum RN, Miller LA, Gaggini LC, et al. Comparative trial of dapsone versus trimethoprim/sulfamethoxazole for primary prophylaxis of *Pneumocystis carinii* pneumonia. J Acquir Immune Defic Syndr Hum Retrovirol 1992;5:341–347.

551. Salmon-Ceron D, Fontbonne A, Saba J, et al. Lower survival in AIDS patients receiving dapsone compared with aerosolized pentamidine for secondary prophylaxis of *Pneumocystis carinii* pneumonia. J Infect Dis 1995;172:656–664.

552. Girard PM, Landman R, Gaudebout C, et al. Dapsone-pyrimethamine compared with aerosolized pentamidine as primary prophylaxis against *Pneumocystis carinii* pneumonia and toxoplasmosis in HIV infection. N Engl J Med 1993;328:1514–1520.

553. Opravil M, Hirschel B, Lazzarin A, et al. Once-weekly administration of dapsone/pyrimethamine vs. aerosolized pentamidine as combined prophylaxis for *Pneumocystis carinii* pneumonia and toxoplasmic encephalitis in human immunodeficiency virus–infected patients. Clin Infect Dis 1995;20:531–541.

554. Torres RA, Barr M, Thorn M, et al. Randomized trial of dapsone and aerosolized pentamidine for the prophylaxis of *Pneumocystis carinii* pneumonia and toxoplasmic encephalitis. Am J Med 1993; 95:573–583.

555. Opravil M, Hirschel B, Luthy R. Does dapsone increase mortality when given for prophylaxis of *Pneumocystis carinii* pneumonia? AIDS 1996;10:1045–1046.

556. Ionnidis JPA, Cappelleri JC, Skolnik PR, et al. A meta-analysis of the relative efficacy and toxicity of *Pneumocystis carinii* prophylactic regimens. Arch Intern Med 1996;156:177–188.

557. Gottlieb MS, Knight S, Mitsuyasu R, et al. Prophylaxis of *Pneumocystis carinii* infections in AIDS with pyrimethamine–sulfadoxine. Lancet 1984;2:398–399.

558. Centers for Disease Control. Revised recommendations for preventing malaria in travelers to areas with chloroquine-resistant *Plasmodium falciparum*. MMWR Morb Mortal Wkly Rep 1985;34:185–195.

15

TOXOPLASMOSIS IN THE SETTING OF AIDS

Oliver Liesenfeld, Sin-Yew Wang, and Jack S. Remington

In 1968, Vietzke and his colleagues at the National Institutes of Health in Bethesda, Maryland reported the first series of patients with malignancy in whom *Toxoplasma gondii* was the cause of encephalitis (1). Five years thereafter, Carey and associates at the Memorial Sloan–Kettering Cancer Center reported a series of 14 patients with neoplastic diseases, in whom toxoplasmosis developed with particular predilection for the central nervous system (CNS) (2). In 1979, McLeod and associates reported a case in a patient who had undergone heart transplantation and who had the then unique finding of a brain abscess caused by *T. gondii* (3). Not until the advent of AIDS was the full impact of this protozoan infection in the immunocompromised host fully appreciated.

Toxoplasmosis refers to the clinical or pathologic evidence of disease caused by *Toxoplasma gondii*. This usage differentiates toxoplasmosis from *Toxoplasma* infection, which is asymptomatic in at least 90% of children and adults. Chronic (latent) infection is the term used for asymptomatic persistence of *T. gondii* in the cyst form. Reactivation of the chronic infection with resultant toxoplasmosis occurs almost exclusively in patients who are severely immunocompromised and is likely the cause of disease in most patients with AIDS. In the patient with AIDS, toxoplasmosis most commonly involves the brain with encephalitis (4), the lung with pneumonitis (5–7), and the eye with retinochoroiditis (8). Diseases in other organs may occur but are less common. Multiorgan involvement has also been reported in AIDS patients, and it may present with acute respiratory failure and hemodynamic abnormalities that suggest septic shock (5, 9, 10). Toxoplasmic encephalitis (TE) is the most common clinical disease entity caused by toxoplasmosis observed in AIDS patients (4), and it is the most frequent cause of focal intracerebral lesions in patients with AIDS (11–15).

ETIOLOGY AND INCIDENCE

Organism

Toxoplasma gondii is an obligate intracellular protozoan in the phylum Apicomplexa, class Sporozoa, and subclass Coccidia. It is ubiquitous, and natural reservoirs include cats, birds, and domestic animals. The definitive hosts of *T. gondii* are members of the cat family; all other infected animals including humans are secondary hosts. In nature, the parasite exists in two cycles in separate biotypes, an enteroepithelial sexual cycle and an extraintestinal asexual cycle. *T. gondii* exists in three forms: the oocyst (that contains sporozoites), which is the product of the sexual cycle; the tachyzoite, which is the asexual invasive form; and the tissue cyst (that contains bradyzoites), which persists in the chronic (latent) phase of the infection.

OOCYST

The oocyst is ovoid and measures 10×12 mm. The enteroepithelial cycle, which involves gametogony in the small intestine of cats, results in formation of oocysts (discussed later in this section under life cycle). To become infectious, oocysts undergo cellular divisions that result in eight sporozoites. This maturation process occurs after excretion of the oocysts into the environment. Maturation is more rapid at warm temperatures (2 to 3 days at 24°C compared with 14 to 21 days at 11°C) (16). Oocysts may remain viable for as long as 18 months in moist soil. Cats shed oocysts for 1 to 2 weeks after infection, and as many as 10 million may be shed in a single day.

TACHYZOITE

The tachyzoite is the invasive form seen in the acute infection. It is crescent shaped, 3×7 μm in size, and although it has its own Golgi apparatus, ribosomes, and mitochondria, it requires an intracellular habitat to survive. Tachyzoites can be visualized in sections stained with hematoxylin and eosin, but they are better visualized with Wright–Giemsa and immunoperoxidase stains. Interested readers are referred to a review on the cell biology of the parasite (17).

Tachyzoites are destroyed within minutes in gastric juice, but they can survive in tryptic digestive fluid for as long as 3 hours. They have the capacity to infect and multiply within virtually all mammalian cells. In the cytoplasm of the host's cells, tachyzoites multiply every 4 to 6 hours within the

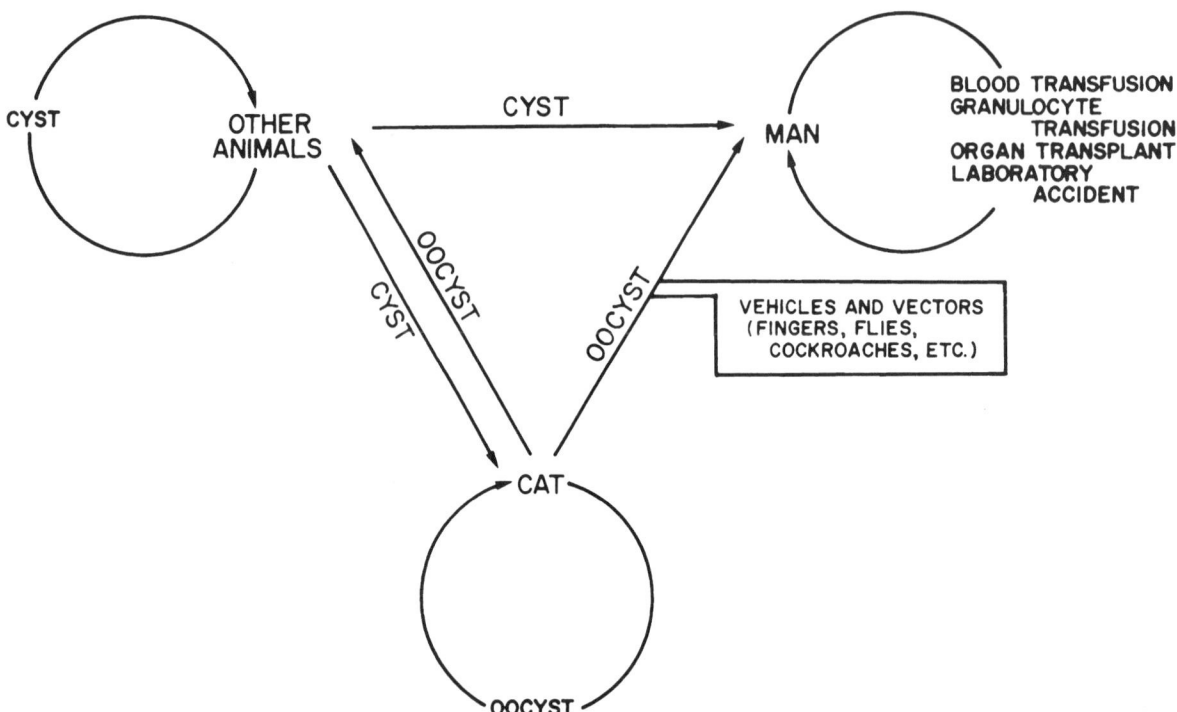

Figure 15.1. Life cycle of *Toxoplasma gondii*.

parasitophorous vacuole, where they form rosettes and pseudocysts. The latter are large numbers of intracellular parasites without a true cyst wall. After repeated replication, tachyzoites disrupt the infected host cell and proceed to infect adjacent cells. When specific humoral immunity has developed, the extracellular tachyzoite, before invasion of contiguous cells, may be lysed by antibody and complement.

CYST

Cysts vary in size (10 to 100 mm in diameter), contain up to several thousand bradyzoites, and most likely persist in tissues for the life of the host. They stain well with periodic acid–Schiff (PAS), Wright–Giemsa, Gomori–methenamine silver, and immunoperoxidase stains. They may be found in any organ but are most readily demonstrable in myocardium, striated skeletal muscle, and the CNS (18). Cysts express stage-specific antigens (19–22) and, when compared to the tachyzoite, are resistant to pepsin–hydrochloric acid and trypsin (23). Evidence indicates that individual bradyzoites may escape from cysts without total cyst wall disruption. Such bradyzoites may proceed to invade contiguous cells and thereby may result in the "daughter cysts" so commonly seen in tissue sections. The mechanism involved in transformation of the actively replicating tachyzoite stage to the slowly dividing bradyzoite and formation of the cyst is unknown.

Toxoplasma cysts are found in brains of experimentally infected mice as early as the first week of infection (24). Whether a subpopulation of tachyzoites is already primed for the switch to bradyzoites or whether invasion of slowly dividing cells by any tachyzoite will trigger the switch to bradyzoites (without predisposition to switch) is unknown. Thus, a portion of the cyst wall is formed from the host cell, and this may explain the lack of inflammation around cysts in otherwise normal tissue. Using electron microscopy, two groups of investigators have published contrasting data on whether tissue cysts are solely intracellular (25, 26) or whether they can persist extracellularly (27). This issue is of major importance because the site in which the cyst resides is critical for drug design against this form of the parasite.

Toxoplasma gondii cysts in meat are rendered nonviable by γ irradiation (greater than 25 rad), by heating the center of the meat to more than 61°C for 4 minutes (28), or by freezing to −20°C for 24 hours and then thawing (29).

LIFE CYCLE

Infection in animals is acquired by ingestion of *Toxoplasma gondii* cysts or oocysts or through transplacental transmission (Fig 15.1). After ingestion, the outer wall of the cysts or oocysts is disrupted by enzymatic degradation, and the components of the infective stage (bradyzoites and sporozoites, respectively) are liberated into the intestinal lumen, where they rapidly invade and multiply as tachyzoites within surrounding cells. Thereafter, spread of tachyzoites occurs by disruption of infected cells followed by invasion of contiguous cells and through the blood within cells.

The sexual cycle occurs throughout the small intestine in members of the cat family. Gametocytes appear in the small intestine from 3 to 15 days after infection, and the zygote is formed by the fusion of the male microgamete and female macrogamete. A protective wall is formed around the zygote (then termed an oocyst), which is then excreted into the environment, where sporulation occurs.

In other tissues of the cat and in secondary hosts, cysts are formed, and this form persists for life. After development of specific cellular and humoral immunity, tachyzoites are no longer demonstrable. Immunity in the immunocompetent host is lifelong. Reinfection, which likely occurs in humans, does not appear to result in clinically apparent disease (30).

DIFFERENT STRAINS OF *TOXOPLASMA GONDII*

Evidence that more than one strain of *Toxoplasma gondii* exists has been based on differences in virulence of different isolates for laboratory animals and with generation time in tissue culture (30–32). Efforts to explain these differences in virulence using protein and antigen analyses have been unrevealing (33, 34). In contrast, "virulent" strains of *T. gondii* have been differentiated from nonvirulent strains by isoenzyme patterns (35) and restriction fragment length polymorphisms (36). Population genetics analysis based on the latter technique in both animals and humans indicated that *T. gondii* consists of three clonal lineages, designated types I, II, and III (37). More than 70% of cases of toxoplasmosis in AIDS patients were associated with type II strains; type I strains were mostly found associated with congenital infection (37). More recently, DNA fingerprinting has been reported to allow unambiguous strain identification for epidemiologic studies (38).

HOST–PARASITE RELATIONSHIP

Unlike most nonviral intracellular pathogens including *Listeria*, *Mycobacteria*, and *Leishmania*, *Toxoplasma* is unique in that it infects virtually all cells, rather than solely macrophages. A review of the numerous advances in our knowledge of the biology of *T. gondii* is beyond the scope of this chapter; for further information on the subject, the reader is referred to recent reviews (17, 39, 40).

Specific Immunity

Because immunocompetent individuals with recently acquired *Toxoplasma gondii* infection do not usually suffer apparent clinical illness, the immune response clearly is critical for prevention of development of TE. The occurrence of TE in patients with defects in T-cell–mediated immune mechanisms (41) and experiments in murine models of the disease have revealed that T-cell–mediated immunity is of primary importance in resistance against *T. gondii* (30, 42–44). Although CD8+ T cells appear most important in murine models, both CD4+ and CD8+ T cells play substantial roles (44, 45) and in vivo act in concert with other effector cells including macrophages, natural killer (NK), and lymphokine-activated killer (LAK) cells in conferring protection. CD8+ T cells may confer their resistance through direct cytotoxic activity against *T. gondii*–infected cells (45, 46) or by secretion of cytokines such as interferon-γ (IFN-γ) (44, 45). Depletion of CD4+ T cells in acute experimental murine infection inhibits development of cell-mediated and humoral immune responses to the parasite and prevents cure of the disease by antimicrobial agents that are otherwise effective in the intact animal (46, 47). The role of the recently described superantigen of *T. gondii* is unclear (48, 49). Expression of heat shock proteins was demonstrated to be closely correlated with protection against infection with *T. gondii*; γ/δ T cells play a critical role in expression of this protein (50, 51). A relative increase in the percentage of γ/δ T cells has been observed in the peripheral blood of patients during the acute stage of the infection (52, 53). Subauste and associates demonstrated that human γ/δ T cells are preferentially expanded in vitro in response to *T. gondii*, are cytotoxic against cells infected with *T. gondii*, and produce IFN-γ (54).

Infection with *Toxoplasma gondii* triggers production of immunoglobulin G (IgG), IgM, IgA, and IgE antibodies against multiple proteins of the tachyzoite. Infection with oocysts results in development of antibodies against the oocyst and sporozoite forms (55). Specific antibody in the presence of complement lyses extracellular tachyzoites (56) and forms the basis of the Sabin–Feldman dye test (57). In murine models of toxoplasmosis, humoral immunity by itself does not provide significant protection against virulent strains of *T. gondii*, but it does give limited protection against less virulent challenge (30, 58–60). Thus, together with cellular immunity, antibodies probably play an important role in resistance against *T. gondii*.

Cytokines

The role of cytokines has been extensively investigated in murine models of the disease. IFN-γ is the major mediator of host resistance against *Toxoplasma gondii*. In vivo administration of IFN-γ in mice protects against lethal infection (61) and reduces the severity of encephalitis (62). The importance of endogenous IFN-γ was demonstrated in chronically infected mice when administration of monoclonal antibody against IFN-γ resulted in encephalitis similar to that seen in AIDS (63). In studies using gene-targeted "knockout-mice," interleukin-4 (IL-4) and IL-6 have been reported to protect against TE (64) (Suzuki and associates, unpublished data). A role for tumor necrosis factor-α (TNF-α) in *Toxoplasma* infections has been recently described; TNF-α is required for certain of the anti-*Toxoplasma* activity of IFN-γ activated macrophages (65, 66). TNF-α is important for nitric oxide production, an inhibitor of *T. gondii*, and for the ability of IFN-γ to activate macrophages to inhibit replication of *T. gondii*. Treatment of mice with anti-TNF-α was shown to increase the severity of TE (67). The results described previously suggest that it is not the inability to produce protective cytokines, including IFN-γ and TNF-α, that correlates with susceptibility to TE in these mouse models. Rather, other cytokines possibly antagonize the protective activity of IFN-γ and TNF-α and thereby determine susceptibility to TE (68). Increased levels of the downregulatory

IL-10 (mRNA) were found in brains of mice with TE (67), and the presence of IL-10 in brains of mice with TE has been demonstrated using immunohistochemistry (69). Tumor growth factor-β (TGF-β) mRNA is expressed in brains of mice with TE (70), and murine microglia can be activated by IFN-γ plus TGF-β to inhibit multiplication of *T. gondii* (71). IL-12 has been shown to be important in resistance against *T. gondii* during the early, but not the chronic, stage of infection (72, 73). Deckert-Schlüter and associates reported that the interaction between adhesion molecules including VLA-4 and VCAM-1 may play an important role in lymphocyte entry into the brain during murine TE (74).

Nonspecific Effector Cells

Toxoplasma gondii enters conventional phagocytic cells by direct invasion or phagocytosis, and the organisms are killed by monocytes, neutrophils, and certain macrophages. Depending on the anatomic site, macrophages may inhibit or kill the parasite or may require activation by cytokines to achieve this goal (75–78). NK and LAK cells have the capacity to lyse *T. gondii*-infected cells (79), and NK cells have been reported to kill the parasite directly (80). In mice with severe combined immunodeficiency (SCID), which lack T and B lymphocytes but possess a NK-cell–dependent mechanism of resistance to *T. gondii*, the importance of proinflammatory (IL-12, IFN-γ, and TNF-α) and down-regulatory (IL-10 and TGF-β) cytokines has been documented (81, 82). Furthermore, NK cells can be triggered to kill *T. gondii* through a *Toxoplasma* antibody-dependent mechanism mediated by a specific receptor (CD16) on the surface of NK cells (83).

Epidemiology and Incidence

Infection in humans is found throughout the world. Prevalence rates are lower at high altitudes, in cold regions, and in hot and arid climates. The incidence increases with age, and in virtually all populations studied, no differences in incidence occur between the sexes. The most common route of infection is by oral ingestion of undercooked or raw meat that contains tissue cysts (84, 85) or of food and water contaminated with oocysts (86, 87). Previous studies have demonstrated that viable tissue cysts are present in commercial cuts of pork (88, 89) and lamb (90, 91). The importance of beef in the transmission of *Toxoplasma gondii* is not yet resolved, but most likely it only plays a minor role (92). Transplacental transmission or peripartum transmission may occur in pregnant women who acquire the infection during gestation (93). The frequency with which this occurs in women with AIDS who are chronically infected with *T. gondii* is under study (see the discussion in this chapter on congenital toxoplasmosis). Such vertical transmission rarely occurs in chronically infected immunocompetent women, but it may occur if they are severely immunosuppressed (93). Less commonly, infection may be acquired by blood transfusion (94), by transplanted organs to previously uninfected patients (95–99), by and laboratory accidents (100, 101).

In the United States, TE has been reported in 1 to 5% of patients with AIDS (102, 103). However, the routine use of prophylactic drug regimens in many countries has resulted in a marked decrease in the incidence of this disease in AIDS patients (104, 105). For example, in the study reported by Oksenhendler and associates (105), only 3 (3.8%) of 80 patients receiving trimethoprim–sulfamethoxazole (TMP–SMZ) (in most cases at a dose of more than 560 to 2800 mg per week) for primary prophylaxis of toxoplasmosis developed TE, whereas 72 (17.2%) of 419 patients without TMP–SMZ did develop TE. TE was reported to be the index AIDS diagnosis in 44 to 58% of HIV-positive patients with TE (102, 103, 106). These figures are higher in geographic locales that have populations with a higher prevalence of *Toxoplasma* seropositivity. Such surveillance data likely underestimate the true prevalence of toxoplasmosis in AIDS because they frequently do not include all AIDS-related illnesses in a single patient. In the AIDS population in the United States, TE and toxoplasmosis involving other organs are almost always due to reactivation of a chronic (latent) infection that results from the progressive immune dysfunction in these patients (12). Thus, the incidence of TE is directly related to or directly correlates with the prevalence of *Toxoplasma* antibodies in a given population and with the stages of HIV infection in individuals in that population. In the United States, *Toxoplasma* seropositivity among HIV-infected patients varies from 10 to 45% (93, 107, 108). In contrast, the seropositivity rate is approximately 50 to 78% in certain areas of Western Europe and Africa (109, 110). Factors responsible for these different seroprevalence rates include increased exposure to areas soiled by infected cat feces and culinary habits that favor consumption of raw or undercooked meat. Investigators estimate that 20 to 47% of HIV-infected, *Toxoplasma*-seropositive individuals will ultimately develop TE (111–113). Thus, in geographic locales with a high seroprevalence, 25 to 50% of all AIDS patients who do not receive appropriate prophylactic drugs will develop TE (111–114). For example, in France, TE was the AIDS-defining diagnosis in 16% of patients reported with AIDS (115), and 37% of AIDS patients had evidence of TE at autopsy (116).

Within the United States, differences are significant both in the incidence of TE in different geographic regions and among various ethnic groups (103, 106). Toxoplasmosis in AIDS patients was reported to occur three times more frequently in Florida than in other areas of the United States (103), and in persons of Haitian origin with AIDS in Florida, 12 to 40% developed TE (103, 117). These differences in incidence rates reflect regional and ethnic population differences in prevalence of *Toxoplasma* seropositivity (93, 107).

Of interest is the low reported incidence of TE from Africa despite *Toxoplasma* seroprevalence rates of 32 to 75%. Lack of autopsy data and lack of neuroimaging studies may contribute to the low incidence reported. Investigators have also suggested that, because of poor access to medical care, many HIV-infected patients in Africa succumb to infection with

Table 15.1. Effect of CD4 T-Cell Number on Incidence of Toxoplasmic Encephalitis (TE)

	No. Patients	Incidence (%) of TE at Months		
		6	12	18
CD4 T cells/mm^3				
< 50	77	8	33	45
50–99	54	11	14	25
100–149	64	2	10	12
≥ 150	85	2	8	16

(Adapted from Leport C, Chêne G, Moriat P, et al. Pyrimethamine for primary prophylaxis of toxoplasmic encephalitis in patients with human immunodeficiency virus: a double-blind, randomized trial. J Infect Dis 1996; 173:91–97.)

organisms such as *Mycobacterium tuberculosis* before they develop the opportunistic infections associated with the advanced stage of HIV infection, including toxoplasmosis. However, in one autopsy series of 175 patients with AIDS-defining disorders from the Ivory Coast, the prevalence of TE was 21% (118).

The risk of toxoplasmosis can be stratified further in patients who have antibodies against both HIV and *Toxoplasma* by their CD4+ T-cell count. In a study in France, when CD4+ T-cell counts were higher than 100/mm^3, 18% of patients developed toxoplasmosis by 12 months and 28% by 18 months. In contrast, the figures were 47 and 70%, respectively, if the CD4+ T-cell counts were less than 100/mm^3 (Table 15.1) (119).

NEWLY ACQUIRED TOXOPLASMA INFECTION

In a longitudinal study in France, 72 HIV-infected, *Toxoplasma*-seronegative patients were followed for a median of 28 months; 5.5% of these patients seroconverted, thereby placing them at risk for development of TE (120). In a Swiss study, seroconversion occurred in 4% of patients who had a median follow-up of 16 months (121). A study from the United States reported asymptomatic seroconversion in 2% of such patients after a mean follow-up of 2 years (122). These data highlight the importance of educating *Toxoplasma*-seronegative patients on how they can prevent acquisition of new infection and suggests the need for periodic serologic evaluation (Table 15.2; see also the discussion of prevention later in this chapter).

PATHOPHYSIOLOGY AND PATHOLOGY

Pathophysiology

Neurologic manifestations dominate the clinical picture of toxoplasmosis in AIDS patients. Most of our knowledge of the pathophysiology of TE comes from autopsy studies and experimental infections in animals. Disruption of cysts in the brain or other tissues allows for escape of individual or multiple bradyzoites. This appears to occur as an intermittent but rare event without apparent clinical disease in chronically infected immunocompetent mice (123) and probably in humans as well. One sees a marked influx of inflammatory cells during the early stages of cyst disruption with development of a microglial nodule indicating a prompt immune reaction (123).

The cell-mediated immune response is of major importance in host resistance against *Toxoplasma gondii* (30, 124, 125), and the advent of AIDS, with its associated immunologic abnormalities including T-cell, macrophage, and NK-cell dysfunctions, has demonstrated that an intact immune system is required to maintain the chronic infection in a quiescent state. Because TE in AIDS patients is almost always a result of reactivation of a chronic infection, investigators have postulated that intermittent cyst disruption or leakage of parasites out of cysts occurs in the CNS and the defective cellular immunologic response in these individuals results in uncontrolled proliferation of tachyzoites and progressive encephalitis. The spontaneous and simultaneous development of multiple lesions in the brain and the successful isolation of the parasite from the blood of 14 to 38% of patients with TE (126–128) suggest that hematogenous spread of the parasite caused by reactivation outside the CNS also occurs in some cases (4, 129, 130).

As is true for AIDS patients with TE, those with pulmonary (5, 6) or ocular toxoplasmosis (8, 131, 132) have serologic evidence of a previous infection. Thus, reactivation is also the likely mechanism of the disease in these patients. In immunocompetent patients, reactivation of retinochoroiditis is most often secondary to congenital infection, it frequently recurs, and it is characterized by the presence of

Table 15.2. Measures to Prevent Toxoplasmosis in the HIV-Infected Patient

Identification of HIV-infected individuals at risk by serologic screening for *Toxoplasma* IgG antibodies
Primary prophylaxis for the seropositive patient with CD4 lymphocyte count < 200/mm^3 [a]
Prevention of new infection[b]
  Wash fruits and vegetables before consumption.
  Refrain from skinning animals.
  Avoid mucous membrane contact when handling raw meat.
  Wash hands thoroughly after contact with raw meat.
  Kitchen surfaces and utensils that have come in contact with raw meat should be washed.
  Cook meat to well done. (Meat that is smoked or cured in brine is noninfectious.)
  Avoid ingestion of dried meat.
  Avoid contact with materials potentially contaminated with cat feces, especially handling of cat litter and gardening. Gloves are advised when these activities are necessary.
  Disinfect cat litter with near boiling water for 5 minutes before handling.

[a] Because approximately 90% of patients who develop toxoplasmic encephalitis do so when their CD4 lymphocyte count is less than 200/mm^3, we recommend instituting primary prophylaxis at this stage. (See text and Table 15.8 for the regimens that have been reported to be efficacious.)
[b] Whether reinfection by *T. gondii* in the HIV-infected and *Toxoplasma*-seropositive patient poses any risk of toxoplasmosis is unknown. Until such data become available, we recommend that preventive measures be used by all HIV-infected patients.
(Adapted from Remington JS, McLeod R, Desmonts G. Toxoplasmosis. In: Remington JS, Klein JO, eds. Infectious diseases of the fetus and newborn infant. Philadelphia: WB Saunders, 1995:140–267.)

active retinochoroiditis around old scars. In contrast, lesions of retinochoroiditis in AIDS patients are often multiple, are large (8), and are rarely associated with preexisting scars (8, 132, 133). The multiplicity of lesions and their lack of association with preexisting lesion or scars support the contention that they are most likely secondary to hematogenous spread rather than to local reactivation of infection from an area around a previous scar (8, 132, 133).

As mentioned earlier, both cyst numbers in the brain (134–136) and development of TE (134, 137, 138) in inbred strains of mice are under genetic control. Because not all AIDS patients who have *Toxoplasma* antibodies develop TE, similar genetic susceptibility may be important in humans as well. Suzuki and associates recently reported the first evidence for genetic regulation of susceptibility to TE in AIDS patients (139). HLA-DQ3 appeared to be a genetic marker of susceptibility, whereas HLA-DQ1 was found to be a genetic marker of resistance to development of TE in AIDS patients (139). Coinfection with other opportunistic pathogens may also be important in predisposing to reactivation. Such reactivation has been described in *T. gondii*–infected mice after acute infection with murine cytomegalovirus (CMV) (140).

Histopathologic Findings

CENTRAL NERVOUS SYSTEM

In patients with AIDS, toxoplasmosis most commonly presents as a disease involving the CNS (4). Extracerebral involvement, both symptomatic and asymptomatic, is found less commonly, either in combination with cerebral manifestations or as the sole manifestation (Table 15.3) (7).

The presence of multiple brain abscesses is the hallmark of TE in AIDS patients (Fig 15.2 and Color plate 1). These abscesses have three characteristic zones (117). The central zone is avascular and contains amorphous material with few organisms. When present, vessels in this zone are occluded and necrotic. The intermediate zone is hyperemic with a prominent inflammatory infiltrate. One sees scattered areas of necrosis with numerous intracellular and extracellular tachyzoites at the margins of necrotic foci. Perivascular cuffing by lymphocytes, plasma cells, and macrophages is also present. In the outer, peripheral zone, more *Toxoplasma* cysts are present with few tachyzoites; necrosis is usually rare, and vascular lesions are minimal. In the areas around the abscesses, edema, vasculitis, hemorrhage, and cerebral infarction secondary to vascular involvement may also be present (141, 142).

Widespread, poorly demarcated, and confluent areas of necrosis with minimal inflammatory response are seen in some patients (142). A "diffuse form" of TE has been described with histopathologic findings of widespread microglial nodules without abscess formation in the gray matter of the cerebrum, cerebellum, and brainstem (117, 143). In these patients, involvement by *Toxoplasma gondii* was confirmed by immunoperoxidase stains that demonstrated cysts and tachyzoites. In diffuse TE, the clinical course progresses rapidly to death. Investigators have postulated that, in such cases, the lack of characteristic findings on computed tomography (CT) or magnetic resonance imaging (MRI) scans is due to insufficient time for abscesses to form before death occurs. Leptomeningitis is infrequent and, when present, occurs over adjacent areas of encephalitis.

Identification of tachyzoites is pathognomonic of active infection, but visualization is difficult in sections stained with hematoxylin and eosin (see Fig 15.2 and Color plate 2) (12). The use of immunoperoxidase staining improves identification of both cyst and tachyzoite forms and highlights the presence of *Toxoplasma gondii* antigens (144, 145). Important associated features in TE are the presence of arteritis, perivascular cuffing, and astrocytosis (145). Because these findings also may be present in patients with viral encephalitis, immunoperoxidase staining is important for differentiating these pathologic processes.

In most autopsy series, the near universal involvement of the cerebral hemispheres includes a remarkable predilection for involvement of the basal ganglia (see Fig 15.2 and Color plate 1) (13, 142). The distribution of lesions in the CNS in a pathology study of 46 patients was as follows: cerebral hemispheres, 91%; basal ganglia, 78%; cerebellum, 51%; and brainstem, 31% (13). Involvement of the choroid plexus was found in 9 of 17 patients (146). Concurrent diseases of the CNS with lymphoma, progressive multifocal leukoencephalopathy (PML), and coinfection with other opportunistic pathogens including CMV, *Cryptococcus neoformans*, *Aspergillus* species, and *M. tuberculosis* may occur, but these infections are uncommon (13).

Once therapy is instituted, the abscesses gradually become organized over a period of several weeks, with well-demarcated areas of central necrosis surrounded by a rim of lipid-laden macrophages (14). Cysts and tachyzoites are less numerous at this stage. After several months of treatment, the abscesses are smaller (less than 5 mm in diameter) and are

Table 15.3. Sites of Extracerebral Toxoplasmosis in 176 HIV-Infected Patients with a Single Extracerebral Location of *Toxoplasma gondii*

Site[a]	No. Patients (%)	Cerebral Toxoplasmosis (%)
Eyes	99 (50)	51 (51)
Lung	52 (26)	17 (33)
Bone marrow	6 (3)	1 (17)
Heart	6 (3)	1 (17)
Bladder	2 (1)	0
Conus medullaris	1 (0.5)	1
Liver	1 (0.5)	1
Lymph nodes	1 (0.5)	0
Rhinopharynx	1 (0.5)	0
Skin	1 (0.5)	0
Blood	6 (3)	0

[a] Parasite demonstrated by histologic examination or isolation.
(Adapted from Rabaud C, May T, Amiel C, et al. Extracerebral toxoplasmosis in patients infected with HIV. Medicine 1994;73:306–314.)

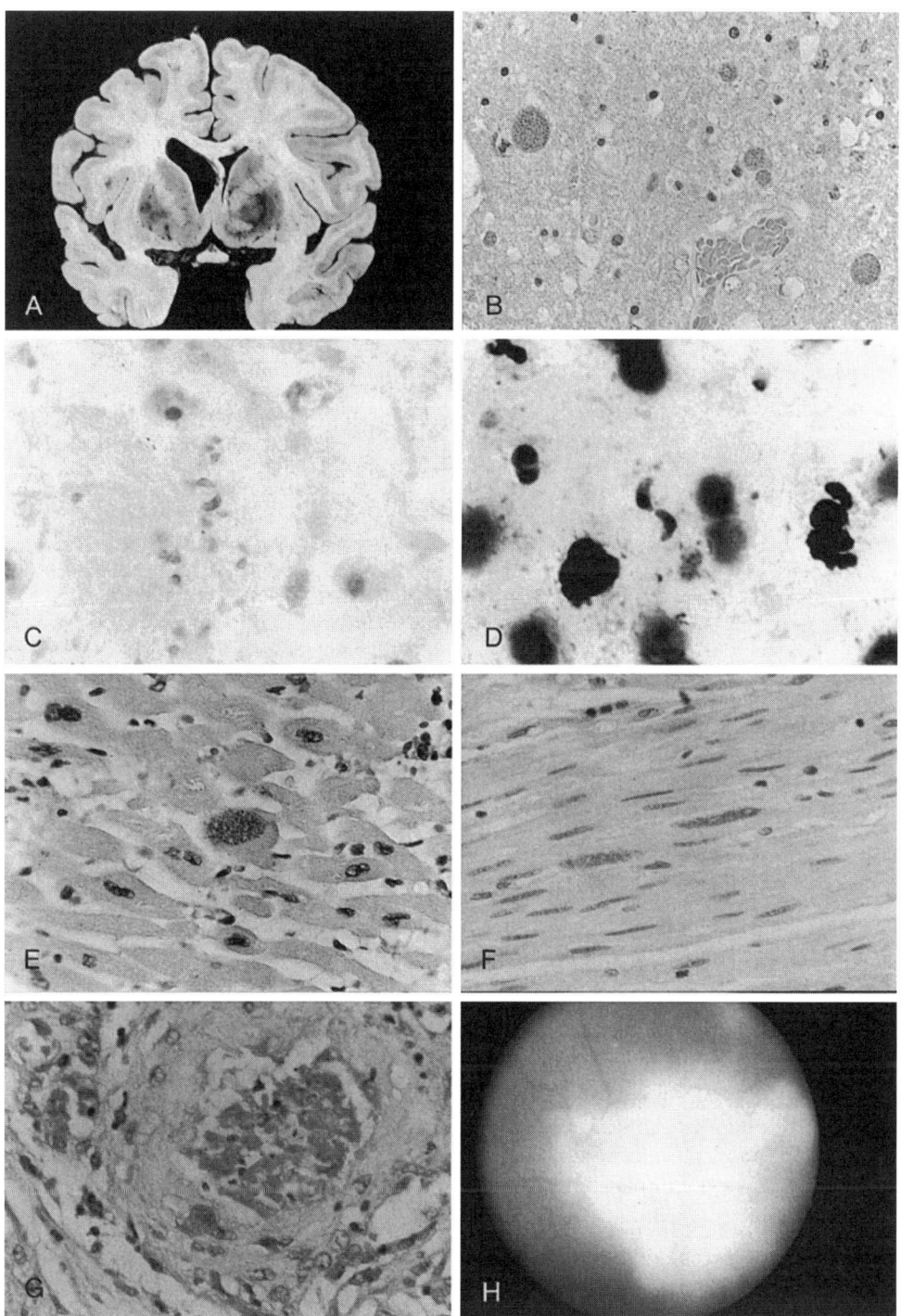

Figure 15.2. A. Toxoplasmic encephalitis. Coronal section of the brain demonstrating multiple cerebral abscesses in the basal ganglia from toxoplasmic encephalitis (Courtesy of Dr. Frances Conley, Stanford, CA). B. Toxoplasmic encephalitis. Note the necrotic area *(arrow)* and the numerous cysts of different sizes (hematoxylin–eosin) (Courtesy of Dr. Seitz, Bonn, Germany). C. Pulmonary toxoplasmosis. Cross section of the lung with tachyzoites in the alveolar space demonstrated by the immunoperoxidase stain *(arrow)* (Courtesy of Dr. Linnea Garcia, Boston, MA). D. Pulmonary toxoplasmosis. *T. gondii* tachyzoites in the bronchoalveolar lavage (BAL) specimen. The BAL fluid was concentrated by centrifugation, and smears were made from the sediment and were stained with Giemsa (From Schnapp L, Geaghan S, Campagna A, et al. *Toxoplasma gondii* pneumonitis in patients with the human immunodeficiency virus. Arch Intern Med 1992;152:1073–1076). E. Myocardial involvement by *T. gondii* *in a patient who died of toxoplasmosis.* A well-demarcated *Toxoplasma* cyst within a myocardial fiber can be seen (hematoxylin–eosin stain). Note the absence of an inflammatory reaction (Courtesy of Dr. Frances Conley, Stanford, CA). F. Esophageal involvement by *T. gondii* from a patient who died of disseminated toxoplasmosis. Cross section of the esophagus. Parasites are seen within cysts in the muscularis layer. Cellular reaction to the presence of the intracellular parasites is minimal (hematoxylin–eosin stain) (Courtesy of Dr. Linnea Garcia, Boston, MA). G. Testicular toxoplasmosis. Cross section of the testis depicting orchitis with a *T. gondii* cyst *(arrow)* (hematoxylin–eosin stain) (Courtesy of Dr. Linnea Garcia, Boston, MA). H. Fundoscopic findings in an adult patient with toxoplasmic retinochoroiditis. The yellow-white areas of retinitis with fluffy borders are characteristic. Note the vitreous haze and absence of hemorrhage (Courtesy of Dr. Peter Egbert, Stanford, CA). (See color section).

observed as cystic spaces that contain lipid-laden and occasionally hemosiderin-filled macrophages with surrounding gliosis (14, 142). In the surrounding brain tissue, rare *Toxoplasma* cysts, but not tachyzoites, may be present.

In one report, the spinal cord was involved at autopsy in 6% of patients with CNS toxoplasmosis (142). In view of the propensity of *Toxoplasma gondii* to cause severe neurologic disease in the CNS, the reason for the relative sparing of the spinal cord is unclear. Spinal cord involvement results in necrotizing myelitis (147). Antemortem diagnosis has been established from biopsy samples by visualization of tachyzoites (148–150).

LUNGS

Pulmonary involvement by *Toxoplasma gondii* has been increasingly recognized in AIDS patients (5, 6) and is second only to TE in these patients. Histologic examination reveals a spectrum of findings that includes interstitial pneumonitis, necrotizing pneumonitis, and areas of consolidation (6, 151, 152). Tachyzoites may be observed in alveolar lining cells or alveolar macrophages or lying free in alveoli (see Fig 15.2 and Color plate 3). Fibrinous or fibrinopurulent exudate may be present. Tachyzoites are easily visualized by appropriate staining (153, 154) (see Fig 15.2 and Color plate 4), and *T. gondii* DNA has been detected in bronchoalveolar lavage (BAL) fluid by polymerase chain reaction (PCR) amplification (155–157). Pleural involvement may result in pleural effusion, and tachyzoites have been demonstrated in pleural fluid (6).

EYE

Histopathologic findings in AIDS patients with toxoplasmic retinochoroiditis reveal segmental panophthalmitis with areas of coagulative necrosis involving all layers of the retina (131). Cysts and tachyzoites are seen in the areas of necrosis. The inflammatory response may be minimal. Clusters of organisms have been seen around retinal blood vessels, and retinal vessels that contain fibrin thrombi are seen adjacent to areas of necrotic retina (131). The lesions may be multifocal (17 to 50%) (131, 132) and bilateral (18 to 40%) (8, 132).

HEART

Involvement of the heart has frequently been reported in autopsy series, but in most patients, this involvement is clinically inapparent (158, 159). In an autopsy study of AIDS patients in France, cardiac involvement by *Toxoplasma gondii* was present in 13% (159). Of those with cardiac involvement seen histologically, only 13% had cardiac symptoms, whereas 87% had CNS symptoms. Myocarditis is the most common form of involvement with *T. gondii* and occurs in as many as 73% of cases that come to autopsy (159). Histologic examination usually demonstrates focal necrosis with edema and an inflammatory infiltrate (160–162). Myocarditis with abscess formation has also been observed (160, 163), as has pericarditis with pericardial effusion (164). Tachyzoites may be present in the myocardium without any histologic evidence of an inflammatory response (165) (see Fig 15.2 and Color plate 5).

SKELETAL MUSCLE

In a study from France, skeletal muscle involvement by *Toxoplasma gondii* was found in 4.3% of autopsies in AIDS patients and in 4% of HIV-infected patients who presented with neuromuscular symptoms (166). The parasite has been isolated from skeletal muscle biopsies (128, 166). Histologic sections and electron microscopy demonstrate necrotic muscle fibers with an inflammatory reaction that varies remarkably among patients. Extracellular tachyzoites have not been visualized (166). Intramyocytic cysts are usually observed at sites away from the areas of necrosis and inflammation.

INTESTINAL TRACT

Histologic features of involvement of the gastrointestinal tract may vary from parasitized cells without any pathologic changes to focal and widespread inflammation with necrosis (165, 167, 168). The entire gastrointestinal tract from esophagus (see Fig 15.2 and Color plate 6) to colon may be involved. Even in the same patient, the cellular reaction to the presence of tachyzoites may vary in different parts of the gastrointestinal tract. Hemorrhagic gastritis and colitis with virtually no inflammatory reaction in the infected esophagus (see Fig 15.2 and Color plate 6) and small intestine have been described (165).

TESTIS

On histopathologic examination, one may see extensive destruction of the architecture with abundant necrotic foci and degenerative seminiferous tubules (see Fig 15.4 and Color plate 7) (169, 170). Organisms are often difficult to identify because of the marked inflammatory infiltrate. Tachyzoites have been visualized by immunoperoxidase stain (169) and electron microscopy (170).

OTHER ORGAN INVOLVEMENT

Given the propensity of *Toxoplasma gondii* to infect virtually any cell and tissue, involvement of numerous other organs has been described. These organs include liver (5, 171, 172), pancreas (169, 173), prostate (169), adrenals (167–169, 174), kidneys (173, 175), bone marrow (128, 165, 175), bladder (176, 177), and thyroid (165). The histologic findings vary from tissues that are parasitized but have no other pathologic abnormalities to tissues with marked inflammatory infiltrates with focal or widespread necrosis.

CLINICAL MANIFESTATIONS

The clinical manifestations of toxoplasmosis in AIDS patients are most frequently associated with involvement of the CNS, lungs, and eyes. Clinical manifestations secondary to involvement of other organs are uncommon. In view of the frequency of multiple organ involvement in patients who die of TE, it is remarkable that clinical signs referable to those organs are so infrequently reported. However, patients with disseminated toxoplasmosis have been reported to present acutely with a picture of septic shock (5, 9, 10), septic shock with adult respiratory distress syndrome (5, 178), or disseminated intravascular coagulation (5, 10). Because the lung is frequently involved in these patients, this clinical presentation is described in the section of this chapter on pulmonary manifestations.

Neurologic Manifestations

Because these patients frequently have multifocal involvement of the CNS, one may see a wide spectrum of clinical findings (Table 15.4), including alteration of mental status, seizures, motor weakness, cranial nerve disturbances, sensory abnormalities, cerebellar signs, meningismus, movement disorders, and neuropsychiatric manifestations. The characteristic presentation is usually one of subacute onset with focal neurologic abnormalities in 58 to 89% of patients (14, 103, 179–181). The clinical presentation may, however, be more abrupt, with seizures in 15 to 25% of cases. The most common focal neurologic manifestations are hemiparesis and abnormalities of speech. Cranial nerve lesions often occur secondary to brainstem involvement (182).

As many as two-thirds of patients with TE may exhibit generalized cerebral dysfunction including disorientation, decrease in mentation, lethargy, and coma. In recent years, earlier recognition and diagnosis of TE reduced the number of patients comatose at initial presentation. Uncommon manifestations of TE include parkinsonism (183), focal dystonia (184), rubral tremors (185) and hemichorea–hemiballismus (14, 186), panhypopituitarism (187), diabetes insipidus (12, 188), and the syndrome of inappropriate antidiuretic hormone secretion (SIADH) (189). Neuropsychiatric symptoms including paranoid psychosis, dementia, anxiety, and agitation may dominate the clinical picture (14, 190). In addition to seizures, two other neurologic manifestations have been described that present acutely. They are cerebral hemorrhage (141, 191) and diffuse TE (116, 143). Both may be rapidly fatal (116, 143, 191). The term "diffuse TE" has been used because of the widespread involvement of the brain at autopsy. Diffuse TE is associated with generalized cerebral dysfunction without focal signs or symptoms. CT scans reveal cerebral atrophy or normal findings. The clinical course is rapidly progressive and results in death within several days (116, 143).

Spinal cord involvement by *Toxoplasma gondii* in AIDS patients manifests as motor or sensory disturbances of single or multiple limbs, bladder and bowel dysfunctions, and local pain (192). Cervical myelopathy (193), thoracic myelopathy (147), and conus medullaris syndromes (148–150) have all been described (148–150). Each of the three patients reported in the literature with conus medullaris syndrome had hemophilia A and transfusion-related HIV infection (148–150).

The major differential diagnoses for TE are CNS lymphoma, PML, and involvement of the CNS with other infectious agents including viruses (CMV, herpes simplex virus, varicella-zoster virus, HIV), fungi (*Aspergillus* species, *Cryptococcus neoformans*, *Candida* species, *Coccidioides immitis*), and bacteria (*Mycobacterium tuberculosis* and those bacterial pathogens that commonly cause brain abscesses in immunocompetent individuals). Neuroimaging studies are important in differentiating many of these conditions from TE and are discussed further in the section of this chapter on

Table 15.4. Clinical Presentation of Toxoplasmic Encephalitis Reported in Patients with AIDS

Signs and Symptoms	Percentage Reported by Reference (%)				
	Navia et al (14)	Porter and Sande (103)	Renold et al (180)	Pedrol et al (179)	Cohn et al (181)
Fever	56	47	41	51	78
Headache	56	55	49	38	67
Disorientation	56	52	15	36	NA
Lethargy	52	43	12	NA	NA
Coma	30	3	5	2	3
Behavioral/psychomotor	30	42	37	NA	NA
Meningismus	NA	10	16	4	14
Focal deficits	89	69	76	67	69
Hemiparesis	52	39	49	NA	NA
Cranial nerve palsy	7	28	17	NA	NA
Visual abnormalities	7	7	8	NA	NA
Speech difficulties	26	8	6	NA	NA
Extrapyramidal deficits	7	NA	1	NA	NA
Cerebellar deficits	30	30	9	NA	NA
Seizures	15	29	24	26	25
Other	NA	NA	NA	NA	NA
No CNS signs	4	NA	NA	2	NA

NA, not available.

neuroradiologic findings. Cerebral microsporidiosis in a patient with AIDS has been reported (194). It presented with headache, visual and cognitive impairment, nausea, and vomiting, and a CT scan of the brain showed multiple hypodense lesions of up to 2 cm in diameter (194). It seems likely that this condition will be confused with TE and lymphoma in the future.

Pulmonary Manifestations

Pulmonary disease resulting from toxoplasmosis has been increasingly reported and recognized (5, 6). The diagnosis was established by isolation or identification of *Toxoplasma gondii* tachyzoites in cytocentrifuge preparations of BAL fluid (see Fig 15.2 and Color plate 4) (5, 6, 153, 154). In a study in France, 5% of BAL fluids submitted for histologic or isolation studies were positive for *T. gondii* (195). The most common clinical syndrome is a prolonged febrile illness with cough and dyspnea that is clinically indistinguishable from *Pneumocystis carinii* pneumonia (PCP). Associated extrapulmonary disease is present in 50% of patients (5). A clinical picture consistent with septic shock and associated adult respiratory distress syndrome has been described (5). Patients have developed TE after successful treatment of pulmonary toxoplasmosis when therapy was discontinued (6). Because the clinical presentation is similar to that seen in patients with PCP, pulmonary toxoplasmosis is one of the differential diagnoses when induced sputum specimens or BAL fluid samples do not reveal *P. carinii*. Even when treated, mortality from pulmonary toxoplasmosis in these patients has been reported to be as high as 35% (196). Other pathogens that may cause a similar clinical and radiologic picture include *Mycobacterium tuberculosis, Cryptococcus neoformans, Coccidioides immitis,* and *Histoplasma capsulatum*. Radiologic features of pulmonary toxoplasmosis are discussed later in this chapter.

Ocular Manifestations

Ocular disease resulting from toxoplasmosis is seen infrequently in AIDS patients (8, 197, 198). Ocular pain and loss of visual acuity are common presenting complaints, and fundoscopic examination typically reveals findings consistent with necrotizing retinochoroiditis. The lesions are yellow-white areas of retinitis with fluffy borders (see Fig 15.2 and Color plate 8). In reported series, the lesions were multifocal in 17 to 50% (131, 132), bilateral in 18 to 40% (8, 132), and had optic nerve involvement in approximately 10% (8, 132) of patients. Large areas of retinal necrosis in the posterior pole or peripapillary zones may be present (199). Overlying vitreal inflammation varies from mild localized vitreal haze to extensive vitreous inflammation (8, 132). These lesions have rarely been associated with vasculitis or hemorrhage, (8, 132) and in AIDS patients they have not been associated with preexisting scars (discussed in the section of this chapter on pathophysiology). The presence of concurrent TE in AIDS patients with ocular toxoplasmosis has ranged from 29 to 63% (8, 131, 132).

Ocular toxoplasmosis is the second most common retinal infection in AIDS; the most common is due to CMV retinitis (132). When compared with cases of CMV retinitis, lesions of toxoplasmic retinochoroiditis usually occur at the posterior pole, are more fluffy and edematous, and have ill-defined margins. In addition, the lesions in toxoplasmosis are usually nonhemorrhagic (see Fig 15.2 and Color plate 8) (8, 132). When fluorescein angiography is performed in patients with toxoplasmic retinochoroiditis, fluorescence begins at the periphery and progresses into the center. In CMV retinitis, initial hyperfluorescence in the center progresses to the periphery (132). Other differential diagnoses of the retinal lesions include lesions resulting from syphilis, herpes simplex, varicella-zoster, lymphoma, *Pneumocystis carinii,* and fungal infections. The diagnosis of toxoplasmic retinochoroiditis is based primarily on morphologic findings on fundoscopy and is supported by a prompt response to anti-*Toxoplasma* therapy. Definitive diagnosis has been established by demonstration of the organism by retinal biopsy (131), by isolation of the parasite from a vitreous aspirate (199), and by PCR on the vitreous fluid (200, 201).

Cardiac Manifestations

In contrast to the frequent involvement of the heart in autopsy series (158, 159), clinical disease referable to the heart is unusual, or the extracardiac manifestations, in particular encephalitis, dominate the clinical course (165, 166). Tachycardia (10), cardiac failure from toxoplasmic myocarditis (160, 163, 202), and cardiac tamponade (163) have been described. To date, conduction abnormalities and arrhythmias have not been described in AIDS patients with toxoplasmic myocarditis.

Manifestations of Other Organ Involvement

Clinical manifestations secondary to involvement of other organs by *Toxoplasma gondii* occur infrequently. Endocrine and metabolic syndromes including panhypopituitarism (187), diabetes insipidus (12, 188), and SIADH (189) secondary to involvement of the CNS have been reported. Orchitis presents as tender testicular swelling (169, 170). Gastrointestinal complaints including abdominal pain and ascites may be secondary to involvement of the stomach, peritoneum, or pancreas (168, 203). Diarrhea secondary to involvement of the intestinal tract has been reported (165, 167, 204). Acute hepatic failure was reported in one patient 1 week after he discontinued his maintenance therapy with pyrimethamine for TE (171). Acute pancreatitis (205) and cystitis with bladder wall thickening (176) have also been noted. In one study, skeletal muscle involvement by *T. gondii* (isolation or histopathologic examination) was reported in 4% of HIV-infected individuals who presented with neuromuscular symptoms including weakness, myalgia, and wasting (166). Each of the patients in this study had other organ involvement by *T. gondii* (166). Widespread erythematous blanching skin papules were reported in one patient with disseminated toxoplasmosis (206), in whom tachyzoites were identified on bone marrow biopsy; skin biopsy; revealed perivascular infiltrate without organisms. The rash resolved on therapy for toxoplasmosis (206).

Congenital Toxoplasmosis

In the immunocompetent woman, infection with *Toxoplasma gondii* before pregnancy poses little or no risk of congenital infection (93). In contrast, in the HIV-infected woman, the latent infection may reactivate and result in congenital transmission of the infection. Thus, the increasing incidence of HIV infection in women of childbearing age poses a unique problem. Women who are seronegative for *T. gondii* are at risk of acquiring the acute infection during pregnancy and its attendant risk of the fetus. If these women are seropositive, they are at risk on reactivation of their infection and congenital transmission. Management of women acutely infected during pregnancy is discussed elsewhere (93). Unfortunately, at present we do not have sufficient data to be able to quantify the risk of congenital transmission by HIV-infected mothers who have chronic *Toxoplasma* infection. Preliminary data from a prospective study in Miami by Mitchell and his colleagues revealed a transmission rate for congenital toxoplasmosis in women dually infected with HIV and *T. gondii* that was significantly higher when compared with non–HIV-infected, *Toxoplasma*-seropositive pregnant women (207). All infants with congenital toxoplasmosis born to mothers who were HIV-infected were also infected with HIV. These results suggest that factors predisposing to vertical transmission of HIV also favor transmission of *Toxoplasma* and, perhaps, vice versa. In a study from Europe, none of 71 children born to HIV-positive mothers at risk for the development of TE developed toxoplasmosis (208). One HIV-infected child acquired toxoplasmosis postnatally (208). A low rate of transmission was also reported in the United States (209). However, in these studies, most mothers did not present in the advanced stages of their HIV-infection (208, 209).

In one report (210), the third and fifth children of a woman coinfected with HIV and *Toxoplasma* died of HIV infection and toxoplasmosis. Her first two children were perinatally infected with HIV and died of AIDS, whereas the fourth child was not infected with either HIV or *Toxoplasma*. The woman died 8 months after the birth of her fifth child without ever having developed symptomatic toxoplasmosis. This tragic case clearly illustrates how little we understand about the risk of transmission in mothers who are dually infected.

To date, we are aware of only a limited number of cases of congenital toxoplasmosis in HIV-infected children. The initial clinical presentation of congenital toxoplasmosis in the HIV-infected infant is similar to that in the non–HIV-infected infant, but it appears to run a more progressive course. At birth, most of the infants were asymptomatic. In ensuing months, however, they failed to gain weight or to develop appropriately. Fever, hepatosplenomegaly, retinochoroiditis, seizures, and other neurologic signs developed (211). Most had multiorgan involvement including CNS, cardiac, and pulmonary disease. Before death, and even at autopsy, it is difficult to separate the role of *Toxoplasma gondii* from potential contributions of other pathogens present concurrently such as CMV, hepatitis B virus, *Candida*, and HIV (211). Even when *T. gondii* is detected histologically at autopsy, the relative contribution of *T. gondii* to organ dysfunction and death is often difficult to determine.

DIAGNOSIS

Tests currently available and suggested for the diagnosis of toxoplasmosis in the AIDS patient are listed in Table 15.5. At this time, the clinical usefulness of serologic tests is primarily to identify those HIV-infected patients who are at risk of development of TE and to determine in the AIDS patient with focal lesions in the brain whether TE is likely. *For this reason, all HIV-positive individuals should have an IgG* Toxoplasma *serology performed and the results placed in their medical chart.*

Tests for Antibody

In adults with AIDS and toxoplasmosis, readily available serologic tests have not proved useful in the diagnosis of acute infection in most cases. The usefulness of these tests in the newborn coinfected with HIV and *Toxoplasma gondii* has not yet been defined, but some of these infants exhibit antibody responses similar to those seen in infants infected with *T. gondii* alone.

Different classes of specific *Toxoplasma* antibodies may be detected by various methods including the Sabin–Feldman dye test (IgG), indirect fluorescent antibody (IFA) test (IgG, IgM), agglutination test (IgG), enzyme-linked immunosorbent assay (ELISA) (IgG, IgM, IgA, IgE), immunosorbent

Table 15.5. Laboratory Tests for Diagnosis of Toxoplasmosis in AIDS Patients

Peripheral blood	
Serology	
Specific toxoplasma IgG, IgE, and IgA antibodies[a] differential agglutination test	
Isolation studies	Mouse inoculation or tissue culture
PCR	Multicopy gene preferable
Bronchoalveolar lavage fluid/cerebrospinal fluid	
Histology	Wright–Giemsa and immunoperoxidase stain of cytocentrifuge preparation
Isolation studies	Mouse inoculation or tissue culture
PCR	Multicopy gene preferable
Tissue biopsy sample	
Isolation	Mouse inoculation or tissue culture
Histology	Hematoxylin and eosin, immunoperoxidase stain
PCR	Multicopy gene preferable

[a]In unusual cases, the infection is newly acquired and acute *Toxoplasma* serology results can be demonstrated.
PCR, polymerase chain reaction.

agglutination assay (ISAGA) (IgM, IgA, IgE), immunoblotting (IgG, IgM, IgA), indirect hemagglutination (IHA), and complement fixation (CF) tests. The last two are rarely used in the United States. Results of serologic tests vary among different laboratories, and many commercial kits are poorly standardized and give unacceptable false-positive and false-negative results (212). In the presence of equivocal results, serum should be sent to a reference laboratory for confirmation.

IgG ANTIBODIES

The dye test is the current standard by which all other tests are evaluated. It is sensitive and specific, measures principally IgG antibodies, and is available in only a few research laboratories in the United States. Dye test titers appear 1 to 2 weeks after infection, peak to often more than 1:1000 in 6 to 8 weeks, and then gradually decline over months or years (93). Titers usually persist for life. The more readily available IgG–IFA test measures the same antibodies as the dye test. Titers in the IFA and dye tests are comparable when the tests are performed in a reference laboratory. Unfortunately, some commercially available test kits are improperly standardized with unacceptable sensitivity and specificity.

Ninety-seven to 100% of AIDS patients with TE have detectable IgG (12, 14, 111). IgG *Toxoplasma* antibody titers are significantly higher in AIDS patients with TE than in those without TE (111). A wide range of IgG antibody titers has been reported in AIDS patients with pulmonary (5, 6) and ocular (8) toxoplasmosis. HIV-infected individuals have significantly higher *Toxoplasma* IgG titers than do individuals without HIV infection (213, 214); this most likely reflects their hypergammaglobulinemia (215). Studies by Derouin and associates (216) and by Hellerbrand and colleagues (217) found that, in AIDS patients with CD4 counts of less than $200/\mu L$ and less than $150/\mu L$, respectively, high IgG *Toxoplasma* antibody titers are associated with a greater likelihood of their developing TE.

Demonstration of significant rises in serum IgG antibody titers in patients with TE is uncommon (11, 218, 219). Detection of *Toxoplasma* IgG antibodies in serum identifies those HIV-infected patients who are at risk of developing toxoplasmosis (4); their absence in patients with signs and symptoms of toxoplasmosis strongly suggests another cause (14, 181).

The commercially available agglutination test uses formalin-fixed whole tachyzoites to detect IgG. Of interest is a modification of the whole-cell agglutination technique (220) with which significantly higher antibody titers were found in AIDS patients with TE than in controls (221). IgG antibodies in sera of AIDS patients with TE recognize multiple *Toxoplasma gondii* antigens on protein blots, but no pattern was found useful for the diagnosis of TE (222, 223). Antibodies measured by IHA and CF tests appear later in acute infection and differ from those detected by the IFA and dye test (93); their usefulness in AIDS patients has not been reported.

IgM ANTIBODIES

In the immunologically intact host, IgM antibodies appear early and are demonstrable within 1 to 2 weeks after infection (93). They decrease sooner in acute infection than IgG antibodies. In some patients, IgM antibodies may persist for 1 year or longer after infection but usually only at lower titers (93, 224). Detection of IgM antibodies by ELISA is more sensitive and specific than with the IgM–IFA test. Rheumatoid factor (RF) and antinuclear antibodies (ANA) may cause false-positive reactions in the IgM–IFA test (225) unless sera are pretreated to remove IgG antibodies. The IgM–ISAGA avoids false-positive results caused by RF and ANA and is more sensitive than the IgM–ELISA for detection of specific IgM in congenitally infected infants. The presence of IgM antibodies using the IgM–ISAGA has been reported in AIDS patients with TE (219). In our laboratory, false-positive results have been observed in *Toxoplasma* antibody-positive AIDS patients with no clinical evidence of toxoplasmosis. IgM antibodies measured by ELISA are rarely detected in AIDS patients with TE (12, 213, 218, 226).

IgA ANTIBODIES

Specific IgA antibodies may be detected in the sera of acutely infected adults and congenitally infected infants using ELISA or ISAGA (227, 228). IgA antibodies as measured by ELISA are rarely detectable in sera of AIDS patients with TE (228, 229). In a limited number of AIDS patients with toxoplasmosis, immunoblotting (230) and ISAGA were more sensitive for detection of IgA antibodies. In one series of patients with AIDS-related toxoplasmosis, specific IgA antibodies were detected in 38% of patients and thus had a low sensitivity (226). Further studies on the utility of these IgA antibody tests for diagnosis of toxoplasmosis in AIDS are needed.

IgE ANTIBODIES

Specific IgE antibodies may be detected in sera of acutely infected adults (231, 232), congenitally infected infants (231–233), and children with congenital toxoplasmic retinochoroiditis (234). The presence of *Toxoplasma* IgE antibody measured by ISAGA was reported in patients with TE (231, 232). We have demonstrated IgE antibodies by ELISA in approximately 35% of AIDS patients with TE and consider that this test serves as a useful serologic marker for TE in this population (232).

Although no single test is sufficiently sensitive or specific for the serologic diagnosis of TE, when we use a panel of serologic tests in our laboratory that includes the dye test, agglutination test, IgE ISAGA, and IgE ELISA, a diagnosis can be made in more than 70% of cases.

Antigen Detection

Experimental methods for detection of *Toxoplasma gondii* antigens in sera and other body fluids are promising (235).

T. gondii antigens have been detected in urine of patients with TE (236), and in our laboratory, antigenemia has been demonstrated in up to 20% of AIDS patients with TE.

Polymerase Chain Reaction

Recent advances in our knowledge of the genome of *Toxoplasma gondii* have allowed for study of PCR amplification for detection of *T. gondii* DNA in body fluids and tissues. This method has proved valuable for establishing the diagnosis of toxoplasmosis in AIDS patients.

Using the 35-fold copy B1 gene as a target, PCR has been used with success in diagnosis of congenital (237, 238), ocular, and disseminated toxoplasmosis (239). In AIDS patients with toxoplasmosis, PCR has enabled detection of *Toxoplasma gondii* DNA in brain tissue (240), cerebrospinal fluid (CSF) (200, 241–246), BAL (155–157), and blood (127, 130, 246–248). Sensitivity of PCR in CSF varies between 11 and 77% (200, 241, 246, 249) whereas the specificity was close to 100% in all these studies. Therapy for TE appeared to influence the sensitivity in that it was higher in CSF samples collected within the first week of treatment (243, 244, 250). The sensitivity of PCR on whole blood or buffy coat ranged from 13 to 86.6% (245, 247, 248). PCR on blood appears to be a valuable tool primarily in patients with disseminated disease caused by *T. gondii* (245, 247).

When PCR is used, we recommend that the specimen be split in separate aliquots to allow repeated testing to be performed on independent aliquots. This protocol allows one to reconfirm ambiguous results and to avoid potential misinterpretation. Although positive results have been obtained using single-copy genes including P30 as targets for PCR amplification, multicopy genes including the B1 gene appear to result in greater sensitivity.

Isolation of Toxoplasma

Mouse inoculation is the most sensitive method for isolation of *Toxoplasma gondii*. Unfortunately, results may not be available for 3 to 6 weeks, and animal facilities are frequently not available to clinical microbiology laboratories. Most strains isolated from AIDS patients with TE are avirulent for mice, and for this reason, positive isolation requires demonstration of *T. gondii* antibodies and *T. gondii* cysts in brains of the inoculated mice.

Numerous reports note successful isolations of *Toxoplasma gondii* from clinical samples from AIDS patients, using tissue culture, a useful but less sensitive alternative to mouse inoculation. Isolation can often be documented within 4 to 5 days of inoculation of the cultures (128, 129, 172, 251, 252). In a recent study in HIV-infected patients, *T. gondii* was isolated by tissue culture from 7% of biologic samples, including brain, striated muscle, liver, pericardium, pleura, bone marrow aspirates, BAL fluid, vitreous body, and blood (128). Brain tissue for isolation studies is rarely available because brain biopsy is uncommonly performed in AIDS patients with suspected TE (discussed later in this chapter under approach to management).

Toxoplasma gondii has been isolated from AIDS patients with cerebral, pulmonary, and ocular toxoplasmosis by inoculation of their buffy coat or peripheral blood mononuclear cells onto tissue culture (126, 128, 129). Isolation from blood has been reported in 14 to 38% of AIDS patients with toxoplasmosis (126, 128). Parasitemia appears to occur more frequently when toxoplasmosis involves extraneural sites (128). Once specific therapy is begun, parasitemia as determined by isolation studies rapidly resolves (128). *T. gondii* can be isolated from BAL fluid in as high as 86% of patients with pulmonary toxoplasmosis (153). Given the difficulty in differentiating pulmonary toxoplasmosis from PCP by clinical and radiologic criteria, attempts at isolation of the parasite and its demonstration by histologic studies (discussed in the next section) are important for establishing the diagnosis.

Histology

Demonstration of the tachyzoite form in any tissue or body fluid is proof of active infection. Tachyzoites are demonstrated by immunoperoxidase, Wright–Giemsa, PAS, and eosin–methylene blue stains. They are often difficult to visualize in tissue sections stained with hematoxylin and eosin. Reliance on histologic diagnosis is of particular importance when toxoplasmosis is considered in the differential diagnosis of dysfunction of extraneural organs, particularly in the presence of clinical evidence of involvement of the lung, myocardium, spinal cord, skeletal muscle, or gastrointestinal tract. Histologic features of toxoplasmosis are reviewed earlier in this chapter under histopathologic findings.

Other Laboratory Abnormalities

In AIDS patients with TE, minor abnormalities in clinical chemistries and hematologic parameters are common but are nonspecific (103). Many of these patients suffer from more than one disease process, involvement of more than one organ system and are receiving multiple drugs which may cause hematopoietic, renal or hepatic abnormalities. Thus, it may be difficult to differentiate abnormalities that are due to toxoplasmosis from those caused by coexisting disease processes. Disorders of sodium may suggest SIADH, diabetes insipidus, or abnormalities of the pituitary–adrenal axis. Abnormalities in serum creatine phosphokinase, aldolase, and aspartate aminotransferase should prompt consideration of toxoplasmic myocarditis (160) or myositis (166). Similarly, abnormalities in liver enzymes may indicate toxoplasmic hepatitis.

Most AIDS patients with TE are in the advanced stages of immunocompromise. CD4+ T-cell counts predict the development of toxoplasmosis (discussed in the section of this chapter on epidemiology and incidence). In AIDS patients with TE, the median CD4+ T-cell count has been observed to be approximately $50/mm^3$ (103, 105, 112, 253). Ninety percent of patients with TE have CD4+ T-cell counts below $200/mm^3$, 80 to 84% have counts below $100/mm^3$ (254,

255), and 49% have counts below 50/mm³ (255). In one study, all patients with pulmonary toxoplasmosis had CD4+ T-cell counts below 100/mm³ (5).

Cerebrospinal Fluid

PCR on CSF has proved useful for the diagnosis of TE in patients with AIDS (200, 241–246). Other findings in the CSF of patients with TE and AIDS are nonspecific. Mild mononuclear pleocytosis and mild to moderate elevations of CSF protein may be present (14, 179, 180, 213). Hypoglycorrhachia is uncommon (14, 111, 179, 180, 213). The presence of intrathecal production of *Toxoplasma* IgG antibodies may provide useful information for the diagnosis of TE (256, 257) and may be calculated by the following ratio:

$$\frac{CSF\ Sabin-Feldman\ dye\ test\ titer}{Serum\ dye\ test\ titer} \times \frac{Total\ serum\ IgG}{Total\ CSF\ IgG}$$

A ratio greater than 1 indicates intrathecal production of antibody and is associated with TE. Whether this method is as useful when serologic methods other than the dye test are used has not been shown. A rise in IgG antibody titers on serial CSF specimens has been reported (213). Although elevation of adenosine deaminase has been reported (258), the clinical utility of this test in TE remains to be shown.

Brain Biopsy

For discussion of brain biopsy, see the section of this chapter on management of a patient with suspected toxoplasmosis.

Radiology

NEURORADIOLOGIC FINDINGS

CT findings demonstrate multiple bilateral lesions in the cerebral hemispheres in 70 to 80% of patients with TE (15, 142, 259–262). Single lesions may be present (259, 260, 263). Of 31 AIDS patients with biopsy or autopsy-proved TE, 81% had multiple lesions, and 94% of the lesions demonstrated contrast ring enhancement (259). CT underestimates the number of lesions found at autopsy (14). Characteristic lesions are hypodense, exhibit contrast ring enhancement, tend to occur at the corticomedullary junction, and frequently involve the basal ganglia (Fig 15.3) (259, 260, 263, 264). The ring enhancement is usually located within a region of edema and encircles hypodense centers (260, 264). Use of delayed double-dose contrast imaging may improve visualization of ring enhancement of the lesions (259, 264). Lack of enhancement in the presence of an enlarging hypodense lesion has been reported to be a poor prognostic sign (264).

The lesions of TE on MRI scan are seen as high signal abnormalities on T2-weighted imaging (Fig 15.4). Deep lesions vary in size from 1 to 3 cm in diameter and in the center demonstrate complex patterns of high and low signal intensities. Peripheral lesions are smaller (1 cm in diameter or less), with uniform high signal intensity. "Target" lesions, which occur infrequently, are areas of smooth high signal intensity that surround isodense central regions. MRI scan, with its greater sensitivity, is helpful in establishing the presence of multiple lesions not seen by CT scans (260, 265–267). This is particularly true for the smaller lesions at the corticomedullary junction that often are not seen on CT scans. A gadolinium-enhanced MRI scan may demonstrate focal lesions resulting from TE in patients in whom the initial CT scan was reported to be normal (265). Based on these observations, MRI scanning should be used when feasible as the initial neuroradiologic test and especially in those patients with single lesions seen on CT scans.

Even in the presence of characteristic lesions on CT or MRI scanning, the findings are not pathognomonic of TE. Multifocal lesions that demonstrate ring enhancement on CT scans may be present in as many as 40% of cases of CNS lymphoma in AIDS patients.

Findings on CT scan have revealed improvement in approximately 80 to 90% of patients after 2 to 3 weeks of treatment (103, 260). Early signs of improvement include reduction in areas of contrast enhancement, reduced edema, and reduction of the mass effect (260, 263). Reduction in the size of the lesion is the most reliable indicator of a favorable response (263). Complete resolution takes from 6 weeks to 6 months, and peripheral lesions resolve more rapidly than do deep-seated ones (263). On MRI scans, smaller lesions at the corticomedullary junction or those with a "target" appearance on T2-weighted imaging usually resolve in 3 to 5 weeks without any demonstrable abnormality (263). Lesions that cause a mass effect and have complex central signal resolve more slowly and usually leave a small residual lesion (Fig 15.5) (263). Radiologic response to therapy lags behind the clinical response. Correlation is better between the clinical and radiologic responses at the end of acute therapy (255). Early in therapy and especially during the first 2 weeks, a disparity between these two responses may occasionally be observed when the patient improves clinically despite disease progression evident on neuroradiologic studies.

Patients with diffuse TE may have CT scans that are reported either as normal or as showing cerebral atrophy only (116, 143). Whether gadolinium-enhanced MRI scans would detect abnormalities not seen by CT scans in these patients is unknown. Hemorrhagic lesions may also be seen but are uncommon (141, 188, 191).

When toxoplasmosis involves the spinal cord, CT and MRI scans usually demonstrate localized cord enlargement consistent with an intramedullary lesion (147–150, 192). These findings may mimic an intramedullary tumor and may be severe enough to cause total obstruction of dye flow (147). Gadolinium-enhanced MRI scans usually demonstrate an intramedullary, brightly enhancing lesion at the site of cord enlargement (147, 148).

The major differential diagnosis for both single and multiple lesions in the brain by neuroradiologic imaging is CNS lymphoma. Based on neuroimaging studies alone of 274 AIDS patients with TE, CNS lymphoma, or PML, the probability of TE in the presence of multiple lesions was 0.63

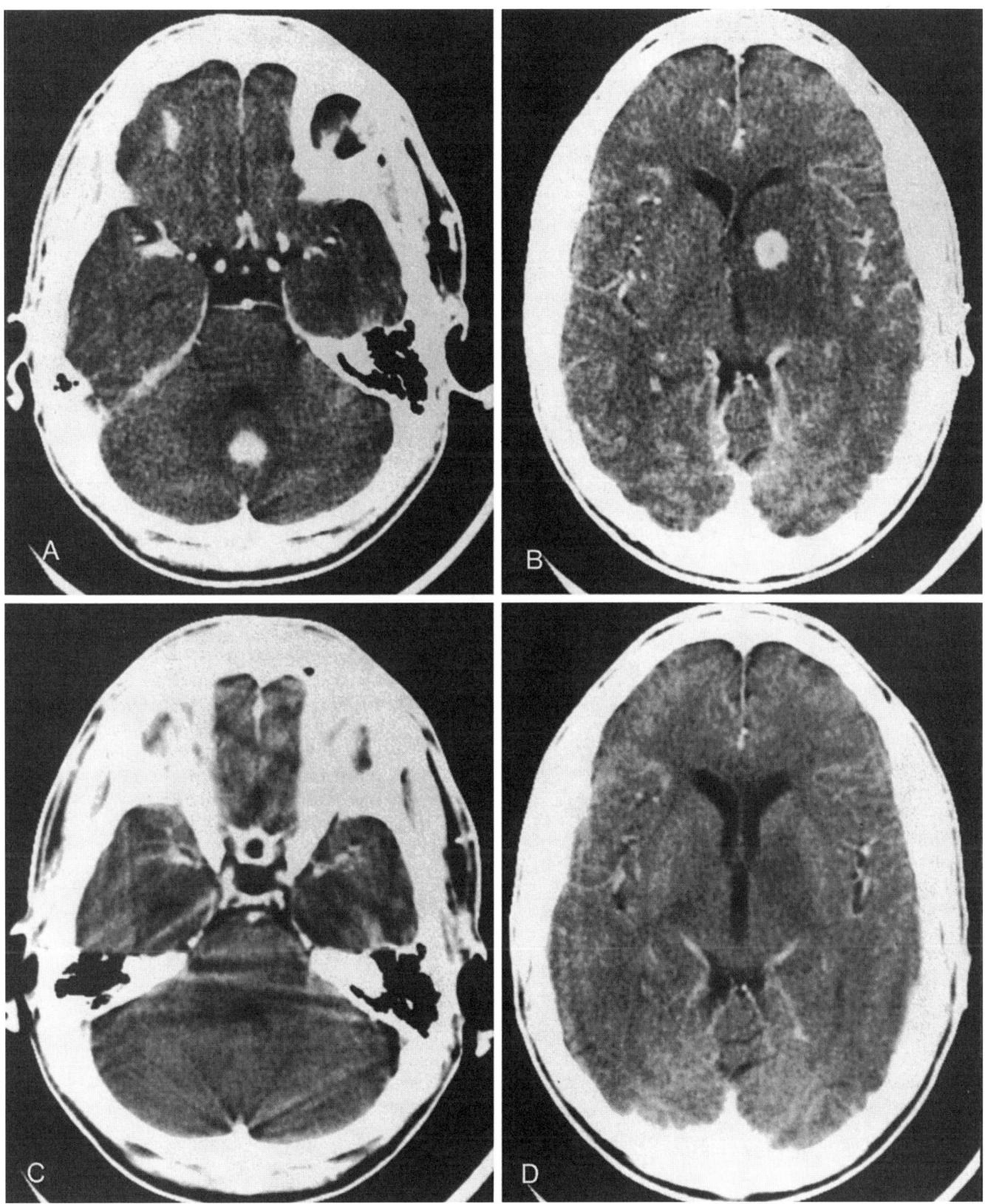

Figure 15.3. Neuroradiologic findings of toxoplasmic encephalitis (TE). CT scan findings of TE. **A and B.** Postcontrast CT scan showed nodular contrast-enhancing lesions in the vermis just posterior to the fourth ventricle **(A)** and in the left basal ganglia region **(B)**. Both lesions enhanced homogeneously and were surrounded by low-density vasogenic edema. **C and D.** Postcontrast CT scan performed 12 days later after appropriate antibiotic therapy showed complete resolution of the abnormal contrast enhancement; no residual abnormalities were noted in the vermis **(C)**, and only low residual density was noted in the left basal ganglia region **(D)**. The mass effect had also resolved. (Courtesy of Dr. Dieter Enzmann, Stanford, CA.)

for CT and 0.60 for MRI; the corresponding probability for single lesions was 0.36 for CT and 0.34 for MRI (268). In the presence of multiple lesions, the probability of CNS lymphoma was 0.23 for CT and 0.19 for MRI. In contrast, in the presence of single lesions, the probability of CNS lymphoma was increased to 0.40 for CT and 0.56 for MRI. These data underscore the increased frequency of conditions other than TE when only a solitary lesion is present. Other infectious agents also warrant consideration (discussed in the section of this chapter on neurologic manifestations). This situation emphasizes the importance of obtaining a definitive diagnosis by brain biopsy or aspirate in the patient with a solitary lesion (4, 267). Preliminary reports of the use of thallium-201 single photon emission CT for rapid differential diagnosis of TE and primary CNS lymphoma have appeared (269, 270).

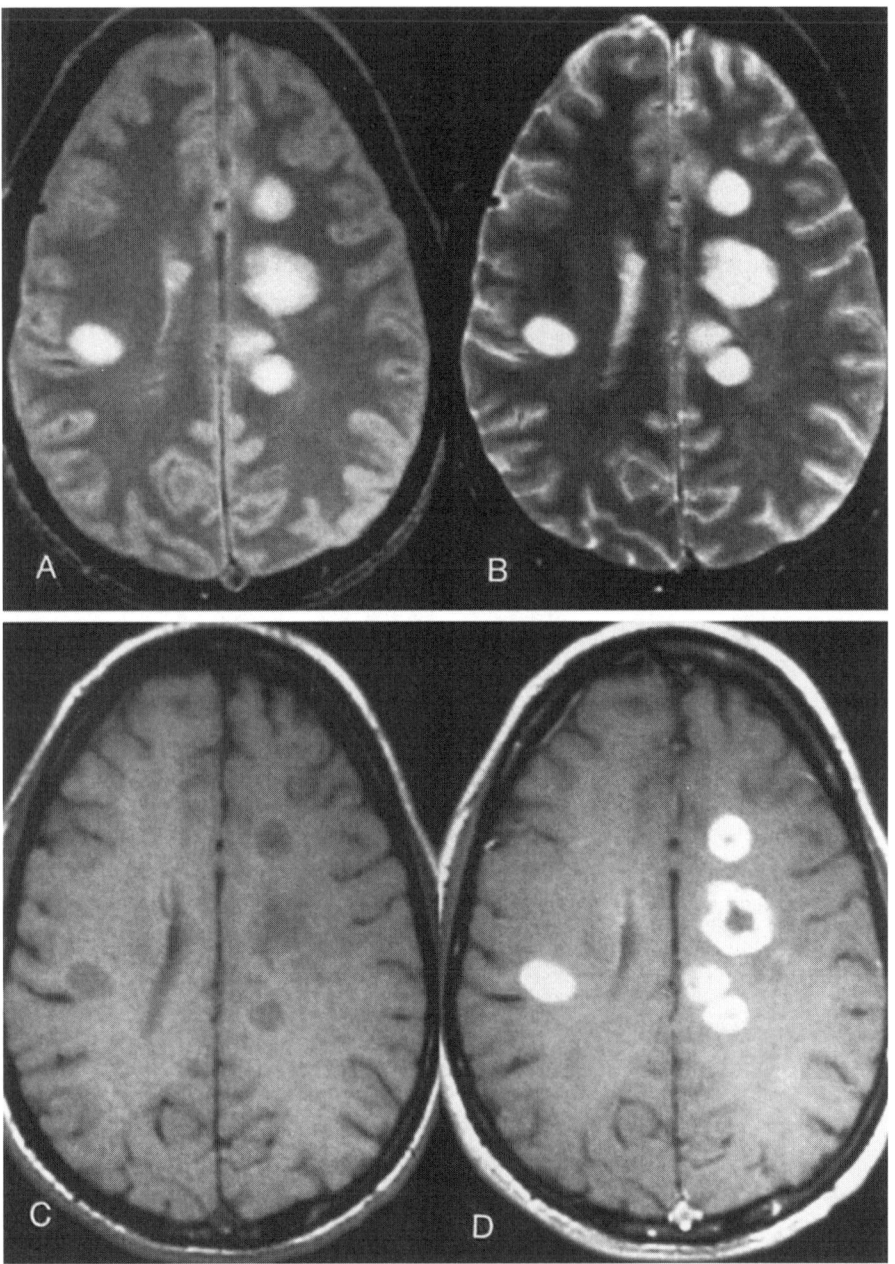

Figure 15.4. MR findings of toxoplasmic encephalitis (TE). **A and B.** The T_2-weighted (T_2W) images were performed using a first (TE, 30) **(A)** and second (TE, 80) **(B)** echo. On both these images, CNS toxoplasmosis appears as abnormal high density (i.e., white). Multiple round, nodular lesions were noted in both hemispheres deep in the white matter. The multiplicity and distribution of these lesions were typical; an atypical feature was the relative lack of surrounding vasogenic edema (see Fig 15.5). **C and D.** T_1-weighted (T_1W) images were used in combination with the contrast agent gadolinium–diethylene triamine pentaacetic acid (GdDPTA) to demonstrate abnormalities in the blood–brain barrier. The precontrast T_1W image **(C)** showed these lesions as low signal intensity compared with normal white matter. On the postcontrast T_1W scan **(D)**, abnormal contrast accumulation was seen as high signal intensity. These lesions showed either ring or nodular patterns of enhancement with GdDTPA **(D).**

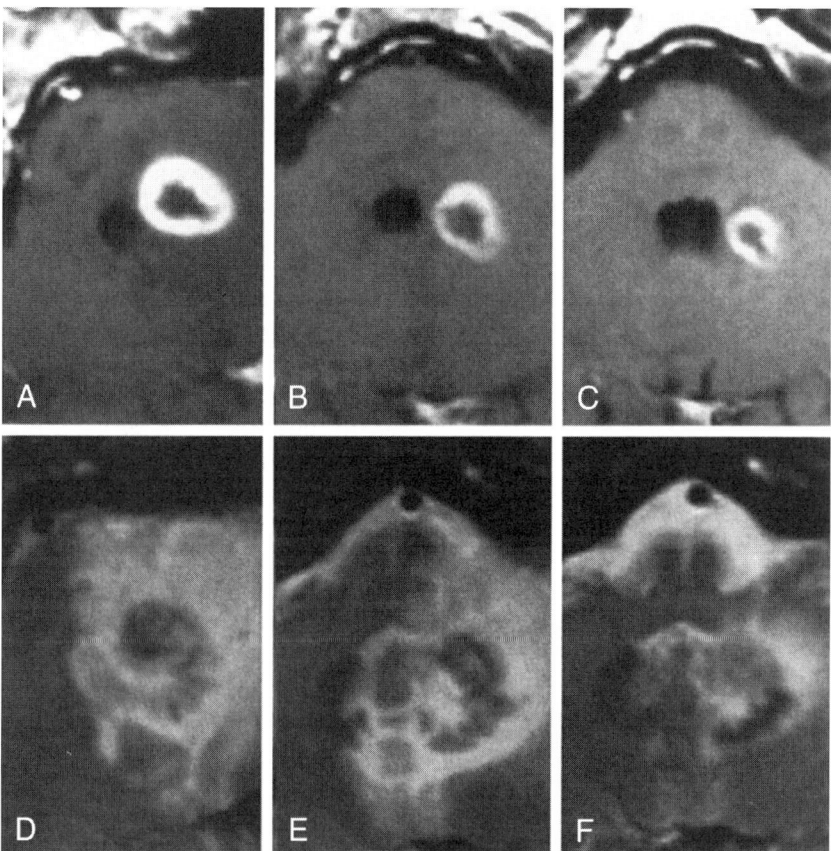

Figure 15.5. Brainstem toxoplasmosis showing the response to appropriate antibiotic treatment on both postcontrast T_1- and T_2-weighted (T_1W and T_2W) images. **A to C.** The upper row of serial postcontrast T_1W scans demonstrates decreasing ring enhancement in the brainstem adjacent to the fourth ventricle indicative of a resolving toxoplasmosis abscess. **D to F.** The lower row of concomittant T_2W images shows the decreasing size of the abscess that is of relative low signal intensity and also the regression of surrounding vasogenic edema, depicted as high signal intensity around the abscess. This amount of surrounding vasogenic edema is typical of toxoplasmosis lesions.

CHEST X-RAY FINDINGS

The most common chest radiographic findings in patients with pulmonary toxoplasmosis are bilateral interstitial infiltrates (5, 6) which may be indistinguishable from PCP. Bilateral hilar adenopathy (6), pleural effusion (6), and nodular (5, 6, 271), cavitatory, and alveolar infiltrates have also been described (5, 6). Coarse nodular infiltrates together with the presence of pleural effusion or hilar adenopathy are uncommon in PCP and should alert the clinician to consider pulmonary toxoplasmosis (271).

TREATMENT

Antimicrobial Agents

Whereas various antimicrobial agents and regimens have been used for treatment of toxoplasmosis in AIDS patients, few studies have adequately defined those that are optimal. An attempt is made here to focus on those agents and regimens for which data are adequate and to identify those for which the data appear promising but are incomplete (272). Outcomes in therapeutic trials depend on the compliance of the patient and on the patient's ability to tolerate the prescribed drug. Thus, figures provided by various authors on efficacy of primary prophylaxis and maintenance therapy should be interpreted with these limitations in mind (273). Adverse reactions occur frequently in AIDS patients treated for TE. A complete description of the side effects caused by antimicrobial agents that have been used is beyond the scope of this chapter. The most common side effects, in particular those that occur in AIDS patients, are mentioned. Readers are encouraged to refer to the package inserts of each antimicrobial agent for a complete description of possible adverse effects.

STANDARD ANTIMICROBIAL AGENTS

Pyrimethamine

Pyrimethamine is a dihydrofolate reductase inhibitor with remarkable activity against *Toxoplasma gondii*. In a murine model of acute toxoplasmosis, 100% survival was associated with serum pyrimethamine levels higher than 0.5 mg/L, whereas survival was 55 and 0% when serum levels were 0.37 mg/L and less than 0.1 mg/L, respectively (274). The optimum dose of pyrimethamine for treatment of TE has been difficult to determine because serum levels vary among patients and within the same patient on different days (275–277). Based on pharmacokinetic studies, a loading dose of 200 mg orally as a single dose (278–280), followed by 50 to 75 mg per day (1 to 1.25 mg/kg per day), is recommended for adults (280). In a recent study, peak and trough serum levels in patients given 100 mg orally every other day were 1.92 ± 0.43 and 1.34 ± 0.35 mg/L, respectively (276). In the same study, peak and trough levels in patients given 50 mg daily were 1.24 ± 0.22 and 0.82 ± 0.19 mg/L, respectively. Whether serum levels in patients with TE are critical in determining outcome of therapy has not been determined. Studies in patients with leukemia and in AIDS patients have determined that the concentration of pyrimethamine in the CSF is 10 to 25% of the serum levels (281, 282). From studies in patients undergoing neurosurgery, investigators demonstrated that levels of pyrimethamine in brain tissue were higher at 24 hours than at 12 and 48 hours. The concentrations in the brain tissue were 1.56 ± 0.84 and 0.67 ± 0.09 µg/g after an oral dose of 100 mg and 50 mg, respectively (276). The half-life of pyrimethamine was calculated to be 40 hours in brain tissue and 28 hours in serum (276).

Side effects of pyrimethamine are common and may lead to discontinuation of therapy. They present most frequently as (dose-related) bone marrow suppression and skin rash (283–286). Patients who experienced rash when treated with pyrimethamine as prophylactic therapy appeared to be at higher risk for TE (286). To ameliorate the bone marrow suppressive effect, 10 to 20 mg per day of oral folinic acid (leucovorin) is recommended for AIDS patients who receive 50 to 75 mg per day of pyrimethamine. Folinic acid may also be administered by the intramuscular or intravenous routes. Up to 50 mg per day of oral folinic acid has been used for patients suspected of having pyrimethamine-induced hematologic toxicity (287). At the lower doses, folinic acid does not appear to inhibit the action of pyrimethamine on *Toxoplasma gondii*; whether the higher doses will affect its efficacy is not known.

Sulfonamides

Sulfonamides inhibit the dihydrofolic acid synthetase of *Toxoplasma gondii* and interfere with the parasite's ability to use *p*-aminobenzoic acid. Of the sulfonamides tested in vivo in animal models, sulfadiazine, sulfamethazine, and sulfamerazine had the greatest efficacy (288). The combination of pyrimethamine and sulfadiazine blocks folate metabolism at two sequential levels and has been shown to be synergistic in vitro (289) and in animal models (290, 291) of toxoplasmosis. At present, this combination is considered the therapeutic regimen of choice. For acute therapy, the recommended dose of sulfadiazine in the combination is 4 to 6 g per day (100 to 150 mg/kg per day) by the oral route. The combination of sulfadiazine at 2 g per day and pyrimethamine 25 mg per day has also been used with some success for maintenance therapy (179, 181, 218, 292, 293). Trisulfapyrimidines, which contain sulfadiazine, may be used at the same dose as sulfadiazine. The most common side effects associated with sulfadiazine in AIDS patients include skin rashes, which may be life-threatening (181), crystal-induced nephrotoxicity (294, 295), and hematologic toxicity (296). Crystal-induced nephrotoxicity manifested by flank pain, crystalluria, hematuria, and renal impairment is reversible if treated promptly with hydration, alkalinization of urine, and dose reduction of sulfadiazine (294, 295). Worsening encephalopathy, hallucinations, or new onset of neuropsychiatric manifestations may be sulfadiazine induced. This possibility must be considered in the patient with such signs who is nonresponsive to otherwise appropriate *Toxoplasma* treatment (297, 298). The presence of drug rash to sulfonamides does not necessarily preclude its use at lower daily doses for maintenance therapy (299). Some investigators have reported the success of desensitization to sulfadiazine in the management of patients with TE who have suffered untoward reactions to the drug (300–303).

Clindamycin

Treatment with clindamycin significantly reduced mortality, tachyzoite numbers, and brain inflammation in murine models of toxoplasmosis (304, 305). Its mechanism of action on *Toxoplasma gondii* is unknown. The earliest studies in AIDS patients, although uncontrolled, revealed efficacy when the drug was combined with pyrimethamine (114, 306). Clindamycin in combination with pyrimethamine has been effective in prospective studies, and its efficacy and toxicity were reported comparable to those of pyrimethamine–sulfadiazine when used for the treatment of TE (254, 255, 307, 308). The consensus of a panel of experts was to use clindamycin, 600 mg every 6 hours, as the oral dose and the same dose for the intravenous form of the drug (280). An intravenous dose of 1200 mg every 6 hours has been used (254). Adverse reactions associated with clindamycin in these studies were rash, nausea, vomiting, and diarrhea. Skin rash occurred at a frequency similar to that seen with the pyrimethamine–sulfadiazine combination (254). Myopathy with typical electromyographic findings and elevated serum creatine phosphokinase levels have been described in an AIDS patient (309).

EXPERIMENTAL AND INVESTIGATIONAL THERAPY

The high incidence of untoward side effects associated with the previously recommended regimens, the concern for eventual emergence of drug-resistant strains of *Toxoplasma gondii*, and the hope for discovery of a single drug that will be effective for treatment and for prophylaxis have stimulated interest in searching for new antimicrobials and new regimens against *T. gondii*. The principal sites of the tachyzoite that are targeted by antimicrobial agents are inhibition of metabolism, protein synthesis, and ribonucleic acid synthesis.

T. gondii has been reported to have a plastid (310). Further characterization of the plastid's functions may lead to the design of new drugs that block the plastid with minimal side effects for humans.

In reviewing studies on the use of antimicrobial agents in laboratory animal models, two considerations are important. Readers are cautioned in regard to extrapolation of results derived from animal models to results that could occur in patients with AIDS. In addition, different strains of *Toxoplasma gondii* differ in their susceptibility to any given antimicrobial agent (272, 311).

Inhibitors of Folate Metabolism

These agents have been most extensively investigated because *Toxoplasma gondii* totally depends on its host cell for its supply of purines.

Trimethoprim and Trimethoprim–Sulfamethoxazole. TMP has activity against *Toxoplasma gondii*, but its ability to inhibit parasite replication was less than for comparable concentrations of pyrimethamine (312). In experimental toxoplasmosis, both in vitro and in vivo data have demonstrated the greater efficacy of the combination of pyrimethamine–sulfadiazine when compared with TMP–SMX (312, 313). Retrospective studies have suggested that the combination is effective for the treatment of TE in AIDS patients (314–316). In these studies, the dose of TMP in the combination was 6.6 or 20 mg/kg per day delivered orally or intravenously in four divided doses. Because experimental data demonstrate lesser efficacy of the TMP–SMX combination, and because more data are available on the use of pyrimethamine–sulfadiazine in treatment of TE, we prefer the latter at present.

Trimetrexate. Trimetrexate has greater in vitro inhibitory activity against *Toxoplasma gondii* than pyrimethamine or TMP (317, 318). One clinical study of trimetrexate used alone as salvage therapy demonstrated initial clinical response but subsequent relapse while patients were still receiving the drug (319).

Piritrexin. Piritrexin is lipid soluble and has activity against murine toxoplasmosis (320). When combined with sulfadiazine, it significantly protected against death in infected mice (320). It has not been tested in humans with TE.

Dapsone

Dapsone inhibits dihydropteroate synthase of the parasite (321) and significantly reduced mortality in murine toxoplasmosis (321–323). When used at an oral dose of 100 mg per day in combination with oral pyrimethamine at 25 mg per day, dapsone has been reported to be effective for the treatment of TE (324). It has also been used for primary prophylaxis and maintenance therapy (secondary prophylaxis) for toxoplasmosis in AIDS patients. Adverse reactions are frequent and include skin rash, hematologic abnormalities, fever, and nausea (325–328).

Pyrimethamine–Sulfadoxine (Fansidar)

Fansidar, administered intramuscularly (the intramuscular preparation is not available in the United States), has been reported to have effected both clinical and radiologic response in 80% of AIDS patients with TE (329). This combination has also been efficacious for primary prophylaxis and maintenance therapy when taken orally at doses of one tablet once each week (330) or three tablets every second week (331). Adverse reactions are common and include skin rashes, Stevens–Johnson syndrome, and hematologic and gastrointestinal side effects. These adverse effects have prompted physicians to discontinue the drug in up to 39% of patients (331).

Macrolides–Azalides and Ketolides

The newer macrolide–azalide antibiotics with efficacy in murine models of toxoplasmosis are azithromycin (332), clarithromycin (333), and roxithromycin (334, 335). Given the potent inhibitory activity of these drugs on prokaryotic protein synthesis, investigators have postulated that this mechanism accounts for the anti-*Toxoplasma* activity of this group of antibiotics (336). A remarkable difference exists in susceptibility of different strains of *T. gondii* to these agents in animal models (332). Azithromycin has activity against both tachyzoite and cyst forms (332, 337). Initial analysis of data from a recent trial (ACTG 156) that investigated the use of azithromycin (900 to 1500 mg every day) plus pyrimethamine (25 to 50 mg) for treatment of TE revealed a response rate of 31% (338). In this study, 9% of patients were classified as potential responders, 50% as relapses and induction failures, and another 9% had an indeterminate response. It is evident from this study that azithromycin is effective (when used in combination with pyrimethamine) for treatment of some cases of TE in AIDS patients. Until the data analysis is completed, a final conclusion in regard to the effectiveness of the azithromycin–pyrimethamine combination cannot be made. A single case report described the dramatic response to azithromycin in a patient with TE who was allergic to sulfonamide and pyrimethamine and in whom clindamycin and doxycycline were not effective (339).

Promising results have been reported in a pilot study for the treatment of TE in AIDS patients with the combination of pyrimethamine, 75 mg per day, and clarithromycin, 1 g every 12 hours by the oral route: 62% of patients had a complete and 23% a partial clinical response; 15% died by week 3 of therapy (340). When patients were evaluated at 3 and 6 weeks of treatment, the radiologic response did not correlate with the clinical response. Adverse events associated with therapy in this study included nausea and vomiting (38%), skin rash (38%), hepatic enzyme abnormalities (24%), hematologic abnormalities (31%), and hearing loss (15%). Twenty-seven percent of the surviving patients stopped receiving clarithromycin because of drug toxicity that resulted in thrombocytopenia or liver enzyme abnormalities. More recently, ketolides have been shown to possess excellent in vitro activity against *Toxoplasma gondii* and have provided remarkable protection against death in infected mice (FG Araujo, unpublished data).

Tetracyclines

Both doxycycline (341) and minocycline (342, 343) have efficacy in murine toxoplasmosis. Their mechanism of action on *Toxoplasma gondii* is unknown. Doxycycline was used successfully in two AIDS patients with TE when it was administered at 300 mg per day intravenously in three divided doses (344). When doxycycline was used orally at doses of 100 mg twice a day in six patients intolerant to pyrimethamine–sulfadiazine, five patients had associated neurologic and radiologic recurrences while receiving the drug (345). Further study of the tetracyclines in the treatment of toxoplasmosis is likely to involve their use in combination with other antimicrobials.

Atovaquone

Atovaquone has been approved for use in patients with mild to moderate PCP. Atovaquone has been reported to have potent in vitro activity against both tachyzoite and cyst forms (337, 346). It significantly reduced mortality in murine toxoplasmosis and had remarkable, although differing, activity against different strains of *Toxoplasma gondii* (346). Atovaquone has been used in AIDS patients with TE with encouraging results. In studies that included small numbers of patients (347, 348), clinical response rates of 75 and 66% were reported with atovaquone. In a large series of patients with AIDS-related TE, use of atovaquone as salvage therapy was successful in 37% of those intolerant to standard therapy (349). Unfortunately, relapse occurred in approximately 50% of patients in whom atovaquone was used for acute therapy and continued alone as maintenance therapy (347, 349). Seventeen (26%) of 65 patients treated with atovaquone as a single agent for maintenance therapy of TE experienced a relapse (350). The combination of pyrimethamine and atovaquone may prove more useful (351). Serum levels of atovaquone in patients treated with TE were not predictive of clinical response or failure (348). Bioavailability of the drug is improved when the medication is ingested with food. The reliability of absorption of this drug continues to be a problem. Survival time was significantly better among those patients with higher steady-state plasma concentrations of the drug (349). Although a new formulation of atovaquone is reported to achieve higher plasma concentrations, prospective trials are needed to compare the efficacy of this drug with that obtained in standard drug regimens. This drug should never be used alone for the treatment of the acute infection, but rather it should be used in combination with drugs such as pyrimethamine. Use of atovaquone with or without pyrimethamine in AIDS patients with TE has been well tolerated. The adverse events observed in these studies included hepatic enzyme abnormalities (50%), rash (25%), nausea (21%), and diarrhea (19%) (348). Between 3 and 10% of patients treated with atovaquone were reported to discontinue the drug because of rash, hepatic enzyme abnormalities, nausea, or vomiting (348, 350, 351). Leukopenia associated with the combination of pyrimethamine and atovaquone has responded to folinic acid (leucovorin) and granulocyte colony-stimulating factor therapy (351).

Other Antimicrobial Agents

Other antimicrobial agents that have demonstrable activity against *Toxoplasma gondii* include arprinocid, a purine analog (352), qinghaosu (353), and pentamidine (354). Arprinocid has not been used in humans; the latter two agents are of particular interest because of the considerable experience with their use in other infectious diseases. The antimetabolite 5-fluorouracil has in vitro activity against *T. gondii* (355) and at doses approximately 10-fold less than those used for cancer chemotherapy. Two reports have noted the successful use of the combination of 5-fluorouracil and clindamycin for treatment of TE in AIDS patients. Severe toxicity was not observed (356, 357). Rifabutin, a derivative of rifamycin, has shown remarkable activity against acute toxoplasmosis in mice (358) and rifapentine, another derivative of rifamycin, was noted to be active in vitro and in vivo against *T. gondii* (359). Recently, the fluoroquinolones trovafloxacin (360) and levafloxacin (AA Khan, unpublished data) have been shown to be effective against *T. gondii* in vitro. Trovafloxacin has also been demonstrated to protect mice against death (360).

Combination Antimicrobial Therapy

Monotherapy for treatment of TE in AIDS patients is usually associated with initial clinical improvement followed by relapse even while the drug is being continued (347, 361). *Therefore, until clear evidence to the contrary exists, we recommend that acute and maintenance therapies should include at least two drugs.* Drug combinations other than those described previously that have demonstrated remarkable and even synergistic activity in murine toxoplasmosis include pyrimethamine–dapsone (362), clarithromycin–minocycline (363), pyrimethamine–azithromycin (364), azithromycin–sulfadiazine (365), clarithromycin–sulfadiazine (366), clarithromycin–pyrimethamine (366), atovaquone–pyrimethamine and atovaquone–sulfadiazine (367, 368), and rifabutin–atovaquone, and rifabutin–sulfadiazine (369).

Immunotherapy: Cytokines

Because of the severely impaired immune function in patients with AIDS, immunotherapy has been proposed as adjunctive treatment for life-threatening toxoplasmosis. Thus far, most experimental studies have focused on administration of biologic response modifiers in murine models of toxoplasmosis. Those with reported success include IFN-γ (61, 62, 370), IFN-β (371), IL-2 (372), TNF-α (373), IL-1 (373), and IL-12 (73). Of particular interest is IFN-γ, which has previously been identified as an important mediator of resistance against *Toxoplasma gondii* (370). In AIDS patients with TE, serum IFN-γ levels were significantly lower than in immunocompetent patients with toxoplasmic lymphadenopathy (374). In addition, treatment of monocytes and monocyte-derived macrophages of AIDS patients with IFN-γ enhanced their activity against *Toxoplasma* (375–377). This in vitro effect on monocytes has been confirmed in vivo in AIDS patients treated with IFN-γ (378). In murine models of toxoplasmosis, administration of IFN-γ in concert with antimicrobial agents has resulted in synergistic or additive toxoplasmacidal activity. These regimens include IFN-γ in combination with roxithromycin (379), pyrimethamine (364), azithromycin (380), and clindamycin (381). The combination of IL-12 plus atovaquone or IL-12 plus clindamycin has also proved useful in a mouse model of acute toxoplasmosis in mice (382).

Management of a Patient with Suspected Toxoplasmosis

APPROACH TO MANAGEMENT

Toxoplasmic Encephalitis

The empiric treatment of TE based on characteristic clinical and neuroradiologic findings evolved when it became apparent that the definitive diagnosis could be made only by brain biopsy and that TE was the most common cause of focal brain lesions in patients on CT or MRI scans (4, 14). In the presence of a compatible clinical syndrome, a positive *Toxoplasma* IgG serologic test, and multiple ring-enhancing lesions on CT or MRI, the predictive value for TE is approximately 80% (181). This percentage was sufficiently high to warrant suggestions for empiric therapy (4, 12, 14, 181, 260, 383). Numerous retrospective and prospective analyses have reported the efficacy of such a management strategy. Clinical trials of new treatment regimens have used clinical response to therapy as presumptive of a diagnosis of TE.

The algorithm shown in Figure 15.6 details a suggested approach to the management of a patient with suspected TE. These guidelines are not meant to be restrictive; individual circumstances and clinical judgment must be considered. As discussed earlier, MRI scans are significantly more sensitive for demonstration of CNS lesions of TE when compared with CT scans. The presence of multiple lesions on neuroimaging studies increases the probability of TE versus other causes of CNS lesions in AIDS. This crucial distinguishing point directly influences clinical decision making because it favors empiric treatment for TE.

In the presence of a single lesion on MRI, the probability of CNS lymphoma is at least equal to or higher than the probability of TE (268). Other disease processes including tuberculomas, cryptococcomas, and aspergillomas must also be considered, and in such cases, emphasis should be placed on careful examination for an extraneural lesion that could explain the cause of the CNS findings. In an AIDS patient with clinical signs referable to the CNS, if the initial CT scan was normal or showed only cerebral atrophy, MRI scanning, with its greater sensitivity, may detect significant lesions.

In regard to what can be expected in relation to clinical and radiologic response, a study in which a detailed graded neurologic assessment was performed prospectively on patients treated empirically for TE demonstrated that, of the 49 eligible patients, 71% had a complete or partial response. Using the neurologic assessment, 86% of the responders had clear evidence of clinical improvement by day 7 and, 91% had improved clinically by day 14 (255). Neurologic improvement precedes radiologic improvement (255). Early improvement of the radiologic abnormalities in a patient receiving high-dose corticosteroids should not be confused as necessarily being a response to specific therapy. The 29% classified as nonresponders all either experienced progression of their baseline neurologic abnormalities or developed new ones within the first 10 days of empiric therapy. Headaches and seizures tended to be insensitive indicators of response to therapy because both responders and nonresponders resolved these abnormalities.

In regard to the questions whether and when brain biopsy is indicated, AIDS patients who are compliant with primary prophylaxis against toxoplasmosis (discussed in the section of this chapter on primary prophylaxis) and who present with focal lesions on neuroimaging studies should be considered candidates for brain biopsy at initial presentation rather than receiving empiric *Toxoplasma* therapy. Brain biopsy and neuroradiologic imaging should also be considered in patients who deteriorate clinically by 7 days or who do not improve clinically by 10 days of empiric therapy. A recent study revealed that, of AIDS patients with CNS mass lesions who did not improve by 7 days of therapy, 36% had CNS lymphoma, 24% had PML, and 8% had TE (384). Lack of response to empiric therapy does not exclude the diagnosis of TE because concurrent disease processes from other infections and lymphoma may be present (385). In addition, in some patients, despite treatment with what is considered an optimal regimen, toxoplasmosis continues apparently unabated and results in death (254).

In retrospective studies, the decision to administer empiric therapy has resulted in delay in diagnosis of another treatable infection in 2 to 5% of patients (179, 181). Thus, given the morbidity associated with brain biopsy, the reluctance of neurosurgeons to perform the procedure, and possible sampling error, attempts at antemortem histologic diagnosis of TE should be considered primarily for patients who present with a single lesion on MRI scan and for those who fail to respond to empiric treatment and those who have no demonstrable antibodies to *Toxoplasma gondii* (386).

Extraneural Toxoplasmosis

Data on the outcome of treatment of AIDS patients with toxoplasmosis outside the CNS are limited; available information on therapy of ocular (8, 131, 132) and pulmonary involvement (5, 6) indicates that these forms of toxoplasmosis are also responsive to treatment. A favorable response to therapy in cases of ocular toxoplasmosis has been the rule (8, 131, 132), and therapy was successful in 50 to 77% of patients with pulmonary toxoplasmosis (5, 6, 196).

USE OF ANTIMICROBIAL THERAPY

Antimicrobial therapy for toxoplasmosis in AIDS patients is for the acute (primary) stage, maintenance treatment (secondary prophylaxis), and primary prophylaxis. Acute therapy is that administered during the acute symptomatic phase of the disease. *Because relapse occurs frequently after discontinuation of primary therapy, maintenance therapy is continued for the life of the patient.* Primary prophylaxis against toxoplasmosis in AIDS patients is discussed in the section on prevention. *Until further data become available, antimicrobial agents should not be used alone for acute or maintenance therapy.* As yet no convincing data from prospective carefully designed trials are available to allow recommendations regarding single drug use for primary prophylaxis.

Acute or Primary Therapy

Acute therapy should be administered for at least 3 weeks (280). For more severely ill patients who have not achieved a complete clinical or neuroradiologic response, a course of 6 weeks or more is recommended. Most investigators agree that the combination of pyrimethamine–sulfadiazine is the therapy of choice for AIDS patients with toxoplasmosis and is the standard by which most experimental regimens are compared. In retrospective studies, this regimen was associated with a clinical response in 68 to 95% of patients with TE (11, 14, 103, 180, 218). Unfortunately, up to 40% of patients treated with this regimen developed side effects of sufficient severity to require discontinuation of their therapy (103, 180, 218). The regimen of pyrimethamine–clindamycin appears comparable in efficacy to pyrimethamine–sulfadiazine (254, 307, 308). Unfortunately, both regimens are also

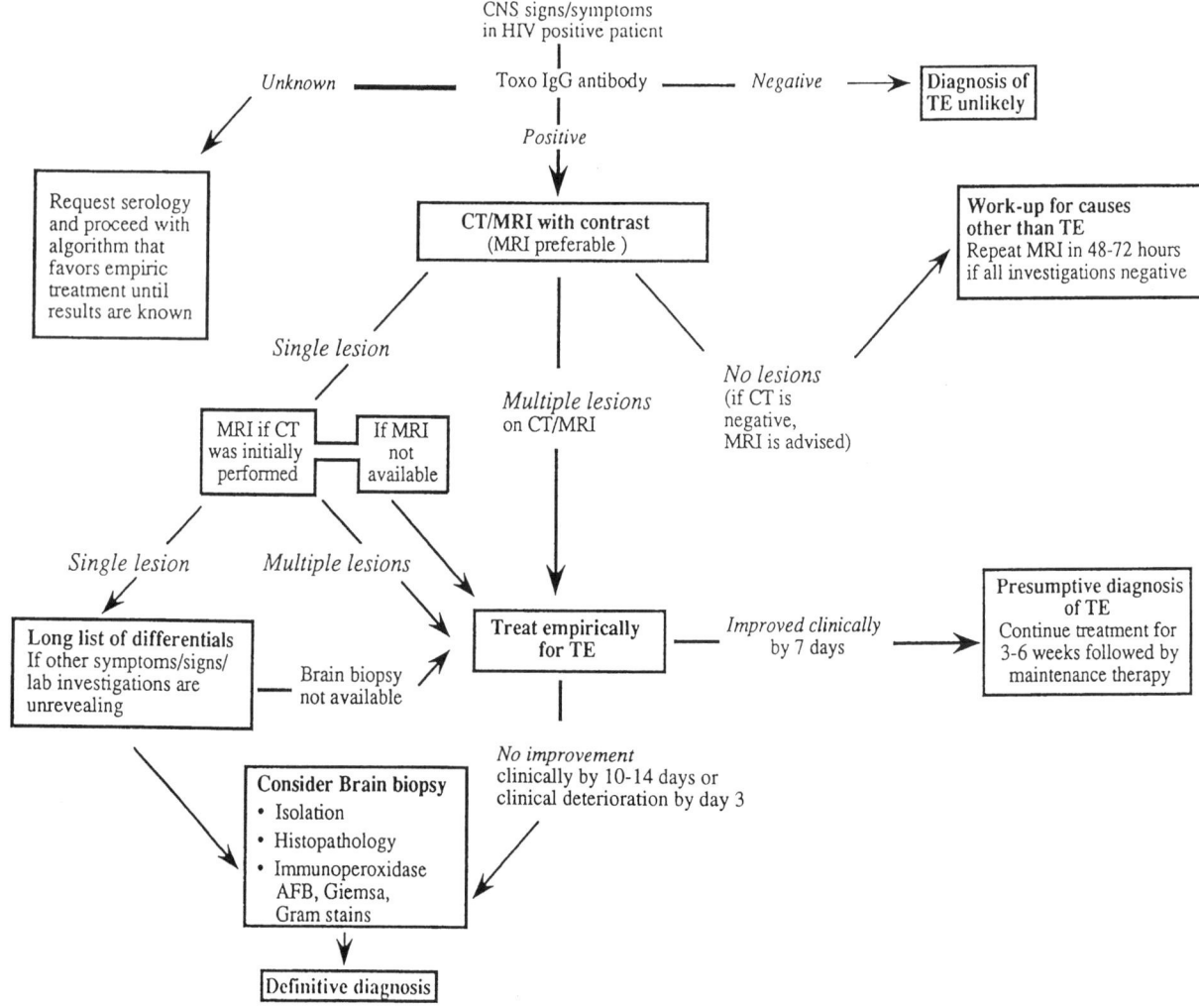

Figure 15.6. Guidelines for management of suspected toxoplasmic encephalitis.

Table 15.6. Guidelines for Acute/Primary Therapy of Toxoplasmic Encephalitis in Patients with AIDS

Drug	Dosage Schedule
Standard regimens	
Pyrimethamine	Oral, 200 mg loading dose, then 50 to 75 mg once daily
Folinic acid (leucovorin)[a]	Oral, IV, or IM, 10–20 mg once daily (up to 50 mg once daily)
plus	
Sulfadiazine	Oral, 1–1.5 g q6h
or	
Clindamycin	Oral or IV, 600 mg q6h (up to IV 1200 mg q6h)
Possible alternative regimens[b]	
Trimethoprim–sulfamethoxazole[c]	Oral or IV, 5 mg (trimethoprim component)/kg q6h
Pyrimethamine and folinic acid	As in standard regimens plus one of the following
Clarithromycin	Oral, 1 g q12h
Atovaquone	Oral, 750 mg q6h
Azithromycin[d]	Oral, 1200–1500 mg once daily
Dapsone	Oral, 100 mg once daily

[a]The dose of folinic acid can be titrated based on the hemogram to reduce pyrimethamine associated myelotoxicity; up to 50 mg/day has been used.
[b]These agents have been used in clinical studies with small numbers of patients and have response rates lower than the standard regimens (see text for references). They should be used only in patients who are intolerant of the standard regimens. Alternative agents must be used in combination with another antimicrobial agent (most frequently, pyrimethamine with folinic acid) that has proved clinical activity against *Toxoplasma gondii*.
[c]In a small study, trimethoprim–sulfamethoxazole at a dose of 6.6 mg (trimethoprim component)/kg per day has been reported to have similar efficacy to 20 mg trimethoprim/kg per day. Further studies are required to determine the optimal dosage schedule (see text).
[d]The dosages given here are those that appear to have been effective in a small number of patients.

comparable in their incidence of toxicity. Pyrimethamine–clindamycin may be regarded as a suitable alternative in those patients who are unable to tolerate pyrimethamine–sulfadiazine.

The standard and alternative regimens used for acute therapy and their dosage schedules are listed in Table 15.6. The reader is referred to the section of this chapter on experimental and investigational antimicrobial agents for further information on the drugs listed in the alternative regimens.

Maintenance Therapy or Secondary Prophylaxis

Relapse of TE will occur in approximately 50% (179, 218) to 80% (181) of patients within several months of discontinuing therapy for TE. After an initial 3 to 6 weeks of primary therapy, all patients must receive lifelong maintenance therapy to prevent relapse.

At the time of writing this chapter, no single regimen both is efficacious and has an acceptable adverse reaction profile. Relapse of TE occurs in approximately 20 to 30% of patients who are receiving maintenance therapy; some of these relapses are likely the result of noncompliance and patient intolerance to the prescribed regimen (273); these factors should be considered when interpreting reports of data on efficacy or lack thereof with different maintenance regimens (180, 387, 388). Because the regimens, dosages, and dosing intervals have not been studied in systematic fashion, it is difficult to provide unqualified recommendations. Rather, we have provided the reader with dosing schedule reported as having a favorable effect (Table 15.7).

A higher relapse rate with the use of pyrimethamine–clindamycin compared with pyrimethamine–sulfadiazine as secondary prophylaxis has been reported by several investigators (180, 308, 385, 387–389). These data have prompted a panel of experts to recommend at least 1200 mg per day of clindamycin in divided doses when pyrimethamine–clindamycin is used for secondary prophylaxis (280). At present, the combination of pyrimethamine–sulfadiazine has been associated with reports of the lowest relapse rate and is recommended. When daily therapy with pyrimethamine–sulfadiazine was compared with a twice-weekly regimen for prevention of recurrence of TE, the latter was found less effective (179, 293, 390, 391). Patients receiving the pyrimethamine–sulfadiazine combination most likely do not require another regimen for PCP prophylaxis. Whereas 25% of patients receiving pyrimethamine–clindamycin subsequently developed PCP (392), no patient receiving pyrimethamine–sulfadiazine developed PCP (293, 392). Unfortunately, because of drug toxicity, many patients are unable to continue receiving the combination of pyrimethamine–sulfadiazine for maintenance therapy.

Table 15.7. Guidelines for Maintenance Therapy/Secondary Prophylaxis of Toxoplasmic Encephalitis in Patients with AIDS[a]

Recommended regimens	
Pyrimethamine	Oral, 25–50 mg once daily
Folinic acid (leucovorin)	Oral, 10–20 mg once daily
plus	
Sulfadiazine[b]	Oral, 1 g q6h
or	
Clindamycin[c]	Oral, 450–600 mg q6h
Pyrimethamine–sulfadoxine[d] (Fansidar)	Oral, 1 tablet 3 times a week
Alternative regimens[e]	
Pyrimethamine	Oral, 50 mg once daily
Folinic acid (leucovorin)	Oral, 10 to 20 mg once daily
Pyrimethamine with folinic acid plus one of the following	As in recommended regimens
Dapsone	Oral, 100 mg twice a week
Atovaquone	Oral, 750 mg q6h
Clarithromycin	Oral, 1000 mg q12h
Azithromycin[f]	Oral, 1200–1500 mg once daily

[a]At the time of writing this chapter, an optimum regimen for maintenance therapy that is both efficacious and that has an acceptable adverse reaction profile has not been described.
[b]Intermittent dosing of pyrimethamine–sulfadiazine or pyrimethamine–clindamycin 2 days a week maintenance therapy at doses similar to primary therapy has been reported with varying efficacy when compared to daily dosing (see text for references).
[c]Use of pyrimethamine–clindamycin for maintenance therapy is associated with a higher relapse rate when compared with pyrimethamine–sulfadiazine.
[d]One tablet of Fansidar contains 25 mg pyrimethamine and 500 mg sulfadoxine (see text for references).
[e]These alternative regimens described for maintenance therapy have been used only in small numbers of patients. Most of these patients were intolerant of standard therapy for acute disease and were therefore placed on one of the alternative regimens. They were then continued on these alternative regimens (see text for references).
[f]The doses given for maintenance therapy are the same as those given for acute therapy in Table 15.6.

Encouraging results have been reported with other drug combinations. These include Fansidar and pyrimethamine–dapsone administered on an intermittent schedule (two to three times a week) (325, 328, 393). The long half-life of these agents allows for the longer dosing interval.

When pyrimethamine was used alone as maintenance therapy at 50 mg per day (292, 394) and 100 mg per day (292), the relapse rates were 10 to 28% and 5%, respectively. The efficacy of TMP–SMZ for maintenance therapy has not been sufficiently investigated. Further studies are required before specific recommendations can be made for other drug combinations.

ADJUNCTIVE THERAPY

Corticosteroids

Corticosteroids are frequently administered to patients with TE for reduction of cerebral edema and raised intracranial pressure, as well as when a mass effect causes a midline shift. The clinical response and survival in those patients with biopsy-proved TE who received corticosteroids in addition to antimicrobial therapy were no different than in those who received antimicrobial agents alone (181). A recent study confirmed no significant difference in the response rate and the time to response in patients who received corticosteroids when compared with those who did not (255). Other investigators have recommended the use of corticosteroids specifically in patients with acute TE who exhibit deteriorating levels of consciousness (115). Corticosteroid therapy should be reduced rapidly once clinical response is achieved, and in most instances, no more than 2 weeks of therapy is required (115). Corticosteroid use may also complicate interpretation of empiric therapy for presumed TE because partial clinical and radiologic improvement may result from the reduction in edema and the inflammatory response. Such improvement may also be observed in patients with CNS lymphoma. Corticosteroids are not required or advocated in toxoplasmic retinochoroiditis because histopathologic examination shows little intraretinal inflammation in the lesions (8, 131, 132).

Anticonvulsant Therapy

Seizures occur in 15 to 35% of patients with TE (12, 14, 103, 179, 181, 218). Anticonvulsant therapy should only be administered when seizures have occurred. Because of their numerous side effects and drug interactions, these agents should not be administered prophylactically. One retrospective study demonstrated a poorer outcome for those patients who received anticonvulsant therapy compared with those who did not (181). Whether this result represents a true drug effect or a selection bias (given that those receiving anticonvulsant therapy are likely to be more severely ill) is unclear.

Outcome

TE is uniformly fatal if left untreated. Clinical response to either of the standard antimicrobial regimens (see Table 15.5) is to be expected in 68 to 95% of patients (12, 14, 103, 179, 181, 218). Factors reported to be associated with a poorer outcome include depression of consciousness at presentation (254), fever higher than 38.4°C (103), presence of multiple lesions on neuroimaging studies (254, 255), previous opportunistic infections (103), and use of anticonvulsant therapy (181). In some studies, the median survival for patients from the time of acute therapy was 224 to 490 days (103, 181, 395). Even with appropriate antimicrobial treatment, as many as 40% of patients continued to have neurologic sequelae (179).

Prevention

Most AIDS patients at risk for development of TE can be clearly identified. They are those with preexisting IgG *Toxoplasma* antibodies. Thus, serologic testing for *Toxoplasma* antibodies should be performed in all HIV-infected patients. Patients with high IgG *Toxoplasma* antibody titers are at greater risk of developing TE (216, 217).

Prevention in HIV-infected patients involves two major strategies (see Table 15.1). The first is directed at instituting primary prophylaxis to patients who are *Toxoplasma* seropositive. The second is directed especially at those patients who are *Toxoplasma* seronegative and hence uninfected. In these latter individuals, education on how to avoid acquisition of primary infection is needed. In different geographic locales, reported annual seroconversion rates vary from 1 to 3% in these patients (120–122). Consideration should be given to repeat serologic testing for *Toxoplasma* IgG antibodies at least yearly to identify those who inadvertently become infected. We recommend that this be carried out until data from multiple geographic areas and in different ethnic groups are available to negate the value of such testing.

PRIMARY PROPHYLAXIS

Despite the availability of effective antimicrobial regimens, toxoplasmosis has been associated with a mortality rate as high as 70% by 12 months after the diagnosis of TE (105). TMP–SMZ (104, 396–399), pyrimethamine–dapsone (104, 326, 328, 393), and Fansidar (330, 331) have been reported to be effective. Dosage schedules are shown in Table 15.8.

In single studies, roxithromycin, administered at 300 mg three times a week (400), was reported to be effective. Some investigators have studied pyrimethamine for primary prophylaxis and have come to different conclusions regarding dosing and efficacy (119, 284, 401). In one such study, pyrimethamine actually was associated with a higher death rate (284), whereas in another study, no such correlation was found (119). Patients who developed a rash while they were receiving prophylactic therapy with pyrimethamine were also noted to be at higher risk of TE (286). At this time, pyrimethamine for primary prophylaxis cannot be recommended. Clarithromycin (402, 403) and spiramycin (404) have been reported to be ineffective for primary prophylaxis when used alone. A randomized, placebo-controlled trial demonstrated that, when clindamycin was administered at

Table 15.8. Regimens That Have Been Reported to Have Efficacy for Primary Prophylaxis of Toxoplasmic Encephalitis in AIDS Patients

Drug	Dosage Schedule	Reference
For toxoplasma-seropositive HIV-infected individuals[a]		
Trimethoprim–sulfamethoxazole	Oral, 1 DS tab once daily[b]	(347)
	Oral, 2 DS tab twice a week	(346)
Pyrimethamine[c]/dapsone	Oral pyrimethamine, 50 mg once a week, plus oral dapsone 50 mg once daily	(135)
	Oral pyrimethamine, 25 mg twice a week, plus oral dapsone, 100 mg twice a week	(293)
	Oral pyrimethamine, 75 mg once a week, plus oral dapsone, 200 mg once a week	(29)
Pyrimethamine/sulfadoxine (Fansidar)	Oral Fansidar, 3 tablets every 2 weeks	(296)
	Oral Fansidar, 1 tablet twice a week	(124)
For toxoplasma-seropositive HIV-infected pregnant women (no published data exist on the efficacy of primary prophylaxis in this population)[d]		
Spiramycin	Oral, 1000 mg q8h	

[a]Different dosage schedules have been reported. The dosages given are those from studies in which numbers of patients enrolled were adequate and the data were well described. Although in many of the studies, more frequent dosing schedules may have offered a trend toward better efficacy, this advantage may be offset by increased adverse reactions.
[b]One DS (double-strength) tablet of trimethoprim–sulfamethoxazole contains 160 mg trimethoprim and 800 mg sulfamethoxazole. Pyrimethamine/sulfadoxine is usually administered as tablets of Fansidar, each of which contains 25 mg pyrimethamine and 500 mg sulfadoxine.
[c]It is recommended that 10 to 20 mg folinic acid (leucovorin) be administered together with each dose of 25 to 75 mg pyrimethamine.
[d]Although at present no data exist on the efficacy of prophylaxis against congenital transmission in this group of patients, we consider it prudent to recommend spiramycin because preliminary studies by Mitchell and his colleagues suggest that the transmission rate for congenital toxoplasmosis in these women is remarkably and significantly higher when compared with non–HIV-infected, toxoplasma-seropositive women.

600 mg per day for primary prophylaxis, it was associated with an unacceptably high rate of gastrointestinal disease, in particular diarrhea, a finding suggesting that poor patient tolerance will prevent its further study for this purpose (405).

In some studies of TMP–SMX (396), pyrimethamine–dapsone (326), and Fansidar (330, 331) for primary prophylaxis, discontinuation of therapy as a result of adverse effects was reported in 29 to 39% of the patients. Thus, on an intent-to-treat basis, these regimens are not satisfactory for a significant number of AIDS patients.

Approximately 90% of patients who developed TE did so when their CD4+ T-cell counts were below $200/mm^3$. For this reason, we recommend instituting primary prophylaxis at this stage.

The pregnant woman who is dually infected with HIV and *Toxoplasma* poses a unique problem (discussed in the section of this chapter on congenital toxoplasmosis). Whether therapy is necessary or effective in preventing recrudescence of chronic *Toxoplasma* infection in the asymptomatic HIV-infected pregnant woman is not known. Although no information is currently available on the use of prophylaxis against congenital infection in this group of women, the high congenital transmission rate strongly suggests that intervention to reduce this transmission is necessary. Until more data are available, we recommend that these women receive oral spiramycin, 1 g every 8 hours, throughout their pregnancy if their CD4+ T-cell counts are below $200/mm^3$.

MEASURES TO PREVENT NEWLY ACQUIRED INFECTION

Education on the modes of transmission of *Toxoplasma gondii* infection and preventive measures are crucial for the HIV-infected patient who is *Toxoplasma* seronegative, and such an approach is recommended for the *Toxoplasma*-seropositive patient as well (see Table 15.1). The case reports of disseminated toxoplasmosis (165) and diffuse TE (116, 143) in AIDS patients who were either seronegative or had positive IgM titers most likely represent acute, recently acquired infections with devastating consequences. All meat and eggs should be cooked to "well done" (at least to 60°C) before ingestion. Only meat cooked to well done should be eaten. Tissue cysts in meat that is smoked or cured in brine will have been rendered noninfective (406), but ingestion of dried meat should be avoided. Freezing to −20°C for 24 hours also kills tissue cysts, but most commercially available meats have not been frozen to such temperatures. Patients should refrain from skinning animals, and hands should be washed after handling uncooked meat. Fruits and vegetables should be washed to remove oocysts. Contact with cat feces and cat litter removal must be avoided. Gloves should be worn when gardening.

Acknowledgments

We wish to acknowledge the thoughtful contributions from Benjamin Luft, Charles Mitchell, and Dieter Enzmann, who generously provided us with their unpublished data and insights into this fascinating protozoan infection in AIDS.

References

1. Vietzke WM, Gelderman AH, Grimley PM, et al. Toxoplasmosis complicating malignancy: experience at the National Cancer Institute. Cancer 1968;21:816–827.
2. Carey RM, Kimball AC, Armstrong D, et al. Toxoplasmosis: clinical experiences in a cancer hospital. Am J Med 1973;54:30–38.
3. McLeod R, Berry PF, Marshall WHJ, et al. Toxoplasmosis presenting as brain abscesses: diagnosis by computerized tomography and cytology of aspirated purulent material. Am J Med 1979;67:711–714.
4. Luft BJ, Remington JS. Toxoplasmic encephalitis in AIDS (AIDS commentary). Clin Infect Dis 1992;15:211–222.
5. Oksenhendler E, Cadranel J, Sarfati C, et al. *Toxoplasma gondii* pneumonia in patients with the acquired immunodeficiency syndrome. Am J Med 1990;88:5-18N–5-21N.
6. Schnapp L, Geaghan S, Campagna A, et al. *Toxoplasma gondii* pneumonitis in patients infected with the human immunodeficiency virus. Arch Intern Med 1992;152:1073–1076.
7. Rabaud C, May T, Amiel C, Katlama C, et al. Extracerebral toxoplasmosis in patients infected with HIV. Medicine 1994;73:306–314.

8. Friedman AH, Orellana J, Gagliuso DJ, et al. Ocular toxoplasmosis in AIDS patients. Trans Am Ophthalmol Soc 1990;88:63–88.
9. Lucet J-C, Bailly M-P, Bedos J-P, et al. Septic shock due to toxoplasmosis in patients infected with the human immunodeficiency virus. Chest 1993;104:1054–1058.
10. Albrecht H, Skörde J, Arasteh K, et al. Disseminated toxoplasmosis in AIDS patients: report of 16 cases. Scand J Infect Dis 1995;27:71–74.
11. Luft BJ, Remington JS. AIDS commentary: toxoplasmic encephalitis. J Infect Dis 1988;157:1–6.
12. Luft BJ, Brooks RG, Conley FK, et al. Toxoplasmic encephalitis in patients with acquired immune deficiency syndrome. JAMA 1984;252:913–917.
13. Levy RM, Bredesen DE, Rosenblum ML. Neurological manifestations of the acquired immunodeficiency syndrome (AIDS): experience at UCSF and review of the literature. J Neurosurg 1985;62:475–495.
14. Navia BA, Petito CK, Gold JW, et al. Cerebral toxoplasmosis complicating the acquired immune deficiency syndrome: clinical and neuropathological findings in 27 patients. Ann Neurol 1986;19:224–238.
15. Handler M, Ho V, Whelan M, et al. Intracerebral toxoplasmosis in patients with acquired immune deficiency syndrome. J Neurosurg 1983;59:994–1001.
16. Frenkel JK, Dubey JP, Miller NL. *Toxoplasma gondii* in cats: faecal stages identified as coccidian oocysts. Science 1970;167:893–896.
17. Pfefferkorn ER. Cell biology of *Toxoplasma gondii*. In: Wyler DJ, ed. Modern parasite biology: cellular, immunological, and molecular aspects. New York: WH Freeman, 1990:26–50.
18. Remington JS, Cavanaugh EN. Isolation of the encysted form of *Toxoplasma gondii* from human skeletal muscle and brain. N Engl J Med 1965;273:1308–1310.
19. Kasper LH. Identification of stage-specific antigens of *Toxoplasma gondii*. Infect Immun 1989;57:668–672.
20. Weiss L, LaPlace D, Tanowitz H, et al. Identification of *Toxoplasma gondii* bradyzoite-specific monoclonal antibodies [letter]. J Infect Dis 1992;166:213–215.
21. Bohne W, Hessemann J, Gross U. Induction of bradyzoite-specific *Toxoplasma gondii* antigens in gamma interferon–treated mouse macrophages. Infect Immun 1993;61:1141–1145.
22. Tomavo S, Fortier B, Soete M, et al. Characterization of bradyzoite-specific antigens of *Toxoplasma gondii*. Infect Immun 1991;59:3750–3753.
23. Jacobs L, Remington JS, Melton ML. The resistance of the encysted form of *Toxoplasma gondii*. J Parasitol 1960;46:11–21.
24. Dubey JP, Frenkel JK. Feline toxoplasmosis from acutely infected mice and the development of *Toxoplasma* cysts. J Protozool 1976;23:537–46.
25. Ferguson DJ, Hutchison WM. An ultrastructural study of the early development and tissue cyst formation of *Toxoplasma gondii* in the brains of mice. Parasitol Res 1987;73:483–91.
26. Sims TA, Hay J, Talbot IC. An electron microscope and immunohistochemical study of the intracellular location of *Toxoplasma* tissue cysts within the brains of mice with congenital toxoplasmosis. Br J Exp Pathol 1989;70:317–325.
27. Pavesio C, Chiappino M, Setzer P, et al. *Toxoplasma gondii:* differentiation and death of bradyzoites. Parasitol Res1992;78:1–9.
28. Dubey J, Kotula A, Sharar A, et al. Effect of high temperature on infectivity of *Toxoplasma gondii* tissue cysts in pork. J Parasitol 1990;76:201.
29. Dubey JP. Long-term persistence of *Toxoplasma gondii* in tissues of pigs inoculated with *T. gondii* oocysts and effect of freezing on viability of tissue cysts in pork. Am J Vet Res 1988;49:910–913.
30. Krahenbuhl JL, Remington JS. The immunology of toxoplasma and toxoplasmosis. In: Cohen S, Warren KS, eds. Immunology of parasitic infections. 2nd ed. London: Blackwell Scientific Publications, 1982:356–421.
31. Kaufman HE, Remington JS, Jacobs L. Toxoplasmosis: the nature of virulence. Am J Ophthalmol 1958;46:255–260.
32. Kaufman HE, Melton ML, Remington JS, et al. Strain differences of *Toxoplasma gondii*. J Parasitol 1959;45:189–190.
33. Handman E, Goding JW, Remington JS. Detection and characterization of membrane antigens of *Toxoplasma gondii*. J Immunol 1980;124:2578–2583.
34. Bulow R, Boothroyd JC. Protection of mice from fatal *Toxoplasma gondii* infection by immunization with p30 antigen in liposomes. J Immunol 1991;147:3496–3500.
35. Dardé M, Bouteille B, Pestre-Alexandre M. Isoenzyme analysis of 35 *Toxoplasma gondii* isolates and the biological and epidemiological implications. J Parasitol 1992;78:786–794.
36. Sibley LD, Boothroyd JC. Virulent strains of *Toxoplasma gondii* comprise a single clonal lineage. Nature 1992;359:82–85.
37. Howe DK, Sibley DL. *Toxoplasma gondii* comprises three clonal lineages: correlation of parasite genotype with human disease. J Infect Dis 1995;172:1561–1566.
38. Messina M, Kim S, Sibley LD. A family of dispersed DNA elements that contain GAA repeats in *Toxoplasma gondii*. Mol Biochem Parasitol 1996;81:247–252.
39. Wong S, Remington JS. Biology of *Toxoplasma gondii*. AIDS 1993;7:299–316.
40. McLeod R, Mack D, Brown C. *Toxoplasma gondii*: new advances in cellular and molecular biology. Exp Parasitol 1991;72:109–121.
41. Israelski DM, Remington JS. Toxoplasmosis in the non-AIDS immunocompromised host. In: Remington J, Swartz M, eds. Current clinical topics in infectious diseases. Vol. 13. London: Blackwell Scientific Publications, 1993:322–356.
42. Suzuki Y, Remington JS. Dual regulation of resistance against *Toxoplasma gondii* infection by Lyt-2+ and Lyt-1+, L3T4+ T cells in mice. J Immunol 1988;140:3943–3946.
43. Nagasawa H, Manabe T, Maekawa Y, et al. Role of L3T4$^+$ and Lyt-2$^+$ T cell subsets in protective immune responses of mice against infection with a low or high virulent strain of *Toxoplasma gondii*. Microbiol Immunol 1991;35:215–222.
44. Gazzinelli RT, Hakim FT, Hieny S, et al. Synergistic role of CD4+ and CD8+ T lymphocytes in IFN-γ production and protective immunity induced by an attenuated *Toxoplasma gondii* vaccine. J Immunol 1991;146:286–292.
45. Subauste CS, Koniaris AH, Remington JS. Murine CD8+ cytotoxic T lymphocytes lyse *Toxoplasma gondii*–infected cells. J Immunol 1991;147:3955–3959.
46. Hakim FT, Gazzinelli RT, Denkers E, et al. CD8+ T cells from mice vaccinated against *Toxoplasma gondii* are cytotoxic for parasite-infected or antigen-pulsed host cells. J Immunol 1991;147:2310–2316.
47. Murray H, Teitelbaum R, Hariprashad J. Response to treatment for an intracellular infection in a T cell–deficient host: toxoplasmosis in nude mice. J Infect Dis 1993;167:1173–1177.
48. Denkers E, Caspar P, Sher A. *Toxoplasma gondii* possesses a superantigen activity that selectively expands murine T cell receptor Vβ5-bearing CD8+ lymphocytes. J Exp Med 1994;180:985–994.
49. Denkers EY. A *Toxoplasma gondii* superantigen: biological effects and implications for the host–parasite interaction. Parasitol Today 1996;12:362–366.
50. Nagasawa H, Oka M, Maeda K, et al. Induction of heat shock protein closely correlates with protection against *Toxoplasma gondii* infection. Proc Natl Acad Sci U S A 1992;89:3155–3158.
51. Hisaeda H, Nagasawa H, Maeda K, et al. γδ T cells play an important role in hsp65 expression and in acquiring protective immune responses against infection with *Toxoplasma gondii*. J Immunol 1995;154:244–251.
52. de Paoli P, Basaglia G, Gennari D, et al. Phenotypic profile and functional characteristics of human gamma and delta T cells during acute toxoplasmosis. J Clin Microbiol 1992;30:729–731.
53. Scalise F, Gerli R, Castellucci G, et al. Lymphocytes bearing the γδ T-cell receptor in acute toxoplasmosis. Immunology 1992;76:668–670.
54. Subauste CS, Chung JY, Do D, et al. Preferential activation and expansion of human peripheral blood γδ T cells in response to *Toxoplasma gondii* in vitro and their cytokine production and cytotoxic

activity against *T. gondii*–infected cells. J Clin Invest 1995;96: 610–619.
55. Kasper LH, Ware PL. Recognition and characterization of stage-specific oocyst/sporozoite antigens of *Toxoplasma gondii* by human antisera. J Clin Invest 1985;75:1570–1577.
56. Schreiber RD, Feldman HA. Identification of the activator system for antibody to *Toxoplasma* as the classical complement pathway. J Infect Dis 1980;141:366–369.
57. Sabin AB, Feldman HA. Dyes as microchemical indicators of a new immunity phenomenon affecting a protozoan parasite *(Toxoplasma)*. Science 1948;108:660–663.
58. Foster BG, McCulloch WF. Studies of active and passive immunity in animals inoculated with *Toxoplasma gondii*. Can J Microbiol 1968;14: 103–110.
59. Pavia CS. Protection against experimental toxoplasmosis by adoptive immunotherapy. J Immunol 1986;137:2985–2990.
60. Johnson AM, McDonald PJ, Neoh SH. Monoclonal antibodies to *Toxoplasma* cell membrane surface antigens protect mice from toxoplasmosis. J Protozool 1983;30:351–356.
61. McCabe RE, Luft BJ, Remington JS. Effect of murine interferon gamma on murine toxoplasmosis. J Infect Dis 1984;150:961–962.
62. Suzuki Y, Conley FK, Remington JS. Treatment of toxoplasmic encephalitis in mice with recombinant gamma interferon. Infect Immun 1990;58:3050–3055.
63. Suzuki Y, Conley FK, Remington JS. Importance of endogenous IFN-γ for prevention of toxoplasmic encephalitis in mice. J Immunol 1989;143:2045–2050.
64. Suzuki Y, Yang Q, Yang S, et al. IL-4 is protective against development of toxoplasmic encephalitis. J Immunol 1996;157:2564–2569.
65. Sibley LD, Adams LB, Fukutomi Y, et al. Tumor necrosis factor-α triggers antitoxoplasmal activity of IFN-γ primed macrophages. J Immunol 1991;147:2340–2345.
66. Langermans J, van der Hulst M, Nibbering P, et al. IFN-γ induced L-arginine-dependent toxoplasmastatic activity in murine peritoneal macrophages is mediated by endogenous tumor necrosis factor. J Immunol 1992;148:568–574.
67. Gazzinelli R, Eltoum I, Wynn T, et al. Acute cerebral toxoplasmosis is induced by in vivo neutralization of TNF-α and correlates with the down-regulated expression of inducible nitric oxide synthase and other markers of macrophage activation. J Immunol 1993;151: 3672–3681.
68. Hunter CA, Remington JS. Immunopathogenesis of toxoplasmic encephalitis. J Infect Dis 1994;170:1057–1067.
69. Hunter CA, Litton MJ, Remington JS, et al. Immunocytochemical detection of cytokines in the lymph nodes and brains of mice resistant or susceptible to toxoplasmic encephalitis. J Infect Dis 1994;170: 939–945.
70. Hunter CA, Roberts CW, Murry M, et al. Detection of cytokine mRNA in the brains of mice with toxoplasmic encephalitis. Parasite Immunol 1992;14:405–413.
71. Chao CC, Hu S, Gekker G, et al. Effects of cytokines on multiplication of *Toxoplasma gondii* in microglial cells. J Immunol 1993;150: 3404–3410.
72. Gazzinelli R, Wysocka M, Hayashi S, et al. Parasite-induced IL-12 stimulates early IFN-γ synthesis and resistance during acute infection with *Toxoplasma gondii*. J Immunol 1994;153:2533–2543.
73. Hunter CA, Candolfi E, Subauste C, et al. Studies on the role of interleukin-12 in acute murine toxoplasmosis. Immunology 1995;84: 16–20.
74. Deckert-Schlüter M, Schlüter D, et al. Differential expression of ICAM-1, VCAM-1 and their ligands LFA-1, Mac-1, CD43, VLA-4, and MHC class II antigens in murine *Toxoplasma* encephalitis: a light microscopic and ultrastructural immunohistochemical study. J Neuropathol Exp Neurol 1994;53:457–468.
75. Nakayama I. Effects of immunization procedures in experimental toxoplasmosis. Keio J Med 1965;14:63–72.
76. Stadtsbaeder S, Nguyen BT, Calvin-Preval MC. Respective role of antibodies and immune macrophages during acquired immunity against toxoplasmosis in mice. Ann Immunol (Paris) 1975;126c: 461–474.
77. Vischer WA, Suter E. Intracellular multiplication of *Toxoplasma gondii* in adult mammalian macrophages cultivated in vitro. Proc Soc Exp Biol Med 1954;86:413–419.
78. Remington JS, Krahenbuhl JL, Mendenhall JW. A role for activated macrophages in resistance to infection with *Toxoplasma*. Infect Immun 1972;6:829–834.
79. Subauste CS, Dawson L, Remington JS. Human lymphokine-activated killer cells are cytotoxic against cells infected with *Toxoplasma gondii*. J Exp Med 1992;176:1511–1519.
80. Dannemann BR, Morris VA, Araujo FG, et al. Assessment of human natural killer and lymphokine-activated killer cell cytotoxicity against *Toxoplasma gondii* trophozoites and brain cysts. J Immunol 1989;143: 2684–2691.
81. Sher A, Oswald I, Hieny S, et al. *Toxoplasma gondii* induces a T-independent IFN-γ response in natural killer cells that requires both adherent accessory cells and tumor necrosis factor-α. J Immunol 1993;150:3982–3989.
82. Hunter CA, Subauste C, Van Cleave V, et al. Production of gamma interferon by natural killer cells from *Toxoplasma gondii*–infected SCID mice: regulation by interleukin-10, interleukin-12, and tumor necrosis factor alpha. Infect Immun 1994;62:2818–2824.
83. Erbe DV, Pfefferkorn ER, Fanger MW. Functions of the various human IgG Fc receptors in mediating killing of *Toxoplasma gondii*. J Immunol 1991;146:3145–3151.
84. Frenkel JK. Toxoplasmosis: parasite life cycle pathology and immunology. In: Hammond DM, Long PL, eds. The coccidia. Baltimore: University Park Press, 1973:343–410.
85. Kean BH, Kimball AC, Christenson WN. An epidemic of acute toxoplasmosis. JAMA 1969;208:1002–1004.
86. Frenkel JK, Dubey JP. Toxoplasmosis and its prevention in cats and man. J Infect Dis 1972;126:664–73.
87. Benenson MW, Takafuji ET, Lemon SM, et al. Oocyst-transmitted toxoplasmosis associated with ingestion of contaminated water. N Engl J Med 1982;307:666–669.
88. Jacobs L. The interrelation of toxoplasmosis in swine, cattle, dogs and man. Public Health Rep 1957;72:872–882.
89. Dubey JP, Murrell KD, Fayer R, et al. Distribution of *Toxoplasma gondii* tissue cysts in commercial cuts of pork. J Am Vet Med Assoc 1986;188:1035–1037.
90. Jacobs L, Remington JS, Melton ML. A survey of meat samples from swine, cattle, and sheep for the presence of encysted *Toxoplasma*. J Parasitol 1960;46:23–28.
91. Dubey JP, Kirkbride CA. Economic and public health considerations of congenital toxoplasmosis in lambs. J Am Vet Med Assoc 1989;195: 1715–1716.
92. Dubey JP. Status of toxoplasmosis in cattle in the United States. J Am Vet Med Assoc 1990;196:257–259.
93. Remington JS, Klein JO. Infectious diseases of the fetus newborn infant. 4th ed. Philadelphia: WB Saunders, 1995.
94. Siegel SE, Lunde MN, Gelderman AH, et al. Transmission of toxoplasmosis by leukocyte transfusion. Blood 1971;37:388–394.
95. Reynolds ES, Walls KW, Pfeiffer RI. Generalized toxoplasmosis following renal transplantation: report of a case. Arch Intern Med 1966;118:401–405.
96. Anthony CW. Disseminated toxoplasmosis in a liver transplant patient. J Am Med Wom Assoc 1972;27:601–603.
97. Stinson EB, Bieber CP, Griepp RB, et al. Infectious complications after cardiac transplantation in man. Ann Intern Med 1971;74: 22–36.
98. Ryning FW, McLeod R, Maddox JC, et al. Probable transmission of *Toxoplasma gondii* by organ transplantation. Ann Intern Med 1979; 90:47–49.
99. Luft BJ, Naot Y, Araujo FG, et al. Primary and reactivated *Toxoplasma* infection in patients with cardiac transplants: clinical spectrum and problems in diagnosis in a defined population. Ann Intern Med 1983;99:27–31.

100. Neu HC. Toxoplasmosis transmitted at autopsy. JAMA 1967;202: 284–285.
101. Remington JS, Gentry LO. Acquired toxoplasmosis: infection versus disease. Ann N Y Acad Sci 1970;174:1006–1017.
102. Levy RM, Janssen RS, Bush TJ, et al. Neuroepidemiology of acquired immunodeficiency syndrome. J Acquir Immune Defic Syndr 1988;1: 31–40.
103. Porter SB, Sande M. Toxoplasmosis of the central nervous system in the acquired immunodeficiency syndrome. N Engl J Med 1992;327: 1643–1648.
104. Podzamczer D, Salazar A, Jiménez J, et al. Intermittent trimethoprim–sulfamethoxazole compared with dapsone–pyrimethamine for the simultaneous primary prophylaxis of pneumocystis pneumonia and toxoplasmosis in patients infected with HIV. Ann Intern Med 1995;122:755–761.
105. Oksenhendler E, Charreau I, Tournerie C, et al. *Toxoplasma gondii* in advanced HIV infection. AIDS 1994;8:483–487.
106. Moore RD, Chaisson R, McArthur J. Natural history of central nervous system *Toxoplasmosis* [abstract]. In: 8th International Conference on AIDS. Amsterdam, Congrex Holland, 1992.
107. Luft BJ, Castro KG. An overview of the problem of toxoplasmosis and pneumocystosis in AIDS in the USA: implication for future therapeutic trials. Eur J. Clin Microbiol Infect Dis 1991;10:178–181.
108. Mathews W, Fullerton S. Use of a clinical laboratory database to estimate *Toxoplasma* seroprevalence among human immunodeficiency virus–infected patients. Arch Pathol Lab Med 1994;118:807–810.
109. Clumeck N. Some aspects of the epidemiology of toxoplasmosis and pneumocystosis in AIDS in Europe. Eur J Clin Microbiol Infect Dis 1991;10:177–178.
110. Zumla A, Savva D, Wheeler RB, et al. *Toxoplasma* serology in Zambian and Ugandan patients infected with the human immunodeficiency virus. Trans Roy Soc Trop Med Hyg 1991;85:227–229.
111. Grant IH, Gold JWM, Rosenblum M, et al. *Toxoplasma gondii* serology in HIV-infected patients: the development of central nervous system toxoplasmosis. AIDS 1990;4:519–521.
112. Matheron S, Dournon E, Garakhanian S, et al. Prevalence of toxoplasmosis in 365 AIDS and ARC patients before and during zidovudine treatment [abstract]. In: 6th International Conference on AIDS. San Francisco: University of California at San Francisco, 1990.
113. Zangerle R, Allerberger F, Pohl P, et al. High risk of developing toxoplasmic encephalitis in AIDS patients seropositive to *Toxoplasma gondii*. Med Microbiol Immunol 1991;180:59–66.
114. Pohle HD, Ruf B, Eichenlaub D, et al. CNS-toxoplasmosis in AIDS patients: incidence and results of treatment with pyrimethamine and macrolide antibiotics. Paper presented at the 4th International Conference on AIDS, Stockholm, Sweden, 1988.
115. Leport C, Remington JS. *Toxoplasmose* au cours du SIDA. Presse Med 1992;21:1165–1171.
116. Khuong MA, Matheron S, Marche C, et al. Diffuse toxoplasmic encephalitis (DTE) without abscess in AIDS patients [abstract]. Paper presented at the 30th Interscience Conference on Antimicrobial Agents and Chemotherapy, Atlanta, GA, 1990.
117. Post MJ, Chan JC, Hensley GT, et al. Toxoplasmosis encephalitis in Haitian adults with acquired immunodeficiency syndrome: a clinical-pathologic-CT correlation. Am J Neuroradiol 1983;4:155–162.
118. Lucas S, Hounnou A, Peacock C, et al. The mortality and pathology of HIV infection in a West African city. AIDS 1993;7:1569–1579.
119. Leport C, Chêne G, Morlat P, et al. Pyrimethamine for primary prophylaxis of toxoplasmic encephalitis in patients with human immunodeficiency virus infection: a double-blind, randomized trial. J Infect Dis 1996;173:91–97.
120. Partisani M, Candolfi E, De Mautort E, et al. Seroprevalence of latent *Toxoplasma gondii* infection in HIV-infected individuals and long-term follow up of *Toxoplasma* seronegative subjects. In: Program and Abstracts of the 7th International Conference on AIDS, Florence, Italy, 1991. Rome: International Conference on AIDS, 1991.
121. Sugar A, Zufferey J, Rudaz P, et al. Serology of latent toxoplasmic infection and cerebral toxoplasmosis in patients from the Swiss HIV Cohort Study [abstract]. In: 8th International Conference on AIDS. Amsterdam: Congrex Holland, 1992.
122. Wallace MR, Rossetti RJ, Olson PE. Cats and toxoplasmosis risk in HIV-infected adults. JAMA 1993;269:76–77.
123. Ferguson DJ, Hutchison WM, Pettersen E. Tissue cyst rupture in mice chronically infected with *Toxoplasma gondii*. Parasitol Res 1989;75: 599–603.
124. Johnson LL. SCID mouse models of acute and relapsing chronic *Toxoplasma gondii* infections. Infect Immun 1992;60:3719–3724.
125. Frenkel JK, Nelson BM, Arias SJ. Immunosuppression and toxoplasmic encephalitis: clinical and experimental aspects. Hum Pathol 1975;6:97–111.
126. Tirard V, Niel G, Rosenheim M, et al. Diagnosis of toxoplasmosis in patients with AIDS by isolation of the parasite from the blood. N Engl J Med 1991;324:632.
127. Lavareda DS, Maslo C, Depouy-Camet J, et al. PCR in blood for diagnosis of toxoplasmosis in AIDS patients. Paper presented at the 3rd European Conference Clinical Aspects and Treatment of HIV Infection, Paris, 1992.
128. Derouin F, Garin Y. Isolement de *Toxoplasma gondii*. Presse Med 1992;21:10–13.
129. Hofflin JM, Remington JS. Tissue culture isolation of *Toxoplasma* from blood of a patient with AIDS. Arch Intern Med 1985;145: 925–926.
130. Lamoril J, Molina J-M, Gouvello AD, et al. Detection by PCR of *Toxoplasma gondii* in blood in the diagnosis of cerebral toxoplasmosis in patients with AIDS. J Clin Pathol 1996;49:89–92.
131. Holland G, Engstrom R Jr, Glasgow B, et al. Ocular toxoplasmosis in patients with acquired immunodeficiency syndrome. Am J Ophthalmol 1988;106:653–667.
132. Cochereau-Massin I, LeHoang P, Lautier-Frau M, et al. Ocular toxoplasmosis in human immunodeficiency virus–infected patients. Am J Ophthalmol 1992;114:130–135.
133. Smith RE. Toxoplasmic retinochoroiditis as an emerging problem in AIDS patients [editorial]. Am J Ophthalmol 1988;106:738–739.
134. Suzuki Y, Joh K, Orellna MA, et al. A gene(s) within the H-2D region determines the development of toxoplasmic encephalitis in mice. Immunology 1991;74:732–739.
135. Brown CR, McLeod R. Class I MHC genes and CD8+ T cells determine cyst number in *Toxoplasma gondii* infection. J Immunol 1990;145:3438–3441.
136. Brown C, Hunter C, Estes R, et al. Definitive identification of a gene that confers resistance against *Toxoplasma* cyst burden and encephalitis. Immunology 1995;85:419–428.
137. Freund Y, Sgarlato G, Jacob C, et al. Polymorphisms in the tumor necrosis factor α (TNF-α) gene correlate with murine resistance to development of toxoplasmic encephalitis and with levels of TNF-α mRNA in infected brain tissue. J Exp Med 1992;175:683–688.
138. Brown C, Estes R, Beckmann E, et al. Definitive identification of a gene that confers resistance against toxoplasmosis. In: 47th Annual Meeting Opportunistic Protozoan Pathogens. Cleveland: Society of Protozoologists, 1994.
139. Suzuki Y, Wong S-Y, Grumet FC, et al. Evidence for genetic regulation of susceptibility to toxoplasmic encephalitis in AIDS patients. J Infect Dis 1996;173:265–268.
140. Pomeroy C, Filice G, Hitt J, et al. Cytomegalovirus-induced reactivation of *Toxoplasma gondii* in mice: lung lymphocyte phenotypes and suppressor function. J Infect Dis 1992;166:677–81.
141. Casado-Naranjo I, Lopez-Trigo J, et al. Hemorrhagic abscess in a patient with the acquired immunodeficiency syndrome. Neuroradiology 1988;31:289.
142. Strittmatter C, Lang W, Wiestler OD, et al. The changing pattern of human immunodeficiency virus associated cerebral toxoplasmosis: a study of 46 postmortem cases. Acta Neuropathol 1992;83:475–481.
143. Gray F, Gherardi R, Wingate E, Wingate J, et al. Diffuse "encephalitic" cerebral toxoplasmosis in AIDS. J Neurol 1989;236:273–277.
144. Conley FK, Jenkins KA, Remington JS. *Toxoplasma gondii* infection of the central nervous system: use of the peroxidase-antiperoxidase

method to demonstrate toxoplasma in formalin fixed, paraffin embedded tissue sections. Hum Pathol 1981;12:690–698.
145. Moskowitz LB, Hensley GT, Chan JC, et al. Brain biopsies in patients with acquired immune deficiency syndrome. Arch Pathol Lab Med 1984;108:368–371.
146. Falangola M, Petito C. Choroid plexus infection in cerebral toxoplasmosis in AIDS patients. Neurology 1993;43:2035–2040.
147. Herskovitz S, Siegel SE, Schneider AT, et al. Spinal cord toxoplasmosis in AIDS. Neurology 1989;39:1552–1553.
148. Harris TM, Smith RR, Bognanno JR, et al. Toxoplasmic myelitis in AIDS: gadolinium-enhanced MR. J Comput Assist Tomogr 1990;14:809–811.
149. Kayser C, Campbell R, Sartorious C, et al. Toxoplasmosis of the conus medullaris in a patient with hemophilia A–associated AIDS. J Neurosurg 1990;73:951–953.
150. Overhage JM, Greist A, Brown DR. Conus medullaris syndrome resulting from *Toxoplasma gondii* infection in a patient with the acquired immunodeficiency syndrome. Am J Med 1990;89:814–815.
151. Catterall JR, Hofflin JM, Remington JS. Pulmonary toxoplasmosis. Am Rev Respir Dis 1986;133:704–705.
152. Pomeroy C, Filice GA. Pulmonary toxoplasmosis: a review. Clin Infect Dis 1992;14:863–870.
153. Derouin F, Sarfati C, Beauvais B, et al. Laboratory diagnosis of pulmonary toxoplasmosis in patients with acquired immunodeficiency syndrome. J Clin Microbiol 1989;27:1661–1663.
154. Bottone EJ. Diagnosis of acute pulmonary toxoplasmosis by visualization of invasive and intracellular tachyzoites in Giemsa-stained smears of bronchoalveolar lavage fluid. J Clin Microbiol 1991;29:2626–2627.
155. Roth A, Roth B, Höffken G, et al. Application of the polymerase chain reaction to diagnosis of pulmonary toxoplasmosis in immunocompromised patients. Eur J Clin Microbiol Infect Dis 1992;11:1177–1181.
156. Lavrard I, Chouaid C, Roux P, et al. Pulmonary toxoplasmosis in HIV-infected patients: usefulness of polymerase chain reaction and cell culture. Eur Respir J 1995;8:697–700.
157. Bretagne S, Costa J-M, Fleury-Feith J, et al. Quantitative competitive PCR with bronchoalveolar lavage fluid for diagnosis of toxoplasmosis in AIDS patients. J ClinMicrobiol 1995;33:1662–1664.
158. Roldan EO, Moskowitz L, Hensley GT. Pathology of the heart in acquired immunodeficiency syndrome. Arch Pathol Lab Med 1987;111:943–946.
159. Hofman P, Drici M-D, Gibelin P, et al. Prevalence of *Toxoplasma* myocarditis in patients with the acquired immunodeficiency syndrome. Br Heart J 1993;70:376–381.
160. Cappell MS, Mikhail N, Ortega A. *Toxoplasma* myocarditis in AIDS. Am Heart J 1992:1728–1729.
161. Scully RE, Mark EJ, McNeely WF, et al. Case records of the Massachusetts General Hospital: weekly clinicopathological exercises. N Engl J Med 1992;327:790–799.
162. Tschirhart D, Klatt E. Disseminated toxoplasmosis in the acquired immunodeficiency syndrome. Arch Pathol Lab Med 1988;112:1237–1241.
163. Adair OV, Randive N, Krasnow N. Isolated *Toxoplasma* myocarditis in acquired immune deficiency syndrome. Am Heart J 1989;118:856–857.
164. Guerot E, Aissa F, Kayal S, et al. Toxoplasma pericarditis in acquired immunodeficiency syndrome. Intensive Care Med 1995;21:229–230.
165. Garcia LW, Hemphill RB, Marasco WA, et al. Acquired immunodeficiency syndrome with disseminated toxoplasmosis presenting as an acute pulmonary and gastrointestinal illness. Arch Pathol Lab Med 1991;115:459–463.
166. Gherardi R, Baudrimont M, Lionnet F, et al. Skeletal muscle toxoplasmosis in patients with acquired immunodeficiency syndrome: a clinical and pathological study. Ann Neurol 1992;32:535–542.
167. Pauwels A, Meyohas MC, Eliaszewicz M, et al. *Toxoplasma* colitis in the acquired immunodeficiency syndrome. Am J Gastroenterol 1992;87:518–519.
168. Smart PE, Weinfeld A, Thompson NE, et al. Toxoplasmosis of the stomach: a cause of antral narrowing. Radiology 1990;174:369–370.
169. Crider SR, Horstman WG, Massey GS. *Toxoplasma* orchitis: report of a case and a review of the literature. Am J Med 1988;85:421–424.
170. Nistal M, Santana A, Paniaqua R, et al. Testicular toxoplasmosis in two men with the acquired immunodeficiency syndrome (AIDS). Arch Pathol Lab Med 1986;110:744–746.
171. Brion J-P, Pelloux H, Le Marc'hadour F, et al. Acute toxoplasmic hepatitis in a patient with AIDS. Clin Infect Dis 1992;15:183–184.
172. Calico I, Caballero E, Martinez O, et al. Isolation of *Toxoplasma gondii* from immunocompromised patients using tissue culture [letter]. Infection 1991;19:340–342.
173. Bergin C, Murphy M, Lyons D, et al. Toxoplasma pneumonitis: fatal presentation of disseminated toxoplasmosis in a patient with AIDS. Eur Respir J 1992;5:1018–1020.
174. Groll A, Schneider M, Althoff PH, et al. Morphology and clinical significance of AIDS-related lesions in the adrenals and pituitary. Dtsch Med Wochenschr 1990;115:483–488.
175. Brouland JP, Audouin J, Hofman P, et al. Bone marrow involvement by disseminated toxoplasmosis in acquired immunodeficiency syndrome: the value of bone marrow trephine biopsy and immunohistochemistry for the diagnosis. Hum Pathol 1996;27:302–306.
176. Hofman P, Quintens H, Michiels J-F, et al. *Toxoplasma* cystitis associated with acquired immunodeficiency syndrome. Urology 1993;42:589–592.
177. Gluckman G, Werboff L. Toxoplasmosis of the bladder: case report and review of the literature. J Urol 1994;151:1629–1630.
178. Gandhi S, Lyubsky S, Jimenez-Lucho V. Adult respiratory distress syndrome associated with disseminated toxoplasmosis. Clin Infect Dis 1994;19:169–171.
179. Pedrol E, Gonzales-Clemente JM, Gatell JM, et al. Central nervous system toxoplasmosis in AIDS patients: efficacy of an intermittent maintenance therapy. AIDS 1990;4:511–517.
180. Renold C, Sugar A, Chave J-P, et al. Toxoplasma encephalitis in patients with the acquired immunodeficiency syndrome. Medicine 1992;71:224–239.
181. Cohn J, McMeeking A, Cohen W, et al. Evaluation of the policy of empiric treatment of suspected *Toxoplasma* encephalitis in patients with the acquired immunodeficiency syndrome. Am J Med 1989;86:521–527.
182. Hamed LM, Schatz NJ, Galetta SL. Brainstem ocular motility defects and AIDS. Am J Ophthalmol 1988;106:437–442.
183. Carrazana EJ, Rossitch EJ, Samuels MA. Parkinsonian symptoms in a patient with AIDS and cerebral toxoplasmosis. J Neurol Neurosurg Psychiatry 1989;52:1445–1446.
184. Tolge CF, Factor SA. Focal dystonia secondary to cerebral toxoplasmosis in a patient with acquired immune deficiency syndrome. Mov Disord 1991;6:69–72.
185. Koppel BS, Daras M. "Rubral" tremor due to midbrain *Toxoplasma* abscess. Mov Disord 1990;5:254–256.
186. Sanchez-Ramos JR, Factor SA, Weiner WJ, et al. Hemichorea–hemiballismus associated with acquired immune deficiency syndrome and cerebral toxoplasmosis. Mov Dis 1989;4:266–273.
187. Milligan SA, Katz MS, Craven PC, et al. Toxoplasmosis presenting as panhypopituitarism in a patient with the acquired immune deficiency syndrome. Am J Med 1984;77:760–764.
188. Wijdicks EFM, Borleffs JCC, Hoepelman AIM, et al. Fatal disseminated hemorrhagic toxoplasmic encephalitis as the initial manifestation of AIDS. Ann Neurol 1991;29:683–686.
189. Farkash AE, Maccabee PJ, Sher JH, et al. CNS toxoplasmosis in acquired immune deficiency syndrome: a clinical-pathological-radiological review of 12 cases. J Neurol Neurosurg Psychiatry 1986;49:744–748.
190. Arendt G, Hefter H, Figge C, et al. Two cases of cerebral toxoplasmosis in AIDS patients mimicking HIV-related dementia. J Neurol 1991;238:439–442.

191. Chaudhari AB, Singh A, Jindal S, et al. Hœmorrhage in cerebral toxoplasmosis: a report on a patient with the acquired immunodeficiency syndrome. S Afr Med J 1989;76:272–274.
192. Vyas R, Ebright JR. Toxoplasmosis of the spinal cord in a patient with AIDS: case report and review. Clin Infect Dis 1996;23:1061–1065.
193. Mehren M, Burns PJ, Mamani F, et al. Toxoplasmic myelitis mimicking intramedullary spinal cord tumor. Neurology 1988;38:1648–1650.
194. Weber R, Deplazes P, Flepp M, et al. Cerebral microsporidiosis due to *Encephalitozoon cuniculi* in a patient with human immunodeficiency virus infection. N Engl J Med 1997;336:474–478.
195. Derouin F, Sarfati C, Beauvais B, et al M. Prevalence of pulmonary toxoplasmosis in HIV-infected patients. AIDS 1990;4:1036.
196. Rabaud CTM, Lucet JC, Leport C, et al. Pulmonary toxoplasmosis in patients infected with human immunodeficiency virus: a French national study. Clin Infect Dis 1996;23:1249–1254.
197. Schuman JS, Friedman AH. Retinal manifestations of the acquired immune deficiency syndrome (AIDS): cytomegalovirus, *Candida albicans, Cryptococcus,* toxoplasmosis and *Pneumocystis carinii.* Trans Ophthalmol Soc U K 1983;103:177–190.
198. Friedman AH. The retinal lesions of the acquired immune deficiency syndrome. Trans Am Ophthalmol Soc 1984;82:447–491.
199. Heinemann MH, Gold JM, Maisel J. Bilateral toxoplasma retinochoroiditis in a patient with acquired immune deficiency syndrome. Retina 1986;6:224–227.
200. Dupon M, Cazenave J, Pellegrin J-L, et al. Detection of *Toxoplasma gondii* by PCR and tissue culture in cerebrospinal fluid and blood of human immunodeficiency virus–seropositive patients. J Clin Microbiol 1995;33:2421–2426.
201. Verbraak FD, Galema M, Hans van den Horn G, et al. Serological and polymerase chain reaction-based analysis of aqueous humour samples in patients with AIDS and necrotizing retinitis. AIDS 1996;10:1091–1099.
202. Grange F, Kinney EL, Monsuez J-J, et al. Successful therapy for *Toxoplasma gondii* myocarditis in acquired immuniodeficiency syndrome. Am Heart J 1990;120:443–444.
203. Israelski DM, Skowron G, Leventhal JP, et al. *Toxoplasma* peritonitis in a patient with acquired immunodeficiency syndrome. Arch Intern Med 1988;148:1655–1657.
204. Yang M, Path MCR, Perez E. Disseminated toxoplasmosis as a cause of diarrhea. South Med J 1995;88:860–861.
205. Hofman P, Michiels J, Mondain V, et al. Pancréatite aiguë toxoplasmique. Gastroenterol Clin Biol 1994;18:895–897.
206. Hirschmann JV, Chu AC. Skin lesions with disseminated toxoplasmosis in a patient with the acquired immunodeficiency syndrome [letter]. Arch Dermatol 1988;124:1446–1447.
207. Mitchell CD, Lewis L, McLellan S, et al. Increased risk of congenital toxoplasmosis (Ct) among infants born to mothers infected with HIV-1 and *Toxoplasma gondii* [abstract]. In: Program and Abstracts of 3rd Conference on Retroviruses and Opportunistic Infections, Washington, DC, 1996.
208. European Collaborative Study Group. Low incidence of congenital toxoplasmosis in children born to women infected with human immunodeficiency virus. Eur J Obstet Gynecol Reprod Biol 1996;68:93–96.
209. Minkoff H, Remington JS, Holman S, et al. Vertical transmission of toxoplasma by human immunodeficiency virus-infected women. Am J Obstet Gynecol 1997;176:555–559.
210. Mitchell CD, Erlich SS, Mastrucci MT, et al. Congenital toxoplasmosis occurring in infants perinatally infected with human immunodeficiency virus 1. Pediatr Infect Dis J 1990;9:512–518.
211. Miller MJ, Remington JS. Toxoplasmosis in infants and children with HIV infection or AIDS. In: Pizzo PA, Wilfert CM, eds. Pediatric AIDS: the challenge of HIV infection in infants, children, and adolescents. Baltimore: Williams & Wilkins, 1990:299–307.
212. Liesenfeld O, Press C, Montoya JG, et al. False-positive results in immunoglobulin M (IgM) toxoplasma antibody tests and importance of confirmatory testing: the *Platelia toxo* IgM test. J Clin Microbiol 1997;35:174–178.
213. Wong B, Gold JWM, Brown AE, et al. Central-nervous-system toxoplasmosis in homosexual men and parenteral drug abusers. Ann Intern Med 1984;100:36–42.
214. Israelski DM, Chmiel JS, Poggensee L, et al. Prevalence of *Toxoplasma* infection in a cohort of homosexual men at risk of AIDS and toxoplasmic encephalitis. J Acquir Immune Defic Syndr 1993;6:414–418.
215. Candolfi E, Partisani M, De Mautort E, et al. Serologic prevalence of toxoplasma infection in 346 individual infected with HIV in East France. Presse Med 1992;21:394–395.
216. Derouin F, Leport C, Pueyo S, et al. Predictive value of *Toxoplasma gondii* antibody titres on the occurrence of toxoplasmic encephalitis in HIV-infected patients. AIDS 1996;10:1521–1527.
217. Hellerbrand C, Goebel FD, Disko R. High predictive value of *Toxoplasma gondii* IgG antibody levels in HIV-infected patients for diagnosis of cerebral toxoplasmosis. Eur J Clin Microbiol Infect Dis 1996;15:869–872.
218. Haverkos HW. Assessment of therapy for toxoplasma encephalitis: the TE Study Group. Am J Med 1987;82:907–14.
219. Holliman RE. Clinical and diagnostic findings in 20 patients with toxoplasmosis and the acquired immune deficiency syndrome. J Med Microbiol 1991;35:1–4.
220. Dannemann BR, Vaughan WC, Thulliez P, et al. Differential agglutination test for diagnosis of recently acquired infection with *Toxoplasma gondii.* J Clin Microbiol 1990;28:1928–1933.
221. Suzuki Y, Israelski DM, Dannemann BR, et al. Diagnosis of toxoplasmic encephalitis in patients with acquired immunodeficiency syndrome by using a new serologic method. J Clin Microbiol 1988;26:2541–2543.
222. Weiss LM, Udem SA, Tanowitz H, et al. Western blot analysis of the antibody response of patients with AIDS and toxoplasma encephalitis: antigenic diversity among *Toxoplasma* strains. J Infect Dis 1988;157:7–13.
223. Hassl A, Aspöck H. Antigens of *Toxoplasma gondii* recognized by sera of AIDS patients before, during, and after clinically important infections. Int J Med Microbiol 1990;272:514–525.
224. Remington JS, McLeod R. Toxoplasmosis. In: Gorbach SL, Bartlett JG, Blacklow NR, eds. Infectious diseases. Philadelphia: WB Saunders, 1992:1328–1343.
225. Araujo FG, Barnett EV, Gentry LO, et al. False-positive anti-*Toxoplasma* fluorescent-antibody tests in patients with antinuclear antibodies. Appl Microbiol 1971;22:270–275.
226. Pinon JM, Foudrinier F, Mougheto G, et al. Evaluation of risk and diagnostic value of quantitative assays for anti-*Toxoplasma gondii* immunoglobulin A (IgA), IgE, and IgM and analytical study of specific IgG in immunodeficient patients. J Clin Microbiol 1995;33:878–884.
227. Pinon JM, Thoannes H, Pouletty PH, et al. Detection of IgA specific for toxoplasmosis in serum and cerebrospinal fluid using a non-enzymatic IgA-capture assay. Diagn Immunol 1986;4:223–227.
228. Stepick-Biek P, Thulliez P, Araujo FG, et al. IgA antibodies for diagnosis of acute congenital and acquired toxoplasmosis. J Infect Dis 1990;162:270–273.
229. Sulahian A, Nugues C, Garin Y, et al. Serodiagnosis of toxoplasmosis in patients with acquired or reactivating toxoplasmosis and analysis of the specific IgA antibody response by ELISA agglutination and immunoblotting. Immunol Infect Dis 1993;3:63–69.
230. Gross U, Roos T, Appoldt D, et al. Improved serological diagnosis of *Toxoplasmosis gondii* Infection by detection of immunoglobulin A (IgA) and IgM antibodies against P30 by using the immunoblot technique. J Clin Microbiol 1992;30:1436–1441.
231. Pinon JM, Toubas D, Marx C, et al. Detection of specific immunoglobulin E in patients with toxoplasmosis. J Clin Microbiol 1990;28:1739–1743.
232. Wong SY, Hadju M-P, Ramirez R, et al. The role of specific immunoglobulin E in diagnosis of acute *Toxoplasma* infection and toxoplasmosis. J Clin Microbiol 1993;31:2952–2959.
233. Pinon JM, Thoannes H, Gruson N. An enzyme-linked immunofiltration assay used to compare infant and maternal antibody profiles in toxoplasmosis. J Immunol Meth 1985;77:15–23.

234. Poirriez J, Toubas D, Marx-Chemia C, et al. Isotypic characterization of anti-*Toxoplasma gondii* antibodies in 18 cases of congenital toxoplasmic chorioretinitis. Acta Ophthalmol 1988;67:164–168.
235. Araujo FG, Remington JS. Antigenemia in recently acquired acute toxoplasmosis. J Infect Dis 1980;141:144–50.
236. Huskinson J, Stepick-Biek P, Remington JS. Detection of antigens in urine during acute toxoplasmosis. J Clin Microbiol 1989;27:1099–1101.
237. Grover CM, Thulliez P, Remington JS, et al. Rapid prenatal diagnosis of congenital *Toxoplasma* infection by using polymerase chain reaction and amniotic fluid. J Clin Microbiol 1990;28:2297–2301.
238. van de Ven E, Melchers W, Galama J, et al. Identification of *Toxoplasma gondii* infections by B1 gene amplification. J Clin Microbiol 1991;19:2120–2124.
239. Brezin AP, Egwuagu CE, Burnier M, et al. Identification of *Toxoplasma gondii* in paraffin-embedded sections by the polymerase chain reaction. Am J Ophthalmol 1990;110:599–604.
240. Holliman RE, Johnson JD, Savva D. Diagnosis of cerebral toxoplasmosis in association with AIDS using the polymerase chain reaction. Scand J Infect Dis 1990;22:243–244.
241. Parmley SF, Goebel FD, Remington JS. Detection of *Toxoplasma gondi* DNA in cerebrospinal fluid from AIDS patients by polymerase chain reaction. J Clin Microbiol 1992;30:3000–3002.
242. Schoondermark-van de Van E, Galama J, Kraaijeveld C, et al. Value of the polymerase chain reaction for the detection of *Toxoplasma gondii* in cerebrospinal fluid from patients with AIDS. Clin Infect Dis 1993;16:661–6.
243. Novati R, Castagna A, Morsica G, et al. Polymerase chain reaction for *Toxoplasma gondii* DNA in the cerebrospinal fluid of AIDS patients with focal brain lesions. AIDS 1994;8:1691–1694.
244. Cingolani A, De Luca A, Ammassari A, et al. Detection of *T. gondii*–DNA by PCR in AIDS-related toxoplasmic encephalitis. J Eukaryot Microbiol 1996;43:118S–119S.
245. Robert F, Ouatas T, Blanche P, et al. Evaluation retrospective de la detection de *Toxoplasma gondii* par reaction de polymerisation en chaine chez des patients sidéens. Presse Med 1996;25:541–545.
246. Foudrinier F, Aubert D, Puygauthier-Toubas D, et al. Detection of *Toxoplasma gondii* in immunodeficient subjects by gene amplification: influence of therapeutics. Scand J Infect Dis 1996;28:383–386.
247. Khalifa K, Roth A, Roth B, et al. Value of PCR for evaluating occurrence of parasitemia in immunocompromised patients with cerebral and extracerebral toxoplasmosis. J Clin Microbiol 1994;32:2813–2819.
248. Dupouy-Camet J, Lavareda de Souza L, Maslo C, et al. Detection of *Toxoplasma gondii* in venous blood from AIDS patients by polymerase chain reaction. J Clin Microb 1993;31:1866–1869.
249. Eggers C, Grob U, Klinker H, et al. Limited value of cerebrospinal fluid for direct detection of *Toxoplasma gondii* in toxoplasmic encephalitis associated with AIDS. J Neurol 1995;242:644–649.
250. Cinque P, Scarpellini P, Vago L, et al. Diagnosis of central nervous system complications in HIV-infected patients: cerebrospinal fluid analysis by the polymerase chain reaction. AIDS 1997;11:1–17.
251. Derouin F, Mazeron MC, Garin YJ. Comparative study of tissue culture and mouse inoculation methods for demonstration of *Toxoplasma gondii*. J Clin Microbiol 1987;25:1597–1600.
252. Derouin F, Garin Y, Beauvais B, et al. Tissue culture isolation of *T. gondii* for diagnosis of toxoplasmosis in AIDS patients. Paper presented at the 3rd European Conference Clinical Aspects and Treatment of HIV Infection, Paris, 1992.
253. Dannemann BR, McCutchan JA, Israelski DM, et al. Treatment of acute toxoplasmosis with intravenous clindamycin. Eur J Clin Microbiol Infect Dis 1991;10:193–195.
254. Dannemann BR, McCutchan JA, Israelski DA, et al. Treatment of toxoplasmic encephalitis in patients with AIDS: a randomized trial comparing pyrimethamine plus clindamycin to pyrimethamine plus sulfadiazine. Ann Intern Med 1992;116:33–43.
255. Luft BJ, Hafner R, Korzun AH, et al. Toxoplasmic encephalitis in patients with the acquired immunodeficiency syndrome. N Engl J Med 1993;329:995–1000.
256. Potasman I, Resnick L, Luft BJ, et al. Intrathecal production of antibodies against *Toxoplasma gondii* in patients with toxoplasmic encephalitis and the acquired immunodeficiency syndrome (AIDS). Ann Intern Med 1988;108:49–51.
257. Orefice G, Carrieri PB, de Marinis T, et al. Use of the intrathecal synthesis of antitoxoplasma antibodies in the diagnositc assessment and in the follow-up of AIDS patients with cerebral toxoplasmosis. Acta Neurol (Napoli) 1990;12:79–81.
258. Pedro-Botet J, Soriano JC, Tomás S, et al. Adenosine deaminase in cerebrospinal fluid of cerebral toxoplasmosis in AIDS. Infection 1991;19:13–17.
259. Post MJ, Kursunoglu SJ, Hensley GT, et al. Cranial CT in acquired immunodeficiency syndrome: spectrum of diseases and optimal contrast enhancement technique. AJNR Am J Neuroradiol 1985;6:743–754.
260. Levy RM, Rosenbloom S, Perrett LV. Neuroradiologic findings in AIDS: a review of 200 cases. AJNR Am J Neuroradiol 1986;147:977–983.
261. Whelan MA, Kricheff II, Handler M, et al. Acquired immunodeficiency syndrome: cerebral computed tomographic manifestations. Radiology 1983;149:477–484.
262. Weisberg LA, Greenberg J, Stazio A. Computed tomographic findings in cerebral toxoplasmosis in adults. Comput Med Imaging Graph 1988;12:379–383.
263. De La Paz R, Enzmann D. Neuroradiology of acquired immunodeficiency syndrome. In: Rosenblum ML, ed. AIDS and the nervous system. New York: Raven Press, 1988:121–154.
264. Post MJ, Chan JC, Hensley GT, et al. *Toxoplasma* encephalitis in Haitian adults with acquired immunodeficiency syndrome: a clinical-pathologic-CT correlation. AJR Am J Roentgenol 1983;140:861–868.
265. Jarvik JG, Hesselink JR, Kennedy C, et al. Acquired immunodeficiency syndrome: magnetic resonance patterns of brain involvement with pathologic correlation. Arch Neurol 1988;45:731–736.
266. Kupfer MC, Zee C-S, Colletti PM, et al. MRI evaluation of AIDS-related encephalopathy: toxoplasmosis vs lymphoma. Magn Reson Imaging 1990;8:51–57.
267. Ciricillo SF, Rosenblum ML. Use of CT and MR imaging to distinguish intracranial lesions and to define the need for biopsy in AIDS patients. J Neurosurg 1990;73:720–724.
268. Ciricillo SF, Rosenblum ML. Imaging of solitary lesions in AIDS [letter]. J Neurosurg 1991;74:1029.
269. Lorberboym M, Estok L, Machac J, et al. Rapid differential diagnosis of cerebral toxoplasmosis and primary central nervous system lymphoma by Thallium-201 SPECT. J Nucl Med 1996;37:1150–1154.
270. Barker DE, Trepashko D, DeMarais P, et al. Utility of thallium brain SPECT in the exclusion of CNS lymphoma in AIDS [abstract]. Paper presented at the 4th Annual Conference on Retroviruses and Opportunistic Infections, Washington, DC, 1996.
271. Goodman PC, Schnapp LM. Pulmonary toxoplasmosis in AIDS. Radiology 1992;184:791–793.
272. Araujo FG, Remington JS. Recent advances in the research for new drugs for treatment of toxoplasmosis. Int J Antimicrob Agents 1992;1:153–164.
273. Van Delden C, Gabriel V, Sudre P, et al. Reasons for failure of prevention of *Toxoplasma* encephalitis. AIDS 1996;10:509–513.
274. Weiss L, Luft B, Tanowitz H, et al. Pyrimethamine concentrations in serum during treatment of acute murine experimental toxoplasmosis. Am J Trop Med Hyg 1992;46:288–291.
275. Leport C, Meulemans A, Dameron G, et al. Levels of pyrimethamine in serum of AIDS patients treated for toxoplasmic encephalitis [abstract]. Paper presented at the 4th European Congress of Clinical Microbiology, Nice, France, 1989.
276. Leport C, Meulemans A, Robine D, et al. Levels of pyrimethamine in serum and penetration into brain tissue in humans. AIDS 1992;6:1040–1041.
277. Klinker H, Langmann P, Richter E. Plasma pyrimethamine concentrations during long-term treatment for cerebral toxoplasmosis in

patients with AIDS. Antimicrob Agents Chemother 1996;40: 1623–1627.
278. Kaufman HE, Caldwell LA. Pharmacological studies of pyrimethamine (Daraprim) in man. Arch Ophthalmol 1959;61:885–890.
279. Weiss LM, Harris C, Berger M, et al. Pyrimethamine concentrations in serum and cerebrospinal fluid during treatment of acute *Toxoplasma* encephalitis in patients with AIDS. J Infect Dis 1988;157: 580–583.
280. Remington JS, Vilde JL, Antunes F, et al. Clindamycin for toxoplasmosis encephalitis in AIDS [letter]. Lancet 1991;338:1142–1143.
281. Geils GF, Scott CW, Baugh CM, et al. Treatment of meningeal leukemia with pyrimethamine. Blood 1971;38:131–137.
282. Stickney DR, Simmons WS, DeAngelis RL, et al. Pharmacokinetics of pyrimethamine (PRM) and 2,4-diamino-5-(3′,4′-dichlorophenyl)-6-methylpyrimidine (DMP) relevant to meningeal leukemia. Proc Am Assoc Cancer Res 1973;14:52.
283. Kaufman HE, Geisler PH. The hematologic toxicity of pyrimethamine (Daraprim) in man. Arch Ophthalmol 1960;64:140–146.
284. Jacobson M, Besch C, Child C, et al. Primary prophylaxis with pyrimethamine for toxoplasmic encephalitis in patients with advanced human immunodeficiency virus disease: results of a randomized trial. J Infect Dis 1994;169:384–394.
285. Jacobson JM, Davidian M, Rainey PM, et al. Pyrimethamine pharmacokinetics in human immunodeficiency virus-positive patients seropositive for *Toxoplasma gondii*. Antimicrob Agents Chemother 1996; 40:1360–1365.
286. Rousseau F, Pueyo S, Morlat P, et al. Increased risk of toxoplasmic encephalitis in human immunodeficiency virus-infected patients with pyrimethamine-related rash. Clin Infect Dis 1997;24:396–402.
287. Leport C, Raffi F, Matheron S, et al. Treatment of central nervous system toxoplasmosis with pyrimethamine-sulfadiazine combination in 35 patients with the acquired immunodeficiency syndrome: efficacy of long-term continuous therapy. Am J Med 1988;84:94–100.
288. Eyles DE, Coleman N. The relative activity of the common sulfonamides against toxoplasmosis in the mouse. Am J Trop Med Hyg 1953;2:54–63.
289. Cook MK, Jacobs L. In vitro investigations on the action of pyrimethamine against *Toxoplasma gondii*. J Parasitol 1958;44:280–288.
290. Eyles DE, Coleman N. Synergistic effect of sulfadiazine and Daraprim against experimental toxoplasmosis in the mouse. Antibiot Chemother 1953;3:483–490.
291. Eyles DE, Coleman N. An evaluation of the curative effects of pyrimethamine and sulfadiazine, alone and in combination, on experimental mouse toxoplasmosis. Antibiot Chemother 1955;5:529–539.
292. Maslo C, Matheron S, Saimot AG. Cerebral toxoplasmosis: assessment of maintenance therapy. In: 7th International Conference on AIDS. Amsterdam: Congrex Holland, 1992.
293. Podzamczer D, Miró J, Bolao F, et al.. Twice-weekly maintenance therapy with sulfadiazine–pyrimethamine to prevent recurrent toxoplasmic encephalitis in patients with AIDS. Ann Intern Med 1995; 123:175–180.
294. Carbone LG, Bendixen B, Appel GB. Sulfadiazine-associated obstructive nephropathy occurring in a patient with the acquired immunodeficiency syndrome. Am J Kidney Dis 1988;12:72–75.
295. Sahai J, Heimberger T, Collins K, et al. Sulfadiazine-induced crystalluria in a patient with the acquired immunodeficiency syndrome: a reminder [letter]. Am J Med 1988;84:791–792.
296. Torroba AL, Hermida DJ, Ezpeleta BC, et al. Metahemoglobinemia secundaria al tratamiento de infecciones oportunistas en pacientes con SIDA. Rev Clin Esp 1988;182:289–90.
297. Young C. Acute encephalopathy associated with sulfadiazine in a patient with AIDS-related complex. J Infect Dis 1989;160:163–164.
298. Reboli AC, Mandler HD. Encephalopathy and psychoses associated with sulfadiazine in two patients with AIDS and CNS toxoplasmosis. Clin Infect Dis 1992;15:556–557.
299. Israelski DM, Remington JS. AIDS-associated toxoplasmosis. In: Sande MA, Volberding PA, eds. The medical management of AIDS. 3rd ed. Philadelphia: WB Saunders, 1992:319–345.
300. Tenant-Flowers M, Boyle MJ, Carey D, et al. Sulphadiazine desensitization in patients with AIDS and cerebral toxoplasmosis. AIDS 1991;5:311–315.
301. Torgovnick J, Arsura E. Desensitization to sulfonamides in patients with HIV infection. Am J Med 1990;88:548–549.
302. Gluckstein D, Ruskin J. Rapid oral desensitization to trimethoprim–sulfamethoxazole (TMP–SMZ): use in prophylaxis for *Pneumocystis carinii* pneumonia in patients with AIDS who were previously intolerant to TMP–SMZ. Clin Infect Dis 1995;20:849–853.
303. Piketty C, Gilquin J, Kazatchkine M. Efficacy and safety of desensitization to trimethoprim–sulfamethoxazole in human immunodeficiency virus-infected patients. J Infect Dis 1995;172:611.
304. Araujo FG, Remington JS. Effect of clindamycin on acute and chronic toxoplasmosis in mice. Antimicrob Agents Chemother 1974; 5:647–51.
305. Hofflin JM, Remington JS. Clindamycin in a murine model of toxoplasmic encephalitis. Antimicrob Agents Chemother 1987;31: 492–496.
306. Rolston KV, Hoy J. Role of clindamycin in the treatment of central nervous system toxoplasmosis. Am J Med 1987;83:551–554.
307. Katlama C. Evaluation of the efficacy and safety of clindamycin plus pyrimethamine for induction and maintenance therapy of toxoplasmic encephalitis in AIDS. Eur J Clin Microbiol Infect Dis 1991;10: 189–91.
308. Katlama C, De Wit S, O'Doherty E, et al. Pyrimethamine–clindamycin vs. pyrimrthamine–sulfadiazine as acute and long-term therapy for toxoplasmic encephalitis in patients with aids. Clin Infect Dis 1996; 22:268–275.
309. Coppola S, Angarano G, Monno L, et al. Adverse effects of clindamycin in the treatment of cerebral toxoplasmosis in AIDS patients [abstract]. In: Program and Abstracts of 7th International Conference on AIDS, Florence, Italy, 1991. Rome: International Conference on AIDS, 1991.
310. Köhler S, Delwiche CF, Denny PW, et al. A plastid of probable green algal origin in apicomplexan parasites. Science 1997;275: 1485–1489.
311. Araujo FG, Shepard RM, Remington JS. In vivo activity of the macrolide antibiotics azithromycin, roxithromycin and spiramycin against *Toxoplasma gondii*. Eur J Clin Microbiol Infect Dis 1991;10: 519–524.
312. Grossman PL, Remington JS. The effect of trimethoprim and sulfamethoxazole on *Toxoplasma gondii* in vitro and in vivo. Am J Trop Med Hyg 1979;28:445–455.
313. Feldman HA. Effects of trimethoprim and sulfisoxazole alone and in combination on murine toxoplasmosis. J Infect Dis 1973;128: S774–S776.
314. Solbreux P, Sonnet J, Zech F. A retrospective study about the use of cotrimoxazole as diagnostic support and treatment of suspected cerebral toxoplasmosis in AIDS. Acta Clin Belg 1990;45:85–96.
315. Canessa A, Del Bono V, De Leo P, et al. Cotrimoxazole therapy of *Toxoplasma gondii* encephalitis in AIDS patients. Eur J Clin Microbiol Infect Dis 1992;11:125–130.
316. Herrera G, Villalta O, Visona K. Trimethoprim–sulfametoxazole treatment of toxoplasma encephalitis in AIDS patients [abstract]. In: Programs and abstracts of 7th International Conference on AIDS, Florence, Italy, 1991. Rome: International Conference on AIDS, 1991.
317. Allegra CJ, Kovacs JA, Drake JC, et al. Potent in vitro and in vivo antitoxoplasma activity of the lipid-soluble antifolate trimetrexate. J Clin Invest 1987;79:478–482.
318. Kovacs JA, Allegra CJ, Chabner BA, et al. Potent effect of trimetrexate, a lipid-soluble antifolate, on *Toxoplasma gondii*. J Infect Dis 1987; 155:1027–1032.
319. Masur H, Polis M, Tuazon C, et al. Salvage trial of trimetrexate–leucovorin for the treatment of cerebral toxoplasmosis in patients with AIDS. J Infect Dis 1993;167:1422–1426.
320. Araujo FG, Guptill DR, Remington JS. In vivo activity of piritrexin against *Toxoplasma gondii*. J Infect Dis 1987;156:828–830.

321. Allegra CJ, Boarman D, Kovacs JA, et al. Interaction of sulfonamide and sulfone compounds with *Toxoplasma gondii* dihydropteroate synthase. J Clin Invest 1990;85:371–379.
322. Eyles DE, Coleman N. An evaluation of the effect of sulfones on experimental toxoplasmosis in the mouse. Antibiot Chemother 1957; 7:578–585.
323. Derouin F, Picketty C, Chastang C, et al. Anti-*Toxoplasma* effects of dapsone alone and combined with pyrimethamine. Antimicrob Agents Chemother 1991;35:252–255.
324. Ward DJ. Dapsone/pyrimethamine for the treatment of *Toxoplasmic Encephalitis* [abstract]. In: 7th International Conference on AIDS. Amsterdam: Congrex Holland, 1992.
325. Opravil M, Hirschel B, Lazzarin A, et al. Once-weekly administration of dapsone/pyrimethamine vs. aerosolized pentamidine as a combined prophylaxis for *Pneumocystis carinii* pneumonia and toxoplasmic encephalitis in human immunodeficiency virus-infected patients. Clin Infect Dis 1995;20:531–541.
326. Girard P-M, Landman R, Gaudebout C, et al. Dapsone–pyrimethamine compared with aerosolized pentamidine as a primary prophylaxis against *Pneumocystis carinii* pneumonia and toxoplasmosis in HIV infection. N Engl J Med 1993;328:1514–1520.
327. Clotet B, Sirera G, Romeu J, et al. Twice weekly dapsone–pyrimethamine for preventing primary and secondary pneumocystis carinii pneumonia (PCP): its role in the prevention of cerebral toxoplasmosis [abstract]. In: Program and Abstracts of 7th International Conference on AIDS, Florence, Italy, 1991. Rome: International Conference on AIDS, 1991.
328. Torres R, Barr M, Thorn M, et al. Randomized trial of dapsone and aerosolized pentamidine for the prophylaxis of *Pneumocystis carinii* pneumonia and toxoplasmic encephalitis. Am J Med 1993;95:573–583.
329. Paulic P, Pestre P, Bonnet E, et al. Treatment of brain toxoplasmosis by Fansidar [abstract]. In: 6th International Conference on AIDS. San Francisco: University of California at San Francisco, 1990.
330. Köppen S, Grunewald T, Jautzke G, et al. Prevention of *Pneumocystis carinii* pneumonia and toxoplasmic encephalitis in human immunodeficiency virus infected patients: a clinical approach comparing aerosolized pentamidine and pyrimethamine/sulfadoxine. Clin Invest 1992;70:508–512.
331. Partisani M, De Mautort E, Hassairi N, et al. Primary prophylaxis of cerebral toxoplasmosis with pyrimethamine-sulfadoxine in human immunodeficiency virus-infected individuals seropositive to *Toxoplasma* [abstract]. In: 8th International Conference on AIDS. Amsterdam: Congrex Holland, 1992.
332. Araujo FG, Guptill DR, Remington JS. Azithromycin, a macrolide antibiotic with potent activity against *Toxoplasma gondii*. Antimicrob Agents Chemother 1988;32:755–757.
333. Chang HR, Rudareanu FC, Pechere JC. Activity of A-56268 (TE-031), a new macrolide, against *Toxoplasma gondii* in mice. J Antimicrob Chemother 1988;22:359–361.
334. Luft BJ. In vivo and in vitro activity of roxithromycin against *Toxoplasma gondii* in mice. Eur J Clin Microbiol 1987;6:479–481.
335. Chang HR, Pechere JC. Activity of roxithromycin against *Toxoplasma gondii* in murine models. J Antimicrob Chemother 1987;20:69–74.
336. Derouin F, Chastang C. Activity in vitro against *Toxoplasma gondii* of azithromycin and clarithromycin alone and with pyrimethamine. J Antimicrob Chemother 1990;25:708–711.
337. Huskinson-Mark J, Araujo FG, Remington JS. Evaluation of the effect of drugs on the cyst form of *Toxoplasma gondii*. J Infect Dis 1991;164:170–177.
338. Remington JS. Macrolides, azalides, and streptogramins in treatment of opportunistic infections in immunocompromised patients. In: Zinner ST, Young LS, Acar JF, et al., eds. Expanding indications for the new macrolides, azalides, and streptogramins. New York: Marcel Dekker, 1997:189–204.
339. Farthing C, Rendel M, Currie B, et al. Azithromycin for cerebral toxoplasmosis. Lancet 1992;339:437.
340. Fernandez-Martin J, Leport C, Morlat P, et al. Pyrimethamine–clarithromycin combination for therapy of acute *Toxoplasma* encephalitis in patients with AIDS. Antimicrob Agents Chemother 1991; 35:2049–2052.
341. Chang HR, Comte R, Pechere JC. In vitro and in vivo effects of doxycycline on *Toxoplasma gondii*. Antimicrob Agents Chemother 1990;34:775–780.
342. Tabbara KF, Sakuragi S, O'Connor GR. Minocycline in the chemotherapy of murine toxoplasmosis. Parasitology 1982;84:297–302.
343. Chang HR, Comte R, Piguet P-F, et al. Activity of minocycline against *Toxoplasma gondii* infection in mice. J Antimicrob Chemother 1991; 27:639–645.
344. Pope-Pegram L, Gathe J Jr, Bohn B, et al. Treatment of presumed central nervous system toxoplasmosis with doxycycline [abstract]. In: Program and Abstracts of 7th International Conference on AIDS, Florence, Italy, 1991. Rome: International Conference on AIDS, 1991.
345. Turett G, Pierone G, Masci J, et al. Failure of doxycycline in the treatment of cerebral toxoplasmosis [abstract]. In: 6th International Conference on AIDS. San Francisco: University of California at San Francisco, 1990.
346. Araujo FG, Huskinson J, Remington JS. Remarkable in vitro and in vivo activities of the hydroxynaphthoquinone 566C80 against tachyzoites and tissue cysts of *Toxoplasma gondii*. Antimicrob Agents Chemother 1991;35:293–299.
347. Kovacs JA. Efficacy of atovaquone in treatment of toxoplasmosis in patients with AIDS. Lancet 1992;340:637–638.
348. Clumeck N, Katlama C, Ferrero T, et al. Atovaquone (1.4 hydroxynaphtoquione, 566C80) in the treatment of acute cerebral toxoplasmosis (CT) in AIDS Patients (P) [abstract]. Paper presented at the 32nd Interscience Conference on Antimicrobial Agents and Chemotherapy, Anaheim, CA, 1992.
349. Torres R, Weinberg W, Stansell J, et al. Atovaquone for salvage treatment and suppression of toxoplasmic encephalitis in patients with AIDS. Clin Infect Dis 1996;24:422–429.
350. Katlama C, Mouthon B, Gourdon D, et al. Atovaquone as long-term suppressive therapy for toxoplasmic encephalitis in patients with AIDS and multiple drug intolerance. AIDS 1996;10:1107–1112.
351. Kovacs JA, Polis MA, Blair B, et al. Evaluation of azithromycin or the combination of 566C80 and pyrimethamine in the treatment of toxoplasmosis [abstract]. In: 8th International Conference on AIDS. Amsterdam: Congrex Holland, 1992.
352. Luft BJ. Potent in vivo activity of arprinocid, a purine analogue, against murine toxoplasmosis. J Infect Dis 1986;154:692–694.
353. Ou-yang K, Krug EC, Marr JJ, et al. Inhibition of growth of *Toxoplasma gondii* by qinghaosu and derivatives. Antimicrob Agents Chemother 1990;34:1961–1965.
354. Lindsay DS, Blagburn BL, Hall JE, et al. Activity of pentamidine and pentamidine analogs against *Toxoplasma gondii* in cell cultures. Antimicrob Agents Chemother 1991;35:1914–1916.
355. Harris C, Salgo MP, Tanowitz HB, et al. In vitro assessment of antimicrobial agents against *Toxoplasma gondii*. J Infect Dis 1988; 157:14–22.
356. Eliaszewicz M, Kirstetter M, Meyohas M, et al. Treatment of cerebral toxoplasmosis by clindamycin and 5-fluorouracil [abstract]. In: 5th International Conference on AIDS: the scientific and social challenge. Montreal, Quebec, Canada, 1989. Ottawa: International Development Research Center, 1989.
357. Dhiver C, Milandre C, Poizot-Martin I, et al. 5-Fluro-uracil-clindamycin for treatment of cerebral toxoplasmosis. AIDS 1993;7:143–144.
358. Araujo FG, Slifer T, Remington JS. Rifabutin is active in murine models of toxoplasmosis. Antimicrob Agents Chemother 1994;38:570–575.
359. Araujo FG, Khan AA, Remington JS. Rifapentine is active in vitro and in vivo against *Toxoplasma gondii*. Antimicrob Agents Chemother 1996;40:1335–1337.

360. Khan AA, Slifer T, Araujo FG, et al. Trovafloxacin is active against *Toxoplasma gondii*. Antimicrob Agents Chemother 1996;40:1855–1859.
361. Polis MA, Masur H, Tuazon C, et al. Salvage trial of trimetrexate-leucovorin for treatment of cerebral toxoplasmosis in AIDS patients [abstract]. Clin Res 1989;37:437A.
362. Beverley JKA, Fry BA. Sulphadimidine, pyrimethamine and dapsone in the treatment of toxoplasmosis in mice. Br J Pharmacol 1957;12:189–193.
363. Araujo FG, Prokocimer P, Remington JS. Clarithromycin-minocycline is synergistic in a murine model of toxoplasmosis [letter]. J Infect Dis 1992;165:788.
364. Derouin F, Almadany R, Chau F, et al. Synergistic activity of azithromycin and pyrimethamine or sulfadiazine in acute experimental toxoplasmosis. Antimicrob Agents Chemother 1992;36:997–1001.
365. Araujo FG, Lin T, Remington JS. Synergistic combination of azithromycin and sulfadiazine for treatment of toxoplasmosis in mice. Eur J Microbiol Infect Dis 1992;11:71–72.
366. Araujo FG, Prokocimer P, Lin T, et al. Activity of clarithromycin alone or in combination with other drugs for treatment of murine toxoplasmosis. Antimicrob Agents Chemother 1992;36:2454–2457.
367. Araujo FG, Remington JS. Recent advances in the search for new drugs for treatment of toxoplasmosis. Int J Antimicrob Agents 1992;1:153–164.
368. Araujo FG, Lin T, Remington JS. The activity of atovaquone (566C80) in murine toxoplasmosis is markedly augmented when used in combination with pyrimethamine or sulfadiazine. J Infect Dis 1993;167:494–497.
369. Araujo FG, Suzuki Y, Remington JS. Use of rifabutin in combinations with atovaquone, clindamycin, pyrimethamine or sulfadiazine for treatment of toxoplasmic encephalitis in mice. Eur J Clin Microbiol Infect Dis 1996;15:394–397.
370. Suzuki Y, Orellana MA, Schreiber RD, et al. Interferon-γ: the major mediator of resistance against *Toxoplasma gondii*. Science 1988;240:516–518.
371. Orellana MA, Suzuki Y, Araujo FG, et al. Role of beta interferon in resistance to *Toxoplasma gondii* infection. Infect Immun 1991;59:3287–3290.
372. Sharma SD, Hofflin JM, Remington JS. In vivo recombinant interleukin 2 administration enhances survival against a lethal challenge with *Toxoplasma gondii*. J Immunol 1985;135:4160–4163.
373. Chang HR, Grau GE, Pechere JC. Role of TNF and IL-1 in infections with *Toxoplasma gondii*. Immunology 1990;69:33–37.
374. Canessa A, Del Bono V, Miletich F, et al. Serum cytokines in toxoplasmosis: increased levels of interferon-γ in immunocompetent patients with lymphadenopathy but not in AIDS patients with encephalitis [letter]. J Infect Dis 1992;165:1168–1170.
375. Murray HW, Gellene RA, Libby DM, et al. Activation of tissue macrophages from AIDS patients: in vitro response of AIDS alveolar macrophages to lymphokines and interferon-gamma. J Immunol 1985;135:2374–2377.
376. Murray HW, Scavuzzo D, Jacobs JL, et al. In vitro and in vivo activation of human mononuclear phagocytes by interferon-gamma: studies with normal and AIDS monocytes. J Immunol 1987;138:2457–2462.
377. Delemarre F, Stevenhagen A, Kroon F, et al. Effect of IFN-γ on the proliferation of *Toxoplasma gondii* in monocytes and monocyte-derived macrophages from AIDS patients. Immunology 1994;83:646–650.
378. Delemarre F, Stevehagen A, Snijders F, et al. Restoration of the toxoplasmastiatic activity of monocytes from AIDS patients during in vivo treatment with Interferon-γ. J Infect Dis 1993;168:516–517.
379. Hofflin JM, Remington JS. In vivo synergism of roxithromycin (RU 965) and interferon against *Toxoplasma gondii*. Antimicrob Agents Chemother 1987;31:346–348.
380. Araujo FG, Remington JS. Synergistic activity of azithromycin and gamma interferon in murine toxoplasmosis. Antimicrob Agents Chemother 1991;35:1672–1673.
381. Israelski DM, Remington JS. Activity of gamma interferon in combination with pyrimethamine or clindamycin in treatment of murine toxoplasmosis. Eur J Clin Microbiol Infect Dis 1990;9:358–360.
382. Araujo FG, Hunter CA, Remington JS. Treatment with interleukin 12 in combination with atovaquone or clindamycin significantly increases survival of mice with acute toxoplasmosis. Antimicrob Agents Chemother 1997;41:188–190.
383. Wanke C, Tuazon CU, Kovacs A, et al. *Toxoplasma* encephalitis in patients with acquired immune deficiency syndrome: diagnosis and response to therapy. Am J Trop Med Hyg 1987;36:509–516.
384. Chappell ET, Guthrie BL, Orenstein J. The role of stereotactic biopsy in the management of HIV-related focal brain lesions. Neurosurgery 1992;30:825–829.
385. Levy RM, Bredesen DE. Central nervous system dysfunction in acquired immunodeficiency syndrome. J Acquir Immune Defic Syndr 1988;1:41–64.
386. Mathews C, Barba D, Fullerton SC. Early biopsy versus empiric treatment with delayed biopsy of non-responders in suspected HIV-associated cerebral toxoplasmosis: a decision analysis. AIDS 1995;9:1243–1250.
387. Leport C, Raguin G, Vilde JL. Toxoplasmosis in AIDS [abstract]. In: 17th International Congress of Chemotherapy, Berlin, 1991. Munich: Futuramed, 1991.
388. Madlener J, Enzensberger W, Herdt P, et al. Neurological outcome and follow-up after successful treatment of CNS toxoplasmosis [abstract] In: 8th International Conference on AIDS. Amsterdam: Congrex Holland, 1992.
389. Leport C, Bastuji-Garin S, Perronne C, et al. An open study of the pyrimethamine-clindamycin combination in AIDS patients with brain toxoplasmosis [letter]. J Infect Dis 1989;160:557–558.
390. Fong IW, Glazer S, Fletcher D, et al. Recurrence of CNS toxoplasmosis in AIDS patients of chronic suppressive treatment [abstract]. In: 8th International Conference on AIDS. Amsterdam: Congrex Holland, 1992.
391. Daniel P. Randomized daily vs. twice-weekly maintenance therapy with sulfadiazine–pyrimethamine for cerebral toxoplasmosis in AIDS patients: preliminary results [abstract]. In: 8th International Conference on AIDS. Amsterdam, 1992.
392. Heald A, Flepp M, Chave J-P, et al. Treatment for cerebral toxoplasmosis protects against *Pneumocystis carinii* pneumonia in patients with AIDS. Ann Intern Med 1991;115:760–763.
393. Clotet B, Sirera G, Romeu J, et al. Twice-weekly dapsone–pyrimethamine for preventing PCP and cerebral toxoplasmosis. AIDS 1991;5:601–2.
394. de Gans J, Portegies P, Reiss P, et al. Pyrimethamine alone as maintenance therapy for central nervous system toxoplasmosis in 38 patients with AIDS. J Acquir Immune Defic Syndr 1992;5:137–142.
395. Moore RD, Chaisson RE. Natural history of opportunistic disease in an HIV-infected urban clinical cohort. Ann Intern Med 1996;124:634–642.
396. Carr A, Tindall B, Brew BJ, et al. Low-dose trimethoprim–sulfamethoxazole prophylaxis for toxoplasmic encephalitis in patients with AIDS. Ann Intern Med 1992;117:106–111.
397. Michelet C, Raffi F, Besnier J, et al. Cotrimoxazole (CMX) versus aerosolized pentamidine (AP) for primary prophylaxis of *Pneumocystis carinii* pneumonia (PCP). In: 33rd International Conference on Antimicrobial Agents and Chemotherapy. New Orleans: American Society of Microbiology, 1993.
398. Antinori A, Murri R, Ammassari A, et al. Aerosolized pentamidine, cotrimoxazole and dapsone–pyrimethamine for primary prophylaxis of *Pneumocystis carinii* pneumonia and toxoplasmic encephalitis. AIDS 1995;9:1343–1350.
399. Bozzette SA, Finkelstein DM, Spector SA, et al. A randomized trial of three antipneumocytstis agents in patients with advanced human immunodeficiency virus infection. N Engl J Med 1995;332:693–699.

400. Durant J, Hazime F, Carles M, et al. Prevention of *Pneumocystis carinii* pneumonia and of cerebral toxoplasmosis by roxithromycin in HIV-infected patients. Infection 1995;23:S33–S38.
401. Klinker H, Langmann P, Richter E. Pyrimethamine alone as prophylaxis for cerebral toxoplasmosis in patients with advanced HIV infection. Infection 1996;4:324–328.
402. Ruf B, Schurmann D, Pohle H. Failure of clarithromycin in preventing toxoplasmic encephalitis in AIDS patients [letter]. J Acquir Immune Defic Syndr 1992;5:530–531.
403. Raffi F, Struillou L, Ninin E, et al. Breakthrough cerebral toxoplasmosis in patients with AIDS who are being treated with clarithromycin. Clin Infect Dis 1995;20:1076–1077.
404. Leport C, Vilde JL, Katlama C, et al. Failure of spiramycin to prevent neurotoxoplasmosis in immunosuppressed patients [letter]. JAMA 1986;255:2290.
405. Jacobson M, Besch C, Child C, et al. Toxicity of clindamycin as prophylaxis for AIDS-associated toxoplasmic encephalitis. Lancet 1992;339:333–334.
406. Work K. Resistance of *Toxoplasma gondii* encysted in pork. Acta Pathol Microbiol Scand 1968;73:85–92.

16
TUBERCULOSIS

Robert W. Shafer and Jose G. Montoya

Before the first AIDS cases were diagnosed in 1981, one-third of the world's population was estimated to be infected with *Mycobacterium tuberculosis* (1). Each year 8 to 10 million persons developed active disease, and nearly 3 million persons died of tuberculosis (TB) (1). As many as 7% of all deaths and 26% of preventable deaths in developing countries were caused by TB (1, 2). Nonetheless, before the emergence of the human immunodeficiency virus (HIV), most *M. tuberculosis* infections were successfully dealt with by the host immune response and remained latent for the lifetime of the human host (3). With host and pathogen in a standoff, the elimination of TB from parts of the industrialized world was considered an achievable goal, and inroads into TB control had been made in many developing nations (1, 2, 4).

The HIV pandemic has changed the epidemiology and natural history of TB in many parts of the world. HIV infection is the strongest risk factor for the progression of latent *Mycobacterium tuberculosis* infection to active TB (5–7). Conversely, TB is the most common life-threatening HIV-related infection worldwide and is often the sentinel illness of HIV infection (8, 9). The HIV pandemic has stalled the elimination of TB in the United States and has created a dire situation in many of the most heavily afflicted countries (8, 10–14). The World Health Organization (WHO) Tuberculosis Programme estimated that by the end of 1997 more than 15 million persons worldwide were coinfected with both *M. tuberculosis* and HIV (Table 16.1 and Fig 16.1).

PATHOGENESIS

Mycobacterium Tuberculosis Infection

TB differs from all other HIV-related infections in that it is communicable through the airborne route. *Mycobacterium tuberculosis* infection is acquired by inhaling infectious airborne particles small enough (approximately 1 to 5 μm) to reach the alveolar air spaces. The probability of infection depends on the intensity of exposure and probably also on the effectiveness of innate and acquired host defenses. Alveolar macrophages from some individuals may have a high degree of innate mycobacterial resistance, and in these individuals, tubercle bacilli are presumably destroyed before infection is established (3, 15). In other individuals, inhaled mycobacteria survive phagocytosis, replicate, and spread to regional lymph nodes and throughout the body. Although investigators have reported functional macrophage defects (16, 17) and abnormal lung surfactant (18) in HIV-infected individuals, no data show that HIV-infected persons are more susceptible than HIV-seronegative persons to becoming infected with *M. tuberculosis* after similar exposures.

Immunologic Response to *Mycobacterium Tuberculosis*

The cell-mediated immune response to *Mycobacterium tuberculosis* is characterized by complex interactions among different subsets of lymphocytes and monocyte–macrophage cells (19). After ingesting mycobacteria, macrophages produce many monokines, including interleukin-10 (IL-10), IL-12, tumor necrosis factor-α (TNF-α), IL-1, IL-6, and transforming growth factor-β (TGF-β) (20–22). *M. tuberculosis*–specific precursor T-cell lymphocytes (CD4+ T cells, CD8+ T cells, and γδ T cells) are stimulated to proliferate and secrete lymphokines. These lymphokines, in turn, recruit circulating monocytes and induce their maturation into macrophages with enhanced phagocytic and microbicidal activity. In the ensuing granulomatous response, tubercle bacilli are killed by repeated cycles of phagocytosis, cytolysis, and exposure to microbicidal products.

As more is learned about the immune response to *Mycobacterium tuberculosis* from in vitro and animal models, the apparent division of labor among different cell types has become blurred. For example, T-cell subsets, such as CD4+ cells, CD8+ cells, and γδ cells not only are a source of antigen-specific cytokine production, but also serve as cytotoxic effector cells against *M. tuberculosis*–infected macrophages (23, 24). In addition to presenting antigens to T lymphocytes, macrophages also secrete cytokines with immunoregulatory properties (21). Nonetheless, CD4+ T cells play a dominant role in the cellular immune response against *M. tuberculosis* (3, 19, 21). Adoptive transfer of CD4+ T cells from sensitized to naive mice confers protection against *M. tuberculosis* infection (25), whereas mice depleted of CD4+ T cells are not able to contain mycobacterial infections (26, 27).

Table 16.1 Estimated Numbers of Adults Infected with Tuberculosis (TB) and HIV at the End of 1997

Region	HIV Infected (thousands)	TB Infected (%)	HIV/TB Infected Number (thousands)	HIV/TB Infected Percentage of total (%)
Sub-Saharan Africa	19,830	59	11,700	76.30
North Africa and Middle East	203	37	75	0.49
Latin America and Caribbean	1,585	29	460	3.00
South and Southeast Asia	5,911	48	2,837	18.50
East Asia and Pacific	437	31	135	0.88
Australia and New Zealand	12	7	1	0.01
North America	851	7	60	0.39
Western Europe	525	8	42	0.27
Eastern Europe and Central Asia	145	16	23	0.15
All Regions	**29,499**		**15,333**	**100.00**

(Data from Tuberculosis Programme, World Health Organization, Geneva.)

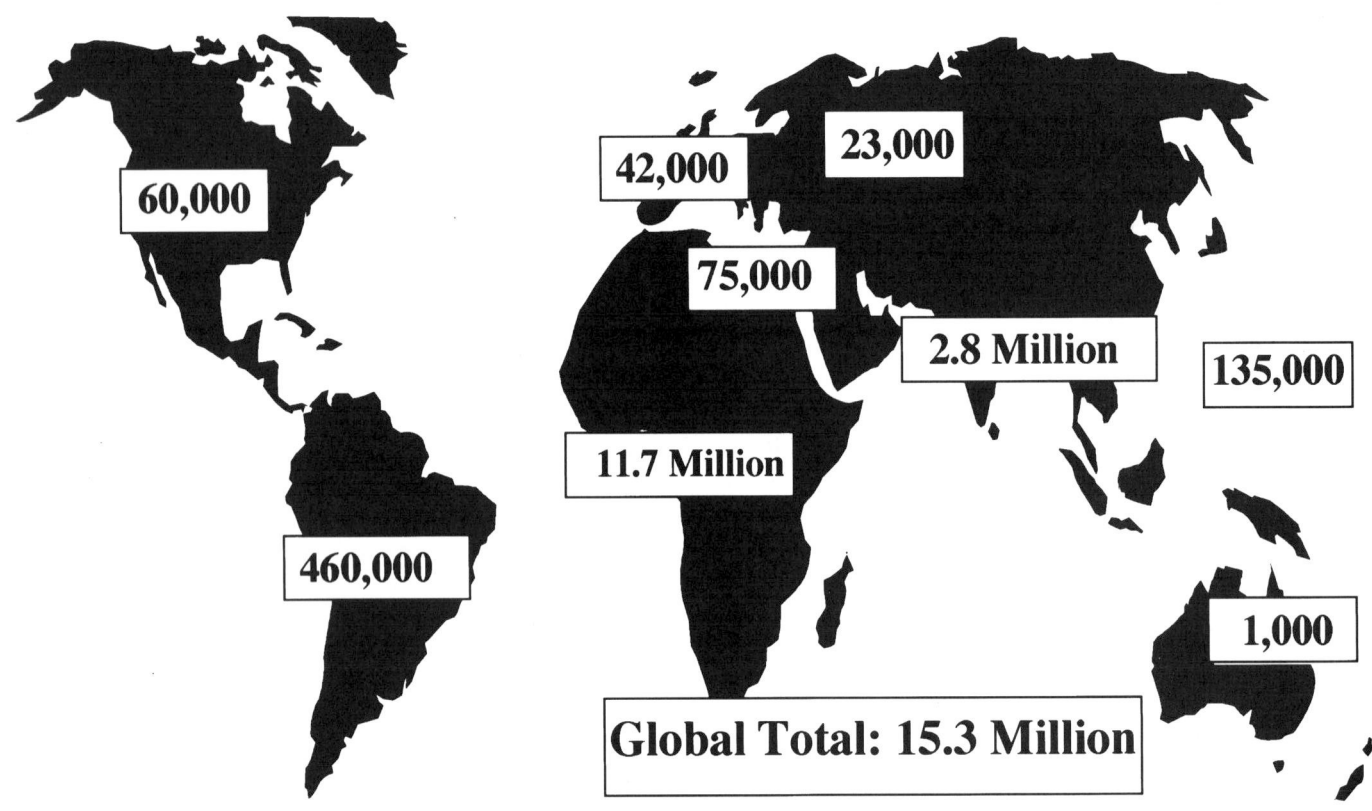

Figure 16.1. Estimated cumulative number of individuals who have been infected with TB and HIV since the beginning of the AIDS pandemic, 15- to 49-year-old group, at the end of 1997. (Courtesy of Tuberculosis Programme, World Health Organization, Geneva.)

Development of Active Tuberculosis

The immunologic response to *Mycobacterium tuberculosis* is frequently not sterilizing, and surviving but dormant organisms often cause latent infection. A process of active immunosurveillance maintains the latency of dormant foci. Clinical disease occurs when the mycobacterial replication that follows initial infection cannot be controlled (progressive primary TB) or when latent organisms overcome immunologic control (reactivation TB). Approximately 5% of immunologically normal adults who become infected with *M. tuberculosis* develop progressive primary TB within 2 years of initial infection. In another 5%, TB reactivates later in life (5).

HIV-induced CD4+ T-lymphocyte depletion in humans leads to a defective immunologic response to *Mycobacterium tuberculosis* (28–31). HIV-infected persons with latent *M. tuberculosis* infection are at high risk of reactivation TB, and those with recently acquired *M. tuberculosis* are at high risk of progressive primary TB. Active TB develops at an annual rate of 5 to 12% in HIV-infected persons with previous *M. tuberculosis* infection (32–38) (Table 16.2). The risk of TB is more than 25 to 30 times higher among HIV-infected persons than among HIV-seronegative controls (32–34).

In most studies, the risk of TB in HIV-infected persons is several times higher for persons whose tuberculin skin tests are positive than for those with negative skin tests (32, 36–38), a finding suggesting that, in these studies, reactivation of latent *Mycobacterium tuberculosis* is the most common mechanism leading to active TB. However, rapid progression from recent *M. tuberculosis* infection to active TB (progressive primary TB) has also frequently been demonstrated, particularly in HIV-infected persons exposed to *M. tuberculosis* during institutional outbreaks (39–48). HIV-infected persons are so vulnerable to progressive primary TB that active disease may develop within weeks of exposure to *M. tuberculosis*. In addition, in patients with advanced HIV infection, previous *M. tuberculosis* infection is not always protective, and exogenous reinfection with a different strain of *M. tuberculosis* may occur (49).

HIV-infected patients with TB are usually less immunocompromised than HIV-infected patients with other AIDS-defining opportunistic infections, and their CD4+ T-lymphocyte counts are generally in the range of 150 to 350 cells/mm^3 (50–61). However, TB also may occur in HIV-infected persons with marked CD4+ T-lymphocyte depletion, particularly as a result of newly acquired *Mycobacterium tuberculosis* infection. In both situations, the severity of TB correlates with the degree of CD4+ T-cell depletion.

Infectiousness

Most studies have shown that HIV-infected patients with TB have fewer acid-fast bacilli in their sputum and less frequent pulmonary cavitation than HIV-seronegative TB patients (50, 53, 62–64). Indeed, the frequency of positive acid-fast sputum smears and of pulmonary cavitation decreases with increasing immunosuppression. In addition, tuberculin skin test reactivity rates among contacts of HIV-infected patients with TB are generally lower than among contacts of HIV-seronegative TB patients (65–69).

Therefore, on an individual basis, HIV-infected patients with active TB are usually less infectious than HIV-negative individuals with active TB. However, a group of HIV-infected individuals exposed to a source of *Mycobacterium tuberculosis* is more likely to generate new *M. tuberculosis* infections than a group of similarly exposed HIV-negative individuals. This is because HIV-infected individuals infected with *M. tuberculosis* are more likely to develop active TB and to become additional sources of transmission.

Impact on the Course of HIV Infection

Findings from several studies suggest that active TB may accelerate HIV-induced immunologic deterioration. First, active TB is associated with transient CD4+ T-lymphocyte depression (70, 71). Second, TB results in immune stimula-

Table 16.2 Incidence of Tuberculosis (TB) in HIV-Seropositive (HIV+) and HIV-Seronegative (HIV−) Persons in Various Studies

No. and Type of Participants (Reference)	Months of Follow-up (Median)	No. of TB Cases	Incidence of TB (% per Year)
HIV-seropositive persons in HIV-seronegative controls			
Intravenous drug users, New York City (32)			
49 HIV+/PPD+	22	7	7.9
166 HIV+/PPD−	21	1	0.3
62 HIV−/PPD+	23	0	NA
236 HIV−/PPD−	23	0	NA
Women of childbearing age, Zaire (33)[a]			
249 HIV+	30	19	3.1
310 HIV−	32	1	0.1
Women of childbearing age, Rwanda (34)[a]			
401 HIV+	24	20	2.5
917 HIV−	26	2	0.1
HIV-seropositive persons, categorized according to tuberculin skin test results			
Intravenous drug users, New York City (32)			
166 PPD−	21	1	0.3
49 PPD+	22	7	7.9
Multicenter study, Italy (38)			
849 PPD−	19	6	0.5
1,649 Anergic[b]	15	62	3.0
197 PPD+	17	15	5.4
Natural history study, Spain (36)			
87 PPD−	16	0	NA
235 Anergic	16	8	2.6
87 PPD+	18	11	8.4
Natural history study, Spain (37)			
154 PPD−	29	19	5.4
112 Anergic	17	20	12.4
84 PPD+	30	24	10.4

NA, Not applicable; PPD+, tuberculin skin test (purified protein derivative)–positive; PPD−, tuberculin skin test–negative.
[a]Tuberculin skin testing was not performed in these studies.
[b]Anergy was determined with use of multiple puncture skin tests.

tion and the increased production of cytokines, such as TNF (3, 72, 73), which increase HIV replication in vitro (74, 75). Third, in one study, HIV-infected patients with TB appeared to have a higher risk of opportunistic infections and death than HIV-infected patients with similar CD4+ T-cell counts but without TB (76). Fourth, a 5- to 160-fold increase in plasma HIV-1 RNA levels was observed in HIV-infected individuals during the acute phase of TB (77). Finally, in one study, isoniazid preventive therapy for HIV-infected patients not only reduced the risk of active TB, but also appeared to delay the onset of other opportunistic infections and death (35). However, despite these suggestive findings, no prospectively controlled data show that *Mycobacterium tuberculosis* infection worsens the prognosis of HIV infection.

EPIDEMIOLOGY

Between 1985 and 1992, the number of reported TB cases in the United States increased by 19% (78) (Fig 16.2). During this interval, an estimated 52,000 more cases occurred than would have been expected had the downward trend of 1981 to 1984 continued (78, 79) (see Fig 16.2). Between 1992 and 1996, reported TB cases decreased an average of 6% per year (80–82) (see Fig 16.2). Epidemiologic evidence suggests that HIV has played an important role in the resurgence of TB in the United States and that recently introduced improvements in TB control measures in state and local health departments played a role in the decline in cases between 1992 and 1996 (82).

Between 1985 and 1992, the largest increases in TB occurred in demographic groups and locations with the highest HIV prevalence (83). Between 1980 and 1992, the number of cases of TB increased more than 150% in New York City, and between 1984 and 1990, TB incidence increased 40 to 50% in California, Florida, and New Jersey (84, 85). Among 25- to 44-year-old persons, TB incidence increased 52%, with most of the increase occurring among African–American and Hispanic persons (11, 83, 86). Moreover, in the locations and groups experiencing the greatest increases in TB cases, the prevalence of HIV among TB patients has been high. Studies of TB patients in New York City, Miami, San Francisco, and Seattle have reported HIV prevalence of 30 to 50% (53, 54, 87–89).

Between 1981 and 1991 at least 11,299 patients with AIDS in the United States also had TB (90). Persons with AIDS were 59 times more likely to be found to have TB than the rest of the population, and persons with TB were 204 times more likely to be found to have AIDS than the rest of the population (90). In New York City in 1995, 33% of the 2445 new cases of TB were reported as HIV seropositive, 31% were reported as HIV seronegative, and the remainder had an unreported or unknown HIV serostatus (91, 92).

Transmission of *Mycobacterium Tuberculosis*

In the 1970s and 1980s, fiscal constraints led to cutbacks in many TB control programs (88, 93). At the same time, the overlapping social problems of homelessness, substance abuse, and poverty increased in populations affected by both TB and HIV and limited the success of TB control in these groups. Between 1988 and 1992, TB outbreaks occurred as persons with HIV and persons with active TB were brought together in health care facilities, homeless shelters, and correctional facilities (39–48, 94–98).

Studies using restriction fragment length polymorphism (RFLP) analysis have suggested that perhaps one-third of TB cases in New York City and San Francisco during the early 1990s resulted from recently transmitted infections (99, 100). TB among HIV-infected homeless persons became common (88, 100–102), and the number of TB cases increased sharply in the correctional systems of New York, California, New Jersey, and several other states (103–106). Thus an increase in *Mycobacterium tuberculosis* transmission during the late 1980s and early 1990s also contributed to the resurgence of TB.

The outbreaks also demonstrated the potential for *Mycobacterium tuberculosis* to spread among HIV-infected persons in institutionalized settings (Fig 16.3). In one outbreak, a single, highly drug-resistant organism was isolated from 30 HIV-infected inmates who had been incarcerated in more than 20 different prisons (98, 107). Indeed, that same strain was associated with 112 TB cases in New York City in 1992 (108). During recent TB outbreaks, many exposed persons (e.g., health care workers and prison inmates) had tuberculin skin test conversions, and some developed active TB (45–48, 95, 98, 109–112).

Between 1985 and 1991, TB incidence increased 36% among children from birth to 4 years old (83), with the largest increase occurring in New York City (113). TB cases in children are strong evidence of recent TB transmission. Indeed, some pediatric cases reflect transmission from HIV-

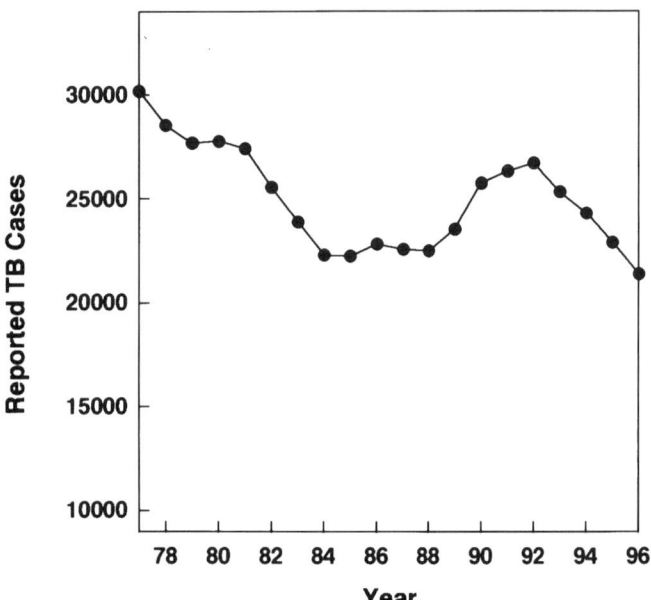

Figure 16.2. Yearly incidence of TB in the United States from 1978 to 1996. (Adapted from Centers for Disease Control and Prevention. Tuberculosis morbidity: United States, 1996. MMWR Morb Mortal Wkly Rep 1997;46:695–699.)

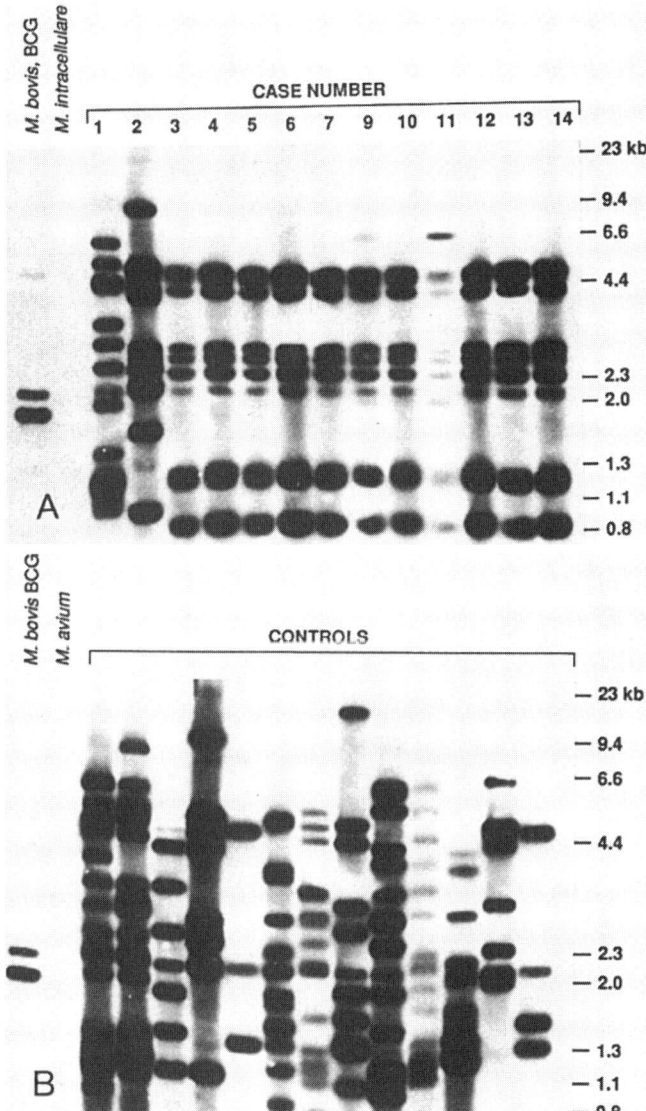

Figure 16.3. Restriction-length fragment polymorphisms (RFLPs) of *M. tuberculosis* isolates obtained from HIV-infected residents of a congregate living site (A) and of random TB patients identified in the same city (B). (From Daley CL, Small PM, Schecter GF, et al. An outbreak of tuberculosis with accelerated progression among persons infected with the human immunodeficiency virus: an analysis using restriction-fragment-length polymorphisms. N Engl J Med 1992;326:231–235.)

infected adults, and some cases reflect the high risk of progressing to active TB among children coinfected with HIV and *Mycobacterium tuberculosis* (114–118).

Tuberculosis and HIV Outside the United States

Even before the AIDS pandemic, the countries of sub-Saharan Africa suffered disproportionately from TB. Approximately 50% of adults in sub-Saharan Africa are estimated to be infected with *Mycobacterium tuberculosis*, and the incidence of active TB may be as high as 200 per 100,000 persons (1, 12, 13). In some urban areas, 10 to 30% of adults are HIV-seropositive (119, 120), and more than 6 million Africans are estimated to be coinfected with HIV and *M. tuberculosis* (8, 13, 14) (see Table 16.1). Nationwide notification rates and hospital-based studies suggest that the incidence of TB has more than doubled since the early 1980s in those countries with the highest rates of HIV infection (8, 119–125). In some African cities, 60 to 80% of hospital beds are occupied by HIV-infected patients, and TB is present in about half these patients (9, 121, 122, 126–131).

Historically, the largest number of TB cases has occurred in Asia, where HIV is spreading rapidly. Already, more than 2.2 million adults in Southeast Asia are estimated to be coinfected with HIV and TB (see Table 16.1 and Fig 16.1) (14, 132–134). Because of the rapid spread of HIV in Thailand, India, and Myanmar (Burma), the number of TB cases in Asia attributable to HIV may, by the year 2000, approximate the number of such cases in sub-Saharan Africa (13).

More than 400,000 adults in Latin America and the Caribbean islands are estimated to be coinfected with HIV and TB (see Table 16.1). TB has been reported in 26 to 60% of Haitian persons with AIDS (135–137) and in 7 to 28% of Latin American persons with AIDS (14, 138). In Spain and Italy, the incidence of TB appears to have increased as a result of TB among HIV-infected intravenous drug users (139). TB has been reported in more than 30% of persons with AIDS in Spain (139–142) and in 2 to 13% of HIV-infected persons in other Western European countries (56, 57, 139, 143, 144).

Drug-Resistant Tuberculosis

Resistance of *Mycobacterium tuberculosis* to drugs is caused by mutations in genes encoding the targets of anti-TB therapy (145–150). These mutations occur with a predictable frequency of one in 10^5 to 10^8 organisms (151). When anti-TB drugs are used in combination, the growth of mutant *M. tuberculosis* organisms resistant to any single drug is prevented by the other drugs in the combination. However, when organisms are exposed to only one effective drug because of incomplete or erratic anti-TB therapy, drug resistance may develop. Once *M. tuberculosis* becomes resistant to one drug, continued treatment or the addition of a single active drug may result in organisms resistant to additional drugs (152). If *M. tuberculosis* becomes resistant to both isoniazid and rifampin, termed multidrug-resistant TB (MDR TB), treatment becomes much more difficult and expensive (153, 154). Patients with MDR TB have a high mortality and may become chronically ill and persistently infectious.

The prevalence of MDR TB in the United States increased from 0.5% in 1982 to 1986 to 3.5% during the first 3 months of 1991 and 1992 (155, 156). The highest rates of MDR TB were reported from New York City, New Jersey, and Florida (155, 157). The increase in MDR TB was one of the factors leading to improved funding of control measures and to the mandatory reporting of drug-susceptibility results (158). Between 1993 and 1996, nationwide rates of MDR TB decreased to 2.2%, with most of the decrease attributable to a marked reduction in MDR TB in New York City (158, 159).

Table 16.3 Outbreaks of Multidrug-Resistant Tuberculosis (MDR TB) Involving HIV-Infected Persons[a]

Setting (Reference)	Comments
United States 1988–1992	
>5 hospitals in New York City (42–44, 48, 94)	Of >200 patients with TB, >80% HIV infected; mean incubation, 1–3.5 mo in the different hospital outbreaks; multiple failures in infection control contributing to transmission
Prison system, New York State (NYS) (98, 108)	38 of 39 inmates HIV+; 29 inmates infected with a strain resistant to isoniazid, rifampin, ethambutol, streptomycin, ethionamide, rifabutin, and kanamycin (strain W); inmates with MDR TB living in 23 of the 68 NYS prisons while potentially infectious (12 transferred through 20 prisons while ill with MDR TB); TST conversions in ≥30% of exposed inmates in 1 prison, 60 staff members in another prison, and in >50 health-care workers; in 1992, strain W isolated from 112 cultures in 21 hospitals (22% of MDR TB in NYC)
Hospital and clinic, Miami (47, 96)	62 HIV-infected patients with MDR TB over 3-yr period
Substance-abuse treatment facility, Michigan (97)	At least 15 and possibly as many as 31 exposed clients and staff with TST conversions
TB ward, New York City (49)	4 HIV-infected patients hospitalized with drug-susceptible TB reinfected with an MDR TB strain with active TB within 2–9 mo of initial hospitalization
Worldwide 1991–present	
Hospital in Madrid, Spain (174)	MDR TB diagnosed in 47 HIV-infected patients hospitalized in an HIV ward and in 1 HIV-infected health care worker; of 48 cases, 47 deaths; mean interval from diagnosis of MDR TB to death, 78 days.
Hospital in Buenos Aires, Argentina (163)	MDR TB (resistance documented to isoniazid, rifampin, and at least 3 other drugs) infecting >100 HIV-infected patients over a 1½-y period
Hospital in Milano, Italy (175)	More than 31 HIV-infected patients diagnosed with MDR TB; median CD4+ count, 18; median survival, 13 wk
Hospital in Rosario, Argentina (167)	34 HIV-infected patients diagnosed with MDR TB; average CD4+ count, 188; average survival, 4 wk
Hospital in London, United Kingdom (173)	8 HIV-infected patients developed MDR TB (resistant to isoniazid, rifampin, pyrazinamide, clofazimine, and ethionamide); median interval from infection to active disease, 8 wk; at 6-mo follow-up, 1 patient dead of TB meningitis
Hospital in Madrid, Spain (171)	4 HIV-infected children with advanced disease diagnosed with MDR TB and all 4 children died; median survival from time of diagnosis, 11 wk

[a]In addition to these outbreaks are at least two nosocomial outbreaks of MDR *M. tuberculosis bovis,* characterized by person-to-person transmission among HIV-infected persons (257, 259).

Data regarding institutional outbreaks (Table 16.3) have demonstrated the high rate of disease progression among HIV-infected persons who become infected with *Mycobacterium tuberculosis* strains that are already multidrug resistant (i.e., initial drug resistance). Several reports have noted acquired rifampin resistance among HIV-infected persons receiving treatment for drug-susceptible TB (160, 161). However, most cases of MDR TB among HIV-infected persons have been due to initial drug resistance, and HIV-related immunosuppression only rarely increases the likelihood that drug resistance will develop in a person infected with drug-susceptible *M. tuberculosis* (i.e., acquired drug resistance) (162–164).

In many developing countries, the rate of primary isoniazid resistance is higher than 10%, and in those countries using rifampin, MDR TB is observed with increased frequency (165–171). Areas where the prevalence of HIV is also increasing will have progressively more contacts between patients with MDR TB and HIV in both community and institutional settings. Indeed, several large outbreaks of MDR TB among HIV-infected persons have already been reported outside the United States in hospitals that were unprepared for nosocomial airborne infections (163, 164, 166–175) (see Table 16.3).

CLINICAL FEATURES

In HIV-infected patients with TB, immunodeficiency is associated with increased dissemination of *Mycobacterium tuberculosis,* increased number and severity of symptoms, and rapid progression to death unless treatment is begun. Fever, weight loss, and other constitutional symptoms almost always occur. Cough, chest pain, and other respiratory symptoms are also common because most patients have some degree of pulmonary involvement. Shaking chills, hypotension, and acute respiratory distress may occur in patients with disseminated TB (64, 176–178). Localized signs and symptoms depend on the organs involved and on coexisting HIV-related complications.

Sites of Disease

Pulmonary TB occurs in 70 to 90% of patients with TB, including most of those with extrapulmonary TB (6, 7, 57, 60, 61, 179–181). The frequency of extrapulmonary TB ranges from 40 to 80% and increases with the severity of immunosuppression and the extent of diagnostic evaluation. Disseminated disease and lymphadenitis are the most common forms of extrapulmonary TB (64). *Mycobacterium tuberculosis* bacteremia, extremely unusual in patients without HIV infection, has been noted in up to 20 to 40% of HIV-infected patients with TB (182–185).

The cervical, supraclavicular, and axillary lymph nodes are the most common sites of peripheral TB lymphadenitis (29, 56, 64, 186–190). The intrathoracic and intraabdominal lymph nodes, rare sites of TB in patients without HIV infection, are commonly involved in HIV-infected patients with advanced immunodeficiency (64, 191). Tuberculous lymph nodes in HIV-infected patients have an increased tendency to caseate and may predispose to abscesses, fistulas, and unusual sites of infection (64, 192, 193). Tuberculous retroperitoneal lymph nodes may erode into the stomach or pancreas; mediastinal lymph nodes may erode into the esophagus, trachea, or bronchi; and mesenteric lymph nodes may erode into the lower intestine (64, 194–198).

Central nervous system involvement occurs in 5 to 10% of HIV-infected patients with TB (58, 64, 140, 141, 181, 199, 200). Most HIV-infected patients with central nervous system TB have meningitis, but tuberculomas are also common (201–203). Urine cultures are positive for most patients with disseminated TB, but localized renal TB is rarely diagnosed (58, 64, 199). Pleural disease and pericardial disease are commonly recognized forms of extrapulmonary TB in HIV-infected African patients (204–208). TB of the skin and soft tissues may result from hematogenous seeding or contiguous organ involvement (64, 176, 193, 209–211).

Radiographic Findings

Chest radiographs of HIV-infected patients with TB and advanced immunosuppression are notable for a nonapical distribution of infiltrates, infrequent cavitation, and an increased frequency of intrathoracic adenopathy, miliary infiltrates, and pleural effusions (6, 7, 62, 212–214) (Fig 16.4). Apical fibrocavitary infiltrates, the classic finding in adults with reactivation TB, occur predominantly in HIV-infected patients with TB who are not severely immunodeficient. Localized alveolar infiltrates may be confused with bacterial pneumonia, and diffuse interstitial infiltrates may mimic *Pneumocystis carinii* pneumonia. The occurrence of hilar or mediastinal adenopathy, which is noted in about one-third of HIV-infected patients with TB, suggests the diagnosis of TB because intrathoracic adenopathy occurs rarely with other HIV-related pulmonary complications. Miliary infiltrates and pleural effusions occur in more than 10% of HIV-infected patients with TB and often develop during diagnostic evaluation. A normal chest radiograph does not preclude the diagnosis of pulmonary TB because radiographic findings may lag behind rapidly evolving active TB (64, 214, 215).

In patients with intrathoracic adenopathy, computed tomography scans usually demonstrate clusters of enlarged lymph nodes, often containing low-density centers consistent with caseous necrosis (64, 213, 216) (Fig 16.5A). In patients with disseminated TB, abdominal sonography and computed tomography scans may demonstrate intraabdominal lymphadenopathy and focal hepatic and splenic lesions (64, 141, 192, 217–219) (see Fig 16.5B).

Tuberculin Skin Testing and Histopathology

The sensitivity of tuberculin skin testing in HIV-infected patients is inversely related to the degree of immunosuppression. Among HIV-infected patients with active TB, tuberculin reactions are at least 10 mm in 40 to 60% of those with otherwise asymptomatic HIV infection but in only 10 to 30% of those with symptomatic HIV infection (6, 7, 50, 53, 54, 64, 89, 199, 220, 221). Data are not available on the frequency of a 5 mm or greater tuberculin reaction, which is

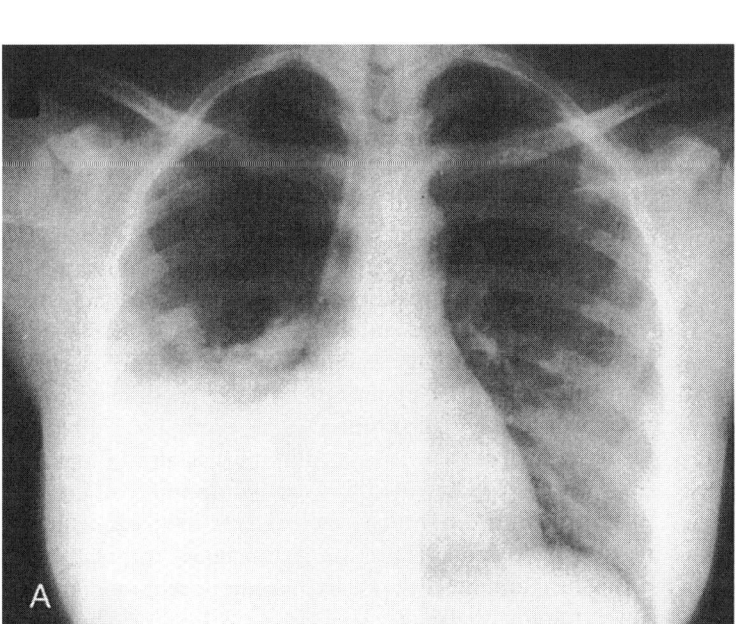
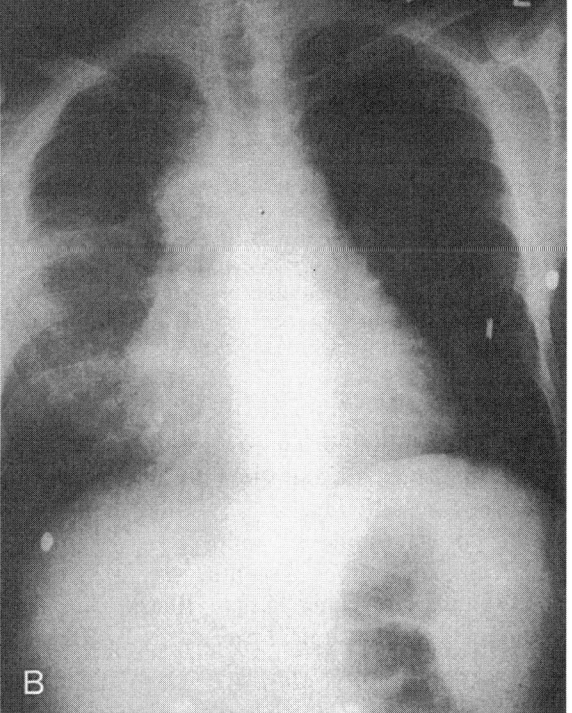

Figure 16.4. Chest radiographs of patients with TB and HIV infection. A. Right lower lobe infiltrate and pleural effusion. **B.** Right middle lobe infiltrate and widening of the mediastinum due to subcarinal, right paratracheal, and hilar lymphadenopathy (Courtesy of Bernard Suster, M.D., Saint Luke's Roosevelt Medical Center, New York, NY.).

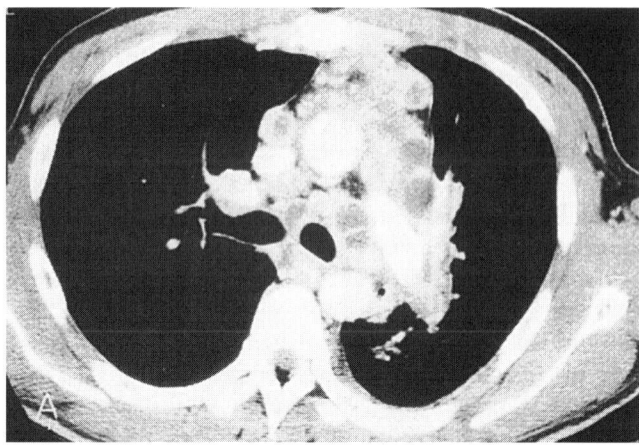

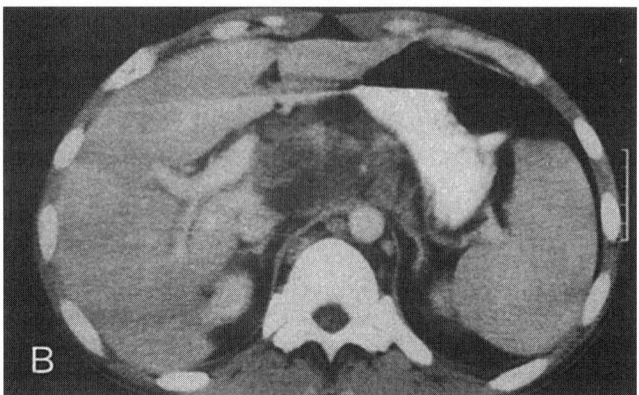

Figure 16.5. Computed tomography scans of patients with TB and HIV infection. **A.** Chest scan demonstrating multiple enlarged necrotic mediastinal lymph nodes. **B.** Abdominal scan demonstrating a large necrotic periportal lymph node. (Courtesy of Bernard Suster, MD, Saint Luke's Roosevelt Medical Center, New York.)

diagnostic tests is usually the most common reason for diagnostic delays.

TB should be considered in HIV-infected persons with unexplained fever, constitutional symptoms, cough, pulmonary infiltrates, lymphadenopathy, meningitis, brain abscess, pericarditis, pleural effusions, or intraabdominal, musculoskeletal, or cutaneous abscesses. The probability of active TB is increased among patients who have a history of TB, whose tuberculin skin test is positive, or who have emigrated from a country or belong to a group with a high prevalence of TB (e.g., racial and ethnic minorities, homeless persons, intravenous drug users, alcoholics, and correctional facility inmates). In areas where nosocomial outbreaks have occurred, recent hospitalization should also be considered a risk factor for TB.

The chest radiograph may show a classic reactivation pattern (apical fibrocavitary disease or miliary infiltrate), an "atypical" pattern (intrathoracic adenopathy, with or without single or multilobar infiltrates, or pleural effusion), or evidence of past infection (calcified lymph node or lung nodule or pleural or parenchymal fibrosis). Although the sensitiv-

the currently recommended cutoff in HIV-infected patients with active TB.

The histopathologic features of TB in HIV-infected patients also depend on the degree of host immunity. Biopsy specimens from patients with early immunodeficiency tend to have granulomas composed of lymphocytes, epithelioid cells, and giant cells (29, 64, 222, 223), whereas those from more immunocompromised patients tend to contain necrosis, polymorphonuclear cells, and macrophages (64, 186, 224, 225) (Fig 16.6). This histologic picture of TB contrasts with that of *Mycobacterium avium* complex, in which granulomas are either absent or small and nonnecrotizing (226).

DIAGNOSIS

Because the clinical features of HIV-infected patients with TB are often nonspecific, diagnosis can be difficult. Many HIV-infected patients with TB have died or have been hospitalized for a prolonged period before TB has been diagnosed (64, 121, 179, 227–229). The decreased tuberculin reactivity, atypical radiographic presentations, and confusion with other HIV-related infections have often hindered the diagnosis of TB in HIV-infected patients. However, failure to suspect TB and to order the appropriate

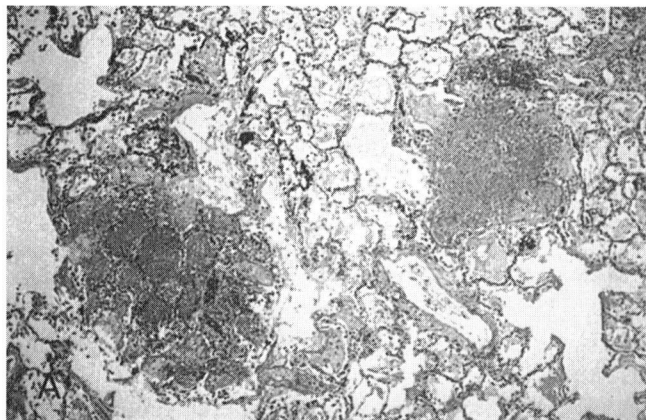

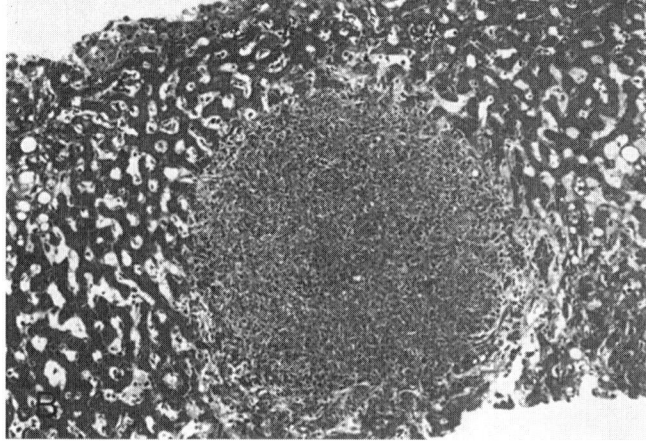

Figure 16.6. Biopsy specimens of lung (A) and liver (B) from patients with TB and HIV infection. Both specimens demonstrate focal areas of necrosis and cellular debris without lymphocytes, epithelioid cells, or giant cells. Both specimens contained many acid-fast bacilli on Fite stain. (Courtesy of Ross Hill, MD, State University of New York, Health Science Center at Brooklyn, New York.)

ity of the tuberculin skin test decreases with declining immunity, a positive test in a symptomatic person with advanced HIV infection suggests active TB (61, 73, 230–232).

Acid-fast bacilli are found on microscopic examination of sputum specimens from 40 to 67% of HIV-infected patients with TB; *Mycobacterium tuberculosis* is recovered from 74 to 95% in culture (50, 53, 56, 57, 63, 64, 141, 199, 227, 233–235) (Table 16.4). If adequate sputum specimens cannot be obtained, sputum should be induced with nebulized hypertonic saline (236). Acid-fast staining and culture of gastric washings are also useful, particularly for infants and children. Fiberoptic bronchoscopy with bronchoalveolar lavage and transbronchial biopsy is indicated in patients with progressive unexplained pulmonary disease (237–240). During bronchoscopy, specimens from enlarged mediastinal lymph nodes may be obtained by endobronchial needle aspiration.

Lymphatic, central nervous system, pericardial, pleural, and musculoskeletal TB may be suggested by physical examination. New signs often develop during diagnostic evaluation and may direct further tests or indicate new complications. Enlarged, tender, or fluctuant lymph nodes should be aspirated percutaneously. In some series, as many as 90% of suspicious lymph nodes contain acid-fast bacilli (58, 64, 141, 199, 227, 241, 242) (see Table 16.4). One large study suggests that the diagnosis of TB can also frequently been made by aspirating lymph nodes 2 cm or larger even if they are nonfluctuant and symmetric (243). Among patients with disseminated TB, biopsies of skin lesions have revealed acid-fast bacilli or granulomas (176, 210, 211, 244).

Blood and urine should be cultured for mycobacteria; however, patients with *Mycobacterium tuberculosis* bacteremia require treatment before the time it usually takes for these cultures to become positive (182, 183). Although acid-fast bacilli are often seen in the buffy coat smears of patients with disseminated *M. avium complex* infection (245), only one report of a positive buffy coat smear in an HIV-infected patient with *M. tuberculosis* has been published (246). Some investigators have reported that most HIV-infected patients with extrapulmonary TB have positive urine cultures for *M. tuberculosis*, and in several cases, the diagnosis of TB has been based on the finding of acid-fast bacilli in smears of concentrated urine (58, 64, 141, 199, 247) (see Table 16.4). Although cerebrospinal fluid and pleural fluid are generally abnormal in patients with involvement of these sites, stains for acid-fast bacilli are usually negative.

Biopsy of the bone marrow or liver may be effective in diagnosing disseminated TB in the absence of localized findings (57, 64, 248, 249) (see Table 16.4). Abdominal sonography or computed tomography should be considered in difficult cases because these tests may demonstrate necrotic lymph nodes that provide a high diagnostic yield when aspirated percutaneously (64, 192, 217). Neuroimaging studies may be helpful in the diagnosis of central nervous system TB; radiographic clues include multiloculated abscess, cisternal enhancement, basal ganglia infarction, and communicating hydrocephalus, which are not findings associated with toxoplasma encephalitis or central nervous system lymphoma (203, 250) (Fig 16.7).

The rapidly progressive nature of TB in HIV-infected patients requires that the diagnosis of suspected TB be pursued expeditiously. For patients whose initial evaluation is nondiagnostic, including acid-fast bacillus stains of sputum and other readily obtainable specimens, invasive procedures must be considered. For patients who are at high risk of TB

Table 16.4 Diagnostic Yield of Clinical Specimens from HIV-Infected Patients With Tuberculosis (TB)

Specimen	Percentage of patients for whom findings are positive (%)	
	Microscopy[a]	Culture
Sputum	40–67	74–95
Bronchoscopy		
Bronchoalveolar lavage	7–20	52–89
Transbronchial biopsy	10–39	42–85
Urine	22	45–77
Blood	NA[b]	26–64
Lymph nodes	37–90	40–95
Bone marrow	18–52	25–67
Liver biopsy	78	56–78
Cerebrospinal fluid	0–27	NA[b]
Pleural specimens		
Pleural fluid	3–6	NA[b]
Pleural biopsy	52–55	NA[b]

[a]Acid-fast bacilli seen on smears or granulomas seen on histopathologic specimens.
[b]Not available. Blood smears have rarely been examined for HIV-infected patients with TB. The yields of cultures of cerebrospinal fluid and pleural specimens are not shown because most reports present data regarding only *Mycobacterium tuberculosis*–positive cultures of these specimens.

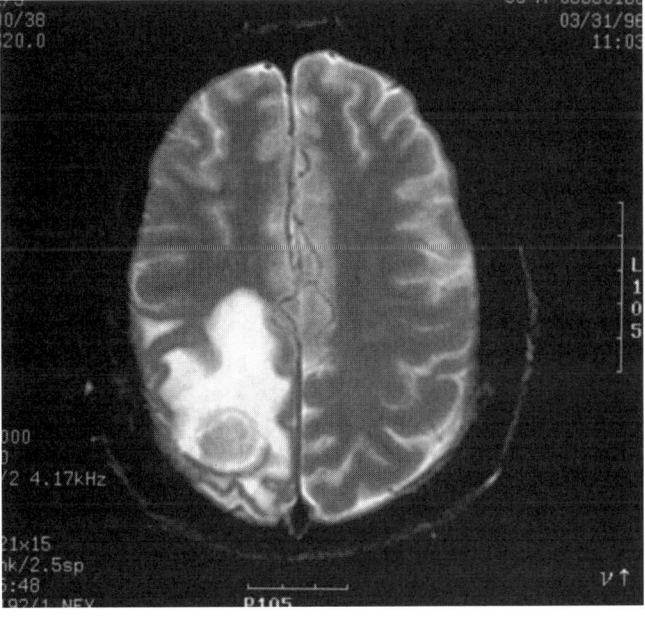

Figure 16.7. Magnetic resonance imaging findings of a tuberculoma in a patient with HIV infection. T_2-weighted images demonstrate a $3.0 \times 2.5 \times 2.5$ cm ring enhancing lesion within the right parietal lobe with extensive vasogenic edema and central necrosis. Culture of brain biopsy specimen revealed *M. tuberculosis*. (Courtesy of Dennis Israelsky, MD, Stanford University Medical Center, Stanford, CA.)

or whose conditions are deteriorating rapidly, empiric anti-TB therapy should be started. Because sputum, urine, and blood cultures are most likely positive in patients with fulminant TB, specimens for these cultures should be obtained before empiric therapy is begun to provide later confirmation of the diagnosis and to provide an *Mycobacterium tuberculosis* isolate for drug-susceptibility testing. The role of DNA amplification tests in assisting the diagnosis of TB is reviewed in the next section.

MICROBIOLOGY

The rapid progression of TB among HIV-infected individuals and the increase in prevalence of drug-resistant TB underscore the importance of rapidly identifying and determining the drug susceptibility of *Mycobacterium tuberculosis* strains. The preferred method for examining clinical specimens for acid-fast bacilli is fluorochrome staining because it is more rapid and slightly more sensitive than the Ziehl–Neelsen and Kinyoun stains (251). Radiometric culture methods using liquid media, such as BACTEC (Becton Dickinson Diagnostic Instruments Systems, Sparks, MD), are recommended because they detect mycobacterial growth in 1 to 4 weeks, an average of 10 days before colonies can be seen on solid media (251, 252). Solid culture media, however, should be used in conjunction with liquid media to detect mixed mycobacterial infections.

Traditional methods for determining the species of mycobacterial isolates (e.g., on the basis of the growth rate, colonial morphology, pigmentation, and biochemical profile) are unacceptably slow for identifying *Mycobacterium tuberculosis*. A nucleic acid hybridization assay (Gen-Probe, Inc., San Diego, CA) can identify *M. tuberculosis* complex organisms within several hours after growth is detected (253). Rapid hybridization assays also are available to identify *M. avium*, *M. intracellulare*, and several other nontuberculous mycobacteria. Because mixed mycobacterial infections occur, a positive hybridization assay for another species, such as *M. avium*, does not exclude the simultaneous presence of *M. tuberculosis* (95, 254).

Mycobacterium bovis and *M. bovis* bacille Calmette-Guérin (BCG) belong to the *M. tuberculosis* complex and have been isolated from HIV-infected persons (255–259). *M. bovis* has caused both isolated cases and nosocomial outbreaks of TB among HIV-infected individuals, whereas disseminated BCG has been reported after BCG vaccination (260). Infections with these organisms often have different epidemiologic implications than infections with *M. tuberculosis*, and differentiating these organisms from *M. tuberculosis* requires classic biochemical tests.

High-performance liquid chromatography (HPLC), a popular method in some reference laboratories, can reliably identify most *Mycobacterium* species in less than 4 hours on the basis of mycolic acid profile (253). HPLC is particularly useful in identifying mixed and unusual mycobacterial infections, which are more common in HIV-infected patients (261–264).

Several gene amplification techniques can detect *Mycobacterium tuberculosis* nucleic acid within hours directly from clinical specimens. Assays using the polymerase chain reaction (PCR; Roche Amplicor MTB, Roche Diagnostic Systems, Branchburg, NJ) or transcription-mediated amplification (TMA; Gen-Probe Amplified Mycobacterium Direct Test, San Diego, CA) have been evaluated extensively on clinical samples (253, 265–273). In reference laboratories, both tests are highly specific (>95%) and are more sensitive than staining for acid-fast bacilli (271–276).

The PCR and TMA assays have been approved by the United States Food and Drug Administration (FDA) to confirm the diagnosis of *Mycobacterium tuberculosis* in patients whose respiratory samples contain acid-fast bacilli (265, 266). Although PCR and TMA are not FDA approved for making the diagnosis of TB in patients with negative AFB smears, these assays may be useful in patients with diagnostically difficult cases, particularly if two separate assays are positive.

Initial *Mycobacterium tuberculosis* isolates from all patients should be submitted for antimicrobial susceptibility testing (156, 251). Radiometric methods using liquid media can be used to test susceptibility to isoniazid, rifampin, ethambutol, pyrazinamide, and streptomycin and usually yield results 4 to 7 days after the initial detection of mycobacterial growth (251). The rapid identification of rifampin resistance by direct DNA amplification methods is often possible because specific *rpo*b gene mutations are found in more than 90% of rifampin-resistant isolates. Because rifampin resistance is often a surrogate for multidrug resistance, genetic screening for rifampin resistance may be useful in specific outbreak situations (277–281).

TREATMENT

Effectiveness of Therapy in HIV-Infected Patients

HIV-related initial immunosuppression by itself does not interfere with the effectiveness of TB therapy. Defervescence, sputum conversion, and resolution of chest radiograph abnormalities occur as rapidly in HIV-infected patients as in patients without HIV infection (64, 199, 228, 282–288). Most early deaths among HIV-infected patients with TB have resulted from undiagnosed TB or from nontuberculous HIV-related complications (64, 199, 228, 288–290).

Most TB treatment failures in HIV-infected patients have resulted from drug resistance or poor adherence to therapy. In addition, anecdotal cases of treatment failure attributed to undrained tuberculous abscesses (291–293) or malabsorption of anti-TB drugs (294–298) have been reported. Indeed, several reports note acquired rifampin resistance among HIV-infected patients with TB together with data linking these cases to possible drug malabsorption (160, 161, 297).

In most studies of HIV-infected patients completing 6 to 9 months of standard anti-TB treatment (with regimens including at least isoniazid and rifampin), less than 5% of patients followed for more than 1 year after the completion of therapy had recurrent TB, and, of these, some adhered poorly to therapy (57, 199, 228, 285, 286, 299–301). On the basis of these studies, the most recent Centers for Disease Control and Prevention (CDC)/American Thoracic Society (ATS) guidelines recommended similar treatment regimens for HIV-infected and HIV-negative TB patients, with the caveat that the response to therapy of HIV-infected TB patients should be followed more closely, and therapy should be prolonged for patients with a slow or suboptimal response (302, 303).

However, in the only completed prospective randomized study of HIV-infected patients with TB, 9% of those receiving therapy for 6 months relapsed over a 2-year period, compared with only 2% of those receiving treatment for 12 months (288). In addition, in a retrospective study of 189 HIV-infected patients followed for a median of about 2.5 years, the relapse rate was 24% (10 of 41) in patients receiving 6 months of therapy compared with 3.4% (5 of 148) receiving 9 months of therapy (304). Because HIV-infected patients are living longer because of improved medical management, studies are urgently needed to assess the risk of relapse more than 1 to 2 years after the completion of anti-TB therapy and to determine whether a subset of patients is at increased risk of relapse as a result of anti-TB drug malabsorption.

Treatment Recommendations

A four-drug regimen consisting of isoniazid, rifampin, pyrazinamide, and either ethambutol or streptomycin is recommended as initial therapy. This four-drug regimen is recommended because significant levels of isoniazid resistance (more than 4%) are present in 41 of 50 states (82, 158, 303) (Table 16.5). Initiating anti-TB therapy with four drugs reduces the likelihood of drug failure and the emergence of additional resistance in patients primarily infected with drug-resistant organisms. In addition, four-drug regimens reduce infectiousness more rapidly than do three-drug regimens (303). Treatment of drug-susceptible TB should be continued for a total of 6 to 9 months (see Table 16.5).

To assess the probability of drug resistance, all patients should be questioned thoroughly about previous preventive or curative therapy for TB and exposure to known cases of TB. The possibility of resistance to any drug the patient has received should be considered, and results of past susceptibility testing of isolates from the patient or from known contacts should be sought. In some cases, emigration from certain developing countries could also be considered a risk factor for drug resistance (165).

Patients with drug-resistant TB should receive supervised therapy managed in consultation with clinicians who are experienced in treating such cases (303). Resistance to either isoniazid or rifampin can usually be overcome by the substitution of other first-line drugs (see Table 16.5). The duration of therapy is usually determined by the extent of drug resistance, the severity of TB, the severity of immunodeficiency, and the response to therapy.

If resistance to both isoniazid and rifampin is suspected, the initial drug regimen should include isoniazid, rifampin, pyrazinamide, and three drugs to which local MDR TB strains are susceptible (303) (see Table 16.5). HIV-infected patients with MDR TB who are treated initially with at least two to three anti-TB drugs to which the causative organism is susceptible improve clinically, become noninfectious, and survive longer than patients treated with fewer effective drugs (96, 305–308). Continued treatment should

Table 16.5 Treatment Regimens for HIV-Infected Adults with Tuberculosis (TB)

Clinical Circumstances and Treatment Considerations	Initial Therapy[a]	Continuation Phase
DOT	INH, RIF, PZA, and SM or EMB daily for 2 wk followed by 2–3 × wk for 6 wk or INH, RIF, PZA and SM or EMB 3 × for 6 mo	INH, RIF 2–3 × wk to complete 6 mo of treatment
DOT not considered necessary to ensure patient's compliance	INH, RIF, PZA, and SM or EMB daily (pending susceptibility data) and then INH, RIF, PZA to complete 8 wk of therapy with these 3 drugs	INH, RIF daily to complete 6 mo of treatment
Resistance (or intolerance) to INH[b]		RIF, EMB, PZA × 18 mo (and ≥12 mo after culture conversion)
Resistance (or intolerance) to RIF[b]		INH, EMB, PZA × 18 mo (and ≥12 mo after culture conversion)
Possible or confirmed resistance to both INH and RIF (MDR TB)[b]	INH, RIF, PZA, and EMB or SM, plus additional second-line drugs or a quinolone antibiotic, so patient receives ≥3 drugs to which local MDR TB strains are likely to be susceptible	≥3 drugs to which patient's *Mycobacterium tuberculosis* strain is susceptible; appropriate duration of therapy not known

DOT, directly observed therapy; INH, isoniazid, 5 mg/kg (maximum [max], 300 mg) for daily therapy or 15 mg/kg (max, 900 mg) for intermittent therapy; RIF, rifampin, 10 mg/kg (max. 600 mg) for daily and intermittent therapy; PZA, pyrazinamide, 15–30 mg/kg (max, 2 g) for daily therapy or 50–70 mg/kg (max. 8–9 g/wk) for intermittent therapy; EMB, ethambutol, 15–25 mg/kg (max, 2.5 g) for daily therapy or 25–50 mg/kg (max, 2.5 g) for intermittent therapy; SM, streptomycin, 15 mg/kg (max, 1 g) for daily therapy or 25–30 mg/kg (max. 1–1.5 g) for intermittent therapy; MDR TB, multidrug-resistant TB.
[a]In areas where surveillance for drug-resistant TB has documented drug resistance rates <4%, INH, RIF, and PZA alone may be used for initial therapy.
[b]All patients with drug-resistant TB should receive DOT; MDR TB should be treated in consultation with physicians experienced at treating such patients.
(Data from references 153, 302, and 303.)

be guided by the results of anti-TB drug susceptibility testing.

For patients with MDR TB, one needs to determine susceptibilities to the second-line anti-TB drugs and to the quinolones. The optimal drugs for treating MDR TB include the other first-line anti-TB drugs (ethambutol, streptomycin, and pyrazinamide) and the quinolones (ofloxacin, ciprofloxacin, and levofloxacin) (153, 154, 309, 310). Administration of aminosalicylic acid, ethionamide, and cycloserine may need to be initiated in the hospital to permit observation of toxicity, intolerance, and initial response (153). Resectional surgery should be considered for patients with extensive drug resistance, localized disease, and good cardiopulmonary reserve (311). Although HIV-infected patients with MDR TB show improvement with appropriate therapy and become noninfectious (225, 305–308, 312), whether discontinuing anti-TB treatment exposes such patients to a high risk of relapse is not yet known.

Nonadherence and Directly Observed Therapy

Although generally highly efficacious, therapy for TB requires a prolonged course of multiple medications that often have side effects. Because patients with TB often no longer feel ill after the first few weeks of treatment, continuing anti-TB therapy may become a low priority for them. Although persons leading disadvantaged and disorganized lives, such as homeless persons and substance abusers, are less likely than others to complete therapy, nonadherence occurs in individuals from all backgrounds (313), and failure to complete anti-TB therapy has been common in many parts of the United States (314).

Adherence can be improved by enablers such as transportation and short waiting times, incentives such as meals or money, and a trusting relationship between patient and health care provider. The use of formulations with multiple drugs of demonstrated bioavailability such as Rifater (isoniazid, rifampin, and pyrazinamide, Marion Merrell Dow, Kansas City, MO), and Rifamate (isoniazid and rifampin, Marion Merrel Dow) may enhance adherence and, by preventing discontinuation of any one of the component drugs, may reduce the likelihood that drug resistance will develop (315, 316).

However, the best way to ensure adherence is to supervise the administration of therapy directly. Directly observed therapy (DOT), administered two or three times per week, has been highly successful in many different settings (303, 317). The costs of supervision are more than offset by savings resulting from the decreased risk of treatment failure, relapse, drug resistance, and secondary spread (317–320). The use of DOT reduced the risk of relapse and drug resistance in Tarrant County, Texas from 1986 to 1992 (318). The increased use of DOT in New York City and Baltimore has been responsible in part for large decreases in the number of TB cases recently observed in those cities (319, 320). Although the efficacy of intermittent (twice or thrice weekly) DOT has been established primarily among patients without HIV infection, additional data suggest that HIV-infected patients with TB also respond well to supervised intermittent therapy (228, 285, 288, 303).

Drug Toxicity and Interactions

In some initial studies, as many as 20% of HIV-infected TB patients treated with standard chemotherapy experienced an adverse reaction that prompted a change in therapy (55, 57, 199). Most of the reactions occurred within the first 2 months of treatment and consisted of mild rash or hepatitis, usually attributed to rifampin. However, most subsequent studies have not found an increase in anti-TB drug toxicity in HIV-infected patients (56, 64, 89, 228, 285, 288, 299).

With the recent introduction of many new antiretroviral drugs and improvement in HIV treatment, pharmacokinetic interactions between anti-TB and anti-HIV drugs now present the major challenge to treating HIV-infected TB patients (Table 16.6). The rifamycins (rifampin and, to lesser extent, rifabutin) are potent inducers of the hepatic cytochrome P450 enzyme system and reduce the activity of several drugs commonly used in HIV-infected patients by accelerating their metabolism (321). The drugs most commonly affected include several anti-HIV drugs (e.g., the protease inhibitors, the nonnucleoside reverse transcriptase [RT] inhibitors, and zidovudine, formerly known as azidothymidine or AZT) and other drugs commonly used in HIV infection (e.g., the antifungal azoles, methadone, and oral contraceptives) (321–324).

Coadministration of rifamycin drugs and each of the protease inhibitors leads to subtherapeutic protease inhibitor levels and to potentially toxic rifamycin drug levels (322–325). With recent studies showing that the most successful anti-HIV regimens include a protease inhibitor and two RT inhibitors, optimal treatment of HIV and TB at the same time has become difficult. Because active TB poses the greater immediate threat to HIV-infected patients and their contacts, optimal TB treatment must be the focus of the initial therapeutic efforts. Moreover, HIV-infected patients with TB are generally cured with 6 months of TB therapy, whereas the duration of treatment for HIV is indefinite. The exclusion of rifamycins from the anti-TB regimen to allow the use of protease inhibitors is not recommended because treatment of TB without rifampin (or rifabutin) requires at least 18 months of therapy, prolongs the duration of infectivity, and increases the likelihood of treatment failure (290, 302, 324, 326–328).

For HIV-infected individuals with TB who do not yet have advanced immunodeficiency, the most reasonable management strategy is probably to complete TB treatment with a regimen containing rifampin before starting anti-HIV therapy (324). Although treatment with RT inhibitors is not contraindicated in this setting, many HIV treatment experts believe that treatment with RT inhibitors alone is suboptimal and may promote the development of HIV resistance to the

Table 16.6 Drug Interactions between Antituberculosis and Antiretroviral Agents

Primary Drug	Drugs Affected	Effect	Mechanism	Comment
Rifampin	Protease inhibitors; ritonavir, saquinavir, indinavir, nelfinavir	Protease inhibitor concentrations are decreased by 70–90% to subtherapeutic levels	Induction of cytochrome P450 enzymes	All combinations of rifampin and currently available protease inhibitors contraindicated because of the reduction in protease inhibitor activity and an increase in rifampin levels to potentially toxic levels
	Zidovudine	Zidovudine concentrations are decreased by 50%	Induction of glucuronidation	No consensus on whether to increase dose of zidovudine in persons receiving rifampin
	Delavirdine	Delavirdine concentrations reduced by 90+% to subtherapeutic levels	Induction of cytochrome P450 enzymes	Combination of rifampin and delavirdine is contraindicated
Rifabutin	Protease inhibitors: ritonavir, saquinavir, indinavir, nelfinavir	Concentrations of indinavir and nelfinavir are reduced by about 30%. Concentrations of ritonavir and saquinavir are reduced by more than 50%.	Induction of cytochrome P450 enzymes	Rifabutin can be administered with indinavir or nelfinavir; however, indinavir and nelfinavir (as well as saquinavir and ritonavir) induce a complementary increase in rifabutin levels; therefore, rifabutin should be used at half-dose (150 mg per day) and rifabutin levels should be monitored; some investigators also recommend increasing the dosage of indinavir and nelfinavir
Nevirapine	Rifampin, rifabutin	Rifampin and rifabutin levels are decreased	Induction of cytochrome P450 enzymes	Combination of nevirapine and rifampin or rifabutin is not recommended
Didanosine	Quinolone antibiotics	Quinolone concentrations are reduced	Chelation of quinolones by cations present in the didanosine buffer	Administer didanosine 6 hours before or 2 hours after the quinolone antibiotic

RT inhibitors. This could then preclude the possibility of ever completely suppressing HIV replication with currently available drugs.

For HIV-infected individuals with TB who are extremely immunocompromised and cannot risk a delay in anti-HIV treatment, simultaneous treatment of HIV and TB requires modifying the anti-HIV and anti-TB regimens, as well as carefully monitoring the clinical and bacteriologic response to anti-TB and anti-HIV therapy. The TB regimen should be modified by substituting rifabutin (a less potent inducer of the hepatic P450 enzyme pathway) for rifampin and by prolonging therapy to at least 9 months. The dose of rifabutin should be lowered from 300 to 150 mg per day, and serum levels of this drug should be monitored. The HIV regimen should be modified by avoiding ritonavir (the most potent inhibitor of the P450 enzyme pathway among the protease inhibitors) and saquinavir. Therefore, an anti-HIV drug regimen consisting of two nucleoside analog RT inhibitors and either indinavir or nelfinavir can be used.

Treatment in Developing Countries

In resource-poor developing countries, limited funds have often forced TB control programs to use suboptimal treatment regimens. In most of sub-Saharan Africa, standard therapy has often consisted of isoniazid, thiacetazone, and streptomycin for 2 months, followed by isoniazid and thiacetazone for 10 months. Unfortunately, this regimen fails in more than 10% of fully compliant HIV-seronegative patients with TB (1) and is even less effective for HIV-infected patients (290, 326–328). Furthermore, 10 to 20% of HIV-infected patients receiving thiacetazone develop severe and occasionally fatal cutaneous hypersensitivity reactions (204, 329–331).

The increased proportion of TB patients worldwide with HIV, the poor treatment success rates in many regions (332), and the increase in drug-resistant TB have prompted the WHO to recommend short-course DOT with rifampin-containing regimens (9). Although only 10% of TB patients worldwide currently have access to short-course DOT (333), the WHO has launched a campaign to obtain additional funding from governmental and nongovernmental agencies to expand DOT programs. At a cost of $11 to $40 United States dollars per TB patient, short-course DOT, although highly cost-effective, is not affordable in many countries.

PREVENTION

Preventive Therapy

Preventive therapy with isoniazid decreases the risk of active TB in HIV-infected persons latently infected with *Mycobacterium tuberculosis* (32, 35, 36, 38, 300, 334–336). In a controlled trial in Haiti, the TB incidence over a 3-year period was more than fivefold lower among tuberculin-reactive HIV-infected patients receiving isoniazid for 12 months than among tuberculin-reactive HIV-infected patients receiving placebo (35). In a controlled trial in Zambia, an unsupervised 6-month course of isoniazid decreased the risk of active TB, although, the incidence of TB among isoniazid recipients gradually increased during the postprophylaxis period (334).

Because HIV-infected persons with latent *Mycobacterium tuberculosis* infection have an extraordinary risk of reactivation, and preventive therapy can reduce that risk, identifying individuals dually infected with *M. tuberculosis* and HIV is critically important. Tuberculin skin testing is therefore recommended for all HIV-infected persons, and preventive therapy should be available to persons at high risk of dual infection (337, 338).

Patients whose tuberculin skin test is positive require a chest radiograph and careful assessment to exclude both pulmonary and extrapulmonary TB, because administration of isoniazid alone to patients with active TB selects for isoniazid-resistant strains. After active TB is excluded, all HIV-infected persons whose tuberculin skin test is positive should receive isoniazid for 12 months unless such treatment is medically contraindicated (302).

Because TB may develop in HIV-infected persons after exogenous reinfection (49), preventive therapy after new exposure to an infectious case of TB should be considered even in persons who have previously been treated for active TB or received prophylaxis for latent TB. HIV-infected persons who have been significantly exposed to an infectious case of MDR TB should receive preventive therapy with a combination of two or three drugs to which the multidrug-resistant organism is susceptible (302, 339).

To improve the sensitivity of tuberculin skin testing in HIV-infected individuals, the CDC and ATS recommend that, in this population, an induration larger than 5 mm should be considered positive (302, 340). However, even with this cutoff, the sensitivity of tuberculin skin testing for detecting latent *Mycobacterium tuberculosis* infection is probably reduced in HIV-infected persons. In several studies, HIV-infected persons have been less likely than matched HIV-seronegative controls to have positive tuberculin skin tests (102, 341–345) (Table 16.7).

Tuberculin skin testing should be done as early as possible in the course of HIV infection because the sensitivity of tuberculin testing declines as immunodeficiency increases (221). The yield of tuberculin skin testing may also be increased if patients with negative tests are retested after at least 7 days (346). Moreover, HIV-infected patients in a risk group for TB who are initially tuberculin negative should have a repeat skin test performed several months after starting anti-HIV therapy because the immunologic improvement associated with such therapy may increase the sensitivity of tuberculin skin testing.

Some experts have recommended that HIV-infected persons with negative tuberculin tests be tested for skin-test anergy with at least two control antigens, such as mumps, tetanus toxoid, or *Candida* antigens, and that those who do not have at least a 3-mm induration to any control antigen (anergic patients) be considered for preventive therapy if they belong to a group with an estimated prevalence of *Mycobacterium tuberculosis* of at least 10% (36, 37, 335, 347). A multicenter clinical trial in the United States randomized approximately 500 HIV-infected anergic patients, considered at risk for TB, to either isoniazid for 6 months or placebo. After a mean 33 months of follow-up, TB developed in 3 of 260 patients receiving isoniazid as compared with 6 of 257 patients receiving placebo (348). Thus, isoniazid prophylaxis did not provide significant clinical benefit in this study. The results of this study, however, cannot be extrapolated to all anergic HIV-infected patients. First, the median CD4 count of patients in this study was 240 cells/μL (range, 100 to 417), and at this level of moderate immunodeficiency, a negative tuberculin test is more reliable than a negative test in patients with more advanced immunodeficiency. Second, the risk of latent *M. tuberculosis* in the population studied is probably lower than in contacts of persons with active TB or in patients from countries with a high prevalence of *M. tuberculosis* infection.

Although more than 95% of dually infected individuals live in developing countries, widescale TB preventive therapy in some of these locations has not been feasible (349). For example, the Pan American Health Organization recom-

Table 16.7 Results of Tuberculin Skin Tests (TSTs) of Asymptomatic HIV-Seropositive (HIV+) Persons and HIV-Seronegative (HIV−) Controls

Subjects (Study Location and Period) (Reference)	TST Cutoff[a] (mm)		Percentage of Subjects for Whom TST Was Positive (%)		P value
	HIV+	HIV−	HIV+	HIV−	
Postpartum women (Uganda, 1988–1989) (341)	3	3	48	82	< .01
Adult residents (Haiti, 1990–1991) (342)	10	10	52	63	< .01
	5	5	65	67	NS
Injection drug users (Baltimore, 1990) (343)	5	10	14	25	.02
	2	10	20	25	NS
Homeless adults (San Francisco, 1990–1992) (102)	5	10	19	37	< .01
Intravenous drug users and homosexual men (Pulmonary Complications of HIV Study Group, United States, 1988–1990) (344)	5	10	6	10	.09

[a]Minimum diameter of induration at skin test site required for test to be considered positive.
NS, not significant.

mends preventive therapy for HIV-infected persons with positive tuberculin skin tests in all areas and for all HIV-infected persons in areas of high TB transmission (350). However, in sub-Saharan Africa, facilities for diagnosing HIV infection are not routinely available, and TB control programs are designed primarily for treating active TB. Because preventive therapy could have a major impact on TB control in this region, studies of the operational aspects of such therapy are being conducted (127, 349, 351–354).

Bacille Calmette-Guérin Vaccination

BCG, a live attenuated strain of *Mycobacterium bovis*, is used throughout the developing world for vaccinating newborns against *M. tuberculosis*. Although BCG vaccine does not prevent *M. tuberculosis* infection, it reduces the risk of active TB, particularly the serious forms of extrapulmonary TB such as meningitis, in infants and young children (355). BCG does not appear to prevent the activation of latent TB induced by HIV-related immunodeficiency (34).

Because BCG is a live vaccine, its safety is a concern in areas where HIV is prevalent. Reported complications include local ulcers, regional suppurative adenitis, and disseminated BCG infection (255). Such complications occurred in infants weeks to months after vaccination (356, 357) and in adults years after childhood vaccination (358) and within weeks after vaccination during adulthood (359). Although complications developed in 13% of vaccinated infants in one institution (360), serious BCG complications have not been observed as frequently in other studies (361–364).

Because most developing countries have no practical means of diagnosing HIV infection in newborns and because TB transmission to children is common in these countries, the WHO recommends that all infants in Africa without symptomatic HIV infection continue to receive BCG vaccine (365). The putative benefits of BCG among infants without HIV infection, and possibly among HIV-infected infants who are not yet immunocompromised, are thought to outweigh the low risk of BCG-related complications in HIV-infected infants.

Infection Control

The large number of recent institutional outbreaks and the increase in cases of MDR TB have led to a reassessment of TB prevention in high-risk environments, and new infection control guidelines were published in 1994 (366). However, analysis of recent outbreaks demonstrated that transmission resulted from inadequate implementation of previously recommended preventive measures, rather than from the inadequacy of existing infection control guidelines (44, 79, 367–369). In some cases, TB diagnosis was delayed because of insufficient clinical evaluation. In other cases, lapses in infection control procedures facilitated transmission.

Current guidelines for preventing TB transmission within institutions emphasize a hierarchy of three strategies. Most important is rapidly to identify, isolate, and treat persons with TB. The second is to use environmental controls to minimize the density of infectious droplet nuclei in areas containing persons with TB. The third is to protect institutional workers who have contact with persons with infectious TB. The intensity of control measures necessary in each institution depends on the number of TB patients cared for and indicators of nosocomial transmission, such as tuberculin skin-test conversion rates among health care workers (366).

Guidelines for preventing nosocomial TB transmission are not specific to HIV-infected persons. However, HIV-infected patients often undergo cough-inducing procedures (e.g., sputum induction, bronchoscopy, and the administration of aerosolized pentamidine), and screening for active TB before cough-inducing procedures is an important part of managing HIV-infected patients. In addition, HIV-infected health care workers need to be informed of their increased risk of developing active TB should they become infected with *Mycobacterium tuberculosis*, so they can follow appropriate preventive measures and consider voluntary work reassignment (111, 112, 366).

RESEARCH AND PUBLIC HEALTH PRIORITIES

Basic research is yielding many practical tools for controlling TB. Gene amplification techniques have led to rapid tests for diagnosing TB. The identification of an *Mycobacterium tuberculosis* insertion sequence (IS6110) has led to a method for fingerprinting *M. tuberculosis* strains (370, 371). The development of a reporter mycobacteriophage has led to a rapid screening test for evaluating anti-TB compounds (372, 373). Advances in understanding the targets of anti-TB drug therapy can be applied to the rapid assessment of drug resistance and to the rational design of new anti-TB compounds (374, 375). Progress in identifying the determinants of mycobacterial virulence and the correlates of human immunity should lead to a more effective vaccine than BCG.

Still, the experience of the past decade demonstrates that if existing TB control strategies are aggressively applied, they will be successful in controlling HIV-associated TB (61). If recent gains made against the resurgence of TB in the United States are sustained, the incidence of TB in this country will continue to decline. In contrast, the number of HIV-infected persons with TB and MDR TB in many countries is increasing rapidly. Scientific research may eventually provide new tools for TB control in these countries. However, in the next few years, the global TB/HIV epidemic will be contained only by the expansion of local TB programs and by the introduction of new resources and political resolve into international public health.

References

1. Murray CJ, Styblo K, Rouillon A. Tuberculosis in developing countries: burden, intervention and cost. Bull Int Union Tuber Lung Dis 1990;65:6–24.
2. Kochi A. The global tuberculosis situation and the new control strategy of the World Health Organization. Tubercle 1991;72:1–6.
3. Haas DW, Des Prez RM. *Mycobacterium tuberculosis*. In: Mandell G, Douglas R, Bennett J, eds. Principles and practice of infectious diseases, vol. 3. New York: Churchill Livingstone, 1995:2213–2243.

4. Centers for Disease Control and Prevention. A strategic plan for the elimination of tuberculosis in the United States. MMWR Morb Mortal Wkly Rep 1989;38:1–25.
5. Rieder HL, Cauthen GM, Comstock GW, et al. Epidemiology of tuberculosis in the United States. Epidemiol Rev 1989;11:79–98.
6. Barnes PF, Bloch AB, Davidson PT, et al. Tuberculosis in patients with human immunodeficiency virus infection. N Engl J Med 1991;324:1644–1650.
7. Hopewell PC. Impact of human immunodeficiency virus infection on the epidemiology, clinical features, management, and control of tuberculosis. Clin Infect Dis 1992;15:540–547.
8. Narain JP, Raviglione MC, Kochi A. HIV-associated tuberculosis in developing countries: epidemiology and strategies for prevention. Tuber Lung Dis 1992;73:311–321.
9. Raviglione MC, Narain JP, Kochi A. HIV-associated tuberculosis in developing countries: clinical features, diagnosis, and treatment. Bull WHO 1992;70:515–526.
10. Centers for Disease Control and Prevention. Tuberculosis and human immunodeficiency virus infection: recommendations of the Advisory Committee for the Elimination of Tuberculosis (ACET). MMWR Morb Mortal Wkly Rep 1989;38:236–238, 243–50.
11. American Thoracic Society. Control of tuberculosis in the United States. Am Rev Respir Dis 1992;146:1623–1633.
12. Sudre P, ten Dam G, Kochi A. Tuberculosis: a global overview of the situation today. Bull WHO 1992;70:149–159.
13. Dolin PJ, Raviglione MC, Kochi A. Global tuberculosis incidence and mortality during 1990–2000. Bull WHO 1994;72:213–220.
14. Raviglione MC, Snider DE, Kochi A. Global epidemiology of tuberculosis: morbidity and mortality of a worldwide epidemic. JAMA 1995;273:220–226.
15. Stead WW. Genetics and resistance to tuberculosis: could resistance be enhanced by genetic engineering? Ann Intern Med 1992;116:937–941.
16. Meltzer MS, Skillman DR, Gomatos PJ, et al. Role of mononuclear phagocytes in the pathogenesis of human immunodeficiency virus infection. Annu Rev Immunol 1990;8:169–194.
17. Rose RM. Immunology of the lung in HIV infection: the pathophysiologic basis for the development of tuberculosis in the AIDS setting. Bull Int Union Tuber Lung Dis 1991;66:15–20.
18. Downing JF, Pasula R, Wright JR, et al. Surfactant protein A promotes attachment of *Mycobacterium tuberculosis* to alveolar macrophages during infection with human immunodeficiency virus. Proc Natl Acad Sci U S A 1995;92:4848–4852.
19. Orme IM, Andersen P, Boom WH. T cell response to *Mycobacterium tuberculosis*. J Infect Dis 1993;167:1481–1497.
20. Toossi Z, Kleinhenz ME, Ellner JJ. Defective interleukin 2 production and responsiveness in human pulmonary tuberculosis. J Exp Med 1986;163:1162.
21. Boom WH. The role of T-cell subsets in *Mycobacterium tuberculosis* infection. Infect Agents Dis 1996;5:73–81.
22. Toossi Z, Gogate P, Shiratsuchi H, et al. Enhanced production of TGF-beta by blood monocytes from patients with active tuberculosis and presence of TGF-beta in tuberculous granulomatous lung lesions. J Immunol 1995;154:465.
23. De Libero G, Flesch I, Kaufmann SH. Mycobacteria-reactive Lyt-2+ T cell lines. Eur J Immunol 1988;18:59–66.
24. Tsukaguchi K, Balaji KN, Boom WH. CD4+ alpha beta T cell and gamma delta T cell responses to *Mycobacterium tuberculosis*: similarities and differences in Ag recognition, cytotoxic effector function, and cytokine production. J Immunol 1995;154:1786–1796.
25. Orme IM, Collins FM. Protection against *Mycobacterium tuberculosis* infection by adoptive immunotherapy: requirement for T cell-deficient recipients. J Exp Med 1983;158:74–83.
26. Pedrazzini T, Hug K, Louis JA. Importance of L3T4+ and Lyt-2+ cells in the immunologic control of infection with *Mycobacterium bovis* strain bacillus Calmette-Guérin in mice: assessment by elimination of T cell subsets in vivo. J Immunol 1987;139:2032–2037.
27. Muller I, Cobbold SP, Waldmann H, et al. Impaired resistance to *Mycobacterium tuberculosis* infection after selective in vivo depletion of L3T4+ and Lyt-2+ T cells. Infect Immun 1987;55:2037–2041.
28. Forte M, Maartens G, Rahelu M, et al. Cytolytic T-cell activity against mycobacterial antigens in HIV. AIDS 1992;6:407–411.
29. Shen JY, Barnes PF, Rea TH, et al. Immunohistology of tuberculous adenitis in symptomatic HIV infection. Clin Exp Immunol 1988;72:186–189.
30. Saltini C, Amicosante M, Girardi E, et al. Early abnormalities of the antibody response against *Mycobacterium tuberculosis* in human immunodeficiency virus infection. J Infect Dis 1993;168:1409–1414.
31. Zhang M, Gong J, Iyer DV, et al. T cell cytokine responses in persons with tuberculosis and human immunodeficiency virus infection. J Clin Invest 1995;94:2435–2442.
32. Selwyn PA, Hartel D, Lewis VA, et al. A prospective study of the risk of tuberculosis among intravenous drug users with human immunodeficiency virus infection. N Engl J Med 1989;320:545–550.
33. Braun MM, Badi N, Ryder RW, et al. A retrospective cohort study of the risk of tuberculosis among women of childbearing age with HIV infection in Zaire. Am Rev Respir Dis 1991;143:501–504.
34. Allen S, Batungwanayo J, Kerlikowske K, et al. Two-year incidence of tuberculosis in cohorts of HIV-infected and uninfected urban Rwandan women. Am Rev Respir Dis 1992;146:1439–1444.
35. Pape JW, Jean SS, Ho JL, et al. Effect of isoniazid prophylaxis on incidence of active tuberculosis and progression of HIV infection. Lancet 1993;342:268–272.
36. Guelar A, Gatell JM, Verdejo J, et al. A prospective study of the risk of tuberculosis among HIV-infected patients. AIDS 1993;7:1345–1349.
37. Moreno S, Baraia-Etxaburu J, Bouza E, et al. Risk for developing tuberculosis among anergic patients infected with HIV. Ann Intern Med 1993;119:194–198.
38. Antonucci G, Girardi E, Raviglione MC, et al. Risk factors for tuberculosis in HIV-infected persons: a prospective cohort study. JAMA 1995;274:143–148.
39. Di Perri G, Cruciani M, Danzi MC, et al. Nosocomial epidemic of active tuberculosis among HIV-infected patients. Lancet 1989;2:1502–1504.
40. Centers for Disease Control and Prevention. *Mycobacterium tuberculosis* transmission in a health clinic: Florida, 1988. MMWR Morb Mortal Wkly Rep 1989;38:256–258, 263–264.
41. Daley CL, Small PM, Schecter GF, et al. An outbreak of tuberculosis with accelerated progression among persons infected with the human immunodeficiency virus: an analysis using restriction-fragment-length polymorphisms. N Engl J Med 1992;326:231–235.
42. Edlin BR, Tokars JI, Grieco MH, et al. An outbreak of multidrug-resistant tuberculosis among hospitalized patients with the acquired immunodeficiency syndrome. N Engl J Med 1992;326:1514–1521.
43. Pearson ML, Jereb JA, Frieden TR, et al. Nosocomial transmission of multidrug-resistant *Mycobacterium tuberculosis*: a risk to patients and health care workers. Ann Intern Med 1992;117:191–196.
44. Dooley SW, Jarvis WR, Martone WJ, et al. Multidrug-resistant tuberculosis [editorial]. Ann Intern Med 1992;117:257–259.
45. Iseman MD. A leap of faith: what can we do to curtail intrainstitutional transmission of tuberculosis? Ann Intern Med 1992;117:251–253.
46. Dooley SW, Villarino ME, Lawrence M, et al. Nosocomial transmission of tuberculosis in a hospital unit. JAMA 1992;267:2632–2634.
47. Beck-Sague C, Dooley SW, Hutton MD, et al. Hospital outbreak of multidrug-resistant *Mycobacterium tuberculosis* infections: factors in transmission to staff and HIV-infected patients. JAMA 1992;268:1280–1286.
48. Coronado VG, Beck-Sague CM, Hutton MD, et al. Transmission of multidrug-resistant *Mycobacterium tuberculosis* among persons with human immunodeficiency virus infection in an urban hospital: epidemiologic and restriction fragment length polymorphism analysis. J Infect Dis 1993;168:1052–1055.

49. Small PM, Shafer RW, Hopewell PC, et al. Exogenous reinfection with multidrug-resistant *Mycobacterium tuberculosis* in patients with advanced HIV infection. N Engl J Med 1993;328:1137–1144.
50. Rieder HL, Cauthen GM, Bloch AB, et al. Tuberculosis and acquired immunodeficiency syndrome: Florida. Arch Intern Med 1989;149:1268-1273.
51. Centers for Disease Control and Prevention. Tuberculosis and acquired immunodeficiency syndrome: New York City. MMWR Morb Mortal Wkly Rep 1987;36:785–790, 795.
52. Stoneburner R, Laroche E, Prevots R, et al. Survival in a cohort of human immunodeficiency virus–infected tuberculosis patients in New York City. Implications for the expansion of the AIDS case definition. Arch Intern Med 1992;152:2033–2037.
53. Shafer RW, Chirgwin KD, Glatt AE, et al. HIV prevalence, immunosuppression, and drug resistance in patients with tuberculosis in an area endemic for AIDS. AIDS 1991;5:399–405.
54. Theuer CP, Hopewell PC, Elias D, Set al. Human immunodeficiency virus infection in tuberculosis patients. J Infect Dis 1990;162:8–12.
55. Korzeniewska-Kosela M, FitzGerald JM, Vedal S, et al. Spectrum of tuberculosis in patients with HIV infection in British Columbia: report of 40 cases. Can Med Assoc J 1992;146:1927–1934.
56. Dupon M, Ragnaud JM. Tuberculosis in patients infected with human immunodeficiency virus 1: a retrospective multicentre study of 123 cases in France. Q J Med 1992;85:719–730.
57. Perronne C, Ghoubontni A, Leport C, et al. Should pulmonary tuberculosis be an AIDS-defining diagnosis? Tuber Lung Dis 1992;73:39–44.
58. Llibre JM, Tor J, Manterola JM, et al. Risk stratification for dissemination of tuberculosis in HIV-infected patients. Q J Med 1992;82:149–157.
59. Mukadi Y, Perriens JH, St Louis ME, et al. Spectrum of immunodeficiency in HIV-1-infected patients with pulmonary tuberculosis in Zaire. Lancet 1993;342:143–146.
60. Jones BE, Young SM, Antoniskis D, et al. Relationship of the manifestations of tuberculosis to CD4 cell counts in patients with human immunodeficiency virus infection. Am Rev Respir Dis 1993;148:1292–1297.
61. Shafer RW, Edlin BR. Tuberculosis in patients infected with human immunodeficiency virus: perspective on the past decade. Clin Infect Dis 1996;22:683–704.
62. Pitchenik AE, Rubinson HA. The radiographic appearance of tuberculosis in patients with the acquired immune deficiency syndrome (AIDS) and pre-AIDS. Am Rev Respir Dis 1985;131:393–396.
63. Klein NC, Duncanson FP, Lenox TH, et al. Use of mycobacterial smears in the diagnosis of pulmonary tuberculosis in AIDS/ARC patients. Chest 1989;95:1190–1192.
64. Shafer RW, Kim DS, Weiss JP, Quale JM. Extrapulmonary tuberculosis in patients with human immunodeficiency virus infection. Medicine 1991;70:384–397.
65. Cauthen GM, Dooley SW, Onorato IM, et al. Transmission of *Mycobacterium tuberculosis* from tuberculosis patients with HIV infection or AIDS. Am J Epidemiol 1996;144:69–77.
66. Manoff SB, Cauthen GM, Stoneburner RL, et al. TB patients with AIDS: Are they more likely to spread TB? [abstract 4621] In: Program and abstracts of the 4th International Conference on AIDS. Stockholm: Swedish Ministry of Health and Social Affairs, 1988:216.
67. Klausner JD, Ryder RW, Baende E, et al. *Mycobacterium tuberculosis* in household contacts of human immunodeficiency virus type 1-seropositive patients with active pulmonary tuberculosis in Kinshasa, Zaire. J Infect Dis 1993;168:106–111.
68. Elliott AM, Hayes RJ, Halwiindi B, et al. The impact of HIV on infectiousness of pulmonary tuberculosis: a community study in Zambia. AIDS 1993;7:981–987.
69. Nunn P, Mungai M, Nyamwaya J, et al. The effect of human immunodeficiency virus type-1 on the infectiousness of tuberculosis. Tuber Lung Dis 1994;75:25–32.
70. Shiratsuchi H, Tsuyuguchi I. Analysis of T cell subsets by monoclonal antibodies in patients with tuberculosis after in vitro stimulation with purified protein derivative of tuberculin. Clin Exp Immunol 1984;57:271–278.
71. Onwubalili JK, Edwards AJ, Palmer L. T4 lymphopenia in human tuberculosis. Tubercle. 1987;68:195–200.
72. Schauf V, Rom WN, Smith KA, et al. Cytokine gene activation and modified responsiveness to interleukin-2 in the blood of tuberculosis patients. J Infect Dis 1993;168:1056–1059.
73. Wallis RS, Vjecha M, Amir-Tahmasseb M, et al. Influence of tuberculosis on human immunodeficiency virus (HIV-1): enhanced cytokine expression and elevated beta 2-microglobulin in HIV-1-associated tuberculosis. J Infect Dis 1993;167:43–48.
74. Toossi Z, Sierra-Madero JG, Blinkhorn RA, et al. Enhanced susceptibility of blood monocytes from patients with pulmonary tuberculosis to productive infection with human immunodeficiency virus type 1. J Exp Med 1993;177:1511–1516.
75. Lederman MM, Georges DL, Kusner DJ, et al. *Mycobacterium tuberculosis* and its purified protein derivative activate expression of the human immunodeficiency virus. J Acquir Immune Defic Syndr 1994;7:727–733.
76. Whalen C, Horsburgh CR, Hom D, et al. Accelerated course of human immunodeficiency virus infection after tuberculosis. Am J Respir Crit Care Med 1995;151:129–135.
77. Goletti D, Weissman D, Jackson RW, et al. Effect of *Mycobacterium tuberculosis* on HIV replication: role of immune activation. J Immunol 1996;157:1271–1278.
78. Centers for Disease Control and Prevention. Tuberculosis morbidity: United States, 1992. MMWR Morb Mortal Wkly Rep 1993;42:696–697, 703,704.
79. Ellner JJ, Hinman AR, Dooley SW, et al. Tuberculosis symposium: emerging problems and promise. J Infect Dis 1993;168:537–551.
80. Centers for Disease Control and Prevention. Expanded tuberculosis surveillance and tuberculosis morbidity: United States, 1993. MMWR Morb Mortal Wkly Rep 1994;43:361–366.
81. Centers for Disease Control and Prevention. Tuberculosis morbidity: United States, 1994. MMWR Morb Mortal Wkly Rep 1995;44:387–395.
82. Centers for Disease Control and Prevention. Tuberculosis morbidity: United States, 1996. MMWR Morb Mortal Wkly Rep 1997;46:695–699.
83. Cantwell MF, Snider DE Jr, Cauthen GM, et al. Epidemiology of tuberculosis in the United States, 1985 through 1992. JAMA 1994;272:535–539.
84. Centers for Disease Control and Prevention. Tuberculosis data in the United States: final data, 1990. MMWR Morb Mortal Wkly Rep 1990;40:23–27.
85. New York City Department of Health, Bureau of Tuberculosis Control. Tuberculosis in New York City, 1992: information summary. New York: New York City Department of Health, Bureau of Tuberculosis Control, 1993.
86. Centers for Disease Control and Prevention. Prevention and control of tuberculosis in U.S. communities with at-risk minority populations: recommendations of the Advisory Council for the Elimination of Tuberculosis. MMWR Morb Mortal Wkly Rep 1992;41:1–11.
87. Onorato IM, McCray E. Prevalence of human immunodeficiency virus infection among patients attending tuberculosis clinics in the United States. J Infect Dis 1992;165:87–92.
88. Brudney K, Dobkin J. Resurgent tuberculosis in New York City: human immunodeficiency virus, homelessness, and the decline of tuberculosis control programs. Am Rev Respir Dis 1991;144:745–749.
89. Pitchenik AE, Burr J, Suarez M, et al. Human T-cell lymphotropic virus-III (HTLV-III) seropositivity and related disease among 71 consecutive patients in whom tuberculosis was diagnosed: a prospective study. Am Rev Respir Dis 1987;135:875–879.

90. Burwen DR, Bloch AB, Griffin LD, et al. National trends in the concurrence of tuberculosis and acquired immunodeficiency syndrome. Arch Intern Med 1995;155:1281–1286.
91. Telzak EE. Tuberculosis and human immunodeficiency virus infection. Med Clin North Am 1997;81:345–360.
92. New York City Department of Health, Bureau of Tuberculosis Control. Tuberculosis in New York City, 1995: information summary. New York: New York City Department of Health, 1995.
93. Bloom BR, Murray CJ. Tuberculosis: commentary on a reemergent killer. Science 1992;257:1055–1064.
94. Centers for Disease Control and Prevention. Outbreak of multidrug-resistant tuberculosis at a hospital: New York City, 1991. MMWR Morb Mortal Wkly Rep 1993;42:427, 433–434.
95. Pierce JR, Sims SL, Holman GH. Transmission of tuberculosis to hospital workers by a patient with AIDS. Chest 1992;101:581–582.
96. Fischl MA, Uttamchandani RB, Daikos GL, et al. An outbreak of tuberculosis caused by multiple-drug-resistant tubercle bacilli among patients with HIV infection. Ann Intern Med 1992;117:177–183.
97. Centers for Disease Control and Prevention. Transmission of multidrug-resistant tuberculosis from an HIV-positive client in a residential substance-abuse treatment facility: Michigan. MMWR Morb Mortal Wkly Rep 1991;40:129–131.
98. Valway SE, Greifinger RB, Papania M, et al. Multidrug-resistant tuberculosis in the New York State prison system, 1990–1991. J Infect Dis 1994;170:151–156.
99. Small PM, Hopewell PC, Singh SP, et al. The epidemiology of tuberculosis in San Francisco: a population-based study using conventional and molecular methods. N Engl J Med 1994;330:1703–1709.
100. Alland D, Kalkut G, Moss AR, et al. Transmission of tuberculosis in New York City: an analysis by DNA fingerprinting and conventional epidemiological methods. N Engl J Med 1994;330:1710–1716.
101. Torres RA, Mani S, Altholz J, Brickner PW. Human immunodeficiency virus infection among homeless men in a New York City shelter: association with *Mycobacterium tuberculosis* infection. Arch Intern Med 1990;150:2030–2036.
102. Zolopa AR, Hahn JA, Gorter R, et al. HIV and tuberculosis infection in San Francisco's homeless adults: prevalence and risk factors in a representative sample. JAMA 1994;272:455–461.
103. Braun MM, Truman BI, Maguire B, et al. Increasing incidence of tuberculosis in a prison inmate population: association with HIV infection. JAMA 1989;261:393–397.
104. Centers for Disease Control and Prevention. Prevention and control of tuberculosis in correctional institutions: recommendations of the Advisory Committee for the Elimination of Tuberculosis. MMWR Morb Mortal Wkly Rep 1989;38:313–320, 325.
105. Bellin EY, Fletcher DD, Safyer SM. Association of tuberculosis infection with increased time in or admission to the New York City jail system. JAMA 1993;269:2228–2231.
106. Glaser JB, Greifinger RB. Correctional health care: a public health opportunity. Ann Intern Med 1993;118:139–145.
107. Ikeda RM, Birkhead GS, DiFerdinando GT, et al. Nosocomial tuberculosis: an outbreak of a strain resistant to seven drugs. Infect Control Hosp Epidemiol 1995;16:152–159.
108. Moss AR, Alland D, Telzak E, et al. A city-wide outbreak of a multiple-drug-resistant strain of *Mycobacterium tuberculosis* in New York. Int J Tuber Lung Dis 1997;1:115–121.
109. Centers for Disease Control and Prevention. Meeting the challenge of multidrug-resistant tuberculosis: summary of a conference. MMWR Morb Mortal Wkly Rep 1992;41: 51–57.
110. Edlin BR, Valway SE, Onorato IM. Clusters of multidrug-resistant tuberculosis [letter]. Ann Intern Med 1993;118:77.
111. Sepkowitz KA. AIDS, tuberculosis, and the health care worker. Clin Infect Dis 1995;20:232–242.
112. Menzies D, Fanning A, Yuan L, et al. Tuberculosis among health care workers. N Engl J Med 1995;332:92–98.
113. New York City Department of Health, Bureau of Tuberculosis Control. Tuberculosis in New York City, 1990: information summary. New York: New York City Department of Health, 1995.
114. Jones DS, Malecki JM, Bigler WJ, et al. Pediatric tuberculosis and human immunodeficiency virus infection in Palm Beach County, Florida. Am J Dis Child 1992;146:1166–1170.
115. Bakshi SS, Alvarez D, Hilfer CL, et al. Tuberculosis in human immunodeficiency virus-infected children: a family infection. Am J Dis Child 1993;147:320–324.
116. Khouri YF, Mastrucci MT, Hutto C, et al. *Mycobacterium tuberculosis* in children with human immunodeficiency virus type 1 infection. Pediatr Infect Dis J 1992;11:950–955.
117. Moss WJ, Dedyo T, Suarez M, et al. Tuberculosis in children infected with human immunodeficiency virus: a report of five cases. Pediatr Infect Dis J 1992;11:114–116.
118. Gutman LT, Moye J, Zimmer B, et al. Tuberculosis in human immunodeficiency virus–exposed or -infected United States children. Pediatr Infect Dis J 1994;13:963–968.
119. Perriens JH, Mukadi Y, Nunn P. Tuberculosis and HIV infection: implications for Africa. AIDS 1991;5(Suppl 1):S127–S133.
120. Goodgame RW. AIDS in Uganda: clinical and social features. N Engl J Med 1990;323:383–389.
121. De Cock KM, Soro B, Coulibaly IM, et al. Tuberculosis and HIV infection in sub-Saharan Africa. JAMA 1992;268:1581–1587.
122. Snider DE Jr, La Montagne JR. The neglected global tuberculosis problem: a report of the 1992 World Congress on Tuberculosis. J Infect Dis 1994;169:1189–1196.
123. Okot-Nwang M, Wabwire-Mangen F, Kagezi VB. Increasing prevalence of tuberculosis among Mulago Hospital admissions, Kampala, Uganda (1985–1989). Tuber Lung Dis 1993;74:121–125.
124. Batungwanayo J, Taelman H, Dhote R, et al. Pulmonary tuberculosis in Kigali, Rwanda: impact of human immunodeficiency virus infection on clinical and radiographic presentation. Am Rev Respir Dis 1992;146:53–56.
125. Nunn P, Gathua S, Kibuga D, et al. The impact of HIV on resource utilization by patients with tuberculosis in a tertiary referral hospital, Nairobi, Kenya. Tuber Lung Dis 1993;74:273–279.
126. Abouya YL, Beaumel A, Lucas S, et al. *Pneumocystis carinii* pneumonia: an uncommon cause of death in African patients with acquired immunodeficiency syndrome. Am Rev Respir Dis 1992;145:617–620.
127. Bermejo A, Veeken H, Berra A. Tuberculosis incidence in developing countries with high prevalence of HIV infection. AIDS 1992;6:1203–1206.
128. Reeve PA. HIV infection in patients admitted to a general hospital in Malawi. BMJ 1989;298:1567–1568.
129. Lucas SB, Hounnou A, Peacock C, et al. The mortality and pathology of HIV infection in a west African city. AIDS 1993;7:1569–1579.
130. Cantwell MF, Binkin NJ. Tuberculosis in sub-Saharan Africa: a regional assessment of the impact of the human immunodeficiency virus and National Tuberculosis Control Program quality. Tuber Lung Dis 1996;77:220–225.
131. Cantwell MF, Binkin NJ. Impact of HIV on tuberculosis in sub-Saharan Africa: a regional perspective. Int J Tuber Lung Dis 1997;1:205–214.
132. Jain MK, John TJ, Keusch GT. A review of human immunodeficiency virus infection in India. J Acquir Immune Defic Syndr 1994;7:1185–1194.
133. Kaur A, Babu PG, Jacob M, et al. Clinical and laboratory profile of AIDS in India. J Acquir Immune Defic Syndr 1992;5:883–889.
134. Solomon S, Anuradha S, Rajasekaran S. Trend of HIV infection in patients with pulmonary tuberculosis in South India. Tuber Lung Dis 1995;76:17–19.
135. Vieira J, Frank E, Spira TJ, et al. Acquired immune deficiency in Haitians: opportunistic infections in previously healthy Haitian immigrants. N Engl J Med 1983;308:125–129.
136. Pape JW, Liautaud B, Thomas F, et al. Characteristics of the acquired immunodeficiency syndrome (AIDS) in Haiti. N Engl J Med 1983; 309:945–950.

137. Pitchenik AE, Cole C, Russell BW, et al. Tuberculosis, atypical mycobacteriosis, and the acquired immunodeficiency syndrome among Haitian and non-Haitian patients in south Florida. Ann Intern Med 1984;101:641–645.
138. Jessurun J, Angeles-Angeles A, Gasman N. Comparative demographic and autopsy findings in acquired immune deficiency syndrome in two Mexican populations. J Acquir Immune Defic Syndr 1990;3:579–583.
139. Raviglione MC, Sudre P, Rieder HL, et al. Secular trends of tuberculosis in western Europe. Bull WHO 1993;71:297–306.
140. Bouza E, Martin-Scapa C, Bernaldo de Quiros JC, et al. High prevalence of tuberculosis in AIDS patients in Spain. Eur J Clin Microbiol Infect Dis 1988;7:785–788.
141. Laguna F, Adrados M, Diaz F, et al. AIDS and tuberculosis in Spain: a report of 140 cases. J Infect 1991;23:139–144.
142. Vall Mayans M, Maguire A, Miret M, et al. The spread of AIDS and the re-emergence of tuberculosis in Catalonia, Spain. AIDS 1997;11:499–505.
143. Antonucci G, Girardi E, Armignacco O, et al. Tuberculosis in HIV-infected subjects in Italy: a multicentre study: the Gruppo Italiano di Studio Tubercolosi e AIDS. AIDS 1992;6:1007–1013.
144. Yates MD, Pozniak A, Grange JM. Isolation of mycobacteria from patients seropositive for the human immunodeficiency virus (HIV) in south east England: 1984–1992. Thorax 1993;48:990–995.
145. Zhang Y, Heym B, Allen B, et al. The catalase-peroxidase gene and isoniazid resistance of *Mycobacterium tuberculosis*. Nature 1992;358:591–593.
146. Telenti A, Imboden P, Marchesi F, et al. Detection of rifampicin-resistance mutations in *Mycobacterium tuberculosis*. Lancet 1993;341:647–650.
147. Banerjee A, Dubnau E, Quemard A, et al. inhA, a gene encoding a target for isoniazid and ethionamide in *Mycobacterium tuberculosis*. Science 1994;263:227–230.
148. Honore N, Cole ST. Streptomycin resistance in mycobacteria. Antimicrob Agents Chemother 1994;38:238–242.
149. Sullivan EA, Kreiswirth BN, Palumbo L, et al. Emergence of fluoroquinolone-resistant tuberculosis in New York City. Lancet 1995;345:1148–1150.
150. Altamirano M, Marostenmaki J, Wong A, et al. Mutations in the catalase-peroxidase gene from isoniazid-resistant *Mycobacterium tuberculosis* isolates. J Infect Dis 1994;169:1162–1165.
151. Iseman MD. Evolution of drug-resistant tuberculosis: a tale of two species. Proc Natl Acad Sci U S A. 1994;91:2428–2429.
152. Mahmoudi A, Iseman MD. Pitfalls in the care of patients with tuberculosis. Common errors and their association with the acquisition of drug resistance. JAMA 1993;270:65–68.
153. Iseman MD. Treatment of multidrug-resistant tuberculosis. N Engl J Med 1993;329:784–791.
154. Goble M, Iseman MD, Madsen LA, et al. Treatment of 171 patients with pulmonary tuberculosis resistant to isoniazid and rifampin. N Engl J Med 1993;328:527–532.
155. Bloch AB, Cauthen GM, Onorato IM, et al. Nationwide survey of drug-resistant tuberculosis in the United States. JAMA 1994;271:665–671.
156. Centers for Disease Control and Prevention. National action plan to combat multidrug-resistant tuberculosis. MMWR Morb Mortal Wkly Rep 1992;41:5-48.
157. Frieden TR, Sterling T, Pablos-Mendez A, et al. The emergence of drug-resistant tuberculosis in New York City. N Engl J Med 1993;328:521–526.
158. Moore M, Onorato IM, McCray E, et al. Trends in drug-resistant tuberculosis in the United States, 1993-1996. JAMA 1997;278:833–837.
159. Fujiwara PI, Larkin C, Frieden TR. Directly observed therapy in New York City: history, implementation, results, and challenges. Clin Chest Med 1997;18:135–148.
160. Bradford WZ, Martin JN, Reingold AL, et al. The changing epidemiology of acquired drug-resistant tuberculosis in San Francisco, USA. Lancet 1996;348:928–931.
161. Nolan CM, Williams DL, Cave MD, et al. Evolution of rifampin resistance in human immunodeficiency virus-associated tuberculosis. Am J Respir Crit Care Med 1995;152:1067–1071.
162. Shafer RW, Small PM, Larkin C, et al. Temporal trends and transmission patterns during the emergence of multidrug-resistant tuberculosis in New York City: a molecular epidemiological assessment. J Infect Dis 1995;171:170–176.
163. Ritacco V, Di Lonardo M, Reniero A, et al. Nosocomial spread of human immunodeficiency virus–related multidrug resistant tuberculosis in Buenos Aires. J Infect Dis 1997;176:637–642.
164. Nolan CM. Nosocomial multidrug-resistant tuberculosis-global spread of the third epidemic. J Infect Dis 1997;176:748–751.
165. Cohn DL, Bustreo F, Raviglione MC. Drug-resistant tuberculosis: review of the worldwide situation and the WHO/IUATLD Global Surveillance Project. International Union Against Tuberculosis and Lung Disease. Clin Infect Dis 1997;24(Suppl 1):S121–S130.
166. Phadtare JM, Saple DG, Banka RB. Multiple drug resistance tuberculosis and mycobacteriosis in HIV infection. Presented at the 11th International Conference on AIDS, Vancouver, British Columbia, Canada, 1996.
167. Arbulu MM, Weisburd G, Biglione J, et al. Multidrug resistant tuberculosis in AIDS patients in the infectious diseases service sala I Poli I: Carrasco-Rosario, Argentina. Presented at the 11th International Conference on AIDS, Vancouver, British Columbia, Canada, 1996.
168. Gonzalez ML, Palmero D, Alberti F, et al. Nosocomial outbreak of multi-drug resistant tuberculosis among AIDS patients in Buenos Aires, Argentina. Presented at the 11th International Conference on AIDS, Vancouver, British Columbia, Canada, 1996.
169. Masini R, Metta H, Corti M, et al. Nosocomial outbreak of multidrug resistant tuberculosis: evaluation of control measures. Presented at the 11th International Conference on AIDS, Vancouver, British Columbia, Canada, 1996.
170. Shetty K, Bhave G, Salvi V. Comparative study of drug resistance pattern in HIV positive and HIV negative cases of tuberculosis. Presented at the 11th International Conference on AIDS, Vancouver, British Columbia, Canada, 1996.
171. Mellado M, M-Fontelos P, Clleruelo M, et al. Nosocomial outbreak of multidrug resistant tuberculosis in HIV infected children. Presented at the 11th International Conference on AIDS, Vancouver, British Columbia, Canada, 1996.
172. Kritski AL, Rodrigues de Jesus LS, Andrade MK, et al. Retreatment tuberculosis cases: factors associated with drug resistance and adverse outcomes. Chest 1997;111:1162–1167.
173. Easterbook P, Bell A, Hannan M, et al. Nosocomial outbreak of multidrug resistant tuberculosis in a London HIV unit: outbreak investigation and clinical follow-up. Presented at the 11th International Conference on AIDS, Vancouver, British Columbia, Canada, 1996.
174. Centers for Disease Control and Prevention. Multidrug-resistant tuberculosis outbreaks on an HIV ward: Madrid, Spain, 1991–1995. MMWR Morb Mortal Wkly Rep 1996;45:330–333.
175. Volonterio A, Orcese C, Caggese L, et al. Clinical aspects of an outbreak of multidrug-resistant human tuberculosis in advanced HIV infection. Presented at the 11th International Conference on AIDS, Vancouver, British Columbia, Canada, 1996.
176. Gachot B, Wolff M, Clair B, et al. Severe tuberculosis in patients with human immunodeficiency virus infection. Intensive Care Med 1990;16:491–493.
177. Ahuja SS, Ahuja SK, Phelps KR, et al. Hemodynamic confirmation of septic shock in disseminated tuberculosis. Crit Care Med 1992;20:901–903.
178. Vadillo M, Corbella X, Carratala J. AIDS presenting as septic shock caused by *Mycobacterium tuberculosis*. Scand J Infect Dis 1994;26:105–106.

179. Sunderam G, McDonald RJ, Maniatis T, et al. Tuberculosis as a manifestation of the acquired immunodeficiency syndrome (AIDS). JAMA 1986;256:362–366.
180. Chaisson RE, Schecter GF, Theuer CP, et al. Tuberculosis in patients with the acquired immunodeficiency syndrome: clinical features, response to therapy, and survival. Am Rev Respir Dis 1987;136:570–574.
181. Soriano E, Mallolas J, Gatell JM, et al. Characteristics of tuberculosis in HIV-infected patients: a case-control study. AIDS 1988;2:429–432.
182. Shafer RW, Goldberg R, Sierra M, et al. Frequency of *Mycobacterium tuberculosis* bacteremia in patients with tuberculosis in an area endemic for AIDS. Am Rev Respir Dis 1989;140:1611–1613.
183. Barber TW, Craven DE, McCabe WR. Bacteremia due to *Mycobacterium tuberculosis* in patients with human immunodeficiency virus infection: a report of 9 cases and a review of the literature. Medicine 1990;69:375–383.
184. Clark RA, Blakley SL, Greer D, et al. Hematogenous dissemination of *Mycobacterium tuberculosis* in patients with AIDS. Rev Infect Dis 1991;13:1089–1092.
185. Bouza E, Diaz-Lopez MD, Moreno S, et al. *Mycobacterium tuberculosis* bacteremia in patients with and without human immunodeficiency virus infection. Arch Intern Med 1993;153:496–500.
186. Nambuya A, Sewankambo N, Mugerwa J, et al. Tuberculous lymphadenitis associated with human immunodeficiency virus (HIV) in Uganda. J Clin Pathol 1988;41:93–96.
187. Hewlett D Jr, Duncanson FP, Jagadha V, et al. Lymphadenopathy in an inner-city population consisting principally of intravenous drug abusers with suspected acquired immunodeficiency syndrome. Am Rev Respir Dis 1988;137:1275–1279.
188. Shriner KA, Mathisen GE, Goetz MB. Comparison of mycobacterial lymphadenitis among persons infected with human immunodeficiency virus and seronegative controls. Clin Infect Dis 1992;15:601–605.
189. Pithie AD, Chicksen B. Fine-needle extrathoracic lymph-node aspiration in HIV-associated sputum-negative tuberculosis. Lancet 1992;340:1504–1505.
190. Bem C, Patil PS, Elliott AM, et al. The value of wide-needle aspiration in the diagnosis of tuberculous lymphadenitis in Africa. AIDS 1993;7:1221–1225.
191. Fee MJ, Oo MM, Gabayan AE, et al. Abdominal tuberculosis in patients infected with the human immunodeficiency virus. Clin Infect Dis 1995;20:938–944.
192. Radin DR. Intraabdominal *Mycobacterium tuberculosis* vs *Mycobacterium avium-intracellulare* infections in patients with AIDS: distinction based on CT findings. AJR Am J Roentgenol 1991;156:487–491.
193. Lupatkin H, Brau N, Flomenberg P, et al. Tuberculous abscesses in patients with AIDS. Clin Infect Dis 1992;14:1040–1044.
194. Brody JM, Miller DK, Zeman RK, Ket al. Gastric tuberculosis: a manifestation of acquired immunodeficiency syndrome. Radiology 1986;159:347–348.
195. Wasser LS, Shaw GW, Talavera W. Endobronchial tuberculosis in the acquired immunodeficiency syndrome. Chest 1988;94:1240–1244.
196. de Silva R, Stoopack PM, Raufman JP. Esophageal fistulas associated with mycobacterial infection in patients at risk for AIDS. Radiology 1990;175:449–453.
197. Allen CM, Craze J, Grundy A. Tuberculous broncho-oesophageal fistula in the acquired immunodeficiency syndrome. Clin Radiol 1991;43:60–62.
198. Jaber B, Gleckman R. Tuberculous pancreatic abscess as an initial AIDS-defining disorder in a patient infected with the human immunodeficiency virus: case report and review. Clin Infect Dis 1995;20:890–894.
199. Small PM, Schecter GF, Goodman PC, et al. Treatment of tuberculosis in patients with advanced human immunodeficiency virus infection. N Engl J Med 1991;324:289–294.
200. Berenguer J, Moreno S, Laguna F, et al. Tuberculous meningitis in patients infected with the human immunodeficiency virus. N Engl J Med 1992;326:668–672.
201. Bishburg E, Sunderam G, Reichman LB, et al. Central nervous system tuberculosis with the acquired immunodeficiency syndrome and its related complex. Ann Intern Med 1986;105:210–213.
202. Dube MP, Holtom PD, Larsen RA. Tuberculous meningitis in patients with and without human immunodeficiency virus infection. Am J Med 1992;93:520–524.
203. Whiteman M, Espinoza L, Post JD, et al. Central nervous system tuberculosis in HIV-infected patients: clinical and radiographic findings. Am J Neuroradiol 1995;16:1319–1327.
204. Elliott AM, Luo N, Tembo G, et al. Impact of HIV on tuberculosis in Zambia: a cross sectional study. BMJ 1990;301:412–415.
205. Cegielski JP, Ramiya K, Lallinger GJ, et al. Pericardial disease and human immunodeficiency virus in Dar es Salaam, Tanzania. Lancet 1990;335:209–212.
206. Batungwanayo J, Taelman H, Allen S, et al. Pleural effusion, tuberculosis and HIV-1 infection in Kigali, Rwanda. AIDS 1993;7:73–79.
207. Pozniak AL, Weinberg J, Mahari M, et al. Tuberculous pericardial effusion associated with HIV infection: a sign of disseminated disease. Tuber Lung Dis 1994;75:297–300.
208. Maher D, Harries AD. Tuberculosis pericardial effusion: a prospective clinical study in a low-resource setting: Blantyre, Malawi. Int J Tuber Lung Dis 1997;1:358–364.
209. Lin RY, Schwartz RA, Lambert WC. Cutaneous-pericardial tuberculous fistula in an immunocompromised host. Int J Dermatol 1986;25:456–458.
210. Stack RJ, Bickley LK, Coppel IG. Miliary tuberculosis presenting as skin lesions in a patient with acquired immunodeficiency syndrome. J Am Acad Dermatol 1990;23:1031–1035.
211. Rohatgi PK, Palazzolo JV, Saini NB. Acute miliary tuberculosis of the skin in acquired immunodeficiency syndrome. J Am Acad Dermatol 1992;26:356–359.
212. Long R, Maycher B, Scalcini M, et al. The chest roentgenogram in pulmonary tuberculosis patients seropositive for human immunodeficiency virus type 1. Chest 1991;99:123–127.
213. Saks AM, Posner R. Tuberculosis in HIV positive patients in South Africa: a comparative radiological study with HIV negative patients. Clin Radiol 1992;46:387–390.
214. Greenberg SD, Frager D, Suster B, et al. Active pulmonary tuberculosis in patients with AIDS: spectrum of radiographic findings (including a normal appearance). Radiology 1994;193:115–119.
215. Pedro-Botet J, Gutierrez J, Miralles R, et al. Pulmonary tuberculosis in HIV-infected patients with normal chest radiographs. AIDS 1992;6:91–93.
216. Pastores SM, Naidich DP, Aranda CP, et al. Intrathoracic adenopathy associated with pulmonary tuberculosis in patients with human immunodeficiency virus infection. Chest 1993;103:1433–1437.
217. Hulnick DH, Megibow AJ, Naidich DP, et al. Abdominal tuberculosis: CT evaluation. Radiology 1985;157:199–204.
218. Pedro-Botet J, Maristany MT, Miralles R, et al. Splenic tuberculosis in patients with AIDS. Rev Infect Dis 1991;13:1069–1071.
219. Wolff MJ, Bitran J, Northland RG, et al. Splenic abscesses due to *Mycobacterium tuberculosis* in patients with AIDS. Rev Infect Dis 1991;13:373–375.
220. Long R, Scalcini M, Manfreda J, et al. Impact of human immunodeficiency virus type 1 on tuberculosis in rural Haiti. Am Rev Respir Dis 1991;143:69–73.
221. Huebner RE, Schein MF, Bass JB. The tuberculin skin test. Clin Infect Dis 1993;17:968–975.
222. Jagadha V, Andavolu RH, Huang CT. Granulomatous inflammation in the acquired immune deficiency syndrome. Am J Clin Pathol 1985;84:598–602.
223. Nichols L, Florentine B, Lewis W, et al. Bone marrow examination for the diagnosis of mycobacterial and fungal infections in the acquired immunodeficiency syndrome. Arch Pathol Lab Med 1991;115:1125–1132.
224. Hill AR, Premkumar S, Brustein S, et al. Disseminated tuberculosis in the acquired immunodeficiency syndrome era. Am Rev Respir Dis 1991;144:1164–1170.

225. Fischl MA, Daikos GL, Uttamchandani RB, et al. Clinical presentation and outcome of patients with HIV infection and tuberculosis caused by multiple-drug-resistant bacilli. Ann Intern Med 1992;117:184–190.
226. Young LS. *Mycobacterium avium* complex infection. J Infect Dis 1988;157:863–867.
227. Kramer F, Modilevsky T, Waliany AR, et al. Delayed diagnosis of tuberculosis in patients with human immunodeficiency virus infection. Am J Med 1990;89:451–456.
228. Alwood K, Keruly J, Moore-Rice K, et al. Effectiveness of supervised intermittent therapy for tuberculosis in HIV-infected patients. AIDS 1994;8:1103–1108.
229. Miralles P, Moreno S, Perez-Tascon M, et al. Fever of uncertain origin in patients infected with the human immunodeficiency virus. Clin Infect Dis 1995;20:872–875.
230. Colebunders RL, Lebughe I, Nzila N, et al. Cutaneous delayed-type hypersensitivity in patients with human immunodeficiency virus infection in Zaire. J Acquir Immune Defic Syndr 1989;2:576–578.
231. Espinal MA, Reingold AL, Koenig E, et al. Screening for active tuberculosis in HIV testing centre. Lancet 1995;345:890–893.
232. Girardi E, Antonucci G, Ippolito G, et al. Association of tuberculosis risk with the degree of tuberculin reaction in HIV-infected patients: the Gruppo Italiano di Studio Tuberculosi e AIDS. Arch Intern Med 1997;157:797–800.
233. Long R, Scalcini M, Manfreda J, et al. The impact of HIV on the usefulness of sputum smears for the diagnosis of tuberculosis. Am J Public Health 1991;81:1326–1328.
234. Elliott AM, Namaambo K, Allen BW, et al. Negative sputum smear results in HIV-positive patients with pulmonary tuberculosis in Lusaka, Zambia. Tuber Lung Dis 1993;74:191–194.
235. Barnes PF, Steele MA, Young SM, et al. Tuberculosis in patients with human immunodeficiency virus infection: how often does it mimic *Pneumocystis carinii* pneumonia? Chest 1992;102:428–432.
236. Parry CM, Kamoto O, Harries AD, et al. The use of sputum induction for establishing a diagnosis in patients with suspected tuberculosis in Malawi. Tuber Lung Dis 1995;76:72–76.
237. Salzman SH, Schindel ML, Aranda CP, et al. The role of bronchoscopy in the diagnosis of pulmonary tuberculosis in patients at risk for HIV infection. Chest 1992;102:143–146.
238. Kennedy DJ, Lewis WP, Barnes PF. Yield of bronchoscopy for the diagnosis of tuberculosis in patients with human immunodeficiency virus infection. Chest 1992;102:1040–1044.
239. Miro AM, Gibilara E, Powell S, et al. The role of fiberoptic bronchoscopy for diagnosis of pulmonary tuberculosis in patients at risk for AIDS. Chest 1992;101:1211–1214.
240. Calpe JL, Chiner E, Laramendi CH. Endobronchial tuberculosis in HIV-infected patients. AIDS 1995;9:1159–1164.
241. Modilevsky T, Sattler FR, Barnes PF. Mycobacterial disease in patients with human immunodeficiency virus infection. Arch Intern Med 1989;149:2201–2205.
242. Llatjos M, Romeu J, Clotet B, et al. A distictive cytologic pattern for diagnosing tuberculous lymphadenitis in AIDS. J Acquir Immune Defic Syndr 1993;6:1335–1338.
243. Bem C, Patil PS, Bharucha H, et al. Importance of human immunodeficiency virus–associated lymphadenopathy and tuberculous lymphadenitis in patients undergoing lymph node biopsy in Zambia. Br J Surg 1996;83:75–78.
244. Bassiri A, Chan NB, McLeod A, et al. Disseminated cutaneous infection due to *Mycobacterium tuberculosis* in a person with AIDS. Can Med Assoc J 1993;148:577–578.
245. Eng RH, Bishburg E, Smith SM, et al. Diagnosis of *Mycobacterium* bacteremia in patients with acquired immunodeficiency syndrome by direct examination of blood films. J Clin Microbiol 1989;27:768–769.
246. Biron F, Reveil JC, Penalba C, et al. Direct visualization of *Mycobacterium tuberculosis* in a blood sample from an AIDS patient [letter]. AIDS 1990;4:259.
247. Fournier AM, Dickinson GM, Erdfrocht IR, et al. Tuberculosis and nontuberculous mycobacteriosis in patients with AIDS. Chest 1988;93:772–775.
248. Comer GM, Mukherjee S, Scholes JV, et al. Liver biopsies in the acquired immune deficiency syndrome: influence of endemic disease and drug abuse. Am J Gastroenterol 1989;84:1525–1531.
249. Prego V, Glatt AE, Roy V, et al. Comparative yield of blood culture for fungi and mycobacteria, liver biopsy, and bone marrow biopsy in the diagnosis of fever of undetermined origin in human immunodeficiency virus–infected patients. Arch Intern Med 1990;150:333–336.
250. Whiteman ML. Neuroimaging of central nervous system tuberculosis in HIV-infected patients. Neuroimaging Clin North Am 1997;7:199–214.
251. Tenover FC, Crawford JT, Huebner RE, et al. The resurgence of tuberculosis: is your laboratory ready? J Clin Microbiol 1993;31:767–770.
252. Roberts GD, Koneman EW, Kim YK. *Mycobacterium*. In: Balows A, Hausler W, Herrman K, et al, eds. Manual of Clinical Microbiology, vol. 5. Washington, DC: American Society for Microbiology, 1991:304–339.
253. Shinnick TM, Good RC. Diagnostic mycobacteriology laboratory practices. Clin Infect Dis 1995;21:291–299.
254. Lombardo PC, Weitzman I. Isolation of *Mycobacterium tuberculosis* and *M. avium* complex from the same skin lesions in AIDS [letter]. N Engl J Med 1990;323:916–917.
255. Weltman AC, Rose DN. The safety of Bacille Calmette-Guérin vaccination in HIV infection and AIDS. AIDS 1993;7:149–157.
256. Dankner WM, Waecker NJ, Essey MA, et al. *Mycobacterium bovis* infections in San Diego: a clinicoepidemiologic study of 73 patients and a historical review of a forgotten pathogen. Medicine 1993;72:11–37.
257. Guerrero A, Cobo J, Fortun J, et al. Nosocomial transmission of *Mycobacterium bovis* resistant to 11 drugs in people with advanced HIV-1 infection. Lancet 1997;350:1738–1742.
258. Torriani FJ, Havlir DV, Hwang J, et al. A ten year review of *Mycobacterium tuberculosis* and *Mycobacterium bovis* infections in adults coinfected with HIV in San Diego. Presented at the 4th Conference on Retroviruses and Opportunistic Infections, Washington, DC, 1997.
259. Blazquez J, Espinosa de Los Monteros LE, Samper S, et al. Genetic characterization of multidrug-resistant *Mycobacterium bovis* strains from a hospital outbreak involving human immunodeficiency virus-positive patients. J Clin Microbiol 1997;35:1390–1393.
260. Talbot EA, Perkins MD, Fagundes S, et al. Disseminated bacille Calmette-Guérin disease after vaccination: case report and review. Clin Infect Dis 1997;24:1139–1146.
261. Horsburgh CR, Selik RM. The epidemiology of disseminated nontuberculous mycobacterial infection in the acquired immunodeficiency syndrome (AIDS). Am Rev Respir Dis 1989;139:4–7.
262. Levine B, Chaisson RE. *Mycobacterium kansasii*: a cause of treatable pulmonary disease associate with advanced human immunodeficiency virus (HIV) infection. Ann Intern Med 1991;114:861–868.
263. Shafer RW, Sierra MF. *Mycobacterium xenopi, Mycobacterium fortuitum, Mycobacterium kansasii*, and other nontuberculous mycobacteria in an area endemic for AIDS. Clin Infect Dis 1992;15:161–162.
264. Bottger EC, Teske A, Kirschner P, et al. Disseminated *Mycobacterium genavense* infection in patients with AIDS. Lancet 1992;340:76–80.
265. Workshop ATS. Rapid diagnostic tests for tuberculosis: what is the appropriate use? Am J Respir Crit Care Med 1997;155:1804–1814.
266. Barnes PF. Rapid diagnostic tests for tuberculosis: progress but no gold standard [editorial; comment]. Am J Respir Crit Care Med 1997;155:1497–1498.
267. Brisson-Noel A, Gicquel B, Lecossier D, et al. Rapid diagnosis of tuberculosis by amplification of mycobacterial DNA in clinical samples. Lancet 1989;2:1069–1071.
268. Eisenach KD, Sifford MD, Cave MD, et al. Detection of *Mycobacterium tuberculosis* in sputum samples using a polymerase chain reaction. Am Rev Respir Dis 1991;144:1160–1163.

269. Schluger NW, Condos R, Lewis S, Rom WN. Amplification of DNA of *Mycobacterium tuberculosis* from peripheral blood of patients with pulmonary tuberculosis. Lancet 1994;344:232–233.
270. Noordhoek GT, Kolk AH, Bjune G, et al. Sensitivity and specificity of PCR for detection of *Mycobacterium tuberculosis*: a blind comparison study among seven laboratories. J Clin Microbiol 1994;32:277–284.
271. Bodmer T, Gurtner A, Schopfer K, et al. Screening of respiratory tract specimens for the presence of *Mycobacterium tuberculosis* by using the Gen-Probe amplified *Mycobacterium tuberculosis* direct test. J Clin Microbiol 1994;32:1483–1487.
272. Pfyffer GE, Kissling P, Wirth R, et al. Direct detection of *Mycobacterium tuberculosis* complex in respiratory specimens by a target-amplified test system. J Clin Microbiol 1994;32:918–923.
273. D'Amato RF, Wallman AA, Hochstein LH, et al. Rapid diagnosis of pulmonary tuberculosis using Roche AMPLICOR *Mycobacterium tuberculosis* PCR test. J Clin Microbiol 1995;33:1832–1834.
274. Clarridge JE, 3d, Shawar RM, Shinnick TM, et al. Large-scale use of polymerase chain reaction for detection of *Mycobacterium tuberculosis* in a routine mycobacteriology laboratory. J Clin Microbiol 1993;31:2049–2056.
275. Miller N, Hernandez SG, Cleary TJ. Evaluation of gen-probe amplified *Mycobacterium tuberculosis* direct test and PCR for direct detection of *Mycobacterium tuberculosis* in clinical specimens. J Clin Microbiol 1994;32:393–397.
276. Vuorinen P, Miettinen A, Vuento R, et al. Direct detection of *Mycobacterium tuberculosis* complex in respiratory specimens by Gen-Probe Amplified Mycobacterium Direct Test and Roche Amplicor *Mycobacterium tuberculosis* Test. J Clin Microbiol 1995;33:1856–1859.
277. Nachamkin I, Kang C, Weinstein MP. Detection of resistance to isoniazid, rifampin, and streptomycin in clinical isolates of *Mycobacterium tuberculosis* by molecular methods. Clin Infect Dis 1997;24:894–900.
278. Telenti A. Genetics of drug resistance in tuberculosis. Clin Chest Med 1997;18:55–64.
279. Telenti A, Honore N, Bernasconi C, et al. Genotypic assessment of isoniazid and rifampin resistance in *Mycobacterium tuberculosis*: a blind study at reference laboratory level. J Clin Microbiol 1997;35:719–723.
280. Nash KA, Gaytan A, Inderlied CB. Detection of rifampin resistance in *Mycobacterium tuberculosis* by use of a rapid, simple, and specific RNA/RNA mismatch assay. J Infect Dis 1997;176:533–536.
281. Rossau R, Traore H, De Beenhouwer H, et al. Evaluation of the INNO-LiPA Rif. TB assay, a reverse hybridization assay for the simultaneous detection of *Mycobacterium tuberculosis* complex and its resistance to rifampin. Antimicrob Agents Chemother 1997;41:2093–2098.
282. Brindle RJ, Nunn PP, Githui W, et al. Quantitative bacillary response to treatment in HIV-associated pulmonary tuberculosis. Am Rev Respir Dis 1993;147:958–961.
283. Cohn DL. Treatment and prevention of tuberculosis in HIV-infected persons. Infect Dis Clin North Am 1994;8:399–412.
284. Grosset JH. Treatment of tuberculosis in HIV infection. Tuber Lung Dis 1992;73:378–383.
285. Jones BE, Otaya M, Antoniskis D, et al. A prospective evaluation of antituberculosis therapy in patients with human immunodeficiency virus infection. Am J Respir Crit Care Med 1994;150:1499–1502.
286. Kassim S, Sassan-Morokro M, Ackah A, et al. Two-year follow-up of persons with HIV-1- and HIV-2-associated pulmonary tuberculosis treated with short-course chemotherapy in West Africa. AIDS 1995;9:1185–1191.
287. Ackah AN, Coulibaly D, Digbeu H, et al. Response to treatment, mortality, and CD4 lymphocyte counts in HIV-infected persons with tuberculosis in Abidjan, Cote d'Ivoire. Lancet 1995;345:607–610.
288. Perriens JH, St. Louis ME, Mukadi YB, et al. Pulmonary tuberculosis in HIV-infected patients in Zaire: a controlled trial of treatment for either 6 or 12 months. N Engl J Med 1995;332:779–784.
289. Flora GS, Modilevsky T, Antoniskis D, et al. Undiagnosed tuberculosis in patients with human immunodeficiency virus infection. Chest 1990;98:1056–1059.
290. Nunn P, Brindle R, Carpenter L, et al. Cohort study of human immunodeficiency virus infection in patients with tuberculosis in Nairobi, Kenya. Analysis of early (6-month) mortality. Am Rev Respir Dis 1992;146:849–854.
291. Duncanson FP, Hewlett D Jr, Maayan S, et al. *Mycobacterium tuberculosis* infection in the acquired immunodeficiency syndrome: a review of 14 patients. Tubercle 1986;67:295–302.
292. Johnson SC, Stamm CP, Hicks CB. Tuberculous psoas muscle abscess following chemoprophylaxis with isoniazid in a patient with human immunodeficiency virus infection. Rev Infect Dis 1990;12:754–756.
293. Shafer RW, Jones WD. Relapse of tuberculosis in a patient with the acquired immunodeficiency syndrome despite 12 months of antituberculous therapy and continuation of isoniazid. Tubercle 1991;72:149–151.
294. Berning SE, Huitt GA, Iseman MD, et al. Malabsorption of antituberculosis medications by a patient with AIDS [letter]. N Engl J Med 1992;327:1817–1818.
295. Peloquin CA, MacPhee AA, Berning SE. Malabsorption of antimycobacterial medications [letter]. N Engl J Med 1993;329:1122–1123.
296. Gordon SM, Horsburgh CR Jr, Peloquin CA, et al. Low serum levels of oral antimycobacterial agents in patients with disseminated *Mycobacterium avium* complex disease. J Infect Dis 1993;168:1559–1562.
297. Patel KB, Belmonte R, Crowe H. Drug malabsorption and resistant tuberculosis in HIV-infected patients [letter]. N Engl J Med 1995;332:336–337.
298. Sahai J, Gallicano K, Swick L, et al. Reduced plasma concentrations of antituberculosis drugs in patients with HIV infection. Ann Intern Med 1997;127:289–293.
299. Schurmann D, Bergmann F, Jautzke G, et al. Acute and long-term efficacy of antituberculous treatment in HIV-seropositive patients with tuberculosis: a study of 36 cases. J Infect 1993;26:45–54.
300. Pitchenik AE, Fertel D. Medical management of AIDS patients: tuberculosis and nontuberculous mycobacterial disease. Med Clin North Am 1992;76:121–171.
301. Shafer RW, Bloch AB, Larkin C, et al. Predictors of survival in HIV-infected tuberculosis patients. AIDS 1996;10:269–272.
302. American Thoracic Society and Centers for Disease Control and Prevention. Treatment of tuberculosis and tuberculosis infection in adults and children. Am J Resp Crit Care Med 1994;149:1359–1374.
303. Centers for Disease Control and Prevention. Initial therapy for tuberculosis in the era of multidrug resistance. Recommendations of the Advisory Council for the Elimination of Tuberculosis. MMWR Morb Mortal Wkly Rep 1993;42:1-8.
304. Pulido F, Pena JM, Rubio R, et al. Relapse of tuberculosis after treatment in human immunodeficiency virus-infected patients. Arch Intern Med 1997;157:227–232.
305. Turett GS, Telzak EE, Torian LV, et al. Improved outcome of HIV-infected patients with multidrug-resistant tuberculosis in a nonoutbreak setting at an inner-city hospital in New York City. Clin Infect Dis 1995;21:1238–1244.
306. Salomon N, Perlman DC, Friedmann P, et al. Predictors and outcome of multidrug-resistant tuberculosis. Clin Infect Dis 1995;21:1245–1252.
307. Lockhart B, Sharp V, Squires K, et al. Improved outcome of MDR TB in patients receiving a five or more drug initial therapy [abstract PO-B07-1163]. In: Abstracts of the 9th International Conference on AIDS. Berlin: Institute for Clinical and Experimental Virology of the Free University of Berlin, 1993:329.
308. Edlin BR, Attoe LS, Grieco MH, et al. Recognition and treatment of primary multidrug-resistant tuberculosis in HIV-infected persons [abstract WS-B09-6]. In: Abstracts of the 9th International Conference on AIDS. Berlin: Institute for Clinical and Experimental Virology of the Free University of Berlin, 1993:52.
309. Rastogi N, Labrousse V, Goh KS. In vitro activities of fourteen antimicrobial agents against drug susceptible and resistant clinical

isolates of *Mycobacterium tuberculosis* and comparative intracellular activities against the virulent H37Rv strain in human macrophages. Curr Microbiol 1996;33:167–175.
310. Rastogi N, Goh KS, Bryskier A, et al. In vitro activities of levofloxacin used alone and in combination with first- and second-line antituberculous drugs against *Mycobacterium tuberculosis*. Antimicrob Agents Chemother 1996;40:1610–1616.
311. Iseman MD, Madsen L, Goble M, et al. Surgical intervention in the treatment of pulmonary disease caused by drug-resistant *Mycobacterium tuberculosis*. Am Rev Respir Dis 1990;141:623–625.
312. Park MM, Davis AL, Schluger NW, et al. Outcome of MDR-TB patients, 1983–1993: prolonged survival with appropriate therapy. Am J Respir Crit Care Med 1996;153:317–324.
313. Sumartojo E. When tuberculosis treatment fails: a social behavioral account of patient adherence. Am Rev Respir Dis 1993;147:1311–1320.
314. Bloch AB, Brown ED, Hayden CH, et al. Completion of tuberculosis therapy in the United States [abstract]. Am J Crit Care Resp Med 1995;151:A555.
315. International Union Against Tuberculosis and Lung Disease/Tuberculosis Programme of the World Heath Organization. The promise and reality of fixed-dose combinations with rifampicin. Tuber Lung Dis 1994;75:180–181.
316. Moulding T, Dutt AK, Reichman LB. Fixed-dose combinations of antituberculous medications to prevent drug resistance. Ann Intern Med 1995;122:951–954.
317. Iseman MD, Cohn DL, Sbarbaro JA. Directly observed treatment of tuberculosis. We can't afford not to try it. N Engl J Med 1993;328:576–578.
318. Weis SE, Slocum PC, Blais FX, et al. The effect of directly observed therapy on the rates of drug resistance and relapse in tuberculosis. N Engl J Med 1994;330:1179–1184.
319. Frieden TR, Fujiwara PI, Washiko RM, et al. Tuberculosis in New York City: turning the tide. N Engl J Med 1995;333:229–233.
320. Chaulk CP, Moore-Rice K, Rizzo R, et al. Eleven years of community-based directly observed therapy for tuberculosis. JAMA 1995;274:945–951.
321. Strayhorn VA, Baciewicz AM, Self TH. Update on rifampin drug interactions. III. Arch Intern Med 1997;157:2453–2458.
322. Piscitelli SC, Flexner C, Minor JR, et al. Drug interactions in patients infected with human immunodeficiency virus. Clin Infect Dis 1996;23:685–693.
323. Barry M, Gibbons S, Back D, et al. Protease inhibitors in patients with HIV disease: clinically important pharmacokinetic considerations. Clin Pharmacokinet 1997;32:194–209.
324. Centers for Disease Control and Prevention. Clinical update: impact of HIV protease inhibitors on the treatment of HIV-infected tuberculosis patients with rifampin. MMWR Morb Mortal Wkly Rep 1996;45:921–925.
325. Jacobs DS, Piliero PJ, Kuperwaser MG, et al. Acute uveitis associated with rifabutin use in patients with human immunodeficiency virus infection. Am J Opthalmol 1994;118:716–722.
326. Perriens JH, Colebunders RL, Karahunga C, et al. Increased mortality and tuberculosis treatment failure rates among human immunodeficiency virus (HIV) seropositive compared with HIV seronegative patients with pulmonary tuberculosis treated with "standard" chemotherapy in Kinshasa, Zaire. Am Rev Respir Dis 1991;144:750–755.
327. Hawken M, Nunn P, Gathua S, et al. Increased recurrence of tuberculosis in HIV-1-infected patients in Kenya. Lancet 1993;342:332–337.
328. Okwera A, Whalen C, Byekwaso F, et al. Randomised trial of thiacetazone and rifampicin-containing regimens for pulmonary tuberculosis in HIV-infected Ugandans. Lancet 1994;344:1323–1328.
329. Nunn P, Kibuga D, Gathua S, et al. Cutaneous hypersensitivity reactions due to thiacetazone in HIV-1 seropositive patients treated for tuberculosis. Lancet 1991;337:627–630.
330. Pozniak AL, MacLeod GA, Mahari M, et al. The influence of HIV status on single and multiple drug reactions to antituberculous therapy in Africa. AIDS 1992;6:809–814.
331. Chintu C, Luo C, Bhat G, et al. Cutaneous hypersensitivity reactions due to thiacetazone in the treatment of tuberculosis in Zambian children infected with HIV-I. Arch Dis Child 1993;68:665–668.
332. Raviglione MC, Dye C, Schmidt S, et al. Assessment of worldwide tuberculosis control. Lancet 1997;350:624–629.
333. Grange JM, Zumla A. Making DOTS succeed. Lancet 1997;350:157.
334. Wadhawan D, Hira S, Mwansa N, et al. Preventive tuberculosis chemotherapy with isoniazid among patients infected with HIV-1 [abstract PO-B07-11]. In: Abstracts of the 9th International Conference on AIDS. Berlin: Institute for Clinical and Experimental Virology of the Free University of Berlin, 1993:53.
335. Selwyn PA, Sckell BM, Alcabes P, et al. High risk of active tuberculosis in HIV-infected drug users with cutaneous anergy. JAMA 1992;268:504–509.
336. Moreno S, Miralles P, Diaz MD, et al. Isoniazid preventive therapy in human immunodeficiency virus-infected persons: long-term effect on development of tuberculosis and survival. Arch Intern Med 1997;157:1729–1734.
337. Centers for Disease Control and Prevention. Screening for tuberculosis and tuberculosis infection in high-risk populations. MMWR Morb Mortal Wkly Rep 1995;44:19–34.
338. Centers for Disease Control and Prevention. Tuberculosis prevention in drug-treatment centers and correctional facilities: selected U.S. sites, 1990–1991. MMWR Morb Mortal Wkly Rep 1993;42:210–213.
339. Centers for Disease Control and Prevention. Management of persons exposed to multidrug-resistant tuberculosis. MMWR Morb Mortal Wkly Rep 1992;41:61–71.
340. Centers for Disease Control and Prevention. Screening for tuberculosis and tuberculous infection in high-risk populations: recommendations of the Advisory Committee for Elimination of Tuberculosis. MMWR Morb Mortal Wkly Rep 1990;39:1–7.
341. Centers for Disease Control and Prevention. Tuberculin reactions in apparently healthy HIV-seropositive and HIV-seronegative women: Uganda. MMWR Morb Mortal Wkly Rep 1990;39:638–639, 645–646.
342. Johnson MP, Coberly JS, Clermont HC, et al. Tuberculin skin test reactivity among adults infected with human immunodeficiency virus. J Infect Dis 1992;166:194–198.
343. Graham NM, Nelson KE, Solomon L, et al. Prevalence of tuberculin positivity and skin test anergy in HIV-1-seropositive and -seronegative intravenous drug users. JAMA 1992;267:369–373.
344. Markowitz N, Hansen NI, Wilcosky TC, et al. Tuberculin and anergy testing in HIV-seropositive and HIV-seronegative persons. Ann Intern Med 1993;119:185–193.
345. MacGregor RR, Dunbar D, Graziani AL. Tuberculin reactions among attendees at a methadone clinic: relation to infection with the human immunodeficiency virus. Clin Infect Dis 1994;19:1100–1104.
346. Webster CT, Gordin FM, Matts JP, et al. Two-stage tuberculin skin testing in individuals with human immunodeficiency virus infection. Am J Respir Crit Care Med 1995;151:805–808.
347. Centers for Disease Control and Prevention. Purified protein derivative (PPD)-tuberculin anergy and HIV infection: guidelines for anergy testing and management of anergic persons at risk of tuberculosis. MMWR Morb Mortal Wkly Rep 1991;40:27–32.
348. Gordin FM, Matts JP, Miller C, et al. A controlled trial of isoniazid in persons with anergy and human immunodeficiency virus infection who are at high risk for tuberculosis. Terry Beirn Community Programs for Clinical Research on AIDS. N Engl J Med 1997;337:315–320.
349. Walley J, Porter J. Chemoprophylaxis in tuberculosis and HIV infection: is it feasible in developing countries? [editorial] BMJ 1995;310:1621–1622.
350. Organization PAH. Association between HIV and tuberculosis: technical guide. Bull Pan Am Health Org 1993;27:297–310.

351. Heymann SJ. Modelling the efficacy of prophylactic and curative therapies for preventing the spread of tuberculosis in Africa. Trans R Soc Trop Med Hyg 1993;87:406–411.
352. Aisu T, Raviglione MC, van Praag E. Preventive chemotherapy for HIV-associated tuberculosis in Uganda: a feasibility study [abstract WS-B09-3]. In: Abstracts of the 9th International Conference on AIDS. Berlin: Institute for Clinical and Experimental Virology of the Free University of Berlin, 1993:52.
353. De Cock KM, Grant A, Porter JDH. Preventive therapy for tuberculosis in HIV-infected persons: international recommendations, research, and practice. Lancet 1995;345:833–836.
354. O'Brien RJ, Perriens JH. Preventive therapy for tuberculosis in HIV infection: the promise and the reality. AIDS 1995;9:665–673.
355. Colditz GA, Brewer TF, Berkey CS, et al. Efficacy of BCG vaccine in the prevention of tuberculosis: meta-analysis of the published literature. JAMA 1994;271:698–702.
356. Blanche S, Le Deist F, Fischer A, et al. Longitudinal study of 18 children with perinatal LAV/HTLV III infection: attempt at prognostic evaluation. J Pediatr 1986;109:965–970.
357. Ninane J, Grymonprez A, Burtonboy G, et al. Disseminated BCG in HIV infection. Arch Dis Child 1988;63:1268–1269.
358. Armbruster C, Junker W, Vetter N, et al. Disseminated bacille Calmette-Guérin infection in an AIDS patient 30 years after BCG vaccination [letter]. J Infect Dis 1990;162:1216.
359. Centers for Disease Control and Prevention. Disseminated *Mycobacterium bovis* infection from BCG vaccination of a patient with acquired immunodeficiency syndrome. MMWR Morb Mortal Wkly Rep 1985;34:227-228.
360. Besnard M, Sauvion S, Offredo C, et al. Bacillus Calmette-Guérin infection after vaccination of human immunodeficiency virus–infected children. Pediatr Infect Dis J 1993;12:993–997.
361. Lallemant-Le Coeur S, Lallemant M, Cheynier D, et al. Bacillus Calmette-Guérin immunization in infants born to HIV-1–seropositive mothers. AIDS 1991;5:195–199.
362. Centers for Disease Control and Prevention. BCG vaccination and pediatric HIV infection-Rwanda, 1988–1990. MMWR Morb Mortal Wkly Rep 1991;40:833–836.
363. Ryder RW, Oxtoby MJ, Mvula M, et al. Safety and immunogenicity of bacille Calmette-Guérin, diphtheria-tetanus-pertussis, and oral polio vaccines in newborn children in Zaire infected with human immunodeficiency virus type 1. J Pediatr 1993;122:697–702.
364. O'Brien KL, Ruff AJ, Louis MA, et al. Bacille Calmette-Guérin complications in children born to HIV-1–infected women with a review of the literature. Pediatrics 1995;95:414–418.
365. World Health Organization. BCG immunization and paediatric HIV infection. Wkly Epidemiol Rec 1992;67:129–132.
366. Centers for Disease Control and Prevention. Guidelines for preventing the transmission of *Mycobacterium tuberculosis* in health-care facilities, 1994. MMWR Morb Mortal Wkly Rep 1994;43(No. RR-13):1–132.
367. Castro KG. Tuberculosis as an opportunistic disease in persons infected with human immunodeficiency virus. Clin Infect Dis 1995;21(Suppl 1):S66–S71.
368. Blumberg HM, Watkins DL, Berschling JD, et al. Preventing the nosocomial transmission of tuberculosis. Ann Intern Med 1995;122:658–663.
369. McGowan JE. Nosocomial tuberculosis: new progress in control and prevention. Clin Infect Dis 1995;21:489–505.
370. Hermans PWM, van Soolingen D, Dale JW, et al. Insertion element IS986 from *Mycobacterium tuberculosis*: a useful tool for the diagnosis and epidemiology of tuberculosis. J Clin Microbiol 1990;28:2051–2058.
371. Casper C, Singh SP, Rave S, et al. The transcontinental transmission of tuberculosis: a molecular epidemiological assessment. Am J Public Health 1996;86:551–553.
372. Jacobs WR Jr, Barletta RG, Udani R, et al. Rapid assessment of drug susceptibilities of *Mycobacterium tuberculosis* by means of luciferase reporter phages. Science 1993;260:819–822.
373. Cooksey RC, Crawford JT, Jacobs WR, et al. A rapid method for screening antimicrobial agents for activities against a strain of *Mycobacterium tuberculosis* expressing firefly luciferase. Antimicrob Agents Chemother 1993;37:1348–1352.
374. Dessen A, Quemard A, Blanchard JS, et al. Crystal structure and function of the isoniazid target of *Mycobacterium tuberculosis*. Science 1995;267:1638–1641.
375. Musser JM. Antimicrobial agent resistance in mycobacteria: molecular genetic insights. Clin Microbiol Rev 1995;8:496–514.
376. Spellman CW, Matty KJ, Weis SE. A survey of drug-resistant *Mycobacterium tuberculosis* and its relationship to HIV infection. AIDS 1998;12:191–195.

17

NONTUBERCULOUS (ATYPICAL) MYCOBACTERIA

Lowell S. Young

"Atypical mycobacteria" is a term coined during the decades of the 1940s and 1950s to designate those organisms that stood apart from the *Mycobacterium tuberculosis* complex and the etiologic agent of Hansen's disease, *M. leprae*. Among the earliest "atypicals" were organisms that belonged to the group known as *M. intracellulare* or the "Battey bacillus," a group of acid-fast staining respiratory pathogens causing a clinical picture virtually indistinguishable from pulmonary tuberculosis (1). As organisms were gradually added to the atypical group, the well-known classification of Runyon and colleagues became widely accepted (2). Table 17.1 summarizes the Runyon classification. This microbiologic framework still used by microbiologists classifies organisms by their growth patterns and their pigmentation in the presence or absence of light. An alternative term now believed to be more appropriate is "nontuberculous" mycobacteria (3).

For the purposes of this review, and placing the problem of nontuberculous mycobacteria in clinical perspective, the classic microbiologic groupings are of limited usefulness. From a clinical perspective and to assist in differential diagnostic approaches, the classification of disease patterns with specific nontuberculous mycobacterial species summarized in Table 17.2 is likely to be more useful. For instance, a rapidly growing acid-fast bacillus (recovery in 7 days) cultured from sputum is more likely to be *Mycobacterium chelonae* than *M. kansasii* or *M. avium*. A slow-growing organism from a skin lesion is more likely to be *M. ulcerans* than *M. marinum*.

From the beginning of first clinical descriptions of the acquired immunodeficiency syndrome (AIDS), clinicians recognized the strong association between impaired cellular immunity and infection with organisms characteristically viewed as "intracellular pathogens." The expectation that mycobacteria would play an important role complicating impaired cell-mediated immunity was quickly borne out in publications after the classic paper of Gottlieb and colleagues (4). A year after the initial description of AIDS in refereed text, Zakowski and colleagues called attention to the important role of atypical organisms as an end-stage complication of HIV disease (5). Indeed, this association has persisted to this day. Important epidemiologic studies indicate that the nontuberculous mycobacteria and *Mycobacterium avium* complex organisms in particular are an important component of the spectrum of opportunistic infections complicating AIDS (6–8). Furthermore, although initially, clinical results in treatment of systemic *M. avium* infections were poor overall, the last decade has witnessed an impressive array of clinical reports indicating that 1) this particular nontuberculous mycobacterium is common in patients with advanced AIDS, 2) aggressive treatment with either single-drug or multidrug regimens can reduce or suppress bacteremia and can ameliorate symptoms of the disease, 3) treatment may prolong survival, 4) significant improvement in quality of life has been associated with effective treatment, and 5) prophylaxis trials with one of several agents can reduce the incidence of bacteremia and prophylaxis can prolong survival (9). Thus, clinicians dealing with a patient with AIDS should familiarize themselves with the diagnostic approaches and the increasing number of therapeutic agents available for treatment or prophylaxis of the nontuberculous mycobacteria, and specifically *M. avium*. Most of this chapter concentrates on the *M. avium* complex because of the predominant role of this group of nontuberculous mycobacterium causing disease in AIDS patients (see later). Many of the other mycobacteria besides *M. tuberculosis* appear to be of environmental origin, replicate within an intracellular milieu, and express clinical disease in a manner analogous to *M. avium* (3).

INCIDENCE AND EPIDEMIOLOGY

The relative distribution of nontuberculous mycobacterial organisms recovered from blood cultures of AIDS patients is summarized in Table 17.3, based on information gathered by the United States Centers for Disease Control (10). From a clinical viewpoint, some time may elapse between recovery of an acid-fast bacillus and species identification. If the isolate is from blood or is respiratory in origin, emphasis must be placed on rapid identification because the epidemiologic implications in a hospital setting are obvious (tuberculosis versus nontuberculous mycobacteria). In centers caring for AIDS patients in which clinical tuberculosis is uncommon, acid-fast isolates from blood or tissue probably belong to the *Mycobacterium avium* complex.

Table 17.3 reflects the common observation that organisms belonging to the *Mycobacterium avium* complex are the most commonly recovered organisms from disseminated, bacteremic infections. In a prospective, natural history study by Nightingale and colleagues, the incidence of this infection as determined by serial monthly blood cultures increased linearly at a rate of approximately 25% each year after a patient's first AIDS-defining opportunistic event (11). This information is graphically depicted in Figure 17.1. Viewed in terms of the immunologic status of the patient, the incidence of *M. avium* bacteremia increased exponentially as the CD4 lymphocyte count approached zero. At CD4 counts less than 100 cells/mm^3 of blood, the likelihood of *M. avium* bacteremia during the following year approached 80%. Thus, Nightingale and colleagues, in publishing one of the largest natural history studies of *M. avium* complicating AIDS, viewed systemic disease to be a virtual inevitability if patients with AIDS live long enough.

In a correlative study involving cohorts from another medical center, Chaisson and associates noted that *Mycobacterium avium* disease developed within 1 year in approximately 8% of patients with CD4 lymphocyte counts below 100 cells/mm^3 at baseline, but in virtually no patients with counts above this level (12). Overall, one can conclude that patients will eventually develop *M. avium* bacteremia when their CD4 counts are less than 50 cells/mm^3 unless they receive prophylaxis. Our own experience from the era before the introduction of protease inhibitor therapy against human immunodeficiency virus (HIV) is that more than 80% of patients followed carefully from the time of diagnosis of clinical AIDS to death will develop *M. avium* infections of the blood if appropriate diagnostic studies are undertaken in patients who are not receiving prophylaxis. In the observational cohort study described by Chaisson and colleagues, *M. avium* disease was a significant independent predictor of death (12). This also correlates with the observations of Horsburgh and colleagues, who matched patients for comparable low CD4 counts and found that those individuals

Table 17.1. Classification of Mycobacteria

Group	Representative Species of Mycobacteria
Typical, slow-growing, strict pathogens	*M. tuberculosis*, *M. bovis*, *M. leprae*
Photochromogens	*M. kansasii*
	M. marinum
Scotochromogens	*M. scrofulaceum*
	M. szulgai
	M. xenopi
Nonphotochromogens	*M. avium* } *M. avium* complex
	M. intracellulare
	M. malmoense
	M. haemophilum
Rapidly growing organisms	*M. fortuitum*
	M. chelonae

Data from Wolinsky E. Nontuberculous mycobacteria and associated diseases. Am Rev Respir Dis 1979;119:107–159; Runyon EH. Ten mycobacterial pathogens. Tubercle 1974;55:235–240.

Table 17.3. Mycobacterial Species Causing Disseminated Nontuberculous Mycobacterial Infection Reported in AIDS Patients

Species	Number (%)
M. avium complex	1,906 (96.1)
M. kansasii	57 (2.9)
M. gordonae	11 (0.6)
M. fortuitum	5 (0.3)
M. chelonae	5 (0.3)
Total	1,984[a] (100.0)

[a]A total of 285 isolates were reported without speciation.
(From Horsburgh CR Jr, Selik RM. The epidemiology of disseminated nontuberculous mycobacterial infections in AIDS. Am Rev Respir Dis 1989; 139:4–7.)

Table 17.2. Clinical Disease and the Nontuberculous Mycobacteria Recovered from Humans

Clinical Disease	Common Etiologic Species	Growth Rate	Morphologic Growth Features[a]
Pulmonary	*M. avium* complex	Slow (> 7 d)	Usually not pigmented
	M. kansasii	Slow	Photochromogen
	M. chelonae subspecies	Rapid (< 7 d)	Not pigmented
	M. xenopi	Slow	Pigmented
Lymphadenitis	*M. avium* complex	Slow	Usually not pigmented
	M. scrofulaceum	Slow	Scotochromogen
Cutaneous	*M. marinum*	Rapid	Photochromogen; requires low temperatures (28 to 30° C) for isolation
	M. fortuitum	Rapid	Not pigmented
	M. chelonae	Rapid	Not pigmented
	M. ulcerans	Slow	Usually a scotochromogen: requires low temperatures for isolation
Disseminated	*M. avium* complex	Slow	Isolates from patients with AIDS, often pigmented (80%)
	M. genovense	Very slow (> 6 wk)	Growth better in broth than in agar
	M. kansasii	Slow	Photochromogen
	M. chelonae	Rapid	Not pigmented
	M. haemophilum	Slow	Not pigmented; requires hemin, often needs low temperatures and carbon dioxide to grow
	M. malmoense	Very slow (> 6 wk)	Prefers low pH

[a]Photochromogen: isolate is buff colored in the dark but turns yellow with brief exposure to light. Scotochromogen: isolate is yellow orange or orange even when grown in the dark.

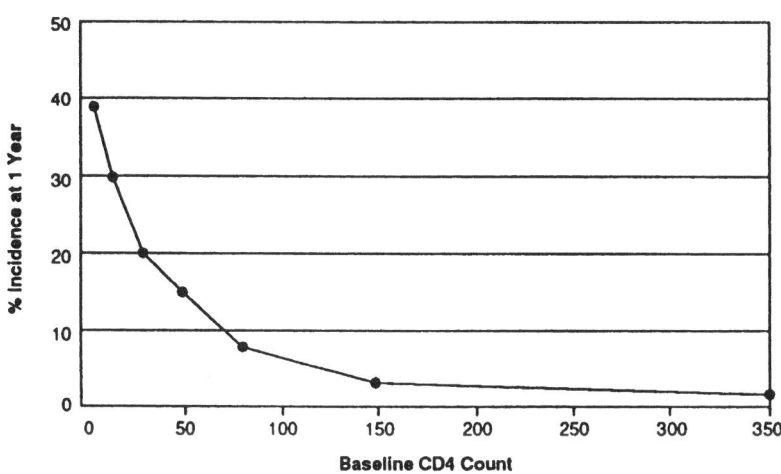

Figure 17.1. Product limit incidence of *Mycobacterium avium-intracellulare* complex bacteremia at 1 year after baseline CD4 cell count was drawn, stratified by baseline CD4 cell count. (From Nightingale SD, Bryd LT, Southern PM, et al. Incidence of *Mycobacterium avium-intracellulare* complex bacteremia in human immunodeficiency virus–positive patients. J Infect Dis 1992;165:1982–1985.)

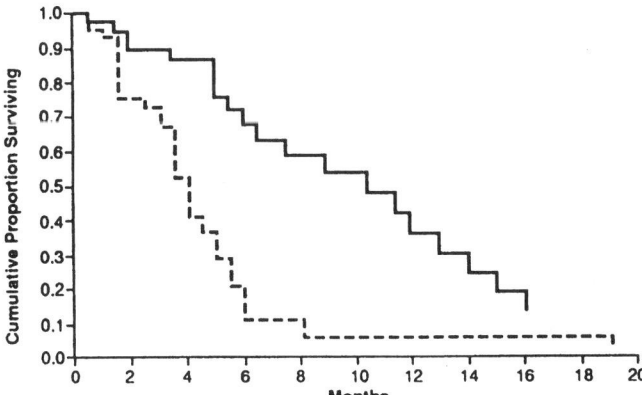

Figure 17.2. Survival pf patients with untreated disseminated *Mycobacterium avium* complex infection *(dotted line)* and control patients *(solid line)*; $P<.0001$. (Adapted from Horsburgh CR Jr, Havlik JA, Ellia DA, et al. Survival of patients with acquired immune deficiency syndrome and disseminated *Mycobacterium avium* complex infection with and without antimycobacterial chemotherapy. Am Rev Respir Dis 1991;144:557–559.)

who had documented *M. avium* bacteremia had significantly decreased life expectancy (13) (Fig 17.2).

Unlike pulmonary tuberculosis or disseminated tuberculosis that originates from an initial pulmonary focus, *Mycobacterium avium* and other nontuberculous mycobacteria appear to be acquired from the environment (3, 9, 10). In contrast to tuberculosis, of which humans are the exclusive reservoir and in which spread of disease occurs among humans, nontuberculous mycobacteria are ubiquitous and are commonly isolated from soil, plants, house dust, and water, including both salt water and potable urban water supplies (3). As the name implies, *M. avium* organisms can be isolated from birds, but other sources in nature such as swine, cattle, and nonhuman primates, as well as pasteurized milk and eggs, may be the source.

In terms of route of acquisition, two routes are plausible and are supported by epidemiologic evidence. Because organisms are present in water or dust, acquisition by the respiratory route is possible. In studies by Jacobson and colleagues, the isolation of *Mycobacterium avium* from respiratory secretions and particularly from materials obtained during bronchoscopic evaluation of lung infiltrates had a positive predictive value for the development of systemic disease (14). Progression to dissemination has occurred with equal frequency in patients with positive respiratory or stool isolates during a mean observation period of 5 months. Another study indicated that almost 75% of AIDS patients develop *M. avium*–positive blood cultures after the isolation of the organisms from respiratory or stool sources (15). The most common route of infection of the human host appears to be the gastrointestinal tract. Isolation of organisms or the detection of acid-fast forms in stool may be the harbinger of systemic disease (6, 16). The isolation of *M. avium* from any source in the gastrointestinal tract appears to have a positive predictive value, particularly the isolation of organisms from gastric washings or intubated small intestine as well as stool. Symptoms such as diarrhea are common, but clearly other causes of gastroenteritis besides *M. avium* exist.

From the viewpoint of infection-control measures, the implications of these conclusions are obvious. Nontuberculous organisms can be assumed to be of environmental origin and do not spread from patient to patient or from patient to health care worker. Specific isolation measures are not necessary, as is with *Mycobacterium tuberculosis*.

PATHOGENESIS, PATHOLOGY, AND IMMUNE RESPONSE

Colonization of mucosal surfaces, more likely the intestinal tract than respiratory mucosa, precedes the development of *Mycobacterium avium* bacteremia. Various cases of localized gastrointestinal disease have been reported with superficial lesions observed in the esophagus, duodenum, and both the small and large intestines (17, 18). Primary pneumonia, bronchitis, or other respiratory manifestations of the *M. avium* complex are uncommon, but massive involvement of the gastrointestinal submucosa with bacilli-filled macrophages or "foam cells" is typical (17, 18). The reactive process involves Peyer's patches and mesenteric lymph nodes. Thus, histopathologic studies suggest that the disease then spreads from the gut to the local lymph nodes and may cause inflammatory retroperitoneal lymphadenitis, which can be massive and can displace visceral organs. Bacteremia eventually develops, and striking involvement of the liver, spleen, and other components of the reticuloendothelial system is a prominent part of the histologic picture. In these organs, microscopic sections reveal large numbers of macrophages or tissue histiocytes with large numbers of intracellular bacilli as well.

Mycobacterium avium isolates recovered from AIDS patients readily survive within macrophages and are resistant to oxidative bactericidal mechanisms within macrophages. The host defects associated with survival within cells such as macrophages have not been specifically and reproducibly defined (19). Although investigators appreciate that activated macrophages in cooperation with cell-mediated or T-lymphocyte immunity are important for killing intracellular organisms such as mycobacteria, the specific defects predisposing to survival and proliferation of *M. avium* are still poorly understood. One observation is that macrophages from HIV-infected patients or HIV-infected macrophages manifest impaired killing of mycobacteria (20), but this finding has not been consistently observed. However, peripheral blood mononuclear phagocytes from AIDS patients are not functionally impaired, as measured by the ability to respond to cytokine stimulation.

Phagocytosis and processing of antigens by macrophages as well as the effects of cytotoxic and helper T cells, natural killer (NK) cells, lymphokine-activated killer (LAK) cells, and γ/δ cells may be important components of host resistance (21, 22). Cytokine activation may also result in intracellular killing, but conflicting and contradictory results have been reported about the protective roles of interferon-γ and tumor necrosis factor (23, 24). To date, almost all studies of phagocytic cell function represent populations harvested from the peripheral blood of subjects, whether or not these cells have been "naturally infected" by HIV in patients with AIDS or infected in the laboratory. Therefore, studies on these populations may represent an important selection bias and may have little relation, mechanistically or immunologically, to host defense cells at the active site of an infectious process. Overall, the pathogenesis of *Mycobacterium avium* infection in AIDS patients appears to be multifactorial. Defects in antigen recognition, host-cell activation, and intracellular killing within macrophage sanctuaries are likely to be the critical factors predisposing to the development of disseminated disease. Although AIDS patients are also likely to have B-cell defects (resulting in impaired synthesis of specific antibody), no evidence indicates that humoral antibodies provide protection.

CLINICAL MANIFESTATIONS AND COURSE OF DISEASE

The presentation of *Mycobacterium avium* complex disease in patients with AIDS differs from that in patients without AIDS. The "classic" nontuberculous presentation is that of a pulmonary infection occurring in individuals with

Table 17.4. *Mycobacterium avium* Clinical Syndrome in AIDS Patients

"Early" symptoms (CD4 lymphocyte count > 100 cells/mm^3)
  Fever
  Lymphadenopathy
  Lung infiltrates
"Late" symptoms (CD4 lymphocyte count < 100 cells/mm^3)
  Fatigue, malaise
  Fever
  High fever, chills, drenching night sweats
  Weight loss
  Diarrhea
  Organomegaly
  Abdominal pain
  Anorexia
Laboratory findings in the "late" syndrome
  Anemia
  Liver function abnormalities, especially elevated alkaline phosphatase
  Neutropenia
  Granulomas in bone marrow, liver

chronic obstructive pulmonary disease. Most patients are elderly, they may have diffuse lung infiltrates or relatively segmental or lobar involvement, and occasionally they have cavitary pneumonia. Symptoms include cough, low-grade fever, bronchospasm, and hemoptysis. A report by Prince and colleagues indicated that the histologic process consisted of granulomatous infiltration with caseous necrosis, a finding similar to that seen in patients with tuberculosis (25). Among the clinical signs and symptoms, fever and weight loss were uncommon, whereas cough with diffuse pneumonitic involvement was more typical.

Occasionally, *Mycobacterium avium* disease occurs in AIDS patients with high CD4 counts (more than 200 cells/mm^3). Individuals present with fleeting lung infiltrates. They produce sputum or induced cough specimens that grow *M. avium*. These patients have transient fevers, but they seem to contain their infections promptly. Occasionally, an HIV-seropositive patient develops lymphadenitis of the cervical and supraclavicular regions and has a diagnostic biopsy. Acid-fast organisms in these lesions initially can be mistaken for *M. tuberculosis*. This scrofula-like pattern is uncommon, but it may recur. Treatment of this disease is easy in comparison with that of disseminated *M. avium* infections.

Far more typically, disseminated *Mycobacterium avium* disease is a "late" opportunistic infection. By late, we are referring to a CD4 count usually less than 100 cells/mm^3 and often less than 50 cells/mm^3. Before to the universal acceptance of anti-*Pneumocystis* prophylaxis, most of these patients had an AIDS-defining illness that included *P. carinii* pneumonia. Localized oropharyngeal infections such as those due to *Candida* are common, and patients may have run the gamut of toxoplasmosis, cryptococcosis, or cytomegalovirus disease before developing evidence of disseminated *M. avium* infection. Table 17.4 is an enumeration of the most typical symptoms reported by patients with a "late" clinical syndrome.

Almost all bacteremic patients have had severe fatigue and chronic malaise. Significant loss of weight, defined as loss of 20% of normal weight or more, is paralleled by the clinical appearance of wasting. Initial fevers may be variable in intensity and intermittent, but if untreated, this clinical state evolves from recurrent low-grade fevers to fevers exceeding 105 to 106°F that are preceded by severe rigors. Even when the fevers and rigors are suppressed by antipyretic treatment, patients report drenching night sweats that may compel them to change bed clothing or bed sheets several times during the night. Mild to severe diarrhea also commonly accompanies these symptoms. Obviously, the association between symptoms and disease is a retrospective association. If one were to look prospectively at a group of HIV-positive patients with CD4 counts lower than 50 cells/mm^3 for fevers that exceed 103°F associated with severe rigors and night sweats, with negative conventional bacteriologic cultures of blood, and with no obvious illness involving the lung or central nervous system, the likelihood of finding *Mycobacterium avium* in the blood would exceed 75%. When bacteremia develops, multiple organs are involved. Although bone, meninges, and skin are uncommon areas of involvement in bacteremic patients, isolation of *M. avium* from bone marrow, spleen, liver, lungs, and any highly vascularized organ may parallel isolation from blood.

The clinical course of the disease reflects the aggressiveness with which the diagnosis is pursued and the willingness of clinicians to administer treatment as well as the patient's willingness to accept treatment. When the diagnosis has been made early and effective treatment with combinations of drugs (discussed later) is instituted, life expectancy after the documentation of organisms in the blood may exceed 1 year and can approach 2 years. As documented by Horsburgh and colleagues, median survival after first positive blood culture in the untreated patient is 4 to 5 months (13). This projection must be made with caution, and survival may depend on whether or not the patient develops other opportunistic infections or cancer (and clearly such observations were made before the introduction of protease inhibitor therapy). The 4 or 5 months of survival projected by Horsburgh and others (11–14) are accompanied by severe symptoms and a progressive downhill course (11, 12). Laboratory findings include anemia, leukopenia, and elevated liver function tests. The most consistent abnormality is an elevated serum alkaline phosphatase. Although patients are usually anemic because of various clinical factors, a precipitous decline in hemoglobin and hematocrit often heralds the onset of bacteremic *Mycobacterium avium* disease.

DIAGNOSIS

Detection of *Mycobacterium avium* complex infection is now readily accomplished by modern laboratory techniques (26). The easiest system to use is the culture of blood with long observation time (3 to 4 weeks), but culture of bone marrow or exudates, abscesses, lymph nodes, liver, and spleen readily yields organisms. Recovery of *M. avium* from stool, duodenal biopsies or aspirates, bronchial washings, or other respiratory tract sources should be interpreted with caution because the presence of organisms could reflect colonization. However, in the patient with a CD4 count less than 100/mm^3, the recovery of organisms from these sites may be a harbinger of systemic infection (14–16). In a patient with symptoms, the recovery of organisms from these sites (from which they may be labeled as possible contaminants) must be viewed with concern, and repeat studies and careful clinical observation are warranted.

Among the most useful tools are the commercial systems that provide rapid detection of mycobacterial growth and some quantitation of the level of bacteremia. The essential steps that improve the recovery of mycobacteria involve lysis of leukocytes and concentration by centrifugation. Leukocyte lysis that releases intracellular organisms may be accomplished by a hypotonic agent such as distilled water or chemical agents. Then, to facilitate detection of growth, radiometric devices (BACTEC-II instrument, Becton Dickinson, Baltimore, MD) measure the generation of radioactive carbon-14 from an appropriate substrate long before visible turbidity (the usual standard for determining blood culture positivity) is obvious to the laboratory technologist. Routine blood cultures rely on observation of growth as manifested by turbidity, whereas radiometric detection of growth is based on counting of radioactive carbon-14 detectable at an earlier stage. Even routine blood culture media can support the growth of atypical organisms such as *Mycobacterium avium*, but this requires the observation of routine blood culture bottles for many weeks, a technique not widely practiced by most diagnostic laboratories. For institutions that do not have a heavy volume of mycobacterial blood cultures, careful and close cooperation between the clinician and the diagnostic laboratory may facilitate the selection of procedures or careful monitoring approaches that can lead to earlier diagnosis.

Once a mycobacterium is isolated from blood or body fluids, the organism must be speciated. The epidemiologic differences between *Mycobacterium tuberculosis* and the *M. avium* complex are obvious. Sufficient growth must be available: specific DNA probes can be used on organisms concentrated from broth culture, but the availablility of single-colony growth from solid media is preferable for speciation techniques. This procedure is costly but necessary if a potential exists for the isolate to be *M. tuberculosis*. Presumptive identification may also be accomplished using growth characteristics in the BACTEC-II medium, colonial morphology, microscopic appearance, and some biochemical reactions, but the results may not be as reliable as those obtained with DNA probes.

The issue of in vitro susceptibility testing is controversial yet evolving. Thus, routine testing of organisms, particularly single agents, has no established value, and the use of tests of combinations of therapy cannot be recommended for the routine management of a patient with documented infection (26, 27). The reason for the current state of ignorance in this area is that results of in vitro tests vary widely, depending on the antimicrobial agent tested, the choice of media, incubation conditions, the test system, and even the pH of the test media (28). Results may vary for macrolides and aminoglycosides, which are two of the most clinically useful classes of agents. Although proposals for standardization of in vitro testing have been made, the evolution of treatment may be such that these tests will be largely of academic interest rather than of practical value in the management of the patient. Even today, the choice of therapies for atypical mycobacterial disease must be based on the likely susceptibility of organisms. A few selected reference laboratories may be chosen if in vitro susceptibility results must be obtained in the management of a specific clinical problem, but even those results must be interpreted with caution. If any agents are to be tested, they should include an aminoglycoside, ethambutol, a macrolide, rifabutin, and possibly a quinolone. Investigators are interested in nonculture methods for identifying microbes, but at present no method of sensitive antigen detection or nucleic acid amplification can be recommended for routine use (26).

DECISION TO TREAT

As implied in the introduction to this chapter, the treatment of nontuberculous mycobacterial disease was initially controversial (7). In the early years of the AIDS epidemic, the survival time between diagnosis and death was short. Most of the early treatment studies did not have the additional added benefit of concomitant antiretroviral chemotherapy.

We and others have published anecdotal, noncomparative studies that demonstrate that treatment regimens are effective in terms of fever and other critical symptoms (29–34). In clinical decision making, certain factors must be weighed. We believe, as published previously, that the presence of two or more serious opportunistic infections other than *Mycobacterium avium*, such as concurrent pneumocystosis and cytomegalovirus disease, usually augurs poorly for a successful outcome in treating *M. avium* symptoms. Multiple drug therapy is difficult in terms of the toxicity of the individual agents and potential side effects, and the presence of other opportunistic infections is a marker of advanced immune deficiency that is likely to be unremitting, unless treatment is simultaneously initiated with a potent antiretroviral regimen. Treatment of patients who have other opportunistic infections is far less likely to improve symptoms than treatment of patients in whom no *other* proved cause of symptoms such as fever and weight loss is evident.

Another factor that weighs in clinical decision making has to do with the status of critical organ function. Agents such as aminoglycosides and macrolides, as well as the rifamycins, maybe toxic to renal and hepatic function, respectively. Impairment of any of the solid organ functions reduces the likelihood of treatment success. Perhaps the overriding factor in a decision to give treatment is the patient's attitude toward the disease. Some individuals may not wish to participate in an aggressive chemotherapeutic regimen that requires administration of multiple, potentially toxic agents. Highly motivated patients are those who are most likely to accept and tolerate complicated treatment regimens.

A growing clinical literature emphasizes that aggressive treatment of *Mycobacterium avium* disease has a beneficial impact on symptoms that is paralleled by a reduction in mycobacteremia. Studies such as those published by the California Collaborative Treatment Group, our own studies with azithromycin, and clinical studies using clarithromycin emphasize the correlation between clinical improvement and reduction in mycobacteremia (35–42). Still, no prospective randomized comparative trial of treatment versus placebo with follow-up of patients for more than a half a year has been conducted.

SPECIFIC RECOMMENDATIONS FOR TREATMENT

Table 17.5 summarizes the major therapeutic agents available for treatment of nontuberculous mycobacterial disease in general and *Mycobacterium avium* in particular. Summarized are specific agents' doses and important adverse reactions. Experience in pediatric patients is limited, so extrapolation of adult dosing regimens to this younger patient population should be undertaken with care. Before the initiation of treatment, at least two blood cultures should be positive in patients who are HIV positive. Furthermore, supporting laboratory data should be present such as complete blood counts and liver function tests. More than 80% of patients with disseminated *M. avium* disease have hemoglobin values lower than 10 g/dL or hematocrit of less than 30%. More than 90% of patients with *M. avium* bacteremia have elevated serum alkaline phosphatase values. The likelihood of true bacteremia or sustained bacteremia correlates strongly with symptoms of fever, night sweats, weight loss (greater than 15%), and persistent diarrhea. Selection of specific agents should consider the available drugs, drug toxicities, and interactions with other agents that patients may be simultaneously taking. Clearly, simplification of multidrug regimens is merited. Some suggestion exists that agents effective against *M. avium* may be beneficial against multiple opportunistic pathogens.

Currently, our recommendation is that the essential component of any anti-*Mycobacterium avium* chemotherapeutic regimen is a macrolide, either azithromycin or clarithromycin. Both have been shown to be effective as monotherapy in quantitative reduction of bacteremia or sterilization of blood cultures, but the danger lies in the emergence of resistance (39). Either macrolide must be given with at least one other agent, and the easiest and least expensive is ethambutol (Table 17.6). No trials have randomized patients receiving macrolide plus ethambutol regimens to a third drug versus a placebo, but investigators generally believe that critically ill patients with *M. avium* bacteremia may benefit from a third agent. Selecting that third agent could be challenging because the added benefit of drugs such as rifabutin, clofa-

Table 17.5. Antimycobacterial Agents Commonly Used to Treat *Mycobacterium avium* Complex Infection[a]

Agent	Adult Dose	Pediatric Dose	Adverse Effects
Aminoglycosides			
Amikacin	10–15 mg/kg QD (or in divided doses)	10–15 mg/kg QD (or in divided doses)	Ototoxicity, nephrotoxicity
Streptomycin	15–20 mg/kg QD	15–20 mg/kg QD	—
Liposomal gentamicin[b]	5 mg/kg QD	—	—
Macrolides			
Azithromycin	500 mg QD[c]–600 mg QD[d]	10–20 mg/kg daily	Diarrhea, nausea, vomiting, abdominal pain, headache, dizziness, elevations in hepatic enzymes, hearing loss
Clarithromycin	500 mg BID	15–30 mg/kg	Same as above
Quinolones			
Ciprofloxacin	500–750 mg BID	20–30 mg/kg daily in divided doses	Anorexia, nausea, vomiting, abdominal pain, diarrhea, rash, joint pain, mental status changes, headache, anxiety
Levofloxacin	500 mg QD	No recommendation	Same as above
Sparfloxacin	400 mg, then 200 mg QD	No recommendation	Same as above, plus phototoxicity (red rash), prolonged QT interval
Rifamycins			
Rifampin	10 mg/kg QD	No recommendation	Anorexia, nausea, vomiting, diarrhea, rash, myalgias, arthralgias, orange urine
Rifabutin	450–600 mg QD[c]	No recommendation	Leukopenia, thrombocytopenia, rash, nausea, flatulence, transaminase elevations, myositis
Clofazimine	100–200 mg QD	No recommendation	Skin discoloration, ichthyosis, anorexia, nausea, vomiting, abdominal pain, peripheral neuropathy, rarely ocular changes
Ethambutol	15 mg/kg QD	10–25 mg/kg daily	Anorexia, nausea, vomiting, diarrhea, rash, mental status changes, retrobulbar neuritis

[a]All drugs given orally, except aminoglycosides (IV or IM). Some of the quinolones are available for IV use.
[b]Investigational.
[c]May administer in divided doses BID.
[d]600 mg dose is lactose free.

Table 17.6. Recommendations for Treatment of *Mycobacterium avium* Bacteremia in AIDS Patients[a]

Severe symptomatic disease and poor oral intake:
  Intravenous: amikacin plus rifampin
  Oral: ethambutol plus a macrolide (either azithromycin or clarithromycin)
Symptomatic disease, adequate oral intake
  Essential: macrolide plus ethambutol
  Possibly beneficial: clofazimine, rifabutin
  If diarrhea present: ciprofloxacin, levofloxacin, sparfloxacin
"Breakthrough" bacteremia after treatment or prophylaxis
  Continue macrolide plus ethambutol
  Add at least two of the following:
    Amikacin
    Rifabutin
    A fluoroquinolone (levofloxacin or sparfloxacin)
    Clofazimine

[a]The value of in vitro *M. avium* susceptibility testing has not been established. If available, such information is of potential usefulness in selecting alternative therapy.

zimine, or quinolone can only be inferred, and the evidence supporting a therapeutic benefit from clofazimine is marginal (40, 43). A recent French study comparing clarithromycin plus clofazimine with clarithromycin–ethambutol–rifabutin found the three-drug regimen to be statistically superior in limiting the emergence of clarithromycin resistance (44). Concern, however, has been expressed about a clarithromycin–rifabutin interaction that may effectively reduce clarithromycin serum levels (45). Ethambutol appears consistently to add to the activity of a macrolide in experimental infection (46).

Some patients in the past were so critically ill with *Mycobacterium avium* disease that oral absorption of drugs was questionable. In this case, intravenous amikacin and rifampin may be the most expeditious way to achieve an induction of remission (47, 48). As soon as oral agents can be tolerated, a macrolide plus ethambutol should be given. As far as the role of quinolones is concerned, no single-agent trial has demonstrated a therapeutic benefit. Nonetheless, they may have a slight effect on the gastrointestinal phase of the disease (quinolones are taken orally and achieve high gut concentrations). The most active quinolones appear to be sparfloxacin and levofloxacin, followed by ofloxacin and ciprofloxacin, but none has been specifically licensed by the United States Food and Drug Administration for treatment of mycobacterial disease (49).

With aminoglycoside administration, we have learned that drug should preferably be given over several hours, and streptomycin has always been recommended for intramuscular injection. The latter may be poorly tolerated. If aminoglycosides are given intravenously, they should be given slowly (over a 2- to 3-hour period) because bolus injections of drugs such as amikacin are likely to result in rapid rises and declines in aminoglycoside levels in young patients with good renal function (most of drug appears within the urine during the next 4 hours). An agent such as amikacin can be given in a dose of 5 mg/kg intravenously every 12 hours in a 2- to

3-hour infusion, and, once remission is achieved, the maintenance dose of 10 mg/kg daily can be given intramuscularly or intravenously. The longer infusion time permits greater distribution to the extravascular fluid compartment, and organisms such as mycobacteria may have a prolonged postantibiotic effect (18 hours or more) when exposed to drugs such as amikacin. Both amikacin and gentamicin have been encapsulated within liposomes for enhanced delivery to the reticuloendothelial system. Human trials have been reported, but the treatment remains experimental (50).

At present, clinical responses with combination therapies may be observed in up to 90% of patients. A response is defined in terms of defervescence, improvement in well-being, and a slowing of weight loss, although recovery of weight or weight gain is uncommon unless a newer and more effective antiretroviral regimen is simultaneously given. If the patient has not improved in terms of fever, night sweats, and recurrent chills within 3 weeks, one should consider modifying the regimen. Modifications usually involve additions of therapy rather than deletions or substitutions. Although in the past we believed that systemic nontuberculous mycobacterial disease required lifelong therapy, such a concept is being questioned in light of the sustained rises in CD4 counts achieved by new antiretroviral regimens. Often, an induction regimen of two to four drugs can be simplified if patients have a good therapeutic effect (response to infection and an enduring rise in CD4 counts).

Little information is available on management of "breakthrough" *Mycobacterium avium* bacteremia in which the isolate proves resistant to azithromycin or clarithromycin. The macrolide has been continued in one reported study (51), and additional agents such as amikacin, a quinolone, and rifabutin have been added. Most patients experienced a decrease in bacteremia in the latter study. The results of antimicrobial susceptibility testing may be helpful in choosing one and preferably two new agents in the face of "breakthrough" bacteremia. The most active quinolones against *M. avium* licensed in the United States are probably sparfloxacin and levofloxacin.

AIDS patients are clearly prone to multiple causes of diarrhea. When diarrhea precedes the initiation of systemic *Mycobacterium avium* treatment, the diarrhea may well be a manifestation of mycobacterial disease and not a side effect of treatment. If diarrhea follows the onset of anti-*M. avium* treatment and is associated with nausea, vomiting, and gastrointestinal symptoms, a macrolide side effect should be considered. Management of this problem is vexing, but the macrolide may be divided into multiple doses, or one of the lactose-free preparations may be considered for use. Clearly, if diarrhea has started after administration of the anti-*M. avium* regimen, a stool smear to detect acid-fast bacilli should be performed to determine whether the diarrhea is associated with the presence of acid-fast bacteria in stool. Routine culturing of stool for acid-fast bacilli is to be discouraged.

PREVENTION OF SYSTEMIC *MYCOBACTERIUM AVIUM* COMPLEX DISEASE

The last half-decade has seen progress in the identification of regimens that significantly prevent systemic *Mycobacterium avium* disease but with varying degrees of protection. These are targeted for patient populations with CD4 counts less than $50/mm^3$.

Initial studies with rifabutin in a daily dose of 300 mg per day demonstrated an efficacy of approximately 50% in reduction of *Mycobacterium avium* bacteremia (intention to treat analysis) (52). Breakthrough bacteremias were documented, but organisms were more likely than not to remain susceptible to rifabutin. The inference has been made that such breakthroughs have resulted from poor patient compliance or poor absorption of the drug rather than from true prophylactic failure.

Additional clinical trials have been executed in which azithromycin (1200 mg weekly) and clarithromycin (500 mg twice daily) have been assessed as monoprophylaxis and in combination. In the clarithromycin prophylaxis trials, compared with placebo, a significant reduction in *Mycobacterium avium* complex bacteremia was documented (approximately 70%) but with breakthrough bacteremias associated with macrolide-resistant organisms (53). Attempts have been made to combine these macrolides with rifabutin, and macrolide efficacy may be greater. Combination of rifabutin with clarithromycin has shown variable results, and the failure to demonstrate striking benefit may be due to drug interactions (rifabutin triggers the cytochrome P450 hepatitic microsome system to accelerate metabolism of clarithromycin) (44). Azithromycin does not appear to be associated with such an interaction, but even when azithromycin was combined with rifabutin, the improvement, which was a further decrease in incidence of *M. avium* complex bacteremia, was marginal and was associated with far more side effects and increased cost (54). Thus, combination drug prophylaxis is not recommended. Of interest in the clarithromycin placebo-controlled trials was the demonstration, for the first time in a prospective study, of a survival benefit to prophylaxis (53). In the macrolide prophylaxis trials, evidence showed an overall reduction in bacterial pneumonias, sinusitis, and *Pneumocystis* pneumonia as well. Other studies have demonstrated that even an agent such as erythromycin when given with a sulfonamide has an added prophylactic effect against *P. carinii* disease.

At present, clinicians should assume that patients who have received macrolide (azithromycin or clarithromycin prophylaxis) and who then go on to experience breakthrough bacteremia have macrolide-resistant organisms. At such a point, it would be desirable to add at least two active agents, and intravenous amikacin may well be the only drug of comparable effect to clarithromycin or azithromycin in terms of quantitative reduction of bacterial load (55). Both ethambutol and rifabutin may be given with amikacin. Rifamycins, like rifabutin, enhance the metabolism of protease inhibitors, and this factor limits rifamycin prophylaxis in patients with advanced HIV disease. Patients who are receiving protease inhibitors should not be given rifabutin unless the protease inhibitor is shown to be free of interactions with rifabutin.

A summary of the most recent guidelines of the United States Public Health Service/Infectious Disease Society of America for the prevention of opportunistic infection in persons infected with HIV contains specific recommendations for prophylaxis with azithromycin, clarithromycin, and rifabutin. These guidelines set the threshold for implementation of the recommendation at a CD4 count of 50 cells/mm^3 (56).

OVERALL PROGNOSIS

Overall, the prognosis after the documentation of *Mycobacterium avium* in blood cultures has generally been regarded as poor. Survival figures of 4 to 5 months have been quoted, but the outlook appears to be improving (13, 57, 58). Survival beyond 1 year has become common, with the new macrolides being an instrumental part of a multidrug therapeutic regimen. With combination antiretroviral therapy leading to undetectable HIV levels in plasma and sustained rises in CD4 counts above 100 cells/mm^3, the numbers of admissions to acute-care hospitals for treatment of *M. avium* bacteremia has declined. Ultimately, survival seems related to the net effect of all HIV disease management rather than to the abrogation of a single opportunistic infection. In other words, the nature of the underlying antiretroviral therapy and the measures taken to prevent or aggressively treat all major opportunistic infections all contribute to survival.

MYCOBACTERIAL INFECTIONS OTHER THAN WITH *MYCOBACTERIUM AVIUM*

Table 17.3 indicates that systemic infections due to the *Mycobacterium avium* complex comprise most mycobacterial processes occurring in AIDS patients. Perhaps the only other entity to provide a therapeutic challenge is infection with *M. kansasii*. *M. kansasii* infections are still primarily pulmonary, although systemic disease has been observed. In vitro susceptibility tests as summarized in Table 17.7 may be of some use in guiding therapy of *M. kansasii* pulmonary infections (27). As with *M. avium*, we consider the need for treatment to be lifelong in the patient with AIDS whose CD4 lymphocyte count does not rise. The selection of agents may be modified by organ toxicity and by the results of any in vitro studies that become available. Systemic disease may well respond to the same agents that have proved useful against *M. avium*: specifically, intravenous amikacin (if required by the patient's limited oral intake) and a macrolide, but the drugs of first choice are isoniazid, rifampin, and ethambutol. Convincing trials of pulmonary disease caused by *M. kansasii* show that treatment makes a difference in overall outcome, but the experience in treating *M. kansasii* in AIDS patients is limited.

Mycobacterium gordonae may be isolated from respiratory secretions, but rarely has it been convincingly identified as the sole cause of a pulmonary infection. This organism tends to be more susceptible to conventional antituberculous agents than either *M. avium* or *M. kansasii*. Often, isolation of *M. gordonae* from respiratory secretions does not correlate with any objective pulmonary disease.

Table 17.3 probably underestimates the importance of the so-called "rapidly growing" mycobacteria, *Mycobacterium fortuitum–M. chelonae*. The in vitro antibiotic susceptibility of this group of organisms varies, and active agents include cefoxitin and amikacin (for *M. fortuitum*). Quinolones may also be active against *M. fortuitum*. The clinical presentations involve either abscesses or cellulitis, particularly if associated with a foreign body. Surgical drainage of superficial or subcutaneous abscesses may be important in the clinical management of these patients. Information on the duration of treatment in AIDS patients for documented abscesses and cellulitis is limited because of the paucity of carefully studied cases. However, treatment duration should probably range over several weeks, accompanied by objective evidence of a resolution of the cellulitic process before treatment is stopped.

Mycobacterium haemophilum is a slow-growing mycobacterial species that has special requirements including hemin, low incubation (30 to 32°C) temperature, and carbon dioxide for optimal growth. The organism has been isolated from both immunocompromised patients and AIDS patients, and it may be missed if the special media and conditions used to grow this organism are not used. So far, *M. haemophilum* appears to be susceptible to conventional antimycobacterial agents, and in this regard, in vitro susceptibility testing (as for *M. tuberculosis*) may be of use as an initial guideline to treatment.

Mycobacterium malmoense was initially a nontuberculous mycobacterium described as a cause of pulmonary disease. It can affect immunocompetent patients, but more recently it has been strongly associated with the AIDS epidemic. It is a slow-growing organism and replicates at low temperatures in an acid environment. Chemotherapy of this agent with drugs similar in their activity against the *M. avium* complex is currently recommended.

Table 17.7. **Standard Drug Susceptibilities of the Commonly Pathogenic Nontuberculous Mycobaceria Using the Current Drug Concentrations Recommended for *Mycobacterium tuberculosis***

Species	Susceptible	Resistant	Intermediate
M. kansasii	RMP, EMB	PZA	INH, SM
M. marinum	RMP, EMB	INH, PZA	SM
M. avium complex	None	INH, RMP, SM, PZA	Cycloserine, EMB
M. fortuitum	None	INH, RMP, EMB	Capreomycin
M. chelonae		SM, PZA	

EMB, ethambutol; *INH*, isoniazid; *PZA*, pyrazinamide; *RMP*, rifampin; *SM*, streptomycin.
(Adapted from Wallace RJ Jr, Obrein R, Glassroth J, et al. Diagnosis and treatment of disease caused by nontuberculous mycobacteria. Am Rev Respir Dis 1990; 142:940–953.)

Mycobacterium genovense was first isolated from an AIDS patient during the present decade. Initially, it was associated with a diffuse or disseminated infectious process and an inability to culture the organism on routine mycobacterial laboratory media. Subsequently, it was shown to be a unique species that grows in liquid (BACTEC-II) systems after 5 weeks of incubation and is difficult to subculture onto solid media. Growth is slow and sparse, yet the susceptibility of this agent appears to be similar to that of the *M. avium* complex. Thus, regimens similar to those recommended for treatment of *M. avium* disease should be used to treat bacteremic *M. genovense* disease.

Various other nontuberculous mycobacteria have been discovered and distinguished by their 16S rRNA gene sequences. Many of these organisms appear to be saprophytic, but because of the severe immune deficiency in AIDS patients, it would not be surprising if other species of nontuberculous mycobacteria were to be associated with individuals who are HIV positive and have low CD4 counts. Advanced immune suppression appears to be the single unifying predisposing factor for clinical disease in patients with severely compromised cell-mediated immunity.

In conclusion, the widespread availability of protease inhibitors beginning in 1996 and the tendency to use such agents in combination with at least two reverse transcriptase inhibitors have had a significant impact on the incidence of systemic *Mycobacterium avium* disease in AIDS patients. Significant rises in CD4 counts have been repeatedly documented, and the magnitude of these changes has resulted in stable CD4 lymphocyte counts well above those thresholds at which prophylaxis of *M. avium* disease has been recommended. Cases of dissemination or bacteremic disease have clearly been documented when CD4 counts are higher than $75/mm^3$, but they are uncommon. Thus, an unanswered question is the degree of reconstitution achieved with improving antiretroviral therapy. A corollary to this issue is whether patients should be maintained on anti-*M. avium* prophylaxis, as well as other prophylactic measures, if they have dramatic and sustained improvements in CD4 counts. No recommendation can be made at this time, but those individuals who appear to have a CD4 count in excess of 150 cells/mm^3 for more than 6 months are unlikely to benefit from continued anti-*M. avium* complex prophylaxis.

Equally compelling is the issue of whether patients who have documented infections of the blood should continue to receive treatment after more than a year. Investigators previously believed that the therapy of *Mycobacterium avium* complex disease should be lifelong, but sustained remissions have been amply documented, and protocols are underway to assess the wisdom of discontinuing all treatment after a defined interval of systemic therapy. The essential factor leading to a decision to stop therapy should be a sustained rise in CD4 lymphocyte counts to levels considerably above the threshold of increased risk. Development of resistance or selection of resistance during therapy, particularly monotherapy with macrolides, is a real problem, and thus no monotherapeutic treatment protocols can be sanctioned for long duration. In view of the breakthrough of bacteremias with resistant organisms amply documented in the clarithromycin trials, the search for new agents active against *M. tuberculosis* and nontuberculous mycobacteria must continue. A priority must still be placed on finding treatments, specifically new agents, that achieve high concentration in infected cells, particularly macrophages, and have a rapid bactericidal effect. Although targeted drug delivery through liposomal or similar preparations is shown to be of benefit and feasibility in early human clinical trials, the high cost and impracticability of intravenous medication for long periods have limited widespread introduction. Similarly, some recombinant cytokine preparations have been shown both in vitro and in animals to confer some benefit, yet they are not a practical alternative to prophylaxis measures, nor can they be routinely incorporated into treatment regimens. Pilot studies with innovative biotherapeutic agents are warranted.

References

1. Wolinsky E. Nontuberculous mycobacteria and associated diseases. Am Rev Respir Dis 1979;119:107–159.
2. Runyon EH. Ten mycobacterial pathogens. Tubercle 1974;55:235–240.
3. Falkinham JO III. Epidemiology of infection by nontuberculous mycobacteria. Clin Microbiol Rev 1996;9:177–215.
4. Gottlieb MS, Schroff R, Schanker HM, et al. *Pneumocystis carinii* pneumonia and mucosal candidiasis in previously healthy homosexual men: evidence of a new acquired cellular immunodeficiency. N Engl J Med 1981;305:1425–1431.
5. Zakowski P, Fliegel S, Berlin OGW, et al. Disseminated *Mycobacterium avium-intracellulare* infection in homosexual men dying of acquired immunodeficiency. JAMA 1982;248:2980–2982.
6. Young LS, Inderlied CB, Berlin OG, et al. Mycobacterial infections in AIDS patients, with an emphasis on the *Mycobacterium avium* complex. Rev Infect Dis 1986;8:1024–1033.
7. Young LS. *Mycobacterium avium* complex infection. J Infect Dis 1988;157:863–867.
8. Horsburgh CR Jr. *Mycobacterium avium* complex infection in the acquired immunodeficiency syndrome. N Engl J Med 1991;324:1332–1338.
9. Phair JP. Clinical challenges of *Mycobacterium avium*. Am J Med 1997;102:1–55.
10. Horsburgh Jr. CR, Selik RM. The epidemiology of disseminated nontuberculous mycobacterial infections in AIDS. Am Rev Respir Dis 1989;139:4–7.
11. Nightingale SD, Byrd LT, Southern PM, et al. Incidence of *Mycobacterium avium-intracellulare* complex bacteremia in human immunodeficiency virus-positive patients. J Infect Dis 1992;165:198–1985.
12. Chaisson RE, Moore RD, Richman DD, et al. Incidence and natural history of *Mycobacterium avium* complex infection in advanced HIV disease treated with zidovudine. Am Rev Respir Dis 1991;143:A278.
13. Horsburgh CR Jr, Havlik JA, Ellia DA, et al. Survival of patients with acquired immune deficiency syndrome and disseminated *Mycobacterium avium* complex infection with and without antimycobacterial chemotherapy. Am Rev Respir Dis 1991;144:557–559.
14. Jacobson MA, Hopewell PC, Yajko M, et al. Natural history of disseminated *Mycobacterium avium* complex infection in AIDS. J Infect Dis 1991;164:994–998.
15. Chin DP, Hopewell PC, Yajko DM, et al. *Mycobacterium avium* complex in the respiratory or gastrointestinal tract and the risk of

M. avium complex bacteremia in patients with human immunodeficiency virus infection. J Infect Dis 1994;169:289–295.
16. Damsker B, Bottone EJ. *Mycobacterium avium–Mycobacterium intracellulare* from the intestinal tracts of patients with acquired immunodeficiency syndrome: concepts regarding acquisition and pathogenesis. J Infect Dis 1985;151:179–181.
17. Gray JR, Rabeneck L. Atypical mycobacterial infection of the gastrointestinal tract in AIDS patients. Am J Gastroenterol 1989;84:1521–1524.
18. Roth RI, Owen RL, Keren DF, et al. Intestinal infection with *Mycobacterium avium* in acquired immune deficiency syndrome (AIDS): pathological and clinical comparison with Whipple's disease. Dig Dis Sci 1985;30:497–504.
19. Bermudez LE, Young LS. Oxidative and non-oxidative intracellular killing of *Mycobacterium avium* complex. Microb Pathog 1989;7:289–298.
20. Kallenius G, Koivula T, Rydgard KJ, et al. Human immunodeficiency virus type 1 enhances growth of *Mycobacterium avium* in human macrophages. Infect Immun 1992;60:2453–2458.
21. Bermudez LE, Kolonoski P, Young LS. Natural killer cell activity and macrophage-dependent inhibition of growth or killing of *Mycobacterium avium* complex in a mouse model. J Leukoc Biol 1990;47:135–141.
22. Bermudez LE, Young LS. Natural killer cell-dependent mycobacteriostatic and mycobactericidal activity in human macrophages. J Immunol 1991;146:265–270.
23. Black CM, Bermudez LEM, Young LS, et al. Co-infection of macrophages modulates interferon gamma and tumor necrosis factor-induced activation against intracellular pathogens. J Exp Med 1990;172:977–980.
24. Bermudez LE, Young LS. Recombinant granulocyte-macrophage colony-stimulating factor activates human macrophages to inhibit growth or kill *Mycobacterium avium* complex. J Leukoc Biol 1990;48:57–73.
25. Prince DS, Peterson DD, Steiner RM, et al. Infection with *Mycobacterium avium* complex in patients without predisposing conditions. N Engl J Med 1989;321:863–868.
26. Inderlied CB. Microbiology and minimum inhibitory concentration testing for *Mycobacterium avium* complex prophylaxis. Am J Med 1997:102:2–10.
27. Wallace Jr. RJ, Obrein R, Glassroth J, et al. Diagnosis and treatment of disease caused by nontuberculous mycobacteria. Am Rev Repir Dis 1990;142:940–953.
28. Inderlied CB, Young LS, Yamada JK. Determination of in vitro susceptibility of *Mycobacterium avium* complex isolates to antimicrobial agents by various methods. Antimicrob Agents Chemother 1987;31:1697–1702.
29. Baron EJ, Young LS. Amikacin, ethambutol, and rifampin for treatment of disseminated *Mycobacterium avium intracellulare* infections in patients with acquired immune deficiency syndrome. Diagn Microbiol Infect Dis 1986;5:215–220.
30. Hawkins CC, Gold JWM, Whimby E, et al. *Mycobacterium avium* complex infections in patients with the acquired immunodeficiency syndrome. Ann Intern Med 1986;105:184–188.
31. Masur HC, Tuazon C, Gill V, et al. Effect of combined clofazimine and ansamycin therapy on *Mycobacterium avium-intracellulare* bacteremia in patients with AIDS. J Infect Dis 1987;155:127–129.
32. Agins BD, Berman DS, Spicehandler D, et al. Effect of combined therapy with ansamycin, clofazimine, ethambutol, and isoniazid for *Mycobacterium avium* infection in patients with AIDS. J Infect Dis 1989;159:784–787.
33. Hoy J, Mijch A, Sandland M, et al. Quadruple-drug therapy for *Mycobacterium avium-intracellulare* bacteremia in AIDS patients. J Infect Dis 1990;161:801–805.
34. Koletar SL. Treatment of *Mycobacterium avium* in human immunodeficiency virus-infected individuals. Am J Med 1997;102:16–21.

35. Dautzenberg B, Truffot C, Legris S, et al. Activity of clarithromycin against *Mycobacterium avium* infection in patients with the acquired immune deficiency syndrome. Am Rev Respir Dis 1991;144:564–569.
36. Young LS, Wiviott L, Wu M, et al. Azithromycin for treatment of *Mycobacterium avium-intracellulare* complex infection in patients with AIDS. Lancet 1991;338:1107–1109.
37. deLalla F, Maserati R, Scapellini P, et al. Clarithromycin–ciprofloxacin–amikacin for therapy of *M. avium* bacteremia in patients with AIDS. Antimicrob Agents Chemotherapy 1992;36:1567–1569.
38. Kemper CA, Meng TC, Nussbaum J, et al. Treatment of *Mycobacterium avium* complex bacteremia in AIDS with a four-drug oral regimen: rifampin, ethambutol, clofazimine and ciprofloxacin. Ann Intern Med 1992;116:466–472.
39. Chaisson RE, Benson CA, Dube MP, et al. Clarithromycin therapy for bacteremic *Mycobacterium avium* complex disease: a randomized, double-blind, dose-ranging study in patients with AIDS. Ann Intern Med 1994;121:905–911.
40. Shafran SD, et al. A comparison of two regimens for the treatment of *Mycobacterium avium* complex bacteremia in AIDS: rifabutin, ethambutol, and clarithromycin versus rifampin, ethambutol, clofazimine, and ciprofloxacin. N Engl J Med 1996;335:377–383.
41. Jacobsen MA, Yajko D, Northfelt D, et al. Randomized, placebo-controlled trial of rifampin, ethambutol, and ciprofloxacin for AIDS patients with disseminated *Mycobacterium avium* complex infection. J Infect Dis 1993;168:112–119.
42. Sullam PM, Gordin FM, Wynne BA, et al. Efficacy of rifabutin in the treatment of disseminated infection due to *Mycobacterium avium* complex. Clin Infect Dis 1994;19:84–86.
43. Kemper CA, Havlir D, Haghighat D, et al. The individual microbiologic effect of three antimycobacterial agents, clofazimine, ethambutol, and rifampin, on *Mycobacterium avium* complex bacteremia in patients with AIDS. J Infect Dis 1994;170:157–164.
44. May T, Brel F, Beuscart C, et al. Comparison of combination therapy regimens for treatment of human immunodeficiency virus-infected patients with disseminated bacteremia due to *Mycobacterium avium*. Clin Infect Dis 1997;25:621–629.
45. Wallace RJ Jr, Brown BA, Griffith DE, et al. Reduced serum levels of clarithromycin in patients treated with multidrug regimens including rifampin or rifabutin for *Mycobacterium avium–M. intracellulare* infection. J Infect Dis 1995;171:747–750.
46. Bermudez LE, Nash KA, Petrofsky M, et al. Effect of ethambutol on emergence of clarithromycin-resistant *Mycobacterium avium* complex in the beige mouse model. J Infect Dis 1996;174:1218–1222.
47. Chiu J, Nussbaum J, Bozzette S, et al. Treatment of disseminated *Mycobacterium avium* complex infection in AIDS with amikacin, ethambutol, rifampin, and ciprofloxacin. Ann Intern Med 1990;113:358–361.
48. Benson CA, Kessler HA, Pottage JC, et al. Successful treatment of acquired immunodeficiency syndrome-related *Mycobacterium avium* complex disease with a multiple drug regimen including amikacin. Arch Intern Med 1991;1512:582–585.
49. Bermudez LE, Inderlied CB, Kolonoski P, et al. Activities of bay Y 3118, levofloxacin, and ofloxacin alone or in combination with ethambutol against *Mycobacterium avium* complex in vitro, in human macrophages, and in beige mice. Antimicrob Agents Chemother 1996;40:546–551.
50. Nightingale SD, Saletan SL, Swenson CD, et al. Liposome-encapsulated gentamicin treatment of *Mycobacterium avium–Mycobacterium intracellulare* complex bacteremia in AIDS patients. Antimicrob Agents Chemother 1993;37:1869–1872.
51. Dube MP, Sattler FR, Torriani F, See D, et al. A randomized evaluation of ethambutol for prevention of relapse and drug resistance during treatment of *Mycobacterium avium* complex bacteremia with clarithromycin-based combination therapy. J Infect Dis 1997; 173:1225–1232.
52. Nightingale SD, Cameron DW, Gordin FM, et al. Two controlled trials of rifabutin prophylaxis against *Mycobacterium avium* complex infection in AIDS. N Engl J Med 1993;219:828–833.

53. Pierce M, Crampton S, Henry D, et al. A randomized trial of clarithromycin as prophylaxis against disseminated *Mycobacterium avium* complex infection in patients with advanced acquired immunodeficiency syndrome. N Engl J Med 1996;335:384–391.
54. Havlir DV, Dube MP, Sattler FR, et al. Prophylaxis against disseminated *Mycobacterium avium* complex with weekly azithromycin, daily rifabutin, or both. N Engl J Med 1996;335:392–398.
55. Benson CA. Critical drug interactions with agents used for prophylaxis and treatment of *Mycobacterium avium* complex infections. Am J Med 1997;102:32–36.
56. USPHS/IDSA Prevention of Opportunistic Infections Working Group. USPHS/IDSA guidelines for the prevention of opportunistic infections in persons infected with human immunodeficiency virus. MMWR Morb Mortal Wkly Rep 1997;46:1–46.
57. Ives DV, Davis RB, Currier JS. Impact of clarithromycin and azithromycin on patterns of treatment and survival among AIDS patients with disseminated *Mycobacterium avium* complex. AIDS 1995;9:261–266.
58. Horsburgh CR Jr. Advances in the prevention and treatment of *Mycobacterium avium* disease. N Engl J Med 1996;335:428–429.

18
SYPHILIS

Daniel M. Musher and Robert E. Baughn

Sexually transmitted diseases are highly associated with one another, as was demonstrated with tragic consequences by John Hunter, the famous eighteenth-century Scottish surgeon who inoculated himself with urethral exudate from a patient with gonorrhea and developed not only gonorrhea but also a fatal case of syphilis. Because of uncertainties in diagnosing infection caused by *Treponema pallidum* and the fact that human immunodeficiency virus (HIV) infection can span a full decade with recognition for only some fraction of that time, it is difficult to know the precise frequency with which the two coexist. Certainly, most persons who are at risk for one of these two diseases are at risk for the other, and a high degree of association has been amply documented (1–3). Our experience has been that most men whose HIV infection results from a homosexual or bisexual lifestyle have had a diagnosis of syphilis, however made, some time in the past. This association is present, albeit less strikingly so, among women whose HIV infection results from prostitution. The information is less certain (4) for those who acquired HIV infection as a complication of intravenous drug abuse, although, in practice, the distinction is arbitrary because of the high degree of association between the use of illicit drugs and prostitution, in which the latter becomes the means for supporting the former. A special relationship between syphilis and HIV infection has been documented (5) in which the presence of a chancre enhances the transmissibility of HIV.

Problems addressed in this chapter include the impact of HIV infection on: 1) the natural history of syphilis and its clinical manifestations; 2) the diagnosis of syphilis; and 3) the response of syphilis to antibiotic treatment. In addition, we discuss possible approaches to treating syphilis in HIV-infected persons.

NATURAL HISTORY OF SYPHILIS AND NEUROSYPHILIS

The initial sign or lesion of syphilis, called a primary chancre, appears 2 to 3 weeks after treponemes have been inoculated, usually into an unrecognized break in the skin. Such inoculation inevitably results from intimate, nearly always venereal, human contact (6). Infection by *Treponema pallidum* is always generalized; widespread hematogenous dissemination can be documented a few days before the chancre appears. In fact, in experimentally infected animals, treponemes can be recovered from lymph nodes, liver, and spleen soon after the initial time of infection. Three to 8 weeks after the chancre first appears, lesions of disseminated infection develop. The skin is the principal target organ, reflecting the propensity of *T. pallidum* to proliferate more readily at temperatures several degrees below 37°C; in rabbits, the most reliable experimental models for syphilis, lesions appear only where the fur has been shaved. In this stage of syphilis, the skin, lymph nodes, liver, and bones are regularly involved. In the absence of treatment, the initial chancre resolves over 2 to 5 weeks; thus, in some patients with secondary syphilis, a primary chancre can still be detected if its presence is sought. Because of this widespread involvement, we prefer the term *disseminated* syphilis to *secondary* syphilis, but the latter is too thoroughly entrenched in medical parlance to be replaced. The incubation period of disseminated syphilitic lesions is prolonged beyond the 2 to 3 weeks observed in primary syphilis, and the lesions do not have the appearance of syphilitic chancres; the reason for this difference is that an immune response has already occurred. When rabbits are injected intravenously with 5×10^7 viable *T. pallidum*, they develop lesions in shaved areas that actually resemble primary chancres; this occurs because lesions appear before the animals have had time to develop immunity.

For reasons that shall become apparent, involvement of the central nervous system (CNS) is most relevant to the relationship between syphilis and HIV infection. Treponemes can be identified in the cerebrospinal fluid (CSF) in more than one-quarter of persons with disseminated (secondary) syphilis, and another one-quarter have abnormalities in the CSF that are consistent with syphilitic involvement (7–10). This CNS infection produces no symptoms, and the involvement is detected only if routine lumbar punctures are done.

In the absence of treatment, secondary syphilis is brought under control by a poorly understood interaction between humoral and cell-mediated immune mechanisms. Skin lesions disappear, and evidence of involvement of other organs diminishes, although *Treponema pallidum* remains recoverable, for example, by aspirating lymph nodes and injecting the material intradermally in rabbits. This stage, which lasts from several years to a lifetime, is called latent syphilis. When no treatment is given, about one-third of patients develop a late (or tertiary) form of syphilis; nearly one-third of these (7 to 10%) have neurosyphilis (9, 11, 12). Thus, in the absence of treatment, the brain serves as a reservoir for treponemes, and active syphilitic infection of the CNS may recur years after this disease has seemingly been brought under control.

In the first part of the twentieth century, treatment with neoarsphenamine regularly arrested early syphilis and caused rapid resolution of lesions. Tertiary syphilis continued to occur many years later, but only in about 5% of adequately treated patients, with neurosyphilis appearing in half these cases. To grasp fully the relationship between syphilis and HIV infection, one must realize that treponemes could still be found in lymph nodes of subjects who had been treated with and seemingly cured by arsphenamine, whose serum Venereal Disease Research Laboratory (VDRL) reaction had become negative and who did not go on to develop tertiary syphilis. Early in the twentieth century, authorities agreed that natural immune mechanisms worked together with antimicrobial therapy to arrest syphilis (13). Those persons whose syphilis had been treated at an earlier stage, such as in its primary stage, had a higher likelihood of late relapse after treatment than those whose syphilis had progressed to latency before treatment.

With the onset of the penicillin era, therapy was simplified, and its duration was reduced from 18 months to 1 to 3 weeks. Adequate doses of penicillin uniformly produced a clinical cure of early syphilis, and neurosyphilis rarely occurred after such therapy (14–16). In countries where socialized medicine makes it possible to retrieve all relevant data, persons who have been found to have neurosyphilis have not received an effective course of penicillin therapy (17). Nevertheless, strong evidence indicates that treponemes are not eradicated; that is, a biologic cure has not been produced, even by penicillin therapy. Lymph nodes from treated persons as well as from rabbits that were infected with *Treponema pallidum*, allowed to progress to latent infection, and then treated with huge doses of penicillin continue to harbor viable organisms (12).

SYPHILIS AND HIV INFECTION

A disease such as HIV infection, which causes striking suppression of nearly every aspect of the immune response, is expected to alter the natural history of other infections. From that point of view, it is surprising that syphilis in its early stages is not more notably altered by concurrent HIV infection than appears to be the case. Certainly, in experimentally infected rabbits, immunosuppression by corticosteroids causes more exuberant lesions to appear, and athymic mice develop syphilitic lesions, whereas normal ones do not. Only two kinds of differences have been documented in carefully executed studies: 1) HIV-infected patients are more likely to have persistent chancres and to present with disseminated (secondary) then with primary syphilis, without regard to the patient's sexual preference (13); 2) rapid plasma reagin (RPR) titers may be higher in HIV-infected persons (14–16), although this finding may be confined to first episodes of recognized syphilis (15); higher levels of RPR may relate to a higher likelihood of "biologic false-positive" RPR test results (17). In addition to these findings from well-controlled studies are numerous anecdotal reports of florid cases of primary and secondary syphilis and individual cases with the diagnosis of lues maligna or "quaternary" syphilis in HIV-infection, but these reports have not been documented in comparative prospective studies, a finding suggesting that, even if the association is real, the incidence is rare.

One possible explanation for the finding that early syphilis is not more florid in HIV-infected persons is that the lesions in early syphilis may result, at least in part, from deposition of immune complexes in walls of vessels, thus reflecting the host response as much as the presence of infecting organisms (18). In fact, a worrisome possibility, albeit entirely unproved to date, is that active syphilis in some HIV-infected individuals is overlooked because an inadequate immune response prevents both the appearance of lesions and the development of antibody that could react in serologic tests.

NEUROSYPHILIS AND HIV INFECTION

In contrast, in the case of neurologic involvement, HIV infection appears to exert a profound impact on the manifestations of syphilis (19–24). By 1970, newly diagnosed cases of proved neurosyphilis had come to be uncommon at large teaching hospitals. In striking contrast, beginning in the mid-1970s and continuing to the present, cases of meningitis, cranial nerve abnormalities, or cerebrovascular accidents due to syphilis have become commonplace. A review of the medical literature through 1990 (21) revealed 42 reported cases in which neurosyphilis was proved to coexist with HIV infection (Table 18.1). Five of the 42 patients had abnormal CSF but were otherwise free of neurologic symptoms and were classified as asymptomatic. Acute syphilitic meningitis was present in 24 patients, 9 of whom presented with symptoms and signs of meningitis (fever, headache, stiffness of the neck, or confusion) and 15 with cranial nerve abnormalities but without meningeal signs. Five of those in whom

Table 18.1. Reported Cases of Neurosyphilis in HIV-Infected Patients[a]

Cases	No.
Asymptomatic neurosyphilis	5
Acute syphilitic meningitis	25
Meningitis	9
Cranial nerve dysfunction	15
Polyradiculopathy	1
Meningovascular syphilis	11
General paresis	1

[a]Cases collected from the English-language literature toward the end of 1990, and most cited individually in reference 19.
(Adapted from Musher DM. Syphilis, neurosyphilis, penicillin and AIDS. J Infect Dis 1991;163:1201–1206.)

meningitis predominated also had cranial nerve abnormalities. Optic neuritis or neuroretinitis, most common, was diagnosed in 11 cases; presenting symptoms included blurred vision and blindness. Six patients had involvement of the otic or vestibular branch of cranial nerve VIII; these patients presented with deafness, loss of balance, or both. Individual cases showed involvement of cranial nerves III, IV and VI, V, or VII; many of those patients who had second or eighth nerve abnormalities had other cranial nerves involved as well. One patient had polyradiculopathy. Eleven patients with meningovascular syphilis had symptoms and signs of a cerebrovascular accident that varied depending on the location of the lesion and the presence or absence of infarction. In most patients, computed tomography confirmed the presence of lesions, and in 2 individuals, angiography demonstrated multiple areas of narrowing (beading) of the cerebral arteries. Two patients who originally presented with syphilitic meningitis but were not treated developed strokes resulting from progression of untreated neurosyphilis. Finally, 1 patient had general paresis.

Some abnormality of the CSF was demonstrated in 38 of 39 patients in whom a spinal tap was performed, and for any given parameter (white blood count, protein, glucose), 30 to 80% of CSFs were abnormal. The percentage of abnormal results and the median of abnormal values are shown in Table 18.2. The true incidence of a negative VDRL reaction in the CSF may even be higher than the 21% shown in Table 18.2, reflecting the tendency to report only inarguable cases in the medical literature. These data show that a near-normal CSF analysis cannot absolutely exclude the possibility that an individual patient has neurosyphilis, a worrisome situation but one that has not changed since the preantibiotic era.

These manifestations of neurosyphilis in HIV-infected patients are similar to those of meningeal or meningovascular syphilis, which also presents with meningitis, cranial nerve abnormalities, and strokes (12). Early meningeal syphilis was a rare form of infection in the prepenicillin era; it was diagnosed in only 80 among several thousand cases of syphilis by Merritt and his colleagues in the 1930s (25). Ehrlich had called this form of infection "neurorecurrence" because most cases occurred within 1 year after patients had received inadequate doses of therapy. The analogy between giving inadequate antimicrobial therapy to immunologically normal hosts and administering adequate antibiotic therapy to immunologically suppressed hosts is obvious. Meningovascular syphilis was the earliest form of tertiary syphilis to appear, often occurring 5 years after the initial infection. In contrast, tertiary neurosyphilis usually appeared 15 to 20 years after the primary infection and presented with well-known and progressive syndromes, such as tabes dorsalis or paresis, that reflected parenchymal invasion. These observations explain the emphasis on the rapid progression to neurologic disease caused by syphilis in HIV-infected persons (19). Comparative studies (23, 24) show that early neurosyphilis predominates in HIV-infected persons, whereas late neurosyphilis predominates in those who are not infected with HIV.

Four additional points must be made about the relation between HIV infection and syphilis. First, of 42 reported patients with concurrent neurosyphilis and HIV infection, 17 had acquired immunodeficiency syndrome (AIDS), 4 had AIDS-related complex, and 14 had only serologic evidence of HIV infection. The numbers of CD4 cells often were not reported; our later experience has shown that, although in most patients this number is less than $200/mm^3$, in others it may exceed $500/mm^3$. This observation emphasizes that, early in the course of HIV infection, subtle abnormalities in the host's immunologic capacity occur, increasing susceptibility to typical human pathogens such at *Treponema pallidum* and *Mycobacterium tuberculosis,* unlike the later course, in which a much greater degree of damage has been done to the immune system and infections from less pathogenic organisms such as *Pneumocystis carinii* or *Mycobacterium avium* predominate. Second, in 11 of 25 patients (44%) for whom data were available, the diagnosis of HIV infection first was made at the time of presentation for neurosyphilis. Thus, neurosyphilis may be a sentinel infection in the recognition of HIV infection. Considering its rarity in the non–HIV-infected population, the diagnosis of neurosyphilis should automatically lead to evaluation of the patient for HIV infection, although, as noted earlier, such an evaluation should already have been done in a patient who has a sexually transmitted disease. Third, 16 of the 42 reported HIV-infected patients had previously been treated with penicillin for syphilis. Five of these 16 (31%) developed early neurosyphilis within 6 months of having received a recommended course of therapy, usually 2.4 million units of benzathine penicillin, a relapse rate inconceivable in the penicillin era. Finally, as tragically documented in several reported cases and amply confirmed in our experience, the failure to treat asymptomatic neurosyphilis in HIV-infected persons may be followed by rapid progression to symptomatic neurosyphilis, often meningovascular infection manifested as a stroke.

The extraordinary prevalence of asymptomatic neurosyphilis in HIV-infected patients has been documented in other ways. Even in the absence of a prospective search, Katz and Berger (20) found that 1.5% of all patients attending a clinic for HIV-related disease had been diagnosed as having neurosyphilis. Finding neurosyphilis in a measurable percentage of any patient group in the United States in the 1980s was

Table 18.2. Cerebrospinal Fluid Abnormalities in 42 Reported Cases of Coexisting Syphilis and HIV Infection

	Cells	Protein	Glucose	VDRL
Abnormal/reported	29/34	28/34	11/32	31/39
Median abnormal values	173	125	37	1:4
Range abnormal values[a]	8–2,000	46–1,000	11–42	Weakly reactive, 1:16

[a]Normal values taken from Jaffe HW, Kabins SA. Examination of cerebrospinal fluid in patients with syphilis. Rev Infect Dis 1982;4(Suppl):S842–847.
(Adapted from Musher DM, Hamill RJ, Baughn RE. Effect of human immunodeficiency virus (HIV) infection on the course of syphilis and on the response to treatment. Ann Intern Med 1990;113:872–881.)

simply amazing. In a retrospective study, these same investigators (23) found that more than half of all cases of neurosyphilis occur in HIV-infected persons. Two clinics that provide care for HIV-infected patients have shown that of the 5 to 10% of all patients who have serum RPR reactive at 1:4 or greater, as many as 10 to 50% have CSF abnormalities suggestive or diagnostic of neurosyphilis (26, 27). For example, in our clinic (27), 13 asymptomatic HIV-infected patients with serum RPR 1:4 or greater submitted to a lumbar puncture. The CSF was abnormal in 7, all of whom were characterized by a reactive VDRL; 5 of the 7 had 6 white blood cells/mm^3 or greater, and 6 had at least 46 mg protein/dL. Thus, an alarming proportion of HIV-infected persons who have a serum RPR 1:4 or greater in the absence of CNS symptoms have asymptomatic neurosyphilis. Consistent with the results of earlier reports, nearly half these patients had received 1 to 3 doses of benzathine penicillin in the preceding 2 years. None had any history suggestive of recent untreated syphilis, and many did not even have a new exposure. Thus, these cases are thought to reflect reactivation, either of latent disease or of prolonged, smoldering infection that has persisted, despite seemingly appropriate therapy.

SEROLOGIC TESTS FOR SYPHILIS IN HIV IHFECTION

Because of the severity of the immunosuppression caused by HIV infection, investigators have been concerned that serologic tests to diagnose syphilis may not be reliable in HIV-infected subjects. In a few reported cases, antibody to cardiolipin, as measured by RPR or VDRL test, was undetectable despite active secondary disease (28–30). In most instances, however, RPR tests are positive, often at a higher titer than is seen in non–HIV-infected individuals, as pointed out earlier, presumably reflecting polyclonal activation of the immune system. The finding of especially high RPR titers has led to renewed concern about the prozone phenomenon, particularly in congenital syphilis. Several reports have described newborn infants with congenital syphilis whose mothers were said to have a nonreactive RPR test on undiluted serum, but who actually had such high titers that the undiluted sample was negative because of the prozone. Physicians must be reminded that most laboratories no longer perform dilutions on routine RPR determinations, and a specific request that they be done should accompany all sera from patients who are thought to have syphilis, as well as in screening patients who may be in a high-risk category.

Regarding antitreponemal antibody, microhemagglutinating antibody to *Treponema pallidum* (MHA-TP) reactivity may be lost with progression of HIV infection (31), although the relation of negative serologic tests to the activity of syphilis is uncertain. This result does suggest that one may not be able to rely on a negative MHA-TP test to exclude the possibility of prior *T. pallidum* infection in patients with AIDS.

THERAPY

Until recently, no prospective study evaluated treatment options in HIV versus non–HIV-infected patients. Numerous anecdotal reports described treatment failures (21, 32); such reports had not appeared in the decade preceding the emergence of HIV infection. One small prospective study (15) had shown no apparent difference in failure rate. The United States Public Health Service Centers for Disease Control (CDC) has continued to recommend a single dose of 2.4 million units of benzathine penicillin for early (primary or secondary) syphilis, based on the finding that documentation of failures is largely anecdotal. A recent, multicenter, prospective study (16) supports this approach. In 103 HIV-infected patients with early syphilis, 1 patient had a relapse after treatment with a single dose of benzathine penicillin, versus none of 450 non–HIV-infected patients.

We believe that it still may be reasonable to administer two or three doses of benzathine penicillin at weekly intervals based on the number of documented failures, a number that, even though anecdotal, far exceeds what could have been expected in the pre-HIV era. Further defending this approach may be studies showing a delayed resolution of lesions (16), a slower decline in RPR (16, 32) (although this result was not supported in Hutchinson [13]), and a higher rate of serologic failure (16) in HIV-infected persons. Finally, some association may exist in a patient's mind between the intensity of therapy and the need for follow-up studies that would support the use of additional injections.

If latent syphilis is diagnosed and the absence of neurosyphilis is confirmed by lumbar puncture, we recommend three doses of benzathine penicillin, each of 2.4 million units, at weekly intervals. If a lumbar puncture is not done because the patient refuses, our recommendations for treatment are, in fact, no different, although the degree of vigilance on the part of the physician must be increased by the lack of knowledge of the patient's clinical status.

It may seem intuitively obvious that HIV-infected patients with asymptomatic neurosyphilis (CSF abnormalities suggestive of neurosyphilis in the absence of symptoms or signs of disease) should receive more intensive therapy, but it needs to be stated at the outset that the limited available data (27) do not clearly support this intuitive view. Daily administration of 600,000 units of procaine penicillin for 10 to 14 days together with probenecid provided definitive treatment for symptomatic neurosyphilis in the pre-AIDS era, and one has no reason to believe that this regimen would be less adequate than any other in HIV-infected patients. (In fact, three doses of benzathine penicillin were also recommended as appropriate therapy for neurosyphilis; daily procaine penicillin was given by the cautious physician who wished to be more certain of efficacy.) We are inclined to avoid possible complications of probenecid (said to be more prevalent in AIDS patients than in the population at large) by omitting this drug and, instead, increasing the dosage of penicillin to 1.2 million units daily. Furthermore, it may be advisable to treat the patient for a total of 14 days rather than 10 days.

Another approach in the patient with asymptomatic neurosyphilis is to give ceftriaxone daily for 10 to 14 days; at least, data are available on the outcome of this regimen. In a retrospective study (27), 1 g of this drug, given daily for 14 days, effectively treated 6 of 7 patients who had documented asymptomatic neurosyphilis. No evidence indicated that doubling the dose was associated with a better outcome. No comparison with daily procaine penicillin was included, and there even was the suggestion that 3 weekly doses of benzathine penicillin were as effective as 14 daily doses of ceftriaxone. These points show that: 1) daily administration of procaine penicillin is likely to be as effective as ceftriaxone and much less costly; 2) the possibility that 3 doses of benzathine penicillin may be as effective has not been excluded; and 3) good prospective studies are needed to compare these various regimens.

In cases of symptomatic neurosyphilis, nearly all authorities recommend prolonged, high-dose antibiotic therapy such as 12 to 24×10^6 units of aqueous penicillin daily for 10 days, although some failures have already been reported (34), and daily administration of 1 or 2 g ceftriaxone or 1.2 million units of procaine penicillin may be just as effective. Until a prospective comparison has been made, it is unclear whether treatment with daily procaine penicillin, intravenous penicillin, or daily ceftriaxone is preferable. Because the basic problem appears to be the host, not the antibiotic dose, we believe that once-daily administration of procaine penicillin or ceftriaxone is an entirely acceptable initial approach that may eventually be proved as effective as 24 million units of daily penicillin with its mandatory hospitalization (35).

CEREBROSPINAL FLUID EXAMINATION IN SYPHILIS

Should the CSF be examined in every patient who has syphilis and concurrent HIV infection? This approach was taken routinely in the prepenicillin era to monitor therapy and to ensure that neurosyphilis did not develop. Opposing this approach is the argument that treponemes may be present or abnormalities may be detected by conventional means in the CSF of up to 40% of patients with secondary syphilis, yet, in the past, these findings did not require an altered approach to penicillin therapy. It is also true, although perhaps it has been overstated, that CSF abnormalities may be present because of the HIV infection itself, which would confound the situation. Finally, lumbar puncture takes time and requires a suitable facility, a problem for some clinics that provide care to HIV-infected persons.

Favoring the routine use of lumbar puncture in HIV-infected persons, especially those with latent syphilis, is the observation that, when such a study is done, many of these patients have evidence of CNS disease. Of all the infections that AIDS patients may develop, neurosyphilis may still be among the more readily treatable. Furthermore, repeated lumbar puncture provides a means for following the results of treatment; for this reason, repeated CSF examination was considered so valuable in the prepenicillin era. Even this last point, however, may be overstated inasmuch as repeated determinations of serum RPR may give equally good insight into response or failure; lumbar puncture could then be reserved for those patients who have serologic evidence of treatment failure or of relapse. Data on the predictive value of routine or other serologic tests in this situation are not available. Thus, the question whether CSF analysis should be performed routinely in every HIV-infected person who has a reactive VDRL remains unanswered, although we believe that it certainly should be done in patients who do not show an appropriate serologic response to therapy. Perhaps some serologic test eventually will enable these diagnostic distinctions to be made.

FOLLOW-UP CARE

These considerations indicate that repeated, close evaluation of HIV-infected syphilitic patients, perhaps with repeated examination of CSF, is crucial to providing good long-range care. This is precisely what was done in the prepenicillin era, when less effective antimicrobial agents were used to treat syphilis in immunologically normal hosts. During the penicillin era, but before the advent of HIV infection, individual practitioners could be less rigid about their serologic monitoring after treatment. This approach is clearly not acceptable with HIV-infected persons.

Some physicians have wondered whether, after the initial course of treatment for uncomplicated early syphilis, continuous suppressive antibiotic therapy should be given to HIV-infected subjects to prevent a relapse. Several reasons exist for not doing so. First, the rate at which neurosyphilis develops after treatment with benzathine penicillin is unclear; if the rate is as low as 1 to 2%, further thought must be given to the question whether another prophylactic drug should be given to HIV-infected persons to prevent the development of a syndrome of neurosyphilis that may be readily recognized and treated. Second, drug levels in the CNS—the area that needs to be targeted with therapy—are likely to be so low with long-term oral therapy that neurologic disease may progress notwithstanding, although opposing this notion is that normal hosts tended to develop early neurosyphilis in the prepenicillin era only when therapy was discontinued altogether. At present, we do not recommend prescribing continuous antibiotic prophylaxis for HIV-infected persons after therapy for neurosyphilis.

In summary, *Treponema pallidum*, a unique pathogenic bacterium, causes infection that, in its early stages, disseminates widely throughout the body, including the CNS. Infection is followed first by the appearance of lesions at the initial site of inoculation and then by widespread systemic disease that is eventually brought under control by the host's immune response. Latency ensues, but, in the absence of treatment, tertiary syphilis appears in about one-third of infected persons, one-quarter of whom develop neurosyphilis. Treatment of syphilis with neoarsphenamine reduced the rate of late neurosyphilis to about 5%, and treatment with penicillin reduced it further, perhaps to the vanishing point.

Treponemes are probably not eradicated by such therapy, and the presumption is that continued action of an intact immune system maintains the infection in check.

By its remarkable effects on the immune system, infection with HIV unleashes syphilis in the area that is most carefully protected from eradication of treponemes, namely, the CNS. A syndrome of early neurosyphilis has been frequently observed, manifested by cranial nerve abnormalities, meningitis, and stroke in young adults with HIV infection. Definitive schedules for treating early syphilis or early neurosyphilis in the HIV-infected patient have not yet been determined, and unfortunately, only the most rudimentary studies are, to our knowledge, in progress. The notions that "more is better" and "most is best" are not supported by available data. In the absence of information on the best way to treat syphilis in HIV-infected persons, each physician must select a practical regimen that seems likely to be effective and then rigorously must monitor the efficacy by repeated serologic tests, perhaps also with repeated CSF analysis, especially if CSF abnormalities have been demonstrated.

References

1. Nelson KE, Vlahov D, Cohn S, et al. Sexually transmitted diseases in a population of intravenous drug users: association with seropositivity to the human immunodeficiency virus (HIV). J Infect Dis 1991;164: 457–463.
2. Weisfuse IB, Greenberg BL, Back SD, et al. HIV-1 infection among New York City inmates. AIDS 1991;5:1133–1138.
3. Pereira LH, Embil JA, Haase DA, et al. Prevalence of human immunodeficiency virus in the patient population of a sexually transmitted disease clinic: association with syphilis and gonorrhea. Sex Transm Dis 1992;19:115–120.
4. Robles RR, Colon HM, Sahai H, et al. Behavioral risk factors and human immunodeficiency virus (HIV) prevalence among intravenous drug users in Puerto Rico. Am J Epidemiol 1992;135:531–540.
5. Hook EW III, Cannon RO, Nahmias AJ, et al. Herpes simplex virus infection as a risk factor for human immunodeficiency virus infection in heterosexuals. J Infect Dis 1992;165:251–255.
6. Musher DM, Knox JM. Syphilis and yaws. In: Schell RF, Musher DM, eds. Pathogenesis and immunology of treponemal infections. New York: Marcel Dekker, 1983:101–120.
7. Chesney AM, Kemp JE. Incidence of *Spirochaeta pallida* in cerebrospinal fluid during early stage of syphilis. JAMA 1924; 83:1725–1728.
8. Stokes JH. Modern clinical syphilology: diagnosis–treatment–case study. Philadelphia: WB Saunders, 1934.
9. Kampmeier RH. Essentials of syphilology. Philadelphia: JB Lippincott, 1943.
10. Lukehart SA, Hook EW III, Baker-Zander SA, et al. Invasion of the central nervous system by *Treponema pallidum:* implications for diagnosis and treatment. Ann Intern Med 1988;109:855–862.
11. Gjestland T. The Oslo study of untreated syphilis: an epidemiologic investigation of the natural course of syphilitic infection based upon a re-study of the Boeck–Bruusgaard material. Acta Dermatol Venereol 1955;35(Suppl 34):1–368, i–lvi, list of tables and figures.
12. Swartz MN, Healy BP, Musher DM. Late syphilis. In: Sexually transmitted diseases. 3rd ed.
13. Hutchinson CM, Hook EW III, Shepherd M, et al. Altered clinical presentation of early syphilis in patients with human immunodeficiency virus infection. Ann Intern Med 1994;121:94–99.
14. Hutchinson CM, Rompalo AM, Reichard CA, et al. Characteristics of patients with syphilis attending Baltimore STD clinics. Arch Intern Med 1991;151:511–516.
15. Gourevitch MN, Selwyn PA, Davenny K, et al. Effects of HIV infection on the serologic manifestations and response to treatment of syphilis in intravenous drug users. Ann Intern Med 1993;118:350–355.
16. Rolfs RT, Joesoef MR, Hendershot EF, et al. Treatment of early syphilis in HIV-infected and uninfected persons: a randomized trial of enhanced therapy that included examination of cerebrospinal fluid. N Engl J Med 1997.
17. Augenbraun MH, DeHovitz JA, Feldman J, et al. Biological false-positive syphilis test results for women infected with human immunodeficiency virus. Clin Infect Dis 1994;19:1040–1044.
18. Jorizzo JL, McNeely MC, Baughn RE, et al. Role of circulating immune complexes in human secondary syphilis. J Infect Dis 1986;153: 1014–1022.
19. Johns DR, Tierney M, Felsenstein D. Alterations in the natural history of neurosyphilis by concurrent infection with the human immunodeficiency virus. N Engl J Med 1987;316:1569.
20. Katz DA, Berger JR. Neurosyphilis in acquired immunodeficiency syndrome. Arch Neurol 1989;46:895–898.
21. Musher DM, Hamill RJ, Baughn RE. Effect of human immunodeficiency virus (HIV) infection on the course of syphilis and on the response to treatment. Ann Intern Med 1990;113:872–881.
22. Musher DM. Syphilis, neurosyphilis, penicillin and AIDS. J Infect Dis 1991;163:1201–1206.
23. Katz DA, Berger JR, Duncan RC. Neurosyphilis: a comparative study of the effects of infection with human immunodeficiency virus. Arch Neurol 1993;50:243–249.
24. Flood JM, Weinstock HS, Guroy ME, et al. Neurosyphilis during the AIDS epidemic, San Francisco, 1985–1989. In: Program Abstracts of the 31st Interscience Conference on Antimicrobial Agents and Chemotherapy, abstract 334:154.
25. Merritt HH, Adams RD, Solomon HC. Neurosyphilis. Oxford: Oxford University Press, 1946.
26. Holtom PD, Larsen RA, Leal ME, et al. Prevalence of neurosyphilis in human immunodeficiency virus–infected patients with latent syphilis. Am J Med 1992;93:9–12.
27. Dowell ME, Ross PG, Musher DM, et al. Response of latent syphilis or neurosyphilis to ceftriaxone therapy in persons infected with human immunodeficiency virus. Am J Med 1992; 93:481–488.
28. Hicks CB, Benson PM, Lupton GP, et al. Seronegative secondary syphilis in a patient infected with the human immunodeficiency virus (HIV) with Kaposi sarcoma: a diagnostic dilemma. Ann Intern Med 1987;107:492–495.
29. Passo MS, Rosenbaum JT. Ocular syphilis in patients with human immunodeficiency virus infection. Am J Ophthalmol 1988;106:1–6.
30. Radolf JD, Kaplan RP. Unusual manifestations of secondary syphilis and abnormal humoral immune response to *Treponema pallidum* antigens in a homosexual man with asymptomatic human immunodeficiency virus infection. J Am Acad Dermatol 1988;18: 423–428.
31. Johnson PDR, Graves SR, Stewart L, et al. Specific syphilis serological tests may become negative in HIV infection. AIDS 1991;5: 419–424.
32. Malone JL, Wallace MR, Hendrick BB, et al. Syphilis and neurosyphilis in a human immunodeficiency virus type-1 seropositive population: evidence for frequent serologic relapse after therapy. Am J Med 1995;99:55–63.
33. Telzak EE, Greenberg MS, Harrison J, et al. Syphilis treatment response in HIV-infected individuals. AIDS 1991;5:591–595.
34. Gordon SM, Eaton ME, George R, et al. The response of symptomatic neurosyphilis to high-dose intravenous penicillin G in patients with human immunodeficiency virus infection. N Engl J Med 1994;331: 1469–1473.
35. Musher DM, Baughn RE. Neurosyphilis in HIV-infected persons. N Engl J Med 1994;331:1516–1517.

19
BACILLARY ANGIOMATOSIS

Jeffery S. Loutit

Bacillary angiomatosis is a descriptive term first applied by LeBoit (1). The term describes the characteristic pattern, noted on pathology specimens, of vascular proliferation along with the bacillary forms observed using special stains and electron microscopy. Stoler and colleagues, in 1983, first described a case with many of the salient features of bacillary angiomatosis (2).

Not until the late 1980s were the causative agents of bacillary angiomatosis identified. The two organisms implicated are *Bartonella* (formerly *Rochalimaea*) *henselae* and *Bartonella* (formerly *Rochalimaea*) *quintana*, both members of the tribe Rickettsiales. Successful cultivation of these microorganisms in the laboratory has permitted the spectrum of disease attributed to *Bartonella* species to be expanded (Table 19.1). This spectrum now encompasses bacillary angiomatosis with cutaneous and/or visceral organ involvement, relapsing fever with bacteremia, endocarditis, trench fever, and bacillary peliosis hepatis. In addition, cat-scratch disease has been added to the list of syndromes caused by *B. henselae*.

Antibody detection assays have added to our diagnostic capabilities and our understanding of the epidemiology of these organisms. This chapter describes these new advances, as well as the classification, clinical presentations, epidemiology, microbiology, diagnosis, and treatment of *Bartonella* species in human immunodeficiency virus (HIV)-infected patients.

HISTORY

The first case of bacillary angiomatosis was described by Stoler and colleagues. The patient was a 32-year-old man whose CD4 count was $40/mm^3$ and who initially presented with odynophagia secondary to both esophageal *Candida albicans* and herpes simplex. He later developed multiple, firm, indurated, nontender subcutaneous nodules varying in size from 2 to 6 cm. Histologic examination of these nodules revealed a proliferation of histiocytic and endothelial cells within a framework of poorly formed capillary channels. Warthin–Starry silver stain revealed a diffuse infiltration of small bacillary forms, the presence of which was confirmed by transmission electron microscopy; however, all cultures of these lesions were negative. Empiric oral erythromycin resulted in resolution of the nodules. The nodules were believed to represent an atypical granulation tissue with neutrophilic infiltration associated with a culturally undefined bacterial infection in a patient with acquired immunodeficiency syndrome (AIDS). After describing this case of what was later to be named bacillary angiomatosis, Stoler and colleagues postulated a diverse list of microorganisms as possible etiologic agents (2).

In 1987, Cockerell and colleagues (3) reported five HIV-positive patients presenting with vascular neoplasms involving the skin, larynx, gastrointestinal tract, peritoneum, and diaphragm. The term epithelioid hemangioma was used to describe the characteristic cuboidal endothelial cells noted in the pathology samples. These were the first reported cases of bacillary angiomatosis involving organ systems other than the skin.

In 1988, LeBoit and coworkers examined the skin biopsies of seven HIV-positive men with bacillary angiomatosis. Despite the pathologic differences, these investigators speculated that the cat-scratch disease agent could be the causative agent of bacillary angiomatosis based on staining reactions, electron microscopy, and reaction with antiserum to the cat-scratch bacillus. They also noted the marked similarity, based on clinical appearance and histologic features, between their cases and verruga peruana, a chronic cutaneous manifestation of infection with *Bartonella bacilliformis*. This disease, which is endemic to some areas of Peru and other South American countries, is rarely seen in the United States. Therefore, although *B. bacilliformis* and the organism seen within bacillary angiomatosis lesions have different staining and electron microscopic characteristics, these investigators postulated that the two bacterial agents could be identical (4). When the nucleotide base sequence of the 16S ribosomal RNA genes of *B. bacilliformis* and *B. henselae* were subsequently determined, it became apparent that each was a unique species within a single genus (5, 6).

In December, 1990, three simultaneous reports (7–9) and a subsequent letter (10) helped to identify the etiologic agent of bacillary angiomatosis. Slater and coworkers described the cultivation of a motile, curved, Gram-negative bacillus in the blood cultures of five patients. Two of these patients were HIV positive, one was a bone marrow transplant recipient, and two were reportedly immunocompetent. None of the patients had lesions of cutaneous bacillary angiomatosis. The

Table 19.1. Disease Presentations Linked to *Bartonella* Species

Bartonella henselae
  Cat-scratch disease
  Bacillary angiomatosis
  Bacillary peliosis hepatis
  Bacteremia or fever
  Endocarditis
  Necroinflammatory parenchymal nodules
  HIV dementia (?)
Bartonella quintana
  Bacillary angiomatosis
  Bacillary peliosis hepatis
  Bacteremia or fever
  Endocarditis
Bartonella bacilliformis
  Oroya fever
  Verruga peruana
Bartonella elizabethae
  Endocarditis or bacteremia
Bartonella clarridgeiae
  Bacteremia
  Cat-scratch disease

---

organisms isolated from the blood of these five patients were identical on the basis of phenotypic characteristics, fatty acid, and restriction enzyme analysis. By fatty acid analysis, the organism was most closely related to *B. quintana*, but it was shown not to be *B. quintana* by restriction enzyme analysis (7).

At the same time, Perkocha and colleagues described a new clinical syndrome called bacillary peliosis hepatis, which involved replacement of normal liver and splenic parenchyma with cystic blood-filled spaces (8). All patients were HIV infected and several had AIDS. Bacterial forms resembling those seen in cutaneous bacillary angiomatosis were revealed by Warthin–Starry silver staining, although no bacteria could be isolated by culture.

Relman and colleagues simultaneously reported the identification of the etiologic agent of bacillary angiomatosis by applying a newly described method for the identification of unculturable organisms (9). This method used the polymerase chain reaction (PCR) and oligonucleotide primers complementary to the 16S ribosomal RNA genes of eubacteria (a group encompassing all human pathogens and commensals). The 16S ribosomal gene fragment was amplified directly from tissue samples obtained from patients with localized or disseminated bacillary angiomatosis. DNA sequence of these fragments was determined and analyzed to determine the degree of phylogenetic relatedness to other known organisms. Tissue from these patients yielded a unique 16S gene sequence that contained DNA with 98.3% homology with *Bartonella quintana*. This study demonstrated that the causative organism of bacillary angiomatosis was a newly identified species of rickettsia most closely related to *B. quintana*. Follow-up work linking these articles provided evidence that a new rickettsial species was the cause of bacillary angiomatosis, bacillary peliosis hepatis, and fever with bacteremia in immunocompetent and immunocompromised patients (10). The organism was subsequently named *Rochalimaea henselae*, in honor of Diane Hensel, who contributed much to its successful isolation and identification (11). Further analysis of the 16S rRNA sequences of *B. bacilliformis* and *R. henselae* determined that these organisms were in the same genus (6, 12); therefore *R. henselae* was renamed *B. henselae*.

Isolation of *Bartonella henselae* from tissue in the laboratory has been difficult. Koehler and colleagues were the first to report the isolation and propagation of *B. henselae* from the bacillary angiomatosis skin lesion of an HIV-positive patient. In addition, they isolated *B. quintana* from three other HIV-infected patients, all of whom had typical bacillary angiomatosis skin lesions (13). Therefore, these additional data indicated that bacillary angiomatosis can be caused by both *B. henselae* and *B. quintana*. The ability to grow these organisms made it possible to develop serologic tests and further refine PCR methods for the identification of these organisms in tissues.

Regnery and colleagues developed an indirect fluorescent antibody (IFA) assay for *Bartonella henselae* (14). This IFA assay, and PCR analysis of the cat-scratch disease skin test material, indicated clearly that *B. henselae* is the cause of cat-scratch disease (15).

Dolan and colleagues were the first to isolate *Bartonella henselae* from the lymph nodes of two patients with classic cat-scratch disease lymphadenitis (16). This finding was followed by work from Anderson and colleagues, who found *B. henselae*–specific nucleic acid sequences in 21 of 25 involved lymph nodes from patients with cat-scratch disease (17).

These observations confirmed Leboit and colleagues' original hypothesis (4), namely, that cat-scratch disease and bacillary angiomatosis are caused by the same organism, and the agent of bacillary angiomatosis is closely linked to the causative agent of verruga peruana. A newly described *Bartonella* species, *B. clarridgeiae*, has been isolated from the blood of an HIV-positive male and his cat (18). In addition, this organism has been isolated from the blood of a kitten implicated in a classic case of cat-scratch disease (19). The extent of infection caused by this organism is unknown at this time.

EPIDEMIOLOGY

Cases of bacillary angiomatosis have been reported from all areas of the United States, with most cases reported from areas where HIV infection is most prevalent, including New York City, San Francisco, Florida, and Texas. In addition, cases from continental Europe, the United Kingdom, and Africa have been described.

Preliminary estimates of the prevalence of antibodies to *Bartonella* sp. among healthy humans range from 4 to 6% (14, 20). Despite the advent of serologic testing for *Bartonella* sp., the incidence of bacillary angiomatosis in the HIV-positive population remains unknown. In a recent study in Houston, 2 (1%) of 204 blood cultures from HIV-positive patients were positive for *Bartonella* sp. (18). In another study from Bahrain, *B. henselae* antibody was found in the serum of 16% of HIV-infected patients and only 3.5% of controls (21). Although the disease is uncommon, most patients who develop bacillary angiomatosis are infected with HIV. However, bacillary angiomatosis and fever with bacteremia secondary to *Bartonella* sp. have also been described in patients with immunosuppression from other causes (22–24) and even in immunocompetent individuals (7, 25–28).

Approximately 90% of all reported cases of bacillary angiomatosis are men. Forty percent are white, 40% are black, and 20% are Hispanic (29). Tappero and colleagues (30) performed a case-control study of 48 patients with histologically confirmed bacillary angiomatosis or bacillary peliosis, 6 HIV-negative and 42 HIV-positive, and 94 HIV-positive controls matched for clinic site. Thirty percent of the patients had no history of cat exposure. However, on bivariate analysis, only a recent cat bite or scratch was associated with disease. Patients were as likely as controls to have an AIDS-defining diagnosis.

Mohle-Boetani and colleagues (31) performed a case-control study consisting of 42 HIV-positive patients with histologically confirmed bacillary angiomatosis and 84 HIV-positive controls matched for clinic site. The cases and controls were similar with respect to sex (95% male), age (37 years), race (97% white), ethnicity (79% non-Hispanic), and HIV risk factors (21% injection drug users). Of 42 HIV-positive case patients, 31% presented with superficial skin lesions, 24% had subcutaneous nodules or masses, 21% had asymmetric lymphadenopathy without cutaneous or subcutaneous lesions, and 24% had abdominal symptoms and fever. The median time from development of symptoms to evaluation by a physician was 4 weeks for patients with cutaneous lesions. The median CD4 lymphocyte count among case patients was $21/mm^3$, compared with $186/mm^3$ for controls. Case patients were more likely to be classified as having AIDS (94% versus 54%).

The link between bacillary angiomatosis and cats is becoming stronger. Koehler and colleagues were able to demonstrate *Bartonella henselae* bacteremia in 7 cats, all of which had had close contact with patients with bacillary angiomatosis. These investigators were also able to demonstrate the presence of *B. henselae* in fleas from the cats by both PCR and culture (32). Now that the etiologic agents of bacillary angiomatosis have been identified as members of the tribe Bartonellaceae, arthropod-borne transmission seems likely. Extensive work has been devoted to determining the epidemiology of *B. henselae* among cats and humans throughout the United States. In a study of 39 consecutive patients with cat-scratch disease, 21 of 31 kittens associated with these cases had positive blood cultures and elevated antibody titers to *B. henselae*. All kittens had fleas or had recently been treated for flea infestation. These data, added to the growing literature, support the contention that many patients with cat-scratch disease have close association with flea-infested kittens. The kittens are usually symptom free but bacteremic with *B. henselae* (20, 32). Adult cats are less commonly implicated as a source of cat-scratch disease, but experimental infection with *B. henselae* and *B. quintana* of pathogen-free cats demonstrated that cats can be persistently bacteremic but asymptomatic for many months (33). Further studies of the prevalence of *B. henselae* antibodies in cats have demonstrated that the southeastern United States, coastal California, the Pacific Northwest, and the south central plains have the highest prevalence, ranging from 36 to 54%. These areas of high prevalence are regions of increased warmth and humidity and closely correlate with the distribution in the United States of the cat flea, *Ctenocephalides felis felis*. Further study will be necessary to confirm the role of the cat flea as a vector of *B. henselae*.

Chomel and colleagues found that 39% of a nonrandom sample of 205 cats were bacteremic with *Bartonella henselae*. Cats that were impounded or were less than 1 year of age were more likely to be bacteremic. Bacteremic cats were more likely than nonbacteremic cats to be flea infested. The lack of *B. henselae* antibody was highly predictive of the absence of bacteremia, and these investigators suggested that seronegative cats may be more appropriate pets for immunocompromised individuals (34).

Bartonella quintana antibody is prevalent in the serum of homeless persons, with a seroprevalence of 16% observed in a group of hospitalized homeless patients. The prevalence of antibodies to *B. quintana* in these patients was significantly associated with the presence of body lice and exposure to cats. The prevalence of HIV infection in these patients was not reported (35). A study from Baltimore, Maryland, revealed that among urban intravenous drug users, the incidence of antibodies to *B. elizabethae*, *B. henselae*, and *B. quintana* was 33%, 11%, and 10% respectively. Patients who were HIV antibody positive had a significant inverse association of antibody prevalence to *B. henselae* and *B. quintana* and CD4 lymphocyte count (36).

Although most patients report cat contact, cat bite, or cat scratch, cases have been described in association with tick bites (7, 26) and even a parakeet scratch (25). *Bartonella quintana* is transmitted by the human body louse in cases of trench fever, but no evidence suggested louse-borne transmission of *B. quintana* infection in the HIV-positive cases reported by Koehler and colleagues (13).

MICROBIOLOGY AND DIAGNOSIS

Slater and associates reported the first successful cultivation of *Bartonella henselae* in the laboratory and provided phenotypic characterization (7). Non-*bacilliformis* species of *Bartonella* are slow-growing, weakly Gram-negative rods that can be cultivated on artificial media. To date, the best method for culturing the organisms from blood appears to be a lysis-centrifugation system with plating onto appropriate media. Conventional, semiautomated blood culture systems have not yielded positive growth-index readings and have required special stains and subcultures to detect isolates.

If a physician suspects non-*bacilliformis Bartonella* sp. bacteremia, the laboratory must be informed so the lysis-centrifugation–processed blood can be placed on enriched media. The cultures are incubated at 35°C in a humidified atmosphere containing 5% carbon dioxide on either blood or chocolate agar, for at least 14 days. Colonies are detected in 5 to 15 days. The organisms grow best on fresh media. Growth is not observed on heme-compound negative agar. The organism can also be grown on brain–heart infusion agar and trypticase–soy agar supplemented with 5% rabbit blood. Optimum temperature is 35 to 37°C, except for *B. bacilliformis*, which grows best at 25 to 30°C. On subculture, *B. henselae* and *B. quintana* isolates do not grow anaerobically or at temperatures of 25 or 42°C (7, 11, 37).

Alternatives to the lysis-centrifugation blood culture method include biphasic, broth, and cell culture systems, but these have not enhanced primary recovery of the organisms. Routine acridine orange staining at 8 days of semiautomated blood culture bottles has been proposed (38). Spach and his colleagues grew *Bartonella quintana* from the blood of several patients after 1 week of incubation with this method, but subculturing was still required (39).

Koehler and her colleagues have isolated *Bartonella henselae* and *B. quintana* from cutaneous bacillary angiomatosis skin lesions. These investigators plated homogenized skin biopsy specimens from four HIV-positive patients onto culture media that included fresh chocolate agar, trypticase soy agar with 5% defibrinated sheep blood, and heart infusion agar with 5% rabbit blood. The plates were incubated at 36°C in a sterile candle jar for 3 to 4 weeks. The skin biopsy samples were also inoculated onto tissue culture monolayers of bovine pulmonary artery endothelial cells and were incubated at 36° in 6% carbon dioxide and 85% humidity. The supernatants from these tissue culture monolayers were inoculated onto the foregoing agars after turbidity was noted. *B. henselae* was isolated from one skin biopsy sample by direct plating. Growth of *B. henselae* was not observed on the endothelial cell monolayers. *B. quintana* was grown from one biopsy specimen by direct plating and from three skin samples after cocultivation with an endothelial cell monolayer (13).

Dolan and colleagues were the first to grow *Bartonella henselae* from the lymph nodes of two patients with cat-scratch disease. They used CDC anaerobic plates, consisting of sheep blood with added hemin and L-cysteine (BDMS, Cockeysville, MD), and chocolate agar. Growth was observed at day 13 and 33 in the two cases reported. Growth was slower on chocolate agar. Fatty acid analysis and restriction fragment length polymorphism analysis of PCR-amplified citrate synthetase gene DNA from both of the lymph node isolates confirmed the organism to be *B. henselae* (16).

Despite this information, *B. henselae* and *B. quintana* have rarely been isolated from infected tissue when similar methods of direct plating have been used. A new chemically defined medium developed by Wong and colleagues is cell and extract free. It has been used to isolate *Bartonella* species from the blood of one cat and from the lymph nodes of three patients with cat-scratch disease (40). Whether this new medium will enhance the primary detection of *Bartonella* sp. is unknown.

The colonies of non-*bacilliformis Bartonella* sp. from primary isolation are either whitish, raised, dry, autoadherent, and embedded in the agar or small, tan, and moist-appearing. With multiple passages, the colonies become less adherent, less dry, and larger, and colonies are often observed after only 3 to 4 days of incubation. *B. henselae* is usually more heterogeneous, often with a larger proportion of the rough morphology. *B. quintana* often has predominantly smooth colonies.

Microscopically, *Bartonella henselae* is a small, curved, Gram-negative bacillus, measuring 2 by 0.6 μm. It displays twitching motility when mounted in saline (11, 37). These features, along with the prolonged period required for primary isolation and negative catalase and oxidase reactions, are sufficient for a presumptive identification of non-*bacilliformis Bartonella* sp.

Distinguishing *B. henselae* from *B. quintana* is more difficult because they are closely related, both biochemically and on the basis of DNA hybridization. The Microscan rapid anaerobic panel (Baxter, Sacramento, CA) has been used with some success for this purpose (41). Fatty acid analysis may be the most useful method for distinguishing *Bartonella* spp., but many laboratories do not have the necessary capabilities to perform this test (7). PCR–restriction fragment length polymorphism (RFLP) analysis of a portion of the citrate synthetase gene, useful for identifying rickettsial genotypes and species, is able to differentiate *B. henselae* from *B. quintana* and *B. vinsonii* (11). Investigators have encountered some difficulty applying this method to all *Bartonella* sp. Therefore, other recommended methods have been the PCR–RFLP analysis of the 16S rRNA gene (42) and 16S-23S rRNA intergenic spacer region (43), as well as the repetitive element PCR with primers based on repetitive palindromic DNA sequences (44).

Because of difficulties in growing *Bartonella* sp. from tissue and blood, other methods such as DNA amplification, serologic testing, and immunocytochemical staining are used (45). One method suggested for identifying *Bartonella* sp. from blood cultures in patients with suspected infectious endocarditis or bacteremia includes acridine orange and Gram staining followed by PCR–RFLP analysis of the blood culture bottle supernatant (46). PCR detection of *B. henselae* DNA from lymph nodes of patients with cat-scratch disease using degenerate primers has been successful. The sensitivity was reported as 84%. Three specimens were PCR negative, serology positive. The reason for the discrepancy in these samples is unclear, but it may reflect tissue DNA degradation or the presence of an amplification inhibitor (47).

PCR detection of *Bartonella* sequences from numerous tissues has expanded our knowledge of the disease processes caused by these organisms. However, because of technical difficulties, most clinical laboratories are using serologic testing as the mainstay for diagnosis. Both immunofluorescence assays and enzyme immunoassays are used to diagnose *B. henselae* infection, particularly for cat-scratch disease. An IFA assay for serum immunoglobulin G (IgG) directed against *B. henselae*, *B. quintana*, and *B. elizabethae* sp. is available. A titer of more than 1:64 or a fourfold rise in titer is considered significant. Published data indicate that in cat-scratch disease this test has a sensitivity and specificity of 88 and 94%, respectively, based on confirmatory pathologic data and a compatible clinical picture (14). In a retrospective review of cat-scratch disease, the foregoing sensitivity and specificity were confirmed (48); however, in a prospective study, only 67% of case patients were seropositive (49). This decrease in sensitivity may reflect the less rigorous definition of cat-scratch disease used by these investigators. At this time, no similar data on the utility of this test in HIV-positive patients are available.

Antibody responses in humans are often cross-reactive among *Bartonella quintana*, *B. henselae*, and *B. elizabethae*, thereby at times making a definitive diagnosis difficult (50). An enzyme-linked immunosorbent assay for *B. henselae* IgG, IgM, and IgA antibodies is available. It is reportedly more sensitive than the IFA detection method, but it has been less extensively validated (51).

HISTOPATHOLOGY

Several extensive reviews of the histopathologic picture of bacillary angiomatosis have been published (1, 52–54). Regardless of the site of involvement, the basic histologic architecture of bacillary angiomatosis consists of lobular proliferation of blood vessels producing neovascularization, as shown in Figure 19.1.

Superficial skin lesions involve the upper dermis. Of particular note are the following features: thinning of the overlying epidermis with occasional focal ulceration, epithelial collarettes, and edematous stroma with ectatic vessels. In both superficial and deep cutaneous lesions, a lobular pattern

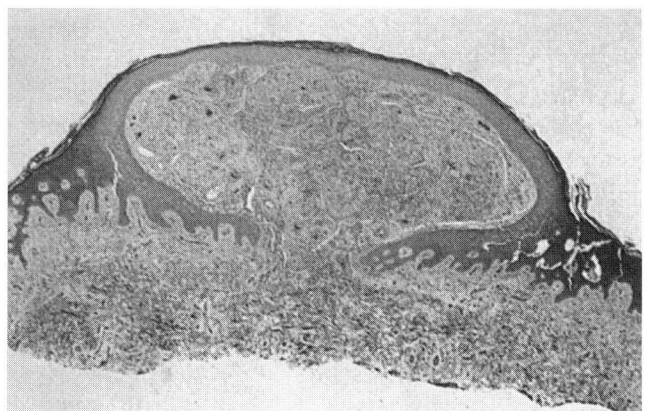

Figure 19.1. Superficial cutaneous lesion of bacillary angiomatosis resembling pyogenic granuloma on low-power microscopy. Note the lobular proliferation of capillaries with edematous stroma and a collarette of epithelium. (×50)

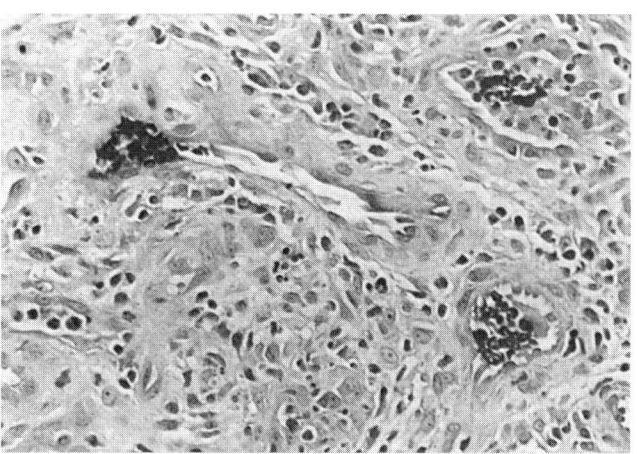

Figure 19.2. Higher magnification of superficial bacillary angiomatosis skin lesion demonstrating multiple blood vessels with cuboidal endothelial cells present interstitially. (×400)

of vascular proliferation with small capillaries arranged around ectatic ones, with edema, mucin, or fibrotic stroma surrounding the lobules, produces a characteristic histopathologic pattern. Although the superficial lesions are usually loose and edematous, deep lesions are frequently dense and compact (52).

Vascular lobules are composed of endothelial cells (Fig. 19.2) with varying appearance, ranging from only a slight protuberance into the vascular lumen to a cuboid. Vascular channels are seen singly, in small groups, or in areas of solid proliferation. Foci of endothelial cell necrosis containing neutrophils and sometimes macrophages are often observed. In most cases, clusters of neutrophils and neutrophilic debris are seen adjacent to the capillaries and are scattered throughout the lesion. The presence of neutrophils adjacent to the blood vessels may be an important clue to the diagnosis of bacillary angiomatosis. Abscesses, on rare occasions, may be seen within and outside the vascular lobules.

Clumps of granular purplish material that correspond to clusters of bacilli are seen interstitially between vessels in almost all specimens, more frequently in dense, cellular areas. These clumps may be confused with fibrin deposition; therefore, either silver staining or electron microscopy should be performed to confirm their nature. Silver stains, including the Warthin–Starry, Dieterle's stain, and Steiner's stain enable one to identify bacillary angiomatosis bacteria, although the first is more sensitive (Fig. 19.3). Warthin–Starry staining is technically difficult to perform and is not specific for the agents of bacillary angiomatosis; other bacteria, including spirochetes and strains of *Nocardia*, *Legionella*, and *Campylobacter* also react. Conventional stains such as acid-fast, Giemsa, periodic acid–Schiff, and the Brown–Brenn modification of Gram's stain fail to demonstrate the bacillus; however, these stains should be used on appropriate specimens because concomitant infection with other organisms, such as *Mycobacterium avium intracellulare* and the agent of bacillary angiomatosis, has been

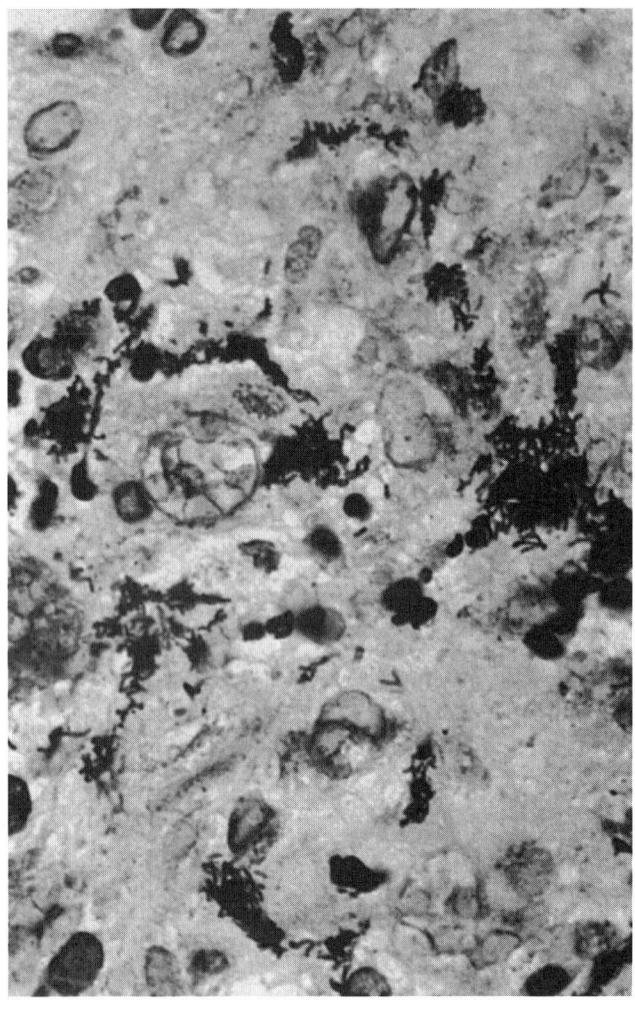

Figure 19.3. Warthin–Starry stain of superficial bacillary angiomatosis skin lesion demonstrating large numbers of extracellular bacilli.

described (55). By electron microscopy, the bacilli possess a trilaminar cell wall and contain electron-dense granular material. The microorganisms are usually observed in clumps, are found in close association with neutrophil aggregates, and are more prominent in the more cellular areas of vascular proliferation (53).

The histologic features of bacillary angiomatosis and its differential diagnosis have been well characterized by LeBoit and associates (1). The histologic differential diagnosis of cutaneous bacillary angiomatosis includes pyogenic granuloma (lobular capillary hemangioma), histiocytoid (epithelioid) hemangioma, verruga peruana (vasoproliferative stage of bartonellosis), epithelioid hemangioendothelioma, acquired tufted angioma, papular angiokeratoma, angiosarcoma, and Kaposi's sarcoma.

Lymph node involvement is characterized by coalescing nodules of proliferated vessels in the cortical and paracortical areas (53). Several features should alert the pathologist to the possibility of bacillary angiomatosis in a vasoproliferative lesion of a lymph node. These include abundant eosinophilic or amphophilic interstitial material (clumps of bacteria), pronounced stromal edema, neutrophilic infiltration, which is not always present, and plump endothelial cells with pale, finely vacuolated cytoplasm with well-formed vessels as contrasted with Kaposi's sarcoma. Uninvolved parenchyma can show follicular hyperplasia, plasmacytosis, or sinus histiocytosis (54).

Liver and spleen involvement with bacillary angiomatosis can be manifested as the appearance of discrete nodules of vascular proliferation or as peliosis. Peliosis is characterized by cystic, blood-filled spaces within the liver parenchyma rimmed by fibromyxoid tissue containing inflammatory cells, dilated capillaries, and clumps of bacilli (8). Portal areas are expanded with entrapment of portal vessels and bile ductules (53).

PATHOGENESIS

Hypotheses about the manner in which infection with *Bartonella* species produces the characteristic lesions associated with bacillary angiomatosis and cat-scratch disease must consider the state of the human host immune defenses. Infection by *B. henselae* in the patient with HIV disease elicits an angiogenic response, accompanied by acute and chronic inflammation associated with many microorganisms, whereas infection in immunocompetent individuals may lead to either chronic bacteremia or typical cat-scratch disease. The pathologic response to the organism in cat-scratch disease is typically granuloma formation and microabscesses, without evidence of neovascularization. As opposed to bacillary angiomatosis, the number of microorganisms that can be visualized by Warthin–Starry stain in tissue samples of cat-scratch disease is usually low. Although most cases of bacillary angiomatosis occur in patients with HIV infection, the virus itself is not a necessary cofactor, inasmuch as *Bartonella* infection in other immunocompromised patients also elicits an identical pathologic response. Most HIV-infected patients with bacillary angiomatosis have low CD4 counts, and many have AIDS, a finding suggesting that the T-lymphocytic response to infection may determine, in part, whether angiogenesis occurs. However, concomitant infection with opportunists such as cytomegalovirus, herpes simplex, *Pneumocystis carinii,* and *Toxoplasma* may also play a role in promoting angiogenesis, possibly mediated by cytokines and growth factors stimulated by these infectious agents.

Laboratory studies on the genetic and molecular basis of angiogenesis caused by *Bartonella* sp. are in their infancy, and little is known about bacterial factors that could contribute to endothelial cell proliferation. Because *B. bacilliformis* infection produces an identical histopathologic response, a few investigators have examined the ability of this species to induce neovascularization or endothelial cell proliferation (56, 57). *Bartonella henselae* has also been shown to induce endothelial cell proliferation, but the identification of the bacterial factors responsible for this proliferation is ongoing (58).

CLINICAL MANIFESTATIONS

Bacillary angiomatosis affects most organs particularly, the skin, lymph nodes, and liver and/or spleen.

Cutaneous Manifestations

Although as many as 50% of patients with bacillary angiomatosis may not have cutaneous involvement, this is the most commonly published presentation. Skin lesions of bacillary angiomatosis are diverse, presenting as erythematous papules, subcutaneous nodules, or hyperpigmented plaques (59). The most common appearance is of an enlarging red-purple papule, often surrounded by a collarette of scale (Fig. 19.4). These papules range in size from a few millimeters to several centimeters and may become pedunculated as they grow. They range in number from single to multiple (greater than 100), are often friable, and are occasionally tender. Some lesions may resolve spontaneously without antibiotic therapy. The lesions are easily removed by curettage, and bleeding is easily controlled with pressure or topical anticoagulants (60). With resolution, slight hyperpigmentation, induration, and atrophy may remain.

The clinical differential diagnosis of cutaneous bacillary angiomatosis includes Kaposi's sarcoma, pyogenic granuloma, simple hemangioma, and angiokeratoma. Thus, the definitive diagnosis of bacillary angiomatosis should be made histologically. Distinguishing solitary lesions of bacillary angiomatosis from pyogenic granuloma may be clinically difficult; however, multiple lesions are common in bacillary angiomatosis and bartonellosis, as opposed to the other pathologic processes included in the differential diagnosis (22).

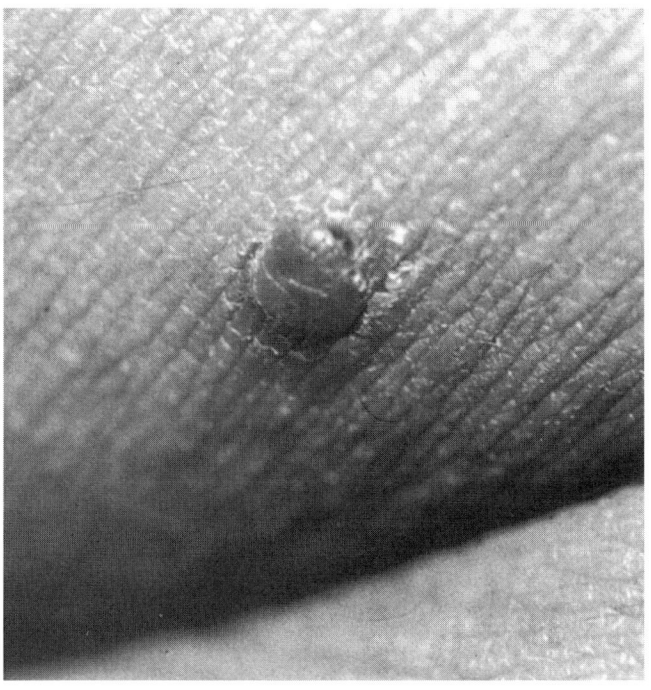

Figure 19.4. Superficial skin lesion of bacillary angiomatosis.

The next most common presentation is a flesh-colored nodule in the deeper subcutaneous tissue that may vary in size (up to 10 cm) and number. Underlying cortical bone involvement has been described with these nodules (7, 59, 61). One often sees minimal epidermal change or hyperpigmentation; however, overlying skin changes resembling cellulitis have been observed (7). These nodules may be tender, but they rarely ulcerate or bleed.

The least common presentation is manifested as indurated, hyperpigmented plaques that are often oval and several centimeters in diameter. These plaques, which may be hyperkeratotic, are typically found on the extremities (62).

Musculoskeletal Manifestations

Inflammatory arthritides have been well described in HIV-positive patients such as psoriatic arthritis, Reiter's syndrome, and undifferentiated spondyloarthropathies. Other types of skeletal involvement are uncommon (63). Several reports have described bacillary angiomatosis in bone. Baron and colleagues described six HIV-positive patients with focal bone pain and skin lesions consistent with bacillary angiomatosis (61). Most of these patients had osteolytic lesions on plain radiographs, consisting of either well-circumscribed lytic areas or ill-defined regions of cortical destruction with periosteal reaction and an adjacent soft tissue mass. Of the three patients who had biopsies, two had typical histopathologic changes of bacillary angiomatosis, and the other had fibrosis. Dramatic improvement and resolution occurred with antibiotic therapy. Further reports have described individual cases of bone involvement with similar presentations. (7, 59, 64–66). Because lytic bone disease from other causes in patients with AIDS is so uncommon, bacillary angiomatosis should be strongly considered in any HIV-positive patient with lytic bone lesions on radiographs (61).

Skeletal muscle involvement in bacillary angiomatosis has been described. An HIV-positive man presented with a left lateral wall chest mass that, on resection, revealed large areas of vascular tumor within dense fibrous tissue. Warthin–Starry staining and electron microscopy revealed clusters of small extracellular bacteria (67). Two other cases of bacillary angiomatosis involving muscle have been described (68, 69).

Mucous Membrane Manifestations

Mucosal lesions involving the oral, nasal, conjunctival, laryngeal, and anal mucosa have been well described, although these are not common presentations of bacillary angiomatosis (3, 61, 65, 70). Van der Wouw and colleagues (65) described a patient who presented with hoarseness and multiple red nodules on his pharynx, epiglottis, and vocal cords. Laryngeal occlusion by multiple angiomas was also the cause of death in one of the patients described by Cockerell and associates (3).

Documented gastrointestinal involvement of bacillary angiomatosis has been infrequently reported (71–75), but gastrointestinal hemorrhage may occur. Asymptomatic gastrointestinal mucosal lesions are probably more common than recognized or reported. Involvement of the female genital tract has also been described, in a 32-year-old women with AIDS who presented with red-purple nodules of the vulva and cervix (76).

Bone Marrow Manifestations

Although rare, case reports describing bone marrow involvement with bacillary angiomatosis have been published. The pancytopenia reportedly responds rapidly to antibiotic therapy (23, 77, 78).

Pulmonary Manifestations

Pulmonary involvement with bacillary angiomatosis is uncommon. Szaniawski and colleagues (60) reported a patient with a pulmonary infiltrate and skin lesions consistent with bacillary angiomatosis. Bronchial mucosal biopsy revealed epithelioid cells and vascular spaces. Polypoid endobronchial lesions of the trachea and regional bronchi have been noted on bronchoscopy; histopathologic examination of tissue samples showed changes typical of bacillary angiomatosis (72, 79). Pleural effusions that have responded to therapy for cutaneous and visceral bacillary angiomatosis have been noted (23), but in most cases confirmatory thoracenteses or pleural biopsies have not been performed.

Hepatosplenic Manifestations

Many reports of bacillary angiomatosis affecting the liver and spleen (8, 80, 81) with or without cutaneous involvement have been published. The spectrum of bacillary angiomatosis involving the liver and spleen varies from simple hepatosplenomegaly noted on clinical examination to bacillary peliosis hepatis found on biopsy. The actual incidence of liver involvement is unknown. Many patients who present with cutaneous bacillary angiomatosis have symptoms of fever, malaise, night sweats, and abdominal pain. Although examination may reveal hepatosplenomegaly and the alkaline phosphatase levels may be elevated, whether these findings reflect a true pathologic process is unclear. In many cases, the liver or spleen is not visualized or sampled for biopsy, but the abnormalities resolve with appropriate antibiotics.

Before the AIDS epidemic, peliosis of internal organs, characterized by cystic, blood-filled spaces throughout the tissue parenchyma, was rare. Most cases were associated with chronic debilitating illnesses such as tuberculosis, malignancy, and the systemic use of anabolic steroids and various other compounds. Since the advent of AIDS, increasing reports of peliosis, most commonly involving the liver, without evidence of bacillary forms on ultrastructural studies (82, 83), have been published.

Perkocha and colleagues published a series of cases of patients with bacillary peliosis hepatis. These investigators studied the liver tissue of eight HIV-infected patients with peliosis hepatis, two of whom had cutaneous bacillary angiomatosis, and of four HIV-negative patients who also had peliosis hepatis. Bacteria morphologically identical by Warthin–Starry staining and electron microscopy to those found in cutaneous bacillary angiomatosis were seen in the liver tissue in each of the HIV-infected patients but not in those who were HIV negative. Two patients also had peliosis of the spleen. Clinically, most of the patients with bacillary peliosis hepatis had weight loss, fever, abdominal pain, hepatosplenomegaly, elevated alkaline phosphatase levels, and normal or slightly elevated bilirubin and aminotransferase levels (8).

The largest study of bacillary peliosis is by Mohle-Boetani and colleagues. They compared 42 case patients with histologically confirmed bacillary peliosis with 84 control patients. Cutaneous and subcutaneous lesions of bacillary angiomatosis were found in only 55% of case patients. Case patients were more likely to present with fever and anorexia and to have lymphadenopathy and hepatosplenomegaly on examination. Case patients were likely to have lower CD4 lymphocyte counts, high alkaline phosphatase levels, and anemia (84).

Slater and his colleagues reported an immunosuppressed patient who, after an allogeneic renal transplantation, had peliosis, angiogenesis, and pyogranulomatous inflammation in her liver and spleen. *Bartonella henselae* was isolated from her spleen (85).

Biliary tract involvement is uncommon; only a single case report of biliary obstruction secondary to extrahepatic lymph node enlargement in conjunction with peripheral lymph node involvement with epithelioid angiomatosis has been described (86).

Fever and Bacteremia

Fever with bacteremia from *Bartonella henselae* has been well described (7, 37). As mentioned earlier, in one study, 1% of all blood cultures from HIV-positive patients tested positive for *Bartonella* sp. (18). Special techniques are required for isolation of *Bartonella* sp. and are not routine for most clinical microbiology laboratories. Therefore, bacteremia with *Bartonella* sp. remains a relatively unreported finding. In one study, *B. henselae* was isolated from the blood of nine patients. Four of the nine were HIV positive; one had AIDS. Two patients were recipients of allogeneic transplants and were receiving immunosuppressive agents; three were immunocompetent. An epidemiologic link could not be found among these nine patients. All the HIV-infected patients presented with malaise, fatigue, weight loss, and recurring fevers. Response to antimicrobial agents was variable, as was the relapse of symptoms after cessation of antibiotics. In general, the non–HIV-infected patients had an abrupt onset of a febrile illness with a rapid response to short courses (less than 10 days) of antimicrobial treatment and no subsequent relapses. One of the five HIV-negative patients relapsed clinically and bacteriologically after two short courses of therapy but responded to 2 weeks of chloramphenicol followed by 2 weeks of erythromycin (7).

Clinical relapses after treatment have been described in immunocompetent men with persistent *Bartonella henselae* bacteremia. One patient had persistent bacteremia despite being asymptomatic (11).

Bartonella quintana has long been known as a cause of bacteremia, which in some cases may persist for longer than 1 year (87). Spach and colleagues recently described 10 patients with *B. quintana* bacteremia. All were chronic alcoholics, and 8 were homeless; none were known to have HIV infection or immunosuppression. Other than fever, no consistent symptoms or abnormalities were noted on examination. Only 1 patient had lice, 3 reported a cat scratch, and 5 patients had scabies infestation, but none reported flea bites. Patients who underwent follow-up and who resolved their bacteremia in general received ceftriaxone initially, followed by azithromycin or erythromycin for at least 4 weeks. Two of these patients had endocarditis (88).

The initial report of *Bartonella* sp. as a cause of endocarditis was published in 1993 (39). Since then, further reports of endocarditis caused by *B. henselae* (89), *B. quintana* (90, 91), and *B. elizabethae* (92) have been published. Most cases have occurred in immunocompetent males who presented with fever and malaise. Most patients with endocarditis have required valve replacement and have been treated with a 6- to 9-month antibiotic course, usually with erythromycin or azithromycin.

If the diagnosis of *Bartonella* sp. bacteremia or endocarditis is suspected, the lysis-centrifugation blood culture system should be used, or blind subcultures of routine semiautomated blood culture bottles to appropriate agar should be performed at 7 to 14 days.

Central Nervous System Manifestations

Direct neurologic involvement has rarely been described in bacillary angiomatosis, although mental status changes and acute psychiatric illness have been reported in patients with cutaneous bacillary angiomatosis (23, 77, 93, 94). Spach and colleagues (95) described the first case of confirmed central nervous system involvement with bacillary angiomatosis. A 49-year-old HIV-positive man presented with seizures and a temporal lobe contrast-enhancing mass on computed tomography. Pyrimethamine–sulfadiazine plus acyclovir was started without response. An initial biopsy was unrevealing, but a repeat biopsy, performed several months later because of neurologic deterioration, revealed a lymphocyte-rich inflammatory infiltrate, prominent microvasculature with plump atypical endothelial cells, reactive gliosis, and a positive Warthin–Starry stain. Skin lesions typical of bacillary angiomatosis were also present. Erythromycin was started, and the patient's mental status improved with resolution of the brain lesion over the next 5 months. The investigators believed that this patient likely suffered from central nervous system involvement by the organism causing bacillary angiomatosis on the basis of typical pathologic features of the brain lesions; characteristic bacilli observed in the brain, and skin lesions with a positive Warthin–Starry stain; no alternative cause of the lesions was found despite an extensive search and the response of the brain and skin lesions to erythromycin.

HIV-Associated Dementia

The link between cat-scratch disease, bacillary angiomatosis, *Bartonella henselae*, and AIDS encephalopathy was postulated in 1992 by Patnaik and colleagues (96). They argued that: 1) *B. henselae* is associated with cat-scratch disease, bacillary angiomatosis, and bacillary peliosis hepatis, and 2) encephalopathy occurs in cat-scratch disease. They postulated, therefore, that *B. henselae* may be a cause of AIDS encephalopathy. Evidence of intrathecal *B. henselae* antibody production was observed in some patients (30%) with HIV encephalopathy after comparison of antibody levels in the serum and cerebrospinal fluid (97). In a follow-up study, this same group found an association between an acute decline in neuropsychological testing and the presence of *Bartonella*-reactive IgM antibodies in the serum, but not IgG antibodies. Four percent of those cases with HIV-associated dementia had IgM antibodies to *B. henselae* (98). The significance of these observations remains unclear and will require strong epidemiologic investigation in conjunction with further serologic testing to confirm any association between *B. henselae* and HIV-associated neurologic disease.

TREATMENT

All patients with recognized bacillary angiomatosis should be treated. Spontaneous resolution of superficial skin papules has been reported, but patients can develop dissemination and serious consequences. No controlled trials have been performed; therefore, treatment decisions must rely on anecdotal evidence of treatment response. Therapeutic end points remain undefined and relapse is common.

Anecdotal evidence strongly favors the use of erythromycin or a tetracycline derivative. Erythromycin remains the drug of choice, at a dose of 500 mg four times per day for at least 4 weeks, usually 8 weeks. Longer courses are necessary if recurrence occurs after discontinuation of therapy and also in patients with bacteremia or endocarditis. The newer macrolides such as azithromycin have also been used with success (99).

Responses to other antibiotics have been reported. Of these, doxycycline is most commonly used. Other agents reported to have been successful include isoniazid and rifampicin in combination, vancomycin, trimethoprim–sulfamethoxazole, ciprofloxacin, and a combination of ciprofloxacin and gentamicin. Inhibitors of cell-wall synthesis, such as the penicillins and cephalosporins, uniformly fail to cure bacillary angiomatosis, although in vitro testing indicates that both *Bartonella quintana* and *B. henselae* are sensitive to these antibiotics (100, 101). Jarisch-Herxheimer–like reactions occurring soon after the administration of doxycycline or erythromycin have been reported. (13).

Currently, susceptibility testing is not standardized for either *Bartonella henselae* or *B. quintana* and is difficult to perform. Musso and colleagues, using macrophage-like cells and a human endothelial cell line, determined that aminoglycosides were the only bactericidal agents against *B. henselae* (102). Although aminoglycosides have seldom been used for treatment of bacillary angiomatosis, these data may indicate the usefulness of these agents, perhaps in combination with other antimicrobials, in serious *B. henselae* infections such as endocarditis. The Etest method, which uses a plastic strip impregnated with an antibiotic concentration gradient, may be useful in performing susceptibility testing. Results using this method compare well with agar dilution methods. Although in vitro results of *Bartonella* susceptibility testing may not necessarily correlate with clinical response the Etest may be a simpler way of performing the testing (103).

PREVENTION

All cat owners and physicians should be aware of the risks associated with close cat contact. In particular, immunocompromised individuals should take particular precautions to diminish the risk of cat-scratch disease or bacillary angiomatosis. It does not seem reasonable to prevent patients from having cat contact because many patients derive great pleasure from that contact. In addition, because transmission can occur with just close contact, recommending declawing of cats does not seem reasonable. Common sense rules should apply: 1) wash hands after animal contact and keep all wounds and abrasions as clean as possible; 2) avoid cats younger than 1 year of age because they are more prone to "carry" the organism; 3) keep cats as free from fleas as possible, although the role of fleas in transmission of *Bartonella henselae* has not been fully delineated (104). Serologic testing of cats to determine their possible exposure to *B. henselae* may become routine in the future. A negative antibody status is strongly predictive of negative blood cultures and suggests that the risk of transmission is lower. However, the incidence of bacillary angiomatosis and cat-scratch disease is so low that screening of all cats is unlikely to be cost-effective.

Acknowledgments

The author wishes to thank the American Foundation for AIDS Research and the Center for AIDS Research and the Beckman Director's Fund, Stanford University, for support.

References

1. LeBoit PE, Berger TG, Egbert BM, et al. Bacillary angiomatosis: the histopathology and differential diagnosis of a pseudoneoplastic infection in patients with human immunodeficiency virus disease. Am J Surg Pathol 1989;13:909–920.
2. Stoler MH, Bonfiglio TA, Steigbigel RT, et al. An atypical subcutaneous infection associated with acquired immunodeficiency syndrome. Am J Clin Pathol 1983;80:714–718.
3. Cockerell CJ, Whitlow MA, Webster GF, et al. Epithelioid angiomatosis: a distinct vascular disorder in patients with the acquired immunodeficiency syndrome or AIDS-related complex. Lancet 1987; 2:654–656.
4. LeBoit PE, Berger TG, Egbert BM, et al. Epithelioid haemangioma-like vascular proliferation in AIDS: manifestation of cat-scratch disease bacillus infection? Lancet 1988;1:960–963.
5. Birtles RJ, Harrison TG, Taylor AG. The causative agent of bacillary angiomatosis. N Engl J Med 1991;325:1447.
6. Relman DA, Lepp PW, Sadler KN, et al. Phylogenetic relationships among the agent of bacillary angiomatosis, *Bartonella bacilliformis,* and other alpha-proteobacteria. Mol Microbiol 1992; 6:1801–1807.
7. Slater LN, Welch DF, Hensel D, et al. A newly recognized fastidious Gram-negative pathogen as a cause of fever and bacteremia. N Engl J Med 1990;323:1587–1593.
8. Perkocha LA, Geaghan SM, Benedict Yen TS, et al. Clinical and pathological features of bacillary peliosis hepatis in association with human immunodeficiency virus infection. N Engl J Med 1990; 323:1581–1586.
9. Relman DA, Loutit JS, Schmidt TM, et al. The agent of bacillary angiomatosis: an approach to the identification of uncultured pathogens. N Engl J Med 1990;323:1573–1580.
10. Relman DA, Falkow S, LeBoit PE, et al. The organism causing bacillary angiomatosis, peliosis hepatis, and fever and bacteremia in immunocompromised patients. N Engl J Med 1991;324:1514.
11. Regnery RL, Anderson BE, Clarridge JE, et al. Characterization of a novel *Rochalimaea* species, *R. henselae* sp. nov., isolated from blood of a febrile, human immunodeficiency virus-positive patient. J Clin Microbiol 1992;30:265–274.
12. Brenner DJ, O'Connor SP, Winkler HH, et al. Proposals to unify the genera *Bartonella* and *Rochalimaea*, with descriptions of *Bartonella quintana* comb. nov., *Bartonella vinsonii* comb. nov., *Bartonella henselae* comb. nov., and *Bartonella elizabethae* comb. nov., and to remove the family *Bartonellaceae* from the order *Rickettsiales*. Int J Syst Bacteriol 1993;43:777–786.
13. Koehler JE, Quinn FD, Berger TG, et al. Isolation of *Rochalimaea* species from cutaneous and osseus lesions of bacillary angiomatosis. N Engl J Med 1992;327:1625–1631.
14. Regnery RL, Olson JG, Perkins BA, et al. Serologic response to *Rochalimaea henselae* antigen in suspected cat scratch disease. Lancet 1992;339:1443–1445.
15. Anderson B, Kelly C, Threlkel R, et al. Detection of *Rochalimaea henselae* in cat-scratch disease skin test antigens. J Infect Dis 1993; 168:1034–1036.
16. Dolan MJ, Wong MT, Regnery RL, et al. Syndrome of *Rochalimaea henselae* adenitis suggesting cat scratch disease. Ann Intern Med 1993;118:331–336.
17. Andersen B, Sims K, Regnery R, et al. Detection of *Rochalimaea henselae* DNA in specimens from cat scratch disease patients by PCR. J Clin Microbiol 1194;32:942–948.
18. Clarridge JE, Raich TJ, Pirwani D, et al. Strategy to detect and identify Bartonella species in routine clinical laboratory yields *Bartonella henselae* from human immunodeficiency virus-positive patient and unique *Bartonella* strain from his cat. J Clin Microbiol 1995;33: 2107–2113.
19. Kordick DL, Hilyard EJ, Hadfield TL, et al. *Bartonella clarridgeiae,* a newly recognized zoonotic pathogen causing inoculation papules, fever, and lymphadenopathy (cat scratch disease). J Clin Microbiol 1997;35:1813–1818.
20. Zangwill KM, Hamilton DH, Perkins BA, et al. Cat scratch disease in Connecticut: epidemiology, risk factors, and evaluation of a new diagnostic test. N Engl J Med 1993;329:8–13.
21. Yousif A, Farid I, Baig B, et al. Prevalence of *Bartonella henselae* antibodies among human immunodeficiency virus–infected patients from Bahrain. Clin Infect Dis 1996;23:398–399.
22. Webster GF, Cockerell CJ, Whitlow MA, et al. Epithelioid angiomatosis: a variant of Kaposi's sarcoma. Lancet 1987; 2:1215.
23. Kemper CA, Lombard CM, Deresinski SC, et al. Visceral bacillary epithelioid angiomatosis: possible manifestations of disseminated cat-scratch disease in the immunocompromised host. A report of two cases. Am J Med 1990;89:216–222.
24. Omura EF, Omura GA. Human immunodeficiency virus–associated skin lesions. JAMA 1989;261:991.

25. Cockerell CJ, Bergstresser PR, Myrie-Williams C, et al. Bacillary epithelioid angiomatosis occurring in an immunocompetent individual. Arch Dermatol 1990;126:787–790.
26. Lucey D, Dolan MJ, Wayne Moss C, et al. Relapsing illness due to *Rochalimaea henselae* in immunocompetent hosts: implication for therapy and epidemiological associations. Clin Infect Dis 1992; 14:683–688.
27. Tappero JW, Koehler JE, Berger TG, et al. Bacillary angiomatosis and bacillary splenitis in immunocompetent adults. Ann Intern Med 1993;118:363–365.
28. Smith KJ, Skelton HG, Tuur S, et al. Bacillary angiomatosis in an immunocompetent child. Am J Dematopathol 1996;18:597–600.
29. Spach DH. Bacillary angiomatosis. Int J Dermatol 1992;31:19–24.
30. Tappero JW, Mohle-Boetani J, Koehler JE, et al.. The epidemiology of bacillary angiomatosis and bacillary peliosis. JAMA 1993;269: 770–775.
31. Mohle-Boetani J, Reingold A, LeBoit P, et al. Bacillary angiomatosis: spectrum of disease and clinical characteristics in HIV-positive patients. In: Abstracts of the 32nd Interscience Conference of Antimicrobial Agents and Chemotherapy. Anaheim, CA: American Society for Microbiology, 1992.
32. Koehler JE, Glaser CA, Tappero JW. *Rochalimaea henselae* infection:a new zoonosis with the domestic cat as the reservoir. JAMA 1994;271: 531–535.
33. Regnery RL, Rooney JA, Johnson AM, et al. Experimentally induced *Bartonella henselae* infections followed by challenge exposure and antimicrobial therapy in cats. Am J Vet Res 1996;57:1714–1719.
34. Chomel BR, Abbot RC, Kasten RW, et al. *Bartonella henselae* prevalence in domestic cats in California: risk factors and association between bacteremia and antibody titers. J Clin Microbiol 1995;33: 2445–2450.
35. Brouqui P, Hopikian P, Dupont HT, et al. Survey of the seroprevalence of *Bartonella quintana* in homeless people. Clin Infect Dis 1996;23: 756–759.
36. Comer JA, Fln C, Regnery RL, et al. Antibodies to *Bartonella* species in inner-city intravenous drug users in Baltimore, MD. Arch Intern Med 1996;156:2491–2495.
37. Welch DF, Pickett DA, Slater LN, et al. *Rochalimaea henselae* sp. nov., a cause of septicemia, bacillary angiomatosis, and parenchymal bacillary peliosis. J Clin Microbiol 1992;30:275–280.
38. Larson AM, Dougherty MJ, Nowowiejski, et al. Detection of *Bartonella (Rochalimaea) quintana* by routine acridine orange staining of broth blood cultures. J Clin Microbiol 1994;32:1492–1496.
39. Spach DH, Callis KP, Paauw DS, et al. Endocarditis caused by *Rochalimaea quintana* in a patient with human immunodeficiency virus. J Clin Microbiol 1993;31:692 694.
40. Wong MT, Thornton DC, Kennedy RC, et al. A chemically defined liquid medium that supports primary isolation of *Rochalimaea (Bartonella) henselae* from blood and tissue specimens. J Clin Microbiol 1995;33:742–744.
41. Welch DF, Hensel DM, Pickett DA, et al. Bacteremia due to *Rochalimaea henselae* in a child: practical identification of isolates in the clinical laboratory. J Clin Microbiol 1993;31:2381–2386.
42. Birtles RJ. Differentiation of *Bartonella* species using restriction endonuclease analysis of PCR-amplified 16S rRNA genes. FEMS Microbiol Lett 1995;129:261–266.
43. Roux V, Raoult D. Inter-and intraspecies identification of *Bartonella (Rochalimaea)* species. J Clin Microbiol 1995;33:1573–1579.
44. Rodriguez-Barradas MC, Hamill RJ, Houston ED, et al. Genomic fingerprinting of *Bartonella* species by repetitive element PCR for distinguishing species and isolates. J Clin Microbiol 1995;33:1089–1093.
45. Kyung-Whan M, Reed JA, Welch DF, et al. Morphologically variable bacilli of cat scratch disease are identified by immunoncytochemical labelling with antibodies to *Rochalimaea henselae*. Am J Clin Pathol 1994;101:607–610.
46. Joblet C, Roux, V, Drancourt M, et al. Identification of *Bartonella (Rochalimaea)* species among fastidious Gram-negative bacteria on the basis of the partial sequence of the citrate-synthase gene. J Clin Microbiol 1995;33:1879–1883.
47. Anderson B, Sims K, Regnery R, et al. Detection of *Rochalimaea henselae* DNA in specimens from cat scratch disease patients by PCR. J Clin Microbiol 1994;32:942–948.
48. Dalton MJ, Robinson LE, Cooper J, et al. Use of *Bartonella* antigens for serologic diagnosis of cat-scratch disease at a national referral center. Arch Intern Med 1995;155:1670–1676.
49. Hamilton DH, Zangwill KM, Hadler JL, et al. Cat-scratch disease: Connecticut, 1992–1993. J Infect Dis 1995;172:570–573.
50. Waldvogel K, Regnery RL, Anderson BE, et al. Disseminated cat-scratch disease: detection of *Rochalimaea henselae* in affected tissue. Eur J Pediatr 1994;153:23–27.
51. Barka NE, Hadfield T, Patnaik M, et al. EIA for detection of *Rochalimaea henselae*-reactive IgG, IgM, and IgA antibodies in patients with suspected cat scratch disease. J Infect Dis 1993;167: 1503–1504.
52. Cockerell CJ, LeBoit PE. Bacillary angiomatosis: a newly characterized pseudoneoplastic, infectious, cutaneous vascular disorder. J Am Acad Dermatol 1990;22:501–512.
53. Tsang WYW, Chan JKC. Bacillary angiomatosis: a new disease with a broadening clinicopathologic spectrum. Histol Histopathol 1992; 7:143–152.
54. Chan JKC, Lewin KJ, Teitelbaum S, et al. Histopathology of bacillary angiomatosis of lymph node. Am J Surg Pathol 1991;15:430–437.
55. Sagerman PM, Relman DA, Niroomand F, et al. Localization of *Mycobacterium avium*-intracellulare within a skin lesion of bacillary angiomatosis in a patient with AIDS. Diagn Mol Pathol 1992;1: 212–216.
56. Garcia FU, Wojta J, Broadley KN, et al. *Bartonella bacilliformis* stimulates endothelial cells in vitro and is angiogenic in vivo. Am J Pathol 1990;136:1125–1135.
57. Garcia FU, Wojta J, Hoover RL. Interactions between live *Bartonella bacilliformis* and endothelial cells. J Infect Dis 1992;165:1138–1141.
58. Conley T, Slater L, Hamilton K. *Rochalimaea* species stimulates human endothelial cell proliferation and migration in vitro. J Lab Clin Med 1994;124:521–528.
59. Koehler JE, LeBoit PE, Egbert BM, et al. Cutaneous vascular lesions and disseminated cat-scratch disease in patients with the acquired immunodeficiency syndrome (AIDS) and AIDS-related complex. Ann Intern Med 1988;109:449–455.
60. Szaniawski WK, Don PC, Bitterman SR, et al. Epithelioid angiomatosis in patients with AIDS. J Am Acad Dermatol 1990; 23:41–48.
61. Baron AL, Steinbach LS, LeBoit PE, et al. Osteolytic lesions and bacillary angiomatosis in HIV infection: radiologic differentiation from AIDS-related Kaposi sarcoma. Radiology 1990;177:77–81.
62. Webster GF, Cockerell CJ, Friedman-Kein AE. The clinical spectrum of bacillary angiomatosis. Br J Dermatol 1992;126:535–541.
63. Brancato LJ, Itescu S, Winchester R. Reiter's syndrome and related rheumatic conditions in HIV infection. J Musculoskel Med 1989; 6:14–32.
64. Conrad SE, Jacobs D, Gee J, et al. Pseudoneoplastic infection of bone in acquired immunodeficiency syndrome. J Bone Joint Surg Am 1991;73:774–777.
65. Van der Wouw PA, Hadderingh RJ, Reiss P, et al. Disseminated cat-scratch disease in a patient with AIDS. AIDS 1989;3:751–753.
66. Olive A, Tena X, Raventos A, et al. Bone bacillary angiomatosis in an HIV-infected patient. Br J Rheumatol 1996;35:901–904.
67. Schinella RA, Greco MA. Bacillary angiomatosis presenting as a soft-tissue tumor without skin involvement. Hum Pathol 1990;21: 567–569.
68. Whitfield MJ, Kaveh S, Koehler JE, et al. Bacillary angiomatosis associated with myositis in a patient infected with human immunodeficiency virus. Clin Infect Dis 1997;24:562–564.

69. Sanchez MA, Rorat E. Fine needle aspiration diagnosis of intramuscular bacillary angiomatosis: a case report. Acta Cytol 1996;40: 751–755.
70. Vickery CL, Dempewolf S, Porubsky ES, et al. Bacillary angiomatosis presenting as a nasal mass with epistaxis. Otolaryngol Head Neck Surg 1996;114:443–446.
71. Tuur S, Macher AM, Angritt P, et al. AIDS case for diagnosis series. Milit Med 1988;153:M57–M64.
72. Slater LN, Min KW. Polypoid endobronchial lesions: a manifestation of bacillary angiomatosis. Chest 1992;102:972–974.
73. Huh YB, Rose S, Schoen RE, et al. Colonic bacillary angiomatosis. Ann Intern Med 1996;124:735–737.
74. Chang AD, Drachenberg CI, James SP. Bacillary angiomatosis associated with extensive esophageal polyposis: a new mucocutaneous manifestation of acquired immunodeficiency disease (AIDS). Am J Gastroenterol 1996;91:2220–2223.
75. Koehler JE, Cederberg L. Intra-abdominal mass associated with gastrointestinal hemorrhage: a new manifestation of bacillary angiomatosis. Gastroenterology 1995;109:2011–2014.
76. Long SR, Whitfield MJ, Eades C, et al. Bacillary angiomatosis of the cervix and vulva in a patient with AIDS. Obstet Gynecol 1996;88: 709–711.
77. Schwartzman WA, Marchevsky A, Meyer RD. Epithelioid angiomatosis or cat-scratch disease with splenic and hepatic abnormalities in AIDS: case report and review of the literature. Scand J Infect Dis 1990;22:121–133.
78. Milam MW, Balerdi MJ, Toney JF, et al. Epithelioid angiomatosis secondary to disseminated cat-scratch disease involving the bone marrow and skin in a patient with acquired immunodeficiency syndrome. Am J Med 1990;88:180–183.
79. Foltzer MA, Guiney WB Jr, Wager GC, et al. Bronchopulmonary bacillary angiomatosis. Chest 1993;104:973–975.
80. Steeper TA, Rosenstein H, Weiser J, et al. Bacillary epithelioid angiomatosis involving the liver, spleen, and skin in an AIDS patient with concurrent Kaposi's sarcoma. Am J Clin Pathol 1992;97: 713–718.
81. Schlossberg D, Morad Y, Krouse TB, et al. Culture-proved disseminated cat-scratch disease in acquired immunodeficiency syndrome. Arch Intern Med 1989;149:1437–1439.
82. Welch K, Finkbeiner W, Alpers CE, et al. Autopsy findings in the acquired immune deficiency syndrome. JAMA 1984;252:1152–1159.
83. Scoazec J, Marche C, Girard P, et al. Peliosis hepatis and sinusoidal dilatation during infection by the human immunodeficiency virus (HIV). Am J Pathol 1988;131:38–47.
84. Mohle-Boetani JC, Koehler JE, Berger TG, et al. Bacillary angiomatosis and bacillary peliosis in patients infected with human immunodeficiency virus: clinical characteristics in a case-control study. Clin Infect Dis 1996;22:794–800.
85. Slater LN, Welch DF, Kyung-Whan M. *Rochalimaea henselae* causes bacillary angiomatosis and peliosis hepatis. Arch Intern Med 1992; 152:602–606.
86. Krekorian TD, Radner AB, Alcorn JM, et al. Biliary obstruction caused by epithelioid angiomatosis in a patient with AIDS. Am J Med 1990;89:820–822.
87. Vinson JW, Varela G, Molina-Pasquel C. Trench fever. III. Induction of clinical disease in volunteers inoculated with *Rickettsia quintana* propagated on blood agar. Am J Trop Med Hyg 1969;18:713–722.
88. Spach DH, Kanter AS, Dougherty MJ, et al. *Bartonella* (*Rochalimaea*) *quintana* bacteremia in inner-city patients with chronic alcoholism. N Engl J Med 1995;332:424–428.
89. Holmes AH, Greenough TC, Balady GJ, et al. *Bartonella henselae* endocarditis in an immunocompetent adult. Clin Infect Dis 1995;21: 1004–1007.
90. Spach DH, Kanter AS, Daniels NA, et al. *Bartonella* (*Rochalimaea*) species as a cause of apparent "culture-negative" endocarditis. Clin Infect Dis 1995;20:1044–1047.
91. Drancourt M, Mainardi JL, Brouqui P, et al. *Bartonella* (*Rochalimaea*) *quintana* endocarditis in three homeless men. N Engl J Med 1995; 332:419–423.
92. Daly JS, Worthington MG, Brenner DJ, et al. *Rochalimaea elizabethae* sp. nov. isolated from a patient with endocarditis. J Clin Microbiol 1993;31:872–881.
93. Szaniawski WK, Don PC, Bitterman SR, et al. Epithelioid angiomatosis in patients with AIDS. J Am Acad Dermatol 1990;23:41–48.
94. Baker J, Ruiz-Rodriguez R, Whitfield M, et al. Bacillary angiomatosis: a treatable cause of acute psychiatric symptoms in human immunodeficiency virus infection. J Clin Psychiatry 1995;56:161–166.
95. Spach DH, Panther LA, Thorning DR, et al. Intracerebral bacillary angiomatosis in a patient infected with human immunodeficiency virus. Ann Intern Med 1992;116:740–742.
96. Patnaik M, Schwartzman WA, Barks NE, et al. Possible role of *Rochalimaea henselae* in pathogenesis of AIDS encephalopathy [letter]. Lancet 1992;340:971.
97. Schwartzman WA, Patnaik M, Barka NE, et al. *Rochalimaea* antibodies in HIV-associated neurologic disease. Neurology 1994;44:1312–1316.
98. Schwartzman WA, Patnaik M, Angulo FJ, et al. *Bartonella* (*Rochalimaea*) antibodies, dementia, and cat ownership among men infected with human immunodeficiency virus. Clin Infect Dis 1995;21: 954–959.
99. Guerra LG, Neira CJ, Boman D, et al. Rapid response of AIDS-related bacillary angiomatosis to azithromycin. Clin Infect Dis 1993;17: 264–266.
100. Maurin M, Raoult D. Antimicrobial susceptibility of *Rochalimaea quintana*, *Rochalimaea vinsonii*, and the newly recognized *Rochalimaea henselae*. J Antimicrob Chemother 1993;32(4):587–594.
101. Meyers WF, Grossman DM, Wisseman CL. Antibiotic susceptibility patterns in *Rochalimaea quintana*, the agent of trench fever. J Antimicrob Chemother 1984;25:690–693.
102. Musso D, Drancourt M, Raoult D. Lack of bactericidal effect of antibiotics except aminoglycosides on *Bartonella* (*Rochalimaea*) *henselae*. J Antimicrob Chemother 1995;36:101–108.
103. Wolfson C, Branley J, Gottlieb T. The Etest for antimicrobial susceptibility testing of *Bartonella henselae*. J Antimicrob Chemother 1996;38:963–968.
104. Groves MG, Harrington KS. *Rochalimaea henselae* infections: newly recognized zoonoses transmitted by domestic cats. JAMA 1994;204: 267–271.

20

TROPICAL DISEASES IN THE HIV-INFECTED TRAVELER

Robert C. Bollinger and Thomas C. Quinn

As in other areas, the clinical manifestations of the human immunodeficiency virus (HIV) infection in tropical countries are diverse and frequently reflect many other endemic infections within each region. The most common coinfection observed in patients with HIV infection in tropical countries is tuberculosis. The World Health Organization reported that more than 5 million persons are estimated to be dually infected with HIV and *Mycobacterium tuberculosis*, with most of these individuals residing in Asia and sub-Saharan Africa (1). The incidence of tuberculosis in patients with HIV infection in the United States has been estimated to be 0.7 cases per 100 person-years, with increased incidence in patients with lower CD4 counts and those living in areas of higher tuberculosis prevalence (2). In developing countries, particularly sub-Saharan Africa, reactivated pulmonary tuberculosis is perhaps one of the earliest and most common opportunistic infections in HIV infection (3). In Burundi, 55% of tuberculosis patients were HIV seropositive; in Zaire, 38% of patients hospitalized with tuberculosis were HIV seropositive; and in Kampala, Uganda, 66% of newly diagnosed tuberculosis patients were HIV positive (3–6). As a consequence, tuberculosis has emerged as a strong predictor of underlying HIV disease among hospitalized patients in many of these countries (7).

Progressive weight loss, commonly known as Slim disease, is perhaps the most common sign of HIV infection in Africa. Weight loss, anorexia, intermittent or persistent fever, and diarrhea are observed in more than 80% of patients with acquired immunodeficiency syndrome (AIDS) in this region (8). Studies in Zaire and Uganda have found that the most commonly identified pathogens responsible for Slim disease are *Isospora, Cryptosporidium, Salmonella, Shigella,* and *Campylobacter* species (8, 9).

In addition, many of the other opportunistic infections seen in HIV-infected individuals residing in more temperate countries are also observed in tropical countries, but at different frequencies (10). For example, although *Pneumocystis carinii* pneumonia and disseminated *Mycobacterium avium* complex infection are common in developed countries, they are rare in tropical countries. Thus, the exposure of HIV-infected individuals to pathogens in their country of residence as well as to pathogens endemic to countries where they may travel broadens the differential diagnosis of infection. In addition, some opportunistic infections, such as *Penicillium* and *Leishmania* infections, may present a greater risk to HIV-infected individuals in tropical countries (11, 12). Finally, because of their underlying immunosuppression, the clinical presentation of many common diseases in HIV-infected individuals may be exacerbated or slow to respond to therapy, thereby further complicating the individual's underlying disease process.

Ten to 12 million United States residents travel to developing countries each year. With the increasing prevalence of HIV infection worldwide, greater numbers of seropositive individuals who engage in international travel for business or pleasure will be exposed to the risk of acquiring travelers' diseases. In addition, only 3% of the 15 million immigrants to the United States since 1970 have been European. Therefore, an understanding of the special risks that HIV-infected individuals may encounter during international travel should begin with a review of the common causes of travelers' disease in general. In 1984, a study of more than 10,000 short-term travelers was undertaken in Switzerland (13). A summary of the results of their study and a review of the medical literature up to 1987 are shown in Table 20.1. These data are notable for the absence of unusual or exotic tropical infections. This finding illustrates that short-term travelers to developing countries rarely acquire helminth infections or other exotic tropical diseases. However, long-term residents such as Peace Corps volunteers and missionaries are at a greater risk of acquiring endemic infections, similar to other residents of developing countries.

The most common ailment observed during or after travel is diarrhea, which affects 30 to 50% of visitors to developing countries. The highest risk appears to be in Asia, Africa, Latin America, and the Middle East. Fever in the returning traveler, although less prevalent than diarrhea, also presents a particular diagnostic dilemma.

Certain other infections endemic to the developing world have been associated with a higher prevalence or a more

Table 20.1 Relevant Infections in 7,886 Short-Term Visitors to Developing Countries

Illness	Definite	Possible
Giardiasis	34	4
Hepatitis (all)	23	4
Hepatitis A	8	—
Hepatitis B	2	—
Hepatitis, other	13	4
Amebiasis	22	8
Gonorrhea	17	6
Salmonellosis	6	1
Malaria	5	7
Helminthic infection	5	2
Syphilis	2	—
Shigellosis	1	—

Column header: Diagnosis of Illness in Travelers to Developing Countries

(From Steffen R, Richenbach M, Wilhelm U, et al. Health problems after travel to developing countries. J Infect Dis 1987;156:84–91.)

progressive disease in HIV-infected patients. These infections are described in this chapter, and recommendations regarding vaccination, malaria and diarrhea prophylaxis, and special concerns for HIV-infected travelers are provided.

CLINICAL PRESENTATION AND TREATMENT

With increasing immunosuppression, some HIV-infected travelers may be at greater risk of acquiring certain diseases of the tropics. Some of these infections may have a more progressive course or may be more resistant to treatment in the HIV-seropositive individual (Table 20.2). This section includes a description of the clinical presentation and response to therapy for both common and rare tropical diseases that may be encountered in the HIV-infected traveler.

Traveler's Diarrhea

Up to 50% of travelers to developing countries experience an episode of diarrhea. This usually occurs within the first week of travel, persists for 3 to 4 days, and is often associated with nausea, abdominal pain, and fever (14–16). In up to 50% of cases of traveler's diarrhea, a specific pathogen cannot be identified (4). *Salmonella* spp., *Campylobacter jejuni*, and enterotoxigenic *Escherichia coli* are the most common specific pathogens associated with traveler's diarrhea. Diarrhea due to *Campylobacter* infection, salmonellosis, shigellosis, cryptosporidiosis, microsporidiosis, and *Isospora* infection may be associated with a worse clinical presentation in the HIV-infected individual (see Table 20.2). In contrast, other common causes of traveler's diarrhea including *Entamoeba histolytica*, enterotoxigenic *E. coli*, and *Giardia* do not appear to present a greater risk for the HIV-infected individual.

Although enterotoxigenic and enteroinvasive *Escherichia coli* has been reported to be one of the most common cause of traveler's diarrhea, HIV coinfection has not been associated with a higher prevalence or a more prolonged or progressive illness, except for bacteremia in the case of enteroinvasive *E. coli* (17). The most common parasitic cause of traveler's diarrhea is *Giardia lamblia*. Although *Giardia* is a well-described cause of traveler's diarrhea (18), and it has been described in HIV-infected patients with diarrhea (19), it is not thought to represent a significant problem and would not be expected to cause a more pathogenic disease or be more resistant to therapy in the HIV-infected patient.

Infection with *Entamoeba histolytica* has also been described in returning travelers and is more prevalent in homosexual men (20, 21). Although *E. histolytica* has been associated with diarrhea in HIV-infected patients (22) and in rare instances has been associated with fulminant invasive colitis (23), studies have suggested that the prevalence of invasive amebiasis is not increased in patients with AIDS (24). Pathogenic *E. histolytica* or invasiveness appears to be related more to the virulence factors within certain strains of *E. histolytica* than to the underlying immunocompetence of the host.

In contrast, *Cryptosporidium* is one of the most important causes of diarrhea in AIDS patients worldwide. It has been implicated as a cause of 10 to 20% of cases of culture-negative diarrhea in AIDS patients in the United States (19, 25) and in up to 55% of cases of diarrhea in the developing world (26, 27). In addition, *Cryptosporidium* has been implicated as an important nosocomial infection in AIDS patients (28). Although *Cryptosporidium* is a common cause of mild, self-limited diarrhea in the immunologically normal host (29, 30) and has been described as a cause of traveler's diarrhea (31), the parasite causes a severe, chronic diarrheal illness in AIDS patients. After an incubation period of 2 to 14 days, a clinical syndrome develops characterized by chronic, often voluminous, watery diarrhea, severe abdominal pain, weight loss, anorexia, malaise, low-grade fever, and often electrolyte imbalance (32, 33). Stool examination is usually positive in infected patients, but an average of three specimens may be required before oocysts are identified, and concentration techniques may be required to optimize detection in some patients (34, 35). (See Chapter 21 for further discussion of treatment.)

Of the bacterial agents, *Mycobacterium avium* complex is the most frequently identified cause of chronic diarrhea in HIV infection (20, 36 ,37). Although this pathogen is a frequent cause of systemic opportunistic infection in AIDS,

Table 20.2 Common Clinical Problems of HIV-Infected Travelers

Potentially severe or prolonged course in HIV-infected individuals
  Campylobacter jejuni infection
  Salmonella species infection
  Shigella species infection
  Cryptosporidium infection
Clinical course similar in HIV-infected and uninfected individuals
  Entamoeba histolytica infection
  Giardia lamblia infection
  Hepatitis A
  Enterotoxigenic *Escherichia coli* infection
  Malaria
  Viral influenza

typically associated with chronic fever and weight loss (38), it is not believed to be an important cause of traveler's diarrhea. However, other bacterial agents, in particular *Salmonella* spp., *Shigella flexneri*, and *Campylobacter jejuni*, which can all be associated with traveler's diarrhea, produce a more severe diarrheal illness and may be more resistant to therapy in the HIV-infected patient (13, 14, 39) (see Table 20.2). *Salmonella* spp. are the most important to consider, because they are 20-fold more common in patients with AIDS than in the general population (40, 41). Salmonellosis often presents early in HIV infection as enteric fever, with the acute onset of abdominal pain and watery diarrhea (42–46). *Salmonella* bacteremia is 100-fold more common in AIDS patients and often presents without intestinal symptoms (40). Chronic infection and relapse with typhoidal and nontyphoidal salmonellosis is well described in HIV-infected patients throughout the world (45, 47–49). *Salmonella* enteritis and bacteremia should be suspected in any HIV-infected patient or traveler who presents with the acute onset of abdominal pain and fever. Occasionally, patients develop an acute abdomen and bowel perforation before the onset of diarrhea. Thus, a high index of suspicion should be maintained to identify and manage this treatable and dangerous pathogen. Therapeutic options include amoxicillin, ciprofloxacin, and trimethoprim–sulfamethoxazole. Because of the high relapse rate in HIV-infected patients, long-term secondary prophylaxis with ciprofloxacin or amoxicillin may be required.

Other bacterial causes of acute and chronic diarrhea that may affect the HIV-infected traveler include *Shigella flexneri*, which causes an intestinal illness ranging from mild diarrhea to severe dysentery (50, 51). Bloody diarrhea, fever, abdominal cramps, and bacteremia may occur, and relapsing infections have been described. *Campylobacter jejuni* causes a persistent and severe diarrheal illness in patients with AIDS. Although it may be associated with abdominal pain and severe symptoms, the diarrhea is typically a self-limited illness in immunocompetent persons and travelers (49, 52–54). Recurrent bacteremia and antibiotic-resistant organisms have been described, and although stool cultures are usually positive, chronic *C. jejuni* infection may require culture of biopsy specimens if multiple stool cultures are negative (53). Shigellosis may be treated with ampicillin or sulfamethoxazole–trimethoprim. Ciprofloxacin should only be used for resistant strains. *Campylobacter* is usually sensitive to erythromycin, doxycycline, or ciprofloxacin. Although not classically considered as a cause of traveler's diarrhea, *Clostridium difficile* should also be considered, particularly if the patient has been taking antibiotics for either prophylaxis or treatment of another condition. Diagnosis is confirmed by a positive stool *C. difficile* toxin assay. Treatment consists of oral vancomycin or metronidazole.

Certain rare clinical causes of traveler's diarrhea may be exacerbated in the HIV-infected individual, including isosporiasis and microsporidiosis (Table 20.3). Although *Isospora belli* is a rare pathogenic parasite in the normal host (55), isosporiasis is a common problem in AIDS patients, particularly in the developing world (56–58). As with *Cryptosporidium* infection, the clinical manifestations of

Table 20.3 Rare Clinical Problems in Travelers Exacerbated in HIV-Infected Individuals

Coccidiodomycosis
Hepatitis B
Histoplasmosis
Isosporiasis
Leishmaniasis
Measles
Microsporidiosis
Syphilis
Tuberculosis

I. belli infection include bloodless, watery diarrhea, crampy abdominal pain, weight loss, anorexia, and fever (57). Patients may also present with steatorrhea, in contrast to cryptosporidiosis, and eosinophilia. *Isospora* is typically concentrated in the small intestine, but dissemination of this organism has been described in AIDS (59). The diagnosis is established by identification of the large oval oocysts in stool with a modified Kenyan acid fast stain (60). Unlike *Cryptosporidium* infection, effective therapy for *Isospora* infection is available for AIDS patients. Isosporiasis responds to trimethoprim–sulfamethoxazole therapy (two double-strength tablets twice a day for 2 to 4 weeks), and secondary prophylaxis is recommended with trimethoprim–sulfamethoxazole or pyrimethamine–sulfadoxine to prevent recurrence (58, 61).

Enterocytozoon bienseusi is a newly identified species of the phylum Microspora that has been associated with a chronic diarrhea syndrome in AIDS similar to that seen with *Cryptosporidium* and has rarely been associated with diarrhea in the immunologically normal host. This important enteric pathogen in HIV-infected patients is a ubiquitous, small, intracellular, spore-forming protozoan that has been identified in up to 64% of AIDS patients with chronic, unexplained diarrhea (36, 62–65). The typical clinical syndrome of chronic, watery diarrhea, weight loss, and malaise is similar to that of cryptosporidiosis (66). The diagnosis of microsporidiosis is difficult because of the small size and poor staining qualities of these organisms. Although definitive diagnosis has required electron microscopic evaluation of small bowel biopsy specimens (36, 62), light microscopic examination of duodenal biopsy specimens has shown recent promise (66, 67). As for cryptosporidiosis, therapeutic options for microsporidian infection are limited primarily to symptomatic and supportive care. Evidence suggests that metronidazole may result in symptomatic improvement, although therapeutic efficacy has not been clearly established, and metronidazole therapy does not result in clearance of the organism (65).

Febrile Illnesses

As mentioned in the introduction, fever is a common problem in the returning traveler (11). The differential diagnosis of fever in these patients can generally be separated into the causes of fever with a short incubation (1 to 4 weeks) or those with a long incubation (4 weeks or

Table 20.4 Differential Diagnosis of Fever in the Traveler

Short incubation (less than 4 weeks)
Brucellosis
Dengue
Enteric fever[a]
Hepatitis A[a]
Influenza[a]
Legionnaires disease
Malaria[a]
Measles
Relapsing fever
Rickettsial disease
Strongyliodiasis
Tularemia
Yellow fever

Long incubation (4 weeks or longer)
Amebiasis[a]
Brucellosis
Filariasis
Hepatitis B
Katayama syndrome
Leishmaniasis
Leptospirosis
Malaria[a]
Melioidosis
Paragonimiasis
Rabies
Strongyloidiasis
Trypanosomiasis
Tuberculosis

[a]Common

longer) (Table 20.4). Malaria, influenza, hepatitis B virus, and typhoid fever are the most common causes of fever with a short incubation period in travelers. Other rare causes of fever have also been reported, including dengue and various rickettsioses. Fever with long incubation is more typically related to malaria or amebiasis in the returning traveler. The most commonly associated condition in a returning traveler with fever is acute respiratory tract infection. Although the causes of traveler-associated respiratory tract infections and fever have not been adequately investigated, viral influenza infection has been documented (68, 69). Prospective studies have not shown an increased morbidity from influenza in HIV-infected patients (70). However, secondary bacterial infections, particularly with *Streptococcus pneumoniae*, are common in HIV-infected persons (71–73).

Insect-borne infections are rare in short-term travelers, except in those who travel to malaria-endemic regions. To date, little evidence has demonstrated that malaria is more common in patients with HIV infection (74–76), despite anecdotal case reports of severe malaria associated with HIV infection (77). Dengue, filariasis, and yellow fever are rare in travelers, and no convincing evidence to date indicates that the HIV-infected traveler is at greater risk.

Hepatitis A is a disease with worldwide distribution. Although it is rarely fatal, it is a common cause of morbidity in developing nations and in returning travelers (11). Immune globulin provides protection against the clinical disease for 4 to 6 months for most travelers (78). HIV-infected individuals do not have a greater risk of infection with hepatitis A virus or a more severe disease. Hepatitis B virus infection is rare in travelers and would only be expected to occur in those at risk from parenteral needle exposure, from blood transfusions, or through sexual contact. However, individuals with HIV infection are more likely to become hepatitis B virus carriers if they are subsequently infected, and they have been found to have higher concentrations of circulating hepatitis B virus (79, 80).

Penicillium marneffei is a dysmorphic fungus that can cause human infection in both healthy and compromised hosts. In endemic countries of Southeast Asia, particularly Thailand, systemic infection with *Penicillium* is the third most common opportunistic infection in HIV-infected patients (81). HIV-infected travelers to Thailand, particularly if they are exposed to rural agricultural areas infested by bamboo rats, are at risk for acquiring *Penicillium* infection. More than 90% of HIV-infected patients with *Penicillium* infection present with fever. Anemia, weight loss, generalized papular skin lesions, diarrhea, and cough, associated with a diffuse reticulonodular pattern on chest radiograph, are common. Diagnosis typically requires biopsy of skin, bone marrow, or lymph nodes. The organism can also be isolated by blood culture. Presumptive diagnosis is made by microscopic identification of a nonbudding yeast with characteristic clear central septation. Mortality in untreated HIV-infected individuals approaches 75%. A therapeutic response of greater than 70% is typically found with amphotericin or itraconazole. Relapse after initial treatment is also not uncommon.

Coccidioidomycosis is a fungal infection that is usually benign and self-limited. It is occasionally acquired by aerosol in travel to endemic areas of Mexico and occasionally Central America. In immunosuppressed patients, including those with HIV, disseminated coccidioidomycosis has been reported (82). The incidence of coccidioidomycosis in patients with AIDS is not much higher than that in the general population, but the risk to HIV-infected travelers is still unclear, because the high incidence of this disease in patients with AIDS may be the result of reactivated latent infection (83). Another endemic mycosis, histoplasmosis, may also present an increased risk for disseminated multisystem disease in persons with HIV who live in or have traveled to endemic areas, which include sub-Saharan and West Africa. Reactivation of latent infection and also primary infection are important modes of acquiring disease in HIV-infected persons. In highly endemic areas, *Histoplasma capsulatum* infection has been reported in up to 27% of AIDS patients, but it is rare in nonendemic areas (84). Disseminated histoplasmosis is not uncommon in infected AIDS patients (84–87).

Measles presents a rare but severe problem for the HIV-infected individual. Outbreaks of measles related to international travel have been reported (88). Persons, including those infected with HIV, vaccinated before 1980 are at greater risk for having primary vaccine failure resulting from vaccination between 12 and 14 months of age or because of less than optimal storage of vaccines before 1979 (89). Between 1980 and 1985, imported measles accounted for up to 7% of the annual cases, and half of these cases were in returning travelers (90). Twenty-seven percent of the imported cases of measles in United States citizens were in children under the age of 16 months, but 17% were in adults over the age of 19 years. One-third of these cases were acquired in Europe and 24% in Asia (90). This finding has resulted in recommendations for revaccination before travel of all persons born after 1956 and vaccinated before 1980 (91). These recommendations apply to both HIV-infected and uninfected individuals. This is particularly important for HIV-infected persons because many HIV-infected individuals fall into the age range of potentially susceptible adults, and HIV-infected persons are at higher risk for more severe and frequently fatal measles as compared with HIV-seronegative individuals (92–94). However, for those persons vaccinated before 1956, evidence suggests that HIV-infected adults retain a high prevalence of measles antibody, and the declining immunity due to progressive HIV infection does not appear to be associated with a lack of antibody or increased susceptibility (95). See later for further discussion of vaccination issues in the HIV-infected patient.

The risk of tuberculosis in short-term travelers is rare. However, individuals with long-term exposure in endemic areas are at increased risk for such infection. In the developing world, tuberculosis is the most common pulmonary infection in HIV-positive patients and is expected to have a dramatic increase in incidence as a result of the HIV epidemic (96, 97). Studies have shown that patients with HIV and tuberculosis have a greater plasma viral load than matched patients with HIV alone. In addition, HIV-infected individuals who develop tuberculosis appear to have a more rapid progression of their HIV disease than HIV-infected individuals without tuberculosis, despite adequate therapy for tuberculosis (98, 99). Extrapulmonary tuberculosis also appears to be more common in patients with HIV-induced immunosuppression (100–102). The need to recognize and diagnose the atypical presentations of *Mycobacterium tuberculosis* in HIV-infected patients has been emphasized by reports of tuberculosis caused by multidrug-resistant bacilli among HIV-infected patients (103–107). Thus, a high index of suspicion for tuberculosis is important in the evaluation of any HIV-infected long-term traveler to an endemic area who presents with fever or nonspecific symptoms.

Leishmaniasis is a parasitic intracellular infection transmitted by sandflies. This infection has been a rare complication of international travel, but in light of reports of *Leishmania* infection in returning servicemen from Operation Desert Storm, exposure to this organism in the appropriate setting may be more prevalent than originally thought (108). This finding has important implications for the HIV-positive traveler, who may visit areas endemic for *Leishmania,* including India and the Middle East. Visceral leishmaniasis (kala-azar) has been reported as a complicating infection in patients with HIV infection who are from the Mediterranean area (109–114). Kala-azar has also been reported in HIV-infected individuals from India and Algeria (111). These anecdotal reports suggest that HIV-infected persons are at a greater risk of visceralization of *Leishmania* infection because of the compromise of their cellular immunity. At-risk travelers should take appropriate precautions to avoid contact with the sandfly vector if traveling in endemic areas.

Sexually Transmitted Diseases

Depending on sexual behavior and sexual contact with high-risk individuals, sexually transmitted diseases may be acquired by the traveler (11, 115). The increased prevalence of genital ulcer disease in the tropics, including chancroid, lymphogranuloma venereum, and granuloma inguinale present an increased risk for HIV acquisition or transmission and, in some cases, have been associated with a more progressive and less responsive infection (Table 20.5). The data on the impact of HIV infection on sexually transmitted diseases are limited. However, some evidence suggests decreased responsiveness to standard therapy for chancroid and syphilis in individuals infected with HIV (116–119). In addition, HIV infection may result in an atypical presentation of chancroid, including larger or extragenital lesions and systemic symptoms (119, 120). The clinical presentation of syphilis may be atypical in the setting of HIV infection, with more rapid progression to neurosyphilis or other tertiary disease more likely (118, 121–123). In HIV-infected patients, herpes infection may present atypically with more extensive and persistent lesions than in HIV-negative individuals and may result in more frequent recurrences (124–126). The incidence of infection with human papillomavirus may be increased in the presence of HIV infection (127, 128). The response to therapy of genital human papillomavirus lesions is also altered in the setting of HIV infection (129–131). Multidrug-resistant gonorrhea is prevalent in many tropical areas, especially Southeast Asia and Africa (132). HIV-infected patients with gonorrhea in Kenya were found to be more likely than HIV-negative patients to be infected with penicillinase-producing gono-

Table 20.5 Association of Sexually Transmitted Diseases and HIV Infection

	Increased Risk for HIV Acquisition	Clinical Course Exacerbated in HIV-Infected Patient
Neisseria gonorrhoeae infection	+/−	+/−
Trichomonas vaginalis infection	+	−
Haemophilus ducreyi infection	+	+
Chlamydia trachomatis infection	+	+/−
Syphilis	+	+
Herpes simplex	+	+
Granuloma inguinale	+	+/−
Human papillomavirus infection	+/−	+
Lymphogranuloma venereum	+	+/−
Hepatitis B	−	+

Table 20.6 Special Problems for the HIV-Infected Traveler

Health insurance
Restricted travel
Treatment issues:
　Availability
　Drug reactions
　Vaccinations

---

cocci (133). In addition, the risk of complications of gonorrhea, including pelvic inflammatory disease and disseminated gonococcal infection, may also be increased in the setting of HIV infection (134).

SPECIAL PROBLEMS

HIV-infected individuals, particularly those receiving antiretroviral therapy or taking *Pneumocystis* prophylaxis, should be conscious of the limited availability of appropriate medical care should they develop complications during their travel (Table 20.6). Many countries have specific foreign entry requirements that restrict travel for HIV-infected tourists as well as long-term inhabitants. An updated list of specific foreign entry requirements for individual countries is available from the United States Department of State Bureau of Consular Affairs (135). Increasing numbers of countries require that visitors be tested for HIV before entry. This is particularly true for students or long-term visitors. The United States Department of State recommends that, before traveling abroad, individuals should check with the embassy of the country to be visited to learn their specific entry requirements and to determine whether HIV testing is required. For some countries, United States test results are acceptable, but testing may be required to be performed on arrival for many applicants for work or residence permits.

TREATMENT AND VACCINATION ISSUES

In many developing countries, most pharmaceutical medications may be obtained, often with unrestricted access. However, the availability of antiretroviral drugs may be limited. HIV-infected individuals are more likely to have drug reactions such as rash, fever, and neutropenia, particularly associated with the use of sulfa drugs including trimethoprim–sulfamethoxazole for treatment or prophylaxis of *Pneumocystis carinii* infection (136, 137). Fatal Stevens–Johnson Syndrome has been documented in patients with AIDS taking pyrimethamine–sulfadoxine for *Pneumocystis* prophylaxis (138). Antibacterials including trimethoprim–sulfamethoxazole have frequently been recommended for prevention or treatment of traveler's diarrhea (139–142). Because of the increased risk of reactions to sulfa drugs and the possibility that short-term treatment for traveler's diarrhea may sensitize an HIV-infected individual to future reactions when trimethoprim–sulfamethoxazole may be required for *Pneumocystis* prophylaxis or treatment, quinolone antibiotics, such as norfloxacin or ciprofloxacin, or doxycycline may be a more appropriate choice for traveler's diarrhea in the HIV-infected patient (140).

Malaria prophylaxis and treatment in the HIV-infected individual present additional potential problems (Table 20.7). The risk of exposure to malaria needs to be evaluated based on the duration of the trip, the time of year, and the destination. More than 70% of imported *Plasmodium falciparum* malaria occurs in United States citizens who travel to sub-Saharan Africa (143, 144). *P. falciparum* is often highly resistant to chloroquine, which has been typically used for prophylaxis and treatment in short-term travelers to endemic areas (143). In addition to reduced efficacy, chloroquine may be relatively contraindicated in the HIV-infected individual because of the theoretic concern that it may cause additional immunosuppression (144). Mefloquine has become available in the United States and is the recommended drug of choice for travelers at risk of chloroquine-resistant *P. falciparum* infection (145). However, no information is available about the safety of mefloquine in the HIV-infected individual. Given its rare but well-described central nervous system toxicity (146), this drug should be used with caution in the HIV-infected person. Doxycycline has some efficacy for treatment of chloroquine-resistant malaria and is usually well tolerated in the HIV-infected individual, and therefore, it may be a more acceptable alternative (145). Few data are available about the side effects of quinine, proquanil, or primaquine in the HIV-infected individual. Primaquine, which is used for treatment of the extraerythrocytic phase of *P. vivax* infection, may exacerbate anemia in HIV-infected individuals, particularly those with glucose-6-phosphate dehydrogenase (G6PD) deficiency (145).

Vaccine Efficacy

The traveler's destination, itinerary, and immunization history help to determine the appropriate recommendations for pretravel vaccination. Because of the immunosuppression associated with HIV infection, the response to vaccination and the risk of side effects, particularly with live virus vaccines, complicate these recommendations. In addition to the quantitative depletion of CD4+ T cells that occurs during the course of HIV-1 infection, qualitative defects also occur in the function of circulating CD4+ T cells. In some studies,

Table 20.7 Malaria Prophylaxis, Treatment, and Potential Adverse Reactions in the HIV-Infected Traveler

Drug	Adverse Effect
Chloroquine	Potential immunosuppression
Quinine	Anemia, thrombocytopenia
Mefloquine	CNS toxicity, possible immunosuppression
Doxycycline	Photosensitivity, skin rash
Proquanil	Limited data available
Primaquine	Anemia in glucose-6-phosphate dehydrogenase deficiency
Sulfadoxine	Toxic epidermal necrosis

[a]Many of these reactions are rare, but the HIV-infected individual should be aware of these reactions, and the drug should be discontinued if they occur.

T-cell proliferative responses to soluble recall antigens are spared until immediately before the onset of AIDS (147, 148). However, the CD4+ T-cell help needed for the in vitro generation of antiinfluenza cytotoxic T-lymphocyte responses is defective in some healthy HIV-positive individuals (149). This functional defect has been attributed in some studies to selected depletion of memory CD4+ T cells that normally accounts for much of this response (150). In addition to the effects on CD4+ T cells, HIV-infected individuals also exhibit B-lymphocyte dysfunction (151). The polyclonal B-cell activation seen in HIV-1 infection is found in conjunction with decreased in vivo humoral responses to specific antigens. Healthy HIV-seropositive individuals fail to produce immunoglobulin in response to pokeweed mitogen and have impaired antibody production after antigenic challenge (152). Responses to pneumococcal vaccine antigens are impaired, as are responses to natural infections with *Giardia lamblia*, *Toxoplasma gondii*, *Coccidioides immitis*, and cytomegalovirus (153–157). This defect in the ability to respond to polysaccharide antigens such as pneumococcal vaccination is more pronounced in patients with with more advanced disease (158). This decreased response associated with more progressive disease has also been seen with inactivated poliomyelitis vaccination (159). In contrast, *Haemophilus influenzae* type B vaccines have been found to induce a reasonable antibody response in HIV-infected individuals (160). In general, the polysaccharide vaccines—*Haemophilus influenzae* B, meningococcus, and pneumococcus—may have reduced immunogenicity in HIV-infected individuals, especially those with AIDS (161), but there is little evidence of significant side effects, and these vaccines are generally well tolerated. Tetanus and diphtheria toxoid boosting is indicated in adults whether they travel or not. Studies in Haiti and Africa have shown that women infected with HIV have the same level of tetanus antibody after vaccination during pregnancy as seronegative women (162, 163). The stage of HIV disease does appear to influence the response to viral influenza vaccination. Symptomatic HIV-infected patients are much less likely to response to influenza A and B vaccines than are seronegative individuals (164–166). However, asymptomatic individuals are just as likely as seronegative persons to acquire protective levels of antibody (164, 166).

The response to measles vaccination in HIV infection has been evaluated primarily in children from developing countries. The response to measles vaccine also appears to be related to the stage of disease in HIV-infected individuals. In general, HIV-infected children have a reduced response to primary immunization with measles vaccine (167, 168). HIV-infected adults who have received primary vaccination with measles, mumps, and rubella (MMR) vaccine during childhood or who have a history of measles infection usually maintain protective levels of measles antibody, and no evidence indicates that this protective antibody is lost (169, 170).

HIV-infected adults appear to have an impaired response to hepatitis B vaccine. This has been found in both plasma-derived and recombinant vaccines (171–174). HIV-infected individuals have a lower seroconversion rate, a reduced antibody response, and an accelerated loss of hepatitis B surface antibody as compared with responses to vaccines in HIV-negative patients (171–175). The response to inactivated polio vaccine in HIV-infected individuals is generally good for those who were previously vaccinated with oral polio vaccine during childhood (159). Symptomatic HIV-positive individuals, however, may be less likely to respond if CD4 cells are particularly low (less than 200/mm^3).

Safety of Vaccination

For any traveler, appropriate vaccination is an important component of the pretravel medical evaluation. For the HIV-infected individual, vaccinations may present a greater risk of side effects, particularly with live viral vaccines. The safety of vaccination in HIV-infected patients has been investigated primarily in children (159, 176, 177). In general, adverse reactions to oral polio vaccination, MMR, measles vaccination, and diphtheria, tetanus, and pertussis (DTP) vaccination are rare in the HIV-infected child (159, 176, 177). Few data are available on the safety of live measles vaccination in HIV-positive adults. However, the safety data in children are reassuring, with no reported complications. No data are available on the safety of oral typhoid or yellow fever vaccination in HIV-infected persons. In general, except for measles vaccination, live attenuated vaccinations such as these should be avoided in the HIV-infected individual. The risk of live attenuated vaccination in HIV infection is best illustrated by the experience with bacille Calmette-Guérin (BCG) and vaccines. An asymptomatic, HIV-infected military recruit developed generalized vaccinia after smallpox vaccination (178). In addition, regional lymphadenitis and disseminated infection have been reported in adults with HIV who were vaccinated with BCG (179, 180).

Killed vaccines and subunit vaccinations appear to be relatively well tolerated, although, as mentioned earlier, they may be less immunogenic in the HIV-infected patient. Transient increases in HIV replication have been described in HIV-infected individuals with pneumococcal, tetanus, and influenza vaccines (181–183). Other studies have suggested that influenza vaccination does not increase HIV-1 viral load (184). To date, no evidence indicates that administration of vaccinations accelerates the progression of HIV disease through T-cell activation and subsequent increased HIV replication. Some studies have shown that clinical disease in HIV-infected individuals who received routine immunizations had no significant clinical deterioration relative to HIV-negative vaccine recipients (185–187).

Recommendations for Vaccination

Because the use of inactivated or subunit vaccines poses no additional risk of adverse events and may be beneficial for the HIV-infected individual, these vaccines should be considered part of routine health maintenance for these patients (Table 20.8). Specifically, *Haemophilus influenzae* B and pneumococcal vaccine should be considered for all HIV-infected individuals. HIV-positive travelers to endemic areas should be given a meningococcal vaccination. Hepatitis B virus vaccine is recommended for HIV-infected individuals, and routine boosting with diphtheria and tetanus toxoids should also be given. For travelers with seasonal exposure, influenza vaccinations should also be considered. Boosting with inactivated poliomyelitis vaccination is recommended for any HIV-infected traveler. All HIV-infected adults born after 1957 who have no evidence of immunity to measles should also receive MMR vaccination.

Except for MMR, the live attenuated vaccines are generally contraindicated in HIV-infected individuals (see Table 20.8). For the HIV-infected traveler, these vaccines include oral typhoid, yellow fever, oral poliomyelitis, and BCG vaccination (188, 189). No information is available concerning the safety and immunogenicity of cholera, Japanese B encephalitis, or preexposure rabies vaccinations in the HIV-infected individual. Because the cholera vaccine is minimally effective, a physician's waiver seems appropriate for the HIV-infected traveler who requires documentation of cholera vaccination for entry.

In conclusion, HIV-infected individuals planning travel to tropical areas should receive a thorough evaluation and comprehensive instruction before their departure (Table 20.9). In addition to a thorough physical examination and documentation of previous vaccination and travel history, certain other issues need to be addressed. Patients should have a CD4 cell count before their departure, to determine their appropriateness for antiretroviral therapy. If indicated, these patients should be given sufficient antiretroviral medication and *Pneumocystis* prophylaxis for the duration of their trip. Evaluation of their purified protein derivative (PPD) status by skin test, including an anergy panel to determine past exposure to tuberculosis, is important before travel and for assessing a posttravel fever. Baseline serology for syphilis is also recommended.

In addition to the standard adult immunizations recommended for the HIV-infected individual, specific recommendations concerning vaccinations depend on the itinerary. In general, it is probably prudent to recommend avoidance of areas endemic for yellow fever, because vaccination is contraindicated. In addition, instruction on the use of a bed net and the avoidance of arthropod vectors should also be given. For travelers to malaria-endemic areas, evaluation for G6PD deficiency may be indicated before departure. Many antimalarial drugs induce hemolytic anemia in the G6PD-deficient patient. This consequence should be particularly avoided in the HIV-infected individual. In addition to the standard instructions for avoidance of high-risk foods, such as undercooked meat and uncooked fresh vegetables, the HIV-infected traveler could be provided with antimicrobials such as ciprofloxacin, norfloxacin, or doxycycline for the treatment of traveler's diarrhea. Given the high incidence of adverse reactions, sulfa drugs such as trimethoprim–sulfamethoxazole should be avoided unless indicated for *Pneumocystis* prophylaxis. Finally, issues of travel restriction, availability of care, and the need for health insurance coverage should be investigated before departure.

Table 20.8 Vaccination for the HIV-Infected Individual

Relatively Safe	Contraindicated
Viral influenza vaccine	Oral poliomyelitis vaccine
Haemophilus influenzae B vaccine	Oral typhoid vaccine
Meningococcal vaccine	Yellow fever vaccine
Pneumococcal vaccine	Bacille Calmette–Guérin vaccine
Hepatitis B virus vaccine	
Inactivated typhoid vaccine	
Tetanus/diphtheria vaccine	
Inactivated poliomyelitis vaccine	
Measles, mumps, and rubella vaccine	

Table 20.9 Checklist for the HIV-Infected Individual Before Travel

1. CD4 cell count
2. Purified protein derivative status/anergy panel
3. Syphilis serology
4. Vaccinations (see Table 20.8)
5. Complete blood count if on zidovudine (CD4 < 500)
6. *Pneumocystis* prophylaxis for those with CD4 < 200
7. Malaria prophylaxis (check glucose-6-phosphate dehydrogenase status)
8. Diarrhea treatment
9. Insurance coverage
10. Travel restrictions
11. Availability of care

References

1. Raviglione MC, Snider DE Jr, Kochi A. Global epidemiology of tuberculosis: morbidity and mortality of a worldwide epidemic [see comments]. JAMA 1995;273:2206–2226.
2. Marches N, Hansen NI, Hopewell PC, et al. Incidence of tuberculosis in the United States among HIV-infected persons. Ann Intern Med 1997;126:123–132.
3. DeCock KM, Soro B, Coulibaly IM, et al. Tuberculosis and HIV infection in sub-Saharan Africa. JAMA 1992;268:1581–1587.
4. Standaert B, Niragira F, Kadenda P, et al. The association of tuberculosis and HIV infection in Burundi. AIDS Res Hum Retroviruses 1989;5:247–251.
5. Colebunders RL, Ryder RW, Nzilambi N, et al. HIV infection in patients with tuberculosis in Kinshasa, Zaire. Am Rev Respir Dis 1989;139:1082–1085.
6. McLeod DT, Neill P, Robertson VJ, et al. Pulmonary diseases in patients infected with the human immunodeficiency virus in Zimbabwe, Central Africa. Trans R Soc Trop Med Hyg 1989;83:694–697.
7. Hellinger J, Marlink R, Kaptue L, et al. Are tuberculosis patients a sentinel' population for HIV epidemic in Africa? Trans R Soc Trop Med Hyg 1990;84:292.
8. Sewankambo N, Mugerwa RD, Goodgame RW, et al. Enteropathic AIDS in Uganda: an endoscopic, histological and microbiological study. AIDS 1987;1:9–13.
9. Colebunders RL, Kimputu L, Gigase P, et al. Persistent diarrhea in Zairian AIDS patients: an etiologic study. Am J Gastroenterol 1987;82:859–864.

10. Kotler DP. Malnutrition and HIV infection and AIDS. AIDS 1989; 3:S175–S180.
11. Alvar J, Canavate C, Gutierrez-Solar B, et al. *Leishmania* and human immunodeficiency virus coinfection: the first 10 years. Clin Microbiol Rev 1997;10:298–319.
12. Chariyalertsak S, Sirisanthana T, Supparatpinyo K, et al. Case-control study of risk factors for *Penicillium marneffei* infection in human immunodeficiency virus-infected patients in northern Thailand. Clin Infect Dis 1997;24:1080–1096.
13. Steffen R, Rickenbach M, Wilhelm U, et al. Health problems after travel to developing countries. J Infect Dis 1987;156:84–91.
14. Mattila L. Clinical features and duration of traveler's diarrhea in relation to its etiology. Clin Infect Dis 1994;19:728–734.
15. Ericsson CD, DuPont HL, Sullivan P, et al. Bicozamycin, a poorly absorbable antibiotic, effectively treats travelers' diarrhea. Ann Intern Med 1983;98:20–25.
16. Dupont HL, Reeves RR, Galindo E, et al. Treatment of travelers' diarrhea with trimethoprim/sulfamethoxazole and with trimethoprim alone. N Engl J Med 1982;307:841–844.
17. Bessesen MT, Wang E, Echeverria P, et al. Enteroinvasive *Escherichia coli*: a cause of bacteremia in patients with AIDS. J Clin Microbiol 1991;29:2675–2677.
18. Merson MH, Morris GK, Sack DA, et al. Travelers' diarrhea in Mexico: a prospective study of physicians and family members attending a congress. N Engl J Med 1976;294:1299–1305.
19. Connolly GM, Forbes A, Gazzard BG. Investigation of seemingly pathogen-negative diarrhoea in patients infected with HIV-1. Gut 1990;31:886–889.
20. Quinn TC, Stamm WE, Goodell SE, et al. The polymicrobial origin of intestinal infections in homosexual men. N Engl J Med 1983;309:603–606.
21. Pearce RB, Abrams DI. *Entamoeba histolytica* in homosexual men. N Engl J Med 1987;316:960–961.
22. Connolly GM, Shanson D, Hawkins, et al. Non-cryptosporidial diarrhoea in human immunodeficiency virus (HIV) infected patients. Gut 1989;30:195–200.
23. Hall-Crags M, Soltzberg DM. Fulminant amebic colitis in a homosexual man. Am J Gastroenterol 1986;81:209–212.
24. Jessurun J, Barrón-Rodríguez LP, Fernández-Tinoco G, et al. The prevalence of invasive amebiasis is not increased in patients with AIDS. AIDS 1992;6:307–309.
25. Garcia LS, Current WL. Cryptosporidiosis: clinical features and diagnosis. Crit Rev Clin Lab Sci 1989;27:439–460.
26. Malbranche R, Arnoux E, Guerin JM, et al. Acquired immunodeficiency syndrome with severe gastrointestinal manifestations in Haiti. Lancet 1983;2:873–878.
27. Colebunders R, Francis H, Mann JM, et al. Persistent diarrhea strongly associated with HIV infection in Kinshasa, Zaire. Am J Gastroenterol 1987;82:859–863.
28. Ravn P, Lundgren JD, Kjaeldgaard P, et al. Nosocomial outbreak of cryptosporidiosis in AIDS patients. BMJ 1991;302:277–280.
29. Current WL, Reese NC, Ernst JV, et al. Human cryptosporidiosis in immunocompetent and immunodeficient persons: studies of an outbreak and experimental transmission. N Engl J Med 1984;388:1252–1257.
30. Wolfson JS, Richter JM, Waldron MA, et al. Cryptosporidiosis in immunocompetent patients. N Engl J Med 1985;312:1278–1282.
31. Sterling CR, Seegar K, Sinclair NA. *Cryptosporidium* as a causative agent of traveler's diarrhea [letter]. J Infect Dis 1986;153:380–381.
32. Soave R, Armstrong D. *Cryptosporidium* and cryptosporidiosis. Rev Infect Dis 1986;8:1012–1023.
33. Janoff EN, Reller LB. *Cryptosporidium* species, a protean protozoan. J Clin Microbiol 1987; 25:967–975.
34. Ma P, Soave R. Three-step stool examination for cryptosporidiosis in 10 homosexual men with protracted watery diarrhea. J Infect Dis 1983;147:824–828.
35. Sterling CR, Arrowwood MJ. Detection of *Cryptosporidium* and cryptosporidiosis. Rev Infect Dis 1986;8:1012.
36. Greenson JK, Belitsos PC, Yardley JH, et al. AIDS enteropathy: occult enteric infections and duodenal mucosal alterations in chronic diarrhea. Ann Intern Med 1991;114:366–372.
37. MacDonell KB, Glassroth J. *Mycobacterium avium* complex and other nontuberculous mycobacteria in patients with HIV infection. Semin Respir Infect 1989;4:123–132.
38. Horsburgh RC. *Mycobacterium avium* complex infection in the acquired immunodeficiency syndrome. N Engl J Med 1991;324:1332–1338.
39. Taylor DN, Echeverria P. Etiology and epidemiology of travelers' diarrhea in Asia. Rev Infect Dis 1986;8:136–142.
40. Celem CL, Chaisson RE, Rutherford GW, et al. Incidence of salmonellosis in patients with AIDS. J Infect Dis 1987;156:998–1001.
41. Sperber SJ, Schleuner CJ. Salmonellosis during infection with human immunodeficiency virus. Rev Infect Dis 1987;9:925–934.
42. Bottone EJ, Wormser GP, Duncanson FP. Non-typhoidal *Salmonella* bacteremia as an early infection in acquired immunodeficiency syndrome. Diagn Microbiol Infect Dis 1984;2:247–250.
43. Jacobs JL, Gold JMWM, Murray HW, et al. *Salmonella* infections in patients with acquired immunodeficiency syndrome. 1985;102:186–188.
44. Smith PD, Macher AM, Bookman MA, et al. *Salmonella typhimurium* enteritis and bacteremia in the acquired immunodeficiency syndrome. Ann Intern Med 1985;102:207–209.
45. Levine WC, Buehler JW, Bean NH, et al. Epidemiology of nontyphoidal *Salmonella* bacteremia during the human immunodeficiency virus epidemic. J Infect Dis 1991;164: 81–87.
46. Gilks CF, Brindle RJ, Otieno LS, et al. Life-threatening bacteriaemia in HIV-1 seropositive adults admitted to hospital in Nairobi, Kenya. Lancet 1990;336:545–549.
47. Glaser JB, Morton-Kute L, Berger SR, et al. Recurrent *Salmonella typhimurium* bacteremia associated with the acquired immunodeficiency syndrome. Ann Intern Med 1985;102:189–193.
48. Mayer KH, Hanson E. Recurrent *Salmonella* infection with a single strain in the acquired immunodeficiency syndrome confirmation by plasmid fingerprinting. Diagn Microbiol Infect Dis 1986;4:71–76.
49. Connolly GM, Forbes A, Gazzard BG. Investigation of seemingly pathogen-negative diarrhoea in patients infected with HIV-1. Gut 1990;31:886–889.
50. Baskin DH, Lax JD, Barenberg D. *Shigella* bacteremia in patients with the acquired immune deficiency syndrome. Am J Gastroenterol 1987;82:338–341.
51. Simor AE, Poon R, Borczyk A. Chronic *Shigella flexneri* infection preceding development of acquired immunodeficiency syndrome. J Clin Microbiol 1989;27:353–355.
52. Dworkin B, Wormser GP, Abdoo RA, et al. Persistence of multiply antibiotic-resistant *Campylobacter jejuni* in a patient with the acquired immunodeficiency syndrome. Am J Med 1986;80:965–970.
53. Perlman DM, Ampel NM, Schifman RB, et al. Persistent *Campylobacter jejuni* infections in patients infected with the human immunodeficiency virus. Ann Intern Med 1988;108:540–546.
54. Connolly GM, Shanson D, Hawkins DA, et al. Non-cryptosporidial diarrhoea in human immunodeficiency virus (HIV) infected patients. Gut 1989;30:195–200.
55. Faust EC, Giraldo LE, Caicedo G, et al. Human isosporosis in the Western Hemisphere. Am J Med 1983;10:343.
56. Dehovitz JA, Pape JW, Boney M. et al. Clinical manifestations and therapy of *Isospora belli* infections in patients with the acquired immunodeficiency syndrome. N Engl J Med 1986;315:87–90.
57. Soave R, Johnson WD Jr. *Cryptosporidium* and *Isospora belli* infections. J Infect Dis 1988;157:225–229.
58. Pape JW, Johnson WD Jr. *Isospora belli* infections. Prog Clin Parasitol 1991;2:119–127.
59. Restrep C, Macher AM, Radny EH. Disseminated extraintestinal isosporiasis in a patient with acquired immunodeficiency syndrome. Am J Clin Pathol 1987;87:536.

60. Ng E, Markell EK, Flemming RL, et al. Demonstration of *Isospora belli* by acid fast stain in a patient with acquired immune deficiency syndrome. J Clin Microbiol 1984;20:384–386.
61. Quinn TC, Stamm WE. Proctitis, proctocolitis, enteritis and esophagitis in homosexual men. In Holmes KK, Mardh PA, Sparling PF, et al., eds. Sexually transmitted diseases. New York: McGraw-Hill, 1990:663–683.
62. Kotler DP, Francisco A, Clayton F, et al. Small intestinal injury and parasitic diseases in AIDS. Ann Intern Med 1990;113:444–449.
63. Shadduck JA. Human microsporidiosis and AIDS. Rev Infect Dis 11:203–207, 1989.
64. Cali A, Owen RL. Intracellular development of *Enterocytozoon*, a unique microsporidian found in the intestine of AIDS patients. J Protozool 1990;37:145–155.
65. Eeftinck Schattenkerk JK, van Gool T, van Ketel RJ, et al. Clinical significance of small-intestinal microsporidiosis in HIV-1-infected individuals. Lancet 1991;337:895–898.
66. Orenstein JM, Chiang J, Steinberg W, et al. Intestinal microsporidiosis as a cause of diarrhea in human immunodeficiency virus-infected patients: a report of 20 cases. Hum Pathol 1990;21:475–481.
67. van Gool T, Hollister WS, Schattenkerk JE, et al. Diagnosis of *Enterocytozoon bieneusi* microsporidiosis in AIDS patients by recovery of spores from faeces. Lancet 1990;336:697–698.
68. Moser MR, Bender TR, Margolis HS, et al. An outbreak of influenza aboard a commercial airliner. Am J Epidemiol 1979;110:1–6.
69. Centers for Disease Control and Prevention. Acute respiratory illness among cruise-ship passengers: Asia. MMWR Morb Mortal Wkly Rep 1988;37:64–66.
70. Cohen JP, Macauley C. Susceptibility to influenza A in HIV-positive patients [letter]. JAMA 1989;261:245.
71. Polosky B, Gold JW, Whambey E, et al. Bacterial pneumonia in patients with acquired immunodeficiency syndrome. Ann Intern Med 1988;85:172–176.
72. Witt DJ, Craven DE, McCabe WR. Bacterial infections in adult patients with the acquired immune deficiency syndrome (AIDS) and AIDS-related complex. Am J Med 1987;82:900–906.
73. Schlamm HT, Yancovitz SR. *Haemophilus influenzae* pneumonia in young adults with AIDS, ARC, or risk of AIDS. Am J Med 1989;86:11–14.
74. Greenberg AE, Nguyen-Dinh P, Mann JM, et al. The association between HIV seropositivity, blood transfusion and malaria in a pediatric population in Kinshasa. JAMA 1988;259:545–549.
75. Nguyen-Dinh P, Greenberg AE, Mann JM, et al. Absence of association between *Plasmodium falciparum* malaria and HIV infection in children in Kinshasa, Zaire. Bull WHO 1987,65:607–613.
76. Nguyen-Dinh P, Greenberg AE, Colebunders RI, et al. HIV infection, AIDS, and *Plasmodium falciparum* in an adult emergency ward population in Kinshasa, Zaire [abstract]. Presented at the Annual Meeting of the American Society of Tropical Medicine and Hygiene, Los Angeles, 1987.
77. Miskovits E, Banhegyi D, Axmann A, et al. Severe cerebral malaria association with HIV infection [abstract 5547]. Presented at the 4th International Conference on AIDS, Stockholm, 1988.
78. Conrad ME, Lemon SM. Prevention of endemic icteric viral hepatitis by administration of immune serum gamma globulin. J Infect Dis 1987;156:56–63.
79. Perrillo RP, Regenstein FG, Roodman ST. Chronic hepatitis B in asymptomatic homosexual men with antibody to the human immunodeficiency virus. Ann Intern Med 1986;105:382–383.
80. Krogsgaard K, Lindhardt BO, Nielson JO, et al. The influence of HTLV-III infection on the natural history of hepatitis B virus infection in male homosexual HbsAG carriers. Hepatology 1987;7:37–41.
81. Supparatpinyo K, Khamwan C, Baosoung V, et al. Disseminated *Penicillium marneffei* infection in southeast Asia. Lancet 1994;344:110–113.
82. Bronnimann DA, Adam RD, Galgiani JN, H et al. Coccidioidomycosis in the acquired immunodeficiency syndrome. Ann Intern Med 1987;106:372–379.
83. Kovacs A, Forthal DN, Kovacs JA, et al. Disseminated coccidioidomycosis in a patient with acquired immune deficiency syndrome. West J Med 1984;140:447–449.
84. Wheat LJ, Connolly-Stringfield PA, Baker RL, et al. Disseminated histoplasmosis in the acquired immune deficiency syndrome: clinical findings, diagnosis and treatment, and review of the literature. Medicine 1990;69:361–374.
85. Johnson PC, Sarosi GA, Septimus EJ, et al. Progressive disseminated histoplasmosis in patients with the acquired immune deficiency syndrome: a report of 12 cases and a literature review. Semin Respir Infect 1986;1:1–9.
86. Bonner JR, Alexander J, Dismukes WE, et al. Disseminated histoplasmosis in patients with the acquired immune deficiency syndrome. Arch Intern Med 1984;199:2178–2181.
87. Mandell W, Goldberg DM, Neu HC. Histoplasmosis in patients with the acquired immune deficiency syndrome. Am J Med 1986;81:974–978.
88. von Reyn CF, Saviteer M. Measles immunization for international travelers [letter]. Ann Intern Med 1989;111:766–767.
89. Centers for Disease Control and Prevention. Measles prevention: supplementary statement. MMWR Morb Mortal Wkly Rep 1989;38:11–14.
90. Marches LE, Tomasi A, Hawkins CE, et al. International measles importations, 1980–1985. Int J Epidemiol 1988;17:187–192.
91. Hill DR, Pearson RD. Measles prophylaxis for international travel. Ann Intern Med 1989;111:699–701.
92. Kemper CA, Zolopa AR, Hamilton JR, et al. Prevalence of measles antibodies in adults with HIV infection: possible risk factors of measles seronegativity. AIDS 1992;6:1321–1325.
93. Kaplan LJ, Daum RS, Smaron M, et al. Severe measles in immunocompromised patients. JAMA 1992;267:1237–1241.
94. Krasinski K, Borkowsky W. Measles and measles immunity in children infected with human immunodeficiency virus. JAMA 1989;261:2512–2516.
95. Mustafa M, Weitman SD, Winick NJ, et al. Measles inclusion body encephalitis in immunocompromised patients: report of diagnosis by PCR and treatment with intravenous ribavirin [abstract 1113]. Presented at the 31st Interscience Conference on Antimicrobial Agents and Chemotherapy, Chicago, 1991.
96. Bernejo A, Veeken H, Bera A. Tuberculosis incidence in developing countries with high prevalence of HIV infection. AIDS 1992;6:1203–1206.
97. Mets T, Ngendahayo P, Van de Perre P, et al. HIV infection and tuberculosis in Central Africa. N Engl J Med 1989;322:542–543.
98. Whalen C, Horsburgh CR, Hom D, et al. Accelerated course of human immunodeficiency virus infection after tuberculosis. Am J Respir Crit Care Med 1995; 151:129–135.
99. Pape JW, Jean SS, Ho JL, et al. Effect of isoniazid prophylaxis on incidence of active tuberculosis and progression of HIV infection [see comments]. Lancet 1993;342:268–272.
100. Shafer RW, Goldberg R, Sierra M, et al. Frequency of *Mycobacterium tuberculosis* bacteremia in patients with tuberculosis in an area endemic for AIDS. Am Rev Respir Dis 1989; 140:1611–1613.
101. Barnes PF, Block AB, Davidson PT, et al. Tuberculosis in patients with human immunodeficiency virus infection. N Engl J Med 1991;324:1644–1650.
102. Chaisson RE, Schechter GF, Theuer CP, et al. Tuberculosis in patients with the acquired immunodeficiency syndrome. Am Rev Respir Dis 1987;136:570–574.
103. Fischl MA, Uttamschandani RB, Daikos GL, et al. An outbreak of tuberculosis caused by multiple-drug-resistant tubercle bacilli among patients with HIV infection. Ann Intern Med 1992;117:177–183.
104. Fischl MA, Daikos GL, Uttamchandani RB, et al. Clinical presentation and outcome of patients with HIV infection and tuberculosis caused by multiple-drug–resistant bacilli. Ann Intern Med 1992;117:184–190.

105. Pearson ML, Jereb JA, Frieden TR, et al. Nosocomial transmission of multidrug-resistant *Mycobacterium tuberculosis*. Ann Intern Med 1992;117:191–196.
106. Edlin BR, Tokars JI, Grieco MH, et al. An outbreak of multidrug-resistant tuberculosis among hospitalized patients with the acquired immunodeficiency syndrome. N Engl J Med 1992;326:1514–1521.
107. Braun MM, Kulburn JO, Smithwick RW, et al. HIV infection and primary resistance to antituberculosis drugs in Abidjan, Côte d'Ivoire. AIDS 1992;6:1327–1330.
108. Centers for Disease Control and Prevention. Viscerotropic leishmaniasis in persons returning from Operation Desert Storm: 1990–1991. MMWR Morb Mortal Wkly Rep 41:132–133.
109. Clauvel JP, Couder LJ, Belmin J, et al. Visceral leishmaniasis complicating acquired immunodeficiency syndrome (AIDS) [letter]. Trans R Soc Trop Med Hyg 1986;80:1010–1011.
110. Montalbán C, Sevilla F, Moreno A, et al. Visceral leishmaniasis as an opportunistic infection in the acquired immunodeficiency syndrome. J Infect Dis 1987;15:247–250.
111. Yebra M, Segovia J, Manzano L, et al. Disseminated-to-skin kala-azar and the acquired immunodeficiency syndrome [letter]. Ann Intern Med 1988;108:490–491.
112. Berenguer J, Moreno S, Cercenado E, et al. Visceral leishmaniasis in patients infected with human immunodeficiency virus (HIV). Ann Intern Med 1989;111:129–132.
113. Medrano FJ, Hernández-Quero J, Jimínez E, et al. Visceral leishmaniasis in HIV-1-infected individuals: a common opportunistic infection in Spain? AIDS 1992;6:1499–1503.
114. Jeannel D, Tuppin P, Brucker G, et al. Leishmaniasis in France [letter]. Lancet 1989;2:804.
115. Wasserheit JN. Epidemiological synergy: interrelationships between human immunodeficiency virus infection and other sexually transmitted diseases. Sex Transm Dis 1992;19:61–77.
116. Cameron DW, Plummer FA, D'Costa LJ, et al. Prediction of HIV infection by treatment failure for chancroid, a genital ulcer disease [abstract 7637]. Presented at the 4th International AIDS Conference, Stockholm, 1988.
117. MacDonald KS, Cameron W, D'Costa LJ, et al. Evaluation of fleroxacin (RO 23-6240) as single-oral-dose therapy of culture-proven chancroid in Nairobi, Kenya. Antimicrob Agents Chemother 1989;33:612–614.
118. Lukehart SA, Hook EW, Baker-Zander SA, et al. Invasion of the central nervous system by *Treponema pallidum*: implications for diagnosis and treatment. Ann Intern Med 1988;109:855–862.
119. Quale J, Teplita E, Augenbraun M. Atypical presentation of chancroid in a patient infected with the human immunodeficiency virus. Am J Med 1990;88:43N–44N.
120. Latif AS. Epidemiology and control of chancroid [abstract 66]. Presented at the 8th International Society for Sexually Transmitted Disease Research, Copenhagen, 1989.
121. Caumes E, Janier M, Janssen F, et al. Atypical secondary syphilis in HIV seropositive patients [abstract W.B.P. 49]. Presented at the 5th International AIDS Conference, Montreal, 1989.
122. Stoumbos VD, Klein ML. Syphilitic retinitis in a patient with acquired immunodeficiency syndrome-related complex. Am J Ophthalmol 1987;103:103–104.
123. Katz DA, Berger JR. Neurosyphilis in acquired immunodeficiency syndrome. Arch Neurol 1989;46:895–897.
124. Quinnan GV, Masur H, Rook AH, et al. Herpesvirus infections in the acquired immune deficiency syndrome. JAMA 1984;252:72–77.
125. Siegal FP, Lopez C, Hammer GS, et al. Severe acquired immunodeficiency in male homosexuals, manifested by chronic perianal ulcerative herpes simplex lesions. N Engl J Med 1981;305:1439–1444.
126. Gold D, Corey L. Acyclovir prophylaxis for herpes simplex virus infection. Antimicrob Agents Chemother 1987;31:361–367.
127. Palefsky J, Gonzales J, Greenblatt RM, et al. Anal intraepithelial neoplasia and anal papillomavirus infection among homosexual males with group IV HIV disease. JAMA 1990;263:2911–2916.
128. Feingold AR, Vermund SH, Burk RD, et al. Cervical cytologic abnormalities and papillomavirus in women infected with human immunodeficiency virus. J Acquir Immune Defic Syndr 1990;3:896–903.
129. McMillan A, Bishop PE. Clinical course of anogenital warts in men infected with human immunodeficiency virus. Genitourin Med 1989;65:225–228.
130. Bishop PE, McMillan A, Fletcher S. Immunological study of condylomata acuminata in men infected with the human immunodeficiency virus. Int J STD AIDS 1990;1:28–31.
131. Rudlinger R, Grob R, Buchmann P, et al. Anogenital warts of the condylomata acuminatum type in HIV-positive patients. Dermatologica 1988;176:277–288.
132. Centers for Disease Control and Prevention. Global distribution of penicillinase-producing *Neisseria gonorrhoeae* (PPNG). MMWR Morb Mortal Wkly Rep 182;31:1–3.
133. Ombette JJ, Ndinya-Achola JO, Maitha G, et al. Prevalence of HIV among men and women with *H. ducreyi* and *Neisseria gonorrhoeae* infection in Nairobi, Kenya [abstract Th.C. 572]. Presented at the 6th International AIDS Conference, San Francisco, 1990.
134. Moyle G, Barton SE, Rowe IF, et al. Gonococcal arthritis caused by auxotype P in a man with HIV infection. Genitourin Med 1990;66:91–92.
135. U.S. Department of State, Bureau of Consular Affairs. Foreign entry requirements. Revised. Washington, DC: Department of State Publication 9940, 1992.
136. Gordin FM, Simon Gl, Wofsy C, et al. Adverse reactions to trimethoprim–sulfamethoxazole in patients with the acquired immune deficiency syndrome. Ann Intern Med 1984;100:495–499.
137. Fischl MA, Dickinson GM, La Voie L. Safety and efficacy of sulfamethoxazole and trimethoprim chemoprophylaxis for *Pneumocystis carinii* pneumonia in AIDS. JAMA 1988;259:1185–1189.
138. Arndt KA, Jick H. Rates of cutaneous reactions to drugs. JAMA 1976;235:915–923.
139. Sack RB. Antimicrobial prophylaxis of travelers' diarrhoea: a summary of studies using doxycycline or trimethoprim and sulfamethoxazole. Scand J Gastroenterol 1983;84(Suppl):111–117.
140. DuPont HL, Galindo E, Evans DG, et al. Prevention of travelers' diarrhea with trimethoprim–sulfamethoxazole and trimethoprim alone. Gastroenterology 1983:84:75–80.
141. DuPont HL, Ericsson CD, Johnson PC, et al. Antimicrobial agents in the prevention of travelers' diarrhea. Rev Infect Dis 1986:8(Suppl 2):S167–S171.
142. Ericsson CD, Johnson PC, DuPont HL, M et al. Ciprofloxacin or trimethoprim–sulfamethoxazole as initial therapy for travelers' diarrhea. Ann Intern Med 1987;106:216–220.
143. Spencer HC. Drug-resistant malaria: changing patterns mean difficult decisions. Trans R Soc Trop Med Hyg 1985;79:748–758.
144. Salmeron G, Lipsky PE. Immunosuppressive potential of antimalarials. Am J Med 1983;75:19–24.
145. Centers for Disease Control and Prevention. Recommendations for the prevention of malaria among travelers. MMWR Morb Mortal Wkly Rep 1990;39:1–10.
146. Sturchler D, Handschin J, Kaiser D, et al. Neuropsychiatric side effects of mefloquine [letter]. N Engl J Med 1990;332:1752–1753.
147. Giorgi JV, Fahey JL, Smith DC, et al. Early effects of HIV on CD4+ lymphocytes in vivo. J Immunol 1987;138:3725–3730.
148. Gurley RJ, Ikeuchi K, Byrn RA, et al. CD4+ lymphocyte function with early human immunodeficiency virus infection. Proc Natl Acad Sci U S A 1989;86:1993–1997.
149. Shearer GM, Bernstein DC, Tung KSK, et al. A model for the selective loss of major histocompatibility complex self-restricted T cell immune responses during the development of acquired immune deficiency syndrome (AIDS). J Immunol 1986;137:2514–2521.
150. van Noesel CJM, Gruters RA, Terpstra FG, et al. Functional and phenotypic evidence for a selective loss of memory T cells in asymptomatic human immunodeficiency virus–infected men. J Clin Invest 1990;86:293–299.

151. Amadori A, Chieco-Bianchi L. B-cell activation and HIV-1 infection: deeds and misdeeds. Immunol Today 1990;11:374–379.
152. Miedema F, Chantal Petit AJ, Terpstra FG, et al. Immunological abnormalities in human immunodeficiency virus (HIV)–infected asymptomatic homosexual men. HIV affects the immune system before CD4+ helper T cell depletion occurs. J Clin Invest 1988;82:1908–1914.
153. Janoff EN, Douglas JM, Gabriel AT, et al. Class-specific antibody response to pneumococcal capsular polysaccharides in men infected with human immunodeficiency virus type 1. J Infect Dis 1988;158:983–989.
154. Janoff EN, Smith PD, Blaser MJ. Acute antibody responses to *Giardia lamblia* are depressed in patients with AIDS. J Infect Dis 1988;157:798–804.
155. Luft DJ, Conley R, Remington J. Outbreak of central nervous system toxoplasmosis in Western Europe and North America. Lancet 1983;1:781–783.
156. Roberts CJ. Coccidioidomycosis in acquired immune deficiency syndrome: depressed humoral as well as cellular immunity. Am J Med 1984;76:734–736.
157. Dylewski J, Chan S, Merigan TC. Absence of detectable IgM antibody during cytomegalovirus disease in patients with AIDS. N Engl J Med 1983;309:493–497.
158. Rodriguez-Barradas MC, Musher DM, Lahart C, et al. Antibody to capsular polysaccharides of *Streptococcus pneumoniae* after vaccination of human immunodeficiency virus–infected subjects with 23-valent pneumococcal vaccine. J Infect Dis 1992;165:553–556.
159. Vardinon N, Handsher R, Burke M, et al. Poliovirus vaccination responses in HIV-infected patients; correlation with T4 cell counts. J Infect Dis 1990;162:238–241.
160. Steinhoff MC, Auerbach BS, Nelson KE, et al. Antibody responses to *Haemophilus influenzae* type b vaccines in men with human immunodeficiency virus infection. N Engl J Med 1991;325:1837–1842.
161. Simberkoff MS, El Sadr W, Schiffman G, et al. *Streptococcus pneumoniae* infections and bacteremia in patients with acquired immune deficiency syndrome, with report of a vaccine failure. Am Rev Respir Dis 1984;130:1174–1176.
162. Halsey NA, Boulos R, Donnenberg AD, et al. Anti-tetanus antibody in umbilical cord blood from HIV-seropositive Haitian women. Presented at the 4th International Conference on AIDS, Stockholm, 1988.
163. Baende E, Ryder R, Halsey N, et al. Equally poor response to tetanus vaccine in HIV seropositive and seronegative mothers in Zaire. Presented at the 5th International AIDS Conference, Montreal, 1989.
164. Nelson KE, Clements ML, Miotti P, et al. The influence of human immunodeficiency virus infection on antibody responses to influenza vaccines. Ann Intern Med 1988;109:383–388.
165. Miotti PG, Nelson KE, Dallabetta GA, et al. The influence of HIV infection on antibody responses to a two-dose regimen of influenza vaccine. JAMA 1989;261:2512–2516.
166. Ragni MV, Ruben FL, Winkelstein A, et al. Antibody responses to immunization of patients with hemophilia with and without evidence of human immunodeficiency virus infection. J Lab Clin Med 1987;109:545–549.
167. Krasinski K, Borkowsky W. Measles and measles immunity in children infected with human immunodeficiency virus. JAMA 1989;261:2512–2516.
168. Oxtoby MS, Mvula M, Ryder R, et al. Measles and measles immunity in African children with HIV. Presented at the 28th Interscience Conference on Antimicrobial Agents and Chemotherapy. Los Angeles, 1988.
169. Kovamees J, Sheshberadaran H, Chiodi F, et al. Accentuated antibody response to paramyxoviruses in individuals infected with human immunodeficiency virus. J Med Virol 1988;26:41–48.
170. Kemper C, Zolopa A, Bhatia G, et al. Measles immunity in HIV infection. Presented at the 7th International Conference on AIDS, Florence, Italy, 1991.
171. Collier AC, Corey L, Murphy VL, et al. Antibody to human immunodeficiency virus and suboptimal response to hepatitis B vaccination. Ann Intern Med 1988;109:101–105.
172. Carne CA, Weller IVD, Waite J, et al. Impaired responsiveness of homosexual men with HIV antibodies to plasma derived hepatitis B vaccine. BMJ 1987;294:866–868.
173. Odaka N, Elred L, Cohn S, et al. Comparative immunogenicity of plasma and recombinant hepatitis B vaccines in homosexual men. JAMA 1988;260:3635–3637.
174. Geseman M, Scheiemann N, Brockmeyer N, et al. Clinical evaluation of a recombinant hepatitis B vaccine in HIV-infected vs. uninfected persons. In: Zuckerman AJ, ed. Viral hepatitis and liver disease. New York: Alan R. Liss, 1988:1076–1078.
175. Hadler SC, Judson FN, O'Malley PM, et al. Studies of hepatitis B vaccine in homosexual men. In: Coursaget P, Tong MJ, eds. Progress in hepatitis B immunization. London: John Libbey Eurotext, 1990:165–175.
176. McLaughlin M, Thomas P, Onorato I, et al. Use of live virus vaccines in HIV-infected children: a retrospective survey. Pediatrics 1988;82:229–233.
177. Dabis F, Msellati P, Lepage P, et al. HIV and adverse reactions following routine childhood immunization in Africa: a cohort study in Kigali, Rwanda. Presented at the 6th International AIDS Conference, San Francisco, 1990.
178. Redfield RR, Wright DC, James WD, et al. Disseminated vaccinia in a military recruit with human immunodeficiency virus disease. N Engl J Med 1987;316:673–676.
179. Armbruster C, Junker W, Vetter N, et al. Disseminated bacille Calmette-Guérin infection in an AIDS patient 30 years after BCG vaccination. J Infect Dis 1990;162:1216.
180. Centers for Disease Control and Prevention. Disseminated *Mycobacterium bovis* infection from BCG vaccination of a patient with acquired immunodeficiency syndrome. MMWR Morb Mortal Wkly Rep 1985;34:227–228.
181. Brichacek B, Swindells S, Janoff EN, et al. Increased plasma human immunodeficiency virus type 1 burden following antigenic challenge with pneumococcal vaccine. J Infect Dis 1996;174:1191–1199.
182. O-Brien WA, Grovit-Ferbas K, Namazi A, et al. Human immunodeficiency virus-type 1 replication can be increased in peripheral blood of seropositive patients after influenza vaccination. Blood 1995;86:1082–1089.
183. Stanley SK, Ostrowski MA, Justement JS, et al. Effect of immunization with a common recall antigen on viral expression in patients infected with human immunodeficiency virus type 1 [see comments]. N Engl J Med 1996;334:1222–1230.
184. Glesby MJ, Hoover DR, Farzadegan H, et al. Effect of influenza vaccination on human immunodeficiency virus type 1 load: a randomized, double-blind, placebo-controlled study. J Infect Dis 1996;174:1332–1336.
185. Huang KL, Ruben FL, Rinaldo CR, et al. Antibody responses after influenza and pneumococcal immunization in HIV-infected homosexual men. JAMA 1987;257:2047–2050.
186. Nelson KE, Clements ML, Miotti P, et al. The influence of human immunodeficiency virus infection on antibody responses to influenza vaccines. Ann Intern Med 1988;109:383–388.
187. Buchbinder S, Hessol N, Lifson A, et al. Does infection with hepatitis B virus or vaccination with plasma-derived hepatitis B vaccine accelerate progression to AIDS? Presented at the 6th International Conference on AIDS, San Francisco, 1990.
188. Immunization Practices Advisory Committee. Typhoid immunization. MMWR Morb Mortal Wkly Rep 1990;39:1–5.
189. Immunization Practices Advisory Committee. Yellow fever vaccine. MMWR Morb Mortal Wkly Rep 1990;39:1–6.

21

INTESTINAL PARASITIC INFECTIONS: CRYPTOSPORIDIOSIS AND MICROSPORIDIOSIS

Rosemary Soave and Elizabeth S. Didier

Cryptosporidium and microsporidia are protozoan parasites that were first described approximately a century ago but were not recognized as pathogens for humans until they were brought to the attention of the medical community by the acquired immunodeficiency syndrome (AIDS). It took the profound immune defect of AIDS to amplify disease caused by these parasites sufficiently that physicians finally took note. Both cryptosporidiosis and microsporidiosis are particularly devastating problems for patients with AIDS because of the absence of consistently effective therapy. The two parasites differ phylogenetically, taxonomically, and in the clinical expression of the disease they cause. Since the early 1980s, a tremendous surge of interest has been expressed in *Cryptosporidium* and microsporidia parasites as evidenced by an explosion of published articles. However, many crucial aspects of the epidemiology and immunopathogenesis of these infections are still unknown. Furthermore, improved methods for rapid, early diagnosis, and effective treatment are badly needed.

CRYPTOSPORIDIOSIS

Historical Highlights

Subsequent to a brief description, in 1895, by Clarke, of a coccidian in the stomach of mice, E.E. Tyzzer, in 1907, named and described, in accurate detail, *Cryptosporidium*, based on his studies of the gastric glands of mice (1, 2). *Cryptosporidium* (which means "little hidden spore" in Greek) was considered rare and both medically and economically insignificant for nearly a half-century. In 1955, the parasite was linked to gastrointestinal disease in young turkeys (3), and in 1971, it was found to be associated with bovine diarrhea (4), thus stimulating veterinary and agricultural interest. The first two cases of human cryptosporidiosis were reported in 1976 (5, 6), but the parasite was not considered important until 1981 to 1982, when it was linked with refractory diarrhea in patients with AIDS (7). Inclusion of chronic cryptosporidial enteritis as an AIDS-defining opportunistic infection resulted in increased detection, greater awareness of its devastating potential for the immunocompromised host, and significant frustration because of the absence of effective therapy (8–14).

In 1993, an estimated 403,000 people in Milwaukee, Wisconsin, became ill from *Cryptosporidium*-contaminated drinking water (15), and interest in detecting, controlling, and understanding the parasite surged over the next 5 years, as evidenced by an avalanche of publications and several workshops (16–21). The threat of *Cryptosporidium* to global health has become a challenge for public health and other government officials, the water industry, and health care providers (21).

With improvement in the management of human immunodeficiency virus (HIV) infection, and especially after the introduction of highly active antiretroviral therapy (HAART), the incidence of cryptosporidial infection, particularly the choleralike illness so often seen in patients with AIDS, has decreased (22, 23). Hopefully, this welcome development will not cause us to be lulled into complacency; indeed, it would be short-sighted to assume that this elusive global menace has been conquered.

Parasite

TAXONOMY AND PHYLOGENY

Cryptosporidium is one of many genera, referred to as coccidians, in the phylum Apicomplexa. Other genera closely related to *Cryptosporidium* include coccidians that can develop entirely in the gastrointestinal tract of vertebrates, *Isospora*, *Cyclospora*, and *Eimeria*, and the tissue cyst-forming coccidia that have an extraintestinal phase, *Sarcocystis* and *Toxoplasma*. *Cryptosporidium* is also related to coccidia found in the blood, the malaria-causing *Plasmodium* sp. and *Babesia* (24, 25).

Approximately 20 species of *Cryptosporidium* have been named after the host in which they were found, but some of these species are now considered to have been misidentified (24–26). Investigators commonly accept that at least two valid species infect birds, *C. baileyi* and *C. meleagridis,* and two infect mammals, *C. muris* and *C. parvum*; *C. parvum* is responsible for clinical illness in humans and in approximately 80 species of mammals.

Study of the molecular biology of *Cryptosporidium* is still in its infancy (27). Using different techniques, at least five, but perhaps up to eight, *C. parvum* chromosomes have been resolved. Phylogenetic relationships between *Cryptosporidium* and other apicomplexans have been studied by analysis of the 18S small subunit ribosomal RNA (srRNA); one study revealed no close relationships with other apicomplexans (28), whereas *Cryptosporidium* appeared most closely related to *Plasmodium* in another study (29). Further analysis of the srRNA nucleotide sequences of *C. parvum* and *C. muris* revealed greater than 99% sequence identity (30–31).

LIFE CYCLE

Cryptosporidium is an intracellular pathogen that infects and reproduces in epithelial cells lining the digestive or respiratory tracts of most vertebrates. The parasite's potential for causing unrelenting enteritis in patients with AIDS stems in part from certain unique features of its life cycle. *Cryptosporidium* completes its life cycle (Fig. 21.1) within a single host (monoxenous life cycle), similar to *Isospora* but unlike *Toxoplasma*. Infection starts with ingestion of the oocyst, generally transmitted by infected feces. After ingestion, the oocyst excysts, usually on exposure to reducing agents such as bile salts and digestive enzymes, but sometimes simply after exposure to warm aqueous solution alone, a characteristic that may explain why primary respiratory infection and autoinfection from endogenous oocysts are possible. Four banana-shaped, motile sporozoites are released and attach to the epithelial cell wall to form a dense five-layer attachment or feeder band (32). *Cryptosporidium* life cycle stages remain at the surface of the host cell, within a parasitophorous vacuole composed of two host cell and two parasite-derived membranes that make *Cryptosporidium* intracellular but extracytoplasmic (25, 32–34). The parasite has also been identified, however, in guinea pigs, in M cell cytoplasm adjacent to Peyer's patches, and in macrophages (32).

The sporozoites undergo merogony, or asexual multiplication, within the host cell, developing first into a trophozoite and then into one of two types of meronts, which release merozoites intraluminally. A type I meront or schizont produces six to eight merozoites that reinvade the host cell and recycle through the asexual portion of the life cycle to produce another meront and a powerful autoinfectious cycle. A type II meront or schizont has four or more merozoites that reinvade the host cell to begin the next reproductive phase, gametogony, or sexual maturation. These merozoites develop into either macrogamonts (ovum equivalent) or microgamonts (sperm equivalent); fertilization follows with zygote formation. The oocyst wall and four new sporozoites (sporogony) are then formed. The oocyst is excreted from the host cell and either excysts immediately within the host intestinal tract, initiating another autoinfectious cycle, or passes into the environment, fully sporulated and infectious. *Cryptosporidium* is the only coccidian oocyst that does not need to complete maturation after excretion. Autoinfection, the repetition of various phases of the life cycle in the same

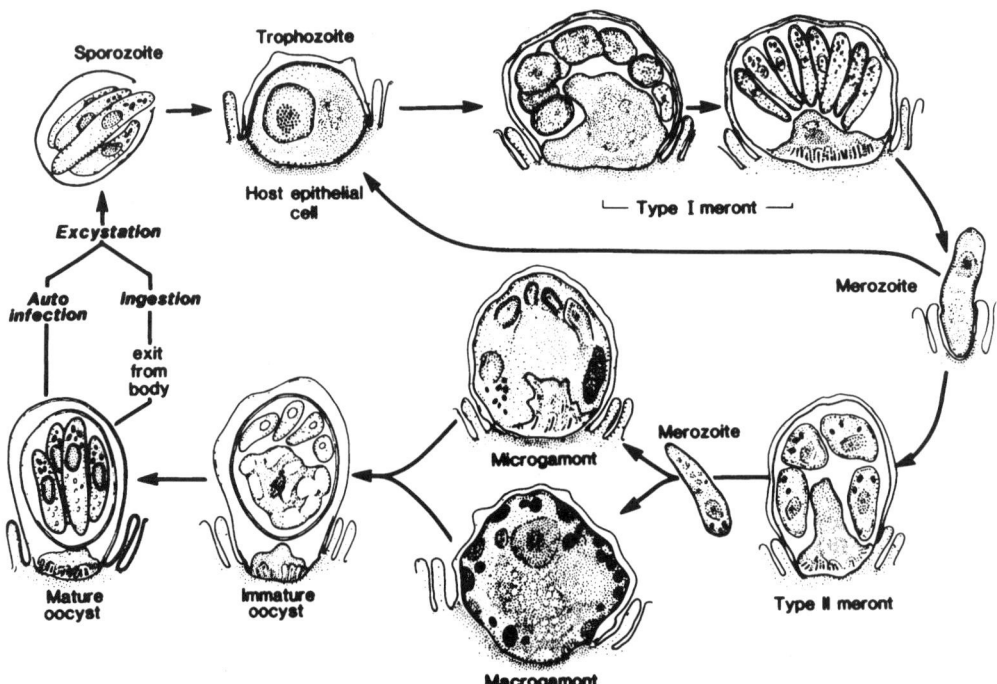

Figure 21.1. Life cycle of *Cryptosporidium*. (From Fayer R, Ungar BLP. *Cryptosporidium spp.* and cryptosporidiosis. Microbiol Rev 1986;50:458–483.)

host, is uncommon among other coccidia (24). Two distinct oocyst forms are believed to exist—80% with a two-layered environmentally resistant wall and 20% with a single-layered membrane that ruptures easily and reinfects the host (13). The time between oocyst ingestion and the excretion of newly developed oocysts varies with *Cryptosporidium* species and host; the experimentally determined prepatent period in humans ranges from 4 to 22 days, and the duration of oocyst excretion is generally 1 to 20 days (35), but it can be as long as 85 days (36).

The autoinfectious life cycle stages, both type 1 meronts and oocysts, are likely responsible for the persistent infections in immunodeficient persons and may also explain why ingestion of only a few oocysts can lead to severe disease regardless of host immune status (35, 37). Furthermore, introduction of this ubiquitous parasite, with its unique reproductive capacity and impressively resistant oocyst form, into people with severely impaired immunity, such as those with AIDS, has perhaps resulted in the creation of a human reservoir for the parasite and a mechanism for its own endless perpetuation.

Epidemiology

GEOGRAPHIC DISTRIBUTION AND PREVALENCE

Cryptosporidium is globally distributed among humans and many species of animals. Since the early 1980s, over 1000 reports have documented cryptosporidial infection in humans in well over 60 countries on all 6 inhabited continents (8–13, 18, 21, 38, 39). Most prevalence data from large-scale geographic surveys rely on examination of fecal specimens from selected, and not necessarily comparable, populations using various diagnostic techniques to detect *Cryptosporidium* oocysts. Accurate prevalence or incidence rates cannot be derived from these data because of bias related to study design, such as criteria for subject selection and diagnostic methods used.

Excluding documented outbreaks, infection rates reported in large-scale surveys conducted since the early 1980s, primarily in children not known to be infected with HIV, generally have ranged between 1 and 3% in the industrialized countries of Europe and North America and between 5 and 10% in less industrialized nations (38, 39, 40–47). More recently, higher infection rates have been reported, including 6%, 10%, and 12% in Spain (48), Italy (49, 50), and Romania (51), and, 26%, 29%, and 45% in Nigeria (52), Mexico (53), and Peru (54), respectively. If this trend toward an increase in infection rates is real, then the relative contribution of factors ranging from better diagnostics to an expanding global reservoir of infection in humans and animals needs to be explored.

In spite of their lack of comparability, review of the many geographically based studies of *Cryptosporidium* oocyst excretion suggests a higher prevalence of infection in children, particularly those less than 2 years of age who reside in less developed countries (38, 39, 40–54). Although infection with this parasite is often said to be seasonal, published reports differ on the season in which infection predominates. (38, 39, 48, 55–57).

Approximately 2.2% of all patients with AIDS and 3.5% of children with AIDS who are reported to the United States Centers for Disease Control and Prevention (CDC) have cryptosporidiosis as their AIDS-defining illness (14, 58–63). Overall, the prevalence of cryptosporidial infection in persons with HIV infection or AIDS ranges from 3 to 20% in the United States and Europe and from 4 to 48% in developing countries (8, 14, 18, 38, 39, 56, 57, 59, 61–78). In studies of hospitalized or severely symptomatic HIV-infected patients in the United States and Europe, between 11 and 21% of AIDS patients with diarrhea excreted *Cryptosporidium* oocysts (14, 59, 61, 62, 64, 65, 70–73). Because diarrhea occurs in approximately one-half of all patients with AIDS each year, the annual rate of cryptosporidial infection among all patients with AIDS is estimated to approach 5 to 15% (59). Worldwide, one sees significant variation in the spectrum of opportunistic infections by geographic area (79). Although the recent decrease in the incidence of cryptosporidial infection in HIV-infected patients (80, 81) has been attributed primarily to enhanced immunity achieved with the use of highly effective antiretroviral regimens (22, 23), a decrease had already been noted between 1983 and 1986 in Los Angeles (66) and since 1988 in the United Kingdom (68, 71).

Despite the decrease in incidence, the impact of cryptosporidial infection on morbidity, mortality, and health care costs continues to be significant (42, 61–63). Cryptosporidial infection was associated with an elevated relative hazard of death in comparison with other AIDS-defining diagnoses in a series from San Francisco (63).

Few reports of cryptosporidial infection in immunocompromised hosts exist other than in HIV-infected persons. In studies of patients with neoplastic disease and diarrhea, rates of cryptosporidial infection ranged from 1.3 to 17% (82–85). Cryptosporidial and microsporidial infection were found in 6.3 and 2.3% of Egyptian patients with varying types of immunocompromise including corticosteroid therapy, renal failure, and malignant disease (86). In a Turkish study, 18.8% of renal transplant recipients were found to have cryptosporidial infection (87).

Seroprevalence studies, in which immunofluorescent antibody (IFA) or enzyme-linked immunosorbent assay (ELISA) techniques were used to detect specific anti-*Cryptosporidium* immunoglobulin M (IgM), IgG, or IgA, suggest that *Cryptosporidium* infections some time in life may, in fact, be more common than surveys of fecal oocyst excretion can demonstrate (8, 38, 39, 69, 77, 88–95). In Australia, Europe, and North America, seroprevalence rates range between 25 and 58%, whereas in Latin America, they are generally higher than 50% and have been found to be as high as 94.6% in Northeast Brazil. In one study, 42.3 and 57.5% of persons studied in China and Brazil, respectively, were seropositive compared with 16.9% of children and young adults in Virginia (93). Results from most studies confirm that seroprevalence rates are higher in developing countries, and these rates increase with increasing age and with certain risk factors including attendance at a day care center (95), exposure to cattle (91), and travel to developing countries (88). Seroprevalence data in patients with AIDS or other types of immunocompromise are limited. Data obtained in two prevalence studies, of a similar population of HIV-infected New York City residents, conducted 5 years apart, reveal a decrease in the incidence of *Cryptosporidium*-positive stools but no change in the seroprevalence rate (69, 81).

TRANSMISSION

Cryptosporidium species are transmitted by ingestion of oocysts that are present in the feces of infected humans or animals. Thus, *Cryptosporidium* is spread from animals to humans, from humans to animals, from person to person, and through ingestion of fecally contaminated water or food or through contact with environmentally infected surfaces.

Factors that facilitate the spread of *Cryptosporidium* include the following: 1) infected humans and animals excrete large numbers of highly infectious oocysts in their stool, and excretion may continue well beyond resolution of clinical symptoms (36); 2) the infective dose of ingested oocysts is low (35); and 3) the oocysts are highly resistant to commonly used disinfectants (25). Furthermore, a lack of host specificity exists among cryptosporidial isolates; well over 80 mammals are known to be infected with *C. parvum*, the species that infects humans. *Cryptosporidium* species that infect birds, reptiles, and fish do not appear to be infectious for humans (18, 25). To date, only one case of infection with an organism resembling *C. baileyi*, a species that commonly infects birds, has been reported in an HIV-infected human (96).

Zoonotic spread of *Cryptosporidium*, from farm and laboratory animals, primarily through occupational exposure has been well documented (8, 10, 13, 18, 38, 39, 59). *Cryptosporidium* is ubiquitous in farm animals; investigators have estimated that more than 50% of dairy cows shed *C. parvum* oocysts in their stool (97). Although the number of humans that have direct contact with cows and other farm animals is limited, inadvertent or indirect exposure may occur. Educational visits to farms and livestock markets have been implicated in the acquisition of cryptosporidial infection by groups of students (98–100). Attendance at riding stables, use of animal manure to fertilize gardens, and drinking unpasteurized milk may be linked to the spread of infection (59, 101). Infected dogs, cats, and other exotic pets have been putative sources in some cases of cryptosporidiosis, but the direction of spread or the presence of a source common to both could not be determined (25, 38, 59, 102–104.). Fomites and rodents are also potential reservoirs for the spread of cryptosporidial infection to humans, but this type of transmission has not been documented (105, 106).

Person-to-person spread, an important mode by which *Cryptosporidium* is transmitted among humans, has been well documented among children and their caretakers in day care centers (107), in members of the household of infected cases (108, 109), and in nosocomial spread among health care workers and their patients (110–114). Sexual practices in which a person has oral contact with fecal material of an infected person constitute a high-risk exposure that has been linked to development of cryptosporidial infection in HIV-infected persons (59, 70–73).

The first documented foodborne outbreak of cryptosporidiosis was recorded in 1993, in Maine, where children who drank fresh-pressed apple cider contaminated by cow manure became ill (115). In at least two subsequent outbreaks, apple cider and chicken salad, respectively, were implicated (116, 117); the former was also associated with *Escherichia coli* 0157:H7 infection (117). Cryptosporidial contamination of food is most likely underrecognized because of difficulties with detection of the parasite in food (118, 119).

Perhaps most troubling has been the spread of *Cryptosporidium* through contaminated water. Numerous well-documented outbreaks of cryptosporidiosis have been attributed to drinking water in the United States, the United Kingdom, and other parts of the world (15, 20, 38, 59, 120–129). Surface water (rivers, lakes, streams), springs, and well and ground water have all been implicated as sources. Although in each of these outbreaks, water utilities met existing government regulations, such as the United States Environmental Protection Agency (USEPA) standards for drinking water quality, it has become apparent that the standards are not adequate to protect consumers from waterborne cryptosporidiosis (20, 120). Outbreaks have also been associated with recreational water exposure, including swimming pools, wave pools, and water slides at amusement parks (130–134). In these cases, disinfection measures that use chlorination are known to be totally inadequate for protection against *Cryptosporidium*.

The largest waterborne outbreak ever recorded in the United States occurred in 1993, when 403,000 persons in Milwaukee, Wisconsin became ill because of *Cryptosporidium*-contaminated drinking water (15, 135). More than 4000 people were hospitalized, and at least 100 deaths occurred, primarily in immunocompromised (HIV-infected) and elderly hosts. The magnitude of this outbreak resulted in heightened public awareness of the potential threat posed by this parasite. The presence of *Cryptosporidium* oocysts in 65 to 97% of surface waters (e.g., rivers, lakes) had already been established (120). However, in 1997, the USEPA began to implement the Information Collection Rule, which requires utilities to test water routinely for *Cryptosporidium*; indeed, the presence of low-level, intermittent contamination has been documented (20, 59, 120, 136). Because the oocysts cannot easily be characterized by species, and viability, and because the number is often so low, the potential threat to the health of the public posed by low-level, endemic contamination has yet to be established. Risk-assessment models and prospective studies are being used to evaluate the risk of infection from low levels of oocysts in water (20, 81, 120, 137–141). Surveillance has been heightened, and cryptosporidiosis is now reportable in 37 states (59, 142). An explosion of interest has occurred in developing methods for detecting *Cryptosporidium* in water, and various kits are now commercially available (120, 142–144). The challenge of developing water treatment and disinfection practices that will make drinking water safe from resistant parasites such as *Cryptosporidium* has become a major priority for the water industry (20, 38, 59, 120, 142, 144). Since the Milwaukee outbreak, numerous workshops and symposia have been convened to address the problems of epidemic and endemic waterborne cryptosporidiosis (20, 142). In 1994, the CDC, in collaboration with other federal agencies, state and local health departments, and other interested parties, created the Working Group on Waterborne Cryptosporidiosis (145). This group meets through regularly scheduled conference calls to exchange ideas, make recommendations, establish guidelines, and address the many issues related to waterborne transmission of *Cryptosporidium* (142, 146).

MOLECULAR EPIDEMIOLOGY

Precise determination of strain variation among cryptosporidial isolates from epidemic and isolated cases would allow for source identification, characterization of risk factors, and linkage with clinical and epidemiologic outcomes. Numerous investigators have used various techniques including antigen–antibody and isoenzyme analysis, two-dimensional gel electrophoresis, and Western blotting to detect differences in isolates from varied geographic areas and from animals and humans (38, 147–150). The typing or fingerprinting of infective organisms using sophisticated molecular techniques is a more powerful tool for characterizing differences among isolates, and these techniques are just beginning to be applied to *Cryptosporidium* (27, 151–157). Various studies, including a molecular analysis of 39 human and bovine *C. parvum* isolates (157), have indicated the presence of two genotypes, thus suggesting the presence of two distinct transmission cycles of *C. parvum* in humans.

DISINFECTION

Infection with *Cryptosporidium* occurs after ingestion of highly resistant oocysts, which can remain viable for many months in the environment and when stored in normal saline at 4°C in a laboratory (13, 25). Oocysts are not easily destroyed by extremes of temperature, but they are sensitive to desiccation and ultraviolet irradiation (25, 158–160). Oocysts can be rendered noninfectious at temperatures at or above 64.2°C for 5 minutes and 74.2°C for 1 minute (25, 160). Although they can withstand freezing at or above −20°C for extended periods, they do not survive at or below −70°C (25, 160, 161). *Cryptosporidium* oocysts are resistant to most commonly used disinfectants (25, 158, 163, 164). Those chemicals that render the oocysts noninfectious must be used at high concentrations or are toxic. Aqueous or gaseous ammonia, hydrogen peroxide, and ozone appear to be the most applicable substances for adequate disinfection (25).

Clinical Features

SUSCEPTIBILITY

Persons of both genders, all ages, and any underlying state of health and immune function are susceptible to infection with *Cryptosporidium*. The true distribution of cryptosporidial infection across different age groups is not known. Although data from epidemiologic surveys suggest that young age (less than 2 years) may be associated with increased susceptibility to infection, possibly because of factors such as immunologic immaturity and lack of hygiene (8, 10, 11, 18, 39–54), cryptosporidiosis probably is underrecognized in other groups such as the elderly (165, 166).

SPECTRUM OF CLINICAL ILLNESS

The spectrum of human illness resulting from cryptosporidial infection is broad; it can vary from a self-limited bout of diarrhea lasting, at most, 1 to 2 weeks, to months of persistent enteritis, complicated by extraintestinal disease. Symptoms can be mild, moderate, severe, or choleralike and fulminant irrespective of illness duration (8–11, 39, 167, 168). Anyone who is exposed to *Cryptosporidium* can become infected, but the determinants of clinical disease are poorly understood. The duration of cryptosporidial disease is determined primarily by host immune function; prolonged infections usually occur in those with immune dysfunction or in extremely young animals (8–11, 39, 167–172). Nutritional status and the absence of mature intestinal flora may also contribute to the duration and severity of the illness, but the role of these factors is not clear (18, 44, 54, 104, 173–179). Parasite virulence factors probably also contribute to modulating illness severity and duration, but they have not yet been characterized. Adding further to the complexity of clinical illness with *Cryptosporidium* is the considerable variation in clinical course; mild transient infections have been documented in immunocompromised hosts (180–182), and severe, protracted illness has been documented during primary HIV infection (183), as well as in apparently immunocompetent children and adults (184–187).

Protracted cryptosporidial infection is most commonly associated with HIV infection, but it also occurs in persons with congenital immunodeficiency, including hypogammaglobulinemia, IgA deficiency, X-linked immunodeficiency with hyper-IgM, interferon-γ (IFN-γ) deficiency (6, 8–12, 169, 170, 188–192), concurrent viral infections (193, 194), thalassemia major (195), and diabetes mellitus (196, 197) and in patients taking exogenous immunosuppressive agents after solid organ and bone marrow transplantation or for neoplastic or other underlying diseases (108, 112, 197–204). Malnourished children are also more susceptible to chronic, severe cryptosporidiosis, and conversely, cryptosporidial infection may exacerbate malnutrition and may delay developmental milestones (54, 104, 173–177). Three reports of cryptosporidial infection in the late stages of pregnancy have been published; although maternal illness was severe and was accompanied by fetal distress and failure to thrive, illness resolved completely in all mothers and babies (205–207).

Cryptosporidial illness was not protracted in immunocompetent hosts with inflammatory bowel disease who became infected during the Milwaukee outbreak (208), nor did it exacerbate inflammatory bowel disease in HIV-infected persons (209). Whether cryptosporidial infection of the immunocompromised host, particularly patients with AIDS, reflects endogenous reactivation of previously acquired infection or whether it always represents de novo acquisition is not known.

Asymptomatic cryptosporidial infection has been well documented in immunocompetent and immunocompromised adults and children in various parts of the world, but the true magnitude of asymptomatic carriage and the patterns and duration of oocyst shedding in the asymptomatic host have not been characterized (11, 39, 49, 100, 107, 210–212). Asymptomatic oocyst shedding is common among day care center attendees (11, 107, 211). Of 154 adult patients in New York City who underwent endoscopy for abdominal symptoms other than diarrhea, 18 had *Cryptosporidium* detected in duodenal aspirates, but only 7 had organisms identified in feces (213); these findings have not been substantiated in subsequent studies (214, 215). Asymptomatic intestinal infections may be underestimated inasmuch as oocysts may be difficult to find when the number shed is modest. Whether such infections are truly asymptomatic or represent oocyst detection sometime after a brief, mild, or atypical clinical illness remains speculative (107, 212). The significance of asymptomatic infection is uncertain beyond the increased potential for inadvertent transmission.

CLINICAL MANIFESTATIONS

In the immunocompetent host, the incubation period for cryptosporidial infection ranges from 2 to 10 days, as documented in several case reports as well as in a human volunteer study of *Cryptosporidium parvum* infection (35, 36, 39, 108, 216). Enteritis is usually explosive in onset, lasts approximately 10 to 14 days, and is followed by complete clinical and parasitologic recovery. Oocyst shedding usually lags behind clinical resolution, sometimes by as much as 1 to 2 months. Recurrent infection was common in individuals who acquired the infection during the Milwaukee outbreak of 1993 (135, 217), but it is otherwise poorly documented.

Unlike in the immunocompetent host, the onset of cryptosporidiosis in the HIV-infected host is usually insidious; diarrheal symptoms may precede detection of the organism by weeks to months. When HIV-infected patients have been exposed to a known source of infection, as occurred in the Milwaukee outbreak (15, 218), or after exposure to contaminated ice from a vending machine in an Italian hospital (112), the mean incubation period (13 days) was slightly longer than that recorded for the immunocompetent host. In HIV-infected adults and children, cryptosporidiosis lasting longer than 30 days is part of the CDC case definition of AIDS, and it usually occurs in patients with CD4 counts below 200 cells/mm^3 (14, 218–225). In these individuals, symptoms may wax and wane in severity, or the illness may escalate unrelentingly as immune function becomes more deranged. Spontaneous remission of cryptosporidiosis has occurred after initiation of antiretroviral or immunomodulatory therapy or at any stage along the spectrum of HIV infection for reasons that have not been explained. Cryptosporidiosis is often a devastating complication for persons with AIDS; it contributes significantly to morbidity and hastens death.

The clinical manifestations of cryptosporidial infection include watery, nonbloody diarrhea that can be voluminous and choleralike, cramping abdominal pain, nausea, vomiting, weight loss, anorexia, urgency, incontinence, flatulence, excessive borborygmi, and fever. Diarrhea, abdominal pain, nausea, and vomiting are the most common complaints.

Cryptosporidiosis has no characteristic laboratory features. Leukocytosis is not a common finding, and eosinophilia, a frequent finding in patients with AIDS, is not specific for cryptosporidial infection (9, 11, 39). Malabsorption of fat, D-xylose, and vitamin B_{12} and other metabolic changes have been noted in association with cryptosporidial infection in AIDS patients (39, 170, 226–230). Abdominal radiographic findings may include prominent mucosal folds, air–fluid levels, distended loops of bowel, and disordered motility; these findings are nonspecific and nondiagnostic. Computed tomographic studies are similarly nonspecific.

Infected persons appear to shed oocysts on a daily basis, and oocyst excretion appears to persist for as long as 1 to 2 months after symptoms resolve (8–11, 36, 39, 169, 230–232). The relationship among the intensity of clinical symptoms, the magnitude of oocyst shedding in stool, and intestinal injury is not clear (226, 233, 234). Severe symptoms are usually associated with a high oocyst burden, but in a study of experimentally infected human volunteers, oocyst excretion in infected but asymptomatic individuals was not significantly lower than oocyst excretion in patients who had diarrhea (233).

The differential diagnosis of enteric cryptosporidiosis in HIV-infected patients includes *Shigella*, *Salmonella*, *Campylobacter*, *Mycobacterium avium* complex, *Clostridium difficile*, *Giardia lamblia*, *Entamoeba histolytica*, *Isospora belli*, *Cyclospora*, microsporidia, and cytomegalovirus. Concomitant infection with one or more of the foregoing pathogens occurs frequently in HIV-infected patients with cryptosporidiosis. Coinfection with cytomegalovirus is common, but dual *Cryptosporidium* and microsporidia infection is documented with increasing frequency (235–238).

Cryptosporidial infection of the gallbladder or biliary tract is the most commonly reported complication of cryptosporidiosis in the HIV-infected individual; it usually occurs when CD4+ counts drop below 50 cells/mm^3 (8–12, 14, 39, 72, 218, 239–249). Conversely, *Cryptosporidium* is a commonly identified pathogen in AIDS patients with cholangiopathy, but its role in causing disease is not always clear (246–248). The true prevalence of this complication cannot be accurately determined because invasive procedures are required for diagnosis. Using both clinical criteria and strict parasitologic diagnosis, between 13 and 82% of AIDS patients with intestinal cryptosporidiosis have been reported to have cryptosporidial cholecystitis or cholangiopathy (218, 221, 242, 243, 246–248, 250). Clinical manifestations of acalculous cholecystitis or biliary cryptosporidiosis include abdominal pain, commonly in the right upper quadrant, fever, nausea, and vomiting. Serum alkaline phosphatase and γ-glutamyl transpeptidase levels are elevated, sometimes markedly, whereas serum transaminase levels are often normal or slightly raised. Jaundice is uncommon, and its presence should prompt a search for other causes of illness.

Sonographic or computed tomographic imaging usually shows an enlarged gallbladder with a thickened wall and dilated or irregular intrahepatic and extrahepatic biliary ducts with a normal or stenotic distal common bile duct. Cholangiography may reveal papillary stenosis or pruning of the intrahepatic bile ducts with beading of the bile ducts and dilatation of the common bile duct (239, 240, 242, 244, 246, 250–253). Biliary cryptosporidiosis may mimic malignancy (254, 255). Definitive diagnosis is made by detection of parasitic forms on histologic examination of the gallbladder, or ampullary tissue, or examination of the bile for oocysts. Oocysts are not necessarily detectable in fecal specimens even when they are present in bile. Concurrent infection with cytomegalovirus, *Enterobacter cloacae*, *Mycobacterium avium* complex, microsporidia, *Isospora*, cytomegalovirus, or fungi has been reported (239, 245, 251, 254). Therapeutic intervention is most often aimed at palliation of the major symptom, abdominal pain. Sphincterotomy, T-tube drainage, and cholecystectomy have been used with variable success (240, 249, 251). Papillotomy is helpful if the patient has obstruction from papillary stenosis, but the benefits are often transient (242, 252). The ultimate prognosis is poor (218, 242, 245, 248). Only 17% of the AIDS patients who developed biliary cryptosporidiosis during the Milwaukee outbreak were alive at the end of 1 year as compared with 52% of the AIDS patients who had cryptosporidiosis without biliary involvement (218).

Pancreatic duct infection or pancreatitis has been described in association with cryptosporidiosis, in immunocompetent and immunocompromised hosts (240, 241, 250, 256–259). As with cholangiopathy, the cause of pancreatitis in AIDS patients is multifactorial and can include drugs, neoplasms, and infection with multiple pathogens (257, 258, 260). Pancreatic abnormalities are often present in patients with cryptosporidial sclerosing cholangitis and may be responsible for the persistent pain that often occurs despite sphincterotomy (250). Other intestinal complications including gastropathy, gastric antral stricture (261–263), toxic megacolon (264), enterovesical fistula (265), and pneumatosis cystoides intestinales (266, 267) have also been reported in AIDS patients with cryptosporidiosis.

Whether detection of *Cryptosporidium* in the respiratory tract reflects true disease, bronchial colonization, or contamination of secretions by aspiration from the intestinal tract is controversial. Approximately 60 cases of pulmonary cryptosporidiosis have been described since 1980 (39, 72, 84, 200, 241, 256, 268–274) and summarized in a review (273). Symptoms associated with respiratory cryptosporidiosis include shortness of breath, hoarseness, wheezing, croup, and, most often, cough (273); severe pulmonary dysfunction has rarely been described (274). In a study of 36 HIV-positive patients with respiratory symptoms, those with and without pulmonary cryptosporidiosis were indistinguishable (270). Not all patients with respiratory tract cryptosporidiosis have diarrhea, and stool examination to detect *Cryptosporidium* is not always performed. Chest radiographic findings include infiltrates or increased bronchial markings, but often the chest radiograph is normal. Organisms have been identified in sputum, tracheal aspirates, bronchoalveolar lavage fluid, brush and lung biopsy specimens, and alveolar exudate, and they have been seen attached to the surface of bronchial mucosal cells or in macrophages. In most instances, other pulmonary pathogens such as cytomegalovirus, *Pneumocystis carinii*, *Mycobacterium tuberculosis*, or atypical mycobacterial species have been concurrently detected, although in a few HIV-infected patients, *Cryptosporidium* was the only pathogen identified, for up to 9 months after initial diagnosis in one case (270, 274). Cryptosporidial laryngotracheitis, sinusitis, and otitis media have also been reported (275–277). *Cryptosporidium* has also been detected in the nasal mucosa of an AIDS patient and in the conjunctiva of rhesus monkeys infected with simian immunodeficiency virus (SIV) (278, 279).

Three immunologically healthy patients with *Cryptosporidium* enteritis concurrently developed reactive arthritis without other obvious causes (280, 281). Each patient had joint involvement (wrists, hands, knees, ankles, feet) within 7 days of *Cryptosporidium* infection, followed by complete spontaneous resolution. A child with Reiter's syndrome and cryptosporidial gastroenteritis has also been reported (282).

No reports of cases of disseminated cryptosporidiosis have been published. One adult patient with leukemia and disseminated candidiasis was found to have *Cryptosporidium* in the intestinal epithelium and respiratory parenchyma at autopsy, as well as in the lumen of submucosal colonic vessels, a finding suggesting possible hematogenous dissemination (283).

Pathology and Pathogenesis

The gross and histopathologic changes associated with cryptosporidial infections in humans are nonspecific. On biopsy or autopsy of immunocompromised patients with cryptosporidiosis, organisms have been found throughout the intestinal tract, from esophagus to rectum and including the appendix, gallbladder, and bile and pancreatic ducts, within colonic blood vessels, and in the respiratory tract, sinuses, and nasal mucosa (8–13, 18, 39, 243, 284). Histopathologic studies of *Cryptosporidium*-infected immunologically healthy patients are limited. Microscopically, endogenous stages of the parasite have been identified within a parasitophorous vacuole inside epithelial cells but in an extracytoplasmic position (32–34) (Fig. 21.2). Histologic changes in the intestinal tract include villus atrophy, blunting,

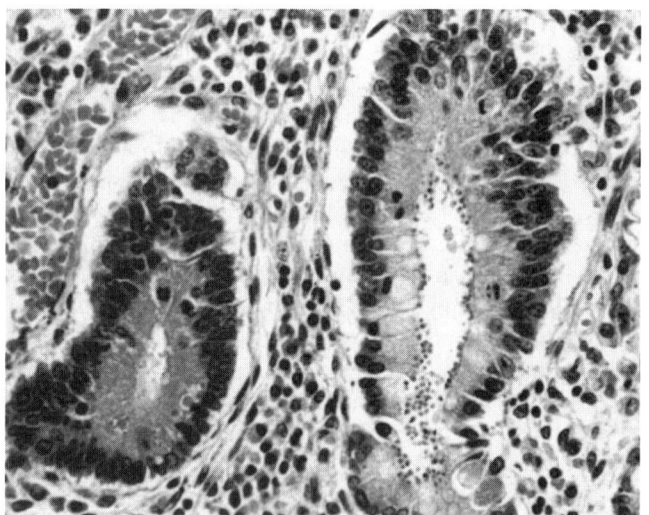

Figure 21.2. Section of human intestinal epithelium from an AIDS patient with overwhelming *Cryptosporidium* infection. Organisms are seen studding the microvillous border (hematoxylin and eosin stain; light microscopic examination). (Courtesy of Dr. Timothy P. Flanigan, the Miriam Hospital, Providence, RI.)

fusion, or loss and crypt hyperplasia. Inflammatory changes include infiltration of the lamina propria with lymphocytes, neutrophils, plasma cells, and macrophages.

Several investigators have sought to correlate morphologic changes with the severity of cryptosporidial illness in immunocompromised adults (226, 227, 234) and immunocompetent children (185). In a study of naturally infected human patients, severe duodenal morphologic abnormalities and diarrhea were associated with high-intensity infection, but diarrhea was also present in patients who had no morphologic abnormalities and low-intensity infection (226, 234). Investigation of the distribution of cryptosporidial organisms in the gastrointestinal tract revealed that illness was more severe in patients with proximal small bowel involvement compared with those who had primarily colonic infection (227). Severe intestinal dysfunction also appears to be associated with crypt rather than villous infection (185, 227).

The pathogenesis of human cryptosporidiosis is poorly understood, but studies have begun to unravel the complex interplay of multiple potential mechanisms that may be operative (285, 286). Severe epithelial cell damage, malabsorption, and reduced sodium chloride absorption in response to prostaglandins, which are believed to act directly on the epithelium and indirectly through enteric nerves, have been documented in perfusion studies of the *Cryptosporidium*-infected piglet model (287–289). The absorption defect and resulting secretory diarrhea may be partially mediated by reactive oxygen metabolites and are reversed with prostaglandin synthesis inhibitors, glutamine, and peptide YY (289, 290). However, solute malabsorption has not been documented in *Cryptosporidium*-infected human patients (226, 227, 291). In vitro studies using cell monolayers and in vivo studies in humans and in the piglet model have revealed the loss of mucosal barrier function (292–295). The voluminous watery diarrhea, often associated with cryptosporidiosis, is reminiscent of cholera and a toxin-mediated process, with hypersecretion of fluids and electrolytes, although cytopathic changes in cell lines have not been demonstrated (292, 293). Enterotoxic activity has been identified in stool from *Cryptosporidium*-infected cattle and humans; whether the activity was due to a parasite-derived enterotoxin or to a host-derived factor such as a secretory hormone is not clear (296, 297). The role of inflammatory cytokines in the pathogenesis of cryptosporidiosis is gaining interest, but studies are as yet inconclusive (298–300).

Immune Response

Most of our current knowledge of the immune response to cryptosporidial infection has been generated over the past 10 years. Significant progress has been made, but the components of host immunity that confer resistance to cryptosporidial infection, limit its spread, and ultimately mediate eradication remain poorly understood (18, 285, 301–303). Because it is beyond the scope of this chapter to present all the studies in great detail, interested readers are referred to published reviews (18, 301).

Infection and clinical illness are generally self-limited in immunocompetent hosts including humans, nonhuman primates, and several animal species, and they are protracted in the immunodeficient host, including those with congenital or acquired, diffuse or selective γ-globulin deficiencies, T-cell abnormalities, or IFN-γ deficiency (8–14, 18, 169, 170, 188–192, 301–304). Thus, both B- and T-lymphocyte–mediated processes are likely involved, and they may be differentially important during extracellular and intracellular portions of the *Cryptosporidium* life cycle.

Specific anticryptosporidial IgG, IgA, IgM, IgE, and secretory IgA have been detected by ELISA, IFA, or Western blot in the serum and secretions of AIDS patients with persistent infection, immunocompetent humans, and animals with natural or experimental infections (8, 18, 38, 39, 69, 77, 88–95, 176, 301, 305–315). Specific antibodies usually appear within 1 to 2 weeks of the onset of *Cryptosporidium* infection and persist for varying lengths of time. The humoral immune response appears to correlate with resolution of infection and oocyst shedding in most immunocompetent mammals, but it does not correlate with oocyst shedding in either patients with AIDS (308) or experimentally infected mice (313, 314). Serum and fecal IgA responses in patients with AIDS appear to be predominantly of the IgA1 subclass (315). This finding warrants further study because most neutralization-sensitive *Cryptosporidium* epitopes are glycoconjugates, and they are more commonly associated with an IgA2 subclass response (18, 301, 306–310, 316–320).

Passively acquired antibodies may play a role in the control of cryptosporidial infection. Several studies have recorded a lower prevalence of infection for breast-fed infants (321, 322), but passive lacteal immunity does not appear to be effective in animals (18, 39, 301, 323). Orally administered hyperimmune bovine colostrum (HBC) confers at least partial protection against *Cryptosporidium* in mice and calves (18, 301), and mixed results have been achieved in humans (324–327).

The presumed role of acquired immunity in limiting cryptosporidial infection has fostered a search for potentially immunogenic *Cryptosporidium* antigens. Many parasitic antigens ranging from less than 14 kd to more than 200 kd have been found to react with serum and fecal antibodies from infected humans and animals (18, 150, 301, 306–310, 316–320). Several immunodominant antigens in the 23- to 35-kd range are recognized by serum IgM or IgG from most infected humans; other antigens are less consistently recognized, and considerable heterogeneity occurs from individual to individual. Further studies are needed to determine the functional significance of the parasite antigens that have been characterized and to identify those that could be species-specific.

Investigators generally have recognized that cell-mediated immunity is important in the control of cryptosporidial infection, but studies of cell immunology are recent. Most of the studies have been conducted in the laboratory rodent model and in naturally or experimentally infected calves (18, 301). Accumulating evidence indicates that control of infection requires the presence of T cells, particularly subpopulations that are T-cell receptor $\alpha\beta+$ or CD4+, and IFN-γ (18, 301, 328–334). The role of other immune factors including inflammatory cells such as macrophages, cytokines other than IFN-γ, and nitric oxide has not yet been clarified (335–337). The relationship between cell-mediated and humoral-mediated responses, particularly at the level of the mucosal immune system of the gut, is beginning to generate considerable interest.

Diagnosis

Diagnosis of *Cryptosporidium* infection is based either on identification of parasite developmental stages in small intestinal biopsy sections or detection of parasite oocysts or antigens in feces or body fluids. On histologic examination of tissue sections, the spherical parasite, found on the brush border of mucosal epithelial surfaces, seems to project into the lumen because of its intracellular but extracytoplasmic position. It appears basophilic with hematoxylin and eosin staining; other tissue stains do not improve its visibility. Electron microscopy, which allows resolution of cellular detail, has been used for initial or confirmatory diagnosis (8, 143, 338–340). However, biopsy specimens necessitate an invasive procedure and are difficult to fix without autolysis or separation of the organism from the cell surface. Furthermore, because parasite distribution is often patchy, unaffected intestinal segments may be sampled; in one study, only 4 of 11 patients shedding *Cryptosporidium* in their feces had organisms identified on biopsy (338).

Detection of cryptosporidial oocysts in feces is rendered difficult by their small size and morphologic similarity to other fecal components such as yeasts. Giemsa-stained *Cryptosporidium* oocysts were identified in the feces of calves in 1978 (341) and in humans in 1980 (342); with this stain, both oocysts, generally 4 to 6 µm in diameter, and similarly sized yeast cells stain purple. Since the early 1980s, numerous methods have been developed for optimal detection of oocysts in stool samples as well as in duodenal aspirates, bile, or respiratory secretions. Approximately 75% of clinical laboratories use a modified acid-fast staining method, which was first described in 1981 (343) and is now considered a mainstay of diagnosis (18, 143, 344, 345). Round oocysts stain red or pink, whereas yeast cells and fecal debris take the color of the blue or green counterstain. Sometimes sporozoites can be clearly seen within the oocyst. The red color, however, may be unevenly distributed because of variable carbol fuchsin uptake by the oocyst wall (8, 143, 344). Size is particularly important in differentiating *Cryptosporidium* oocysts (4 to 6 µm) from other acid-fast organisms such as *Cyclospora* (8 to 10 µm) (346). Although acid-fast staining methods are inexpensive, easy-to-perform, and specific, their sensitivity is low (41 to 67%), especially when diarrheal illness is mild (347, 348). There are numerous alternatives to the acid-fast stain that can be used with bright-field microscopy; examples include various negative stains, the safranin–methylene blue, and the aniline–carbol methyl violet–tartrazine stains (8, 18, 143, 344, 345, 347, 349). Fluorescent staining methods such as acridine orange, auramine–rhodamine, 4′,6-diamidino-2-phenylindole (DAPI), and various others can also be can used (8, 18, 143, 344, 345, 349). Although more sensitive than bright-field stains and thus useful for screening, fluorescent stains lack specificity and neither provide a permanent record nor allow visualization of internal oocyst structure. Attempts have also been made to develop stains that simultaneously detect *Cryptosporidium* and microsporidia (350). Available staining techniques have been reviewed extensively (18, 142, 143).

IFA and antigen-capture enzyme immunoassays (EIA) that use oocyst-reactive monoclonal antibodies are commercially available and widely used in clinical and research laboratories (18, 143, 351–359). These new techniques are more specific and sensitive than any of the staining methods, but they are more costly, and they do not detect other acid-fast organisms such as *Cyclospora* and *Isospora*. Despite the avalanche of new diagnostic methods available for *Cryptosporidium* diagnosis, no consensus exists on the optimal method; most laboratories use the method that works best for them for reasons of easy operation and cost. Irrespective of the method used, accurate diagnosis requires experienced technologists and special care when new techniques are implemented, to avoid costly mistakes such as pseudo-outbreaks of cryptosporidial infection (360, 361).

A technique in which oocysts labeled with a cell wall–specific monoclonal antibody are counted by flow cytometry has been reported to be four times as sensitive as the direct fluorescent antibody assay and useful for detecting as few as 10^3 oocysts/mL of human feces; further studies are needed to determine the usefulness of this method in the diagnostic laboratory (362).

The application of polymerase chain reaction techniques holds promise for the detection of small numbers of oocysts in fecal or environmental samples and for distinguishing specific *Cryptosporidium* species and strain isolates. Several *Cryptosporidium* DNA and RNA segments have been proposed as valuable targets for parasite detection as well as for determination of parasite viability and infectivity (18, 27, 118, 143, 153, 363–366). These advanced methods of detection are useful in working with purified oocyst preparations in the research laboratory, but further work is needed to determine their usefulness when applied to fecal specimens in the clinical laboratory or environmental specimens from the field.

Stool specimens may be examined fresh or after fixation, usually in a formalin-containing preservative. For long-term preservation, fecal samples may be stored in 2.5% (weight/volume) potassium dichromate in which oocysts may remain viable for as long as 6 months. Polyvinyl alcohol–preserved specimens are not acceptable because of interference with acid-fast staining and EIA and because of the environmental hazard created by disposal of mercury-containing compounds (18, 143). Stool-concentration techniques are especially important when processing specimens in which the parasite burden may be low. Most clinical laboratories use formalin–ether or formalin–ethyl acetate sedimentation, although simple sedimentation by centrifugation (10 minutes, 500 g) is also effective. Oocysts can also be concentrated by flotation in Sheather's sucrose solution, zinc sulfate (33% to saturated), or sodium chloride (36% to saturated) (8, 143, 344, 349, 367, 368). Most diagnostic laboratories use at least two separate detection methods on every sample, generally a wet-mount examination of the concentrated specimen followed by a staining procedure for confirmation and permanent record. Traditionally, three negative specimens were considered necessary to confirm a negative result, but more recent data suggest that two examinations suffice for evaluating AIDS patients with diarrhea (369).

Serologic detection is primarily used as an investigational or epidemiologic tool inasmuch as specific anti-*Cryptosporidium* antibodies may persist for variable lengths of time after infection, a feature that limits their application to diagnosis of acute infection. However, in a study in which sera collected from crew members of a Coast Guard cutter involved in an outbreak of waterborne infection were analyzed by immunoblot, 15-, 17-, and 27-kd antigen groups were found in those crew members with documented or suspected infection. Immunoblot analysis was twofold more sensitive in detecting cryptosporidial infection than parasitologic examination of single stool specimens (310). Additional studies are needed to validate the usefulness of serologic assays for diagnosis.

Despite the proliferation of diagnostic techniques, the general consensus is that cryptosporidiosis is underdiagnosed because most people with diarrhea do not seek medical attention, and many clinicians are unaware of the disease (20, 370). When testing is requested, the ability to detect *Cryptosporidium* in stool samples varies with the experience of the technologist and the sensitivity of the methods used. Perhaps the most important factor that contributes to underdiagnosis is the misconception on the part of clinicians that a request for ova and parasite examination includes a specific test for *Cryptosporidium*. In fact, only 5% of clinical laboratories routinely perform specific tests for this parasite; most laboratories look for it only if the clinician requests the test (20, 142, 146, 371).

Treatment

No reproducibly effective palliative or curative therapies exist for cryptosporidiosis in either humans or animals. The disease is self-limited in immunocompetent patients, but it may be severe and prolonged, and dehydration may necessitate hospitalization. When exogenous causes of immunosuppression can be removed, infection resolves in the immunocompromised patient; otherwise, this type of host is at risk for persistent, severe disease.

Preclinical drug development and testing have been limited by difficulties in obtaining adequate supplies of oocysts and by the absence of both reproducible in vitro cultivation systems in which the full *Cryptosporidium* life cycle occurs and in vivo small animal models of clinical disease. In addition, the characterization of differences among cryptosporidial isolates and the impact of these differences on parasite virulence are still unknown. Since the first report of in vitro cultivation of *Cryptosporidium*, well over a decade ago (372), dozens of reports of drug testing in laboratory animal models and in vitro systems have been published. The many models are comprehensively cataloged and are extensively described in several reviews (18, 373–375). Using target animals, laboratory animal models, or in vitro techniques, more than 30 agents have been identified as having potential efficacy against *Cryptosporidium*, but few have undergone evaluation in humans (18, 373). Advances have also been made in the use of molecular biology to identify genes products that may be therapeutic targets, but this work is still in its infancy (27, 150, 155, 156).

The urgent need to develop effective therapy for cryptosporidiosis in patients with AIDS has led to an unprecedented administration of an array of chemotherapeutic, immunomodulating, and palliative agents to this population. A formidable list of approximately 100 ineffective compounds has been generated as the result of anecdotal reports (10). Controlled clinical trials, conducted over the past decade, have led to identification of a few promising agents, including azithromycin, paromomycin, and nitazoxanide, that warrant further study. Furthermore, these trials have provided useful insights for optimizing study design in future clinical investigation of this disease (376). The following is an overview of those agents that have been evaluated for the treatment of cryptosporidiosis in humans.

MACROLIDES

Interest in spiramycin as an anticryptosporidial agent stems from its activity against another apicomplexan, *Toxo-

plasma gondii. Anecdotal reports have been published of both success and failure with use of this agent for cryptosporidial infection (39, 108, 376, 377). Divergent results have also been obtained in prospective and controlled clinical trials (378–382). Two placebo-controlled trials of oral spiramycin in immunocompetent children revealed no difference between spiramycin and placebo, possibly because of inadequate dosing or duration of therapy in one study (381) and a statistically significant decrease in oocyst excretion and diarrhea in the other (382). In a double-blind trial in AIDS patients, 9.0 million IU of oral spiramycin daily was no better than placebo, possibly because of poor absorption of the oral agent (R Soave, unpublished data). However, data obtained from an open-label compassionate-use program that ran concomitantly with the controlled trial revealed a favorable clinical response, as well as parasitologic eradication in 75 and 32%, respectively, of treated AIDS patients (378). To circumvent absorption problems, two doses of intravenous spiramycin were examined in a multicenter, single-blind, placebo-controlled, National Institutes of Allergy and Infectious Diseases–sponsored AIDS Clinical Trials Group (ACTG 113) (383). Five of 31 (18%) patients enrolled had both clinical and parasitologic improvement, and analysis of all treated patients as a group revealed a statistically significant drop in oocyst count while these patients were receiving spiramycin. However, serious toxicity associated with intravenous spiramycin has tempered interest in this compound (384).

Experience with the newer azalide, azithromycin, for cryptosporidiosis in humans includes anecdotal reports (200, 385–387), a placebo-controlled trial (388), and open-label studies (389, 390). Preliminary data from 33 of the 85 AIDS patients randomized to either 900 mg oral azithromycin daily or matching placebo in the multicenter, double-blind trial revealed improvement in bowel movement frequency (not statistically significant) in the azithromycin-treated group and a decrease in stool oocyst counts at day 7 and day 21 that correlated significantly with high serum azithromycin levels (388). In an ongoing compassionate-use program conducted by Pfizer Pharmaceuticals, the first 60 patients enrolled had clinical improvement but marginal reduction of stool oocysts counts (389). Because of the absorption issue in AIDS patients, an investigational, intravenous form of azithromycin was administered to 5 extremely ill patients in whom oral azithromycin had failed. Bowel movement frequency and stool oocyst counts remained unchanged, but serum alkaline phosphatase levels decreased in all 5 patients compared with 4 of 13 untreated controls ($P < .05$) (391). The lactose-free form of azithromycin licensed for use in prophylaxis of *Mycobacterium avium* complex infections was used in the placebo-controlled trial and the compassionate-use program.

The potential anticryptosporidial activity of clarithromycin and other newer macrolides including roxithromycin and dirithromycin is of interest, but these agents have not yet been adequately studied. In a retrospective study of 471 patients with AIDS, none of 63 patients who received clarithromycin prophylaxis for *Mycobacterium avium* complex and 4 of 73 who did not receive clarithromycin developed cryptosporidial enteritis (392). In a subsequent 2-year follow-up of an additional 217 patients receiving clarithromycin 500 mg twice daily as *M. avium* complex prophylaxis, none developed cryptosporidial enteritis (392). A open-label study comparing varying doses of the liquid and tablet forms of clarithromycin for treatment of cryptosporidiosis in AIDS patients is being conducted in New York City. Available data suggest that macrolides warrant further investigation for the treatment of cryptosporidiosis.

PAROMOMYCIN

Paromomycin, also known as aminosidine, is a poorly absorbed, oligosaccharide aminoglycoside that achieves high concentrations in the colon and has been used in the United States for many years in the treatment of amebiasis. Experience with this agent for cryptosporidiosis in patients with AIDS has been mixed, but nonetheless it is widely used. Although reports of dramatic responses to this agent have been numerous, complete clinical and parasitologic resolution is rare, and recurrence, sometimes during therapy, is common among treated AIDS patients (200, 221, 263, 272, 373, 393–397). Promising results were obtained in two small placebo-controlled trials in which 10 and 11 patients were enrolled, respectively (398, 399). However, in an ACTG-sponsored, placebo-controlled trial of 35 AIDS patients with cryptosporidiosis (ACTG 192), no clinical benefit could be attributed to paromomycin (400). Anecdotal reports have noted toxicity, including pancreatitis and vertigo, with the use of this agent in AIDS patients (260, 401). In studies conducted in the 1960s in healthy volunteers, paromomycin treatment was linked to malabsorption (402). Paromomycin is nephrotoxic and ototoxic if the drug is absorbed into the systemic circulation; this does not appear to be a major problem for patients with AIDS despite the frequency of intestinal damage in this population. Inability to reach extraintestinal sites of cryptosporidial infection or to achieve adequate luminal concentrations throughout the intestine may contribute to the limited efficacy of this agent (396, 399, 403, 404). Perhaps, if the agent is administered early in the course of infection, when the parasite burden is low and presumably confined to the intestine, paromomycin activity against *Cryptosporidium* may be optimized. Clearly, the role of paromomycin in the treatment of cryptosporidiosis is problematic and requires further study.

NITAZOXANIDE

Nitazoxanide, a nitrothiazole benzamide derivative with activity against many different bacterial, helminthic, and protozoan pathogens, was synthesized in 1976 by Rossignol and colleagues (405). Data from in vitro studies, and from pilot clinical studies in Mexico and Mali (406), suggest that this agent has anticryptosporidial activity. In an open-label study of 30 AIDS patients with cryptosporidiosis, 68% of 22 subjects, who completed at least 4 weeks of therapy, had a reduction in bowel movement frequency, and 41% had parasitologic improvement (407). No toxicity occurred with doses as high as 2 g per day. An ACTG-sponsored, placebo-controlled trial of nitazoxanide (ACTG 336) is currently ongoing.

BENZENEACETONITRILE DERIVATIVES

Interest in this class of veterinary agents stems from their activity against the coccidian parasite, *Eimeria*. Despite the promising results obtained in a limited number of patients (408, 409), diclazuril sodium was found to be ineffective in a randomized, double-blind, placebo-controlled, dose-escalating trial of 60 patients conducted at 3 centers in New York City (410). Because lack of efficacy was believed to have resulted from poor drug bioavailability, letrazuril, a better absorbed *p*-fluor analog of diclazuril, was synthesized by Janssen. Anecdotal experience and a few prospective, open-label studies of letrazuril in AIDS patients provided mixed results (411–415). No clinical or parasitologic effect was noted in a randomized, double-blind, placebo-controlled treatment trial despite documentation of enhanced bioavailability (ACTG 198) (416). Letrazuril appears to interfere with acid-fast staining techniques used to detect cryptosporidial oocysts in stool; thus, the possibility of false-negative stool results must be entertained when using this agent (416).

OTHER ANTIPROTOZOAN AGENTS

Other agents that have been given for cryptosporidiosis with less than promising results include α-difluoromethylornithine and atovaquone (417–419). Combination therapy with two or more agents has been proposed but not studied in a controlled manner (200, 411).

ANTIRETROVIRAL THERAPY

Anecdotal reports have noted improvement of cryptosporidial diarrhea after the start of treatment with zidovudine, an effect thought to be secondary to enhanced immune function (420, 421). Perhaps the most exciting development has been the observation of resolution of cryptosporidial and microsporidial infection in AIDS patients treated with protease inhibitors and other highly active antiretroviral agents (22–23). Whether the effect is transient or permanent or secondary to augmentation of immune function, direct antimicrobial activity, or some other mechanism is currently unknown.

IMMUNOMODULATORY AGENTS

Biologic immunomodulating agents that have been used for cryptosporidiosis in patients with AIDS or other forms of immune compromise include bovine transfer factor, now called bovine dialyzable leukocyte extract (DLE), normal bovine colostrum (NBC) and HBC, colostral immunoglobulin concentrates, and hyperimmune egg yolks (301).

In a study of 12 patients with AIDS, treatment with DLE, prepared from lymph nodes of *Cryptosporidium*-infected calves (422), resulted in symptomatic improvement (10 patients) and oocyst eradication (7 patients) (423). A similarly treated patient, with congenital dysgammaglobulinemia and biliary cryptosporidiosis, did not show any improvement (424).

HBC (324–327), NBC (324, 425), immunoglobulin-enriched fractions from NBC (426, 427), colostral immunoglobulin concentrates (428), and normal human serum immunoglobulin (429), administered either orally or by direct duodenal infusion to patients with AIDS, leukemia, or hypogammaglobulinemia, have yielded mixed results. Some patients achieved rapid dramatic clinical improvement that lasted up to 3 months, but few had parasitologic responses, and relapses were common. The best results, irrespective of the type of preparation used, have been obtained in children with leukemia or hypogammaglobulinemia (325, 425, 427, 429). Major drawbacks to the use of these agents center on difficulties with production of large quantities of standardized product and product stability as it traverses the stomach. In one study, powdered immunoglobulin concentrate was found to be more efficacious than encapsulated concentrate (428). The use of egg yolks from hyperimmunized hens is an alternative to the production of HBC. Eggs laid by hens hyperimmunized with *Cryptosporidium parvum* oocyst antigens have high titers of anticryptosporidial immunoglobulin, which has produced significant parasite reduction in neonatal mice (430). In an open-label study of hyperimmune egg yolks administered to 24 AIDS patients, 25% had a favorable response (431). Although data from in vitro and in vivo animal studies suggest an important role for cytokines in eradication of *Cryptosporidium*, studies in humans are lacking (200, 432).

SUPPORTIVE THERAPY

Nonspecific antidiarrheal agents, including bismuth subsalicylate (Pepto-Bismol), kaolin and pectin (Kaopectate), diphenoxylate (Lomotil), opiates (tincture of opium, paregoric), and loperamide (Imodium), may be helpful, but their use must be individualized. The safety of these agents in patients with cryptosporidiosis is not known.

Anecdotal reports have suggested that the synthetic cyclic octapeptide analog of somatostatin, octreotide (Sandostatin), is useful in the management of cryptosporidial enteritis (373, 433, 434). However, most of the responders in a prospective, multicenter trial of escalating doses of subcutaneously administered octreotide did not have cryptosporidiosis (435).

Supportive care, with oral or intravenous hydration and sometimes total parenteral nutrition, remains the backbone of therapy. Psychological support is often needed to help patients overcome their anxiety in coping with the debilitating symptoms of diarrheal illness.

Prevention

In the absence of effective therapy for cryptosporidiosis and because of the difficulties with disinfection, prevention of infection is of paramount importance (59, 142, 436). HIV-infected people should be aware of the modes by which *Cryptosporidium* can be transmitted. They include contact with infected adults, diaper-age children, and animals, drinking of contaminated water, contact with contaminated water during recreational activities (swimming), and eating contaminated food.

Good hygiene with enteric precautions including handwashing, use of gloves, and proper disposal of fecal material is essential in preventing person-to-person spread. Newborn or extremely young pets (less than 6 months) may pose a small risk of cryptosporidial infection. The magnitude of the risk of acquiring *Cryptosporidium* from municipally treated drinking water varies by geographic location and is generally uncertain. Current data are inadequate to recommend that all HIV-infected persons avoid tap water. For those who want to take action, the risk of waterborne cryptosporidiosis can be eliminated by boiling, for 1 minute, all water intended for drinking. Household filters and bottled water may serve as alternatives to boiling water, but careful attention must be paid to selecting effective filters and high-quality bottled water. Details necessary for selecting filters and bottled water are available from the CDC (142). Persons avoiding tap water should be aware that using ice cubes or drinking fountain beverages that are made with tap water may pose a risk. HIV-infected persons should minimize their risk of ingesting contaminated water by not swimming in lakes, rivers, swimming pools, or recreational water parks.

MICROSPORIDIOSIS

Microsporidia are obligate intracellular protozoan parasites belonging to the phylum Microspora. More than 1000 species of microsporidia are classified into approximately 100 genera (437, 438). Microsporidia commonly infect arthropods and members of all classes of vertebrates; microsporidiosis has been responsible for significant economic losses in silkworm, honey bee, and salmonid fish industries (437–440). The use of laboratory animals such as rabbits and mice with subclinical microsporidioses has resulted in contamination of passaged cell lines and interference with the interpretation of results of studies with other infectious agents (441). Microsporidia are of growing concern as a cause of opportunistic infections in persons with AIDS (437–440, 442–446). To date, 12 species of microsporidia have been reported to infect humans (Table 21.1).

Parasite

MORPHOLOGY

The mature spores of microsporidian species infecting humans are oval to pyriform and measure 2.0 to 7.0 μm long and 1.5 to 5.0 μm wide. The characteristic that, above all, defines an organism as being a microsporidian is the coiled polar filament within the spore (Fig. 21.3) (437–446). The polar filament originates from the anchoring disc or polar sac at the anterior end of the spore and forms coils in the middle to posterior region of the spore. The polar filament everts during germination and propels the spore contents into the host cell without damaging the host cell membrane (447–449). The number of polar filament coils varies among

Table 21.1. Species of Microsporidia Reported to Infect Humans

Species	Nonhuman Hosts	Clinical Features	Growth in Vitro
Enterocytozoon bieneusi	Pigs, nonhuman primates	Chronic diarrhea, wasting, malabsorption, cholecystitis, cholangitis	No
Encephalitozoon intestinalis (previously *Septata intestinalis*)	—	Chronic diarrhea, keratoconjunctivitis, disseminated infections	Yes
Encephalitozoon hellem	Budgerigars	Keratoconjunctivitis, disseminated infections	Yes
Encephalitozoon cuniculi		Disseminated infections	Yes
Strain I	Rabbits, mice		
Strain II	Mice, blue foxes		
Strain III	Domestic dogs rodents, goats, sheep, swine, horses, foxes, cats, non-human primates[b]		
Nosema connori	—	Disseminated infection	Culture not attempted
Nosema ocularum	—	Keratitis	Culture not attempted
Nosema sp. (species not identified)	—	Keratitis, myositis	Culture not attempted
Vittaforma corneae (previously *Nosema corneum*)	—	Keratitis	Yes
Pleistophora sp.	Fish	Myositis	Culture not attempted
Trachipleistophora hominis	—	Myositis, rhinitis, sinusitis, keratoconjunctivitis	Yes
Microsporidium ceylonensis[a]	—	Keratitis	Culture not attempted
Microsporidium africanum	—	Keratitis	Culture not attempted

[a] Catch-all genus for microsporidia that could not be classified (437).
[b] Hosts infected with unknown strain of *Encephalitozoon cuniculi* (437, 478).

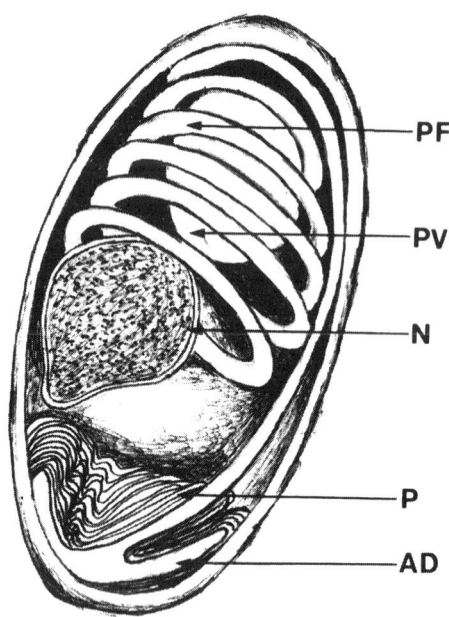

Figure 21.3. Microsporidian spore. The diagram demonstrates the anchoring disc *(AD)*, polaroplast *(P)*, nucleus *(N)*, posterior vacuole *(PV)*, and polar filament *(PF)*.

species; it ranges from 3 to 10 in those species that infect humans (see Table 21.1). At the anterior region of the spore is the anchoring disc, the most carbohydrate-rich structure in the microsporidia (450). Just posterior to the anchoring disc is an array of lamellar membranes called the polaroplast. These membranes also are rich in carbohydrates and are continuous with the outer membrane of the polar filament. The polaroplast forms the outer membrane of the sporoplasm, which is a sac that becomes filled with the spore contents after polar filament extrusion (449). The spore contains either a single nucleus (e.g., *Encephalitozoon, Enterocytozoon, Pleistophora, Trachipleistophora*) or a diplokaryon (e.g., *Nosema, Vittaforma*); the latter consists of two closely aligned nuclei that function as a single unit (437–446). Nuclei divide on mitotic spindles but lack centrioles (437, 439, 444). A posterior vacuole, usually seen in the mature spore, provides a characteristic that is useful in detection of microsporidia in clinical specimens using light microscopy methods (451). The function of the posterior vacuole is unknown, but, along with the polaroplast, it swells just before germination (452–454).

The mature spore is surrounded by an outer electron-dense exospore composed primarily of (glyco)proteins and an inner electron-lucent endospore that contains chitin (437–446). The spore wall affords the microsporidian a level of resistance to environmental influences (454). A plasma membrane encloses the spore contents within the spore wall.

TAXONOMY AND PHYLOGENY

The taxonomy of the microsporidia is primarily based on morphologic characteristics, and, for lack of sufficient information, does not necessarily correlate with the evolution of the microsporidia (438, 455). The microsporidia were assigned to the phylum Microspora by Sprague (456), and they were classified further, in 1980, by the Committee on Systematics and Evolution of the Society of Protozoologists (457). In a complete review of the taxonomy of the microsporidia (438), they are divided into two classes: the Dihaplophasea, which includes species with a diplokaryon during any stage of development, and the Monohaplophasea, which includes species with a single nucleus during all stages of development. These higher categories of microsporidia are grouped according to chromosome cycle. In earlier taxonomic classifications that are still commonly used, the microsporidia were divided into the two orders of Pansporoblastina and Apansporoblastina based on the presence or absence, respectively, of the sporophorous vesicle (437, 439, 445). Families were established on the basis of host–parasite relationships, characteristics of sporogony, and spore morphology. Assignments into genera, species, and strains (subspecies) are still being debated as new information is assimilated. The combined characteristics typically used to classify microsporidia into genera currently include the host type, mode of transmission, host–parasite interface, microsporidian development (merogony and sporogony), and spore morphology (size, nucleus arrangement, turns of the polar filament).

Phylogenetically, microsporidia are considered primitive eukaryotes because they possess nuclei as well as electron-dense ribosomes that resemble those of prokaryotes (458). Vossbrinck and colleagues (459, 460) found that *Varimorpha necatrix* (a microsporidian of butterflies) contains small 70S ribosomes with 16S and 23S subunits, but it lacks a separate 5.8S subunit typically found in eukaryotes. However, the 23S subunit contains sequences of the typical 5.8S subunit. The 16S subunit in microsporidia is smaller than the 18S subunit typically found in eukaryotes, and little homology exists between microsporidian rRNA gene sequence and those of other eukaryotes. Furthermore, microsporidia lack mitochondria, peroxisomes, and a true Golgi apparatus (437, 439, 444, 459, 460). Based on similarities in α- and β-tubulin sequence data, speculation exists that microsporidia may be more closely related to fungi than to protozoa (461).

LIFE CYCLE

The life cycle of microsporidia in mammalian hosts is simple. Infections are believed to occur primarily by ingestion of spores through contaminated urine or feces, and animals can be experimentally infected with *Encephalitozoon cuniculi* by oral inoculation (437, 442). The small intestinal epithelium serves as the primary site of most *Enterocytozoon bieneusi* and *Encephalitozoon intestinalis* infections in humans (462–466). Inhalation probably occurs as well, because organisms (e.g., *Encephalitozoon* spp. and *E. bieneusi*) have been observed in the sputum, bronchoalveolar lavage fluid, and bronchoalveolar epithelium of infected individuals (440). Evidence of transplacental transmission of *E. cuniculi* also has been reported in many animals (437, 441, 442–444), but it occurs more commonly in carnivores than in rodents (437, 442). Transplacental transmission has not been reported in humans, but it has occurred in nonhuman primates (467).

Host cell infection occurs as microsporidian spores germinate by propelling the spore contents through the everting polar filament into the host cell (437–449, 468–470). Organisms also may be internalized by phagocytosis, and macrophages easily become infected with some microsporidia (e.g., *Encephalitozoon* spp.). After the host cell becomes infected, microsporidia enter the proliferative phase, called merogony or schizogony. Parasite division occurs by binary fission (e.g., *Encephalitozoon, Nosema, Vittaforma*), or karyokinesis may occur with delayed cytokinesis, resulting in multinucleated forms called merogonial plasmodia (e.g., *Enterocytozoon, Pleistophora, Trachipleistophora*). Merogony occurs either in direct contact with the host cell cytoplasm (e.g., *Nosema, Enterocytozoon*), within a host cell–derived parasitophorous vacuole (e.g., *Encephalitozoon*), within an amorphous surface coat deposited by the parasites (e.g., *Pleistophora, Trachipleistophora*), or with individual organisms intimately surrounded by endoplasmic reticulum (e.g., *Vittaforma*).

Sporogony is the differentiation of organisms into spores and begins as the outer surface of the developing organism becomes more electron dense (437–449, 468–470). These stages are referred to as sporonts, which still may divide a limited number of times by binary fission (e.g., *Encephalitozoon, Nosema, Vittaforma*). Multinucleated sporonts may develop within what are referred to as sporogonial plasmodia (e.g., *Enterocytozoon, Pleistophora*). *Trachipleistophora* species have multinucleated merogonial plasmodia that undergo plasmotomy to form uninucleated late meronts, so only uninucleated sporonts are seen in this genus.

When sporogony results in the deposition or formation of parasite-generated sporophorous vesicles, the microsporidia are characterized as pansporoblastic (e.g., *Pleistophora, Trachipleistophora*), whereas species that undergo sporogony in the absence of a parasite-derived outer coat are characterized as apansporoblastic (e.g., *Encephalitozoon, Enterocytozoon, Vittaforma, Nosema*). Stages in which organelles can be recognized are referred to as sporoblasts. Smooth and rough endoplasmic reticula increase and produce Golgi-like vesicles that appear to generate the polar filament. Eventually, the spore wall develops a discernible electron-dense exospore and electron-lucent endospore. Mature spores develop from sporoblasts as a result of bisporogony (binary fission), tetrasporogony (in which a second binary fission occurs before the first binary fission was completed), or polysporogony (in which many spores separate from a multinucleated sporogonial plasmodium) (437, 439, 471).

Mature spores are released from infected cells and may infect adjacent cells or disseminate by infecting trafficking macrophages; they may be shed with the stool, urine, or respiratory secretions depending on the site of infection. Whereas meronts, sporonts, and sporoblasts display metabolic activities, little metabolic activity has been detected in mature spores.

Epidemiology

Before the AIDS epidemic, microsporidioses in humans were rare, with only about 10 confirmed cases reported (440). Since the onset of AIDS, prevalence rates in HIV-infected patients with chronic diarrhea and wasting have ranged from 7 to 50% (440). No data are available about the prevalence of disseminated microsporidia infections. Seroprevalence data suggest that microsporidiosis is common in human populations, but the studies are difficult to interpret because *Encephalitozoon cuniculi* was used as the antigen before the other *Encephalitozoon* species or *Enterocytozoon bieneusi* had been identified (440, 444, 472, 473). Interpretation of serologic data continues to be difficult in persons with progressive immunodeficiency; furthermore, *E. bieneusi*, which cannot be cultured, is difficult to obtain in sufficient quantity and purity for use as antigen in serologic assays. Geographically, microsporidia infections are reported worldwide (440, 474).

Human-to-human spread is likely to occur because organisms are shed in the feces, urine, or respiratory secretions of infected individuals (440). Animal reservoirs do exist for species of microsporidia that infect humans, a finding suggesting that microsporidiosis in humans may be zoonotic. *Enterocytozoon bieneusi* has been reported in pigs (475) and monkeys (476). To date, *Encephalitozoon intestinalis* has been reported in humans only, and *Encephalitozoon hellem* was reported in one aviary of budgerigars (477). *Encephalitozoon cuniculi*, on the other hand, has a wide mammalian host range and probably presents the greatest zoonotic risk to humans, even though human infections with *E. cuniculi* are reported less frequently than infections with *E. bieneusi* or *E. intestinalis* (see Table 21.1). Three documented *E. cuniculi* isolates from AIDS patients in the United States were identical to strain III, which was first identified in domestic dogs (478–480); *E. cuniculi* strain I, first identified in rabbits, was detected in HIV-infected patients in Switzerland (481). No direct relationship has been established between any human microsporidian infection and exposure to a zoonotic host, and further studies are needed to determine whether pets, for example, pose a risk to HIV-infected individuals. Insects are common hosts to microsporidia, but to date, no species infecting humans (or mammals, in general) have been identified in insects. Furthermore, speculation exists about whether contaminated water supplies may place individuals at risk for microsporidiosis (482), but again, no microsporidian species infecting humans have been identified in water supplies (440).

Clinical Aspects

The most common microsporidian detected in persons with AIDS is *Enterocytozoon bieneusi*; it is the smallest microsporidian, measuring 1.0 μm × 1.5 μm, and it was first described in a Haitian patient with AIDS living in France (483) (see Table 21.1). *E. bieneusi* infects the enterocytes (most commonly at the microvillous tips of the jejunum) and primarily causes chronic diarrhea with 3 to 10 nonbloody bowel movements of variable volume and consistency that occur at irregular intervals (466). Additional clinical symptoms associated with E. bieneusi infections include abdominal cramping, nausea, weight loss, malabsorption, and zinc deficiency (440, 446, 463, 466, 484). Biliary tract involvement and cholangitis can occur, as well.

Whereas Enterocytozoon bieneusi remains localized primarily to the small intestine and biliary tract, Encephalitozoon species usually disseminate. Encephalitozoon intestinalis is the second most commonly reported microsporidian in AIDS patients; it initially infects enterocytes of the small intestine causing clinical symptoms identical to those associated with E. bieneusi infections (440, 446, 463, 465). Unlike E. bieneusi, E. intestinalis also infects macrophages of the lamina propria and subsequently disseminates widely. Secondary sites include, but are not limited to, epithelial cells of the kidney, bronchial epithelium, sinuses, and cornea (440, 466, 485). Furthermore, dual infections with E. bieneusi and E. intestinalis are known to occur (440, 466).

Two additional species of Encephalitozoon are known to infect humans and have been associated with keratoconjunctivitis, bronchiolitis, sinusitis, nephritis, ureteritis, prostatitis, hepatitis, and peritonitis (440). E. hellem was first described in AIDS patients with keratoconjunctivitis (439, 440) and is morphologically similar to E. cuniculi, which infects a wide range of mammalian hosts, including humans (437, 439, 440, 442–444). As such, cases ascribed to E. cuniculi before 1991 may, in fact, have been due to E. hellem, so some debate exists about the clinical manifestations of infection with each of these species. Clearly, both organisms can infect humans and can result in disseminated infection.

Additional microsporidia have been reported to infect humans, but with less frequency. Nosema species and Vittaforma corneae have been detected in the corneal stroma of non–HIV-infected individuals (437, 440, 470), and disseminated infection with Nosema connori has been documented in a child with thymic deficiency (437, 439, 440). Myositis has been reported in persons infected with either a Pleistophora species or Trachipleistophora hominis (440, 468, 469).

The most consistent risk factor associated with clinical disease in persons with microsporidiosis appears to be the immunologic status of the host. Chronic diarrhea and wasting associated with the presence of microsporidia were most severe in persons with CD4+ T-cell levels lower than $100/mm^3$ (440, 463, 484, 486). Others at risk of significant clinical microsporidiosis are organ transplant recipients receiving immunosuppressing agents (487, 488). Conversely, self-limiting diarrhea has been reported in HIV-infected patients with CD4+ T-cell levels lower than $100/mm^3$ (440) and in non–HIV-infected individuals (489, 490). In other reports, microsporidia were identified in persons with no or intermittent diarrhea, thereby questioning the association between microsporidia and disease (491). In follow up studies, however, "microsporidia were detected in proportionally more of the samples from patients with chronic diarrhea than from patients with nil or intermittent diarrhea" (492, 493). Infections with Nosema and Vittaforma species in non–HIV-infected individuals were primarily limited to the corneal stroma, an immunologically privileged site (440), again suggesting an important role of a competent immune system for preventing disease. Whether clinical disease in an immunodeficient host is the result of de novo exposure to the organism or whether it reflects reactivation of chronic disease as a result of immune dysfunction is unkown.

Immune Responses

Most information about host immune responses against microsporidia is based on experimental infections of laboratory animals (e.g., rabbits and mice) with Encephalitozoon cuniculi. E. cuniculi, the first mammalian microsporidian described, probably has the widest host range among mammals and was the first mammalian microsporidian species grown in culture (437, 439–446). Three types of host–parasite relationships exist in mammals infected with microsporidia. Hosts infected transplacentally (e.g., domestic dogs, blue foxes) generally develop acute and often lethal renal disease. Immunologically competent adult hosts who become infected with microsporidia (e.g., rabbits, rodents) usually develop lifelong chronic subclinical infections. Immunodeficient or immunosuppressed hosts (e.g., athymic and severe combined immune deficiency [SCID] mice, persons with AIDS or organ transplants) infected with microsporidia develop clinically significant infections that may be lethal.

In immunologically competent laboratory animals (mice, rhesus monkeys), IgM responses develop within 2 weeks, whereas IgG levels peak at approximately 5 to 6 weeks and generally persist for the life of the host (441, 494, 495). Antibodies to Encephalitozoon cuniculi have been detected in immunologically competent humans (472, 473), but their presence could not be correlated with true infection because microsporidia were not observed.

Immunodeficient animals such as SCID mice produce no detectable antibodies after infection with Encephalitozoon cuniculi (496). SIV-infected rhesus monkeys who are immunodeficient (CD4+/CD29+ T-cell counts below 10%) at the time of E. cuniculi or E. hellem inoculation fail to produce significant levels of specific antibodies. SIV-infected monkeys inoculated before becoming immunodeficient generate high levels of specific antibodies that decline approximately 1 month before death (495). HIV-infected individuals with proved microsporidia infections, as well as HIV-seronegative individuals with no history of microsporidiosis, produce variable antibody responses to microsporidia (440, 497). The variability is believed to depend, in part, on the immune status of the host at the time of infection with microsporidia. Conversely, casual exposure to microsporidia through ingestion of food or by insect stings, or subclinical infections, may account for antibody responses in immunologically competent persons with no history of microsporidiosis.

Two protective functions have been associated with specific antibodies. Antibodies generated against microsporidia may function as opsonins to facilitate macrophage-mediated phagocytosis (498). In addition, specific murine antibodies raised against *Encephalitozoon cuniculi* fix complement and kill organisms in vitro (499). However, transfer of hyperimmune serum to *E. cuniculi*–infected athymic mice failed to prolong survival (499), a finding suggesting that additional protective mechanisms must exist. Furthermore, antibody responses are likely to have contributed to the immune complex disease observed in *E. cuniculi*-infected blue foxes and domestic dogs (500, 501).

Cell-mediated immune responses are critical in preventing lethal disease in mice. Adoptive transfer of sensitized syngeneic T-cell–enriched spleen cells protect *Encephalitozoon cuniculi*–infected athymic BALB/c or SCID mice (494, 496, 499). Adoptive transfer of naive syngeneic splenic lymphocytes fails to protect athymic mice if given at the same time as the *E. cuniculi* inoculum (499), but it does protect SCID mice if transferred 2 weeks before inoculation with *E. cuniculi* (496). Cytotoxic T cells specific for *E. cuniculi*–infected cells have not been detected, but lymphocytes do appear to release cytokines or other factors that activate macrophages to kill *E. cuniculi* in vitro (499). Murine macrophages activated by incubation with lipopolysaccharide (10 ng/mL) and IFN-γ (100 μm/mL) or tumor necrosis factor-α (TNF-α) (1000 μm/mL) are able to kill or control the growth of *E. cuniculi* in vitro, and this macrophage-mediated killing appears to depend on the generation of nitrogen intermediates (495, 502). IFN-γ receptor knockout BALB/c mice are significantly more susceptible to infection with *E. intestinalis* than wild-type BALB/c mice (503), a finding further indicating an important role for IFN-γ in resistance to microsporidiosis in vivo. Intestinal biopsy specimens were evaluated for cytokine mRNA expression (300). In a comparative study of intestinal biopsy specimens from 13 HIV-infected individuals with either microsporidiosis and diarrhea ($n = 6$) or unknown causes of diarrhea ($n = 7$) and HIV-seronegative individuals, no significant differences were seen in TNF, interleukin-1β (IL-1β), IL-6, IL-8, or IL-10, as determined by cytokine mRNA expression. Comparison between HIV-seronegative individuals with and without microsporidiosis must still be made to rule out cytokine effects resulting from HIV infection.

Diagnosis

Various approaches have been applied to the diagnosis of microsporidiosis. Serologic methods for detecting antibodies to microsporidia (e.g., indirect fluorescent antibody test [IFAT], ELISA) are useful for antemortem diagnosis of microsporidia-infected rodents, rabbits, and dogs (441, 443, 444), but these methods are less reliable in human patients with progressive immunodeficiency such as persons infected with HIV (497). Therefore, detection of microsporidian organisms in stool is required for diagnosis. Transmission electron microscopy is still considered the standard for definitive diagnosis and has been used to identify and characterize the two most important microsporidian species infecting humans, namely, *Enterocytozoon bieneusi* and *Encephalitozoon intestinalis* (462, 464, 465, 483, 504). Transmission electron microscopy, however, is time-consuming, costly, and requires much expertise and specialized equipment.

Microsporidia do not stain well with hematoxylin and eosin, but the presence of cup-shaped indented nuclei in intestinal epithelial cells, as viewed by light microscopy, suggests *Enterocytozoon bieneusi* infection (466). Microsporidia are Gram positive and birefringent under polarizing light (466, 505), and Giemsa-stained microsporidia appear blue with reddish-purple nuclei (466). The Warthin–Starry silver stain has been used to detect microsporidia in tissues; organisms appear grayish black against a yellow background (506). Optical brighteners such as Calcofluor White, Uvitex 2B, or Fungifluor bind to chitin, which is found in the spore wall of microsporidia. Organisms appear as turquoise or white oval halos under ultraviolet light of 395 to 440 nm (507, 508). The modified trichrome stains using 10-fold higher concentrations of Chromotrope 2R were first adapted for detecting microsporidia by Weber and colleagues (451) and were further modified by using a different counterstain and varying the incubation temperature (509, 510). Trichrome-stained microsporidia are pink with a posterior vacuole and have a diagonal pink band, against a green- or blue-counterstained background.

Although *Enterocytozoon bieneusi* is slightly smaller than the other microsporidia that infect humans, species identification is usually not possible with these histochemical staining methods. Species-specific monoclonal and polyclonal antibodies have been used for identifying microsporidia species by IFAT in research laboratories, but these reagents are not commercially available at present (480, 511). Polymerase chain reaction–based methods, with improved sensitivity and specificity, are being developed (512), but currently they are unavailable in most clinical settings.

The choice of method for detecting microsporidia often depends on the type of specimen obtained. Diagnosis of microsporidiosis in tissue can be made using the Brown–Brenn Gram stain, Warthin–Starry silver stain, or fluorescent optical brighteners (166). Giemsa staining (166), and a modified tissue Chromotrope 2R stain (513) have also been successfully used to detect microsporidia in tissue. A diagnostic paradigm has been suggested for detection of microsporidia in stool specimens; first, an optical brightener is used to screen for the presence of microsporidia, and then the modified trichrome stain is used to confirm the presence of microsporidia. Calcofluor White staining is rapid, but false-positive results occur because of the presence of similarly staining yeasts. The modified trichrome blue stain takes longer, but it is more specific in that yeast can be distinguished from microsporidia (514). Gram, Giemsa, and silver stains are not typically used for detecting microsporidia in stool specimens because of high background reactivity. In fluids such as bronchoalveolar lavage or urine, microsporidia can be identified with optical fluorescent brighteners, modified trichrome staining, or Giemsa staining.

Treatment

Some relief of diarrhea has been reported in microsporidia-infected persons treated with metronidazole, octreotide, or trimethoprim–sulfamethoxazole, but the organisms were not eliminated (515, 516). Itraconazole was effective in clearing *Encephalitozoon hellem* in an AIDS patient with keratoconjunctivitis (517). Treatment with atovaquone has been associated with symptom improvement in AIDS patients with microsporidiosis (518). A similar improvement in symptoms has also been reported as a result of regulating dietary intake of fat (519). Albendazole, a benzimidazole derivative given at a dose of 400 mg orally twice a day for 1 month, has resulted in the most marked clinical improvement in patients infected with *Encephalitozoon* species, but it is variably effective in persons with *Enterocytozoon bieneusi* infections (520, 521). Fumagillin, an antibiotic derived from *Aspergillus fumigatus* and known to inhibit angiogenesis and microsporidian growth in vitro, was used successfully in the treatment of patients with microsporidial keratoconjunctivitis (522, 523). Oral fumagillin is not generally used systemically because of toxicity. When this agent was given orally to AIDS patients in France, *E. bieneusi* infections cleared, but thrombocytopenia was a significant side effect (524). An analog of fumagillin, TNP-470 (also named AGM-1470), was less toxic than fumagillin in tumor studies (525), and it was found to inhibit replication of *Encephalitozoon intestinalis* and *Vittaforma corneae* in vitro (526). Pathogenesis of microsporidiosis has been associated with elevated intestinal TNF-α levels; treatment with thalidomide, a TNF inhibitor, resulted in clinical improvement in AIDS patients with microsporidiosis (527). Treatment of HIV-infected patients with combination antiretroviral therapy has led to the resolution of microsporidiosis in several cases, presumably because of enhanced immune function (23, 528).

In conclusion, microsporidia, long recognized as pathogens of animals, are now recognized as human pathogens (529). In immunologically competent animals, microsporidial infections evolve into a balanced host–parasite relationship wherein the host survives with few or no clinical signs of disease and the parasite persists. Conversely, in immunodeficient and immunosuppressed hosts, the host–parasite relationship becomes unbalanced, resulting in clinical signs of disease. The prevalence of chronic subclinical infections, commonly seen in animals, needs further delineation in humans. As diagnostic methods improve, and as more is learned about the epidemiology, immunology, and pathology of microsporidiosis, advances will be made in preventing and controlling these infections in humans.

References

1. Clarke JJ. A study of coccidia in mice. J Microsc Soc 1895;37:277.
2. Tyzzer EE. A sporozoan found in the peptic glands of the common mouse. Proc Soc Exp Biol Med 1907;5:12–13.
3. Slavin D. *Cryptosporidium meleagridis* (sp. nov.). J Comp Pathol 1955;65:262–266.
4. Panciera RJ, Thomassen RW, Garner FM. Cryptosporidial infection in a calf. Vet Pathol 1971;8:479–484.
5. Nime FA, Burek JD, Page DL, et al. Acute enterocolitis in a human being infected with the protozoan *Cryptosporidium*. Gastroenterology 1976;70:592–598.
6. Meisel JL, Perera DR, Meligro C, et al. Overwhelming watery diarrhea associated with *Cryptosporidium* in an immunosuppressed patient. Gastroenterology 1976;70:1156–1160.
7. Centers for Disease Control and Prevention. Cryptosporidiosis: an assessment of chemotherapy of males with acquired immune deficiency syndrome (AIDS). MMWR Morb Mortal Wkly Rep 1982;31:589–592.
8. Fayer R, Ungar BLP. *Cryptosporidium* spp. and cryptosporidiosis. Microbiol Rev 1986;50:458–483.
9. Soave R, Armstrong D. *Cryptosporidium* and cryptosporidiosis. Rev Infect Dis 1986;8:1012–1023.
10. Tzipori S. Cryptosporidiosis in perspective. Adv Parasitol 1988;27:63–129.
11. Crawford FG, Vermund SH. Human cryptosporidiosis. CRC Crit Rev Microbiol 1988;16:113.
12. Dubey JP, Speer CA, Fayer R. Cryptosporidiosis of man and animals. Boca Raton, FL: CRC Press, 1990.
13. Current WL, Garcia LS. Cryptosporidiosis. Clin Microbiol Rev 1991;4:325–358.
14. Petersen C. Cryptosporidiosis in patients infected with the human immunodeficiency virus. Clin Infect Dis 1992;15:903–909.
15. Mackenzie WR, Hoxie NJ, Proctor ME, et al. A massive outbreak in Milwaukee of *Cryptosporidium* infection transmitted through the public water supply. N Engl J Med 1994;331:161–167.
16. Proceedings of the International Workshop. Microsporidiosis and cryptosporidiosis in immunodeficient patients: September 28–October 1, 1993, Ceske Budejovice, Czech Republic. Folia Parasitol (Praha) 1993;40:249–320.
17. Sterling CR. *Cryptosporidium* parvum: a decade of effort. An overview of the Cleveland workshop. J Eukaryot Microbiol 1994;41:68S.
18. O'Donoghue PJ. *Cryptosporidium* and cryptosporidiosis in man and animals. Int J Parasitol 1995; 25:139–195.
19. Mead JR. *Cryptosporidium* workshop overview. J Eukaryot Microbiol 1996;43:90S–91S.
20. Centers for Disease Control and Prevention. Assessing the public health threat associated with waterborne cryptosporidiosis: report of a workshop. MMWR Morb Mortal Wkly Rep 1995;44:1–19.
21. Fayer R. *Cryptosporidium* and cryptosporidiosis. Boca Raton, FL: CRC Press, 1997.
22. Benhamou Y, Bochet MV, Carriere J, et al. Effects of triple antiretroviral therapies including HIV protease inhibitors on chronic intestinal cryptosporidiosis and microsporidiosis in HIV-infected patients [abstract]: abstracts of the 97th Annual Meeting of the American Gastroenterological Association. Gastroenterology 1997;112:A930.
23. Carr A, Marriott D, Field A, et al. Treatment of HIV-1–associated microsporidiosis and cryptosporidiosis with combination antiretroviral therapy. Lancet 1998;351:256–261.
24. Levine ND. Taxonomy and review of the coccidian genus *Cryptosporidium* (Protozoa, Apicomplexa). J Protozool 1984;31:94–98.
25. Fayer R, Speer CA, Dubey. The general biology of *Cryptosporidium*. In: Fayer R, ed. *Cryptosporidium* and cryptosporidiosis. Boca Raton, FL: CRC Press, 1997:1–232.
26. Upton SJ, Current WL. The species of *Cryptosporidium* (Apicomplexa: Cryptosporididae) infecting mammals. J Parasitol 1985;71:625–629.
27. Jenkins MC, Petersen C. Molecular biology of *Cryptosporidium*. In: Fayer R, ed. *Cryptosporidium* and cryptosporidiosis. Boca Raton, FL: CRC Press, 1997:225–232.
28. Johnson AM, Fielke R, Lumb R, et al. Phylogenetic relationships of *Cryptosporidium* determined by ribosomal RNA sequence comparison. Int J Parasitol 1990;20;141–147.
29. Barta JR, Jenkins MC, Danforth HD. Evolutionary relationships of avian *Eimeria* species among other apicomplexan protozoa: monophyly of the Apicomplexa is supported. Mol Biol Evol 1990;345:8.
30. Cai J, Collins MD, McDonald V, et al. PCR cloning and nucleotide sequence determination of the 18S rRNA genes and internal tran-

scribed spacer 1 of the protozoan parasites *C. parvum* and *C. muris*. Biochim Biophys Acta 1992;1131:317.
31. Taghi-Kilani R, Remacha-Moreno M, Wenman WM. Three tandemly repeated 5S ribosomal RNA-encoding genes identified, cloned and characterized from *Cryptosporidium* parvum. Gene 1994;142:253.
32. Marcial MA, Madara JL. *Cryptosporidium*: cellular localization, structural analysis of absorptive cell-parasite membrane-membrane interactions in guinea pigs, and suggestion of protozoan transport by M cells. Gastroenterology 1986;90:583–594.
33. Perrone TL, Dickersin GR. The intracellular location of cryptosporidia. Hum Pathol 1983;14:1092–1093.
34. Pohlenz J, Bemrick WJ, Moon HW, et al. Bovine cryptosporidiosis: a transmission and scanning electron microscopic study of some stages in the life cycle and of the host-parasite relationship. Vet Pathol 1978;15:417–427.
35. Dupont H, Chappell C, Sterling CR, et al. The infectivity of *Cryptosporidium parvum* in healthy volunteers. N Engl J Med 1995;332:855–859.
36. Jokipii L, Jokipii AMM. Timing of symptoms and oocyst excretion in human cryptosporidiosis. N Engl J Med 1986;315:1643–1647.
37. Miller RA, Bronsdon MA, Morton WR. Experimental cryptosporidiosis in a primate model. J Infect Dis 1990;161:312–315.
38. Casemore DP, Wright SE, Coop RL. Cryptosporidiosis: human and animal epidemiology. In: Fayer R. ed. *Cryptosporidium* and cryptosporidiosis. Boca Raton, FL: CRC Press, 1997:65–92.
39. Ungar BLP. Cryptosporidiosis in humans *(Homo sapiens)*. In: Dubey JP, Speer CA, Fayer R. eds. Cryptosporidiosis of man and animals. Boca Raton, FL: CRC Press, 1990:59–82.
40. Fang GD, Lima AA, Martins CV, et al. Etiology and epidemiology of persistent diarrhea in northeastern Brazil: a hospital-based, prospective, case-control study. J Pediatr Gastroenterol Nutr 1995;2:137–144.
41. Franco RM, Cordeiro N da S. Giardiasis and cryptosporidiosis in day-care centers in the municipality Campinas SP. Rev Soc Bras Med Trop 1996;29:585–591.
42. Robertson LJ. Severe giardiasis and cryptosporidiosis in Scotland, UK. Epidemiol Infect 1996;117:551–561.
43. Chacin-Bonilla L, Bonilla MC, Soto-Torres L, et al. *Cryptopsoridium parvum* in children with diarrhea in Zulia State, Venezuela. Am J Trop Med Hyg 1997;56:365–369.
44. Javier Enriquez F, Avila CR, Ignacios Santos J, et al. *Cryptosporidium* infections in Mexican children: clinical, nutritional, enteropathogenic and diagnostic evaluations. Am J Trop Med Hyg 1997;56:254–257.
45. Assefa T, Mohammed H, Abebe A, et al. Cryptosporidiosis in children seen at the children's clinic of Yekatit 12 Hospital, Addis Ababa. Ethiop Med J 1996;34:43–45.
46. Fraser D, Dagan R, Naggan L, et al. Natural history of *Giardia lamblia* and *Cryptosporidium* infections in a cohort of Israeli Bedouin infants: a study of a population in transition. Am J Trop Med Hyg 1997;57:544–549.
47. Brandonisio O, Marangi A, Panaro MA, et al. Prevalence of *Cryptosporidium* in children with enteritis in southern Italy. Eur J Epidemiol 1996;12:187–190.
48. Rodriguez-Hernandez J, Canut-Blasco A, Martin-Sanchez AM. Seasonal prevalences of *Cryptosporidium* and *Giardia* infections in children attending day care centres in Salamanca (Spain) studied for a period of 15 months. Eur J Epidemiol 1996;12:291–295.
49. Pettoello-Mantovani M, Di Martino L, Dettori G, et al. Asymptomatic carriage of intestinal *Cryptosporidium* in immunocompetent and immunodeficient children: a prospective study. Pediatr Infect Dis J 1995;14:1042–1047.
50. Giacometti A, Cirioni O, Balducci M, et al. Epidemiologic features of intestinal parasitic infections in Italian mental institutions. Eur J Epidemiol 1997;13:825–830.
51. Brannan DK, Greenfield RA, Owen WL, et al. Protozoal colonization of the intestinal tract in institutionalized Romanian children. Clin Infect Dis 1996;22:456–461.
52. Okafor JI, Okunji PO. Prevalence of *Cryptosporidium* oocysts in faecal samples of some school children in Enugu State, Nigeria. J Commun Dis 1996;28:49–55.
53. Miller K, Duran-Pinales C, Cruz-Lopez A, et al. *Cryptosporidium parvum* in children with diarrhea in Mexico. Am J Trop Med Hyg 1994;51:322–325.
54. Checkley W, Gilman RH, Epstein LD, et al. Asymptomatic and symptomatic cryptosporidiosis: their acute effect on weight gain in Peruvian children. Am J Epidemiol 1997;145:156–163.
55. Clavel A, Olivares JL, Fleta J, et al. Seasonality of cryptosporidiosis in children. Eur J Clin Microbiol Infect Dis 1996;15:77–79.
56. Moolasart P, Eampokalap B, Ratanasrithong M, et al. Cryptosporidiosis in HIV infected patients in Thailand. Southeast Asian J Trop Med Public Health 1995;26:335–338.
57. Mercado R, Garcia M. Annual frequency of *Cryptosporidium parvum* infections in children and adult outpatients, and adults infected by HIV. Rev Med Chil 1995;123:479–484.
58. Navin TR, Hardy AM. Cryptosporidiosis in patients with AIDS. J Infect Dis 1987;155:150.
59. Juranek DD. Cryptosporidiosis: sources of infection and guidelines for prevention. Clin Infect Dis 1995;21(Suppl 1):S57–S61.
60. Poznansky MC, Coker R, Skinner C, et al. HIV positive patients first presenting with an AIDS defining illness: characteristics and survival. BMJ 1995;15;311:156–158
61. Selik RM, Chu SY, Ward JW. Trends in infectious diseases and cancers among persons dying of HIV infection in the United States from 1987 to 1992. Ann Intern Med 1995;123:933–936.
62. Selik RM, Karon JM, Ward J. Effect of the human immunodeficiency virus epidemic on mortality from opportunistic infections in the United States in 1993. J Infect Dis 1997;176:632–636.
63. Colford JM Jr, Tager IB, Hirozawa AM, et al. Cryptosporidiosis among patients infected with human immunodeficiency virus: factors related to symptomatic infection and survival. Am J Epidemiol 1996;144:807–816.
64. Laughon BE, Druckman DA, Vernon A, et al. Prevalence of enteric pathogens in homosexual men with and without acquired immunodeficiency syndrome. Gastroenterology 1988;94:984–993.
65. Smith PD, Lane HC, Gill VJ, et al. Intestinal infections in patients with the acquired immunodeficiency syndrome. Ann Intern Med 1988;108:328–333.
66. Sorvillo FJ, Lieb LE, Kerndt PR, et al. Epidemiology of cryptosporidiosis among persons with acquired immunodeficiency syndrome in Los Angeles County. Am J Trop Med Hyg 1994;51:326–331.
67. Esfandiari A, Jordan WC, Brown CP. Prevalence of enteric parasitic infection among HIV-infected attendees of an inner city AIDS clinic. Cell Mol Biol (Noisy-le-grand) 1995;41(Suppl 1):S19–S23.
68. Porter K, Fairley CK, Wall PG, et al. AIDS defining diseases in the UK: the impact of PCP prophylaxis and twelve years of change. Int J STD AIDS 1996;7:252–257.
69. Spencer KL, Soave R, Acosta A, et al. Cryptosporidiosis in HIV-infected persons: prevalence in a New York City population. Int J Infect Dis 1997;1:217–221.
70. Pedersen C, Danner S, Lazzarin A, et al. Epidemiology of cryptosporidiosis among European AIDS patients. Genitourin Med 1996;72:128–131.
71. Stuart RL, Hellard ME, Jolley D, et al. Cryptosporidiosis in patients with AIDS. Int J STD AIDS 1997;8:339–341.
72. Lopez-Velez R, Tarazona R, Garcia Camacho A, et al. Intestinal and extraintestinal cryptosporidiosis in AIDS patients. Eur J Clin Microbiol Infect Dis 1995;14:677–681.
73. Jougla E, Pequignot F, Carbon C, et al. AIDS-related conditions: study of a representative sample of 1203 patients deceased in 1992 in France. Int J Epidemiol 1996;25:190–197.
74. Cotte L, Rabodonirina M, Piens MA, et al. Prevalence of intestinal protozoans in French patients infected with HIV. J Acquired Immun Defic Syndr 1993;6:1024.
75. Brandonisio O, Maggi P, Panaro MA, et al. Prevalence of cryptosporidiosis in HIV-infected patients with diarrheal illness. Eur J Epidemiol 1993;9:190.

76. Hunter G, Bagshawe AF, Baboo KS, et al. Intestinal parasites in Zambian patients with AIDS. Trans R Soc Trop Med Hyg 1992;86:543–545.
77. Gomez Morales MA, Atzori C, Ludovisi A, et al. Opportunistic and non-opportunistic parasites in HIV-positive and negative patients with diarrhoea in Tanzania. Trop Med Parasitol 1995;46:109–111.
78. Mengesha B. Cryptosporidiosis among medical patients with the acquired immunodeficiency syndrome in Tikur Anbessa Teaching Hospital, Ethiopia. East Afr Med J 1994;71:376–378.
79. Kaplan JE, Hu DJ, Holmes KK, et al. Preventing opportunistic infections in human immunodeficiency virus-infected persons: implications for the developing world. Am J Trop Med Hyg 1996;55:1–11.
80. Kim LS, Stansell J, Hadley R, et al. Decline in cryptosporidiosis prevalence among patients with AIDS in San Francisco [abstract]: abstracts of the 97th Annual Meeting of the American Gastroenterological Association. Gastroenterology 1997;112:A1013.
81. Roberts HL, Slonim, Y, Soave R, et al. Prevalence of and risk factors for cryptosporidial infection in HIV-infected persons in New York City [abstract 526]. Clin Infect Dis 1997;25:452.
82. Sreedharan A, Jayshree RS, Sridhar H. Cryptosporidiosis among cancer patients: an observation. J Diarrhoeal Dis Res 1996;14:211–213.
83. Tanyuksel M, Gun H, Doganci L. Prevalence of *Cryptosporidium* sp. in patients with neoplasia and diarrhea. Scand J Infect Dis 1995;27:69–70.
84. Gentile G, Venditti M, Micozzi A, et al. Cryptosporidiosis in patients with hematologic malignancies. Rev Infect Dis 1991;13:842–846.
85. Guarner J, Matilde-Nava T, Vilasenor-Flores R, et al. Frequency of intestinal parasites in adult cancer patients Mexico. Arch Med Res 1997;28:219–222.
86. Abaza SM, Makhlouf LM, el-Shewy KA, et al. Intestinal opportunistic parasites among different groups of immunocompromised hosts. J Egypt Soc Parasitol 1995;25:713–727.
87. Ok UZ, Cirit M, Uner A, et al. Cryptosporidiosis and blastocystosis in renal transplant recipients. Nephron 1997;75:171–174.
88. Ungar BLP, Mulligan M, Nutman TB. Serologic evidence of *Cryptosporidium* infection in U.S. volunteers before and after Peace Corps service in Africa. Arch Intern Med 1989;149:894–897.
89. Casemore DP. The antibody response to *Cryptosporidium*: development of a serological test and its use in a study of immunologically normal persons. J Infect 1987;14:125–134.
90. Ungar BLP, Gilman RH, Lanata CF, et al. Seroepidemiology of *Cryptosporidium* infection in two Latin American populations. J Infect Dis 1988;157:551–555.
91. Lengerich EJ, Addiss DG, Marx JJ, et al. Increased exposure to cryptosporidia among dairy farmers in Wisconsin. J Infect Dis 1993;167:1252.
92. Newman RD, Shu-Xian Z, Wuhib T, et al. Household epidemiology of *Cryptosporidium parvum* infection in an urban community in Northeast Brazil. Ann Intern Med 1994;120:500.
93. Zu S-X, Jin-Fen L, Brett LJ, et al. Seroepidemiologic study of *Cryptosporidium* infection in children from rural communities of Anhui, China and Fortaleza, Brazil. Am J Trop Med Hyg 1994;51:1.
94. Groves VJ, Lehmann D, Gilbert GL. Seroepidemiology of cryptosporidiosis in children in Papua New Guinea and Australia. Epidemiol Infect 1994;113:491–499.
95. Kuhls TL, Mosier DA, Crawford DL, et al. Seroprevalence of cryptosporidial antibodies during infancy, childhood, and adolescence. Clin Infect Dis 1994;18:731–735.
96. Ditrich O, Pavlovic L, Sterba J, et al. The first finding of *Crytospridium baileyi* in man. Parasitol Res 1991;180:408–409.
97. Ongerth JE, Stibs HH. Prevalence of *Cryptosporidium* infection in dairy calves in western Washington. Am J Vet Res 1989;50:1069–1070.
98. Miron D, Kenes J, Dagan R. Calves as a source of an outbreak of cryptosporidiosis among young children in an agricultural closed community. Pediatr Infect Dis J 1991;10:438–441.
99. Evans MR, Gardner D. Cryptosporidiosis outbreak associated with an educational farm holiday. Communic Dis Rep Rev 1996;6:R50–R51.
100. Dawson A, Griffin R, Fleetwood A, et al. Farm visits and zoonoses. Communic Dis Rep Rev 1995;5:R81–R86.
101. Laberge I, Griffiths MW, Griffiths MW. Prevalence, detection and control of *Cryptosporidium parvum* in food. Int J Food Microbiol 1996;32:1–26.
102. El-Ahraf A, Tacal JV, Sobih M, et al. Prevalence of cryptosporidiosis in dog and human beings in San Bernardino County, California. J Am Vet Med Assoc 1991;198:631.
103. Causape AC, Quilez J, Sanchez-Acedo C, et al. Prevalence of intestinal parasites, including *Cryptosporidium parvum*, in dogs in Zaragoza city, Spain. Vet Parasitol 1996;67:161–167.
104. Molbak R, Aaby P, Hojlyng N, et al. Risk Factors for *Cryptosporidium* diarrhea in early childhood: a case-control study from Guinea-Bissau, West Africa. Am J Epidemiol 1994;1;139:734–740.
105. Zerpa R, Huicho L. Childhood cryptosporidial diarrhea associated with identification of *Cryptosporidium* sp. in the cockroach *Periplaneta americana*. Pediatr Infect Dis J 1994;13:546–548.
106. Webster JP, Macdonald DW. Cryptosporidiosis reservoir in wild brown rats *(Rattus norvegicus)* in the UK. Epidemiol Infect 1995;115:207–209.
107. Cordell RL, Addiss DG. Cryptosporidiosis in child care settings: a review of the literature and recommendations for prevention and control. Pediatr Infect Dis J 1994;13:310.
108. Collier AC, Miller RA, Meyers JD. Cryptosporidiosis after marrow transplantation: person-to-person transmission and treatment with spiramycin. Ann Intern Med 1984;101:205–206.
109. Soave R, Ma P. Cryptosporidiosis: traveler's diarrhea in two families. Arch Intern Med 1985;145:70–72.
110. Roncoroni AJ, Gomez MA, Mera J, et al. *Cryptosporidium* infection in renal transplant patients. J Infect Dis 1989;160:559.
111. Ravn P, Lundgren JD, Kjaeldgaard P, et al. Nosocomial outbreak of cryptosporidiosis in AIDS patients. Br Med J 1991;302:277–280.
112. Martino P, Gentile G, Caprioli A, et al. Hospital-acquired cryptosporidiosis in a bone marrow transplantation unit. J Infect Dis 1988;158:647–648.
113. Navarrete S, Stetler HC, Avila C, et al. An outbreak of *Cryptosporidium* diarrhea in a pediatric hospital. Pediatr Infect Dis J 1991;10:248–250.
114. Casemore DP, Gardner CA, Mahony CO. Cryptosporidial infection, with special reference to nosocomial transmission of *Cryptosporidium parvum*: a review. Folia Parasitol 1994;41:17–21.
115. Millard PS, Gensheimer KF, Addiss DG, et al. An outbreak of cryptosporidiosis from fresh-pressed apple cider. JAMA 1994;272:1592–1596.
116. Centers for Disease Control and Prevention. Foodborne outbreak of diarrheal illness associated with *Cryptosporidium parvum:* Minnesota, 1995. MMWR Morb Mortal Wkly Rep 1996;45:783–784.
117. Centers for Disease Control and Prevention. Outbreaks of *Escherichia coli* O157:H7 infection and cryptosporidiosis associated with drinking unpasteurized apple cider: Connecticut and New York, October 1996. MMWR Morb Mortal Wkly Rep 1997;46:4–8.
118. Laberge I, Ibrahim A, Barta JR, et al. Detection of *Cryptosporidium parvum* in raw milk by PCR and oligonucleotide probe hybridization. Appl Environ Microbiol 1996;62:3259–3264.
119. Petersen C. *Cryptosporidium* and the food supply [editorial]. Lancet 1995;345:1128–1129.
120. Rose JB, Lisle JT, LeChevallier M. Waterborne cryptosporidiosis: Incidence, outbreaks, and treatment strategies. In: Fayer R. ed. *Cryptosporidium* and cryptosporidiosis. Boca Raton, FL: CRC Press, 1997:93–109.
121. Kramer MH, Herwaldt BL, Craun GF, et al. Surveillance for waterborne-disease outbreaks: United States, 1993-1994. MMWR CDC Surveill Summ 1996;45:1–33.
122. Hayes EB, Matte TD, O'Brien TR, et al. Contamination of a conventionally treated filtered public supply by *Cryptosporidium* associ-

ated with a large community outbreak of cryptosporidiosis. N Engl J Med 1989;320:1372–1376.
123. Dworkin MS, Goldman DP, Wells TG, et al. Cryptosporidiosis in Washington State: an outbreak associated with well water. J Infect Dis 1996;174:1372–1376.
124. Goldstein ST, Juranek DD, Ravenholt O, et al. Cryptosporidiosis: an outbreak associated with drinking water despite state-of-the-art water treatment. Ann Intern Med 1996;124:459–468.
125. Smith HV, Patterson WJ, Hardie R, et al. An outbreak of waterborne cryptosporidiosis caused by post-treatment contamination. Epidemiol Infect 1989;103:703–715.
126. Richardson AJ, Frankenberg RA, Buck AC, et al. An outbreak of waterborne cryptosporidiosis in Swindon and Oxfordshire. Epidemiol Infect 1991;107:485–495.
127. Bridgman SA, Robertson RM, Syed Q, et al. Outbreak of cryptosporidiosis associated with a disinfected groundwater supply. Epidemiol Infect 1995;115:555–566.
128. Maguire HC, Holmes E, Hollyer J, et al. An outbreak of cryptosporidiosis in south London: what value the *p* value? Epidemiol Infect 1995;115:279–287.
129. Kuroki T, Watanabe Y, Asai Y, et al. An outbreak of waterborne cryptosporidiosis in Kanagawa, Japan. Kansenshogaku Zasshi 1996; 70:132–140.
130. Sorvillo FJ, Fujioka K, Nahlen B, et al. Swimming-associated cryptosporidiosis. Am J Public Health 1992;82:742–744.
131. McAnulty JM, Fleming DW, Gonzalez AH. A community-wide outbreak of cryptosporidiosis associated with swimming at a wave pool. JAMA 1994;272:1597–600.
132. Lemmon JM, McAnulty JM, Bawden-Smith J. Outbreak of cryptosporidiosis linked to an indoor swimming pool. Med J Aust 1996;165:613–616.
133. MacKenzie WR, Kazmierczak JJ, Davis JP. An outbreak of cryptosporidiosis associated with a resort swimming pool. Epidemiol Infect 1995;115:545–553.
134. Centers for Disease Control and Prevention. *Cryptosporidium* infections associated with swimming pools: Dane County, Wisconsin, 1993. JAMA 1994;272:914–915.
135. MacKenzie WR, Schell WL, Blair KA, et al. Massive outbreak of waterborne *Cryptosporidium* infection in Milwaukee, Wisconsin: recurrence of illness and risk of secondary transmission. Clin Infect Dis 1995;21:57–62.
136. LeChevaillier MW, Norton WD. Occurrence of *Giardia* and *Cryptosporidium* in raw and finished drinking water. J Am Water Works Assoc 1996;87:54–68.
137. Gale P. Developments in microbiological risk assessment models for drinking water: a short review. J Appl Bacteriol 1996; 81:403–410.
138. Perz JF, Ennever FK, Le Blancq SM. *Cryptosporidium* in tapwater: comparison of predicted risks to observed levels of disease. Am J Epidem (in press).
139. Sorvillo F, Lieb LE, Nahlen B, et al. Municipal drinking water and cryptosporidiosis among persons with AIDS in Los Angeles County. Epidemiol Infect 1994; 13:313–320.
140. Morris RD, Naumova EN, Levin R, et al. Temporal variation in drinking water turbidity and diagnosed gastroenteritis in Milwaukee. Am J Public Health 1996;86:237–239.
141. Payment P, Richardson L, Siemiatycki J, et al. A randomized trial to evaluate the risk of gastrointestinal disease due to consumption of drinking water meeting current microbiological standards. Am J Public Health 1991;81:703–708.
142. *Working Group on Waterborne Cryptosporidiosis. Cryptosporidium* and water: a public health handbook. Atlanta: Working Group on Waterborne Cryptosporidiosis, 1997.
143. Arrowood MJ. Diagnosis of cryptosporidiosis. In: R Fayer, ed. *Cryptosporidium* and cryptosporidiosis. Boca Raton, FL: CRC Press, 1997:43–64.
144. Rose JB. Environmental ecology of *Cryptosporidium* and public health implications. Annu Rev Public Health 1997;18:135–161.
145. Colley DG. Waterborne cryptosporidiosis threat addressed [news]. Emerg Infect Dis 1995;1:67.
146. Navin TR. Detecting cryptosporidiosis as a cause of diarrheal illness: implications for clinicians [letter]. JAMA 1997;277:1355–1356.
147. Nina JMS, McDonald V, Dyson DA, et al. Analysis of oocyst wall and sporozoite antigens from three *Cryptosporidium* species. Infect Immun 1992;60:1509.
148. Mead JR, Humphreys RC, Sammons DW, et al. Identification of isolate-specific sporozoite proteins of *Cryptosporidium parvum* by two-dimensional gel electrophoresis. Infect Immun 1990;58: 2071–2075.
149. Awad-el-Kariem FM, Robinson HA, Dyson DA, et al. Differentiation between human and animal strains of *Cryptosporidium parvum* using isoenzyme typing. Parasitology 1995;110:129–132.
150. Petersen C. Cellular biology of *Cryptosporidium parvum*. Parasitol Today 1993;9:87–91.
151. Bonnin A, Fourmaux MN, Dubremetz JF, et al. Genotyping human and bovine isolates of *Cryptosporidium parvum* by polymerase chain reaction–restriction fragment length polymorphism analysis by a repetitive DNA sequence. FEMS Microbiol Lett 1996;137:207–211.
152. Spano F, Putignani L, Mclauchlin J, et al. PCR-RFLP analysis of the *Cryptosporidium* oocyst wall protei (COWP) gene discriminates between C. *wrairi* and C. *parvum* isolates of human and animal origin. FEMS Microbiol Lett 1997;150:209–217.
153. Morgan UM, Constantine CC, Forbes DA, et al. Differentiation between human and animal isolates of *Cryptosporidium* parvum using rDNA sequencing and direct PCR analysis. J Parasitol 1997;83: 825–830.
154. Carraway M, Tzipori S, Widmer G. A new restriction fragment length polymorphism from *Cryptosporidium* parvum identifies genetically heterogeneous parasite populations and genotypic changes following transmission from bovine to human hosts. Infect Immun 1997; 9:3958–3960.
155. Caccio S, La Rosa G, Pozio E. The beta-tubulin gene of *Cryptosporidium* parvum. Mol Biochem Parasitol 1997;89:307–311.
156. Vasquez JR, Gooze L, Kim K, et al. Potential antifolate resistance determinants and genotypic variation in the bifunctional dihydrofolate reductase–thymidylate synthase gene from human and bovine isolates of *Cryptosporidium parvum*. Mol Biochem Parasitol 1996;79: 153–165.
157. Peng MM, Xiao L, Freeman AR, et al. Genetic polymorphism among *Cryptosporidium* parvum isolates: evidence of two distinct human transmission cycles. Emerg Infect Dis 1997;3:567–573.
158. Robertson LJ, Campbell AT, Smith HV. Survival of *Cryptosporidium parvum* oocysts under various environmental pressures. Appl Environ Microbiol 1992;58:3494–3500.
159. Campbell AT, Robertson LJ, Snowball MR, et al. Inactivation of oocysts of *Cryptosporidium parvum* by ultraviolet radiation. Water Res 1995;29:2583.
160. Fayer R. Effect of high temperature on infectivity of *Cryptosporidium parvum* oocysts in water. Appl Environ Microbiol 1994;60:2732.
161. Harp JA, Fayer R, Pesch BA, et al. Effect of pasteurization on infectivity of *Cryptosporidium parvum* oocysts in water and milk. Appl Environ Microbiol 1996 62:2866–2868.
162. Fayer R, Graczyk TK, Cranfield MR, et al. Gaseous disinfection of *Cryptosporidium parvum* oocysts. Appl Environ Microbiol 1996;62: 3908–3909.
163. Holton J, Nye P, McDonald V. Efficacy of selected disinfectants against mycobacteria and cryptosporidia. J Hosp Infect 1994;27:504.
164. Venczel LV, Arrowood M, Hurd M, et al. Inactivation of *Cryptosporidium* parvum oocysts and *Clostridium perfringens* spores by a mixed-oxidant disinfectant and by free chlorine. Appl Environ Microbiol 1997;63:1598–1601.
165. Bannister P, Mountford RA. *Cryptosporidium* in the elderly: a cause of life-threatening diarrhea. Am J Med 1989;86:507–508.
166. Neill MA, Rice SK, Ahmad NV, et al. Cryptosporidiosis: an unrecognized cause of diarrhea in elderly hospitalized patients. Clin Infect Dis 1996;22:168–170.

167. Blanshard C, Jackson AM, Shanson DC, et al. Cryptosporidiosis in HIV-seropositive patients. Q J Med 1992;85:813–823.
168. Sanchez-Mejorada G, Ponce-de-Leon S. Clinical patterns of diarrhea in AIDS: etiology and prognosis. Rev Invest Clin 1994;46:187–196.
169. Current WL, Reese NC, Ernst JV, et al. Human cryptosporidiosis in immunocompetent and immunodeficient persons. N Engl J Med 1983;308:1252–1257.
170. Soave R, Danner RL, Honig CL, et al. Cryptosporidiosis in homosexual men. Ann Intern Med 1984;100:504–511.
171. Wolfson JS, Richter JM, Waldron MA, et al. Cryptosporidiosis in immunocompetent patients. N Engl J Med 1985;312:1278–1282.
172. Pitlik SD, Fainstein V, Garza D, et al. Human cryptosporidiosis: spectrum of disease. Arch Intern Med 1983;143:2269–2275.
173. MacFarlane DE, Horner-Bryce J. Cryptosporidiosis in well-nourished and malnourished children. Acta Paediatr Scand 1987;76:474–477.
174. Keren G, Barzilai A, Barzilay Z, et al. Life-threatening cryptosporidiosis in immunocompetent infants. Eur J Pediatr 1987;146:187–188.
175. Sallon S, Deckelbaum RJ, Schmid II, et al. *Cryptosporidium*, malnutrition, and chronic diarrhea in children. Am J Dis Child 1988;142:312–315.
176. Laxer MA, Alcantara AK, Javato-Laxer M, et al. Immune response to cryptosporidiosis in Philippine children. Am J Trop Med Hyg 1990;42:131–139.
177. Bhan MK, Bhandari N, Bhatnagar S, et al. Epidemiology and management of persistent diarrhoea in children of developing countries. Indian J Med Res 1996;104:103–114.
178. Harp JA, Chen W, Harmsen AG. Resistance of severe combined immunodeficient mice to infection with *Cryptosporidium parvum*: the importance of intestinal microflora. Infect Immun 1992;60:3509–3512.
179. Heine J, Pohlenz JFL, Moon HW, et al. Enteric lesions and diarrhea in gnotobiotic calves monoinfected with *Cryptosporidium* species. J Infect Dis 1984;150:768–775.
180. Scaglia M, Senaldi G, DiPerri G, et al. Unusual low grade cryptosporidial enteritis in AIDS. Infection 1986;14:43–44.
181. Saltzberg DM, Kotloff KL, Newman JL, et al. *Cryptosporidium* infection in acquired immunodeficiency syndrome: not always a poor prognosis. J Clin Gastroenterol 1991;13:94–97.
182. Berkowitz CD, Seidel JS. Spontaneous resolution of cryptosporidiosis in a child with acquired immunodeficiency syndrome. Am J Dis Child 1985;139:967.
183. Moss PJ, Read RC, Kudesia G, et al. Prolonged cryptosporidiosis during primary HIV infection. J Infect 1995;30:51–53.
184. Molbak K, Lisse IM, Hojlyng N, Aaby P. Severe cryptosporidiosis in children with normal T-cell subsets. Parasite Immunol 1994;16:275–277.
185. Phillips AD, Thomas AG, Walker-Smith JA. *Cryptosporidium*, chronic diarrhea and the proximal small intestinal mucosa. Gut 1992;33:1057–1061.
186. Edelman MJ, Oldfield EC. Severe cryptosporidiosis in an immunocompetent host. Arch Intern Med 1988;148:1873–1874.
187. Guarino A, Spagnuolo MI, Russo S, et al. Etiology and risk factors of severe and protracted diarrhea. J Pediatr Gastroenterol Nutr 1995;20:173–178.
188. Lasser KH, Lewin KJ, Ryning FW. Cryptosporidial enteritis in a patient with congenital hypogammaglobulinemia. Hum Pathol 1979;10:234–240.
189. Weisburger WR, Hutcheon DF, Yardley JH, et al. Cryptosporidiosis in an immunosuppressed renal-transplant recipient with IgA deficiency. Am J Clin Pathol 1979;72:473–478.
190. Jacyna MR, Parkin J, Goldin R, et al. Protracted enteric cryptosporidial infection in selective immunoglobulin A and saccharomyces opsonin deficiencies. Gut 1990;31:714–716.
191. Hayward AR, Levy J, Facchetti F, et al. Cholangiopathy and tumors of the pancreas, liver, and biliary tree in boys with X-linked immunodeficiency with hyper-IgM. J Immunol 1997;15;158:977–983.
192. Gomez Morales MA, Ausiello CM, Guarino A, et al. Severe protracted intestinal cryptosporidiosis associated with interferon gamma deficiency: pediatric case report. Clin Infect Dis 1996;22:848–850.
193. De Mol P, Mukashema S, Bogaerts J, et al. *Cryptosporidium* related to measles diarrhea in Rwanda. Lancet 1894;2:42–43.
194. Stehr-Green JK, Juranek DJ, McCaig L, et al. Chickenpox and infection with cryptosporidiosis. Am J Dis Child 1986;140:1213.
195. Gledhill JA, Porter J. Diarrhoea due to *Cryptosporidium* infection in thalassaemia major. BMJ 1990;301:212–213.
196. Trevino-Perez S, Luna-Castanos G, Matilla-Matilla A, et al. Chronic diarrhea and *Cryptosporidium* in diabetic patients with normal lymphocyte subpopulation: 2 case reports. Gac Med Mex 1995;131:219–222.
197. Chan AW, MacFarlane IA, Rhodes JM. Cryptosporidiosis as a cause of chronic diarrhoea in a patient with insulin-dependent diabetes mellitus. J Infect 1989;19:293.
198. Vajro P, di Martino L, Scotti S, et al. Intestinal *Cryptosporidium* carriage in two liver-transplanted children. J Pediatr Gastroenterol Nutr 1991;12:139.
199. Blakey JL, Bishop RF, Barnes GL, et al. Infectious diarrhea in children undergoing bone-marrow transplantation. Aust N Z J Med 1989;19:31–36.
200. Nachbaur D, Kropshofer G, Feichtinger H, et al. Cryptosporidiosis after CD34-selected autologous peripheral blood stem cell transplantation (PBSCT): treatment with paromomycin, azithromycin and recombinant human interleukin-2. Bone Marrow Transplant 1997;19:1261–1263.
201. Holley HP, Thiers BH. Cryptosporidiosis in a patient receiving immunosuppressive therapy: possible activation of a latent infection. Dig Dis Sci 1986;31:1004–1007.
202. Mead GM, Sweetenham JW, Ewins DL, et al. Intestinal cryptosporidiosis: a complication of cancer treatment. Cancer Treat Rep 1986;70:769–770.
203. Foot ABM, Oakhill A, Mott MG. Cryptosporidiosis and acute leukemia. Arch Dis Child 1990;65:236–237.
204. Miller RA, Holmberg RE, Clauson CR. Life-threatening diarrhea caused by *Cryptosporidium* in a child undergoing therapy for acute lymphoblastic leukemia. J Pediatr 1983;103:256–259.
205. Lahdevirta J, Jokipii AAM, Sammalkorpi K, et al. Perinatal infection with *Cryptosporidium* and failure to thrive. Lancet 1987;1:48–49.
206. Dale BA, Gordon S, Thomson R, et al. Perinatal infection with *Cryptosporidium*. Lancet 1987;1:1042–1043.
207. Leek S. Case study: cryptosporidiosis complicating pregnancy and the puerperium. Midwives Chron 1987;100: 72–74.
208. Manthey MW, Ross AB, Soergel KH. Cryptosporidiosis and inflammatory bowel disease: experience from the Milwaukee outbreak. Dig Dis Sci 1997;42:1580–1586.
209. Yoshida EM, Chan NH, Herrick RA, et al. Human immunodeficiency virus infection, the acquired immunodeficiency syndrome, and inflammatory bowel disease. J Clin Gastroenterol 1996;23:24–28.
210. Janoff EN, Limas C, Gebhard RL, et al. Cryptosporidial carriage without symptoms in the acquired immunodeficincy syndrome. Ann Intern Med 1990;112:75.
211. Crawford FG, Vermund SH, Ma JY, et al. Asymptomatic cryptosporidiosis in a New York City day care center. Pediatr Infect Dis 1988;7:806–807.
212. Vuorio AF, Jokipii AMM, Jokipii L. *Cryptosporidium* in asymptomatic children. Rev Infect Dis 1991;13:261–264.
213. Roberts WG, Green PH, Ma J, et al. Prevalence of cryptosporidiosis in patients undergoing endoscopy: evidence for an asymptomatic carrier state. Am J Med 1989;87:537–539.
214. Ramirez FC, Claridge JE, Heiser MC, et al. A study of the frequency of recovery of unexpected *Giardia lamblia* and *Cryptosporidium* from duodenal aspirates taken during routine upper endoscopy. Am J Gastroenterol 1993;88:552.
215. Ravera M, Reggiori A, Cocozza E. Prevalence of *Cryptosporidium parvum* in AIDS and immunocompetent patients in Uganda [letter]. Int J STD AIDS 1994;5:302.

216. Ma P, Kauffman DL, Helmick CG et al. Cryptosporidiosis in tourists returning from the Caribbean. N Engl J Med 1985;312:647–648.
217. Soave R. Waterborne cryptosporidiosis: setting the stage for control of an emerging pathogen. Clin Infect Dis 1995;21:63–64.
218. Vakil NB, Schwartz SM, Buggy BP, et al. Biliary cryptosporidiosis in HIV-infected people after the waterborne outbreak of cryptosporidiosis in Milwaukee. N Engl J Med 1996;334:19–23.
219. Flanigan T, Whalen C, Turner J, et al. *Cryptosporidium* infection and CD4 counts. Ann Intern Med 1992;116:840–842.
220. Crowe SM, Carlin JB, Stewart KI, et al. Predictive value of CD4 lymphocyte numbers for the development of opportunistic infections and malignancies in HIV-infected persons. J Acquir Immune Defic Syndr 1991;4:770–776.
221. Hashmey R, Smith NH, Cron S, et al. Cryptosporidiosis in Houston, Texas: a report of 95 cases. Medicine 1997;76:118–139.
222. Pozio E, Rezza G, Boschini A, et al. Clinical cryptosporidiosis and human immunodeficiency virus (HIV)–induced immunosuppression: findings from a longitudinal study of HIV-positive and HIV-negative former injection drug users. J Infect Dis 1997;176:969–975.
223. Guarino A, Castaldo A, Russo S, et al. Enteric cryptosporidiosis in pediatric HIV infection. J Pediatr Gastroenterol Nutr 1997;25:182–187.
224. Nicholas SW. The opportunistic and bacterial infections associated with pediatric human immunodeficiency virus disease. Acta Paediatr Suppl 1994;400:46–50.
225. Moore RD, Chaisson RE. Natural history of opportunistic disease in an HIV-infected urban clinical cohort. Ann Intern Med 1996;124:633–642.
226. Goodgame RW, Kimball K, Ou CN, et al. Intestinal function and injury in acquired immunodeficiency syndrome-related cryptosporidiosis. Gastroenterology 1995;108:1075–082.
227. Clayton F, Heller T, Kotler DP. Variation in the enteric distribution of cryptosporidia in acquired immunodeficiency syndrome. Am J Clin Pathol 1994;102:420–425.
228. Bartlett JG, Belitsos PC, Sears C, et al. AIDS enteropathy. Clin Infect Dis 1992;15:726–735.
229. Sciarretta G, Bonazzi L, Monti M, et al. Bile acid malabsorption in AIDS-associated chronic diarrhea: a prospective 1-year study. Am J Gastroenterol 1994;89:379–381.
230. Sharpstone DR, Ross HM, Gazzard BG. The metabolic response to opportunistic infections in AIDS. AIDS 1996;10:1529–1533.
231. Baxby D, Hart CA, Blundell N. Shedding of oocysts by immunocompetent individuals with cryptosporidiosis. J Hyg 1985;95:703–709.
232. Stehr-Green JK, McCaig L, Remsen HM, et al. Shedding of oocysts in immunocompetent individuals infected with *Cryptosporidium*. Am J Trop Med Hyg 1987;36:338–342.
233. Chappell CL, Okhuysen PC, Sterling CR, et al. *Cryptosporidium parvum*: intensity of infection and oocyst excretion patterns in healthy volunteers. J Infect Dis 1996;173:232–236.
234. Genta RM, Chappell CL, White AC Jr, et al. Duodenal morphology and intensity of infection in AIDS-related intestinal cryptosporidiosis. Gastroenterology 1993;105:1769–1775.
235. Wuhib T, Silva TM, Newman RD, et al. Cryptosporidial and microsporidial infections in human immunodeficiency virus-infected patients in northeastern Brazil. J Infect Dis 1994;170:494–497.
236. Garcia L, Shimizu R, Bruckner D. Detection of microsporidial spores in fecal specimens from patients diagnosed with cryptosporidiosis. J Clin Microbiol 1994;32:1739–1741.
237. Cornet M, Romand S, Warszawski J, et al. Factors associated with microsporidial and cryptosporidial diarrhea in HIV infected patients. Parasite 1996;3:397–401.
238. Kotler D, Orenstein J. Prevalence of intestinal microspoiridiosis in HIV-infected individuals referred for gastroenterological evaluation. Am J Gastroenterol 1994;89:1988–2002.
239. Blumberg RS, Kelsey P, Perrone T, et al. Cytomegalovirus- and *Cryptosporidium*-associated acalculous gangrenous cholecystitis. Am J Med 1984;76:1118–1123.
240. Margulis SJ, Honig CL, Soave R, et al. Biliary tract obstruction in the acquired immunodeficiency syndrome. Ann Intern Med 1986;105:207–210.
241. Gross TL, Wheat J, Bartlett M, et al. AIDS and multiple system involvement with *Cryptosporidium*. Am J Gastroenterol 1986;81:456–458.
242. Cello JP. Acquired immunodeficiency syndrome cholangiopathy: spectrum of disease. Am J Med 1989;86:539–546.
243. Godwin TA. Cryptosporidiosis in the acquired immunodeficiency syndrome: a study of 15 autopsy cases. Hum Pathol 1991;22:1215–1224.
244. Bouche H, Housset C, Dumont JL, et al. AIDS-related cholangitis: diagnostic features and course in 15 patients. J Hepatol 1993;17:34.
245. Forbes A, Blanshard C, Gazzard B. Natural history of AIDS related sclerosing cholangitis: a study of 20 cases. Gut 1993;34:116–121.
246. Benhamou Y, Caumes E, Gerosa Y, et al. AIDS-related cholangiopathy: critical analysis of a prospective series of 26 patients. Dig Dis Sci 1993;38:1113–1118.
247. French AL, Beaudet LM, Benator DA, et al. Cholecystectomy in patients with AIDS: clinicopathologic correlations in 107 cases. Clin Infect Dis 1995;21:852–858.
248. Ducreux M, Buffet C, Lamy P, et al. Diagnosis and prognosis in AIDS-related cholangitis. AIDS 1995;9:875–880.
249. Leiva JI, Etter EL, Gathe J Jr, et al. Surgical therapy for 101 patients with acquired immunodeficiency syndrome and symptomatic cholecystitis. Am J Surg 1997;174:414–416.
250. Teare JP, Daly CA, Rodgers C, et al. Pancreatic abnormalities and AIDS related sclerosing cholangitis. Genitourin Med 1997;73:271–273.
251. Farman J, Brunetti J, Baer JW, et al. AIDS-related cholangiopancreatographic changes. Abdom Imaging 1994;19:417–422.
252. Teixidor HS, Godwin TS, Ramirez EA. Cryptosporidiosis of the biliary tract in AIDS. Radiology 1991;180:51–56.
253. Brunetti JC, Van Heertum RL, Kempf JS, et al. Tc-99m DISIDA hepatobiliary scintigraphy in AIDS cholangitis. Clin Nucl Med 1994;19:36–42.
254. Hasan FA, Jeffers LJ, Dickenson, et al. Hepatobiliary cryptosporidiosis and cytomegalovirus infection mimicking metastatic cancer to the liver. Gastroenterology 1991;100:1743–1748.
255. Kline TJ, De las Morenas T, O'Brien M, et al. Squamous metaplasia of extrahepatic biliary system in an AIDS patient with cryptosporidia and cholangitis. Dig Dis Sci 1993;38:960–962.
256. Kocochis SA, Cibull ML, Davis TE, et al. Intestinal and pulmonary cryptosporidiosis in an infant with severe combined immune deficiency. J Pediatr Gastroenterol Nutr 1984;3:149–157.
257. Cappell MS, Hassan T. Pancreatic disease in AIDS: a review. J Clin Gastroenterol 1993;17:254–263.
258. Dowell SF, Holt EA, Murphy FK. Pancreatitis associated with human immunodeficiency virus infection: a matched case-control study. Tex Med 1996;92:44–49.
259. Parenti DM, Steinberg W, Kang P. Infectious causes of acute pancreatitis. Pancreas 1996;13:356–371.
260. Tan WW, Chapnick EK, Abter EI, et al. Paromomycin-associated pancreatitis in HIV-related cryptosporidiosis. Ann Pharmacother 1995;29:22–24.
261. Massimillo AJ, Chang J, Freedman L, et al. *Cryptosporidium* gastropathy: presentation of a case and review of the literature. Dig Dis Sci 1995;40:186–190.
262. Ventura G, Cauda R, Larocca LM, et al. Gastric cryptosporidiosis complicating HIV infection: case report and review of the literature. Eur J Gastroenterol Hepatol 1997;9:307–310.
263. Forester G, Sidhom O, Nahass R, et al. AIDS-associated cryptosporidiosis with gastric stricture and a therapeutic response to paromomycin. Am J Gastroenterol 1994;89:1096–1098.
264. Connolly GM, Gazzard BG. Toxic megacolon in cryptosporidiosis. Postgrad Med J 1987;63:1103–1104.
265. Meyers SA, Kuhlman JE, Fishman EK. Enterovesical fistula in a patient with cryptosporidiosis and AIDS. Clin Imaging 1990;14:143–145.

266. Collins CD, Blanshard C, Cramp M, et al. Case report: pneumatosis intestinalis occurring in association with cryptosporidiosis and HIV infection. Clin Radiol 1992;46:410–411.
267. Samson VE, Brown WR. Pneumatosis cystoides intestinalis in AIDS-associated cryptosporidiosis: more than an incidental finding? J Clin Gastroenterol 1996;22:311–312.
268. Forgacs P, Tarshis A, Ma P, et al. Intestinal and bronchial cryptosporidiosis in an immunodeficient homosexual man. Ann Intern Med 1983;99:793–794.
269. Ma P, Villaneuva TG, Kaufmann, et al. Respiratory cryptosporidiosis in the acquired immunodeficiency syndrome. JAMA 1984;252:1298–1301.
270. Hojlyng N, Jensen BN. Respiratory cryptosporidiosis in HIV-positive patients. Lancet 1987;1:590–591.
271. Travis WD, Schmidt K, MacLowry JD, et al. Respiratory cryptosporidiosis in a patient with malignant lymphoma. Arch Pathol Lab Med 1990;114:519–522.
272. Mohri H, Fujita H, Asakura Y, et al. Case report: inhalation therapy of paromomycin is effective for respiratory infection and hypoxia by *Cryptosporidium* with AIDS. Am J Med Sci 1995;309:60–62.
273. Clavel A, Arnal AC, Sanchez EC, et al. Respiratory cryptosporidiosis: case series and review of the literature. Infection 1996;24:341–346.
274. Meynard JL, Meyohas MC, Binet D, et al. Pulmonary cryptosporidiosis in the acquired immunodeficiency syndrome. Infection 1996;24:328–331.
275. Harari MD, West B, Dwyer B. *Cryptosporidium* as a cause of laryngotracheitis in an infant. Lancet 1983;1:207.
276. Davis JJ, Heyman MB. Cryptosporidiosis and sinusitis in an immunodeficient adolescent. J Infect Dis 1988;158:649.
277. Dunand VA, Hammer SM, Rossi R, et al. Parasitic sinusitis and otitis in patients infected with human immunodeficiency virus: report of five cases and review. Clin Infect Dis 1997;25:267–272.
278. Giang TT, Pollack G, Kotler DP. Cryptosporidiosis of the nasal mucosa in a patient with AIDS [letter]. AIDS 1994;8:555–556.
279. Baskin GB. Cryptosporidiosis of the conjunctiva in SIV-infected rhesus monkeys. Parasitology 1996;82:630–632.
280. Hay EM, Winfield J, McKendrick MW. Reactive arthritis associated with *Cryptosporidium* enteritis. Br Med J 1987;295:248.
281. Shepherd RC, Smail PJ, Sinha GP. Reactive arthritis complicating cryptosporidial infection. Arch Dis Child 1989;64:743–744.
282. Cron RQ, Sherry DD. Reiter's syndrome associated with cryptosporidial gastroenteritis. J Rheumatol 1995;22:1962–1963.
283. Gentile G, Baldasarri L, Caprioli A, et al. Colonic vascular invasion as a possible route of extraintestinal cryptosporidiosis. Am J Med 1987;82:574–575.
284. Lefkowitch JS, Krumholz S, Feng-Chen KC, et al. Cryptosporidiosis of the human small intestine: a light and electron microscopic study. Hum Pathol 1984;15:746–752.
285. Zu S-X, Fang G-D, Fayer R, et al. Cryptosporidiosis: pathogenesis and immunology. Parasitol Today 1992;8:24–27.
286. Clark DP, Sears CL. The pathogenesis of cryptosporidiosis. Parasitol Today 1996;12:221–225.
287. Argenzio RA, Liacos JA, Levy ML et al. Villous atrophy, crypt hyperplasia, cellular infiltration, and impaired glucose-NA absorption in enteric cryptosporidiosis of pigs. Gastroenterology 1990;98:1129–1140.
288. Argenzio RA, Armstrong M, Rhoads JM. Role of the enteric nervous system in piglet cryptosporidiosis. J Pharmacol Exp Ther 1996;279:1109–1115.
289. Argenzio RA, Rhoads JM. Reactive oxygen metabolites in piglet cryptosporidiosis. Pediatr Res 1997;41:521–526.
290. Argenzio RA, Armstrong M, Blikslager A, et al. Peptide YY inhibits intestinal Cl^- secretion in experimental porcine cryptosporidiosis through a prostaglandin-activated neural pathway. J Pharmacol Exp Ther 1997;283:692–697.
291. Kelly P, Thillainayagam AV, Smithson J, et al. Jejunal water and electrolyte transport in human cryptosporidiosis. Dig Dis Sci 1996;41:2095–2099.
292. Adams RB, Guerrant RL, Zu S, et al. *Cryptosporidium parvum* infection of intestinal epithelium: morphologic and functional studies in an in vitro model. J Infect Dis 1994;169:170–177.
293. Griffiths JK, Moore R, Dooley S, et al. *Cryptosporidium parvum* infection of Caco-2 cell monolayers induces an apical monolayer defect, selectively increases transmonolayer permeability, and causes epithelial cell death. Infect Immun 1994;62:4506–4514.
294. Planchon SM, Martins CA, Guerrant RL, et al. Regulation of intestinal epithelial barrier function by TGF-beta 1: evidence for its role in abrogating the effect of a T cell cytokine. J Immunol 1994;153:5730–5739.
295. Moore R, Tzipori S, Griffiths JK, et al. Temporal changes in permeability and structure of piglet ileum after site-specific infection by *Cryptosporidium parvum*. Gastroenterology 1995;108:1030–1039.
296. Guarino A, Canani RB, Pozio E, et al. Enterotoxic effect of stool supernatant of *Cryptosporidium* infected calves on human jejunum. Gastroenterol 1994;106:28–34.
297. Guarino A, Canani RB, Casola A, et al. Human intestinal cryptosporidiosis: secretory diarrhea and enterotoxic activity in Caco-2 cells. J Infect Dis 1995;171:976–983.
298. Kandil HM, Berschneider HM, Argenzio RA. Tumour necrosis factor alpha changes porcine intestinal ion transport through a paracrine mechanism involving prostaglandins. Gut 1994;35:934–940.
299. Sharpstone DR, Rowbottom AW, Nelson MR, et al. Faecal tumour necrosis factor-alpha in individuals with HIV-related diarrhoea. AIDS 1996;10:989–994.
300. Snijders F, van Deventer SJ, Bartelsman JF, et al. Diarrhoea in HIV-infected patients: no evidence of cytokine-mediated inflammation in jejunal mucosa. AIDS 1995;9:367–373.
301. Riggs MW. Imunology: host response and development of passive immunotherapy and vaccines. In: Fayer R, ed. *Cryptosporidium* and cryptosporidiosis. Boca Raton, FL :CRC Press, 1997;129–162.
302. Heyworth MF. Immunology of *Giardia* and *Cryptosporidium* infections. J Infect Dis 1992;166:465–472.
303. Flanigan TP. Human immunodeficiency virus infection and cryptosporidiosis: protective immune responses. Am J Trop Med Hyg 1994;50(5 Suppl):29–35.
304. Nachbaur D, Kropshofer G, Feichtinger H, et al. Cryptosporidiosis after CD34-selected autologous peripheral blood stem cell transplantation (PBSCT): treatment with paromomycin, azithromycin and recombinant human interleukin-2. Bone Marrow Transplant 1997;19:1261–1263.
305. Ungar BLP, Soave R, Fayer R, et al. Enzyme immunoassay detection of immunoglobulin M and G antibodies to *Cryptosporidium* in immunocompetent and immunocompromised persons. J Infect Dis 1986;153:570–578.
306. Kassa M, Comby E, Lemeteil D, et al. Characterization of anti-*Cryptosporidium* IgA antibodies in sera from immunocompetent individuals and HIV-infected patients. J Protozool 1991;38:179s–180s.
307. Cozon G, Biron F, Jeannin M, et al. Secretory IgA antibodies to *Cryptosporidium parvum* in AIDS patients with chronic cryptosporidiosis. J Infect Dis 1994;169:696–699.
308. Benhamou Y, Kapel N, Hoang C, et al. Inefficacy of intestinal secretory immune response to *Cryptosporidium* in acquired immunodeficiency syndrome. Gastroenterology 1995;108:627–635.
309. Kuhls TL, Mosier DA, Crawford DL, et al. Seroprevalence of cryptosporidial antibodies during infancy, childhood, and adolescence. Clin Infect Dis 1994;18:731–735.
310. Moss DM, Bennett SN, Arrowood MJ, et al. Kinetic and isotype analysis of specific immunoglobulins from crew members with cryptosporidiosis on a U.S. Coast Guard cutter. J Eukaryot Microbiol 1994;41:52S.
311. Kapel N, Meillet D, Buraud M, et al. Determination of anti-*Cryptosporidium* coproantibodies by time-resolved immunofluorometric assay. Trans R Soc Trop Med Hyg 1993;87:330–332.

312. de Graaf DC, Peeters JE. Specific interferon-gamma, IgA and IgM responses after experimental infection of neonatal calves with *Cryptosporidium parvum*. Int J Parasitol 1997;27:131–134.
313. Tarazona R, Lally NC, Dominguez-Carmona M, et al. Characterization of secretory IgA responses in mice infected with *Cryptosporidium parvum*. Int J Parasitol 1997;27:417–423.
314. Taghi-Kilani R, Sekla L, Hayglass KT. The role of humoral immunity in *Cryptosporidium* spp infection: studies with B cell–depleted mice. J Immunol 1990;145:1571.
315. Favennec L, Comby E, Ballet JJ, et al. Serum IgA antibody response to *Cryptosporidium parvum* is mainly represented by IgA1 [letter]. J Infect Dis 1995;171:256.
316. Riggs MW, Stone AL, Yount PA, et al. Protective monoclonal antibody defines a circumsporozoite-like glycoprotein exoantigen of *Cryptosporidium parvum* sporozoites and merozoites. J Immunol 1997;158:1787–1795.
317. Répérant JM, Naciri M, Iochmann S, et al. Major antigens of *Cryptosporidium parvum* recognized by serum antibodies from different infected animal species and man. Vet Parasitol 1994;55;1.
318. Mead JR, Arrowood MJ, Sterling CR. Antigens of *Cryptosporidium* sporozoites recognized by immune sera of infected animals and humans. J Parasitol 1988;74:135–143.
319. Lumb R, Lanser JA, O'Donoghue PJ. Electrophoretic and immunoblot analysis of *Cryptosporidium* oocysts. Immunol Cell Biol 1988;66:369–376.
320. Tilley M, Upton SJ, Fayer R, et al. Identification of a 15-kilodalton surface glycoprotein on sporozoites of *Cryptosporidium parvum*. Infect Immun 1991;59:1002–1007.
321. Hojlyng N, Molbak K, Jepsen S. *Cryptosporidium* spp., a frequent cause of diarrhea in Liberian children. J Clin Micro 1986; 23:1109–1113.
322. Mata L. *Cryptosporidium* and other protozoa in diarrheal disease in less developed countries. Pediatr Infect Dis 1986;5:S117–S130.
323. Moon HW, Woodmansee DB, Harp JA, et al. Lacteal immunity to enteric cryptosporidiosis in mice: immune dams do not protect their suckling pups. Infect Immun 1988;56:649–653.
324. Saxon A, Weinstein W. Oral administration of bovine colostrum anti-cryptosporidia antibody fails to alter the course of human cryptosporidiosis. J Parasitol 1987;73:413–415.
325. Tzipori S, Robertson D, Chapman C. Remission of diarrhea due to cryptosporidiosis in an immunodeficient child treated with hyperimmune bovine colostrum. BMJ 1986;293:1276–1277.
326. Ungar BLP, Ward DJ, Fayer RF, et al. Cessation of *Cryptosporidium*-associated diarrhea in an acquired immunodeficiency patient after treatment with hyperimmune bovine colostrum. Gastroenterology 1990;98:486–489.
327. Nord J, Ma P, DiJohn D, et al. Treatment with bovine hyperimmune colostrum of cryptosporidial diarrhea in AIDS patients. AIDS 1990;4:581–584.
328. Culshaw RJ, Bancroft GJ, McDonald V. Gut intraepithelial lymphocytes induce immunity against *Cryptosporidium* infection through a mechanism involving gamma interferon production. Infect Immun 1997;65:3074–3079.
329. Abrahamsen MS, Lancto CA, Walcheck B, et al. Localization of α/β and γ/δ T lymphocytes in *Cryptosporidium parvum*–infected tissues in naive and immune calves. Infect Immun 1997;65:2428–2433.
330. Harp JA, Sacco RE. Development of cellular immune functions in neonatal to weanling mice: relationship to *Cryptosporidium parvum* infection. J Parasitol 1996;82:245–249.
331. Pasquali P, Fayer R, Almeria S, et al. Lymphocyte dynamic patterns in cattle during a primary infection with *Cryptosporidium parvum*. J Parasitol 1997;83:247–250.
332. Wyatt CR, Brackett EJ, Perryman LE, et al. Activation of intestinal intraepithelial T lymphocytes in calves infected with *Cryptosporidium parvum*. Infect Immun 1997;65:185–190.
333. Waters WR, Palmer MV, Ackermann MR, et al. Accelerated inflammatory bowel disease of TCR-alpha–deficient mice persistently infected with *Cryptosporidium parvum*. J Parasitol 1997;83:460–464.
334. Theodos CM, Sullivan KL, Griffiths JK, et al. Profiles of healing and nonhealing *Cryptosporidium parvum* infection in C57BL/6 mice with functional B and T lymphocytes: the extent of gamma interferon modulation determines the outcome of infection. Infect Immun 1997;65:4761–4769.
335. Martinez F, Rosales MJ, Diaz J, et al. The effects of IFN-gamma activated mouse peritoneal and alveolar macrophages on *Cryptosporidium parvum* development. Vet Parasitol 1997;68:305–308.
336. Laurent F, Eckmann L, Savidge TC, et al. *Cryptosporidium parvum* infection of human intestinal epithelial cells induces the polarized secretion of C-X-C chemokines. Infect Immun 1997;65:5067–5073.
337. Urban JF, Fayer R, Chen SJ, et al. Il-12 protects immunocompetent and immunodeficient neonatal mice against infection with *Cryptosporidium parvum*. J Immunol 1996;156:263–268.
338. Connolly GM, Ellis DS, Williams JE, et al. Use of electron microscopy in examination of faeces and rectal and jejunal biopsy specimens. J Clin Pathol 1991;4:313–316.
339. Boldorini R, Tosoni A, Mazzucco G, et al. Intracellular protozoan infection in small intestinal biopsies of patients with AIDS: light and electron microscopic evaluation. Pathol Res Pract 1996;192:249–259.
340. Wilcox CM, Schwartz DA, Cotsonis G, et al. Chronic unexplained diarrhea in human immunodeficiency virus infection: determination of the best diagnostic approach. Gastroenterology 1996;110:30–37.
341. Pohlenz J, Moon HW, Cheville NF, et al. Cryptosporidiosis as a probable factor in neonatal diarrhea of calves. J Am Vet Med Assoc 1978;172:452–457.
342. Tzipori S, Angus KW, Gray EW, et al. Vomiting and diarrhea associated with cryptosporidial infection. N Engl J Med 1980;303:818.
343. Henriksen SA, Pohlenz JFL. Staining of *Cryptosporidia* by a modified Ziehl-Neelsen techniques. Acta Vet Scand 1981;22:594–596.
344. Ma P, Soave R. Three-step stool examination for cryptosporidiosis in 10 homosexual men with protracted watery diarrhea. J Infect Dis 1983;147:824–828.
345. Garcia LS, Bruckner DA, Brewer TC, et al. Techniques for the recovery and identification of *Cryptosporidium* oocysts from stool specimens. J Clin Microbiol 1983;18:185–190.
346. Soave R. Cyclospora: an overview. Clin Infect Dis 1996;23:429–435.
347. MacPherson DW, McQueen R. Cryptosporidiosis: multiattribute evaluation of six diagnostic methods. J Clin Microbiol 1993;31:198–202.
348. Weber R, Bryan RT, Bishop HS, et al. Threshold of detection of *Cryptosporidium* oocysts in human stool specimens: evidence for low sensitivity of current diagnostic methods. J Clin Microbiol 1991;29:1323–1327.
349. Garcia LS, Bruckner DA. Diagnostic medical parasitology. 2nd ed. Washington DC: American Society for Microbiology, 1993:528–532.
350. Ignatius R, Lehmann M, Miksits K, et al. A new acid-fast trichrome stain for simultaneous detection of *Cryptosporidium parvum* and microsporidial species in stool specimens. J Clin Microbiol 1997;35:446–449.
351. Arrowood MJ, Sterling CR. Comparison of conventional staining methods and monoclonal antibody-based methods for *Cryptosporidium* oocyst detection. J Clin Microbiol 1989;27:1490–1495.
352. Grigoriew GA, Walmsley S, Law L, et al. Evaluation of the MeriFluor immunofluorescent assay for the detection of *Cryptosporidium* and *Giardia* in sodium acetate formalin-fixed stools. Diagn Microbiol Infect Dis 1994:19:89.
353. Stazzone AM, Slaats S, Mortagy A, et al. Frequency of *Giardia* and *Cryptosporidium* infections in Egyptian children as determined by conventional and immunofluorescence methods. Pediatr Infect Dis J 1996;15:1044–1046.
354. Newman RD, Jaeger KL, Wuhib T, et al. Evaluation of an antigen capture enzyme-linked immunosorbent assay for detection of *Cryptosporidium* oocysts. J Clin Microbiol 1993;31:2080–2084.
355. Dagan R, Fraser D, El-On J, et al. Evaluation of an enzyme immunoassay for the detection of *Cryptosporidium* spp. in stool

specimens from infants and young children in field studies. Am J Trop Med Hyg 1995;52:134–138.
356. Parisi MT, Tierno PM Jr. Evaluation of new rapid commercial enzyme immunoassay for detection of *Cryptosporidium* oocysts in untreated stool specimens. J Clin Microbiol 1995;33:1963–1965.
357. Kehl KC, Cicrello H, Havens PL. Comparison of four different methods for detection of *Cryptosporidium* species. J Clin Microbiol 1995;33:416–418.
358. Graczyk TK, Cranfield MR, Fayer R. Evaluation of commercial enzyme immunoassay (EIA) and immunofluorescent antibody (FA) test kits for detection of *Cryptosporidium* oocysts of species other than *Cryptosporidium parvum*. Am J Trop Med Hyg 1996;54:274–279.
359. Garcia LS, Shimizu RY. Evaluation of nine immunoassay kits (enzyme immunoassay and direct fluorescence) for detection of *Giardia lamblia* and *Cryptosporidium parvum* in human fecal specimens. J Clin Microbiol 1997;35:1526–1529.
360. Casemore DP. A pseudo-outbreak of cryptosporidiosis. Communic Dis Rep Rev 1992;2:R66–R67.
361. Centers for Disease Control and Prevention. Outbreaks of pseudo-infection with Cyclospora and *Cryptosporidium*: Florida and New York City, 1995. MMWR Morb Mortal Wkly Rep 1997;46:354–358.
362. Valdez LM, Dang H, Okhuysen PC, et al. Flow cytometric detection of *Cryptosporidium* oocysts in human stool samples. J Clin Microbiol 1997;35:2013–2017.
363. Laxer MA, Timblin BK, Patel RJ. DNA sequences for the detection of *Cryptosporidium parvum* by the polymerase chain reaction. Am J Trop Med Hyg 1991;45:688–694.
364. Balatbat AB, Jordan GW, Tang YJ, et al. Detection of *Cryptosporidium parvum* DNA in human feces by nested PCR. J Clin Microbiol 1996;34:1769–1772.
365. Mayer CL, Palmer CJ. Evaluation of PCR, nested PCR, and fluorescent antibodies for detection of *Giardia* and *Cryptosporidium* species in wastewater. Appl Environ Microbiol 1996;62:2081–2085.
366. Deng MQ, Cliver DO, Mariam TW. Immunomagnetic capture PCR to detect viable *Cryptosporidium parvum* oocysts from environmental samples. Appl Environ Microbiol 1997;63:3134–3138.
367. Clavel A, Arnal A, Sanchez E, et al. Comparison of 2 centrifugation procedures in the formalin-ethyl acetate stool concentration technique for the detection of *Cryptosporidium* oocysts. Int J Parasitol 1996;26:671–672.
368. Weber R, Bryan RT, Juranek DD. Improved stool concentration procedure for detection of *Cryptosporidium* oocysts in fecal specimens. J Clin Microbiol 1992;30:2869–2873.
369. Blackman E, Binder S, Gaultier C, et al. Cryptosporidiosis in HIV-infected patients: diagnostic sensitivity of stool examination, based on number of specimens submitted. Am J Gastroenterol 1997;92: 451–453.
370. Morin CA, Roberts CL, Mshar PA, et al. What do physicians know about cryptosporidiosis? A survey of Connecticut physicians. Arch Intern Med 1997;157:1017–1022.
371. Roberts CL, Morin C, Addiss DG, et al. Factors influencing *Cryptosporidium* testing in Connecticut. J Clin Microbiol 1996;34:2292–2293.
372. Current WL, Haynes TB. Complete development of *Cryptosporidium* in cell culture. Science 1984;224:603–605.
373. Blagburn B, Soave R. Prophylaxis and chemotherapy: human and animal. In: Fayer R, ed. *Cryptosporidium* and cryptosporidiosis. Boca Raton, FL: CRC Press, 1997:111–128.
374. Upton SJ. In vitro cultivation. In: Fayer R, ed. *Cryptosporidium* and cryptosporidiosis. Boca Raton, FL: CRC Press, 1997:181–207.
375. Lindsay DS. Laboratory models of cryptosporidiosis. In: Fayer R, ed. *Cryptosporidium* and cryptosporidiosis. Boca Raton, FL: CRC Press, 1997:209–223.
376. Laughon BE, Allaudeen HS, Becker JM, et al. Summary of the workshop on furture directions in discovery and development of therapeutic agents for opportunistic infections associated with AIDS. J Infect Dis 1991;164:244–251.
377. Portnoy D, Whiteside, ME, Buckley E, et al. Treatment of intestinal cryptosporidiosis with spiramycin, Ann Intern Med 1984;101:202.
378. Moskovitz BL, Stanton TL, Kusmierek JJE. Spiramycin therapy for cryptosporidial diarrhea in immunocompromised patients. J Antimicrob Chemother 1988;22(Suppl B):89.
379. Connolly GM, Dryden MS, Shanson DC, et al. Cryptosporidial diarrhea in AIDS and its treatment. Gut 1988;29:593.
380. Woolf GM, Townsend M, Guyatt G, et al. Treatment of cryptosporidiosis with spiramycin in AIDS. An "N of 1" trial. J Clin Gastroenterol 1987;9:632.
381. Wittenberg DF, Miller NM, van den Ende J. Spiramycin is not effective in treating *Cryptosporidium* diarrhea in infants: results of a double-blind randomized trial. J Infect Dis 1989;159:131.
382. Saez-Llorens X, Odio CM, Umana MA, et al. Spiramycin vs. placebo for treatment of acute diarrhea caused by *Cryptosporidium*. Pediatr Infect Dis J 1989;8:136.
383. Soave R, Petillo J, Dieterich DT, et al. Single-blind efficacy evaluation of intravenous spiramycin in patients with AIDS-related cryptosporidial diarrhea (submitted).
384. Weikel C, Lazenby A, Belitsos P, et al. Intestinal injury associated with spiramycin therapy of *Cryptosporidium* infection in AIDS. J Protozool 1991;38:147S.
385. Vargas SL, Shenep JL, Flynn PM, et al. Azithromycin for the treatment of severe *Cryptosporidium* diarrhea in two children with cancer. J Pediatr 1993;123:154–156.
386. Bessette RE, Amsden GW. Treatment of non-HIV cryptosporidial diarrhea with azithromycin. Ann Pharmacother 1995;29:991–993.
387. Hicks P, Zwiener RJ, Squires J, et al. Azithromycin therapy for *Cryptosporidium parvum* infection in four children infected with human immunodeficiency virus. J Pediatr 1996;129:297–300.
388. Soave R, Havlir D, Lancaster D, et al. Azithromycin therapy of AIDS-related cryptosporidial diarrhea: a multi-center, placebo-controlled, double-blind study [abstract 193]. In: 33rd Interscience Conference on Antimicrobial Agents and Chemotherapy. Washington, DC: American Society for Microbiology, 1993.
389. Dunne MW, Williams DJ, Young LS. Azithromycin and the treatment of opportunistic infections. Rev Contemp Pharmacother 1994;5: 373–381.
390. Blanshard C, Shanson DC, Gazzard BG. Pilot studies of azithromycin, letrazuril and paromomycin in the treatment of cryptosporidiosis. Int J STD AIDS 1997;8:124–129.
391. Friedman CR, Soave R, Bremer S. Intravenous azithromycin for cryptosporidiosis in AIDS (submitted).
392. Jordan WC. Clarithromycin prophylaxis against *Cryptosporidium* enteritis in patients with AIDS. J Natl Med Assoc 1996;88:425–427.
393. Bissuel F, Cotte L, Rabodonirina M, et al. Paromomycin: an effective treatment for cryptosporidial diarrhea in patients with AIDS. Clin Infect Dis 1994;18:447–449.
394. Scaglia M, Atzori C, Marchetti G, et al. Effectiveness of aminosidine (paromomycin) sulfate in chronic *Cryptosporidium* diarrhea in AIDS patients: an open, uncontrolled, prospective clinical trial [letter]. J Infect Dis. 1994;170:1349–1350.
395. Flanigan TP, Ramratnam B, Graeber C, et al. Prospective trial of paromomycin for cryptosporidiosis in AIDS. Am J Med 1996;100: 370–372.
396. Armitage K, Flanigan T, Carey J, et al. Treatment of cryptosporidiosis with paromomycin: a report of five cases. Arch Intern Med 1992;152: 2497–2499.
397. Danziger LH, Kanyok TP, Novak RM. Treatment of cryptosporidial diarrhea in an AIDS patients with paromomycin. Ann Pharmacother 1993;27:1460–1462.
398. Kanyok TP, Novak RM, Danziger LH. Preliminary results of a randomized, blinded, control study of paromomycin vs placebo for the treatment of cryptosporidial diarrhea in AIDS patients [abstract 5969]. In: 9th International Congress on AIDS, Berlin, 1993.
399. White AC Jr, Chappell CL, Hayat CS, et al. Paromomycin for cryptosporidiosis in AIDS: a prospective, double-blind trial. J Infect Dis 1994;170:419–424.
400. Hewitt RG, Yiannoutsos CT, Carey J, et al. A double-blind, placebo-controlled trial of paromomycin for the treatment of cryptosporidiosis

in patients with advanced HIV disease and CD4 counts under 150 (ACTG 192). In: Proceedings of the 4th Conference on Retroviruses and Opportunistic Infections. Washington DC: American Society of Microbiology, 1997:65.
401. Wallace MR, Nguyen MT, Newton JA. Use of paromomycin for the treatment of cryptosporidiosis in patients with AIDS [letter; comment]. Clin Infect Dis 1993;17:1070–1071.
402. Keusch GT, Troncale FJ, Buchman RD. Malabsorption due to paromomycin. Arch Intern Med 1970;125:273–276.
403. Bissuel F, Cotte L, de Montclos M, et al. Absence of systemic absorption of oral paromomycin during long-term, high-dose treatment for cryptosporidiosis in AIDS [letter]. J Infect Dis 1994;170:749–750.
404. Ritchie DJ, Becker ES. Update on the management of intestinal cryptosporidiosis in AIDS, Ann Pharmacother 1994;28:767.
405. Rossignol JF, Maisonneuve H, Cho YW. Nitroimidazoles in the treatment of trichomoniasis, giardiasis and amoebiasis. Int J Clin Pharmacol Ther Toxicol 1984;22:63–72.
406. Doumbo O, Rossignol JF, Pichard E, et al. Nitazoxanide in the treatment of cryptosporidial diarrhea and other intestinal parasitic infections associated with acquired immunodeficinecy syndrome in tropical Africa. Am J Trop Med Hyg 1997; 56:637–639.
407. Davis LJ, Soave R, Dudley RE, et al. Nitazoxanide for AIDS-related cryptosporidial diarrhea: an open-label safety, efficacy and pharmacokinetic study [abstract LM50]. In: Proceedings of the 36th Interscience Conference on Antimicrobial Agents and Chemotherapy. Washington, DC: American Society for Microbiology, 1996.
408. Connolly GM., Youle M, Gazzard BG. Diclazuril in the treatment of severe cryptosporidial diarrhea in AIDS patients. AIDS 1990;4:700.
409. Menichetti F, Moretti MV, Marroni M, et al. Diclazuril for cryptosporidiosis in AIDS [letter]. Am J Med 1991;90:271–272.
410. Soave R, Dieterich D, Kotler D, et al. Oral disclazuril for cryptosporidiosis [abstract Th.B. 519]. In: 6th International Conference on AIDS, San Francisco, 1990.
411. Hamour AA, Bonington A, Hawthorne B, et al. Successful treatment of AIDS-related cryptosporidial sclerosing cholangitis. AIDS 1993;7:1449–1451.
412. Harris M, Deutsch G, Maclean JD, et al. A phase I study of letrazuril in AIDS-related cryptosporidiosis. AIDS 1994;8:1109–1113.
413. Loeb M, Walach C, Phillips J, et al. Treatment with letrazuril of refractory cryptosporidial diarrhea complicating AIDS. J Acquir Immune Defic Syndr Hum Retrovirol 1995;10:48–53.
414. Guillem S, Gomez M, Romeu J, et al. Letrazuril for treatment of severe cryptosporidial diarrhea in AIDS [abstract PoB3257]. In: 8th International Conference on AIDS/III STD World Congress, Amsterdam, 1992.
415. Murdoch DA, Bloss DE, Glover SC. Successful treatment of cryptosporidiosis in an AIDS patient with letrazuril [letter]. AIDS 1993;7:1279–1280.
416. Soave R, Dieterich D, Lew E, et al. Letrazuril for AIDS-related cryptosporidial diarrhea: a multi-center, pharmacokinetic study and double-blind, placebo-controlled trial (submitted).
417. Gutteridge WE. 566C80, an antimalarial hydroxynaphthoquinone with broad spectrum: experimental activity against opportunistic parasitic infections of AIDS patients. J Protozool 1991;38:141S–143S.
418. Rolston KVI, Fainstein V, Bodey GP. Intestinal cryptosporidiosis treated with efluornithine: a prospective study among patients with AIDS. J Acquir Immune Defic Syndr 1989;2:426–430.
419. Soave R, Sjoerdsma A, Cawein MJ. Treatment of cryptosporidiosis in AIDS patients with DFMO [abstract 30]. In: 1st International Conference on AIDS, Atlanta, 1985.
420. Chandrasekar PH. "Cure" of chronic cryptosporidiosis during treatment with azidothymidine in a patient with acquired immunodeficiency syndrome. Am J Med 1987;83:187.
421. Greenberg RE, Mir R, Bank S, et al. Resolution of intestinal cryptosporidiosis after treatment of AIDS with AZT. Gastroenterology 1989;97:1327–1330.
422. Louie E, Borkowsky W, Klesius PH, et al. Treatment of *Cryptosporidium* with oral bovine transfer factor. Clin Immunol Immunopathol 1987;44:329–334.
423. McMeeking A, Borkowsky W, Klesius PH, et al. A controlled trial of bovine dialyzable leukocyte extract for cryptosporidiosis in patients with AIDS. J Infect Dis 1990;161:108–112.
424. Chng HH, Shaw D, Klesius P, et al. Inability of oral bovine transfer factor to eradicate cryptosporidial infection in a patient with congenital dysgammaglobulinemia. Clin Immunol Immunopathol 1989;50:402–406.
425. Heaton P. Cryptosporidiosis and acute leukemia. Arch Dis Child 1990;65:813–814.
426. Plettenberg A, Stoehr A, Sterlbrink HJ, et al. A preparation from bovine colostrum in the treatment of HIV-positive patients with chronic diarrhea. Clin Invest 1993;71:42.
427. Shield J, Melville C, Novelli V, et al. Bovine colostrum immunoglobulin concentrate for cryptosporidiosis in AIDS. Arch Dis Child 1993;69:451.
428. Greenberg PD, Cello JP. Treatment of severe diarrhea caused by *Cryptosporidium parvum* with oral bovine immunoglobulin concentrate in patients with AIDS. J Acquir Immune Defic Syndr Hum Retrovirol 1996;13:348–354.
429. Borowitz SM, Saulsbury FT. Treatment of chronic cryptosporidial infection with orally administered human serum immune globulin. J Pediatr 1991;119:593–595.
430. Cama VA, Sterling CR. Hyperimmune hens as a novel source of anti-*Cryptosporidium* antibodies suitable for passive immune transfer. J Protozool 1991;38;42S.
431. Soave R, Davis LJ, Cama VA, et al. Hyperimmune egg yolks for the treatment of cryptosporidiosis in patients with AIDS (submitted).
432. Kern P, Toy J, Dietrich M. Preliminary clinical observation with recombinant interleukin-2 in patients with AIDS or LAS. Blut 1985;50:1–6.
433. Fanning M, Monte M, Sutherland LR, et al. Pilot study of Sandostatin (octreotide) therapy of refractory HIV-associated diarrhea. Dig Dis Sci 1991;36:476–480.
434. Kreinik G, Burstein O, Landor M, et al. Successsful management of intractable cryptosporidial diarrhea with intravenous octreotide, a somatostatin analogue. AIDS 1991;5:765–767.
435. Cello JP, Grendell JH, Basuk P, et al. Effect of octreotide on refractory AIDS-associated diarrhea: a prospective, multicenter clinical trial. Ann Intern Med 1991;115:705–710.
436. United States Public Health Service/Infectious Disease Society of America (USPHS/IDSA) Prevention of Opportunistic Infections Working Group. 1997 USPHS/IDSA guidelines for the prevention of opportunistic infections in persons infected with human immunodeficiency virus: disease-specific recommendations. Clin Infect Dis 1997;25(Suppl 3):S313–S335.
437. Canning EU, Lom J. The microsporidia of vertebrates. New York: Academic Press, 1986.
438. Sprague V, Becnel JJ, Hazard EI. Taxonomy of phylum Microspora. Crit Rev Microbiol 1992;18:285–395.
439. Canning EU, Hollister WS. Human infections with microsporidia. Rev Med Microbiol 1992;3:35–42.
440. Weber R, Bryan RT, Schwartz DA, et al. Human microsporidial infections. Clin Microbiol Rev 1994;7:426–461.
441. Shadduck JA, Pakes SP. Spontaneous diseases of laboratory animals which interfere with biomedical research: encephalitozoonosis (nosematosis) and toxoplasmosis. Am J Pathol 1971;64:657–671.
442. Canning EU, Hollister WS. Microsporidia of mammals: widespread pathogens or opportunistic curiosities? Parasitol Today 1987;3:267–273.
443. Shadduck JA. Human microsporidiosis and AIDS. Rev Infect Dis 1989;11:203–207.
444. Shadduck JA, Greeley E. Microsporidia and human infections. Clin Microbiol Rev 1989;2:158–165.

445. Bryan RT, Cali A, Owen RL, et al. Microsporidia: opportunistic pathogens in patients with AIDS. In: Sun T, ed. Progress in clinical parasitology. Philadelphia: Field and Wood 1990:1–26.
446. Orenstein JM. Microsporidiosis in the acquired immunodeficiency syndrome. J Parasitol 1991;77:843–864.
447. Weidner E. Ultrastructural study of microsporidian invasion into cells. Z Parasitenk 1972;40:227–242.
448. Weidner E, Byrd W. The microsporidian spore invasion tube. II. Role of calcium in the activation of invasion tube discharge. J Cell Biol 1982;93:970–975.
449. Weidner E, Byrd W, Scarborough A, et al. Microsporidian spore discharge and the transfer of polaroplast organelle membrane into plasma membrane. J Protozool 1984;31:195–198.
450. Desportes-Livage I, Chilmonczyk S, Hedrick R, et al. Comparative development of two microsporidian species: *Enterocytozoon bieneusi* and *Enterocytozoon salmonis*, reported in AIDS patients and salmonid fish, respectively. J Eukaryot Microbiol 1996;43:49–60.
451. Weber R, Bryan RT, Owen RL, et al. Improved light-microscopical detection of microsporidia spores in stool and duodenal aspirates. N Engl J Med 1992;326:161–166.
452. Lom J, Vavra J. The mode of sporoplasm extrusion in microsporidian spores. Acta Protozool 1963;1:81–89.
453. Undeen AH. A proposed mechanism for the germination of microsporidian (Protozoa: Microspora) spores. J Theor Biol 1990;142:223–235.
454. Undeen AH, Frixione E. The role of osmotic pressure in the germination of *Nosema algerae* spores. J Protozool 1990;37:561–567.
455. Baker MD, Vossbrinck CR, Didier ES, et al. Small subunit ribosomal DNA phylogeny of various microsporidia with emphasis on AIDS related forms. J Eukaryot Microbiol 1996;42:564–570.
456. Sprague V. Need for drastic revision of the classification of subphylum Amoebagena. Progr Protozool (Int Congr Protozool) 1969;3:372.
457. Levine ND, Corliss JO, Cox FEG, et al. A newly revised classification of the protozoa. J Protozool 1980;27:37–58.
458. Curgy JJ, Vavra J, Vivares C. Presence of ribosomal RNAs with prokaryotic properties in microsporidia, eukaryotic organisms. Biol Cell 1980;38:49–52.
459. Vossbrinck CR, Woese CR. Eukaryotic ribosomes that lack a 5.8S RNA. Nature 1986;320:287–288.
460. Vossbrinck CR, Maddox JV, Friedman S, et al. Ribosomal RNA sequence suggests microsporidia are extremely ancient eukaryotes. Nature 1987;326:411–414.
461. Edlind TD, Li J, Visvesvara GS, et al. Phylogenetic analysis of β-tubulin sequences from amitochondrial protozoa. Mol Phylogenet Evol 1986;5:359–367.
462. Orenstein JM, Chiang J, Steinberg W, et al. Intestinal microsporidiosis as a cause of diarrhea in human immunodeficiency virus-infected patients: a report of 20 cases. Hum Pathol 1990;21:475–481.
463. Kotler DP, Francisco A, Clayton F, et al. Small intestinal injury and parasitic diseases in AIDS. Ann Intern Med 1990;113:444–449.
464. Cali A, Owen RL. Intracellular development of *Enterocytozoon*, a unique microsporidian found in the intestine of AIDS patients. J Protozool 1990;37:145–155.
465. Orenstein JM, Tenner M, Cali A, et al. A microsporidian previously undescribed in humans, infecting enterocytes and macrophages, and associated with diarrhea in an acquired immunodeficiency syndrome patient. Hum Pathol 1992;23:722–728.
466. Kotler DP, Orenstein JM. Microsporidia. In: Blaser MJ, Smith PD, Ravdin JI, et al., eds. Infections of the gastrointestinal tract. New York: Raven Press, 1995:1129–1140.
467. Zeman DH, Baskin GB. *Encephalitozoon*osis in squirrel monkeys (*Saimiri sciureus*). Vet Pathol 1985;22:24–31.
468. Field AS, Marriott DJ, Milliken ST, et al. Myositis associated with a newly described microsporidian, *TrachiPleistophora hominis*, in a patient with AIDS. J Clin Microbiol 1996;34:2803–2811.
469. Hollister WS, Canning EU, Weidner E, et al. Development and ultrastructure of *TrachiPleistophora hominis* n.g., n.sp. after in vitro isolation from an AIDS patient and inoculation into athymic mice. Parasitology 1996;112:143–154.
470. Silveira H, Canning EU. *Vittaforma corneae* n.comb. for the human microsporidium *Nosema corneum* Shaddduck, Meccoli, Davis & Font, 1990, based on its ultrastructure in the liver of experimentally infected athymic mice. J Eukaryot Microbiol 1995;42:158–165.
471. Van Gool T, Canning EU, Gilis H, et al. *Septata intestinalis* frequently isolated from stool of patients with a new cultivation method. Parasitology 1994;109:281–289.
472. Bergquist R, Morfeldt-Masson L, Pehrson PO, et al. Antibody against *Encephalitozoon cuniculi* in Swedish homosexual men. Scand J Infect Dis 1984;16:389–391.
473. Hollister WS, Canning EU, Wilcox A. Evidence for widespread occurrence of antibodies to *Encephalitozoon cuniculi* (microspora) in man provided by ELISA and other serological tests. Parasitology 1991;102:33–43.
474. Albrecht H. Redefining AIDS: towards a modification of the current AIDS case definition. Clin Infect Dis 1997;24:64–74.
475. Deplazes P, Mathis A, Mueller C, et al. Molecular epidemiology of *Encephalitozoon cuniculi* and first detection of *Enterocytozoon bieneusi* in faecal samples in pigs. J Eukaryot Microbiol 1996;43:93S.
476. Mansfield KG, Carville A, Shvetz D, et al. Identification of an *Enterocytozoon bieneusi*-like microsporidian parasite in simian-immunodeficiency virus–inoculated macaques with hepatobiliary disease. Am J Pathol 1997;150:1395–1405.
477. Black SS, Steinohrt LA, Bertucci DC, et al. *Encephalitozoon hellem* in budgerigars (*Melopsittacus undulatus*). Vet Pathol 1997;34:189–198.
478. Didier ES, Vossbrinck CR, Baker MD, et al. Identification and characterization of three *Encephalitozoon cuniculi* strains. Parasitology 1995;111:411–422.
479. Didier ES, Visvesvara GS, Baker MD, et al. A microsporidian isolated from an AIDS patient corresponds to the *Encephalitozoon cuniculi* strain III originally isolated from domestic dogs. J Clin Microbiol 1996;34:2835–2837.
480. Mertens RB, Didier ES, Fishbein MC, et al. Disseminated *Encephalitozoon cuniculi* microsporidiosis in an AIDS patient: report of a case with brain, heart, kidneys, trachea, adrenals, urinary bladder, spleen, and lymph node involvement. Mod Pathol 1997;10:68–77.
481. Deplazes P, Mathis A, Baumgartner R, et al. Immunologic and molecular characteristics of *Encephalitozoon*-like microsporidia isolated from humans and rabbits indicate that *Encephalitozoon cuniculi* is a zoonotic parasite. Clin Infect Dis 1996;22:557–559.
482. Weiss LM. And now microsporidiosis. Ann Intern Med 1995;123:954–956.
483. Desportes I, Le Charpentier Y, Galian A, et al. Occurrence of a new microsporidian, *Enterocytozoon bieneusi* n.g., n.sp., in the enterocytes of a human patient with AIDS. J Protozool 1985;32:250–254.
484. Lambl BB, Federman M, Pleskow D, et al. Malabsorption and wasting in AIDS patients with microsporidia and pathogen-negative diarrhea. AIDS 1996;10:739–744.
485. Lowder CY, McMahon JT, Meisler DM, et al. Microsporidial kerato-conjunctivitis cause by *Septata intestinalis* in a patient with acquired immunodeficiency syndrome. Am J Ophthalmol 1996;121:715–717.
486. Asmuth DM, DeGirolami PC, Federman M, et al. Clinical features of microsporidiosis in patients with AIDS. Clin Infect Dis 1994;18:819–825.
487. Rabodonirina M, Bertocchi M, Desportes-Livage I, et al. *Enterocytozoon bieneusi* as a cause of chronic diarrhea in a heart–lung transplant recipient who was seronegative for human immunodeficiency virus. Clin Infect Dis 1996;23:114–117.
488. Kelkar R, Sastry PS, Kulkarni SS, et al. Pulmonary microsporidial infection in a patient with CML undergoing allogeneic marrow transplant. Bone Marrow Transpl 1997;19:179–182.
489. Sandfort J, Hannemann A, Gelderblom H, et al. *Enterocytozoon bieneusi* infection in an immunocompetent patient who had acute diarrhea and who was not infected with the human immunodeficiency virus. Clin Infect Dis 1994;19:514–516.

490. Sowerby TM, Conteas CN, Berlin OGW, et al. Microsporidiosis in patients with relatively preserved CD4 counts. AIDS 1995;9:975–984.
491. Rabeneck L, Gyorkey F, Genta RM, et al. The role of microsporidia in the pathogenesis of HIV-related chronic diarrhea. Ann Intern Med 1993;119:895–899.
492. Rabeneck L, Genta RM, Gyorkey F, et al. Observations on the pathological spectrum and clinical course of microsporidiosis in men infected with the human immunodeficiency virus: follow-up study. Clin Infect Dis 1995;20:1229–1235.
493. Clarridge JE, Karkhanis S, Rabeneck L, et al. Quantitative light microscopic detection of *Enterocytozoon bieneusi* stool specimens: a longitudinal study of human immunodeficiency virus–infected microsporidiosis patients. J Clin Microbiol 1996;34:520–523.
494. Schmidt EC, Shadduck JA. Murine *Encephalitozoonosis* model for studying the host–parasite relationship of a chronic infection. Infect Immun 1983;40:936–942.
495. Didier ES., Varner PW, Didier PJ, et al. Experimental microsporidiosis in immunocompetent and immunodeficient mice and monkeys. Fol Parasitol (Praha) 1994;41:1–11.
496. Hermanek J, Koudela B, Kucerova A, et al. Prophylactic and therapeutic immune reconstitution of SCID mice infected with *Encephalitozoon cuniculi*. Fol Parasitol (Praha) 1993;40:287–291.
497. Didier ES, Kotler DP, Dieterich DT, et al. Serological studies in human microsporidia infections. AIDS 1993;7:S8–S11.
498. Niederkorn JY, Shadduck JA. Role of antibody and complement in the control of *Encephalitozoon cuniculi* infection by rabbit macrophages. Infect Immun 1980;17:995–1002.
499. Schmidt EC, Shadduck JA. Mechanisms of resistance to the intracellular protozoan *Encephalitozoon cuniculi* in mice. J Immunol 1984;133:2712–2719.
500. Arnesen K, Nordstoga K. Ocular *Encephalitozoonosis (Nosematosis)* in blue foxes, polyarteritis nodosa and cataract. Acta Ophthalmol 1977;55:641–651.
501. Stewart CG, Reyers F, Snyman H. The relationship in dogs between primary renal disease and antibodies to *Encephalitozoon cuniculi*. J S Afr Vet Assoc 1986;59:19–21.
502. Didier ES. Nitrogen intermediates implicated in the inhibition of *Encephalitozoon cuniculi* (phylum Microspora) replication in murine peritoneal macrophages. Parasite Immunol 1995;17:405–412.
503. Achbarou A, Ombrouck C, Gneragbe T, et al. Experimental model for human intestinal microsporidiosis in interferon gamma receptor knockout mice infected by *Encephalitozoon intestinalis*. Parasite Immunol 1996;18:387–392.
504. Cali A, Kotler DP, Orenstein JM. *Septata intestinalis* n.g., n.sp., an intestinal microsporidian associated with chronic diarrhea and dissemination in AIDS patients. J Protozool 1993;40:101–112.
505. Tiner JD. Birefringent spores differentiate *Encephalitozoon* and microsporidia from coccidia. Vet Pathol 1988;25:227–230.
506. Field A, Hing M, Milliken S, et al. Microsporidia in the small intestine of HIV infected patients: a new diagnostic technique and a new species. Med J Aust 1993;158:390–394.
507. Vavra J, Chalupsky J. Fluorescence staining of microsporidian spores with the brightener Calcofluor white M2R. J Protozool 1982;29(Suppl):503.
508. van Gool T, Snijders F, Reiss P, et al. Diagnosis of intestinal and disseminated microsporidial infections in patients with HIV by a new rapid fluorescence technique. J Clin Pathol 1993;46:694–699.
509. Ryan NJ, Sutherland G, Coughlan K, et al. A new trichrome-blue stain for detection of microsporidial species in urine, stool, and nasopharyngeal specimens. J Clin Microbiol 1993;31:3264–3269.
510. Kokoskin E, Gyorkos T, Camus A, et al. Modified technique for efficient detection of microsporidia. J Clin Microbiol 1994;32:1074–1075.
511. Schwartz DA, Visvesvara GS, Leitch GJ, et al. Pathology of symptomatic microsporidial (*Encephalitozoon hellem*) bronchiolitis in AIDS: a new respiratory pathogen diagnosed from lung biopsy, bronchoalveolar lavage, sputum, and tissue culture. Hum Pathol 1993;24:937–943.
512. Fedorko DP, Hijazi YM. Application of molecular techniques to the diagnosis of microsporidial infection. Emerg Infect Dis 1996;2:183–191.
513. Giang TT, Kotler DP, Garro ML, et al. Tissue diagnosis of intestinal microsporidiosis using chromotrope-2R modified trichrome stain. Arch Pathol Lab Med 1993;117:1249–1251.
514. Didier ES, Orenstein JM, Aldras AM, et al. Comparison of three staining methods for detecting microsporidia in fluids. J Clin Microbiol 1995;33:3138–3145.
515. Simon D, Weiss LM, Tanowitz HB, et al. Light microscopic diagnosis of human microsporidiosis and variable response to octreotide. Gastroenterolgy 1991;100;271–273.
516. Eeftinck Schattenkerk JKM, van Gool T, Bartelsman JF, et al. Metronidazole for microsporidium-associated diarrhoea in symptomatic HIV-1 infection [abstract]. In: Abstracts of the 7th International Conference on AIDS, Forence, Italy, 1991:2267.
517. Yee RW, Tio FO, Martinez A, et al. Resolution of microsporidial epithelial keratopathy in a patient with AIDS. Ophthalmology 1990;98:196–201.
518. Anwar-Bruni DM, Hogan SE, Schwartz DA, et al. Atovaquone is effective treatment for the symptoms of gastrointestinal microsporidiosis in HIV-1–infected patients. AIDS 1996;10:619–623.
519. Wanke CA, Pleskow D, Degirolami PC, et al. A medium chain triglyceride–based diet in patients with HIV and chronic diarrhea reduces diarrhea and malabsorption: a prospective, controlled trial. Nutrition 1996;12:766–771.
520. Blanshard C, Ellis DS, Tovey DG, et al. Treatment of intestinal microsporidiosis with albendazole in patients with AIDS. AIDS 1992;6:311–313.
521. Dieterich DT, Lew E, Kotler DP, et al. Treatment with albendazole for intestinal disease due to *Enterocytozoon bieneusi* in patients with AIDS. J Infect Dis 1994;169:178–183.
522. Shadduck JA. Effect of fumagillin on in vitro multiplication of *Encephalitozoon cuniculi*. J Protozool 1980;27:202–208.
523. Diesenhouse MC, Wilson LA, Corrent GF, et al. Treatment of microsporidial keratoconjunctivitis with topical fumagillin. Am J Ophthalmol 1993;115:293–298.
524. Molina JM, Goguel J, Sarfati C, et al. Potential efficacy of fumagillin in intestinal microsporidiosis due to *Enterocytozoon bieneusi* in patients with HIV-infection: results of a drug screening study. AIDS 1997;11:1603–1610.
525. Ingber D, Fujita T, Kishimoto S, et al. Synthetic analogues of fumagillin that inhibit angiogenesis and suppress tumour growth. Nature 1990;348:555–557.
526. Didier ES. Effects of albendazole, fumagillin, and TNP-470 on microsporidia replication in vitro. Antimicrob Agents Chemother 1997;41:1541–1546.
527. Sharpstone D, Rowbottom A, Francis N, et al. Thalidomide: a novel therapy for microsporidiosis. Gastroenterology 1997;112:1823–1829.
528. Goguel J, Katlama C, Sarfati C, et al. Remission of AIDS-associated intestinal microsporidiosis with highly active antiretroviral therapy. AIDS 1997;11:1658–1659.
529. Shadduck JA, Storts R, Adams LG. Selected examples of emerging and reemerging infectious diseases in animals. Am Soc Microbiol News 1996;62:586–588.

22
FUNGI

William G. Powderly

Fungal infections are a common complication of human immunodeficiency virus (HIV) disease, although they vary in their severity from mild discomfort associated with mucosal thrush to life-threatening fungal meningitis. This chapter reviews the clinical features and treatment of the various opportunistic fungal infections.

CANDIDIASIS

Microbiology and Epidemiology

In 1981, the first reports of the acquired immunodeficiency syndrome (AIDS) included patients with *Pneumocystis* pneumonia and mucosal candidiasis (1, 2). Since those reports, oropharyngeal *Candida* infection has been found to affect most HIV-infected patients at some point during the course of their illness. The yeast, *C. albicans,* is the strain most commonly associated with disease in HIV-positive patients (3–5). Other strains such as *C. tropicalis, C. parapsilosis, C. krusei,* and *Torulopsis glabrata* have been implicated in oral disease in HIV-positive patients, most often in patients with advanced HIV disease who have received suppressive azole antifungal therapy (6, 7). *Candida* organisms are ubiquitous in nature and can be isolated from soil, hospital environments, and food (8). Additionally, the skin and mucosal surfaces of humans are colonized at a variable rate (8). Most HIV-positive patients become colonized with *Candida,* especially in the oral cavity, at rates that increase with decreasing CD4 counts (4, 9). The relation of colonization with *Candida* to the subsequent development of infection is not clear. Host factors important in the defense of *Candida* infections include salivary flow rates, epithelial barrier, antimicrobial constituents of saliva, microbial interactions, and local immunity (10, 11). Dental hygiene, smoking, and medication also affect the rate of *Candida* colonization. Several studies suggest abnormalities in some anti-*Candida* host defense mechanisms in HIV-infected persons (9, 10, 12–14). In addition to the well-characterized defect in cell-mediated immunity associated with HIV infection, local oral defense mechanisms appear to be impaired (12). Decreased salivary flow rates and changes in the levels and function of antimycotic factors, such as immunoglobulin A, lysozyme, lactoperoxidase, histatins, and lactoferrin, have been demonstrated in HIV-infected patients. The relation of these abnormalities to *Candida* infection is unknown.

Mucosal candidiasis is common in HIV-infected individuals. In women, *Candida* infection of the vulvovaginal area is commonly associated with HIV infection (15), and recurrent vaginitis often precedes oral candidiasis (16) and may be the first indicator of immune dysfunction (17). In several studies of women with HIV infection, recurrent vaginal candidiasis was the most common clinical event associated with HIV infection, occurring in 32 to 45% of women at some time during the course of their HIV disease. The incidence of oropharyngeal *Candida* infection in HIV-infected individuals varies from 7 to 93%, depending on the method of the study and the degree of immunodeficiency of the study population (3, 4, 18). In one study, 92% of patients with a CD4 count higher than 300 cells/mm^3 had evidence of oral candidiasis (13). Evidence from several studies suggests that 30 to 50% of patients experience at least one recurrence of oral candidiasis (19–21). Esophageal candidiasis is one of the most common gastrointestinal infections in AIDS (22); its frequency varies widely, occurring in 10 to 30% of patients in the United States, and it has been reported to occur in as many as 80% of patients with acquired immune deficiency syndrome (AIDS) in developing countries (23, 24).

The individual *Candida* strains affecting HIV-positive patients are not different from those in other immunosuppressed hosts (25–29), and each patient appears to be infected with a unique individual strain (26–29). Furthermore, no detectable differences are noted in the virulence of strains isolated from HIV-positive versus HIV-negative patients. Studies in patients with recurrent oropharyngeal infection (28–30) suggest two patterns of recurrences: those with the same strain of *C. albicans* and those with either a new strain of *C. albicans* or a new species of *Candida*. The latter phenomenon is more likely to occur in patients with low CD4 lymphocyte counts who have received suppressive azole antifungal therapy (30). Patients receiving fluconazole suppressive therapy are more likely to have infection caused by species such as *C. (Torulopsis) glabrata*, *C. parapsilosis*, and *C. krusei* (7).

Progression of HIV infection has been clearly associated with the occurrence of oral candidiasis, which may be a sentinel event presenting months or years before more severe opportunistic disease. Furthermore, oral candidiasis has been clearly shown to be an independent prognostic marker of the risk of progression to overt AIDS. In 1984, Klein and associates reported that 59% (13 of 22) of a cohort with oral candidiasis and a reversed T4/T8 level progressed to AIDS at a median of 3 months compared with none of 20 control patients (31). The association between the occurrence of oral candidiasis and an increased risk of progression to AIDS has been verified repeatedly in other studies (32–35) and remains true even with effective antiretroviral therapy (36). Whether the prevalence of oral candidiasis in these individuals correlates with HIV viral load has yet not been demonstrated.

Unlike mucosal candidiasis, systemic candidiasis is rare in patients with AIDS; candidemia is reported in about 1% of patients (37), although autopsy studies suggest that this number may be an underestimate of the true problem (38). Candidemia usually occurs in patients with other risk factors for invasive candidiasis, such as neutropenia, parenteral nutrition, broad-spectrum antibacterial therapy, or corticosteroid use (39). Invasive *Candida* infection such as endocarditis may also occur in intravenous drug users, primarily as a consequence of the drug use, rather than as a specific HIV-related illness. The rarity of systemic candidiasis in spite of heavy mucosal colonization is believed to be primarily due to adequate neutrophil function in most HIV-positive patients, although some data suggest that humoral immune responses may also protect patients with HIV infection from invasive candidiasis (40).

Clinical Manifestations and Diagnosis

Symptoms of oropharyngeal candidiasis include burning pain, altered taste sensation, and difficulty in swallowing liquids and solids. However, many patients are asymptomatic. The oral manifestations of candidiasis have been classified into four distinct categories (3, 4): pseudomembranous candidiasis (thrush), acute atrophic candidiasis (erythematous), chronic atrophic candidiasis (e.g., angular cheilitis), and chronic hyperplastic candidiasis (leukoplakia). The pseudomembranous form is characterized by the occurrence of painless, white spots on the tongue, gums, buccal membranes, or throat. Plaques are composed of necrotic material, desquamated parakeratotic epithelia, and hyphae and yeast cells that do not penetrate beyond the stratum spinosum. These plaques are easily removable. The erythematous form occurs as red patches affecting the tongue, buccal membranes, and gums.

The chronic forms of oral candidiasis are less common in HIV-infected patients. Angular cheilitis presents as painful white or red fissuring at the corners of the mouth. Leukoplakias are chronic, discrete lesions that vary in size and appearance and cannot be scraped away.

Vaginal candidiasis generally presents as a creamy-white abnormal vaginal discharge. Symptoms include vaginal or vulvar pruritus, burning pain, and dyspareunia. On examination, the vagina may appear erythematous, and pseudomembranous plaques are often seen.

The diagnosis of mucosal candidiasis is usually made on clinical appearance alone. Cultures often demonstrate *Candida* species, but alone are not diagnostic inasmuch as colonization with yeast is common. Scrapings of active lesions, examined with 10% potassium hydroxide, demonstrate characteristic pseudohyphae and budding yeast. The appearance of the lesion and the presence of hyphae are sufficient for diagnosis, and culture is usually unnecessary unless the lesions fail to clear with appropriate antifungal therapy.

Aphthous ulcerations and herpes virus infections are the most common lesions confused with candidiasis; however, these lesions are usually more painful. Epstein–Barr viral infection causing oral hairy leukoplakia is sometimes confused with oral candidiasis. Culture or histologic examination of the lesion is the best way to differentiate hairy leukoplakia from candidiasis. Other fungal infections, such as histoplasmosis, can also present with oral lesions that may be confused with candidiasis (41).

Patients with esophageal candidiasis develop ulcers and erosions on the esophagus and experience odynophagia or dysphagia, although as many as 40% of patients may have no symptoms. The onset of severe dysphagia in a patient with oral candidiasis should raise the possibility of esophageal involvement (42). The combination of oral candidiasis and esophageal symptoms tends to be both specific and sensitive in predicting esophageal involvement (43). This suggests that a presumptive diagnosis of esophageal candidiasis can be made clinically in most cases, thus avoiding invasive procedures in most patients. Patients can then be treated empirically with antifungal therapy, and endoscopy with biopsy of the esophagus can be reserved for those patients who fail to respond, to evaluate for the presence of other diagnoses such as herpetic or cytomegalovirus esophagitis, idiopathic ulceration, or resistant candidiasis (44, 45).

Other organ involvement occurs rarely. A few patients develop bronchopulmonary candidiasis, presumably as an extension of oropharyngeal disease. Invasive candidiasis usually presents with fever, and involvement of the skin, lungs, liver, kidneys, and central nervous system all are described (39).

Treatment

Most patients with localized mucosal candidiasis (either oropharyngeal or vaginal) respond well to antifungal therapy. Various options—both local and systemic—are available for the treatment of oral candidiasis (Table 22.1). In general, most patients respond to topical therapy initially, and systemic therapy is usually reserved for treatment failures or noncompliant patients. Of the local therapies, troches generally are used more effectively by patients than suspensions. Clinical responses (i.e., resolution of burning, pain, erythema, and visible thrush) occur in 90 to 100% of patients generally within 7 days of starting treatment. Mycologic responses are not usually as high and *Candida* can still be cultured from the oral cavity in many patients. Not surpris-

Table 22.1. Therapeutic Options for Oral and Esophageal Candidiasis

Agent	Formulation	Dosage[a]
Nystatin	Oral suspension	400,000–600,000 (4–6 mL) 4 times daily
	Pastille	1–2 pastilles 4 times daily
Clotrimazole	Troche	10 mg (1 troche) 5 times daily
Ketoconazole	Tablet	200 mg daily
		400–600 mg daily[b]
Fluconazole	Tablet	50–100 mg daily
		200–400 mg daily[b]
	Oral suspension	100–200 mg daily
Itraconazole	Capsule	100 mg daily
		200–400 mg daily[b]
	Oral suspension	100–200 mg daily
Amphotericin B	Oral suspension	100 mg 4 times daily
	IV infusion	0.3–0.5 mg/kg daily

[a]Dosage is the usual dose for the typical patient. The average duration of therapy is 7–14 days. Individual patients may require higher doses or more prolonged treatment.
[b]Esophageal disease.

ingly, the relapse rate has ranged from 20 to 60% in published reports (10, 19, 46).

Several studies have been conducted comparing topical and systemic therapy (20, 46, 47). In general, clinical response rates are similar, although signs and symptoms of disease tend to respond more rapidly with systemic treatment. Patients treated locally are less likely to have mycologic clearance at the end of the treatment. Probably as a consequence, patients with topical therapy tend to have clinical relapses more rapidly, although overall recurrence rates are similar.

Some patients have more refractory oropharyngeal disease and require systemic therapy. Studies comparing systemic treatments usually find them to be similar in clinical effectiveness (46, 48). Response rates of 75 to 100% are generally reported. The relapse rates with systemic therapies also appear to be equivalent. From a practical standpoint, in patients with advanced disease, fluconazole and itraconazole (especially the oral suspension, which is more bioavailable and appears to be more effective than the capsule) may be preferable to ketoconazole. The absorption of ketoconazole depends on gastric acidity, and achlorhydria can be a problem in patients with advanced AIDS (49).

Treatment of esophageal candidiasis requires systemic antifungal therapy. A multicenter, double-blind, randomized study (50) comparing fluconazole, 100 mg daily, and ketoconazole, 200 mg daily, demonstrated a clear-cut superiority of fluconazole in this disease; 81% of patients randomized to fluconazole experienced resolution of symptoms, compared with 66% of patients assigned to ketoconazole. Endoscopic responses were also significantly more frequent in the fluconazole-treated patients. More recent trials comparing fluconazole and itraconazole have found them to be equivalent in activity in treating *Candida* esophagitis (51). In general, larger doses (fluconazole, 100 to 200 mg daily; itraconazole, 200 mg daily; or ketoconazole, 400 mg daily for 14 to 28 days) than those needed for oropharyngeal disease are used to treat esophageal infection. Oral azole treatment may be ineffective in advanced disease. In this circumstance, systemic amphotericin B, 20 to 30 mg per day for 7 to 14 days, may be necessary.

Amphotericin B, 0.5 mg/kg per day, is the therapy of choice for invasive systemic candidiasis. However, because systemic disease is often a terminal event in a patient with advanced HIV disease, the prognosis is generally poor.

Although the triazole antifungals are highly effective, clinical failures are seen, and there are increasing reports of clinical and mycologic resistance to fluconazole (52–56). This is seen especially in patients with advanced HIV disease with low CD4 counts who have had multiple episodes of candidiasis treated with fluconazole (56). Up to 5% of patients with advanced HIV disease are estimated to develop azole-refractory candidiasis (57). Consensus methodology for the performance of in vitro susceptibility testing for *Candida* using the azole antifungals has been developed (58). This has been successfully correlated with outcome for patients with AIDS and oropharyngeal candidiasis. Isolates with a minimum inhibitory concentration (MIC) of up to 8 μg/mL to fluconazole are regarded as susceptible; isolates whose MIC is at least 64 μg/mL are regarded as resistant. Isolates with intermediate MICs are termed as having reduced susceptibility because infection caused by these isolates may respond to higher doses of fluconazole (up to 800 mg). Similar data have been generated using itraconazole (58).

Therapy of fluconazole-refractory thrush may be difficult. Some fluconazole-resistant isolates retain sensitivity to itraconazole and ketoconazole. Fluconazole resistance may be mediated in some cases by increased efflux of fluconazole from the fungal cell (59); this mechanism appears limited to fluconazole. Therapy with ketoconazole or itraconazole is usually not effective in patients whose isolates are completely resistant in vitro; however, in vitro susceptibility does not always imply therapeutic efficacy. Itraconazole capsules are rarely effective, although the cyclodextrin oral suspension formulation of itraconazole has reported response rates of 50 to 60% (60, 61). This benefit was short-lived if some form of long-term maintenance therapy was not given. The oral suspension of amphotericin B is also effective in patients with fluconazole-resistant disease (62). Intravenous amphotericin B should be used initially in patients with severe disease, especially esophagitis, and in patients in whom treatment with azoles has failed. A short course of therapy at low doses (0.3 mg/kg for 7 to 14 days) is usually effective, although relapses are common without some form of maintenance therapy. Anecdotally, some cases refractory to amphotericin B have been seen. Improved antiretroviral therapy with the protease inhibitors has been reported to lead to clearance of refractory thrush (63). Although such agents are not always successful, if the patient has antiretroviral options, these should be considered in the setting of resistant candidiasis.

Prophylaxis of Oropharyngeal Candidiasis

Recurrent disease may be sufficiently severe in some patients to warrant consideration of long-term suppression; fluconazole, 100 to 200 mg per day, has proved successful in suppressing recurrent candidiasis (64). In a large clinical trial of fungal prophylaxis that compared the effectiveness of fluconazole, 200 mg daily, with clotrimazole troches in patients with CD4 counts lower than 200 cells/mm^3, only 10% of patients assigned to fluconazole developed candidiasis, compared with almost 50% in the clotrimazole-treated group (65). Fluconazole was particularly beneficial in preventing esophageal disease.

However, suppressive therapy for oral candidiasis is not universally accepted. Many physicians prefer to treat each episode as it occurs, given that oropharyngeal disease is usually mild and has low morbidity. The improved quality of life associated with suppression of candidiasis should be weighed against the risk (usually low) of toxicity or drug interaction and the risk of developing resistant disease. The issue may be clearest for patients with esophageal candidiasis, in whom the risk of recurrence is almost 100% (66), and thus, long-term maintenance therapy is justified.

CRYPTOCOCCOSIS

Microbiology and Epidemiology

Cryptococcus neoformans is an encapsulated yeastlike fungus that is an important cause of infection and mortality in patients with AIDS (67, 68). *C. neoformans* has four serotypes, and, based on serotypes and mating characteristics, the organism has been classified into two varieties: *C. neoformans* var. *neoformans* (serotypes A and D) and *C. neoformans* var. *gatti* (serotypes B and C). *C. neoformans* var. *neoformans* is ubiquitous in nature and can be isolated from many environmental sources, particularly from soil and the excreta of pigeons and other birds. The environmental niche of *C. neoformans* var. *gatti* was identified when the organism was isolated from the bark of the eucalyptus tree, *Eucalyptus camaldulensis* (69). Although *C. neoformans* var. *gatti* can cause infection in other hosts, it has only rarely been implicated in disease among patients with AIDS, and *C. neoformans* var. *neoformans* is almost exclusively associated with infection in patients with AIDS (70, 71). This is true even in those parts of the world where *C. neoformans* var. *gatti* is a frequent cause of infection in HIV-negative hosts (e.g., southern California, central Africa, and Australia) (72, 73).

Although little direct proof exists, cryptococcosis is presumed to be a primary infection rather than reactivation of previously acquired disease. The organism is assumed to gain access to the host by the respiratory route and generally is controlled there by an intact cell-mediated immune system. Sensitized T cells activate neutrophils and macrophages to ingest and kill cryptococci (74–76). However, in the presence of immunodeficiency, *C. neoformans* disseminates widely, especially to the central nervous system. Of patients with AIDS who are infected with *C. neoformans*, 70 to 90% develop meningitis. However, acute cryptococcal infection of almost every other organ has been described, with the lung, liver, skin, lymph nodes, and adrenals most commonly infected.

In the United States, cryptococcosis is rarely the first opportunistic infection in a patient with AIDS: fewer than 2% of patients with AIDS reported to the United States Centers for Disease Control and Prevention (CDC) presented with cryptococcosis as their first infection. However, such data clearly underestimate the incidence of this infection. About 5 to 10% of patients with AIDS develop cryptococcal meningitis (77); in about 40%, it is the AIDS-defining illness (78–81). Cryptococcal infection in AIDS is always associated with profound immunodeficiency, with the CD4 almost invariably less than 100 cells/mm^3 (82). In addition, simultaneous occurrence of cryptococcosis and other opportunistic infection, especially *Pneumocystis* pneumonia, is not unusual in patients with AIDS. Although the data are incomplete, African-Americans appear to be of greater risk of cryptococcal infection (81). In Western Europe and Australia, the incidence of cryptococcosis is similar to that of the United States. However, cryptococcal meningitis appears to be a more common opportunistic disease in sub-Saharan Africa, occurring in 15 to 30% of patients (83).

Clinical Features

In patients with AIDS, the most common manifestation (70 to 90%) of cryptococcal infection is that of subacute meningitis or meningoencephalitis (67, 77–80). Most patients (75%) present with fever, malaise, and headache, and they are generally symptomatic for 2 to 4 weeks before presentation. Overt meningeal symptoms and signs, such as neck stiffness or photophobia, are unusual, occurring in only about 25% of patients (79), and consequently all patients suspected of having cryptococcal infection should be evaluated for meningeal involvement. Nausea and vomiting occur in about 40%. Some patients (30%) also have symptoms compatible with encephalopathy, such as lethargy, altered mentation, personality changes, and memory loss. Cryptococcomas (large cryptococcal granulomas within the brain) are rare in patients with AIDS. Although abnormalities on brain imaging computed tomography (CT) scans or magnetic resonance imaging are seen in up to 20% of patients, focal neurologic signs or seizures are unusual and occur in only about 10% of patients (79). CT abnormalities attributable to cryptococcosis include meningeal enhancement and, rarely, ring-enhancing lesions from cryptococcomas. However, anatomic abnormalities in the brain parenchyma are usually attributable to other HIV-associated problems (79).

Infection of the lungs is also frequent, and symptoms of pulmonary cryptococcosis may be the initial manifestation of disease (84–87). Patients typically present in a subacute fashion with fever, cough, dyspnea, and hypoxemia. Chest radiographs typically show bilateral alveolar or interstitial pneumonitis, although focal or nodular patterns, pleural effusions, and lymphadenopathy have also been described

(84). Concomitant opportunistic infections, especially with *Pneumocystis carinii,* occur in about 15 to 35% of patients (79, 80, 84). Unlike in HIV-negative patients, in whom pulmonary cryptococcosis tends to be localized to the lung, most patients with AIDS and pulmonary cryptococcosis have disseminated disease, and 60 to 70% of such patients have concomitant meningeal involvement (84). Consequently, all patients should be evaluated for meningitis (87).

Cutaneous involvement is common, and although several types of skin lesions including papules, nodules, and ulcers have been described (88, 89), the most common form is that resembling molluscum contagiosum. As many as 70% of patients with cryptococcosis are fungemic (79), and, not surprisingly, reports exist of disease in virtually every organ, including cryptococcal myocarditis (90, 91), arthritis (92), choroiditis (93), and gastroenteritis (94). Of particular interest is infection of the prostate because evidence indicates that this organ may serve as a nidus for relapse in patients who have been apparently successfully treated with antifungal therapy (95, 96).

A few patients (4 to 8%) present only with fungemia and symptoms such as fever and malaise. In occasional patients, all cultures are negative but serum cryptococcal antigen is positive (97). Generally, such patients should be assumed to have systemic infection and should be treated accordingly.

Diagnosis

Infection with *C. neoformans* is diagnosed by culturing the organism from clinical specimens or by demonstrating compatible yeast forms on histopathologic examination. Blood and cerebrospinal fluid should always be tested, and if extraneural disease is suspected, specimens should be obtained from other potentially infected sites (e.g., skin, bronchial lavage, liver, lymph nodes, and urine). Special stains using mucicarmine should be obtained to confirm cryptococcosis because histopathologic examination is the only means of diagnosis. The organism should be grown on Sabouraud's agar or other selective fungal media, and specimens should be incubated for up to 14 days, especially if the patient received some prior therapy. Culture of *C. neoformans* from any site should be regarded as significant and an indication for further evaluation and initiation of therapy.

The latex agglutination test for cryptococcal polysaccharide antigen is also highly sensitive and specific in the diagnosis of infection with *C. neoformans,* although cross-reactivity with the skin fungus *Trichosporon beigelii* can cause false-positive test results in some situations (98). The serum antigen may be a useful initial screening test in febrile patients. In a large retrospective review, 98% of patients with culture-proved cryptococcal meningitis had a positive serum cryptococcal antigen (79). A positive cryptococcal antigen titer of greater than 1:8 should be regarded as presumptive evidence of cryptococcal infection. Although the measurement of cryptococcal antigen in serum and cerebrospinal fluid is useful diagnostically, whether these measurements are useful in patients who are being treated for cryptococcal meningitis is less clear (99, 100). Changes in serum cryptococcal titers do not correlate with response, and although an unchanged or increased cerebrospinal fluid antigen titer has been shown to correlate with clinical and mycologic failure to respond to treatment, its utility in management is uncertain.

If meningitis is suspected, a lumbar puncture should be performed to obtain cerebrospinal fluid. The normal response to infection is usually blunted in patients with AIDS. The opening pressure may be elevated in patients with cryptococcal meningitis, finding reflecting concomitant raised intracranial pressure. Cerebrospinal fluid analysis characteristically shows numerous organisms and few lymphocytes. In a large study of 89 patients (79), only 21% of patients had more than 20 white blood cells/mL cerebrospinal fluid. India ink stain of the cerebrospinal fluid is positive in about 75% of cases, and about 75% of patients with either pulmonary or meningeal cryptococcosis have positive blood cultures. Antigen titers in the blood and cerebrospinal fluid are usually high and may be greater than 1:10,000, levels rarely seen in other patient populations. Indeed, a prozone phenomenon (i.e., an apparently negative test because of extremely high titers) may be observed when serum fluid antigen testing is performed (101).

Prognostic Factors

The acute mortality (during induction therapy) of AIDS-associated cryptococcosis is 10 to 25% (79, 80, 102), and the 12-month survival of all patients is 30 to 60% (79, 103). Patients without meningeal involvement do not appear to fare any better than those with meningitis (79). In patients with meningitis, the most important predictor of early mortality is the mental status of the patient at presentation. In a large therapeutic trial (102), patients with any alteration in mental status (confusion, lethargy, or obtundation) were far more likely to die than patients who had normal mentation. Other factors that appeared predictive of mortality during treatment included a cerebrospinal fluid cryptococcal antigen titer less than 1:1054, a low cerebrospinal fluid leukocyte count (less than 20 cells/mm^3), and age less than 35 years. In other studies, abnormal mental status, positive extraneural cultures for *C. neoformans,* high cerebrospinal fluid cryptococcal antigen titers, low cerebrospinal fluid leukocyte counts, and hyponatremia have been identified as poor prognostic signs (79, 104). With the increasing use of fluconazole as therapy for cryptococcal meningitis, susceptibility to this antifungal agent among cryptococci may be important prognostically. In a study evaluating fluconazole and flucytosine as treatment, the in vitro susceptibility of cryptococci to fluconazole was a factor predictive of subsequent clinical response (105).

Treatment

The treatment goals in patients with AIDS and cryptococcosis differ from those for other hosts. In AIDS, complete cure is unlikely, and the primary objectives are control of infection, decrease in early mortality, prevention of relapse, and maintenance of the patient's quality of life. Consequently, although the combination of amphotericin B and flucytosine for 4 to 6 weeks has been established as effective for cryptococcal meningitis in HIV-negative patients (106, 107), it is not the regimen of choice in patients with AIDS. Initial experience in AIDS-associated cryptococcosis treated with amphotericin B (with or without flucytosine) suggested that the outcome was similar to that seen in other immunocompromised hosts with an acute mortality rate of 10 to 40% and an overall rate of sterilization of the cerebrospinal fluid of 40 to 60%. The major limitation of the combination of amphotericin B and flucytosine in patients with AIDS has been toxicity, although cases of amphotericin B–resistant cryptococcal infection have been reported (108). Amphotericin B is associated with significant infusion-associated morbidity (especially bacterial superinfection) and nephrotoxicity; flucytosine is associated with myelosuppression and gastrointestinal toxicity. Because of high rates of dose-limiting neutropenia, the usefulness of flucytosine in patients with AIDS has been questioned. Retrospective analysis of one series concluded that the addition of flucytosine offered no therapeutic benefit and was associated with considerably more toxicity, especially cytopenias (79). A more recent prospective placebo-controlled trial that evaluated an initial course of amphotericin B plus flucytosine for 2 weeks found no significant difference in wither mycologic response or toxicity when flucytosine was added (109); however, additional analyses suggested that patients who received flucytosine as initial therapy were significantly less likely to have later relapse (110). Other groups have reported successful use of flucytosine in selected patients for at least 4 weeks of combination therapy (104).

Initial experience with the triazole antifungals, fluconazole and itraconazole (111, 112), suggested that both agents, in doses of 200 to 400 mg per day, were effective in treating patients with AIDS and acute cryptococcal meningitis, with response rates of approximately 60% in patients who had received no prior therapy. In addition, both fluconazole and itraconazole have been used successfully in patients in whom amphotericin B treatment failed or who developed dose-limiting amphotericin B toxicity (113, 114). Several randomized prospective studies evaluating triazole antifungals alone or compared with amphotericin B for initial therapy of cryptococcal meningitis have been reported and are summarized in Table 22.2 (102, 104, 115, 116). In all these studies, the triazole antifungals were associated with clinical and mycologic success rates of approximately 50%.

Most prospective studies of amphotericin B report response rates of 70 to 80% or higher (104, 115). In one large trial, only 40% of patients treated with amphotericin B had complete clinical and mycologic responses (102). This study has been criticized mainly because of the relatively low dosages of amphotericin (on average 0.45 mg/kg per day). In this trial, the cerebrospinal fluid was sterilized more rapidly in those receiving amphotericin B (median time to

Table 22.2. Randomized Comparative Trials of Traizole Antifungals as Initial Treatment of Cryptococcal Meningitis in AIDS

	Response Rate[a]			
	ACTG–MSG (102) (n = 194)	Larsen et al. (104) (n = 21)	de Gans et al. (115) (n = 28)	Moskovitz et al. (116) (n = 66)
Amphotericin B[b]	40%	100%	100%	—
Fluconazole	34%	43%	—	41%
Itraconazole	—	—	50%	38%

ACTG–MSG, AIDS Clinical Trials Group and Mycoses Study Group.
[a]Response is defined as mycologic clearance and clinical improvement by the end of treatment, 6–10 weeks, depending on study.
[b]5-Flucytosine was used in combination with amphotericin B in the studies of Larsen et al. and De Gans et al, and in 14% of patients in the ACTG–MSG study.

negative culture was 16 days for amphotericin B–treated patients and 30 days for fluconazole-treated patients), although the differences between the two treatment groups were not significant. A more rapid cerebrospinal fluid clearance with amphotericin B was also noted in the study of Larsen and associates (104), wherein the mean duration of positive cerebrospinal fluid cultures was 15.6 days in the amphotericin B–treated patients compared with 40.6 days in the fluconazole-treated group.

To determine whether initial intensive amphotericin B for a short period followed by oral triazole therapy could be effective, the Mycoses Study Group and the AIDS Clinical Trials Group (MSG–ACTG) studied initial amphotericin B therapy, 0.7 mg/kg per day (with or without concomitant flucytosine, 25 mg/kg four times daily) for 2 weeks, followed by an 8-week "consolidation" period of therapy with high doses of triazoles, either fluconazole 400 mg daily or itraconazole 400 mg daily (109). The results of this trial are the most successful reported to date. The acute mortality (death in the first 2 weeks) in this trial was 6%, and the overall mortality was 8%. A trend approached significance for a better microbiologic outcome (clearance of organisms from the cerebrospinal fluid) at 2 weeks for patients assigned to receive flucytosine and at 10 weeks for patients assigned to fluconazole. Furthermore, the high-dose amphotericin B regimen was well tolerated, and flucytosine appeared to add little additional toxicity.

Further support for this approach to patient management comes from an Italian study in which all patients were treated with 14 days of high-dose amphotericin B, 1 mg/kg per day, followed by maintenance fluconazole or itraconazole (117). Of 31 patients treated in this fashion, 29 (94%) responded to therapy, and no deaths from cryptococcosis occurred.

Thus, the bulk of current evidence tends to favor the use of amphotericin B as initial treatment for cryptococcal meningitis, especially for those patients with prognostic features that place them at higher risk of early death. Patients should therefore receive an initial period of amphotericin B, 0.7 mg/kg, plus flucytosine for 2 to 3 weeks, followed by triazole therapy, either fluconazole or itraconazole, 400 mg daily, for a further 8 to 10 weeks.

Much of the mortality associated with acute cryptococcal meningitis occurs in the first 2 weeks after diagnosis. One issue that appears to contribute to this increased mortality is intracranial hypertension, which is reflected by raised opening pressure when a lumbar puncture is performed and may threaten both life and vision (118–120). This condition can be present at diagnosis or may develop on therapy. Data from the MSG–ACTG trial indicate that elevated intracranial pressures at baseline are associated with a high risk of early death (109). Although this observation does not prove that lowering such pressures will actually improve patients' outcome, the emerging consensus is that management of elevated intracranial pressure is a critical component of therapy in such patients. Possible approaches to patients with symptomatic intracranial hypertension include mechanical drainage, using an intraventricular shunt, lumbar drain, or daily lumbar punctures (removing 25 to 30 mL of cerebrospinal fluid), and using acetazolamide to inhibit cerebrospinal fluid production. The use of corticosteroids in this setting is controversial and cannot be routinely recommended.

Interest has been expressed in alternatives to amphotericin B. Alternative formulations of amphotericin B have been developed primarily to reduce associated toxicities. One small trial suggested that amphotericin B lipid complex (ABLC) was considerably less toxic than standard amphotericin B deoxycholate and also suggested that ABLC had some activity in patients with cryptococcal meningitis, although the study was too small to assess comparative effectiveness (121). A preliminary report of liposomal amphotericin B in 26 patients with cryptococcosis indicated a mycologic and clinical response rate of approximately 60%, with minimal toxicity (122). A small comparative trial suggested possible superiority of liposomal amphotericin B (123). Larger trials are required to determine the role of these formulations.

Preliminary data are also available on the use of higher doses of fluconazole and of the alternative combination therapy of flucytosine plus a triazole (124, 125). In a series of studies conducted by the California Collaborative Treatment Group (126, 127), the combination of fluconazole with flucytosine as primary treatment resulted in response rates of 60 to 80%, especially at daily doses of fluconazole of 800 mg or greater. Although toxicity from flucytosine was considerable, most patients were reported to tolerate at least 2 weeks of treatment. A few patients have been successfully treated with the combination of itraconazole and flucytosine (128). These data clearly suggest that this combination merits more extensive investigation and may emerge as a useful oral alternative to parenteral amphotericin B–based regimens.

Suppressive Treatment

Management of cryptococcal disease in patients with AIDS is further complicated by the finding that, as with most other opportunistic infections, curative therapy is unusual, and long-term suppressive therapy is likely to be necessary. Relapse rates of 50 to 60% (80) and a shorter life expectancy (79) have been reported in patients who did not receive long-term suppressive therapy. Relapse probably represents failure to eradicate infection rather than a new primary infection. For example, a persistent urinary focus of infection (presumably of prostatic origin) has been reported in approximately 20% of patients completing therapy with amphotericin B (95).

Fluconazole is the suppressive treatment of choice. The California Collaborative Treatment Group compared fluconazole with placebo in a select population of patients who had been treated for acute cryptococcal meningitis with amphotericin B (129). Fluconazole was superior to placebo, with 3% of fluconazole patients and 37% of placebo patients relapsing at any site. Fifteen percent of patients in the placebo arm developed meningitis compared with none in the fluconazole group. An ACTG study compared fluconazole, 200 mg per day, with weekly infusions of amphotericin B, 1 mg/kg, in 189 patients followed for a median of 286 days (103). Relapse rates were 2% (3 of 111) for fluconazole and 17% (14 of 78) for amphotericin B. No difference was seen in overall survival between the 2 groups, but fluconazole was better tolerated. In this study, all patients were treated initially with at least 15 mg/kg of amphotericin B. Higher relapse rates (23%) have been reported when fluconazole alone was also used as primary treatment (111). Fluconazole was also significantly superior to itraconazole in a trial of maintenance therapy conducted by the MSG, in which the relapse rate with itraconazole was 28% compared with 2% for fluconazole maintenance (110).

Relapse usually presents with clinically evident disease, usually with fever, and with recurrence of headache for most patients with meningitis. Routine monitoring by measurement of serum cryptococcal antigen is not useful in predicting relapse (99, 100, 130). Azole resistance among cryptococci is unusual (131, 132). Relapse of cryptococcal meningitis in patients taking fluconazole has not generally been associated with resistant isolates (133). Indeed, the available evidence indicates that most patients are infected with their original strain, a finding suggesting that adherence to therapy may be a critical factor in relapse (133).

Prevention

Several studies have suggested that fluconazole can prevent many cases of cryptococcal meningitis in patients with AIDS (65, 134). Indeed, the declining incidence of this infection has been attributed to widespread use of fluconazole (135, 136). A randomized trial comparing fluconazole, 200 mg per day, with clotrimazole troches for prevention of fungal infections in patients with CD4 counts lower than 200 cells/mm^3 demonstrated a 2-year rate of invasive fungal infection of 2.8% in the fluconazole group compared with 9.1% in the clotrimazole group, with a sevenfold reduction in the risk of cryptococcosis (65). Prospective trials evaluating daily doses of 100 mg or weekly doses of 400 mg of fluconazole also showed a low incidence of cryptococcal infection (137, 138). These prospective trial data are supported by other retrospective or case-controlled analyses of the effect of exposure to fluconazole on the risk of developing cryptococcal meningitis (139, 140). In a placebo-controlled prospective trial (141), itraconazole, 200 mg per day, reduced the occurrence of cryptococcal meningitis from 5.5 to 0.7%. In most studies, maximal risk of cryptococcosis (and thus benefit of prophylaxis) occurs when the CD4 count is less than 50 cells/mm^3 (133). In spite of the clear evidence of a protective effect, the overall utility of routine use of azoles as primary prophylaxis in advanced HIV disease is unclear. Considerable concern exists that prolonged usage of fluconazole may result in acquired resistance to this agent, especially in *Candida* species. At this point, no standard recommendation is available on the use of fluconazole as primary prophylaxis (142).

HISTOPLASMOSIS

Microbiology and Epidemiology

The dimorphic fungus, *Histoplasma capsulatum*, is distributed worldwide, but it is endemic in certain areas of North and South America. In the United States, infection has been noted primarily in the Mississippi and Ohio River valleys, where the mycelial form can be found readily in the environment, particularly associated with bird roosts, chicken coops, and caves (143). Infection results when spores of *H. capsulatum* are inhaled into the lung; conversion to the yeast form then occurs at body temperature. In most cases, effective cell-mediated immunity limits such acute infection to a mild respiratory illness.

Histoplasmosis is a common complication of AIDS in areas where *Histoplasma capsulatum* is endemic (144–146). Indeed, histoplasmosis has been reported in certain parts of the endemic area to be the second or third most frequent opportunistic infection in HIV-positive patients. However, many cases of histoplasmosis in AIDS have now been reported in patients living in parts of the world where the fungus is not endemic (144). Most cases of histoplasmosis in such patients are assumed to represent reactivation of previously acquired disease, and preliminary evidence based on molecular typing supports this hypothesis (147). However, the epidemiology of histoplasmosis in the endemic area is less clear-cut. Some investigators have argued that the high incidence of AIDS-associated histoplasmosis in cities such as Indianapolis, coincident with outbreaks of the disease in the general population, indicates that primary infection accounts for much of the disease in the endemic area (148). However, because some patients with histoplasmosis have diffuse pulmonary calcification suggesting prior exposure, other investigators have argued that reactivation may also play a role in histoplasmosis in patients from the endemic area (149).

Clinical Features and Diagnosis

Histoplasmosis in AIDS usually presents as a disseminated infection (144–146). The most common manifestations (and sometimes the only presentations) are fever and weight loss. Respiratory complaints occur in about 50% of cases (145, 146). The chest radiograph is normal in 30 to 40%; most of the remaining patients have diffuse nodular infiltrates (145). Local or generalized lymphadenopathy, hepatosplenomegaly, colonic lesions (150), and skin (151, 152) and oral ulcers (41) also occur. Between 5 and 10% of patients present with an acute illness resembling septic shock with hypotension and evidence of disseminated coagulopathy (145). Central nervous system involvement with meningitis is a rare but important complication (145, 153, 154). Laboratory findings may include anemia, neutropenia, or thrombocytopenia (reflecting bone marrow involvement by the fungus) and elevation of hepatic enzymes. The CD4 lymphocyte count is almost invariably less than 200 cells/mm^3 and usually less than 100 (146).

The diagnosis is usually made by culturing the fungus from blood or other clinical specimens or by histopathologic examination of bone marrow aspirate or biopsy, lavage fluid, or biopsy material from lung or skin lesions. Detection of anti-*Histoplasma capsulatum* antibodies by immunodiffusion or complement fixation is positive in about 70 to 80% of cases (144–146). Detection of *Histoplasma* antigen in either urine or serum is an extremely sensitive and specific method for diagnosing disseminated histoplasmosis (155, 156), but as yet this test is not widely available. Serial monitoring of either serum or urine histoplasma antigen is also useful in assessing response to therapy (156).

Treatment

Amphotericin B (0.5 to 1.0 mg/kg per day for a total dose of 0.5 to 1.0 g) is associated with an overall response rate of about 85 to 90% in patients with disseminated histoplasmosis (145). Itraconazole, 400 mg orally daily, is effective in about 85% of patients with disseminated disease (157); however, patients with severe life-threatening or central nervous system histoplasmosis were excluded from that study, and amphotericin B remains the therapy of choice for patients with complicated cases.

Itraconazole should also be regarded as the suppressive therapy of choice. Two ACTG trials have shown that itraconazole, 200 to 400 mg daily, is highly effective in preventing relapse of histoplasmosis either after primary therapy with amphotericin B (158) or, for milder disease, after primary therapy with itraconazole (159). Weekly or biweekly infusions of amphotericin B (1.0 mg/kg) have been associated with an 80 to 90% relapse-free survival (145, 160), but they may necessitate an indwelling catheter, which has its own complications. Ketoconazole is generally ineffective as suppressive therapy and is not recommended (145). Fluconazole may be effective in some circumstances as suppressive therapy after initial amphotericin alone (161); however, when used as primary therapy, it appears to be less effective than itraconazole, even at high doses (600 to 800 mg per day). In an ACTG–MSG trial (162), fluconazole was associated with a 74% response rate and about a 33% relapse rate during maintenance therapy, and most experts believe that fluconazole should be regarded as second-line therapy for histoplasmosis.

The role of prophylactic therapy is uncertain. The MSG conducted a placebo-controlled trial of itraconazole, 200 mg daily, as prophylaxis for histoplasmosis in patients with CD4 counts lower than 150 cells/mm^3 who resided in an endemic area (141). Histoplasmosis occurred in 2.8% of itraconazole recipients and in 6.8% of patients receiving placebo. The benefit was maximum in patients with CD4 counts lower than 100 cells/mm^3. Thus, itraconazole could be considered as prophylaxis for histoplasmosis in patients residing in an endemic area, especially those with CD4 counts lower than 100 cell/mm^3. Fluconazole may not be effective; breakthrough cases of histoplasmosis have occurred in patients who were receiving fluconazole prophylaxis (133, 134).

COCCIDIOIDOMYCOSIS

Microbiology and Epidemiology

Infection with *Coccidioides immitis* is increasingly common in patients with AIDS in the southwestern United States, where the fungus is endemic, and the infection is occasionally seen elsewhere in patients who have lived in or visited the endemic area (Arizona, New Mexico, southern California, and western Texas). *C. immitis* is a dimorphic fungus that exists in the soil in the mycelial phase. Maturation of the fungus results in formation of hyphae and arthroconidia, which are easily aerosolized and may be inhaled by animal hosts. Once inhaled, the arthrospores stimulate an inflammatory response in the lung. Sixty percent of infected individuals have asymptomatic infections or symptoms of a simple upper respiratory tract infection (144, 163). In most cases, this remains a self-limited illness controlled by cell-mediated immunity. HIV-positive patients develop disseminated disease (164). Carefully performed epidemiologic studies suggest that both primary infection and reactivation of previously acquired coccidioidomycosis occur in HIV-positive patients, as T-cell immunity wanes. Consequently, both previously infected and naive individuals are susceptible to infection (165). The risk of clinical illness from coccidioidomycosis appears to be higher than 10% for exposed individuals living in the endemic area. Almost 40% of the cases of coccidioidomycosis reported to the CDC as AIDS-defining illnesses occurred in counties outside the endemic area (166). Although these individuals probably acquired their infection in the endemic area, coccidioidomycosis needs to be considered in all patients with AIDS who have ever traveled (even for a brief time) to the endemic area. Disease usually occurs when the CD4 count falls below 250 cells/mm^3 (164, 165).

Clinical Features and Diagnosis

Coccidioidomycosis generally involves the lungs. Most patients present with fever, weight loss, cough, and dyspnea, and they characteristically have a diffuse reticulonodular infiltrate on chest radiography (164, 167). Many such patients are also fungemic (168), suggesting they have hematogenously disseminated disease. Other manifestations include generalized lymphadenopathy, skin nodules or ulcers (88, 167), peritonitis (169), and subacute or chronic meningitis (in about 10 to 12% of patients), which manifests as progressive lethargy and fever (164, 167). In contrast to patients with cryptococcal meningitis, patients with coccidioidal meningitis typically have more than 50 lymphocytes/mL of cerebrospinal fluid (164). Focal pulmonary disease occurs in a few patients (167). Some patients may present with fever in association with positive coccidioidal serology without focal lesions (170), and they are presumed to have coccidioidal infection. Estimates of the risk of infection in such individuals approach 70% and suggest that treatment is warranted.

Diagnosis is made by culture of the organism from clinical specimens or by demonstration of the typical spherule on histopathologic examination (171). The spherule can be identified using stains such as Gomori's silver methenamine or Papanicolaou's stain. *Coccidioides immitis* is a highly contagious organism, and the clinical laboratory should be warned of the possibility of positive cultures. Blood cultures may be positive in some patients. Coccidioidal serologic tests may be positive, but as many as one-quarter of patients with disseminated disease have negative serologic tests (172).

Treatment

The treatment of choice remains amphotericin B (144, 167). The outcome of diffuse pulmonary disease appears to be worse than that of other forms of coccidioidomycosis, with a median survival of only 1 month in one large series (167). The triazole antifungals have been used successfully in patients without AIDS, with a 60% response rate (173, 174); however, the published experience with the use of these agents in patients with AIDS is limited. Fluconazole, 400 to 800 mg orally daily, may be an alternative for patients with mild disease. Both itraconazole and fluconazole have been reported to be successful in approximately 80% patients with *Coccidioides immitis* meningitis (175, 176). Patients with coccidioidal meningitis require lifelong therapy (177). The specific experience with coccidioidal meningitis in patients with AIDS is limited.

Prolonged suppressive therapy appears warranted; the triazoles, fluconazole and itraconazole (200 to 400 mg orally daily of either) are preferred. Breakthrough infections have been reported with ketoconazole (178).

PENICILLIOSIS

Penicillium marneffei is a dimorphic fungus endemic in Southeast Asia, especially Vietnam, Thailand (particularly the northern part around Chiang Mai), and the southern part of China. Infection has been seen predominantly in residents of these areas (179, 180). In the Western world, penicilliosis is seen in HIV-positive immigrants from the endemic area as well as in persons who have traveled there (181, 182). Penicilliosis has become an important infection in the endemic area, where it is the second or third most common opportunistic infection and occurs in up to one-third of HIV-infected patients. The organism was first isolated from bamboo rats, which are believed to be an important reservoir of infection because most are chronically infected with the fungus (183). However, the actual route of human infection with this organism is not known.

Penicilliosis in AIDS usually presents as a disseminated infection (180, 181) with fever, anemia, and weight loss, which occur in over 75% of patients. Respiratory complaints (cough, shortness of breath) occur in about half of cases. The chest radiograph in such cases shows diffuse nodular pulmonary infiltrates or cavitary disease. Three-quarters of patients with disseminated disease present with cutaneous involvement, typically multiple papular lesions (184, 185). The diagnosis is usually confirmed by direct microscopy (186) or by culturing the fungus from blood or other clinical specimens, such as skin, bone marrow, or lymph nodes.

Disseminated infection with *Penicillium marneffei* is lethal and always requires antifungal therapy. Amphotericin B, 0.6 to 1.0 mg/kg per day, is regarded as the standard therapy (180, 181). In vitro, *P. marneffei* is susceptible to several to the azole antifungals including itraconazole and ketoconazole, as well as to flucytosine (187). Itraconazole, 200 mg twice daily, appears to be effective in vivo also, and it can be used in patients with mild-to-moderate disease. As with the other endemic mycoses, relapse is common if chronic suppressive therapy is not given, and long-term suppressive therapy, with itraconazole, 200 mg daily, is warranted.

ASPERGILLOSIS

Aspergillosis is a rare complication of AIDS. It is usually seen in patients with advanced disease who have additional risk factors for infection with *Aspergillus*, such as neutropenia, steroid use, alcoholism, broad-spectrum antibacterial therapy, or hematologic malignancy (188–192). Aspergillosis may also be a direct effect of advanced HIV disease, perhaps because of impaired specific macrophage function (193). Most patients present with pulmonary disease, which often disseminates. The usual radiographic patterns are of cavitatory pneumonitis or diffuse infiltrates. Obstructive bronchial lesions have also been described (188). *Aspergillus* infection of the brain and sinuses has also been reported (191, 194), usually presenting with focal central nervous system signs or mental status changes. Cutaneous *Aspergillus* infection has also been described (195, 196).

Disseminated aspergillosis has a poor prognosis. The usual therapy is amphotericin B (1.0 mg/kg per day), although itraconazole may have a role in the treatment of patients intolerant of amphotericin B and for long-term suppression (197). The MSG evaluated itraconazole in patients with aspergillosis and reported a 40% response rate (198), with better outcomes seen in patients with pulmonary disease and the worst outcomes seen with central nervous system disease. Unfortunately, poor responses were seen in patients with AIDS. Amphotericin B lipid complex, 5.0 mg/kg per day, has been evaluated in the treatment of aspergillosis in patients intolerant to regular amphotericin B or in whom such treatment has failed, and the reported response rate of such patients is 30 to 40% (199). Specific experience in patients with AIDS is limited.

OTHER FUNGAL INFECTIONS

Other fungal infections occur in patients with AIDS (200). Blastomycosis is unusual among patients with AIDS, even in the endemic area (midwestern United States). In those cases, the disease has presented with cavitatory pulmonary lesions, skin lesions, and fever (201). Widespread dissemination may occur and is associated with a poor prognosis. In contrast, some patients, usually with less advanced HIV disease, may present with focal pulmonary or skin disease and respond better to antifungal therapy. Amphotericin B is the treatment of choice for disseminated blastomycosis (201), with itraconazole, 200 to 400 mg per day, an alternative for mild disease and long-term suppression (202). Disseminated sporotrichosis (caused by the dimorphic fungus, *Sporothrix schenckii*) has been reported rarely in patients with AIDS (203, 204). The usual presentation is one of diffuse cutaneous disease with polyarthritis. Amphotericin B is the treatment of choice. Itraconazole may also be effective. Invasive mucormycosis also occurs rarely, typically in patients with neutropenia or in intravenous drug users (200, 205). The usual manifestation is with brain or sinus involvement, and the prognosis is poor.

Acknowledgment

This work was supported in part by National Institutes of Health Grant AI-25903.

References

1. Gottlieb MS, Schroff R, Schanker HM, et al. *Pneumocystis carinii* pneumonia and mucosal candidiasis in previously healthy homosexual men: evidence of a new acquired cellular immunodeficiency. N Engl J Med 1981;305:1425–1431.
2. Masur H, Michelis MA, Greene JB, et al. An outbreak of community-acquired *Pneumocystis carinii* pneumonia: initial manifestation of cellular immune dysfunction. N Engl J Med 1981;305:1431–1438.
3. Holmstrup P, Samaranayake LP. Acute and AIDS-related oral candidosis. In: Samaranayake LP, MacFarlane TW, eds. Oral candidosis. London: Wright, 1990:133–155.
4. Pindborg JJ. Oral candidosis in HIV infection. In: Robertson PB, Greenspan JS, eds. Perspectives on oral manifestations of AIDS. Littleton, MA: PSG Publishing, 1988:23–32.
5. Odds FC. *Candida* infections in AIDS patients. Int J STD AIDS 1992;3:157–160.
6. Powderly WG. Mucosal candidiasis caused by non-*albicans* species of *Candida* in HIV-positive patients. AIDS 1992;6:604–605.
7. Maenza JR, Merz WG, Romagnoli MJ, et al. Infection due to fluconazole-resistant *Candida* in patients with AIDS: prevalence and microbiology. Clin Infect Dis 1997;24:28–34.

8. Odds F. *Candida* and candidosis: a review and bibliography. 2nd ed. London: Balliere Tindall, 1988.
9. McCarthy GM. Host factors associated with HIV-related oral candidiasis. Oral Surg Oral Med Oral Pathol 1992;73:181–186.
10. Warnock DW. Immunological aspects of candidosis in AIDS patients. In: vanden Bossche H, Mackenzie DWR, Cauwenbergh G, et al., eds. Mycosis in AIDS patients. New York: Plenum Press, 1990:83–91.
11. Epstein JB, Truelove EL, Izutzu KT. Oral candidiasis: pathogenesis and host defense. Rev Infect Dis 1984;6:96–102.
12. Yeh CK, Fox PC, Ship JA, et al. Oral defense mechanisms are impaired early in HIV-1 infected patients. J Acquir Immune Defic Syndr 1988;1:361–366.
13. McCarthy GM, Mackie ID, Koval J, et al. Factors associated with increased frequency of HIV-related oral candidiasis. J Oral Pathol Med 1991;20:332–336.
14. Crowe SM, Vardaxis NJ, Kent SJ, et al. HIV infection of monocyte-derived macrophages in vitro reduces phagocytosis of *Candida albicans*. J Leuk Biol 1994;56:318–327.
15. Carpenter CCJ, Mayer KH, Fisher A, et al. Natural history of acquired immunodeficiency syndrome in women in Rhode Island. Am J Med 1989;86:771–779.
16. Imam N, Carpenter CCJ, Mayer KH, et al. Hierarchical pattern of mucosal *Candida* infection in HIV-seropositive women. Am J Med 1990;89:142–146.
17. Rhoads JL, Wright DC, Redfield RR, et al. Chronic vaginal candidiasis in women with human immunodeficiency syndrome. JAMA 1987;257:3105–3107.
18. Feigal DW, Katz MH, Greenspan D, et al. The prevalence of oral lesions in HIV-infected homosexual and bisexual men: three San Francisco epidemiological cohorts. AIDS 1991;5:519–525.
19. Bruatto M, Vidotto V, Marinuzzi G, et al. *Candida albicans* biotypes in human immunodeficiency virus type 1-infected patients with oral candidiasis before and after antifungal therapy. J Clin Microbiol 1991;29:726–730.
20. Pons V, Greenspan D, Debruin M. Therapy for oropharyngeal candidiasis in HIV-infected patients: a randomized, prospective multicenter study of oral fluconazole versus clotrimazole troches. The Multicenter Study Group. J Acquir Immune Defic Syndr 1993;6:1311–1316.
21. Fichtenbaum C, Yiannoutsos C, Holland F, et al. Clinical factors associated with recurrent oral candidiasis in HIV infection [abstract]. In: Program and abstracts of the 4th Conference on Retroviruses and Opportunistic Infections. Alexandria, VA: IDSA Foundation for Retrovirology and Human Health, 1997.
22. Moore RD, Chaisson RE. Natural history of opportunistic disease in an HIV-infected urban clinical cohort. Ann Intern Med 1996;124:633–642.
23. Malebranche R, Guerin JM, Laroche AC, et al. Acquired immunodeficiency syndrome with severe gastrointestinal manifestations in Haiti. Lancet 1983;1:873–877.
24. Piot P, Quinn TC, Taelman H, et al. Acquired immunodeficiency syndrome in a heterosexual population in Zaire. Lancet 1984;2:65–69.
25. Whelan WL, Krisch DR, Kwon-Chung KJ, et al. *Candida albicans* in patients with the acquired immunodeficiency syndrome: absence of a novel or hypervirulent strain. J Infect Dis 1990;162:513–518.
26. Powderly WG, Robinson K, Keath EJ. Molecular typing of *Candida albicans* isolated from oral lesions of HIV-infected individuals. AIDS 1992;6:81–84.
27. Schmid J, Odds FC, Wiselka MJ, et al. Genetic similarity and maintenance of *Candida albicans* strains from a group of AIDS patients, demonstrated by DNA fingerprinting. J Clin Microbiol 1992;30:935–941.
28. Miyasaki SH, Hicks JB, Greenspan D, et al. The identification and tracking of *Candida albicans* isolates from oral lesions in HIV-seropositive individuals. J Acquir Immune Defic Syndr 1992;5:1039–1046.
29. Lupetti A, Guzzi G, Paladini A, et al. Molecular typing of *Candida albicans* in oral candidiasis: karyotype epidemiology with human immunodeficiency virus-seropositive patients in comparison with that with healthy carriers. J Clin Microbiol 1995;33:1238–1242.
30. Powderly WG, Robinson K, Keath EJ. Molecular epidemiology of recurrent oral candidiasis in HIV-positive patients: evidence for two patterns of recurrence. J Infect Dis 1993;168:463–466.
31. Klein RS, Harris CA, Small C, et al. Oral candidiasis in high-risk patients as the initial manifestation of the acquired immunodeficiency syndrome. N Engl J Med 1984;311:354–358.
32. Kaslow RA, Phair JP, Friedman HB, et al. Infection with the human immunodeficiency virus: clinical manifestations and their relationship to immune deficiency. Ann Intern Med 1987;107:474–480.
33. Kirby AJ, Munoz A, Detels R, et al. Thrush and fever as measures of immunocompetence in HIV-1-infected men. J Acquir Immune Defic Syndr Hum Retrovirol 1994;7:1242–1249.
34. Katz MH, Greenspan D, Westenhouse J, et al. Progression to AIDS in HIV-infected homosexual and bisexual men with hairy leukoplakia and oral candidiasis. AIDS 1992;6:95–100.
35. Dodd CL, Greenspan D, Katz MH, et al. Oral candidiasis in HIV infection: pseudomembranous and erythematous candidiasis show similar rates of progression to AIDS. AIDS 1991;5:1339–1344.
36. Fischl MA, Richman DD, Hansen N, et al. The safety and efficacy of zidovudine (AZT) in the treatment of patients with mildly symptomatic HIV infection: a double-blind, placebo-controlled trial. Ann Intern Med 1990;112:727–737.
37. Whimbey E, Gold JW, Polsky B, et al. Bacteremia and fungemia in patients with the acquired immunodeficiency syndrome. Ann Intern Med 1986;104:511–514.
38. Wilkes MS, Fortin Ah, Felix JW, et al. Value of necropsy in acquired immunodeficiency syndrome. Lancet 1988;2:85–88.
39. Chu FE, Carrow M, Blevins A, et al. Candidemia in patients with acquired immunodeficiency syndrome. In: vanden Bossche H, Mackenzie DWR, G Cauwenbergh G, et al., eds. Mycosis in AIDS patients. New York: Plenum Press, 1990:75–82.
40. Matthews R, Burnie J, Smith D, et al. *Candida* and AIDS: evidence for protective antibody. Lancet 1988;2:263–266.
41. Eisig S, Boguslaw B, Cooperband B, et al. Oral manifestations of disseminated histoplamosis in the acquired immunodeficiency syndrome: report of two cases and review of the literature. J Oral Maxillofac Surg 1991;49:310.
42. Tavitian A, Raufman J-P, Rosenthal LE. Oral candidiasis as a marker for esophageal candidiasis in the acquired immunodeficiency syndrome. Ann Intern Med 1986;104:54–55.
43. Porro GB, Parente F, Cernuschi M. The diagnosis of esophageal candidiasis in patients with acquired immune deficiency syndrome: is endoscopy always necessary? Am J Gastroenterol 1989;84:143–146.
44. Rabeneck L, Laine L. Esophageal candidiasis in patients infected with the human immunodeficiency virus: a decision analysis to assess cost-effectiveness of alternative management strategies. Arch Intern Med 1994;154:2705–2710.
45. Wilcox CM, Straub RF, Clark WS. Prospective evaluation of oropharyngeal findings in human immunodeficiency virus–infected patients with esophageal ulceration. Am J Gastroenterol 1995;90:1938–1941.
46. Smith DE, Midgley J, Allan M, et al. Itraconazole versus ketoconazole in the treatment of oral and oesophageal candidosis in patients infected with HIV. AIDS 1991;5:1367–1371.
47. Just G, Steinheimer D, Schnellbach M, et al. Treatment of candidosis in AIDS patients. In: vanden Bossche H, Mackenzie DWR, Cauwenbergh G, et al., eds. Mycosis in AIDS patients. New York: Plenum Press, 1990:279–285.
48. De Wit S, Gloossens H, Weerts D, et al. Comparison of fluconazole and ketoconazole for oropharyngeal candidiasis in AIDS. Lancet 1989;1:746–747.
49. Lake-Bakaar G, Tom W, Lake-Bakaar D, et al. Gastropathy and ketoconazole malabsorption in the acquired immunodeficiency syndrome (AIDS). Ann Intern Med 1988;109:471–473.

50. Laine L, Dretletr RH, Conteas CN, et al. Fluconazole compared with ketoconazole for the treatment of *Candida* esophagitis in AIDS. Ann Intern Med 1992;117:655–660.
51. Barbaro G, Barbarini G, Di Lorenzo G. Fluconazole compared with itraconazole in the treatment of esophageal candidiasis in AIDS patients: a double-blind, randomized, controlled clinical study. Scand J Infect Dis 1995;27:613–617
52. Baily GG, Perry FM, Denning DW, et al. Fluconazole-resistant candidosis in an HIV cohort. AIDS 1994;8:787–792
53. Powderly WG. Resistant candidiasis. AIDS Res Hum Retroviruses 1994;10:925–929.
54. Sangeorzan JA, Bradley SF, He X, et al. Epidemiology of oral candidiasis in HIV-infected patients: colonization, infection, treatment, and emergence of fluconazole resistance. Am J Med 1994;97:339–346.
55. Johnson EM, Warnock DW, Luker J, et al. Emergence of azole drug assistance in *Candida* species from HIV-infected patients receiving prolonged fluconazole therapy for oral candidosis. J Antimicrob Chemother 1995;35:103–114.
56. Maenza JR, Keruly JC, Moore RD, et al. Risk factors for fluconazole-resistant candidiasis in human immunodeficiency virus-infected patients. J Infect Dis 1996;173:219–225.
57. Fichtenbaum CJ, Koletar S, Yiannoutsos C, et al. Fluconazole resistant *Candida* in advanced HIV disease [abstract Mo.B.112]. In: Program and abstracts of the 11th International Conference on AIDS. Vancouver: 11th International Conference on AIDS, 1996.
58. Rex JH, Pfaller MA, Galgiani JN, et al. Development of interpretive breakpoints for antifungal susceptibility testing: conceptual framework and analysis of in vitro–in vivo correlation data for fluconazole, itraconazole and candida infections. Clin Infect Dis 1997;24:235–247.
59. Sanglard D, Kuchler K, Ischer F, et al. Mechanisms of resistance to azole antifungal agents in *Candida albicans* isolates from AIDS patients involves specific multidrug transporters. Antimicrob Agents Chemother 1995;39:2378–2386.
60. Cartledge JD, Midgley J, Youle M, et al. Itraconazole cyclodextrin solution: effective treatment for HIV-related candidosis unresponsive to other azole therapy [letter]. J Antimicrob Chemother 1994;33:1071–1073.
61. Philips P, Zemcov J, Mahmood W, et al. Itraconazole cyclodextrin solution for fluconazole-refractory oropharyngeal candidiasis in AIDS: correlation of clinical response with in vitro susceptibility. AIDS 1996;10:1369–1376.
62. Dewsnup DH, Stevens DA. Efficacy of oral amphotericin B in AIDS patients with thrush clinically resistant to fluconazole. J Med Vet Mycol 1994;32:389–393.
63. Zingman BS. Resolution of refractory AIDS-related mucosal candidiasis after initiation of didanosine plus saquinavir [letter]. N Engl J Med 1996;334:1674–1675.
64. Stevens DA, Greene SI, Lang OS. Thrush can be prevented in patients with acquired immunodeficiency syndrome and acquired immunodeficiency syndrome-related complex: randomized, double-blind, placebo-controlled study of 100 mg oral fluconazole daily. Arch Intern Med 1991;151:2458–2464.
65. Powderly WG, Finkelstein D, Feinberg J, et al. A randomized trial comparing fluconazole with clotrimazole troches for the prevention of fungal infections in patients with advanced human immunodeficiency virus infection. N Engl J Med 1995;332:700–705.
66. Laine L. The natural history of esophageal candidiasis after successful treatment in patients with AIDS. Gastroenterology 1994;107:744–746.
67. Dismukes WE. Cryptococcal meningitis in patients with AIDS. J Infect Dis 1988;157:624–628.
68. Powderly WG. Cryptococcal meningitis and AIDS. Clin Infect Dis 1993;17:837–842.
69. Ellis DH, Pfeiffer TJ. Ecology, life cycle, and infectious propagule of *Cryptococcus neoformans*. Lancet 1990;336;923–925.
70. Rinaldi MG, Drutz DJ, Howell A, et al. Serotypes of *Cryptococcus neoformans* in patients with AIDS. J Infect Dis 1986;153:642.
71. Shimizu RY, Howard DH, Clancy MN. The variety of *Cryptococcus neoformans* in patients with AIDS. J Infect Dis 1986;154:1042.
72. Swinne D, Nkurikiyinfura JB, Muyembe TL. Clinical isolates of *Cryptococcus neoformans* from Zaire. Eur J Clin Microbiol 1986;5:50–51.
73. Speed B, Dunt D. Clinical and host differences between infections with the two varieties of *Cryptococcus neoformans*. Clin Infect Dis 1995;21:28–34
74. Fung PYS, Murphy JW. In vitro interactions of immune lymphocytes and *Cryptococcus neoformans*. Infect Immun 1982;36:1128–1138.
75. Kozel TR, Pfrommer GST, Redelman D. Activated neutrophils exhibit enhanced phagocytosis of *Cryptococcus neoformans* opsonized with normal human serum. Clin Exp Immunol 1987;70:238–246.
76. Harrison TS, Kornfeld H, Levitz SM. The effect of infection with human immunodeficiency virus on the anticryptococcal activity of lymphocytes and monocytes. J Infect Dis 1995;172:665–671.
77. Currie BP, Casadevall A. Estimation of the prevalence of cryptococcal infection among patients infected with the human immunodeficiency virus in New York City. Clin Infect Dis 1994 19:1029–1033.
78. Kovacs JA, Kovacs AA, Polis M, et al. Cryptococcosis in the acquired immunodeficiency syndrome. Ann Intern Med 1985;103:533–538.
79. Chuck SL, Sande MA. Infections with *Cryptococcus neoformans* in the acquired immunodeficiency syndrome. N Engl J Med 1989;321:794–799.
80. Clark RA, Greer D, Atkinson W, et al. Spectrum of *Cryptococcus neoformans* infection in 68 patients infected with human immunodeficiency virus. Rev Infect Dis 1990;12:768–777.
81. Pinner RW, Hajjeh R, Powderly WG. Prospects for prevention of cryptococcosis in persons infected with human immunodeficiency virus. Clin Infect Dis 1995;21:S103–S107.
82. Crowe SM, Carlin JB, Stewart KI, et al. Predictive value of CD4 lymphocyte numbers for the development of opportunistic infections and malignancies in HIV-infected persons. J Acquir Immune Defic Syndr 1991;4:770–776.
83. Clumeck N, Van de Perre P, Carael M. The African AIDS experience in contrast with the rest of the world. In: Leoung G, Mills J, eds. Opportunistic infections in patients with the acquired immune deficiency syndrome. New York: Marcel Dekker, 1989:43–56.
84. Clark RA, Greer DL, Valainis GT, et al. *Cryptococcus neoformans* pulmonary infection in HIV-1 infected patients. J Acquir Immune Defic Syndr 1990;3:480–484.
85. Cameron ML, Bartlett JA, Gallis HA, et al. Manifestations of pulmonary cryptococcosis in patients with acquired immunodeficiency syndrome. Rev Infect Dis 1991;13:64–67.
86. Meyohas MC, Roux P, Bollens D, et al. Pulmonary cryptococcosis: localized and disseminated infections in 27 patients with AIDS. Clin Infect Dis 1995;21:628–633.
87. Driver JA, Saunders CA, Heinze-Lacey B, et al. Cryptococcal pneumonia in AIDS: is cryptococcal meningitis preceded by clinically recognizable pneumonia? J Acquir Immune Defic Syndr Hum Retrovirol 1995;9:168–171.
88. Penneys NS. Skin manifestations of AIDS. Philadelphia: JB Lippincott, 1990.
89. Murakawa GJ, Kerschmann R, Berger T. Cutaneous *Cryptococcus* infection and AIDS: report of 12 cases and review of the literature. Arch Dermatol 1996;132:545–548.
90. Lewis W, Lipsick J, Cammarosano C. Cryptococcal myocarditis in acquired immune deficiency syndrome. Am J Cardiol 1985;55:1240–1242.
91. Lafont A, Wolff M, Marche C, et al. Overwhelming myocarditis due to *Cryptococcus neoformans* in an AIDS patient. Lancet 1987;2:1145–1146.
92. Ricciardi DD, Sepkowitz DV, Berkowitz LB, et al. Cryptococcal arthritis in a patient with acquired immune deficiency syndrome: case report and review of the literature. J Rheumatol 1986;13:455–459.

93. Morinelli EN, Dugel PU, Riffenburgh R, et al. Infectious multifocal choroiditis in patients with acquired immune deficiency syndrome. Ophthalmology 1993;100:1014–1021.
94. Bonacini M, Nussbaum J, Ahluwalia C. Gastrointestinal, hepatic, and pancreatic involvement with *Cryptococcus neoformans* in AIDS. J Clin Gastroenterol 1990;12:295–300.
95. Larsen RA, Bozzette S, McCutchan JA, et al., and the California Collaborative Treatment Group. Persistent *Cryptococcus neoformans* of the prostate after successful treatment of meningitis. Ann Intern Med 1989;111:125–128.
96. Ndimbie OK, Dekker A, Martinez AJ, et al. Prostatic sequestration of Cryptococcus neoformans in immunocompromised persons treated for cryptococcal meningoencephalitis. Histol Histopathol 1994;9:643–648.
97. Feldmeser M, Harris C, Reichberg S, et al. Serum cryptococcal antigen in patients with AIDS. Clin Infect Dis 1996;23:827–830.
98. McManus EJ, Jones JM. Detection of a *Trichosporon beigelii* antigen cross reactive with *Cryptococcus neoformans* capsular polysaccharide in serum from a patient with disseminated *Trichosporon* infection. J Clin Microbiol 1985;21:681–685.
99. Powderly WG, Cloud GA, Dismukes WE, et al. Measurement of cryptococcal antigen in serum and cerebrospinal fluid: value in the management of AIDS-associated cryptococcal meningitis. Clin Infect Dis 1994;18:789–792.
100. Powderly WG, Tuazon C, Cloud GA, et al. Serum and CSF cryptococcal antigen in management of cryptococcal meningitis in AIDS [abstract]. In: Program and abstracts of the 4th Conference on Retroviruses and Opportunistic Infections. Alexandria, VA: IDSA Foundation for Retrovirology and Human Health, 1997.
101. Hamilton JR, Noble A, Denning DW, et al. Performance of *Cryptococcus* antigen latex agglutination kits on serum and cerebrospinal fluid specimens of AIDS patients before and after pronase treatment. J Clin Microbiol 1991;29:333–339.
102. Saag MS, Powderly WG, Cloud GA, et al. Comparison of amphotericin B with fluconazole in the treatment of acute AIDS-associated cryptococcal meningitis. N Engl J Med 1992;326:83–89.
103. Powderly WG, Saag MS, Cloud GA, et al. A randomized controlled trial of fluconazole versus amphotericin B as maintenance therapy for prevention of relapse of cryptococcal meningitis in patients with AIDS. N Engl J Med 1992;326:793–798.
104. Larsen RA, Leal M, Chan L. Fluconazole compared with amphotericin B plus flucytosine for cryptococcal meningitis in AIDS. Ann Intern Med 1990;113:183–187.
105. Witt MD, Lewis RJ, Larsen RA et al. Identification of patients with acute AIDS-associated cryptococcal meningitis who can be effectively treated with fluconazole: the role of antifungal susceptibility testing. Clin Infect Dis 1996;22:322–328.
106. Bennett JE, Dismukes WE, Duma RJ, et al. A comparison of amphotericin B alone and combined with flucytosine in the treatment of cryptococcal meningitis. N Engl J Med 1979;301:126–131.
107. Dismukes WE, Cloud G, Gallis H, et al. Treatment of cryptococcal meningitis with combination of amphotericin B and flucytosine for four as compared with six weeks. N Engl J Med 1987;317:334–341.
108. Powderly WG, Keath EJ, Sokol-Anderson M, et al. Amphotericin B resistant *Cryptococcus neoformans* in a patient with AIDS. Infect Dis Clin Pract 1992;1:314–316.
109. Van der Horst CM, Saag MS, Cloud GA, et al. Treatment of AIDS-associated acute cryptococcal meningitis: a four-arm, two step clinical trial. N Engl J Med 1997;337:15–21.
110. Saag MS, NIAID Mycoses Study Group. Comparison of fluconazole versus itraconazole as maintenance therapy of AIDS-associated cryptococcal meningitis. In: 35th Interscience Conference on Antimicrobial Agents and Chemotherapy. Washington, DC: American Society for Microbiology, 1995.
111. Dupont B, Hilmarsdottir I, Datry A, et al. Cryptococcal meningitis in AIDS patients: a pilot study of fluconazole therapy in 52 patients. In: vanden Bossche H, Mackenzie DWR, Cauwenbergh G, et al., eds. Mycosis in AIDS patients. New York: Plenum Press, 1990:287–303.
112. Denning DW, Tucker RM, Hanson LH, et al. Itraconazole therapy for cryptococcal meningitis and cryptococcosis. Arch Intern Med 1989;149:2301–2308.
113. Denning DW, Tucker RM, Hostetler JS, et al. Oral itraconazole therapy of cryptococcal meningitis and cryptococcosis in patients with AIDS. In: vanden Bossche H, Mackenzie DWR, Cauwenbergh G, et al., eds. Mycosis in AIDS patients. New York: Plenum Press, 1990:305–324.
114. Robinson PA, Knirsch AK, Joseph JA. Fluconazole for life-threatening fungal infections in patients who cannot be treated with conventional antifungal therapy. Rev Infect Dis 1990;12(Suppl 3):S349–S363.
115. De Gans J, Portegies P, Tiessens G, et al. Itraconazole compared with amphotericin B plus flucytosine in AIDS patients with cryptococcal meningitis. AIDS 1992;6:185–190.
116. Moskovitz BL, Wiesinger B, Cryptococcal Meningitis Research Group. Randomized comparative trial of itraconazole and fluconazole for treatment of AIDS-related cryptococcal meningitis. In: Abstracts of the 1st National Conference on Human Retroviruses. Washington, DC: American Society for Microbiology, 1994:61.
117. De Lalla F, Pellizzer G, Vaglia A, et al. Amphotericin B as primary therapy for cryptococcosis in AIDS patients: reliability of relatively high doses administered over a relatively short period. Clin Infect Dis 1995;20:263–266.
118. Denning DW, Armstrong RW, Lewis BH, et al. Elevated cerebrospinal fluid pressures in patients with cryptococcal meningitis and acquired immunodeficiency syndrome. Am J Med 1991;91:267–272.
119. Johnston SRD, Corbett EL, Foster O, et al. Raised intracranial pressure and visual complication in AIDS patients with cryptococcal meningitis. J Infect 1992;24:185–189.
120. Malessa R, Krams M, Hengge U. Elevation of intracranial pressure in acute AIDS-related cryptococcal meningitis. Clin Invest 1994;72:1020–1026
121. Sharkey PK, Graybill JR, Johnson ES, et al. Amphotericin B lipid complex compared with amphotericin B in the treatment of cryptococcal meningitis in patients with AIDS. Clin Infect Dis 1996,22:315–321.
122. Coker R, Tomlinson D, Harris J. Successful treatment of cryptococcal meningitis with liposomal amphotericin B after failure of treatment with fluconazole and conventional amphotericin B. AIDS 1991;5:231–232.
123. Leenders ACAP, Reiss P, Portegies P, et al. Liposomal amphotericin B (Ambisome) compared with amphotericin B both followed by oral fluconazole in the treatment of AIDS-associated cryptococcal meningitis. AIDS 1997;11:1463–1471.
124. Berry AJ, Rinaldi MG, Graybill JR. Use of high dose fluconazole as salvage therapy for cryptococcal meningitis in patients with AIDS. Antimicrob Agents Chemother 1992;36:690–692.
125. Haubrich R, Haghighat D, Bozzette SA, et al. High-dose fluconazole for treatment of cryptococcal disease in patients with human immunodeficiency virus infection. J Infect Dis 1994;170:238–242.
126. Larsen RA, Bozzette SA, Jones BE, et al. Fluconazole combined with flucytosine for the treatment of cryptococcal meningitis in patients with AIDS. Clin Infect Dis 1994;19:741–747.
127. Milefchik E, Leal M, Haubrich R, et al. A phase II dose escalation trial of high dose fluconazole with and without flucytosine for AIDS associated cryptococcal meningitis [abstract]. In: Program and abstracts of the 4th Conference on Retroviruses and Opportunistic Infections. Alexandria, VA: IDSA Foundation for Retrovirology and Human Health, 1997.
128. Viviani MA, Tortorano AM, Langer M, et al. Experience with itraconazole in cryptococcosis and aspergillosis. J Infect 1989;18:151–65.
129. Bozzette SA, Larsen R, Chiu J, et al. A controlled trial of maintenance therapy with fluconazole after treatment of cryptococcal meningitis in the acquired immunodeficiency syndrome. N Engl J Med 1991;324:580–584.

130. Nelson MR, Bower M, Smith D, et al. The value of serum cryptococcal antigen in the diagnosis of cryptococcal infection in patients infected with the human immunodeficiency virus. J Infect 1990;21:175–181.
131. Paugam A, Dupouy-Camet J, Blanche P, et al. Increased fluconazole resistance of *Cryptococcus neoformans* isolated from a patient with AIDS and recurrent meningitis Clin Infect Dis 1994;19:975–976.
132. Birley HD, Johnson EM, McDonald P, et al. Azole drug resistance as a cause of clinical relapse in AIDS patients with cryptococcal meningitis. Int J STD AIDS 1995;6:353–355.
133. Brandt ME, Pfaller MA, Hajjeh R, et al. Molecular subtypes and antifungal susceptibilities of serial *Cryptococcus neoformans* isolates in human immunodeficiency virus infected patients. J Infect Dis 1996; 174:812–820.
134. Nightingale SD, Cal SX, Peterson DM, et al. Primary prophylaxis with fluconazole against systemic fungal infections in HIV-positive patients. AIDS 1992;6:191–194.
135. Newton JA Jr, Tasker SA, Bone WD, et al. Weekly fluconazole for the suppression of recurrent thrush in HIV-seropositive patients: impact on the incidence of disseminated cryptococcal infection. AIDS 1995; 9:1286–1287.
136. McNeil JI., Kan VL. Decline in the incidence of cryptococcosis among HIV-infected patients. J Acquir Immune Defic Syndr Hum Retrovirol 1995;9:206–208.
137. Havlir DV, Bozzette SA, McCutchan JA, et al. A double-blind, randomized study of weekly versus daily fluconazole for the prevention of fungal infections in AIDS patients [abstract 568]. In: 3rd Conference on Retroviruses and Opportunistic Infections. Washington DC: American Society for Microbiology, 1996.
138. Singh N, Barnish MJ, Berman S, et al. Low dose fluconazole for primary prophylaxis of cryptococcal infection in AIDS patients with CD4 <100/mm^3: demonstration of efficacy in a prospective, multicenter trial. Clin Infect Dis 1996;23:1282–1286.
139. Quagliarello VJ, Viscoli C, Visconti RI. Primary prevention of cryptococcal meningitis by fluconazole in HIV-infected patients. Lancet 1995;345:548–552.
140. Ammassari A, Linzalone A, Murri R, et al. Fluconazole for primary prophylaxis of AIDS-associated cryptococcosis: a case-control study. Scand J Infect Dis 1995;27:235–237.
141. McKinsey D, Wheat J, Cloud G, et al. Itraconazole is effective primary prophylaxis against systemic fungal infections in patients with advanced HIV infection [abstract LB09]. In: 36th Interscience Conference on Antimicrobial Agents and Chemotherapy. Washington, DC: American Society for Microbiology, 1996.
142. USPHS/IDSA Prevention of Opportunistic Infections Working Group. USPHS/IDSA guidelines for preventing opportunistic infections in persons infected with human immunodeficiency virus: disease-specific recommendations. Clin Infect Dis 1995;21(Suppl 1):S32.
143. Wheat LJ. Histoplasmosis: diagnosis and management. Infect Dis Clin Pract 1992;1:287–290.
144. Wheat J. Histoplasmosis and coccidioidomycosis in individuals with AIDS: a clinical review. Infect Dis Clin North Am 1994;8:467–482.
145. Wheat LJ, Connolly-Stringfield P, Baker RL, et al. Disseminated histoplasmosis in the acquired immune deficiency syndrome: clinical findings, diagnosis and treatment, and review of the literature. Medicine (Baltimore) 1990;69:361–374.
146. Sarosi GA, Johnson PC. Disseminated histoplasmosis in patients with human immunodeficiency virus. Clin Infect Dis 1992;14:S60–S67.
147. Keath EJ, Kobayashi GS, Medoff G. Typing of *Histoplasma* capsulatum by restriction fragment length polymorphisms in a nuclear gene. J Clin Microbiol 1992;30:2104–2107.
148. Dickinson DJ, Durry E, Fleissner ML, et al. Epidemiology of histoplasmosis among AIDS patients during a community-wide outbreak in 1988–90, Marion County (Indianapolis), Indiana. In: Program and abstracts of 31st Interscience Conference on Antimicrobial Agents and Chemotherapy. Anaheim, CA: American Society for Microbiology, 1992.
149. McKinsey DS, Brewer J, Niehart R, et al. Risk factors for histoplasmosis in AIDS: results from an ongoing cohort study [abstract 60]. In: Abstracts of the 1992 IDSA meeting. Anaheim, CA: Infectious Diseases Society of America, 1992:22.
150. Trylesinski A, Carbonnel F, Bouchaud O, et al. Intestinal histoplasmosis in AIDS patients: report of three cases observed in France and review of the literature. Eur J Gastroenterol Hepatol 1995;7: 679–683.
151. Graham BD, McKinsey DS, Driks MR, et al. Colonic histoplasmosis in acquired immunodeficiency syndrome: report of two cases. Dis Colon Rectum 1991;34:185.
152. Cohen PR, Bank DE, Silvers DN, et al. Cutaneous lesions of disseminated histoplasmosis in human immunodeficiency virus-infected patients. J Am Acad Dermatolol 1990;23:422.
153. Anaissie E, Fainstein V, Samo T, et al. Central nervous system histoplasmosis: an unappreciated complication of the acquired immune deficiency syndrome. Am J Med 1988;84:215–219.
154. Wheat LJ, Batteiger BE, Sathapatayavongs B. *Histoplasma capsulatum* infection of the central nervous system. Medicine (Baltimore) 1990; 69:244.
155. Wheat LJ, Kohler RB, Tewari RP. Diagnosis of disseminated histoplasmosis by detection of *Histoplasma capsulatum* antigen in serum and urine specimens. N Engl J Med 1986;314:83–88.
156. Wheat LJ, Connolly-Stringfied P, Kohler RB, et al. *Histoplasma capsulatum* polysaccharide antigen detection in the diagnosis and management of disseminated histoplasmosis in patients with acquired immunodeficiency syndrome. Am J Med 1989;897:396.
157. Wheat LJ, Hafner RE, Korzun A, et al. Itraconazole treatment of disseminated histoplasmosis in patients with the acquired immunodeficiency syndrome. Am J Med 1995 98:336–342.
158. Wheat LJ, Hafner RE, Wulfsohn M, et al. Prevention of relapse of histoplasmosis with itraconazole in patients with the acquired immunodeficiency syndrome. Ann Intern Med 1993;118:610–616.
159. Hecht FM, Wheat LJ, Korzun A, et al. Itraconazole maintenance treatment for histoplasmosis in AIDS: a prospective, multi-center trial. J Acquir Immune Defic Syndr Hum Retrovirol 1997;16: 100–107.
160. McKinsey DS, Gupta MR, Riddlker SA, et al. Long-term amphotericin B therapy for disseminated histoplasmosis in patients with the acquired immunodeficiency syndrome (AIDS). Ann Intern Med 1989;111: 655–659.
161. Norris S, Wheat J, McKinsey D, et al. Prevention of relapse of histoplasmosis with fluconazole in patients with the acquired immunodeficiency syndrome. Am J Med 1994;96:504–508.
162. Wheat J, MaWhinney S, Hafner R, et al. Treatment of histoplasmosis with fluconazole in patients with the acquired immunodeficiency syndrome. Am J Med 1997;103:223–232.
163. Knoper SR, Galgiani JN. Coccidiomycosis. Infect Dis Clin North Am 1988;2:861–876.
164. Galgiani JN, Ampel NM. Coccidioidomycosis in human immunodeficiency virus-infected patients. J Infect Dis 1990;162:1165–1169.
165. Ampel NM, Dols CS, Galgiani JN. Coccidioidomycosis during human immunodeficiency virus infection: results of a prospective study in a coccidioidal endemic area. Am J Med 1993;94:235–240.
166. Jones JL, Fleming PL, Ciesielski CA, et al. Coccidioidomycosis among persons with AIDS in the United States. J Infect Dis 1995;171:961–966.
167. Fish DG, Ampel NM, Galgiani JN, et al. Coccidioidomycosis during human immunodeficiency virus infection: a review of 77 patients. Medicine (Baltimore) 1990;69:384–391.
168. Ampel NM, Ryan KJ, Carry PJ, et al. Fungemia due to *Coccidioides immitis:* an analysis of 16 episodes in 15 patients and review of the literature. Medicine (Baltimore) 1986;65:312–321.
169. Byrne WR, Dietrich RA. Disseminated coccidioidomycosis with peritonitis in a patient with acquired immunodeficiency syndrome: prolonged survival associated with positive skin test reactivity to coccidioidin. Arch Intern Med 1989;149:947–948.

170. Arguinchona HL, Ampel NM, Dols CL, et al. Persistent coccidioidal seropositivity without clinical evidence of active coccidioidomycosis in patients infected with human immunodeficiency virus. Clin Infect Dis 1995;20:1281–1285.
171. Sobonya RE, Barbee RA, Wiens J, et al. Detection of fungi and other pathogens in immunocompromised patients by bronchoalveolar lavage in an area endemic for coccidioidomycosis. Chest 1990;97:1349–1355.
172. Antoniskis D, Larsen RA, Akil B, et al. Seronegative disseminated coccidioidomycosis in patients with HIV infection. AIDS 1990;4:691.
173. Graybill JR, Stevens DA, Galgiani JN, et al. Itraconazole treatment of coccidioidomycosis. Am J Med 1990;89:282–290.
174. Catanzaro A, Fierer J, Friedman PJ. Fluconazole in the treatment of persistent coccidioidomycosis. Chest 1990;97:666–669.
175. Tucker RM, Denning DW, Dupont B, et al. Itraconazole therapy for chronic coccidioidal meningitis. Ann Intern Med 1990;112:108–112.
176. Galgiani JN, Catanzaro A, Cloud GA, et al. Fluconazole therapy for coccidioidal meningitis: the NIAID-Mycoses Study Group. Ann Intern Med 1993;119:28–35.
177. Dewsnup DH, Galgiani JN, Graybill JR, et al. Is it ever safe to stop azole therapy for *Coccidioides immitis* meningitis? Ann Intern Med 1996;124:305–310.
178. Zar FA, Fernandez M. Failure of ketoconazole maintenance therapy for disseminated coccidioidomycosis in AIDS [letter]. J Infect Dis 1991;164:824–825.
179. Supparatpinyo K, Chiewchanvit S, Hirunsri P, et al. *Penicillium marneffei* infection in patients infected with human immunodeficiency virus. Clin Infect Dis 1992;14:871–874.
180. Supparatpinyo K, Khamwan C, Baosoung V, et al. Disseminated *Penicillium marneffei* infection in southeast Asia. Lancet 1994;344:110–113
181. Hilmarsdottir I, Meynard JL, Rogeaux O, et al. Disseminated *Penicillium marneffei* infection associated with human immunodeficiency virus: a report of two cases and a review of 35 published cases. J Acquir Immune Defic Syndr 1993;6:466–471.
182. Jones PD, See J. *Penicillium marneffei* infection in patients infected with human immunodeficiency virus: late presentation in an area of nonendemicity. Clin Infect Dis 1992;15:744.
183. Chariyalertsak S, Sirisanthana T, Supparatpinyo K, et al. Seasonal variation of disseminated *Penicillium marneffei* infections in northern Thailand: a clue to the reservoir? J Infect Dis 1996;173:1490–1493.
184. Borradori L, Schmit JC, Stetzkowski M, et al. Penicilliosis marneffei infection in AIDS. J Am Acad Dermatol 1994;31:843–846.
185. Liu M, Wong CK, Fung CP. Disseminated *Penicillium marneffei* infection with cutaneous lesions in an HIV-positive patient. Br J Dermatol 1994;131:280–283.
186. Supparatpinyo K, Sirisanthana T. Disseminated *Penicillium marneffei* infection diagnosed on examination of a peripheral blood smear of a patient with human immunodeficiency virus infection. Clin Infect Dis 1994;18:246–247.
187. Supparatpinyo K, Nelson KE, Merz WG, et al. Response to antifungal therapy by human immunodeficiency virus-infected patients with disseminated *Penicillium marneffei* infections and in vitro susceptibilities of isolates from clinical specimens. Antimicrob Agents Chemother 1993;37:2407–2411.
188. Denning DW, Follansbee SE, Scolaro M, et al. Pulmonary aspergillosis in the acquired immunodeficiency syndrome. N Engl J Med 1991;324:654–662.
189. Minamoto GY, Barlam TF, Vander Els NJ. Invasive aspergillosis in patients with AIDS. Clin Infect Dis 1992;14:66–74.
190. Pursell KJ, Telzak EE, Armstrong D. *Aspergillus* species colonization and invasive disease in patients with AIDS. Clin Infect Dis 1992;14:141–148.
191. Lortholary O, Meyohas MC, Dupont B, et al. Invasive aspergillosis in patients with acquired immunodeficiency syndrome: report of 33 cases. French Cooperative Study Group on Aspergillosis in AIDS. Am J Med 1993;95:177–187.
192. Khoo SH, Denning DW. Invasive aspergillosis in patients with AIDS. Clin Infect Dis 1994 19(Suppl 1):S41–S48.
193. Roilides E, Holmes A, Blake C, et al. Defective antifungal activity of monocyte-derived macrophages from human immunodeficiency virus-infected children against *Aspergillus fumigatus*. J Infect Dis 1993;168:1562–1565.
194. Carrazana EJ, Rossitch E Jr, Morris J. Isolated central nervous system aspergillosis in the acquired immunodeficiency syndrome. Clin Neurol Neurosurg 1991;93:227–230.
195. Hunt SJ, Nagi C, Gross KG, et al. Primary cutaneous aspergillosis near central venous catheters in patients with the acquired immunodeficiency syndrome. Arch Dermatol 1992;128:1229–1232.
196. Diamond HJ, Phelps RG, Gordon ML, et al. Combined *Aspergillus* and zygomycotic (*Rhizopus*) infection in a patient with acquired immunodeficiency syndrome: presentation as inflammatory tinea capitis. J Am Acad Dermatol 1992;26:1017–1018.
197. Denning DW, Tucker RM, Hanson LH, et al. Itraconazole in opportunistic mycoses: cryptococcosis and aspergillosis. J Am Acad Dermatol 1990;23:602–607.
198. Hiemenz JW, Walsh TJ. Lipid formulations of amphotericin B: recent progress and future directions. Clin Infect Dis 1996;22(Suppl 2):133–144.
199. Denning D, Lee JY, Hostetler JS et al. NIAID Mycoses Study Group Multicenter Trial of Oral Itraconazole Therapy for Invasive Aspergillosis. Am J Med 1994 97:135–144.
200. Cunliffe NA, Denning DW. Uncommon invasive mycoses in AIDS. AIDS 1995;9:411–420.
201. Pappas PG, Pottage JC, Powderly WG, et al. Blastomycosis in patients with the acquired immunodeficiency syndrome. Ann Intern Med 1992;116:847–853.
202. Dismukes WE, Bradsher RW, Cloud GC, et al. Itraconazole therapy for blastomycosis and histoplasmosis. Am J Med 1992;93:489–497.
203. Shaw JC, Levinson W, Montanaro A. Sporotrichosis in the acquired immunodeficiency syndrome. J Am Acad Dermatol 1989;21:1145–1147.
204. Heller HM, Fuhrer J. Disseminated sporotrichosis in patients with AIDS: case report and review of the literature. AIDS 1991;5:1243–1246.
205. Cuadrado LM, Guerro A, Asenjo J, et al. Cerebral mucormycosis in two cases of acquired immunodeficiency syndrome. Arch Neurol 1988;5:109–111.

23

CYTOMEGALOVIRUS INFECTION IN PATIENTS WITH HIV INFECTION

Michael A. Polis and Henry Masur

During the 1990s, when prophylaxis for *Pneumocystis carinii* pneumonia became common, but before the use of protease inhibitor antiretroviral therapy became available, clinical disease due to cytomegalovirus (CMV) was recognized in up to 40% of patients with advanced human immunodeficiency virus (HIV) disease (1–3). Retinitis, colitis, esophagitis, and pneumonitis are the most common presentations, although hepatitis, adrenalitis, and neurologic involvement have all been reported. More than 90% of patients with acquired immunodeficiency syndrome (AIDS) and CMV retinitis initially respond to treatment, but relapse occurs predictably (4–6). CMV infection is an independent predictor of death and contributes significantly to both morbidity and mortality in persons with HIV infection (7).

EPIDEMIOLOGY

CMV is a large, double-stranded DNA virus in the herpesvirus family. In persons who are not infected with HIV, disease due to CMV is most commonly associated with heterophile-negative infectious mononucleosis. In HIV-infected persons, as with most other opportunistic infections associated with HIV infection, CMV disease is due to reactivation of the latent virus in a previously infected host. Although more than 90% of persons with HIV infection have antibodies to CMV indicating prior exposure and infection, the clinical manifestations of CMV disease do not generally present until the CD4 count drops below 100 CD4 cells/μL (3, 5). In one study from Australia, which assessed 31 persons with HIV-infection and CMV retinitis who had CD4 lymphocyte determinations performed within the 2 months before or 1 month after the diagnosis of CMV retinitis, the mean CD4 count was 29 cells/μL, and the median was 17 cells/μL (8). In a multicenter observational cohort of 1002 HIV-infected persons with fewer than 250 CD4 cells/μL who were receiving zidovudine, disease due to CMV developed in 109 persons (7). Kaplan–Meier estimates of the proportion of persons who developed CMV disease was 21.4% at 2 years for persons entering the study with fewer than 100 CD4 cells/μL and 10.3% for persons with initial counts higher than 100 cells/μL. Of the 109 persons who developed CMV disease, 93 (85.3%) were diagnosed with retinitis, 10 (9.2%) with esophagitis, 3 with both retinitis and esophagitis, 8 (7.3%) with colitis, and 1 each with gastritis, hepatitis, and encephalitis. A smaller study of 135 persons with fewer than 250 CD4 cells/μL found the Kaplan–Meier estimate for the development of CMV retinitis to be 42% within 27 months for the group with fewer than 50 CD4 cells/μL (9). Of the total of 26 persons developing CMV retinitis, 24 had fewer than 50 CD4 cells/μL before developing CMV retinitis; the other 2 persons had counts of 60 and 160 CD4 cells/μL 7 and 11 months before the diagnosis, respectively. The mean time from the first CD4 cell count lower than 50 cells/μL until the diagnosis of CMV retinitis was 13.1 months. Although CMV disease may occasionally be the initial opportunistic infection in persons with advanced HIV infection, because of the profound immunocompromised setting required for the establishment of CMV end-organ disease, it more commonly presents after the diagnosis of AIDS has been made, especially since 1993 when the United States Centers for Disease Control and Prevention (CDC) surveillance definition of AIDS was expanded to include individuals with a CD4+ count lower than 200 cells/μL.

Since 1990, when the number of cases of *Pneumocystis carinii* pneumonia reported to the CDC began to decrease because of widespread use of prophylaxis to prevent this disease, cases of CMV retinitis increased. In a prospectively followed cohort of 844 men studied before the development of an AIDS-related opportunistic infection, among the persons who received *Pneumocystis carinii* pneumonia prophylaxis, CMV disease was the initial AIDS-related opportunistic infection in 9.4% of men, compared with 3.1% of men who did not receive this prophylaxis. The lifetime occurrence of CMV disease was 44.9 and 24.8% in those groups, respectively (10). With the caveat that the initial opportunistic infections in persons with HIV infection are reported more frequently than subsequent opportunistic infections (leading to underreporting of CMV disease), since 1993, with a constant surveillance definition, cases of CMV disease reported to the CDC have decreased, from 3677 cases in

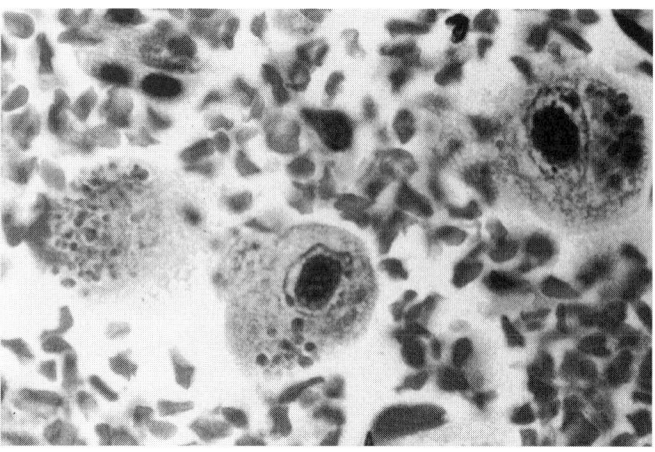

Figure 23.1. Typical "owl's eye" appearance of CMV-infected cells from a lung biopsy. Infected cells show characteristic dense intranuclear and intracytoplasmic inclusion bodies. (See color section.)

1994, to 3105 cases in 1995, to 2592 cases in 1996 (11–14). This change is believed to be due to the increase in use of combination antiretroviral agents, more recently with the addition of protease inhibitor therapy, for HIV infection.

Disease due to CMV in persons with HIV infection is almost invariably the result of reactivation of a previously acquired latent CMV infection. Primary disease from CMV is rarely recognized in persons with HIV infection. More than 90% of persons with AIDS in the United States have evidence of prior infection with CMV (15). Reactivation of the latent infection may result in systemic signs and symptoms such as fever, myalgia, leukopenia, and weight loss, in addition to symptoms attributable to end-organ disease. The diagnosis of CMV in organs such as the liver and lung requires the identification of characteristic histopathologic findings of the pathognomonic "owl's eye" intranuclear and smaller intracytoplasmic inclusion bodies on tissue specimens (Fig. 23.1). Because CMV viremia is common in persons with low CD4 cell counts even in the absence of clinical disease, rare, typical cells containing CMV inclusion bodies may be seen on histopathologic specimens in association with other, more common pathogens. Correspondingly, the diagnosis of CMV disease should only be made when many typical CMV inclusion-containing cells are seen with an associated inflammatory response, in the appropriate clinical setting. In contrast, because of the difficulty in obtaining appropriate tissue specimens, the diagnosis of retinitis due to CMV is not determined by histopathologic findings, but rather, it is based on the characteristic appearance of a hard or fluffy exudate often associated with hemorrhage and perivascular sheathing found in the retina in the appropriate clinical setting (Figs. 23.2 and 23.3).

Commonly, but not invariably, CMV retinitis is associated with CMV viruria and CMV viremia (5). In one study from the National Institutes of Health, 9 of 26 (35%) HIV-infected, CMV-viremic persons with fewer than 200 CD4 cells/µL developed disease due to CMV within 6 months compared with 6 of 74 (8%) persons without CMV viremia (P=.003) (16). Similarly, 13 of 47 (28%) persons who were CMV viruric with fewer than 200 CD4 cells/µL developed CMV within 6 months compared with only 2 of 43 (5%) persons without CMV viruria (P = .008). However, whereas CMV blood and cultures were useful for identifying persons with a high likelihood of developing end-organ disease due to CMV, their positive predictive values were poor and did not prove useful clinically. Positive CMV cultures were more a reflection of the patients' underlying immunologic status and, indeed, were strongly correlated with declining CD4 lymphocyte counts. A similar, prospective study of 28 persons with AIDS and CMV viremia found 50% of these persons developed end-organ disease due to CMV in 16.6 months (17).

Recent data on the use of a qualitative CMV-specific polymerase chain reaction (PCR) on whole blood suggest that this test may be both more sensitive and specific for the development of CMV disease. In a prospective cohort of 97 HIV-infected persons with fewer than 50 CD4+ cells/µL followed every 3 months with CMV PCR, 16 of 27 persons (59%) who were CMV positive by PCR at baseline developed CMV disease within 12 months compared with only 3 of 70 persons (4%) who were initially CMV negative (18). In a cohort of 94 HIV-infected persons without CMV disease at baseline, a qualitative plasma CMV PCR was more sensitive and specific (89 and 75%, respectively) than either urine CMV cultures (85 and 29%, respectively) or leukocyte cultures (38 and 74%, respectively) for the identification of persons developing CMV disease within 12 months (19). Quantitative CMV PCR was able to increase the specificity of the assay further, at some cost to sensitivity. The identification of persons at high risk for the development of CMV disease may allow for the development of preemptive therapeutic strategies to prevent end-organ disease due to CMV, although qualitative and quantitative assays are not yet commercially available.

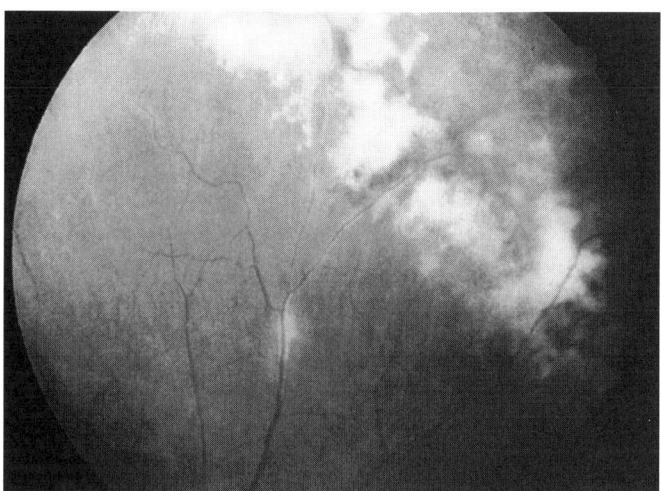

Figure 23.2. CMV retinitis involving the pheripheral retina. The exudate has a fluffy appearance in this example with associated perivascular hemorrhage. Portions of the vasculature near the exudate appear to be sheathed. (See color section.)

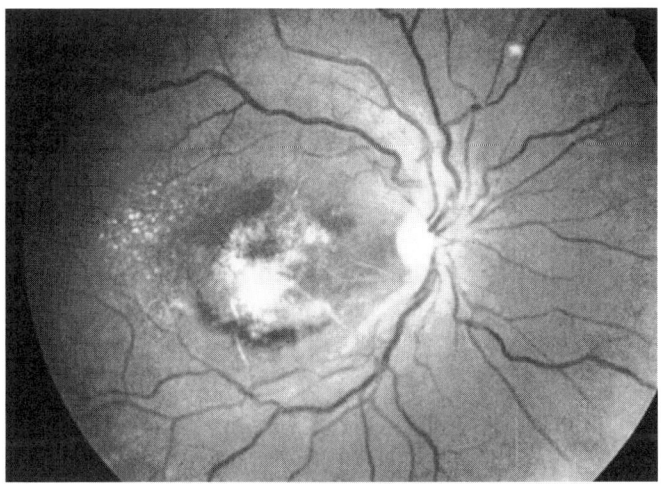

Figure 23.3. Typical zone 1 lesion of CMV retinitis involving the macula of the right eye. The lesion has the appearance of a hard exudate associated with hemorrhage. (See color section.)

ASSOCIATED DISEASES AND CLINICAL MANIFESTATIONS

CMV Retinitis

Retinitis due to CMV results from the hematogenous dissemination of CMV after reactivation of a latent CMV infection (2). Progression of the infection within the retina is generally to contiguous cells. Persons with lesions that first appear near the macula or optic nerve (zone 1) commonly present with complaints of decreased visual acuity or defects in the visual field. Retinal lesions at least 1500 µm from the edge of the optic nerve and at least 3000 µm from the center of the fovea (zones 2 and 3) or anterior to the equator of the eye may be asymptomatic or may present with the complaint of "floaters" or loss of peripheral vision. CMV retinitis is not associated with pain or photophobia.

Visual loss due to CMV retinitis may occur in several ways. First, direct infection of the retinal cells by CMV causes retinal necrosis that may result in a visual field defect or scotoma, depending on where in the retina the lesion occurs. This permanent, irreversible loss of vision is not amenable to therapy and depends on the location and extent of the retinal necrosis. Normal central vision may be preserved if the macula is not involved. Second, retinal involvement of the area near the macula may produce edema in the macula and loss of central visual acuity. The macular edema and loss of visual acuity are potentially reversible if recognized and treated promptly before the retinal cells are infected. Third, after infection with CMV and subsequent retinal necrosis, the retina is left as a thin, atrophic tissue that is susceptible to breaks and detachment (20). Retinal detachment occurs commonly in persons with CMV retinitis and presents with the sudden onset of floaters, flashing lights, loss of visual field, and decreased visual acuity. Retinal detachments can be repaired, but because of the nature of the atrophic retinal tissue, they frequently recur. One series of 145 patients with CMV retinitis found a cumulative probability of retinal detachment of 50% 1 year after diagnosis of CMV retinitis (21).

Because of the difficulty of obtaining retinal tissue for histopathologic examination, the diagnosis of CMV retinitis is made by the appearance of the characteristic perivascular fluffy yellow-white retinal infiltrate often associated with retinal hemorrhage (see Figs. 23.2 and 23.3). The portion of the vessels near the lesion may appear to be sheathed. Occasionally, the lesions may appear granular, rather than fluffy (2). Progression of retinitis is in a characteristic "brushfire" pattern, with a granular, white leading edge advancing before an atrophic, gliotic scar. Progression is irregular and occurs in fits and starts. However, one study using serial, masked retinal photographs found the median progression rate with which disease approached the fovea in 17 untreated patients to be 24.0 µm per day, compared with a median progression rate of 11.5 µm per day in 14 patients treated with ganciclovir (22). Patients with AIDS and CMV retinitis usually have minimal inflammation of the vitreous. CMV retinitis usually presents unilaterally, but, untreated, it becomes bilateral in most cases. The presence of positive blood cultures for CMV is neither necessary nor sufficient to make the diagnosis of CMV retinitis. In one study, although all 24 patients had positive urine cultures for CMV at the time of diagnosis of CMV retinitis, only 15 of 24 (63%) had positive blood cultures (5). The presence of serum antibodies to CMV is of no utility in establishing the diagnosis of CMV retinitis inasmuch as patients with other causes of retinitis usually have immunoglobulin G antibodies to CMV. However, retinitis in a CMV-seronegative individual, rare as it is, should make a diagnosis of CMV retinitis doubtful, but not impossible.

Other ocular lesions in HIV-infected persons are included in the differential diagnosis of CMV retinitis (23). Cotton-wool spots are microinfarctions of the retinal nerve fiber layer that occur commonly in persons with HIV infection and may resemble early CMV retinitis (24). These small, white lesions do not affect vision and spontaneously regress over several weeks. In the setting of an HIV-infected person with fewer than 100 CD4 cells/µL, it is critical to ensure that lesions that appear to be cotton-wool spots regress and do not progress, as would be expected with CMV retinitis. Acute retinal necrosis, caused by herpes zoster, presents with either peripheral retinal vascular occlusion overlying a white, necrotic retina or, when more central vessels are involved, ischemia from central vascular occlusion (25). Intraocular lymphomas may present with small retinochoroidal infiltrates, optic nerve head swelling, and vascular sheathing. Toxoplasmic chorioretinitis may be unifocal or multifocal, but it is usually associated with a moderate-to-severe inflammatory reaction in the vitreous that helps to differentiate it from CMV retinitis (26). *Pneumocystis carinii* chorioretinitis appears as multifocal, white-yellow, raised choroidal lesions with minimal inflammation (27). Other, rare causes of ocular disease in persons with HIV infection include syphilis, *Mycobacterium tuberculosis, Cryptococcus, Candida,* and histoplasmosis (23).

CMV Esophagitis

Esophagitis due to CMV is a common cause of odynophagia in persons with AIDS (28), but it is much less common than *Candida* esophagitis. CMV esophagitis occurs in approximately 10% of persons with AIDS who develop CMV disease (7). The definitive diagnosis of CMV esophagitis is established by biopsy evidence of CMV with an inflammatory response in the appropriate clinical setting. The presence of extensive large, shallow ulcers of the distal esophagus is the hallmark of the disease. Pathologically, the large intranuclear inclusion bodies characteristic of CMV can be seen in the endothelial cells at the edge of the ulcer and are required to confirm the diagnosis (29). Immunohistochemical stains may add to the sensitivity of routine hematoxylin and eosin staining for CMV. Culturing CMV from a biopsy or brushing of the esophagus is not sufficient to establish the diagnosis of CMV esophagitis because many persons with low CD4 counts are viremic and have positive cultures for CMV in the absence of clinical disease (16).

The most common cause of odynophagia in persons with AIDS is *Candida* esophagitis. Dysphagia may be more commonly associated with *Candida* esophagitis and odynophagia with CMV or herpes simplex esophagitis. Other entities in the differential diagnosis of CMV esophagitis include esophagitis due to herpes simplex, reflux or peptic ulcer disease, histoplasmosis, Kaposi's sarcoma, lymphoma, and infection with HIV, *Mycobacterium tuberculosis*, and, rarely, *M. avium-intracellulare* complex, cryptosporidia, and *Pneumocystis carinii* (30). Because of the relative prevalence of *Candida* esophagitis in this population, many clinicians treat esophageal symptoms, especially in the presence of oral thrush, empirically with fluconazole for presumptive *Candida* esophagitis and perform endoscopy only on persons who fail to respond to this therapy (31). Persons with CMV or *Candida* esophagitis typically present with CD4 counts lower than 50 cells/µL, whereas persons with esophageal candidiasis, but not CMV, can present with CD4+ counts between 50 and 400 cells/µL (5, 8).

CMV Colitis

Colitis due to CMV occurs in fewer than 10% of persons with AIDS in whom CMV-induced disease is diagnosed (7). Fever, weight loss, anorexia, abdominal pain, debilitating diarrhea, and malaise are frequently present. Extensive hemorrhage and perforation can be life-threatening complications (32). The symptoms are nonspecific and may be similar to those caused by other gastrointestinal pathogens such as *Cryptosporidium*, microsporidia, *Cyclospora cayetanensis*, *Mycobacterium avium* complex, *Giardia lamblia*, *Entamoeba histolytica*, *Salmonella*, and *Shigella* or gastrointestinal involvement of lymphoma or Kaposi's sarcoma. The radiographic manifestations of CMV colitis are nonspecific and may mimic the findings of other inflammatory bowel conditions, including ulcerative colitis (33). Colonoscopic or rectal biopsy with histopathologic identification of characteristic intranuclear and intracytoplasmic inclusions is required for diagnosis. Identification of CMV by culture or even on histopathologic specimens may not be sufficient to implicate CMV; frequently, multiple pathogens coexist and must be considered in persons with advanced HIV infection (34).

CMV Pneumonitis

Although CMV can be cultured routinely from throat washings, pulmonary secretions, bronchoalveolar lavage specimens, and autopsy lung tissue, CMV is seldom implicated antemortem as an isolated pathogen causing pneumonitis in persons with HIV infection (35). At autopsy, foci of CMV inclusion bodies and pneumonitis can often be found. In one study from San Francisco, although CMV was cultured from bronchial alveolar lavage fluid or transbronchial biopsy specimens in 54 of 111 patients diagnosed with their first episode of *Pneumocystis carinii* pneumonia, the presence of CMV had no impact on the long-term survival, short-term death rate, or length of hospital stay (36). Of 17 persons with biopsy-diagnosed CMV pneumonitis, no clinical, radiographic, or histologic findings distinguished persons with CMV as the sole pathogen from persons with other, concomitant pathogens (37).

CMV pneumonitis generally presents as interstitial pneumonitis in an individual with advanced HIV infection. Shortness of breath, dyspnea on exertion, a nonproductive cough, and hypoxemia are characteristic. Diagnosis of CMV pneumonitis should be made only in the setting of pulmonary infiltrates by the identification of multiple CMV inclusion bodies in lung tissue of appropriate clinical specimens in the absence of other pathogens that are more commonly associated with pneumonitis in this population, such as *Pneumocystis carinii*, *Mycobacterium tuberculosis*, *Histoplasma capsulatum*, *Coccidioides immitis*, *Cryptococcus neoformans*, or bacterial pathogens such as *Streptococcus pneumoniae* or *Haemophilus influenzae*. Treatment should be considered for persons with histologic evidence of CMV infection who do not respond to treatment against other pathogens.

CMV Adrenalitis

CMV involvement of the adrenal glands is frequently reported in autopsy studies of persons with HIV infection; involvement was documented in as many as 64 of 83 (77%) (38) and 42 of 71 (59%) (39) persons in 2 autopsy studies. Patients rarely manifest adrenal insufficiency by laboratory or clinical parameters. The diagnosis of adrenalitis due to CMV is uncommonly made premortem, but hypoadrenalism can occasionally be documented in persons with CMV disease by the cosyntropin stimulation test (1, 40).

CMV Hepatitis and Biliary Disease

Although CMV involvement of the liver and biliary tract may often be seen on autopsy specimens, clinical hepatitis due to CMV is rare in persons with HIV infection (1). Biliary tract or hepatic involvement by CMV may present with right upper quadrant pain and elevated alkaline phosphatase, but infections with *Cryptosporidium* and *Mycobacterium avium-intracellulare* complex are more common with this presentation. In one series of 66 consecutive persons with AIDS and first-episode gastrointestinal CMV disease, 22 patients presented with esophagitis, 28 with colitis, 9 with sclerosing cholangitis, and only 2 with acute hepatitis (41).

CMV Neurologic Disease

CMV has been associated with various neurologic infections in persons with HIV infection, particularly ventriculoencephalitis (42–49) and ascending polyradiculopathy (50–53). Ventriculoencephalitis usually occurs in advanced HIV infection in persons with a prior diagnosis of CMV disease. Patients typically present with lethargy, confusion, and fever, but the clinical presentation may overlap with that of HIV encephalitis. The cerebrospinal fluid (CSF) generally shows a pleocytosis that may be polymorphonuclear, low-to-normal glucose levels, and normal-to-elevated protein levels. Detection of CMV is enhanced by PCR techniques compared with culture (48, 49). Periventricular enhancement of computed tomographic or magnetic resonance images suggests CMV ventriculoencephalitis, rather than HIV-related neurologic disease.

CMV polyradiculopathy is characterized by urinary retention and progressive bilateral leg weakness (50–53). The clinical symptoms generally progress over several weeks to include loss of bowel and bladder control and flaccid paraplegia. A spastic myelopathy has been reported, and sacral paresthesia may occur. The CSF generally shows a pleocytosis that is usually polymorphonuclear, hypoglycorrhachia, and elevated protein levels. Detection of CMV is enhanced by PCR techniques compared with culture. Although CMV is found in the central nervous system in up to 25% of HIV-infected persons in autopsy studies (39, 42, 43), the incidence of CMV-related neurologic disease ante mortem is not well defined.

TREATMENT

Ganciclovir

The first major advance in the treatment for CMV disease was with the use of ganciclovir, an agent highly specific for the human herpesviruses. Ganciclovir is a nucleoside analog whose action depends on inhibition of herpesvirus DNA polymerases. It requires phosphorylation in CMV-infected cells, and most strains of CMV resistant to ganciclovir are unable to phosphorylate ganciclovir. The CMV UL97 open-reading frame codes for a protein kinase capable of phosphorylating ganciclovir in CMV-infected cells (54, 55). Ganciclovir is virustatic against CMV. Thus, when treatment for disease is stopped, viral spread and progression of disease characteristically begin again (3). Lifelong daily therapy is required, most often intravenously through an indwelling catheter. An oral formulation of ganciclovir is available, but it is poorly absorbed and is not as clinically effective as the intravenous formulation (56–58).

When given intravenously by a 1-hour infusion, the standard 5-mg/kg dose of ganciclovir reaches a maximal concentration in the plasma at the end of infusion of approximately 6 µg/mL (24 µM) (57). Trough levels 11 hours after infusion are approximately 1 µg/mL (4 µM). The initial distribution half-life ($t_{1/2}$) is about 0.76 hours, and the terminal elimination $t_{1/2}$ is 3.60 hours (57). Most studies have shown that ganciclovir is less than 10% orally bioavailable and that increasing the dose may not increase plasma concentrations (58). Most studies report that for human CMV isolates, the 50% inhibition (ID_{50}) of viral plaque formation is attained by concentrations of ganciclovir between 0.4 and 11.0 µM (3, 59).

Ganciclovir was approved by the United States Food and Drug Administration (FDA) for the treatment of CMV disease based on a wealth of successful anecdotal data but in the absence of controlled clinical trials (60, 61). The recommended dosage of ganciclovir for the treatment of CMV retinitis in persons with AIDS is 5 mg/kg intravenously twice daily for a 14- to 21-day induction period, followed by a 5-mg/kg daily indefinite maintenance phase. The terms "induction" and "maintenance" may be misnomers inasmuch as progression of CMV retinitis is regularly seen during the maintenance phase with ganciclovir and foscarnet (Table 23.1). Patients having disease progression during the maintenance phase are routinely retreated with the twice-daily regimen. Ganciclovir, at 1000 mg orally thrice daily, is approved for maintenance therapy of CMV retinitis, it but should not be used in persons whose retinitis may be sight-threatening if the disease should progress.

In a compilation of clinical data, treatment with ganciclovir resulted in the improvement or stabilization of CMV retinitis in 80 to 90% of patients (4). The median time to clinical progression, in these uncontrolled studies, appeared to be as long as 145 days from the diagnosis of CMV retinitis, while continuing some maintenance therapy with ganciclovir. One large, uncontrolled series reported the outcomes of 105 immunocompromised (primarily AIDS) patients who were treated with ganciclovir for CMV retinitis. Analysis of a subset of these patients selected for their ability to tolerate a prolonged course of therapy and who had high-dose maintenance therapy (25 to 35 mg/kg per week) after induction therapy showed that mean time to progression of retinitis was 18 weeks. This result, however, is based on subset analysis; these patients were selected for their ability to tolerate a prolonged course of relatively high-dose ganciclovir without the development of neutropenia. The results of other trials indicate that, with standard doses of both agents, no difference in the rate of progression of CMV retinitis occurs in AIDS patients treated with either ganciclovir or foscarnet (5, 6, 62). Clinical examination tends to overestimate the time to progression compared with data based on rigorous photographic end points (4, 56, 63, 64).

Table 23.1 Therapy for Cytomegalovirus Retinitis

Drug	Route	Induction Dose and Frequency	Maintenance Dose and Frequency
Ganciclovir	Intravenous	5 mg/kg q12h for 14 to 21 days	5 mg/kg daily[a], indefinitely
	Oral	None	1000 mg po tid[b], indefinitely
	Intravitreal	400 µg twice weekly for 2 to 3 weeks	400 µg weekly, indefinitely
	Implant	4.5 mg device to be replaced either every 6 to 9 months or for retinitis progression	
Foscarnet	Intravenous	90 mg/kg q12h for 14 to 21 days	90 to 120 mg/kg daily, indefinitely
	Intravitreal	2400 µg twice weekly for 2 to 3 weeks	2400 µg weekly, indefinitely
Cidofovir	Intravenous	5 mg/kg weekly[c] for 2 weeks	5 mg/kg weekly[c], indefinitely
	Intravitreal	20 µg every 5 to 6 weeks[c]	

[a]Higher doses of ganciclovir have been given with colony-stimulating factors.
[b]Maintenance therapy with oral ganciclovir should be restricted to persons without sight-threatening retinitis.
[c]Cidofovir requires the coadministration of probenecid, 2 g orally 3 hours before and 1 g orally 2 hours and 8 hours after administration of cidofovir.

The results of a randomized, controlled trial comparing ganciclovir with delayed therapy using strictly graded photographic end points demonstrated that progression of retinitis while receiving ganciclovir occurred in a median of 50.5 days, compared with the progression on delayed therapy, which occurred in a median of 15 days (6). Similarly, the results of the Studies of the Ocular Complications of AIDS (SOCA) trial demonstrated that the median time to progression of CMV retinitis while on ganciclovir was 56 days (62).

In an open study of ganciclovir for the treatment of CMV esophagitis, of 10 evaluable patients treated with an induction regimen of 2.5 mg/kg intravenously every 8 hours or 5 mg/kg intravenously every 12 hours for 10 days, 5 persons had a good response, 3 had a partial response, and 2 had no response to therapy (28). In general, one sees a high rate of relapse of CMV esophagitis in persons who receive intermittent therapy. The decision about whether to use daily, lifelong treatment or intermittent, high-dose therapy for esophagitis due to CMV needs to be individualized. Maintenance therapy should be considered, particularly after a relapse.

Ganciclovir has been evaluated in a multicenter, double-blind, placebo-controlled trial for the treatment of CMV colitis in persons with AIDS (65). Although the trial lasted only 14 days and was perhaps too short to demonstrate colonic healing and resolution of diarrhea, colonoscopy scores reflecting inflammation and positive cultures for CMV from the colon and urine significantly decreased in patients on the ganciclovir arm of the trial. Most experienced clinicians recommend that treatment for CMV colitis should be given for 3 to 6 weeks. However, unlike in CMV retinitis, because the cells lining the gastrointestinal tract regenerate rapidly, therapy can often wait for the development of moderate-to-severe symptoms to justify the use of systemic therapy associated with some toxicity. As with esophagitis, maintenance therapy is not necessarily required, but it should be strongly considered after a relapse. In a randomized, controlled trial of 48 patients with biopsy-proved gastrointestinal CMV disease comparing intravenous ganciclovir ($n = 22$) with intravenous foscarnet ($n = 26$), 73% of subjects had a good or complete clinical response to a 2- to 4-week trial of either drug, with more than 83% of the subjects demonstrating an endoscopic response (66).

The utility of ganciclovir therapy in the treatment of CMV in other organ systems is largely anecdotal. Although the combination of ganciclovir with high-dose intravenous immunoglobulin has been shown to be more effective than ganciclovir alone in the treatment of CMV pneumonitis in bone marrow transplant recipients (67, 68), this combination has not been shown to be effective in persons with AIDS (69). The response of pneumonitis to intravenous ganciclovir has been reported to be better than 60% (37). The role of maintenance therapy for CMV pneumonitis has not been established. For neurologic disease, initiating therapy promptly is critical for an optimal clinical response, but data on response rates and length of therapy are lacking. CMV viremia may be associated with subclinical involvement of other organ systems. Treatment of symptomatic CMV viremia when no other pathogen has been identified after thorough investigation may occasionally be warranted.

With the increased use of ganciclovir for longer periods resulting from improved survival of persons with AIDS, ganciclovir-resistant CMV has been reported with increasing frequency (70). In one study of 72 CMV-viruric AIDS patients treated with ganciclovir for CMV disease and followed prospectively for the development of ganciclovir-resistant CMV, no resistant strains of CMV were found in 31 randomly chosen patients before therapy or in 7 culture-positive patients treated for less than 3 months (71). After 3 months of therapy, only 20% of persons remained culture positive; 5 of 13 (38%) randomly chosen culture-positive patients, or 8% overall, were found to have ganciclovir-resistant strains with an inhibitory concentration of 50% (IC_{50}) greater than 12 µM. However, decreasing sensitivity of strains of CMV to ganciclovir appears to exist in persons receiving the drug for extended periods suggesting that the progressive shortening of the time between relapses of CMV retinitis may, in part, result from decreasing sensitivity of the virus (72). Low-level ganciclovir resistance (IC_{50} between 8 and 30 µM) is mediated by mutations in the UL97 viral phosphotransferase gene, whereas high-level ganciclovir resistance (IC_{50} greater than 30 µM) is mediated predominantly by combined UL97 and UL54 viral DNA polymerase gene mutations (73).

Neutropenia and thrombocytopenia are the major dose-limiting toxicities of ganciclovir therapy (Table 23.2). Because ganciclovir and zidovudine are both myelosuppressive, it is difficult to administer these agents concurrently (74). In one study, only 18% of 29 persons with CMV disease were able to tolerate full doses of ganciclovir with 600 mg of zidovudine daily (74). In the randomized trial comparing initial therapy with ganciclovir versus foscarnet for the treatment of CMV retinitis, 14 of 127 (11%) patients required switching from ganciclovir to foscarnet, 9 of 14 for progression of retinitis, but only 1 of 14 for drug toxicity (62), a finding demonstrating that ganciclovir is generally well tolerated without the concurrent use of zidovudine. Limited in vitro data suggest that the antiretroviral activity of both zidovudine and didanosine may be antagonized by ganciclovir (75). Whereas the development of ganciclovir has significantly improved the quality of life of many persons with HIV infection and CMV retinitis, this agent's toxicities and the need for daily intravenous infusions or a 12-pill daily oral regimen leave it wanting as an ideal agent for the treatment of CMV retinitis.

Intravitreal injections of ganciclovir have been used for the treatment of CMV retinitis in persons unable or unwilling to tolerate systemic therapy with ganciclovir or foscarnet (see Table 23.1; 76–78). The concentration of ganciclovir in intravitreal fluid immediately after injection has been as high as 65 μM (77). Concentrations greater than the ID_{50} for most strains of CMV can be maintained for 60 hours after a single 400-μg injection (78). Two injections per week are given for 2 to 3 weeks during an induction period, followed by weekly maintenance injections. This alternative therapy appears to be effective in preventing the progression of CMV retinitis without the systemic toxicity of ganciclovir and without toxicity to the retina. Rarely, however, this procedure has been associated with retinal detachment, intraocular infection, intravitreal hemorrhage, and damage to the lens.

GANCICLOVIR INTRAOCULAR DEVICE

Local administration of ganciclovir can also be accomplished by the use of a ganciclovir intraocular device, licensed by the FDA for the treatment of CMV retinitis in 1996. This implant device releases ganciclovir into the vitreous cavity at a rate of approximately 1.40 μg per hour for 6 to 9 months. It is surgically implanted in the affected eye in a simple surgical procedure that does not require an overnight hospital stay. Recovery generally takes several days, but persons may have decreased visual acuity in the implanted eye for 4 weeks (79). In a randomized, controlled clinical trial randomizing patients with peripheral CMV retinitis either to receive immediate implantation of the device or to be closely monitored, the median time to progression of retinitis was 15 days in eyes in the delayed-treatment group ($n = 16$) compared with 226 days in the immediate-treatment group ($n = 14$) ($P < .00001$) (79). In eight persons in whom vitreous levels of ganciclovir were obtained, the mean vitreous drug level was 4.1 μg/mL, roughly four times the concentration obtained with intravenous ganciclovir. The major complications on the trial included the risk of development of CMV retinitis in the fellow eye, estimated at 50% at 6 months, and the development of visceral CMV disease in 31% of patients. Seven late retinal detachments occurred in this study, but because retinal detachment occurs in treated and untreated CMV retinitis (20, 21), no conclusion could be drawn about whether this procedure increases the rate of retinal detachment. Possibly, an increased rate of early, surgically associated retinal detachment may be balanced by a decreased rate of late retinal detachments resulting from better control of CMV retinitis.

A randomized, controlled clinical trial compared the use of intravenous ganciclovir with that of two ganciclovir implant devices releasing ganciclovir at different rates (80). The median time to progression of retinitis was 191 days (71 eyes) and 221 days (75 eyes) with the two implants compared with 71 days (76 eyes) with intravenous ganciclovir ($P<.001$). Extraocular CMV disease occurred more commonly in persons with the implant devices compared with those receiving intravenous ganciclovir (10.3% versus 0%, $P=.04$). Vitreous hemorrhage, generally transient, occurred in 7.8% of eyes. Endophthalmitis was reported in three eyes. Retinal detachments were reported in 11.9% of eyes receiving implants compared with 5.1% of the eyes of persons receiving intravenous ganciclovir. No indication of a significant difference in mortality was noted among the groups in this study (80).

To evaluate the efficacy of oral ganciclovir in combination with the ganciclovir implant to control the development of extraocular and fellow eye CMV disease, a multicenter, three-arm, randomized clinical trial comparing the use of the implant alone versus the implant with coadministration of oral ganciclovir, 1500 mg orally thrice daily, versus standard

Table 23.2 Toxicities of Drugs for Cytomegalovirus Retinitis

Ganciclovir		Foscarnet		Cidofovir	
Neutropenia	++	Nephrotoxicity	++	Iritis	+
Anemia	++	Electrolyte abnormalities	++	Nephrotoxicity	+++
Thrombocytopenia	+++	Gastrointestinal disturbances	++	Hypotony	++++
Catheter-related complications	++	Catheter-related complications	++	Probenecid toxicities	++
Surgical complications (implant)	+	Paresthesias	+		
		Genital (mucosal) ulcerations	+++		

+ to ++++ based on the severity of the symptoms and the requirement to discontinue the drug on the basis of the indicated toxicity.

intravenous ganciclovir was conducted (81). In 377 patients with AIDS and CMV retinitis restricted to a single eye, after 6 months of treatment, the development of extraocular CMV disease or CMV retinitis in the fellow eye was 37.8%, 22.4%, and 17.9% in the 3 groups, respectively, a statistically significant finding comparing either the combination or the intravenous ganciclovir groups with the implant alone group. The rate of development of Kaposi's sarcoma was similarly decreased, occurring in 11.3 %, 2.7%, and 1.5% of the 3 groups, respectively. This is the first time that use of an antiviral agent in a randomized clinical trial decreased the incidence of Kaposi's sarcoma.

Complications associated with the use of the ganciclovir implant are associated with the procedure and include retinal detachment and, rarely, intraocular hemorrhage or infection. The incidence of surgical complications may decrease with increased familiarity with the procedure. Persons may have multiple devices implanted to control CMV retinitis once the ganciclovir is spent. Whether to perform scheduled surgical replacement of these devices at 6 to 9 months after implantation or to replace them once CMV disease progresses is controversial.

Foscarnet

The morbidity and mortality associated with serious CMV infections in organ allograft recipients and especially in AIDS patients prompted a search for effective alternatives to ganciclovir. Foscarnet, or trisodium phosphonoformate hexahydrate, was approved by the FDA in 1991. The recommended regimen for CMV retinitis in persons with AIDS is an intravenous induction period of 90 mg/kg every 12 hours for 2 to 3 weeks, followed by indefinite 90- to 120-mg/kg daily intravenous maintenance (see Table 23.1). As with ganciclovir, the terms "induction" and "maintenance," although commonly used, may be misnomers; both ganciclovir and of foscarnet have a relatively short $t_{1/2}$, and therapeutic drug levels against CMV of both agents may not be maintained during most of the day during the maintenance phase of therapy. This probably accounts for the routine progression of CMV retinitis during the maintenance phase of therapy with either agent. Patients experiencing progression of CMV retinitis during the maintenance phase are routinely retreated with induction doses of foscarnet.

Foscarnet is an antiviral agent with activity against human herpesviruses and HIV type-1 (HIV-1). Foscarnet inhibits DNA polymerases and prevents chain elongation by blocking nucleoside binding sites of all herpesviruses. Specifically, foscarnet prevents the cleavage of pyrophosphate from adenine triphosphate and, unlike ganciclovir, does not require phosphorylation within virally infected cells (3). In addition to having inhibitory activity against the DNA polymerases of herpes simplex 1 and 2 and CMV, foscarnet has activity against the reverse transcriptase of HIV (82–84).

Oral preparations of foscarnet have been poorly tolerated and have resulted in plasma concentrations that are inadequate to inhibit herpesvirus or HIV replication (85). In humans, pharmacokinetic studies have been performed using both intermittent and continuous foscarnet infusions. Administration of 60 mg/kg of foscarnet (or less, depending on creatinine clearance) every 8 hours to eight patients with AIDS and CMV retinitis resulted in a mean plasma $t_{1/2}$ of 4.5 hours and steady-state peak plasma concentrations ranging between 272 and 876 µM, well above the ID_{50} of susceptible viruses. Trough concentrations of 57 to 225 µM were sometimes lower than the ID_{50} of susceptible virus. Plasma clearance was directly related to renal function; two patients with impaired creatinine clearance had delayed clearance and higher plasma concentrations of foscarnet (86).

In another study (87), continuous infusion of foscarnet, 0.14 to 0.19 mg/kg per minute for 8 to 21 days, in 13 patients with HIV infection and generalized lymphadenopathy or AIDS resulted in a mean plasma $t_{1/2}$ of 6.8 hours. At steady state, 79 to 92% of the dose was excreted unchanged in the urine, indicating that foscarnet is not appreciably metabolized and is renally excreted. After 8 days, small amounts of foscarnet could still be measured in the urine of all patients, and in 1 patient, trace amounts were measurable 2.3 years after infusion. Persistent urinary levels are probably due to slow release from bone. CSF levels of foscarnet measured in 5 subjects found a mean ratio of CSF to plasma concentration of 43%. Four of the subjects, however, had elevated CSF protein suggesting a preexisting meningeal barrier defect (87).

Foscarnet also inhibits the reverse transcriptase of HIV and, correspondingly, the replication of HIV (84, 88). Like ganciclovir, foscarnet is only virustatic, and lifelong treatment of disease is generally required. The major toxicities of foscarnet are its effects on renal function and serum electrolytes. The need for the concurrent or preadministration of a saline solution to minimize renal dysfunction requires a longer infusion period than with ganciclovir (89). Therefore, foscarnet should be infused over at least 1 hour with an infusion pump. This is especially true when other nephrotoxic agents are also administered. Frequent monitoring of serum creatinine, creatinine clearance, and serum electrolytes is required.

Uncontrolled trials have demonstrated the efficacy of foscarnet in the treatment of CMV retinitis in AIDS patients (64, 90–92). In a randomized, controlled trial of foscarnet, 24 AIDS patients with CMV retinitis who were not in immediate danger of losing central visual acuity were entered onto a trial with a 1:1 assignment to either an immediate-treatment or a delayed-treatment group (5). Thirteen patients received immediate induction therapy with foscarnet, 60 mg/kg intravenously every 8 hours for 21 days, followed by 90 mg/kg intravenously daily as maintenance therapy, and 11 patients were assigned to delayed therapy. The end point of the trial was defined as the time when any evaluable lesion progressed 750 µm (half the diameter of the optic disc) over a 750-µm front or when any new retinal lesion resulting from CMV appeared. Mean time to progression of retinitis was 13.3 weeks (median, 7.5 weeks) in the foscarnet group versus 3.2 weeks (median, 3 weeks) in the delayed-therapy group from end points determined from retinal photographs taken weekly and read at a masked reading center. Patients on the delayed-therapy arm of the trial received foscarnet when retinitis progressed. This trial design became the model by which other trials of therapeutic agents for CMV retinitis were tested. Persons receiving immediate therapy with foscarnet frequently had conversion of CMV blood and urine cultures from positive to negative, whereas conversion of cultures in those not receiving therapy was rare. Although foscarnet only delayed the progression of retinitis in most patients receiving maintenance therapy, progression could generally be halted by another induction course of foscarnet or by increasing the maintenance dose.

With respect to delay in progression of retinitis, results from the SOCA were almost identical to those of the foscarnet and ganciclovir placebo-controlled trials (5, 6, 62). No difference in the time to progression of CMV retinitis was found between the two arms, with the median time to progression of 59 days on the foscarnet arm and 56 days on the ganciclovir arm.

With increasing use of ganciclovir for longer periods because of better treatment of other AIDS-associated diseases, ganciclovir-resistant strains of CMV are more frequently recognized (71, 72). Treatment with foscarnet has been successful for ganciclovir-resistant CMV retinitis (93). Fewer data are available regarding the development of CMV resistance in patients receiving long-term foscarnet therapy. Unlike ganciclovir, foscarnet does not require viral phosphotransferase to be activated, so low-level ganciclovir resistant isolates are usually sensitive to foscarnet (94). Resistance to foscarnet is mediated largely by mutations in the CMV polymerase gene, but at a site distinct from those that mediate high-level resistance to ganciclovir and cidofovir (95). Most isolates of CMV resistant to ganciclovir and cidofovir are likely to be sensitive to foscarnet.

Clinical trials have demonstrated the clinical utility of foscarnet against gastrointestinal infections from CMV (41, 66, 96). In a study in patients with AIDS, 18 episodes of esophagitis and 27 episodes of colitis were treated with foscarnet, 20 mg/kg over 10 to 30 minutes, followed by a continuous infusion of 200 mg/kg over 24 hours for a total of 3 weeks of therapy (96). Symptoms and mucosal ulcerations resolved in 15 of 16 episodes of esophagitis in which therapy was completed, for a response rate of 94%. Three patients had a relapse of CMV esophagitis at 1, 4, and 7 months after therapy; 2 of these were successfully retreated with foscarnet and remained in remission 9 months later. Eight of the remaining 12 patients died a mean of 5.8 months later without recurrence of esophagitis, a finding suggesting that maintenance therapy may not be necessary for sustained remission of CMV esophagitis.

Of 18 initial episodes of CMV colitis in patients whose therapy was completed, 11 had a complete response, 6 had a partial response, and 1 had no response. In the 6 with partial responses, other pathogens were also present. Therefore, 11 of 12 initial episodes of colitis due to CMV alone responded to foscarnet, for a response rate of 92%. Two patients with relapses responded to either foscarnet or ganciclovir. The 1 case that did not respond to foscarnet also failed to respond to ganciclovir (96). Similar rates of response were found with the intermittent infusions of foscarnet (41).

In comparison, 42 immunocompromised (primarily AIDS) patients treated with ganciclovir for upper (esophagitis and gastritis) and lower (enteritis and colitis) CMV gastrointestinal disease had a response rate of 83%. Some of these patients received maintenance or repeat therapy as a result of disease relapses (4). In a randomized, controlled trial, cited earlier, of 48 patients with biopsy-proved gastrointestinal CMV disease comparing intravenous ganciclovir and foscarnet, clinical and endoscopic responses to a 2- to 4-week trial of either were equivalent (66).

The utility of foscarnet therapy in the treatment of CMV pneumonitis, central nervous system disease, viremia, or other CMV infections is largely anecdotal, but data suggest efficacy rates similar to those for ganciclovir. Although foscarnet has documented efficacy as an antiretroviral agent, the requirement for intravenous administration, its toxicities, and the availability of more potent oral antiretroviral agents make its utility largely of historical interest (5, 62, 97–99).

Foscarnet is less commonly associated with neutropenia and can usually be administered along with zidovudine (see Table 23.2) (5, 62). Elevations in serum creatinine are perhaps the most common laboratory abnormality and occur more frequently when other nephrotoxic agents are administered at the same time. These elevations are usually reversible with reduction or discontinuation of therapy. In one study (89), elevations in serum creatinine of more than 25% over baseline occurred in 66% of 56 episodes of CMV infection treated with foscarnet. Acute renal failure requiring temporary hemodialysis occurred in 1 instance. In this same report, 27 patients were prehydrated with 2.5 L of normal saline per day before and during the administration of foscarnet. Only 1 patient in this group developed an elevated serum creatinine level. Autopsy of 1 patient revealed acute tubular necrosis, a finding suggesting this as one mechanism of foscarnet-associated renal toxicity. Other likely mechanisms for the renal dysfunction include tubulointerstitial nephritis (100) and precipitation of foscarnet crystals in renal glomeruli (101).

In their study of 24 patients treated with foscarnet for CMV retinitis, Palestine and colleagues reported abnormalities in serum electrolytes, neutropenia (more than 500 cells/µL), increased red blood cell transfusion requirements, nausea that required discontinuation of therapy in two instances, and seizures (5). The seizures occurred in the setting of pre-existing toxoplasmic encephalitis in one patient and cryptococcal disease in the other. In a third instance, the patient had a known idiopathic seizure disorder and had a seizure after initiation of foscarnet therapy. The occurrence of seizures in this study suggests that foscarnet may lower the seizure threshold in persons who are already predisposed (5, 62). Seizures have also been reported in several patients with elevated serum levels of foscarnet resulting from the administration of inappropriately large doses. In the randomized trial comparing initial therapy of foscarnet with ganciclovir for the treatment of CMV retinitis, 39 of 107 (36%) patients required switching from foscarnet to ganciclovir, 22 of 39 for drug-related toxicity, and 9 of 39 for progression of retinitis (62), a finding demonstrating that foscarnet is generally less well tolerated than ganciclovir.

In regard to abnormalities in serum electrolytes, one study reported low serum ionized calcium in six patients immediately after foscarnet infusion, although total serum calcium remained normal (102). The combination of foscarnet with intravenous pentamidine was associated with severe hypocalcemia in four patients with AIDS and *Pneumocystis carinii* pneumonia. After discontinuation of one of the drugs, serum calcium returned to normal in three patients, but the fourth patient died with severe hypocalcemia (103).

Other less common adverse experiences associated with foscarnet therapy include penile ulcerations (104, 105), oral ulcerations (105), generalized cutaneous rash (106), and nephrogenic diabetes insipidus (107). As with ganciclovir, whereas the development of foscarnet has improved the quality of life of many persons with HIV infection and CMV retinitis, its toxicities and the need for daily intravenous infusions leave it wanting as an ideal agent for the treatment of CMV retinitis.

Intravitreal injections of foscarnet have also been used for the treatment of CMV retinitis in persons unable or unwilling to tolerate systemic treatment (108). The regimen of two injections, 2400 μg of foscarnet per injection, given for 2 to 3 weeks during an induction period, followed by weekly maintenance injections, is similar to that of ganciclovir. This alternative therapy appears to be as effective and safe as intravitreal ganciclovir in preventing the progression of CMV, but fewer published long-term data are available.

Cidofovir

Because of limited efficacy, the toxicities, and the inconvenience of administration of ganciclovir and foscarnet, other therapeutic agents for the treatment of CMV disease are needed. Cidofovir, a nucleotide analog with activity against all herpesviruses, was licensed for the treatment of CMV retinitis in 1996. Although the terminal $t_{1/2}$ of cidofovir is approximately 2.6 hours, a fraction of the drug appears to be excreted in a slow elimination phase, a finding suggesting that phosphorylated metabolites of cidofovir may have a long intracellular $t_{1/2}$ (109). Early data suggested that clinically tolerated effective doses of cidofovir could be administered as infrequently as every 2 weeks (110, 111). Nephrotoxicity was a relatively common toxicity of cidofovir therapy, so investigators found it necessary to administer saline hydration and large doses of probenecid around the time of infusion of cidofovir to block the uptake of cidofovir by the proximal renal tubular cells (110, 111).

Two randomized, clinical trials have been conducted comparing intravenous cidofovir with deferred therapy in persons with advanced HIV infection and peripheral CMV retinitis (see Table 23.1) (112, 113). In the first trial, using a previously established trial design (5, 6), persons were randomized to receive immediate therapy ($n = 25$) with cidofovir, 5 mg/kg intravenously weekly for 2 weeks for induction therapy, then every 2 weeks for maintenance (with probenecid on the day of infusion, 2 g orally 3 hours before infusion and 1 g 2 hours and 8 hours after infusion), or deferred treatment ($n = 23$) until progression of retinitis. Progression of retinitis was documented by masked reading of retinal photographs. The median time to progression of CMV retinitis was 120 days in the immediate-treatment group compared with 22 days in the deferred-treatment group ($P<.001$). Asymptomatic neutropenia and proteinuria occurred in 15 and 12% of patients, respectively. Cidofovir was discontinued in 10 of 41 patients (24%) because of treatment-limiting nephrotoxicity. Mild-to-moderate constitutional symptoms or episodes of nausea occurred in 23 of 41 patients (56%), but they were treatment limiting in only 3 (7%).

Using similar eligibility criteria, the second trial randomized patients to a deferred-treatment group ($n = 26$), a high-dose–treatment group, using the same dose of cidofovir as in the first trial ($n = 12$), and a low-dose–treatment group receiving cidofovir, 5 mg/kg weekly for 2 weeks, then 3 mg/kg every 2 weeks for maintenance (113). Probenecid was given on the day of cidofovir administration by the same regimen as the first trial. The median time to progression was 21 days in the deferred-treatment group and 64 days in the low-dose–treatment group; it had not been reached in the high-dose–treatment group at the time of data closure. Patients receiving cidofovir on this trial also developed a significant incidence of proteinuria and reactions to probenecid, but findings suggested that the use of probenecid, hydration, and careful monitoring of patients receiving cidofovir may have minimized but not prevented nephrotoxicity (113). Four patients in this trial were noted to have ocular hypotony, defined as a decrease in intraocular pressure by 50% or more from baseline and less than 5 mm Hg.

A recent report raised the concern of the development of iritis in association with the adminstration of cidofovir (114). Iritis, defined as an increase in anterior chamber cells accompanied by photophobia, redness, pain, or blurred vision, occurred in 11 of 43 persons (26%) receiving cidofovir in 3 medical centers. Most patients with iritis were successfully managed with topical corticosteroids and cycloplegics and were able to continue to receive cidofovir. Additionally, 4 of the 11 patients with iritis also developed hypotony. The hypotony was associated with clinically significant events including choroidal or retinal detachments, a macular fold, or a reduction in visual acuity in 5 of the 6 eyes (2 persons had bilateral hypotony). The development of iritis in association with cidofovir was potentially confounded by the use of protease inhibitors in 10 of the 11 persons with iritis, a finding suggesting that the inflammatory response may be a therapeutic response to the institution of potent antiretroviral therapy, rather than a drug toxicity of cidofovir (114).

The data from the two randomized clinical trials suggest that cidofovir is at least as effective as ganciclovir or foscarnet in the control of CMV retinitis, but it has not been compared directly with these agents in controlled clinical trials, and the analysis of the time to progression curves varied among the different studies (5, 6, 112, 113). The incidence of treatment-limiting toxicities of cidofovir (or probenecid) may be greater than those of ganciclovir or foscarnet, but the convenience of an every 2-week therapeutic regimen compared with daily intravenous therapy and the need to maintain a chronic indwelling catheter for ganciclovir or foscarnet is a major advantage of the use of cidofovir (see Table 23.2). Close monitoring of renal function and of ocular pressure is required.

Like ganciclovir and foscarnet, cidofovir has been administered effectively by the intravitreal route (115). Cidofovir, 20 µg intravitreally (with probenecid, as with the intravenous administration of cidofovir), was administered to 32 eyes of 22 patients at 5- to 6-week intervals for a mean follow-up period of 15.3 weeks (range, 5 to 44 weeks). Only 2 of 32 eyes developed progression of CMV retinitis during the study period. Mild iritis developed after 14 of 101 injections (14%) that had been preceded by the administration of probenecid, but the iritis responded within 2 weeks to topical steroids and cycloplegics. Two cases of hypotony (6%) requiring treatment discontinuation and associated with significant visual loss, one irreversible, occurred. Although the administration of cidofovir intravitreally appears efficacious, close monitoring is required. Few clinical data on the efficacy of cidofovir for extraocular CMV disease are available, so treatment of these diseases, especially with the relative inability of cidofovir to suppress CMV viremia (111–113), should be approached with caution.

Salvage Therapy for CMV Retinitis

In spite of continued therapy with prolonged maintenance doses of therapeutic agents, CMV retinitis usually progresses. Simple progressions can be treated with reinduction doses of any of the agents, although successive progressions of retinitis occur at succeedingly shorter intervals. In a CMV retinitis retreatment trial, no benefit appeared to result from switching from ganciclovir to foscarnet or from foscarnet to ganciclovir in individuals who developed early progression of their CMV retinitis (116). Higher doses of ganciclovir have been safely administered, although often in conjunction with colony-stimulating factors to prevent neutropenia. Higher doses of foscarnet and cidofovir are difficult to administer because of the potential to develop nephrotoxicity with these agents.

In persons intolerant to intravenous therapy, the ganciclovir implant may be useful for the treatment of progressive disease. It should be used with caution, however, in individuals who have received intravenous ganciclovir for an extended period and may be resistant to ganciclovir. In these patients, it may be prudent to administer a test dose of intravitreal ganciclovir and to monitor for a response before subjecting them to the surgical procedure of inserting the implant.

Resistance mutations in the CMV polymerase gene causing resistance to ganciclovir overlap those of cidofovir, a finding suggesting that persons with CMV with high-level resistance to ganciclovir may also be resistant to cidofovir. Strains of CMV with low-level resistance to ganciclovir (because of CMV protein kinase gene mutations) are likely to be susceptible to cidofovir (73). Foscarnet may be used for strains of CMV resistant to ganciclovir and cidofovir (95).

Laboratory data have suggested that the coadministration of ganciclovir and foscarnet may have synergistic activity against CMV (117), a finding prompting the initiation of a clinical trial of this combination for persons whose CMV retinitis progressed through continued monotherapy with either ganciclovir or foscarnet (116). In this controlled clinical trial randomizing patients with progressive CMV retinitis to receive high-dose ganciclovir ($n = 94$), high-dose foscarnet ($n = 89$), or a combination regimen of standard doses of ganciclovir and foscarnet ($n = 96$), persons receiving the combination regimen had a longer time to disease progression (median, 4.3 months), compared with persons receiving ganciclovir (2.0 months) or foscarnet (1.3 months) ($P<.001$). Although these patients did not have any significant laboratory toxicities associated with the combination therapy compared with either monotherapy, a significant adverse effect on quality of life was seen in persons receiving combination therapy because of the requirement for two intravenous infusions daily (116).

The combination of the ganciclovir implant and oral ganciclovir has been studied in untreated CMV disease (81), and it may have some merit in the treatment of progressive disease because of the higher vitreal levels obtained with the use of the implant (79). Other therapeutic options, such as intravenous foscarnet or cidofovir combined with oral ganciclovir or the ganciclovir implant or various combinations of intravitreal and systemic therapy, may have merit in special circumstances for individuals with refractory disease, although these combinations have not been studied extensively.

Contribution to Mortality of CMV in Persons with AIDS

In the randomized controlled trial of foscarnet (5), of those persons who had detectable circulating HIV p24 antigen, a presumptive surrogate marker of HIV activity (118), all persons on the immediate-treatment arm of the trial had more than a 50% decrease in circulating p24 antigen by the end of their induction treatment with foscarnet compared with no change in persons randomized to the delayed-treatment arm (5). Persons on the delayed-treatment arm were begun on foscarnet when they reached an end point, and all persons for whom samples were available subsequently had a more than 50% decrease in their p24 antigen levels. Investigators speculated that this anti-HIV effect may have had some positive effect on survival.

With increasing familiarity with the diagnosis of this CMV disease and the availability of ganciclovir to treat this disease, survival after diagnosis of CMV retinitis increased from about 1 to 6 months before 1988 (63, 119–121) to 5 to 13 months for patients diagnosed after 1987 (62, 121, 122). Two of these studies have suggested a survival benefit in patients treated with ganciclovir compared with untreated patients or patients not responding to ganciclovir. Holland and associates reported that patients treated with ganciclovir survived a median of 7 months compared with untreated patients who survived a median of only 2 months (121). Jabs and associates reported that patients who responded to treatment with ganciclovir had a median survival of 10.0 months, compared with a median survival of only 2.3 months among patients who did not have a complete response (123). Long-term survivors (i.e., those responding to ganciclovir) in that study, however, may have been persons who were less immunocompromised at study entry. In studies evaluating the effect of foscarnet on survival, Harb and colleagues (122), in a retrospective study, found no difference in the median survival time from the diagnosis of CMV retinitis between patients treated with ganciclovir (8 months, $n = 56$) and those treated with foscarnet (9 months, $n = 21$). The randomized clinical trial of initial therapy of ganciclovir compared with foscarnet for the treatment of CMV retinitis demonstrated that those persons randomized to the foscarnet arm of the trial ($n = 107$) had a significantly increased survival (12.6 months) compared with those persons randomized to the ganciclovir arm (8.5 months, $n = 127$) (62). This increase in survival, 12.6 months from the diagnosis of CMV retinitis on the foscarnet arm compared with 8.5 months on the ganciclovir arm, could not be entirely attributed to the concurrent use of the specific antiretroviral agents zidovudine, dideoxyinosine, or dideoxycytidine. A subgroup analysis, however, found this increase in survival only among persons with a relatively normal baseline creatinine clearance. A long-term follow-up of the randomized, foscarnet trial independently corroborated the extended survival of foscarnet-treated persons with a median survival of that cohort of 13.5 months (124). Much of this survival difference will change based on the use of the more potent protease inhibitors for HIV infection.

Because of the toxicities of ganciclovir, foscarnet, and cidofovir, less toxic drugs are needed to treat CMV disease. Acyclovir has less in vitro activity against CMV than against HSV or varicella-zoster virus. Although acyclovir has shown some limited benefit in the prevention of CMV infections in renal transplant recipients (125), a pilot trial of high-dose intravenous acyclovir for suppression of CMV retinitis after an induction regimen with ganciclovir failed to show any clinical efficacy (126).

Prophylaxis for CMV Disease

In the first prospective, double-blind study to be completed for the prophylaxis of CMV disease, 725 HIV-infected persons with advanced HIV infection were randomized to receive either oral ganciclovir (1 g orally, three times daily) or placebo (127). At 18 months, CMV disease, retinitis, and colitis occurred in 39%, 39%, and 4%, respectively, in persons receiving placebo, but in only 20%, 18%, and 2%, respectively, of patients treated with ganciclovir. A second study failed to show that oral ganciclovir was beneficial, but this study was limited by lack of routine ophthalmologic examinations and, perhaps, a lower rate of ascertainment of end points (128). Oral ganciclovir therapy, however, has the disadvantage of requiring the administration of 12 capsules per day at an annual wholesale acquisition cost of more than $17,000 (129). The United States Public Health Service and the Infectious Diseases Society of America recommend that prophylaxis with oral ganciclovir be considered an option for HIV-infected patients who are CMV seropositive and have fewer than 50 CD4+ cells/µL, but it should not be considered the standard of care (129).

SCREENING FOR AND PREVENTION OF CMV DISEASE

No consensus exists regarding the screening of persons for CMV disease. This disease rarely occurs in persons with more than 100 CD4 cells/µL (7–9, 11), so screening these persons would appear not to be cost- or time-effective. Screening blood and urine cultures for CMV has poor specificity and poor sensitivity for the detection of persons who will subsequently develop CMV disease (16, 17). CMV PCR assays may improve sensitivity and specificity, although these assays are not yet routinely available (18, 19). The early diagnosis of CMV colitis or esophagitis before the onset of moderate-to-severe symptoms is unlikely to be of benefit to most patients because, given the toxicities of the agents available for treatment, most patients tolerate mild disease before beginning therapy. Additionally, because the cells that line the colon and esophagus reproduce rapidly, later treatment with ganciclovir or foscarnet usually produces no permanent morbidity.

The early diagnosis of CMV retinitis is more important. Because retinal cells do not regenerate, delay in diagnosis can lead to spread of the disease and permanent loss of vision. Early diagnosis is critical in the management of CMV retinitis. Many experts recommend a baseline dilated ophthalmologic examination by the time the CD4 count falls below 100 cells/µL. Because most persons with CMV retinitis present with some symptoms, either vision changes or "floaters," it is most important to query patients about any subtle visual changes, to discuss with susceptible persons early signs of CMV disease, and to bring these signs to the attention of the health care provider. Some experienced clinicians recommend that patients test their own visual fields using standard grids, and others have dilated ophthalmologic examinations performed on their patients with low CD4 counts every 2 to 3 months. Whether these routines are better than close questioning about visual symptoms is unknown.

PROSPECTS FOR THE FUTURE

What lies in the future? Clearly, more efficacious and more easily tolerated therapies for the treatment of CMV disease are required. Oral administration of the valine ester prodrug of ganciclovir has been shown to produce plasma levels of ganciclovir equivalent to the intravenous administration of ganciclovir and has been promising in clinical trials (130). Lobucavir, a cyclobutyl guanosine analog (131), 1263W94, a benzimidazole riboside compound (132), and adefovir, a nucleotide analog are also in clinical trials (133). Fomivirsen, an oligonucleotide antisense compound that is administered intravitreally, is in phase III clinical trials for persons with CMV retinitis intolerant of or with CMV resistant to other therapies (134).

What will happen to the incidence of CMV disease in the new era of combination therapy with potent protease inhibitors for HIV infection? Early data from a large, urban clinical cohort in the United States and data from multiple sites in France suggest that the incidence of CMV disease, as well as that of other opportunistic infections, is decreasing (135, 136). This finding is echoed in data on CMV retinitis reported to the CDC (11–14).

Although it is reasonably well established that the incidence of CMV disease is decreasing, at least in the short term, in response to the use of potent antiretroviral therapy, what is the effect of these agents on the course of established CMV disease? Preliminary reports suggest that the use of these agents may modulate the course of CMV retinitis (137–139). Some individuals with advanced HIV infection and CMV retinitis whose CD4+ cell counts increased after the initiation of potent antiretroviral therapy have subsequently discontinued their maintenance CMV therapy and have had not had progression of disease for up to 12 months (137–139). The subset of patients who may have their maintenance anti-CMV therapy withdrawn, however, has not been defined, and investigations such as these in which an adverse outcome may result in loss of vision should best be done in the context of a carefully monitored clinical trial.

In summary, end-organ disease from CMV occurs late in the course of HIV infection. With improvements in the treatment and prophylaxis of *Pneumocystis carinii* pneumonia, toxoplasmic encephalitis, disseminated disease from *Mycobacterium avium-intracellulare* complex, and treatment for HIV infection itself, more persons with HIV infection are living longer to develop CMV disease. More recently, increased use of both combination antiretroviral therapy and protease inhibitors in these combinations for the treatment of HIV infection may be decreasing the incidence of opportunistic infections, including CMV, in persons with advanced HIV infection. Three agents, ganciclovir, foscarnet, and cidofovir, have been licensed for the treatment of CMV retinitis. All three agents are effective, but oral therapy with ganciclovir is of limited utility, and parenteral administration of one or more of these agents, with attendant toxicities, is generally required. Progression of CMV disease generally occurs in spite of current maintenance regimens with all these agents. Although major positive advances clearly have been made in reducing the morbidity and mortality resulting from CMV infection, better orally bioavailable and less toxic agents are needed for the treatment of CMV disease in persons with AIDS.

References

1. Jacobson MA, Mills J. Serious cytomegalovirus disease in the acquired immunodeficiency syndrome (AIDS). Ann Intern Med 1988;108:585–594.
2. Bloom JN, Palestine AG. The diagnosis of cytomegalovirus retinitis. Ann Intern Med 1988;109:963–969.
3. Drew WL. Cytomegalovirus infection in patients with AIDS. Clin Infect Dis 1992;14:608–615.
4. Buhles WC, Mastre BJ, Tinker AJ, et al. Ganciclovir treatment of life- or sight-threatening cytomegalovirus infection: experience in 314 immunocompromised patients. Rev Infect Dis 1988;10(Suppl 3):S495–S504.
5. Palestine AG, Polis MA, De Smet MD, et al. A randomized, controlled trial of foscarnet in the treatment of cytomegalovirus retinitis in patients with AIDS. Ann Intern Med 1991;115:665–673.
6. Spector SA, Weingeist T, Pollard RB, et al. A randomized, controlled study of intravenous ganciclovir therapy for with cytomegalovirus peripheral retinitis in patients with AIDS. J Infect Dis 1993;168:557–563.
7. Gallant JE, Moore RD, Richman DD, et al. Incidence and natural history of cytomegalovirus disease in patients with advanced human immunodeficiency virus disease treated with zidovudine. J Infect Dis 1992;166:1223–1227.
8. Crowe SM, Carlin JB, Stewart KI, et al. Predictive value of CD4 lymphocyte numbers for the development of opportunistic infections and malignancies in HIV-infected persons. J Acquir Immune Defic Syndr 1991;4:770–776.
9. Pertel P, Hirschtick R, Phair J, et al. Risk of developing cytomegalovirus retinitis in persons infected with the human immunodeficiency virus. J Acquir Immune Defic Syndr 1992; 5:1069–1074.
10. Hoover DR, Saah AJ, Bacellar H, et al. Clinical manifestations of AIDS in the era of *Pneumocystis* prophylaxis. N Engl J Med 1993;329:1922–1926.
11. Centers for Disease Control and Prevention (CDC). HIV/AIDS surveillance report. Atlanta: CDC, 1993;5:1–33.
12. Centers for Disease Control and Prevention (CDC). HIV/AIDS surveillance report. Atlanta: CDC, 1994;6:1–39.
13. Centers for Disease Control and Prevention (CDC). HIV/AIDS surveillance report. Atlanta: CDC, 1995;7:1–39.
14. Centers for Disease Control and Prevention (CDC). HIV/AIDS surveillance report. Atlanta: CDC, 1996;8:1–39.
15. Jacobson MA, Mills J. Serious cytomegalovirus disease in the acquired immunodeficiency syndrome (AIDS): clinical findings, diagnosis, and treatment. Ann Intern Med 1988;108:585–594.
16. Zurlo JJ, O'Neill D, Polis MA, et al. Lack of clinical utility of cytomegalovirus blood and urine cultures in patients with HIV infection. Ann Intern Med 1993;118:12–17.
17. Salmon D, Lacassin F, Harzic M, et al. Predictive value of cytomegalovirus viraemia for the occurrence of CMV organ involvement in AIDS. J Med Virol 1990;32:160–163.
18. Bowen EF, Sabin CA, Wilson P, et al. Cytomegalovirus (CMV) viraemia detected by polymerase chain reaction identifies a group of HIV-positive patients at high risk of CMV disease. AIDS 1997;11:889–893.
19. Shinkai M, Bozzette SA, Powderly W, et al. Utility of urine and leukocyte cultures and plasma DNA polymerase chain reaction for identification of AIDS patients at risk for developing human cytomegalovirus disease. J Infect Dis 1997;175:302–308.
20. Freeman WR, Henderly DE, Wan WL, et al. Prevalence, pathophysiology, and treatment of rhegmatogenous retinal detachment in treated cytomegalovirus retinitis. Am J Ophthalmol 1987;103:527–536.

21. Jabs DA, Enger C, Haller J, et al. Retinal detachments in patients with cytomegalovirus retinitis. Arch Ophthalmol 1991; 109:794–799.
22. Holland G, Shuler JD. Progression rates of cytomegalovirus retinopathy in ganciclovir-treated and untreated patients. Arch Ophthalmol 1992;110:1435–1442.
23. de Smet MD. Differential diagnosis of retinitis and choroiditis in patients with acquired immunodeficiency syndrome. Am J Med 1992;92(Suppl 2A):17S–21S.
24. O'Donnell JJ, Jacobson MA. Cotton-wool spots and cytomegalovirus in AIDS. Int Ophthalmol Clin 1987;29:105–107.
25. Engstrom RE, Holland GN, Margolis TP, et al. The progressive outer retinal necrosis syndrome: a variant of necrotizing herpetic retinopathy in patients with AIDS. Ophthalmology 1994;101:1488–1502.
26. Holland GN, Engstrom RE, Glasgow BJ, et al. Ocular toxoplasmosis in patients with the acquired immunodeficiency syndrome. Am J Ophthalmol 1988;106:653–657.
27. Dugel PU, Rao NA, Forester DJ. *Pneumocystis carinii* choroiditis after long-term aerosolized pentamidine therapy. Am J Ophthalmol 1990; 110:113–117.
28. Wilcox CM, Diehl DL, Cello JP, et al. Cytomegalovirus esophagitis in patients with AIDS: a clinical, endoscopic, and pathologic correlation. Ann Intern Med 1990;113:589–593.
29. Dieterich DT, Wilcox CM. Diagnosis and treatment of esophageal diseases associated with HIV infection. Am J Gastroenterol 1996;91:2265–2269.
30. Wilcox CM. Esophageal disease in the acquired immunodeficiency syndrome: etiology, diagnosis, and management. Am J Med 1992;92:412–421.
31. Porro GB, Parente F, Cernuschi M. The diagnosis of esophageal candidiasis in patients with acquired immune deficiency syndrome: is endoscopy always necessary? Am J Gastroenterol 1989;84:143–146.
32. Dieterich DT, Rahmin M. Cytomegalovirus colitis in AIDS: presentation in 44 patients and a review of the literature. J AIDS 1991; 4(Suppl 1):S29-S35.
33. Frager DH, Frager JD, Wolf EL, et al. Cytomegalovirus colitis in acquired immune deficiency syndrome: radiologic spectrum. Gastrointest Radiol 1986;11:241–246.
34. Smith PD, Lane HC, Gill VJ, et al. Intestinal infections in patients with the acquired immunodeficiency syndrome (AIDS). Ann Intern Med 1988;108:328–333.
35. Wallace JM, Hannah J. Cytomegalovirus pneumonitis in patients with AIDS. Findings in an autopsy series. Chest 1987;82:198–203.
36. Jacobson MA, Mills J, Rush J, et al. Morbidity and mortality of patients with AIDS and first-episode *Pneumocystis carinii* pneumonia unaffected by concomitant pulmonary cytomegalovirus infection. Am Rev Respir Dis 1991;144:6–9.
37. Rodriguez-Barradas MC, Stool E, Musher DM, et al. Diagnosing and treating cytomegalovirus pneumonia in patients with AIDS. Clin Infect Dis 1996;23:76–81.
38. Bricaire F, Marche C, Zoubi D, et al. Adrenocortical lesions and AIDS [letter]. Lancet 1988;1:881.
39. McKenzie R, Travis WD, Dolan SA, et al. The causes of death in patients with human immunodeficiency virus infection: a clinical and pathologic study with emphasis on the role of pulmonary diseases. Medicine (Baltimore) 1991;70:326–343.
40. Greene LW, Cole W, Greene LB, et al. Adrenal insufficiency as a complication of the acquired immunodeficiency syndrome. Ann Intern Med 1984;101:497–498.
41. Blanshard C. Treatment of HIV-related cytomegalovirus disease of the gastrointestinal tract with foscarnet. J Acquir Immun Defic Syndr 1992;5(Suppl 1):S25–S28.
42. Petito CK, Cho ES, Lemann W, et al. Neuropathology of acquired immunodeficiency syndrome (AIDS): an autopsy review. J Neuropathol Exp Neurol 1986;45:635–646.
43. Morgello S, Cho ES, Nielsen S, et al. Cytomegalovirus encephalitis in acquired immunodeficiency syndrome: an autopsy study of 30 cases and a review of the literature. Hum Pathol 1987;18:289–297.
44. Price TA, Digioia RA, Simon GL. Ganciclovir treatment of cytomegalovirus ventriculitis in a patient infected with human immunodeficiency virus. Clin Infect Dis 1992;15:606–608.
45. Kalayjian RC, Cohen ML, Bonomo RA, et al. Cytomegalovirus ventriculoencephalitis in AIDS: a syndrome with distinct clinical and pathological features. Medicine (Baltimore) 1993;72:67–77.
46. Holland NR, Power C, Mathews VP, et al. Cytomegalovirus encephalitis in acquired immunodeficiency syndrome (AIDS). Neurology 1994;44:507–514.
47. Arribas JR, Storch GA, Clifford DB, et al. Cytomegalovirus encephalitis. Ann Intern Med 1996;125:577–587.
48. Arribas JR, Clifford DB, Fichtenbaum CJ, et al. Level of cytomegalovirus (CMV) DNA in cerebrospinal fluid of subjects with AIDS and CMV infection of the central nervous system. J Infect Dis 1995;172: 527–531.
49. Wolf DG, Spector SA. Diagnosis of human cytomegalovirus central nervous system disease in AIDS patients by DNA amplification from cerebrospinal fluid. J Infect Dis 1992;166:1412–1415.
50. Behar R, Wiley C, McCutchan JA. Cytomegalovirus polyradiculopathy in acquired immune deficiency syndrome. Neurology 1987;37: 557–561.
51. McCutchan JA. Cytomegalovirus infections of the nervous system in patients with AIDS. Clin Infect Dis 1995;20:747–754.
52. Olney RK. Acute lumbosacral polyradiculopathy in acquired immunodeficiency syndrome: experience in 23 patients. Ann Neurol 1994; 35:53–58.
53. Miller RF, Fox JD, Thomas P, et al. Acute lumbosacral polyradiculopathy due to cytomegalovirus in advanced HIV disease: CSF findings in 17 patients. J Neurol Neurosurg Psychiatry 1996;61:456–460.
54. Littler E, Stuart AD, Chee MS. Human cytomegalovirus UL97 open reading frame encodes a protein that phosphorylates the antiviral nucleoside analogue ganciclovir. Nature 1992;358:160–162.
55. Sullivan V, Talarico CL, Stanat SC, et al. A protein kinase homologue controls phosphorylation of ganciclovir in human cytomegalovirus-infected cells. Nature 1992;358:162–164.
56. Drew WL, Ives D, Lalezari JP, et al. Oral ganciclovir as maintenance treatment for cytomegalovirus retinitis in patients with AIDS. N Engl J Med 1995;333:615–620.
57. Sommadossi JP, Bevan R, Ling T, et al. Clinical pharmacokinetics of ganciclovir in patients with normal and impaired renal function. Rev Infect Dis 1988;10(Suppl 3):S507–S514.
58. Jacobson MA, DeMiranda P, Cederberg DM et al. Human pharmacokinetics and tolerance of oral ganciclovir. Antimicrob Agents Chemother 1987;31:1251–1254.
59. Faulds D, Heel RC. Ganciclovir: a review of its antiviral activity, pharmacokinetic properties and therapeutic efficacy in cytomegalovirus infections. Drugs 1990;4:597–638.
60. Masur H, Lane HC, Palestine A, et al. Effect of 9-(1,3,-dihydroxy-2-propoxymethyl) guanine on serious cytomegalovirus disease in eight immunosuppressed homosexual men. Ann Intern Med 1986; 104:41–44.
61. Collaborative DHPG Treatment Study Group. Treatment of serious cytomegalovirus infections with 9-(1,3,-dihydroxy-2-propoxymethyl) guanine in patients with AIDS and other immunodeficiencies. N Engl J Med 1986;314:801–805.
62. Studies of the Ocular Complications of AIDS Research Group, AIDS Clinical Trials Group. Mortality in patients with the acquired immunodeficiency syndrome treated with either foscarnet or ganciclovir for cytomegalovirus retinitis. N Engl J Med 1992;326: 213–220.
63. Palestine AG, Rodrigues MM, Macher AM, et al. Ophthalmic involvement in acquired immunodeficiency syndrome. Ophthalmology 1984;91:1092–1099.
64. Jacobson MA, O'Donnell JJ, Mills J. Foscarnet treatment of cytomegalovirus retinitis in patients with the acquired immunodeficiency syndrome. Antimicrob Agents Chemother 1989;33:736–741.

65. Dieterich DT, Kotler DP, Busch DF, et al. Ganciclovir treatment of cytomegalovirus colitis in AIDS: a randomized, double-blind, placebo-controlled multicenter study. J Infect Dis 1993;167:278–282.
66. Blanshard C, Benhamou Y, Dohin E, et al. Treatment of AIDS-associated gastrointestinal cytomegalovirus infection with foscarnet and ganciclovir: a randomized comparison. J Infect Dis 1995;172:622–628.
67. Emanuel D, Cunningham I, Jules-Elysee K, et al. Cytomegalovirus pneumonia after bone-marrow transplantation successfully treated with the combination of ganciclovir and high-dose intravenous immune globulin. Ann Intern Med 1988;109:777–782.
68. Reed EC, Bowden RA, Dandliker PS, et al. Treatment of cytomegalovirus pneumonia with ganciclovir and intravenous cytomegalovirus immunoglobulin in patients with bone marrow transplants. Ann Intern Med 1988;109:783–788.
69. Jacobson MA, O'Donnell JJ, Rousell R, et al. Failure of adjunctive cytomegalovirus intravenous immune globulin to improve efficacy of ganciclovir in patients with acquired immunodeficiency syndrome and cytomegalovirus retinitis: a phase I study. Antimicrob Agents Chemother 1990;34:176–178.
70. Erice A, Chou S, Biron KK, et al. Progressive disease due to ganciclovir-resistant cytomegalovirus in immunocompromised patients. N Engl J Med 1989;320:289–293.
71. Drew WL, Miner RC, Busch DF, et al. Prevalence of resistance in patients receiving ganciclovir for serious cytomegalovirus infection. J Infect Dis 1991;163:716–719.
72. Studies of the Ocular Complications of AIDS (SOCA) in collaboration with the AIDS Clinical Trials Group. Cytomegalovirus (CMV) culture results, drug resistance, and clinical outcome in patients with AIDS and CMV retinitis treated with foscarnet or ganciclovir. J Infect Dis 1997;176:50–58.
73. Smith IL, Cherrington JM, Jiles RE, et al. High-level resistance of cytomegalovirus to ganciclovir is associated with alterations in both the UL97 and DNA polymerase genes. J Infect Dis 1997;176:69–77.
74. Hochster H, Dieterich D, Bozzette S, et al. Toxicity of combined ganciclovir and zidovudine for cytomegalovirus disease associated with AIDS. Ann Intern Med 1990;113:111–117.
75. Medina DJ, Hsiung GD, Mellors JW. Ganciclovir antagonizes the anti-human immunodeficiency virus activity of zidovudine and didanosine in vitro. Antimicrob Agents Chemother 1992;36:1127–1130.
76. Cantrill HL, Henry K, Melroe NH, et al. Treatment of cytomegalovirus retinitis with intravitreal ganciclovir: long-term results. Ophthalmology 1989;69:367–374.
77. Henry K, Cantrill H, Fletcher C, et al. Use of intravitreal ganciclovir (dihydroxy propoxymethyl guanine) for cytomegalovirus retinitis in a patient with AIDS. Am J Ophthalmol 1987;103:17–23.
78. Schulman J, Peyman GA, Horton MR, et al. Intraocular 9-([2-hydroxy-1-(hydroxymethyl)ethoxy]methyl) guanine levels after intravitreal and subconjunctival administration. Ophthalmic Surg 1986;17:429–432.
79. Martin DF, Parks DJ, Mellow SD, et al. Treatment of cytomegalovirus retinitis with an intraocular sustained-release ganciclovir implant. Arch Ophthalmol 1994;112:1531–1539.
80. Musch DC, Martin DF, Gordon JF, et al. Treatment of cytomegalovirus retinitis with a sustained-release ganciclovir implant. N Engl J Med 1997;337:83–90.
81. Martin D, Kuppermann B, Wolitz R, et al. Combined oral ganciclovir (GCV) and intravitreal GCV implant for treatment of patients with cytomegalovirus (CMV) retinitis: a randomized, controlled study [abstract]. In: Program and abstracts of the 37th Interscience Conference on Antimicrobial Agents and Chemotherapy. Washington, DC: American Society for Microbiology, 1997:LB-9.
82. Ostrander M, Cheng Y-C. Properties of herpes simplex virus type 1 and type 2 DNA polymerase. Biochim Biophys Acta 1980; 609:232–245.
83. Eriksson B, Öberg B, Wahren B. Pyrophosphate analogues as inhibitors of DNA polymerases of cytomegalovirus, herpes simplex virus and cellular origin. Biochim Biophys Acta 1982;696:115–123.
84. Sandstrom EG, Byington RE, Kaplan JC, et al. Inhibition of human T-cell lymphotrophic virus type III in vitro by phosphonoformate. Lancet 1985;1:1480–1482.
85. Sjövall J, Karlsson A, Ogenstad S, et al. Pharmacokinetics and absorption of foscarnet after intravenous and oral administration to patients with human immunodeficiency virus. Clin Pharmacol Ther 1988; 44:65–73.
86. Aweeka F, Gambertoglio J, Mills J, et al. Pharmacokinetics of intermittently administered intravenous foscarnet in the treatment of acquired immunodeficiency syndrome patients with serious cytomegalovirus retinitis. Antimicrob Agents Chemother 1989;33:742–745.
87. Sjövall J, Bergdahl S, Movin G, et al. Pharmacokinetics of foscarnet and distribution to cerebrospinal fluid after intravenous infusion in patients with human immunodeficiency virus infection. Antimicrob Agents Chemother 1989;33:1023–1031.
88. Oberg B. Antiviral effects of phosphonoformate (PFA, foscarnet sodium). Pharmacol Ther 1989;19:387–415.
89. Deray G, Martinez F, Katlama C, et al. Foscarnet nephrotoxicity: mechanism, incidence, and prevention. Am J Nephrol 1989;9:316–321.
90. Walmsley SL, Chew E, Read SE, et al. Treatment of cytomegalovirus retinitis with trisodium phosphonoformate hexahydrate (foscarnet). J Infect Dis 1988;157:569–572.
91. Lehoang P, Girard B, Robinet M, et al. Foscarnet in the treatment of cytomegalovirus retinitis in acquired immune deficiency syndrome. Ophthalmology 1989;96:865–874.
92. Fanning MM, Read SE, Benson M, et al. Foscarnet therapy of cytomegalovirus retinitis in AIDS. J Acquir Immune Defic Syndr 1990; 3:472–479.
93. Jacobson MA, Drew WL, Feinberg J, et al. Foscarnet therapy for ganciclovir-resistant cytomegalovirus retinitis in patients with AIDS. J Infect Dis 1991;163:1348–1351.
94. Erice A, Gil-Roda C, Perez JL, et al. Antiviral susceptibilities and analysis of UL97 and DNA polymerase sequences of clinical cytomegalovirus isolates from immunocompromised patients. J Infect Dis 1997;175:1087–1092.
95. Baldanti F, Underwood MR, Stanat SC, et al. Single amino acid changes in the DNA polymerase confer foscarnet resistance and slow-growth phenotype, while mutations in the UL97-encoded phosphotransferase confer ganciclovir resistance in three double-resistant human cytomegalovirus strains recovered from patients with AIDS. J Virol 1996;70:1390–1395.
96. Nelson MR, Connolly GM, Hawkins DA, et al. Foscarnet in the treatment of cytomegalovirus infection of the esophagus and colon in patients with the acquired immune deficiency syndrome. Am J Gastroenterol 1991;86:876–881.
97. Farthing CF, Dalgleish AG, Clark A, et al. Phosphonoformate (foscarnet): a pilot study in AIDS and AIDS related complex. AIDS 1987;1:21–25.
98. Jacobson MA, Crowe S, Levy J, et al. Effect of foscarnet therapy on infection with human immunodeficiency virus in patients with AIDS. J Infect Dis 1988;158:862–865.
99. Jacobson MA, van der Horst C, Causey DM, et al. In vivo antiretroviral effect of combined zidovudine and foscarnet therapy for human immunodeficiency virus infection (ACTG Protocol 053). J Infect Dis 1991;163:1219–1222.
100. Nyberg G, Blohmé I, Persson H, et al. Foscarnet-induced tubulointerstitial nephritis in renal transplant patients. Transplant Proc 1990; 22:241.
101. Beaufils H, Deray G, Katlama C, et al. Foscarnet and crystals in glomerular capillary lumens [letter]. Lancet 1990;1:755.
102. Jacobson MA, Gambertoglio JG, Aweeka FT, et al. Foscarnet-induced hypocalcemia and effects of foscarnet on calcium metabolism. J Clin Endocrinol Metab 1991;72:1130–1135.

103. Youle MS, Clarbour J, Gazzard B, et al. Severe hypocalcaemia in AIDS patients treated with foscarnet and pentamidine. Lancet 1988;1:1455–1456.
104. Van Der Pijl JW, Frissen PHJ, Reiss P, et al. Foscarnet and penile ulceration. Lancet 1990;1:286.
105. Gilquin J, Weiss L, Kazatchkine MD. Genital and oral erosions induced by foscarnet. Lancet 1990;1:287.
106. Green ST, Nathwani D, Goldberg DJ, et al. Generalised cutaneous rash associated with foscarnet usage in AIDS. J Infect 1990;21:227–228.
107. Farese RV, Schambelan M, Hollander H, et al. Nephrogenic diabetes insipidus associated with foscarnet treatment of cytomegalovirus retinitis. Ann Intern Med 1990;112:955–956.
108. Díaz-Llopis M, Chipont E, Sanchez S, et al. Intravitreal foscarnet for cytomegalovirus retinitis in a patient with acquired immunodeficiency syndrome. Am J Ophthalmol 1992;114:742–747.
109. Cundy KC, Petty BG, Flaherty J, et al. Clinical pharmacokinetics of cidofovir in human immunodeficiency virus-infected patients. Antimicrob Agents Chemother 1995;115:686–688.
110. Lalezari JP, Drew WI, Glutzer E, et al. (S)-1-[3-Hydroxy-2-(phosphonylmethoxy)propyl]cytosine (cidofovir): results of a phase I/II study of a novel antiviral nucleotide analogue. J infect Dis 1995;171:788–796.
111. Polis MA, Spooner KM, Baird BF, et al. Anticytomegaloviral activity and safety of cidofovir in patients with human immunodeficiency virus infection and cytomegalovirus viruria. Antimicrob Agents Chemother 1995;39:882–886.
112. Lalezari JP, Stagg RJ, Kuppermann BD, et al. Intravenous cidofovir for peripheral CMV retinitis in patients with AIDS. Ann Intern Med 1997;126:257–263.
113. Studies of the Ocular Complications of AIDS Research Group in collaboration with the AIDS Clinical Trials Group. Parenteral cidofovir for cytomegalovirus retinitis in patients with AIDS: the HPMPC peripheral cytomegalovirus retinitis trial. Ann Intern Med 1997;126:264–274.
114. Davis JL, Taskintuna I, Freeman WR, et al. Iritis and hypotony after treatment with intravenous cidofovir for cytomegalovirus retinitis. Arch Ophthalmol 1997;115:733–737.
115. Rahhal FM, Arevalo JF, Chavez de la Paz E, et al. Treatment of cytomegalovirus retinitis with intravitreaous cidofovir in patients with AIDS: a preliminary report. Ann Intern Med 1996;125:98–103.
116. The Studies of Ocular Complications of AIDS Research Group, AIDS Clinical Trials Group. Combination foscarnet and ganciclovir therapy vs. monotherapy for the treatment of relapsed cytomegalovirus retinitis in patients with AIDS: the Cytomegalovirus Retreatment Trial. Arch Ophthalmol 1996;114:23–33.
117. Manischewitz JF, Quinnan GV Jr., Lane HC, et al. Synergistic effect of ganciclovir and foscarnet on cytomegalovirus replication in vitro. Antimicrob Agents Chemother 1990;34:373–375.
118. Fahey JL, Taylor JMG, Detels R, et al. The prognostic value of cellular and serologic markers in infection with human immunodeficiency virus type 1. N Engl J Med 1990;322:166–172.
119. Henderly DE, Freeman WR, Causey DM, et al. Cytomegalovirus retinitis and response to therapy with ganciclovir. Ophthalmology 1987;94:425–434.
120. Jacobson MA, O'Donnell JJ, Porteous D, et al. Retinal and gastrointestinal disease due to cytomegalovirus in patients with the acquired immune deficiency syndrome: prevalence, natural history, and response to ganciclovir therapy. Q J Med 1988;254:473–486.
121. Holland GN, Sison RF, Jatulis DE, et al. Survival of patients with the acquired immune deficiency syndrome after development of cytomegalovirus retinopathy. Ophthalmology 1990;97:204–211.
122. Harb GE, Bacchetti P, Jacobson MA. Survival of patients with AIDS and cytomegalovirus disease treated with ganciclovir or foscarnet. AIDS 1991;5:959–965.
123. Jabs DA, Enger C, Bartlett JG. Cytomegalovirus retinitis and acquired immunodeficiency syndrome. Ophthalmology 1989;107:75–80.
124. Polis MA, De Smet MD, Baird BF, et al. Increased survival of a cohort of patients with acquired immunodeficiency syndrome and cytomegalovirus retinitis who received sodium phosphonoformate (foscarnet). Am J Med 1993;94:185–190.
125. Balfour HH Jr., Chace BA, Stapleton JT, et al. A randomized placebo-controlled trial of oral acyclovir for the prevention of cytomegalovirus disease in recipients of renal allografts. N Engl J Med 1989;320:1381–1387.
126. Sha BE, Benson CA, Deutsch TA, et al. Suppression of cytomegalovirus retinitis in persons with AIDS with high-dose intravenous acyclovir. J Infect Dis 1991;164:777–780.
127. Spector SA, McKinley GF, Lalezari JP, et al. Oral ganciclovir for the prevention of cytomegalovirus disease in persons with AIDS. N Engl J Med 1996;334:1491–1497.
128. Brosgart CL, Craig C, Hillman D, et al. A randomized placebo-controlled trial of the safety an efficacy of oral ganciclovir for prophylaxis of CMV retinal and gastrointestinal mucosal disease in HIV-infected individuals with severe immunosuppression [abstract]. In: Program and abstracts of the 35th Interscience Conference on Antimicrobial Agents and Chemotherapy. Washington, DC: American Society for Microbiology, 1995:A27.
129. Centers for Disease Control and Prevention. 1997 USPHS/IDSA guidelines for the prevention of opportunistic infections in persons infected with human immunodeficiency virus. MMWR Morb Mortal Wkly Rep 1997;46:1–46.
130. Brown F, Arum I, Francis G, et al. Ganciclovir prodrug (RS-79070)—multiple dose, dose-ranging study with effect of food [abstract]. In: Program and abstracts of the 4th Conference on Retroviruses and Opportunistic Infections. Washington, DC: Infectious Diseases Society of America, 1997:LB19.
131. Dunkle LM, Petty B, Reynolds L, et al. Lobucavir: a promising broad-spectrum antiviral agent [abstract Th.B.943]. In: Supplement to abstracts of the 11th International Conference on AIDS, Vancouver, 1996.
132. Wang LH, Lyogendran S, Weller S, et al. A phase I trial evaluating the tolerability and pharmacokinetics (PK) of 1263W94 following single oral administration of escalating doses in normal healthy volunteers [abstract]. In: Program and abstracts of the 36th Interscience Conference on Antimicrobial Agents and Chemotherapy. Washington, DC: American Society for Microbiology, 1996:H28.
133. Xiong XF, Chen MS. Inhibition of human cytomegalovirus DNA polymerase by PMEA and PMPA deiphosphates [abstract]. In: Program and abstracts of the 36th Interscience Conference on Antimicrobial Agents and Chemotherapy. Washington, DC: American Society for Microbiology, 1996: abstract H29.
134. Hutcherson SL, Palestine AG, Cantrill HL, et al. Antisense oligonucleotide safety for CMV retinitis in AIDS patients [abstract]. In: Program and abstracts of the 35th Interscience Conference on Antimicrobial Agents and Chemotherapy. Washington, DC: American Society for Microbiology, 1995:H136.
135. Moore RD, Keruly JC, Chaisson RE. The effectiveness of combination antiretroviral therapy in clinical practice [abstract]. In: Program and abstracts of the Infectious Diseases Society of America 35th Annual Meeting. Alexandria, VA: Infectious Diseases Society of America, 1997:213.
136. Baril L, Jouan M, Caumes E, et al. The impact of highly active antiretroviral therapy on the incidence of CMV disease in AIDS patients [abstract]. In: Program and abstracts of the 37th Interscience Conference on Antimicrobial Agents and Chemotherapy. Washington, DC: American Society for Microbiology, 1997:1–31.
137. Whitcup SM, Fortin E, Nussenblatt RB, et al. Therapeutic effect of combination antiretroviral therapy on cytomegalovirus retinitis. JAMA 1997;277:1519–1520.
138. Torriani FJ, MacDonald JC, Karevellas M, et al. Lack of progression after discontinuation of maintenance therapy (MT) for cytomegalo-

virus retinitis (CMVR) in AIDS patients responding to highly active antiretroviral therapy (HAART) [abstract]. In: Program and abstracts of the 37th Interscience Conference on Antimicrobial Agents and Chemotherapy. Washington, DC: American Society for Microbiology, 1997:1–33.

139. Tural C, Sirera G, Andreu D, et al. Long lasting remission of cytomegalovirus retinitis without maintenance therapy in HIV+ patients [abstract]. In: Program and abstracts of the 37th Interscience Conference on Antimicrobial Agents and Chemotherapy. Washington, DC: American Society for Microbiology, 1997:1–36.

24

HERPES SIMPLEX AND VARICELLA-ZOSTER VIRUS INFECTIONS IN HIV-INFECTED INDIVIDUALS

Sharon Safrin

HERPES SIMPLEX VIRUS INFECTION

Epidemiology

An ancient disease first described in the fifth century B.C. (1), herpes simplex virus (HSV) infection remains highly prevalent in the general population. The seroprevalence of HSV-1 infection in the United States is estimated at approximately 70%, whereas studies show a 32% rise in the seroprevalence of HSV-2 infection between 1976 to 1980 and 1989 to 1991, from 16 to 22% (2, 3). Although the prevalence of HSV-1 antibody increases incrementally with age and is associated with conditions of crowding, the prevalence of HSV-2 antibody rises only after puberty and is correlated with the number of sexual partners (4). Rates of HSV-2 antibody are generally higher in women than in men (2–4) and in African-Americans compared with whites (2, 3), but rates are particularly high in homosexual or bisexual men with human immunodeficiency virus (HIV) infection (68 to 77%) (5–7). Data suggest comparably high rates in other HIV-infected populations, including HIV-infected women and heterosexual men (8). The frequency of HSV-1 infection in HIV-infected persons has not been well studied.

Pathogenesis

Direct inoculation of the virus through mucous membrane contact results in intraaxonal transport along sensory nerves to the nerve cell bodies in the corresponding dorsal nerve root or trigeminal ganglia, where latency is established. On reactivation, triggered by incompletely understood stimuli, virus replication is initiated. Transport occurs by efferent nerves to mucocutaneous surfaces, where virus replication continues, and clinically apparent lesions may result. In contrast to varicella-zoster infection (see later), no evidence suggests the presence of viremia during uncomplicated primary HSV infection in immunocompetent persons.

Both cell-mediated and humoral immune defenses may modulate the frequency and duration of clinical recurrences. Immunosuppressed patients, particularly those with impaired cell-mediated immunity, tend to manifest a greater frequency and severity of HSV infection (9). Other factors associated with higher rates of recurrence after a symptomatic first episode of genital herpes include a longer duration of the primary episode, male gender, and HSV-2 origin (10).

Mucocutaneous HSV lesions are less prone to resolve spontaneously in HIV-infected individuals than in immunocompetent patients, particularly if these lesions are untreated (11, 12). The case definition of acquired immunodeficiency syndrome (AIDS) was revised by the United States Centers for Disease Control and Prevention in 1987 to include chronic mucocutaneous HSV lesions persisting for more than 1 month in the absence of other causes of immunodeficiency or in the presence of serum antibody against HIV (13). Perhaps the tendency for chronicity increases as the severity of HIV-associated impairment of immune defenses progresses. Although a retrospective study at San Francisco General Hospital found that neither frequency nor duration of HSV recurrences was prolonged in a sample of patients with AIDS, another study suggested that the frequency of HSV recurrences as a cause of cutaneous ulcerations rises sharply as CD4 cell counts fall below $50/mm^3$ (14).

Clinical Manifestations

A vesiculoulcerative lesion may occur at any mucocutaneous site. Although HSV-1 most commonly causes lesions in the mouth or on the lips, and HSV-2 causes lesions in genital and perianal areas, either virus may cause lesions at any location, based on the site of primary mucocutaneous inoculation. HSV-1, for instance, is the cause of primary genital lesions in at least 15% of cases, and HSV-2 may cause herpetic whitlow through self-inoculation. Recent reports suggest that genital herpes infections caused by HSV-1 may be increasing (15). Primary episodes have a longer duration, both clinically and virologically, than recurrent outbreaks, regardless of site; in persons with genital herpes, a primary episode averages 16 to 19 days, whereas a recurrent episode lasts approximately 9 to 10 days (9).

The typical clinical presentation of HSV infection has been challenged by the recognition that up to half the persons with serum antibody to HSV-2 have no history of genital outbreaks (16). In addition, subclinical shedding of HSV, in the absence of clinically overt lesions, is far more common than previously appreciated: in one study of 100 immunocompetent women with recurrent genital herpes who were followed-up for approximately 3 months, 51% of women had at least 1 episode of subclinical shedding, and 33% of all culture-positive days occurred in the absence of lesions (17). Thus, both transmission and acquisition of HSV infection may, in fact, be asymptomatic, thus propagating continued spread. Two reports suggest that mucocutaneous shedding of HSV from anogenital sites occurs with increased frequency in HIV-infected persons, as well as at multiple anatomic sites, thus potentially incurring greater risks for transmission (18, 19).

Anogenital outbreaks of HSV in patients with HIV infection are common, perhaps because of the high prevalence of HSV-2 infection (5–7) and the inability of host defenses to prevent reactivation. In addition to painful or itchy lesions in the perianal area, involvement of the distal rectum may result in painful defecation, tenesmus, discharge, or constipation (20). Fever, inguinal adenopathy, and signs of sacral neuropathy may also be present in patients with proctitis (20). Sigmoidoscopic findings include friable mucosa with vesicular or pustular lesions or diffuse ulceration.

No evidence indicates that complications of HSV infection, such as ocular keratitis, encephalitis, or aseptic meningitis, are more frequent in patients with HIV infection. However, esophageal involvement by HSV occurs in HIV-infected host, as in other immunocompromised hosts, causing dysphagia or odynophagia (21). In these patients, concomitant perioral HSV lesions are often absent (21). Therefore, differentiation from other causes of esophagitis (e.g., *Candida*, cytomegalovirus) requires endoscopic visualization and sampling of the lesion for culture and histopathologic examination.

Diagnosis

The virus culture remains the standard for the diagnosis of active HSV infection. Specimens, obtained by unroofing the vesicular or crusted lesion or swabbing the base of the ulcer with a cotton-tipped or Dacron swab, should be forwarded in appropriate transport media to the clinical virology laboratory, where they are inoculated onto tissue culture cell lines (e.g., Vero or foreskin fibroblast cells). On detection of characteristic changes in cell morphology resulting from cytopathic effect, generally within 24 to 72 hours, the virus type (i.e., HSV-1 versus HSV-2) can be confirmed with the use of specific fluorescein-conjugated monoclonal antibodies.

Alternatives to virus culture include direct antigen detection (by immunofluorescent, immunoperoxidase, or enzyme-linked immunoassay techniques) and the Tzanck smear. Antigen staining requires the presence of infected cells obtained directly from the clinical lesion. Although more advantageous in regard to the rapidity of results and increased availability to office-based physicians, sensitivity and specificity depend on the adequacy of the specimen obtained. Therefore, several slides should be prepared to maximize diagnostic accuracy. In the Tzanck smear, multinucleated giant cells are visualized on Giemsa or Wright staining of scrapings from the base of an herpetic ulcer; however, this examination is nonspecific in that it does not differentiate between HSV and varicella-zoster virus (VZV) infection.

Detection of HSV by the polymerase chain reaction method has proved useful for the diagnosis of herpes simplex encephalitis (22) and for increased sensitivity in the monitoring of cutaneous virus shedding (23). This technique is also available for the diagnosis of mucocutaneous HSV infection.

The development of type-specific serologic techniques for the detection of antibodies to HSV-1 and HSV-2 has facilitated epidemiologic assessment of the prevalence of these infections. However, the detection of serum antibody to HSV-1 or HSV-2 is not generally of use in the individual patient, given the high prevalence rates in HIV-infected populations and the inability of the test to determine the duration of seropositivity or the presence of active infection. Currently commercially available tests do not reliably differentiate between HSV-1 and HSV-2. The Western blot (immunoblot) and an enzyme immunoassay for antibody to HSV glycoprotein G (24) are available in reference or research laboratories. A direct comparison of these techniques in immunocompetent individuals failed to detect any differences in overall sensitivity (24); in patients with AIDS, however, the glycoprotein assay had inferior sensitivity for the detection of serum antibody to HSV-2 (25).

Treatment

Currently available antiviral therapies have been shown to be effective in decreasing the duration of symptoms and of virus shedding in outbreaks of HSV. However, current treatment modalities are limited by their virustatic nature, which fails to eradicate virus that is latent in the paraspinous ganglia. Because HSV infections have a propensity for recurrence, current management techniques are palliative rather than curative.

The "first-generation" antivirals, developed in the 1950s, included 5-iododeoxyuridine (IUdR), trifluorothymidine (TFT), and cytosine arabinoside (ara-C). These agents are nonselective in their inhibition of cellular DNA and thus are too toxic for systemic use (26); however, both TFT and IUdR are used topically for the treatment of herpes keratitis. Adenine arabinoside (vidarabine, ara-A) was licensed as a parenteral agent for the treatment of neonatal HSV infection in the mid-1970s. Vidarabine was the first antiviral drug used successfully to treat HSV encephalitis.

Acyclovir, released in the United States in 1982, is an acyclic guanosine analog formulated in intravenous, oral, and topical preparations. Activation by phosphorylation is required for intracellular antiviral activity and is accomplished in part by a virus-specified thymidine kinase. The induction of thymidine kinase synthesis during infection of cells by HSV renders acyclovir an unusually specific antiviral agent. Its lack of toxicity to host cells is exemplified by the 3000-fold difference between the minimum inhibitory concentration of drug that inhibits replication by 50% (ID_{50}) for Vero cells (300 FM) and for HSV-1 (0.1 FM) (26). After monophosphorylation by the virus-specified thymidine kinase, diphosphorylation and triphosphorylation are accomplished by cellular enzymes; acyclovir triphosphate then inhibits virus replication by competitive inhibition with cellular deoxyguanosine triphosphate for DNA polymerase. The DNA template primer that contains acyclovir monophosphate has a much greater potency of inhibition against the DNA polymerase of HSV-1 and HSV-2 than the cellular α or β DNA polymerases (26), binding viral DNA polymerase irreversibly and preventing further DNA elongation. In addition to this mechanism of anti–herpes virus activity, the incorporation of acyclovir triphosphate into the growing viral DNA chain results in chain termination.

Because acyclovir is not phosphorylated efficiently by the host cellular kinase, it is minimally toxic to host cells and therefore has a high therapeutic:toxic ratio. When given in high doses intravenously, however, acyclovir has been associated with both neurologic toxicity and renal insufficiency, the latter caused by precipitation of the drug in the renal tubules.

Treatment trials using acyclovir for herpes labialis in the immunocompetent host have shown only a modest benefit. Results of studies using acyclovir ointment have had variable results; use of oral acyclovir (400 mg five times daily) shortened lesion duration compared with placebo by approximately 27% (27). For prophylaxis, topical acyclovir is poorly effective, whereas daily acyclovir (400 mg orally twice daily) decreased the number of recurrent episodes by about half (28).

Case reports have been published of chronic orofacial HSV infection in both HIV-infected and non–HIV-infected immunocompromised individuals (29, 30). Such lesions may respond to acyclovir if the drug is administered in adequate doses early in the course. Thus, it is important to consider the diagnosis of HSV in patients with multiple ulcers of the palate, alveolar ridge, or oral mucosa. Once chronic, such lesions may become resistant to acyclovir (31–34).

Placebo-controlled trials have established the clinical and virologic efficacy of both intravenous (5 mg/kg every 8 hours) and oral (200 mg five times daily) acyclovir for 5 to 10 days in the treatment of primary and recurrent genital herpes (35, 36), resulting in significantly reduced virus shedding and a shortening of lesion healing time. However, the magnitude of effect of acyclovir for the treatment of primary genital infections is substantially greater than that in recurrent HSV infection, particularly in the immunocompetent host. Results of treatment trials using topical acyclovir ointment (5%) have not shown substantial clinical benefit. No evidence indicates that acyclovir treatment of a first episode affects the establishment of latency or the frequency of recurrence (10). A placebo-controlled study of oral acyclovir therapy for first-episode HSV proctitis (400 mg five times daily for 10 days) showed significant reduction in the duration of rectal lesions and of virus shedding, but no effect on clinical symptoms (37).

Although the first agent shown to be clinically useful in the treatment of herpes simplex encephalitis was vidarabine (15 mg/kg/day), subsequent studies demonstrated the superior efficacy and lesser toxicity of intravenous acyclovir (10 mg/kg every 8 hours) (38). The clinical presentation of acute encephalitis, with fever, headache, and altered mentation, often with focal neurologic signs, should prompt consideration of this diagnosis.

Long-term suppressive use of acyclovir has also been shown to be effective; in a controlled trial of 144 immunocompetent patients with frequently recurring genital herpes, administration of 400 mg acyclovir twice daily increased the proportion of patients who were free of recurrence in a 1-year period compared with placebo (44% versus 2%) and decreased the mean number of recurrences per year (1.8 versus 11.4) (39). Suppressive therapy does not completely eradicate recurrent episodes, even in immunocompetent hosts. Isolates recovered from "breakthrough" HSV episodes during suppressive therapy are typically not resistant to acyclovir in vitro; thus, the reason for sporadic breakthrough is unclear. A dose of acyclovir, 400 mg twice daily, is the recommended chemosuppressive regimen (40). However, certain patients with frequent recurrences may require higher doses for adequate suppression (41). The safety of the use of suppressive acyclovir for up to 7 consecutive years has been reported.

A placebo-controlled crossover trial of acyclovir chemosuppression (400 mg orally twice daily) in immunocompetent women demonstrated its effectiveness in decreasing subclinical shedding rates of HSV, by 94% (42). A comparably designed trial demonstrated an 86% reduction in the rate of subclinical anogenital shedding in HIV-infected individuals, as compared with placebo (43).

Two other agents are now licensed for the treatment of recurrent genital herpes in the United States, famciclovir (dose, 125 mg orally twice daily) and valacyclovir (dose, 500 mg orally twice daily). Famciclovir is a prodrug of the guanosine analog penciclovir (44). Like acyclovir, it is activated through phosphorylation by the virus-specified thymidine kinase, thereafter inhibiting viral DNA synthesis by competitively inhibiting DNA polymerase. Oral bioavailability is substantially greater than that of acyclovir, and its intracellular half-life is 10 to 20 times longer. A randomized, double-blind comparison of several doses of patient-initiated famciclovir compared with placebo revealed significant benefits on time to healing, time to cessation of virus shedding, and reduction in pain (45). Valacyclovir is a prodrug of acyclovir, achieving serum levels three to five times that achieved with oral acyclovir in humans (46). A randomized double-blind trial comparing two doses of valacyclovir with placebo for therapy of recurrent genital herpes in immunocompetent adults showed significant benefits (47). For chemosuppression of genital recurrent herpes, the recommended dosing regimens are famciclovir, 250 mg twice daily, or valacyclovir, 250 mg twice daily, 500 mg once daily, or 1000 mg once daily (40).

Neither famciclovir nor valacyclovir is approved for use in immunocompromised patient populations, because of the lack of adequate study to date.

Patients who are immunosuppressed as a result of hematologic malignancy or organ transplantation generally respond well to standard doses of acyclovir for episodes of mucocutaneous HSV. The need for higher doses of acyclovir in HIV-infected patients has been sporadically suggested, but not well documented. Although chronicity of herpetic lesions has been reported in patients with HIV infection (11, 12), whether this is a more frequent occurrence than in other immunosuppressed patients is unclear (48). Development of chronic HSV lesions that are resistant to acyclovir, however, seems clearly to occur most frequently in patients with AIDS. Therefore, those patients in whom HSV lesions do not respond appropriately to acyclovir in standard doses should receive higher doses (e.g., 400 to 800 mg five times daily) promptly, to avoid potential subtherapeutic dosing and resultant exertion of a selective pressure that would facilitate the emergence of acyclovir-resistant mutants (49).

Although resistance to acyclovir is readily induced in the laboratory by serial passage of the virus in the presence of the drug, prior exposure is not a prerequisite to the development of resistance: in one study, 6 of 97 isolates of HSV-2 from persons who had never received acyclovir were resistant in vitro (50). Whereas the presence of acyclovir-resistant mutants within a clinical lesion, believed to arise by spontaneous mutation at a rate of approximately 1 in 10,00 virus replications (51), typically does not impair healing within the immunocompetent host, the eventual dominance of such strains within the lesions of immunocompromised patients may result in chronic, nonhealing ulcerations (31–34). Nevertheless, not until the onset of the AIDS epidemic did such lesions become a clinically significant problem (31, 52–55).

A growing body of evidence suggests the presence of a mixed population of acyclovir-susceptible and acyclovir-resistant mutants within mucocutaneous ulcerative lesions (51, 56). Three mechanisms of resistance have been described (57): marked deficiency or absence of the virus-specified thymidine kinase, alteration in substrate specificity of the thymidine kinase, and alteration in the substrate specificity of the viral DNA polymerase. Most clinical isolates derived from patients with acyclovir-resistant HSV infection have shown deficient activity of thymidine kinase, although occasional thymidine kinase–altered (58) and DNA polymerase mutants (56, 59) have been described as well.

HIV-infected patients with acyclovir-resistant HSV infection have advanced HIV disease, based on either clinical diagnoses of AIDS-related conditions or on diminished CD4 cell counts. Lesions are often perirectal, but they may occur on any mucocutaneous surface. A single case of central nervous system involvement from acyclovir-resistant HSV infection, manifesting as fatal meningoencephalitis, has been described (53). In this patient, a thymidine kinase–deficient HSV-2 isolate was recovered from a chronic perianal lesion as well as from the spinal fluid and brain tissue; restriction endonuclease analysis of viral DNA suggested that they were the same strain.

The prevalence of acyclovir-resistant HSV has not been fully studied. A single study in a tertiary care center showed 7 of 207 (3.4%) HSV isolates to be resistant to acyclovir; all 7 were from lesions of immunocompromised patients (60). One isolate of the 14 (7.1%) that were recovered from HIV-infected patients in this study was shown to be resistant to acyclovir. Preliminary data from a separate study of 205 HIV-infected patients found the prevalence of in vitro acyclovir resistance to be 2.9% (S Safrin, unpublished data). The efficacy of transmission of acyclovir-resistant strains compared with that of acyclovir-susceptible HSV has not been analyzed.

Although antiviral susceptibility testing of HSV virus has been performed for decades, multiple methods are used by reference laboratories, with a lack of standardization. The neutral red dye uptake (61), plaque reduction (61), and DNA hybridization (62) assays are the most common. A three-way comparison of these methods using 30 HSV isolates found that susceptibility determinations to acyclovir and foscarnet were comparable once adjustments to the threshold definitions of in vitro resistance were made for each assay (63). The plaque reduction assay is perhaps the most widely accepted method, however, because of validation of in vitro results with clinical response to therapy in a large sample of patients (64). Additionally, the thymidine kinase phenotype of an HSV isolate can be specifically determined using plaque autoradiography (65).

Although prior exposure to acyclovir, on either a long-term or an intermittent basis, is typically present in the histories of patients with acyclovir-resistant HSV infection, the specific factors that predict this outcome in the minority of HIV-infected persons have been difficult to pinpoint. Nevertheless, resistant HSV infection fortunately has remained a rare complication of AIDS, despite the growing numbers of patients with AIDS who have depressed CD4 cell counts.

Treatment options for the patient with acyclovir-resistant HSV infection are limited. Thymidine kinase–deficient or thymidine kinase–altered mutants are cross-resistant with ganciclovir and penciclovir/famciclovir (54, 66). Unlike the pyrimidine nucleoside agents, vidarabine is converted to a triphosphate entirely by cellular enzymes and thus circumvents the need for activation by thymidine kinase (26). However, trials of vidarabine therapy in patients with acyclovir-resistant HSV have not been successful (12, 31, 52). In addition, a multicenter randomized prospective trial comparing vidarabine with foscarnet for the treatment of HIV-infected patients with acyclovir-resistant HSV failed to demonstrate clinical or virologic efficacy of this agent (55). In addition, vidarabine therapy was associated with unexpectedly frequent and severe neurologic toxicity in patients in this trial, resulting in premature termination of the study (55).

The lack of efficacy of vidarabine in treatment of acyclovir-resistant infection despite in vitro susceptibility is not well understood. Vidarabine is approximately 100-fold less active against HSV in vitro than acyclovir (26), perhaps in part because of its rapid deamination by adenosine deaminase in vivo to the much less active metabolite ara-hypoxanthine. Conceivably, therefore, the optimal dosage of vidarabine for antiherpes activity may be greater than the conventionally administered dosages of 10 to 15 mg/kg daily; higher doses, however, are contraindicated by both hematologic and neurologic toxicities.

Foscarnet is a pyrophosphate analog that directly inhibits viral DNA polymerase, thus retaining activity against thymidine kinase–deficient or thymidine kinase–altered strains of acyclovir-resistant HSV (67). After a series of uncontrolled studies and case reports that suggested its efficacy for the therapy of patients with acyclovir-resistant HSV infection (31, 34, 68), a randomized multicenter study comparing foscarnet (40 mg/kg every 8 hours) with vidarabine (15 mg/kg/day) showed superior efficacy as well as lesser serious toxicity in patients receiving foscarnet (55). In this study, the median time to complete healing (13.5 versus 38.5 days) and the median time to cessation of viral shedding (6 versus 17 days) were significantly shorter in patients randomized to receive foscarnet than in those assigned to vidarabine ($P=.001$, $P=.006$, respectively).

Potential toxicities of foscarnet therapy include nephrotoxicity, electrolyte disturbances (hypocalcemia and hypercalcemia, hypophosphatemia and hyperphosphatemia), anemia, seizures, and genital drug eruptions (67). Controlled rates of infusion, saline prehydration, serial titration of dose according to calculated creatinine clearance, and avoidance of concomitant administration of nephrotoxic agents diminish the frequency of these complications.

Recurrence of acyclovir-resistant HSV infection is common, if not ubiquitous; in this sense, therefore, treatment for the condition is palliative rather than curative. In one series, each of 17 patients followed longitudinally after healing of acyclovir-resistant HSV disease developed a recurrence, at a median of 42.5 days after discontinuation of foscarnet (range, 14 to 191) (55). Foscarnet-resistant HSV infection has been reported in several patients (56, 69); such patients typically have been exposed to foscarnet on a recurrent intermittent or long-term basis for the treatment of either acyclovir-resistant HSV or cytomegalovirus infection. Clearly, therefore, alternative agents are needed for the treatment of this disorder, both to offer topical rather than parenteral treatment modalities and to afford a greater choice of agents should resistance to one or more occur during therapy.

Several other agents have been evaluated for this indication. Neither BW 348U87, a ribonucleotide reductase inhibitor combined with acyclovir (70), nor SP-303, a bioflavonoid compound (71), had significant clinical or virologic activity against acyclovir-resistant HSV infection when evaluated in open-label studies. Continuous infusion of acyclovir, with targeting of specific serum levels of acyclovir using serial monitoring by high-pressure liquid chromatography assay, resulted in complete healing of acyclovir-resistant HSV lesions after approximately 6 weeks in a total of five patients with AIDS (72, 73). The topical application of TFT, a nucleoside analog currently licensed as an ophthalmic solution for the treatment of patients with herpes keratitis, was successful in isolated case reports (74, 75); in a separate study of three patients, the combination of trifluridine with interferon-α resulted in healing of lesions (76). In an open-label study of thrice-daily application of trifluridine in AIDS patients with acyclovir-unresponsive mucocutaneous HSV infection, 7 of 24 evaluable patients (29%) had complete healing at a median of 7.1 weeks (77). A total of 14 patients (58%) had at least a 50% decrease in the size of their lesions, at a median of 2.4 weeks. Cessation of virus shedding and reduction in pain were not studied (77). The major limitation in the utility of this treatment is its current formulation, because a liquid solution is difficult to apply and adhere.

Cidofovir, (S)-1-(3-hydroxy-2-[phosphonylmethoxy] propyl)cytosine, formerly HPMPC, is a nucleotide analog with potent activity against HSV (including thymidine kinase–deficient and DNA polymerase mutant acyclovir-resistant strains) as well as other herpesviruses (78, 79). Several case reports have described healing in patients with acyclovir-resistant HSV lesions in response to therapy with either parenteral or topical cidofovir (80–82). In a completed randomized, placebo-controlled trial, 30 AIDS patients with acyclovir-unresponsive HSV infection applied cidofovir gel (0.3 or 1% strengths) or placebo once daily for 5 consecutive days. Cidofovir treatment was associated with statistically significant benefits on complete healing of lesions (30% versus 0%), shrinkage of lesions by 50% or more (50% versus 0%), cessation of virus shedding (87% versus 0%), and mean decrease in pain score, when compared with placebo (83). Twenty-five percent of 20 cidofovir-treated patients manifested application site reactions, compared with 20% of 10 placebo-treated patients.

A second agent studied for this indication is topical foscarnet cream (1%), which was applied five times daily to the acyclovir-resistant HSV lesions of 20 HIV-infected patients (84). After a mean of 35 days of treatment, 45% of lesions were healed, and an additional 25% showed at least a 50% decrease in size (84). However, 50% of treated patients developed either skin ulcerations or application site reactions.

Prevention and Immunity

Candidate HSV vaccines are currently under investigation. The trials perhaps furthest along in clinical evaluation are both of recombinant HSV-2 subunit glycoprotein derivatives combined with immunogenic adjuvants, developed by Chiron Corporation and SmithKline Beecham, respectively.

Both have appeared to be safe and immunogenic to date (85, 86); results regarding their efficacy as preventive and therapeutic modalities against HSV infection are expected within the next 1 to 2 years from multicenter, placebo-controlled phase III trials.

VARICELLA-ZOSTER VIRUS INFECTION

Epidemiology

Varicella tends to occur in children aged 1 to 15 years and has infected over 90% of individuals in the United States by age 15 years (87). Peak incidence of the 3.8 million cases in the United States yearly is in the late winter and early spring. The infection is highly communicable, with a secondary attack rate of up to 90% after a median incubation period of 14 days (87). The incubation period may be shortened in immunosuppressed patients.

In contrast, the probability of an outbreak of zoster increases with age and is most common in the elderly. An estimated 1.5 million cases of zoster occurred yearly in the United States before the onset of the AIDS epidemic (annual incidence, 0.14%; estimated lifetime risk, 10 to 20%). A report by Friedman-Kien and colleagues in 1986 noted that 8% of AIDS patients with Kaposi's sarcoma had a history of herpes zoster, a frequency sevenfold greater than that of age-matched controls (88). A study in San Francisco found an age-adjusted relative risk of 17 when comparing HIV-positive with HIV-seronegative homosexual men (89). Zoster can precede the diagnosis of AIDS by several years. As such, it is one of the AIDS-associated opportunistic pathogens that spans several stages of HIV-related immunosuppression, occurring both early and late. No evidence indicates that zoster induces or is associated with a more rapid progression of HIV infection (89).

Pathogenesis

The etiologic link between varicella and herpes zoster was first proposed in 1892 by the Viennese physician Von Bokay and ultimately was confirmed with the use of restriction endonuclease techniques in 1984 (90). The appearance of the typical rash of varicella follows asymptomatic viremia by 1 to 11 days in both immunocompetent and immunocompromised hosts (87). The appearance of T-lymphocyte proliferation to VZV antigen is correlated with milder illness if occurring early, as well as with rapid termination of viremia. The early production of VZV-specific immunoglobulin G (IgG) or IgM antibodies does not correlate with the clinical course of the infection (91). Transmission is primarily by inhalation of infectious respiratory secretions, although spread by direct mucous membrane contact has also been documented. Airborne transmission of infection in hospitals, resulting in nosocomial spread of infection, has also been described (87).

Although the mechanism is incompletely understood, lifelong latency of VZV appears to be established in the dorsal root ganglia; viral DNA has been recovered from both trigeminal and thoracic ganglia in seropositive individuals. Evidence suggests that the virus becomes latent in many ganglia after primary infection, and more than one region of the viral genome is present during latency (92). Cell-mediated immune mechanisms play a critical role in maintaining dormancy of the virus, and investigators have postulated that the increased incidence of zoster with advancing age corresponds to an immune senescence. Additionally, it appears that lifetime reexposure to VZV, either by vaccination or by close exposure to varicella, decreases the risk of zoster (93). Although humoral immunity may play a role as well, investigators have shown that zoster can occur despite substantial titers of VZV-specific antibody, and it is not more severe or prevalent in agammaglobulinemic patients (87). Although most episodes of zoster are caused by reactivation of latent virus, reports of small outbreaks have demonstrated that exogenous acquisition of zoster is possible as well.

Clinical Manifestations

Patients with varicella manifest macular, papular, vesicular, and crusted lesions diffusely after a prodrome of fever, malaise, arthralgias, or myalgias. In immunocompetent children, new lesions typically form for approximately 4 days; most crusting is completed by day 6 (87). Varicella in adults is associated with a more severe and prolonged course, as well as a 25-fold increased risk for mortality. Descriptions of primary varicella in HIV-infected persons are limited to date, but complications, including cutaneous bacterial superinfection, otitis media, pneumonia, and meningoencephalitis, appear to occur more frequently than in immunocompetent children (94–96). Additionally, reactivations resulting in zoster outbreaks appear to be of increased frequency in HIV-infected children compared with rates in leukemic children or in HIV-infected adults (97).

Herpes zoster, or shingles, generally begins with unilateral pain or dysesthesias that precede the appearance of rash by 1 to 4 days. Clusters of vesicles on an erythematous base subsequently erupt in a dermatomal distribution, evolving from a maculopapular appearance to vesicles and pustules over the course of 4 to 14 days. Full healing typically occurs within 4 weeks, although cutaneous scarring is common. The thoracic dermatome is most frequently involved. Rarely, the rash fails to appear after the typical prodrome ("zoster sine herpete").

Several authors have described cutaneous zoster infection in HIV-infected individuals as being more frequent, severe, or prolonged (30, 88, 98–101). Additionally, reports have noted an increased propensity to cutaneous dissemination (98, 101) and to recurrent zoster (102) in HIV-infected persons. Atypical cutaneous manifestations of zoster in the HIV-infected patient include hyperkeratotic (99, 103) or necrotic (101) skin lesions. Visceral dissemination of VZV causing hepatitis or pneumonitis in patients with AIDS has not been described.

Involvement of the ophthalmic branch of the trigeminal cranial nerve, known as herpes zoster ophthalmicus, is associated with corneal involvement in approximately 50% (90). Uveitis and scleritis may also occur. Several authors have suggested that this syndrome is more frequent in patients with HIV infection (104). The acute retinal necrosis syndrome, with involvement of the retina by VZV causing arteritis and necrosis, is bilateral in approximately one-third of patients and results in retinal detachment in up to three-fourths of patients (105, 106). A unique type of necrotizing retinitis caused by VZV, called rapidly progressive outer retinal necrosis, has also been described in patients with AIDS (107, 108) and is poorly responsive to therapy. In addition, optic neuritis resulting from VZV has been described (109).

Neurologic complications include myelitis, meningoencephalitis, and segmental motor paralysis. Several authors have described encephalitis of delayed or chronic onset in patients with HIV infection (110–112). In addition, contralateral hemiplegia may develop because of cerebral arteritis or infarction (112). The Ramsay Hunt syndrome, a motor neuropathy associated with cephalic zoster, consists of cutaneous lesions in the external auditory canal and hearing loss and vertigo resulting from involvement by the virus of the seventh and eighth cranial nerves. The risk of postherpetic neuralgia, usually defined as pain persisting for more than 1 month after the onset of zoster, increases with age (113). Although the incidence of postherpetic neuralgia appears to be increased in patients with ophthalmic zoster, no evidence suggests an increased incidence in immunocompromised patients (113).

Laboratory Diagnosis

Virus culture has a lower yield and requires a longer incubation for VZV than for HSV, requiring a total of 2 weeks of observation before being considered negative. Balfour has suggested that the aspiration of vesicles with a tuberculin syringe, the rubbing of the base of the lesion with the bevel of the syringe, the inoculation of the specimen onto human foreskin fibroblast monolayers within 15 minutes of collection, and the incubation of cell culture tubes at 36°C in 5% carbon dioxide increase the yield of virus culture for VZV (90).

Although culture of VZV is the current standard, the yield is suboptimal. Alternatives to virus culture include direct fluorescent antigen staining of a swab from the base of the lesion and a Tzanck smear. The former appears to be both sensitive and specific, whereas the latter is sensitive but does not enable one to distinguish between VZV and HSV infection.

Treatment

Acyclovir, acting by selective inhibition of virus DNA polymerase, has been shown to be effective for the treatment of varicella in both immunocompromised and immunocompetent children (114); this drug decreases morbidity from visceral dissemination in the former group and limits the duration of clinical illness in the latter. In addition, acyclovir has accelerated healing in adults and adolescents with varicella (115, 116). Initiation of therapy within 24 hours of the onset of rash appears to be necessary for optimal efficacy. Given that inhibitory concentrations of acyclovir against VZV are approximately 10-fold higher than against HSV, either intravenous (10 mg/kg every 8 hours) or high-dose oral (800 mg four to five times daily) acyclovir is required.

Acyclovir has been shown to shorten the period of virus shedding and to accelerate the time to healing of zoster in both immunocompetent (117–119) and immunocompromised (120) patients when compared with placebo. When compared with vidarabine, an antiviral agent licensed for the treatment of herpes zoster in immunosuppressed hosts, acyclovir was shown to be more effective in preventing cutaneous dissemination and in accelerating clinical and virologic healing in immunocompromised patients (121). However, in a study by Whitley and associates, acyclovir (10 mg/kg every 8 hours) and vidarabine (10 mg/kg/day) appeared to have equivalent efficacy and safety in immunosuppressed patients with cutaneously disseminated zoster, although patients treated with acyclovir were able to be discharged from the hospital sooner than those treated with vidarabine (122). Despite the absence of reported cases of visceral dissemination of zoster in HIV-infected individuals, as occurs in immunosuppressed patients with hematologic malignancies, acyclovir is frequently prescribed in HIV-infected patients to limit the duration of symptoms and virus shedding of the infection.

Two other agents are now licensed in the United States for the treatment of zoster infection: famciclovir (500 mg orally three times daily for 7 days) and valacyclovir (1 g orally three times daily for 7 days). Famciclovir is a prodrug of the guanosine analog penciclovir. Like acyclovir, it is activated through phosphorylation by the virus-specified thymidine kinase, thereafter inhibiting viral DNA synthesis by competitively inhibiting DNA polymerase (44). Oral bioavailability is substantially greater than that of acyclovir, and its intracellular half-life is 10 to 20 times longer. A randomized comparison with placebo in 419 immunocompetent adults with uncomplicated herpes zoster demonstrated accelerated lesion healing and a reduced duration of virus shedding (123). Although the proportion of patients with postherpetic neuralgia was unaffected by treatment, its time to resolution was approximately 2-fold greater than that in the placebo group (123). Valacyclovir is a prodrug of acyclovir, achieving serum levels 3 to 5 times those achieved with oral acyclovir in humans (46). A randomized double-blind trial comparing valacyclovir with acyclovir for therapy of uncomplicated zoster in immunocompetent adults showed comparable effects on lesion healing and cessation of virus shedding, as well as similar proportions of patients with postherpetic neuralgia, but a statistically significant reduction in the median duration of zoster-associated pain (124). Neither famciclovir nor valacyclovir is approved for use in immunocompromised patient populations, because of the lack of adequate study to date.

The decision whether to prescribe an antiviral agent depends on the immune status of the patient and severity of illness. In the HIV-infected patient, it is prudent to treat all episodes of varicella to limit morbidity or mortality. In the HIV-infected patient with zoster, initiation of therapy limits the duration of the acute episode; prevention of postherpetic neuralgia is likely as well, although its prevalence is uncommon in this young patient population. Visceral dissemination to internal organs has not been reported in patients with AIDS, such that treatment to prevent this complication is unlikely to have a high yield. Therefore, the decision to initiate antiviral therapy should be individualized and should depend on such factors as the extent and number of cutaneous lesions, as well as the time since the onset of the outbreak. Administration of acyclovir, or of alternative antiviral agents, is more routinely recommended for the treatment of herpes zoster ophthalmicus in HIV-infected patients, to reduce the risk of ocular complications (125).

The issue of adjunctive corticosteroid use for the treatment of zoster is still controversial. Although two randomized, placebo-controlled trials of acyclovir therapy with and without corticosteroids showed no significant effect on the duration of zoster-associated pain (126, 127), one showed an accelerated time to resolution of acute neuritis and of resumption of normal activities (127). Corticosteroid therapy should be reserved for persons older than 50 years who are at the highest risk of chronic pain, however, and it should be administered carefully if at all to immunocompromised persons.

The first report of acyclovir-resistant VZV infection occurred in a 4-year-old girl with congenital HIV infection in 1988 (128). Subsequently, several case reports of acyclovir-resistant VZV infection in HIV-infected patients have been published (99, 100, 103, 129–135); patients have been both children (103, 135) and adults (99, 100, 129–134) with advanced AIDS. A history of prior treatment with acyclovir, generally for a first episode of either varicella or zoster, is common, although not universal. In at least two patients described to date, resistance to acyclovir occurred during first exposure to acyclovir for the treatment of zoster (100, 131). Although most instances have been limited to cutaneous involvement, recent reports of acyclovir-resistant outer retinal necrosis (132) and meningoradiculoneuritis (133) are of concern.

Most reports of acyclovir-resistant VZV infection have described characteristic, atypical morphologies of cutaneous lesions, described as hyperkeratotic, verrucous, or "poxlike" (99, 100, 103, 129, 130, 134, 135). Some patients, however, have had typical vesiculoulcerative lesions resistant to acyclovir (131); conversely, some hyperkeratotic lesions have responded completely to treatment with acyclovir (130, 131). Therefore, such morphology probably reflects the chronicity of the lesions rather than the acyclovir-susceptibility phenotype. The presence of hyperkeratotic or heaped-up lesions, however, should serve as a stimulus for aggressive attempts at diagnosis and management, and susceptibility testing should be performed to assess resistance to acyclovir in patients whose response to treatment with optimal doses of acyclovir is less than expected.

Investigation of the mechanism of acyclovir resistance in VZV has generally revealed deficient or altered activity of the viral thymidine kinase, with nucleotide substitutions, deletions, or insertions within the thymidine gene (136, 137). Such isolates typically are cross-resistant to penciclovir (famciclovir) with retained susceptibility to foscarnet (136). Additionally, alteration in DNA polymerase has been suggested in a clinical isolate from one patient by concomitant resistance to both acyclovir and foscarnet (131).

Given the infrequency of acyclovir-resistant VZV infection to date, treatment trials have been limited. However, acyclovir-resistant clinical isolates of zoster have shown susceptibility in vitro to vidarabine (98) and to foscarnet (103, 129–133, 136, 137). Therapy with vidarabine has been unsuccessful in at least four patients described to date (99, 103, 128, 130), despite apparent susceptibility in vitro. The explanation for this failure is unclear, although findings have been similar in patients with acyclovir-resistant HSV infection treated with vidarabine (55). Foscarnet, a pyrophosphate analog, has in vitro activity against VZV (138, 139), although its potency is less than that of either acyclovir or vidarabine. In a series of five patients with AIDS and acyclovir-resistant VZV infection, therapy with foscarnet evoked complete healing in three patients after 14, 21, and 26 days, respectively (131). Another patient achieved nearly complete healing after 21 days of therapy. A fifth patient failed to have evidence of clinical or virologic response to foscarnet and discontinued the drug on day 14 of therapy because of gastrointestinal intolerance (131). Other reports have also described clinical responsiveness to foscarnet in patients with acyclovir-resistant VZV infection (129). However, intolerance to foscarnet may be dose limiting. An additional problem is recurrent VZV infection: in one series, two of four patients with resistant VZV infection who achieved complete healing with foscarnet had recurrent episodes of zoster just 7 and 14 days after discontinuation of foscarnet, respectively. Fortunately, in vitro testing demonstrated susceptibility to acyclovir in both patients, a finding suggesting that the phenotype of the virus latent in the ganglion had not been altered at the time when the cutaneous lesion became resistant to acyclovir. In another patient, however, foscarnet-resistant VZV infection emerged during long-term suppressive foscarnet therapy for cytomegalovirus retinitis (140). As with acyclovir, therefore (69), foscarnet-resistant infection may become a problem in patients exposed to the drug on a long-term basis or recurrently.

Evaluation of alternative agents to parenteral foscarnet for the treatment of patients with acyclovir-resistant VZV infection continues. TFT has in vitro activity against VZV (141); in one report, topical application of 1% TFT ophthalmic solution, in conjunction with intralesional injection of interferon-α2b, resulted in regression of the lesion (134). Cidofovir, by virtue of its lack of requirement for activation through phosphorylation by the virus-specified thymidine kinase, is likely to retain activity against acyclovir-resistant strains of VZV. Its clinical activity for this indication, however, has not yet been studied.

Prevention and Immunity

An episode of varicella generally confers lifelong immunity in the immunocompetent person, but reinfections may occur on exposure. Symptomatic reinfections may be more common in immunosuppressed individuals, and recurrences of zoster appear to be more common in HIV-infected patients than in others (96).

A live attenuated varicella (Oka strain) vaccine, developed by Takahashi and colleagues in 1974, has been licensed for use in the United States (142). Routine single-dose subcutaneous vaccination of children younger than 13 years of age should be performed, with expected seroconversion rates to protective levels of 97% (142). Susceptible persons 13 years old and older should received two doses of the vaccine, separated by 4 to 8 weeks; expected seroconversion rates are 99%. Vaccination is particularly advised for adults in the following categories: health care workers, employees at high-transmission settings such as day-care, inmates of correctional institutions, military personnel, family contacts of immunocompromised persons, nonpregnant women of childbearing age, and international travelers (142). Administration of this live, attenuated virus vaccine is contraindicated in immunocompromised individuals, including those with HIV infection (142). Although rates of zoster after vaccination have not yet been adequately studied, they are expected to be lower in adult vaccinees than in unvaccinated adults (142).

Varicella-zoster immune globulin (VZIG) should be administered to susceptible individuals after close contact with patients with varicella or zoster who are at high risk of complicated infection. When a patient's prior history of varicella is unknown, it is prudent to remember that 85 to 90% of adults in the United States are immune. Nevertheless, in the immunosuppressed patient with no history of varicella, administration of VZIG should be considered if respiratory or cutaneous contact was significant. VZIG needs to be administered as early as possible after exposure to be effective, so awaiting results of serum antibody testing to VZV before administering it is not recommended.

References

1. Hutfield DC. History of herpes genitalis. Br J Vener Dis 1966;42: 263–268.
2. Johnson RE, Nahmias AJ, Magder LS, et al. A seroepidemiologic survey of the prevalence of herpes simplex virus type 2 infection in the United States. N Engl J Med 1989;321:7–12.
3. Fleming DT, McQuillan GM, Johnson RE, et al. Herpes simplex virus type 2 in the United States, 1976 to 1994. N Engl J Med 1997;337:1105.
4. Siegel D, Golden E, Washington AE, et al. Prevalence and correlates of herpes simplex infections: the population-based AIDS in multiethnic neighborhoods study. JAMA 1992;268:1702–1708.
5. Safrin S, Ashley R, Houlihan C, et al. Clinical and serologic features of herpes simplex virus infection in patients with AIDS. AIDS 1991;5: 1107–1110.
6. Holmberg SD, Stewart JA, Gerber R, et al. Prior herpes simplex virus type 2 infection as a risk factor for HIV infection. JAMA 1988;259: 1048–1050.
7. Stamm WE, Handsfield H, Rompalo AM, et al. The association between genital ulcer disease and acquisition of HIV infection in homosexual men. JAMA 1988;260:1429–1433.
8. Hook EW III, Cannon RO, Nahmias AJ, et al. Herpes simplex virus infection as a risk factor for human immunodeficiency virus infection in heterosexuals. J Infect Dis 1992;165:251–255.
9. Corey L, Spear PG. Infections with herpes simplex viruses [Second of two parts]. N Engl J Med 1986;314:749–756.
10. Benedetti J, Corey L, Ashley R. Recurrence rates in genital herpes after symptomatic first-episode infection. Ann Intern Med 1994; 121:847–854.
11. Armstrong D, Gold JWM, Dryjanski J, et al. Treatment of infections in patients with the acquired immunodeficiency syndrome. Ann Intern Med 1985;103:738–743.
12. Siegal FP, Lopez C, Hammer GS, et al. Severe acquired immunodeficiency in male homosexuals, manifested by chronic perianal ulcerative herpes simplex lesions. N Engl J Med 1981;305:1439–1444.
13. Centers for Disease Control. Revision of the CDC surveillance case definition for AIDS. MMWR Morb Mortal Wkly Rep 1987; 36(Suppl):1S–15S.
14. Bagdades EK, Pillay D, Squire SB, et al. Relationship between herpes simplex virus ulceration and CD4+ cell counts in patients with HIV infection. AIDS 1992;6:1317–1320.
15. Wilson P, Cropper L, Sharp I. Apparent increase in the prevalence of herpes simplex virus type 1 genital infections among women [letter]. Genitourin Med 1994;70:228.
16. Langenberg A, Benedetti J, Jenkins J, et al. Development of clinically recognizable genital lesions among women previously identified as having "asymptomatic" herpes simplex virus type 2 infection. Ann Intern Med 1989;110:882–887.
17. Wald A, Zeh J, Selke S, et al. Virologic characteristics of subclinical and symptomatic genital herpes infections. N Engl J Med 1995; 333:770–775.
18. Augenbraun M, Feldman J, Chirgwin K, et al. Increased genital shedding of herpes simplex virus type 2 in HIV-seropositive women. Ann Intern Med 1995;123:845–847.
19. Schacker T, Collier A, Corey L. Frequent subclinical herpes simplex virus (HSV) shedding from multiple anatomic sites in HIV-infected people. In: 1st National Conference on Human Retroviruses [abstract 547]. Alexandria, VA: Infectious Diseases Society of America for the Foundation for Retrovirology and Human Health, 1993.
20. Goodell SE, Quinn TC, Mkrtichian E, et al. Herpes simplex virus proctitis in homosexual men: clinical, sigmoidoscopic and histopathological features. N Engl J Med 1983;308:868–871.
21. Genereau T, Lortholary O, Bouchaud O, et al. Herpes simplex esophagitis in patients with AIDS: report of 34 cases. Clin Infect Dis 1996;22:926–931.
22. Rowley AH, Whitley RJ, Lakeman FD, et al. Rapid detection of herpes-simplex-virus DNA in cerebrospinal fluid of patients with herpes simplex encephalitis. Lancet 1990;335:440–441.
23. Cone RW, Hobson AC, Palmer J, et al. Extended duration of herpes simplex virus DNA in genital lesions detected by the polymerase chain reaction. J Infect Dis 1991;164:757–760.
24. Ashley RL, Militoni J, Lee F, et al. Comparison of Western blot (immunoblot) and glycoprotein G-specific immunodot enzyme assay for detecting antibodies to herpes simplex virus types 1 and 2 in human sera. J Clin Microbiol 1988;26:662–667.
25. Safrin S, Arvin A, Mills J, et al. Comparison of the Western immunoblot assay and a glycoprotein G enzyme immunoassay for detection of serum antibodies to herpes simplex virus type 2 in patients with AIDS. J Clin Microbiol 1992;30:1312–1314.

26. Elion GB. Mechanism of action, spectrum and selectivity of nucleoside analogs. In: Mills J, Corey L, eds. Directions for clinical application and research. New York: Elsevier, 1986:118–137.
27. Spruance SL, Stewart JCB, Rowe NH, et al. Treatment of recurrent herpes simplex labialis with oral acyclovir. J Infect Dis 1990;161: 185–190.
28. Rooney JF, Straus SE, Mannix ML, et al. Oral acyclovir to suppress frequently recurrent herpes labialis: a double-blind, placebo-controlled trial. Ann Intern Med 1993;118:268–272.
29. Cohen SG, Greenberg MS. Chronic oral herpes simplex virus infection in immunocompromised patients. Oral Surg 1985;59:465–471.
30. Quinnan GV, Masur H, Rook AH, et al. Herpesvirus infections in the acquired immune deficiency syndrome. JAMA 1984;252:72–77.
31. Safrin S, Assaykeen T, Follansbee S, et al. Foscarnet therapy for acyclovir-resistant mucocutaneous herpes simplex virus infection in 26 AIDS patients: preliminary data. J Infect Dis 1990;161:1078–1084.
32. Crumpacker CS, Schnipper LE, Marlowe SI, et al. Resistance to antiviral drugs of herpes simplex virus isolated from a patient treated with acyclovir. N Engl J Med 1982;306:343–346.
33. Westheim AI, Tenser RB, Marks JG Jr. Acyclovir resistance in a patient with chronic mucocutaneous herpes simplex infection. J Am Acad Dermatol 1987;5:875–880.
34. Vinckier F, Boogaerts M, De Clerck D, et al. Chronic herpetic infection in an immunocompromised patient: report of a case. J Oral Maxillofac Surg 1987;45:723–728.
35. Mindel A, Adler MW. Intravenous acyclovir treatment for primary genital herpes. Lancet 1982;1:697–700.
36. Nilsen AE, Aasen T, Halsos AM, et al. Efficacy of oral acyclovir in the treatment of initial and recurrent genital herpes. Lancet 1982; 2:571–573.
37. Rompalo AM, Mertz GJ, Davis LG, et al. Oral acyclovir for treatment of first-episode herpes simplex virus proctitis. JAMA 1988;259: 2879–2881.
38. Whitley RJ, Alford CA, Hirsch MS, et al. Vidarabine versus acyclovir therapy in herpes simplex encephalitis. N Engl J Med 1986;314: 144–149.
39. Kaplowitz LG, Baker D, Gelb L, et al. Prolonged continuous acyclovir treatment of normal adults with frequently recurring genital herpes simplex virus infection. JAMA 1991;265:747–751.
40. Centers for Disease Control and Prevention. 1998 Guidelines for treatment of sexually transmitted diseases. MMWR Morb Mortal Wkly Rep 1998;47:23.
41. Mindel A, Carney O, Freris M, et al. Dosage and safety of long-term suppressive acyclovir therapy for recurrent genital herpes. Lancet 1988;I:926–928.
42. Wald A, Zeh J, Barnum G, et al. Suppression of subclinical shedding of herpes simplex virus type 2 with acyclovir. Ann Intern Med 1996;124:8–15.
43. Schacker T, Shaughnessy M, Barnum G, et al. Efficacy of famciclovir for suppressing HSV-2 infections among HIV+ persons [abstract]. In: 3rd Conference on Retroviruses and Opportunistic Infections. Alexandria, VA: Infectious Diseases Society of America for the Foundation for Retrovirology and Human Health, 1996.
44. Perry CM, Wagstaff AJ. Famciclovir: a review of its pharmacological properties and therapeutic efficacy in herpesvirus infections. Drugs 1995;50:396–415.
45. Sacks SL, Aoki FY, Diaz-Mitorna F, et al. Patient-initiated, twice-daily oral famciclovir for early recurrent genital herpes: a randomized, double-blind multicenter trial. JAMA 1996;276:44–49.
46. Beutner KR. Valacyclovir: a review of its antiviral activity, pharmacokinetic properties, and clinical efficacy. Antiviral Res 1995;28: 281–290.
47. Spruance SL, Tyring SK, DeGregorio B, et al. A large-scale, placebo-controlled, dose-ranging trial of peroral valaciclovir for episodic treatment of recurrent herpes genitalis. Arch Intern Med 1996;156: 1729–1735.
48. Kalb RE, Grossman ME. Chronic perianal herpes simplex in immunocompromised hosts. Am J Med 1986;80:486–490.
49. Balfour HH Jr, Benson C, Braun J, et al. Management of acyclovir-resistant herpes simplex and varicella-zoster virus infections. J Acquir Immune Defic Syndr 1994;7:254–260.
50. McLaren C, Corey L, Dekket C, et al. In vitro sensitivity to acyclovir in genital herpes simplex viruses from acyclovir-treated patients. J Infect Dis 1983;148:868–875.
51. Parris DS, Harrington JE. Herpes simplex virus variants resistant to high concentrations of acyclovir exist in clinical isolates. Antimicrob Agents Chemother 1982;22:71–77.
52. Norris SA, Kessler HA, Fife KH. Severe progressive herpetic whitlow caused by an acyclovir-resistant virus in a patient with AIDS. J Infect Dis 1987;157:209–210.
53. Gateley A, Gander RM, Johnson PC, et al. Herpes simplex virus 2 meningoencephalitis resistant to acyclovir in a patient with AIDS. J Infect Dis 1990;161:711–715.
54. Erlich KS, Mills J, Chatis P, et al. Acyclovir-resistant herpes simplex virus infections in patients with the acquired immunodeficiency syndrome. N Engl J Med 1989;320:293–296.
55. Safrin S, Crumpacker C, Chatis P, et al. A controlled trial comparing foscarnet with vidarabine for acyclovir-resistant mucocutaneous herpes simplex in the acquired immunodeficiency syndrome. N Engl J Med 1991;325:551–555.
56. Sacks SL, Wanklin RJ, Reece DE, et al. Progressive esophagitis from acyclovir-resistant herpes simplex: clinical roles for DNA polymerase mutants and viral heterogeneity. Ann Intern Med 1989;111:893–899.
57. Balfour HH. Resistance of herpes simplex to acyclovir. Ann Intern Med 1983;98:404–406.
58. Ellis MN, Keller PM, Fyfe JA, et al. Clinical isolate of herpes simplex virus type 2 that induces a thymidine kinase with altered substrate specificity. Antimicrob Agents Chemother 1987;31:1117–1125.
59. Parker AC, Craig JIO, Collins P, et al. Acyclovir-resistant herpes simplex virus infection due to altered DNA polymerase. Lancet 1987;2:1461.
60. Englund JA, Zimmerman ME, Swierkosz EM, et al. Herpes simplex virus resistant to acyclovir: a study in a tertiary care center. Ann Intern Med 1990;112:416–422.
61. McLaren C, Ellis MN, Hunter GA. A colorimetric assay for the measurement of the sensitivity of herpes simplex viruses to antiviral agents. Antiviral Res 1983;3:223–234.
62. Swierkosz EM, Scholl DR, Brown JL, et al. Improved DNA hybridization method for detection of acyclovir-resistant herpes simplex virus. Antimicrob Agents Chemother 1987;31:1465–1469.
63. Safrin S, Phan L, Elbeik T. A comparative evaluation of three methods of antiviral susceptibility testing of clinical herpes simplex virus isolates. Clin Diagn Virol 1995;4:81–91.
64. Safrin S, Elbeik T, Phan L, et al. Correlation between response to acyclovir and foscarnet therapy and in vitro susceptibility result for isolates of herpes simplex virus from human immunodeficiency virus–infected patients. Antimicrob Agents Chemother 1994;38: 1246–1250.
65. Martin JL, Ellis MN, Keller PM, et al. Plaque autoradiography assay for the detection and quantitation of thymidine kinase–deficient and thymidine kinase–altered mutants of herpes simplex virus in clinical isolates. Antimicrob Agents Chemother 1985;28:181–187.
66. Safrin S, Phan L. In vitro activity of penciclovir against clinical isolates of acyclovir-resistant and foscarnet-resistant herpes simplex virus. Antimicrob Agents Chemother 1993;37:2241–2243.
67. Chrisp P, Clissold SP. Foscarnet: a review of its antiviral activity, pharmacokinetic properties and therapeutic use in immunocompromised patients with cytomegalovirus retinitis. Drugs 1991;41:104–129.
68. Erlich KS, Jacobson MA, Koehler JE, et al. Foscarnet therapy for severe acyclovir-resistant herpes simplex virus type-2 infections in patients with the acquired immunodeficiency syndrome (AIDS): an uncontrolled trial. Ann Intern Med 1989;110:710–713.
69. Safrin S, Kemmerly S, Plotkin B, et al. Foscarnet-resistant herpes simplex virus infection in patients with AIDS. J Infect Dis 1994;169: 193–196.

70. Safrin S, Schacker T, Delehanty J, et al. Topical treatment of infection with acyclovir-resistant mucocutaneous herpes simplex virus with the ribonucleotide reductase inhibitor 348U87 in combination with acyclovir. Antimicrob Agents Chemother 1993;37:975–979.
71. Safrin S, McKinley G, McKeough M, et al. Treatment of acyclovir-unresponsive cutaneous herpes simplex virus infection with topically applied SP-303. Antiviral Res 1994;25:185–192.
72. Fletcher CV, Englund JA, Bean B, et al. Continous infusion of high-dose acyclovir for serious herpesvirus infections. Antimicrob Agents Chemother 1989;33:1375–1378.
73. Engel JP, Englund JA, Fletcher CV, et al. Treatment of resistant herpes simplex virus with continuous-infusion acyclovir. JAMA 1990;263:1662–1664.
74. Murphy M, Morley A, Eglin RP, et al. Topical trifluridine for mucocutaneous acyclovir-resistant herpes simplex II in AIDS patient [letter]. Lancet 1992;340:1040.
75. Amin AR, Robinson MR, Smith DD, et al. Trifluorothymidine 0.5% ointment in the treatment of aciclovir-resistant mucocutaneous herpes simplex in AIDS. AIDS 1996;10:1051–1053.
76. Birch CJ, Tyssen DP, Tachedjian G, et al. Clinical effects and in vitro studies of trifluorothymidine combined with interferon-α for treatment of drug-resistant and -sensitive herpes simplex virus infections. J Infect Dis 1992;166:108–112.
77. Kessler HA, Hurwitz S, Farthing C, et al. Pilot study of topical trifluridine for the treatment of acyclovir-resistant mucocutaneous herpes simplex disease in patients with AIDS (ACTG 172). J Acquir Immun Defic Syndr Hum Retrovirol 1996;12:147–152.
78. Hitchcock MJM, Jaffe HS, Martin JC, et al. Cidofovir, a new agent with potent anti-herpesvirus activity. Antiviral Chem Chemother 1996;7:115–127.
79. Mendel DB, Barkhimer DB, Chen MS. Biochemical basis for increased susceptibility to cidofovir of herpes simplex viruses with altered or deficient thymidine kinase activity. Antimicrob Agents Chemother 1995;39:2120–2122.
80. Snoeck R, Andrei G, De Clercq E, et al. A new topical treatment for resistant herpes simplex infections. N Engl J Med 1993;329:968–969.
81. Snoeck R, Andrei G, Gerard M, et al. Successful treatment of progressive mucocutaneous infection due to acyclovir- and foscarnet-resistant herpes simplex virus with (S)-1-(3-hydroxy-2-phosphonylmethoxypropyl)cytosine (HPMPC). Clin Infect Dis 1994;18:570–578.
82. Lalezari JP, Drew WL, Glutzer E, et al. Treatment with intravenous (S)-1-[3-hydroxy-2-(phosphonylmethoxy)propyl]-cytosine of acyclovir-resistant mucocutaneous infection with herpes simplex virus in a patient with AIDS. J Infect Dis 1994;170:570–572.
83. Lalezari JP, Drew WL, Glutzer E, et al. (S)-1-[3-Hydroxy-2-(phosphonylmethoxy)propyl]cytosine (cidofovir): results of a phase I/II study of a novel antiviral nucleotide analogue. J Infect Dis 1995;171:788–796.
84. Hardy D, Javaly K, Wohlfeiler M, et al. Phase I, pilot study of the safety and efficacy of foscarnet (PFA) cream for treatment (Rx) of acyclovir-unresponsive (ACV-R) herpes simplex (HSV) [abstract 167]. In: the 3rd Conference on Retroviruses and Opportunistic Infections. Alexandria, VA: Infectious Diseases Society of America for the Foundation for Retrovirology and Human Health, 1996.
85. Langenberg AGM, Burke RL. Adair SF, et al. A recombinant glycoprotein vaccine for herpes simplex type 2: safety and efficacy. Ann Intern Med 1995;122:889–898.
86. Leroux-Roels G, Moreau E, Desombere I, et al. Persistence of humoral and cellular immune response and booster effect following vaccination with herpes simplex (gD2t) candidate vaccine with MPL [abstract H57]. In: 34th Interscience Conference on Antimicrobial Agents and Chemotherapy. Washington, DC: American Society for Microbiology, 1994.
87. Straus SE, Ostrove JM, Inchauspe G, et al. Varicella-zoster virus infections. Ann Intern Med 1988;108:221–237.
88. Friedman-Kien AE, Lafleur FL, Gendler E, et al. Herpes zoster: a possible early clinical sign for development of acquired immunodeficiency syndrome in high-risk individuals. J Am Acad Dermatol 1986;14:1023–1028.
89. Buchbinder SP, Katz MH, Hessol NA, et al. Herpes zoster and human immunodeficiency virus infection. J Infect Dis 1992;166:1153–1156.
90. Balfour HH Jr. Varicella zoster virus infections in immunocompromised hosts. Am J Med 1988;85:68–73.
91. Arvin AM, Koropchak CM, Bryan RG, et al. Early immune response in healthy and immunocompromised subjects with primary varicella-zoster virus infection. J Infect Dis 1986;154:422–426.
92. Mahalingam R, Wellish M, Wolf W, et al. Latent varicella-zoster viral DNA in human trigeminal and thoracic ganglia. N Engl J Med 1990;323:627–631.
93. Gershon AA, LaRussa P, Steinberg S, et al. The protective effect of immunologic boosting against zoster: an analysis in leukemic children who were vaccinated against chickenpox. J Infect Dis 1996;173:450–453.
94. Jura E, Chadwick EG, Josephs SH, et al. Varicella-zoster virus infections in children infected with human immunodeficiency virus. Pediatr Infect Dis J 1989;8:586–590.
95. Srugo I, Israele V, Wittek AE, et al. Clinical manifestations of varicella-zoster virus infections in human immunodeficiency virus–infected children. Am J Dis Child 1993;147:742–745.
96. von Seidlein L, Gillette SG, Bryson Y, et al. Frequent recurrences and persistence of varicella-zoster virus infections in children infected with human immunodeficiency virus type 1. J Pediatr 1996;128:52–57.
97. Gershon A, Mervish N, Larussa P, et al. Varicella-zoster virus infections in HIV-infected children [abstract 119]. In: 34th annual meeting of the Infectious Diseases Society of America. Alexandria, VA: Infectious Diseases Society of America, 1996.
98. Gilson IH, Barnett JH, Conant MA, et al. Disseminated ecthymatous herpes varicella-zoster virus infection in patients with acquired immunodeficiency syndrome. J Am Acad Dermatol 1989;20:637–642.
99. Hoppenjans WB, Bibler MR, Orme RL, et al. Prolonged cutaneous herpes zoster in acquired immunodeficiency syndrome. Arch Dermatol 1990;126:1048–1050.
100. Janier M, Hillion B, Baccard M, et al. Chronic varicella zoster infection in acquired immunodeficiency syndrome. J Am Acad Dermatol 1988;18:584–585.
101. Cohen PR, Beltrani VP, Grossman ME. Disseminated herpes zoster in patients with human immunodeficiency virus infection. Am J Med 1988;84:1076–1080.
102. Glesby MJ, Moore RD, Chaisson RE, et al. Herpes zoster in patients with advanced human immunodeficiency virus infection treated with zidovudine. J Infect Dis 1993;168:1264–1268.
103. Jacobson MA, Berger TG, Fikrig S, et al. Acyclovir-resistant varicella zoster virus infection after chronic oral acyclovir therapy in patients with the acquired immunodeficiency syndrome (AIDS). Ann Intern Med 1990;112:187–191.
104. Sandor E, Croxson TS, Millman A, et al. Herpes zoster ophthalmicus in patients at risk for AIDS [letter]. N Engl J Med 1984;310:1118–1119.
105. Jabs DA, Schachat AP, Liss R, et al. Presumed varicella zoster retinitis in immunocompromised patients. Retina 1987;7:9–13.
106. Sellitti TP, Huang AJW, Schiffman J, et al. Association of herpes zoster ophthalmicus with acquired immunodeficiency syndrome and acute retinal necrosis. Am J Ophthalmol 1993;116:297–301.
107. Forster DJ, Dugel PU, Frangieh GT, et al. Rapidly progressive outer retinal necrosis in the acquired immunodeficiency syndrome. Am J Ophthalmol 1990;110:341–348.
108. Margolis TP, Lowder CY, Holland GN, et al. Varicella-zoster virus retinitis in patients with the acquired immunodeficiency syndrome. Am J Ophthalmol 1991;112:119–131.
109. Litoff D, Catalano RA. Herpes zoster optic neuritis in human immunodeficiency virus infection. Arch Ophthalmol 1990;108:782–783.

110. Gilden DH, Murray RS, Wellish M, et al. Chronic progressive varicella-zoster virus encephalitis in an AIDS patient. Neurology 1988;38:1150–1153.
111. Ryder JW, Croen K, Kleinschmidt-DeMasters BK, et al. Progressive encephalitis three months after resolution of cutaneous zoster in a patient with AIDS. Ann Neurol 1986;19:182–188.
112. Veenstra J, van Praag RME, Krol A, et al. Complications of varicella zoster virus reactivation in HIV-infected homosexual men. AIDS 1996;10:393–399.
113. Kost RG, Straus SE. Postherpetic neuralgia—Pathogenesis, treatment and prevention. N Engl J Med 1996;355:32–42.
114. Dunkle LM, Arvin AM, Whitley RJ, et al. A controlled trial of acyclovir for chickenpox in normal children. N Engl J Med 1991;325:1539–1544.
115. Wallace MR, Bowler WA, Murray NB, et al. Treatment of adult varicella with oral acyclovir: a randomized, placebo-controlled trial. Ann Intern Med 1992;117:358–363.
116. Balfour HH, Rotbart HA, Feldman S, et al. Acyclovir treatment of varicella in otherwise healthy adolescents. J Pediatrics 1992;120:627–633.
117. Peterslund NA, Ipsen J, Schonheyder H, et al. Acyclovir in herpes zoster. Lancet 1992;1:827–830.
118. Bean B, Braun C, Balfour HH Jr. Acyclovir therapy for acute herpes zoster. Lancet 1992;1:118–121.
119. McKendrick MW, McGill JI, White JE, et al. Oral acyclovir in acute herpes zoster. Br Med J (Clin Res) 1986;293:1529–1532.
120. Balfour HH Jr, Bean B, Laskin OL, et al. Acyclovir halts progression of herpes zoster in immunocompromised patients. N Engl J Med 1983;308:1448–1453.
121. Shepp DH, Dandliker PS, Meyers JD. Treatment of varicella-zoster virus infection in severely immunocompromised patients: a randomized comparison of acyclovir and vidarabine. N Engl J Med 1986;314:208–212.
122. Whitley RJ, Gnann JW Jr, Hinthorn D, et al. Disseminated herpes zoster in the immunocompromised host: a comparative trial of acyclovir and vidarabine. J Infect Dis 1992;165:450–455.
123. Tyring S, Barbarash RA, Nahlik JE, et al. Famciclovir for the treatment of acute herpes zoster: effects on acute disease and postherpetic neuralgia: a randomized, double-blind, placebo-controlled trial. Ann Intern Med 1995;123:89–96.
124. Beutner KR, Friedman DJ, Forszpaniak C, et al. Valaciclovir compared with acyclovir for improved therapy for herpes zoster in immunocompetent adults. Antimicrob Agents Chemother 1995;39:1546–1553.
125. Cobo M. Reduction of the ocular complications of herpes zoster ophthalmicus by oral acyclovir. Am J Med 1988;85(Suppl 2A):90–93.
126. Wood MJ, Johnson RW, McKendrick MW, et al. A randomized trial of acyclovir for 7 days or 21 days with and without prednisolone for treatment of acute herpes zoster. N Engl J Med 1994;330:896–900.
127. Whitley RJ, Weiss H, Gnann JW, et al. Acyclovir with and without prednisone for the treatment of herpes zoster. Ann Intern Med 1996;125:376–383.
128. Pahwa S, Biron K, Lim W, et al. Continuous varicella-zoster infection associated with acyclovir resistance in a child with AIDS. JAMA 1988;260:2879–2882.
129. Smith KJ, Kahlter DC, Davis C, et al. Acyclovir-resistant varicella zoster responsive to foscarnet. Arch Dermatol 1991;127:1069–1071.
130. Linnemann CC, Biron KK, Hoppenjans WG, et al. Emergence of acyclovir-resistant varicella zoster virus in an AIDS patient on prolonged acyclovir therapy. AIDS 1990;4:577–579.
131. Safrin S, Berger TG, Gilson I, et al. Foscarnet therapy in five patients with AIDS and acyclovir-resistant varicella-zoster virus infection. Ann Intern Med 1991;115:19–21.
132. Wunderli W, Miner R, Wintsch J, et al. Outer retinal necrosis due to a strain of varicella-zoster resistant to acyclovir, ganciclovir, and sorivudine [letter]. Clin Infect Dis 1996;22:864–865.
133. Snoeck R, Gerard M, Sadzot-Delvaux C, et al. Meningoradiculitis due to acyclovir-resistant varicella-zoster virus in a patient with AIDS [letter]. J Infect Dis 1993;168:1330–1331.
134. Rossi S, Whitfeld M, Berger TG. The treatment of acyclovir-resistant herpes zoster with trifluorothymidine and interferon alfa. Arch Dermatol 1995;131:24–26.
135. Lyall EGH, Ogilvie MM, Smith NM, et al. Acyclovir resistant varicella zoster and HIV infection. Arch Dis Child 1994;70:133–135.
136. Talarico CL, Phelps WC, Biron KK. Analysis of the thymidine kinase genes from acyclovir-resistant mutants of varicella-zoster virus isolated from patients with AIDS. J Virol 1993;67:1024–1033.
137. Boivin G, Edelman CK, Pedneault L, et al. Phenotypic and genotypic characterization of acyclovir-resistant varicella-zoster viruses isolated from persons with AIDS. J Infect Dis 1994;170:68–75.
138. Baba M, Konno K, Shigeta S, et al. Inhibitory effects of selected antiviral compounds on newly isolated clinical varicella-zoster virus strains. Tohoku J Exp Med 1986;148:275–283.
139. Preblud SR, Arbeter AM, Proctor EA, et al. Susceptibility of vaccine strains of varicella-zoster virus to antiviral compounds. Antimicrob Agents Chemother 1984;25:417–421.
140. Fillet AM, Visse B, Caumes E, et al. Foscarnet-resistant multidermatomal zoster in a patient with AIDS. Clin Infect Dis 1995;21:1348–1349.
141. Shigeta S, Yokota T, Iwabuchi T, et al. Comparative efficacy of antiherpes drugs against various strains of varicella-zoster virus. J Infect Dis 1983;147:576–584.
142. Centers for Disease Control and Prevention. Prevention of varicella. MMWR Morb Mortal Wkly Rep 1996;45:1–36.

25

PROGRESSIVE MULTIFOCAL LEUKOENCEPHALOPATHY

Joseph R. Berger and Eugene O. Major

Progressive multifocal leukoencephalopathy (PML) was first crystallized as a distinct entity by Aström, Mancall, and Richardson in 1958 (1). The syndrome was identified chiefly on the basis of its unique pathologic features of demyelination, abnormal oligodendroglial nuclei, and giant astrocytes. In their review of the literature, these authors discovered prior descriptions of this entity dating to 1930 (2). By 1984, a comprehensive review of PML found only a total of 230 reported cases in the literature (3), of which 69 cases were pathologically confirmed and 40 cases were both virologically and pathologically confirmed. In this series, only 2 of the 230 cases were associated with the acquired immunodeficiency syndrome (AIDS) (4, 5). This number represented 3.0% of all cases in which an underlying disease was identified (3). PML occurring in association with AIDS was reported within 1 year (4) of the initial recognition of AIDS in 1981 (6–8). Since then, this formerly rare disease has become remarkably common. In a study from southern Florida, a 12-fold increase in incidence was observed when the 4-year interval from 1981 to 1984 was compared with the interval from 1991 to 1994 (9). In this study, AIDS-related cases of PML were 50 times more common than those associated with other causes of immunosuppression (9).

The initial description of this illness by Hallervorden was in a monograph entitled "Eigennartige und nicht rubriziebare Prozess" ("Unique and Nonclassifiable Processes") (2). He described two patients, one with tuberculosis and the other without recognized underlying systemic disease, who exhibited multifocal neurologic symptoms associated with discrete areas of demyelination accompanied by bizarre enlarged astrocytes (2). The monograph contained no description of the third histopathologic hallmark of PML, namely, the enlarged oligodendroglial nuclei. With respect to this unusual illness and the others described in his monograph, Hallervorden expressed the opinion that this disease and so many other rare diseases were often excluded from "comprehensive surveys as worthless curiosities" (2). However, he correctly asserted that the value of these unusual cases was often in uncovering unexpected relationships, as proved clearly to be the case with PML.

ETIOLOGY AND PATHOGENESIS

PML is a demyelinating disease of the central nervous system (CNS) that results from infection of oligodendrocytes with JC virus (JCV), a papovavirus. Evidence of a viral origin was initially provided by electron microscopic studies demonstrating papovavirus-like particles in the nuclei of abnormal oligodendrocytes (10–12) approximately a decade after its initial clinical and pathologic description (1, 13–15). This observation was subsequently confirmed by viral isolation. In 1971, Padgett and associates isolated a human polyomavirus (double-stranded DNA–containing virus with an icosahedral symmetry) from long-term cultures composed chiefly of glial cells (14). This virus was capable of hemagglutination of human type O erythrocytes, allowing for determination of antibody in patients. In most cases of PML in which virologic confirmation has been obtained, JCV is the cause. In only three cases has another papovavirus, SV40, been implicated (16–18), and a third papovavirus, BK virus, has not been proved to be neuropathogenic. The cases attributed to SV40 have not been well characterized, and, in some instances, reexamination of these brain tissues by in situ DNA hybridization has revealed JCV, not SV40 (19).

We are only now beginning to understand the pathogenesis of this disease. Chiefly, two reasons explain the improved understanding of PML after two decades of investigation. First, the incidence of PML has increased because of AIDS, and, consequently, investigators have had more opportunity to study the disease. Second, highly sensitive molecular techniques have been developed that allow detection of a few copies of a viral genome including advances in in situ hybridization and amplication of viral genomes using polymerase chain reaction (PCR; 20–27). Application of these techniques to tissues available from patients with PML has focused investigations on determining mechanisms of viral multiplication (23, 28, 29), cellular control over viral gene expression (30, 31), and delivery of virus to the CNS (27, 32). Information now forthcoming helps to explain how the etiologic virus, JCV, can be such a widespread infectious agent in the population by antibody measures yet target such a highly specialized cell in the nervous system, the myelinating oligodendrocyte. Before describing our current understanding of viral pathogenesis, a brief description of the biology and molecular regulation of JCV follows.

Biology of JC Virus

JCV belongs to the *Polyomavirus* genus in the Papovavirus family, represented also by another human polyomavirus, BKV, which shares more than 70% nucleotide homology with JCV (32). BKV, however, has not been associated with PML or other neurologic diseases but causes a serious viral infection in kidney tissue in renal transplant patients (34–36). JCV has a simple DNA genome of 5.1 kilobases in a double-stranded, supercoiled form, encapsidated in an icosahedral protein structure measuring 40 nm in diameter (Fig. 25.1). The DNA codes for two nonstructural proteins. One protein is the large T, which is a multifunctional protein. Three capsid proteins (VP1, VP2, VP3) are present (Fig. 25.2). The T protein is a DNA binding protein and is responsible for initiation of viral DNA replication, transcription including the capsid proteins, and interaction with cellular proteins such as p53 and retinoblastoma protein. In certain rodent and nonhuman primate cells, JCV T-protein expression is consistent with malignant transformation or tumor induction, particularly of astroglial cells into astrocytomas (11, 37–41). In these cells, only the T protein, named for its tumor-promoting function, is expressed. There is little evidence in human gliomas of the presence of JC virions or free or integrated JCV DNA (42, 43). One recent report, however, has described JCV T protein in an oligoastrocytoma in an immunocompetent patient (44). The mRNAs responsible for these proteins are transcribed from opposite strands of the DNA genome (T or capsid protein) and in opposite directions starting from near the viral origin of replication. Cellular splicing accounts for another nonstructural protein, t, from the same DNA strand as the T protein. The smaller t protein does not seem to play a *major* role in the multiplication of the virus and consequently is not considered important for pathogenicity.

Approximately 200 nucleotide base pairs of noncoding sequence are located between the 2 coding sequence areas. This region of the genome contains the signals for DNA replication as well as for promotion and enhancement of transcription (33, 45). It is termed the *regulatory region* and is considered the primary area of the genome responsible for the cellular tropism of JCV (46, 47). This is also the region of the viral genome found in the brain tissue of many PML patients that demonstrates the most sequence variability resulting from deletions and rearrangements perhaps acquired during propagation in brain or in extraneural host tissues (48, 49).

The observation that JCV was a neurotropic virus exclusive to glial cells was derived largely from the initial descriptions of JCV host range. From its first isolation in cultures derived from human fetal brain (10, 14), early studies of JCV host range emphasized the almost exclusive nature of growth in glial cells. JCV does not usually infect neurons in PML brain tissue or in cultures from either human adult or fetal brain, but it does infect both oligodendrocytes and astrocytes (50–52). Experiments using infectious clones of viral DNA reinforced a glial specific host range for transcription of JCV (33, 53). Other studies used recombinant DNA constructs of the viral regulatory sequences linked to a reporter gene, chloramphenicol acetyl transferase (CAT), to achieve a quantitative measurement of transcriptional activity. Activity of the CAT gene was greatest in human glial cells (54). Considering that JCV could induce a malignant transformation in rodent and monkey glial cells but did not multiply in glial cells of these animals, it was known that viral DNA replication was controlled at the species level. Unlike with many other human viral pathogens, susceptibility to JCV infection is not associated with viral attachment to specific cell receptors and penetration, but rather, it is controlled by cell type–specific factors for transcription and species-specific factors for replication (55). These studies have since directed experiments to delineate the molecular factors responsible for JCV growth and have begun to promote an understanding of its pathogenesis at the molecular level.

Molecular Control of JCV Gene Expression

To explain the neurotropism of JCV for glial cells, experiments concentrated on identifying nuclear DNA binding proteins that selectively interacted with the regulatory region of the genome. Such proteins, it is assumed, would bind specific *cis*-acting nucleotide base pairs (np) for control of JCV transcription. Using techniques of gel retention,

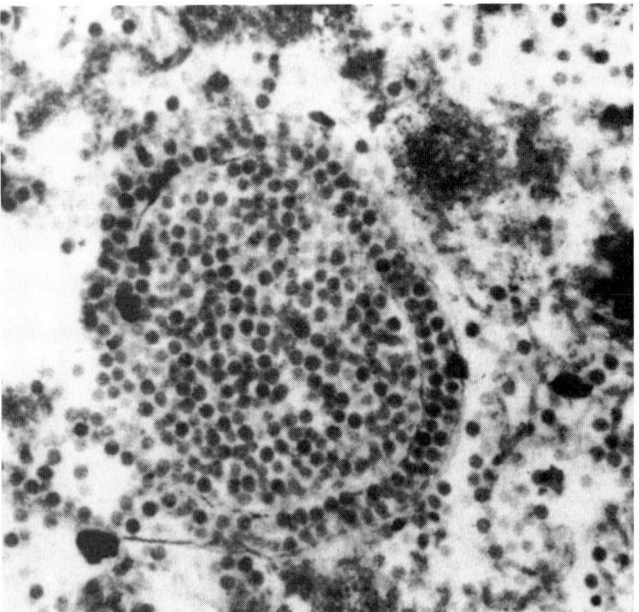

Figure 25.1. Electron micrograph of brain tissue from a patient with progressive multifocal leukoencephalopathy showing the assempy of JC virion particles in the nucleus of an infected oligodendrocyte. (From Major EO, Amemiya K, Tornatore CS, et al. Pathogenesis and molecular biology of progressive multifocal leukoencephalopathy, the JC virus–induced demyelinating disease of the human brain. Clin Microbiol Rev 1992;5:49–73.)

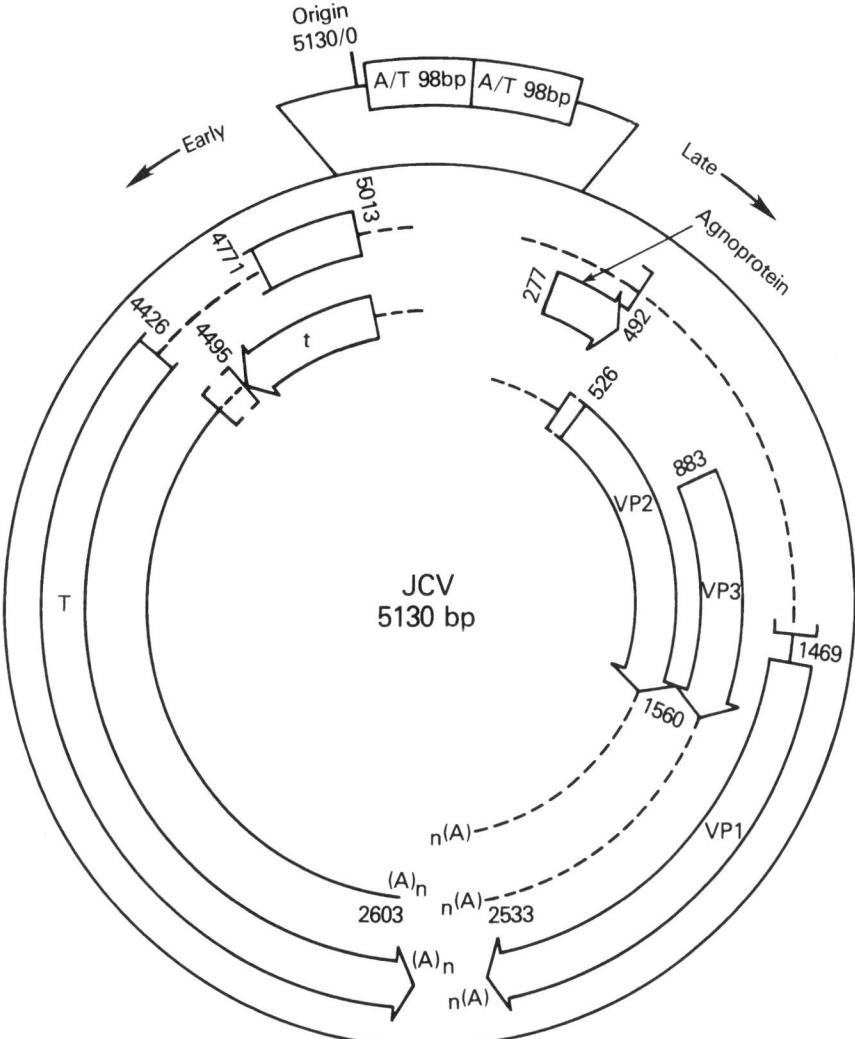

Figure 25.2. Schematic diagram of the JC virus genome. The circular map shows the beginning and end of the putative open-reading frames. Two open-reading frames (*T* and *t*) are shown in the early region on the *left* side, and four open-reading frames (*agnoprotein, VP1, VP2,* and *VP3*) are shown in the late region on the *right* side. The relative positions of the origin of DNA replication and the 98-bp repeat units in the noncoding region are indicated at the *top*. (From Major EO, Amemiya K, Tornatore CS, et al. Pathogenesis and molecular biology of progressive multifocal leukoencephalopathy, the JC virus–induced demyelinating disease of the human brain. Clin Microbiol Rev 1992;5:49–73.)

protein–DNA cross-linking and DNase footprint analysis as *cis*-acting DNA sequences were identified in the regulatory region at nt 33-58 on the viral genome map (56). Because the regulatory region comprises direct tandem repeats of 98 nucleotide pairs each, these binding sites exist twice, as expected, in both repeats. Two other series of nucleotide pairs were also identified as binding sites for nuclear proteins, located to either side of np 33-58 (57). One of these areas, directly next to the sequences necessary for DNA replication, in the direction of the T-protein coding region, is rich in repeated AT sequences that are known to function as RNA start sites (30, 45, 58, 59). The protein that binds these sequences is the TFIID transcription factor represented in almost all eukaryotic cells (60). The other protein-binding site covers an area that includes the transcriptional enhancer for JCV because its sequence is similar, but not identical, to sequences previously described for this function (61). However, nuclear extracts from nonpermissive cells demonstrated some binding to these regions. The functional consequence of this binding appeared to downregulate JCV activity in these cells (31). Therefore, it seems that some proteins positively regulate JCV expression and some block expression in a cell type–specific manner. The region of the regulatory sequences most efficiently bound by protein factor from permissive glial cells was the area of nt 33-58. This area covers the consensus sequence for the binding of nuclear factor 1 (NF-1), a protein that functions in both transcriptional control and replication of DNA. Several reports from independent laboratories have identified an NF-1–like protein found in glial cells that binds to this region (30, 56, 62, 63). A specific class of NF-1, NF-1/D or X, is highly expressed in human glial cells and correlates with susceptibility to JCV infection (64, 65). Another report identified a cDNA for a glial specific factor, GF1, that may also be related to NF-1 and that binds to this region (66). Further implications of NF-1 in JCV regulation come from experiments using purified NF-1 proteins, not simply nuclear extracts, that would compete with extracts for binding to the target sequences in the JCV promoter/enhancer region (30, 67). Additional DNase footprinting data resolved another protein binding immediately adjacent to the NF-1 binding site. This site has been identified as the binding domain for the c-jun protein or *activator protein* (AP-1), another ubiquitous transcription factor. The combination of binding sites for NF-1 and c-jun separated by only a few nucleotides appears to be a common feature for expressions of many brain-specific genes such as glial fibrillary acidic protein (GFAP), neurofilament, human and mouse MBP, S100b, proteolipid protein, and proenkephalin (30). Whether direct interaction occurs between these proteins is not known. Because both NF-1 and c-jun proteins are found in many other cells besides glial cells, these data suggest a family of such proteins. Glial cell susceptibility to JCV infection may be determined by the presence of specific members of this family of transcription proteins that are only present in permissive cells. Cells that are not permissive to JCV infection probably do not have these same protein factors or have other proteins that bind the JCV regulatory sequences and block transcription (30, 31).

Molecular Interactions Between JCV and HIV-1

Because of the increased incidence of PML in AIDS patients, suggestions of direct interactions between JCV and human immunodeficiency virus type 1 (HIV-1) have been tested. The JCV T protein can transactivate the HIV-1 long terminal repeat units (LTR), and the reverse, the transactivator protein of HIV-1, *tat*, can increase transcription from the JCV regulatory region (68). Further studies in glial cell cultures showed that this effect can be specific to the promotion of the JCV late MRNA synthesis, the coding sequences for capsid proteins (69). In this same series of experiments, the JCV T protein was able to stimulate the HIV-1 regulatory sequences, the viral LTR found at the 5′ and 3′ ends of the genome, in either glial or nonglial cells. Novel experiments, however, were done in which both the HIV-1 TAT sequences and a clone that contained the JCV promotor and the *tat* response element, TAR, were introduced into cells normally nonpermissive to JCV. The cells that received both DNA clones showed a high degree of expression from the JCV promoter. The transactivation by *tat* was at the transcriptional level. These data showed that the JCV promoter/enhancer can be functional in nonpermissive cells if specific transcriptional proteins are appropriately regulated (70). As yet, no clear data show that both HIV-1 and JCV infect the same cells in AIDS patients with PML. The white matter lesions from such patients' brain tissue frequently are distinct, but they can also be in close proximity (71). The HIV-1 *tat* protein has been shown to diffuse in cell cultures and can be taken up by neighboring cells (72, 73). Whether a similar mechanism for distribution of *tat* to JCV-infected cells occurs in vivo remains to be observed or tested. Direct or indirect interactions between these two viruses may take place outside the nervous system before entry to the brain. The most likely location for this to take place would be cells of the immune system. HIV-1 chiefly infects macrophages, monocytes, and T and B lymphocytes. In addition to glial cells, JCV has been found in uroepithelial cells in the urinary tract (74, 75), in B lymphocytes in bone marrow and spleen (31), and in peripheral blood lymphocytes (26, 76). Further studies of potential viral interactions at the molecular level are underway in several laboratories.

Molecular Pathogenesis of PML

The clinical descriptions of the course of PML and the identification of JCV in oligodendrocytes were well documented from the first recognition of the disease (11, 15, 77). The explanation of how JCV enters the brain and initiates infection, however, came much later. Current evidence implicates viral latency in lymphocytes in bone marrow or other lymphoid tissues that can be activated during immune suppression and can enter the peripheral blood (33, 77, 78). Circulating infected lymphocytes may be able to cross the blood–brain barrier and to pass infection to astrocytes at the border of vessels that, in turn, augment infection through multiplication eventually to infect oligodendrocytes. Using in situ DNA hydridization, JCV-infected cells are frequently found near blood vessels in the brain, in B lymphocytes in bone marrow (32), and in brain (29). JCV infection has also been documented in hematopoietic stem cells, in CD34+, and in normal B lymphocytes in culture (78). In a report of 19 patients with biopsy-proved PML, more than 90% had JCV DNA in peripheral blood lymphocytes using the PCR technology (26). The number of patients with PML with viral DNA in their peripheral blood lymphocyte circulation has been widely reported, with the percentage ranging from 45 to 90% (79, 80). These studies were done using a series of paired primers representative of three regions of the viral genome to eliminate possible nonspecific amplification of closely related DNA sequences. Data derived from other groups of individuals without PML revealed that 60% of HIV-1 seropositive individuals, 30% of renal transplant recipients, and approximately 5% of normal, healthy volunteers also had JCV DNA in their peripheral circulation. The group whose immune systems may be compromised through immunosuppressive therapies or other diseases would be considered at risk for the development of PML.

Approximately 5 to 10% of the population excrete JCV in urine detected by either PCR or virus isolation; this group includes pregnant women, older individuals, and some organ transplant patients (20, 81–83). These observations have led to the suggestion of the kidney as the site of viral latency. The DNA sequence of the regulatory region from the kidney or urine in these individuals is different from the sequence found in the brain of patients with PML (84). Because the regulatory DNA sequence chiefly governs infectivity of JCV, certain JCV isolates or clones of DNA have been studied. The most prominent DNA sequence arrangement found related to the kidney has been described as an archetype sequence (85). The archetype sequence contains 187 nucleotide pairs with no tandem repeats, but it does contain the origin of viral replication and the TATA sequence as an RNA start site. It also contains a 23-nucleotide pair insert next to the TATA site that is found in many regulatory region sequences from PML brain (49, 86). These sequences probably serve as a functional binding site for the Sp1 DNA transcription factor (86, 87). To convert the archetype sequence to that most often found in PML brain tissue, however, would require deletions, substitutions, and duplications (84, 88). Currently, no evidence of any biologic activity for the archetype sequence or virus isolates that contain these sequences exists. Several regulatory region sequences have been identified from JCV DNA in peripheral blood of patients with PML that are not related to the archetype but are closely related to sequences found in PML brain (26). Further examination of the distribution and importance of the archetype sequence is needed to understand its role in pathogenesis of PML. However, the existence of many variations of the DNA sequence of the regulatory region of JCV highlights the genome diversity of JCV. These data, however, have identified several regions within the regulatory sequences that are always represented and, by inference, are thought to be critical for viral multiplication and perhaps pathogenicity. The origin of replication, the TATA sequence, the 23-nucleotide insert, and sequences found just next to this insert that extend to nucleotides 58-68 are heavily represented in DNA sequences in PML brain (26, 49, 84, 85). These sequences are responsible for the duplication of the viral genome (the origin), the initiation of RNA synthesis (TATA sequences), and transcriptional control (the putative NF-1 binding and possibly the c-jun binding sites).

As mentioned earlier, present evidence suggest that lymphoid organs, particularly bone marrow, may harbor JCV in a latent state and, on activation, may carry virus to the brain. If this is correct, then these cells must also have nuclear DNA binding proteins that recognize these important sites on the JCV regulatory region. Using both gel retention assays and DNase footprinting experiments, investigators described several human B-cell lines as permissive for JCV multiplication and possessing DNA binding proteins that recognized the same sequences on the JCV genome as the highly permissive human glial cells (89). Although these proteins may not be identical, they may represent similar members of an entire family of transcription factors such as NF-1, Sp1, c-jun, and perhaps others not identified as yet.

ASSOCIATION WITH AIDS

The incidence of PML in conditions associated with cellular immunodeficiency (see later) other than AIDS is difficult to assess, but, as suggested by Stoner and colleagues, it does not appear to approach the 4 to 5% incidence observed with HIV-1 infection (90). This apparent increased incidence of PML with HIV-1 infection is the result of a combination of cellular immunodeficiency and CNS inflammation (typically subclinical) resulting from HIV-1 infection. The cellular immunosuppression leads to the expression of JCV in B lymphocytes, and the HIV-1–associated CNS inflammation results in a facilitation of the entry of these cells in to the CNS. PML is the result of subsequent infection of glial cells by JCV.

Early after HIV-1 infection, and often long before the development of significant immunosuppression, evidence of HIV-1 infection of the CNS is present, including recovery of HIV-1 from the cerebrospinal fluid (CSF) (91), intrathecal synthesis of antibody to HIV-1 (92), and abnormalities of the CSF (93–95). HIV-1 has been demonstrated by PCR in the brain of a patient who died within 15 days of infection (96). Viral cultures (91, 97), immunostaining (98), and in situ hybridization (99) confirm the presence of HIV-1 infection in the brain. The infection of the CNS with HIV-1 has been postulated to result from trafficking into the brain of HIV-1 infected monocytes/macrophages, which then establish residence within the brain (100). Some evidence shows an activated state of cellular and humoral immunity in the HIV-1–infected CNS despite a coexistent systemic immune deficiency. Cells expressing major histocompatibility complex (MHC) class I and class II antigens, the prerequisite for antigen presentation to the immunocompetent T cells, are increased in CNS tissue derived from AIDS patients compared with normal CNS tissue (101, 102). B-cell activation in the CNS compartment, perhaps, in part, a response to increased levels of interleukin-6 (IL-6, B-cell stimulatory factor-2) (103), is evidenced by the intrablood–brain barrier production of antibodies to HIV-1 antigens (92). Although the predominant cell types comprising cellular infiltrates observed in the tissue of HIV-1 encephalitis are macrophages and microglia (59, 102, 104), some T cells and B cells have been demonstrated by immunohistochemical technique (101, 102). In addition, several cytokines have been demonstrated in CNS tissue from AIDS patients using immunohistochemical techniques: tumor necrosis factor-α (TNF-α) (101–104), IL-1b, IL-6, and interferon-γ (102).

The selective homing of B lymphocytes to the various lymphoid organs (peripheral lymph nodes, Peyer's patches) is a dynamic process. The migration of B cells into nonlymphoid tissues has been less well characterized. Entry of B cells into such organs as the brain may result from both selective homing and less specific mechanisms. Cytokines released from macrophages and T cells may be chemotactic for B cells (105, 106), may increase the adherence of endothelial cells for B cells (107), or may alter the blood–brain barrier to allow passage of various inflammatory cells into the brain parenchyma (108). TNF-α, IL-1, IL-4, and interferon-γ, cytokines produced by macrophages and other inflammatory cells, such as T cells (109), have been demonstrated to increase the adhesion of vascular endothelium for B lymphocytes (107, 110, 111). The overall environment of "immune activation" described in the CNS (102) possibly results in chemoattraction, enhanced adhesion of B cells to brain endothelia, and activation of B cells latently infected by JCV.

The increased B-cell adhesion to brain endothelia is likely to result from elaboration of IL-1 and TNF-α described in the brains of HIV-1–infected individuals. The stimulation of B cells (112, 113) is possibly mediated by IL-6, IL-4 (B-cell stimulatory factor-1), and other substances, such as, transforming growth factor-β (TGF-β), a cytokine with potent chemotactic activity that has been demonstrated immunohistochemically in CNS tissue from patients with AIDS (114). The adhesion of circulating lymphocytes to target tissue vasculature precedes their subsequent migration into the organ.

Under physiologic conditions, lymphocyte traffic into the brain is limited. Two explanations have been proposed to explain the low lymphocyte traffic into CNS: adhesion of lymphocytes to cerebral endothelium is low, or the tight junctions restrict transendothelial migration of any adherent cells. These proposals are not mutually exclusive. Probably, the entry of JCV-infected B lymphocytes into the brain is facilitated by an upregulation of adhesive molecules on brain endothelial cells in response to HIV-1 infection of the CNS. Possibly JCV antigen–specific lymphocytes appear in the CNS early, rarely migrating far from the vasculature. Because monocytes and astrocytes can present antigen in situ, the antigen-specific B cells are further activated at this site, most likely in an antigen-specific manner. The cytokines secreted locally by microglial cells and monocytes activate the endothelium and surrounding perivascular cells, leading to the expression of adhesion molecules. For example, because of the expression of an avidly binding form of lymphocyte function–associated antigen-1, activated B cells are preferentially recruited to tissue expressing intracellular adhesion molecule-1 (ICAM-1) or other ligands and present in PML. Astrocytes in culture, and maybe in vivo as well, express ICAM, particularly human fetal astrocytes in culture. Lesions of PML, like those of multiple sclerosis and experimental allergic encephalitis, are centered on blood vessels and are formed by a specific subset of inflammatory cells.

EPIDEMIOLOGY OF JCV INFECTION

The ability of JCV to cause hemagglutination of type O erythrocytes has enabled the performance of antibody studies to determine evidence of prior infection. To date, no disease has been convincingly associated with acute infection, although Blake and colleagues have reported chronic meningoencephalitis occurring with acute JCV infection in a 13-year-old girl (115). The acute infection in this patient was identified by a rise of immunoglobulin M (IgM) titers to JCV and not by viral isolation (115). Viral spread is speculated to be by respiratory means. Between the ages of 1 and 5 years, approximately 10% of children demonstrate antibody to JCV, and by age 10, 40 to 60% of the population does so (116–118). JCV can infect tonsillar stromal cells, and evidence suggests that JCV DNA can be found in 30% of normal tonsil tissue (EO Major et al., unpublished data). By adulthood, this figure rises almost sevenfold (117) (Fig. 25.3). Seroconversion rates to JCV have exceeded 90% in some urban areas (117).

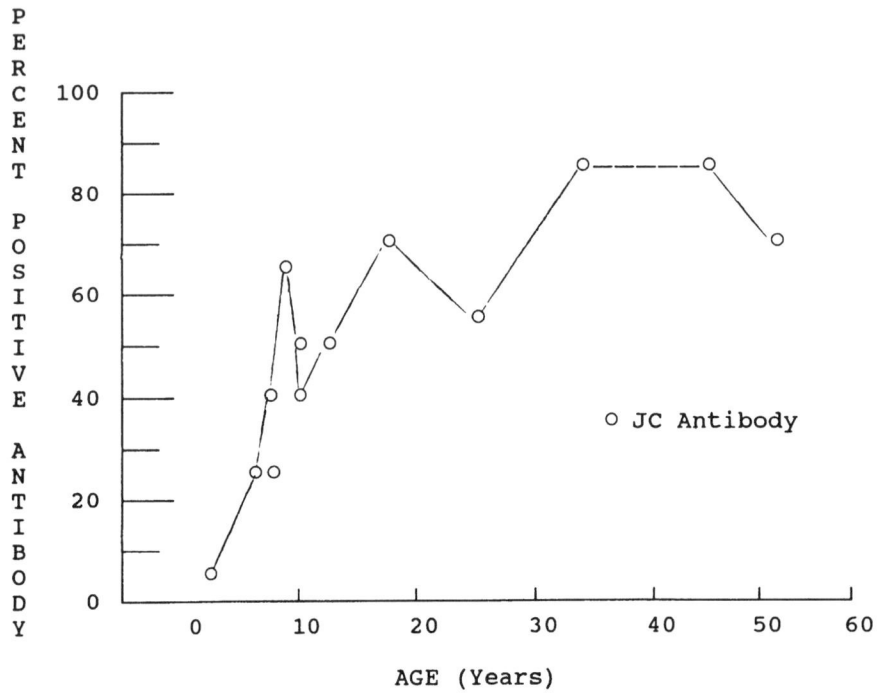

Figure 25.3. Progressive multifocal leukoencephalopathy. The prevalence of anti-JC virus antibody. (Modified from Brooks BR, Walker DL. Progressive multifocal leukoencephalopathy. Neurol Clin 1984;2:299–313.)

The high prevalence of antibodies in the adult population and the rarity of PML in children support the contention that PML is the consequence of reactivation of JCV in individuals who become immunosuppressed. Additionally, high titers of IgM antibody specific for JCV would be anticipated in patients with PML if it were the result of acute infection. However, antibody studies reveal that the sera of only 1 of 21 patients with PML had IgM specific for JCV, whereas 20 of 21 had IgG antibody specific for JCV (119). Some investigators have argued that the latter study does not exclude the possibility of PML as the result of acute JCV infection because many of these patients were studied late in the course of their disease (120). Evidence also indicates that the CSF of some patients contains anti-JCV antibodies from intrathecal antibody synthese (T Weber et al., unpublished data).

HOST FACTORS AND UNDERLYING DISEASES

Although most people have antibodies to JCV by adulthood, only rarely is the disease observed in the absence of underlying cellular immunosuppression. Furthermore, it is rarely observed in childhood. Until the AIDS epidemic, the most common underlying illnesses were lymphoproliferative diseases (3). Since the recognition of the AIDS epidemic in 1981, increasing numbers of individuals with PML have been recognized. PML has been estimated to occur in association with AIDS in 55 to 85% of all current cases (77).

In vitro studies of lymphocyte proliferation to mitogen reveal a blunted response in patients with PML (121). The production of leukocyte migration inhibitory factor from lymphocytes in response to JCV antigens in patients with PML is absent, whereas the production of this factor is normal in patients without PML. This observation suggests that a specific deficiency in cellular immune response to JCV antigen is superimposed on generalized cellular immunodeficiency.

The first three patients described by Aström, Mancall and Richardson (1), in their seminal description of PML, had either chronic lymphocytic leukemia or lymphoma, and, until the early part of the last decade, most patients with PML had lymphoproliferative disorders as the underlying cause of their immunosuppression. In a review of 69 pathologically confirmed cases and 40 virologically and pathologically confirmed cases of PML performed in 1984, Brooks and Walker found lymphoproliferative diseases as the underlying illness in 62.2%, myeloproliferative diseases in 6.5%, carcinomatous disease in 2.2%, and acquired immunodeficiency chiefly from autoimmune disorders and immunosuppressive therapy, but also the result of AIDS, in 10.9% (3). No underlying disease was recognized in 5.6%. In this series, AIDS-related cases accounted for approximately 30% of the cases of PML associated with acquired causes of immunodeficiency and for only 3.0% of the total cases. Data regarding the converse, namely, the frequency of each of these illnesses or conditions of immunologic embarrassment complicated by PML, are either unavailable or difficult to obtain.

Perhaps the most severe states of prolonged cellular immunodeficiency accompany renal and other organ transplantation. Two reviews did not mention PML as a complication (122, 123). In a study of 36 long-term survivors of renal transplantation, PML was not observed (124). In a study of 21 patients who were preselected because of the development of neurologic complications after bone marrow transplantation, only 1 patient had PML (125). Of 156 patients who either had tissue-diagnosed PML or met strict clinical criteria for the diagnosis in a study from southern Florida spanning 14 years (9), only 2 were unassociated with HIV infection, an adolescent with Wiskott–Aldrich syndrome and a young woman with Hodgkin's disease.

AIDS has changed the relative frequency with which PML is observed. A study of PML among patients with AIDS in the San Francisco Bay area estimated a prevalence of PML of 0.3% (126). The findings of these investigators suggested that PML in HIV-infected patients was underestimated by as much as 50% (126). The incidence of this disease is substantially higher and probably approaches 4 to 5% in developed countries. In a study on the epidemiology of PML in the United States (127), mortality data indicated that 0.72% of persons with AIDS reported to the Centers for Disease Control and Prevention from 1981 through June 1990 had PML. However, relying on reported mortality data to estimate the rate of PML or other diseases associated with AIDS is likely to be misleading (128). Inaccurate diagnosis and incomplete reporting may affect case ascertainment.

Other studies indicate that the rate of PML in AIDS is substantially higher. In a retrospective, hospital-based, clinical study (129), PML occurred in approximately 4% of patients hospitalized with AIDS. More recent analysis of this experience indicates little change in that rate. Autopsy series have revealed a similar rate. In a combined series of 7 neuropathologic studies comprising a total of 926 patients with AIDS (130), 4.0% had PML. Similarly, a neuropathology series from Switzerland detected PML in more than 7% of their patients who died of AIDS (131). However, estimating incidence from these studies also has drawbacks because of selection bias. A pathologic study performed on 548 consecutive, unselected autopsies on patients with AIDS by the Broward County (Florida) medical examiner (L. Tate, unpublished data) revealed that 29 (5.3%) had PML confirmed at autopsy. HIV-1 has changed the demography of PML as well as increased its prevalence. Instead of affecting chiefly elderly patients (3), it has become a disease of persons between the ages of 20 and 50 years (9). Despite its rarity in younger age groups, it is also observed in HIV-1-infected children (132, 133).

A possibility exists that PML is more common among some risk groups (gay and bisexual men) than others (parenteral drug abusers). Whether this observation is correct remains to be determined. However, an increasing frequency of PML appears to have been observed since the inception of the AIDS epidemic, and prolonged survival in the face of severe cellular immunosuppression is likely fundamental to this observation.

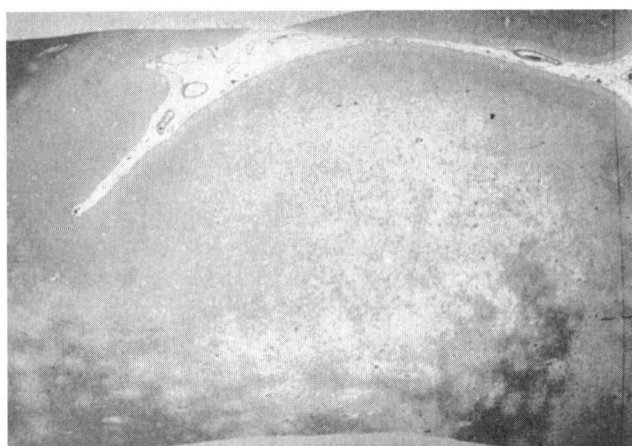

Figure 25.4. Demyelination with progressive multifocal leukoencephalopathy. Demyelination of subcortical white matter is observed on luxol fast blue-hematoxylin and eosin stain.

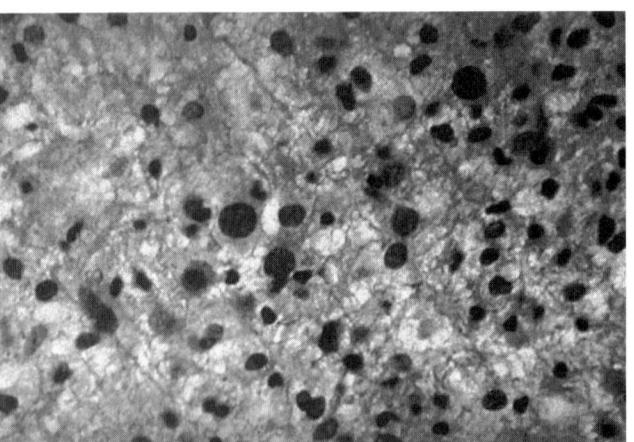

Figure 25.5. Multiple dense, enlarged oligodendroglial nuclei in a region of demyelination.

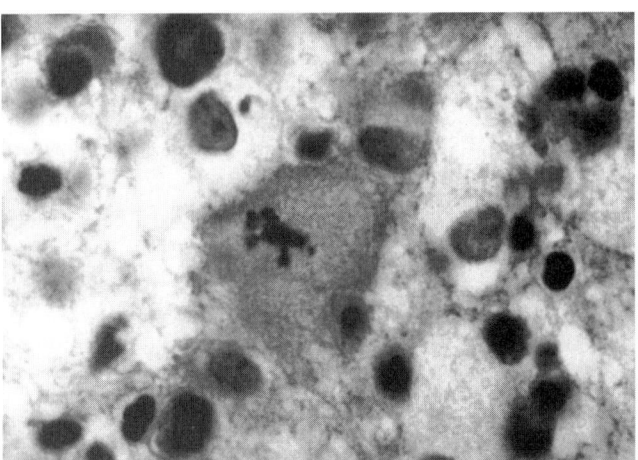

Figure 25.6. Enlarged, bizarre astrocyte from a region of demyelination that is in the process of mitosis.

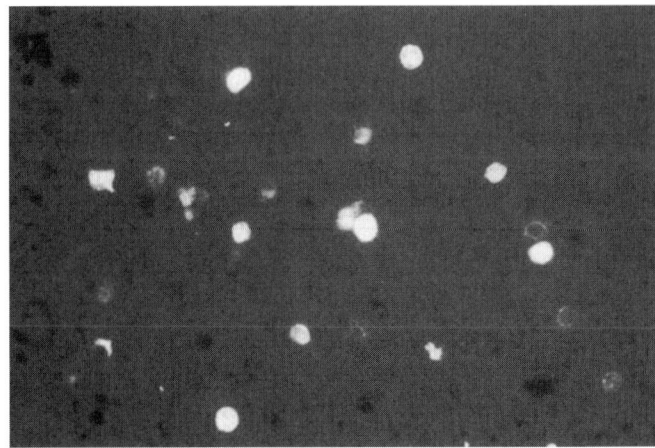

Figure 25.7. In situ hybridization for JC virus (JCV). In situ hybridization for JCV DNA reveals the involvement of the nuclei of multiple oligodendroglial cells.

PATHOLOGY

Macroscopically, the cardinal feature of PML is demyelination. Demyelination may, on rare occasion, be unifocal, but it typically occurs as a multifocal process. These lesions may occur in any location in the white matter; however, they have a predilection for the parietooccipital regions and are infrequently observed in the spinal cord (134). The lesions range in size from 1 mm to several centimeters (1, 126); larger lesions are not infrequently the result of coalescence of multiple smaller lesions.

The histopathologic hallmarks of PML are a triad (1, 126) of multifocal demyelination (Fig. 25.4), hyperchromatic, enlarged oligodendroglial nuclei (Fig. 25.5), and enlarged bizarre astrocytes with lobulated hyperchromatic nuclei. The latter may be seen to undergo mitosis (Fig. 25.6) and may appear malignant. Electron microscopic examination reveals JCV in the oligodendroglial cells. These virions measure 28 to 45 nm in diameter and appear singly or in dense crystalline arrays (10, 11). Less frequently, the virions are detected in reactive astrocytes, and they are uncommonly observed in macrophages that are engaged in removing the affected oligodendrocytes (135, 136). The virions are generally not seen in the large, bizarre astrocytes (137). In situ hybridization for JCV antigen allows for detection of the virion in the infected cells (Figs. 25.7 and 25.8). In rare instances, JCV can be identified in cerebral and cerebellar cortex and may be associated with an unusual clinical presentation associated with the gray matter involvement (138).

CLINICAL DISEASE

Signs and Symptoms

The clinical hallmark of PML is the presence of focal neurologic disease associated with radiographic evidence of white matter disease in the absence of mass effect. Emphasis needs to be placed on the focal features of this disease, particularly those that are apparent on clinical examination. The presentation of AIDS patients with PML does not appear to be substantially different from that of patients with PML complicating other immunosuppressive conditions (9, 130, 139). Table 25.1 displays the relative frequencies of signs and symptoms associated with PML observed in the pre-AIDS era.

The most common initial symptoms are weakness, speech abnormalities, and cognitive disturbances (9), each seen in approximately 40% of patients. In one study (9), headache occurred in 32% of patients, but it is generally not regarded as a significant feature of PML. Gait disturbances, sensory loss, and visual impairment are seen in approximately 20 to 30% of patients (9). Seizures and symptoms implicating brainstem disease are less common (9). The signs observed on physical examination parallel the symptoms reported. Weakness is detected in over half the patients at the time of presentation. Weakness is typically hemiparesis, but monoparesis, hemiplegia, and quadriparesis may be observed. By the time of diagnosis, weakness is present in 50% (9) to more than 80% of patients (3). Gait abnormalities, cognitive problems, and language disorders (dysarthria and dysphasia) are observed in about one-quarter of patients at the time of presentation (9). Limb and trunk ataxia resulting most often from cerebellar involvement is detected in as many as 10% of patients. On occasion, the ataxia may be the result of severe impairment in position sense (sensory ataxia). Extrapyramidal disease, at least at onset, is rare. However, bradykinesia and rigidity may be detected in a some patients with advanced disease (135, 139). Dystonia and severe dysarthria have been observed as a consequence of lesions in the basal ganglia (140, 141). Not unexpectedly, lesions of PML in the basal ganglia chiefly reflect involvement of medullated fibers coursing through this region, rather than involvement of the deep gray matter (142).

Neuro-ophthalmic symptoms occur in 50% of patients with PML and are the presenting manifestation in 30 to 45% (3, 143). The most common visual deficits are homonymous hemianopia or quadrantanopia resulting from lesions of the optic radiations (143). Cortical blindness may eventuate in these patients as the disease progresses. Cortical blindness is present at the time of diagnosis in 5 to 8% of patients (3). Other ophthalmic manifestations include optic aphasia, alexia without agraphia, and, on rare occasion, ocular motor abnormalities (143); this last group occurs as a result of demyelinating lesions in the brainstem. Both supranuclear and nuclear cranial nerve palsies may be seen (143). Visual blurring without further specification has also been described. Although optic atrophy has been reported as a consequence of PML (3), it has never been confirmed histopathologically (143). In several reported cases, coexistent diseases could explain the optic nerve involvement (143, 144).

The spectrum of cognitive changes observed is broad. Unlike the slowly evolving, global dementia of HIV-related cognitive/motor disorder (AIDS dementia complex), the mental impairments of PML are often more rapidly advancing and typically occur in conjunction with focal neurologic deficits. Among the abnormalities seen are personality and behavioral changes, motor impersistence, memory impairment, dyslexia, dyscalculia, and the alien hand syndrome. Global dementia in the absence of focal neurologic disease is rarely the presenting manifestation of PML. Disturbances of language that may be observed include both dysarthria and aphasia.

Sensory disturbances occur with PML, but they are distinctly less common than impairment of strength or visual function. Approximately 10% of patients exhibit a sensory deficit (3). Rarer clinical manifestations include headache, seizures, and vertigo.

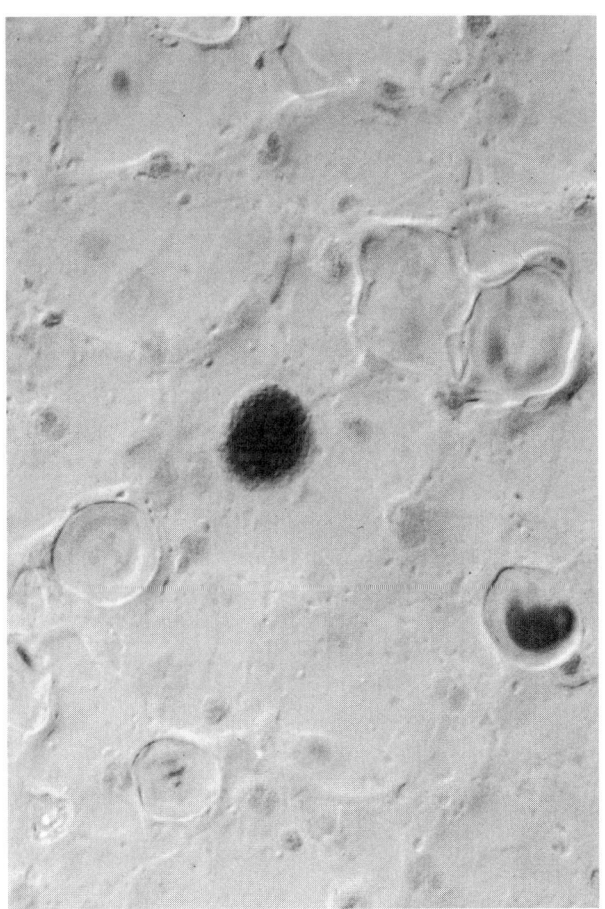

Figure 25.8. JC virus (JCV) DNA in the bone marrow of a patient with progressive multifocal leukoencephalopathy (PML). Detection of JCV DNA in a bone marrow aspirate of a patient with PML using in situ DNA hybridization with a biotinylated viral probe. The hybridization signal is a brown precipitate in the cell nucleus generated by diaminobenzidene oxidation in the presence of strepavidin–biotin horseradish peroxidase.

Prognosis

In AIDS patients, as in those with other underlying diseases, PML usually progresses inexorably to death within a mean of 4 months (129). However, rare cases of recovery of clinical and radiographic manifestations have been reported (145). Survival for longer than 12 months with partial or complete recovery from neurologic deficit was observed in 4 of 72 pathologically proved cases (9). The longest survival in this cohort was 92 months; the patient died of disseminated lymphoma, without any evidence of recurrent PML (9). In 1 patient with biopsy-proved disease, no evidence of PML was evident at autopsy 3 years after presentation (9). The explanation of this recovery remains a conundrum. Factors that may be associated with this benign course seem to include the following: PML as the heralding manifestation of AIDS, high or climbing CD4 T-lymphocyte counts, contrast enhancement of the lesions on radiographic studies, and an inflammatory infiltrate on histopathologic examination. Fong and Toma noted that survival for patients with CD4 T-lymphocyte counts of at least 90 cells/mm^3 at the time of presentation was 9.4 ± 8.7 months, whereas survival for patients with lower counts was 3.6 ± 1.8 months (146). Similarly, these investigators detected a significantly better prognosis when PML was the initial AIDS-defining illness (146).

Radiographic Imaging

The diagnosis of PML is strongly supported by radiographic imaging, but confirmation requires brain biopsy. Computed tomography (CT) of the brain reveals hypodense lesions of the affected white matter (Fig. 25.9) that generally do not enhance with contrast and exhibit no mass effect. These lesions may have a "scalloped" appearance as a result of the subcortical arcuate fibers lying directly beneath the cortex (142). Cranial magnetic resonance imaging (MRI) shows a hyperintense lesion on T_2-weighted images in the affected regions (Fig. 25.10). As with CT, contrast enhancement is an exception; however, contrast enhancement has been observed with both brain imaging techniques in approximately 5 to 10% of pathologically confirmed cases of PML (142). The enhancement observed is typically faint and peripheral. The lesions of PML have a predilection for the parietooccipital lobes, but lesions may occur virtually anywhere. In a review of 47 cases of biopsy-proved or autopsy-proved PML, we found involvement of the basal ganglia, external capsule, and posterior fossa structures (cerebellum

Table 25.1. Signs and Symptoms of Progressive Multifocal Leukoencephalopathy (Percentage of Cases)

Signs and Symptoms	Sign or Symptom Present at Onset (%)		New Sign or Symptom Present at Time of Diagnosis (%)[a]	
Mental deficits	36.1[b]	(37.5)[b]	27.5	(20.0)
Decreased attention only	2.9		0.0	
Decreased memory only	4.3	(2.5)	0.0	
Confusion only	7.2	(12.5)	2.9	(7.5)
Personality change	10.1	(20.0)	0.0	
Dementia	11.6	(2.5)	24.6	(12.5)
Speech deficits	17.3	(15.0)	10.1	(10.0)
Dysarthria	7.2		1.4	
Dysphasia/aphasia	10.1	(15.0)	8.7	(10.0)
Visual deficits	34.7	(45.0)	11.6	(12.5)
Visual blurring	7.2		0.0	
Diplopia	1.4	(2.5)	0.0	
Homonymous hemianopia	23.2	(42.5)	5.8	(5.0)
Cortical blindness	2.9		5.8	(7.5)
Optic atrophy	0.0		1.4	
Motor weakness	33.3	(20.0)	85.4	(75.0)
Monoparesis or hemiparesis	33.3	(20.0)	68.1	(60.0)
Monoplegia or hemiplegia	0.0		13.0	(15.0)
Quadriplegia	0.0		4.3	
Tone alterations	2.8		8.6	
Bradykinesia/akinesia	1.4		1.4	
Rigidity/parkinsonism	1.4		7.2	
Sensory deficits	5.8	(5.0)	11.6	(5.0)
Face, arm numbness	5.8	(5.0)	0.0	
Hemisensory deficit	0.0		11.6	(5.0)
Incoordination	13.0	(10.0)	18.8	
Arm, leg ataxia	10.1	(7.5)	15.9	
Cerebellar dysarthria	2.9	(2.5)	2.9	
Miscellaneous	17.3	(7.5)	8.6	
Headache	7.2	(5.0)	0.0	
Vertigo	4.3		0.0	
Seizures	5.8	(2.5)	7.2	
Coma	0.0		1.4	
No presenting signs or symptoms	1.4		1.4	

[a]Signs or symptoms not present at onset, which developed during progression of disease.
[b]Percentage of cases in pathologically confirmed cases (percentage of cases in virologically and pathologically confirmed cases).
(From Brooks BR, Walker DL. Progressive multifocal leukoencephalopathy. Neurol Clin 1984:2:299–313.)

Cerebrospinal Fluid and Other Studies

Routine analyses of the CSF specimens are nondiagnostic and generally reflect abnormalities expected in the face of HIV-1 infection. The CSF protein may be elevated and myelin basic protein may be detected as a consequence of PML. PCR is becoming increasingly valuable as a diagnostic tool (27, 150–152). Studies have found sensitivities and specificities of CSF PCR for JCV between 43 to 92% and 92 to 100%, respectively (150–152). These values heavily depend on the primer used (152), and nested PCR is more sensitive than standard PCR (153). Positive and negative predictive values for CSF PCR for JCV approach 90% (150).

The electroencephalogram may show focal slowing, but, like other studies, it is also nondiagnostic. For the present, diagnostic certainty depends on the demonstration of typical histopathologic abnormalities at brain biopsy and on detection of the virus. The histopathologic changes include demyelination and the presence of oligodendrocytes with large intranuclear inclusions and of large, bizarre astrocytes with hyperchromatic nuclei. JCV can be demonstrated with electron microscopy or with immunofluorescence or immunocytochemistry.

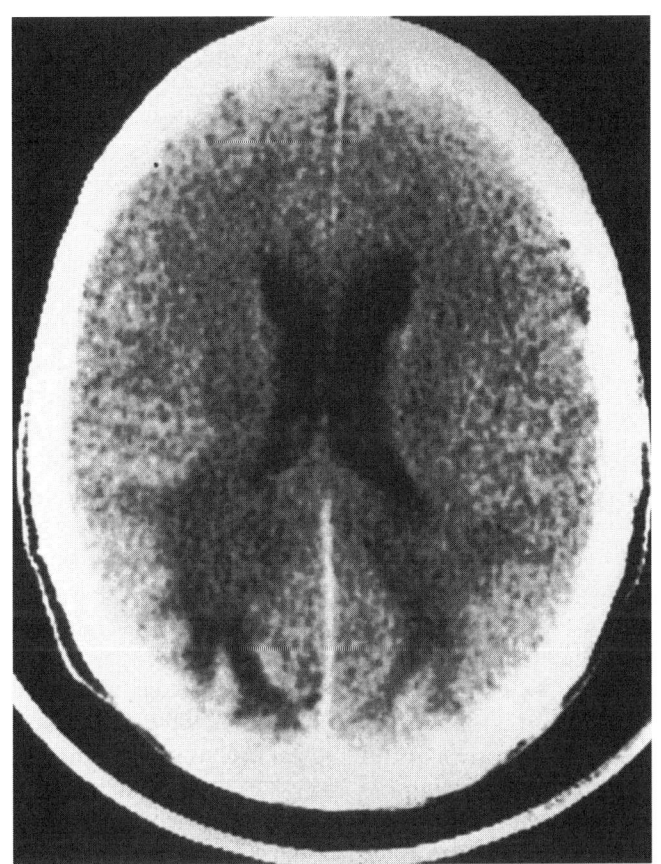

Figure 25.9. Computed tomographic image of the brain reveals bilateral hypodense lesions in the parietooccipital lobes.

and brainstem) (Fig. 25.11) (142). One-third of our patients had involvement of the posterior fossa, and in 5 to 10% of patients, the disease activity was isolated to these structures (142, 145).

Other disorders may cause white matter disease in association with HIV infection. The demyelination observed with HIV-associated cognitive/motor disorder (AIDS dementia complex) may be radiographically indistinguishable from that of PML. Clinically, however, PML is associated with focal neurologic disease and is more rapidly progressive. Radiographic distinctions include a greater propensity of PML lesions to involve the subcortical white matter, its hypointensity on T_1-weighted images, and its rare enhancement (142). Cytomegalovirus may also cause demyelinating lesions. Typically, these lesions are located in the periventricular white matter and centrum seimovale (147). Subependymal enhancement is also observed as a consequence of cytomegalovirus infection (146).

Studies suggest that magnetic resonance spectroscopy may be diagnostically valuable in PML. Proton (hydrogen-1) magnetic resonance spectroscopy shows a significantly different biochemical profile with regard to N-acetyl compounds, total creatine pool, choline-containing compounds, myoinositol, and lactate for PML in comparison with other focal, AIDS-related brain lesions, including toxoplasmosis, brain lymphoma, and cryptococcomas (148, 149).

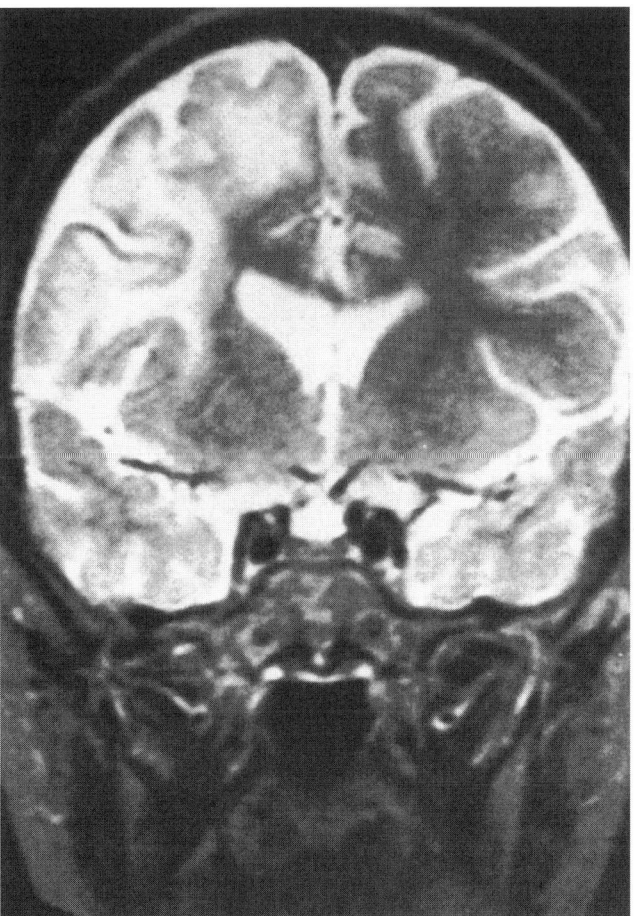

Figure 25.10. Cranial magnetic resonance image reveals a hyperintense signal of the frontal lobe on a T_2-weighted image.

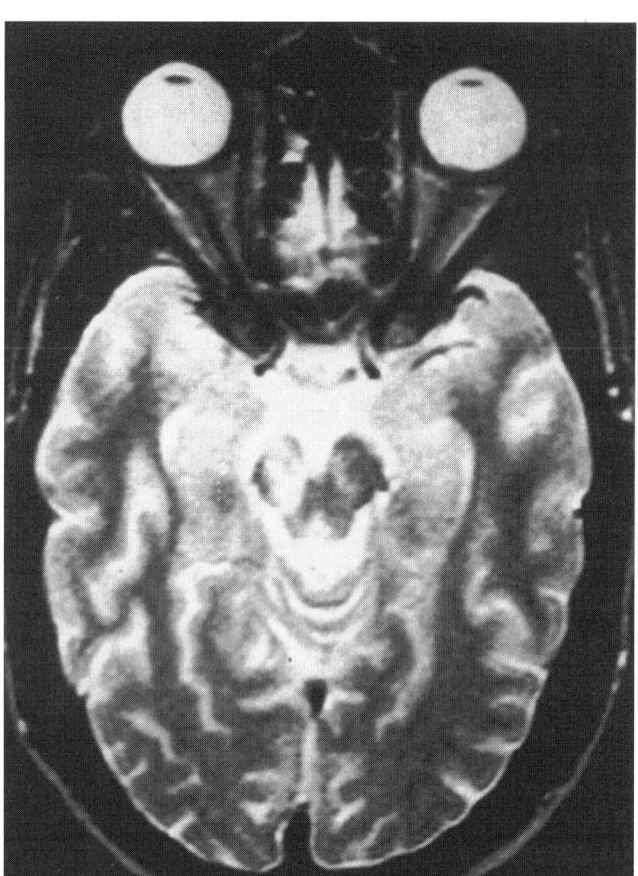

Figure 25.11. Cranial magnetic resonance image of the posterior fossa reveals a hyperintense signal in the midbrain on a T_2-weighted image.

TREATMENT

*"Diseases desperate grown, by desperate appliances are reliev'd,
Or not at all."*

William Shakespeare—Hamlet iii.9

Effective therapy of PML, whether specific antiviral therapy directed at JCV or attempts to enhance cellular immunity, remains elusive. On the basis of anecdotal reports and small series, various treatment regimens have been proposed (Table 25.2). No randomized, double-blind therapeutic regimen has yet been conducted; however, the observation that PML may remain stable for long periods or may even remit in the rare patient (151, 154–159) clearly indicates that the illness is potentially treatable. The rarity of PML before the AIDS epidemic precluded practical therapeutic trials.

Nucleoside analogs exhibit established efficacy in the treatment of some viral diseases. Their mechanism of action is the interference with the synthesis of DNA. Several nucleoside analogs have been used in the treatment of PML with varying degrees of success. Early experience with cytosine arabinoside (ARA-C, cytarabine), a drug chiefly used in the treatment of myeloproliferative disorders, was mixed (160–162). Bauer and colleagues reported rapid and sustained improvement in neurologic symptoms with ARA-C administered intravenously as 60 mg/m^2/day and intrathecally as 10 mg/m^2 (161). The patient described by Marriott and associates showed more delayed, but similarly sustained improvement after ARA-C, 2 mg/kg/day on 5 consecutive days every 3 weeks (163). Similar anecdotal reports of various degrees of improvement have been reported by others (17, 162, 164–167). These regimens used either intrathecal or intravenous administration of ARA-C. A study of intrathecal ARA-C administered as 10 mg/m^2 daily for 3 days with repeat dosing at variable intervals in 26 AIDS patients with PML revealed a salutory effect of 60% that was sustained in 50% for up to 2 years and was transient (less than 6 months) in the remainder (168). The reports of ARA-C efficacy in PML need to be tempered by the reports of its lack of benefit. Some case reports suggest a total lack of efficacy of this agent administered either solely intravenously (160, 169) or in combination with intrathecal therapy (170). Despite these clinical observations regarding the potential efficacy of ARA-C in PML and in vitro data by Major and colleagues demonstrating that 1-β-D-arabinofuranoside at a concentration of 25 μg/mL of culture effectively suppresses JCV replication in human fetal brain tissue infected with JCV (171), a study by the Neurological AIDS Research Consortium of the National Institutes of Health AIDS Clinical Trials Group failed to find any benefit from either intrathecal or intravenous ARA-C administration in comparison with placebo.

Other nucleoside analogs do not appear to have had the same success of ARA-C in the treatment of PML. Wolinsky and associates noted the failure of a 14-day course of adenosine arabinoside (ARA-A; vidarabine), 20 mg/kg/day, in two patients with PML (172). Similar failures of adenosine arabinoside therapy in the treatment of PML have also been described (18, 173). Tarsy and colleagues had no success with a combination of prednisone and intrathecal idoxuridine (5-iodo-2′-deoxyuridine), 2 mg/kg every 12 hours (174).

Table 25.2. Therapies for Progressive Multifocal Leukoencephalopathy

Nucleoside analogs
   Cytosine arabinoside
   Adenine arabinoside
   Iododeoxyuridine
   Zidovudine
Immunomodulatory agents
   Interferon-α
   Interferon-β
   Transfer factor
   Levamisole
   Tilorone
Others
   Corticosteroids
   Heparin
   Antisense oligonucleotides (proposed)

(Adapted from Frankel AD, Pabo CO. Cellular uptake of the tat protein from human immunodeficiency virus. Cell 1988;55:1189–1193.)

Because of their antiviral activity, presumably the result of their ability to stimulate natural killer (NK) cells (175), interferons have been proposed as potential therapeutic agents in the treatment of PML. Interferon-α has established efficacy in the treatment of other papovavirus-related diseases (176). In an open-label trial of the safety and efficacy of recombinant interferon-α2a administered as 3 million units subcutaneously daily with a gradual increment (typically by 3 million units every third day) in the treatment of HIV-associated PML, 2 of 17 patients survived for longer than 1 year (177). No patient had a dramatic reversal in neurologic function. However, a retrospective analysis of the response to therapy in a sizeable group of HIV-infected patients with PML treated with interferon-α suggests that further studies with this agent may be valuable (J McArthur, unpublished data). In 1 patient, combined therapy of intravenous adenine arabinoside and interferon-β (178) showed no efficacy, but intrathecal interferon-β, 1 million units weekly for a total of 19 weeks and monthly thereafter, was associated with modest improvement in her clinical picture and MRI findings (178).

The rationale for the use of low-dose heparan sulfate as an adjunct in the treatment of PML is based on the model of the pathogenesis of PML suggested by Houff and colleagues (32), which postulates that PML is the result of activated JCV infected B lymphocytes crossing the blood–brain barrier and initiating new areas of neuroglial infection throughout the course of the disease. Heparan sulfate has been shown to prevent activated lymphocytes from crossing the blood–brain barrier in animal models by stripping the lymphocyte glycoprotein cell-surface receptors for cerebrovascular endothelial cells. This therapy has no demonstrated efficacy in established disease and is theoretically of value for prophylaxis.

Other agents, either alone or in combination with nucleoside analogs, have been tried in treatment of PML. Tarsy and colleagues administered prednisone in combination with idoxuridine (174), and Van Horn and associates administered corticosteroids, adrenocorticotropin, and transfer factor with cytosine arabinoside without success (170). Theoretically, recovery of the underlying immunologic disorder should be associated with recovery from PML. Selhorst and associates reported a stabilization of the neurologic deficits in a patient treated with tilorone, an immune enhancer (179). Conversely, Dawson and colleagues noted no improvement after cessation of immunosuppressive therapy in a patient with PML and myasthenia gravis (180). One report suggests that PML in association with HIV infection may respond to zidovudine (181). A dramatic improvement followed the administration of zidovudine, 200 mg every 4 hours, and worsening followed a reduction in dose to 200 mg every 8 hours. A return to prior higher zidovudine doses resulted in neurologic stablity (181). Zidovudine may affect levels of the *tat* protein that have been demonstrated to transactivate JCV (69). In our experience, zidovudine use in AIDS-associated PML, even in high doses (1000 mg/day or more), has been devoid of benefit. Recent anecdotal reports suggest that highly active antiretroviral therapy may result in regression of PML and may improve survival (182, 183).

References

1. Aström KE, Mancall EL, Richardson EP Jr. Progressive multifocal leukoencephalopathy: a hitherto unrecognized complication of chronic lymphocytic leukemia and lymphoma. Brain 1958;81: 93–111.
2. Hallervorden J. Eigennartige und nicht rubriziebare Prozesse. In:Bumke O, ed. Handbuch der Geiteskrankheiten. vol. 2. Die Anatomie der Psychosen. Berlin: Springer, 1930:1063–1107.
3. Brooks BR, Walker DL. Progressive multifocal leukoencephalopathy. Neurol Clin 1984;2:299–313.
4. Miller JR, Barrett RE, Britton CB, et al. Progressive multifocal leukoencphalopathy in a male homosexual with T-cell immune deficiency. N Engl J Med 1982;307:1436–1438.
5. Bedri J, Weinstein W, Degregorio P, et al. Progressive multifocal leukoencephalopathy in acquired immunodeficiency syndrome. N Engl J Med 1983;309:492–493.
6. Gottlieb MS, Schroff R, Schranker HM, et al. *Pneumocystis carinii* pneumonia and mucosal candidiasis in previously healthy homosexual men. N Engl J Med 1981;305:1425–1431.
7. Masur H, Michelis MA, Greene JB, et al. An outbreak of community-acquired *Pneumocystis carinii* pneumonia: initial manifestation of cellular immune dysfunction. N Engl J Med 1981;305:1439–1444.
8. Siegal FP, Lopez C, Hammer GS, et al. Severe acquired immunodeficiency in male homosexuals manifested by chronic perianal ulcerative herpes simplex lesions. N Engl J Med 1981;305:1431–1438.
9. Berger JR, Pall L, Lanska D, Whiteman M. Progressive multifocal leukoencephalopathy in patients with HIV infection. J Neurovirol (in press).
10. ZuRhein GM, Chou SM. Particles resembling papovirions in human cerebral demyelinating disease. Science 1965;148:1477–1479.
11. ZuRhein GM. Polyoma-like virions in a human demyelinating disease. Acta Neurol Pathol (Berl) 1967;8:57–68.
12. Silverman L, Rubinstein LJ. Electron microscopic observation on a case of progressive multifocal leukoencephalopathy. Acta Neuropathol (Berl) 1965;5:215–224.
13. Cavanaugh JB, Greenbaum D, Marshall A, et al. Cerebral demyelination associated with disorders of the reticuloendothelial system. Lancet 1959;2:524–529.
14. Padgett BL, ZuRhein GM, Walker DL, et al. Cultivation of papova-like virus from human brain with progressive multifocal leukoencephalopathy. Lancet 1971;1:1257–1260.
15. Richardson EP Jr. Progressive multifocal leukoencephalopathy. N Engl J Med 1961;265:815–823.
16. Narayan O, Penney JB, Johnson RT, et al. Etiology of progressive multifocal leukoencephalopathy. Identification of papovavirus. N Engl J Med 1973;289:1278–1282.
17. Peters ACB, Versteeg J, Bots GTA, et al. Progressive multifocalleukoencephalopathy: immunofluorescent demonstration of SV4 antigen in CSF cells and response to cytarabine therapy. Arch Neurol 1980;37:497–501.
18. Walker DL: Progressive multifocal leukoencephalopathy: an opportunistic viral infection of the central nervous system. In: Vinken PJ, Bruyn GW, eds. Handbook of Clinical Neurology. vol. 34. Amsterdam: Elsevier/North Holland, 1978:307–329.
19. Stoner G, Ryschkewitsch C. Evidence of JC virus in two progressive multifocal leukoencephalopathy (PML) brains previously reported to be infected with SC40. J Neuropathol Exp Neurol 1991;50:342.
20. Arthur RR, Dagostin S, Shah K. Detection of BK virus and JC virus in urine and brain tissue by the polymerase chain reaction. J Clin Microbiol 1989;27:1174–1179.
21. Henson J, Rosenblum M, Furneaux H: A potential diagnostic test for PML: PCR analysis of JC Virus DNA. Neurology 1991;41(Suppl):338.
22. Henson J, Rosenblum M, Armstrong R, et al. Amplification of JC virus DNA from brain and cerebrospinal fluid of patients with progressive multifocal leukoencephalopathy. Neurology 1991;41:1967–1971.
23. Lynch KJ, Frisque RJ: Factors contributing to the restricted DNA replicating activity of JC virus. Virology 1991;180:306–317.

24. Houff SA, Katz D, Kufta C, et al. A rapid method for in situ hybridization for viral DNA in brain biopsies from patients with acquired immunodeficiency syndrome (AIDS). AIDS 1989;3: 843–845.
25. Telenti A, Aksamit AJ, Proper J, et al. Detection of JC virus DNA by polymerase chain reaction in patients with progressive multifocal leukoencephalopathy. J Infect Dis 1990;162:858–861.
26. Tornatore C, Berger JR, Houff S, et al. Detection of JC virus DNA in peripheral lymphocytes from patients with and without progressive multifocal leukoencephalopathy. Ann Neurol 1992;31:454–462.
27. Weber T, Turner RW, Ruf B, et al. JC virus detected by polymerase chain reaction in cerebrospinal fluid of AIDS patients with progressive multifocal leukoencephalopathy. In: Berger JR, Levy RL, eds. Neurological and neuropsychological complications of HIV infection: proceedings from the Satellite Meeting of the International Conference on AIDS, Monterey, CA, 1990:100.
28. Lynch KJ, Frisque RJ. Identification of critical elements with the JC virus DNA replication origin. J Virol 1990;64:5812–5822.
29. Major EO, Amemiya K, Elder G, et al. Glial cells of the human developing brain and B cells of the immune system share a common DNA binding factor for recognition of the regulatory sequences of the human polyomavirus, JCV. J Neurosci Res 1990;27:461–471.
30. Amemiya K, Traub R, Durham L, et al. Adjacent nuclear factor-1 and activator protein binding sites in the enhancer of the neurotropic JC virus. J Biol Chem 1992; 267:14,204–14,211.
31. Tada H, Lashgari M, Rappaport J, et al. Cell type-specific expression of JC virus early promoter by positive and negative regulation. J Virol 1989;63:463–466.
32. Houff SA, Major EO, Katz D, et al. Involvement of JC virus-infected mononuclear cells from the bone marrow and spleen in the pathogenesis of progressive multifocal leukoencephalopathy. N Engl J Med 1988;318:301–305.
33. Frisque RJ, Martin JD, Padgett BL, et al. Infectivity of the DNA from four isolates of JCV. J Virol 1979;32:476–482.
34. Gardner S, MacKenzie E, Smith C, et al. Prospective study of the human polyomaviruses BK and JC and cytomegalovirus in renal transplant recipients. J Clin Pathol 1984;37:578–586.
35. Gardner SD, Field AM, Coleman DV, et al. New human papovavirus (BK) isolated from urine after renal transplantation. Lancet 1971;1: 1253–1257.
36. Tooze J. Human papovaviruses. In: J. Tooze, ed. Molecular biology of tumor viruses. vol. 2. DNA tumor viruses. Cold Spring Harbor, NY: Cold Spring Harbor Laboratory, 1980:205–296.
37. London WT, Houff SA, Madden DL, et al. Brain tumors in owl monkeys inoculated with a human polyomavirus (JC virus). Science 1978;201:1246–1249.
38. London WT, Houff SA, McKeever PE, et al. Viral-induced astrocytomas in squirrel monkeys. Prog Clin Biol Res 1982;105:227–237.
39. Major EO, Vacante DA, Traub TG, et al. Owl monkey astrocytoma cells in culture spontaneously produce infectious JC virus which demonstrates altered biological properties. J Virol 1987;53:306–311.
40. Padgett BL, Walker DL, ZuRhein GM, et al. Differential neuro-oncogenicity of strains of JC virus, a human polyoma virus, in newborn Syrian hamsters. Cancer Res 1977;37:718–720.
41. Walker DL, Padgett BL, ZuRhein GM, et al. Human papovavirus (JC): induction of brain tumors in hamsters. Science 1973;181: 674–676.
42. Dorries K, Loeber G, Meixensbarger J. Association of polyomaviruses JC, SV40, and BK with human brain tumors. Virology 1987;160: 268–270.
43. Major EO, Vacante DA, Houff S: Human papovaviruses: JC virus, progressive multifocal leukoencephalopathy, and model systems for tumors of the central nervous system, In: Spector S, Bendinelli M, Friedman H, eds. Neuropathogenic viruses and immunity. New York: Plenum Press, 1992:207–229.
44. Rencic A, Gordon J, Otte J, et al. Detection of JC virus DNA sequence and expression of the viral oncoprotein, tumor antigen, in brain of immunocompetent patient with oligoastrocytoma. Proc Natl Acad Sci U S A 1996;93:7352–7357.
45. Frisque R, Bream G, Cannella M. Human polyomavirus JC virus genome. J Virol 1984;51:458–469.
46. Khalili E, Rappaport J, Khoury G. Nuclear factors in human brain cells bind specifically to the JCV regulatory region. EMBO J 1988;7:1205–1210.
47. Vacante DA, Traub R, Major EO. Extension of JC virus host range to monkey cells by insertion of a simian virus 40 enhancer into the JC virus regulatory region. Virology 1988;170:353–361.
48. Dorries K. Progressive multifocal leukoencephalopathy: analysis of JC virus DNA from brain and kidney tissue. Virus Res 1984;1:25–38.
49. Martin JD, King DM, Slauch JM, et al. Differences in regulatory sequences of naturally occurring JC virus variants. J Virol 1985;53: 306–311.
50. Aksamit AJ, Proper J. JC virus replicates in primary adult astrocytes in culture. Ann Neurol 1988;24:471.
51. Major EO, Vacante DA: Human fetal astrocytes in culture support the growth of the neurotropic human polyomavirus, JCV. J Neuropathol Exp Neurol 1989;48:425–436.
52. Wroblewska Z, Wellish M, Gilden D. Growth of JC virus in adult human brain cell cultures. Arch Virol 1980;65:141–148.
53. Martin JD, Padgett BL, Walker DL. Characterization of tissue culture induced heterogenicity in DNAs of independent isolates of JC virus. J Gen Virol 1983;64:2271–2280.
54. Kenney SV Natarajan, Strike D, et al. JC virus enhancer-promotor active in human brain cells. Science 1984;226:1337–1339.
55. Feigenbaum L, Khalili K, Major EO, et al. Regulation of the host range of human papovavirus JCV. Proc Natl Acad Sci U S A 1987;84:3695–3698.
56. Raj, GV, Khalili K. Transcriptional regulation: lessons from the human neurotropic polyomavirus, JCV. Virology 1995;213: 283–291.
57. Amemiya K, Traub R, Durham L, et al. Interaction of a nuclear factor-1-like protein with the regulatory region of the human polyomavirus JC virus. J Biol Chem 1989; 264:7025–7032.
58. Miyamura T, Jikuya H, Soeda E, et al. Genomic structure of human polyomavirus JC: nucleotide sequence of the region containing replication origin and small T antigen gene. J Virol 1983;45:73–79.
59. Nandi A, Dos G, Salzman NP: Characterization of a surrogate TATA box promoter that regulates in vitro transcription of the simian virus 40 major late gene. Mol Cell Biol 1985;5:591–594.
60. Dynan W, Tjian R. Control of eukaryotic RNA synthesis by sequence specific DNA binding proteins. Nature 1985;316:774–778.
61. Gruss P, Khoury G. The SV 40 tandem repeats as an element of the early promotor. Proc Natl Acad Sci U S A 1981;78:943–947.
62. Sumner C, Shinohara T, Durham L, et al. Expression of multiple classes of the nuclear factor-1 family in the developing human brain: differential expression of two classes of NF-1 genes. J Neurovirol 1996: 2:87–100.
63. Shinohara T, Nagashima K, Major EO. Propagation of the human polyomavirus, JCV in human neuroblastoma cell lines. Virology 1997;228:269–277.
64. Ahmed S, Rappaport J, Tada H, et al. A nuclear protein derived from brain cells stimulates transcription of the human neurotropic virus promoter, JCVE, in vitro. J Biol Chem 1990;265:13899–13905.
65. Tamura T, Inoue T, Nagata K, et al. Enhancer of human polyoma JC virus contains nuclear factor 1-binding sequences: analysis using mouse brain nuclear extracts. Biochem Biophys Res Commun 1988; 157:419–425.
66. Kerr D, Khalili K. A recombinant cDNA derived from human brain encodes a DNA binding protein that stimulates transcription of the human neurotropic virus JCV. J Biol Chem 1991;286:15876–15881.
67. Sock E, Wegner M, Grummt F. DNA replication of human polyomavirus JC is stimulated by NF-1 in vivo. Virology 1991;182:298–308.
68. Gendelman H, Phelps W, Feigenbaum L, et al. Trans-activation of the human immunodeficiency virus long terminal repeat by DNA viruses. Proc Natl Acad Sci U S A 1986;83:9759–9763.

69. Tada H, Rappaport J, Lashgari M, et al. Trans-activation of the JC virus late promoter by the tat protein of type 1 human immunodeficiency virus in glial cells. Proc Natl Acad Sci U S A 1990;87:3479–3483.
70. Remenick J, Radonovich M, Brady J: Human immunodeficiency virus tat transactivation: induction of a tissue specific enhancer in a non-permissive cell line. J Virol 1991;65:5641–5646.
71. Wiley CA, Grafe M, Kennedy C, et al. Human immunodeficiency virus (HIV) and JC virus in acquired immunodeficiency syndrome (AIDS) patients with progressive multifocal leukoencephalopathy. Acta Neuropathol 1988;76:338–346.
72. Frankel AD, Pabo CO. Cellular uptake of the tat protein from human immunodeficiency virus. Cell 1988;55:1189–1193.
73. Helland D, Welles J, Caputo A, et al. Transcellular transactivation by the human immunodeficiency virus type 1 tat protein. J Virol 1991;65:4547–4549.
74. Beckman A, Shah KV. Propagation and primary isolation of JCV and BKV in urinary epithelial cell cultures. In: Sever JL, Madden D, eds. Polyomaviruses and human neurological diseases. New York: Alan R. Liss, 1983:3–14.
75. Fareed GC, Takemoto KK, Gimbrone MA: Interaction of simian virus 40 and human papovaviruses, BK and JC, with human endothelial cells, In: Schlessinger D, ed. Microbiology. Washington, DC: American Society for Microbiology, 1978:427–431.
76. Tornatore C, Berger J, Winfield D, et al. Detection of JC viral genome in the lymphocytes of non-PML HIV positive patients: association with B cell lymphopenia. Presented at the American Academy of Neurology meeting, San Diego, 1992.
77. Major EO, Amemiya K, Tornatore C, et al. Pathogenesis and molecular biology of progressive multifocal leukoencephalopathy, the JC virus-induced demyelinating disease of the human brain. Clin Microbiol Rev 1992;5:49–73.
78. Monaco MCG, Atwood WJ, Gravell M, et al. JC virus infection of hematopoietic progenitor cells, primary B lymphocytes, and tonsillar stromal cells: Implications for viral latency. J Virol 1996;70:7004–7012.
79. Weber T, Turner RW, Frye S, et al. Progressive multifocal leukoencephalopathy diagnosed by amplification of JC virus-specific DNA from cerebrospinal fluid. AIDS 1994;8:49–57.
80. Dorries K, Vogel E, Gunther S, et al. Infection of human polyomavirus JC and BK in peripheral blood leukocytes from immunocompetent individuals. Virology 1994;198:59–70.
81. Coleman DV, Wolfendale MR, Daniel DA, et al. A prospective study of human polyomavirus infection in pregnancy. J Infect Dis 1980;142:1–8.
82. Flaegstad T, Sundsfjord A, Arthur RR, et al. Amplification and sequencing of the control regions of BK and JC virus from human urine by polymerase chain reaction. Virology 1991;180:553–560.
83. Myers C, Frisque RJ, Arthur RR. Direct isolation and characterization of JC virus from urine samples of renal and bone marrow transplant patients. J Virol 1989;63:444–4449.
84. Yogo Y, Kitamura T, Sugimoto C, et al. Sequence rearrangement in JC virus DNAs molecularly cloned from immunosuppressed renal transplant patients. J Virol 1991;65:2422–2428.
85. Yogo T, Kitamura T, Sugimoto C, et al. Isolation of a possible archetypal JC virus DNA sequence from nonimmunocompromised individuals. J Virol 1990;64:3139–3143.
86. Henson J, Saffer J, Furneaux H. The transcription factor Sp1 binds to the glial specific JC virus promotor and is selectively expressed in glial cells in human brain. Ann Neurol 1992;32:72–77.
87. Briggs M, Kadonaga J, Bell S, et al. Purification and biochemical characterization of the promoter specific transaction factor, Sp1. Science 1986;234:47–52.
88. Tominaga T, Yogo Y, Kitamura T, et al. Persistence of archetypal JC virus DNA in normal renal tissue derived from tumor bearing patients. Virology 1992;186:736–741.
89. Atwood W, Amemiya K, Traub R, et al. Interactions of the human polyomavirus, JCV, with human B lymphocytes. Virology 1992;190:716–723.
90. Stoner GL, Ryschkewitsch CF, Walker DL, et al. JC papovavirus large tumor (T)-antigen expression in brain tissue of acquired immune deficiency syndrome (AIDS) and non-AIDS patients with progressive multifocal leukoencephalopathy. Proc Natl Acad Sci U S A 1986;23:2271–2275.
91. Ho DD, Rota TR, Schooley RT, et al. Isolation of HTLV-III from cerebrospinal fluid and neural tissues of patients with neurologic syndromes related to the acquired immunodeficiency syndrome. N Engl J Med 1985;313:1493–1497.
92. Resnick L, Berger JR, Shapshak P, et al. Early penetration of the blood–brain barrier by HIV. Neurology 1988;38:9–14.
93. Marshall DW, Brey RL, Cahill WT, et al. Spectrum of cerebrospinal fluid findings in various stages of human immunodeficiency virus infection. Arch Neurol 1988;45:954–958.
94. Elovaara I, Iivanainen M, Valle S-L, et al. CSF protein and cellular profiles in various stages of HIV infection related to neurological manifestations. J Neurol Sci 1987;78:331–342.
95. Hollander H. Cerebrospinal fluid normalities and abnormalities in individuals infected with human immunodeficiency virus. J Infect Dis 1988;158:855–858.
96. Davis L, Hjelle BL, Miller VE, et al. Early viral invasion of brain in iatrogenic human immunodeficiency virus infection [abstract]. Ann Neurol 1991;30:314.
97. Levy JA, Shimabukuro J, Hollander H, et al. Isolation of AIDS associated retroviruses from cerebrospinal fluid and brain of patients with neurological symptoms. Lancet 1985;2:586–588.
98. Ward JM, O'Leary TJ, Baskin GB, et al. Immunohistochemical localization of human and simian immunodeficiency viral antigens in fixed tissue sections. Am J Pathol 1987;127:199–205.
99. Shaw GM, Harper ME, Hahn BH, et al. HTLV-III infection in brains of children and adults with AIDS encephalopathy. Science 1985;227:177–182.
100. Koenig S, Gendelman HE, Orenstein JM, et al. Detection of AIDS virus in macrophages in brain tissue from AIDS patients with encephalopathy. Science 1986;233:1089–1093.
101. Vazeux R, Brousse N, Jarry A, et al. AIDS subacute encephalitis, identification of HIV-infected cells. Am J Pathol 1987;126:403–410.
102. Tyor WR, Glass JD, Griffin JW, et al. Cytokine expression in the brain during the acquired immunodeficiency syndrome. Ann Neurol 1992;31:349–360.
103. Gallo P, Frei K, Rordorf C, et al. Human immunodeficiency virus type 1 (HIV-1) infection of the central nervous system: an evaluation of cytokines in cerebrospinal fluid. J Neuroimmunol 1989;23:109–116.
104. Kure K, Lyman WD, Weidenheim KM, et al. Cellular localization of an HIV-1 antigen in subacute AIDS encephalitis using an improved double labeling immunohistochemical method. Am J Pathol 1990;136:1085–1092.
105. Yoshioka M, Nakamura S, Nagano I, et al. The detection of cytokines in the AIDS brain. Presented at the American Academy of Neurology meeting, San Diego, 1992.
106. Oppenheim JJ. Lymphokines. In: Oppenheim JJ, Rosenstreich DL, Potter M, eds. Cellular functions in immunity and inflammation. New York: Elsevier/North Holland, 1981:259–282.
107. Cavender DE, Haskard DO, Joseph B, et al. Interleukin 1 increases the binding of human B and T lymphocytes to endothelial cell monolayers. J Immunol 1986;136:203–207.
108. Brightman MW, Reese TS. Junctions between intimately apposed cell membranes in the vertebrate brain. J Cell Biol 1969;40:648–677.
109. Durum SK, Oppenheim JJ. Macrophage-derived mediators: interleukin 1, tumor necrosis factor, interleukin 6, interferon, and related cytokines. In: Paul WE, ed. Fundamental immunology. 2nd ed. New York: Raven Press, 1989:639–661.
110. Bevilacqua MP, Pober JS, Wheeler ME, et al. Interleukin-1 acts on cultured human vascular endothelium to increase the adhesion of

polymorphonuclear leukocytes, monocytes, and related leukocyte cell lines. J Clin Invest 1985;76:2003–2011.
111. Pryce G, Male DK, Sarkar C. Control of lymphocyte migration into brain: selective interactions of lymphocyte subpopulation with brain endothelium. Immunology 1991;72:393–398.
112. Kishimoto T. The biology of interleukin-6. Blood 1989;74:1–10.
113. Snapper CM, Findelman FD. Regulation of IgG1 and IgE production by interleukin 4. Immunol Rev 1988;102:51–75.
114. Wahl SM, Allen JV, McCartney-Franscis N, et al. Macrophage- and astrocyte-derived transforming growth factor beta as a mediator of central nervous system dysfunction in acquired immune deficiency syndrome. J Exp Med 1991;173:981–991.
115. Blake K, Pillay D, Knowles W, et al. JC virus associated meningoencephalitis in an immunocompetent girl. Arch Dis Child 1992;67:956–957.
116. Taguchi F, Kajioka J, Miyamura T. Prevalence rate and age of acquisition of antibodies aganist JC virus and BK virus in human sera. Microbiol Immunol 1982;26:1057–1064.
117. Walker DL, Padgett BL. The epidemiology of human polyomaviruses. In Sever JL, Madden D, eds. Polyomaviruses and human neurological disease. New York: Alan R. Liss, 1983:99–106.
118. Walker DL, Padgett BL. Progressive multifocal leukoencephalopathy. In Fraenkel-Conrat H, Wagner RR, eds. Comprehensive virology. New York: Plenum, 1983.
119. Padgett BL, Walker DL. Virologic and serologic studies of progressive multifocal leukoencephalopathy, In Sever J, Madden DL, eds. Polyomaviruses and human neurological disease. New York: Alan R. Liss, 1983.
120. Gibson PE, Field AM, Gardner SD, et al. Occurrence of IgM antibodies against BK and JC polyomaviruses during pregnancy. J Clin Pathol 1981;34:674–679.
121. Willoughby E, Price RW, Padgett BL, et al. Progressive multifocal leukoencephalopathy (PML): in vitro cell-mediated immune responses to mitogens and JC virus. Neurology 1980;30:256–262.
122. Harmon WE. Opportunistic infections in children following renal transplantation. Pediatr Nephrol 1991;5:118–125.
123. Yoshimura N, Oka T. Medical and surgical complications of renal transplantion: diagnosis and management. Med Clin North Am 1990;74:1025–1037.
124. Divakar D, Bailey RR, Lynn KL, et al. Long term complications following renal transplantation. N Z Med J 1991;104:352–354.
125. Diener HC, Ehninger G, Schmidt H, et al. Neurologic complications after bone marrow transplantation. Nervenarzt 1991;62:2221–2225.
126. Gillespie SM, Chang Y, Lemp G, et al. Progressive multifocal leukoencephalopathy in persons infected with human immunodeficiency virus, San Francisco, 1981–1989. Ann Neurol 1991;30:597–604.
127. Holman RC, Janssen RS, Buehler JW, et al. Epidemiology of progressive multifocal leukoencephalopathy in the United States: analysis of national mortality and AIDS surveillance data. Neurology 1991;41:1733–1736.
128. Moriyama IM. Problems in measurement of accuracy of cause-of-death statistics. Am J Public Health 1989;79:1349–1350.
129. Berger JR, Kaszovitz B, Post MJ, et al. Progressive multifocal leukoencephalopathy associated with human immunodeficiency virus infection: a review of the literature with a report of sixteen cases. Ann Intern Med 1987;107:78–87.
130. Kure K, Llena JF, Lyman WD, et al. Human immunodeficiency virus-1 infection of the nervous system: an autopsy study of 268 adult, pediatric and fetal brains. Hum Pathol 1991;22:700–710.
131. Lang W, Miklossy J, Deruaz JP, et al. Neuropathology of the acquired immune deficiency syndrome (AIDS): a report of 135 consecutive autopsy cases from Switzerland. Acta Neuropathol 1989;77:379–390.
132. Berger JR, Scott S, Albrecht J, et al. Progressive multifocal leukoencephalopathy in HIV-infected children. AIDS 1992;2:837–841.
133. Wrozlek MA, Brudkowska J, Kozlowski, et al. Opportunistic infections of the central nervous system in children with HIV infection: report of 9 autopsy cases and review of literature. Clin Neuropathol 1995;14:1
134. Bauer W, Chamberlin W, Horenstein S. Spinal demyelination in progressive multifocal leukoencephalopathy. Neurology 1969;19:287.
135. Richardson EP Jr. Progressive multifocal leukoencephalopathy. In: Vinken PJ, Bruyn GW, eds. Handbook of clinical neurology. vol 9. Multiple sclerosis and other demyelinating diseases. New York: Elsevier/North Holland, 1970:485–499.
136. Mazlo M, Herndon RM. Progressive multifocal leukoencephalopathy: ultrastructural findings in two brain biopsies. Neuropathol Appl Neurobiol 1977;3:323–339.
137. Mazlo M, Tariska I. Are astrocytes infected in progressive multifocal leukoencephalopathy. Acta Neuropathol (Berl) 1982;56:45–51.
138. Sweeney BJ, Manji H, Miller RF, et al. Cortical and subcortical JC virus infection: two unusual cases of AIDS associated progressive multifocal leukoencephalopathy. J Neurol Neurosurg Psychiatry 1994;57:994–997.
139. Krupp LB, Lipton RB, Swerdlow ML, et al. Progressive multifocal leukoencephalopathy: clinical and radiographic features. Ann Neurol 1985;17:344–349.
140. Richardson EP Jr. Our evolving understanding of progressive multifocal leukoencephalopathy. Ann N Y Acad Sci 1974;230:358–364.
141. Singer C, Berger JR, Bowen BC, et al. Akinetic-rigid sydnrome in a 13 year old female with HIV related progressive multifocal leukoencephalopathy. Mov Disord 1993;8:113–116.
142. Whiteman M, Post MJD, Berger JR, et al. PML in 47 HIV+ patients. Radiology 1993;187:233–240.
143. Omerud LD, Rhodes RH, Gross SA, et al. Ophthalmologic manifestations of acquired immune deficiency syndrome–associated progressive multifocal leukoencephalopathy. Ophthalmology 1996;103:899–906.
144. Headington JT, Umiker WO. Progressive multifocal leukoencephalopathy. a case report. Neurology 1962;12:434–439.
145. Berger JR, Mucke L. Prolonged survival and partial recovery in AIDS-associated progressive multifocal leukoencephalopathy. Neurology 1988;38:1060–1065.
146. Fong IW, Toma E. The natural history of progressive multifocal leukoencephalopathy in patients with AIDS: Canadian PML Study Group. Clin Infect Dis 1995;20:1305–1310.
147. Sze G, Zimmermann RD. The magnetic resonance imaging of infectious and inflammatory disease. Radiol Clin North Am 1988;26:839–859.
148. Chang L, Miller BL, McBride D, et al. Brain lesions in patients with AIDS: H-1 MRI spectroscopy. Radiology 1995;197:525–531.
149. Bowen BC, Post MJD. Intracranial infections. In: Atlas SW, ed. Magnetic resonance imaging of the brain and spine. New York. Raven Press, 1991:501–538.
150. Fong IW, Britton CB, Luinstra KE, et al. Diagnostic value of detecting JC virus DNA in cerebrospinal fluid of patients with progressive multifocal leukoencephalopathy. J Clin Microbiol 1995;33:484–486.
151. McGuire D, Barhite S, Hollander H, et al. JC virus DNA in cerebrospinal fluid of human immunodeficiency viurs-infected patients: predictive value for progressive multifocal leukoencephalopathy. Ann Neurol 1995;37:935–399.
152. Weber T, Turner RW, Frye S, et al. Specific diagnosis of progressive multifocal leukoencephalopathy by polymerase chain reaction. J Infect Dis 1994;169:1138–1141.
153. de Luca A, Cingolani A, Linzalone A, et al. Improved detection of JC virus DNA in cerebrospinal fluid for diagnosis of AIDS-related progressive multifocal leukoencephalopathy. J Clin Microbol 1996;34:1343–1346.
154. Padgett BL, Walker DL. Virologic and serologic studies of progressive multifocal leukoencephalopathy. Prog Clin Biol Res 1983;105:107–117.
155. Price RW, Nielsen S, Horten B, et al. Progressive multifocal leukoencephalopathy: a burnt-out case. Ann Neurol 1983;13:485–490.
156. Kepes JJ, Chou SM, Price LW Jr. Progressive multifocal leukoencephalopathy with 10 year survival in a patient with nontropical sprue: report of a case with unusual light and electron microscopic features. Neurology 1975;25:1006–1012.

157. Stam FC. Multifocal leukoencephalopathy with slow progression and very long survival. Psychiatr Neurol Neuorchir 1966;69:453–459.
158. Sima AAF, Finkelstein SD, McLachlan DR. Multiple malignant astrocytomas in a patient with spontaneous progressive multifocal leukoencephalopathy. Ann Neurol 1983;14:183–188.
159. Embry JR, Silva FG, Helderman JH, et al. Long term survival and late development of bladder cancer in renal transplant patient with progressive multifocal leukoencephalopathy. J Urology 1988;139:580–581.
160. Castleman B, Scully RE, McNeely BJ. Weekly clinicopathological exercises, case 19-1972. N Engl J Med 1972;286:1047–1054.
161. Bauer WR, Turci AP Jr, Johnson KP. Progressive multifocal leukoencephalopathy and cytarabine. JAMA 1973;226:174–176.
162. Major EO, Curfman BL. Viral induced demyelination leading to progressive multifocal leukoencephalopathy; the involvement of both immune and nervous system target cells. In: Remington J, Peterson PK, eds. Defense of the brain. Oxford: Blackwell Science, 1997.
163. Conomy JP, Beard NS, Matsumoto H, et al. Cytarabine treatment of progressive multifocal leukoencephalopathy. JAMA 1974;229:1313–1316.
164. Marriott PJ, O'Brien MD, MacKenzie IC, et al. Progressive multifocal leukoencephalopathy: remission with cytarabine. J Neurol Neurosurg Psychiatry 1975;38:205–209.
165. Buckman R, Wiltshaw E. Progressive multifocal leukoencephalopathy successfully treated with cytosine arabinoside. Br J Haematol 1976;34:153–154.
166. O'Riordan T, Daly PA, Hutchinson M, et al. Progressive multifocal leukoencephalopathy—remission with cytarabine. J Infect 1990;20:51–54.
167. Rockwell D, Ruben FL, Winkelstein A, et al. Absence of immune deficiencies in a case of progressive multifocal leukoencephalopathy. Am J Med 1976;61:433–436.
168. Portegies P, Algra PR, Hollar CEM, et al. Response to cytarabine in progressive multifocal leucoencephalopathy in AIDS. Lancet 1991;337:680–681.
169. Britton CB, Romagnoli M, Sisti M, et al. Progressive multifocal leukoencephalopathy and response to intrathecal ARA-C in 26 patients [abstract]. In: Proceedings of the 4th Neuroscience of HIV Infection Conference, Amsterdam, 1992:40.
170. Smith CR, Sima AAF, Salit IE, et al. Progressive multifocal leukoencephalopathy: failure of cytarabine therapy. Neurology 1982;32:200–203.
171. Van Horn G, Bastien FO, Moake JL: Progressive multifocal leukoencephalopathy: failure of response to transfer factor and cytarabine. Neurology 1978;28:794–797.
172. Wolinsky JS, Johnson KP, Rand K, et al. Progressive multifocal leukoencephalopathy: clinical patholgoical correlates and failure of a drug trial in two patients. Trans Am Neurol Assoc 1976;101:81–82.
173. Rand KH, Johnson KP, Rubenstein LJ, et al. Adenine arabinoside in the treatment of progressive multifocal leudkoencephaloapthy: use of virus containing cells in the urine to assess response to therapy. Ann Neurol 1977;1:458–462.
174. Tarsy D, Holden EM, Segarra JM, et al. 5-iodo-2'-deoxyuridine (IUDR: NSC-39661) given intraventricularly in the treatment of progressive multifocal leukoencephalopathy. Cancer Chemother Rep Part 1. 1973;57:73–78.
175. Tyring SK, Cauda R, Ghanta V, et al. Activation of natural killer cell function during interferon-alpha treatment of patients with condyloma acuminatum is predictive of clinical response. J Biol Regul Homeost Agents 1988;2:63–66.
176. Weck PK, Buddin DA, Whisnant JK. Interferons in the treatment of genital human papillomavirus infections. Am J Med 1988;85:159–164.
177. Berger JR, Pall L, McArthur J, et al. A pilot study of recombinant alpha 2A interferon in the treatment of AIDS-related progressive multifocalcal leukoencephalopathy [abstract] Neurology 1992;42(Suppl 3):257.
178. Tashiro K, Doi S, Moriwaka F, et al. Progressive multifocal leucoencephalopathy with magnetic resonance imaging verification and therapeutic trials with interferon. J Neurol 1987;234:427–429.
179. Selhorst JB, Ducy KF, Thomas JM, et al. Remission and immunologic reversals [abstract]. Neurology 1978;28:337.
180. Dawson DM: Progressive multifocal leukoencephalopathy in myasthenia gravis. Ann Neurol 1982;11:218–219.
181. Conway B, Halliday WC, Brunham RC. Human immunodeficiency virus-associated progressive multifocal leukoencephalopathy: apparent response to 3'-azido-3'-deoxythymidine. Rev Infect Dis 1990;12:479–482.
182. Baqi M, Kucharczyk W, Walmsley SL. Regression of progressive multifocal leukoencephalopathy with highly active antiretroviral therapy [letter]. AIDS 1997;11:1526–1527.
183. Baldweg T, Catalan J. Remission of progressive multifocal leukoencephalopathy after antiretroviral therapy. Lancet 1997;349:1554–1555.

26

KAPOSI'S SARCOMA AND CLOACOGENIC CARCINOMA: VIRUS-INITIATED MALIGNANCIES

Steven A. Miles

KAPOSI'S SARCOMA

Before 1981, Kaposi's sarcoma (KS) was a rare tumor occurring largely in men of Eastern European or Mediterranean descent, children in Central Africa, and recipients of solid organ transplants (1). The rapid increase in incidence of KS in 1981 heralded the onset of the acquired immunodeficiency syndrome (AIDS) epidemic in the United States (2). This tumor was more aggressive than its classic counterpart and was one of the main manifestations of AIDS. Initial outbreaks were identified in California and New York. Subsequently, it spread to most major cities within the United States. A large discrepancy remains in the frequency of KS among persons with human immunodeficiency virus (HIV) infection (3). The major cities in the United States have a higher incidence, and cities involved in the secondary wave of the HIV epidemic have a lower incidence. In addition, men who have sex with men appear to be at highest risk of KS. Injection drug users, persons with hemophilia, and recipients of blood or blood products, as well as children born to mothers infected with HIV, appear to be at low risk for the development of this cancer (4, 5). This finding is in contrast to non–Hodgkin's lymphoma, which occurs at approximately the same rate in persons belonging to all risk groups for the acquisition of HIV infection.

When KS complicates HIV infection, it has a more aggressive clinical course than in patients with the classic form of this disease (1, 6). It frequently involves the skin of the upper body, mucous membranes, lymph nodes, gastrointestinal tract, lungs, and other organs. Involvement of the liver, spleen, bone marrow, and brain is rare (7–9). Despite the widespread manifestations of KS, death from KS is rare. Tremendous advances have been made in understanding the pathogenesis of KS as a result of the AIDS epidemic. Significant insights into the epidemiology, clinical features (Figs. 26.1–26.5), and etiology have occurred.

History

KS was initially described by Morris Kaposi in 1872. He described the disease as "idiopathic, multiple-pigmented, hemioangiosarcomas of the skin" (10). The disorder was called "Kaposi's sarcoma" at the suggestion of Kobner, although Dr. Kaposi believed the more accurate description was the term "sarcoma idiopathicum multiplex hemorrhagicum." Over the next 15 years, KS was recognized in multiple countries culminating in the description of a disseminated form by Kaposi himself in 1887. The initial case, described in an African patient, occurred in 1914 (11). Only 20 years later was it recognized as a common malignant disease in Africa, when Smith and Elmes reviewed more than 500 tumors and found that approximately 2% were consistent with KS. Subsequently, African KS has been characterized into nodular, infiltrative, florid, and lymphadenopathic forms (1).

The introduction of immunosuppressive drugs and, in particular, the widespread use of corticosteroids, resulted in a dramatic increase in the incidence of KS (12, 13). This occurred largely in Italian renal transplant recipients, but it was observed in other settings (14, 15).

Epidemiology

KS is the most common cancer occurring in persons with HIV infection (3). The risk of KS in these patients is approximately 7000 times the risk of KS in the uninfected population (3, 16–18). Within populations of HIV-infected individuals, men who have sex with men are at the highest risk for acquisition of disease. This is followed by injection drug users, persons with hemophilia, and recipients of blood and blood products (5). Women whose partners are bisexual are also at risk for the acquisition of KS-associated herpesvirus (KSHV) infection and resultant KS (4). In contradistinction to classic KS, epidemic KS is more common in whites than in blacks, and the average age of diagnosis is 35 years. Since 1989, the incidence of KS has declined steadily (19). This

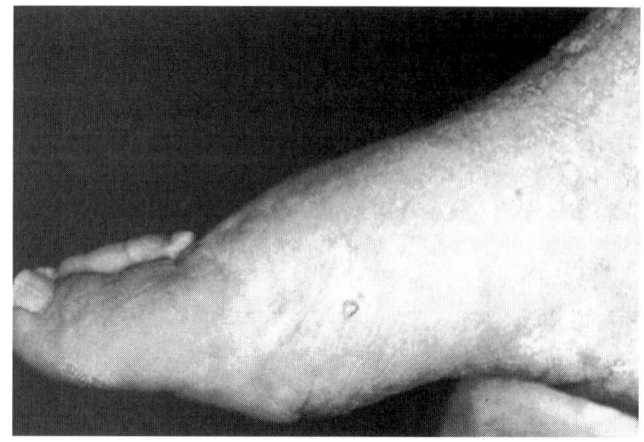

Figure 26.1. Kaposi's sarcoma lesions on the lower extremities. (See color section.)

change has been attributed to safer sex practices with decreased exposure to various herpesviruses including cytomegalovirus (20). With the advent of more potent antiretroviral therapy came a dramatic decline in the incidence of KS from 1995 through 1996 (21). Previously, the incidence was approximately 10% of all AIDS cases. With the introduction of more potent therapies, this incidence has decreased in excess of 50%. As demonstrated in numerous clinical studies, antiretroviral therapy has its most pronounced effect on the incidence of KS and on several opportunistic infections.

Etiology

The cause of KS remains controversial despite several major advances in the last 4 years. Initial studies had focused on genetic and environmental factors as well as infectious agents that could play a role in the development of KS. In the case of African KS, investigators assumed that repeated antigenic stimulation from various parasitic, viral, and bacterial infections led to immune suppression and the development of the disease (22–25). This was also offered as an explanation for the development of disease in classic KS and in KS in transplant recipients (26, 27). In both these situations, the waning immune system, either the result of immunosenescence or exogenous immunosuppressants, was thought to be a contributory factor.

ROLE OF GENETICS

Some early studies in patients with HIV identified an HLA subtype, HLA-DR5, as being increased in frequency in individuals with KS (28, 29). However, persons of Eastern European and Italian descent have a marked increase in the frequency of HLA-DR5, and, as a consequence, this marker may have been cosegregating with the known ethnic predilection for the development of KS (30, 31). Larger studies have demonstrated an increased frequency of HLA-DR1 in persons of Northern European descent (30). However, neither of these observations has withstood rigorous analysis when control of ethnic origin was considered (32, 33).

Nonetheless, specific genetic factors may be associated with the development of KS, as clearly demonstrated by the male predilection in various populations. Whether this is related to specific HLA subtypes or whether it is related to a mild general defect in immune surveillance such as X-linked immunodeficiency syndrome is unknown. Studies are currently under way to evaluate this possibility.

ROLE OF SEXUAL PRACTICES

Intensive study of the sexual histories of men who have developed KS has persistently demonstrated that specific sexual practices may be associated with the development of the disease (34, 35). In particular, the use of nitrate derivatives (36) has been linked to KS, along with oral–fecal contact (34). Both these observations have been controversial because subsequent studies have variably confirmed or refuted these linkages. In addition, although these sexual practices could explain the excess incidence of KS in men with HIV infection, they clearly do not explain the development of KS in endemic populations, nor do they explain the development of KS in classic cases. Thus, other factors must be involved in the genesis of this disease.

ROLE OF HIV

Significant attention has been played to the role of HIV infection in the development of KS. Investigators have postulated that HIV may have both indirect and direct roles. HIV infects CD4+ T cells, which are important for T-helper and suppressor functions within the immune system (37). In advanced stages of HIV infection, a dramatic decline in these cells can lead to severe immunologic defects and the development of numerous opportunistic infections. In addition to a direct immunologic defect in tumor recognition, HIV infection is associated with the perturbation of numerous cytokines. These include interleukin-6 (IL-6) (38, 39), tumor necrosis factor-α (TNF-α) (40), IL-1β (41, 42), IL-8 (43), and various chemokines (44). Laboratory studies have

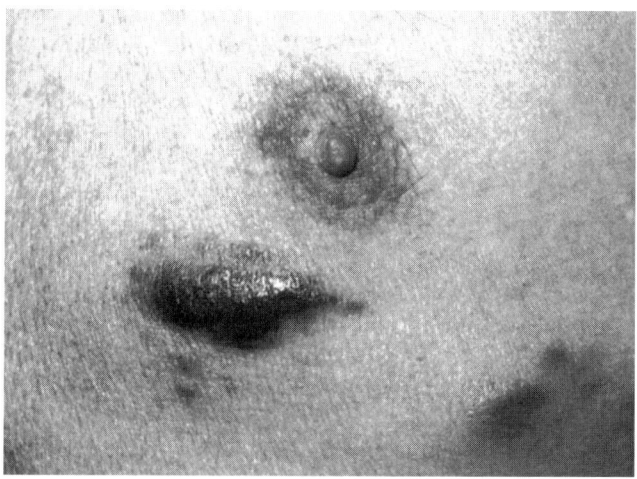

Figure 26.2. Nodular lesion of Kaposi's sarcoma on the chest of a patient with AIDS. (See color section.)

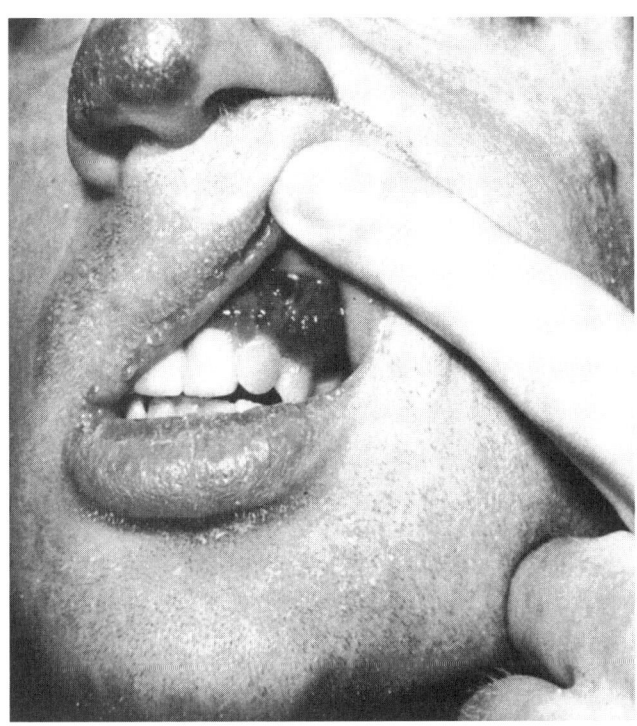

Figure 26.3. Kaposi's sarcoma infiltrating the mucous membrane and the gum in a patient with AIDS. (See color section.)

All this evidence suggests a clear role for HIV in the dramatic incidence of KS observed in the early 1980s. Whether acting through a direct or an indirect mechanism, HIV must be involved in increasing the risk of KS in HIV-infected individuals. However, patients with classic KS, renal transplant recipients, patients with endemic KS, and the rare cases of KS in HIV-negative homosexual men (52) clearly demonstrate that HIV is not the causative factor for the development of KS.

ROLE OF KSHV

Numerous other infectious agents have been postulated as etiologic agents for KS. Over the years, these have included cytomegalovirus (53), human papillomavirus (54), and *Mycoplasma*-like organisms (55). In 1994, Chang and colleagues changed the entire view of KS with the remarkable finding of herpeslike DNA viral sequences in most of KS lesions studied (56). Using representational display, these investigators found two stretches of DNA homologous to γ herpesviruses. Sequencing demonstrated that these were unique, and subsequent studies found these sequences in most KS lesions (57). This includes lesions from HIV-infected individuals, classic KS cases, endemic African cases, and cases in solid organ transplant recipients (58). This work has been confirmed by numerous authors worldwide and is a nearly universal finding (59).

demonstrated that any or all of these cytokines can contribute to the proliferation of explanted KS lesion–derived cells (45). Thus, through at least two different indirect mechanisms, HIV could contribute to the overall pathogenesis of KS.

In addition, some investigators have postulated that HIV may have a direct role in the pathogenesis of KS. Initial studies using HIV *tat* transgenic mice demonstrated that male mice were at increased risk for the development of angiosarcomas (46). These sarcomas had many of the histologic features of human KS. However, subsequent attempts to repeat these experiments have largely resulted in failure. Nonetheless, laboratory studies demonstrate that HIV *tat* has the ability to act as an attachment factor for normal endothelial cells as well as for smooth muscle cells (47). Either of these cells may be the original progenitor for KS. In addition to binding to the RGD sequence of $\alpha_V \beta_3$ integrin receptors (vitronectin) (47), *tat* may have a direct mitogenic effect on KS lesion–derived cells. Moreover, HIV *tat* transactivates the human IL-6 promoter and results in a dramatic upregulation of human IL-6 (48–50). IL-6 independently is a mitogen for these same cells (45), and thus HIV *tat* may indirectly be increasing the proliferation of KS-derived cells through an IL-6–mediated mechanism. Finally, basic fibroblast growth factor, another potent mitogen for endothelial cells, can work with cooperation with HIV *tat* to induce angiosarcoma-like lesions in nude mice (51). These effects can be blocked with antibodies to basic fibroblast growth factor or the omission of HIV *tat* protein. Thus, a human cytokine coupled with HIV *tat* protein has the ability to induce lesions reminiscent of KS directly in animal models.

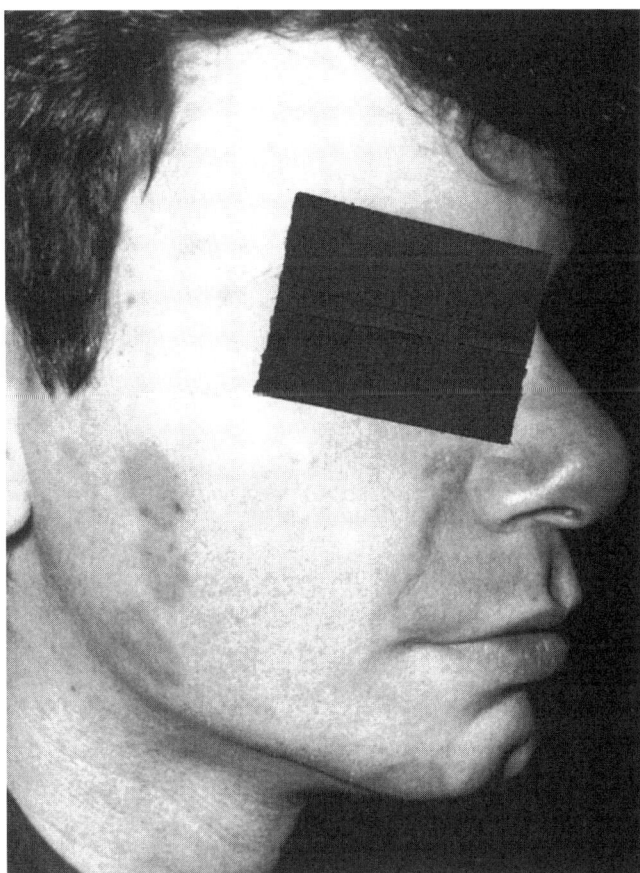

Figure 26.4. Kaposi's sarcoma lesions on the face. (See color section.)

The virus has been isolated, grown to large quantities in cell culture, used to prepare serologic tests (60), and completely sequenced (61, 62). KSHV for human herpesvirus 8 (HHV-8) is a member of the γ herpesvirus family; its most closely related virus is Herpesvirus saimiri. The approximately 134,000-kilobase pair genome contains more than 80 open-reading frames. In addition to the normal structural G, H, and B surface glycoproteins, the virus contains novel open-reading frames that have homology to human cytokines (61, 63–66). This includes homologs to human IL-6, human IL-8 receptor, human macrophage inhibitory proteins α and β, human cyclin D protein, and human bcl-2. In addition, there appears to be an acute transforming region referred to as the K1 product, as well as an interferon-related factor 1 homolog that appears to be functional (67). Thus, like many herpesviruses, KSHV appears to have captured certain human cytokine analogs that are undoubtedly important in the pathogenesis of disease caused by this virus.

Serologic studies using either latent nuclear antigen (60, 68–70) or recombinant enzyme-linked immunosorbent (ELISA) assays based on open-reading frame 65 (ORF65) (71), have demonstrated that most individuals with HIV-related KS are seropositive for KSHV. The highest titers of antibodies to KSHV are found in patients with classic disease. Low frequencies of antibodies are found in injection drug users, persons with hemophilia, and blood or blood product recipients who are also infected with HIV (72). The apparent serologic epidemiology of KSHV mirrors the clinical manifestation and frequency of incidence of KS within the HIV-infected population. Furthermore, a review of participants in the San Francisco Men's Health Study showed that 38% were seropositive for KSHV at baseline in 1984, and 50% of these developed KS within 10 years; KS did not develop in participants who were KSHV at baseline (71a). Thus, a strong linkage exists among exposure to KS, herpesvirus, and the development of KS.

ROLE OF CYTOKINES

As previously mentioned, numerous investigators have identified a role for various cytokines as increasing the proliferation of KS-derived lesions. Initial studies focused on TNF-α and IL-1β (73). Both are autocrine growth factors for these cells. Subsequent studies identified a major role for IL-6 (45), as well as for basic fibroblast growth factor (74) and vascular endothelial cell growth factor (VEGF) (43). In virtually all these studies, the cytokine and its homologous receptor are found on the spindle cells. Most studies have demonstrated that blocking the effects of the cytokine with either neutralizing antibodies or soluble receptors decreases the proliferation of cells. In addition, downregulation of endogenous production of these cytokines through use of corticosteroids, antisense oligonucleotides, or other agents decreases basal proliferation of cells. For example, IL-6 is produced in large amounts by AIDS-KS lesion–derived cells (45). Treatment of these cells with TNF-α or IL-1β induces IL-6 and subsequent proliferation of cells (75). These effects can be blocked through the use of antisense oligonucleotides directed at the first coding region for human IL-6 (45). In addition, these antisense oligonucleotides can decrease basal proliferation of KS-derived cells. Oncostatin-M, a member of the IL-6 family, induces production of IL-6 and is a mitogen for AIDS-KS–derived cells (76, 77). These effects can also be blocked through the use of soluble IL-6 gp130 receptors, IL-6 antisense oligonucleotides, or IL-6 neutralizing monoclonal antibodies (78).

In a similar manner, VEGF is produced in large amounts by AIDS-KS–derived cells (43). The AIDS-KS cells possess both the Flt-1 and KDR receptors. The effects of VEGF can be blocked by antisense oligonucleotides directed at VEGF. These inhibitory effects can be reversed by exogenous VEGF. In addition, an immunotoxin directed at VEGF receptors is lytic for AIDS-KS–derived cells in culture (43).

Patients with HIV infection have varying levels of circulating human cytokines. In general, patients with KS have increased levels of IL-6 (38, 39), VEGF, basal fibroblast growth factor, and human IL-8 (79). In some studies, IL-6 levels have been associated with the selective development of KS in HIV-infected individuals controlling for other factors (38). However, in larger studies, this observation has not been confirmed (39) In situ analysis using riboprobes for human cytokines has demonstrated production of basic fibroblast growth factor, IL-6, and VEGF in KS cells (80, 81). Receptors for human IL-6, platelet-derived growth factor, and VEGF have been demonstrated on these same cells (80, 81). In several instances, either messenger RNA for these

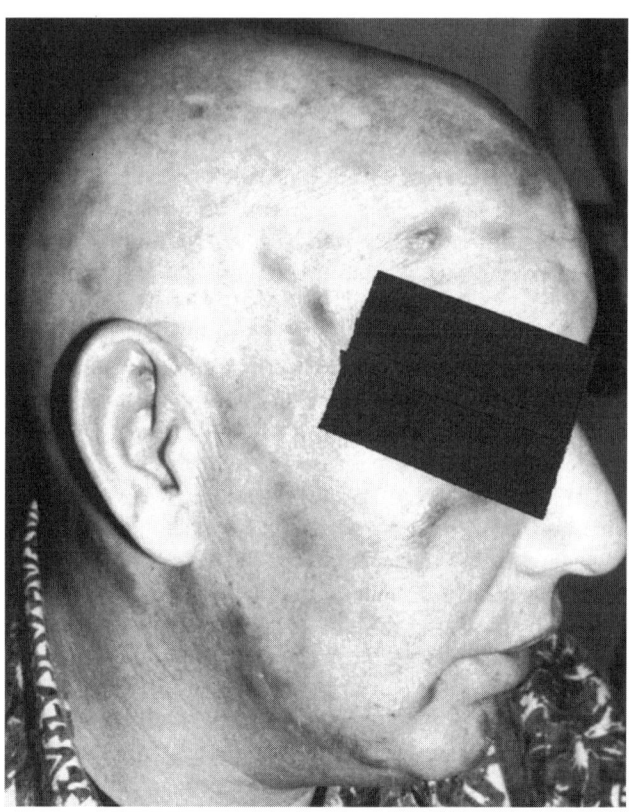

Figure 26.5. Kaposi's sarcoma lesions on the face. (See color section.)

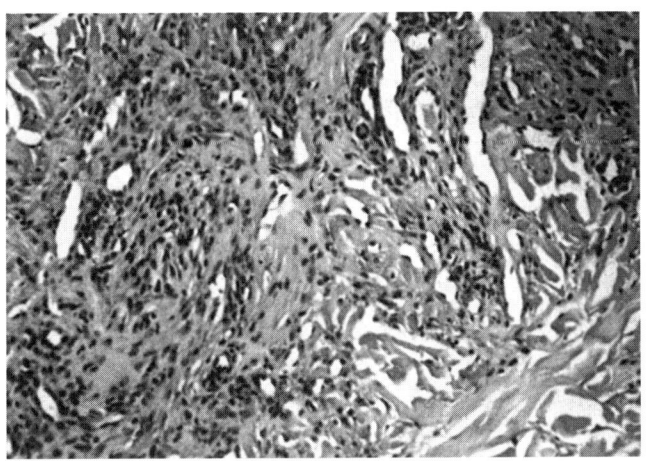

Figure 26.6. Histopathologic features of Kaposi's sarcoma tumor. (See color section.)

human cytokines or protein has been directly identified using reverse transcription–polymerase chain reaction (RT-PCR) or Western blot analysis of KS lesions (80).

Given the observation that KSHV encodes its own viral IL-6, cytokines do appear to play an integral role in the development of the KS lesion. Two of the virally encoded proteins, the macrophage inhibitory protein-1α (82) and interferon-related factor (83) homologs, directly induce angiosarcomas when genetically introduced into NIH 3T3 cells and placed in nude mice. Thus, KS herpesvirus could potentially directly cause KS. Whether KSHV alone induces the appearance of the lesion and is solely responsible for its pathogenesis or whether KSHV directly or indirectly induces other human cytokines largely responsible for the lesion remains controversial. Nonetheless, a clear interaction may exist between KSHV and various human cytokines in the production of the lesion we recognize as KS.

Histopathology

Characteristic histopathologic features of KS tumors include interweaving bands of spindle cells and vascular structures imbedded in the network of collagen and in reticular fibers (Fig. 26.6). The process is believed to begin in the dermis. Results of immunohistochemical staining using antibodies to factor VIII–related antigen and *Ulex europaeus* lectins in KS tissue have shown that both vascular and lymphatic endothelial make up the vessels of the tumor. Cleftlike spaces appear between the spindle cells or fragile capillaries. Significant nuclear pleomorphism may be seen in spindle cells. Histologic features of KS vary, depending on the quantity and characteristics of the spindle cells, vascular structures, fibrosis, and nuclear pleomorphism. The presence of extravasated red blood cells and hemosiderin between the spindle cells is a helpful microscopic feature. The mononuclear infiltrate varies in composition of lymphocytes, histiocytes, and plasma cells. The chronologic changes occur in histopathologic features of KS as lesions progress from macular to plaque and tumor stage. Macular lesions, which represent an early stage, are evident by abundant vessels mixed with the normal superficial vascular plexus within the dermis. The infiltrate is usually sparse and mixed. Plasma cells are seen around the dilated vasculature. Neutrophils are absent. Mitosis and nuclear atypia are rare.

The plaque stages involves entire dermis and at times extends into the adipose tissue. One sees more spindle cells and more extravasated red blood cells between the collagen bundles. Phagocytosized hemosiderin is more evident. Nuclear atypia and mitosis may still be rare. In the nodular and tumor stage, one sees marked increase in spindle cells, extravasated red blood cells, nuclear atypia, pleomorphism, and mitosis. There is an increased number of reticulum fibers but reduced collagen formation. Foot stain, which contains reticulum, aids in their recognition.

Lymph node involvement shows replacement of normal structure with histologic components of KS tumor, as described previously. The pathologic features of AIDS-related KS are similar to those of classic KS.

Immunohistochemical stains for CD34 and CD31 are usually positive for the spindle cells. In addition, large quantities of IL-6, VEGF, and basic fibroblast growth factor are seen in most sections (81). In situ hybridization for KSHV identifies KSHV sequences in the perivascular lining endothelial cells (84). Using in situ hybridization for the human cyclin-D homolog demonstrates widespread KSHV involvement in most spindle cells (85).

Clinical Manifestations

KS generally manifests with one or more multiple red or violaceous macule papules or nodules. The lesions in patients with HIV infection can be found on any part of the body. A predilection exists for involvement of surfaces that undergo trauma, including the feet, the tip of the nose, and the roof of the hard palate. Progression of each lesion generally involves enlargement of the original red macule. This macule gradually extends in diameter, often with an associated echymotic halo. Ultimately, the macular lesion rises vertically in size and develops into a large nodule. These nodules are generally violaceous. They often occur in patches following a distribution of Koebner's lines. Large areas of involvement can coalesce to form a large plaque of disease. These plaques, in turn, can ulcerate, erode, and involve into fungating lesions.

The lesions of AIDS-related KS, in contrast to those of classic KS, tend to be smaller initially and frequently involve the mucous membranes, lymph nodes, and gastrointestinal tract (see Figs. 26.1 to 26.5). Occasionally, the first manifestation of disease is in the lymph nodes or the gastrointestinal tract. The most common extracutaneous site is the gastrointestinal tract, although lesions may be seen in the lung, liver, spleen, adrenal gland, pancreas, bone, bone marrow, and testes. KS has rarely been identified in the brain, where it is generally not found in the parenchyma, but rather in the surrounding vasculature.

At times, clinicians have difficulty in distinguishing between symptoms related to HIV infection and those of KS.

Even in cases of infiltration of vital organs by KS, in general, these lesions do not cause significant physiologic change. Signs and symptoms such as fever, weight loss, anorexia, and malaise are generally due to other opportunistic infections and are rarely related to KS. Lymphadenopathy may be secondary to HIV infection, an opportunistic infection, infiltration by KS, and, in rare cases, lymphoma.

Lymphatic involvement of any form of KS may cause lymphatic obstruction leading to edema and is a significant cause of clinical morbidity. A case in point is ocular involvement of AIDS-related KS. Ocular KS lesions often develop after the occurrence of KS on the extremities, but conjunctival tumors have been reported in the absence of other manifestations. KS can involve the ocular adnexa including eyelids, conjunctiva, lacrimal glands, and orbit. Ophthalmic lesions are usually slowly progressive, but in rare cases they have a rapidly progressive course. With extensive tissue involvement or edema secondary to lymphatic obstruction, visual function may be impaired.

Pulmonary involvement may cause shortness of breath and dyspnea on exertion. Rarely does it present as hemoptysis. Blood loss, vomiting, anemia, diarrhea, weight loss, or persistent mucous discharge from the rectum may be manifestations of gastrointestinal involvement. Most times, pulmonary KS is difficult to distinguish clinically and radiographically from *Pneumocystis carinii* pneumonia. Gallium scanning is uniformly negative in individuals with KS (6, 87). The finding of an isolated or bilateral pleural effusion is usually indicative of KS. These effusions are uniformly bloody. The finding of a pleural effusion in *Pneumocystis carinii* pneumonia is rare.

Course of Disease and Prognosis

The course of KS ranges from a few rare isolated KS lesions that can be surgically removed to cases of rapid disseminated disease resulting in fatal pulmonary complications. The rate of progression is related to the underlying immune defect, successful treatment of HIV infection, and the development of other opportunistic infection.

Commonly, KS initially presents after the development of an opportunistic infection. Despite an alarming increase in the number of lesions over a short period, this can quiesce with successful treatment of the opportunistic infection and underlying HIV infection. In some instances, successful treatment of HIV can result in regression or disappearance of KS (88, 89), although this situation appears rare in patients with advanced AIDS-related KS (21). The development of concurrent opportunistic infections frequently exacerbates KS. Clinicians who are treating HIV-infected individuals and who observe a rapid increase in the rate of progression of KS should be vigilant to the identification of an underlying opportunistic infection.

Survival in epidemic KS largely depends both on the stage of disease and on the underlying deficit and HIV RNA copy number. Large studies have demonstrated that survival of patients with KS has generally increased in proportion to the increase of survival seen with other individuals with HIV infection (90). Individuals who present with KS as an initial manifestation generally live longer than those who present with other opportunistic infections. However, this finding may signify that KS can present at all stages of HIV disease, including conditions with normal CD4 counts. Median survival reported in older studies ranged from 13 to 29 months (79). More recent reports with the advent of antiretroviral therapy suggest that survival may be at least twice as long and perhaps significantly longer. Other reports note regression of KS with intensive anti-HIV therapy as well as use of antiherpes medications (88). As more potent antiherpes become available (91), perhaps regression of clinical KS will be achieved with a combination of antiretroviral and antiherpes medications.

Diagnosis

Diagnosis of fully developed KS is generally made on clinical grounds. Even early lesions of KS are often obvious to those familiar with HIV disease. However, the clinician should confirm the clinical impression with a histopathologic documentation. Punch biopsy of any accessible cutaneous lesion can be readily performed. Cautery can be achieved with the use of silver nitrate. This results in little morbidity and an excellent cosmetic result. Lymph node biopsies are warranted in patients with clinically significant lymphadenopathy. The clinician should exclude the presence of a coexisting lymphoma that may also be related to KSHV infection. Lesions in the gastrointestinal tract can be diagnosed by endoscopic visualization and biopsy. Esophagogastroduodenoscopy, sigmoidoscopy, and colonoscopy are recommended for patients who present with extensive disease or gastrointestinal complaints. Pulmonary KS is generally confirmed by bronchoscopic evaluation and transbronchial biopsy. In the case of pleural effusion, the pleural biopsy and cytologic examination may identify KS spindle cells. Staining with CD34 monoclonal antibodies can be useful in this setting. Sometimes, an open lung biopsy is necessary, given the differential diagnosis.

Differential Diagnosis

Although the diagnosis of KS can be made clinically and confirmed by histologic examination, the differential diagnosis can be considered. The clinical appearance of KS lesions may be confused with other cutaneous entities. Some of the differential diagnoses include malignant melanoma, angiomas, cutaneous angiosarcomas, spindle cell hemangioendothelioma, angiolipoma, dermatofibromas, pyogenic granulomas, anthropod bites, glomus tumors, and sarcoid nodules. More extensive disease may bear notable similarity to lichen planus, sarcoidosis, urticaria pigmentosa, papular urticaria, eruptive xanthomas, disseminated secondary syphilis, and angiosarcomas. Attention should be paid to a more recently described entity, bacillary angiomatosis, which cllinically resembles KS nodules (92, 93). On histologic examination, the two disorders are readily distinguishable. Bacillary angiomatosis responds to macrolide antibiotics. Both entities can be found in the same individual.

Staging

Staging classifications have traditionally been used in cancer patients. The staging takes into account the anatomic distribution of the tumor, including the primary site and any evidence of metastatic spread. Such formulations aid in the clinical management of patients and allowing physicians to decide on the best treatment plan based on stage of disease. Staging also assists in determining the probable prognosis of the patient. In KS, such staging mechanisms do not appear to be effective (94).

In large part, KS presents as multicentric disease, and its rate of progression is largely related to the degree of underlying immune suppression. In addition, the tumor does not metastasize in a traditional manner and frequently has exacerbations related to opportunistic infections. However, several groups have made attempts to introduce staging classifications for KS. Chachoua and Krigel and their colleagues proposed a classification system that categorized AIDS-related KS by primary type of lesion, extent of tumor, and presence or absence of constitutional symptoms (95). Stage 1 represents cutaneous, locally indolent; stage 2, cutaneous, locally aggressive with or without regional lymph nodes; stage 3, generalized mucocutaneous or lymph node involvement; stage 4, visceral. This group further subcategorized patients based on constitutional symptoms on presentation. Thus, subtype A includes no systemic signs or symptoms, and subtype B has the following systemic signs: more than 10% weight loss or fevers (higher than 100EF orally) unrelated to an identifiable source of infection lasting more than 2 weeks. Disease progression, survival, or prognosis can be determined from this classification system.

A more modern staging system was proposed by Mitsuyasu (94). It delineates stage by amount of tumor, location of lesions, and clinical symptoms: stage 1, limited cutaneous (fewer than 10 lesions or 1 anatomic area); stage 2, disseminated cutaneous (more than 10 lesions or more than 1 anatomic area); stage 3, visceral only (gastrointestinal, lymph nodes); stage 4, cutaneous and visceral, or pulmonary KS. Again, each stage is subtyped. Subtype A represents no systemic signs or symptoms, whereas subtype B involves fever (more than 37.8EC unrelated to identifiable infection) lasting longer than 2 weeks or weight loss (more than 10% of body weight). Prognosis, survival, and response to therapy are not addressed in this classification staging system, either.

Mitsuyasu analyzed stage of KS, therapeutic modality, and subsequent response in a retrospective study of AIDS-KS patients treated with recombinant interferon-α. Response to therapy did not correlate with stage of disease. Both stage 1 and stage 3 patients were found to have improved survival compared with patients in stage 2 or stage 4. Contrary to what is seen in most major cancers, visceral involvement was not associated with the worst prognostic outcome. However, response to therapy with recombinant interferon did correlate with subtype. Patients with subtype A had a more favorable response compared with subtype B patients (94).

As discussed earlier, the major prognostic determinant in AIDS-related KS is the underlying degree of immune deficiency as reflected in the absolute number of CD4 cells. In addition, more recent studies suggest that HIV RNA copy number may also provide additional information in subclassifying patients with regard to survival and prognosis. Because KS is rarely a cause of death, immune suppression and viral replication may be the primary determinants of survival.

An attempt to provide a prognostic classification, which took into consideration underlying immune deficits, was proposed by Krown and associates (96). This system involves defining the extent of tumor involvement, the degree of immune suppression, and any evidence of systemic symptoms. Patients are divided into "good-risk" and "poor-risk" categories according to the extent of tumor (T), the severity of immunosuppression (I) (CD4 greater than or equal to or less than $200/mm^3$), and the presence of other systemic HIV-1–associated illness (S). An analysis of this system of classification using 294 consecutive patients enrolled in 8 AIDS Clinical Trials Group (ACTG)–sponsored therapeutic trials for AIDS-related KS showed that the estimated median survival was shorter for patients in the poor-risk category for each of the TIS factors (T0, 27 months versus T1, 15 months, $P<.001$; I0, 40 months versus I1, 13 months, $P<.001$; S0, 22 months versus S1, 16 months, $P=.040$). The stage of tumor (T) and immune status (I) were significant independent predictors of survival and demonstrated that the survival is not independent of the extent of tumor. An interaction was also noted between poor immune function and tumor stage ($P=.025$). Subgroup analyses suggest that other cutoffs for poor immune function (e.g., CD4 up to $100/mm^3$) and exposure to chemotherapy may improve the predictive value of the model (97).

Treatment

Numerous treatment modalities have been recommended for treatment of patients with AIDS-related KS. However, the introduction of liposomal anthracyclines and the discovery that taxane derivatives are highly effective in the treatment of KS have led to a complete rethinking of treatment recommendations for patients.

The fundamental basis for treatment of patients with AIDS-related KS is suppression of HIV replication. Clinicians encountering patients with new-onset KS or worsening KS should first think of inadequate suppression of HIV replication. Numerous clinical studies demonstrate that aggressive antiretroviral therapy can decrease the incidence of KS, slow the rate of progression of KS, and, in rare instances, result in regression of preexistent disease (98, 99). Thus, the initial evaluation of patients should include monitoring of CD4+ T cells and HIV RNA. If the patient does not have near-complete suppression of HIV replication as demonstrated by undetectable HIV RNA, strong consideration should be given to improvement or change in antiretroviral regimen. In addition, if a patient has complete suppression of HIV RNA and slowly improving or increased CD4+ T cells, an extensive evaluation for detection of occult opportunistic infections that may stimulate existing KS should be undertaken. These should include blood cultures for *Mycobacterium avium* and cytomegalovirus and a chest radiograph to exclude *Pneumocystis carinii* pneumonia and other pathogens. Patients with headaches should undergo a lumbar puncture with studies for cryptococcal meningitis. In addition, patients with fevers should have additional studies including those for *Mycobacterium tuberculosis*, cryptococcal antigen, and toxoplasmosis antibody, as indicated.

Patients with adequate suppression of HIV replication and no evidence of an opportunistic infection, and new-onset KS or advancing disease, are candidates for KS-specific therapy. Treatment for such individuals depends on the extent of disease at presentation.

Patients who have recent-onset disease and few lesions can often be adequately treated with antiretroviral agents and topical cryotherapy using liquid nitrogen (100, 101). Lesions can be removed with cryotherapy on virtually any part of the body including the eyelid, eyebrows, conjunctiva, sclera, oropharynx, all mucous membranes, and the shaft and glans of the penis, as well as the perirectal area and the skin. Treatment should aim for a freeze time for the lesion of approximately 20 to 30 seconds. It is not necessary to remove all the KS at a single treatment. Repeated cryotherapy on the same lesion can be performed every 2 to 4 weeks until successful debulking has occurred. It is important not to overtreat with cryotherapy because the resulting cosmetic defect can be as disfiguring as the original lesion.

Other local therapies are more costly and, in some instances, less effective than cryotherapy. These include laser therapy using an argon laser, as well as carbon dioxide lasers. The carbon dioxide laser results in tissue vaporization, and these vapors may contain infectious particles of numerous viruses. Thus, some concerns exist about its safety. The argon laser emits a blue-green light that is absorbed by melanin and oxygenated hemoglobin causing photocoagulation. However, laser treatment is largely impractical because each session requires a long time to treat the numerous lesions. In addition, the patient is often left with a pigmented stain that is as unsightly as the original lesion.

Interlesional treatment with vinblastine or vincristine has been widely used in the last 5 years (102–104). However, this approach has fallen out of favor as more effective antiretroviral therapy and use of local cryotherapy have gained acceptance. Treatment with injections of vinblastine generally uses 0.1 mL per lesion of a 0.1-mg/mL vinblastine solution. Vinblastine injections cause significant local erythema, ulceration, and pain. It is often difficult to control the extent of local tissue destruction. Therefore, vinblastine and laser therapy have less desirable cosmetic results.

Radiation therapy has been used successfully in the treatment of both classic and AIDS-associated KS. These tumors are exquisitely sensitive to radiation therapy, and rarely do treatments require more than 200 cGy per lesion. In addition, patients can often be treated with an electron beam that has less penetration into the skin. Like cryotherapy, radiation therapy can be administered to any part of the body, including treatment of areas often problematic with other forms of treatment. These include areas on the feet that impede mobility and lymph nodes that obstruct lymphatic drainage and cause swelling. Radiation therapy has also been useful in the treatment of periorbital and eyelid tumors that cause edema and visual impairment (105). Patients who have obstructing lesions of the oral pharynx or the gastrointestinal tract can similarly be treated with radiation therapy (106). Patients and therapists must understand that radiation treatment often leaves a hyperpigmented area equal in size to the former lesion or an area of depigmentation around the lesion from the radiation. Thus, although the texture of the skin after radiation therapy returns to normal, the cosmetic result is not as acceptable as with cryotherapy.

Virtually every type of radiation therapy has been used in the treatment of KS. These approaches include orthovoltage, megavoltage, kilovoltage, and electron and photon beams. The selection and type of radiation therapy depend on the size, location, and symptoms associated with treatment. In patients with advanced KS in whom multiple other regimens have failed, fractionated single-dose hemibody radiation can be used. In a report from the New York University Medical Center, 15 patients with KS were treated in this manner for progressive disease (107). All cutaneous disease demonstrated partial regression, and complete regression was noted in 9 patients. Similarly, studies have been performed using electron beam for radiation therapy. In study by Nisce and Safai (108) of a cohort of 38 patients with AIDS-related KS who had previously had chemotherapy, immunotherapy, or hormonal therapy, 11 received total or subtotal electron beam therapy; the treatment involved 40 cGy weekly for 6 weeks. Twenty-seven patients received local radiation therapy at a dose of 200 to 300 cGy for 2 to 3 weeks. Significant amelioration of pain and edema resulted, and in a patient with hemoptysis due to KS, the problem resolved.

Despite the long-standing history and excellent results observed with radiation therapy, the long-term consequences of repeated treatment diminish enthusiasm for the use of this treatment modality. First, patients often require retreatment not only of the original treatment area but also of adjacent involved areas of the skin. Matching the radiation therapy ports is important and is often difficult to accomplish. Although patients who have received 200 cGy can receive additional radiation therapy, if two or more of these fields overlap, skin necrosis often occurs. In addition, radiation therapy causes sclerosis of lymphatics. This effect, coupled with the natural tendency of KS to induce significant edema because of VEGF secretion or obstruction of lymphatics, has long-term consequences. These include severe lymphedema and limb anasarca. Some of the worst long-term results of radiation therapy are seen in patients who have received radiation to the pelvis or groin for extensive disease. These individuals usually have severe, persistent refractory lower extremity edema.

Thus, for patients with limited cutaneous involvement, the ideal treatment remains cryotherapy. Patients who have more than a few lesions should be treated with systemic antineoplastic agents.

CHEMOTHERAPY

The use of liposomal anthracyclines and paclitaxel for the treatment of KS represents a significant milestone in the management of this disease. To date, more than 1000 patients with AIDS-related KS have been treated with liposomal anthracyclines in various clinical settings and clinical trials. Currently, two products are licensed for use in the United States: liposomal doxorubicin (Doxil) and liposomal daunorubicin (DaunoXome). These agents have unique pharmacokinetics, tissue distribution, clinical activity, and toxicities compared with their native counterparts.

Liposomal doxorubicin has two-compartment linear pharmacokinetics (109) and unique tissue accumulation (110). In a phase I studies, lesion response was significantly related to both the average daily maximum doxorubicin concentration ($C_{max,avg}$) and dose intensity. This property is strikingly different from conventional doxorubicin (109). In another phase I study, 18 patients with AIDS-related KS were randomly assigned to receive either standard doxorubicin or pegylated (PEG)-liposomal doxorubicin. Clearance of PEG-liposomal doxorubicin was 0.034 to 0.108 L/m^2 per hour, and the volume of distribution (V_d) was 2.2 to 4.4 L/m^2. The half-lives of the initial decline in the plasma concentration-time curve and of the terminal decline were 3.77 and 41.3 hours, respectively. Seventy-two hours after administration, the doxorubicin levels in the lesions of patients receiving PEG-liposomal doxorubicin were 5.2 to 11.4 times greater than those found in patients given comparable doses of standard doxorubicin (110).

Several phase II studies of liposomal doxorubicin have been reported. In the largest reported trial, 238 patients were treated biweekly with 10, 20, or 40 mg/m^2 liposomal doxorubicin (111). Tumor response was assessed according to ACTG criteria before each cycle. The best response was achieved after a mean of 2.3 cycles (range, 1 to 20). Fifteen patients (6.3%) had a complete response, 177 (74.4%) had a partial response, 44 (18.5%) had stable disease, and 2 (0.8%) had disease progression. Liposomal doxorubicin was well tolerated: 10 patients discontinued therapy because of adverse events, in 4 cases because of neutropenia. Grade 3 or 4 neutropenia occurred after 281 of 2023 cycles (13.9%), but it involved 137 of 240 patients (57.1%) for whom data were available (111).

Similarly, the pharmacokinetic profile of liposomal daunorubicin differs from the free drug daunorubicin. In a phase I study of liposomal daunorubicin, 40 patients with advanced AIDS-related KS were treated with doses of 10, 20, 30, and 40 mg/m^2 given once every 3 weeks, and 40, 50, and 60 mg/m^2 given once every 2 weeks. The area under the plasma concentration curve (AUC) ranged from 16.9 to 375.3 mg/mL per hour. The α half-life ranged from 7.8 to 8.3 hours at 10 to 60 mg/m^2, respectively. Both pharmacokinetic profiles were significantly better than with free daunorubicin. Liposomal daunorubicin was well tolerated with no significant alopecia, mucositis, or vomiting. Neutropenia (less than 1000/μL) occurred in 17% of cycles and was severe (less than 500/μL) in 2%. Like liposomal doxorubicin, liposomal daunorubicin has altered tissue distribution. Even after cumulative doses higher than 1000 mg/m^2, no significant declines in cardiac function were seen (112).

In a phase II study of patients with no prior anthracycline chemotherapy, 30 patients with AIDS-related KS were treated with liposomal daunorubicin at a dose of 40 mg/m^2 intravenously once every 2 weeks. Twenty-two patients (73%) achieved a partial response. Median time to treatment response was 30 days (range, 15 to 202). For patients with a partial response, median time to treatment failure was 153 days (range, 15 to 558). Patients received a median of 10 cycles (range, 1 to 44). Adverse events were minimal. The most common side effect was granulocytopenia, seen in 16 patients (53%) (113).

Both liposomal preparations have been studied in comparative phase III studies against standard therapy. Liposomal doxorubicin (20 mg/m^2 every 3 weeks) was compared with a combination of bleomycin (15 IU/m^2) and vincristine (2 mg) every 3 weeks in 241 patients for 6 cycles. A total of 121 patients received liposomal doxorubicin, and 120 patients received the bleomycin–vincristine combination. Liposomal doxorubicin was more effective (response rate [partial response plus complete response], 58.7% versus 23.3%, $P<.001$) and was better tolerated with fewer adverse events (10.7% versus 26.7%), and more patients receiving liposomal doxorubicin completed the course of therapy (55.4% versus 30.8%). Treatment with bleomycin and vincristine was associated with a significantly higher incidence of peripheral neuropathy ($P<.001$), whereas liposomal doxorubicin was more commonly associated with neutropenia and delays in receiving treatment ($P\leq.001$) (114).

Lipsomal daunorubicin was compared with observation in patients with early KS. Twenty-nine AIDS patients with fewer than 20 cutaneous lesions of KS, no visceral involvement, and CD4 cell counts lower than 400/μL were randomized to 12 weeks of observation or liposomal daunorubicin (40 mg/m^2) every 2 weeks. Six patients in the treatment arm had a response (40%) versus none in the observation arm. Six patients (40%) randomized to liposomal daunorubicin had disease progression during chemotherapy, whereas 10 (72%) in the observation arm of the trial progressed. Neutropenia was the main toxicity (14% of treatment cycles) (115).

Liposomal doxorubicin (20 mg/m^2) was also compared with ABV (doxorubicin [Adriamycin] 20 mg/m^2, bleomycin 10 mg/m^2 and vincristine 1 mg) in 258 patients at 25 treatment centers. Liposomal doxorubicin was more effective (response rate, 45.9%; 95% confidence interval [CI], 37 to 54% versus 24.8%; 95% CI, 17 to 32%; $P<.001$), more rapid to act (median time to response, 39 versus 50 days; $P=.014$; log rank), and equal in duration of response and time to disease progression. Liposomal doxorubicin was associated with significantly less nausea and vomiting, hair loss, peripheral neuropathy, and mucositis, and it had a similar degree of leukopenia. Liposomal daunorubicin (40 mg/m^2) was also compared with a less potent ABV regimen (doxorubicin 10 mg/m^2, bleomycin 10 mg/m^2, and vincristine 1 mg) in 232 patients. Liposomal daunorubicin provided similar efficacy, median time to treatment failure, and overall survival to this lower-dose regimen. However, liposomal daunorubicin was associated with significantly less alopecia and neuropathy ($P<.0001$), but with more episodes of grade 4 neutropenia ($P=.021$) (116).

Clearly, these liposomal anthracycline preparations are more effective and better tolerated than their free drug counterparts. In addition, they are more effective than older combinations of chemotherapy including ABV, vinblastine alternating with vincristine, and vincristine and bleomycin–based regimens. The lack of hair loss and other systemic toxicities represents a tremendous advance in tolerance and cosmesis for patients receiving these agents. Because they are well tolerated, these liposomal preparations represent the most appropriate first-line therapy for patients with advancing KS despite adequate antiretroviral therapy.

Similarly, treatment of refractory KS with paclitaxel represents a significant improvement in the therapy of patients with advanced disease. In a pioneering study, 29 patients with advanced HIV-associated KS were treated with 135 mg/m^2 over 3 hours every 3 weeks without filgrastim support. The dose was increased as tolerated to a maximum of 175 mg/m^2. Patients who failed to respond or in whom disease progressed received filgrastim support or paclitaxel administered over 96 hours. Of 28 assessable patients, 20 had major responses (71.4%; 95% CI, 51.3 to 86.8%). Each of the 5 patients with pulmonary KS responded, as did all 4 assessable patients who had previously received anthracycline therapy for KS. Of 6 patients who went on to receive a 96-hour infusion of paclitaxel, 5 had major responses. Neutropenia was the most frequent dose-limiting toxicity (117).

The preliminary observation of the high-level activity of paclitaxel in AIDS-related KS was confirmed in two additional controlled trials (118, 119). A pilot study with a lower dose but higher intensity of paclitaxel for the treatment of AIDS-related KS was reported. The dose of paclitaxel was 100 mg/m^2 infused over 3 hours every 2 weeks. A total of 34 male patients were treated in the study. Twenty patients had more than 50 lesions, 79% had symptomatic edema, and 34% had symptomatic visceral disease. The median CD4+ cell count was 5/mm^3, with a range of 0 to 230 cells/mm^3. Twenty patients (59%) had received prior multiagent chemotherapy with ABV, 9 (26%) patients had received bleomycin and vincristine, and 5 (15%) had taken liposomal daunorubicin. Fourteen patients (41%) had received more than 2 prior chemotherapy regimens (118).

Of the 30 patients evaluable for response, 16 (53%) showed partial remission and 14 had stable disease. Symptomatic relief of tumor-associated edema occurred in 25 of the 26 patients. All patients had severe alopecia. Other side effects reported included rash, fatigue, nausea, and myalgias. Unlike in the prior study, no drug fever or eosinophilia was observed. Grade 3 or 4 neutropenia, defined as an absolute neutrophil count (ANC) less than 750 cells/mm^3, was relatively uncommon. However, most of the patients in this study received granulocyte colony-stimulating factor before entry into the study.

A third trial of paclitaxel in chemotherapy-naive patients has been reported. The same regimen (paclitaxel at 100 mg/m^2 infused over 3 hours) was used. Twenty patients were included in the study. Seventeen patients had more than 50 lesions, and 85% of the patients had CD4+ cell count less than 100 cells/mm^3. Of the 19 patients evaluable, 1 (5%) had a pathologic complete response, 1 (5%) had a clinical complete response, 12 (60%) had a partial response, and 5 (25%) had stable disease. Overall, a response rate of 70% was observed in this group of chemotherapy-naive patients (118).

It may be possible to use an even less intense regimen of paclitaxel than previously used. Mega and colleagues (119) presented their preliminary results of a low-dose, low-intensity regimen using paclitaxel at 30 mg/m^2 infused over 3 hours every week. Only 4 patients were treated, and all showed flattening of cutaneous lesions and regression of tumor-associated edema. Although the mean ANC at study entry was 1300 cells/mm^3, no patients developed grade 3 or 4 neutropenia after a mean of 4.6 cycles of treatment.

Paclitaxel appears to be more effective than liposomal anthracyclines in the treatment of KS, given the high response rate in patients with late stage disease and in anthracycline therapy failures. If this is true, why not use paclitaxel as initial therapy? The answer lies in the major difference in toxicity between the two regimens. Whereas liposomal anthracyclines cause bone marrow suppression and limited other toxicities, paclitaxel causes severe hair loss, nausea, vomiting, body aches, and pancytopenia. Thus, from the standpoint purely of tolerance, the liposomal anthracyclines remain the drugs of choice as initial therapy. Although it may be possible to examine lower doses of paclitaxel in the future, especially in association with protease inhibitors that block cytochrome p450 CYP3A function, those studies remain to be completed. From the patient's perspective, hair loss is a significant disadvantage to the use of all taxoids. As a result of the introduction of liposomal anthracyclines and taxoids for the treatment of KS, other forms of combination chemotherapy are not recommended for use at this time.

INTERFERONS

The immunomodulatory, antineoplastic, and antiviral effects of interferons have made them prime candidates for investigation and treatment of AIDS-related KS. Their immunomodulatory effects include enhancements of natural killer cell activity, T-cell–mediated cytotoxicity, and macrophage activation. Three recombinant interferon-α preparations are currently in use for the treatment of KS. These are interferon α2a and α2b and "consensus" interferon. Clinical studies have been largely accomplished with the α2a and α2b compounds (120–123). Studies involving the use of interferon-β have shown some clinical activity (124). However, this activity appears to be substantially less than that of the interferon-α products. Interferon-γ has little activity in this disorder (125). As a consequence, treatment with interferon preparations is recommended only for the α2a, α2b, and "consensus" interferon preparations.

Initial studies with interferon-α were performed before the introduction of antiretroviral therapy for HIV (120). Doses as high as 50 million IU subcutaneously three times a week were used during "induction." The original FDA-approval for interferon by the United States Food and Drug Administration included dose recommendations of up to 36 million IU three times a week. These doses are poorly tolerated by most patients, but responses upwards of 30 to 35% have been observed (120). As monotherapy, interferon-α works best in patients who have CD4 counts higher than 200/mm^3 at the time of treatment. Side effects generally seen with higher doses include severe fever, fatigue, chills, nausea, anorexia, weight loss, diarrhea, increased liver functions tests (usually transient during the first 2 months), and cytopenias.

Newer protocols involve the gradual introduction of interferon-α starting at 1 million IU per evening. This dose is increased to 3, 6, and finally 9 million IU per evening over a period of 2 months. Nonsteroidal anti-inflammatory medications and acetaminophen are used prophylactically to prevent the anticipated fevers, chills, and myalgias. These regimens are well tolerated by most patients. When planning anti-KS therapy, clinicians should recognize that the efficacy of interferon is not related to the extent of clinical disease. Patients with widespread disseminated disease can have complete clinical responses, as demonstrated by Krown and colleagues (120), Oettgen, Real, and Krown (126), and Mitsuyasu (94).

The potential for enhancing the effects of interferon-α with antiretroviral therapy was tried. Clinical studies have demonstrated that interferon-α with dideoxycytidine (ddC, zalcitabine) or dideoxyinosine (ddI, didanosine) can result in a greater response rate at lower overall doses of interferon-α (127). Responses can be seen at doses of interferon-α as low as 3 million IU per night and in patients with low CD4 cell counts (lower than 100 CD4 cells/mm^3) (127). In addition, patients who have recovered immune function as a result of antiretroviral therapy appear to have an increased response rate to interferon-α. As a result, clinical trials are ongoing using three- and four-drug antiretroviral regimens with interferon-α preparations. The dose-limiting effects of interferon-α preparations include neutropenia, anemia, transient chemical hepatitis, and constitutional symptoms of fever, malaise, myalgias, and fatigue.

Investigators have also tried using interferon-α after chemotherapy to extend the benefit of chemotherapy. Initial studies in the absence of antiretroviral therapy failed. Patients who received interferon-α after induction ABV chemotherapy generally had treatment failures at a rate similar to those receiving placebo (128). Reports by several clinicians demonstrate that patients who previously received long-term treatment with liposomal anthracycline preparations, including patients with pulmonary disease, can have stable disease when treated with aggressive antiretroviral regimens. This finding led to clinical studies investigating the induction of tumor response by liposomal anthracycline or paclitaxel-containing regimens followed by the use of interferon-α in combination with antiretroviral therapy.

ANTIHERPES MEDICATIONS

The association of KSHV with KS led to the speculation that treatment of the underlying viral infection may result in tumor regression. Three retrospective studies demonstrated that patients who have HIV infection have a greater than 50% decline in the incidence of KS if they have received either ganciclovir- or foscarnet-containing regimens (129–131). No reduction in KS is seen in patients receiving acyclovir (129). For example, Jones and colleagues (131) retrospectively reviewed patients with HIV infection and found that patients who received foscarnet or ganciclovir had a reduced relative risk of KS compared with individuals who did not receive these medications. Glesby and associates (130) reviewed 935 men in the Multicenter AIDS Cohort Study (MACS). These investigators found that the relative risk of development of KS over the period of observation was reduced by 46% in men with cytomegalovirus disease who received ganciclovir (relative risk [RR], 0.56; 95% CI, 0.22 to 1.44; $P=.23$) and by 60% (RR, 0.40; 95% CI, 0.051 to 3.10; $P=.38$) in men who received foscarnet (130). A third report confirmed these two other studies and showed a risk reduction of 61% in 3688 patients with HIV infection who had received foscarnet (RR, 0.38; 95% CI, 0.15 to 0.95; $P=.038$) and 61% (RR, 0.39; 95% CI, 0.19 to 0.84; $P=.015$) in patients who had received ganciclovir. No reduction in incidence was seen in patients who received acyclovir (RR, 1.10; 95% CI, 0.88 to 1.38; $P=.40$) (129). Thus, the in vitro activity of antiherpes medications against KSHV appears to mirror the clinical utility of these agents in preventing the development of KS (91). Given new assays to detect KSHV exposure (132), the in vitro studies suggest the exciting possibility of providing once-daily oral prophylaxis with a medication such as lobucavir (91) to those HIV-infected patients at highest risk for developing KS.

These observations gave rise to widespread introduction of antiherpes medications as a treatment for KS. Unfortunately, these agents have uniformly been unsuccessful. Treatment of individuals with KS with foscarnet or ganciclovir does not result in clinical regression of KS. Preliminary results of a placebo-controlled study of oral ganciclovir in patients with HIV and KS suggested a decrease in the rate of progression of KS, primarily manifested as a decreased incidence in the frequency of subsequent treatment with chemotherapy. However, this finding has not been confirmed in other larger observational cohorts.

Nonetheless, in vitro data clearly suggest that some antiherpes medications could inhibit KSHV transmission or reactivation. These include foscarnet, ganciclovir, lobucavir, PMEA, and cidofovir (91). Acyclovir and penciclovir have no activity in these assays (91). Because some of these medications, such as lobucavir and PMEA, are administered orally once a day medications, the exciting possibility exists for providing KS prophylaxis to patients who have had prior exposure to KSHV. At the current time, antiherpes medications are not recommended for the routine treatment of preexisting KS.

INVESTIGATIONAL AGENTS

Currently, investigators are looking at new treatment modalities for AIDS-related KS that may be less toxic and more specific for the pathogenesis of KS. These treatment methods target molecules or mechanisms that may be involved in proliferation of the lesion. Such modalities include manipulators or various growth factors as well as antibodies, therapeutic soluble receptor molecules, and angiogenesis inhibitors. Several angiogenic compounds have been investigated with limited benefit. These include pentosan polysulfate, synthetic heparin substitutes, recombinant platelet factor 4, and angiogenesis inhibitors such as TNP 470. Although the results of these early studies have been largely disappointing, many potential targets for inhibition of angiogenesis remain.

Studies have suggested that a novel compound, SU4512, may have activity in AIDS-related KS. This agent blocks the effects of VEGF, a cytokine well recognized for its role in the pathogenesis of KS. Additional studies are planned for this agent, along with other inhibitors such as endothelin and angioinhibin.

I anticipate that several molecularly designed therapeutic modalities will demonstrate activity against KS. The ability to identify patients at risk for this disease, to provide prophylaxis with a long-acting oral antiherpes medication such as lobucavir or PMEA, and to treat patients with KS with novel pathogenesis-directed therapies should result in the arrest and eradication of this tumor. This is an exciting area of active research.

CLOACOGENIC CARCINOMA

The incidence of anorectal carcinoma in homosexual men with HIV infection has increased dramatically (3, 133). The rates appear to have increased significantly in most major cities. However, even before the introduction of HIV infection, the incidence of cloacogenic carcinoma appeared to be increasing (134). Cloacogenic epithelium is found in the transitional zone between the anus and the colonic mucosa. It arises from the same embryonic tissue as the cervix. Repeated trauma to the cervix and infection with human papillomavirus are believed to be causal factors in cervical carcinoma. A history of trauma, cervical cancer, and the practice of anal intercourse are believed to be associated with transitional cell and squamous cell carcinoma of the anus.

Papillomavirus infection, especially with subtypes 16 and 18, is also causally linked to this neoplasm (135, 136). Venereal warts are seen with a higher incidence in patients with anal carcinoma than in patients with carcinoma of the colon or rectum. Papillomavirus proteins have been found in anorectal carcinoma and condoloma of homosexual men (135). The incidence of anal dysplasia is high, as noted by anal Papanicolaou (Pap) smears (137, 138). The role of HIV virus in the pathogensis of neoplasm has not been defined. Investigators have suggested that HIV may contribute by transactivating the promoter for human papillomavirus E6 and E7 proteins (135). This could result in an increase in cervical intraepithelial neoplasia associated with papillomaviruses along with anogenital carcinoma.

Because of the clear association among human papillomavirus, anal dysplasia, and an increase in the incidence of cloacogenic carcinoma in HIV-infected homosexual men, it is easy to speculate that these processes are linked (135, 137, 139). However, despite the widespread finding of anal dysplasia in anal Pap smears, cloacogenic carcinoma remains rare (3, 133). Thus, additional factors are necessary before the transition to malignancy. As a consequence, recommendations for the detection and management of anal dysplasia remain controversial (136, 138). The management of patients with rectal warts and anal dysplasia is also unsettled. One group recommends aggressive surgical resection of all involved tissue, and others recommend watchful waiting. At the current time, a digital rectal examination and visual inspection of the anal area are recommended for routine health maintenance in persons with HIV infection. Anal Pap smears are not recommended as routine practice in the USPHS HIV management guidelines. However, these recommendations may change as our understanding of the pathogenesis of this disease improves.

Anal pain and bleeding are the most common symptoms of minimally invasive anal cancer and anal carcinoma in situ. Anal irritation, burning, or pruritus occur more frequently in patients with carcinoma in situ, whereas anal ulcers, masses, or abscesses are more frequent in patients with minimally invasive cancer (140). The recommendation for treatment of cloacogenic carcinoma is combined chemotherapy and radiation therapy. External beam radiation therapy with 45 Gy to the tumor and pelvic as well as inguinal lymphatic drainage is recommended. In tumors larger than T2 N0 lesions, an additional boost of 9 Gy should be given. Chemotherapy should consist of 5-fluorouracil, 1000 mg/m^2 per 24 hours on days 1 to 4 for two cycles, and mitomycin C, either 15 mg/m^2 on day 1 in the first week, or 2 doses of 10 mg/m^2 on day 1 in the first and fifth week, of radiation therapy (141). An alternative regimen consists of a combined approach using low-dose radiation therapy (30 Gy in 15 fractions delivered 5 days per week) and chemotherapy. The chemotherapy is 5-fluorouracil, 1000 mg/m^2 delivered on days 1 to 4 and 29 to 32 as a continuous infusion over 96 hours, and mitomycin C, 10 mg/m^2 delivered as a bolus injection on day 1 (142, 143). Surgical resection of the involved areas with an abdominoperineal approach is not recommended at this time.

References

1. Friedman-Kien AE, Saltzman BR. Clinical manifestations of classical, endemic African, and epidemic AIDS-associated Kaposi's sarcoma. J Am Acad Dermatol 1990;22:1237–1250.
2. Friedman-Kien AE. Disseminated Kaposi's sarcoma syndrome in young homosexual men. J Am Acad Dermatol 1981;5:468–471.
3. Biggar RJ, Rabkin CS. The epidemiology of AIDS-related neoplasms. Hematol Oncol Clin North Am 1996;10:997–1010.
4. Rabkin CS, Biggar RJ, Baptiste MS, et al. Cancer incidence trends in women at high risk of human immunodeficiency virus (HIV) infection. Int J Cancer 1993;55:208–212.
5. Rabkin CS, Goedert JJ, Biggar RJ, et al. Kaposi's sarcoma in three HIV-1-infected cohorts. J Acquir Immune Defic Syndr 1990;3(Suppl 1):S38–S43.
6. Krigel RL, Friedman-Kien AE. Epidemic Kaposi's sarcoma. Semin Oncol 1990;17:350–360.
7. Nguyen C, Lander P, Begin LR, et al. AIDS-related Kaposi sarcoma involving the tarsal bones. Skeletal Radiol 1996;25:100–102.
8. Ahluwalia C, Bernstein-Singer M, Beckstead J, et al. Kaposi's sarcoma in the bone marrow of a patient with AIDS. Am J Clin Pathol 1991;95:561–564.
9. Meyers SA, Kuhlman JE, Fishman EK. Kaposi sarcoma involving bone: CT demonstration in a patient with AIDS. J Comput Assist Tomogr 1990;14:161–162.
10. Kaposi M. Idiopathisches multiples Pigmensarkom der Haut. Arch Dermatol Syphilol 1872;4:265–273.
11. Hallenberger O. Multiple angiosarkome der Haut bein einem Kammerrunneger. Arch Schiffs Trop Hgy 1914;18:647.
12. Ledley GS, Sulica VI, Kao GF. Kaposi's sarcoma in a renal transplant patient receiving cyclosporine. Am J Med Sci 1987;294:211–213.
13. Penn I. Kaposi's sarcoma in immunosuppressed patients. J Clin Lab Immunol 1983;12:1–10.
14. Qunibi WY, Barri Y, Alfurayh O, et al. Kaposi's sarcoma in renal transplant recipients: a report on 26 cases from a single institution. Transplant Proc 1993;25:1402–1405.
15. Lesnoni LP, Masini C, Nanni G, et al. Kaposi's sarcoma in renal-transplant recipients: experience at the Catholic University in Rome, 1988–1996. Dermatology 1997;194:229–233.
16. Biggar RJ, Curtis RE, Cote TR, et al. Risk of other cancers following Kaposi's sarcoma: relation to acquired immunodeficiency syndrome. Am J Epidemiol 1994;139:362–368.
17. Rabkin CS, Biggar RJ, Horm JW. Increasing incidence of cancers associated with the human immunodeficiency virus epidemic. Int J Cancer 1991;47:692–696.
18. Rabkin CS, Blattner WA. HIV infection and cancers other than non Hodgkin lymphoma and Kaposi's sarcoma. Cancer Surv 1991;10:151–160.
19. Des JD, Stoneburner R, Thomas P, et al. Declines in proportion of Kaposi's sarcoma among cases of AIDS in multiple risk groups in New York City [letter]. Lancet 1987;2:1024–1025.
20. Drew WL, Mills J, Hauer LB, et al. Declining prevalence of Kaposi's sarcoma in homosexual AIDS patients paralleled by fall in cytomegalovirus transmission [letter]. Lancet 1988;1:66.
21. Carr A, Milliken S, Lewis C, et al. A pilot phase II safety and activity study of ritonavir in the treatment of HIV-associated cutaneous Kaposi's sarcoma. In: 4th Conference on Retroviruses and Opportunistic Infections. Washington, DC: American Society for Microbiology, 1997.
22. Stein ME, Spencer D, Ruff P, et al. Endemic African Kaposi's sarcoma: clinical and therapeutic implications: 10-year experience in the Johannesburg Hospital (1980–1990). Oncology 1994;51:63–69.
23. Melbye M, Kestens L, Biggar RJ, et al. HLA studies of endemic African Kaposi's sarcoma patients and matched controls: no association with HLA-DR5. Int J Cancer 1987;39:182–184.
24. Abramson C. Podiatric implications of acquired immunodeficiency syndrome. J Am Podiatr Med Assoc 1986;76:124–136.
25. Wahman A, Melnick SL, Rhame FS, et al. The epidemiology of classic, African, and immunosuppressed Kaposi's sarcoma. Epidemiol Rev 1991;13:178–199.
26. Bismuth H, Samuel D, Venancie PY, et al. Development of Kaposi's sarcoma in liver transplant recipients: characteristics, management, and outcome. Transplant Proc 1991;23:1438–1439.
27. Huang YQ, Buchbinder A, Li JJ, et al. The absence of Tat sequences in tissues of HIV-negative patients with epidemic Kaposi's sarcoma. AIDS 1992;6:1139–1142.
28. Kaloterakis A, Papasteriades C, Filiotou A, et al. HLA in familial and nonfamilial Mediterranean Kaposi's sarcoma in Greece. Tissue Antigens 1995;45:117–119.
29. Prince HE, Schroff RW, Ayoub G, et al. HLA studies in acquired immune deficiency syndrome patients with Kaposi's sarcoma. J Clin Immunol 1984;4:242–245.
30. Mann DL, Murray C, O'Donnell M, et al. HLA antigen frequencies in HIV-1–related Kaposi's sarcoma. J Acquir Immune Defic Syndr 1990;3(Suppl 1):S51–S55.
31. Bartholomew C, Wilson V, Cleghorn F. Absence of HLA DR5 and Kaposi's sarcoma in Trinidad and Tobago. In: 5th International Conference on AIDS, San Francisco, 1989.
32. Tzfoni EE, Scherman L, Battat S, et al. No HLA antigen is significant in classic Kaposi's sarcoma [see comments]. J Am Acad Dermatol 1993;28:118–119.
33. Strichman-Almashanu L, Weltfriend S, Gideoni O, et al. No significant association between HLA antigens and classic Kaposi sarcoma: molecular analysis of 49 Jewish patients. J Clin Immunol 1995;15:205–209.
34. Beral V, Bull D, Darby S, et al. Risk of Kaposi's sarcoma and sexual practices associated with faecal contact in homosexual or bisexual men with AIDS [see comments]. Lancet 1992;339:632–635.
35. Armenian HK, Hoover DR, Rubb S, et al. Composite risk score for Kaposi's sarcoma based on a case-control and longitudinal study in the Multicenter AIDS Cohort Study (MACS) population. Am J Epidemiol 1993;138:256–265.
36. Haverkos H, Drotman DP. The search for a cofactor in AIDS-related Kaposi's sarcoma (KS): assessment of nitrite inhalant use in studies of homosexual men with AIDS. In: 5th International Conference on AIDS, San Francisco, 1989.
37. Rosenberg ZF, Fauci AS. Immunopathogenesis of HIV infection. FASEB J 1991;5:2382–2390.
38. Breen EC, Rezai AR, Nakajima K, et al. Infection with HIV is associated with elevated IL-6 levels and production. J Immunol 1990;144:480–484.
39. Dourado I, Martinez-Maza O, Kishimoto T, et al. Interleukin 6 and AIDS-associated Kaposi's sarcoma: a nested case control study within the Multicenter AIDS Cohort Study. AIDS Res Hum Retroviruses 1997;13:781–788.
40. Ammann AJ, Palladino MA, Volberding P, et al. Tumor necrosis factors alpha and beta in acquired immunodeficiency syndrome (AIDS) and AIDS-related complex. J Clin Immunol 1987;7:481–485.
41. Belec L, Meillet D, Hernvann A, et al. Differential elevation of circulating interleukin-1 beta, tumor necrosis factor alpha, and interleukin-6 in AIDS-associated cachectic states. Clin Diagn Lab Immunol 1994;1:117–120.
42. Kreuzer KA, Dayer JM, Rockstroh JK, et al. The IL-1 system in HIV infection: peripheral concentrations of IL-1beta, IL-1 receptor antagonist and soluble IL-1 receptor type II. Clin Exp Immunol 1997;109:54–58.
43. Thierry AR, Zeman RA, Hung JW, et al. In vitro and in vivo inhibition of tumorigenicity of neoplastic Kaposi's sarcoma cell line (KS Y-1) by liposomal IL-6, IL-8 and VEGF antisense oligodeoxynucleotides [abstract]. Proc Annu Meet Assoc Cancer Res 1995;36:A2461.
44. Gallo RC. Novel biological means of control of HIV and AIDS. In: 11th Conference on AIDS, Vancouver, 1996:8.
45. Miles SA, Rezai AR, Salazar-Gonzalez JF, et al. AIDS Kaposi sarcoma-derived cells produce and respond to interleukin 6. Proc Natl Acad Sci U S A 1990;87:4068–4072.

46. Vogel J, Hinrichs SH, Reynolds RK, et al. The HIV *tat* gene induces dermal lesions resembling Kaposi's sarcoma in transgenic mice. Nature 1988;335:606–611.
47. Barillari G, Gendelman R, Gallo RC, et al. The Tat protein of human immunodeficiency virus type 1, a growth factor for AIDS Kaposi sarcoma and cytokine-activated vascular cells, induces adhesion of the same cell types by using integrin receptors recognizing the RGD amino acid sequence. Proc Natl Acad Sci U S A 1993;90:7941–7945.
48. Ambrosino C, Ruocco MR, Chen X, et al. HIV-1 Tat induces the expression of the interleukin-6 (IL6) gene by binding to the IL6 leader RNA and by interacting with CAAT enhancer-binding protein beta (NF-IL6) transcription factors. J Biol Chem 1997;272:14,883–14,892.
49. Rautonen J, Rautonen N, Martin NL, et al. HIV type 1 Tat protein induces immunoglobulin and interleukin 6 synthesis by uninfected peripheral blood mononuclear cells. AIDS Res Hum Retroviruses 1994;10:781–785.
50. Scala G, Ruocco MR, Ambrosino C, et al. The expression of the interleukin 6 gene is induced by the human immunodeficiency virus 1 TAT protein. J Exp Med 1994;179:961–971.
51. Ensoli B, Gendelman R, Markham P, et al. Synergy between basic fibroblast growth factor and HIV-1 Tat protein in induction of Kaposi's sarcoma. Nature 1994;371:674–680.
52. Huang YQ, Buchbinder A, Li JJ, et al. The absence of Tat sequences in tissues of HIV-negative patients with epidemic Kaposi's sarcoma. AIDS 1992;6:1139–1142.
53. Andersen CB, Karkov J, Bjerregaard B, et al. Cytomegalovirus infection in classic, endemic and epidemic Kaposi's sarcoma analyzed by in situ hybridization. APMIS 1991;99:893–897.
54. Huang YQ, Li JJ, Rush MG, et al. HPV-16-related DNA sequences in Kaposi's sarcoma [see comments]. Lancet 1992;339:515–518.
55. Lo SC, Lange M, Wang R, et al. Development of Kaposi's sarcoma is associated with serologic evidence of mycoplasma penetrans infection: retrospective analysis of a prospective cohort study of homosexual men. In: 1st National Conference on Human Retroviruses and Related Infections, Washington, DC, 1993:145.
56. Chang Y, Cesarman E, Pessin MS, et al. Identification of herpesvirus-like DNA sequences in AIDS-associated Kaposi's sarcoma [see comments]. Science 1994;266:1865–1869.
57. Su IJ, Huang LM, Wu SJ, et al. Detection and sequence analysis of a new herpesvirus-like agent in AIDS and non-AIDS Kaposi's sarcoma in Taiwan. J Formos Med Assoc 1996;95:13–18.
58. Chang Y, Ziegler J, Wabinga H, et al. Kaposi's sarcoma-associated herpesvirus and Kaposi's sarcoma in Africa: Uganda Kaposi's Sarcoma Study Group. Arch Intern Med 1996;156:202–204.
59. Su IJ, Hsu YS, Chang YC, et al. Herpesvirus-like DNA sequence in Kaposi's sarcoma from AIDS and non-AIDS patients in Taiwan [letter]. Lancet 1995;345:722–723.
60. Gao SJ, Kingsley L, Li M, et al. KSHV antibodies among Americans, Italians and Ugandans with and without Kaposi's sarcoma [see comments]. Nature Med 1996;2:925–928.
61. Russo JJ, Bohenzky RA, Chien MC, et al. Nucleotide sequence of the Kaposi sarcoma-associated herpesvirus (HHV8). Proc Natl Acad Sci U S A 1996;93:14,862–14,867.
62. Moore PS, Gao SJ, Dominguez G, et al. Primary characterization of a herpesvirus agent associated with Kaposi's sarcomae [published erratum appears in J Virol 1996;70:9083]. J Virol 1996;70:549–558.
63. Nicholas J, Ruvolo V, Zong J, et al. A single 13-kilobase divergent locus in the Kaposi sarcoma-associated herpesvirus (human herpesvirus 8) genome contains nine open reading frames that are homologous to or related to cellular proteins. J Virol 1997;71:1963–1974.
64. Nicholas J, Ruvolo VR, Burns WH, et al. Kaposi's sarcoma-associated human herpesvirus-8 encodes homologues of macrophage inflammatory protein-1 and interleukin-6. Nature Med 1997;3:287–292.
65. Cheng EH, Nicholas J, Bellows DS, et al. A Bcl-2 homolog encoded by Kaposi sarcoma-associated virus, human herpesvirus 8, inhibits apoptosis but does not heterodimerize with Bax or Bak. Proc Natl Acad Sci U S A 1997;94:690–694.
66. Cesarman E, Nador RG, Bai F, et al. Kaposi's sarcoma–associated herpesvirus contains G protein-coupled receptor and cyclin D homologs which are expressed in Kaposi's sarcoma and malignant lymphoma. J Virol 1996;70:8218–8223.
67. Gao SJ, Boshoff C, Jayachandra S, et al. KSHV ORF K9 (vIRF) is an oncogene which inhibits the interferon signaling pathway. Oncogene 1997;15:1979–1985.
68. Olsen SJ, Parravicini C, Moroni M, et al. Antibodies against KSHV-related antigens and development of KS in Italian patients receiving organ allograft transplantation. In: 4th Conference on Retroviruses and Opportunistic Infections. Washington, DC: American Society for Microbiology, 1997.
69. Rigsby MO, Heston L, Grogan E, et al. Antibodies to Butyrate inducible antigens of Kaposi's sarcoma-associated herpesvirus (KSHV) in (HIV-1) infected patients. In: 3rd Conference on Retroviruses and Opportunistic Infections. Washington, DC: American Society for Microbiology, 1996:165.
70. Gao SJ, Kingsley L, Hoover DR, et al. Seroconversion to antibodies against Kaposi's sarcoma–associated herpesvirus-related latent nuclear antigens before the development of Kaposi's sarcoma. N Engl J Med 1996;335:233–241.
71. Simpson GR, Schulz TF, Whitby D, et al. Prevalence of Kaposi's sarcoma associated herpesvirus infection measured by antibodies to recombinant capsid protein and latent immunofluorescence antigen [see comments]. Lancet 1996;348:1133–1138.
71a. Martin JN, Ganem DE, Osmond DH, et al. Sexual transmission and the natural history of human herpesvirus 8 infection. N Engl J Med 1998;338:948–54.
72. Kedes DH, Operskalski E, Busch M, et al. The seroepidemiology of human herpesvirus 8 (Kaposi's sarcoma-associated herpesvirus): distribution of infection in KS risk groups and evidence for sexual transmission [see comments] [published erratum appears in Nature Med 1996;2:1041]. Nature Med 1996;2:918–924.
73. Ensoli B, Nakamura S, Salahuddin SZ, et al. AIDS-Kaposi's sarcoma-derived cells express cytokines with autocrine and paracrine growth effects. Science 1989;243:223–226.
74. Samaniego F, Markham PD, Gendelman R, et al. Inflammatory cytokines induce endothelial cells to produce and release basic fibroblast growth factor and to promote Kaposi's sarcoma–like lesions in nude mice. J Immunol 1997;158:1887–1894.
75. Miles SA. Kaposi sarcoma: a cytokine-responsive neoplasia? Cancer Treat Res 1992;63:129–140.
76. Miles SA, Martinez-Maza O, Rezai A, et al. Oncostatin M as a potent mitogen for AIDS-Kaposi's sarcoma–derived cells. Science 1992;255:1432–1434.
77. Amaral MC, Miles S, Kumar G, et al. Oncostatin-M stimulates tyrosine protein phosphorylation in parallel with the activation of p42MAPK/ERK-2 in Kaposi's cells: evidence that this pathway is important in Kaposi cell growth. J Clin Invest 1993;92:848–857.
78. Yang J, Hagan MK, Offermann MK. Induction of IL-6 gene expression in Kaposi's sarcoma cells. J Immunol 1994;152:943–955.
79. Miles SA, Magpantay L. Angiogenic cytokine levels in patients with AIDS-KS (in press).
80. Cornali E, Zietz C, Benelli R, et al. Vascular endothelial growth factor regulates angiogenesis and vascular permeability in Kaposi's sarcoma. Am J Pathol 1996;149:1851–1869.
81. Sturzl M, Brandstetter H, Roth WK. Kaposi's sarcoma: a review of gene expression and ultrastructure of KS spindle cells in vivo. AIDS Res Hum Retroviruses 1992;8:1753–1763.
82. Boshoff C, Endo Y, Collins PD, et al. Angiogenic and HIV-inhibitory functions of KSHV-encoded chemokines. Science 1997;278:290–294.
83. Zimring JC, Goodbourn S, Offermann MK. Human herpesvirus 8 encodes an interferon regulatory factor (IRF) homolog that represses IRF-1–mediated transcription. J Virol 1998;72:701–707.
84. Friedman-Kien AE, Li JJ, Jensen P, et al. Herpes-like virus (HHV-8) DNA sequences in various types of immunocompromised patients

with Kaposi's sarcoma. In: 11th Conference on AIDS, Vancouver, 1996:8.
85. Orenstein JM, Alkan S, Blauvelt A, et al. Visualization of human herpesvirus type 8 in Kaposi's sarcoma by light and transmission electron microscopy. AIDS 1997;11:F35–F45.
86. Moser E, Tatsch K, Kirsch CM, et al. Value of ^{67}gallium scintigraphy in primary diagnosis and follow-up of opportunistic pneumonia in patients with AIDS. Lung 1990;168(Suppl):692–703.
87. Del val Gomez MA, Castro BJ, Gallardo FG, et al. Thallium and gallium scintigraphy in pulmonary Kaposi's sarcoma in an HIV-positive patient [see comments]. Clin Nucl Med 1994;19:467–468.
88. Murphy M, Armstrong D, Sepkowitz KA, et al. Regression of AIDS-related Kaposi's sarcoma following treatment with an HIV-1 protease inhibitor [letter]. AIDS 1997;11:261–262.
89. Langford A, Ruf B, Kunze R, et al. Regression of oral Kaposi's sarcoma in a case of AIDS on zidovudine (AZT). Br J Dermatol 1989;120:709–713.
90. Miles SA, Wang H, Elashoff R, et al. Improved survival for patients with AIDS-related Kaposi's sarcoma. J Clin Oncol 1994;12:1910–1916.
91. Panyutich EA, Said JW, Miles SA. Detection of putative Kaposi's sarcoma herpesvirus (HHV-8) in human endothelial cells cocultivated with HHV-8 producing cell line. In: 4th Conference on Retroviruses and Opportunistic Infections. Washington, DC: American Society for Microbiology, 1997.
92. Caldwell BD, Kushner D, Young B. Kaposi's sarcoma versus bacillary angiomatosis. J Am Podiatr Med Assoc 1996;86:260–262.
93. Kostianovsky M, Lamy Y, Greco MA. Immunohistochemical and electron microscopic profiles of cutaneous Kaposi's sarcoma and bacillary angiomatosis. Ultrastruct Pathol 1992;16:629–640.
94. Mitsuyasu RT. Clinical variants and staging of Kaposi's sarcoma. Semin Oncol 1987;14:13–18.
95. Chachoua A, Krigel R, LaFleur F, et al. Prognostic factors and staging classification of patients with epidemic Kaposi's sarcoma. J Clin Oncol 1989;7:774–780.
96. Krown SE, Metroka C, Wernz JC. Kaposi's sarcoma in the acquired immune deficiency syndrome: a proposal for uniform evaluation, response, and staging criteria. AIDS Clinical Trials Group Oncology Committee. J Clin Oncol 1989;7:1201–1207.
97. Krown SE, Testa M, Huang J. Validation of the AIDS Clinical Trials Group (ACTG) staging classification for AIDS-associated Kaposi's sarcoma (AIDS/KS) [abstract]. Proc Annu Meet Am Soc Clin Oncol 1996;15:A844.
98. Conant MA, Opp KM, Poretz D, et al. Reduction of Kaposi's sarcoma lesions following treatment of AIDS with ritonovir [letter]. AIDS 1997;11:1300–1301.
99. Workman C, Lewis C, Smith DO. Resolution of Kaposi's sarcoma associated with saquinavir therapy: case report. In: 11th International Conference on AIDS, Vancouver, 1996:303.
100. Tappero JW, Berger TG, Kaplan LD, et al. Cryotherapy for cutaneous Kaposi's sarcoma (KS) associated with acquired immune deficiency syndrome (AIDS): a phase II trial. J Acquir Immune Defic Syndr 1991;4:839–846.
101. Kaliebe T, Schmitz T, Schroder U, et al. Cryotherapy of AIDS-related Kaposi's sarcoma. In: 9th International Conference on AIDS, Berlin, 1993:402–1601.
102. Conant MA, Galzagorry G, Illeman M. Intralesional vinblastine (Velban) treatment of lesions of Kaposi's sarcoma. In: 5th International Conference on AIDS, San Francisco, 1989.
103. Epstein JB, Scully C. Intralesional vinblastine for oral Kaposi sarcoma in HIV infection [letter]. Lancet 1989;2:1100–1101.
104. Nichols M, Flaitz C, Hicks J. Intraoral Kaposi's sarcoma in AIDS and intralesional vinblastine treatment. In: 9th International Conference on AIDS, Berlin, 1993:63–64.
105. Zidar BL. Images in clinical medicine. Periorbital edema in Kaposi's sarcoma [see comments]. N Engl J Med 1995;332:1204.
106. Fogel SC, Gillaspy ML. Radiation treatment of oral epidemic Kaposi's sarcoma lesions: potential adverse effects. J Assoc Nurses AIDS Care 1996;7:25–30.
107. Cooper JS, Fried PR, Laubenstein LJ. Initial observations of the effect of radiotherapy on epidemic Kaposi's sarcoma. JAMA 1984;252:934–935.
108. Nisce LZ, Safai B. Radiation therapy of Kaposi's sarcoma in AIDS: Memorial Sloan-Kettering experience. Front Radiat Ther Oncol 1985;19:133–137.
109. Amantea MA, Forrest A, Northfelt DW, et al. Population pharmacokinetics and pharmacodynamics of pegylated-liposomal doxorubicin in patients with AIDS-related Kaposi's sarcoma. Clin Pharmacol Ther 1997;61:301–311.
110. Northfelt DW, Martin FJ, Working P, et al. Doxorubicin encapsulated in liposomes containing surface-bound polyethylene glycol: pharmacokinetics, tumor localization, and safety in patients with AIDS-related Kaposi's sarcoma. J Clin Pharmacol 1996;36:55–63.
111. Goebel FD, Goldstein D, Goos M, et al. Efficacy and safety of Stealth liposomal doxorubicin in AIDS-related Kaposi's sarcoma: the International SL-DOX Study Group. Br J Cancer 1996;73:989–994.
112. Gill PS, Espina BM, Muggia F, et al. Phase I/II clinical and pharmacokinetic evaluation of liposomal daunorubicin. J Clin Oncol 1995;13:996–1003.
113. Girard PM, Bouchaud O, Goetschel A, et al. Phase II study of liposomal encapsulated daunorubicin in the treatment of AIDS-associated mucocutaneous Kaposi's sarcoma. AIDS 1996;10:753–757.
114. Stewart S, Jablonowski H, Goebel FD, et al. Randomized comparative trial of pegylated liposomal doxorubicin versus bleomycin and vincristine in the treatment of AIDS-related Kaposi's sarcoma: International Pegylated Liposomal Doxorubicin Study Group. J Clin Oncol 1998;16:683–691.
115. Uthayakumar S, Money-Kyrle J, Muyshondt C, et al. DaunoXome (liposomal daunorubicin) in early Kaposi's sarcoma: a cross-over trial versus observation [abstract]. In: Anticancer Treatment: 6th International Congress, Paris, 1996:100.
116. Gill PS, Wernz J, Scadden DT, et al. Randomized phase III trial of liposomal daunorubicin versus doxorubicin, bleomycin, and vincristine in AIDS-related Kaposi's sarcoma. J Clin Oncol 1996;14:2353–2364.
117. Welles L, Saville MW, Lietzau J, et al. Phase II trial with dose titration of paclitaxel for the therapy of human immunodeficiency virus-associated Kaposi's sarcoma. J Clin Oncol 1998;16:1112–1121.
118. Gill PS, Tulpule A, Reynolds T, et al. Paclitaxel (TAXOL) in the treatment of relapsed or refractory advanced AIDS-related Kaposi's sarcoma. Proc Annu Meet Am Soc Clin Oncol 1996;15:854.
119. Mega A, Akhtar MS, Safran H, et al. Low dose weekly paclitaxel for HIV-associated Kaposi's sarcoma. Proc Annu Meet Am Soc Clin Oncol 1996;15:859.
120. Krown SE, Real FX, Krim M, et al. Recombinant leukocyte A interferon in Kaposi's sarcoma. Ann N Y Acad Sci 1984;437:431–438.
121. Krown SE, Paredes J, Bundow D, et al. Interferon-alpha, zidovudine, and granulocyte-macrophage colony-stimulating factor: a phase I AIDS Clinical Trials Group study in patients with Kaposi's sarcoma associated with AIDS. J Clin Oncol 1992;10:1344–1351.
122. Krown SE, Gold JW, Niedzwiecki D, et al. Interferon-alpha with zidovudine: safety, tolerance, and clinical and virologic effects in patients with Kaposi sarcoma associated with the acquired immunodeficiency syndrome (AIDS) [published erratum appears in Ann Intern Med 1990;113:334]. Ann Intern Med 1990;112:812–821.
123. Evans LM, Itri LM, Campion M, et al. Interferon-alpha 2a in the treatment of acquired immunodeficiency syndrome-related Kaposi's sarcoma. J Immunother 1991;10:39–50.
124. Miles SA, Wang HJ, Cortes E, et al. Beta-interferon therapy in patients with poor-prognosis Kaposi sarcoma related to the acquired immunodeficiency syndrome (AIDS): a phase II trial with preliminary evidence of antiviral activity and low incidence of opportunistic infections. Ann Intern Med 1990;112:582–589.

125. Martinez-Maza O, Mitsuyasu RT, Miles SA, et al. Gamma-interferon–induced monocyte major histocompatibility complex class II antigen expression individuals with acquired immune deficiency syndrome. Cell Immunol 1989;123:316–324.
126. Oettgen HF, Real FX, Krown SE. Treatment of AIDS-associated Kaposi's sarcoma with recombinant alpha interferon. Immunobiology 1986;172:269–274.
127. Fischl MA, Richman DD, Saag M, et al. Safety and antiviral activity of combination therapy with zidovudine, zalcitabine, and two doses of interferon-alpha2a in patients with HIV: AIDS Clinical Trials Group Study 197. J Acquir Immune Defic Syndr Hum Retrovirol 1997;16:247–253.
128. Gill PS, Rarick MU, Espina B, et al. Advanced acquired immune deficiency syndrome-related Kaposi's sarcoma: results of pilot studies using combination chemotherapy. Cancer 1990;65:1074–1078.
129. Mocroft A, Youle M, Gazzard B, et al. Anti-herpesvirus treatment and risk of Kaposi's sarcoma in HIV infection: Royal Free/Chelsea and Westminster Hospitals Collaborative Group. AIDS 1996;10:1101–1105.
130. Glesby MJ, Hoover DR, Weng S, et al. Use of antiherpes drugs and the risk of Kaposi's sarcoma: data from the Multicenter AIDS Cohort Study. J Infect Dis 1996;173:1477–1480.
131. Jones JL, Hanson DL, Chu SY, et al. AIDS-associated Kaposi's sarcoma [letter; comment]. Science 1995;267:1078–1079.
132. Rabkin CS, Schulz T, Lennette ET, et al. Interlaboratory correlation of current HHV-8 serologic tests. In: 4th Conference on Retroviruses and Opportunistic Infections. Washington, DC: American Society for Microbiology, 1997.
133. Chadha M, Rosenblatt EA, Malamud S, et al. Squamous-cell carcinoma of the anus in HIV-positive patients. Dis Colon Rectum 1994;37:861–865.
134. Melbye M, Rabkin C, Frisch M, et al. Changing patterns of anal cancer incidence in the United States, 1940–1989. Am J Epidemiol 1994;139:772–780.
135. Palefsky JM, Holly EA, Hogeboom CJ, et al. Virologic, immunologic, and clinical parameters in the incidence and progression of anal squamous intraepithelial lesions in HIV-positive and HIV-negative homosexual men. J Acquir Immune Defic Syndr Hum Retrovirol 1998;17:314–319.
136. Breese PL, Judson FN, Penley KA, et al. Anal human papillomavirus infection among homosexual and bisexual men: prevalence of type-specific infection and association with human immunodeficiency virus. Sex Transm Dis 1995;22:7–14.
137. Sayers SJ, McMillan A, McGoogan E. Anal cytological abnormalities in HIV-infected homosexual men. Int J STD AIDS 1998;9:37–40.
138. Palefsky JM, Holly EA, Hogeboom CJ, et al. Anal cytology as a screening tool for anal squamous intraepithelial lesions. J Acquir Immune Defic Syndr Hum Retrovirol 1997;14:415–422.
139. Palefsky JM, Holly EA, Ralston ML, et al. Anal squamous intraepithelial lesions in HIV-positive and HIV-negative homosexual and bisexual men: prevalence and risk factors. J Acquir Immune Defic Syndr Hum Retrovirol 1998;17:320–366.
140. Forti RL, Medwell SJ, Aboulafia DM, et al. Clinical presentation of minimally invasive and in situ squamous cell carcinoma of the anus in homosexual men. Clin Infect Dis 1995;21:603–607.
141. Hocht S, Wiegel T, Kroesen AJ, et al. Low acute toxicity of radiotherapy and radiochemotherapy in patients with cancer of the anal canal and HIV-infection. Acta Oncol 1997;36:799–802.
142. Peddada AV, Smith DE, Rao AR, et al. Chemotherapy and low-dose radiotherapy in the treatment of HIV-infected patients with carcinoma of the anal canal. Int J Radiat Oncol Biol Phys 1997;37:1101–1105.
143. Smith DE, Shah KH, Rao AR, et al. Cancer of the anal canal: treatment with chemotherapy and low-dose radiation therapy. Radiology 1994;191:569–572.

27
OVERVIEW OF AIDS-RELATED LYMPHOMAS: A PARADIGM OF AIDS MALIGNANCIES

Judith E. Karp

Acquired immunodeficiency syndrome (AIDS), caused by the retrovirus known as human immunodeficiency virus (HIV), has been recognized for almost two decades. During this time, much progress has been made in dissecting the molecular complexities of HIV and in translating basic virologic and immunologic discoveries into clinical practice. For instance, the findings regarding the chemokines and their receptors have shed important light on the molecular mechanisms by which HIV gains cellular entry (1–4), and, in turn, they may provide new targets for blocking HIV infection and thus preventing HIV disease (5–8). With regard to therapy, the advent of multitargeted antiretroviral therapy, such as the combination of one of the new protease inhibitors with the "mainstay" dideoxynucleosides (9), holds promise with respect to deterring or, in some cases, reversing progressive HIV disease. Many of these discoveries are summarized in other chapters.

Yet, as we approach the third decade of the AIDS pandemic and AIDS-targeted scientific pursuits, we still face many challenges. In particular, certain types of malignancies and their incidence rates are increasing in AIDS, perhaps as the development of effective antiretroviral therapies and prophylaxis against opportunistic infections leads to prolonged survival in what would otherwise be a lethal immunocompromised state. Indeed, the net prolongation of survival in the face of impaired immunity may drive the increasing incidence of malignancies in AIDS patients. This linkage is exemplified by the striking relationship between profound cellular immunodeficiency, manifested by the depletion of CD4 lymphocytes, and the development of non–Hodgkin's lymphomas (NHLs), particularly when the CD4 count falls below $50/mm^3$ (10).

The predisposition to develop neoplasia was perhaps first clearly detected in patients with genetically determined disorders of cellular and humoral immunity, in particular ataxia–telangiectasia (11) and Wiskott–Aldrich syndrome (12), and then, not surprisingly, in patients receiving immunosuppressive therapies for autoimmune disorders or transplantation (13–16). This propensity is now mirrored in the AIDS setting. The malignancies arising in the context of insufficient immune function are frequently of lymphoid origin, most commonly B cell, but epithelial (namely, anogenital cancers, including cervical cancer in women) and endothelial-related cancers (in particular, Kaposi's sarcoma [KS]) certainly occur as well.

The common themes underlying the emergence and perpetuation of the diverse malignancies arising in these heterogenous immunocompromised states include several factors, namely, the absence of protective immune surveillance to recognize and eradicate abnormal clones, disruption of the normal balance between cell proliferation and differentiation that partly may be augmented by abnormal growth factor expression, and chronic antigenic stimulation, sometimes accompanied by infection with "oncogenic" pathogens, that leads to expansion of one or more cell cohorts. In addition, the unique immunologic milieu induced by HIV infection likely has a formative role in the pathogenesis and pathophysiology of AIDS-related lymphomas. This environment is characterized by defects in immune regulation, loss of specific immune cell subsets, presence of abnormal cytokine levels, changes in the architecture of germinal centers and other lymphoid tissues, and aberrant immune surveillance. Any or all of these factors may contribute in a pivotal way to the high incidence and distinctive characteristics of AIDS-associated lymphoma. The dysregulation may lead to an increase in the rate of generation of transformed lymphocytes or to enhanced capacity of these cells to escape surveillance and cause disease.

The process of tumorigenesis consists of multiple steps and the interaction of several diverse factors, some known and some not, to which the immunodeficiency and HIV-host interactions present in the AIDS setting add extra dimensions of complexity. Despite our growing molecular understanding of many of these determinants, we still have few established

Table 27.1. Selected Potential Factors in the Pathogenesis of AIDS Malignancies

Pathogenic Factor	Lymphoma	Kaposi's Sarcoma	Anogenital Cancers
Virus	KSHV/HHV-8	KSHV-HHV-8	HPV
	EBV	(EBV)?	HSV-2
	HIV	HIV	HIV
Host gene activation	c-myc	b-FGF	c-myc
	bcl-6	NFκB	MDR
	bcl-2	K-fgf/hst?	
	ras		
	NFκB?		
Tumor suppressor inactivation	p53, rb gene mutations		p53, RB protein modifications
	p53 protein modification		
	RB protein phosphorylation	RB protein phosphorylation	
	6q gene deletions		
Cytokines			
Host origin	IL-6, IL-10, IL-14	IL-1, IL-6, IL-8	IL-6?
		FGFs, VEGF	
		PDGF	
		Oncostatin M	
		TNF	
		HGF/SF	
Viral origin	IL-8 receptor	Extracellular Tat	
	IL-6	IL-8 receptor	
	IL-10 (BCRF-1)	(IL-6)	

EBV, Epstein–Barr virus; b-FGF, basic fibroblast growth factor; HGF/SF, hepatocyte growth factor/scatter factor; HIV, human immunodeficiency virus; HPV, human papillomavirus; HSV, herpes simplex virus; IL, interleukin; K-fgf/hst, Kaposi's-associated fibroblast growth factor; KSHV/HHV-8, Kaposi's sarcoma herpesvirus/human herpesvirus-8; MDR, multidrug resistance; NKκB, nuclear factor κ B; PDGF, platelet-derived growth factor; rb, retinoblastoma gene; RB, retinoblastoma protein; TNF, tumor necrosis factor; VEGF, vascular endothelial growth factor.

facts regarding AIDS-related malignancies. For the purposes of this discussion, we focus on the molecular dissection of AIDS-associated lymphomas as a template for delineating the diverse factors that perhaps have the greatest impact, singly or collectively, on the pathogenesis of all AIDS-related malignancies. Certain selected factors for some of these malignancies are depicted in Table 27.1.

This chapter is intended to provide an overview of selected mechanisms that modulate the balance between lymphohematopoietic cell proliferation, differentiation, survival and death. The perturbation and dysregulation of these mechanisms by genetic lesions or inflammatory stimuli including infectious pathogens, in turn, lead to immunodeficiency and cancer. The uncovering of these important determinants may ultimately lead to targeted molecular strategies that may be applicable to the therapy and prevention of AIDS-related malignancies and of cancers in general.

PATHOGENESIS OF AIDS LYMPHOMAS: MULTIPLE INTERACTIVE FACTORS

Epidemiology and Clinical Manifestations

Soon after AIDS was recognized as a new disease, investigators observed that persons with AIDS or at risk of AIDS had a high incidence of NHLs, generally of B-cell origin, of high grade, and tending to occur in extranodal sites. Yet, even before AIDS, NHLs have been an increasing problem. The incidence of NHL in both men and women in the United States and in other Western countries has been steadily rising over the past two decades, and it is still largely unexplained. This increase in NHL has not been accompanied by a comparable incidence of Hodgkin's disease (HD). However, HD can certainly occur at an increased frequency and with increased aggressiveness in the setting of HIV infection acquired by diverse routes of transmission (discussed in more detail later).

The United States has had an approximate 76% increase in incidence and a 36% increase in the death rate of NHL since the early 1970s (17). In fact, in 1996, roughly 53,000 cases of NHL were expected to occur in the United States alone, so this disease entity can no longer be considered minor or rare. In the last 10 to 15 years, a significant new component of this increase has reflected the emergence of lymphomas associated with AIDS (18–21). The National Cancer Institute's (NCI's) Surveillance, Epidemiology, and End Results (SEER) Program has been able to track this unexpected increase in incidence of specific types of NHL (17). The connection between AIDS and NHL was first reported in 1982. Beginning approximately in 1983, a sharp rise in the numbers of NHL has been detected exclusively for men of ages 20 to 54 years, most particularly in the cohort of men from San Francisco (17, 20). In an analysis of almost 100,000 unselected AIDS patients spanning from 1981 to 1989, approximately 3% had NHL, a 60-fold increase relative to that expected for the general population (22).

Primary central nervous system (CNS) lymphoma may occur with striking frequency in either large cell immunoblastic or small noncleaved cell types, usually as mass lesions, but on occasion as a more diffuse leptomeningeal process (23). Five of 8 patients with AIDS-related NHL at the NCI described by Pluda and colleagues (19) and 10 of 24 such patients from a multicenter study described by Moore and associates (24) had primary CNS involvement. Further, in an autopsy series of 101 AIDS patients during 1981 to 1987, lymphomas were detected in 20, 5 of which were located in the brain and 8 of which (including 4 of the brain tumors) were detected only at autopsy (25). More recently, Cote and colleagues examined AIDS and cancer registries from 9 state and local health departments in terms of demographics, histologic features, and clinical outcomes of brain lymphomas occurring from 1980 to 1989 (26). This analysis revealed a 9-fold increase in the incidence of brain lymphomas during the decade, with most of that increase occurring in the setting of AIDS, and an incidence of brain lymphomas in persons with AIDS that was an astounding 3600-fold higher than that of the general population. Patients with brain lymphomas and AIDS had a devastating prognosis, with a median survival of 2 months, whereas patients with non–AIDS-related brain lymphomas survived a median of 5 to 7 months, and those with AIDS but without brain lymphomas had a median survival of 14 months (26).

The increase in AIDS-related NHL is predominantly in high-grade B-cell types, with large cell immunoblastic and small noncleaved cell lymphomas (SNCLs) comprising about 70% of AIDS-related NHL, and the intermediate-grade diffuse large cell lymphomas (DLCLs) making up the remaining 30% (18, 19). A significant proportion of AIDS-related lymphomas have both the histologic features and the cytogenetic pattern characteristic of Burkitt's lymphoma (19, 22). AIDS lymphomas resemble NHL occurring in other severely immunocompromised settings by their frequent involvement of extranodal sites, particularly gastrointestinal tract and brain, and by the high incidence of stage IV disease, especially in the Burkitt's type, in which bone marrow infiltration is common (19–21). Like other NHLs arising from a background of chronic immunosuppression and unlike NHLs that occur outside a known immunosuppressed state, AIDS-related lymphomas demonstrate a high frequency of multiclonality.

For several years, Yarchoan, Pluda, and colleagues have followed a group of patients on long-term studies of antiretroviral therapy, including the first patients to receive the dideoxynucleoside reverse transcriptase inhibitors zidovudine (formerly known as AZT), dideoxycytidine (ddC), or didanosine (ddI) (10, 19, 27–29). In these cohorts, the risk for development of NHL has not been uniform over time but, rather, has appeared to increase at around 2 years after therapy for full-blown AIDS. This finding is worth noting because studies that do not contain more than a 2-year follow-up will not detect this association accurately. Indeed, 8 of 55 patients on protocols of zidovudine alone or with ddC developed NHL, yielding a rate of 29% after 3 years on therapy (19), and 4 of 61 patients receiving ddI developed NHL, yielding a rate of 9.5% after 3 years (27). Taking together the 116 zidovudine- and ddI-treated AIDS patients, the estimated probability of developing NHL is 8% after 2 years and 19% after 3 years of antiretroviral therapy (27). In these closely followed cohorts of patients, in whom consistent and frequent observations were made over an extended period, virtually all who developed NHL did so with CD4 counts lower than $50/mm^3$ for 12 months or more (median 18) before NHL emerged. Thus, the depth of immunocompromise, as specifically reflected by a CD4 cell count lower than $50/mm^3$, appears to be a singularly critical factor in the emergence of these "opportunistic" NHLs in the setting of AIDS (10, 19, 27). Certainly, lymphomas can and do occur in patients with CD4 counts higher than $50/mm^3$; however, the risk is significantly elevated once this threshold is crossed. In addition, patients with high serum levels of the B-cell stimulating cytokine interleukin (IL)-6 appear to be at increased risk for NHL development (28). Ultimately, prevention of NHL development may hinge on an ability to restore, or at least maintain, immune function at a critical protective level.

Hodgkin's Disease and HIV Infection

HD has been noted to occur in both men and women with active HIV infection. The experiences in regions, such as some segments of southern Europe, including Italy, Spain, and parts of France, where HIV infection is acquired predominantly through intravenous drug use suggest, but certainly do not prove, an association between HD and illicit drug use (30, 31). In the United States, however, where approximately 75 to 80% of all HIV-infected patients are homosexual men, it appears that HD occurs in both populations in roughly proportional frequency (32, 33). These differences in geographically distinct populations merit further study. HIV-infected women also can develop HD (32). Nonetheless, the relative distributions of HD and NHL in the setting of HIV infection suggest that if lymphoma is going to occur, intravenous drug users are more likely to develop HD, whereas the homosexual population is at greater risk of developing NHL (31). Along these lines, a San Francisco-based study detected a 5-fold increased incidence of HD in HIV-infected homosexual men relative to non–HIV-infected counterparts (34); yet, this increase was less than the almost 38-fold increase in NHLs in the HIV-infected cohort. Nevertheless, the clinical features of HIV-associated HD in the intravenous drug use and homosexual populations are similar. The predominant histologic subtypes seen are mixed cellularity and lymphocyte depletion, and more than 80% of HIV-associated HD patients present with stage III or IV disease.

Complete remissions are generally achieved only when HIV infection has not progressed to full-blown AIDS, and favorable survival estimates relate to preservation of CD4 count higher than $400/mm^3$. Overall, complete remission rates in response to cyclic multiagent chemotherapy (47%) and median survival (14 months) are inferior to results obtained in non–HIV-associated HD, in part because of a striking incidence and mortality from opportunistic infections.

The presence of Epstein–Barr virus (EBV) genomic material (both DNA and mRNA) in Reed–Sternberg cells in biopsied lymph node tissue (35–37) suggests that, akin to a substantial proportion of NHL (both AIDS- and non–AIDS-related), EBV may serve as either a direct etiologic agent or a viral "cofactor" promoting the development of HD in some instances. The central pathogenic role of EBV is substantiated by the analysis of 114 Italian patients with AIDS-related HD (38), in which 80% of HIV-infected HD patients had evidence of monoclonal EBV infection with both type 1 and type 2 EBV, in contrast to only 38% of non–HIV-associated HD patients. These findings provide a parallel between HD and NHL arising in the setting of AIDS, and they begin to clarify the potential linkage of EBV to the genesis or perpetuation of HD as well as of B-cell NHL. The pathogenic effects of EBV in both non-AIDS and AIDS lymphomas are discussed later.

Molecular Genetics of AIDS-Related Lymphomas

Lymphohematopoietic malignancies are characterized by the clonal expansion of cells that have been arrested at a specific developmental stage of maturation. The capacity for self-renewal is preserved, but the capacity for terminal differentiation is blocked. In this regard, in addition to T-cell destruction, HIV infection may also be associated with an intrinsic impairment in B-cell maturation. This impairment relates in part to a clonal defect in rearrangements of a subfamily of the genes encoding the variable region of the immunoglobulin heavy chain (V_H), specifically the V_H3L subfamily (39). The clonal defect occurs in B cells within lymph node germinal centers and results in a B-cell maturation arrest that, in turn, leads to a deficit in memory B cells. This impaired B-cell differentiation is accompanied by an increase in circulating levels of IL-6 (40), which may provide a chronic proliferative stimulus for the arrested B-cell clone and thereby may drive expansion of certain B-cell clones. The clonal defect and chronic IL-6–based stimulation (perhaps a compensatory attempt to "override" the maturation blockade and to "push" the arrested clone toward a more differentiated state) may serve as a framework on which malignant B-cell transformation is built.

One pathogenic mechanism underlying the malignant transformation of lymphoid precursors in general and of B cells specifically is the translocation of a normal growth-promoting gene (or so-called "protooncogene") to the lineage-specific antigen receptor genes; in the case of B cells, these are the immunoglobulin genes (41). The juxtaposition of the protooncogene segment with the immunoglobulin gene, in particular its transcriptionally active enhancer sequences, results in deregulation of the translocated growth-promoting gene that, by virtue of overexpression, now functions as a true oncogene. One classic example of oncogene activation resulting from this type of chromosomal rearrangement occurs in Burkitt's lymphoma, in which the c-*myc* gene, located on the long arm of chromosome 8 (8q24) (42), is disrupted and translocated to the immunoglobulin gene heavy-chain locus on 14q32. Certain mechanisms exist by which c-*myc* activation can ensue, all of which may operate to some degree in t(8;14) (43–45). Transcriptional activation of c-*myc* can occur from juxtaposition to immunoglobulin gene enhancer sequences or from the action of long-range enhancers on chromosome 14, without requiring literal proximity of c-*myc* and enhancers.

The translocation and recombination of 8q24 and 14q32 typify Burkitt's lymphoma, in both its endemic (African) and sporadic (American) forms. However, the c-*myc* gene may behave differently in the two variants (44–46). In the endemic form, the breakpoint on chromosome 8q24 is outside the 5′ regulatory region of c-*myc*, and the c-*myc* gene is translocated intact (unrearranged), albeit frequently altered with point mutations, to the joining (J_H) segment of the immunoglobulin gene (44, 46). In this variant, inactivation of the 5′ regulatory sequences of the c-*myc* gene locus can occur mainly through point mutations within its first exon (45) or by separation of the regulatory region from the rest of the gene. In contrast, in the sporadic form, the c-*myc* gene is disrupted within its 5′ portion and is separated from its regulatory (or so-called "repressor") region. The first c-*myc* exon is translocated in a truncated form to the nonswitch (J_H) region or, in some instances, to a break in the switch region of the heavy-chain gene (S_μ) of 14q32 (43, 45). Translocation to the J_H region results in transcription activation (often long-range) by immunoglobulin gene enhancer sequences; alternatively, translocation of the disrupted c-*myc* gene to S_μ is accompanied by c-*myc* gene inversion or true rearrangement, which results in direct oncogene overexpression. The net result of c-*myc* translocation to the immunoglobulin gene locus for either the endemic or the sporadic type is the abrogation of the effects of negative regulatory elements on c-*myc* transcription. More than transcriptional activation or amplification of c-*myc* per se, these gene rearrangements result in constitutive c-*myc* expression and a failure of the normal control mechanisms that, in turn, leads to a net overexpression of the c-myc mRNA- and DNA-binding phosphoprotein (42, 43, 46, 47).

Indeed, c-*myc* mutations or rearrangements occur in 50 to 70% of all AIDS-related NHLs (43, 47, 48). In addition, the continuing molecular dissection of AIDS-associated lymphomas has uncovered a diversity of genetic lesions, many of which play formative roles in lymphomagenesis arising from various backgrounds (not just AIDS) and some of which are distinctive. Mutations of the classic tumor suppressor gene *p53* can be detected in roughly 50 to 70% of AIDS-related Burkitt's lymphomas (and in about 40% non–AIDS-related Burkitt's lymphomas), often linked to c-*myc* rearrangement and activation (48–50). In addition, losses of one or more segments of the long arm of chromosome 6 (6q21-23 and 6q25-27)—sites of multiple putative tumor suppressors—occur in about 20% of all lymphomas, including those associated with AIDS (48). Moreover, mutations of *ras* oncogenes are detectable in about 10 to 15% of AIDS-related Burkitt's lymphomas, a finding that contrasts with the absence of *ras* mutations in the non-HIV setting (48).

Rearrangements of the *bcl-6* gene located on chromosome 3q27, a zinc finger transcription factor–encoding gene that is rearranged in 30 to 40% of DLCLs arising in nonimmunosuppressed hosts, are evident in roughly 20% of AIDS-related DLCLs (both large noncleaved and immunoblastic variants), but not in SNCLs (51). The association of aberrant *bcl-6* expression with DLCL is consistent with the finding that normal *bcl-6* expression is localized within germinal center B cells (52, 53), from which DLCLs are derived, and that the BCL-6 protein may play a pivotal role in germinal center development and maturation of immune responses. The *bcl-6* lesions are independent of the presence or absence of EBV and are not accompanied by alterations in c-*myc* and *p53*. Continued elucidation of the multiple factors and genetic alterations that may contribute to lymphomagenesis in the HIV-infected state should provide a scientific scaffold for design of molecularly targeted therapies, definition of individual risk, and design of prevention strategies.

Additionally, HIV, like other retroviruses, possibly may play a direct etiologic role in certain cases of AIDS-related lymphomagenesis. Although at least 90% of AIDS-related NHLs are of B-cell origin, the incidence of rare T-cell lymphomas appears to be increasing. Molecular analyses of four such T-cell tumors reveal the presence of monoclonal HIV–long terminal repeat sequences integrated within the human *fur* gene, located just upstream of the tyrosine kinase–encoding *fes* oncogene on chromosome 15 (54). Perhaps like other retroviruses, HIV could theoretically drive malignant transformation by several mechanisms, such as insertional mutagenesis and upregulation of oncogene expression, disturbance of normal DNA repair mechanisms, and clonal selection.

Epstein–Barr Virus: Multiple Mechanisms for Malignant Transformation

The role of EBV in B-cell lymphomagenesis has been established for endemic (African) Burkitt's lymphoma and has been postulated for many of the non–Burkitt's B-cell malignancies that arise in the setting of chronic immunosuppression. One mechanism by which EBV may accomplish such B-cell growth dysregulation is through the activation of EBV latent genes encoding at least six transcriptionally active viral nuclear antigens (EBNAs) and two or more signal-transducing latent membrane proteins (LMPs). These proteins enhance the survival and self-renewal capacity of both EBV-infected host cells and viral genome (55). Their actions with respect to B cells, that is, blocking one form of programmed cell death known as apoptosis and extending B-cell longevity, may mimic that of *bcl-2*, an antiapoptosis oncogene that is overexpressed in diverse leukemias, lymphomas, and epithelial malignancies (56). Of particular relevance in this context is the demonstration that EBNA-2, and especially LMP, can induce the expression of *bcl-2* in Burkitt's lymphoma cell lines (*bcl-2* is not commonly detected in vivo) (57, 58), a finding supporting the notion that EBV may immortalize or enhance the survival of B cells through *bcl-2* upregulation and abrogation of apoptosis. Along these lines, the EBV gene BHRF1, a homologue of *bcl-2*, appears to be transcribed in certain EBV-associated B-cell lymphomas, specifically in the malignant cells themselves (59), a finding lending credence to a hypothesized interconnection among EBV, net *bcl-2* expression, and B-cell lymphomagenesis. However, at least in the immunocompromised milieu of posttransplantation lymphoproliferative disorders, *bcl-2* expression is not coupled to BHRF1, but rather, it appears to be linked to LMP1 (60). This finding suggests that EBV infection can culminate in prolonged B-cell survival in vivo by at least two distinctive, noncompetitive mechanisms operating in concert or independently, namely, the viral induction of host *bcl-2* expression and the direct activity of a *bcl-2*-like viral gene.

Additional mechanisms by which EBV gene products may subvert host cell machinery include the induction of B-cell surface antigens that enhance both viral and B-cell activation, namely, CD21, which is a receptor for EBV that is involved in EBV internalization, B-cell activation, and possible EBV-induced autostimulation, and CD23, which is the low-affinity IgE receptor also known as B-cell–activating factor) (61). EBV may also influence the expression of certain lymphocyte adhesion molecules that play significant roles in immune responses requiring cell–cell contact, including cytotoxic T lymphocyte (CTL) recognition (62). Another mechanism of EBV-induced B-cell stimulation may operate through BCRF-1, an EBV-encoded protein that shares structural and functional homology with IL-10 (63). IL-10 is discussed later, in the context of AIDS-related lymphomagenesis.

The EBV-linked lymphoproliferative malignancies that arise in the setting of chronic, profound immunosuppression are often characterized by the presence of multiple neoplastic clones and by an immunoblastic large cell morphology with plasmacytoid features (14, 16, 64–67). In this situation, EBV may provoke polyclonal B-cell activation that, in the absence of normal T-cell controls, permits unopposed B-cell expansion with increased numbers of cells susceptible to destabilizing genetic events such as chromosomal breaks and recombinations. The etiologic effects of EBV have been demonstrated by inducing lymphomas in mice with severe combined immunodeficiency (SCID) that have been reconstituted with EBV-negative human peripheral or nodal lymphocytes (SCID/hu chimeric mice) and subsequently infected with EBV (68) or with peripheral blood lymphocytes from EBV-seropositive donors (69). Of note is the absence of c-*myc* and *bcl-2* translocations or rearrangements. This animal model parallels the large cell immunoblastic B-cell lymphomas that occur in humans with severe immunodeficiency such as those seen after organ transplantation (14, 16, 64, 65) and in primary CNS lymphomas, which are now recognized as an AIDS-associated lesion (26, 66, 70). In the human tumors, as in the SCID/hu mouse model, EBV genome is present in tumor cells; the tumors, often of multiclonal origin, develop from a background polyclonal activation that is likely a consequence of EBV infection. The

SCID mouse is a template for the preclinical development of innovative strategies for therapy and prevention of diverse lymphoproliferative malignancies, in particular AIDS-related lymphomas (see later).

One intriguing mechanism by which EBV may escape immune surveillance is hypermethylation of CpG sites within the EBV latency C promoter (71). The C promoter drives the transcription and net expression of antigenic (or immunodominant) viral EBNAs, against which CD8+ CTLs are directed. The hypermethylation occurs in the region of the promoter, which binds the host cellular transcriptional protein known as CBF2 and prevents CBF2 binding to the target DNA sequences. The abrogation of CBF2 binding inhibits transcriptional activation of the C promoter, with the eventual failure to express those antigens that should generate an EBV-targeted cellular immune response. This mechanism appears to operate in both EBV-associated HD and in Burkitt's lymphomas and is likely responsible for the failure to detect expression of immunodominant EBNAs (EBNA-2, -3A, -3B, and -3C) in these diseases. Provocatively, the hypermethylation can be reversed by 5-azacytidine, an inhibitor of DNA methyltransferase (72). Robertson and colleagues have demonstrated that 5-azacytidine treatment of a Burkitt's lymphoma–derived cell line in which the C promoter is silenced by hypermethylation results in reversal of hypermethylation and resultant activation of C promoter-driven EBNA-2 expression (73). Such modulation of viral gene expression is now being translated into clinical practice, using 5-azacytidine to test the hypothesis that treatment directed against EBV genome hypermethylation and the resultant reinstitution of EBV antigen expression may, in turn, enhance the susceptibility of EBV to immunologic attack.

Several investigators have demonstrated the close relationship between primary CNS lymphomas and EBV infection in this clinical setting (66, 70, 74–76), in which EBV gene sequences and EBER protein (signifying latent EBV infection) are detectable in virtually 100%, and LMP can be found in roughly 40 to 60% of HIV-related primary CNS lymphoma (75, 76). This linkage is not so rigorous for systemic NHLs, although EBV DNA and RNA sequences have been detected in roughly 50% (but up to 80% in some series) of AIDS-related lymphomas (66, 70, 74, 77). As a case in point, Shibata and Levine and their colleagues in Los Angeles have detected the EBV genome, in monoclonal form, in 66% of the systemic B-cell NHLs arising in the setting of AIDS (77). EBV genomic expression in these NHLs was found to be distinctive, with coexpression of both EBNA-1 (as in Burkitt's lymphomas) and LMP. Along these lines, Camilleri-Broet and associates detected the expression of both LMP1 and bcl-2 in 10 of 11 EBV-positive primary CNS lymphomas (74). In counterpoint, although 46 of 57 (80%) of the systemic NHLs examined in this series were linked to EBV, only 21 (46%) of the EBV-positive tumor cell cohorts expressed LMP1, and a mere 3 systemic tumors, all extranodal, expressed bcl-2 (74).

In a series from Shiramizu and colleagues in San Francisco (70), roughly 40% of all AIDS-related B-cell NHLs were found to contain EBV gene sequences, especially in monoclonal tumors; it is particularly noteworthy that *all* CNS tumors were EBV positive, whereas only one-third of the systemic NHLs contained detectable EBV genomic material. In this population, c-*myc* rearrangements were linked exclusively to monoclonal NHLs. Continued observation of this cohort has revealed that the most common lymphoma was a polyclonal, high-grade systemic B-cell NHL without detection of EBV infection or c-*myc* rearrangements (78). The polyclonal NHLs occurred in the setting of a higher CD4 count, and, in response to chemotherapy, patients with polyclonal disease, especially those with CD4 counts of $200/mm^3$ or more, enjoyed a longer survival (more than 50% alive at 26^+ to 65^+ months) relative to those who had monoclonal tumors and CD4 counts less than $200/mm^3$ (median survival 3.5 months). The presence of EBV conferred a strikingly poor prognosis, independent of clonality status, with overall median survival of 3.2 months for those with EBV-positive disease versus 9 months for those with EBV-negative tumors.

Although EBV is often accompanied by alterations and deregulation of c-*myc*, no inextricable linkage exists between EBV and c-*myc* perturbations in AIDS-associated NHLs (66, 79, 80). For instance, Meeker and associates found that primary CNS lymphomas may contain the EBV genome without accompanying c-*myc* gene rearrangements (66). More commonly, however, when dissociation of EBV and c-*myc* exists, c-*myc* mutations or rearrangements occur in the absence of detectable EBV sequences (79, 80). Most of these non-EBV, non–Burkitt's NHLs have c-*myc* rearrangements and 14q32 switch region breaks that mimic the "sporadic Burkitt's" type, but "endemic-type" breakpoints in both c-*myc* and 14q32 occur in approximately 25% of non-EBV AIDS-associated NHLs and are accompanied by similar point mutations in the first *myc* exon (43). Along this line, mutations in the coding region of c-*myc* occur in roughly one-third of AIDS-related NHLs, predominantly but not exclusively in SNCLs, in the absence of EBV, and they are linked to the presence of the translocation involving c-*myc* and the immunoglobulin gene locus (79). In all, whatever the specific breakpoints and mechanisms of deregulation, the prevalence of molecular abnormalities in c-*myc* structure and function is consistent with the notion that c-*myc* has a central role in the malignant transformation and clonal expansion of B-cell lymphomas in AIDS.

KSHV/HHV-8: A New Herpesvirus with Etiologic Implications for AIDS Malignancies

A new inroad into understanding the pathogenesis of lymphoproliferative malignancies and KS has been forged, with the discovery of DNA sequences from a putative new herpesvirus, KSHV/HHV-8 (*K*aposi's *s*arcoma *h*erpes*v*irus/*h*uman *h*erpes*v*irus-*8*), that are linked to KS and body cavity lymphomas arising in various settings, including

AIDS (81–83). The sequences (called KS330$_{233}$) were initially identified through studies of tissues obtained from AIDS patients with KS (81–84), and they were detected in more than 90% of AIDS-KS tissues, in 15% of non-KS tissues from AIDS patients, and in few non-KS, non-AIDS tissues (84). The initial clinical and molecular epidemiologic observations have been extended with the findings that 95% of all KS lesions examined from AIDS patients, as well as lesions from patients with "classic" (Mediterranean) KS and HIV-negative homosexual men with KS, contain the sequences (82, 85). KSHV/HHV-8 sequences have been detected in peripheral blood mononuclear cells in more than 50% of patients with KS, but in only 8% of HIV-infected patients without KS (86). Further, KSHV/HHV-8 has been detected before the clinical development of KS and has predicted the eventual emergence of KS. Taken together, these findings add credence to the notion that KSHV/HHV-8 may be a true etiologic agent in KS.

The emerging story of KSHV/HHV-8 and its potential etiologic role in tumorigenesis becomes even more complex with the finding of a specific linkage between KSHV and NHLs occurring in body cavities, namely, the pleura, pericardium, and peritoneum (83, 87–89). These "primary effusion lymphomas" can occur in both the presence and absence of HIV infection (88, 89), and they have a clinically distinctive presentation as localized effusions without contiguous tumor masses. Morphologically, they possess features of both immunoblastic and anaplastic large cell lymphomas, and immunophenotypically, they express the "hematopoietic" antigen CD45 and a panoply of activation antigens (HLA-DR, CD30, CD38, CD71), but they do not express characteristic B-cell or T-cell differentiation antigens. Nonetheless, the genotype of these primary effusion lymphomas is consistent with a B-cell malignancy, because they contain clonal immunoglobulin heavy-chain rearrangements. In addition, evidence for an accompanying clonal EBV infection occurs frequently. However, unlike with other aggressive NHL variants arising in the setting of HIV infection, no accompanying c-*myc* rearrangements occur, nor are there any consistent mutations, translocations, or rearrangements in *bcl-2, bcl-6, p53,* or *ras* (88). Finally, the detection of KSHV/HHV-8 sequences in the peripheral blood and lymph nodes of patients with multicentric Castleman's disease—a polyclonal lymphoproliferative disorder accompanied by vascular hyperplasia that can arise in the setting of HIV infection and can be associated with the development of KS and NHLs (90–92)—further substantiates the postulated etiologic role of KSHV/HHV-8 in both vascular and lymphoid neoplasias.

The unique genomic sequences of KSHV/HHV-8 bear significant homology to genes encoding the minor capsid and tegument proteins of two Gammaherpesviriae, EBV and Herpesvirus saimiri (HVS) (81, 82). Both EBV and HVS exhibit oncogenic activity. As detailed later, EBV is pathogenically linked to an interesting spectrum of malignancies including lymphomas, nasopharyngeal carcinomas, and smooth muscle tumors arising in HIV-infected children and immunocompromised organ transplant recipients (47, 93–95). HVS induces a fatal, polyclonal T-cell lymphoproliferative disease in "nonimmune" primates, much as EBV causes B-cell lymphoproliferative disorders in humans (96). Of particular interest is the presence of a gene in HVS that has homology with the *bcl-1* oncogene (97) encoding the cell cycle–promoting protein cyclin D$_1$, which is often overexpressed in some intermediate lymphomas and is amplified in certain epithelial cancers (esophageal, breast, bladder, and non–small cell lung cancers) (98). Molecular dissection of HHV-8 has uncovered the presence of gene sequences that are structurally similar to those encoding D-type cyclins, with production of a protein that functions like a D cyclin (phosphorylates and inactivates the tumor suppressor retinoblastoma, or RB, protein) and the detection of cyclin D–encoding gene transcripts in biopsy tissues from KS and primary effusion lymphoma (99). Taken together, these data support the hypothesis that the net overexpression of a D-type cyclin plays a formative role in the pathogenesis and pathophysiology of the vascular and lymphoid neoplasms associated with KSHV/HHV-8. KSHV/HHV-8 also bears genomic similarity to EBV by encoding proteins that influence human cell cycle progression and cell survival, for example, BCL-2, human cytokines such as IL-6, chemokines such as macrophage inflammatory proteins and the receptor for the chemokine IL-8, and certain cell-surface adhesion molecules (100). The KSHV-related IL-6 gene is of particular interest, because it appears to be preferentially expressed in KSHV/HHV-8–infected hematopoietic cells, compatible with the notion that viral IL-6 could have a special pathogenic role in the emergence and perpetuation of KSHV-related primary effusion lymphomas. Thus, KSHV/HHV-8, like EBV and other "oncogenic" viruses, seems likely to produce a panoply of factors with a broad diversity of molecular mechanisms, each of which, alone or in concert with other viral and host cell proteins, can perturb cellular homeostasis and predispose to the survival and expansion of a malignant clone.

Cytokines in the Pathogenesis and Pathophysiology of AIDS Lymphomas

The production of hematopoietic and immunomodulatory cytokines in response to infection may contribute to the development of lymphomas in many settings, in particular the immunocompromised host and perhaps especially the HIV-infected individual. The major cellular sources of cytokine production are T cells, monocytes, and bone marrow stromal cells, all of which can be infected by HIV and can perturb net cytokine production (101). In this regard, HIV-related changes in IL-6 production may be especially relevant to both "premalignant" polyclonal B-cell expansion and to eventual malignant transformation in AIDS-related (and non–AIDS-related) lymphomas.

IL-6 has major effects on the proliferation, differentiation, and net expression of multiple arms of the immune system, including B cells and cytotoxic T cells (102). As mentioned earlier, the increase in serum IL-6 levels that accompanies the HIV-associated clonal VH3L defect in B-cell maturation occurs early in HIV infection, even before subclinical evidence for cellular immune impairment (39), a finding suggesting that the compensatory increase in circulating IL-6 levels also occurs early in HIV infection and thus can drive B-cell proliferation over a long period. Further, IL-6 may augment HIV replication and thus disease progression in an autocrine loop through its enhancement of T-cell and monocyte growth (101). Additionally, the production of IL-6 from HIV-infected monocytes promotes the proliferation of activated B cells, such as by EBV, thereby driving immunoglobulin synthesis and causing the nonspecific hyperimmunoglobulinemia commonly seen in early HIV infection (101, 103).

Based on its proliferative targets, IL-6 is one logical candidate for the promotion of malignant transformation in B-cell precursors. It is provocative that, in the zidovudine-treated AIDS patients in the NCI series, those patients who eventually developed B-cell NHL had elevated serum IL-6 levels at the time of study entry, with continued IL-6 increases over time (28). The hypothetic linkage between IL-6 and B-cell dyscrasias is further supported by data suggesting that IL-6 is implicated in the pathogenesis of multiple myeloma through its activity as an autocrine growth factor for malignant plasma cells (102). Along these lines, Emilie and coworkers (104), examining high-grade B-cell NHLs, found striking expression of both IL-6 and IL-6 receptor predominantly in the non–Burkitt's, immunoblastic subset, which has a prominent plasmacytoid phenotype, independent of HIV or EBV positivity. In addition, Jucker and associates found HD and Reed–Sternberg cells to express both IL-6 and IL-6 receptors (105), and Leger-Ravet and associates documented high levels of intranodal IL-6 expression in Castleman's disease (106), both by intrafollicular dendritic cells and interfollicular cohorts associated with blood vessels. Thus, IL-6, acting in autocrine or paracrine fashion, may be pivotal in the emergence or perpetuation of multiple lymphoid dyscrasias.

In addition to mechanisms that directly stimulate B-cell expansion, suppression of T-helper cell antiviral or cytotoxic surveillance activities can permit the establishment of malignant clones. IL-10, so-called cytokine synthesis inhibitory factor, is such a suppressor of T-cell function and, as such, may be a particularly important cytokine in AIDS lymphoma pathogenesis (47, 107, 108). IL-10 is produced by the activated T_H2 subset of helper T cells, which regulate antibody production and also produce IL-4, IL-5, and IL-6 (109, 110). IL-10 shares significant homology with the EBV protein BCRF-1 and impairs the ability of the T_H1 subset of CD4+ helper T cells to synthesize interferon-γ and IL-2, both of which exert antiviral activity against EBV and are crucial to the generation of cytotoxic CD8+ T cells (63, 109). Thus, by suppressing T_H1 cytokine synthesis and concomitantly enhancing B-cell survival, excess or unopposed IL-10 may permit viral replication (particularly EBV and possibly also HIV) to go unchecked; this, in turn, promotes the cascade of events that culminate in the establishment of clonal B-cell malignancy. EBV-positive Burkitt's lymphoma cell lines, in particular those derived from AIDS patients, are capable of producing IL-10 in a constitutive fashion (107). The link between tumor cell IL-10 expression and EBV positivity, in particular LMP-1 expression, has been documented in HD (111) and in multiple variants of AIDS-related NHLs as well (107, 108). Moreover, in a SCID/hu chimeric mouse in vivo, in which the SCID mouse is repopulated with peripheral blood lymphocytes from EBV+ individuals, the resultant EBV+ tumor cells (of human origin) produce both IL-10 and the IL-10 receptor, with resultant autocrine growth stimulation that results from IL-10–driven B-cell proliferation and a separate but concomitant IL-10–induced abrogation of apoptosis (112). Intriguingly, IL-10–producing lines also secrete IL-6, which provides yet an additional mechanism by which IL-10 may promote B-cell proliferation and immortalization (108). The potential central role of IL-10 in AIDS-related lymphomagenesis suggests that it could be an important molecular target for inhibition by drugs designed to block the interactions of IL-10 with other cytokine-producing cells, namely, T_H1 cells and monocytes.

Opportunities for Therapeutic Innovation

The molecular dissection of the etiology and pathogenesis of lymphomas arising in the setting of HIV infection and severe immunocompromise is providing an increasing diversity of mechanisms that may serve as potential targets for therapy and prevention. Some of the innovative strategies being designed currently and prospectively to target such pivotal pathways are listed in Table 27.2. This discussion focuses on just a few of the selected molecularly directed approaches that exploit one or more of the complex mechanisms contributing to AIDS-related lymphomagenesis.

Like other lymphomas arising in immunodeficient hosts, AIDS-related lymphomas are a resilient, clinically aggressive therapeutic challenge, presenting as histologically high-grade tumors with multiorgan involvement and a substantial tumor burden. CNS tumor is especially common and, partly because it is a protected "sanctuary" site, a frequent site of relapse. HIV-related bone marrow suppression, which is likely a consequence of direct progenitor cell infection or stromal cell infection with attendant suppression of hematopoietic growth factors (113), and the presence of multiple chronic opportunistic infections act in concert to limit the ability of the host to tolerate full cytotoxic therapy. Moreover, the absence of any antitumor immunity permits the expansion of tumor cells remaining after therapy to proceed unchecked.

As a result, multidrug regimens effective in de novo NHL have met with variable results in AIDS-associated lymphomas. The combinations of alternating noncross-resistant agents that reproducibly achieve complete remission rates of 70 to 90%, median disease-free survivals longer than 3 to 5 years, and median overall survivals exceeding 5 to 7 years in

Table 27.2. Molecularly Targeted Approaches to Therapy and Prevention of AIDS-Related Lymphoproliferative Malignancies

Cytotoxic therapies
   New mechanisms (e.g., paclitaxel and other tubulin-directed agents, camptothecins)
   Novel delivery systems (e.g., liposomal anthracyclines)
   Mechanisms to overcome drug resistance
Cytokine-based (biomodulatory) therapies
   IL-2, IL-12, Interferon
   Anti–IL-6, anti–IL-10, antitumor necrosis factor
Immune–based therapies
   Monoclonal antibodies, including immunotoxins and radioimmunoconjugates
   Vaccines (anti-idiotype, antiviral)
Immunorestorative approaches
   Bone marrow transplantation
   Stem cell reconstitution (gene-altered)
   Adoptive immunotherapy (HIV, EBV, CMV)
Antiviral strategies
   New virocidal agents (including anti-KSHV)
   Antiviral immunity (e.g., adoptive immunotherapy, immunomodulation, vaccines)
   Modulation of EBNA gene expression (alteration of gene methylation)
   Antiretroviral targets (e.g., reverse transcriptase, protease, nucleocapsid protein, integrase)
Gene-targeted approaches
   Antisense (host and viral genomes)
   Ribozymes

CMV, cytomegalovirus; EBNA, Epstein–Barr nuclear antigen; EBV, Epstein–Barr virus; HIV, human immunodeficiency virus; IL, interleukin; KSHV, Kaposi's sarcoma herpesvirus.

patients with advanced stage, aggressive NHLs (114) have yielded remission rates of 20 to 50%, with overall survivals far less than 1 year for AIDS-associated lymphomas (115). The complexities of the lymphomas arising in the setting of HIV infection may suggest that multimodality approaches that target multiple aspects of lymphoma pathogenesis and pathophysiology are necessary to achieve long-lasting improvements in clinical results. Such approaches could combine potentially active cytotoxic agents with marrow-protective hematopoietic growth factors and antiretroviral agents (29, 113, 116–119). A clinical trial by Sparano and colleagues exemplifies this concept by combining systemic cytoreductive therapy (consisting of 96-hour infusion of cyclophosphamide, doxorubicin, and etoposide), CNS-directed prophylaxis (cytosine arabinoside and methotrexate), antiretroviral therapy (ddI), and hematologic support (granulocyte colony-stimulating factor) (119). Paradoxically, although ddI was given throughout chemotherapy, the investigators detected an increase in circulating HIV, a finding that could in theory reflect a liberation of HIV virions that were trapped in dendritic cells or in germinal centers before cytotoxic therapy. Nonetheless, HIV disease has not appeared to accelerate in these patients, and the multimodality approach has resulted in a complete remission rate of approximately 60%, with a median duration of remission lasting 18 months and a median survival of 2 years for those achieving remission (119).

As emphasized earlier in this chapter, IL-6 is probably a critical factor in the genesis and clonal expansion of diverse AIDS-related malignancies, particularly NHLs and also HD and AIDS-KS. It is thus logical to search for therapeutic agents that could inhibit net IL-6 activity, such as retinoic acid, pentoxifylline, anti–IL-6 antibodies, IL-6–based immunotoxins, or other molecular modifications that could block IL-6 binding and signaling. For example, studies in multiple myeloma (in part, an IL-6–driven B-cell malignancy) demonstrate that retinoic acid can downregulate IL-6 receptor expression on myeloma cell surface (both the α and gp130, or β, chains) and also can downregulate the production of IL-6 by both myeloma and bone marrow stromal cells, thus inhibiting IL-6–mediated autocrine and paracrine growth stimulation (120, 121). This mechanism of inhibition may also apply to AIDS-KS, which, like multiple myeloma, appears to be driven by IL-6 in autostimulatory fashion through upregulation of tumor cell IL-6 receptors. Along similar lines, the methylxanthine pentoxifylline inhibits intracellular HIV replication by inhibiting tumor necrosis factor (TNF)-α synthesis (122). Because IL-6 expression is linked to TNF production through an autocrine loop, it is intriguing to speculate that pentoxifylline could provide both antiretroviral and anti–IL-6 effects in one or more AIDS-related malignancies (123).

With regard to the immune targeting of IL-6 and its receptor, Kreitman and colleagues developed an immunotoxin by coupling IL-6 to a mutant *Pseudomonas* exotoxin (IL-6–PE^{4E}) that is selectively cytotoxic to approximately 50% of fresh myeloma cell populations (124). Along this line, treatment of patients with advanced myeloma using a murine anti–IL-6 monoclonal antibody demonstrates marked inhibition of myeloma cell proliferation and overall IL-6 production in roughly 50% of the patients studied thus far (125). Another murine anti–IL-6 monoclonal antibody has been tested recently in a small series of patients with AIDS-related NHLs, with evidence of disease stabilization and clinical improvement of 2 to 7 months' duration in about 50% of the study cohort (126). These or related monoclonal antibody–based constructs could afford a molecularly targeted approach to AIDS and non-AIDS lymphomas (and malignancies such as KS) in which the malignant clone expresses both IL-6 and the IL-6 receptor and is, to a meaningful extent, chronically driven by IL-6.

The intriguing finding that IL-4, another lymphokine produced by $T_H 2$ cells and involved in overall B-cell proliferation and differentiation, can induce a "shift" in overall cellular cytokine synthesis (127) raises the possibility that IL-4 could downregulate IL-6 production in a therapeutically advantageous fashion. IL-4 may also have salutary effects on any existing cytotoxic T lymphocytes, although most cases of AIDS-related NHL arise late in the course of HIV infection, when few functional T cells remain (10, 118). The "reciprocal" relationship between IL-4 and IL-6 is supported by the findings that IL-4 blocks IL-6 production by adherent bone marrow cell populations from patients with multiple myeloma, possibly by downregulating IL-6 gene transcription; the consequent inhibition of IL-6 expression results in growth suppression of the IL-6–responsive malignant plasma cell population (128). Similarly, Defrance and colleagues demonstrated that IL-4 inhibits the proliferation of fresh B-NHL cells (129), in part by inhibiting their responsiveness to IL-2 and likely also by interrupting IL-6 activity. The potential role of IL-4 in the therapy of lymphoproliferative malignancies is currently under clinical investigation in both AIDS and non-AIDS settings.

The SCID mouse repopulated with peripheral blood lymphocytes from EBV+ individuals provides an elegant model of IL-2–based immunotherapy for EBV-induced, B-cell lymphoproliferative tumors that, in turn, has served as the foundation for an innovative clinical approach in AIDS-related NHLs (112, 130, 131). In the SCID/hu chimera, low-dose IL-2 prevents the establishment of fatal EBV+ "lymphomatous" disease, an effect that is mediated by natural killer (NK) and CD8+ T cells (130, 131). As noted earlier, the human tumor cells generate copious amounts of IL-6 and IL-10, both of which are downregulated by IL-2 (112). In the clinic, the administration of low-dose IL-2 after the chemotherapy-induced partial or complete responses prevented or forestalled relapse or disease progression for up to 1 year in the majority of patients with HIV-related NHLs, even when the CD4 count was less than $100/mm^3$ (131). These exciting observations in AIDS-related NHL are the basis for a confirmatory national trial to define the impact of daily, postchemotherapy, low-dose IL-2 given as "maintenance" immunotherapy on duration of response, viral load and replicative activity, cellular and humoral immunologic parameters, and opportunistic complications.

The SCID mouse also serves as a fertile testing ground for immunoconjugates directed against malignant B-cell populations. As a case in point, an in vivo model of human CNS leukemia has been established, using an SCID mouse engrafted with CNS-infiltrating human pre–B-cell acute lymphoblastic leukemia cells (132). In this model, the intrathecal administration of an immunotoxin composed of the B43 (anti-CD19) monoclonal antibody coupled to pokeweed antiviral protein results in marked diminution of CNS leukemia and prolongation of survival, far superior to that seen with the commonly used antileukemia drug methotrexate. Systemic administration was not effective against the CNS lesions, because the immunotoxin is not able to cross the blood–brain barrier. This innovative adaptation of the SCID model may have important parallels for CNS lymphomas, and it may provide a unique opportunity to identify active agents and to design new strategies for this devastating type of AIDS-related lymphoma.

The modality of adoptive immunotherapy, developed first as an anticancer strategy, has important potential as an immunorestorative approach in both herpesvirus and retrovirus infections. Immunorestorative approaches may be critical to the ability to achieve and, perhaps more pertinently, to sustain an antitumor response. This likely holds true for all AIDS-related and many non–AIDS-related malignancies. To this end, Riddell and colleagues demonstrated the ability to restore immunity to cytomegalovirus in immunosuppressed bone marrow transplant (BMT) patients through the in vivo administration and subsequent expansion of allogeneic, in vitro–propagated, cytomegalovirus-specific CTLs (133). The principles of this "adoptive transfer" are being exploited to confer virus-specific immunity directed against HIV infection through developmental clinical trials of autologous adoptive transfer of HIV-specific CD8+ T cells in patients with AIDS (134, 135).

Adoptive immunotherapy is also being tested for the EBV-related lymphoproliferative disorders that arise after allogeneic BMT, especially T-cell–depleted BMT in combination with anti–T-cell approaches to prevent graft-versus-host disease (136, 137). In this clinical setting, infusions of unirradiated CD3+ T-cell populations isolated from the peripheral blood of the BMT recipient's EBV-exposed donor induced complete remissions of 10 to 16 months' duration in three of five patients with post-BMT B-cell DLCLs containing EBV DNA (137). The lymphomas arose from donor cells (138), in keeping with the notion that the marked suppression of T-cell–based immune surveillance permitted expansion and dysregulation of an EBV-infected B-cell clone, a situation that bears great similarity to AIDS. In another series, Heslop and associates documented the ability of adoptively transferred, donor-derived, EBV-specific CTLs to confer long-lasting immunity to EBV, with the capacity to respond to EBV challenge in vitro and in vivo for up to 18 months (136). Thus, the EBV-targeted adoptive immunotherapy approach could have important implications for the therapy and prevention of the high-grade EBV+ lymphomas that arise in progressive HIV infection.

EBV provides a spectrum of antiviral and immunologic targets for exploitation in AIDS lymphomas. One such target is the expression of immunodominant EBV antigens, for instance, EBNA-2, discussed earlier in this chapter. To exploit this finding, a trial of 5-aza-2′-ddC in EBV+ AIDS-related lymphomas (primary CNS lymphoma and Burkitt's lymphoma) is being conducted (71, 73). This trial, which is based on the detection of hypermethylation-induced viral gene's silencing in diverse malignant lymphoid cell cohorts and the ability of 5-azacytidine to reinstitute gene expression by a process of demethylation in vitro and in vivo in a SCID/hu model of EBV+ lymphoproliferative disease, is testing the hypothesis that 5-azacytidine will uncover latent EBV antigens that could be critical for stimulating a host immune response (71, 73). Another target is the EBV nuclear antigen EBNA-1, which is not highly antigenic but is responsible for EBV replication and lymphocyte immortalization by EBV as well as the maintenance of EBV in the latent episomal state. Antisense constructs to the EBNA-1 gene inhibit proliferation of EBV-immortalized B cells (138), a finding that could have future implications for gene-targeted antiviral therapy.

FUTURE DIRECTIONS: PREVENTION

As with all malignancies, the most effective strategies are those targeted at prevention. The ability, early in the course of active HIV infection, to interfere with mechanisms that promulgate B-cell hyperproliferation and clonal expansion—especially growth factors (IL-6 and IL-10, in particular) and concomitant viral infections (EBV and KSHV/HHV-8, as examples, and perhaps especially KSHV/HHV8)—could decrease the occurrence or prolong the time to development of AIDS-related malignancies. Ultimately, however, the key strategies will be those directed toward maintaining the CD4 cell count at a level that prevents the establishment and perpetuation of transformed clones. From the studies of Yarchoan and colleagues (10, 118), the critical level for NHL development in particular appears to be a CD4 count of approximately $50/mm^3$. In a sense, this implies a considerable redundancy and safety factor for effective immune surveillance, and it offers an achievable goal for current therapeutic strategies. In this regard, the potential to restore some immune responsiveness through adoptive transfer technologies or cytokine-based immunomodulatory therapies is provocative, particularly if therapy is implemented before irrevocable immune cell depletion ensues. However, until such time as effective regeneration of the immune system is achievable, the identification of factors that portend a significant risk of cancer in an HIV-infected individual and the development of antiretroviral strategies that confer long-term suppression of HIV activity and relative preservation of immune function, perhaps in combination with specific antigrowth factor or other antiviral therapies, will remain essential to the ultimate prevention of all malignancies that arise as a consequence of HIV-induced immunosuppression.

References

1. Alkhatib G, Combadiere C, Broder CC, et al. CC CKR5: A RANTES, MIP-1α, MIP-1β receptor as a fusion cofactor for macrophage-tropic HIV-1. Science 1996;272:1955–1958.
2. Bates P. Chemokine receptors and HIV-1: an attractive pair? Cell 1996;86:1–3.
3. Cocchia F, DeVico AL, Garzino-Demo A, et al. Identification of RANTES, MIP-1α, and MIP-1β as the major HIV-suppressive factors produced by CD8+ T cells. Science 1995;270:1811–1815.
4. Feng Y, Broder CC, Kennedy PE, et al. HIV-1 entry cofactor: functional cDNA cloning of a seven transmembrane, G protein-coupled receptor. Science 1996;272:872–877.
5. Cocchia F, DeVico AL, Garzino-Demo A, et al. The V3 domain of the HIV-1 gp120 envelope glycoprotein is critical for chemokine-mediated blockade of infection. Nature Med 1996;2:1244–1247.
6. Dean M, Carrington M, Winkler C, et al. Genetic restriction of HIV-1 infection and progression to AIDS by a deletion allele of the CKR5 structural gene. Science 1996;273:1856–1862.
7. Huang Y, Paxton WA, Wolinsky SM, et al. The role of a mutant CCR5 allele in HIV-1 transmission and disease progression. Nature Med 1996;2:1240–1243.
8. Liu R, Paxton WA, Choe S, et al. Homozygous defect in HIV-1 coreceptor accounts for resistance of some multiply-exposed individuals to HIV-1 infection. Cell 1996;86:367–377.
9. Collier AC, Coombs RW, Schoenfeld DA, et al. Treatment of human immunodeficiency virus infection with saquinavir, zidovudine, and zalcitabine. N Engl J Med 1996;334:1011–1017.
10. Yarchoan R, Venzon DJ, Pluda JM, et al. CD4 count as a mortality risk indicator in human immunodeficiency virus (HIV)–infected patients receiving antiretroviral therapy: experience in a research hospital. Ann Intern Med 1991;115:184–189.
11. Waldmann TA, Misiti J, Nelson DL, et al. Ataxia–telangiectasia: a multisystem hereditary disease with immunodeficiency, impaired organ maturation, x-ray hypersensitivity, and a high incidence of neoplasia. Ann Intern Med 1983;99:367–379.
12. Cotelingham JD, Witebsky FG, Hsu SM, et al. Malignant lymphoma in patients with the Wiskott–Aldrich syndrome. Cancer Invest 1985;3:515–522.
13. Cockburn ITR, Krupp P. The risk of neoplasms in patients treated with cyclosporine A. J Autoimmun 1989;2:723–731.
14. Knowles DM, Cesarman E, Chadburn A, et al. Correlative, morphologic and molecular genetic analysis demonstrates three distinct categories of posttransplantation lymphoproliferative disorders. Blood 1995;85:552–565.
15. Lebland V, Sutton L, Dorent R, et al. Lymphoproliferative disorders after organ transplantation: a report of 24 cases observed in a single center. J Clin Oncol 1995;13:961–968.
16. Penn I. Tumors arising in organ transplant recipients. Adv Cancer Res 1978;28:31–61.
17. Division of Cancer Prevention and Control, National Cancer Institute. Cancer statistics review 1973–1993. Bethesda, MD: National Institutes of Health, 1996;96–2789.
18. Knowles DM, Chamulak GA, Subar M, et al. Lymphoid neoplasia associated with the acquired immunodeficiency syndrome (AIDS). Ann Intern Med 1988;108:744–753.
19. Pluda JM, Yarchoan R, Jaffe ES, et al. Development of non-Hodgkin's lymphoma in a cohort of patients with severe immunodeficiency virus (HIV) infection on long-term antiretroviral therapy. Ann Intern Med 1990;113:276–282.
20. Rabkin CS, Biggar RJ, Horm JW. Increasing incidence of cancers associated with the human immunodeficiency virus epidemic. Int J Cancer 1991;47:692–696.
21. Ziegler JL, Beckstead JA, Volberding PA, et al. Non–Hodgkin's lymphoma in 90 homosexual men: relation to generalized lymphadenopathy and the acquired immunodeficiency syndrome. N Engl J Med 1984;211:565–570.
22. Beral V, Peterman T, Berkelman R, et al. AIDS-associated non–Hodgkin lymphoma. Lancet 1991;337:805–809.
23. Gill PS, Levine AM, Meyer PR, et al. Primary central nervous system lymphoma in homosexual men: clinical, immunologic and pathologic features. Am J Med 1985;78:742–748.
24. Moore RD, Kessler H, Richman DD, et al. Non–Hodgkin's lymphoma in patients with advanced HIV infection treated with zidovudine. JAMA 1991;265:2208–2211.
25. Wilkes MS, Fortin AH, Felix JC, et al. Value of necropsy in acquired immunodeficiency syndrome. Lancet 1988;2:85–88.
26. Cote TR, Manns A, Hardy CR, et al. Epidemiology of brain lymphoma among people with or without acquired immunodeficiency syndrome. J Natl Cancer Inst 1996;88:675–679.
27. Nguyen B-Y, Yarchoan R, Wyvill KM, et al. Five-year follow-up of a phase I study of didanosine in patients with advanced human immunodeficiency virus infection. J Infect Dis 1995;171:1180–1189.
28. Pluda JM, Venzon DJ, Tosato G, et al. Parameters affecting the development of non–Hodgkin's lymphoma in patients with severe human immunodeficiency virus infection receiving antiretroviral therapy. J Clin Oncol 1993;11:1099–1107.
29. Yarchoan R, Pluda JM, Perno C-F, et al. Anti-retroviral therapy of HIV infection: current strategies and challenges for the future. Blood 1991;78:859–884.
30. Garnier G, Taillan B, Michiels JF. HIV-associated Hodgkin's disease. Ann Intern Med 1991;115:233.
31. Monfardini S, Tirelli U, Vaccher E, et al. Hodgkin's disease in 63 intravenous drug users infected with human immunodeficiency virus. Ann Oncol 1991;2(Suppl):201–205.
32. Ames ED, Conjalka MS, Goldberg AF, et al. Hodgkin's disease and AIDS. Hematol Oncol Clin North Am 1991;5:343–356.
33. Gold JE, Altarac D, Ree HJ, et al. HIV-associated Hodgkin disease: a clinical study of 18 cases and review of the literature. Am J Hematol 1991;36:93–99.

34. Hessol NA, Katz MH, Liu JY, et al. Increased incidence of Hodgkin disease in homosexual men with HIV infection. Ann Intern Med 1992;117:309–311.
35. Brousset P, Chittal S, Schlaifer D, et al. Detection of Epstein–Barr virus messenger RNA in Reed–Sternberg cells of Hodgkin's disease by in situ hybridization with biotinylated probes on specially processed modified acetone methyl benzoate xylene (Mod AMex) sections. Blood 1991;77:1781–1786.
36. Herbst H, Steinbrecher E, Niedobitek G, et al. Distribution and phenotype of Epstein–Barr virus–harboring cells in Hodgkin's disease. Blood 1992;80:484–491.
37. Knecht H, Odermatt BF, Bachmann E, et al. Frequent detection of Epstein–Barr virus DNA by the polymerase chain reaction in lymph node biopsies from patients with Hodgkin's disease without genomic evidence of B- or T-cell clonality. Blood 1991;78:760–767.
38. Tirelli U, Errante D, Dolcetti R, et al. Hodgkin's disease and human immunodeficiency virus infection: clinicopathologic and virologic features of 114 patients from the Italian Cooperative Group on AIDS and tumors. J Clin Oncol 1995;13:1758–1767.
39. Berberian L, Valles-Ayoub Y, Sun N, et al. A VH clonal deficit in human immunodeficiency virus–positive individuals reflects a B-cell maturational arrest. Blood 1991;78:175–179.
40. Breen EC, Rezai AR, Nakajima K, et al. Infection with HIV is associated with elevated IL-6 levels and production. J Immunol 1990;144:480–484.
41. Waldmann TA, Korsmeyer SJ, Bakhshi A, et al. Molecular genetic analysis of human lymphoid neoplasms: immunoglobulin genes and the c-*myc* oncogene. Ann Intern Med 1985;102:497–510.
42. Dalla-Favera R, Bregni M, Erikson J, et al. Human c-*myc* oncogene is located on the region of chromosome 8 that is translocated in Burkitt lymphoma cells. Proc Natl Acad Sci U S A 1982;79:7824–7827.
43. Ladanyi M, Offitt K, Jhanwar SC, et al. MYC rearrangement and translocations involving band 8q24 in diffuse large cell lymphomas. Blood 1991;7:1057–1063.
44. Pellici PG, Knowles DM, Magrath I, et al. Chromosomal breakpoints and structural alterations of the c-*myc* locus differ in endemic and sporadic forms of Burkitt lymphoma. Proc Natl Acad Sci U S A 1986;83:2984–2988.
45. Shiramizu B, Barriga F, Neequaye J, et al. Patterns of chromosomal breakpoint locations in Burkitt's lymphoma: relevance to geography and Epstein–Barr virus association. Blood 1991;77:1516–1526.
46. Croce CM, Nowell PC. Molecular basis of human B cell neoplasia. Blood 1985;65:1–7.
47. Karp JE, Broder S. Acquired immunodeficiency syndrome and non–Hodgkin's lymphomas. Cancer Res 1991;51:4743–4756.
48. Ballerini P, Gaidano G, Gong JZ, et al. Multiple genetic lesions in acquired immunodeficiency syndrome–related non–Hodgkin's lymphoma. Blood 1993;81:1166–1176.
49. De Re V, Carbone A, De Vita S, et al. p53 protein over-expression and p53 gene abnormalities in HIV-1 related non–Hodgkin's lymphomas. Int J Cancer 1994;56:662–667.
50. Edwards RH, Raab-Traub N. Alterations of the p53 gene in Epstein–Barr virus–associated immunodeficiency-related lymphomas. J Virol 1994;68:1309–1315.
51. Gaidano G, Lo Coco F, Ye BH, et al. Rearrangements of the *BCL6* gene in acquired immunodeficiency syndrome–associated non–Hodgkins lymphoma: association with diffuse large-cell subtype. Blood 1994;84:397–402.
52. Cattoretti G, Chang C-C, Cechova K, et al. BCL-6 protein is expressed in germinal-center B cells. Blood 1995;86:45–53.
53. Onizuka T, Moriyama M, Yamochi T, et al. BCL-6 gene product, a 92- to 98-kD phosphoprotein, is highly expressed in germinal center B cells and their neoplastic counterparts. Blood 1995;86:28–37.
54. Shiramizu B, Herndier BG, McGrath MS. Identification of a common clonal human immunodeficiency virus integration site in human immunodeficiency virus–associated lymphomas. Cancer Res 1994;54:2069-2072.
55. Gregory CD, Dive C, Henderson S, et al. Activation of Epstein–Barr virus latent genes protects human B cells from death by apoptosis. Nature 1991;349:612–614.
56. Yang E, Korsmeyer SJ. Molecular thanatopsis: a discourse on the BCL2 family and cell death. Blood 1996;88:386–401.
57. Finke J, Fritzen R, Ternes P, et al. Expression of *bcl-2* in Burkitt's lymphoma cell lines: induction by latent Epstein–Barr virus genes. Blood 1992;80:459–469.
58. Henderson S, Rowe M, Gregory C, et al. Induction of *bcl-2* expression by Epstein–Barr virus latent membrane protein 1 protects infected B cells from progammed cell death. Cell 1991;65:1107–1115.
59. Oudejans JJ, van den Brule AJC, Jiwa NM, et al. BHRF1, the Epstein–Barr virus (EBV) homologue of the BCL-2 proto-oncogene, is transcribed in EBV-associated B-cell lymphomas and in reactive lymphocytes. Blood 1995;86:1893–1902.
60. Murray PG, Swinnen LJ, Constandinou CM, et al. BCL-2 but not its Epstein–Barr virus–encoded homologue, BHRF1, is commonly expressed in posttransplantation lymphoproliferative disorders. Blood 1995;87:706–711.
61. Calender A, Cordier M, Billaud M, et al. Modulation of cellular gene expression in B lymphoma cells following in vitro infection by Epstein–Barr virus (EBV). Int J Cancer 1990;46:658–663.
62. Inghirami G, Grignani F, Sternas L, et al. Down-regulation of LFA-1 adhesion receptors by c-*myc* oncogene in human B lymphoblastoid cells. Science 1990;250:682–686.
63. Moore KW, Vieira P, Fiorentino DF, et al. Homology of cytokine synthesis inhibitory factor (IL-10) to the Epstein–Barr virus gene BCRF1. Science 1990;248:1230–1234.
64. Antin JH, Bierer BE, Smith BR, et al. Selective depletion of bone marrow T lymphocytes with anti-CD5 monoclonal antibodies: effective prophylaxis for graft-versus-host disease in patients with hematologic malignancies. Blood 1991;78:2139–2149.
65. Hanto DW, Frizzera G, Gajl-Peczalska KJ, et al. Epstein–Barr virus–induced B-cell lymphoma after renal transplantation. N Engl J Med 1982;306:913–918.
66. Meeker TC, Shiramizu B, Kaplan L, et al. Evidence for molecular subtypes of HIV-associated lymphoma: division into peripheral monoclonal, polyclonal and central nervous system lymphoma. AIDS 1991;5:669–674.
67. Shearer WT, Ritz J, Finegold MJ, et al. Epstein–Barr virus–associated B-cell proliferations of diverse clonal origins after bone marrow transplantation in a 12-year-old patient with severe combined immunodeficiency. N Engl J Med 1985;312:1151–1159.
68. Cannon MJ, Pisa P, Fox RI, et al. Epstein–Barr virus induces aggressive lymphoproliferative disorders of human B cell origin in SCID/hu chimeric mice. J Clin Invest 1990;85:1333–1337.
69. Rowe M, Young LS, Crocker J, et al. Epstein–Barr virus (EBV)–associated lymphoproliferative disease in the SCID mouse model: implications for the pathogenesis of EBV-positive lymphomas in man. J Exp Med 1991;173:147–158.
70. Shiramizu B, Herndier B, Meeker T, et al. Molecular and immunophenotypic characterization of AIDS-associated: Epstein–Barr virus–negative, polyclonal lymphoma. J Clin Oncol 1992;10:383–389.
71. Robertson KD, Manns A, Swinnen LJ, et al. CpG methylation of the major Epstein–Barr virus latency promoter in Burkitt's lymphoma and Hodgkin's disease. Blood 1996;88:3129–3136.
72. Jutterman R, Li E, Jaenisch R. Toxicity of 5-aza-2′-deoxycytidine to mammalian cells is mediated primarily by covalent trapping of DNA methyltransferase rather than DNA demethylation. Proc Natl Acad Sci U S A 1994;91:11797–11801.
73. Robertson KD, Hayward DJ, Ling PD, et al. Transcriptional activation of the EBV latency C promoter following 5-azacytidine treatment: evidence that demethylation at a single CpG site is crucial. Mol Cell Biol 1995;15:6150–6159.
74. Camilleri-Broet S, Davi F, Feuillard J, et al. High expression of latent membrane protein 1 of Epstein–Barr virus and BCL-2 oncoprotein in acquired immunodeficiency syndrome–related primary brain lymphomas. Blood 1995;86:432–435.

75. Hamilton-Dutoit SJ, Raphael M, Audouin J, et al. In situ demonstration of Epstein–Barr virus small RNAs (EBER-1) in acquired immunodeficiency syndrome–related lymphomas: correlation with tumor morphology and primary site. Blood 1993;82:619–624.
76. MacMahon EME, Glass JD, Hayward D, et al. Epstein–Barr virus in AIDS-related primary central nervous system lymphoma. Lancet 1991;338:969–973.
77. Shibata D, Weiss LM, Hernandez AM, et al. Epstein–Barr virus–associated non–Hodgkin's lymphoma in patients infected with the human immunodeficiency virus. Blood 1993;81:2102–2109.
78. Kaplan LD, Shiramizu B, Herndier B, et al. Influence of molecular characteristics on clinical outcome in human immunodeficiency virus–associated non–Hodgkin's lymphoma: identification of a subgroup with favorable clinical outcome. Blood 1995;85:1727–1735.
79. Bhatia K, Spangler G, Gaidano G, et al. Mutations in the coding region of *c-myc* occur frequently in acquired immunodeficiency syndrome–associated lymphomas. Blood 1994;84:883–888.
80. Subar M, Neri A, Inghirami G, et al. Frequent *c-myc* oncogene activation and infrequent presence of Epstein–Barr virus genome in AIDS-associated lymphoma. Blood 1988;72:667–671.
81. Chang Y, Cesarman E, Pessin MS, et al. Identification of herpesvirus-like DNA sequences in AIDS-associated Kaposi's sarcoma. Science 1994;266:1865–1869.
82. Moore P, Chang Y. Detection of herpesvirus-like DNA sequences in Kaposi's sarcoma in patients with and without HIV infection. N Engl J Med 1995;332:1181–1185.
83. Cesarman E, Chang Y, Moore PS, et al. Kaposi's sarcoma–associated herpesvirus-like DNA sequences in AIDS-related body-cavity–based lymphomas. N Engl J Med 1995;332:1186–1191.
84. Ambroziak JA, Blackbourn DJ, Herndier BG, et al. Herpes-like sequences in HIV-infected and uninfected Kaposi's sarcoma patients. Science 1995;268:582–583.
85. Schalling M, Ekman M, Kaaya EE, et al. A role for a new herpes virus (KSHV) in different forms of Kaposi's sarcoma. Nature Med 1995;1:707–708.
86. Whitby D, Howard MR, Tenant-Flowers M, et al. Detection of Kaposi's sarcoma associated with herpesvirus in peripheral blood of HIV-infected individuals and progression to Kaposi's sarcoma. Lancet 1995;346:799–802.
87. Nador RG, Cesarman E, Chadburn A, et al. Primary effusion lymphoma: a distinct clinicopathologic entity associated with the Kaposi's sarcoma–associated herpes virus. Blood 1996;88:645–656.
88. Said JW, Chien K, Takeuchi S, et al. Kaposi's sarcoma–associated herpesvirus (KSHV or HHV8) in primary effusion lymphoma: ultrastructural demonstration of herpesvirus in lymphoma cells. Blood 1996;87:4937–4943.
89. Said JW, Tasaka T, Takeuchi S, et al. Primary effusion lymphoma in women: report of two cases of Kaposi's sarcoma herpes virus–associated effusion-based lymphoma in human immunodeficiency virus–negative women. Blood 1996;88:3124–3128.
90. Karcher DS, Alkan S. Herpes-like DNA sequences, AIDS-related tumors, and Castleman's disease [letter]. N Engl J Med 1995;333:797–798.
91. Dupin N, Gorin I, Deleuze J, et al. Herpes-like DNA sequences, AIDS-related tumors, and Castleman's disease [letter]. N Engl J Med 1995;333:798.
92. Soulier J, Grollet L, Oksenhendler E, et al. Kaposi's sarcoma–associated herpesvirus-like DNA sequences in multicentric Castleman's disease. Blood 1995;86:1276–1280.
93. Levine AM: AIDS-related malignancies: the emerging epidemic. J Natl Cancer Inst 1993;85:1382–1396.
94. Lee ES, Locker J, Nalesnik M, et al. The association of Epstein–Barr virus with smooth muscle tumors occurring after organ transplantation. N Engl J Med 1995;332:19–25.
95. McClain KL, Leach CT, Jenson HB, et al. Association of Epstein–Barr virus with leiomyosarcomas in young people with AIDS. N Engl J Med 1995;332:12–18.
96. Chu EW, Rabson AS. Chimerism in lymphoid cell culture lines derived from lymph node of marmoset infected with Herpesvirus saimiri. J Natl Cancer Inst 1972;48:771–775.
97. Nicholas J, Cameron KR, Honess RW. Herpesvirus saimiri encodes homologues of G protein–coupled receptors and cyclins. Nature 1992;355:362–365.
98. Motokura T, Arnold A: Cyclin D and oncogenesis. Curr Opin Genet Devel 1993;3:5–10.
99. Chang Y, Moore PS, Talbot SJ, et al. Cyclin encoded by KS herpsevirus. Nature 1996;382:410.
100. Moore PS, Boshoff C, Weiss RA, et al. Molecular mimicry of human cytokine and cytokine response pathway genes by KSHV. Science 1996;274:1739-1744.
101. Birx DL, Redfield RR, Tencer K, et al. Induction of interleukin-6 during human immunodeficiency virus infection. Blood 1990;76:2303–2310.
102. Kishimoto T, Akira S, Narazaki M, et al. Interleukin-6 family of cytokines and gp130. Blood 1995;86:1243–1254.
103. Yarchoan R, Redfield RR, Broder S. Mechanisms of B cell activation in patients with acquired immunodeficiency syndrome and related disorders. J Clin Invest 1986;78:439–447.
104. Emilie D, Coumbaras J, Raphael M, et al. Interleukin-6 production in high grade B lymphomas: correlation with the presence of malignant immunoblasts in acquired immunodeficiency syndrome and in human immunodeficiency syndrome virus–seronegative patients. Blood 1992;80:498–504.
105. Jucker M, Abts H, Li W, et al. Expression of interleukin-6 and interleukin-6 receptor in Hodgkin's disease. Blood 1991;77:2413–2418.
106. Leger-Ravet MB, Peuchmaur M, et al. Interleukin-6 gene expression in Castleman's disease. Blood 1991;78:2923–2930.
107. Benjamin D, Knobloch TJ, Dayton MA. Human B-cell interleukin-10: B-cell lines derived from patients with acquired immunodeficiency syndrome and Burkitt's lymphoma constitutively secrete large quantities of interleukin-10. Blood 1992;80:1289–1298.
108. Masood R, Zhang Y, Bond MW, et al. Interleukin-10 is an autocrine growth factor for acquired immunodeficiency syndrome–related B-cell lymphoma. Blood 1995;85:3423–3430.
109. Fiorentino DF, Zlotnik A, Vieira P, et al. IL-10 acts on the antigen-presenting cell to inhibit cytokine production by T$_H$1 cells. J Immunol 1991;146:3444–3451.
110. Salgame P, Abrams JS, Clayberger C, et al. Differing lymphokine profiles of functional subsets of human CD4 and CD8 T cell clones. Science 1991;254:279–282.
111. Herbst H, Foss H-D, Samol J, et al. requent expression of interleukin-10 by Epstein–Barr virus–harboring tumor cells of Hodgkin's disease. Blood 1996;87:2918–2929.
112. Baiocchi RA, Ross ME, Tan JC, et al. Lymphomagenesis in the SCID-hu mouse involves abundant production of human interleukin-10. Blood 1995;85:1063–1074.
113. Scadden DT, Zeira M, Woon A, et al. Human immunodeficiency virus infection of human bone marrow stromal fibroblasts. Blood 1990;76:317–322.
114. Aisenberg AC. Coherent view of non–Hodgkin's lymphoma. J Clin Oncol 1995;13:2656–2675.
115. Raphael BG, Knowles DM. Acquired immunodeficiency syndrome-associated non–Hodgkin's lymphoma. Semin Oncol 1990;17:361–366.
116. Kaplan LD, Kahn JO, Crowe S, et al. Clinical and virologic effects of recombinant human granulocyte–macrophage colony-stimulating factor in patients receiving chemotherapy for human immunodeficiency virus–associated non–Hodgkin's lymphoma: results of a randomized trial. J Clin Oncol 1991;9:929–940.
117. Perno C-F, Cooney DA, Gao W-Y, et al. Effects of bone marrow stimulatory cytokines on human immunodeficiency virus replication and the antiviral activity of dideoxynucleosides in cultures of monocytes/macrophages. Blood 1992;80:995–1003.

118. Yarchoan R, Mitsuya H, Broder S. The immunology of HIV infection: implications for therapy. AIDS Res Hum Retroviruses 1992; 8:1023–1031.
119. Sparano JA, Wiernik PH, Hu X, et al. Pilot trial of infusional cyclophosphamide, doxorubicin, and etoposide plus didanosine and filgrastim in patients with human immunodeficiency virus–associated non–Hodgkin's lymphoma. J Clin Oncol 1996;14:3026–3035.
120. Ogata A, Nishimoto N, Shima Y, et al. Inhibitory effects of all-*trans* retinoic acid on the growth of freshly isolated myeloma cells via interference with interleukin-6 signal transduction. Blood 84:3040, 1994.
121. Sidell N, Taga T, Hirano T, et al. Retinoic acid-induced growth inhibition of a human myeloma cell line via down-regulation of IL-6 receptors. J Immunol 1991;146:3809–3814.
122. Fazely F, Dezube BJ, Allen-Ryan J, et al. Pentoxifylline (Trental) decreases the replication of the human immunodeficiency virus type 1 in human peripheral blood mononuclear cells and in cultured T cells. Blood 1991;77:1653–1656.
123. Dezube BJ: Pentoxifylline for the treatment of infection with human immunodeficiency virus. Clin Infect Dis 1994;18:285–287.
124. Kreitman RJ, Siegall CB, FitzGerald DJP, et al. Interleukin-6 fused to a mutant form of *Pseudomonas* exotoxin kills malignant cells from patients with multiple myeloma. Blood 1992;79:1775–1780.
125. Bataille R, Barlogie B, Lu ZY, et al. Biologic effects of anti-interleukin-6 murine monoclonal antibody in advanced multiple myeloma. Blood 1995;86:685.
126. Emilie D, Wijdenes J, Gisselbrecht C, et al. Administration of an antiinterleukin-6 monoclonal antibody to patients with acquired immunodeficiency syndrome and lymphoma: effect on lymphoma growth and on B clinical symptoms. Blood 1994;84: 2472–2479.
127. teVelde AA, Huijbens RJF, Heije K, et al. Interleukin (IL)-4 inhibits secretion of IL-1β, tumor necrosis factor-α and IL-6 by monocytes. Blood 1990;76:1392–1397.
128. Herrmann F, Andreeff M, Gruss H-J, et al. Interleukin-4 inhibits growth of multiple myelomas by suppressing interleukin-6 expression. Blood 1991; 78:2070–2074.
129. Defrance T, Fluckiger A-C, Rossi J-F, et al. Antiproliferative effects of interleukin-4 on freshly isolated non–Hodgkin malignant B-lymphoma cells. Blood 1992; 79:990–996.
130. Baiocchi RA, Caligiuri MA. Low-dose interleukin 2 prevents the development of Epstein–Barr virus (EBV)–associated lymphoproliferative disease in *scid/scid* mice reconstituted i. p. with EBV-seropositive human peripheral blood lymphocytes. Proc Natl Acad Sci U S A 1994; 91:5577–5581.
131. Bernstein ZP, Porter MM, Gould M, et al. Prolonged administration of low-dose interleukin-2 in human immunodeficiency virus–associated malignancy results in selective expansion of innate immune effectors without significant clinical toxicity. Blood 1995;86:3287–3294.
132. Gunther R, Chelstrom LM, Tuel-Ahlgren L, et al. Biotherapy for xenografter human central nervous system leukemia in mice with severe combined immundoeficiency using B43 (anti-CD19)–pokeweed antiviral protein immunotoxin. Blood 1995;85:2537v2545.
133. Riddell SR, Watanabe KS, Goodrich JM, et al. Restoration of viral immunity in immunodeficient humans by the adoptive transfer of T cell clones. Science 1992;257:238–241.
134. Bex F, Hermans P, Sprecher S, et al. Syngeneic adoptive transfer of antihuman immunodeficiency virus-1 (HIV-1)–primed lymphocytes from a vaccinated HIV-seronegative individual to his HIV-1–infected identical twin. Blood 1994;84:3317–3326.
135. Riddell SR, Elliott M, Lewinsohn DA, et al. T-cell mediatd rejection of gene-modified HIV-specific cytotoxic T lymphocytes in HIV-infected patients. Nature Med 1996;2:216–223.
136. Heslop HE, Ng CYC, Li C, et al. Long-term restoriation of immunity against Epstein–Barr virus infection by adoptive transfer of gene-modified virus-specific T lymphocytes. Nature Med 1996;2:551–555.
137. Papadopoulos EB, Ladanyi M, Emanuel D, et al. Infusions of donor leukocytes to treat Epstein–Barr virus–associated lymphoproliferative disorders after allogeneic bone marrow transplantation. N Engl J Med 1994;330:1185–1191.
138. Roth G, Curiel T, Lacy J. Epstein-Barr viral nuclear antigen-1 antisense oligodexoynucleotide inhibits proliferation of Epstein–Barr virus–immortalized B cells. Blood 1994;84:582–587.

28
CLINICAL ASPECTS OF AIDS-RELATED LYMPHOMA

Richard F. Ambinder and Ian W. Flinn

PRESENTATION AND DIAGNOSTIC WORKUP

Both non–Hodgkin's and Hodgkin's lymphomas are increased in incidence in patients with human immunodeficiency virus (HIV) infection, although the increase in non–Hodgkin's lymphomas is much greater, and only aggressive B-cell non–Hodgkin's lymphomas have been recognized as acquired immunodeficiency syndrome (AIDS)–defining illnesses. The clinical presentation of non–Hodgkin's lymphoma and Hodgkin's disease in patients with HIV is varied, but it includes local mass effect, symptoms of organ infiltration, and constitutional symptoms such as weight loss, fever, and night sweats. Constitutional symptoms occur much more commonly in HIV-infected patients with lymphoma than in their non–HIV-infected counterparts, although how frequently these symptoms are direct manifestations of lymphoma rather than of opportunistic infection remains uncertain (1–5).

Extranodal sites are the most frequent locus of both non–Hodgkin's and Hodgkin's lymphoma in patients with HIV infection, and this finding represents a substantial difference from lymphoma patients without HIV infection (3, 5–8).

Common extranodal sites of involvement are the central nervous system, the gastrointestinal tract, and the liver. Extranodal sites of involvement that are virtually only found in patients infected by HIV include the common bile duct, the heart, and the rectum. Similarly, Hodgkin's disease can involve brain and skin at presentation in HIV-infected patients (9, 10). Primary effusion lymphomas may arise in pleural, pericardial, or peritoneal cavities and are often not associated with any "solid" tumor mass (11, 12).

Diagnosis of lymphoma, with the possible exception of primary central nervous system lymphoma, always requires biopsy. Imaging studies of the chest and abdomen are often useful in identifying lesions likely to yield diagnostic material. Even with such studies, lymphoma in the gastrointestinal tract occasionally is detected only endoscopically. Enlarged accessible peripheral lymph nodes may reflect only persistent generalized lymphadenopathy, and biopsy of a node that shows hyperplasia alone does not exclude the possibility of lymphoma elsewhere. Whenever possible, lymph node biopsies should be performed on asymmetrically enlarged nodes. Bone marrow biopsy sometimes yields a diagnosis even in the absence of cytopenias and should be routinely considered before more invasive open procedures.

The type of biopsy performed is determined in part by the location of the pathologic lesion. Lesions normally devoid of lymphoid tissue such as the brain are adequately assessed by needle biopsy, whereas lymph node lesions may require an open biopsy, to allow assessment of the architecture. Particularly, when only small amounts of tissue are available, characterization of clonality by evaluation of κ and λ immunoglobulin expression using flow cytometry may be useful in establishing a diagnosis. However, failure to identify a clonal population, either by flow cytometry or by Southern blot hybridization, to detect immunoglobulin gene rearrangements does not exclude lymphoma. Indeed, series of patients with lymphoma have been reported in whom clonality could not be demonstrated in most lesions (13).

Once a diagnosis of lymphoma has been established, staging is completed with imaging studies of the brain, thorax, abdomen, and pelvis and with a bone marrow biopsy. In the absence of contraindications, lumbar puncture is performed to evaluate possible meningeal involvement and often to administer an initial dose of prophylactic intrathecal chemotherapy (14).

HISTOLOGY

Whereas non–Hodgkin's lymphomas, in general, include both indolent and aggressive, follicular and diffuse, B- and T-cell tumors, the increased incidence of non–Hodgkin's lymphomas in patients with HIV is mainly an increase in aggressive B-cell tumors with diffuse architecture. Histologically, 30 to 40% are diffuse small noncleaved, 20 to 30% are diffuse large cell of the immunoblastic subtype, and 30 to 40% are other types of diffuse large cell lymphomas (3, 4, 6, 8).

Most of these tumors express B-cell surface markers CD19, CD20, and CD22, although primary effusion lymphomas often exhibit an indeterminate phenotype with expression of lymphoid activation markers (8). Anaplastic large cell lymphomas with bizarre, pleomorphic, malignant cells that sometimes resemble Reed–Sternberg cells and that mark with CD30 are also recognized (15). T-cell lymphomas have also been described (16).

Hodgkin's disease in HIV-infected patients is similarly skewed to particular histologic subtypes relative to Hodgkin's disease in the non–HIV-infected population. Mixed cellularity and lymphocyte-depleted subtypes are the most common, and lymphocyte-predominant Hodgkin's disease is virtually unknown (5, 17, 18).

Diffuse immunoblastic and diffuse large cell lymphoma histologic patterns and isolated extranodal disease (stage Ie) seem to occur later in the HIV disease process. Thus, in the era before highly active antiretroviral therapy, the median CD4 count in patients with Burkitt's lymphoma was 270/µL, whereas it was 99/µL for diffuse immunoblastic and diffuse large cell lymphomas (19). In parallel fashion, among patients with lymphoma as an AIDS-defining event, Burkitt's lymphoma accounted for 47% of lymphomas occurring as the first manifestation of AIDS, whereas it accounted for only 13% of non–Hodgkin's lymphomas that developed after another AIDS-related event. Isolated extranodal lymphomas were diffuse immunoblastic or large cell in histologic pattern (97%) and were associated with a median CD4 count of 70/µL. Primary central nervous system lymphomas represents the extreme end of this spectrum and are associated with a particularly low CD4 count. In a recent cooperative group series, the median was less than 10/µl (RF Ambinder, et al, unpublished data).

DIAGNOSIS OF PRIMARY CENTRAL NERVOUS SYSTEM LYMPHOMA

Intracranial mass lesions in HIV-infected patients warrant special discussion with regard to diagnosis. Primary central nervous system lymphoma in non–HIV-infected patients is a rare entity. The incidence of this lymphoma is increased several thousandfold in HIV-infected patients and accounts for approximately 15% of non–Hodgkin's lymphomas (20). However, the most common intracranial mass lesions in HIV-infected patients are associated with toxoplasmosis rather than with lymphoma. These two disease processes cannot be differentiated on clinical grounds and show substantial overlap radiographically. Focal or multifocal ring enhancing lesions on computed tomography or magnetic resonance imaging are common in both diseases. The morbidity and occasional mortality of biopsy, as well as the poor prognosis of primary central nervous system lymphoma even with treatment, have led to reluctance to perform biopsy of suspicious lesions (21, 22). One widely accepted approach has been to treat patients empirically for toxoplasmosis and to pursue biopsy only if the disease progresses during anti-*Toxoplasma* therapy (23). Although this approach spares many patients from undergoing biopsy, it also delays definitive diagnosis and may ultimately contribute to the poor clinical outcome. Thus, much interest has been expressed in alternative diagnostic techniques.

Positron emission tomography (PET) with fluorine-18-fluoro-2-deoxyglucose (FDG) has shown promise in this regard. Primary central nervous system lymphoma has is a metabolically active FDG-avid tumor (24). FDG-PET has been able to differentiate between lymphoma and most infectious intracranial lesions accurately in three studies, although progressive multifocal leukoencephalopathy is also metabolically active (25–27). A more widely available imaging technique, single-photon emission computed tomography (SPECT) with thallium-201, is also promising. In several studies in HIV-infected patients, this technique has generally identified patients with primary central lymphoma, but it has also occasionally mislabeled patients with infectious lesions (28–33).

Several groups have investigated the utility of polymerase chain reaction (PCR) for Epstein–Barr (EBV) DNA in cerebrospinal fluid in the diagnosis of AIDS-related primary central nervous system lymphoma. This approach is based on the uniform association of EBV with this tumor (34). Although EBV DNA is occasionally detected in cerebrospinal fluid in other settings, such as acute infectious mononucleosis with neurologic manifestations, EBV DNA is rarely detected in the cerebrospinal fluid of HIV-infected patients without lymphoma, and investigators from several institutions have found it to be a useful diagnostic adjunct (35, 36).

These various noninvasive or minimally invasive tests may complement each other. In the presence of characteristic lesion or lesions on imaging studies, a positive thallium scan, and positive EBV DNA PCR from cerebrospinal fluid, biopsy is probably unnecessary. If imaging studies are consistent with lymphoma but lumbar puncture is prohibited because of concerns with high intracranial pressure and possible herniation, then biopsy should be undertaken, but delay of an empiric trial of anti-*Toxoplasma* therapy is unnecessary. In centers where FDG-PET is available, this method may provide an alternative to EBV PCR.

PROGNOSTIC INDICATORS

Various prognostic indicators for non–Hodgkin's lymphoma patients were identified in the era before highly active antiretroviral therapy. These indicators include the absolute CD4 count, the performance status, the presence of bone marrow involvement, and a history of a previous AIDS-defining illness (3, 37).

Age, serum lactate dehydrogenase, and histologic subtype may also affect survival (7, 38). EBV-associated lymphomas have a poorer prognosis. A particularly favorable "polyclonal" lymphoma variant has been described, but the existence of this entity remains controversial (39). The largest prognostic analysis was conducted using patients treated on the randomized AIDS Clinical Trials Group trial comparing low-dose and standard-dose therapy, as discussed later. In univariate and multivariate analysis, four adverse prognostic factors emerged: age greater than 35 years, intravenous drug use, CD4 counts less than 100/μL, and stage III or IV disease (40).

Similar prognostic factors have been identified in HIV-associated Hodgkin's disease. Absolute CD4 count of 250 cells/μL or greater and the absence of prior AIDS diagnosis are favorable (41). It seems likely that HIV load will emerge as an important prognostic factor for both non–Hodgkin's and Hodgkin's lymphoma, but this has not yet been documented.

TREATMENT

Early experience with aggressive lymphoma regimens underscored the toxicity of chemotherapy and the extra sensitivity of HIV-infected patients to various complications of therapy. Multivariate analysis of an early study showed the poorest survival in patients treated with the highest doses of cyclophosphamide (3). Reports of opportunistic infection and treatment delays from other investigators reinforced the notion that chemotherapy for HIV-associated lymphoma is a double-edged sword whose antitumor effects must be balanced against immunosuppressive effects. Trials with a low-dose regimen showed that reduced-dose chemotherapy was sometimes efficacious in achieving lasting remission (42). Ultimately, a randomized phase III trial was carried out comparing full-dose methotrexate, bleomycin, doxorubicin, cyclophosphamide, vincristine, and dexamethasone (m-BACOD) with reduced-dose m-BACOD (Table 28.1) (43). No differences in overall and disease-free survivals were found. However, there was a decrease in the percentage of patients developing grade 3 or higher toxicity associated with the use of lower doses of chemotherapy (50% versus 71%, $P<.008$).

The appropriate interpretation of this randomized controlled trial is complicated by several factors (44, 45). First, m-BACOD chemotherapy has largely been abandoned in the treatment of aggressive lymphoma because it has been associated with increased toxicity relative to other regimens without increased efficacy (46). Thus, whether full-dose treatment with another standard regimen such as cyclophosphamide, doxorubicin, vincristine, and prednisone (CHOP) would have also been associated with increased toxicity without an increase in overall or disease-free survival is not clear. Second, the availability of highly active antiretroviral therapy may profoundly alter the balance with regard to toxicities that could be anticipated in association with cytotoxic chemotherapy (47). Third, the benefits of dose-reduced therapy may only apply to patients with low CD4 counts. Higher CD4 counts are associated with higher remission rate and higher disease-free survival (48). Given that therapy in many patients with AIDS-associated lymphoma is failing, with tumor relapse, and that dose intensity is an important prognostic factor in the treatment of lymphoma in general (49, 50), it seems likely that at least a subset of patients will benefit from standard-dose therapy.

An alternative therapy using higher doses in a 96-hour infusional regimen of cyclophosphamide, doxorubicin, and etoposide (CDE) was piloted with an impressive median survival of 18 months (see Table 28.1) (51, 52). A disadvantage associated with this regimen is the requirement for placement of a central venous catheter. Another intensive therapy, modified LNH84, was studied by the French–Italian Cooperative Group in patients with good performance status and no prior opportunistic infections (7). Overall median survival was 9 months, but an even more highly selected subset of patients with good prognostic factors had a 50% survival rate at 2 years. An all-oral regimen consisting of CCNU, etoposide, cyclophosphamide, and procarbazine proved both convenient to deliver and relatively inexpensive; this regimen achieved complete remissions in 39% of patients, with a median survival of 7 months (53).

Therapy for HIV-infected patients with Hodgkin's disease has generally been similar to therapy for patients without HIV. However, because most patients have advanced stage lymphoma at the time of presentation, the use of radiation as sole therapy has been limited (17, 41). With chemotherapy alone or combined modality therapy, median survival was 15 months in both series.

Myeloid growth factors have become standard in conjunction with cytotoxic chemotherapy in the treatment of AIDS-related lymphomas. Granulocyte–macrophage colony-stimulating factor (GM-CSF) and G-CSF both diminish the severity and duration of neutropenia, but their impact on survival has not yet been demonstrated (54, 55).

The results of treatment of primary central nervous system lymphoma have been generally disappointing. Whole-brain irradiation is the mainstay of treatment. Tumor responses, improvement in neurologic function, quality of life, and survival are all suggested by retrospective studies, but long-term survival is rare (56–58). Experience in combining chemotherapy with radiation therapy is limited; occasional patients have survived beyond a year (59). Virtually all these patients had CD4 counts greater than 200 cell/μL and therefore were unusual; in this disease, the CD4 count is generally less than 30/μL. An Eastern Cooperative Oncol-

Table 28.1. Results of Treatment of AIDS-Related Lymphoma

Chemotherapy	CR (%)	Median Survival	Patients	Reference
m-BACOD	52	31 wk	81	43
Modified m-BACOD	41	35 wk	94	
CDE	58	18.4 mo	25	52
ACVB and LNH84	63	9 mo	141	7
Oral agents	39	7 mo	18	53

ACVB, doxorubicin, cyclophosphamide, vincristine, and bleomycin; CDE, cyclophosphamide, doxorubicin, and etoposide; CR, clinical response; m-BACOD, methotrexate, bleomycin, doxorubicin, cyclophosphamide, vincristine, and dexamethasone.

ogy Group trial combining radiation and chemotherapy in a group of patients with a median CD4 count less than 10 cells/μL achieved a median survival of less than 3 months.

NEW APPROACHES

In contrast to Kaposi's sarcoma (KS), in which several agents have been approved specifically for the treatment of this tumor, treatment of lymphoma in HIV-infected patients has relied on agents generally used in the treatment of lymphoma. As noted earlier, studies to date have focused on appropriate dosing of chemotherapeutic agents and characterization of supportive care options during therapy, but treatments have not specifically targeted HIV-associated lymphomas. Liposomal anthracyclines that have established activity against KS are better tolerated and are more effective than their nonliposomal anthracyclines. This property may relate to better localization to highly vascular KS lesions or to different pharmacokinetic profiles. The possible benefits of liposomal formulations in the treatment of lymphoma in HIV-infected patients are under investigation. Newer, less myelosuppressive chemotherapeutic agents such as mitoguazone may also find a role in treatment of HIV-associated lymphoma (60). Humanized monoclonal antibodies targeting B cells with or without radioligands (61) and immune reconstitution with interleukin-2 and other cytokines are areas of interest (62, 63). The consistent association of EBV with a subset of HIV-associated lymphomas has raised the possibility that these EBV-associated tumors could be specifically targeted. However, antiherpesviral agents such as acyclovir and ganciclovir, which are effective in the treatment of oral hairy leukoplakia, a nonneoplastic disease associated with lytic viral replication (64), have not any reported impact on EBV-associated malignant processes in HIV-infected patients. Several interesting preclinical models using gene therapy approaches have been developed, but serious obstacles related to gene delivery prevent their implementation at present (65–68). Finally, adoptive cellular immunotherapy with T cells specifically targeting EBV-infected cells is promising. This approach is useful in the prophylaxis and treatment of EBV-associated B-cell lymphoproliferative disease in bone marrow transplant recipients (69, 70). We anticipate that, over the next several years, dramatic advances will be seen as new modalities for immune reconstitution and immune-mediated killing of tumor cells, including cytokines, humanized monoclonal antibodies, and T-cell infusions, find their place in therapy. In addition, progress in antiretroviral therapy promises to make standard therapies more tolerable and allow approaches that involve dose-escalation rather than dose reduction.

References

1. Levine AM, Gill PS, Meyer PR, et al. Retrovirus and malignant lymphoma in homosexual men. JAMA 1985;254:1921–1925.
2. Gill PS, Levine AM, Krailo M, et al. AIDS-related malignant lymphoma: results of prospective treatment trials. J Clin Oncol 1987;5:1322–1328.
3. Kaplan LD, Abrams DI, Feigal E, et al. AIDS-associated non–Hodgkin's lymphoma in San Francisco. JAMA 1989;261:719–724.
4. Lowenthal DA, Straus DJ, Campbell SW, et al. AIDS-related lymphoid neoplasia: the Memorial Hospital experience. Cancer 1988; 61:2325–2337.
5. Tirelli U, Spina M, Vaccher E, et al. Clinical evaluation of 451 patients with HIV related non–Hodgkin's lymphoma: experience on the Italian cooperative group on AIDS and tumors (GICAT). Leuk Lymphoma 1995;20:91–96.
6. Ziegler JL, Beckstead JA, Volberding PA, et al. Non–Hodgkin's lymphoma in 90 homosexual men. N Engl J Med 1984;311:565–570.
7. Gisselbrecht C, Oksenhendler E, Tirelli U, et al. Human immunodeficiency virus–related lymphoma treatment with intensive combination chemotherapy. French–Italian Cooperative Group. Am J Med 1993; 95:188–196.
8. Knowles DM, Chamulak GA, Subar M, et al. Lymphoid neoplasia associated with the acquired immunodeficiency syndrome (AIDS): the New York University Medical Center experience with 105 patients (1981–1986). Ann Intern Med 1988;108:744–753.
9. Hair LS, Rogers JD, Chadburn A, et al. Intracerebral Hodgkin's disease in a human immunodeficiency virus–seropositive patient. Cancer 1991; 67:2931–2934.
10. Shaw MT, Jacobs SR. Cutaneous Hodgkin's disease in a patient with human immunodeficiency virus infection. Cancer 1989;64:2585–2587.
11. Nador RG, Cesarman E, Chadburn A, et al. Primary effusion lymphoma: a distinct clinicopathologic entity associated with the Kaposi's sarcoma–associated herpes virus. Blood 1996;88:645–656.
12. Cesarman E, Nador RG, Aozasa K, et al. Kaposi's sarcoma–associated herpesvirus in non-AIDS related lymphomas occurring in body cavities. Am J Pathol 1996;149:53–57.
13. Meeker TC, Shiramizu B, Kaplan L, et al. Evidence for molecular subtypes of HIV-associated lymphoma: division into peripheral monoclonal, polyclonal and central nervous system lymphoma. AIDS 1991; 5:669–674.
14. Levine AM. Acquired immunodeficiency syndrome–related lymphoma. Blood 1992;80:8–20.
15. Chadburn A, Cesarman E, Jagirdar J, et al. CD30 (Ki-1) positive anaplastic large cell lymphomas in individuals infected with the human immunodeficiency virus. Cancer 1993;72:3078–3090.
16. Lust JA, Banks PM, Hooper WC, et al. T-cell non–Hodgkin lymphoma in human immunodeficiency virus-1-infected individuals. Am J Hematol 1989;31:181–187.
17. Rubio R. Hodgkin's disease associated with human immunodeficiency virus infection: a clinical study of 46 cases. Cooperative Study Group of Malignancies Associated with HIV Infection of Madrid. Cancer 1994; 73:2400–2407.
18. Andrieu JM, Roithmann S, Tourani JM, et al. Hodgkin's disease during HIV-1 infection: the French registry experience. French Registry of HIV-associated Tumors. Ann Oncol 1993;4:635–641.
19. Roithmann S, Toledamo M, Tourani JM, et al. HIV-associated non–Hodgkin's lymphomas: clinical characteristics and outcome. The experience of the French Registry of HIV-associated tumors. Ann Oncol 1991;2:289–295.
20. Cote TR, Manns A, Hardy CR, et al. Epidemiology of brain lymphoma among people with or without acquired immunodeficiency syndrome: AIDS/Cancer Study Group. J Natl Cancer Inst 1996;88:675–679.
21. Donahue BR, Sullivan JW, Cooper JS, et al. Additional experience with empiric radiotherapy for presumed human immunodeficiency virus–associated primary central nervous system lymphoma. Cancer 1995;76: 328–332.
22. Corn BW, Trock BJ, Curran WJ. Management of primary central nervous system lymphoma for the patient with acquired immunodeficiency syndrome: confronting a clinical catch-22. Cancer 1995;76: 163–166.
23. Galetto G, Levine A. AIDS-associated primary central nervous system lymphoma: Oncology Core Committee, AIDS Clinical Trials Group. JAMA 1993;269:92–93.

24. Rosenfeld SS, Hoffman JM, Coleman RE, et al. Studies of primary central nervous system lymphoma with fluorine–18-fluorodeoxyglucose positron emission tomography. J Nucl Med 1992;33:532–536.
25. Hoffman JM, Waskin HA, Schifter T, et al. FDG-PET in differentiating lymphoma from nonmalignant central nervous system lesions in patients with AIDS. J Nucl Med 1993;34:567–575.
26. Villringer K, Jager H, Dichgans M, et al. Differential diagnosis of CNS lesions in AIDS patients by FDG-PET. J Comput Assist Tomogr 1995;19:532–536.
27. Heald AE, Hoffman JM, Bartlett JA, et al. Differentiation of central nervous system lesions in AIDS patients using positron emission tomography (PET). Int J STD AIDS 1996;7:337–346.
28. O'Malley JP, Ziessman HA, Kumar PN, et al. Diagnosis of intracranial lymphoma in patients with AIDS: value of 201Tl single-photon emission computed tomography. AJR Am J Roentgenol 1994;163:417–421.
29. Ruiz A, Ganz WI, Post MJ, et al. Use of thallium-201 brain SPECT to differentiate cerebral lymphoma from toxoplasma encephalitis in AIDS patients. AJNR Am J Neuroradiol 1994;15:1885–1894.
30. Lorberboym M, Estok L, Machac J, et al. Rapid differential diagnosis of cerebral toxoplasmosis and primary central nervous system lymphoma by thallium-201 SPECT. J Nucl Med 1996;37:1150–1154.
31. Naddaf SY, Akisik MF, Aziz M, et al. Comparison between ^{201}Tl-chloride and ^{99}Tc(m) sestamibi SPET brain imaging for differentiating intracranial lymphoma from non-malignant lesions in AIDS patients. Nucl Med Commun 1998;19:47–53.
32. D'Amico A, Messa C, Castagna A, et al. Diagnostic accuracy and predictive value of ^{201}Tl SPET for the differential diagnosis of cerebral lesions in AIDS patients. Nucl Med Commun 1997;18:741–750.
33. Fisher DC, Chason DP, Mathews D, et al. Central nervous system lymphoma not detectable on single-photon emission CT with thallium 201. AJNR Am J Neuroradiol 1996;17:1687–1690.
34. MacMahon EME, Glass JD, Hayward SD, et al. Epstein–Barr virus in AIDS-related primary central nervous system lymphoma. Lancet 1991;338:969–973.
35. De Luca A, Antinori A, Cingolani A, et al. Evaluation of cerebrospinal fluid EBV-DNA and IL-10 as markers for in vivo diagnosis of AIDS-related primary central nervous system lymphoma. Br J Haematol 1995;90:844–849.
36. Roberts TC, Storch GA. Multiplex PCR for diagnosis of AIDS-related central nervous system lymphoma and toxoplasmosis. J Clin Microbiol 1997;35:268–269.
37. Levine AM, Sullivan-Halley J, Pike MC, et al. Human immunodeficiency virus-related lymphoma: prognostic factors predictive of survival. Cancer 1991;68:2466–2472.
38. Vaccher E, Tirelli U, Spina M, et al. Age and serum lactate dehydrogenase level are independent prognostic factors in human immunodeficiency virus-related non-Hodgkin's lymphomas: a single-institute study of 96 patients. J Clin Oncol 1996;14:2217–2223.
39. Kaplan LD, Shiramizu B, Herndier B, et al. Influence of molecular characteristics on clinical outcome in human immunodeficiency virus-associated non-Hodgkin's lymphoma: identification of a subgroup with favorable clinical outcome. Blood 1995;85:1727–1735.
40. Straus DJ. HIV-associated lymphomas. Curr Opin Oncol 1997;9:450–454.
41. Tirelli U, Errante D, Dolcetti R, et al. Hodgkin's disease and human immunodeficiency virus infection: clinicopathologic and virologic features of 114 patients from the Italian cooperative group on AIDS and tumors. J Clin Oncol 1995;13:1758–1767.
42. Levine AM, Wernz JC, Kaplan L, et al. Low-dose chemotherapy with central nervous systm prophylaxis and zidovudine maintenance in AIDS-related lymphoma. JAMA 1991;266:84–88.
43. Kaplan LD, Straus DJ, Testa MA, et al. Low-dose compared with standard-dose m-BACOD chemotherapy for non-Hodgkin's lymphoma associated with human immunodeficiency virus infection: National Institute of Allergy and Infectious Diseases AIDS Clinical Trials Group. N Engl J Med 1997;336:1641–1648.
44. Sparano J. Chemotherapy for AIDS-related lymphomas. N Engl J Med 1997;337:1173–1174.
45. Wilson WH. Chemotherapy for AIDS-related lymphomas. N Engl J Med 1997;337:1172–1173.
46. Fisher RI, Gaynor ER, Dahlberg S, et al. Comparison of a standard regimen (CHOP) with three intensive chemotherapy regimens for advanced non-Hodgkin's lymphoma. N Engl J Med 1993;328:1002–1006.
47. Tan B, Ratner L. The use of new antiretroviral therapy in combination with chemotherapy. Curr Opin Oncol 1997;9:455–464.
48. Levine AM. Lymphoma in acquired immunodeficiency syndrome. Semin Oncol 1990;17:104–112.
49. Kwak LW, Halpern J, Olshen RA, et al. Prognostic significance of actual dose intensity in diffuse large-cell lymphoma: results of a tree-structured survival analysis. J Clin Oncol 1990;8:963–977.
50. Meyer RM, Hryniuk WM, Goodyear MD. The role of dose intensity in determining outcome in intermediate-grade non-Hodgkin's lymphoma. J Clin Oncol 1991;9:339–347.
51. Sparano JA, Wiernik PH, Strack M, et al. Infusional cyclophosphamide, doxorubicin, and etoposide in human immunodeficiency virus- and human T-cell leukemia virus type I–related non-Hodgkin's lymphoma: a highly active regimen. Blood 1993;81:2810–2815.
52. Sparano JA, Wiernik PH, Hu X, et al. Pilot trial of infusional cyclophosphamide, doxorubicin, and etoposide plus didanosine and filgrastim in patients with human immunodeficiency virus-associated non-Hodgkin's lymphoma. J Clin Oncol 1996;14:3026–3035.
53. Remick SC, McSharry JJ, Wolf BC, et al. Novel oral combination in the treatment of intermediate-grade and high-grade AIDS-related non-Hodgkin's lymphoma. J Clin Oncol 1993;11:1691–1702.
54. Kaplan LD, Kahn JO, Crowe S, et al. Clinical and virologic effects of recombinant human granulocyte–macrophage colony-stimulating factor in patients receiving chemotherapy for human immunodeficiency virus-associated non-Hodgkin's lymphoma: results of a randomized trial. J Clin Oncol 1991;9:929–940.
55. Gabarre J, Lepage E, Thyss A, et al. Chemotherapy combined with zidovudine and GM-CSF in human immunodeficiency virus–related non-Hodgkin's lymphoma. Ann Oncol 1995;6:1025–1032.
56. Baumgartner JE, Rachlin JR, Beckstead JH, et al. Primary central nervous system lymphomas: natural history and response to radiation therapy in 55 patients with acquired immunodeficiency syndrome. J Neurosurg 1990;73:206–211.
57. Goldstein JD, Dickson DW, Moser FG, et al. Primary central nervous system lymphoma in acquired immune deficiency syndrome: a clinical and pathologic study with results of treatment with radiation. Cancer 1991;67:2756–2765.
58. Nisce LZ, Kaufmann T, Metroka C. Radiation therapy in patients with AIDS-related central nervous system lymphomas. JAMA 1992;267:1921–1922.
59. Forsyth PA, Yahalom J, Deangelis LM. Combined-modality therapy in the treatment of primary central nervous system lymphoma in AIDS. Neurology 1994;44:1473–1479.
60. Levine AM, Tulpule A, Tessman D, et al. Mitoguazone therapy in patients with refractory or relapsed AIDS-related lymphoma: results from a multicenter phase II trial. J Clin Oncol 1997;15:1094–1103.
61. Maloney DG, Grillo-Lopez AJ, White CA, et al. IDEC-C2B8 (Rituximab) anti-CD20 monoclonal antibody therapy in patients with relapsed low-grade non-Hodgkin's lymphoma. Blood 1997;90:2188–2195.
62. Bernstein ZP, Porter MM, Gould M, et al. Prolonged administration of low-dose interleukin-2 in human immunodeficiency virus-associated malignancy results in selective expansion of innate immune effectors without significant clinical toxicity. Blood 1995;86:3287–3294.
63. Mazza P, Bocchia M, Tumietto F, et al. Recombinant interleukin-2 (rIL-2) in acquired immune deficiency syndrome (AIDS): preliminary report in patients with lymphoma associated with HIV infection. Eur J Haematol 1992;49:1–6.

64. Resnick L, Herbst JS, Ablashi DV, et al. Regression of oral hairy leukoplakia after orally administered acyclovir therapy. JAMA 1988; 259:384–388.
65. Franken M, Estabrooks A, Cavacini L, et al. Epstein–Barr virus–driven gene therapy for EBV-related lymphomas. Nature Med 1996;2:1379–1382.
66. Rogers RP, Ge JQ, Holley-Guthrie E, et al. Killing Epstein–Barr virus–positive B lymphocytes by gene therapy: comparing the efficacy of cytosine deaminase and herpes simplex virus thymidine kinase. Hum Gene Ther. 1996;7:2235-2245.
67. Gutierrez MI, Judde JG, Magrath IT, et al. Switching viral latency to viral lysis: a novel therapeutic approach for Epstein–Barr virus–associated neoplasia. Cancer Res 1996;56:969–972.
68. Judde JG, Spangler G, Magrath I, et al. Use of Epstein–Barr virus nuclear antigen-1 in targeted therapy of EBV-associated neoplasia. Hum Gene Ther 1996;7:647–653.
69. Heslop HE, Ng CY, Li C, et al. Long-term restoration of immunity against Epstein-Barr virus infection by adoptive transfer of gene-modified virus-specific T lymphocytes. Nature Med 1996;2:551–555.
70. Rooney CM, Smith CA, Ng CY, et al. Use of gene-modified virus-specific T lymphocytes to control Epstein–Barr virus–related lymphoproliferation. Lancet 1995;345:9–13.

29
OCULAR SEQUELAE

James P. Dunn and Gary N. Holland

The ocular sequelae of human immunodeficiency virus (HIV) infection can be particularly devastating because of their impact on a patient's quality of life. The majority of patients with acquired immunodeficiency syndrome (AIDS) will develop one or more ophthalmic disorders during the course of their illness, and 20 to 40% are at risk for severe vision loss from ocular infections. The importance of ophthalmic disease in the AIDS epidemic is reflected in the finding that fear of blindness has been stated to be the leading cause of suicide among patients with AIDS (1).

Most ocular tissues are easily observed, and even tiny foci of disease in the eye can cause profound visual symptoms. Ophthalmic lesions therefore are often an early marker for multifocal disease and disseminated infections. The same degree of disease in many other organs would remain clinically silent.

Ophthalmic diseases pose a unique diagnostic challenge to clinicians. Although tissues such as the retina can be observed, they are not easily accessible in most cases for culture or other diagnostic tests. Retinal biopsies are reserved only for selected cases, usually when visual function has already been lost as a result of infection or retinal detachment, and diagnosis is important for treatment of similar disease in the other eye. The widespread availability of polymerase chain reaction techniques has led to the more frequent use of vitreous humor biopsies, which are safer and easier to perform, for diagnosis of atypical viral retinopathies (2). Nevertheless, in most cases of intraocular disease, ophthalmologists depend to a great extent on the clinical appearance and course of lesions in making a diagnosis. Complicating these clinical diagnoses is the finding that the immunosuppression associated with HIV infection alters the typical clinical characteristics of many well-known ophthalmic diseases such as ocular toxoplasmosis.

The early and accurate diagnosis of ophthalmic disease is critical. Not only may lesions be early markers for potentially life-threatening disseminated diseases, but also preservation of sight requires immediate treatment in many cases. Retinal tissue that is destroyed cannot be regenerated, and even mild damage to many structures such as the retina, optic nerve, or cornea can cause profound vision loss.

HIV INFECTION

HIV has been recovered from most ocular tissues, but its ability to cause clinically apparent ocular disease as a direct result of ocular infection remains a subject of debate. Occasionally, HIV-infected patients have chronic iridocyclitis that cannot be attributed to any secondary intraocular infection or systemic inflammatory disease (3). The iridocyclitis resolves rapidly in some patients with zidovudine therapy, a finding suggesting a direct relationship with HIV. Alternatively, inflammation could be the result of an unidentified infectious agent of low virulence that is successfully suppressed with improvement in the patient's immune function.

Other AIDS patients who have no evidence of secondary intraocular infections have decreased vision, vitreous inflammatory reactions, constricted visual fields, and reduced or extinguished electroretinograms. Investigators have theorized that these findings may represent other manifestations of direct infection with HIV. Such cases are rare, and most HIV-infected patients do not have intraocular inflammation. When inflammation is seen, opportunistic infections, such as toxoplasmosis, syphilis, or fungal endophthalmitis or drug-induced uveitis (rifabutin, cidofovir) should be considered first; only after these conditions are ruled out should HIV-induced uveitis be considered.

Investigators have hypothesized that HIV acts as a cofactor in retinal infections. HIV and cytomegalovirus (CMV) have been found in the same retinal cells at autopsy (4). Interactions between the two viruses, which are known to occur in vitro, may enhance the activity of CMV in coinfected cells and may be one reason that CMV retinitis is more severe in some patients.

The secondary disorders that make up the bulk of the ophthalmic manifestations of AIDS fall into four major categories: lesions attributed to vascular disease of the retina and other tissues, infections, neoplasms, and neuro-ophthalmic signs of intracranial disease (Table 29.1).

VASCULAR DISEASE

The most common ocular lesions in HIV-infected patients are "cotton-wool" spots (5, 6). They are discrete areas of retinal opacification, usually located around the optic disc or along the major vascular arcades in the posterior pole (Fig. 29.1). They correspond to areas of nerve fiber layer swelling caused by retinal ischemia (7), and they are the most common manifestation of a diffuse retinal microvasculopathy that probably occurs in all HIV-infected persons. Trypsin digest preparations of affected retina show loss of pericytes and microaneurysm formation. Ultrastructural studies show swollen endothelial cells, occluded vascular lumina, and thickened vascular basal lamina (8). These findings are strikingly similar to vascular changes in diabetic retinopathy.

Microvascular abnormalities can also be seen in the bulbar conjunctiva, and they indicate that vascular damage is widespread in patients with HIV infection (9). Changes, which are most apparent in the inferior, perilimbal bulbar conjunctiva, consist of dilated capillaries, isolated vascular fragments, vessel segments of irregular caliber, and sludging of blood flow. Ischemic optic neuropathy, although seen infrequently among HIV-infected patients, appears to be more common than in same-aged persons in the general population. This condition may be the result of similar microvascular disease in

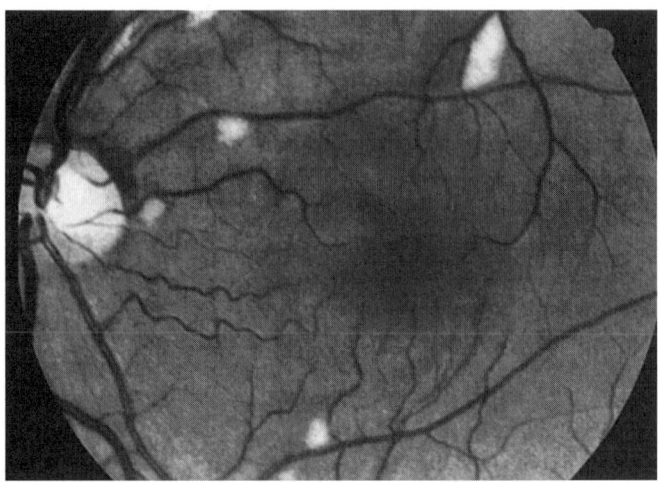

Figure 29.1. Cotton-wool spots.

Table 29.1 Ophthalmic Disorders Associated with HIV Infection

Vasculopathy
  Microvasculopathy
    Retina
      Cotton-wool spots
      Retinal hemorrhages
      Microaneurysms
      Ischemic maculopathy
    Conjunctiva
      Changes in vessel structure (dilated capillaries, microaneurysms, isolated vascular fragments, vessel segments of irregular caliber)
      Altered blood flow ("sludging")
    Optic nerve
      Ischemic optic neuropathy
  Large vessel disease
    Retina
      Central retinal vein occlusion
      Branch retinal vein occlusion
Opportunistic infectious diseases (see Table 29.2)
Neoplasms
  Kaposi's sarcoma
    Eyelids
    Conjunctiva
    Orbit (rare)
  Lymphoma
    Intraocular
      Large cell
      Small cell, noncleaved
    Orbital
      Burkitt's lymphoma
      Small cell, noncleaved
Neuro-ophthalmic signs of intracranial disease
  Cranial nerve palsies
  Eye movement abnormalities
  Visual field defects
  Occipital blindness
  Papilledema
  Pupillary abnormalities
  Optic atrophy

the optic nerve. Ischemic optic neuropathy results in pale optic discs and visual field loss. Infectious and neoplastic causes must always be ruled out before attributing optic neuropathy to microvascular disease, however.

Various causes have been hypothesized for the microvasculopathy and retinal ischemia; they include damage caused by HIV infection of endothelial cells (10), deposition of immune complexes (8), and alterations in blood flow (9). The vasoconstrictor cytokine endothelin-1 has been associated with both retinal microvasculopathy and conjunctival blood-flow sludging (11). Microvasculopathy is neither the result of opportunistic infections of involved tissues nor of immunosuppression alone (7). HIV infection of the endothelial cells with subsequent vascular occlusion does not fully explain all findings of the condition, nor does it account for the marked similarity between HIV-associated retinal microvasculopathy and that seen in diabetes mellitus or some connective tissue disorders like systemic lupus erythematosus. In addition, infection of endothelial cells is not a consistent finding in patients with retinal microvasculopathy (12).

Immunoglobulin deposition has been noted in arteriolar walls of patients with AIDS (8). The presence of polyclonal B-cell activation, hypergammaglobulinemia, and circulating immune complexes characterizes not only AIDS but also collagen vascular diseases that have similar microvasculopathies. One report noted an increased rate of microvasculopathy in patients coinfected with hepatitis C (13); the authors of this report attributed the finding to hypergammaglobulinemia and increased serum viscosity in these patients.

Engstrom and associates found an association between fibrinogen levels and both conjunctival microvasculopathy and cotton-wool spots in HIV-infected patients (9). The cause of the increased fibrinogen is unknown. The authors theorized that increased fibrinogen causes increased red cell aggregation and blood flow sludging; this abnormality, in turn, causes vascular hypoxia that contributes to the development of the microvasculopathy. In their studies, circulating immune complex levels did not correlate strongly with microvasculopathy. The cause is probably multifactorial. Other, less frequent disorders presumed to be manifestations of the microvasculopathy include posterior flame-shaped retinal hemorrhages, peripheral blot retinal hemorrhages, and microaneurysms.

Cotton-wool spots rarely produce gross visual disturbances and therefore are of little clinical significance to the individual patient. These lesions are, however, more common in patients with AIDS than in those with asymptomatic HIV infections (6, 14), and therefore, they may represent a nonspecific sign of severe immunosuppression. Investigators have thus suggested that these lesions represent a poor prognostic sign. Cotton-wool spots are more common in men who acquired HIV infection through sex with other men than in men with comparable CD4+ T-lymphocyte counts who became infected through other routes (15). No association, however, has ever been identified between retinal microangiopathy and any specific AIDS-related infection or neoplasm.

Although cotton-wool spots are generally considered asymptomatic lesions, some investigators suspect that the underlying retinal microvascular disease may lead to diffuse retinal dysfunction with subtle visual changes. It may be a contributing factor to the finding of axonal loss in optic nerves of patients with AIDS and associated defects in color vision, contrast sensitivity, and visual field loss among individuals infected with HIV (16–18).

Retinal microvasculopathy may be a marker for vascular disease in nonocular tissues. A relationship has been found between the presence of the cotton-wool spots and alterations in cognitive functioning (19). Changes were most apparent on neuropsychological examinations that test short-term memory. Investigators also found a relationship between the number of cotton-wool spots on ophthalmoscopic examination and reduced cerebral blood flow, as measured by technetium-99m-hexamethyl propyleneamine oxime single photon emission tomography, which may help to explain the cognitive abnormalities (20).

Some investigators have hypothesized that retinal microvascular damage may facilitate the development of opportunistic infections of the retina by trapping blood-borne infectious agents in the retinal circulation or by facilitating access of these agents to various retinal cells through damaged vessel walls (7, 8, 21).

Central or branch retinal vein occlusions are believed by many investigators to be more frequent in HIV-infected patients than in similar-aged individuals in the general population. These occlusions are not usually associated with evidence of other retinal or optic nerve disorders. These cases indicate that large vessel disease can occur as well as microvasculopathy. Abnormal blood flow may be a common factor in these various disorders (22).

Perivascular sheathing not associated with infectious retinitis is another vascular abnormality associated with AIDS. It has not turned out to be a common manifestation of the syndrome in the United States, but it is common in Africa, particularly in African children with AIDS (23). The cause of this disorder and the reason for its geographic distribution are not known.

OPPORTUNISTIC INFECTIONS

More than a dozen infectious agents have been reported to cause ocular disease in patients with HIV infection (Table 29.2). Certain pathogens are tissue specific in the infections they cause, but most structures of the eye and ocular adnexa are susceptible to infection by one or more agents. Infections of the retina and choroid are the most common and most important (24). Information about these infections that is pertinent to the general care of patients is summarized here.

Infections of the Retina and Choroid

Infections of the retina and choroid vary in prevalence, but all can lead to loss of vision or blindness. With the exception of CMV retinitis, all tend to be much less common than systemic diseases caused by the same organisms (8). As a group, all infections other than CMV retinitis probably account for 5% or less of retinal infections seen in HIV-infected patients. Most of the reported retinal and choroidal infections are not unique to HIV-infected patients. Many, however, were so rare before the AIDS epidemic that they would not have been encountered by most ophthalmologists.

CYTOMEGALOVIRUS

Because the United States Centers for Disease Control and Prevention (CDC) do not keep statistics on CMV

Table 29.2 Infectious Agents Associated with Ophthalmic Disease in HIV-Infected Patients

Infections of the retina and choroid
   Candida albicans
   Cryptococcus neoformans
   Cytomegalovirus
   Endogenous bacteria
   Fusarium species
   Herpes simplex virus
   Histoplasma capsulatum
   Mycobacterium avium complex
   Mycobacterium tuberculosis
   Nocardia species
   Pneumocystis carinii
   Sporothrix schenckii
   Staphylococcus aureus
   Toxoplasma gondii
   Treponema pallidum
   Varicella-zoster virus
Infections of the ocular surface and adnexae
   Bacteria (most commonly *Pseudomonas* species and *Staphylococcus aureus*)
   Acanthamoeba species
   Candida albicans
   Chlamydia trachomatis, serotype L2 (lymphogranuloma venereum)
   Cytomegalovirus
   Herpes simplex virus
   Microsporidia
   Molluscum contagiosum
   Varicella-zoster virus

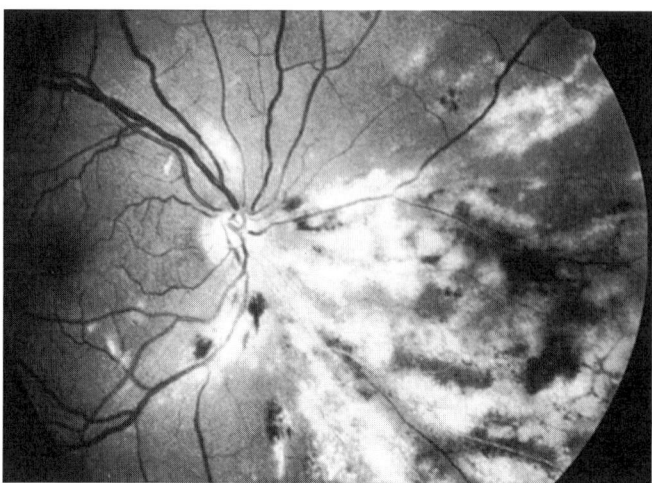

Figure 29.2. Cytomegalovirus retinopathy. The infection is characterized by retinal opacification (whitening) with a dry-appearing, granular border corresponding to areas of retinal necrosis. Scattered hemorrhage is present in the lesion.

retinitis, the exact prevalence of the disease is not known. Most ophthalmologists have noted a drop in the incidence of CMV retinitis since the early 1990s, possibly related to the use of more effective antiretroviral drugs or to changes in the demographics of HIV infection. Nevertheless, CMV retinitis is far more common in patients with AIDS than in other immunocompromised patients infected with CMV, such as organ or bone marrow transplant recipients. The reasons for the higher prevalence are not known. Possibilities include greater immunosuppression in patients with AIDS, specific immune defects that facilitate CMV infection, more prolonged CMV viremia, or coinfection of retinal cells with HIV. As mentioned earlier, retinal microvasculopathy may also increase the likelihood of CMV infection.

The risk of CMV retinitis is inversely related to CD4+ T-lymphocyte count, with most cases occurring only after the count has fallen below $50/mm^3$ (25). Although CMV retinitis is an index disease for AIDS, only about 2% of patients with AIDS have CMV retinitis as the first and only manifestation of the syndrome (26). In the 1980s, the risk of developing CMV retinitis as the first manifestation of AIDS was reported to be less than 0.5% during the first 7 years after infection with HIV (26). The risk increases, however, to approximately 25% within 4 years after the CD4+ T-lymphocyte count drops below $100/mm^3$ (27). Little is known of other factors that could increase one's risk of retinal infection. Men acquiring HIV infection through sex with other men may have a greater risk of CMV retinitis than men or women acquiring HIV infection through injection drug use (15). Median survival after the diagnosis of CMV retinitis is currently between 7 and 13 months (28, 29), although the use of newer antiretroviral therapy and better treatment of other opportunistic infections possibly will increase survival significantly. Many clinicians have now seen patients who survived for 3 to 4 years after the diagnosis of CMV retinitis.

The diagnosis of CMV retinitis is based on clinical findings. Because of the high prevalence of anti-CMV antibodies in the general population, serologic tests are of little value in diagnosis, as are blood cultures or shedding of virus in urine or other body fluids.

The appearance of CMV retinitis lesions has a spectrum. Variable degrees of retinal whitening or opacification and variable degrees of retinal hemorrhage are noted (Fig. 29.2). One may or may not see sheathing of the retinal vessels. All lesions have an irregular, dry-appearing, granular border, which is the most clinically diagnostic feature of CMV retinitis (Fig. 29.3). Evidence that the rate of lesion enlargement in untreated patients varies with its appearance and location has been limited (30).

Other clinical features that suggest a diagnosis of CMV retinitis include slow progression of all lesions and minimal vitreous humor and anterior chamber inflammatory reactions. The immunodeficiency caused by HIV infection is sometimes cited as the reason that patients do not mount an inflammatory response to CMV retinitis. This concept is far too simplistic; patients with syphilitic or toxoplasmic ocular disease can mount a profound inflammatory response, as described later. Nevertheless, with the introduction of combination antiretroviral therapies, clinicians began to see patients with CMV retinitis who had more profound vitreous inflammatory reactions and an increased rate of complications, such as macular edema and epiretinal membrane formation; these changes presumably result from improved immune function and heightened reactions against CMV in the eye.

The location of lesions has important implications for vision. Those in the macula (roughly that area within the major temporal vascular arcades) and around the optic disc are considered to be an immediate threat to vision, and they are considered to be in "zone 1" of the retina (31). Those lesions outside the major vascular arcades (zones 2 and 3, sometimes referred to as the "peripheral retina") are not immediately threatening to central vision. Nevertheless,

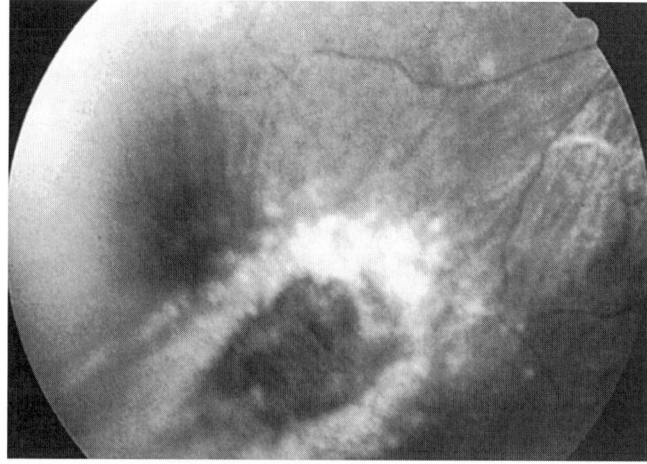

Figure 29.3. A focus of cytomegalovirus retinopathy in the peripheral retina. It has the typical granular border, but less retinal opacification than that seen in Figure 29.1 and no hemorrhage.

electrophysiologic and psychophysical testing suggests that a diffuse dysfunction of the retina exists in patients with CMV retinitis, even when only localized, peripheral lesions are noted clinically (32).

An understanding of the natural history of CMV retinitis is important for making decisions about treatment. Usually, patients have only one or two foci of infection at presentation, and new lesions form infrequently, even without treatment. These isolated lesions expand slowly. Lesions tend to spread more rapidly in an anterior direction (toward the ora serrata) than in a posterior direction (toward the optic disc and macula); untreated lesions expand toward the fovea (center of the macula) at a median rate of only 24 μm per day (30). In addition, CMV retinitis has been considered to spare the fovea; with enlargement, the posterior border of lesions tends to spread circumferentially around the fovea, rather than straight toward it. An untreated lesion in the peripheral retina may therefore pose little threat to central vision for some time after diagnosis, a finding that has raised the possibility of deferring treatment for small lesions outside the major vascular arcades for 1 week to several weeks if necessary for medical reasons or the convenience of the patient. Although lesions continue to enlarge during a period of treatment deferral, they come under control once treatment is started. As yet, no evidence indicates that small amounts of lesion enlargement in the peripheral retina affects final visual outcome, and the risk of rhegmatogenous retinal detachments (33, 34) is probably not altered by short periods of treatment deferral. Although initiation of therapy should not be considered an emergency, most clinicians initiate treatment as soon as possible. Immediate treatment reduces the risk of new ocular lesions and second eye involvement, and it presumably treats clinically inapparent, nonocular sites of CMV infection that could eventually be life-threatening (35).

Currently, three drugs are available for treatment of CMV retinopathy: ganciclovir, foscarnet, and cidofovir (36–46). Patients are given an initial "induction" course of therapy (ganciclovir, 5 mg/kg every 12 hours for 14 days; foscarnet, 90 mg/kg every 12 hours for 14 days; cidofovir, 5 mg/kg once weekly for 2 weeks), designed to inactivate the virus and to prevent further enlargement of lesions. Induction therapy is followed by lifelong "maintenance" therapy (regimens approved by the United States Food and Drug Administration [FDA]: ganciclovir, 5 mg/kg intravenously once daily or 1 g orally three times a day; foscarnet, 90 to 120 mg/kg intravenously daily; cidofovir, 3 to 5 mg/kg intravenously once every 2 weeks) to prevent disease reactivation. Reactivation and progression of lesions eventually occur in almost all patients despite systemic maintenance therapy.

A change in retinal opacification is the most easily recognized effect of treatment, but it is not necessarily a reliable measure of disease control; lesions with little opacity can continue to enlarge. Increasing opacification of the lesion border is believed to be a predictor of eventual lesion enlargement, however (31).

With the availability of these drugs, patients with AIDS now rarely die without any vision as a result of CMV retinitis.

Nevertheless, the best management of CMV retinitis remains controversial. It is difficult to compare many studies in the literature and to determine the relative benefits of the various treatment regimens described. In the early years of the AIDS epidemic, no uniform techniques for the assessment of disease response existed. Many early studies reported an 80 to 100% response rate (primarily reduced retinal opacification) with ganciclovir induction therapy. With a detailed examination of fundus photographs, however, a complete halt to lesion enlargement can be seen to occur in only 50 to 60% of patients at the conclusion of induction therapy (31). In recent years, more objective methods have been developed for clinical studies (31, 47), and investigators are proceeding with carefully designed trials to address management issues.

The efficacy and toxicity of ganciclovir and foscarnet were compared in the Foscarnet–Ganciclovir CMV Retinitis Trial (FGCRT), conducted by the National Institutes of Health (NIH)–funded Studies of the Ocular Complications of AIDS (SOCA) Research Group in a large, prospective, multicenter clinical trial (29). No apparent difference was seen between the two drugs for major clinical end points such as final visual acuity and the time to first disease reactivation and progression (just under 60 days for both drugs). However, a statistically significant difference was noted between treatment groups for patient survival. Those who received foscarnet had a median survival of approximately 12.6 months, whereas those who received only ganciclovir had a median survival of approximately 8.5 months. The cause of the differential survival could not be determined. Possibly, survival was prolonged by foscarnet, because it has antiretroviral activity. The differential survival could also have been attributable, in part, to other factors that were not controlled in the trial. Although analysis did not identify the differential use of other antiretroviral agents as a factor in the survival, patients taking ganciclovir were less able to tolerate zidovudine (48). The development of protease inhibitors and the use of combination antiretroviral therapy for HIV infection probably reduce, or eliminate altogether, any treatment advantage associated with the anti-HIV effect of foscarnet in comparison with ganciclovir (49).

In comparison with ganciclovir, foscarnet therapy was associated with a greater incidence of side effects (primarily renal toxicity) that required discontinuation of drug administration (29). Survival among a subgroup of patients with preexisting renal impairment was actually longer with ganciclovir than with foscarnet in the aforementioned trial. The decision to begin treatment with ganciclovir or foscarnet therefore should be based on nonophthalmic factors.

In several case reports, zidovudine therapy alone appeared to cause inactivation of CMV retinitis (50, 51). The effect was presumably through enhancement of the patients' own immune defenses or by the drug's suppression of HIV, which is known to enhance CMV activity in vitro. Any effect of zidovudine treatment on CMV retinitis may not be apparent for several weeks, and it may be only temporary. In most patients, it does not prevent disease progression. After the introduction of protease inhibitors, it appeared that CMV retinitis lesions did not progress and eventually became inactive in some patients receiving these drugs but no anti-CMV therapy (52); again, this effect, presumably attributable to enhanced immune function, is probably not universal and requires additional study.

The most pressing problem in the management of CMV retinitis is the failure of long-term maintenance therapies. The cause of late disease reactivations is not entirely clear. Both ganciclovir- and foscarnet-resistant viruses have been isolated from patients undergoing drug therapy (53–55), a finding that has led some investigators to advocate switching from ganciclovir to foscarnet or vice versa when reactivation occurs. The correlation between in vitro sensitivity testing and clinical response to treatment does not appear to be close in all patients (53), however. In most cases, the first reactivation of CMV retinitis can again be brought under control by administering induction-level doses of the same drug that is being used for maintenance, a finding that suggests that the drug levels achieved in standard maintenance therapies are simply too low to prevent disease reactivation (56). An inverse relation between ganciclovir dose and CMV viremia in patients receiving maintenance therapy has been shown (57).

The doses of ganciclovir and foscarnet used for maintenance therapy have been limited by their toxicities. Patients tolerate prolonged ganciclovir therapy better with the concurrent use of the leukocyte growth factors sargramostim (granulocyte–monocyte colony-stimulating factor) and filgrastim (granulocyte colony-stimulating factor), which increase a patient's neutrophil count (58). The continued administration of induction-level ganciclovir with the concurrent use of leukocyte growth factors has been proposed as therapy for patients whose lesions reactivate on standard maintenance therapy regimens (59).

In vitro evidence indicates that ganciclovir and foscarnet act synergistically against CMV (60, 61). Both controlled and uncontrolled studies have shown that combination therapy is effective in patients with multiple disease reactivations (59, 62, 63). The Cytomegalovirus Retinitis Retreatment Trial (CRRT) (59) found that the time to subsequent relapse in patients with active CMV retinitis was 4.3 months in patients treated with both foscarnet and ganciclovir, compared with 1.3 months and 2.0 months in patients treated with only foscarnet or ganciclovir, respectively. Side effects were similar in the three treatment groups, but combination therapy was associated with the greatest negative impact of treatment on quality-of-life measures, because of the longer infusion time required for combination therapy.

In contrast to results from the FGCRT, no significant difference in mortality was seen between patients treated with ganciclovir and those treated with foscarnet. Because of the study design, investigators could not determine whether the absence of differential mortality in the CRRT was due to 1) greater use of filgrastim than in the FGCRT, 2) more rapid discontinuation of foscarnet and thus less antiretroviral effect, or 3) the possibility that patients with reactivated CMV retinitis are sicker than those with newly diagnosed retinitis and therefore are less able to tolerate the side effects of foscarnet.

One reason for progression of CMV retinitis is the development of antiviral resistance (54). The prevalence of resistance increases with the duration of therapy (53). Molecular genetic studies indicate that most cases of ganciclovir resistance are due to mutations in the UL97 viral gene, which codes for the initial phosphorylation of the drug (64); without this step, ganciclovir is not taken up into infected cells, where it undergoes additional phosphorylation by cellular enzymes to the active drug, ganciclovir triphosphate. Foscarnet does not require phosphorylation and therefore is not affected by UL97 mutations. Mutations in DNA polymerase may cause resistance to either ganciclovir or foscarnet, however (55, 65). Several studies have suggested that changing therapy to foscarnet in patients with multiple relapses during treatment with ganciclovir or vice versa may improve control of CMV retinitis (66, 67). The failure of this approach in the CRRT may have been due to the low number of previous reactivations in the study (mean, 1.6); reactivations in these patients therefore probably resulted from factors other than antiviral resistance.

Several studies have reported that oral ganciclovir, at a dose of 1 g three times a day, is similar in efficacy to intravenous ganciclovir when used as maintenance therapy (45, 46), and oral ganciclovir was approved by the FDA for maintenance therapy of CMV retinitis in 1995. Most clinicians, however, believe that oral ganciclovir is less effective than intravenous therapy and therefore restrict its use to patients with peripheral CMV retinitis, in whom repeated episodes of disease progression are less likely to affect vision. The reduced efficacy can be attributed to its low bioavailability (about 9%). Patients should first receive induction intravenous ganciclovir at standard dosages for 3 weeks. Side effects of oral and intravenous ganciclovir are similar. The major advantage of oral ganciclovir is the avoidance of a permanent indwelling catheter. Disadvantages include the need to take a total of 12 capsules of the drug daily, a need that may increase noncompliance in patients already taking various pills for prevention and treatment of other HIV-related infections.

Cidofovir is a nucleotide analog with in vitro anti-CMV activity 10- to 100-fold greater than that of ganciclovir or foscarnet. Cidofovir contains a phosphonate group that enables it to bypass the initial virus-dependent phosphorylation required in the metabolism of ganciclovir. Cellular enzymes convert cidofovir to the active diphosphonate form, which, because of its long intracellular half-life, allows maintenance therapy to be given every 2 weeks (68). Permanent indwelling catheters are therefore not needed. Randomized clinical trials have shown that cidofovir is effective in controlling both untreated CMV retinitis and lesions that have reactivated after treatment with other drugs (43, 44). Dosages of both 3 mg/kg and 5 mg/kg intravenously every 2 weeks are effective as maintenance therapy, although the latter is more commonly used by clinicians. Common side effects include neutropenia, proteinuria, and elevation in serum creatinine. Probenecid must be given concurrently to reduce the risk of renal dysfunction, but probenecid's side effects (including fever, nausea, rash, and malaise) occur in over one-half of patients and may be severe enough to necessitate discontinuation of probenecid (and therefore cidofovir). Whether intravenous cidofovir reduces CMV viremia as effectively as ganciclovir or foscarnet is not clear.

Cidofovir may be particularly useful in patients with ganciclovir resistance, because CMV strains with UL97 mutations are usually sensitive to cidofovir (69). Cidofovir resistance as a result of a CMV DNA polymerase mutation has been reported but appears rare; affected patients are also resistant to ganciclovir. Cidofovir was not compared directly with ganciclovir or foscarnet in clinical trials before approval, and it is difficult to compare results with those in historical controls, but this agent appears to be at least as effective as other drugs.

Because of the toxicity and inconvenience of systemic antiviral therapy, local administration of drugs is a subject of continuing interest. Direct injection of ganciclovir (200 µg to 2 mg per injection) and foscarnet (1200 to 2400 µg per injection) into the vitreous humor has been used extensively as an alternative to systemic treatment (70–73). The median time to relapse of CMV retinitis in patients treated with ganciclovir injections (400 µg weekly) was 8 weeks in one series (70). A 2-mg dose of ganciclovir in 0.1 mL appears to be safe and effective, and it lasts for approximately 1 week (73). Higher doses have been associated with severe vision loss from retinal necrosis (74).

The administration of intravitrous injections on a weekly or twice-weekly basis indefinitely to large numbers of patients is impractical. Cidofovir has been investigated as an alternative drug for intravitreous injections. The median time to relapse after a single 20-µg intravitreous injection of cidofovir was 55 days in one study (75). Compared with ganciclovir and foscarnet, intravitreous cidofovir has been associated with more frequent and severe ocular side effects, including iritis and hypotony. The use of oral probenecid appears to reduce the risk of cidofovir-associated iritis significantly (76). Because of the potentially severe toxicities associated with intravitreous injections of cidofovir, clinicians are advised against injecting small volumes of intravenous formulations into the eye (as is done with ganciclovir and foscarnet), and much more work is required beyond the aforementioned pilot studies before cidofovir can be recommended for treatment. The potential complications of intravitreous injections include endophthalmitis, retinal detachment, increased intraocular pressure at the time of injection, and scarring of the injection site, but the rate of clinical problems appears to be low.

A sustained-release ganciclovir intraocular device (77–79), consisting of a 4.5-mg pellet of drug (Vitrasert) was approved by the FDA for treatment of CMV retinitis in 1996. The pellet is surrounded by a drug-permeable polyvinyl alcohol (PVA) coating and a drug-impermeable ethylvinyl acetate coating; by fixing the area of the PVA diffusion port, the constant release rate of the drug is adjusted to approximately 1 µg per hour (80). The device is surgically implanted into the vitreous cavity through a pars plana sclerotomy and is sutured to the sclera. The ganciclovir intraocular device is significantly more effective than intravenous ganciclovir for suppressing virus activity, with a median time to progression of 226 days (80). Multiple devices can be placed in the same eye, and planned exchange of the implant at regular intervals (every 6 to 8 months) has been viewed as a means of achieving sustained control of CMV retinitis without relapse (81). Placement of the device in eyes previously treated for CMV retinitis is less effective, presumably because of the development of some antiviral resistance associated with prior intravenous ganciclovir therapy (82). The implant is usually well tolerated within the eye (83). Disadvantages of the device include risks associated with the procedure: retinal detachment, infection, vitreous hemorrhage, hyphema, and endophthalmitis. In addition, patients often have a temporary decrease in vision postoperatively as a result of surgically induced astigmatism (80). A device designed to last 18 to 24 months is undergoing clinical trials.

On the basis of autopsy studies, CMV retinitis is believed to be a reliable indicator of tissue-invasive infections in other organs as well (8). In most cases, these nonocular sites of infection are not clinically apparent at the time CMV retinitis is diagnosed, but they may eventually be life-threatening. Patients who are treated with intravenous ganciclovir or foscarnet for CMV retinitis have been found to have significantly fewer nonocular CMV infections at autopsy (35). The inherent disadvantage of local therapy for CMV retinitis is the lack of protection against second-eye or extraocular disease. In one controlled study, 31% of patients treated with an intraocular device in one eye developed extraocular CMV disease, and 50% developed contralateral CMV retinitis (80). For this reason, most ophthalmologists also use concomitant oral ganciclovir in patients whose CMV retinitis is treated with local therapy.

Long-term efficacy of a treatment depends on factors other than time to progression as reported in clinical trials; for example, relative rates of retinal detachment influence the success of a treatment for preserving vision. The choice among available therapies should be individualized for patients on the basis of many factors including drug tolerance, estimated survival, lifestyle considerations, and ophthalmologic factors including location and extent of lesions, as well as previous response to antiviral drugs.

Two randomized clinical trials evaluating local versus systemic therapy in patients with CMV retinitis are under way. The first trial compares treatment with intravenous ganciclovir, the ganciclovir intraocular device plus oral ganciclovir, or the device plus placebo. The second trial compares treatment with intravenous cidofovir with the ganciclovir implant plus oral ganciclovir.

Many investigators believe that, clinically, repeated disease reactivations come at increasingly short intervals even with reinduction therapy, a finding suggesting that the disease becomes more difficult to control as the patient's immune defenses wane further. With increasing survival of patients, the clinician must consider the long-term goals of therapy. In most clinical trials, progression of disease is identified by linear advancement of lesion borders into uninfected retina that exceeds an arbitrary threshold, generally 750 µm (31). Although useful in clinical trials, this definition of progression is perhaps too rigid to be used as an indication of clinical treatment failure. For lesions outside the major vascular arcades, small amounts of disease progression over a prolonged period of treatment may be tolerable, especially late in the course of infection. A more realistic goal for long-term therapy in some patients may be simply to protect zone 1 of the retina.

Rhegmatogenous retinal detachment occurs in at least 20% of patients with CMV retinitis. It is generally a late complication (34). Reported risk factors for the development of rhegmatogenous retinal detachments include active CMV retinitis, duration of retinitis, anterior location, and involvement of more than 25% of the peripheral retina (84). Rhegmatogenous retinal detachments must be distinguished from exudative neurosensory detachments, which usually involve the peripapillary or macular region in patients with CMV retinitis in zone 1; such detachments are usually reversible with anti-CMV therapy (85). Rhegmatogenous detachments can be repaired, but final visual acuity is often poor even if the macula is attached and uninfected (86). Furthermore, the most successful technique (vitrectomy and silicone tamponade) results in a hyperopic shift and other optical problems that make visual rehabilitation difficult, even when visual potential is good. Cataracts are also common in eyes that contain silicone oil, and removal of these cataracts requires modification of intraocular lens power calculation for best visual results (87). Despite these limitations, aggressive therapy of retinal detachment is often indicated in patients because the operated eye may ultimately become the better-seeing eye.

Primary prophylaxis against CMV retinitis using oral ganciclovir has been investigated in two large studies. One study found that a dose of 1 g three times a day significantly reduced the risk of CMV retinitis (88), but another found no beneficial effect (89). Methodologic differences between the two studies do not explain the strikingly different findings. Based on the cost of ganciclovir prophylaxis (at least $15,000 per year), the potential toxicity, and the questionable benefit, most clinicians do not currently recommend ganciclovir for primary prophylaxis. Possibly, however, determination of high-risk factors that accurately predict development of CMV retinitis (such as CMV load in the blood) may eventually identify a subset of patients for whom "targeted prophylaxis" is cost-effective.

The major disorders in the differential diagnosis of CMV retinitis include toxoplasmic retinochoroiditis, varicella-zoster virus and herpes simplex virus retinopathies, syphilitic retinitis, and intraocular lymphoma. The distinguishing features of each are discussed later in this section. These disorders can occur concurrently with CMV retinitis, (90–94). In any patient with presumed CMV retinopathy with atypical features or with poor response to therapy, other diagnoses should be considered.

VARICELLA-ZOSTER

Varicella-zoster virus can cause necrotizing retinitis. Although this disorder is far less common than CMV retinitis, it is probably the second most common infection of the retina in HIV-infected patients in the United States. Most patients have a history of dermatomal herpes zoster, but the retinitis may develop concurrently with, or even may precede, cutaneous herpes zoster in any dermatomal distribution. As with CMV retinitis, this infection is rarely the initial manifestation of HIV infection. Affected patients had a mean CD4+ T-lymphocyte count of 21/µL (range, 0 to 130/µL) in one study (95).

Varicella-zoster virus retinitis in HIV-infected patients presents as a distinctive entity referred to by many investigators as the "progressive outer retinal necrosis syndrome." It is characterized clinically by multifocal deep retinal opaque lesions (believed to be retinal edema) throughout the peripheral retina that quickly coalesce to involve the entire retina (95–97) (Fig. 29.4). Perifoveal lesions are also common at presentation. The retina can become completely necrotic over a period of a few days to several weeks. Histopathologic examination reveals full-thickness retinal infection (94), and infection of choroidal cells has been reported (98). Little or no vitreous humor or anterior chamber inflammatory reaction is noted. Vasculitis is not a feature of the syndrome, but patients are left with severe vascular attenuation.

Optic neuropathy may precede the retinopathy (94) and is usually accompanied by headache and eye pain. Optic atrophy may result from infection and necrosis of the nerve. Most patients develop retinal detachments early in the course of the infection. Prophylactic laser retinopexy is usually not effective for reducing the risk of detachment.

The extensive distribution of early infection (including the optic nerve), the rapidity of its progression, and the high rate of retinal detachment make varicella-zoster virus retinitis by

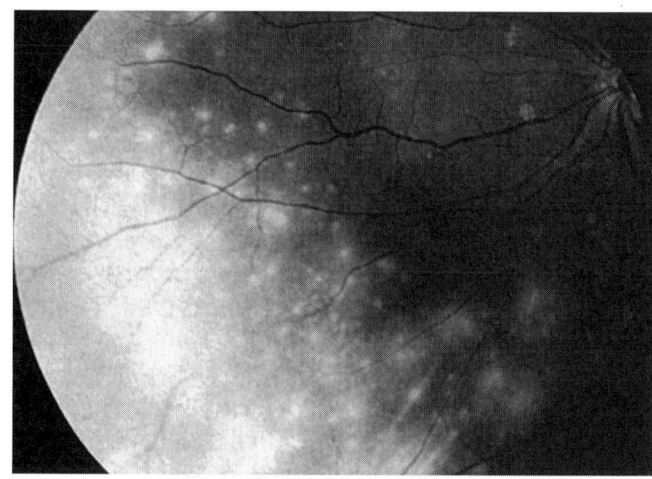

Figure 29.4. Varicella-zoster virus retinopathy. Homogeneous opacification of the largest region is present, as well as multiple small lesions throughout the peripheral retina.

far the most devastating retinal infection associated with HIV disease. Many patients with this infection have no light perception in either eye by the time they die (95).

The results of treatment for varicella-zoster virus retinitis have generally been disappointing. Even with high-dose intravenous acyclovir, disease may progress rapidly (96). The poor response to therapy is presumably due to the severe and widespread disease already present at the time treatment is initiated. More recently, patients with this infection have been treated with combinations of intravenous acyclovir and foscarnet or ganciclovir and foscarnet (99). Experience with these therapies is too limited, however, for the best management of this infection to have been determined. Apparently, even if lesions become inactive with initial therapy, reactivation and progression of disease are common soon after antiviral therapy is stopped (94), unlike with cutaneous herpes zoster lesions. In this respect, varicella-zoster virus retinitis is like CMV retinitis. Maintenance therapy using intravenous antiviral agents is therefore now used in patients who have retained some useful vision.

HERPES SIMPLEX

Herpes simplex virus infections of the retina in HIV-infected patients have been confirmed histologically (100–102). One report noted that HSV-1 infection involved primarily the retinal arterioles, whereas HSV-2 retinitis involved primarily the retinal venules (102). Cases of herpes simplex virus retinitis in patients with AIDS are so rare, however, that the course, prognosis, and response to therapy have not been established.

TOXOPLASMOSIS

Toxoplasma gondii infection of the retina is probably the third most common infection of the retina in patients with AIDS. Its prevalence is not known, but it is seen only occasionally even by clinicians who care for large numbers of patients with AIDS and retinal disease. It is therefore much less common than intracranial toxoplasmosis. When this disorder does occur, however, accurate diagnosis is critical; the infection poses a serious threat to vision, yet it responds well to appropriate treatments in most cases.

In HIV-infected patients, toxoplasmic retinochoroiditis can have various clinical manifestations, including single lesions, multifocal lesions in one or both eyes, and broad areas of retinal necrosis that can be confused with CMV retinitis (91, 93, 103, 104). Although most reported cases have been unilateral (91, 104), bilateral cases are not uncommon (90).

The high prevalence of exposure to *Toxoplasma gondii* in the general population makes the presence of anti-*T. gondii* antibodies of little value in making a diagnosis of ocular infection. Conversely, serologic tests may be negative in biopsy-confirmed toxoplasmic retinitis (105). However, several clinical features seem to be reliable signs of toxoplasmic retinochoroiditis. In cases with full-thickness necrosis, the retina appears to have a thick, wet, and "indurated" appearance with sharply demarcated borders (Fig. 29.5). Usually,

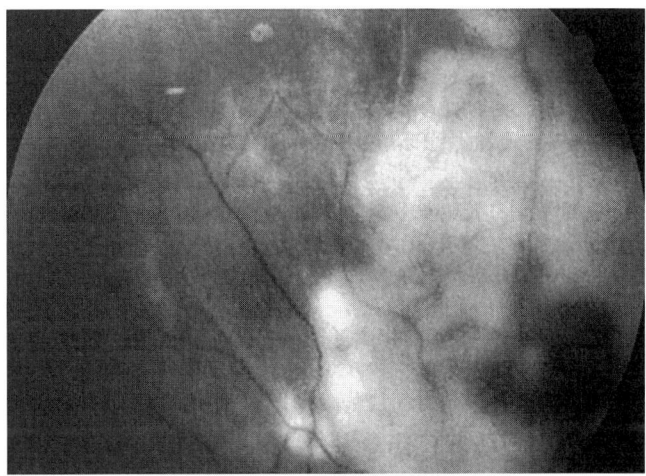

Figure 29.5. **Toxoplasmic retinochoroiditis.** The lesion has a thicker and more densely opaque appearance, and its border is more distinct and less granular than in cytomegalovirus retinopathy. The view is hazy because of vitreous inflammation.

one sees little or no hemorrhage, and prominent vitreous inflammation is often present. Inflammatory vascular sheathing may be noted.

In most cases, a preexisting retinochoroidal scar is not present, a finding that indicates that the majority of AIDS-related cases are not due to reactivation of encysted organisms that persist from a previous infection, as in otherwise healthy individuals. In the general population, ocular toxoplasmosis is, in most cases, believed to be a reactivation of congenital disease. Ocular toxoplasmosis associated with HIV infection can therefore be a great diagnostic challenge to ophthalmologists who are accustomed to its "classic" appearance in immunocompetent hosts: a single, discrete focus of intense retinal inflammation adjacent to a chorioretinal scar. A DNA polymerase chain reaction test that amplifies the B1 gene fragment of the organism has been reported, but its clinical utility for differentiating toxoplasmic retinochoroiditis from other retinal lesions has not been confirmed (105).

A prominent inflammatory reaction in the vitreous humor and anterior chamber has been described in several reports of HIV-associated ocular toxoplasmosis, although other investigators report little associated vitritis or iridocyclitis (90). The difference may be one of interpretation. Although the degree of secondary inflammation may vary and is generally less than that seen in immunocompetent hosts, the inflammatory reactions exceed those that would result from CMV retinitis. Anterior segment inflammation may result in a red, painful eye or the presence of posterior synechiae (adhesions between the iris and lens, causing an irregular pupil), neither of which occurs with CMV retinitis. Toxoplasmic retinopathy may progress to panophthalmitis and orbital cellulitis (106). Miliary toxoplasmic retinitis (105), indicating disseminated disease, may mimic tuberculous or fungal infection.

Patients with suspected ocular toxoplasmosis should be evaluated for systemic toxoplasmosis as well. Investigators have reported that 29 to 50% of patients with ocular toxoplasmosis have central nervous system (CNS) involvement, and ocular disease may be recognized before any neurologic manifestations of intracranial infection (90, 91, 107).

Lesions continue to enlarge without treatment; spontaneous resolution of toxoplasmic retinochoroiditis in HIV-infected patients has not been reported. Progression is generally slow.

All cases of ocular toxoplasmosis in HIV-infected patients should be treated. Various medications have been used, but most investigators believe that pyrimethamine in combination with at least one other antiparasitic agent is the most effective of the currently available treatment for ocular disease (107, 108). Atovaquone has also been used successfully to treat ocular toxoplasmosis in a patient with AIDS (109). Response to antimicrobial therapy can be remarkably fast (90, 91). Patients with red, painful eyes and decreased vision from vitreous inflammatory reations may notice an improvement in just a few days. Lesions generally heal completely within 4 to 6 weeks. Corticosteroids are generally not used in combination with antimicrobial agents for several reasons. Inflammation does not appear to play an important role in tissue destruction, corticosteroids may further impair host defenses, and corticosteroids are generally not necessary for control of vitreous humor and anterior chamber inflammatory reactions.

Toxoplasmic retinochoroiditis will reactivate if treatment is discontinued. Various maintenance therapies have been used successfully, including continued full-dose administration of multiple drugs or single-drug, intermittent therapy. Some investigators continue to administer pyrimethamine because it is considered the most effective treatment, although others prefer not to use it because of its potential for bone marrow suppression and interference with zidovudine therapy (91, 107, 108). Apparently, disease reactivation can be prevented with relatively low-dose therapy that would not be adequate for initial control of lesions. Single-drug therapy with clindamycin or even tetracycline has been reported anecdotally to be successful, but no large series has been studied to confirm the benefits of one drug versus another.

SYPHILIS

Syphilitic retinal disease can take several forms in HIV-infected patients. These patients may have patchy infiltrates, with or without retinal necrosis, that can mimic the more indolent-appearing forms of CMV retinitis. A characteristic subretinal lesion has also been described in other patients with HIV infection and syphilis (110). It is typically a large, nonelevated, subretinal, plaquelike mass found in the macular and juxtapapillary area. The borders of the lesion are distinctly yellow, although the central area may be more faded. Retinal disease may be unilateral or bilateral. Vascular sheathing may be present.

Syphilitic retinal disease is usually accompanied by marked inflammatory reactions in the vitreous humor and anterior chamber (110–112). Posterior synechiae are common. Keratic precipitates may be fine white or granulomatous (large, irregular, and "greasy") in appearance. The associated anterior uveitis is usually bilateral (113).

Investigators generally believe that ocular disease is more common in HIV-infected patients with syphilis than in patients with syphilis who do not have HIV infection, although one study did not find such a difference (113). Other reported ocular manifestations of syphilis in HIV-infected patients have included granulomatous iridocyclitis, vitreous inflammatory reactions, and optic neuritis. In a series of 9 HIV-infected patients with syphilitic eye disease, 4 (5 of 15 eyes) had retinitis or neuroretinitis (111).

Although ocular disease can occur in patients with secondary or early latent syphilis, most reported patients with HIV infection and syphilitic eye disease have had neurosyphilis (111, 113). All patients with suspected ocular syphilis should be evaluated for CNS involvement and should be treated with antibiotic therapy appropriate for neurosyphilis. Both syphilitic retinitis and subretinal placoid lesions regress with therapy. Patients may be left with coarse pigmentary stippling of the fundi, but vision is generally good (110–112).

OTHER INFECTIONS

Metastatic bacterial infections of the retina and choroid have been reported rarely. Metastatic bacterial infections appear to be more common in children than in adults (114). *Nocardia* species can cause focal retinal infiltrates (24). Two patients with focal retinal lesions were found at biopsy to have probable bacterial retinitis, although the bacteria could not be identified (114). *Rhodococcus equi (Corynebacterium equi)* was suspected on the basis of histopathologic findings. Neither patient had signs to suggest a systemic bacterial infection at presentation. Retinal lesions in both patients resolved with systemic doxycycline therapy administered over several months. The lesions were nonspecific in appearance and could have been mistaken for a variety of infections. Infections of indwelling catheters used for long-term intravenous therapy of CMV retinitis occur at a rate of 1 to 1.5 per patient per year, and they may rarely cause disseminated bacterial endophthalmitis (115).

Several fungi can infect the retina or choroid in patients with AIDS. Although none is a common cause of disease, visual outcomes are usually poor, and disease-related mortality is high. Recognition of a metastatic infection is critical because the ocular manifestations may be the first sign of disseminated disease. Most fungal infections of the eye have been published as isolated case reports. *Cryptococcus neoformans* is the fungus most commonly reported as a cause of intraocular infection in patients with AIDS (8, 100, 116–121). Affected patients have higher mean CD4+ T-lymphocyte counts than patients with CMV retinitis (120). Intraocular organisms have been found as incidental findings at autopsy (8), where they are seen within retinal and choroidal vessels without associated inflammation. Infection may result in multifocal, discrete, yellow-white choroidal lesions up to a disc diameter in size with few clinical signs of inflammation (119, 121). Lesions predominantly involving the retina have also been reported (100, 116). Similar choroidal and retinal lesions have been reported rarely as a result of disseminated *Histoplasma capsulatum* infection (122, 123). In the largest series reported to date (120), 26 of 80 patients (32.5%) had papilledema, although optic atrophy was rare. Unilateral or bilateral sixth cranial nerve palsies occurred in 9% of patients.

Cryptococcal lesions have been reported to fade with many weeks of intravenous amphotericin B and oral 5-flucytosine therapy. Some investigators have reported an increased risk of vision loss in patients treated with amphotericin-B, possibly because of optic nerve toxicity of the drug (120).

Because mucocutaneous candidal infections are common in HIV-infected patients, some clinicians incorrectly assume that patients are at high risk for candidal chorioretinitis. In fact, candidemia is uncommon among HIV-infected patients, and intraocular candidal infections are rare. They are probably most common among patients having the same risk factors associated with intraocular candidal infections in immunocompetent patients: intravenous drug use, indwelling catheters, and broad-spectrum antibiotic use (8, 118). Similar risk factors probably account for most other cases of fungal and bacterial chorioretinitis or endophthalmitis.

A case of endophthalmitis caused by *Sporothrix schenckii* has been reported, characterized by a prominent inflammatory reaction without retinal necrosis (124). Patients are also presumably at risk for *S. schenckii* chorioretinitis, inasmuch as it has been reported in other groups. *Fusarium* infections may cause more vascular invasion than *Cryptococcus neoformans* and may result in more fulminant intraocular inflammation (125). Fungal (125) and bacterial endophthalmitides (115, 126) are rare, and whether clinical appearances described in the literature are typical for the reported infection is unknown. These organisms also may coexist with more common pathogens such as CMV retinitis (115, 127).

Although tuberculosis occurs frequently in patients with AIDS, ocular involvement is uncommon, as is true for patients without AIDS who develop pulmonary tuberculosis. Patients with miliary disease are those at highest risk for ocular disease. Multiple yellow-white choroidal infiltrates are the most common finding (128–131). Severe anterior uveitis and vitreous inflammatory reaction may also be present, as may concurrent tuberculous meningitis. The ocular lesions usually heal with combination antituberculosis therapy, leaving behind atrophic chorioretinal scars. Disseminated atypical mycobacterial infections, usually with *Mycobacterium avium* complex, may also result in choroidal granulomas (8, 127).

Choroidal pneumocystosis, which was first described clinically in 1989, is one of the few previously unknown ophthalmic diseases that has emerged as a result of the AIDS epidemic. The typical clinical appearance of lesions is a discrete, yellow-white subretinal plaque 300 to 3000 μm in diameter (132–134). As many as several dozen lesions may be seen in the posterior poles of both eyes, but unilateral and unifocal disease has occurred (135). Lesions are not seen anterior to the equator, and organisms are not found in the retina. Histologically, lesions are collections of *Pneumocystis carinii* organisms surrounded by a frothy material, with few or no inflammatory cells (132, 134). Without treatment, choroidal lesions enlarge slowly, and they can they assume irregular and multilobular shapes (134, 136). Large, geographic yellow-white areas can result from lesion coalescence as disease progresses. A vitreous inflammatory reaction does not occur.

Patients with choroidal pneumocystosis are frequently asymptomatic. Some may complain of intermittent blurring of vision, and Snellen acuity may be reduced a few lines; but even with lesions directly below the fovea, objective visual acuity can be as good as 20/25 (133).

The clinical importance of choroidal pneumocystosis is primarily related to the possibility of its being an early sign of disseminated, life-threatening *Pneumocystis carinii* infection. An association between choroidal pneumocystosis and inhaled pentamidine prophylaxis against pulmonary disease has been emphasized in the literature (136, 137). No evidence, however, shows that inhaled pentamidine directly increases one's risk of choroidal pneumocystosis, as implied by some authors. It may simply be that the use of inhaled pentamidine and other prophylactic agents has increased survival sufficiently to allow the emergence of late, uncommon opportunistic infections. Although choroidal pneumocystosis was not recognized before the widespread use of inhaled pentamidine, cases of the disease in patients without a history of prophylactic treatment have been reported (134, 136). However, inhaled pentamidine offers no protection against extrapulmonary *P. carinii* infections. The incidence of choroidal pneumocystosis fell with the introduction of systemic prophylaxis against *P. carinii* pneumonia.

Choroidal lesions respond to either intravenous pentamidine or trimethoprim–sulfamethoxasole (137). Oral trimethoprim and dapsone have also been used successfully (133). Lesions may resolve within 3 weeks of initiating treatment (137), but regression usually takes many weeks or months (133). Some lesions fade, but do not resolve completely. Without continuous or frequent intermittent suppressive therapy, lesions recur. Average survival after diagnosis of choroidal pneumocystosis was reported to be 4 months in a 1991 report (136).

Patients with choroidal pneumocystosis may have concurrent CMV retinitis. A known association exists between *Pneumocystis carinii* and CMV infections in immunosuppressed patients that results in a higher prevalence of concurrent infection of the same organ than would be expected from chance alone (134). Because these organisms infect different layers of the eye, their association in AIDS patients may simply be coincidental, as a result of severe immunosuppression, rather than reflecting any sort of synergism. Among choroidal infections, pneumocystosis has received the most attention, but clinicians should remember that various choroidal infections, including cryptococcosis and mycobacterial granulomas, can present in a similar manner.

Infections of the Ocular Surface and Adnexa

Severe infections of the ocular surface also occur in HIV-infected patients, although they are less prevalent than CMV retinitis (138, 139). The most common problem is herpes zoster ophthalmicus, characterized by cutaneous lesions in the distribution of the first division of the trigeminal nerve. If the nasociliary branch is involved, patients can develop keratitis and anterior uveitis. Herpes zoster ophthalmicus can be seen early in the course of HIV disease, and it is believed to be a harbinger of further deterioration in the patient's immune status.

Oral acyclovir (800 mg five times a day), used at the onset of skin lesions, has been shown to reduce the severity and incidence of ocular involvement in immunocompetent hosts. Acyclovir presumably has a similarly beneficial effect in patients with HIV infection, although this issue has not been studied specifically. Because of the risk of disseminated varicella-zoster virus infection, many clinicians now treat patients having newly diagnosed herpes zoster ophthalmicus with intravenous acyclovir.

In most cases, herpes zoster keratitis is an immunologic reaction, and virus cannot be recovered from the cornea. Herpes zoster keratitis and anterior uveitis may persist long after cutaneous lesions have resolved. The use of topical corticosteroids may be necessary to control the inflammation associated with these disorders.

Patients with HIV disease can also develop a chronic, productive varicella-zoster virus infection of the corneal epithelium that resembles herpes simplex virus epithelial keratitis (140). This infection was not previously reported in immunocompetent patients. This keratitis occasionally follows herpes zoster ophthalmicus, with isolation of varicella-zoster virus from corneal lesions many weeks after the resolution of cutaneous vesicles. Other patients have no history of cutaneous herpes zoster. Varicella-zoster virus epithelial keratitis in HIV-infected patients responds to topical acyclovir ointment (not commercially available in the United States), but it may not respond to trifluridine solution (Viroptic), the most commonly used topical antiviral agent.

Herpes simplex virus epithelial keratitis has been reported in patients with HIV infection, although it does not appear to be more prevalent among patients with AIDS than in the general population (141). Young and associates reported that herpes simplex virus keratitis tends to be more prolonged and severe in HIV-infected patients (142), with lesions more likely to be adjacent to the corneal limbus. A more recent study found no differences in the clinical presentation and outcome between the two groups, except for a higher recurrence rate in HIV-infected patients (141). Cases appear to respond to conventional antiviral therapies such as topical trifluridine. CMV may cause an epithelial keratitis and stromal keratouveitis that mimics varicella-zoster virus–associated keratitis (143).

Fungal and bacterial corneal ulcers have been reported in patients with AIDS, although they are uncommon (138). Factors predisposing to infectious keratitis in otherwise healthy individuals, such as trauma, epithelial defects, neurotrophic keratitis, or contact lens use, may be absent, and atypical pathogens such as *Candida albicans* and *Bacillus* spp. appear to be more common than in ulcers seen in the general population (144, 145). The natural defenses of normal eyelid function, adequate tear production, and an intact corneal epithelium are critical for reducing the risk of corneal infections in HIV-infected individuals. Patients who wear contact lenses should be instructed carefully in the techniques of meticulous contact lens care. Eyelid abnormalities that result in exposure or trichiasis (rubbing of the eyelashed against the cornea) should be corrected immediately. Other factors such as dry eyes and keratoconjunctivitis sicca, which appear to be more common in HIV-infected individuals (146), may contribute to the risk of infection. The "crack eye syndrome" has been used to describe a constellation of findings, including corneal epithelial defects, punctate keratopathy, and sterile or infectious keratitis, that result from direct toxicity of crack cocaine smoke or the anesthetic effects of the drug (147).

Because of diminished host immune defenses, bacterial and fungal corneal ulcers may be particularly severe. Some patients in whom the spread of infection to other ocular tissues could not be prevented have lost their eyes. Treatment requires the intensive use of appropriate topical antimicrobials, and some ophthalmologists administer intravenous antibiotics as well, a procedure that is usually not done when treating corneal ulcers in otherwise healthy patients. Visual outcome may be compromised by poor compliance with therapeutic regimens and difficulty with consistent medical follow-up, as can occur in some HIV-infected populations or with extremely ill patients.

Corneal microsporidiosis is a rare disorder. *Encephalitozoon* (148–150) and *Septata* (151) are the only genera associated with corneal disease in HIV-infected patients. The parasite causes a diffuse corneal epitheliopathy without associated stromal involvement. Patients present with chronically red and irritated eyes, and the irregular epithelial surface results in a marked drop in vision. Because inflammation is minimal, the cornea appears clear on gross examination.

The source of microsporidial ocular infection is unknown. The superficial location of the organisms in the cornea suggests that direct inoculation may be the route of infection. Topical fumagillin is effective, but it must be continued indefinitely to prevent recurrence (150).

Molluscum contagiosum lesions of the eyelids are seen frequently in HIV-infected patients (152). In otherwise healthy individuals, molluscum contagiosum lesions of the eyelid margin may stimulate follicular conjunctivitis and corneal infiltrates. In HIV-infected patients, keratoconjunctivitis is usually less severe, presumably because of immunodeficiency. Lesions may become large or confluent and may irritate the eye mechanically. Molluscum contagiosum lesions are difficult to eliminate from the eyelid margins. Extremely large lesions can be excised surgically. Cryotherapy is successful in reducing the size of lesions, and it is well tolerated (153). Recurrences are common with both treatment modalities. Molluscum lesions involving the bulbar conjunctiva are rare (154).

Lymphogranuloma venereum (LGV) with ocular involvement has been reported in a patient with AIDS (155). LGV is a known, although rare, cause of Parinaud's oculoglandular syndrome, keratoconjunctivitis, episcleritis, uveitis, papilledema, and retinal hemorrhages. In the reported case, corneal perforation occurred, is a previously unreported sequela of LGV. As with some other HIV-related ocular infections, the prevalence of LGV is not necessarily increased, but the infection can apparently be much more severe when it does occur as a coincident disorder.

NEOPLASMS

Kaposi's sarcoma is the most common tumor to involve the eye in HIV-infected patients. Ocular involvement has been reported to occur in 20% of patients with AIDS-related Kaposi's sarcoma, and, in fact, Kaposi's sarcoma may make its first appearance on or around the eye (156, 157). The eyelids are the most common sites of ophthalmic involvement. Conjunctival tumors are also seen frequently, whereas orbital involvement is rare.

Conjunctival tumors can occur anywhere on the surface of the eye or the inner surface of the eyelids, but they are most common in the inferior fornix (Fig. 29.6). Bilateral disease is frequent. Lesions can be missed if the lower eyelids are not pulled down on examination. They are bright to deep red or violaceous, and initially they may be mistaken for chronic subconjunctival hemorrhages. Conjunctival lesions spread slowly throughout the fornix, but they do not invade the eye, nor do they involve the cornea. Intraocular Kaposi's sarcoma has not been reported. Kaposi's sarcoma therefore presents little or no threat to a patient's vision.

Eyelid and conjunctival tumors are usually asymptomatic, although bulky lesions may cause mild irritation. Conjunctival lesions are primarily a cosmetic problem; eyelid margin tumors are the greatest concern. As they enlarge, eyelid margin tumors can result in entropion formation (inturning of the eyelid) with trichiasis. By abrading the corneal epithelium, trichiasis places the patient at increased risk of a secondary infectious corneal ulcer.

Ophthalmic Kaposi's sarcoma lesions may respond well to systemic chemotherapy. In addition, interferon-α-2a, which inhibits proliferating vascular endothelial cells, has been used both systemically and locally (158). The lesions can also be treated locally with radiation therapy (156, 159), cryotherapy (160), or surgical excision. The most extensive experience has been with radiation therapy. Administration of 2000 to 3000 cGy in 200- to 300-cGy fractions over a 3-week period by means of a 6-MeV linear accelerator (while shielding the eye) or a 100-kVp superficial radiation unit causes total or near total resolution of lesions with minimal side effects. Recurrences, however, are common. More recently, single applications of 800 cGy have been reported to be equally effective (159). Cryotherapy, a circulating liquid nitrogen probe at 300°C with a freeze-thaw-freeze-thaw technique, has been used successfully as alternative local therapy (160). No evidence indicates whether radiation therapy or cryotherapy is safer or more effective for local therapy of Kaposi's sarcoma.

Shuler and associates outlined the indications for treatment of ophthalmic Kaposi's sarcoma lesions and for the use of local therapy (156). Specific treatment of conjunctival lesions is rarely necessary because of their slow growth and lack of invasiveness of these tumors. Occasionally, treatment of conjunctival tumors is indicated; for example, large bulky lesions may be cosmetically disturbing, they may interfere with eyelid function (rare), or they may produce discomfort because of mass effect (the tumors themselves are not painful). Eyelid margin lesions, on the other hand, should be followed closely and treated in many cases to prevent the development of entropion formation with trichiasis or ulceration of the eyelid margin. In recent years, the use of effective systemic chemotherapeutic regimens has meant that eyelid lesions rarely progress to the point of becoming a management problem. Local therapy for ophthalmic lesions is necessary only if systemic therapy is unsuccessful, if systemic therapy cannot be tolerated, if local therapy is needed to supplement systemic therapy when immediate response is needed to prevent complications, or if the patient has isolated ophthalmic lesions that make systemic treatment unnecessary.

Squamous cell carcinoma is the third most common malignancy, after lymphoma, associated with HIV infection, and it may affect the conjunctiva and eyelid (161–166). The frequency of dysplastic and neoplastic conjunctival lesions has increased notably since the onset of the AIDS epidemic (164, 165, 167). Squamous cell carcinoma is typically much faster growing and more invasive in patients with AIDS than in older immunocompetent patients, and it may involve the cornea and sclera (164, 166). Human papillomavirus (HPV) has been identified in some (161, 165), but not other (164), biopsy specimens; it therefore remains unproved whether a breakdown of tumor surveillance associated with HIV infection, allowing sustained HPV proliferation and transforma-

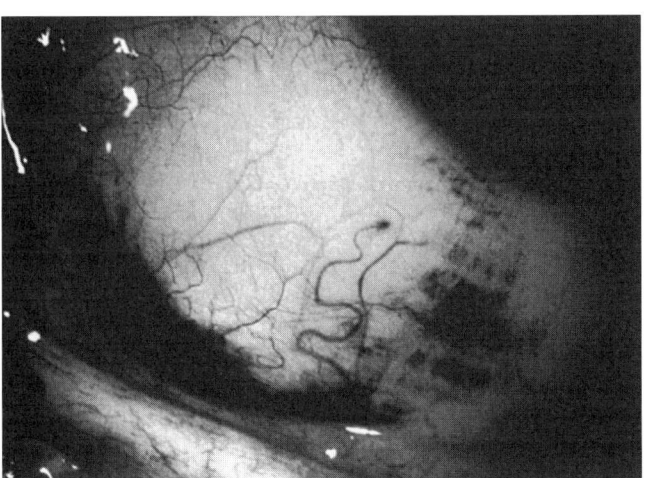

Figure 29.6. Conjunctival Kaposi's sarcoma in the inferior fornix.

tion of infected cells into malignant ones (168), accounts for the increased rate of tumors.

A growing problem in ophthalmology is the occurrence of intraocular and orbital lymphomas among patients with AIDS (92). Large cell (92) and small, noncleaved cell (169, 170) types predominate. Ocular involvement may result from extension of CNS disease (92) or hematogenous dissemination from peripheral locations (170). Intraocular manifestations can include a cellular reaction in the vitreous fluid or an ill-defined subretinal mass. If the retina is involved, the lymphoma can be mistaken for CMV retinitis or other necrotizing viral infections (92, 169, 171), although the progression of lymphoma is generally slower. Proptosis is usually the first manifestation of orbital involvement (172). Bilateral orbital and intraocular involvement has been reported (92, 170). Treatment consists of radiation therapy or systemic chemotherapy, but long-term experience in treating this problem is limited because of the high associated mortality rates.

NEURO-OPHTHALMIC DISORDERS

Patients with intracranial infections and neoplasms may develop various neuro-ophthalmic abnormalities including cranial nerve palsies, abnormal eye movements, visual field defects, papilledema, pupillary abnormalities, cortical blindness, and optic atrophy (173–176). The associated visual symptoms or ophthalmic signs may bring patients to the attention of an ophthalmologist before other neurologic problems develop. A mass lesion on one side of the brain may produce profound homonymous hemianopia on the opposite side, which may be misinterpreted by patients as a problem with the eye on that side only.

Optic neuropathy in patients with AIDS causes rapid vision loss and may be caused by various infectious diseases, including toxoplasmosis (91, 104), CMV optic neuritis or retinitis (177), syphilis (113), or herpes zoster (94). It may be the presenting sign of varicella-zoster virus infection and may precede necrotizing retinitis (94). Patients with CMV retinitis affecting the peripapillary retina are at increased risk for development of CMV encephalitis; in contrast, CNS symptoms are unlikely to be attributable to CMV if the retina is not involved (177). Treatment of herpetic optic neuropathy with corticosteroids in patients with AIDS is contraindicated because these agents may exacerbate viral retinitis (171).

Cryptococcal meningitis is the most common cause of papilledema in patients with AIDS. Patients with cryptococcosis occasionally also develop an unusual syndrome of sudden, severe, bilateral vision loss, with or without papilledema. Its pathogenesis is not fully understood. It occurs in the absence of intraocular *Cryptococcus neoformans* infection and is believed to be the result of a retrobulbar or intracranial process.

Sudden blindness has also been reported as a consequence of rhino-orbitocerebral mucormycosis and occlusive vasculitis of the optic chiasm in a patient with diabetes mellitus and AIDS (178).

Progressive multifocal leukoencephalopathy (PML) is a late complication of AIDS that can present with visual symptoms. Ocular manifestations include progressive retrochiasmal visual field defects, supranuclear and nuclear cranial nerve palsies, occipital blindness, and nystagmus ataxia (176).

Orbital infections caused by various bacterial, fungal, and parasitic infections are uncommon, but they can present with neuroophthalmic signs, as well as with proptosis, eyelid swelling and pain (179). They typically occur late in the course of AIDS and are frequently life-threatening. *Aspergillus fumigatus* appears to be the most common pathogen.

OTHER DISORDERS

In addition to the well-established ophthalmic manifestations of HIV infection discussed earlier are isolated case reports of other ophthalmic disorders in HIV-infected patients. Study of additional cases will be required to determine whether these disorders were simply coincident to the patients' HIV infections or whether they were causally related to their virus-induced immunosuppression. However, any ophthalmic disease, regardless of its underlying cause, clearly can have unusual features in an HIV-infected patient. Reported disorders include bilateral angle-closure glaucoma resulting from ciliochoroidal effusions of unknown cause (180, 181), eosinophilic granuloma involving the cavernous sinus and orbital apex (182), and uveitis associated with Reiter's syndrome.

Drug toxicity may affect the eye. Uveitis has been attributed to rifabutin (183, 184), intravenous infusions and intravitreous injections of cidofovir, and intravitreous injections of fomivirsen. The uveitis associated with rifabutin may be sufficiently severe to cause hypopyon and condensates of inflammatory material in the anterior vitreous body, mimicking infectious endophthalmitis, but it resolves quickly with cessation of the drug and with the use of topical corticosteroids. The cause is not known, although most affected patients are also taking clarithromycin and fluconazole, which increase blood level of the drug. Because of the potential for uveitis in patients treated with rifabutin and a macrolide antibiotic, the drug dose of rifabutin should not exceed 300 mg per day. Atrophy of the peripheral retinal pigment epithelium was noted in 3 of 43 children treated with didanosine, but this condition has not been reported in adults (185).

Corneal and conjunctival diseases of uncertain cause have been reported in several patients without evidence of infection (186). Peripheral corneal ulceration resulting from limbal immune complex deposition, complement activation, and neutrophil invasion has been noted in various immunologic disorders, including rheumatoid arthritis and Mooren's ulcer. The high levels of circulating immune complexes in many patients with AIDS could predispose them to peripheral corneal problems, but additional cases have not been reported. Milder forms of conjunctivitis and keratitis of unknown cause have also been reported (5), and the rate of mild-to-moderate aqueous tear deficiency and staphylococcal blepharitis appears to be high among HIV-infected individuals.

ISSUES REGARDING HIV TRANSMISSION IN THE WORKPLACE

The presence of virus in corneal tissue, tears, and even contact lenses worn by indiviuals with HIV infection raises special concerns about disease transmission. To date, no reports of HIV transmission related to the practice of ophthalmology have been published. Because the actual risk is not fully known, however, universal precautions have been recommended during all examinations of the eye. Infectious disease guidelines also reduce the spread of secondary pathogens, such as herpes simplex virus, that may be present on the ocular surface of patients with AIDS. Handwashing is crucial, but gloves are unnecessary for most ophthalmic examinations. Some ophthalmologists prefer to wear disposable gloves during indirect ophthalmoscopy or other situations in which the eyelids are manipulated and tearing can be expected. Gloves are specifically recommended in such situations if the examiner has open lesions on the hands.

Special emphasis has been placed on the potential for disease transmission by contaminated tonometer tips. Studies have shown that Goldmann tonometer tips can be disinfected against HIV and herpes simplex virus simply by wiping with a 70% isopropyl alcohol swab followed by air drying (187). Only the tip need be treated, thus avoiding dissolution of the side markings. In such disinfection procedures, one must physically wipe any debris from the contaminated device.

The excimer laser, which is used for refractive surgical procedures, aerosolized infectious herpes simplex virus and adenovirus in an experimental model (188), a finding suggesting that transmission of HIV-infected cells in this manner is at least theoretically possible. Measures should be taken by the surgeon and other medical staff to reduce this risk, including the use of gloves, masks, and possibly vacuum evacuators.

Contact lenses are effectively disinfected against HIV with either hydrogen peroxide or thermal disinfection. One or the other of these techniques can be used on any available rigid or soft contact lens; recommendations can be obtained from the manufacturer. The efficacy of various commercially available chemical disinfection systems against HIV in the clinical setting has not been established.

Concern has also been raised about transmission of HIV through corneal transplantation. The transmission of other viruses, such as the agents responsible for rabies and hepatitis B, through corneal transplantation is well documented, but despite intensive study, no evidence suggests that HIV transmission occurs by this route. In 1987, Pepose and associates reported several cases in which corneal donors were found in retrospect to be infected with HIV (189). None of the recipients had developed antibodies to HIV at the time of the report. Many of them are still being followed-up, and none have seroconverted, with follow-up periods as long as 5 years (JS Pepose, unpublished data). Failure to become infected with HIV may reflect the low virus load presented by corneal transplantation, compared with that related to blood transfusion or sexual intercourse.

Although there appears to be little or no risk of HIV transmission by corneal transplantation, many potential donors, including coroners' cases, come from groups at high risk for HIV infection. The Eye Bank Association of America therefore routinely screens all potential donors for HIV antibodies. Because seroconversion may not occur immediately after HIV infection, individuals are not accepted as donors if they are known to have specific risk factors. The CDC has issued guidelines for prophylaxis against HIV infection after accidental needlestick injuries and other occupational exposures to the virus. After the introduction of protease inhibitors, these guidelines were reviewed with reference to occupational risks associated with eye care (190).

In conclusion, with continued spread of the AIDS epidemic and increasing survival of its victims, greater attention is being focused on the ophthalmic manifestations of HIV infection. Based on more than a decade of experience with these disorders, one can draw several important conclusions about their management that are of importance to the primary care provider.

Vision-threatening diseases are usually among the later manifestations of AIDS. Widespread screening and prophylaxis programs for all HIV-infected patients to identify CMV retinitis or other ophthalmic disorders are neither practical nor cost-effective. It is more appropriate for patients and their primary care providers to learn the signs and symptoms of intraocular disease, such as floaters, blind spots, and blurring of vision. Patients who develop these problems should seek help from an ophthalmologist immediately. Currently, prophylaxis against ophthalmic infections is not given in most cases. With regard to ocular surface infections, topical antiviral drugs are too toxic to corneal epithelium for prolonged prophylactic use, and prolonged use of topical antibiotics may select for resistant organisms. Until risk factors for CMV retinitis are better understood, and until more convenient and less toxic anti-CMV drugs become available, prophylaxis against this infection is not practical. However, research may identify risk factors, such as the high levels of CMV in the blood, that will allow prophylaxis in targeted populations.

Because of the blood-retina barrier and the lack of blood vessels in some ocular tissues, many drugs reach sites of infection with difficulty. That fact, in addition to the severe immunosuppression associated with the later stages of AIDS, means that immediate, aggressive, and prolonged therapy is usually required to control HIV-related opportunistic infections of the eye. Because intraocular infections are usually a manifestation of disseminated disease, systemic therapy is an important part of treatment. Early treatment of intraocular infections presumably controls nonocular sites of disease before they become clinical problems (35). For most intraocular infections, long-term low-dose antimicrobial therapy is necessary to prevent reactivation of disease.

Previously rare ocular infections and neoplasms have emerged as frequent manifestations of AIDS. Some, such as the progressive outer retinal necrosis syndrome, choroidal pneumocystosis, and corneal microsporidiosis, were not identified until several years after the start of the epidemic. Therefore, additional rare disorders probably will emerge as the epidemic grows. This review reflects experience through early 1998. As new drugs become available and additional information about these diseases emerges, concepts about their diagnosis and management will undoubtedly change. Of particular importance will be new information suggesting that combination antiretroviral therapies are altering the epidemiology, clinical characteristic course, and response to treatment of CMV retinitis.

References

1. Culbertson WW. Infections of the retina in AIDS. Int Ophthalmol Clin 1989;29:108–118.
2. Knox CM, Chandler D, Short GA, et al. PCR based assays for the diagnosis of viral retinitis: use in diagnostic dilemmas. Ophthalmology 1998;105:37–45.
3. Farrell PL, Heinemann MH, Roberts CW, et al. Response of human immunodeficiency virus-associated uveitis to zidovudine. Am J Ophthalmol 1988;106:7–10.
4. Skolnik PR, Pomerantz RJ, de la Monte SM, et al. Dual infection of retina with human immunodeficiency virus type 1 and cytomegalovirus. Am J Ophthalmol 1989;107:361–372.
5. Holland GN, Pepose JS, Pettit TH, et al. Acquired immune deficiency syndrome: ocular manifestations. Ophthalmology 1983;90:859–873.
6. Jabs DA, Green WR, Fox R, et al. Ocular manifestations of acquired immune deficiency syndrome. Ophthalmology 1989;96:1092–1099.
7. Glasgow BJ, Weisberger AK. A quantitative and cartographic study of retinal microvasculopathy in acquired immunodeficiency syndrome. Am J Ophthalmol 1994;118:46–56.
8. Pepose JS, Holland GN, Nestor MS, et al. Acquired immune deficiency syndrome: pathogenic mechanisms of ocular disease. Ophthalmology 1985;92:472–484.
9. Engstrom RE, Holland GN, Hardy WD, et al. Hemorheologic abnormalities in patients with human immunodeficiency virus infection and ophthalmic microvasculopathy. Am J Ophthalmol 1990;109:153–161.
10. Pomerantz RJ, Kuritzkes DR, de la Monte SM, et al. Infection of the retina by human immunodeficiency virus type I. N Engl J Med 1987;317:1643–1647.
11. Geier SA, Rolinski B, Sadri I, et al. Ocular microangioathy syndrome in patients with AIDS is associated with increased plasma levels of the vasoconstrictor endothelin-1 [German]. Klin Monatsbl Augenheilkd 1995;207:353–360.
12. Faber DW, Wiley CA, Lynn GB, et al. Role of HIV and CMV in the pathogenesis of retinitis and retinal vasculopathy in AIDS patients. Invest Ophthalmol Vis Sci 1992;33:2345–2353.
13. Thierfelder S, Linnert D, Grehn F. Increased prevalence of HIV-related retinal microangiopathy syndrome in patients with hepatitis C. Arch Ophthalmol 1996;114:899.
14. Freeman WR, Chen A, Henderly DE, et al. Prevalence and significance of acquired immunodeficiency syndrome-related retinal microvasculopathy. Am J Ophthalmol 1989;107:229–235.
15. Spaide RE, Gaissinger A, Podhorzer JR. Risk factors for cotton-wool spots and for cytomegalovirus retinitis in patients with human immunodeficiency virus infection. Ophthalmology 1995;102:1860–1864.
16. Quiceno JI, Caparelli E, Sadun AA, et al. Visual dysfunction without retinitis in patients with acquired immunodeficiency syndrome. Am J Ophthalmol 1992;113:8–13.
17. Tenhula WN, Xu S, Madigan MC, et al. Morphometric comparisons of optic nerve axon loss in acquired immunodeficiency syndrome. Am J Ophthalmol 1992;113:14–20.
18. Plummer DJ, Sample PA, Arevalo JF, et al. Visual field loss in HIV-positive patients without infectious retinopathy. Am J Ophthalmol 1996;122:542–549.
19. Geier SA, Perro C, Klauss V, et al. HIV-related ocular microangiopathic syndrome and cognitive functioning. J Acquir Immune Def Syndr 1993;6:252–258.
20. Geier SA, Schielke E, Klauss V, et al. Retinal microvasculopathy and reduced cerebral blood flow in patients with acquired immunodeficiency syndrome. Am J Ophthalmol 1992;113:100–101.
21. Palestine AG, Rodriguez MM, Macher AM, et al. Ophthalmic involvement in acquired immunodeficiency syndrome. Ophthalmology 1984;91:1092–1099.
22. Friedman SM, Margo CE. Bilateral central retinal vein occlusions in a patient with acquired immnodeficiency syndrome. Arch Ophthalmol 1995;113:1184–1188.
23. Kestelyn P, Van de Perre P, Rouvroy D, et al. A prospective study of the ophthalmologic findings in the acquired immune deficiency syndrome in Africa. Am J Ophthalmol 1985;100:230–238.
24. Holland GN. AIDS: retinal and choroidal infections. In: Ryan SJ, Lewis H, eds. Medical and surgical retina: advances, controversies, and management. St. Louis: Mosby–Year Book, 1994:415–433.
25. Pertel P, Hirschtick R, Phair J, et al. Risk of developing cytomegalovirus retinitis in persons infected with the human immunodeficiency virus. J Acquir Immune Def Syndr 1992; 5:1069–1074.
26. Sison RF, Holland GN, MacArthur LJ, et al. Cytomegalovirus retinopathy as the initial manifestation of the acquired immunodeficiency syndrome. Am J Ophthalmol 1991; 112:243–249.
27. Hoover DR, Peng Y, Saah A, et al. Occurrence of cytomegalovirus retinitis after human immunodeficiency virus immunosuppression. Arch Ophthalmol 1996;114:821–827.
28. Holland GN, Sison RF, Jatulis DE, et al. Survival of patients with the acquired immunodeficiency syndrome after development of cytomegalovirus retinopathy. Ophthalmology 1990;97:204–211.
29. Studies of Ocular Complications of AIDS (SOCA) Research Group in collaboration with the AIDS Clinical Trials Group (ACTG). Mortality in patients with the acquired immunodeficiency syndrome treated with either foscarnet or ganciclovir for cytomegalovirus retinitis. N Engl J Med 1992;326:213–220.
30. Holland GN, Shuler JD. Progression rates of cytomegalovirus retinopathy in ganciclovir-treated and untreated patients. Arch Ophthalmol 1992;110:1435–1442.
31. Holland GN, Buhles WC, Mastre B, et al. A controlled retrospective study of ganciclovir treatment for cytomegalovirus retinopathy: use of standardized system for the assessment of disease outcome. Arch Ophthalmol 1989; 107:1759–1766.
32. Latkany PA, Holopigian K, Lorenzo-Latkany M, et al. Electroretinographic and psychophysical findings during early and late stages of human immunodeficiency virus infection and cytomegalovirus retinitis. Ophthalmology 1997;104:445–453.
33. Freeman WR, Henderly DE, Wan WL, et al. Prevalence, pathophysiology, and treatment of rhegmatogenous retinal detachment in treated cytomegalovirus retinitis. Am J Ophthalmol 1987;103:527–536.
34. Jabs DA, Enger C, Haller J, de Bustros S. Retinal detachments in patients with cytomegalovirus retinitis. Arch Ophthalmol 1991; 109:794–799.
35. Morinelli EN, Dugel PU, Lee M, et al. Opportunistic intraocular infections in AIDS. Trans Am Ophthalmol Soc 1992; 90:97–108.
36. Holland GN, Sidikaro Y, Kreiger AE, et al. Treatment of cytomegalovirus retinopathy with ganciclovir. Ophthalmology 1987; 94:815–823.

37. Gross JG, Bozette SA, Mathews WC, et al. Longitudinal study of cytomegalovirus retinitis in acquired immune deficiency syndrome. Ophthalmology 1990;97:681–686.
38. Henderly DE, Freeman WR, Causey DM, et al. Cytomegalovirus retinitis and response to therapy with ganciclovir. Ophthalmology 1987;94:425–434.
39. Jabs DA, Enger C, Bartlett JG. Cytomegalovirus retinitis and acquired immunodeficiency syndrome. Arch Ophthalmol 1989;107:75–80.
40. Jacobson MA, O Donnell JJ, Brodie HR, et al. Randomized prospective trial of ganciclovir maintenance therapy for cytomegalovirus retinitis. J Med Virol 1988;25:339–349.
41. Jacobson MA, O Donnell JJ, Mills J. Foscarnet treatment of cytomegalovirus retinitis in patients with the acquired immunodeficiency syndrome. Antimicrob Agents Chemother 1989;33:736–741.
42. Palestine AG, Polis MA, de Smet MD, et al. A randomized, controlled trial of foscarnet in the treatment of cytomegalovirus retinitis in patients with AIDS. Ann Intern Med 1991;115:665–673.
43. Studies of Ocular Complications of AIDS (SOCA) Research Group in collaboration with the AIDS Clinical Trials Group (ACTG). Cidofovir (HPMPC) for the treatment of cytomegalovirus retinitis in patients with AIDS: the HPMPC peripheral cytomegalovirus retinitis trial. A randomized, controlled trial. Ann Intern Med 1997;126:264–274.
44. Lalezari JP, Stagg RJ, Kuppermann BD, et al. Intravenous cidofovir for peripheral cytomegalovirus retinitis in patients with AIDS: a randomized, controlled trial. Ann Intern Med 1997;126:257–263.
45. Drew WL, Ives D, Lalezari JP, et al. Oral ganciclovir as maintenance treatment for cytomegalovirus retinitis in patients with AIDS. N Engl J Med 1995;333:615–620.
46. Oral Ganciclovir European and Australian Cooperative Study Group. Intravenous versus oral ganciclovir: European/Australian comparative study of efficacy and safety in the prevention of cytomegalovirus retinitis recurrence in patients with AIDS. AIDS 1995;9:471–477.
47. Studies of Ocular Complications of AIDS (SOCA) Research Group in collaboration with the AIDS Clinical Trials Group (ACTG). Studies of ocular complications of AIDS (SOCA) foscarnet-ganciclovir cytomegalovirus retinitis trial. 1. Rationale, design, and methods. Controlled Clin Trials 1992;13:22–39.
48. Hochster H, Dieterich D, Bozzette S, et al. Toxicity of combined ganciclovir and zidovudine for cytomegalovirus disease associated with AIDS. An AIDS clinical trials group study. Ann Intern Med 1990;113:111–117.
49. Jacobson MA. Treatment of cytomegalovirus retinitis in patients with the acquired immunodeficiency syndrome. N Engl J Med 1997;337:105–114.
50. D Amico DJ, Skolnik PR, Kosloff BR, et al. Resolution of cytomegalovirus retinitis with zidovudine therapy. Arch Ophthalmol 1988;106:1168–169.
51. Guyer DR, Jabs DA, Brant AM, et al. Regression of cytomegalovirus retinitis with zidovudine: a clinicopathologic correlation. Arch Ophthalmol 1989;107:868–874.
52. Reed JB, Schwab IR, Gordon J, et al. Regression of cytomegalovirus retinitis associated with protease inhibitor treatment in patients with AIDS. Am J Ophthalmol 1997;124:199–205.
53. Drew WL, Miner RC, Busch DF, et al. Prevalence of resistance in patients receiving ganciclovir for serious cytomegalovirus infection. J Infect Dis 1991;163:716–719.
54. Erice A, Chou S, Biron KK. Progressive disease due to ganciclovir-resistant cytomegalovirus in immunocompromised patients. N Engl J Med 1989;320:289–293.
55. Sullivan V, Coen DM. Isolation of foscarnet-resistant human cytomegalovirus patterns of resistance and sensitivity to other antiviral drugs. J Infect Dis 1991;164:781–784.
56. Arevalo JF, Gonzalez C, Capparelli EV, et al. Intravitreous and plasma concentrations of ganciclovir and foscarnet after intravenous therapy in patients with AIDS and cytomegalovirus retinitis. J Infect Dis 1995;172:951–956.
57. Jennens ID, Lucas CR, Sandland AM, et al. Cytomegalovirus cultures during maintenance DHPG therapy for cytomegalovirus (CMV) retinitis in acquired immunodeficiency syndrome (AIDS). J Med Virol 1990;30:42–44.
58. Hardy D, Spector S, Polsky B, et al. Combination of ganciclovir and granulocyte–macrophage colony-stimulating factor in the treatment of cytomegalovirus retinits in AIDS patients. Eur J Clin Microbiol Infect Dis 1994;13(suppl 2):S34–S40.
59. The Studies of Ocular Complications of AIDS Research Group in collaboration with the AIDS Clinical Trials Group. Combination foscarnet and ganciclovir therapy vs monotherapy for the treatment of relapsed cytomegalovirus retinitis in patients with AIDS: the cytomegalovirus retreatment trial. Arch Ophthalmol 1996;114:23–33.
60. Freitas VR, Fraser-Smith EB, Matthews TR. Increased efficacy of ganciclovir in combination with foscarnet against cytomegalovirus and herpes simplex virus type 2 in vitro and in vivo. Antiviral Res 1989;12:205–212.
61. Manischewitz JF, Quinnan GV Jr, Lane HC, et al. Synergistic effect of ganciclovir and foscarnet on cytomegalovirus replication in vitro. Antimicrob Agents Chemother 1990;34:373–375.
62. Weinberg DV, Murphy R, Naughton K. Combined daily therapy with intravenous ganciclovir and foscarnet for patients with recurrent cytomegalovirus retinitis. Am J Ophthalmol 1994;117:776–782.
63. Kuppermann BD, Flores-Aguilar M, Quiceno JI, et al. Combination ganciclovir and foscarnet in the treatment of clinically resistant cytomegalovirus retinitis in patients with acquired immunodeficiency syndrome. Arch Ophthalmol 1993;111:1359–1366.
64. Sullivan V, Talarico CL, Stanat SC, et al. A protein kinase homologue controls phosphorylation of ganciclovir in human cytomegalovirus-infected cells. Nature 1992;358:162–164.
65. Sullivan V, Biron KK, Talarico C, et al. A point mutation in the human cytomegalovirus DNA polymerase gene confers resistance to ganciclovir and phosphonylmethoxyalkyl derivatives. Antimicrob Agents Chemother 1993;37:19–25.
66. Dunn JP, MacCumber MW, Forman MS, et al. Viral sensitivity testing in patients with cytomegalovirus retinitis clinically resistant to foscarnet or ganciclovir. Am J Ophthalmol 1995;119:587–596.
67. Flores-Aguilar M, Kuppermann BD, Quiceno JI, et al. Pathophysiology and treatment of clinically resistant cytomegalovirus retinitis. Ophthalmology 1993;100:1022–1031.
68. Cundy KC, Petty BG, Flaherty J, et al. Clinical pharmacokinetics of cidofovir in human immunodeficiency virus-infected patients. Antimicrob Agents Chemother 1995;39:1247–1252.
69. Jabs DA, Dunn J, Enger C, et al. Cytomegalovirus retinitis and viral resistance: prevalence of resistance at diagnosis. In: Abstracts of the 11th Conference on AIDS 1996;2:218.
70. Cochereau-Massin I, LeHoang P, Lautier-Frau M, et al. Efficacy and tolerence of intravitreal ganciclovir in cytomegalovirus retinitis in acquired immune deficiency syndrome. Ophthalmology 1991; 98:1348–1355.
71. Heinemann MH. Long-term intravitreal ganciclovir therapy for cytomegalovirus retinopathy. Arch Ophthalmol 1989;107:1767–1772.
72. Diaz-Llopis M, Espana E, Munoz G, et al. High dose intravitreal foscarnet in the treatment of cytomegalovirus retinitis in AIDS. Br J Ophthalomol 1994;78:120–124.
73. Morlet N, Young S, Strachan D, et al. Technique of intravitreal injection. Aust N Z J Ophthalmol 1993;21:130-131.
74. Saran BR, Maguire AM. Retinal toxicity of high-dose intravitreal ganciclovir. Retina 1994;14:248–252.
75. Kirsch LS, Arevalo JF, Chavez-de la Paz E, et al. Intravitreal cidofovir (HPMPC) treatment of cytomegalovirus retinitis in patients with acquired immune deficiency syndrome. Ophthalmology 1995;102:533–543.
76. Chavez-de la Paz E, Arevalo J, Kirsch LS, et al. Anterior nongranulomatous uveitis after intravitreal HPMPC (cidofovir) for the treatment of cytomegalovirus retinitis: analysis and prevention. Ophthalmology 1997;104:539–544.

77. Sanborn GE, Anand R, Torti RE, et al. Sustained-release ganciclovir therapy for treatment of cytomegalovirus retinitis: use of an intravitreal device. Arch Ophthalmol 1992;110:188–195.
78. Anand R. Nightingale SD, Fish RH, et al. Control of cytomegalovirus retinitis using sustained release of intraocular ganciclovir. Arch Ophthalmol 1993;111:223–227.
79. Anand R, Font RL, Rish RH, et al. Pathology of cytomegalovirus retinitis treated with sustained release intravitreal ganciclovir. Ophthalmology 1993;100:1032–1039.
80. Martin DF, Parks DJ, Mellow SD, et al. Treatment of cytomegalovirus retinitis with an intraocular sustained-release ganciclovir implant: a randomized controlled clinical trial. Arch Ophthalmol 1994;112:1531–1539.
81. Morley MG, Duker JS, Ashton P, et al. Replacing ganciclovir implants. Ophthalmology 1995;102:388–392.
82. Marx JL, Kapusta MA, Patel SS, et al. Use of the ganciclovir implant in the treatment of recurrent cytomegalovirus retinitis. Arch Ophthalmol 1996;114:815–820.
83. Charles NC, Steiner GC. Ganciclovir intraocular implant: a clinicopathologic study. Ophthalmology 1996;103:416–421.
84. Freeman WR, Friedberg DN, Berry C, et al. Risk factors for development of rhegmatogenous retinal detachment in patients with cytomegalovirus retinitis. Am J Ophthalmol 1993;116:713–720.
85. Gangan PA, Besen G, Munguia D, et al. Macular serous exudation in patients with acquired immunodeficiency syndrome and cytomegalovirus retinitis. Am J Ophthalmol 1994;118:212–219.
86. Davis JL, Serfass MS, Lai M-Y, et al. Silicone oil in repair of retinal detachments caused by necrotizing retinitis in HIV infection. Arch Ophthalmol 1995;113:1401–1409.
87. Meldrum ML, Aaberg TM, Patel A, Davis J. Cataract extraction after silicone oil repair of retinal detachments due to necrotizing retinitis. Arch Ophthalmol 1996;114:885–892.
88. Spector SA, McKinley GF, Lalezari JP, et al. Oral ganciclovir for the prevention of cytomegalovirus disease in persons with AIDS. N Engl J Med 1996;334:1491–1497.
89. Brosgart CL, Craig C, Hillman D, et al. A randomized, placebo-controlled trial of the sagety and efficacy of oral ganciclovir for prophylaxis of CMV retinal and gastrointestinal mucosal disease in HIV-infected individuals with severe immunosuppression [abstract]. In: Program and Abstracts of the 35th Interscience Conference on Antimicrobial Agents and Chemotherapy. Washington, DC: American Society for Microbiology, 1995:LB-10.
90. Gagliuso DJ, Teich SA, Friedman AH, et al. Ocular toxoplasmosis in AIDS patients. Trans Am Ophthalmol Soc 1990;88:63–86.
91. Holland GN, Engstrom RE, Glasgow BJ, et al. Ocular toxoplasmosis in patients with the acquired immunodeficiency syndrome. Am J Ophthalmol 1988;106:653–667.
92. Schanzer MC, Font RL, O Malley RE. Primary ocular malignant lymphoma associated with the acquired immune deficiency syndrome. Ophthalmology 1991;98:88–91.
93. Elkins BS, Holland GN, Opremcak EM, et al. Ocular toxoplamosis misdiagnosed as cytomegalovirus retinitis in immunocompromised patients. Ophthalmology 1994;101:499–507.
94. Friedlander SM, Rahhal FM, Ericson L, et al. Optic neuropathy preceding acute retinal necrosis in acquired immunodeficiency syndrome. Arch Ophthalmol 1996;114:1481–1485.
95. Engstrom RE Jr, Holland GN, Margolis TP, et al. The progressive outer retinal necrosis syndrome: a variant of necrotizing herpetic retinopathy in patients with AIDS. Ophthalmology 1994;101:1488–1502.
96. Margolis TP, Lowder CY, Holland GN, et al. Varicella zoster virus retinitis in patients with the acquired immunodeficiency syndrome. Am J Ophthalmol 1991;112:119–131.
97. Forster DJ, Dugel PU, Frangieh GT, et al. Rapidly progressive outer retinal necrosis in the acquired immunodeficiency syndrome. Am J Ophthalmol 1990;110:341–348.
98. Greven CM, Ford J, Stanton C, et al. Progressive outer retinal necrosis secondary to varicella zoster virus in acquired immune deficiency syndrome. Retina 1995;15:14–20.
99. Johnston WH, Holland GN, Engstrom RE Jr, et al. Recurrence of presumed varicella zoster virus retinopathy in patients with acquired immunodeficiency syndrome. Am J Ophthalmol 1993;116:42–50.
100. Schuman JS, Orellana J, Friedman AH, et al. Acquired immunodeficiency syndrome (AIDS). Surv Ophthalmol 1987;31:384–410.
101. Pepose JS, Hilborne LH, Cancilla PA, et al. Concurrent herpes simplex and cytomegalovirus retinitis and encephalitis in the acquired immune deficiency syndrome (AIDS). Ophthalmology 1984; 91:1669–1677.
102. Cunningham ET, Short GA, Irvine AR, et al. Acquired immunodeficiency syndrome-associated herpes simplex virus retinitis: clinical description and use of a polymerase chain reaction-based assay as a diagnostic tool. Arch Ophthalmol 1996;114:834–840.
103. Holland GN. Ocular toxoplasmosis in the immunocompromised host. Int Ophthalmol 1989;13:399–402.
104. Grossniklaus HE. *Toxoplasma gondii* retinochoroiditis and optic neuritis in acquired immune deficiency syndrome: report of a case. Ophthalmology 1990;97:1342–1346.
105. Berger BB, Egwuagu CE, Freeman WR, et al. Miliary toxoplasmosis retinitis in acquired immunodeficiency syndrome. Arch Ophthalmol 1993;111:373–376.
106. Bottoni F, Gonnella P, Autelitano A, et al. Diffuse necrotizing retinochoroiditis in a child with AIDS and toxoplasmic encephalitis. Graefes Arch Clin Exp Ophthalmol 1990;228:36–39.
107. Cochereau-Massin I, LeHoang P, Lautier-Frau M, et al. Ocular toxoplasmosis in human immunodeficiency virus-infected patients. Am J Ophthalmol 1992;114:130–135.
108. Engstrom RE, Holland GN, Nussenblatt RB, et al. Current practices in the management of ocular toxoplasmosis. Am J Ophthalmol 1991;111:601–610.
109. Lopez JS, de Smet MD, Masur H, et al. Orally administered 566C80 for treatment of ocular toxoplasmosis in a patient with the acquired immunodeficiency syndrome. Am J Ophthalmol 1992;113:331–333.
110. Gass JDM, Braunstein RA, Chenoweth RG. Acute syphilitic posterior placoid chorioretinitis. Ophthalmology 1990;97:1288–1297.
111. McLeish WM, Pulido JS, Holland S, et al. The ocular manifestations of syphilis in the human immunodeficiency virus type 1-infected host. Ophthalmology 1990;97:196–203.
112. Stoumbos VD, Klein ML. Syphilitic retinitis in a patient with acquired immunodeficiency syndrome-related complex. Am J Ophthalmol 1987;103:103–104.
113. Shalaby I, Dunn JP, Semba RD, et al. Syphilitic uveitis in HIV-infected patients. Arch Ophthalmol 1997;115:469–473.
114. Davis JL, Nussenblatt RB, Bachman DM, et al. Endogenous bacterial retinitis in AIDS. Am J Ophthalmol 1989; 107:613–623.
115. Tufail A, Weisz, Holland GN. Endogenous bacterial endophthalmitis as a complication of intravenous therapy for cytomegalovirus retinitis. Arch Ophthalmol 1996;114:879–880.
116. Denning DW, Armstrong RW, Fishman M, et al. Endophthalmitis in a patient with disseminated cryptococcosis and AIDS who was treated with itraconazole. Rev Infect Dis 1991; 13:1126–1130.
117. Newman NM, Mandel MR, Gullett J, et al. Clinical and histologic findings in opportunistic ocular infections: part of a new syndrome of acquired immunodeficiency. Arch Ophthalmol 1983; 101:396–401.
118. Schuman JS, Friedman AH. Retinal manifestations of the acquired immune deficiency syndrome (AIDS): cytomegalovirus, *Candida albicans, Cryptococcus,* toxoplasmosis, and *Pneumocystis carinii*. Trans Ophthalmol Soc UK 1983;103:177–190.
119. Winward KE, Hamed LM, Glaser JS. The spectrum of optic nerve disease in human immunodeficiency virus infection. Am J Ophthalmol 1989;107:373–380.
120. Kestelyn P, Taelman H, Bogaerts J, et al. Ophthalmic manifestations of infections with *Cryptococcus neoformans* in patients with the acquired immunodeficiency syndrome. Am J Ophthalmol 1993;116:721–727.

121. Carney MD, Combs JL, Waschler W. Cryptococcal choroiditis. Retina 1990;10:27–32.
122. Macher A, Rodrigues MM, Kaplan W, et al. Disseminated bilateral chorioretinitis due to *Histoplasma capsulatum* in a patient with the acquired immunodeficiency syndrome. Ophthalmology 1985; 92: 1159–1164.
123. Specht CS, Mitchell KT, Bauman AE, et al. Ocular histoplasmosis with retinitis in a patient with acquired immune deficiency syndrome. Ophthalmology 1991;98:1356–1359.
124. Kurosawa A, Pollock SC, Collins MP, et al. *Sporothrix schenckii* endophthalmitis in a patient with human immunodeficiency virus infection. Arch Ophthalmol 1988;106:376–380.
125. Glasgow BJ, Engstrom RE, Holland GN, et al. Bilateral endogenous *Fusarium* endophthalmitis associated with acquired immunodeficiency syndrome. Arch Ophthalmol 1996;114:873–877.
126. Walton RC, Wilson J, Chan C-C. Metastatic choroidal abscess in the acquired immunodeficiency syndrome. Arch Ophthalmol 1996;114: 880–881.
127. Morinelli EN, Dugel PU, Riffenburg R, et al. Infectious multifocal choroiditis in patients with acquired immune deficiency syndrome. Ophthalmology 1993;100:1014–1021.
128. Blodi BA, Johnson MW, McLeish WM, et al. Presumed choroidal tuberculosis in a human immunodeficiency virus infected host. Am J Ophthalmol 1989;108:605–607.
129. Croxatto JO, Mestre C, Puente S, et al. Nonreactive tuberculosis in a patient with acquired immune deficiency syndrome. Am J Ophthalmol 1986;102:659–660.
130. Menezo JL, Martinez-Costa R, Marin F, et al. Tuberculous panophthalmitis associated with drug abuse. Intl Ophthalmol 1987;10: 235–240.
131. Muccioli C, Belfort R Jr. Presumed ocular and central nervous system tuberculosis in a patient with the acquired immunodeficiency syndrome. Am J Ophthalmology 1996;121:217–219.
132. Rao NA, Zimmerman PL, Boyer D, et al. A clinical, histopathologic, and electron microscopic study of *Pneumocystis carinii* choroiditis. Am J Ophthalmol 1989;107:218–228.
133. Koser MW, Jampol LM, MacDonell K. Treatment of *Pneumocystis carinii* choroidopathy. Arch Ophthalmol 1990;108:1214–1215.
134. Holland GN, MacArthur LJ, Foos RY. Choroidal pneumocystosis. Arch Ophthalmol 1991;109:1454–1455.
135. Foster RE, Lowder CY, Meisler DM, et al. Presumed *Pneumocystis carinii* choroiditis: unifocal presentation, regression with intravenous pentamidine, and choroiditis recurrence. Ophthalmology 1991;98: 1360–1365.
136. Shami MJ, Freeman W, Friedberg D, et al. A multicenter center study of *Pneumocystis* choroidopathy. Am J Ophthalmol 1991;112:15–22.
137. Dugel PU, Rao NA, Forster DJ, et al. *Pneumocystis carinii* choroiditis after long-term aerosolized pentamidine therapy. Am J Ophthalmol 1990;110:113–117.
138. Shuler JD, Engstrom RE, Holland GN. External ocular disease and anterior segment disorders associated with the acquired immunodeficiency syndrome. Int Ophthalmol Clin 1989;29:98–104.
139. Jabs DA. Ocular manifestations of HIV infection. Trans Am Ophthalmol Soc 1995;93:623–683.
140. Engstrom RE, Holland GN. Chronic herpes zoster virus keratitis associated with the acquired immunodeficiency syndrome. Am J Ophthalmol 1988;105:556–558.
141. Hodge WG, Margolis TP. Herpes simplex virus keratitis among patients who are positive or negative for human immunodeficiency virus: an epidemiologic study. Ophthalmology 1997;104:120–124.
142. Young TL, Robin JB, Holland GN, et al. Herpes simplex keratitis in patients with acquired immune deficiency syndrome. Ophthalmology 1989;96:1476–1479.
143. Wilhelmus KR, Font RL, Lehmann RP, et al. Cytomegalovirus keratitis in acquired immunodeficiency syndrome. Arch Ophthalmol 1996;114:869–872.
144. Aristumuño B, Nirankari VS, Hemady RK, et al. Spontaneous ulcerative keratitis in immunocompromised patients. Am J Ophthalmol 1993; 115:202–208.
145. Hemady RK. Microbial keratitis in patients infected with the human immunodeficiency virus. Ophthalmology 1995;102:1026–1030.
146. Lucca JA, Farris RL, Bielory L, et al. Keratoconjunctivitis sicca in male patients infected with human immunodeficiency virus type 1. Ophthalmology 1990;97:1008–1010.
147. Sachs R, Zagelbaum BM, Hersh PS. Corneal complications associated with the use of crack cocaine. Ophthalmology 1993;100:187–191.
148. Schwartz DA, Visvevara GS, Diesenhouse MC, et al. Pathologic features and immunoflourescent antibody demonstration of ocular microsporidiosis (*Encephalitozoon hellem*) in seven patients with acquired immunodeficiency syndrome. Am J Ophthalmol 1993;115: 285–292.
149. Lowder CY, Meisler DM, McMahon JT, et al. Microsporidia infection of the cornea in a man seropositive for human immunodeficiency virus. Am J Ophthalmol 1990;109:242–244.
150. Diesenhouse MC, Wilson LA, Corrent GF, et al. Treatment of microsporidial keratoconjunctivitis with topical fumagillin. Am J Ophthalmol 1993;115:293–298.
151. Lowder CY, McMahon JT, Meisler DM, et al. Microsporidial keratoconjunctivitis caused by *Septata intestinalis* in a patient with acquired immunodeficiency syndrome. Am J Ophthalmol 1996;121:71–717.
152. Robinson MR, Udell IJ, Garber PF, et al. Molluscum contagiosum of the eyelids in patients with acquired immune deficiency syndrome. Ophthalmology 1992;99:1745–1747.
153. Bardenstein DS, Elmets C. Hyperfocal cryotherapy of multiple *Molluscum contagiosum* lesions in patients with the acquired immune deficiency syndrome. Ophthalmology 1995;102:1031–1034.
154. Charles NC, Friedberg DN. Epibulbar molluscum contagiosum in acquired immune deficiency syndrome; case report and review of the literature. Ophthalmology 1992;99:1123–1126.
155. Buus DR, Pflugfelder SC, Schachter J, et al. Lymphogranuloma venereum conjunctiva with a marginal corneal perforation. Ophthalmology 1988;95:799–802.
156. Shuler JD, Holland GN, Miles SA, et al. Kaposi sarcoma of the conjunctiva and eyelids associated with the acquired immunodeficiency syndrome. Arch Ophthalmol 1989;107:858–862.
157. Kurumety UR, Lustbader JM. Kaposi's sarcoma of the bulbar conjunctiva as an initial clinical manifestation of acquired immunodeficiency syndrome. Arch Ophthalmol 1995;113:978.
158. Hummer J, Gass JDM, Huang AJW. Conjunctival Kaposi's sarcoma treated with interferon alpha-2a. Am J Ophthalmol 1993;116:502–503.
159. Ghabrial R, Quivey JM, Dunn JP, et al. Radiation therapy of acquired immunodeficiency syndrome-related Kaposi's sarcoma of the eyelids and conjunctiva. Arch Ophthalmol 1992;110:1423–1426.
160. Dugel PU, Gill PS, Frangieh GT, et al. Treatment of ocular adnexal Kaposi's sarcoma in acquired immune deficiency syndrome. Ophthalmology 1992;99:1127–1132.
161. MacLean H, Dhillon B, Ironside J. Squamous cell carcinoma of the eyelid and the acquired immunodeficiency syndrome. Am J Ophthalmol 1996;121:219–221.
162. Winward KE, Curtin VT. Conjunctival squamous cell carcinoma in a patient with human immunodeficiency virus infection. Am J Ophthalmol 1989;107:554–555.
163. Margo CE, Mack W, Guffey JM. Squamous cell carcinoma of the conjunctiva and human immunodeficiency virus infection [letter]. Arch Ophthalmol 1996;114:349.
164. Lewallen S, Shroyer KR, Keyser RB, et al. Aggressive conjunctival squamous cell carcinoma in three young Africans. Arch Ophthalmol 1996;114:215–218.
165. Ateenyi-Agaba C. Conjunctival squamous-cell carcinoma associated with HIV infection in Kampala, Uganda. Lancet 1995;345:695–696.
166. Kim RY, Seiff SR, Howes EL Jr, et al. Necrotizing scleritis secondary to conjunctival squamous cell carcinoma in acquired immunodeficiency syndrome. Am J Ophthalmol 1990;109:231–233.

167. Kestelyn P, Stevens AM, Ndayambaje A, et al. HIV and conjunctival malignancies. Lancet 1990;336:51–52.
168. Lane HC, Masur H, Edgar L. Abnormalities of B cell activation and immunoregulation in patients with the acquired immunodeficiency syndrome. N Engl J Med 1983;309:453–458.
169. Matzkin DC, Slamovits TL, Rosenbaum PS. Simultaneous intraocular and orbital non–Hodgkin lymphoma in the acquired immune deficiency syndrome. Ophthalmology 1994;101:850–855.
170. Logani S, Logani SC, Ali BH, et al. Bilateral, intraconal non–Hodgkin's lymphoma in a patient with acquired immunodeficiency syndrome. Am J Ophthalmol 1994;118:401–402.
171. Topilow HW, Ackerman AL, Friedman A. Progressive outer retinal necrosis [letter]. Ophthalmology 1995;102:1737–1738.
172. Antle CM, White VA, Horsman DE, et al. Large cell orbital lymphoma in a patient with acquired immune deficiency syndrome: case report and review. Ophthalmology 1990;97:1494–1498.
173. Friedman DI. Neuro-ophthalmic manifestations of human immunodeficiency virus infection. Neurol Clin 1991;9:55–72.
174. Keane JR. Neuro-ophthalmologic signs of AIDS: 50 patients. Neurology 1991;41:841–845.
175. Mansour AM. Neuro-ophthalmic findings in acquired immunodeficiency syndrome. J Clin Neuro Ophthalmol 1990;10:167–174.
176. Ormerod LD, Rhodes RH, Gross SA, et al. Ophthalmologic manifestations of acquired immune deficiency syndrome–associated progressive multifocal leukoencephalopathy. Ophthalmology 1996;103:899–906.
177. Bylsma SS, Achim CL, Wiley CA, et al. The predictive value of cytomegalovirus retinitis for cytomegalovirus encephalitis in acquired immunodeficiency syndrome. Arch Ophthalmol 1995;113:89–95.
178. Lee BL, Holland GN, Glasgow BJ. Chiasmal infarction and sudden blindness caused by mucormycosis in AIDS and diabetes mellitus. Am J Ophthalmol 1996;122:895–896.
179. Kronish JW, Johnson TE, Gilberg SM, et al. Orbital infections in patients with human immunodeficiency virus infection. Ophthalmology 1996;103:1483–1492.
180. Krzystolik MG, Kuperwasser M, Low RM, et al. Anterior-segment ultrasound biomicroscopy in a patient with AIDS and bilateral angle-closure glaucoma secondary to uveal effusions. Arch Ophthalmol 1996;114:878–879.
181. Williams AS, Williams FC, O Donnell JJ. AIDS presenting as acute glaucoma. Arch Ophthalmol 1988;106:311–312.
182. Gross FJ, Waxman JS, Rosenblatt MA, et al. Eosinophilic granuloma of the cavernous sinus and orbital apex in an HIV-positive patient. Ophthalmology 1989;96:462–467.
183. Saran BR, Maguire AM, Nichols C, et al. Hypopyon uveitis in patients with acquired immunodeficiency syndrome treated for systemic *Mycobacterium avium* complex infection with rifabutin. Arch Ophthalmol 1994;112:1159–1165.
184. Jacobs DS, Piliero PJ, Kuperwaser MG, et al. Acute uveitis associated with rifabutin use in patients with human immunodeficiency virus infection. Am J Ophthalmol 1994;118:716–722.
185. Whitcup SM, Butler KM, Caruso R, et al. Retinal toxicity in human immunodeficiency virus infected children treated with 2′,3′-dideoxyinosine. Am J Ophthalmol 1992;113:1–7.
186. Pflugfelder SC, Saulson R, Ullman S. Peripheral corneal ulceration in a patient with AIDS-related complex. Am J Ophthalmol 1987;104:542–543.
187. Pepose JS, Linette G, Lee SF, et al. Disinfection of Goldmann tonometers against human immunodeficiency virus type 1. Arch Ophthalmol 1989;107:983–985.
188. Moreira LB, Sanchez D, Trousdale MD, et al. Aerosolization of infectious virus by excimer laser. Am J Ophthalmol 1997;123:297–302.
189. Pepose JS, MacRae S, Quinn TC, et al. Serologic markers after the transplantation of corneas from donors infected with human immunodeficiency virus. Am J Ophthalmol 1987;103:798–801.
190. Landers MB, Fraser VJ. Antiviral chemoprophylaxis after occupational exposure to human immunodeficiency virus: why, when, where, and what. Am J Ophthalmol 1997;124:227–233.

30
NEUROLOGIC COMPLICATIONS OF HIV-1 INFECTION AND AIDS

Richard W. Price

The neurologic complications of human immunodeficiency virus type 1 (HIV-1) infection are both common and diverse; for general reviews, see elsewhere (1–5). These complications include various central nervous system (CNS) and peripheral nervous system (PNS) disorders related to several types of underlying pathogenetic processes, with particular complications developing at different stages in the evolving course of systemic HIV-1 infection (Table 30.1). To the neophyte, the spectrum of complications may appear both exotic and bewildering. Yet, as with HIV-1–related diseases of other organ systems, an understanding of the effects of HIV-1 on the host immune system and a working knowledge of the experience that has been accumulated over nearly two decades provide the clinician with a rational and effective framework for neurologic diagnosis. Not only can a diagnosis usually be established rapidly and logically, but also appropriate steps can be taken to arrest, reverse, or palliate many of these diseases, thus significantly reducing their attendant morbidity and disability. This chapter provides a broad overview for approaching neurologic disease in the setting of HIV-1 infection. Because several of the important neurologic diseases complicating acquired immunodeficiency syndrome (AIDS) are considered in greater detail elsewhere (see Chaps. 15, 18, 22, 25, and 29), the emphasis is on general principles of neurologic diagnosis and on the disorders that are not considered in detail elsewhere in this volume.

GENERAL CONSIDERATIONS

The initial approach to neurologic diagnosis emphasizes three principal aspects of the clinical presentation: 1) the *neuroanatomic localization* of the clinical dysfunction; 2) the *temporal profile* of its evolution; and 3) the *phase of the patient's systemic HIV-1 infection* and the presence of other risk factors. The importance of neuroanatomic localization relates to the finding that individual diseases have particular predilections for involvement of certain parts of the nervous system. The neurologic history and examination usually allow an accurate approximation of anatomic localization and, as a result, usually immediately circumscribe the differential diagnosis. This preliminary localization also guides further study, including the selective use of neuroimaging or other laboratory studies.

Neurologists also generally rely heavily on the temporal profile of disease evolution to help categorize the type of underlying disease process, and neurologic disease in the HIV-1 setting is no exception. The time course is determined by the type of pathophysiologic insult. For example, acute events that evolve in the time scale of minutes relate to changes in cellular energy metabolism or membrane integrity. Hence, vascular disorders usually evolve rapidly when a region of the brain is deprived of oxygen, glucose, and other essential metabolic substrates. Seizures have an even faster time frame; they present acutely as a result of sudden alterations in ion flux and neuronal firing. It is obviously important to distinguish these two causes of acute symptoms, inasmuch as seizures relate either to general metabolic disturbance or to a range of microscopic or macroscopic focal brain disorders, whereas strokes or transient ischemic attacks are secondary to embolic or occlusive vascular disease.

However, more common in AIDS patients is a group of brain disorders that evolve subacutely over days to weeks. In broad pathogenetic terms, this temporal profile relates to new genetic replication, transcription, and translation, with resultant alterations in cell proliferation, cell behavior, and intercellular signals. These genetic processes pertain to the invading organisms and the host cell responses, both of which evolve in this time frame. Although these processes are involved in many, indeed most, neurologic complications of HIV-1, variations in this time scale exist and can be useful in differential diagnosis, at least at first encounter. Thus, in the case of focal brain diseases, cerebral toxoplasmosis usually unfolds over a few days, presumably related to the tempo of unrestrained propagation of *Toxoplasma gondii*, whereas primary CNS lymphoma (PCNSL) develops more slowly, in step with the longer doubling time of neoplastic lymphocytes. On the other hand, more indolent disease evolution, typical of degenerative neurologic diseases, is unusual in the AIDS patient, although some cases of AIDS dementia complex (ADC) and peripheral neuropathy can pursue this more chronic, progressive course.

Table 30.1. Some of the Principal Nervous System Complications of HIV-1 Infection

	Central Nervous System	Peripheral Nervous System
Opportunistic Infections		
Common[a]	Cryptococcal meningitis	CMV polyradiculitis
	Cerebral toxoplasmosis	
	Progressive multifocal leukoencephalopathy	
Uncommon	Severe CMV encephalitis	Severe or complicated VZV radiculitis
		CMV mononeuritis multiplex
Rare	Aspergillus fumigatus	
	Nocardia asteroides	
	Mycobacterium tuberculosis	
	Histoplasma capsulatum	
	Herpes simplex virus types 1 and 2	
	Listeria monocytogenes	
Opportunistic Neoplasms		
Common	Primary CNS lymphoma (EBV-related)	
Uncommon	Metastatic systemic lymphoma	Lymphoma-related radiculopathy, cranial neuropathy
Rare	Kaposi's sarcoma	
Autoimmune		
Uncommon		Chronic inflammatory demyelinating polyneuropathy
		Acute demyelinating polyneuropathy (Guillian-Barré)
		Brachial neuropathy
		Cranial neuropathy
		Polymyositis
Rare	Acute encephalitis	Mononeuritis multiplex benign
	Multiple sclerosis-like disease	
Disorders Related to HIV-1 Itself		
Common	Aseptic meningitis	DSPN
	AIDS dementia complex	
	Headache (without meningitis)	
Metabolic and Toxic Disorders		
Common	Hypoxic encephalopathy	Toxic neuropathy (ddI, ddC, d4T)
	"Sepsis" encephalopathy	Myopathy (zidovudine)
Uncommon	Vascular (transient ischemic attack or stroke-like event)	

[a]The terms *common, uncommon,* and *rare* are used in a relative sense and loosely. Thus, *common* implies an incidence of about 5% or more, and the other terms reflect a proportionally lower incidence.
CMV, cytomegalovirus; EBV, Epstein–Barr virus; DSPN, distal sensory polyneuropathy; VZV, varicella-zoster virus.

The temporal profile of clinical presentation also tells the clinician how rapidly to pursue further diagnostic studies. Although the clinically stable patient with sensory neuropathy or with mild, long-standing cognitive complaints can be scheduled for elective diagnostic testing, the patient with fever, hemiparesis, and aphasia, advancing over a matter of hours, needs to be evaluated immediately so appropriate treatment can prevent further progression and more extensive permanent neurologic injury.

The neurologic complications of HIV-1 infection are also stage specific with respect to their development over the course of systemic HIV-1 infection. This is because they are secondary manifestations of the evolving interaction between HIV-1 and host responses. Thus, during the acute seroconversion phase of infection, certain acute or subacute neurologic syndromes have been reported that likely relate to immunopathologic events triggered by viremia and, more particularly, early immune responses. During the clinically latent phase of infection, the nervous system is largely spared; however, autoimmune disorders may occur during this phase, presumably related to perturbed, but not globally suppressed, immune reactions. Evidence of long-term exposure of the CNS to HIV-1 without overt dysfunction can also be detected during this phase. Subsequently, as immune defenses are depleted, evidence of the effect of HIV-1 itself on the CNS (ADC) and on both minor (e.g., herpes zoster) and major (e.g., progressive multifocal leukoencephalopathy [PML]) opportunistic processes is manifested with increasing frequency and severity. A clear knowledge of the patient's immune status provides a guide to these stage-specific disorders and, hence, to the probabilities of differential diagnosis. Although the diagnosis is usually evident from the patient's prior opportunistic diseases and from laboratory assessment of CD4+ T-lymphocyte count, the patient's response to highly active antiretroviral therapy (HAART) can make this assessment more complex. Prophylactic antimicrobial drug therapy can also be an important variable in probability of diagnosis, as discussed later.

With this framework, evaluation of nervous system disease in HIV-1 infection follows the same procedures and logic used for other neurologic diagnoses. A careful history allows preliminary anatomic localization and defines the temporal profile and background context. The neurologic examination refines this localization, and neuroimaging not only confirms it but also provides information regarding the character of the lesion. Until recently, cerebrospinal fluid (CSF) analysis was useful principally in the diagnosis of meningitis and cytomegalovirus (CMV) polyradiculitis. However, use of nucleic acid amplification techniques, including the polymerase chain reaction (PCR), has emerged as a practical clinical tool for specific diagnosis, as described later. In selected patients with peripheral neuropathy, electromyography, nerve conduction studies, and quantitative sensory testing may aid in diagnosis and in accurately following progression or regression of disease.

Using these clinical and laboratory methods, the clinician can establish an accurate neurologic diagnosis in most HIV-1 infected patients. Nonetheless, in some situations, the clinician does not feel secure in understanding CNS or PNS events. Patients are complex, and one still encounters "outliers" with respect to the typicality of clinical presentations of the more common conditions, as well as patients with unusual diseases (e.g., aspergillosis) or with two diseases presenting sequentially or concurrently. For some of these patients, biopsy of brain or nerve is required for definitive diagnosis. Additionally, as treatments become more complicated, new conditions emerge, related either to direct neurotoxicity or to indirect toxic effects (e.g., depression of neutrophil counts, widening the range of opportunistic infections). Thus, the AIDS clinician approaching neurologic complications must always be diagnostically alert and thoughtful. Moreover, because of the functional implications of an impaired nervous system, the clinician must also be humane and view the overall picture to consider the broader goals of medical management. Decisions should be fully rational and targeted to the principal end of relieving suffering and maximizing meaningful neurologic function in accord with the patient's premorbid and current wishes.

NEUROLOGY OF ACUTE HIV-1 INFECTION

Various CNS and PNS disorders can complicate the course of initial HIV-1 infection and seroconversion. These disorders occur at the same time as or shortly after other systemic reactions to primary HIV-1 infection, including fever, and have been reviewed by Brew and Tindall (6). Headache is most common, manifesting in one-third or more of cases, and is accompanied by meningismus or photophobia in a lesser number of patients. More severe neurologic diseases are probably uncommon and have been documented largely in case reports and limited case series. One such disease is encephalitis, with or without notable pleocytosis, which may be severe, with subacute evolution to coma (7). Myelopathy has also been reported (8). More common are various neuropathies. These include cranial neuropathies (most commonly involving one or both facial nerves), brachial plexopathy, or either focal or diffuse (poly-)neuropathies (9–14). Muscle disease with rhabdomyolysis has also been reported in this setting (15, 16). Characteristically, all these disorders are monophasic in their evolution, and most patients recover within several weeks. In a few patients, cognitive or other deficits have persisted. Laboratory evaluation in some of these patients has revealed a minor lymphocyte-predominant pleocytosis in the CSF with a concomitant modest rise in protein. Pathogenetically, these afflictions probably relate to autoimmune or immunopathologic processes and are similar to other postinfectious or parainfectious encephalitides or neuropathies.

NERVOUS SYSTEM DURING THE "CLINICALLY LATENT" PHASE OF SYSTEMIC HIV-1 INFECTION

Asymptomatic HIV-1 Infection of the Nervous System

Current concepts of the pathogenesis of systemic HIV-1 infection emphasize the activity of HIV-1 infection that continues in untreated patients even when they are asymptomatic with relatively well preserved immune defenses (17, 18). This is also the case in the CNS. Evidence of this phenomenon comes chiefly from studies of CSF obtained from neurologically and systemically asymptomatic subjects in whom ongoing infection is most readily detected by quantitative nucleic acid amplification techniques (19–22). Host reactions are also detected commonly and include both specific (intrathecal synthesis of anti–HIV-1 antibodies) and nonspecific (elevated protein, elevated immunoglobulins, and increased cell number) host responses (23–29). Such observations indicate that the CNS is exposed to HIV-1 early and perhaps continuously through the clinically latent period. This also underscores the finding that virus exposure alone is not sufficient to cause CNS disease, inasmuch as these individuals remain neurologically normal even as assessed by refined neuropsychological testing (30, 31). The significance of early exposure to the CNS by HIV-1 with respect to the eventual development of ADC and HIV-1 encephalitis is unknown.

A practical implication of this early exposure to HIV-1 and host CSF response relates to interpretation of CSF findings in these patients. "Background" elevations in protein and cells (usually in the range of 5 to 20 cells/mm^3) must be taken into account when HIV-1–infected patients undergo diagnostic lumbar puncture. Such abnormalities can provoke a false impression of the presence of another disease or of failure to respond fully to therapy, for example, in the case of syphilis.

Multiple Sclerosis-like Disease

CNS disease related to asymptomatic HIV-1 with preserved T-helper lymphocytes is rare. One notable exception is an illness that resembles multiple sclerosis and presents with multifocal deficits that pursue a course of remissions and exacerbations (32–34). The pathologic features are also apparently similar to those of multiple sclerosis. The disorder is speculated to involve an autoimmune process related to alteration of regulatory circuits of the immune system.

Neuropathies

Although neuropathies are also uncommon, they are more frequent than CNS disease in this phase of systemic infection; for review of these early and other later neuromuscular complications, see elsewhere (35). Most notable are the demyelinating polyneuropathies. Patients in this phase of HIV-1 infection are at increased risk of developing either acute or subacute inflammatory demyelinating polyneuropathy (Guillain-Barré syndrome) or more chronic inflammatory demyelinating polyneuropathy (36–38). These disorders resemble the same conditions occurring in non–HIV-1–infected patients, except the CSF more often demonstrates uncharacteristic, albeit still mild, pleocytosis (10 to 50 cells/mm^3). Patients present with progressive, ascending distal and proximal weakness with little or no sensory loss. Reflexes are absent, although this finding may be delayed for several days after the onset of weakness in acute or subacute inflammatory demyelinating polyneuropathy. Pathogenetically, these disorders probably have an autoimmune basis, as suspected in other settings. Experience suggests that patients respond favorably to intravenous immunoglobulin, plasma exchange, or corticosteroid administration, although these therapies have not been rigorously compared in an HIV-1–infected group (39).

Two other, less common, types of neuropathy have been described in this stage of HIV-1 infection. Moulignier and colleagues (40) have characterized a painful polyneuropathy associated with the diffuse infiltrative lymphocytosis syndrome. This disorder is associated with a Sjögren's syndrome-like picture and multivisceral infiltrates of CD8+ T lymphocytes. It also can involve peripheral nerves and can manifest with symmetric or asymmetric painful neuropathy. Both anti–HIV-1 treatment and corticosteroids have been reported to be beneficial. Bradley and Verma (41) reported another cause of painful neuropathy in the transitional phase of infection. This was associated with vasculitis that responded to prednisone therapy. Although this condition may be related to the benign form of mononeuritis multiplex discussed later, its presentation with more symmetric symptoms suggesting polyneuropathy is noteworthy.

NEUROLOGIC COMPLICATIONS OF THE LATE PHASE OF HIV-1 INFECTION

Serious CNS and PNS complications of HIV-1 infection occur principally in patients with severe immunosuppression, and, indeed, their incidence generally parallels the severity of CD4+ cell depletion. As a general guideline, a CD4+ count of less than 200 cells/mm^3 places the individual in the "susceptible" category for development of major opportunistic neurologic diseases, but lower counts (particularly fewer than 50 cells/mm^3) increase this risk greatly. As noted earlier, the effect of HAART therapy and resultant elevations of CD4+ counts on these risks is currently being defined. The following sections discuss these neurologic complications using the neuroanatomic classification of focal and nonfocal brain and spinal cord diseases, meningitis and headache, peripheral neuropathy, and myopathy.

Predominantly Focal Central Nervous System Disorders

Figure 30.1 depicts a general algorithm for evaluation of focal brain lesions. Among these lesions, three predominate and are therefore the usual first focus of diagnostic evaluation: cerebral toxoplasmosis, PCNSL, and PML. Although the individual neurologic symptoms and signs vary among individual patients, depending on the precise location of lesions, all three of these conditions can present with similar symptoms and signs. However, some clinical clues help in their separation: these conditions tend to differ in their temporal evolution, in their general effects on mentation and alertness, and in the concomitant systemic manifestations (Table 30.2). More important, neuroimaging features often allow their distinction (see Table 30.2).

CEREBRAL TOXOPLASMOSIS

Cerebral toxoplasmosis in AIDS almost always relates to activation of dormant *Toxoplasma gondii*, rather than to newly acquired infection (42, 43) (see Chap. 15). Earlier in

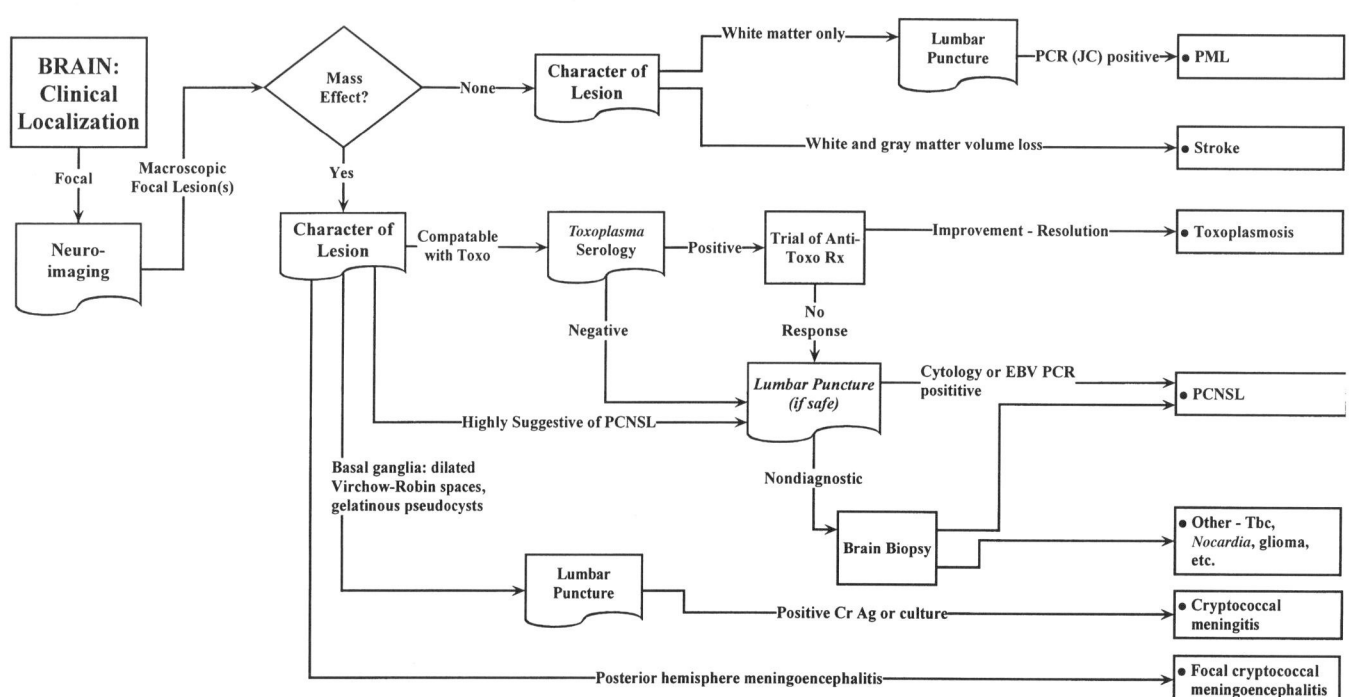

Figure 30.1. General algorithm for diagnostic evaluation of focal brain diseases.

Table 30.2. Comparative Features of the Major Focal CNS Processes in AIDS

	Clinical Features		Neuroradiologic Features		
	Temporal Profile	Level of Alertness	No. of Lesions	Location of Lesions	Type of Lesions
Cerebral toxoplasmosis	Days	Reduced	Multiple	Basal ganglia cortex	Spheric, ring-enhancing Edema Mass effect
Primary CNS lymphoma	Days to weeks	Preserved	One or few	Periventricular, subependymal	Irregular, diffuse Less intensely enhancing Less edema than toxoplasmosis

Progressive multifocal leukoencephalopathy	Weeks to month	Preserved	Multiple	White matter, adjacent to cortex	No mass effect (loss of volume)
					No enhancement
					MRI characteristics:
					  High T_2 signal
					  Low T_1 signal

the epidemic, this disorder was clearly the most common focal cerebral disease and likely remains so in some parts of the developed world, with an earlier incidence ranging from 5 to 20% of patients with late AIDS. In the 1980s, reactivated CNS disease complicated the course of about one-third of AIDS patients with previous exposure to the organism, as evidenced by seropositivity (42). In recent years, this disease has been reduced in both its absolute (likely related partially to the influence of HAART) and relative (related to the widespread use of trimethoprim–sulfamethoxazole prophylaxis against *Pneumocystis* pneumonia) incidence (44–49). The disorder is now less common in the United States than it was 10 years ago, and it may also be less common than PCNSL or PML, although this awaits more extensive surveillance data. Nonetheless, cerebral toxoplasmosis is still an important diagnostic consideration in late HIV-1 infection.

Diagnosis is suspected on the basis of the clinical picture, supported by neuroimaging and serologic findings, and "presumptively" established by a favorable response to a trial of therapy. *Toxoplasma* abscesses characteristically localize to the cerebral cortex or the diencephalic nuclei (basal ganglia and thalamus), less commonly to the cerebellum, and rarely to the brainstem or spinal cord. Clinically, patients usually manifest focal cerebral deficits referable to the location of these abscesses (e.g., hemiparesis, aphasia, ataxia, hemisensory loss, hemianopic visual field loss or seizures, and less commonly with asymmetric movement disorders or ataxia and, rarely, transverse myelitis or cauda equina syndrome) (43, 50–60). Focal deficits evolve over several days. Lethargy is common even with only a few macroscopic lesions. Fever and headache can occur, although less commonly. In addition, unusual patients may present with a diffuse ("encephalitic") form of toxoplasmosis with multiple microabscesses in which the sensorium is altered with minimal focal features (61).

As diagramed in Figure 30.1, neuroimaging is a critical step in pursuing the diagnosis of the focal brain disorders. Both computed tomography (CT) and magnetic resonance imaging (MRI) usually show contrast ring-enhancing spheric lesions in the basal ganglia or cortex (Fig. 30.2) (62, 63). Of these methods, MRI is preferred because of its greater sensitivity. Lesions are usually surrounded by edema and exhibit some mass effect. When the neuroimaging findings are compatible with toxoplasmosis, the next most important variable is the blood anti–*Toxoplasma* serologic study. Because toxoplasmosis almost always represents reactivation of a previously quiescent infection, the presence of serum immunoglobulin G (IgG) antibodies against the organism indicates susceptibility to reactivated infection, and, conversely, the absence of antibody markedly (although not absolutely) decreases the likelihood of cerebral toxoplasmosis. These considerations are independent of changing antibody titers, which can rise, fall, or remain unchanged at the onset of reactivated disease in AIDS patients (43). Whether or not patients are taking prophylactic trimethoprim–sulfamethoxazole also bears on the probability of the diagnosis (46). In general, in patients with suggestive scans (single or multiple ring-enhancing lesions) and positive blood serologic studies, the usual practice is to treat for toxoplasmosis and to establish a *presumptive* diagnosis when patients respond clinically and as demonstrated by neuroimaging. Only when patients fail to respond are other studies, including brain biopsy, undertaken to seek an alternative diagnosis. Fortunately, the efficacy of current anti–*Toxoplasma* therapy is such that when this pathway is followed, biopsy is rarely needed to establish a diagnosis of toxoplasmosis. Specifics of therapy are discussed in detail in Chapter 15. Patients usually respond clinically within a few days and radiographically within a week or so (Fig. 30.3). Concomitant use of *corticosteroids should be avoided* unless cerebral edema is sufficient to threaten brain herniation. Because PCNSL and other inflammatory illnesses may clinically improve with steroids, the use of these agents may obscure the interpretation of the therapeutic trial.

CSF analysis is usually not undertaken because of mass effect and because standard serologic tests and cultures are not helpful. More recently, PCR DNA amplification to detect *Toxoplasma gondii* nucleic acid has been applied to CSF in this setting (46). Although promising and seemingly relatively specific, PCR is not highly sensitive. If this method become widely available, it may prove useful in some patients, although likely most patients will continue to be diagnosed

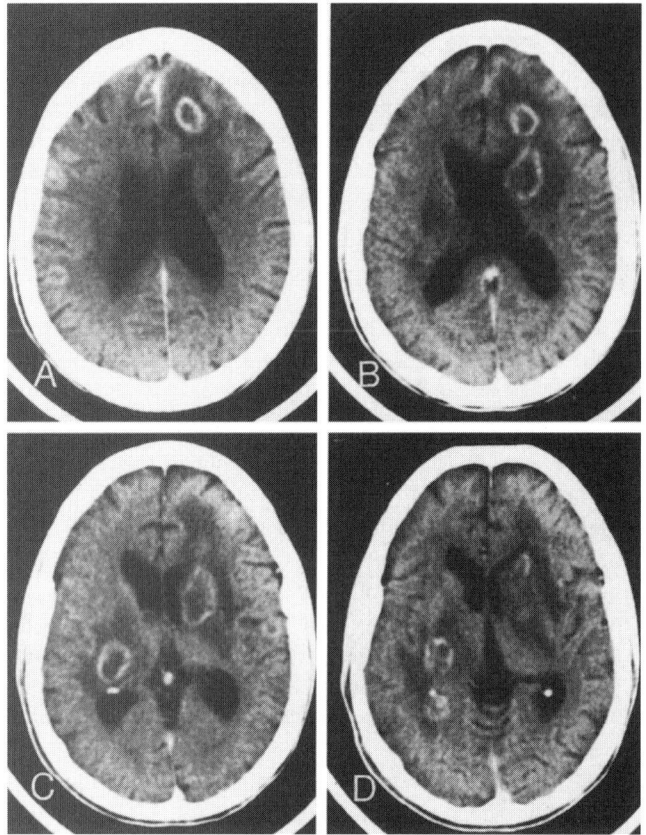

Figure 30.2. **Cerebral toxoplasmosis at presentation.** Computed tomography scans with contract enhancement are from a 33-year-old man with a 3-day history of fever, confusion, somnolence, and a mild left hemiparesis. The scans reveal multpile ring-enhancing lesions in the left basal ganglia, right thalamus, and left frontal white matter. One sees significant associated edema.

by the current sequence of studies and therapeutic trial. Functional neuroimaging using single photon emission CT (SPECT) or positron emission tomography (PET) to examine blood flow or glucose use has been shown to be useful in distinguishing toxoplasmosis lesions ("cold" on these metabolic tests) from those of PCNSL ("hot" by these techniques); however, because these studies provide only a small extra margin of diagnostic information and, in the case of PCNSL, do not substitute for tissue diagnosis, I suspect that their utility will also remain limited, although some other investigators disagree (63–66).

PRIMARY CENTRAL NERVOUS SYSTEM LYMPHOMA

PCNSL is the principal diagnostic alternative to toxoplasmosis to be considered in patients presenting with focal CNS symptoms and signs related to a brain mass lesion (67–75) (see also Chaps. 27 and 28). This disorder is an opportunistic neoplasm of B-cell origin; virtually all contain Epstein–Barr virus (EBV) genetic material. PCNSL occurs late in the course of HIV-1 infection, at the same stage as toxoplasmosis, in patients with marked CD4+ cell depletion. Some clinical differences tend to occur, although these are often too closely overlapping to predict diagnosis in more than half

these patients (see Table 30.2). The tempo of disease evolution is usually slower in PCNSL, with symptoms insidiously worsening over a few weeks rather than within hours or days. The variety of focal deficits attributable to lymphoma reflects their differing neuroanatomic localization. However, because these deficits often occur deep in the brain, patients may present with changes in personality and slowing of intellect and movement accompanied by only mild or unapparent "cortical" deficits such as aphasia. Usually, patients have evidence of asymmetric motor involvement, however, such as hemiparesis. Consciousness is usually preserved, although some patients may appear dull, apathetic, or even lethargic.

Although nearly all PCNSLs are multicentric pathologically, patients often present with a single clinical and radiographic focus (53, 56). These neoplasms tend to involve the periventricular white matter and to extend along the subependymal surface of the lateral ventricles, although they may occur anywhere in the brain. They appear as space-occupying mass lesions with some surrounding edema and are more often more diffusely enhancing than *Toxoplasma* abscesses (Fig. 30.4).

Although the outcome in PCNSL is generally poor, this tumor is generally radioresponsive, at least initially, and some

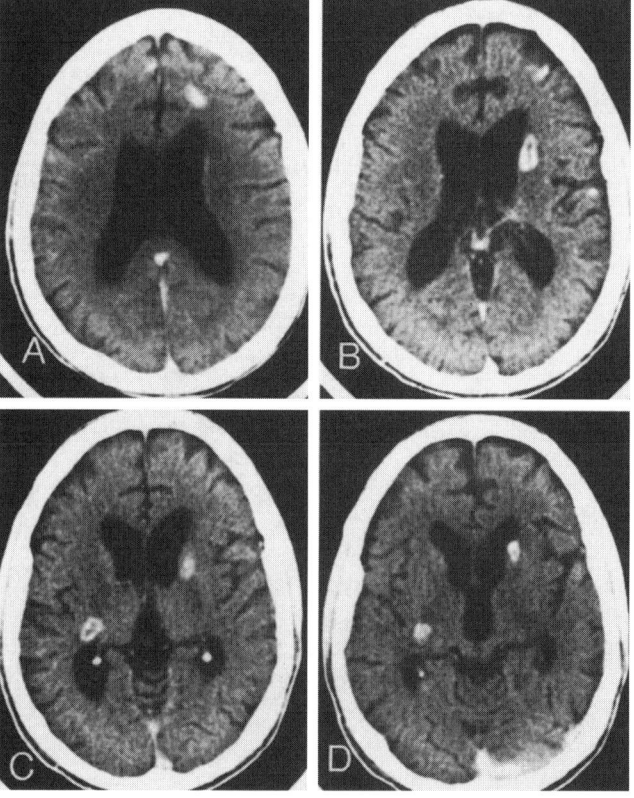

Figure 30.3. **Treated cerebral toxoplasmosis.** Follow-up computed tomography scans with contrast enhancement are from the same patient as in Figure 30.1, after 2 months of antitoxoplasmosis therapy. The patient has improved clinically. The scans demonstrate partial resolution of the lesion. Note both the diminution of size and the greater density of contrast enhancement. No associated edema is present.

patients do remarkably well. For this reason, my colleagues and I have advocated aggressive, early diagnosis when feasible. An important aspect of this approach is to avoid a trial of therapy for toxoplasmosis in those in whom PCNSL is a more likely diagnosis. This approach is outlined in Figure 30.1. If the character of the CNS lesion by neuroimaging suggests PCNSL (periventricular lesion, involvement of the corpus callosum, subependymal spread, diffuse contrast enhancement) or if the blood *Toxoplasma* serologic study is negative, we advocate proceeding directly to lumbar puncture if judged safe with respect to the likelihood of brain herniation. The CSF is then examined for neoplastic cytologic findings and, when available and established as reliable, for EBV sequences by PCR. The latter is relatively new and has been reported to exhibit excellent specificity and sensitivity in this setting (46), although this finding needs to be confirmed by experience in the community setting. If these tests are positive, we consider this adequate for diagnosis and radiation therapy. If this technique is not available or the studies are negative, brain biopsy is then performed for definitive diagnosis. Although this procedure is often feared, it is generally safe and effective in establishing the diagnosis of PCNSL or one of the less common brain lesions (see later). As discussed earlier, metabolic imaging with SPECT or PET may be of ancillary use, but it usually is not a substitute for tissue (or PCR) diagnosis.

The diagnosis of PCNSL should not be delayed or made by exclusion, but rather, it should be pursued rapidly unless the clinician believes that the patient's condition is so severe as to be irreversible. Although previous reports of therapeutic success were all too often short-lived, it also seemed that many of these patients died of other conditions rather than because of a return of their cancer. In the era of HAART, the general prognosis of PCNSL may not be as gloomy as previously. This advance provides further justification for early diagnosis and treatment. The specifics of treatment are discussed elsewhere (see Chaps. 27 and 28).

PROGRESSIVE MULTIFOCAL LEUKOENCEPHALOPATHY

PML is the third major cause of focal CNS disease in AIDS patients (see Chap. 25). PML is an opportunistic infection caused by a human papovavirus, JC virus (named for the initials of the first patient from whom the virus was isolated, at the University of Wisconsin in Madison). In AIDS patients with low CD4+ counts (usually below 200 cells/mm^3), this otherwise innocent virus causes characteristic effects on certain cells of the nervous system. Most notably, oligodendrocytes, which are the source of CNS myelin, support productive-lytic viral infection. Their death leads to demyelination. Astrocytes undergo morphologic changes resembling "transformation," but these cells are not truly neoplastic; neurons are not affected. This topic is discussed in detail in Chapter 25.

Like toxoplasmosis and PCNSL, PML presents with focal symptoms and signs, most commonly aphasia, visual field

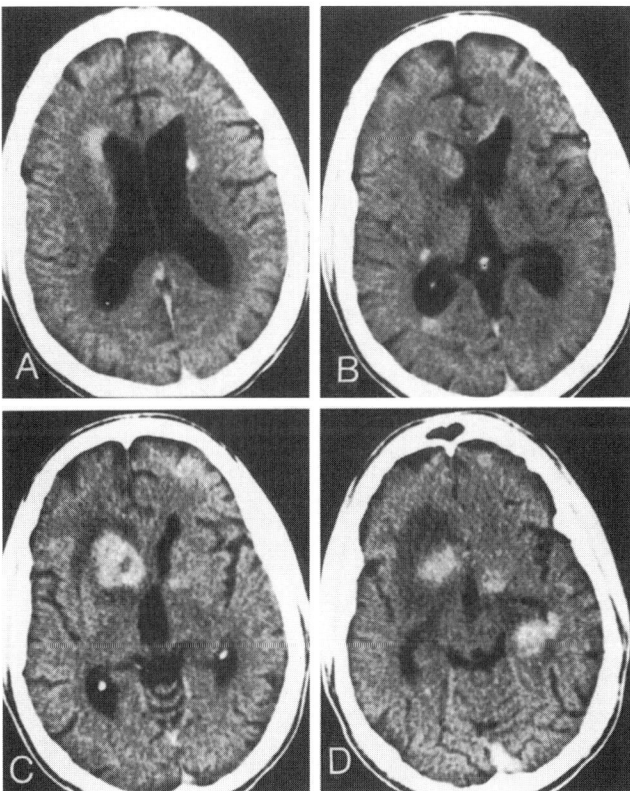

Figure 30.4. Primary central nervous system lymphoma. Computed tomography scans with contrast enhancement are from the same patient as in Figures 30.1 and 30.2, 30.5 months after his original presentation. Clinically, he was increasingly lethargic, with a greater left hemiparesis. The scans reveal a more diffuse, periventricular location of a new mass lesion that proved to be a lymphoma. The lymphoma is more confluently enhancing than lesions of toxoplasmosis.

loss, or one-sided sensory loss related to hemispheric lesions; a few patients may have ataxia related to cerebellar location or brainstem symptoms and signs. PML often differs from the other two common focal disorders in its slower temporal evolution. Onset and progression are more frequently measured in weeks or months, rather than hours or days (see Table 30.2). Patients usually appear systemically well without fever and with fully preserved alertness.

As with the other focal disorders, neuroimaging is critical to diagnosis, and MRI is the preferred modality. Multiple or single (the disorder is commonly unifocal) lesions of the white matter are characteristic (Fig. 30.5) (76, 77). These lesions often begin at the cortical gray–white matter junction and spread concentrically. They characteristically show high signal (white) on T_2-weighted MRI sequences and low signal (black or gray) on T_1-weighted sequences (see Fig. 30.5). They usually do not enhance with contrast, although some can show a delicate, lacy zone of enhancement at the margins of the lesion. One sees loss of tissue rather than mass effect, usually steering diagnosis away from toxoplasmosis or PCNSL (see Fig. 30.1). In this setting and with the appropriate history (insidious onset, continued progression), the experienced clinician can usually be confident of the diagnosis on the basis of these findings. If further certainty is needed,

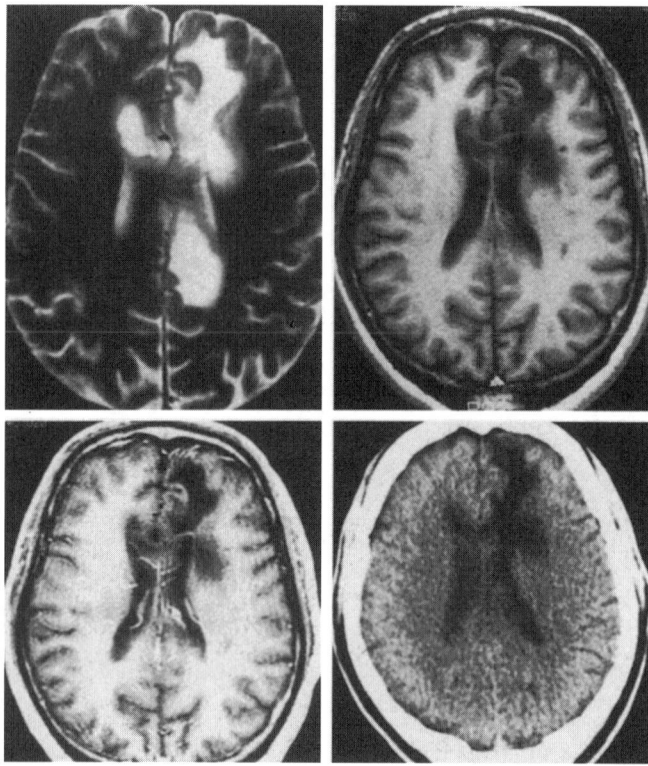

Figure 30.5. Progressive multifocal leukoencephalopathy (PML). The characteristic appearance of PML is demonstrated by several neuroimaging techniques obtained in a 33-year-old man who presented with right leg weakness and aphasia. The *upper left panel* demonstrates the white appearance of involved white matter (increased T_2 signal). The *upper right panel* demonstrates the black appearance of the affected white matter on T_1-weighted images. The *lower left panel* demonstrates the nonenhancing characteristics of PML. The *lower right panel* gives a typical computed tomographic appearance of low attenuation of the white matter. Note the sparing of the medial frontal cortex.

PCR to amplify JC virus sequences in CSF has proved useful (78–81). Although of limited sensitivity (about 60 to 75%), in this setting positive CSF PCR is specific and obviates consideration of brain biopsy. In less typical cases in which PCR is negative or not available, biopsy may be required. Although the histopathologic features are usually adequate to establish a diagnosis, immunohistochemistry and nucleic acid amplification may be helpful in some cases (82).

The most common errors by inexperienced clinicians relate to interpretation of scans without attention to clinical correlates. This problem includes interpretation of larger cavitary PML lesions as cerebral infarcts when the history of slow, steady progression is ignored or of white matter lesions associated with ADC as PML when the character of the clinical picture and the exact nature of the lesions are misinterpreted. The white matter lesions of ADC and HIV-1 encephalitis (see later) are not accompanied by clear focal neurologic deficits, whereas those of PML are. Additionally, PML lesions usually involve the subcortical U fibers, which are spared in ADC. The non-PML white matter lesions also usually are not black in T_2-weighted MRI images.

As discussed elsewhere, current treatment begins with maximizing antiretroviral therapy. Although spontaneous remission of PML was well documented earlier in the epidemic (83), this seems more common in patients begun on HAART after presenting with PML, particularly if CD4+ T-lymphocyte counts are high or respond to therapy (84–88). The simplest interpretation of this and previous observations is that these clinical remissions relate to restoration of the host's immune response to JC virus. Efforts at more directed antiviral therapy have thus far been unsuccessful, most recently in a trial of cytosine arabinoside that failed to show benefit (89). Currently, two drugs with in vitro activity against JC or a related animal papovavirus, cidofovir and topotecan, are being examined in pilot clinical trials; both have support of anecdotal clinical reports.

OTHER DISEASES OF THE CENTRAL NERVOUS SYSTEM

Although much less common than the three conditions discussed earlier, other diseases, infectious and noninfectious, may cause focal CNS disease in AIDS patients, as listed in Table 30.1 or as shown in Figure 30.1. Infectious causes include organisms from various taxonomic groups. In most cases, diagnosis is made by identification of the organism in another tissue (for example, lung) or by direct brain biopsy.

Cryptococcal meningitis is the most common CNS fungal infection (see Chap. 22), but it usually presents without focal abnormalities. Both gelatinous pseudocysts and cryptococcomas can develop as complications (90, 91). The pseudocysts result from expansion of the perivascular (Virchow–Robin) spaces, and although they are usually small (1 to 5 mm in diameter), they can expand into huge, bubbly lesions seemingly displacing the basal ganglia. Deep-seated cryptococcomas (inflammatory granulomas related to this fungus) are uncommon in AIDS, although some inflammation and extracellular organisms are common (92, 93). I have seen several patients with a clinically and radiographically characteristic focal complication of cryptococcal meningitis (94, 95). The lesions are centered in the cerebral sulci, most commonly in the high parietal–occipital region, where they show dense contrast enhancement and underlying edema that extends deep into the underlying white matter. Biopsy shows both inflammation and fungi. Patients present with focal seizures with or without focal neurologic deficits. The neuroimaging appearance is sufficiently characteristic to obviate the need for biopsy.

Invasive *Aspergillus* infection is surprisingly rare, presumably related to preservation of granulocyte defenses in these patients (96–98). When it occurs, it may present as stroke or mass lesion, or a combination of the two. Diagnosis requires high suspicion or biopsy of an extracerebral site or of the brain itself. *Candida* infection of the brain is even rarer, despite the frequency of oral and esophageal infection. The reasons that *Mycobacterium tuberculosis* is only rarely complicated by brain abscess are not clear. Diagnosis may be difficult without biopsy if CNS involvement occurs without documented systemic dissemination, although CSF PCR holds promise of more certain and more timely diagnosis (96–99). The atypical mycobacteria do not cause significant parenchymal brain infections.

Among the viruses, CMV usually causes diffuse microscopic infection with or without major symptoms and signs (see later), but it rarely causes discrete, small, macroscopic, spheric lesions detectable by MRI (100, 101). Varicellazoster virus (VZV) rarely causes multifocal demyelinating lesions reminiscent of PML (102–105), and it may also cause vasculitis presenting as delayed stroke, usually contralateral to a first-division trigeminal nerve eruption (102, 106, 107). VZV myelitis complicating herpes zoster usually presents as a delayed segmental myelopathy at or near the spinal cord level corresponding to the dermatomal rash (108–111). Although herpes simplex virus may also cause encephalitis in AIDS, it is rare, and both the clinical presentation and the pathologic findings may be atypical. The disease may be less fulminate and more diffusely distributed, and it may lack the necrotizing tissue reaction characteristic of the limbic encephalitis found in nonimmunosuppressed patients (112–114).

Although major strokes are rare in AIDS patients, some suffer either small infarcts or episodes consistent with transient ischemic attacks, which are brief acute focal events with complete resolution (115, 116). The pathogenesis of the latter is not always clear. Some may represent nonbacterial thrombotic endocarditis, but this seems less likely when these episodes occur in patients who are otherwise well systemically and when the overall course is self-limited. Autopsy studies have infrequently detected ischemic infarcts. Some may be associated with anticardiolipin antibodies or other serologic abnormalities, but these are of uncertain clinical importance in this setting because they are also present in AIDS patients without stroke. Other causes of stroke in the young (e.g., cocaine use) should also be pursued when appropriate. Hemorrhagic lesions, including subarachnoid hemorrhage, may occur as agonal events.

SEIZURES IN HIV-1 INFECTED PATIENTS

Seizures are the other main cause of acute brain dysfunction and can relate to any of the focal disorders discussed previously as well as to metabolic disturbance (117–119). Hence, the diagnostic evaluation is often similar to that of focal brain disease and includes neuroimaging. In patients with new seizures but without macroscopic focal disease, causes include CMV and, presumably, HIV-1 encephalitis. Both are cryptic and difficult to diagnose with certainty without concomitant clinical abnormalities. Cryptococcal or other meningitides should also be suspected and should lead to lumbar puncture. Metabolic disease (e.g., hypoxia or renal or hepatic failure) or drug toxicity (e.g., meperidine) may also cause seizures in these patients.

Fortunately, in most of these patients, seizures are readily controlled. The choice of anticonvulsant drugs is complicated by the interaction of at least two of the major anticonvulsants, phenytoin and carbamazapine, with some of the protease inhibitors, leading to accelerated metabolism of the latter (altered metabolism of the anticonvulsant also occurs, but can be corrected for by measuring serum drug levels). From the standpoint of seizure control, these two drugs are probably the most favored. The clinician must decide which takes precedence, effectiveness and simplicity of seizure control or potential drug interactions. Alternative anticonvulsant drugs include valproic acid, which has less important interactions. Gabapentin is another alternative with limited drug interactions, but it is generally a less effective anticonvulsant, particularly as monotherapy.

Nonfocal Central Nervous System Disease

Brain disorders without lateralizing or focal features can generally be divided into two broad categories: 1) those with concomitant depression of alertness and cognition; and 2) those with preserved alertness in the face of cognitive impairment, that is, those in patients who can be considered to suffer *dementia* if the disorder is both sufficiently severe and chronic. The first category includes many different conditions, with the metabolic encephalopathies probably the most common. However, disseminated intravascular coagulation, certain sedatives, or other drugs and toxins (e.g., anticonvulsants, narcotics) can cause a similar picture. Because these disorders are not specific to HIV-1 infection, they are beyond the limits of this chapter. Rather, this section focuses on a disorder unique to HIV-1 infection and, more briefly, on one of the more common opportunistic infections causing encephalitis in AIDS, CMV. Brief discussions of headache and meningitis are also included.

AIDS DEMENTIA COMPLEX

The *ADC* syndrome refers to a constellation of cognitive, motor, and behavioral symptoms and signs that, on the basis of its clinical characteristics, is classified among the subcortical dementias (120, 121). It is thought to relate to an effect of HIV-1 itself, rather than to a second opportunistic infection (120–122). Arguing for this pathogenesis is the uniqueness of the syndrome to HIV-1 infection, the failure to implicate another organism, and the pathologic association with brain HIV-1 infection in the severe form of the syndrome. However, the nature of the association between the virus and brain injury remains incompletely understood (4, 123–126).

Clinical Features

Unless patients present with the vacuolar myelopathy variant of the syndrome, the earliest and most prominent symptoms of ADC relate to cognitive difficulty (127, 128). Patients complain of difficulty in concentrating or attending and consequent forgetfulness and trouble in rapidly processing information or performing complex tasks. Normal mental activities take longer, although in mild cases, patients are still able to manage their daily affairs. These symptoms nonetheless intrude on patients' activities, forcing them to reread paragraphs or pages of text or to keep detailed lists of planned activities to an extent well beyond previous levels. When the disease is of greater severity, patients have difficulty in taking care of the checkbook or other affairs, and, finally, patients exhibit more general confusion. The severely affected patient appears befuddled and empty. Concomitant behavioral change usually is notable for a loss of interest and personality animation. This change may be misconstrued as depression, but dysphoria does not color the apathy. Usually, judgment is preserved until late, but some patients may be more agitated and even frankly manic as well.

Early on, examination of cognition may be deceptively normal when routine bedside tests are used, although the examiner usually notes slowness of responses and hesitancy or inaccuracy of complex tasks such as word reversals, serial 7s, or complex commands. When the disease is more severe, Mini-Mental Status (129) scores are below the normal range. The end stage of the disease is characterized by near or absolute mutism.

Although usually not giving rise to early symptoms, subclinical motor abnormalities are the rule on examination and provide a clue to the diagnosis. As with cognition, slowing is the predominant character of motor dysfunction. Rapid alternating movements of the fingers (opposition of thumb and index finger), toe tapping, and ocular saccades are slowed early in the process. Deep tendon reflexes, including the jaw jerk, are usually hyperactive unless the patient has concomitant neuropathy, and even then only the ankle jerks are usually depressed, whereas more proximal reflexes remain overactive. Pathologic release reflexes, particularly the snout response, and later grasps and Babinski signs are also common.

In the variant of ADC characterized pathologically by vacuolar myelopathy, motor abnormalities predominate over cognitive impairment (130). Afflicted patients usually present with gait difficulty, combining both spasticity and ataxia, but with no clear segmental localization and usually with minor distal sensory loss. In addition, these patients often have concomitant distal sensory polyneuropathy, so the aforementioned combination of relatively *hypo*active ankle jerks with brisk knee jerks and other reflexes, along with gait slowing and instability, is common. Likewise, most often it is not a matter of either cognitive difficulty or motor dysfunction, but rather a varying combination of the two. Moreover, although pathologically the spinal cord shows vacuolation principally in the cervical and thoracic cord, the process clearly involves higher pathways, inasmuch as the supraspinal motor abnormalities described previously, such as a hyperactive jaw jerk and release reflexes, are the rule. Other abnormalities noted in some patients include exaggerated "physiologic" or postural tremor, and occasional patients exhibit more striking movement disorders, including myoclonus or chorea.

Because of the frequency of both cognitive and motor impairment and the concomitant involvement of brain and spinal cord, it is useful to combine the entire spectrum into one ADC staging system based on functional capacity in cognitive and motor spheres (Table 30.3) (131, 132). The American Academy of Neurology (AAN) and the World Health Organization (WHO) have proposed an alternative terminology, referring to this broad syndrome as *HIV-1 associated cognitive/motor complex*, with subcategories referring to patients with predominantly cognitive (HIV-1–associated dementia) or myelopathic (HIV-1–associated myelopathy) presentations with sufficient severity to interfere with normal activities of daily living (133, 134). The term *HIV-1–associated minor cognitive/motor disorder* was introduced to designate milder symptoms and signs, and it roughly translates into the ADC stage 1. Fortunately, these two sets of terms can be "translated" because the AAN and WHO definitions are based largely on ADC staging (2).

Childhood AIDS is frequently complicated by a parallel disorder, termed *HIV encephalopathy*, characterized by loss of previously acquired motor and cognitive milestones, spastic paraparesis, or quadriparesis with pseudobulbar palsy and rigidity (135–137). The course may be steadily progressive or static.

Table 30.3. Staging of the AIDS Dementia Complex (ADC)

ADC Stage	Characteristics
0 Normal	Normal mental and motor function
0.5 Equivocal/subclinical	Either minimal or equivocal *symptoms* of cognitive or motor dysfunction characteristic of ADC, or mild signs (snout response, slowed extremity movements), but *without impairment of work or capacity to perform ADL;* normal gait and strength
1 Mild	Unequivocal evidence (symptoms, signs, neuropsychological test performance) of functional intellectual or motor impairment characteristic of ADC, but able to perform *all but the more demanding aspects of work or ADL;* can walk without assistance
2 Moderate	Cannot work or maintain the more demanding aspects of daily life, but able to perform *basic activities of self-care;* ambulatory, but may require a single prop
3 Severe	*Major intellectual incapacity* (cannot follow news or personal events, cannot sustain complex conversation, considerable slowing of all output) *or motor disability* (cannot walk unassisted, requiring walker or personal support, usually with slowing and clumsiness of arms as well)
4 End stage	*Nearly vegetative:* Intellectual and social comprehension and responses are at a rudimentary level. Nearly or absolutely mute; paraparetic or paraplegic with double incontinence

ADL, activities of daily living.

Laboratory Studies

Although ADC is not an opportunistic infection, immunosuppression probably is involved in its development. At least in its severe form, this disorder usually afflicts patients who are immunologically compromised (120, 138). In this sense, immunosuppression appears to have a "permissive effect" on its development, although rare exceptions occur. This observation has both epidemiologic and diagnostic implications. It implies that otherwise asymptomatic seropositive patients with preserved CD4+ counts are unlikely to be cognitively impaired and hence should not be categorically restricted from their livelihood, and the diagnosis of more severe affliction (stage 2 or greater) should be made reluctantly (although it rarely occurs) in the face of CD4+ counts above 200 cells/mm^3.

Neuroimaging studies are useful chiefly to rule out other conditions, but they may also show characteristic abnormalities that support the diagnosis (120, 139–142). These include brain atrophy, although atrophy itself should not be used to make a diagnosis of ADC without the characteristic clinical symptoms and signs. MRI also may detect changes in the white matter or basal ganglia with increased T_2 signal in a focal or more diffuse pattern (Fig. 30.6). Radiographic differentiation of these abnormalities from PML is discussed above.

Routine *CSF examination* also is most useful in differential diagnosis, rather than in directly supporting ADC, because findings in these patients are nonspecific (27, 120, 143). The protein may be normal, but it is usually mildly elevated, whereas the white blood cell counts also may be normal or show mild mononuclear pleocytosis; these elevations in cell count and protein do not distinguish these patients from neurologically normal, HIV-1–infected individuals. Similarly, culture for HIV-1 is not useful because of the high background of culture positivity in asymptomatic patients, as discussed earlier. HIV-1 p24 can also be detected in the CSF of severely affected patients, but in most of these cases, the diagnosis is readily made on clinical grounds (144).

More recently, investigators have shown interest in the issue of whether quantitative assay of HIV-1 RNA (viral load) in the CSF could be useful diagnostically (20, 21, 145). Unfortunately, studies to date suggest that elevations in CSF viral load are not sufficiently specific to use as a diagnostic marker (146). Thus, although CSF viral loads are often elevated in more severe ADC (stages 2 to 4) and, indeed, may be extremely high in some patients (more than 10^5 copies/mL), they may also be high in asymptomatic persons. Although one can show group differences between those with and without ADC, the overlap is such that this test is not diagnostically useful in the individual case. Treatment with HAART results in marked reduction in CSF viral load, just as in the plasma. Whether monitoring this reduction is useful in assessing ADC therapy is uncertain.

Earlier studies have assessed the utility of measuring the concentrations of CSF markers of immune activation in the

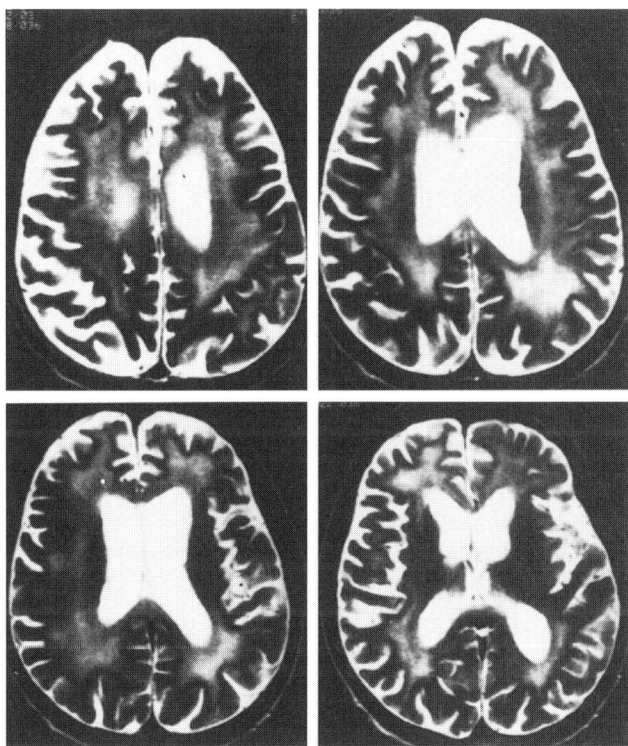

Figure 30.6. HIV-1–related white matter disease. Magnetic resonance imaging (MRI) scans are from a 47-year-old man with abnormal cognition characterized by a generalized psychomotor slowing. He was diagnosed with AIDS dementia complex stage 3.0. MRI is remarkable for diffuse atrophy with widening of the sulci, enlarged sylvian fissures, and enlarged lateral vesicles. Abnormal increased T_2 signal is seen diffusely in the subcortical white matter consistent with HIV-1–related changes.

CSF. These studies suggested that such testing could be useful in some clinical situations. These markers include β_2-microglobulin (β_2M) and neopterin, which can be readily measured in most institutions, and quinolinic acid, which requires more specialized assay (147–150). Although elevation of these markers is nonspecific and occurs in CNS opportunistic infections and in PCNSL, in the absence of these other conditions, increased concentrations support a diagnosis of ADC. For practical purposes, these determinations are most useful in differentiating ADC from psychiatric disease or coincident neurodegenerative diseases.

Formal neuropsychological testing can be useful in some cases by confirming that the pattern of impairment conforms to that of ADC and also by documenting the severity of abnormalities. Formal testing can also provide an accurate quantitative record of performance to follow over time, particularly when therapy of ADC is an issue. The most useful tests are those that emphasize motor speed and agility, as well as concentration and attention (128, 151, 152).

Pathology and Pathogenesis

The pathology of ADC is heterogeneous, an observation that has contributed to the uncertainty regarding pathogenesis (121, 153–157). My colleagues and I have previously divided the most common findings into three pathologic subsets, each with a seeming different relation to HIV-1 brain infection (121). The most distinct of these is multinucleated cell encephalitis. Although this is the only histopathologic feature that is clearly a marker of HIV-1, infection can also be detected in brains of patients without multinucleated cells. Thus, HIV-1 encephalitis encompasses a larger spectrum. Characteristic mononuclear or multinucleated macrophages are located around small blood vessels, but infected macrophages and microglia may be scattered in the brain parenchyma. In situ hybridization and immunohistochemical staining indicate that these cells are transcriptionally and translationally active and presumably producing progeny HIV-1 (158–161). They are occasionally surrounded by microfocal tissue rarefaction. The distribution of these collections is not homogeneous but favors certain regions, including the globus pallidus, other basal ganglia, and deep white matter; Kure and colleagues (162) have pointed out the parallel of the gray matter distribution to that of the pathology of multisystem atrophy. One of the intriguing aspects of brain HIV-1 infection is that productive infection is confined largely, if not exclusively, to cells of bone marrow derivation, rather than to cells of neuroectodermal origin. Macrophages have both CD4 and chemokine receptors, whereas the former is not present on neurons or macroglia (astrocytes and oligodendrocytes). Nonetheless, evidence indicates that astrocytes, endothelial cells, and, more controversially, neurons can support restricted infection with expression of regulatory gene products, but presumably not production of infectious progeny (161, 163). The restricted cell tropism of the major component of infection raises the question of how brain function is disturbed when the major functional elements of the brain undergo much more limited infection.

This central pathogenetic issue is further complicated by the observation that the second major pathologic feature, diffuse myelin pallor, may occur without notable productive HIV-1 infection. This is the most common finding in the brains of patients dying of AIDS, and it correlates to some degree with ADC. The substrate of myelin pallor is not clear, but it is not to be confused with frank demyelination. Rather, it is a loss of myelin staining that may relate best to an increase in interstitial water. This pallor is associated with diffuse astrogliosis and increased microglia (164).

The third major pathologic feature, vacuolar myelopathy, resembles subacute combined degeneration of the spinal cord caused by vitamin B_{12} deficiency, but it is not associated with appreciable vitamin B_{12} abnormality in these patients. Although some controversy exists regarding viral association, the vacuolar pathologic features do not correlate with local productive HIV-1 infection (165, 166), a finding suggesting a different relation to the virus, if any, than occurs in multinucleated cell encephalitis. Indeed, the pathogenesis of this condition remains enigmatic, with speculation centering on some toxic process or cytokine effect.

Eventual understanding of the pathogenesis of the full spectrum of ADC will involve reconciliation of clinical and pathologic observations, on the one hand, with virologic studies, on the other. With regard to the latter, HIV-1 has early access to the CNS, and the CNS is likely either continuously reexposed to the virus or has ongoing persistent local infection. In either case, factors other than simple "opportunity" for CNS infection clearly underlie the development subsequent productive brain infection and brain dysfunction. The three major candidates for important modifying factors are 1) immunosuppression with loss of anti–HIV-1 defenses, 2) immune activation with upregulation of certain cytokines and chemokines, and 3) alterations in the character of the virus. All these factors may well be operant and, indeed, interactive.

The finding that more severe ADC occurs in the setting of immunosuppression suggests that the loss of host defenses against HIV-1 may be important in allowing CNS replication to occur. In this sense, CNS HIV-1 infection may be considered an opportunistic infection that "creates" its own opportunity. Yet immunosuppression and viremia are not the only prerequisites for severe ADC and HIV-1 encephalitis because many patients with high plasma viral loads and low CD4+ cell counts remain neurologically normal.

Because brain infection alone does not appear to explain brain injury, leading hypotheses regarding the links between infection and ADC center on an intermediary role for cytokines and endogenous neurotoxic pathways (4, 125, 167, 168). This linkage is supported by studies of CSF, autopsied brain, and cell culture model systems. These studies have identified certain viral gene products that could act as signal molecules initiating disease. Most attention in this regard has centered on the viral envelope glycoprotein, gp120, as the predominant molecule, although studies have also implicated gp41, and the viral *tat* and *nef* gene products. Putative intermediates in the pathway have included tumor necrosis-α, nitric oxide, and quinolinic acid, among others. The *N*-methyl-D-aspartate (NMDA) glutamine receptor and its effect on intracellular calcium metabolism may provide a common neuropathogenic pathway. The potential importance of understanding these mechanisms is that they may provide targets for therapeutic intervention, so-called adjuvant therapies (122). In fact, this strategy is currently being pursued in clinical trials.

Variation in the infecting virus is the variable that has received most attention in regard to the issue of why individual patients do or do not develop ADC. Studies have established that virus isolates (identified by culture or by PCR amplification and direct cloning) share the biologic property of "macrophage tropism" and, more recently, of CCR5 chemokine receptor use; studies also indicate that brain infection in patients with ADC may be compartmentalized with genetically different predominant populations found in brain (and CSF) compared with blood (169–175). What was initially hypothesized as neurotropism (enhanced capacity to infect the nervous system) involves, at a minimum, the capacity to infect macrophages and microglia that, in turn, relates to chemokine receptor use. Whether other properties more specifically define neurotropism, neurovirulence (capacity to damage the nervous system), or neurotoxicity (elaboration of directly or indirectly toxic gene products) is currently less clear, but these issues are under study both in patients and in animal models, including the primate models of simian immunodeficiency virus (SIV) (176).

Treatment

Although the adjuvant strategies discussed earlier that are aimed at inhibiting secondary neurotoxic pathways have a theoretically attractive role, no established evidence exists of an effective intervention of this type. Rather, the mainstay of treatment is antiviral therapy. Unfortunately, the optimal regimen for ADC is not established, largely because this issue has not yet been addressed with respect to contemporary combination therapy. In fact, evidence of antiviral efficacy derives principally from the experience with zidovudine monotherapy, which has been shown in adult and pediatric studies to prevent and reverse clinically symptomatic ADC and also to reduce the incidence of brain infection (177–184). One therefore needs to extrapolate from these data, which demonstrate that zidovudine monotherapy is helpful, to the suggestion that combination therapy likely would be even more effective as it is in systemic HIV-1 infection. This concept seems reasonable even if not directly proven or supported by controlled observations (185).

An additional issue relates to the importance of antiviral drug penetration into the brain, across the blood–brain barrier. At present, this is not known. Although it seems reasonable that antiviral drugs should reach the site of brain infection, reports have noted neurologic improvement of patients treated with protease inhibitors that penetrate the blood–brain barrier poorly. Given this uncertainty, as well as the limited information on penetration of some of the antiviral drugs, I recommend the following empiric approach in patients with ADC: 1) patients should be treated with aggressive antiretroviral therapy; 2) combinations of three, four, or more drugs should usually be used; 3) these drugs should be chosen first on the basis of whether or not they are likely to be effective in suppressing systemic infection in the individual patient (particularly that the patient's predominating viral quasispecies is unlikely to be resistant to the component drugs) and also whether they will be practically tolerated by the patient; and 4) one should include, if possible, two drugs with appreciable penetration of the blood–brain barrier. Among the nucleoside reverse transcriptase inhibitors (RTIs), zidovudine, stavudine, and abacavir likely have the best penetration, and lamivudine has a lesser extent (186, 187). Nevirapine, a nonnucleoside RTI, also has favorable penetration. Among the protease inhibitors, only indinavir has been reported to penetrate CSF appreciably (188). More precise definition of the penetration of these and other drugs is likely to be available in the near future.

CYTOMEGALOVIRUS ENCEPHALITIS

CMV encephalitis is the most important differential diagnosis in patients with more severe ADC. Although some other conditions can cause subacute progressive cognitive loss, the patient's history and laboratory profile usually allow one to make the distinction. By contrast, diagnosis of CMV can be more difficult, in part because the full spectrum of its clinical presentation is uncertain, but also because its milder form may overlap or may contribute to presentation of ADC. A few features of more severe CMV encephalitis may be helpful in raising one's suspicion of the diagnosis (189–195). These characteristics include lethargy and somnolence or focal features including nystagmus, ataxia, and cranial neuropathies. Neuroimaging features may be more distinct in some patients and may include periventricular signal change or enhancement (196). Although the CSF is usually indistinguishable from that of ADC, some patients have polymorphonuclear pleocytosis. When these clinical and laboratory findings are not present, diagnosis using routine studies is difficult. Fortunately, CSF PCR or bDNA detection of CMV sequences appears to provide a useful adjunct and likely is both sensitive and specific (197–199). Because of the specific treatment implications (see Chap. 23), I generally recommend CMV PCR of the CSF when any of the foregoing features are present or if the patients being evaluated for ADC have other atypical features.

MENINGITIS AND HEADACHE

The most important cause of meningitis in AIDS patients is *Cryptococcus neoformans*, which earlier in the epidemic was estimated to complicate the course in 5 to 15% of AIDS patients (see Chap. 22) (200–202). Clinical presentation varies widely from nearly asymptomatic infection to a more characteristic picture of meningitis with headache, nausea, vomiting, and confusion. Usually, patients have a history of low-grade fever, malaise, and headache in the days or weeks preceding diagnosis. In parallel with the clinical spectrum, the CSF profile varies; it may include no cells and little or no perturbation in the protein or glucose levels, or it may demonstrate a more vigorous mononuclear pleocytosis with a concomitant increase in protein and modest glucose depression. However, irrespective of the cellular and protein profile, the cryptococcal antigen is almost universally positive. Likewise, cryptococcal antigen is almost always present in the serum, thereby providing a screen for patients in whom the diagnostic suspicion is low or for whom a lumbar puncture is contraindicated or refused. Focal complications of cryptococcal meningitis were discussed earlier.

Probably, the second most common type of meningitis in HIV-1–infected patients is the so-called "aseptic meningitis," which is speculated to be caused by HIV-1 itself (203). This occurs most commonly during the period of transition from asymptomatic to symptomatic systemic infection, as the CD4+ count is falling into the AIDS range. Both acute and chronic forms of this condition have been identified. Symptoms are typical of a benign meningitis with headache and photophobia. The CSF demonstrates a mononuclear pleocytosis with mildly elevated protein levels and normal or mildly depressed glucose levels. One reservation about this condition (diagnosed by the coexistence of headache and pleocytosis) concerns its relation to the background, asymptomatic pleocytosis found in other HIV-1–infected individuals. This is further confused by some patients who present with a similar headache, but no cells in the CSF. The latter has been referred to as *HIV headache* (204, 205). At times, this type of headache indicates the onset of systemic infection, such as *Pneumocystis* pneumonia, giving rise to the speculation that systemic cytokine release may be involved in pathogenesis. In other cases, it is an isolated symptom. Is aseptic meningitis really a distinct entity, or does it simply represent the coincidence of background pleocytosis related to HIV-1 infection and headache that involves other mechanisms? Whatever the cause, pleocytosis may respond to HAART, although how this affects headache has not been examined. Otherwise, the treatment of the latter is generally symptomatic and empiric, relying on therapies used in the prevention of migraine (tricyclic antidepressants, calcium channel blockers, and so forth) and analgesics.

Other important causes of meningitis are relatively rare. Although meningitis due to *Mycobacterium tuberculosis* complicates systemic infection in HIV-1–infected patients, it remains surprisingly uncommon and may pursue an atypically indolent clinical course compared with non–HIV-1–infected populations (206) (see Chap. 16). Other fungal infections such as coccidioidomycosis (207–210) and histoplasmosis (210, 211) may cause chronic meningitis in patients with environmental exposure (see Chap. 22). Although it is not strictly an opportunistic infection, the epidemiology of neurosyphilis overlaps with that of HIV-1 infection, and the latter may both confuse diagnosis and alter its course (see Chap. 18) (212).

Peripheral Nervous System Disease in Late HIV-1 Infection

Several types of neuropathy can complicate the late phase of HIV-1 infection (35, 213). The most common of these is the *distal sensory polyneuropathy* (DSPN) (214, 215) This is an axonal neuropathy, and although it is suspected to relate in some fundamental way to HIV-1, its cause and pathogenesis remain unknown. HIV-1 infection has only occasionally been identified in peripheral nerves, and then only in macrophages. Macrophage infection has also been identified in sensory and autonomic ganglia (205, 215–217). The most favored explanation of pathogenesis parallels that proposed for ADC and involves cytokine-mediated neurotoxicity (218).

Afflicted patients usually complain of burning or painful dysesthesia of the feet. In most cases, this problem is mild and tolerable, but in a few patients the pain may be so severe as to preclude walking. Pain and paresthesias usually begin on the underside of the toes or ball of the foot and ascend symmetrically in a circumferential, "stocking" distribution. When they extend to or above the ankle, similar sensations may also manifest in the fingers. Sensory symptoms usually far exceed either sensory or motor dysfunction, and thus walking is altered because of discomfort, rather than because of sensory ataxia. Indeed, impairment in walking is more often related to coincident vacuolar myelopathy than to the neuropathy itself.

A second type of sensory neuropathy that may be difficult to distinguish from the aforementioned "HIV-related" DSPN is the toxic axonal neuropathy caused by some of the antiretroviral nucleosides, including, in order of incidence, zalcitabine (ddC), didanosine (ddI), and stavudine (d4T)—the so-called "d" drugs (219–225). These are dose-related axonal neuropathies that usually present with what some patients relate initially as either "aching" or "bruise-like" discomfort of the feet or the more typical dysesthesias described previously. The neuropathy is speculated to be caused by a toxic effect of these drugs on neuronal mitochondrion DNA polymerase. Unfortunately, laboratory tests, including electromyography, are not usually helpful in distinguishing this condition from HIV-related DSPN, and the clinician must rely on the clinical setting, including onset within weeks or a few months of starting the drugs and remission when the drugs are stopped. If recognized at onset, the toxic neuropathies are reversible; however, improvement may not begin for several weeks.

Otherwise, treatment of both these neuropathies is largely symptomatic and is borrowed from strategies found effective in other painful neuropathies; amitriptyline or another tricyclic antidepressant is usually the most effective medication (226). This agent should be initiated at low doses and gradually escalated. More recently, gabapentin has gained favor, based largely on word-of-mouth reports (227). Other medications are less helpful. Occasional patients may have a lancinating or "stabbing" component of pain that may respond to carbamazepine or phenytoin. I have found neither mexiletine nor capsaicin to be useful.

Far less common, but clinically important because of its devastating morbidity and its potential for treatment, is the *polyradiculopathy* caused by CMV (189, 228, 229) (see Chap. 23). This disorder usually presents subacutely with back and radicular pain involving lumbosacral roots, along with bladder and bowel dysfunction, and ascending weakness and sensory loss. Analysis of CSF shows a characteristic, and pathognomonic in this setting, polymorphonuclear cell–predominant pleocytosis. CMV can be isolated by culture, or more conveniently and sensitively, it can be detected by PCR in the CSF. Early recognition is important because prompt treatment can arrest and, to some extent, reverse the condition (230).

HIV-1 infection can also be complicated by two types of mononeuritis multiplex (affliction of multiple independent nerves) (231). The first of these is a more circumscribed and benign disorder that occurs earlier in infection at the time when CD4+ cells are falling to the range of 200 cells/mm^3; this may relate to vasculitis involving immune complexes or other immunopathologic processes. The second type is more aggressive and can be lethal when untreated. It occurs later in the course, when CD4+ cells are severely depressed, and it presents with patchy neurogenic weakness, often involving nerves supplying the shoulder girdle, although peripheral nerves in any location are at risk. Compelling evidence suggests that this multifocal neuropathy is caused by CMV infection of peripheral nerve (229, 232). Diagnosis may be difficult because CMV PCR of the CSF may not be positive. In these patients, one should rely on clinical recognition, supported by electromyographic documentation to begin empiric anti-CMV therapy. These patients can sustain a gratifying, albeit slow, recovery of function.

Other neuritides include facial palsy with or without aseptic meningitis, herpes zoster, and compression of nerve or invasion by extraspinal, spinal, or meningeal lymphoma. Facial palsy may be clinically indistinguishable from idiopathic Bell's palsy and may have a self-limiting course with good likelihood of significant recovery (233, 234). It is difficult to understand fully why herpes zoster is so common in the middle phases HIV-1 infection but increases neither in frequency nor in severity as immunosuppression worsens; it is usually benign even in the later phases of HIV-1 infection, with recovery accompanied by little or only subclinical sensory and motor deficits (235–240) (see Chap. 24). Postherpetic neuralgia may also occur, as may the CNS complications discussed earlier. Meningeal lymphoma complicates systemic lymphoma and hence may occur both early and late in HIV-1 infection (241–243).

MYOPATHIES

Several myopathies have been identified in AIDS patients, with severities ranging from asymptomatic elevation of serum creatinine kinase to severe proximal weakness (35, 244–246). Unfortunately, a fully satisfying, coherent scheme of classification related to etiology and pathogenesis has not emerged. Histologically, abnormalities may include an inflammatory myopathic process resembling polymyositis as well as noninflammatory disease with or without nemaline rods. How these relate to each other and to the underlying processes responsible remains uncertain. Simpson and colleagues (245) reported seeming therapeutic success with corticosteroid treatment, a finding suggesting immunopathologic processes even without overt inflammatory changes. Whether plasma exchange or intravenous immunoglobulin will also be therapeutically useful and less hazardous awaits study.

Infectious myopathies can also occur. Toxoplasmosis can infect skeletal muscle, either asymptomatically or presenting with weakness and wasting, myalgias, and high serum creatinine kinase levels (247). Concomitant systemic abnormalities may include fever, encephalitis, and multiorgan dysfunction in the setting of marked depression of CD4+ counts. Staphylococcal myositis can also occur in this setting.

Confounding clinical diagnosis in some of these patients is the finding that zidovudine can also cause a toxic myopathy that may be difficult to distinguish clinically from "spontaneous" AIDS-related myopathies (248–251). This drug-related disorder seems to be much less common with present doses of zidovudine compared with earlier years, when this was the sole therapy and was used at higher doses for longer periods. This indolent, slowly progressive disorder causes muscle wasting and proximal weakness. Pathogenetically, it is due to a toxic effect of the nucleoside on muscle mitochondria mediated through an effect on mitochondrial DNA polymerase. Biopsy with light (ragged red fibers) and electron (abnormal mitochondrial morphology) microscopy may be helpful, but it is not invariably diagnostic. An assessment of the patient's response to discontinuation of zidovudine may be necessary to be certain of the drug's role.

References

1. Brew BJ. Medical management of AIDS patients: central and peripheral nervous system abnormalities [review]. Med Clin North Am 1992;76:63–81.
2. Price RW. Management of the Neurological Complications of HIV-1 and AIDS. In: Sande MA, Volberding PA, eds. The medical management of AIDS. 5th ed. Philadelphia: WB Saunders, 1997:197–216.
3. Berger JR, Levy RM. AIDS and the nervous system. 2nd ed. Philadelphia: Lippincott-Raven, 1997.
4. Gendelman HE, Lipton SA, Epstein L, et al. The neurology of AIDS. New York: Chapman & Hall, 1998.
5. Wormser G. AIDS and other manifestations of HIV infection. 2nd ed. New York: Raven Press, 1992.
6. Brew B, Tindall B. Neurological manifestations of primary human immunodeficiency virus-1 infection. In: Berger J, Levy R, eds. AIDS and the nervous system. 2nd ed. Philadelphia: Lippincott-Raven, 1997:517–526.
7. Carne C, Smith A, Elkington S, et al. Acute encephalopathy coincident with seroconversion for anti HTLV-III. Lancet 1985;2:1206.
8. Denning D, Anderson J, Rudge P, et al. Acute myelopathy associated with primary infection with human immunodeficiency virus. BMJ 1987;294:143.
9. Piette A, Tusseau F, Vignon D, et al. Acute neuropathy coincident with seroconversion for anti-LAV/HTLV-III [letter]. Lancet 1986; 1:852.
10. Wiselka M, Nicholson K, Ward S, et al. Acute infection with human immunodeficiency virus associated with facial nerve palsy and neuralgia. J Infect 1987;15:189.
11. Murr AH, Benecke JE Jr. Association of facial paralysis with HIV positivity. Am J Otol 1991;12:450–451.
12. Calabrese L, Proffitt M, Levin K, et al. Acute infection with the human immunodeficiency virus (HIV) associated with acute brachial neuritis and exanthematous rash. Ann Intern Med 1987;107:849.
13. Wechsler AF, Ho DD. Bilateral Bell's palsy at the time of HIV seroconversion. Neurology 1989;39:747–748.
14. Vendrell J, Heredia C, Pujol M, et al. Guillain-Barré syndrome associated with seroconversion for anti-HTLV-III [letter]. Neurology 1987;37:544.
15. del Rio C, Soffer O, Widell JL, et al. Acute human immunodeficiency virus infection temporally associated with rhabdomyolysis, acute renal failure, and nephrosis. Rev Infect Dis 1990;12:282–285.
16. Mahe A, Bruet A, Chabin E, et al. Acute rhabdomyolysis coincident with primary HIV-1 infection [letter]. Lancet 1989;2:1454–1455.
17. Embretson J, Zupancic M, Ribas J, et al. Massive covert infection of helper T lymphocytes and macrophages by HIV during the incubation period of AIDS. Nature 1993;362:359–362.
18. Pantaleo G, Graziosi C, Demarest J, et al. HIV-1 infection is active and progressive in lymphoid tissue during the clinically latent stage of disease. Nature 1993;362:355–358.
19. Rolfs A, Schumacher HC. Early findings in the cerebrospinal fluid of patients with HIV-1 infection of the central nervous system [letter]. N Engl J Med 1990;323:418–419.

20. Ellis RJ, Hsia K, Spector SA, et al. Cerebrospinal fluid human immunodeficiency virus type 1 RNA levels are elevated in neurocognitively impaired individuals with acquired immunodeficiency syndrome: HIV Neurobehavioral Research Center Group [see comments]. Ann Neurol 1997;42:679–688.
21. McArthur JC, McClernon DR, Cronin MF, et al. Relationship between human immunodeficiency virus–associated dementia and viral load in cerebrospinal fluid and brain [see comments]. Ann Neurol 1997;42:689–698.
22. Conrad A, Schmid P, Syndulko K, et al. Quantifying HIV-1 RNA using the polymerase chain reaction on cerebrospinal fluid and serum of seropositive individuals with and without neurologic abnormalities. J Acquir Immune Defic Syndr Hum Retrovirol 1995;10:425–435.
23. Appleman M, Marshall D, Brey R, et al. Cerebrospinal fluid abnormalities in patients without AIDS who are seropositive for the human immunodeficiency virus. J Infect Dis 1988;158:193–199.
24. Marshall D, Brey R, Cahill W, et al. Spectrum of cerebrospinal fluid findings in various stages of human immunodeficiency virus infection. Arch Neurol 1988;45:954–958.
25. Elovaara I, Nykyri E, Poutiainen E, et al. CSF follow-up in HIV-1 infection: intrathecal production of HIV-specific and unspecific IGG, and beta-2-microglobulin increase with duration of HIV-1 infection. Acta Neurol Scand 1993;87:388–396.
26. Elovaara I, Albert PS, Ranki A, et al. HIV-1 specificity of cerebrospinal fluid and serum IgG, IgM, and IgG1-G4 antibodies in relation to clinical disease. J Neurol Sci 1993;117:111–119.
27. Elovaara I, Iivanainen M, Valle S, et al. CSF protein and cellular profiles in various stages of HIV infection related to neurological manifestations. J Neurol Sci 1987;78:331–342.
28. Goudsmit J, Epstein LG, Paul DA, et al. Intra-blood–brain barrier synthesis of human immunodeficiency virus antigen and antibody in humans and chimpanzees. Proc Natl Acad Sci U S A 1987;84:3876–3880.
29. Van Wielink G, McArthur JC, Moench T, et al. Intrathecal synthesis of anti-HIV IgG: correlation with increasing duration of HIV-1 infection. Neurology 1990;40:816–819.
30. Sidtis JJ, Price RW. Early HIV-1 infection and the AIDS dementia complex [comment]. Neurology 1990;40:323–326.
31. Selnes O, Miller E, McArthur J, et al. No evidence of cognitive decline during the asymptomatic stages. Neurology 1990;40:204.
32. Berger J, Sheremata W, Resnick L, et al. Multiple sclerosis-like leukoencephalopathy revealing human immunodeficiency virus infection. Neurology 1989;39:324–329.
33. Gray F, Chimelli L, Mohr M, et al. Fulminating multiple sclerosis-like leukoencephalopathy revealing human immunodeficiency virus infection [see comments]. Neurology 1991;41:105–109.
34. Berger JR, Tornatore C, Major EO, et al. Relapsing and remitting human immunodeficiency virus–associated leukoencephalomyelopathy. Ann Neurol 1992;31:34–38.
35. Simpson D, Tagliati M. Neuromuscular syndromes in human immunodeficiency virus disease. In: Berger J, Levy R, eds. AIDS and the nervous system. 2nd ed. Philadelphia: Lippincott-Raven, 1997:189–221.
36. Cornblath D, McArthur J, Kennedy P, et al. Inflammatory demyelinating peripheral neuropathies associated with human T-cell lymphotropic virus type III infection. Ann Neurol 1986;21:32.
37. Hagberg L, Malmval B, Svennerholm L, et al. Guillain-Barré syndrome as an early manifestation of HIV central nervous system infection. Scand J Infect Dis 1987;18:591.
38. Miller R, Parry G, Pfaeffl W, et al. The spectrum of peripheral neuropathy associated with ARC and AIDS. Muscle Nerve 1988;11:857.
39. Cornblath D, Chaudhry V, Griffin J. Treatment of chronic inflammatory demyelinating polyneuropathy with intravenous immunoglobin. Ann Neurol 1991;30:104–106.
40. Moulignier A, Authier FJ, Baudrimont M, et al. Peripheral neuropathy in human immunodeficiency virus–infected patients with the diffuse infiltrative lymphocytosis syndrome. Ann Neurol 1997;41:438–445.
41. Bradley WG, Verma A. Painful vasculitic neuropathy in HIV-1 infection: relief of pain with prednisone therapy. Neurology 1996;47:1446–1451.
42. Grant I, Gold J, Rosemblum M, et al. *Toxoplasma gondii* serology in HIV-infected patients: the development of central nervous system toxoplasmosis in AIDS. AIDS 1990;4:519.
43. Navia B, Petito C, Gold J, et al. Cerebral toxoplasmosis complicating the acquired immune deficiency syndrome: clinical and neuropathological findings in 27 patients. Ann Neurol 1986;19:224–238.
44. Jacobson MA, Besch CL, Child C, et al. Primary prophylaxis with pyrimethamine for toxoplasmic encephalitis in patients with advanced human immunodeficiency virus disease: results of a randomized trial. Terry Beirn Community Programs for Clinical Research on AIDS. J Infect Dis 1994;169:384–394.
45. Chaisson RE, Gallant JE, Keruly JC, et al. Impact of opportunistic disease on survival in patients with HIV infection. AIDS 1998;12:29–33.
46. Antinori A, Ammassari A, De Luca A, et al. Diagnosis of AIDS-related focal brain lesions: a decision-making analysis based on clinical and neuroradiologic characteristics combined with polymerase chain reaction assays in CSF. Neurology 1997;48:687–694.
47. Bucher HC, Griffith L, Guyatt GH, et al. Meta-analysis of prophylactic treatments against *Pneumocystis carinii* pneumonia and *Toxoplasma* encephalitis in HIV-infected patients. J Acquir Immune Defic Syndr Hum Retrovirol 1997;15:104–114.
48. Powderly WG. Multiple opportunistic infection prophylaxis. AIDS 1996;10(Suppl A):S165–S171.
49. Dunlop O, Rootwelt V, Sannes M, et al. Risk of toxoplasmic encephalitis in AIDS patients: indications for prophylaxis. Scand J Infect Dis 1996;28:71–73.
50. Porter SB, Sande MA. Toxoplasmosis of the central nervous system in the acquired immunodeficiency syndrome [see comments]. N Engl J Med 1992;327:1643–1648.
51. Henin D, Smith TW, De Girolami U, et al. Neuropathology of the spinal cord in the acquired immunodeficiency syndrome. Hum Pathol 1992;23:1106–1114.
52. Holliman RE. Clinical and diagnostic findings in 20 patients with toxoplasmosis and the acquired immune deficiency syndrome. J Med Microbiol 1991;35:1–4.
53. Resnick DK, Comey CH, Welch WC, et al. Isolated toxoplasmosis of the thoracic spinal cord in a patient with acquired immunodeficiency syndrome: case report. J Neurosurg 1995;82:493–496.
54. Luft BJ, Hafner R, Korzun AH, et al. Toxoplasmic encephalitis in patients with the acquired immunodeficiency syndrome: members of the ACTG 077p/ANRS 009 Study Team. N Engl J Med 1993;329:995–1000.
55. Mariuz P, Bosler EM, Luft BJ. Toxoplasmosis in individuals with AIDS [review]. Infect Dis Clin North Am 1994;8:365–381.
56. Dannemann B, McCutchan JA, Israelski D, et al. Treatment of toxoplasmic encephalitis in patients with AIDS: a randomized trial comparing pyrimethamine plus clindamycin to pyrimethamine plus sulfadiazine. The California Collaborative Treatment Group. Ann Intern Med 1992;116:33–43.
57. Maggi P, de Mari M, De Blasi R, et al. Choreoathetosis in acquired immune deficiency syndrome patients with cerebral toxoplasmosis. Mov Disord 1996;11:434–436.
58. Nath A, Jankovic J, Pettigrew LC. Movement disorders and AIDS. Neurology 1987;37:37–41.
59. Koppel BS, Daras M. "Rubral" tremor due to midbrain *Toxoplasma* abscess. Mov Disord 1990;5:254–256.
60. Overhage JM, Greist A, Brown DR. Conus medullaris syndrome resulting from *Toxoplasma gondii* infection in a patient with the acquired immunodeficiency syndrome. Am J Med 1990;89:814–815.
61. Gray F, Gherardi R, Wingate E, et al. Diffuse "encephalitic" cerebral toxoplasmosis in AIDS: report of four cases. J Neurol 1989;236:273.
62. Post MJ, Kursunoglu SJ, Hensley GT, et al. Cranial CT in acquired immunodeficiency syndrome: spectrum of diseases and optimal con-

trast enhancement technique. AJR Am J Roentgenol 1985;145: 929–940.
63. Lorberboym M, Estok L, Machac J, et al. Rapid differential diagnosis of cerebral toxoplasmosis and primary central nervous system lymphoma by thallium-201 SPECT. J Nucl Med 1996;37:1150–1154.
64. Brightbill TC, Post MJ, Hensley GT, et al. MR of *Toxoplasma* encephalitis: signal characteristics on T_2-weighted images and pathologic correlation. J Comput Assist Tomogr 1996;20:417–422.
65. Hoffman JM, Waskin HA, Schifter T, et al. FDG-PET in differentiating lymphoma from nonmalignant central nervous system lesions in patients with AIDS. J Nucl Med 1993;34:567–575.
66. Ruiz A, Ganz WI, Post MJ, et al. Use of thallium-201 brain SPECT to differentiate cerebral lymphoma from toxoplasma encephalitis in AIDS patients [see comments]. AJNR Am J Neuroradiol 1994;15:1885–1894.
67. So Y, Beckstead J, Davis R. Primary central nervous system lymphoma in acquired immune deficiency syndrome: a clinical and pathological study. Ann Neurol 1986;20:566–572.
68. Corn BW, Donahue BR, Rosenstock JG, et al. Palliation of AIDS-related primary lymphoma of the brain: observations from a multi-institutional database. Int J Radiat Oncol Biol Phys 1997;38:601–605.
69. Forsyth PA, DeAngelis LM. Biology and management of AIDS-associated primary CNS lymphomas. Hematol Oncol Clin North Am 1996;10:1125–1134.
70. Ruiz A, Post MJ, Bundschu C, et al. Primary central nervous system lymphoma in patients with AIDS. Neuroimaging Clin North Am 1997;7:281–296.
71. Johnson BA, Fram EK, Johnson PC, et al. The variable MR appearance of primary lymphoma of the central nervous system: comparison with histopathologic features. AJNR Am J Neuroradiol 1997;18:563–572.
72. Chamberlain MC. Long survival in patients with acquired immune deficiency syndrome–related primary central nervous system lymphoma. Cancer 1994;73:1728–1730.
73. Galetto G, Levine A. AIDS-associated primary central nervous system lymphoma: Oncology Core Committee, AIDS Clinical Trials Group. JAMA 1993;269:92–93.
74. Grant JW, Isaacson PG. Primary central nervous system lymphoma. Brain Pathol 1992;2:97–109.
75. Rizzardini G, Boldorini R, Vivirito MC, et al. Primary central nervous system lymphomas in AIDS. Acta Neurol 1990;12:91–94.
76. Trotot PM, Vazeux R, Yamashita HK, et al. MRI pattern of progressive multifocal leukoencephalopathy PML in AIDS: pathological correlations. J Neuroradiol 1990;17:233–254.
77. Thurnher MM, Thurnher SA, Meuhlbauer B, et al. Progressive multifocal leukoencephalopathy in AIDS: initial and follow-up CT and MRI. Neuroradiology 1997;39:611–618.
78. Weber T, Turner RW, Frye S, et al. Progressive multifocal leukoencephalopathy diagnosed by amplification of JC virus-specific DNA from cerebrospinal fluid. AIDS 1994;8:49–57.
79. Hammarin AL, Bogdanovic G, Svedhem V, et al. Analysis of PCR as a tool for detection of JC virus DNA in cerebrospinal fluid for diagnosis of progressive multifocal leukoencephalopathy. J Clin Microbiol 1996;34:2929–2932.
80. Matsiota-Bernard P, De Truchis P, Gray F, et al. JC virus detection in the cerebrospinal fluid of AIDS patients with progressive multifocal leucoencephalopathy and monitoring of the antiviral treatment by a PCR method. J Med Microbiol 1997;46:256–259.
81. McGuire D, Barhite S, Hollander H, et al. JC virus DNA in cerebrospinal fluid of human immunodeficiency virus-infected patients: predictive value for progressive multifocal leukoencephalopathy. Ann Neurol 1995;37:395–399.
82. Ueki K, Richardson EP Jr, Henson JW, et al. In situ polymerase chain reaction demonstration of JC virus in progressive multifocal leukoencephalopathy, including an index case. Ann Neurol 1994;36:670–673.
83. Berger J, Mucke L. Prolonged survival and partial recovery in AIDS-associated progressive multifocal leukoencephalopathy. Neurology 1988;38:1060.
84. Garrels K, Kucharczyk W, Wortzman G, et al. Progressive multifocal leukoencephalopathy: clinical and MR response to treatment. AJNR Am J Neuroradiol 1996;17:597–600.
85. Berger JR, Concha M. Progressive multifocal leukoencephalopathy: the evolution of a disease once considered rare. J Neurovirol 1995;1:5–18.
86. Domingo P, Guardiola JM, Iranzo A, et al. Remission of progressive multifocal leucoencephalopathy after antiretroviral therapy [letter; comment]. Lancet 1997;349:1554–1555.
87. Baldeweg T, Catalan J. Remission of progressive multifocal leucoencephalopathy after antiretroviral therapy [letter; comment]. Lancet 1997;349:1554–1555.
88. Elliot B, Aromin I, Gold R, et al. 2.5-Year remission of AIDS-associated progressive multifocal leukoencephalopathy with combined antiretroviral therapy [letter; see comments]. Lancet 1997;349:850.
89. Hall C, Dafni U, Simpson D, et al. Failure of cytosine arabinoside therapy for human immunodeficiency virus-1 associated progressive multifocal leukoencephalopathy. N Engl J Med (in press).
90. Garcia CA, Weisberg LA, Lacorte WS. Cryptococcal intracerebral mass lesions: CT-pathologic considerations. Neurology 1985;35:731–734.
91. Miszkiel KA, Hall-Craggs MA, Miller RF, et al. The spectrum of MRI findings in CNS cryptococcosis in AIDS. Clin Radiol 1996;51:842–850.
92. Lee SC, Dickson DW, Casadevall A. Pathology of cryptococcal meningoencephalitis: analysis of 27 patients with pathogenetic implications. Hum Pathol 1996;27:839–847.
93. Lee SC, Casadevall A, Dickson DW. Immunohistochemical localization of capsular polysaccharide antigen in the central nervous system cells in cryptococcal meningoencephalitis. Am J Pathol 1996;148:1267–1274.
94. McGuire D, Bromley E, Aberg J, et al. Focal posterior hemisphere invasive cryptococcal encephalitis: a distinct neuroimaging entity complicating cryptococcal meningitis in AIDS [abstract]. Ann Neurol 1997;41:467.
95. Arnder L, Castillo M, Heinz ER, et al. Unusual pattern of enhancement in cryptococcal meningitis: in vivo findings with postmortem correlation. J Comput Assist Tomogr 1996;20:1023–1026.
96. Singh N, Yu VL, Rihs JD. Invasive aspergillosis in AIDS [review]. South Med J 1991;84:822–827.
97. Pursell KJ, Telzak EE, Armstrong D. *Aspergillus* species colonization and invasive disease in patients with AIDS [review]. Clin Infect Dis 1992;14:141–148.
98. Carrazana EJ, Rossitch E Jr, Morris J. Isolated central nervous system aspergillosis in the acquired immunodeficiency syndrome. Clin Neurol Neurosurg 1991;93:227–230.
99. Farrar DJ, Flanigan TP, Gordon NM, et al. Tuberculous brain abscess in a patient with HIV infection: case report and review. Am J Med 1997;102:297–301.
100. Masdeu JC, Small CB, Weiss L, et al. Multifocal cytomegalovirus encephalitis in AIDS. Ann Neurol 1988;23:97–99.
101. Moulignier A, Mikol J, Gonzalez-Canali G, et al. AIDS-associated cytomegalovirus infection mimicking central nervous system tumors: a diagnostic challenge. Clin Infect Dis 1996;22:626–631.
102. Morgello S, Block G, Price R, et al. Varicella-zoster virus leukoencephalitis and cerebral vasculopathy. Arch Pathol Lab Med 1988;112:173.
103. Horten B, Price R, Jimenez D. Multifocal varicella-zoster virus leukoencephalitis temporally remote from herpes zoster. Ann Neurol 1981;9:251.
104. Ryder JW, Croen K, Kleinschmidt-DeMasters BK, et al. Progressive encephalitis three months after resolution of cutaneous zoster in a patient with AIDS. Ann Neurol 1986;19:182–188.

105. Kleinschmidt-DeMasters BK, Amlie-Lefond C, Gilden DH. The patterns of varicella zoster virus encephalitis. Hum Pathol 1996;27:927–938.
106. Eidelberg D, Sotrel A, Horopian D, et al. Thrombotic cerebral vasculopathy associated with herpes zoster. Ann Neurol 1986;19:7.
107. Hilt D, Bucholz D, Krumholz A, et al. Herpes zoster ophthalmicus and delayed contralateral hemiparesis caused by cerebral angitiis: diagnosis and management approaches. Ann Neurol 1983;14:543.
108. Gilden DH, Kleinschmidt-DeMasters BK, Wellish M, et al. Varicella zoster virus, a cause of waxing and waning vasculitis: the New England Journal of Medicine case 5-1995 revisited. Neurology 1996;47:1441–1446.
109. Kenyon LC, Dulaney E, Montone KT, et al. Varicella-zoster ventriculo- encephalitis and spinal cord infarction in a patient with AIDS. Acta Neuropathol (Berl) 1996;92:202–205.
110. Gray F, Baelec L, Lescs MC, et al. Varicella-zoster virus infection of the central nervous system in the acquired immune deficiency syndrome. Brain 1994;117:987–999.
111. Devinsky O, Cho E, Petito C, et al. Herpes zoster myelitis. Brain 1991;114:1181.
112. Gray F, Bâelec L, Geny C, et al. Diagnosis of diffuse encephalopathies in adults with HIV infection. I. Presse Med 1993;22:1226–1231.
113. Hamilton RL, Achim C, Grafe MR, et al. Herpes simplex virus brainstem encephalitis in an AIDS patient. Clin Neuropathol 1995;14:45–50.
114. Chrâetien F, Bâelec L, Hilton DA, et al. Herpes simplex virus type 1 encephalitis in acquired immunodeficiency syndrome. Neuropathol Appl Neurobiol 1996;22:394–404.
115. Engstrom JW, Lowenstein DH, Bredesen DE. Cerebral infarctions and transient neurologic deficits associated with acquired immunodeficiency syndrome. Am J Med 1989;86:528–532.
116. Berger JR, Harris JO, Gregorios J, et al. Cerebrovascular disease in AIDS: a case-control study. AIDS 1990;4:239–244.
117. Holtzman D, Kaku D, So Y. New onset seizures associated with human immunodeficiency virus infection: causation and clinical features in 100 cases. Am J Med 1989;87:173.
118. Wong M, Suite N, Labar D. Seizures in human immunodeficiency virus infection. Arch Neurol 1990;47:640.
119. Van Paesschen W, Bodian C, Maker H. Metabolic abnormalities and new-onset seizures in human immunodeficiency virus-seropositive patients. Epilepsia 1995;36:146–150.
120. Navia B, Jordan B, Price R. The AIDS dementia complex. I. Clinical features. Ann Neurol 1986;19:517–524.
121. Navia B, Cho E-W, Petito C, et al. The AIDS dementia complex. II. Neuropathology. Ann Neurol 1986;19:525–535.
122. Price R. Management of AIDS dementia complex and HIV-1 infection of the nervous system. AIDS 1995;9(Suppl A):S221–S230.
123. Price R, Brew B, Sidtis J, et al. The brain in AIDS: central nervous system HIV-1 infection and AIDS dementia complex. Science 1988;239:586–592.
124. Price RW. Understanding the AIDS dementia complex (ADC): the challenge of HIV and its effects on the central nervous system [review]. Res Publ Assoc Res Nerv Ment Dis 1994;72:1–45.
125. Lipton SA, Gendelman HE. Seminars in medicine of the Beth Israel Hospital, Boston: dementia associated with the acquired immunodeficiency syndrome [review]. N Engl J Med 1995;332:934–940.
126. Epstein LG, Gendelman HE. Human immunodeficiency virus type 1 infection of the nervous system: pathogenetic mechanisms [see comments] [review]. Ann Neurol 1993;33:429–436.
127. Price RW. The AIDS dementia complex and human immunodeficiency virus type 1 infection of the central nervous system. In: Handbook of clinical neurology: systemic diseases. part 3. Amsterdam: Elsevier Science Publishers, 1998.
128. McArthur J, Selnes O. Human immunodeficiency virus-associated dementia. In: Berger J, Levy R, eds. AIDS and the nervous system. 2nd ed. Philadelphia: Lippincott-Raven, 1997:527–567.
129. Folstein M, Folstein S, McHugh P. "Mini-mental status": a practical method for grading the cognitive the cognitive state of patients for the clinician. J Psychiatry Res 1975;12:189–198.
130. Petito C, Navia B, Cho E, et al. Vacuolar myelopathy pathologically resembling subacute combined degeneration in patients with acquired immunodeficiency syndrome (AIDS). N Engl J Med 1985;312:874–879.
131. Price R, Brew B. The AIDS dementia complex. J Infect Dis 1988;158:1079–1083.
132. Price R, Sidtis J. Early HIV infection and the AIDS dementia complex. Neurology 1990;40:323–326 .
133. Janssen RS, Cornblath DR, Epstein LG, et al. Human immunodeficiency virus (HIV) infection and the nervous system: report from the American Academy of Neurology AIDS Task Force [review]. Neurology 1989;39:119–122.
134. World Health Organization. 1990 World Health Organization consultation on the neuropsychiatric aspects of HIV-1 infection. AIDS 1990;4:935–936.
135. Belman A, Ultmann M, Horoupian D, et al. Neurological complications in infants and children with acquired immune deficiency syndrome. Ann Neurol 1985;18:560.
136. Epstein LG, Sharer LR, Joshi VV, et al. Progressive encephalopathy in children with acquired immunodeficiency syndrome. Ann Neurol 1985;17:488–496.
137. Mintz M. Clinical features of HIV infection in children. In: Gendelman H, Lipton S, Epstein L, et al., eds. The neurology of AIDS. New York: Chapman & Hall, 1998:385–407.
138. McArthur JC, Hoover DR, Bacellar H, et al. Dementia in AIDS patients: incidence and risk factors. Multicenter AIDS Cohort Study. Neurology 1993;43:2245–2252.
139. Moeller AA, Backmund HC. Ventricle brain ratio in the clinical course of HIV infection. Acta Neurol Scand 1990;81:512–515.
140. Gelman B, Guinto FJ. Morphometry, histopathology, and tomography of cerebral atrophy in the acquired immunodeficiency syndrome. Ann Neurol 1992;31:32–40.
141. Wilkinson ID, Chinn RJ, Hall-Craggs MA, et al. Sub-cortical white-grey matter contrast on MRI as a quantitative marker of diffuse HIV-related parenchymal abnormality. Clin Radiol 1996;51:475–479.
142. Hall M, Whaley R, Robertson K, et al. The correlation between neuropsychological and neuroanatomic changes over time in asymptomatic and symptomatic HIV-1–infected individuals. Neurology 1996;46:1697–1702.
143. Singer EJ, Syndulko K, Tourtellotte WW. Neurodiagnostic testing in human immunodeficiency virus infection (cerebrospinal fluid). In: Berger JR, Levy RM, eds. AIDS and the nervous system. 2nd ed. Philadelphia: Lippincott-Raven, 1997:255–278.
144. Brew BJ, Paul MO, Nakajima G, et al. Cerebrospinal fluid HIV-1 p24 antigen and culture: sensitivity and specificity for AIDS-dementia complex. J Neurol Neurosurg Psychiatry 1994;57:784–789.
145. Brew B, Pemberton L, Cunningham P, et al. Levels of human immunodeficiency virus type 1 RNA in cerebrospinal fluid correlate with AIDS dementia stage. J Infect Dis 1997;175:963–966.
146. Price RW, Staprans S. Measuring the "viral load" in cerebrospinal fluid in human immunodeficiency virus infection: window into brain infection? [editorial; comment]. Ann Neurol 1997;42:675–678.
147. Brew BJ, Bhalla RB, Paul M, et al. Cerebrospinal fluid beta 2-microglobulin in patients with AIDS dementia complex: an expanded series including response to zidovudine treatment. AIDS 1992;6:461–465.
148. Brew B, Bhalla R, Paul M, et al. Cerebrospinal fluid neopterin in human immunodeficiency virus type 1 infection. Ann Neurol 1990;28:556–560.
149. Heyes M, Saito K, Major E, et al. A mechanism of quinolinic acid formation by brain in inflammatory neurological disease: attenuation of synthesis of L-tryptophan by 6-chlorotryptophan and 4-chloro-3-hydroxyanthraniliate. Brain 1993;116:1425–1450.

150. Heyes MP, Brew BJ, Martin A, et al. Quinolinic acid in cerebrospinal fluid and serum in HIV-1 infection: relationship to clinical and neurological status. Ann Neurol 1991;29:202–209.
151. Price RW, Sidtis JJ. Evaluation of the AIDS dementia complex in clinical trials. J AIDS 1990;3(Suppl 2):S51–S60.
152. Sidtis JJ. Evaluation of the AIDS dementia complex in adults [review]. Res Publ Assoc Res Nerv Ment Dis 1994;72:273–287.
153. Rosenblum M. Infection of the central nervous system by the human immunodeficiency virus type 1: morphology and relation to syndromes of progressive encephalopathy and myelopathy in patients with AIDS. Pathol Annu 1990;25:117–169.
154. Davies J, Everall IP, Weich S, et al. HIV-associated brain pathology in the United Kingdom: an epidemiological study. AIDS 1997;11: 1145–1150.
155. Petito CK. Neuropathology of human immunodeficiency virus: questions and answers [editorial]. Hum Pathol 1996;27:623–624.
156. Budka H. Cerebral pathology in AIDS: a new nomenclature and pathogenetic concepts [review]. Curr Opin Neurol Neurosurg 1992; 5:917–923.
157. Masliah E, Achim CL, Ge N, et al. Cellular neuropathology in HIV encephalitis [review]. Res Publ Assoc Res Nerv Ment Dis 1994;72: 119–131.
158. Pumarole-Sune T, Navia B, Cordon-Cardo C, et al. HIV antigen in the brains of patients with the AIDS dementia complex. Ann Neurol 1987;21:490–496.
159. Kure K, Llena JF, Lyman WD, et al. Human immunodeficiency virus-1 infection of the nervous system: an autopsy study of 268 adult, pediatric, and fetal brains. Hum Pathol 1991;22:700–710.
160. Gray F, Gherardi R, Baudrimont M, et al. Leucoencephalopathy with multinucleated giant cells containing human immune deficiency virus-like particles and multiple opportunistic cerebral infections in one patient with AIDS. Acta Neuropathol (Berl) 1987;73:99–104.
161. Takahashi K, Wesselingh S, Griffin D, et al. Localization of HIV-1 in human brain using polymerase chain reaction/in situ hybridization and immunocytochemistry. Ann Neurol 1996;39:705–711.
162. Kure K, Weidenhiem K, Lyman W, et al. Morphology and distribution of HIV-1 gp41-positive microglia in subacute AIDS encephalitis. Acta Neuropathol (Berl) 1990;80:393–400.
163. Bagasra O, Lavi E, Bobroski L, et al. Cellular reservoirs of HIV-1 in the central nervous system of infected individuals: identification by the combination of in situ polymerase chain reaction and immunohistochemistry. AIDS 1996;10:573–585.
164. Power C, Kong PA, Crawford TO, et al. Cerebral white matter changes in acquired immunodeficiency syndrome dementia: alterations of the blood–brain barrier. Ann Neurol 1993;34:339–350.
165. Rosenblum M, Scheck A, Cronin K, et al. Dissociation of AIDS-related vacuolar myelopathy and productive human immunodeficiency virus type 1 (HIV-1) infection of the spinal cord. Neurology 1989;39:892–896.
166. Petito CK, Vecchio D, Chen YT. HIV antigen and DNA in AIDS spinal cords correlate with macrophage infiltration but not with vacuolar myelopathy. J Neuropathol Exp Neurol 1994;53:86–94.
167. Price R. The cellular basis of central nervous system HIV-1 infection and the AIDS dementia complex: introduction. J Neuro-AIDS 1995;1:1–28.
168. Wesselingh SL, Glass J, McArthur JC, et al. Cytokine dysregulation in HIV-associated neurological disease [review]. Adv Neuroimmunol 1994;4:199–206.
169. Koyangi Y, Miles S, Mitsuyasu R, et al. Dual infection of the central nervous system by AIDS viruses with distinct cellular tropisms. Science 1987;236:819–822.
170. Li Y, Hui H, Burgess CJ, et al. Complete nucleotide sequence, genome organization, and biological properties of human immunodeficiency virus type 1 in vivo: evidence for limited defectiveness and complementation. J Virol 1992;66:6587–6600.
171. Li Y, Kappes JC, Conway JA, et al. Molecular characterization of human immunodeficiency virus type 1 cloned directly from uncultured human brain tissue: identification of replication-competent and -defective viral genomes. J Virol 1991;65:3973–3985.
172. O'Brien W. Genetic and biologic basis of HIV-1 neurotropism. In: Price R, Perry S, eds. HIV, AIDS and the brain. New York: Raven Press, 1994:47–70.
173. He J, Chen Y, Farzan M, et al. CCR3 and CCR5 are co-receptors for HIV-1 infection of microglia. Nature 1997;385:645–649.
174. Lavi E, Strizki JM, Ulrich AM, et al. CXCR-4 Fusin, a co-receptor for the type 1 human immunodeficiency virus HIV-1, is expressed in the human brain in a variety of cell types, including microglia and neurons. Am J Pathol 1997;151:1035–1042.
175. Vallat AV, De Girolami U, He J, et al. Localization of HIV-1 co-receptors CCR5 and CXCR4 in the brain of children with AIDS. Am J Pathol 1998;152:167–178.
176. Sasseville VG, Smith MM, Mackay CR, et al. Chemokine expression in simian immunodeficiency virus-induced AIDS encephalitis. Am J Pathol 1996;149:1459–1467.
177. Schmitt F, Bigleg J, McKinnis R, et al. Neuropsychological outcome of azidothymidine (AZT) in the treatment of AIDS and AIDS-related complex: a double blind, placebo-controlled trial. N Engl J Med 1988;319:1573–1578.
178. Sidtis JJ, Gatsonis C, Price RW, et al. Zidovudine treatment of the AIDS dementia complex: results of a placebo-controlled trial. AIDS Clinical Trials Group. Ann Neurol 1993;33:343–349.
179. Brouwers P, Moss H, Wolters P, et al. Effect of continuous-infusion zidovudine therapy on neuropsychologic functioning in children with symptomatic human immunodeficiency virus infection. J Pediatr 1990;116:980–985.
180. Gray F, Belec L, Keohane C, et al. Zidovudine therapy and HIV encephalitis: a 10-year neuropathological survey. AIDS 1994;8:489–493.
181. Galgani S, Balestra P, Narciso P, et al. Nimodipine plus zidovudine versus zidovudine alone in the treatment of HIV-1–associated cognitive deficits [letter]. AIDS 1997;11:1520–1521.
182. Chiesi A, Vella S, Dally LG, et al. Epidemiology of AIDS dementia complex in Europe: AIDS in Europe Study Group. J Acquir Immune Defic Syndr Hum Retrovirol 1996;11:39–44.
183. Baldeweg T, Catalan J, Lovett E, et al. Long-term zidovudine reduces neurocognitive deficits in HIV-1 infection. AIDS 1995;9:589–596.
184. Portegies P. Review of antiretroviral therapy in the prevention of HIV-related AIDS dementia complex ADC. Drugs 1995;49(Suppl 1):25–31; discussion 38–40.
185. Filippi CG, Sze G, Farber SJ, et al. Regression of HIV encephalopathy and basal ganglia signal intensity abnormality at MR imaging in patients with AIDS after the initiation of protease inhibitor therapy. Radiology 1998;206:491–498.
186. Burger D, Kraaijeveld C, Meenhorst P, et al. Penetration of zidovudine into the cerebrospinal fluid of patients infected with HIV. AIDS 1993;7:1581–1587.
187. Foudraine N, De Wolf F, Hoetelmans R, et al. CSF and serum HIV-RNA levels during AZT/3TC and d4T/3TC treatment. In: 4th Conference on Retroviruses and Opportunistic Infections. Washington, DC: American Society for Microbiology, 1997.
188. Collier A, Marra C, Coombs R. Cerebrospinal fluid (CSF) HIV RNA levels in patients on chronic indinavir therapy [abstract 22]. In: Abstracts of the Infectious Diseases Society of America 35th annual meeting, San Francisco, 1997.
189. Fuller GN. Cytomegalovirus and the peripheral nervous system in AIDS [review]. J Acquir Immune Defic Syndr 1992;5:S33–S36.
190. Holland NR, Power C, Mathews VP, et al. Cytomegalovirus encephalitis in acquired immunodeficiency syndrome (AIDS). Neurology 1994;44:507–514.
191. Kalayjian RC, Cohen ML, Bonomo RA, et al. Cytomegalovirus ventriculoencephalitis in AIDS: a syndrome with distinct clinical and pathologic features [review]. Medicine 1993;72:67–77.
192. Cohen B, Dix R. Cytomegalovirus and other herpesviruses. In: Berger J, Levy R, eds. AIDS and the nervous system. 2nd ed. Philadelphia: Lippincott-Raven, 1997:595–639.

193. McCutchan JA. Clinical impact of cytomegalovirus infections of the nervous system in patients with AIDS. Clin Infect Dis 1995;21(Suppl 2):S196–S201.
194. Setinek U, Wondrusch E, Jellinger K, et al. Cytomegalovirus infection of the brain in AIDS: a clinicopathological study. Acta Neuropathol (Berl) 1995;90:511–515.
195. Salazar A, Podzamczer D, Reane R, et al. Cytomegalovirus ventriculoencephalitis in AIDS patients. Scand J Infect Dis 1995;27:165–169.
196. Clifford DB, Arribas JR, Storch GA, et al. Magnetic resonance brain imaging lacks sensitivity for AIDS associated cytomegalovirus encephalitis. J Neurovirol 1996;2:397–403.
197. Gozlan J, el Amrani M, Baudrimont M, et al. A prospective evaluation of clinical criteria and polymerase chain reaction assay of cerebrospinal fluid for the diagnosis of cytomegalovirus-related neurological diseases during AIDS. AIDS 1995;9:253–260.
198. Arribas JR, Clifford DB, Fichtenbaum CJ, et al. Level of cytomegalovirus CMV DNA in cerebrospinal fluid of subjects with AIDS and CMV infection of the central nervous system. J Infect Dis 1995;172:527–531.
199. Cinque P, Vago L, Dahl H, et al. Polymerase chain reaction on cerebrospinal fluid for diagnosis of virus-associated opportunistic diseases of the central nervous system in HIV-infected patients. AIDS 1996;10:951–958.
200. Chuck S, Sande M. Infections with *Cryptococcus neoformans* in the acquired immunodeficiency syndrome. N Engl J Med 1989;321:794.
201. Powderly WG, Finkelstein D, Feinberg J, et al. A randomized trial comparing fluconazole with clotrimazole troches for the prevention of fungal infections in patients with advanced human immunodeficiency virus infection. NIAID AIDS Clinical Trials Group [see comments]. N Engl J Med 1995;332:700–705.
202. Powderly WG. Cryptococcal meningitis and AIDS [review]. Clin Infect Dis 1993;17:837–842.
203. Hollander H, Stringari S. Human immunodeficiency virus–associated meningitis: clinical course and correlations. Am J Med 1987;83:813–816.
204. Brew BJ, Miller J. Human immunodeficiency virus–related headache. Neurology 1993;43:1098–1100.
205. Holloway RG, Kieburtz KD. Headache and the human immunodeficiency virus type 1 infection. Headache 1995;35:245–255.
206. Bishburg E, Sunderam G, Reichman L, et al. Central nervous system tuberculosis with the acquired immunodeficiency syndrome and its related complex. Ann Intern Med 1986;105:210.
207. Singh VR, Smith DK, Lawerence J, et al. Coccidioidomycosis in patients infected with human immunodeficiency virus: review of 91 cases at a single institution. Clin Infect Dis 1996;23:563–568.
208. Jones JL, Fleming PL, Ciesielski CA, et al. Coccidioidomycosis among persons with AIDS in the United States. J Infect Dis 1995;171:961–966.
209. Mischel PS, Vinters HV. Coccidioidomycosis of the central nervous system: neuropathological and vasculopathic manifestations and clinical correlates. Clin Infect Dis 1995;20:400–405.
210. Wheat J. Histoplasmosis and coccidioidomycosis in individuals with AIDS: a clinical review. Infect Dis Clin North Am 1994;8:467–482.
211. Anaissie E, Fainstein V, Samo T, et al. Central nervous system histoplasmosis: an unappreciated complication of the acquired immunodeficiency syndrome. Am J Med 1988;84:215–217.
212. Marra C. Syphilis, human immunodeficiency virus, and the nervous system. In: Berger J, Levy R, eds. AIDS and the nervous system. 2nd ed. Philadelphia: Lippincott-Raven, 1997:677–691.
213. So Y, Holtzman D, Abrams D, et al. Peripheral neuropathy associated with acquired immunodeficiency syndrome: prevalence and clinical features from a population based survey. Arch Neurol 1988;45:945.
214. Cornblath D, McArthur J. Predominantly sensory neuropathy in patients with AIDS and AIDS-related complex. Neurology 1988;38:794.
215. Rizzuto N, Cavallaro T, Monaco S, et al. Role of HIV in the pathogenesis of distal symmetrical peripheral neuropathy. Acta Neuropathol (Berl) 1995;90:244–250.
216. Dalakas MC, Pezeshkpour GH. Neuromuscular diseases associated with human immunodeficiency virus infection [review]. Ann Neurol 1988;23:S38–S48.
217. Chaunu MP, Ratinahirana H, Raphael M, et al. The spectrum of changes on 20 nerve biopsies in patients with HIV infection. Muscle Nerve 1989;12:452–459.
218. Tyor W, Wesselingh S, Griffin J, et al. Unifying hypothesis for the pathogenesis of HIV-associated dementia complex, vacuolar myelopathy, and sensory neuropathy. J Acquir Immune Defic Syndr Hum Retrovirol 1995;9:379–388.
219. Berger AR, Arezzo JC, Schaumburg HH, et al. 2′,3′-Dideoxycytidine (ddC) toxic neuropathy: a study of 52 patients. Neurology 1993;43:358–362.
220. Fischl MA, Richman DD, Saag M, et al. Safety and antiviral activity of combination therapy with zidovudine, zalcitabine, and two doses of interferon-alpha2a in patients with HIV: AIDS Clinical Trials Group Study 197. J Acquir Immune Defic Syndr Hum Retrovirol 1997;16:247–253.
221. Rana KZ, Dudley MN. Clinical pharmacokinetics of stavudine. Clin Pharmacokinet 1997;33:276–284.
222. Adkins JC, Peters DH, Faulds D. Zalcitabine: an update of its pharmacodynamic and pharmacokinetic properties and clinical efficacy in the management of HIV infection. Drugs 1997;53:1054–1080.
223. Blum AS, Dal Pan GJ, Feinberg J, et al. Low-dose zalcitabine-related toxic neuropathy: frequency, natural history, and risk factors. Neurology 1996;46:999–1003.
224. Fichtenbaum CJ, Clifford DB, Powderly WG. Risk factors for dideoxynucleoside-induced toxic neuropathy in patients with the human immunodeficiency virus infection. J Acquir Immune Defic Syndr Hum Retrovirol 1995;10:169–174.
225. Simpson DM, Tagliati M. Nucleoside analogue–associated peripheral neuropathy in human immunodeficiency virus infection. J Acquir Immune Defic Syndr Hum Retrovirol 1995;9:153–161.
226. Max MB. Treatment of post-herpetic neuralgia: antidepressants. Ann Neurol 1994;35(Suppl):S50–S53.
227. Newshan G. HIV neuropathy treated with gabapentin [letter]. AIDS 1998;12:219–221.
228. Eidelberg D, Sotrel A, Vogel H, et al. Progessive polyradioculopathy in acquired immune deficiency syndrome. Neurology 1986;36:912.
229. Said G, Lacroix C, Chemouilli P, et al. CMV neuropathy in AIDS: a clinical and pathological study. Ann Neurol 1991;29:139.
230. So YT, Olney RK. Acute lumbosacral polyradiculopathy in acquired immunodeficiency syndrome: experience with 23 patients. Ann Neurol 1994;35:53–58.
231. So Y, Olney R. The natural history of mononeuropathy multiplex and simplex in patients with HIV infection [abstract]. Neurology 1991;41(Suppl):374.
232. Roullet E, Assueurs V, Gozlan J, et al. Cytomegalovirus multifocal neuropathy in AIDS: analysis of 15 consecutive cases. Neurology 1994;44:2174–2182.
233. Belec L, Georges AJ, Bouree P, et al. Peripheral facial nerve palsy related to HIV infection: relationship with the immunological status and the HIV staging in Central Africa. Cent Afr J Med 1991;37:88–93.
234. Snider W, Simpson D, Nielson S, et al. Neurological complications of acquired immune deficiency syndrome: analysis of 50 patients. Ann Neurol 1983;14:403–418.
235. Glesby MJ, Moore RD, Chaisson RE. Clinical spectrum of herpes zoster in adults infected with human immunodeficiency virus [see comments]. Clin Infect Dis 1995;21:370–375.
236. Whitley RJ, Gnann JW Jr. Herpes zoster in patients with human immunodeficiency virus infection: an ever-expanding spectrum of disease [editorial]. Clin Infect Dis 1995;21:989–990.
237. Veenstra J, van Praag RM, Krol A, et al. Complications of varicella zoster virus reactivation in HIV-infected homosexual men. AIDS 1996;10:393–399.

238. Johnson KB, Blazes DL, Keith M, et al. Ramsay Hunt syndrome in a patient infected with human immunodeficiency virus [letter; comment]. Clin Infect Dis 1996;22:1128–1129.
239. Cinque P, Bossolasco S, Vago L, et al. Varicella-zoster virus VZV DNA in cerebrospinal fluid of patients infected with human immunodeficiency virus: VZV disease of the central nervous system or subclinical reactivation of VZV infection? Clin Infect Dis 1997;25:634–639.
240. Burke DG, Kalayjian RC, Vann VR, et al. Polymerase chain reaction detection and clinical significance of varicella-zoster virus in cerebrospinal fluid from human immunodeficiency virus–infected patients. J Infect Dis 1997;176:1080–1084.
241. Chand V, Sweeney C, Agger WA. Mental neuropathy in patients with AIDS-associated malignant lymphoma. Clin Infect Dis 1997;24:521–522.
242. Berger JR, Flaster M, Schatz N, et al. Cranial neuropathy heralding otherwise occult AIDS-related large cell lymphoma. J Clin Neuroophthalmol 1993;13:113–118.
243. Levy RM, Bredesen DE, Rosenblum ML. Neurological manifestations of the acquired immunodeficiency syndrome (AIDS): experience at UCSF and review of the literature. J Neurosurg 1985;62:475–495.
244. Dalakas MC, Pezeshkpour GH, Gravell M, et al. Polymyositis associated with AIDS retrovirus. JAMA 1986;256:2381–2383.
245. Simpson DM, Citak KA, Godfrey E, et al. Myopathies associated with human immunodeficiency virus and zidovudine: can their effects be distinguished? Neurology 1993;43:971–976.
246. Masanaes F, Pedrol E, Grau JM, et al. Symptomatic myopathies in HIV-1 infected patients untreated with antiretroviral agents: a clinico pathological study of 30 consecutive patients. Clin Neuropathol 1996;15:221–225.
247. Gherardi R, Baudrimont M, Lionnet F, et al. Skeletal muscle toxoplasmosis in patients with acquired immunodeficiency syndrome: a clinical and pathological study. Ann Neurol 1992;32:535–542.
248. Morgello S, Wolfe D, Godfrey E, et al. Mitochondrial abnormalities in human immunodeficiency virus–associated myopathy. Acta Neuropathol (Berl) 1995;90:366–374.
249. Cupler EJ, Danon MJ, Jay C, et al. Early features of zidovudine-associated myopathy: histopathological findings and clinical correlations. Acta Neuropathol (Berl) 1995;90:1–6.
250. Casademont J, Barrientos A, Grau JM, et al. The effect of zidovudine on skeletal muscle mtDNA in HIV-1 infected patients with mild or no muscle dysfunction. Brain 1996;119:1357–1364.
251. Kieburtz K. HIV or zidovudine myopathy? [letter; comment]. Neurology 1994;44:361;discussion 362–364.

31

CUTANEOUS MANIFESTATIONS OF HIV INFECTION

Clay J. Cockerell and Alvin E. Friedman-Kien

The skin is affected in virtually all patients with human immunodeficiency virus (HIV) infection at some point during the course of their illness (Figs. 31.1 to 31.15). Cutaneous disease may serve as the initial or only problem that these patients may suffer until more serious sequelae develop. Because patients with HIV disease now survive longer, especially with the advent of protease inhibitor therapy, issues related to quality of life are of greater importance.

Various cutaneous disorders may serve as initial clues either to the underlying diagnosis of HIV infection itself or to the existence of one or more serious underlying opportunistic infectious diseases. In the immunocompromised host, they are also often the sources of severe morbidity, both physical and psychological. Clinicians caring for these patients must be well grounded in the diagnosis and treatment of these conditions.

VIRAL INFECTIONS

Acute Exanthem of HIV Disease

The earliest manifestation of HIV infection is an acute viral syndrome often associated with an exanthem, which is sometimes subclinical and often is unnoticed by patients. A fine, morbilliform eruption involving the trunk, chest, back, and upper arms develops within 2 to 4 weeks of infection and is often accompanied by headache, malaise, fever, diarrhea, myalgias, and pharyngitis (1, 2). The acute syndrome generally lasts for 5 to 7 days and usually resolves with complete recovery. Patients are highly infectious during this time. Although the most common manifestation is a pinkish, morbilliform eruption, other manifestations include urticaria, palatal and esophageal ulcers, thrush, and perleche (3, 4).

Histologic evaluation of skin biopsies taken from the morbilliform eruption demonstrates an infiltrate consisting primarily of lymphocytes around blood vessels of the superficial vascular plexus (5). One also sees slight spongiosis and occasional individually necrotic keratinocytes in the epidermis. One study reported a dense infiltrate with epidermal necrosis (6). These findings are similar to those observed in other viral exanthemas as well as in morbilliform drug eruptions.

The differential diagnosis includes other viral exanthemas such as those caused by parvovirus, measles, and rubella. Drug eruptions may also cause similar eruptions and must be excluded. Zidovudine and other antiviral agents have been administered to patients with the acute HIV viral exanthem without repeatable success (7–9).

Herpesvirus Infections

Herpesvirus infections may be seen in 20 to 50% of patients at some point during the course of HIV infection (10). The prevalence of infection with these viruses ranges from between 20 and 40% with herpes simplex virus (HSV) to virtually 100% with varicella-zoster virus (VZV), cytomegalovirus (CMV) (see Fig. 31.1), and Epstein–Barr virus (EBV) (11).

Recurrent oral, labial, and genital herpes simplex infections are commonly seen in both immunocompetent patients as well as in HIV-infected individuals who are relatively immunocompetent. These infections are manifest as painful, grouped vesicles on an erythematous base that rupture and become crusted. Healing is usually complete in less than 2 weeks. Once significant immune suppression supervenes, however, lesions caused by HSV may become progressive and may be manifest by chronic ulcerative mucocutaneous lesions that may last for months (12) (see Fig. 31.3).

Up to 13% of patients who develop the acquired immunodeficiency syndrome (AIDS) have a recent history of herpes zoster (shingles) (see Fig. 31.2) (13). It may precede the development of oral thrush and oral hairy leukoplakia (OHL) by more than 1 year and is predictive of progression from HIV infection to AIDS; it has been associated with progression to AIDS in 23% at 2 years, 46% at 4 years, and 73% at 6 years. Most cases of zoster develop in patients with CD4 lymphocyte counts of between 200 and 500 cells/mm^3. Patients treated with protease inhibitors whose CD4 lymphocyte counts have risen from as low as 1 to 10 cells/mm^3 to these levels have developed zoster, a finding

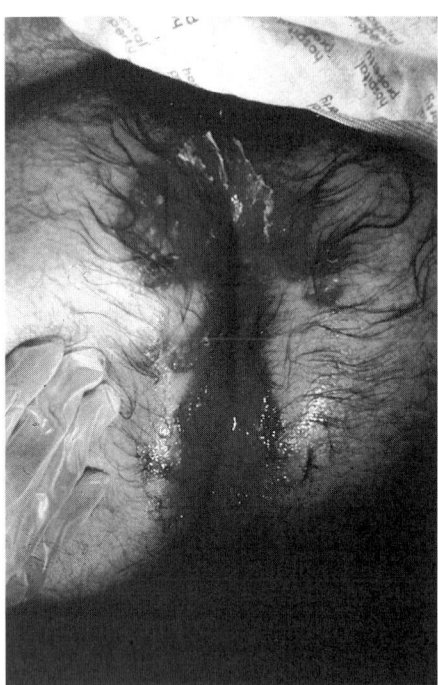

Figure 31.1. Cytomegalovirus (CMV) ulceration in a patient with AIDS. Many ulcerations of the perianal region contain CMV, but only when it is the sole pathogen identified can one state with certainty that it has caused the ulcer. (See color section.)

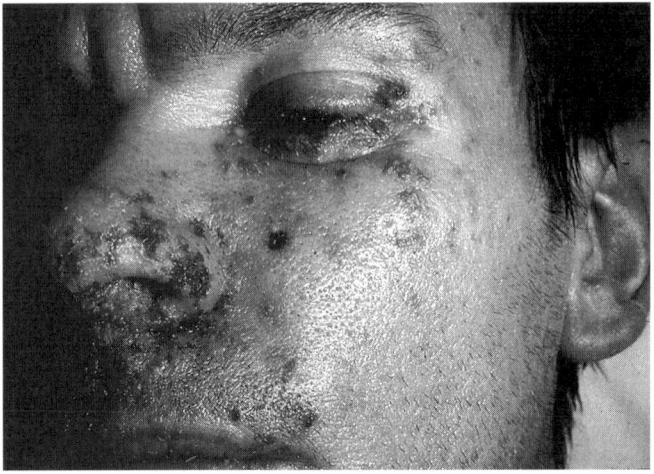

Figure 31.2. Herpes zoster in a young patient should cause concern about the possibility of underlying HIV infection. The ophthalmic branch of the trigeminal nerve is commonly involved, as depicted here. (See color section.)

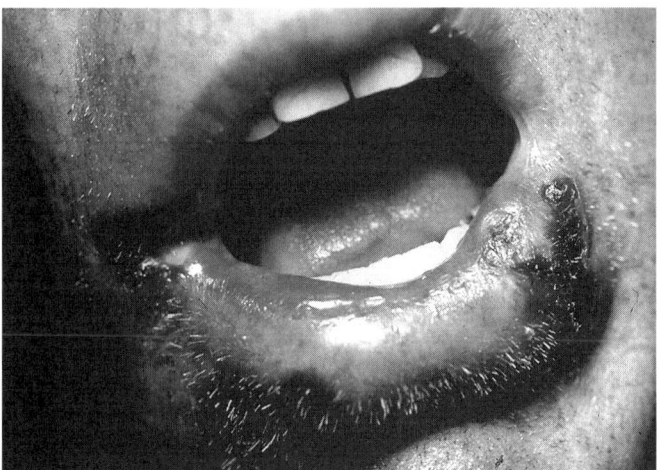

Figure 31.3. Severe necrotizing ulcerations of herpes simplex virus infection in a patient with advanced AIDS. This picture was taken 1 day before the patient's death. (See color section.)

that suggests that the host's immunity may play a specific role in the development of this manifestation.

In addition to zoster, on rare occasions HIV-infected individuals may develop varicella (chickenpox) that, although it most commonly has a benign course, may be associated with pulmonary involvement, which may be fatal (14). If an HIV-infected patient is exposed to VZV for the first time, careful consideration should be given to the use of varicella-zoster immunoglobulin or a prophylactic thymidine kinase inhibitor such as acyclovir, famciclovir, or valacyclovir.

Administration of the newly released VZV vaccine should be considered for HIV-infected individuals who are still relatively immunocompetent and have not had previous infection with this virus.

Infections with VZV in HIV-infected immunocompromised patients are more serious than in the immunocompetent host. Second episodes of varicella, recurrent zoster infections at the same or different sites, and multidermatomal involvement may occur. Dissemination of virus with development of widespread blisters over large areas of the skin may develop concomitant with the characteristic zosteriform group of vesicles (15, 16). Postherpetic neuralgia, manifest as persistent, severe pain in an affected dermatome, commonly develops in these patients. This complication is often difficult to treat. Painful, atrophic scars and persistent ulcerations may also develop after zoster (17, 18). Chronic verrucous lesions that are often resistant to antiviral therapy with acyclovir may also develop (19).

HSV and VZV infections are manifest histologically by intraepidermal acantholytic vesicles associated with characteristic cytopathic effects in epithelial cells. One sees margination of the chromatin with ballooning nuclear degeneration and pinkish intracytoplasmic and intranuclear inclusions known as Cowdry bodies. An inflammatory infiltrate in the dermis consists of lymphocytes, histiocytes, eosinophils, neutrophils, and plasma cells. Careful inspection of dermal inflammatory infiltrates demonstrates perineural and intraneural inflammation associated with degeneration of nerves (20). In immunocompromised patients with either HSV or VZV, extensive cytonecrosis of the epidermis is associated with abundant viral infection of keratinocytes and involvement of hair follicles, sebaceous glands, and other cutaneous adnexae (21). Some lesions may have extensive ulceration, so the herpetically infected cells cannot be visualized with routine microscopy. In these cases, immunoperoxidase stains and DNA probes may be useful in detecting viral antigens. Skin lesions caused by both viruses appear identical histologically.

The treatment of herpesvirus infections is to use one of the thymidine kinase inhibitors, which include acyclovir, famciclovir, and valacyclovir. Of these three commercially available agents, acyclovir was the first to be developed. It is administered at doses ranging from 200 to 1000 mg orally every 4 hours while the patient is awake. Famciclovir offers the advantage of only having to be administered three times daily at doses of 500 mg orally. Valacyclovir is the valine ester of acyclovir and is converted to acyclovir by an enzyme in the small intestine, where it is absorbed and reaches serum levels equivalent to those of intravenously administered acyclovir. Acyclovir-resistant cases of VZV or HSV require treatment with intravenous foscarnet (180 mg/kg per day in two divided doses for 10 to 14 days) (22, 23). On occasion, patients with seemingly resistant zoster or herpes simplex infection may be suffering from atrophic gastritis preventing absorption of acyclovir, so a change to intravenous administration or to valacyclovir may be effective. Other helpful measures may include local care with cool compresses or sitz baths, topical anesthetics such as 2 to 5% lidocaine gel or ointment, and pramoxine ointment or lotion. Sometimes, secondary bacterial infections of the ulcerated skin lesions of shingles may require topical or systemic antibiotics, especially in the immunocompromised host.

Cytomegalovirus

Up to 90% of patients with AIDS may develop acute active CMV infection at some point during their illness (24). When the skin is involved, CMV may cause various different clinical manifestations including ulcerations (see Fig. 31.1), verrucous lesions, and palpable purpuric papules (25, 26). Vesicles, bullae, generalized morbilliform eruptions, and hyperpigmented, indurated plaques have been reported (27, 28). Occasionally, patients develop CMV perianal ulcerations secondary to chronic CMV proctocolitis; these ulcers represent contiguous spread of CMV to the skin from the gastrointestinal tract (29). In spite of the high frequency of CMV viremia in AIDS patients, skin disease caused by CMV is uncommon. Ulcers are often secondarily colonized with the virus, and many patients have combined HSV and CMV infections (30).

Histopathologically, one sees infection of fibroblasts and endothelial cells in the dermis with overlying ulceration. Cutaneous epithelial cells are not infected. Infected cells are enlarged to several times their normal diameter, with purplish intracytoplasmic and intranuclear inclusions having a crystalline shape. A variable degree of inflammation is noted in the dermis. One must ensure that the infection is not "mixed" infection because both HSV and CMV may appear within the same section. Treatment is with intravenous ganciclovir, foscarnet, or the cidofovir.

Oral Hairy Leukoplakia (Epstein–Barr Virus)

With advanced immunodeficiency in HIV-infected patients, latent EBV infection becomes active leading to hairy leukoplakia, Burkitt's lymphoma, or EBV-associated large cell lymphoma. OHL is manifest as one or more whitish plaques usually on the lateral margins of the tongue. The surface is usually corrugated or folded, giving rise to hairlike projections. OHL clinically may simulate other white lesions of the mucous membranes including true premalignant leukoplakia as well as oral candidiasis (thrush) (31). Unlike thrush, the lesion of OHL cannot be easily rubbed off with a tongue depressor, a helpful finding in distinguishing it from candidiasis with which the tongue may be concomitantly infected. The condition is usually asymptomatic, but it may become verrucous and lead to dysphagia. OHL has been correlated with progression from HIV infection to AIDS because 48% of patients with OHL develop AIDS by 16 months and 83% develop OHL by 31 months (32).

Histopathologically, OHL is manifest by epithelial hyperplasia with a verrucous appearance (33). Keratinocytes demonstrate marked ballooning degeneration with pallor. Minimal inflammation is seen in the lamina propria. The differential diagnosis includes other ballooning degenerative lesions of the mouth including chronic maceration and white sponge nevus. Electron microscopy as well as DNA in situ hybridization can be used to demonstrate viral particles in the epithelium (34, 35).

OHL often requires no treatment, but it may respond to treatment with acyclovir at a dose of 200 to 400 mg five times a day, topical podophyllin resin 20% in alcohol applied two to three times daily, or application of topical isotretinoin (Retin-A) gel. Local destructive measures may also be beneficial (36, 37). Unfortunately, the propensity for recurrence when therapy is discontinued is high. Some cases have resolved with administration of protease inhibitors.

Human Papillomavirus Infections

Human papillomavirus (HPV) infections are extremely prevalent in HIV-infected patients. The annual of incidence of condylomata acuminata has been reported to be as high as 106.5 per 100,000 or about 0.1% of the entire population in the United States (38). Infection with this group of viruses is even more prevalent in HIV-infected individuals. Condylomata acuminata have been demonstrated in 20% of HIV-infected homosexual men (39), and 54% of homosexual men with AIDS were shown to have evidence of HPV infection (40). HPV types 16 and 18 are the most common viral isolates from anogenital condylomata. The pathogenesis and relationship between HPV and malignancy are dealt with elsewhere in this text.

Different HPV types tend to be associated with different clinical lesions. HPV types 1, 2, 3, and 4 most commonly cause nongenital lesions such as plantar, common, or flat warts. HPV types 3, 5, 8, and 10 induce epidermodysplasia verruciformis. Mucosal lesions involving the genital, oral, or laryngeal epithelia are caused most commonly by types 6, 11, 16, 18, 31, and 33, some of which are believed to be associated with cervical and rectal malignancies. Bowenoid papulosis, a premalignant condition seen on the genitalia, is almost exclusively associated with HPV types 16 and 18, with 16 the most frequent (41).

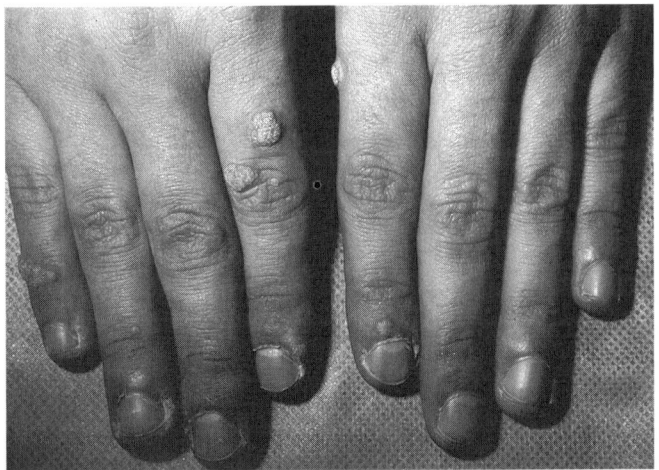

Figure 31.4. Multiple verrucae vulgares on the hands of a patient with otherwise asymptomatic HIV infection. Persistent human papillomavirus infection should cause concern about the possibility of occult HIV disease. (See color section.)

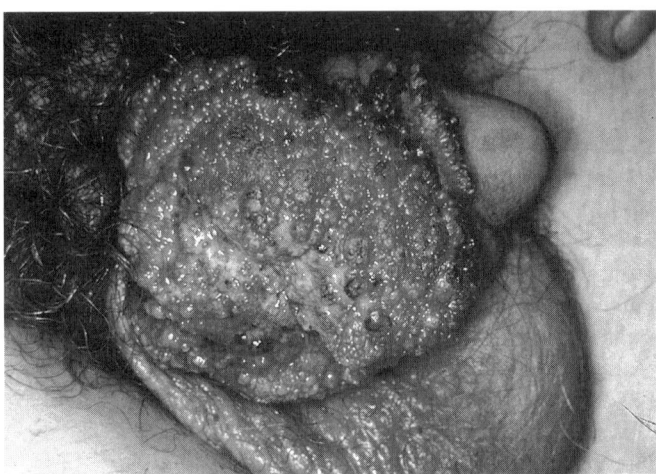

Figure 31.6. Verrucous carcinoma associated with human papillomavirus infection in a patient with AIDS. These lesions are being observed with increasing frequency as a consequence of longer patient survival. (See color section.)

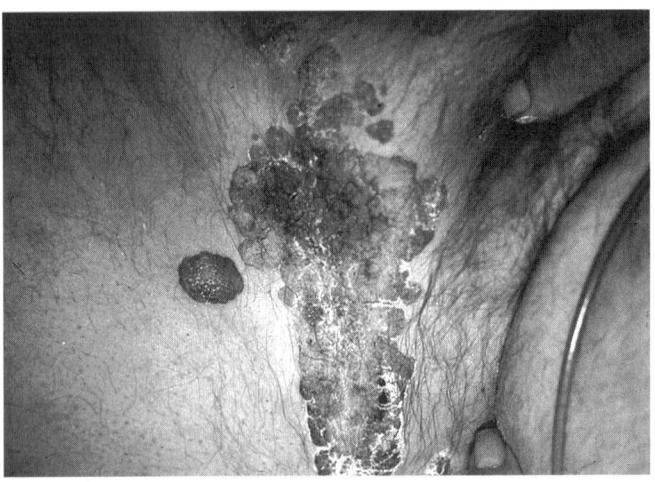

Figure 31.5. Bowenoid papulosis in a patient with HIV infection. This represents a manifestation of squamous cell carcinoma in situ and is caused most commonly by HPV types 16 and 18. Recognition of this disorder is important because it may progress to fully developed squamous cell carcinoma. (See color section.)

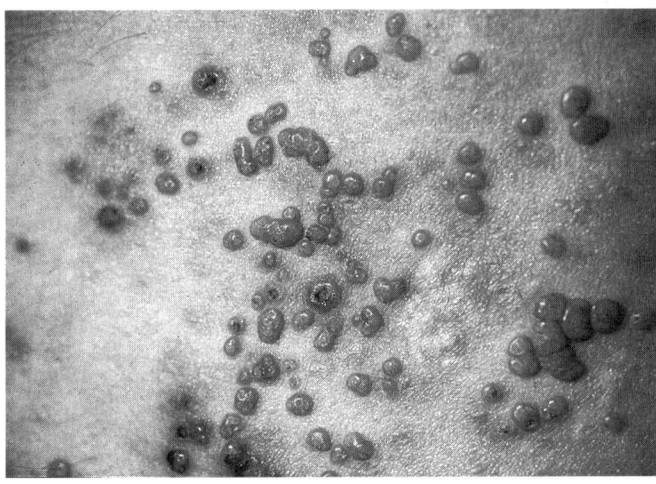

Figure 31.7. Molluscum contagiosum may give rise to multiple lesions, as depicted here. Treatment usually consists of locally destructive measures such as liquid nitrogen cryosurgery. (See color section.)

Patients with HIV disease, especially those who are immunocompromised, may present with multiple verrucae vulgares, especially in periungual locations (see Fig. 31.4). Multiple plantar warts, including mosaic warts, may develop and may lead to pain on walking. Extensive flat and filiform warts on the bearded area of the face manifested by small verrucous papules are also seen in HIV-infected individuals and may be the first sign of HIV infection.

HPV in men can appear on the penis, urethra, scrotum, and perianal, anal, and rectal areas (see Figs. 31.5 and 31.6). Condylomata acuminata are usually recognized as soft, sessile lesions with surfaces that range from smooth to rough with fingerlike projections. Exuberant cauliflowerlike plaques may involve the perianal region as well as flexural areas such as the axillae and angles of the mouth. Extensive perianal condylomata may lead to difficulty with defecation and may cause secondary constipation. Subclinical anal HPV infection is common in homosexual men and presents as diffuse foci of epithelial hyperplasia that are invisible on routine examination (42). Such subclinical infection as well as intraurethral and vaginal condylomata may serve as a major reservoir for HPV, and treatment failure in women may represent reinfection by a male sexual partner with one of these occult forms.

In women, the spectrum of clinical disease induced by HPV is broad. Classic exophytic lesions of condyloma acuminatum of the external genitalia are readily recognized by clinical examination alone. Detection of other intravaginal or cervical forms of HPV infection requires colposcopic and sigmoidoscopic examination. Vulvar condylomata acuminata appear as soft, whitish, sessile tumors with fingerlike projections seen most commonly in moist areas such as in the introitus and on the labia (43). Cervical and intravaginal condylomata acuminata are commonly seen in women with external vulvar condylomata.

Histologically, condylomata acuminata are manifest as dome-shaped papular lesions with acanthosis and koilocytosis. Bowenoid papulosis has architectural features of condyloma, but histologically it shows changes of squamous cell carcinoma in situ. Epidermodysplasia verruciformis appears similar to flat verrucae with characteristic large, bluish-gray keratinocytes in the epidermis. Atypical keratinocytic changes suggestive of evolving carcinoma in situ may be seen as well. Verrucous carcinoma has histologic features similar to those of large condylomata acuminata, except such lesions extend deeply into the dermis.

The differential diagnosis of HPV infection includes other benign epithelial neoplasms including seborrheic keratoses, pyogenic granulomas, nevi, and various other keratoses and acanthomas. Diagnosis is based on clinical features in the context of histopathologic findings. Biopsy is important in any cases that could conceivably represent a malignant HPV-induced condition. In difficult cases, immunoperoxidase stains for HPV antigens, DNA in situ hybridization, and the polymerase chain reaction can be performed to ascertain the type of HPV causing the lesion. Knowledge of the HPV type, however, does not influence the course of the disease or its treatment.

Treatment of HPV infection includes measures that diminish clinical lesions, destruction of premalignant or malignant lesions, reduction of symptoms, and minimizing of transmission to uninfected individuals. Successful therapy depends on the ability of the host's immune status to keep the viral infection in check. Frequent recurrences are probably a consequence of reactivation of latent HPV infection. Unfortunately, no treatment has been shown to eradicate HPV entirely. Destructive measures such as application of topical chemicals, such as salicylic or trichloroacetic acid, cryotherapy with liquid nitrogen, or ablative surgery are standard techniques used for common verrucae. Condylomata acuminata are usually treated by applying topical podophyllin resin 10 to 50% in tincture of benzoin directly to lesions by a physician or an assistant; this substance is washed off in 4 to 6 hours. In extensive cases, the entire penile shaft may be "painted" with the resin. Treatments are administered weekly until resolution or until significant reduction of the number of lesions is noted, at which point, secondary destruction with liquid nitrogen cryosurgery or surgical destruction may be performed. Although this procedure is generally safe, complications of severe necrosis and scarring in the anogenital area, fistula in ano, dermatitis, balanitis, and phimosis may develop, especially if the caustic agent is left on the skin or mucosa for long periods (44). Systemic reactions to podophyllin are rare (45, 46). Podophyllotoxin (Condylox, Oclassen, Ventura, CA), the active ingredient in podophyllin, twice daily for 3 days per week for 3 to 4 weeks can be applied by the patient at home (47). A newer topical agent, imiquimod, is effective when applied two to three times weekly. The only reported side effect of this compound noted to date has been local irritation. Liquid nitrogen cryotherapy, electrodesiccation, and curettage as well as carbon dioxide laser vaporization also may be performed. Care must be taken to avoid adverse consequences of infectious papillomavirus in the laser plume with these latter methods, however (48, 49). Plantar verrucae are generally treated with a topical 40% salicylic acid plaster applied daily with paring of hyperkeratotic areas, although intralesional bleomycin and liquid nitrogen therapy have also been used. Verruca plana and filiform verrucae are treated commonly with topical tretinoin (Retin-A) 0.05% cream or 0.01% gel applied daily and increased two to three times per day depending on the amount of irritation that can be tolerated. Topical 5-fluorouracil cream (Efudex) may be applied once or twice per day and may be used in combination with tretinoin. Light electrodesiccation and liquid nitrogen application may be used as an adjunct therapy. Bowenoid papulosis is generally treated by electrodesiccation and curettage, although liquid nitrogen cryodestruction is also usually effective. Verrucous carcinoma requires excision surgery.

Intralesional interferon-α also may be used to treat condylomata successfully. The intralesional dosage is approximately 500,000 to 1 million IU intralesionally three times a week for 8 to 12 weeks. The frequency of visits and expense are generally prohibitive for this form of therapy except in selected instances (50).

Molluscum Contagiosum

Skin lesions of molluscum contagiosum develop in at least 20% of patients with AIDS (51) (see Fig. 31.7). Most patients are severely immunocompromised at the time of infection, with CD4+ cell counts of less than 200 cells/mm^3. The molluscum contagiosum virus, the largest virus known to afflict humans, is a member of the pox family of viruses. The virus is spread by direct contact and has a tropism for epithelial cells, where it replicates in the cytoplasm and eventually completely fills it with viral particles known as molluscum or Henderson–Patterson bodies. These particles compress the nucleus to the periphery of the cell, which subsequently ruptures so adjacent cells become infected. The epithelia of hair follicles are preferentially infected.

Molluscum contagiosum infection is characterized by dome-shaped, umbilicated translucent papules that may develop on any part of the body, especially the genital areas and the face. The mucosal surfaces are spared. Lesions may number in excess of 100, and individual lesions may become large, often larger than 1 cm in diameter (52). In immunocompetent hosts, lesions generally undergo spontaneous resolution, but in HIV-infected patients, lesions may persist for months to years. As with some other minor viral infections in HIV-infected hosts, when therapy with protease inhibitors is initiated and the CD4 lymphocyte count rises, these infections may undergo regression.

Histologically, ones sees a dome-shaped papule with a central crater, which arises as a consequence of coalescence of numerous hair follicles and adnexal structures infected by the molluscum virus. Identification of the characteristic molluscum body, a 25-μm structure manifested as a pinkish, hyaline-resembling, oval structure within the cytoplasm of suprabasilar keratinocytes or floating free within the central crater, is pathognomonic. These bodies are usually present in large numbers near the surface of the center of fully developed lesions.

In patients with HIV infection, waxy lesions of cryptococcosis, cutaneous pneumocystosis, and other infectious disorders may appear similar to molluscum contagiosum, so a biopsy is often necessary to exclude more serious infections. Solitary molluscum lesions may resemble pyogenic granuloma, keratoacanthoma, or basal cell carcinoma, and they may occasionally be difficult to define.

Treatment of molluscum contagiosum is generally by destructive measures. Cryotherapy is the usual method of treatment and may be successful, especially if the procedure is done every 1 to 2 weeks until lesions have resolved. Lesions are sprayed with liquid nitrogen for 5 to 10 seconds to yield a 15- to 20-second thaw time. Although the method is generally safe, in dark-skinned individuals, dyspigmentation may develop. Unfortunately, discontinuation of therapy is often associated with recurrence. Electrosurgery, application of topical keratolytic preparations, and removal by curettage are other effective therapies.

BACTERIAL INFECTIONS

Folliculitis, Abscesses, Furuncles, Impetigo, and Related Infections

Most banal bacterial infections such as folliculitis and impetigo are caused by staphylococci and streptococci, organisms commonly encountered in immunocompetent hosts (see Figs. 31.8 and 31.9). *Staphylococcus aureus* is the most common cutaneous and systemic bacterial pathogen in HIV-infected adults. The initial site of colonization with *S. aureus* is the nares, and the nasal carriage rate in HIV-infected patients is approximately 50%, twice that of HIV-seronegative individuals (53). Up to 83% of patients with AIDS may suffer from some form of *S. aureus* infection at some point during the course of HIV disease (54). Infection with *Pseudomonas* spp. is also seen with some frequency in patients who are infected with HIV, and up to 8% of all cases of bacteremia in patients with AIDS are due to these organisms (55). Aggressive *Haemophilus influenzae* infection of the head and neck has also been observed (56).

Folliculitis is generally manifested as widely distributed acneiform papules and pustules over the skin (see Fig. 31.9). Lesions may be pruritic and excoriated. Most cases are confined to the skin superficially, but occasionally, sepsis may supervene. In some cases, the bacterial density may increase significantly as a consequence of immunodepression, leading to more deeply seated skin infections such as botryomycosis or ecthyma (57). Botryomycosis is most commonly caused by *Staphylococcus aureus* and represents a manifestation of extension of staphylococcal folliculitis with the formation of bacterial colonies into the dermis (57, 58). Clinically, this is often manifested as a nondescript papule or plaque in the skin that may be surrounded by pustules on the trunk, neck, or extremities. Soft tissue and deeply seated bacterial infections such as cellulitis, pyomyositis, deep soft tissue abscesses, and necrotizing fasciitis may also develop in HIV-infected hosts (58), and these infections are generally manifested by diffuse, red, warm tender areas in the skin. Patients often have extreme toxemia, so early recognition is essential. Streptococcal axillary lymphadenitis presents as diffuse, painful swelling of lymph nodes in the axillae that is usually bilateral (59) (see Fig. 31.8). When the lymph nodes are incised, copious pustular drainage is noted.

Impetigo is manifested as localized or widespread edematous crusted areas of the skin associated with yellowish

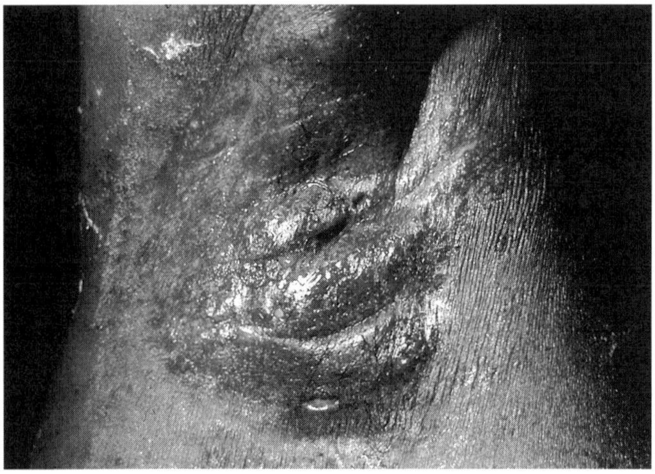

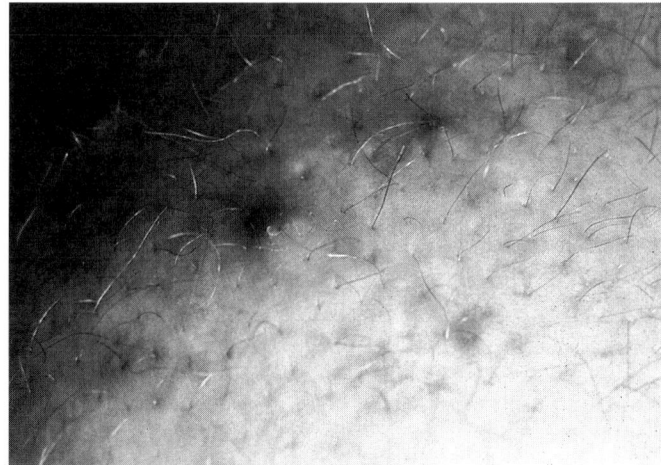

Figure 31.8. Streptococcal axillary lymphadenitis is a newly described manifestation of HIV disease. As patients survive longer with HIV infection, serious complications caused by common pathogens such as *Streptococcus pyogenes* are recognized with greater frequency. (See color section.)

Figure 31.9. Staphylococcal folliculitis and furunculosis may also be a presenting sign of HIV infection, especially when these lesions are refractory to treatment with routine measures. (See color section.)

surface crusts. Although impetigo is seen most commonly on the face in healthy individuals, in patients with HIV disease, it is seen more often in axillary, inguinal, and other intertriginous locations. The infection usually begins with painful red macules that may develop superficial vesicles that rupture, oozing serous and purulent fluid that contains potentially infective HIV. A characteristic honey-colored surface crust usually forms, and satellite lesions may develop. In some cases, intact bullae and pustules may be observed.

Pseudomonas aeruginosa and *P. cepacia* infections, frequently acquired from hot tub use, may cause folliculitis, otitis externa, and ecthyma gangrenosum, both primary and secondary to septicemia (60, 61). The clinical manifestations of these disorders when caused by *Pseudomonas* spp. appear similar to those caused by other pyogenic bacteria, namely, firm erythematous papulopustules or nodules as with localized necrosis. Cultures are essential in making a definitive diagnosis and to ensure the administration of appropriate antibiotic therapy (62).

Histologically, one usually sees suppurative inflammation in the dermis, often centered within and around hair follicles. These lesions may rupture, with secondary granulomatous inflammation. Histologically, impetigo demonstrates a subcorneal pustule with clusters of Gram-positive bacteria seen within the space. Botryomycosis is manifested by diffuse inflammation in the dermis with darkly staining "grains" that represent colonies of bacteria growing in the skin.

Pyogenic bacterial infections generally respond to treatment with dicloxacillin, cephalexin, or ciprofloxacin. Chlorhexidine gluconate washes of the skin and application of topical antibiotics such as polymyxin B sulfate, bacitracin, or mupirocin ointment preparations into the nostrils may help to eradicate bacterial colonization. Unfortunately, in immunocompromised hosts, recurrence is common.

Bacillary Angiomatosis

Bacillary angiomatosis is a bacterial infection caused by organisms of the genus *Bartonella* (formerly *Rochalimaea*), specifically *B. quintana*, and *B. henselae*. One case of endocarditis has been associated with *B. elizabethae* (63). The pathogenesis is not completely known, but investigators have postulated that a vasoproliferative factor either is produced by the bacterium itself or is induced to be formed by the host as a consequence of bacterial infection.

Bacillary angiomatosis has various clinical cutaneous manifestations. Cutaneous vascular lesions are the most common, and of these, small, pinpoint, reddish to purple papules are the earliest lesions. These may resemble pyogenic granulomas and are seen in two-thirds of patients with cutaneous disease (64–66). These papules range in number from one to several thousand and range in size from 1 mm to several centimeters. Lesions may ulcerate and may be covered by a crust. The second most common skin lesion is the subcutaneous nodule that occurs in approximately 50% of patients with skin lesions. Such nodules may be located deep in the subcutis and may extend to involve soft tissue and bone (67). Two cases of deeply seated skeletal muscle pyomyositis have been reported (68). When bone is involved, lesions are generally osteolytic. Nondescript crusted ulcerations, plaques, and cellulitis may also be seen in 5 to 10% of patients (69). Viscera may be involved either as disseminated vascular lesions or as bacillary peliosis hepatis of the liver. Although virtually every organ system may be affected, other than the skin, the liver and spleen are the most common sites of involvement. Liver disease is usually manifested by elevated levels of circulating liver enzymes. Patients with bacillary angiomatosis may develop fever, weight loss, and night sweats (70). These symptoms usually resolve with institution of antibiotic therapy.

Histopathologic findings in bacillary angiomatosis are characterized by a lobular proliferation of capillaries associated with enlarged epithelioid-appearing endothelial cells. The background stroma is usually edematous in superficial lesions and is more compact in deeper ones. Neutrophils and leukocytoclasis are often seen in the interstitium between vessels. The presence of neutrophils in the body of lesions is a valuable finding that permits distinction from ulcerated pyogenic granulomas that may have similar histologic features, although neutrophils are present primarily under areas of ulceration. Granular amphophilic aggregates are characteristically seen adjacent to vessels, often in association with neutrophils, which represent masses of *Bartonella* organisms. These appear black after staining with the Warthin–Starry stain. Electron microscopy is confirmatory. Although the diagnosis can usually be made on the basis of microscopic examination of routine hematoxylin and eosin–stained tissue sections, on occasion, atypia of endothelial cells may be marked, causing histologic confusion with angiosarcoma.

Bacillary angiomatosis must be differentiated from other vascular lesions that develop in patients with HIV infection, especially Kaposi's sarcoma. Generally, the lack of macular and plaque lesions or the presence of lesions oriented along skin lines is helpful in making this distinction. Histopathologic findings are also distinct.

Bacillary angiomatosis responds well to systemic treatment with erythromycin ethyl succinate at doses of 500 mg orally four times daily for 4 weeks to 6 months, depending on the tendency to relapse. Doxycycline hydrochloride, 100 mg orally twice daily, is also effective. Other antibiotics shown to have some efficacy include rifampin, ciprofloxacin, trimethoprim–sulfamethoxazole, and gentamicin. Azithromycin, rozithromycin, and fluoroquinolones such as norfloxacin have also been used with good response. Recent data indicated that trimethoprim–sulfamethoxazole is effective in preventing relapses (T Berger, unpublished data). Because of the widespread administration of this agent to HIV-infected individuals, it is likely responsible in part for the declining incidence of bacillary angiomatosis.

Mycobacterial Infections

Any of the mycobacteria including *Mycobacterium avium-intracellulare* and *M. haemophilum* may induce skin lesions in up to 10% of patients with systemic mycobacterial infections (71–73). This is important because the latter organism is more difficult to culture than other mycobacteria and requires supplementation of media with blood, iron, and other growth factors. Infection with *M. bovis* after bacille Calmette-Guérin vaccination in a patient with HIV infection has also been reported (74).

Mycobacterial skin lesions may assume various different appearances. Small papules and pustules that resemble folliculitis, eruptions that resemble atopic dermatitis, localized cutaneous abscesses, suppurative lymphadenitis, nonspecific ulcerations, palmar and plantar hyperkeratoses, and sporotrichoid nodules all have been reported (75–77). *Mycobacterium marinum* may cause classic swimming pool granulomas in patients with HIV disease manifested as verrucous nodules often with a distribution involving ascending lymph nodes on an extremity. Most reported cases behave in an indolent fashion. Lesions may take the form of painful erythematous papules and nodules on the distal extremities and ears (76).

Histologically, cutaneous mycobacterial infections may assume classic patterns of suppurative granulomatous infiltrates in the dermis associated with pseudocarcinomatous hyperplasia, although other patterns may be observed, including dense areas of suppuration with few if any macrophages. Cutaneous atypical mycobacterial infections demonstrate variable responses to antibiotics, so one must culture the organisms and determine sensitivities.

Syphilis

Syphilis is prevalent in patients with HIV infection, and of all reported cases of syphilis between 1984 and 1993, 25% developed in HIV-infected hosts (78). Other venereal diseases including lymphogranuloma venereum, chancroid, granuloma inguinale, and *Neisseria gonorrhoeae* infection all may develop and may be more severe as a consequence of immunocompromise in these patients.

Syphilis may assume various different clinical manifestations in patients with HIV infection ranging from classic papulosquamous lesions with involvement of the palms, soles, and mucous membranes to unusual forms that may defy diagnosis. Examples of unusual manifestations of syphilis in HIV-infected hosts include rapid progression from the primary chancre through secondary stages to advanced late stage disease over a period of months, lues maligna (syphilitic vasculitis), sclerodermiform lesions, rupial verrucous plaques, extensive oral ulcerations, keratoderma, deep cutaneous nodules, rubeoliform eruptions, and widespread gummas (79–81). Central nervous system disease has been noted more frequently and with greater severity in patients with HIV infection (82), and, as in other forms of syphilis, it may have an accelerated course.

The histopathologic features of cutaneous syphilis are usually similar to those seen in immunocompetent hosts, with the characteristic superficial and deep psoriasiform lichenoid pattern of inflammation associated with plasma cells and histiocytes. However, unusual histologic findings have been described including vasculitis, as well as sparse inflammatory infiltrates with minimal numbers of plasma cells and abundant spirochetes. Plasma cells are seen in virtually all cases, and many of these cells are situated around and within nerves. Direct immunofluorescence studies demonstrate deposition of immunoglobulin, complement, and fibrinogen around blood vessels and at the dermoepidermal junction.

Syphilis may have protean manifestations in patients with HIV infection, just as it may in immunocompetent hosts. The list of diseases that may be simulated includes many other bacterial and fungal infections as well as connective tissue diseases, Kaposi's sarcoma, and lymphoma. Therapy is with penicillin, but higher doses must be used and courses of treatment must be longer than in immunocompetent hosts. Intravenous administration is necessary in patients with central nervous system disease.

PARASITIC INFECTIONS AND ECTOPARASITIC INFESTATIONS

Scabies

Scabies is one of the most frequent skin conditions to develop in patients with HIV infection, and it is the most common ectoparasitic infestation in these individuals. The causative agent is the mite *Sarcoptes scabiei* var. *humanus*. Although data regarding the overall incidence of scabies and HIV infection are not well determined, in one study, it was reported in 20% of patients (83).

Scabies may have various different clinical manifestations in patients with HIV infection. Hyperkeratotic lesions on the palms, soles, trunk, or extremities may develop and may resemble crusted scabies in other settings. In other patients, only scattered pruritic papules accompanied by slight scale of the trunk and extremities may be seen. A widespread papulosquamous eruption that may resemble atopic dermatitis and scalp and facial scaling that may mimic seborrheic dermatitis have also been reported (84–87). Characteristic burrows may be difficult to identify, so all patients with a scaly persistent pruritic eruption should have skin lesions scraped and examined histologically in search of mites of scabies. Severe forms of scabies may be associated with secondary infection, bacteremia, and fatal septicemia, especially in severely compromised hosts (88). Patients complain of intractable pruritus that is worse at night. Usually, contacts are infested, especially in the context of the number of mites present on the skin of these individuals. Patients with crusted scabies usually have a superficial and intermediate-to-deep perivascular and interstitial infiltrate of lymphocytes with numerous eosinophils. The epidermis is hyperplastic, with prominent crusting and many scabitic mites visible in the cornified layer. In patients with postscabetic "id" reactions, spongiotic dermatitis may be noted, and in nodular scabies, a dense mixed inflammatory infiltrate with numerous eosinophils in a nodular configuration resembling pseudolymphoma may be seen. In nodular scabies, few mites are present, and it may be difficult to find them. Scabies in patients with

HIV infection must be distinguished from many other disorders. Norwegian (crusted) scabies may resemble palmoplantar hyperkeratotic disorders such as psoriasis. Diffuse scabies may mimic atopic dermatitis as well as other spongiotic dermatitides such as nummular dermatitis. Occasionally, scabies may involve the scalp with scaling and may simulate seborrheic dermatitis. Nodular scabies may mimic lymphomatoid papulosis as well as other insect bite reactions.

Scabies generally responds to treatment with lindane cream or lotion or 5% permethrin cream applied from head to toe, left in place for 8 to 12 hours and then washed off. The treatment is repeated in 1 week. In some patients, recurrences develop as a consequence of failure to treat under the fingernails and the intertriginous zones, although resistance to scabicidal medications may develop. Some clinicians have recommended alternating treatment with lindane and permethrin. Multiple treatments may be required. One report of the use of oral ivermectin for this disorder is highly encouraging, and the drug has been approved for this indication. Postscabetic id reactions must be treated with antihistamines such as doxepin, 10 to 25 mg orally three or four times daily, with topical application of corticosteroid preparations to diminish inflammation. In cases of nodules, injection of triamcinolone acetonide may be required. Careful laundering of linen and clothing is necessary, and household and other contacts should be treated. In cases of crusted scabies, entire wards of patients may require therapy (89). Adjunctive therapies are also important because pruritus is often severe. Topical application of corticosteroid preparations as well as antipruritic agents containing menthol and phenol, pramoxine, and antihistamines may be required. Five percent doxepin cream (Zonalon) is a valuable antipruritic agent that may be used in patients with refractory pruritus. Exposure to ultraviolet B (UVB) irradiation and to psoralen ultraviolet A (PUVA) is also helpful.

Pneumocystosis

Approximately five cases of cutaneous *Pneumocystis carinii* infection have been reported in patients with HIV infection. *P. carinii* may involve the skin preferentially in patients who use aerosolized pentamidine for prophylaxis of *P. carinii* pneumonia. By creating a more unfavorable environment in the lung, organisms spread more widely to involve visceral organs as well as the skin. The disorder may have several different cutaneous manifestations, the most common of which is friable reddish papules or nodules seen in the ear canal or the nares. Small, translucent papules that resemble molluscum contagiosum, bluish cellulitic plaques, and deeply seated abscesses have also been observed. Histologically, *P. carinii* in the skin resembles that in the lung, with a diffuse infiltrate of foamy-appearing cells that, when stained with Gomori's methenamine silver or Steiner stains, highlight the microorganisms and result in a "teacup and saucer" appearance. Pneumocystosis responds to the usual treatment for *P. carinii* pneumonia, namely, intravenous pentamidine.

Other Parasitic Infestations

Cutaneous strongyloidiasis, caused by the helminth *Strongyloides stercoralis,* has been reported rarely in patients with HIV infection. Clinically, lesions resemble urticaria, figurate erythemas, livedo reticularis, and other causes of cutaneous livedo. Histologically, one sees a diffuse infiltrate of lymphocytes and eosinophils scattered throughout the dermis. If an organism itself is contained within the biopsy specimen, it is located in the upper papillary or reticular dermis. Acanthamebiasis, caused by *Acanthamoeba castellanii* (84, 90–94), part of the normal oral flora, develops when this organism proliferates abnormally and disseminates to the skin and often to the central nervous system in profoundly immunocompromised patients. Clinically, lesions appear as necrotic nodules or painful ulcerations of the skin, often involving the extremities. Histologically, one sees a diffuse infiltrate of amebic cysts and trophozoites throughout the skin, especially around blood vessels and in the subcutaneous fat. Careful inspection is required because these may appear similar to histiocytes or other normal-appearing structures in the skin. Erythrophagocytosis is often noted.

Strongyloidiasis requires treatment with thiabendazole, 25 mg/kg twice daily for 4 to 5 days to several weeks, depending on the immune status of the host. Amebiasis responds to metronidazole, at a dosage of 750 mg orally twice daily for 10 days, but because these patients are often severely immunocompromised, response to therapy may be poor.

SYSTEMIC FUNGAL INFECTIONS

The most common systemic opportunistic fungal infections to involve the skin in HIV-seropositive patients are histoplasmosis and cryptococcosis (see Fig. 31.10). Nearly 20% of HIV-seropositive individuals with disseminated histoplasmosis and up to 10% of those with disseminated cryptococcosis develop mucocutaneous lesions. Systemic and cutaneous coccidioidomycosis are both recognized periodically in HIV-infected patients. HIV-infected hosts with

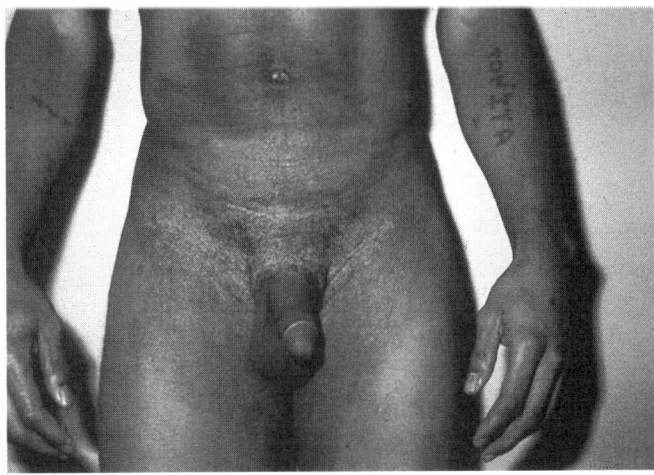

Figure 31.10. Severe dermatophytosis, as depicted here, may also be a presenting sign of HIV disease. (See color section.)

blastomycosis, paracoccidioidomycosis, or sporotrichosis have also been observed.

Mucocutaneous lesions associated with deep systemic fungal infections may assume different forms. The most common lesions are pustules and ulcers, although papules and nodules are also frequently observed. Less often, patches, plaques, and mucosal ulcerations are seen.

Oral thrush involving either the tongue or buccal mucosa, with or without esophageal infection, is the most common manifestation of candidiasis in HIV-seropositive patients (95). Oral candidiasis may be the initial sign of HIV infection in many individuals. Other manifestations that may develop include chronic paronychia and onychodystrophy, chronic refractory vaginal candidiasis, distal urethritis, and persistent monilial infection of the axilla, glans penis, groin, or inframammary area. Disseminated candidiasis in HIV-infected individuals has been reported in a few HIV-infected patients.

Although increasing numbers of HIV-infected patients with coccidioidomycosis are being described, only a few of these individuals have been reported with associated skin lesions (96–98). Some of the manifestations include leukocytoclastic vasculitis, painful erythema of the buttock, and papulopustules on the extremities, chest, back, and palm. Other skin manifestations seen in coccidioidomycosis include ulcers, abscesses, and nodules.

Cryptococcosis

Cryptococcosis is not uncommon in HIV-infected individuals (99–101). The incidence of cutaneous involvement was found to be approximately 6 to 7% when a large series of HIV-infected patients with cryptococcosis was evaluated. Mucocutaneous lesions of cryptococcosis are polymorphous and may appear as erythematous papules, nodules, pustules, or ulcers of the skin and mucosa (102). Cutaneous cryptococcosis, like other opportunistic infections that develop in these patients, may mimic the cutaneous morphology of other disorders such as HSV, cellulitis, or molluscum contagiosum infection, as well as soft tissue hypertrophic lesions such as rhinophyma and Kaposi's sarcoma (103, 104). In addition to simulating Kaposi's sarcoma, *Cryptococcus neoformans* has been demonstrated within lesions of cutaneous Kaposi's sarcoma. Cryptococcosis has a characteristic histopathologic appearance in most cases. Diffuse pallor of the dermis correlates with the mucoid capsular material of the organisms, which are usually present in abundance. Inflammation is usually minimal.

Histoplasmosis

Cutaneous lesions of histoplasmosis may develop in 10 to 17% of patients with systemic infection with *Histoplasma capsulatum* (105). Clinically, the lesions have appeared protean, manifested as cutaneous and mucosal ulcers, erythematous macules and patches, fistulas, papules and nodules, pustules, and verrucous plaques (106–109) (see Fig. 31.11). In some patients with AIDS, *H. capsulatum* in-

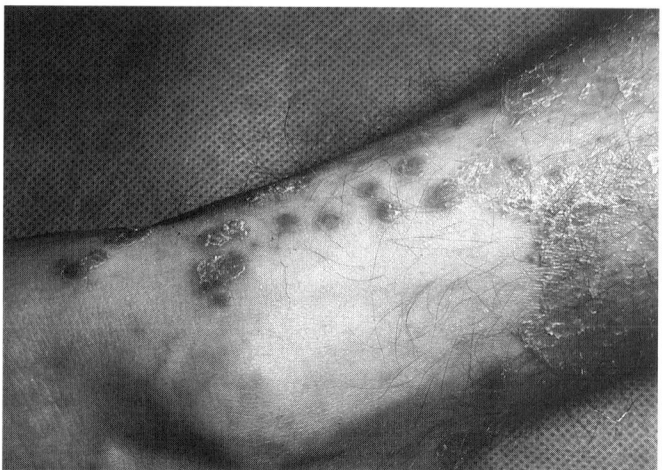

Figure 31.11. Histoplasmosis, a common opportunistic infection in HIV-infected hosts, involves the skin in up to 10% of patients with disseminated disease. Lesions may be nondescript and may mimic other disorders, as in this case, which resembled psoriasis. (See color section.)

fection and Kaposi's sarcoma coexisted in a single skin lesion (109, 110).

Histologically, histoplasmosis exhibits a diffuse dermal infiltrate of histiocytes, neutrophils, and leukocytoclasis. Careful inspection reveals that, although true leukocytoclasia is present in many cases, many of the small particles seen freely in the dermis are fungal organisms. Some cases have been mistakenly diagnosed as leukocytoclastic vasculitis because of these features.

Sporotrichosis

Clinical forms of sporotrichosis include lymphocutaneous, fixed cutaneous, disseminated cutaneous, and systemic. The systemic form may present as either localized pulmonary disease or widespread involvement of numerous organs. In patients with HIV infection, skin lesions may be ulcers, papules, nodules, plaques, or pustules (111–113). These lesions may be widespread, and internal organ involvement may develop that often proves fatal.

In contrast to the situation in immunocompetent patients with sporotrichosis, fungal spores may be numerous, either free in the dermis or within histiocytes, multinucleated giant cells, or abscesses in HIV-infected individuals (114). Although organisms can often be identified on hematoxylin and eosin–stained sections, special stains such as periodic acid–Schiff and Gomori's methenamine silver can be used to facilitate detection. In some cases, especially in relatively immunocompetent hosts, examination of multiple sections taken from the biopsy specimen may be necessary to visualize organisms. *Sporothrix schenckii* grows readily when cultured on Sabouraud's medium.

Blastomycosis

Disseminated blastomycosis is also seen in some patients with HIV infection and AIDS. Widespread verrucous papules, nodules, and plaques have been seen in patients from endemic areas. In one case report, a 30-year-old homosexual HIV-seropositive man had *Blastomyces dermatitidis*–related pustules, nodules, and cutaneous ulcers (115). The condition failed to respond well to treatment and eventually proved fatal.

Other Fungal Infections

In addition to the fungal infections described above, a number of other fungal infections have been recently reported in patients with HIV disease. Disseminated *Scedosporium inflatum*, *Pseudallescheria boydii*, and *Microsporum canis* infections have been recently observed in these patients, as have infections with other saprophytic fungi (116–118). *Aspergillus* infections have been reported with increased frequency. Some of the reported manifestations include facial palsy secondary to mastoid sinus involvement, deep soft tissue and muscular aspergillosis, localized verrucous lesions secondary to cutaneous innoculation or occlusive dressings, and cutaneous spread from visceral foci (119). Zygomycotic infection of the head and neck may develop and may be manifested as local pain, cutaneous necrosis, and necrotizing ulcerations (120, 121). These infections are encountered more frequently as a consequence of better prophylaxis against other opportunistic infections and because of abnormal neutrophil function.

Penicillium marneffei, a fungus endemic to Asia, causes an infection that has been reported with increasing frequency in patients with AIDS in Thailand (122). Seventy-six percent of affected individuals develop skin disease. Some of the cutaneous manifestations include umbilicated papules that may be confused with molluscum contagiosum, ecthymiform lesions, folliculitis, subcutaneous nodules, and morbilliform eruptions. The diagnosis is established by histologic evaluation of skin biopsies and by the performance of cultures.

The treatment of disseminated fungal infections in HIV-infected patients is currently in flux, but trials with newer imidazoles such as fluconazole and itraconazole are promising (123). Nevertheless, until these agents have been used to treat significant numbers of HIV-infected individuals, amphotericin B remains the drug of choice for many.

NONINFECTIOUS SKIN DISORDERS

Seborrheic Dermatitis

Seborrheic dermatitis, the most common skin condition to affect patients with HIV infection, is seen in up to 85% of all HIV-infected individuals at some point during the course of their disease (124). Seborrheic dermatitis most commonly is manifested as slightly indurated, diffuse or confluent, pinkish-red scaly plaques involving the face and scalp (see Fig. 31.12). These may be large, thickened, and heavily crusted and may involve other areas such as the upper anterior chest, back, groin, and extremities. Clinically, seborrheic dermatitis must be distinguished from other papulosquamous dermatoses such as psoriasis, dermatophytosis, and even scabies.

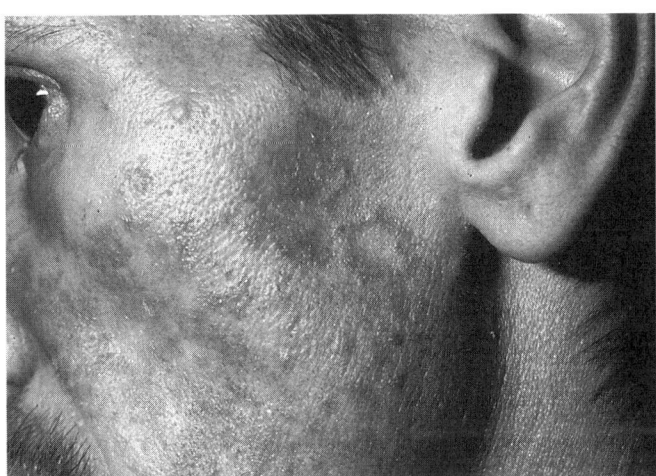

Figure 31.12. **Seborrheic dermatitis, often severe and diffuse, occurs commonly in HIV-infected hosts.** It may serve as an early warning signal of HIV disease. (See color section.)

The histopathologic findings of seborrheic dermatitis are similar to those seen in patients with non–HIV-associated disease, namely, psoriasiform hyperplasia of the epidermis with mounds of parakeratosis containing neutrophils near ostia of hair follicular infundibula. One sees an infiltrate of lymphocytes and scattered plasma cells in the dermis. One finding that is characteristic of seborrheic dermatitis in patients with HIV infection and AIDS and that is not seen generally in patients with non–HIV-associated seborrheic dermatitis is the presence of scattered individually necrotic keratinocytes (125).

Seborrheic dermatitis is generally treated with topical application of corticosteroid preparations and antifungal creams. Exposure to UVB phototherapy is also often effective as an adjunct. The disease may be more difficult to control with routine therapy in HIV-infected individuals, a finding that should serve as a clue that a patient could be immunocompromised.

Psoriasis

Psoriasis develops in 5% of patients with HIV infection (126, 127). Patients with HIV-associated psoriasis may develop arthritis in up to 10% of cases, an incidence that is significantly higher than the 1% of immunocompetent patients with psoriasis who develop psoriatic arthritis. Psoriasis may resemble classic psoriasis found in immunocompetent hosts consisting of reddish plaques with superficial micaceous scale on the extensor surfaces with nail changes of onycholysis, pitting, and subungual hyperkeratosis. In other patients, severe psoriatic arthritis may be seen. Different forms of psoriasis may be found in the same patient such as guttate psoriasis associated with classic psoriasis vulgaris. Severe exfoliative erythroderma may develop, and acral pustular lesions of keratoderma blenorrhagicum coexisting with psoriasis or sebopsoriasis have been noted. Concomitant seborrheic dermatitis of the scalp is almost always seen. HIV-related psoriasis may develop in patients with mild preexisting psoriasis that suddenly undergoes severe exacerbation in patients once AIDS develops, or it may develop spontaneously at some point after HIV seroconversion in an individual who has never before had clinical disease.

Psoriasis has histologic features similar to those seen in non–HIV-infected patients. The pattern is that of marked acanthosis with regular elongation of epidermal retia associated with dilated tortuous blood vessels in the papillary dermis, thin suprapapillary plates, and mounds of parakeratosis containing neutrophils. In pustular cases, spongiform areas in the epidermis containing collections of neutrophils are noted. Psoriasis may have histologic features similar to those of other psoriasiform processes including psoriasiform drug eruptions (109). Other skin disorders that may progress to widespread erythroderma include cutaneous T-cell lymphoma, drug eruptions, and atopic dermatitis, and these conditions must also be excluded.

Psoriasis may undergo partial remission in response to zidovudine therapy, although recurrence is common (127). Spontaneous remission and complete unresponsiveness to all forms of treatment have both been observed in HIV-infected patients. Emollients such as hydrophilic petrolatum applied several times daily, 3 to 5% salicylic acid ointment applied once to twice per day for keratolytic effect, and application of triamcinolone acetonide ointment 0.025 to 0.1% or its equivalent for localized short-term therapy are often partially effective. In many cases, systemic drugs such as etretinate, at a dosage of 1 mg/kg of body weight daily, with or without the addition of dapsone, 100 to 200 mg per day, may be required, as may systemic PUVA therapy.

Methotrexate may be used with extreme caution, beginning at a dose of 5 to 7.5 mg per week and gradually increasing the dose by 2.5 mg per week as needed. Patients must be monitored carefully, however, because this drug may worsen immunodepression. Concomitant administration of trimethoprim-containing compounds is contraindicated because the folate reductase–inhibiting effect is synergistic with that induced by methotrexate (R Auerbach, unpublished data).

Reiter's Syndrome

Reiter's syndrome has been reported in 6 to 10% of HIV-infected patients (128, 129). It is characterized clinically by arthritis (especially sacroiliitis), urethritis, conjunctivitis, and pustular scaling lesions of the glabrous skin, glans penis, and scalp. Debilitating palmoplantar pustular disease is common, and one generally sees striking nail dystrophy associated with periungual erythema, inflammation, and hyperkeratosis with prominent crusting. Reiter's disease has a histologic picture similar to that of pustular psoriasis. Clinically, Reiter's syndrome must be distinguished from other forms of arthritis such as lupus erythematosus and infectious conditions such as arthritis due to disseminated gonococcal infection.

Noninfectious Papular Pruritic Disorders ("Itchy Red Bump Disease")

Pruritic conditions in patients with HIV infection are common, although the precise incidence and prevalence are unknown. Some studies have shown prevalences of up to 20 to 30% (130–132). Some of the disorders include eosinophilic folliculitis, atopic dermatitis, and xerosis. Xerotic dermatitis is commonly found in patients with advanced HIV disease and AIDS and may be seen to some degree in up to 85% of patients.

The pathogeneses of various pruritic dermatoses in patients with HIV infection are not entirely clear. Such patients should be evaluated for the presence of ectoparasites and other pathogens such as scabies and fungi because these may cause itching. Systemic parasites also may lead to itching by inducing urticarial reactions or as a consequence of migration through the skin. Other causes of itchy eruptions include hypersensitivity to medications and underlying atopic dermatitis, both of which should be included in the differential diagnosis. Patients with HIV infection commonly have elevated circulating immunoglobulin E (IgE) antibodies (133). This finding may correlate with an increased frequency of IgE-mediated disorders such as worsened atopic dermatitis and other hypersensitivity disorders. Basophils have been shown to be hyperreleasable in patients with HIV disease, and the mast cells in some patients are presumed to have a lowered threshold for release of histamine (134), with attendant inflammatory reactions and pruritus. Patients with HIV disease may also have direct neural infection with HIV leading to neural irritation and enhanced sensations of itching (135). This condition may result in chronic excoriation, lichen simplex chronicus, and prurigo nodularis. Sometimes, autonomic dysfunction is associated with diminished sweating and sebaceous gland secretion that worsens xerosis and itching. In addition, patients infected with HIV may be under considerable stress, also leading to urticaria and itching. Finally, patients with HIV infection may develop pruritus secondary to underlying circulating pruritogens associated with different systemic disorders. Chronic liver disease or renal disease and systemic lymphoma may be associated with pruritus. All these factors should be considered when dealing with an itchy HIV-infected patient. In our experience, most patients develop pruritus as a consequence of a primary cutaneous disease rather than secondary to an underlying systemic illness.

Prurigo Nodularis

Prurigo nodularis is a reaction pattern that may be associated with many of the aforementioned underlying causes of itching. Patients chronically rub and scratch lesions, resulting in thickening of the skin. Prurigo nodularis appears as hyperpigmented, dome-shaped, verrucous and often crusted papules and nodules that are usually associated with lichen simplex chronicus. Chronic rubbing and scratching induce lesions.

Eosinophilic Folliculitis

Eosinophilic pustular folliculitis is one of the most common pruritic dermatoses to develop in patients with HIV disease (see Fig. 31.13). Patients generally present with widespread excoriated follicular papules that involve the trunk, extremities, and head and neck (131). The clinician must to exclude the diagnosis of scabies, which may look similar. Although the condition is known as eosinophilic pustular folliculitis, intact pustules are a rare finding because patients are usually so uncomfortable that, by the time they present to the dermatologist, lesions have been excoriated vigorously. Many patients have clinical appearances manifested mostly as lichen simplex chronicus and prurigo nodularis. The term "itchy red bumps" has been used to describe the clinical presentation of this disorder. Eosinophilic folliculitis has a characteristic histopathologic appearance that allows the diagnosis to be made in most cases. Characteristically, within the infundibula of hair follicles are clusters of eosinophils that may be numerous. One often sees a perifollicular inflammatory infiltrate of lymphocytes, neutrophils, and some eosinophils, especially when follicles have ruptured. In some cases, the number of eosinophils may be small, in which case differentiation from bacterial folliculitis may be difficult. When long-standing lesions undergo biopsy, the primary finding may be that of lichen simplex chronicus or prurigo nodularis manifested by marked acanthosis and hyperkeratosis with coarse thickened collagen bundles in the papillary dermis.

Eosinophilic pustular folliculitis resembles other pruritic dermatoses that may be found in both HIV-infected individuals and immunocompetent patients. Bacterial folliculitis may be associated with pruritus and has clinical features similar to those of eosinophilic pustular folliculitis. Insect bite reactions, scabies, and dermatitis herpetiformis must all be excluded. In the setting of pruritic dermatosis in an HIV-seropositive patient with skin scrapings that show no evidence of scabies, the diagnosis can generally be assumed to be eosinophilic pustular folliculitis and treated accordingly without a biopsy in most cases.

Therapy of eosinophilic pustular folliculitis has been the subject of several studies because of the frequency of the disorder and the morbidity it induces in HIV-infected individuals. UVB exposure has been shown to be efficacious in relieving the pruritus associated with this condition (132). Patients are generally treated with gradually increasing exposure to UVB, usually administered by phototherapy units. Irradiances beginning at one-third of the minimal erythemogenic dose with gradual increase by one-third to one-half of the previous dose are instituted and are continued until remission is experienced. Because exposure to ultraviolet irradiation may be associated with complications of photosensitivity as well as theoretically causing activation of HIV, indiscriminate use of UVB or sunlight exposure should be avoided (136). Nevertheless, several studies have demonstrated that moderate exposure to UVB is safe in the treatment of HIV-related dermatoses if therapy is administered properly (137). If patients are unable to undergo treatment with UVB for financial or other reasons, excellent relief may be obtained by exposure to natural sunlight. Use of tanning booths that provide ultraviolet A also may be of benefit. In addition to ultraviolet light, administration of itraconazole in doses of 400 mg orally twice daily has been shown to diminish the pruritus of eosinophilic pustular folliculitis (138). The mechanism of action is unknown, but the drug may act by diminishing the concentration of *Pityrosporum* yeasts within follicular infundibula. Oral therapy with isotretinoin has been shown to be efficacious. Other agents such as metronidazole, 250 to 500 mg orally two or three times per day, may be beneficial. Administration of antihistamines, such as doxepin at doses of 10 to 20 mg every 6 hours by mouth, as well as topical application of antipruritic agents such as pramoxine and menthol and phenol-containing lotions may also diminish sensations of itching.

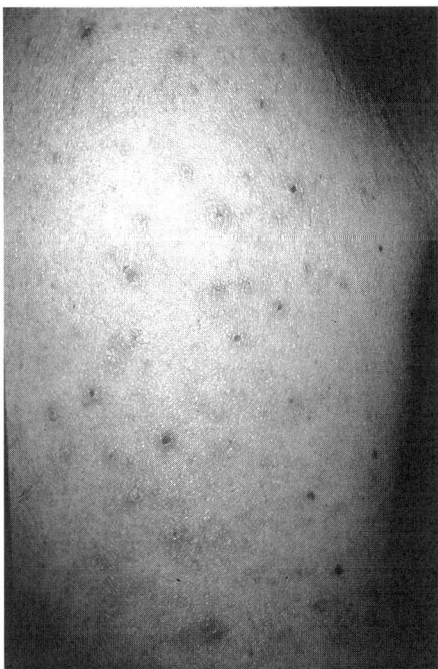

Figure 31.13. **Eosinophilic folliculitis is also commonly found in HIV-infected individuals with advanced immunosuppression.** The condition is usually severely pruritic. (See color section.)

Atopic Dermatitis

Atopic dermatitis is characteristically manifested by erythematous patches and plaques with fine papulovesicles associated with scaling, crusting, and lichen simplex chronicus. Patients often have associated hyperlinear palms, allergic rhinitis, and asthma. HIV-infected individuals who develop atopic dermatitis may manifest severe forms of the disorder with erythroderma. Atopic dermatitis has microscopic features of a superficial perivascular infiltrate of lymphocytes and eosinophils with epidermal hyperplasia and foci of spongiosis. Late lesions have morphologic features that are primarily those of lichen simplex chronicus. Asteatotic dermatitis or xerotic dermatitis shows little inflammation in the dermis with slight epidermal hyperplasia, tiny amounts of spongiosis, and small zones of parakeratosis. Atopic dermatitis must be differentiated from other psoriasiform dermatitides such as psoriasis, cutaneous T-cell lymphoma, and psoriasiform drug eruptions. In general, the presence of severe pruritus and a history of atopy aid in this diagnosis.

Atopic dermatitis usually responds to measures used to treat atopic dermatitis in immunocompetent hosts. These measures consist of avoidance of irritants, application of emollients, and use of topical corticosteroid preparations.

Xerotic Dermatitis

Xerotic dermatitis generally is characterized by diffuse dryness of the skin with hyperpigmented scales and focal crusting (see Fig. 31.14). Many lesions may be fissured and, in some cases, eczema craquele develops. This latter complication may lead to localized infection because the skin is broken, serving as portals of entry for bacteria and fungi. Clinically, xerotic dermatitis is generally characteristic. Other forms of dry, scaly dermatoses such as the characteristic "flaky paint" dermatitis seen with kwashiorkor should be excluded. Because both conditions occur in patients with advanced AIDS, evaluation of nutritional status is essential.

Papular Urticaria

Pinkish-red erythematous papules and plaques initially with little surface change manifest papular urticaria and chronic urticaria. Edema and a *peau d'orange* appearance of the skin are noted. Angioedema may be seen. Although papular urticaria may be excoriated, primary urticaria generally is not.

Chronic Actinic Dermatitis

Chronic actinic dermatitis may be associated with HIV infection and is believed to be related to the exaggerated B-cell immune response that may be present in these individuals. These patients may develop allergies to drugs and other substances, and with alteration of the immune system, underlying allergic phenomena may be recalled. The condition is characteristically manifested by psoriasiform lichenified plaques in the sun-exposed areas of the body, which are often hyperpigmented, scaly, and pruritic (139, 140). Lesions are generally located on the dorsal surfaces of the hands, forearms, face, upper anterior portion of the chest, and posterior portion of the neck. Extensive lichenification is often seen, and patients may have an appearance similar to that described in actinic reticuloid.

Chronic actinic dermatitis is manifested histologically by superficial and often deep psoriasiform dermatitis with an infiltrate of lymphocytes and abundant eosinophils. Some cases may be associated with a bandlike infiltrate and epidermotropism of lymphocytes, many of which may be atypical in appearance, simulating mycosis fungoides. Clinical correlation may be necessary to render a definitive diagnosis. Spongiosis is generally seen, and necrotic keratinocytes may be noted. The diagnosis of chronic actinic dermatitis may be corroborated by phototesting. Thorough questioning is important to elicit a history of recent exposure to potential photoallergens or phototoxins as well as past histories of exposure to such stimuli that may have been reactivated.

Treatment of chronic actinic dermatitis consists of avoidance of photoallergens and phototoxins as well as application of topical corticosteroid preparations. Avoidance of ultraviolet light is also important. In some cases, even visible light may precipitate a flare of the condition, so in these cases, complete light avoidance is essential because even light emitted from television monitors may be sufficient to worsen the condition. Paradoxically, the use of PUVA may "harden" the skin and lead to remission. Administration of hydroxychloroquine (Plaquenil), at doses of 200 mg orally once or twice daily, may also be beneficial. Fortunately, the incidence of this condition, which is often difficult to manage, remains low. Photoexacerbated drug eruptions often appear lichenoid or erythematous, distributed on photoexposed sites.

Porphyria Cutanea Tarda

Porphyria cutanea tarda has been reported in increased incidence in patients with HIV infection. HIV-infected patients are known to produce greater concentrations of porphyrins, possibly as a consequence of abnormal liver function secondary to hepatitis such as hepatitis C. The disorder appears virtually identical to that seen in immunocompetent hosts, with blisters on the dorsal surfaces of the hands and other sun-exposed areas associated with crusting, milia formation, dyspigmentation, and scarring (141–143). In addition, one often sees hyperpigmentation and hypertrichosis of the malar areas of the face. Patients may describe the excretion of dark urine.

Porphyria cutanea tarda has histologic findings similar to those seen in immunocompetent individuals and manifested

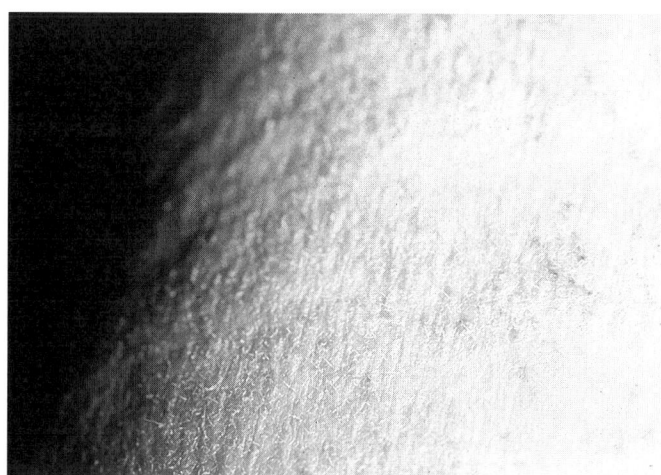

Figure 31.14. Severe widespread xerosis is especially common in patients with end-stage AIDS. The condition may be refractory to treatment with many different emollient regimens. (See color section.)

by a subepidermal blister with minimal inflammation in the dermis. Preservation of dermal papillae, so-called "festooning," is seen, and thick, hyaline, periodic acid–Schiff–positive rims surround blood vessels in the upper dermis. Elongated aggregations of necrotic keratinocytes often present in the epidermis overlying the blister have been referred to as "caterpillar bodies" (144).

Porphyria is diagnosed on the basis of clinical and histologic findings as well as demonstration of elevated urinary uroporphyrins and coproporphyrins. In immunocompetent hosts, the most common treatment is repeated phlebotomy. In patients with HIV infection, who are often anemic, this treatment cannot be used. Low doses of hydroxychloroquine, beginning at 25 mg weekly and increased to 200 mg weekly, may be effective in mobilizing accumulated porphyrin in the liver (Cockerell CJ. Successful treatment of HIV-related porphyria cutanea tarda with low-dose oral hydroxychloroquine [submitted for publication 1996]). (145). Erythropoietin has been shown to be effective in treatment of this disorder by enhancing heme biosynthesis, resulting in mobilization of porphyrins (146). Thus, although this therapy is expensive, it may be the most beneficial form of treatment because it corrects the hematologic deficit as well as the metabolic disorder.

Cutaneous Drug Eruptions

Cutaneous drug-induced eruptions are the most common manifestation of drug hypersensitivity. In one study, 79% of HIV-infected patients had one or more dermatologic diagnoses, many of which included cutaneous reactions to drugs (147). In some studies, 50 to 60% of HIV-positive patients have been shown to develop a cutaneous eruption resulting from trimethoprim–sulfamethoxazole (148). Up to 45% of patients develop morbilliform eruptions, with variable numbers of other reactions being reported. Stevens–Johnson syndrome and toxic epidermal necrolysis occur sporadically (149). Other antibiotics are common offenders because morbilliform eruptions may be seen in 10% of patients taking antituberculous regimens and in 40% of patients treated with amoxicillin–clavulanic acid (150–152).

Trimethoprim–sulfamethoxazole is the best known and most common cause of allergic drug eruption in patients with HIV infection. In some studies, 50 to 60% of HIV-positive patients developed a cutaneous eruption from this agent (148). In most cases, a widespread eruption of fine pink to red macules and papules involving the trunk and extremities develops 8 to 12 days after initiating therapy and reaches maximal intensity 1 to 2 days later. In some cases, desquamation may supervene. The eruption may disappear within 3 to 5 days even though therapy is continued, although in some cases, the eruption may persist for days to weeks after discontinuation of the medication. Cutaneous eruptions from trimethoprim–sulfamethoxazole do not always recur with drug rechallenge in HIV-infected patients; however, if the agent is to be reinstituted, it should be done under controlled circumstances to monitor for possible anaphylactoid reactions. Stevens–Johnson syndrome and toxic epidermal necrolysis may also develop as a consequence of trimethoprim–sulfamethoxazole administration. Stevens–Johnson syndrome is characterized by fever and widespread blisters of the skin and mucous membranes of the eye, mouth, or genitals. Toxic epidermal necrolysis, a more serious manifestation of the same process, involves widespread areas of the skin with confluent bullae that can lead to loss of skin in massive sheets. Thirty-five cases of toxic epidermal necrolysis have been reported in HIV-infected individuals.

Zidovudine may induce several different cutaneous complications. The most common reaction is hyperpigmentation of the nails. Blue to brown–black nail discoloration has been reported to occur in more than 40% of patients (153, 154). It is more common in black patients and usually begins 4 to 8 weeks after initiating treatment, or it may occur as late as 1 year after the start of therapy. Longitudinal streaks are most common, but diffuse pigmentation and transverse bands may occur. The thumbnails are affected most frequently. Zidovudine may also induce hyperpigmentation of the mucous membranes and the skin that may mimic the hyperpigmentation seen with adrenal insufficiency (155, 156). In addition to pigmentary abnormalities, severe exanthematous eruptions may develop within 1 to 2 weeks of the initiation of zidovudine therapy. Lichenoid papular reactions may appear almost identical to lichen planus with whitish, lacy plaques of the mucous membranes as well as polygonal pink papules on flexural surfaces of glabrous skin (157). Lichenoid eruptions from zidovudine must be distinguished from true lichen planus. Zidovudine-induced nail pigmentation must be differentiated from other causes of pigmented bands in the nail plate such as junctional nevi and acrolentiginous melanoma. Other manifestations include acral and periarticular reticulate erythema that may simulate dermatomyositis (158).

The histopathologic features of the common morbilliform drug eruptions typically consist of a superficial perivascular inflammatory infiltrate of lymphocytes with scattered eosinophils associated with vacuolar alteration of the dermoepidermal junction and individually necrotic keratinocytes. The differential diagnosis of morbilliform drug eruptions includes other morbilliform eruptions such as those caused by viruses. In some cases, spongiosis is prominent. Slight parakeratosis may be noted, and scattered plasma cells may be seen. Allergic drug eruptions may also clinically appear as erythema multiform, Stevens–Johnson syndrome, or toxic epidermal necrolysis, all characterized by prominent vacuolar interface changes with extensive keratinocytic necrosis of the epidermis. In toxic epidermal necrolysis, the number of inflammatory cells in the dermis may be minimal, although confluent epidermal necrosis occurs with no parakeratosis, a consequence of the rapidity of progression of the eruption. Urticarial eruptions are usually characterized by mixed infiltrates of inflammatory cells interstitially in the dermis with minimal epidermal change.

Ulcerations caused by foscarnet used for herpesvirus infections may mimic fixed drug eruptions or ulcers of other causes including those induced by infectious agents such as HSV, CMV, and in some cases bacteria and fungi. Toxic epidermal necrolysis is generally characteristic, but it must be distinguished from staphylococcal scalded skin syndrome and toxic streptococcal syndrome. Skin biopsy or frozen section evaluation of the roof of the blister demonstrates confluent epithelial necrosis in erythema multiforme and sloughing of the stratum corneum in staphylococcal scalded skin syndrome.

The most important aspect of the treatment of a cutaneous drug eruption relates to the avoidance of serious complications that may arise if the diagnosis is not made in timely fashion and the offending agent is not withdrawn. The most serious cutaneous complication is toxic epidermal necrolysis. Other complications include systemic toxicity such as hepatotoxicity or renal damage associated with the sulfone syndrome. Toxic epidermal necrolysis may lead to secondary infection with sepsis, volume depletion, and high-output cardiac failure as a consequence of widespread denudation of the skin. Patients who develop this condition must be treated aggressively in intensive care settings. Whether systemic corticosteroids should be used remains controversial.

Hypersensitivity to trimethoprim–sulfamethoxazole has been successfully treated with desensitization. Desensitization to other antibiotics may also be attempted when necessary (159).

Hair and Nail Abnormalities

Certain abnormalities of hair and nails may be encountered in patients with HIV disease. Chronic inflammatory and noninflammatory alopecia has been observed. The hair may become lusterless and dull, and in patients with curly hair, straightening of the hair is often noted (160). Biopsies of the scalp have shown histologic features resembling those of noninflammatory telogen effluvium alopecia as well as dense inflammatory cell infiltrates containing lymphocytes, histiocytes, and plasma cells with destruction of follicles (CJ Cockerell, unpublished data). Diffuse, fine, downy alopecia that may or may not be associated with scaling has also been observed, usually in patients with end-stage AIDS. Finally, patients with HIV infection may develop serious infections with high fevers leading to true telogen effluvium.

In addition to loss of scalp hair, patients may have elongation of the eyelashes, a sign of a prolonged anagen phase. This condition has been termed trichomegaly of the eyelashes (161–163). The cause of this phenomenon is unknown, but in some cases it is associated with the administration of drugs such as recombinant interferon-α. The frequency with which this problem develops is unclear, but it has been reported in as many as 20% of HIV-infected patients in one study (164). Other changes of the hair seen in HIV-infected patients include premature canities and alopecia areata (165, 166).

Nail disorders commonly develop in patients with HIV infection. Patients receiving zidovudine may develop elongated pigmented grayish streaks of multiple nail plates, as mentioned previously. Nail plate thickening with subungual hyperkeratosis and dystrophy may be associated with fungal infections from dermatophytes, *Candida,* and *Scytalidium* spp. and other nondermatophyte fungi. The yellow nail syndrome secondary to metabolic abnormalities, lymphedema, and hypoxia has been reported to develop in HIV-infected patients, as has transverse and longitudinal ridging (167, 168). Diminished thickness of the nail plate may also be seen. Increased nail plate opacity and both Muehrcke's and Terry's nails have been noted. Ridging and nail thickness changes are most likely a consequence of diminished matrix growth with decreased nail plate turnover. Just as in immunocompetent patients, Beau's lines may be seen 2 to 3 months after an episode of a serious infection. Involvement of the periungual tissues by infectious agents, psoriasis, and erythema with features similar to Gottron's papules may also occur.

NEOPLASTIC DISORDERS

Many different neoplasms of the skin are seen in HIV-infected individuals. As patients live for longer periods, the opportunity for these patients to develop these disorders will almost certainly increase. Thus, this issue probably will become a major public health problem in the future. Because visceral and vascular neoplasms, specifically Kaposi's sarcoma (see Chap. 26), are discussed elsewhere in this text, they are not addressed in detail here.

Primary Cutaneous Neoplasms

The incidence of epithelial neoplasms in patients infected with HIV is increased, most commonly in oral, cervical, and anorectal locations. Bowenoid papulosis refers to squamous cell carcinoma in situ that develops as a consequence of infections with HPV types 16 and 18 most commonly (see Fig. 31.6). Lesions often have morphologic features similar to those of condylomata acuminata and may be clinically confused with them. Generally, lesions are brownish, flat-topped papules on the labia or penile skin. Lesions are often hyperpigmented, but in some cases, they clinically resemble condylomata acuminata. Rarely, brownish macules may be the only manifestation of the disease. Epidermodysplasia verruciformis, a premalignant condition associated with HPV infection, has a clinical appearance of widespread warty papules that are either pink or red. In some cases, diffuse erythematous pruritic areas of the skin may be seen (169). Ultraviolet irradiation is a major risk factor for the development of carcinomas in patients with this condition. Biopsies are necessary to establish this diagnosis and demonstrate characteristic vacuolated HPV-infected cells in the epidermis. Basal cell carcinomas have been reported in HIV-seropositive patients, often on unexposed sites. Most have had clinical appearances similar to those seen in immunocompetent hosts although multiple primary nodular or superficial basal cell carcinomas may develop. In rare cases, metastases of basal cell carcinoma occur, probably as a consequence of immunocompromise (170). Most metastases have been to draining lymph nodes and the lung.

Melanoma involving HIV-infected patients has also been observed sporadically. Although no adequate data exist about the relative frequency of this neoplasm in these patients, multiple primary and "early" nodular lesions have been noted. In at least one patient, a highly aggressive, fatal course ensued.

The histopathologic findings of these conditions range from subtle atypical intraepithelial proliferations within stratified squamous epithelium that begin at the basal cell layer to full-thickness involvement of the epithelium by atypical neoplastic keratinocytes. Epithelial retia are expanded and are replaced by atypical cells, many of which are strikingly pleomorphic and in mitosis. In time, bulbous aggregations of neoplastic cells extend from the epithelium into the underlying lamina propria and reticular dermis. Involvement of deeper soft tissues, nerves, and blood vessels may develop in due course. Lesions are often digitated, verrucous, and associated with prominent necrosis.

Bowenoid papulosis is manifested histologically by similar cytologic features, except lesions have a histologic architectural pattern similar to that of condyloma acuminatum. Epidermodysplasia verruciformis is characterized by a diffuse infiltrate of pale-appearing cells in the epidermis that represent koilocytes (171). One also sees dyskeratosis and characteristic structures resembling corps ronds in the stratum corneum.

Squamous cell carcinoma may have clinical and histologic features similar to those of pseudocarcinomatous hyperplasia including that induced by infectious agents. Giant HPV-induced verrucous carcinoma may have histologic features resembling those of giant condylomata. These lesions are similar clinically to the Buschke–Löwenstein variant of verrucous carcinoma. Epidermodysplasia verruciformis may clinically simulate widespread warts or, in some cases, other forms of erythroderma or widespread erythematous scaly dermatoses. Basal cell carcinoma may mimic molluscum contagiosum as well as nondescript papular lesions of opportunistic infections.

Diagnosis is established primarily on the basis of clinical appearance and skin biopsy. Studies have evaluated the efficacy of exfoliative cytology in determining the presence of intraepithelial neoplasia of both cervical and anal areas and have found a high rate of false-negative results when comparing this technique with colposcopically or sigmoidoscopically directed tissue biopsies (172).

Treatment of squamous cell carcinoma usually requires excision or aggressive destructive measures. Cryotherapy, generally used for the management of cervical intraepithelial neoplasia, was shown in one study to have an overall efficacy of 25%, significantly lower than that observed in HIV-seronegative patients (173). Carbon dioxide laser destruction may be more effective in this setting. Bowenoid papulosis, although generally treated with simple cryosurgical destruction or topical application of 5-fluorouracil, should be treated with either electrodesiccation and curettage or other destructive surgical measures with biopsy confirmation of removal, rather than by conservative topical measures. Basal cell carcinoma also should be treated aggressively with destructive measures such as cryosurgery or excision because of the potential for metastasis in HIV-infected immunocompromised hosts. Epidermodysplasia verruciformis may be refractory to all forms of therapy. Any neoplasms that develop should be destroyed or excised. Systemic administration of retinoids such as etretinate or 13,cis-retinoic acid at doses of 1 to 2 mg/kg may be effective in preventing development of carcinomas.

Lymphoreticular Malignancies

Most cases of lymphoma in HIV-infected patients involve visceral sites. When the skin is affected by non–Hodgkin's lymphoma, it is usually manifested as pink to purplish papules or nodules (see Fig. 31.15). Any site may be involved, including the head and neck, trunk, or extremities. Deeply seated soft tissue involvement may expand superficially, forming dome-shaped nodules that often ulcerate. Cutaneous Hodgkin's disease resembles non–Hodgkin's lymphoma either as diffuse nodular lesions or as a "panniculitis." HIV-related cutaneous T-cell lymphoma may have a clinical appearance similar to that of mycosis fungoides manifested as widespread plaques that may progress to erythroderma (174). Human T-cell leukemia/lymphoma virus type 1 (HTLV-1)–associated lymphoma may also resemble mycosis fungoides, although it may have a clinical picture of an acute viral exanthem with an eruption of morbilliform papules and small fine vesicles (175).

When the skin is involved by lymphoma, histologically one generally sees a diffuse infiltrate of atypical lymphoid cells that are monomorphous in appearance. Many of the cells are large, pleomorphic, and in mitosis. The infiltrate tends to be deeply situated, involving the lower portions of the dermis and subcutaneous fat, and one often sees extensive necrosis as well as obliteration of preexisting adnexal structures. Hodgkin's disease involving the skin may appear similar to an inflammatory infiltrate in the skin, although

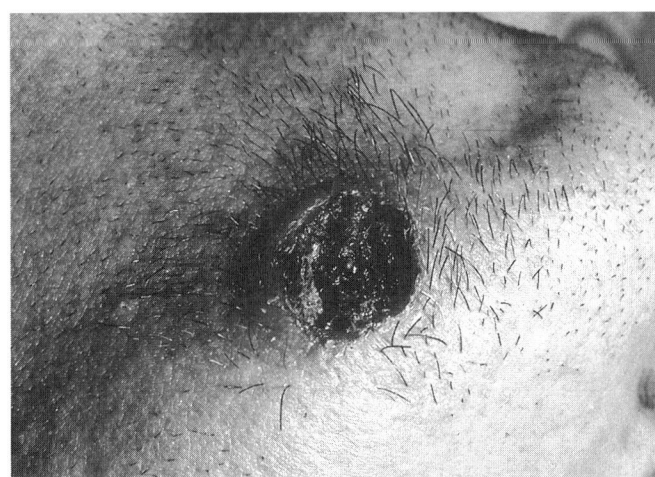

Figure 31.15. Cutaneous lymphoma is encountered with more frequency in these patients. Its presence usually portends a poor prognosis. (See color section.)

the diffuse nature of the infiltrate and the presence of large, atypical cells morphologically resembling Reed–Sternberg cells generally aid in making the diagnosis. Cutaneous T-cell lymphoma is usually manifested histologically by psoriasiform hyperplasia of the epidermis with a bandlike infiltrate of atypical lymphocytes, many having convoluted nuclei with a cerebriform appearance. These cells are also present in the epidermis, where they often form small collections. In some cases, minimal epidermotropism is noted, but the atypical nature of the cells allows the diagnosis to be made. In cases of HTLV-1–associated lymphoma, neoplastic lymphocytes are often large and multilobulated, with a "cloverleaf" appearance. In addition, one usually notes prominent exocytosis, and because of the associated leukemia, atypical lymphoid cells are often seen in blood vessels and lymphatics.

The routine diagnosis of these neoplasms is based on the characteristic clinical appearance taken in the context of the histopathologic features. In many cases, gene rearrangement studies, flow cytometric immunologic analysis, and DNA probes are necessary to characterize and subtype the neoplasm further. Immunophenotyping of mycosis fungoides–like cutaneous T-cell lymphoma in HIV-seropositive patients is usually characterized by an infiltrate of CD8+ lymphocytes, but it may be composed of monoclonal CD4+ cells (175). HTLV-1–associated leukemia or lymphoma is characterized by an infiltrate of CD4+ cells with absent CD2+ and CD7+ antigens (176).

Treatment consists of the usual therapy for systemic lymphoma. Some of the regimens used include methotrexate, prednisone, bleomycin, doxorubicin, cyclophosphamide, and vincristine. Cutaneous T-cell lymphoma may respond to PUVA therapy, total body electron beam, and topical nitrogen mustard. As expected, however, these lymphomas are more aggressive than in patients who are immunocompetent, and survival generally is between 5 and 10 months of diagnosis (177). Because patients are already immunocompromised, administration of many of these agents may cause profound immunocompromise with acceleration of death.

References

1. Tindall B, Barker S, Donovan B, et al. Characterization of the acute clinical illness associated with human immunodeficiency virus infection. Arch Intern Med 1988;148:945–949.
2. Sinicco A, Palestro G, Caramello P, et al. Acute HIV-1 infection: clinical and biologic study of twelve patients. J Acquir Immune Defic Syndr 1990;3:260–265.
3. Kinlock S, de Saussure P, Vanhems P, et al. Primary HIV infection: a prospective and retrospective study [abstract]. In Abstract of the 8th International Conference on AIDS, Amsterdam, 1992.
4. Rabeneck L, Popovic M, Gartner S, et al. Acute HIV infection presenting with painful swallowing and esophageal ulcers. JAMA 1990;263:2318–2322.
5. McMillan A, Bishop PE, Aw D, et al. Immunohistology of the skin rash associated with acute HIV infection. AIDS 1989;3:309–312.
6. Shapiro P. Histologic findings in the acute exanthem of HIV infection. Presented at the meeting of the American Society of Dermatopathology, New Orleans, 1995.
7. Henderson DK, Gerberding JL. Prophylactic zidovudine after occupational exposure to the human immunodeficiency virus: an interim analysis. J Infect Dis 1989;160:321–323.
8. Looke DFM, Grove DI. Failed prophylactic zidovudine after needlestick injury [letter]. Lancet 1990;335:1280.
9. Lange J, Boucher CAB, Hollack CEM, et al. Failure of zidovudine prophylaxis after accidental exposure to HIV-1. N Engl J Med 1990;322:1375–1377.
10. Safran S, Ashley R, Houlihan C, et al. Clinical and serologic features of herpes simplex virus infection in patients with AIDS. AIDS 1991;5:1107–1110.
11. Masur H. Clinical implications of herpes virus infections in patients with AIDS. Am J Med 1992;92:1S–2S.
12. Siegal FP, Lopez C, Hammer GS, et al. Severe acquired immunodeficiency in male homosexuals, manifested by chronic perianal ulcerative herpes simplex lesions. N Engl J Med 1981;305:1439–1444.
13. Friedman-Kien AE, LaFleur FL, Gendler EC, et al. Herpes zoster: a possible early clinical sign for development of acquired immunodeficiency syndrome in high-risk individuals. J Am Acad Dermatol 1986;14;1023–1028.
14. Jura E, Chadwick EG, Josephs HS, et al. Varicella zoster virus infections in children infected with human immunodeficiency virus. Pediatr Infect Dis J 1989;8:586–590.
15. Williamson BC. Disseminated herpes zoster in a human immunodeficiency virus-positive homosexual man without complications. Cutis 1987;40:45–46.
16. Gilson IH, Barnett JH, Conans MA, et al. Disseminated ecthymatous varicella-zoster virus infection in patients with acquired immunodeficiency syndrome. J Am Acad Dermatol 1989;20:637–642.
17. Janier M, Hilion B, Baccard M, et al. Chronic varicella zoster infection in acquired immunodeficiency syndrome [letter]. J Am Acad Dermatol 1988;18:584–585.
18. Cohen PR, Beltranny VP, Grossman ME. Disseminated herpes zoster in patients with immunodeficiency virus infection. Am J Med 1988;84:1076–1080.
19. Jacobson MA, Berger TG, Fikrig S, et al. Acyclovir-resistant varicella zoster virus infection after chronic oral acyclovir therapy in patients with the acquired immunodeficiency syndrome (AIDS). Ann Intern Med 1990;112:187–191.
20. Worrell JT, Cockerell CJ: Histopathology of cutaneous nerves in herpesvirus infections: Society for Investigative Dermatology, May, 1993. Washington, DC: American Society of Dermatopathology, 1992.
21. Smith KJ, Skelton HG, Angritt P. Histopathologic features of HIV-associated skin disease. Dermatol Clin 1991;9:551–578.
22. Hardy WD. Foscarnet treatment of acyclovir-resistant herpes simplex virus infection in patients with acquired immunodeficiency syndrome: preliminary results of a controlled, randomized, regimen-comparative trial. Am J Med 1992;92:30s–35s.
23. Chatis PA, Miller CH, Schrager LE, et al. Successful treatment with foscarnet of an acyclovir-resistant mucocutaneous infection with herpes simplex virus in a patient with acquired immunodeficiency syndrome. N Engl J Med 1989;320:297–300.
24. Klatt EC, Shibata D. Cytomegalovirus infection in the acquired immunodeficiency syndrome. Arch Pathol Lab Med 1988;112:540–544.
25. Lin CS, Pinha PD, Krishnan MN, et al. Cytomegalic inclusion disease of the skin. Arch Dermatol 1981;117:282–284.
26. Feldman PS, Walker AN, Baker R. Cutaneous lesions heralding disseminated cytomegalovirus infections. J Am Acad Dermatol 1982;7:545–548.
27. Muehler-Stamou A, Sen HJ, Emodi G. Epidermolysis in a case of severe cytomegalovirus infection. BMJ 1974;3:609–611.
28. Minars N, Silverman JF, Escobar NR, et al. Fatal cytomegalic inclusion disease: associated skin manifestations in a renal transplant patient. Arch Dermatol 1977;113:1569–1571.
29. Horn TD, Hood AF. Cytomegalovirus is predictably present in perineal ulcers from immunosuppressed patients. Arch Dermatol 1990;126:642–644.

30. Lee JY, Peel R: Concurrent cytomegalovirus and herpes simplex virus infections in skin biopsy specimens from two AIDS patients with fatal CMV infection. Am J Dermatopathol 1989;11:136–143.
31. Greenspan JS, Greenspan D, Lenette ET, et al. Replication of Epstein–Barr virus within epithelial cells of oral "hairy" leukoplakia and AIDS associated lesion. N Engl J Med 1985;313:1564–1571.
32. Greenspan D, Greenspan JS, Overby G, et al. Risk factors for rapid progression from hairy leukoplakia to AIDS: a nested case-control study. J Acquir Immune Defic Syndr 1991;4:652–658.
33. Cockerell CJ. Mucocutaneous signs of AIDS other than Kaposi's sarcoma, In: Friedman-Kien AE, ed. *Color atlas of AIDS.* Philadelphia: WB Saunders, 1989:96.
34. Fowler CD, Reed KD, Brannon RB. Intranuclear inclusions correlate with the ultrastructural detection of herpes-type virions in oral hairy leukoplakia. Am J Surg Pathol 1989;13:114–119.
35. DeSouza YG, Greenspan D, Feltzen JR, et al. Localization of Epstein–Barr virus DNA in the epithelial cells of oral hairy leukoplakia via in situ hybridization of tissue sac [letter]. N Engl J Med 1989;320:1559.
36. Kessler HA, Benson CA, Urbanski P. Regression of oral hairy leukoplakia during treatment with azidothymidine. Ann Intern Med 1988;148:2496–2497.
37. Schofer H, Ochsendorf FR, Elm EB, et al. Treatment of oral hairy leukoplakia in AIDS patients with vitamin A acid (topically) or acyclovir (systemically) [letter]. Dermatologica 1987;174:150–151.
38. Beutner KR, Becker TM, Stone KM. Epidemiology of HPV infections. Dermatol Clin 1991;9:211–218.
39. Mattes WL, Triana A, Shapiro R, et al. Dermatologic findings associated with human immunodeficiency virus infection. J Am Acad Dermatol 1987;17:746–751.
40. Palefsky JM, Gonzales J, Greenblatt RM, et al. Anal intraepithelial neoplasia and anal papillomavirus infection among homosexual males with group IV HIV disease. JAMA 1990;263:2911–2916.
41. Rütlinger R, Buchmann P. HPV 16—positive bowenoid papulosis and squamous cell carcinoma in an HIV-positive man. Dis Colon Rectum 1989;32:1042–1045.
42. Rosemberg SK. Subclinical papilloviral infection of male genitalia. Urology 1985;26:552–557.
43. Campion MJ. Clinical manifestations and natural history of genital human papillomavirus infection: Obstet Gynecol Clin North Am 1987;14:363–388.
44. Melchers W, Van Den Brule A, Walboomers J, et al. Increased detection rate of human papillomavirus in cervical scrapes by the polymerase chain reaction as compared to modified FISH and Southern blot analysis. J Med Virol 1989;27:329–335.
45. Stoeh GP, Peterson AL, Taylor WJ. Systemic complications of local podphyllin therapy. Ann Intern Med 1978;89:362–363.
46. Slater GE, Rumack BH, Peterson RG. Podopyllin poisoning: systemic toxicity following cutaneous application. Obstet Gyencol 1987;52:94–96.
47. Beutner KR, Conant M, Friedman-Kien AE, et al. Patient-applied podofilox for treatment of genital warts. Lancet 1989;1:831–838.
48. Baggish MS. Improved laser techniques for the elimination of genital and extragenital warts. Am J Obstet Gynecol 1985;153:545–550.
49. Sawchuck WS, Weber RJ, Lowry DR, et al. Infectious papillomavirus in the vapor of warts treated with carbon dioxide laser or electrocoagulation: detection and protection. J Am Acad Dermatol 1989;21:41–49.
50. Friedman-Kien AE, Eron LJ, Conant M, et al. Natural interferon alfa for treatment of condylomata acuminata. JAMA 1988;259:533–538.
51. Katzman M, Carey JT, Elmets CA, et al. Molluscum contagiosum and AIDS: clinical and immunologic details of two cases. Br J Dermatol 1987;116:131–138.
52. Fivenson DP, Weltman RE, Gibson SH. Giant molluscum contagiosum presenting as basal cell carcinoma in an AIDS patient [letter]. J Am Acad Dermatol 1988;19:912–914.
53. Ganesh R, Castle D, Gibbon D, et al. Staphylococcal carriage in HIV infection. Lancet 1989;2:558.
54. Nichols SL, Balog K, Silverman M. Bacterial infection and AIDS: clinical pathologic correlations in a series of autopsy cases. Am J Clin Pathol 1989;92:787–790.
55. Pitrack DL, Pall AK, Back PA. Serious *Pseudomonas aeruginosa* infection complicating AIDS. Presented at the 9th International Conference on AIDS, Berlin, 1993.
56. Steinhart R, Reingold AL, Taylor F, et al. Invasive *Haemophilus influenzae* infections in men with HIV infection. JAMA 1992;268:3350–3352.
57. Patterson JW, Kitces EN, Neafie RC. Cutaneous botryomycosis in a patient with acquired immunodeficiency syndrome. J Am Acad Dermatol 1987;16:238–242.
58. Weitzner JM, Dhawan SS, Rosen LB, et al. Successful treatment of botryomycosis in a patient with acquired immune deficiency syndrome. J Am Acad Dermatol 21:1312–1314.
59. Janssen F, Zelinsky-Gurung A, Caumes E, et al. Group A streptococcal cellulitis-adenitis in a patient with the acquired immunodeficiency syndrome. J Am Acad Dermatol 1991;24:363–365.
60. el Baze P, Thyss A, Vinti H, et al. A study of nineteen immunocompromised patients with extensive skin lesions caused by *Pseudomonas aeruginosa* with and without bacteremia. Acta Derm Venereol (Stockh) 1991;71:411–415.
61. Kielhofner M, Atmar RL, Hamill RF, et al. Life-threatening *Pseudomonas aeruginosa* infections in patients with human immunodeficiency virus infection. Clin Infect Dis 1992;14:403–411.
62. Sangeorzan JA, Bradley SF, Kaufman CA. Cutaneous manifestation of *Pseudomonas* infection in the acquired immune deficiency syndrome. Arch Dermatol 1990;126:832–833.
63. Adal K, Cockerell CJ, Petrie WP. Bacillary angiomatosis, cat scratch disease, and other infections due to *Rochalimaea*. N Engl J Med 1994;330:1509–1515.
64. Cockerell CJ, LeBoit PE. Bacillary angiomatosis: a novel pseudoneoplastic, infectious vascular disorder. J Am Acad Dermatol 1990;22:501–519.
65. Cockerell CJ, Whitlow MA, Webster GF, et al. Epithelioid angiomatosis: a distinct vascular disorder in patients with acquired immunodeficiency syndrome or AIDS-related complex. Lancet 1987;329:654–656.
66. LeBoit PE, Berger TG, Egbert BM, et al. Bacillary angiomatosis: the histopathology and differential diagnosis of a pseudoneoplastic infection in patients with human immunodeficiency virus disease. Am J Surg Pathol 1989;13:909–920.
67. Behren AL, Steinbach LS, LeBoit PE, et al. Osteolytic lesions in bacillary angiomatosis in AIDS patients: a basis for radiologic differentiation from Kaposi's sarcoma. Radiology 1990;177:77–81.
68. Berger TG, Taparo JW, Kayman A, et al. Bacillary (epithelioid) angiomatosis and concurrent Kaposi's sarcoma in acquired immunodeficiency syndrome. Arch Dermatol 1989;125:1543–1547.
69. Schwartzman WA, Marchevski A, Meyer RD. Epithelioid angiomatosis or cat-scratch disease with splenic and hepatic abnormalities in AIDS: case report or review of the literature. Scand J Infect Dis 1990;22:121–133.
70. Knobler EH, Silvers DN, Fein KC, et al. Unique vascular skin lesions associated with human immunodeficiency virus. JAMA 1988;260:524–527.
71. Barbaro DJ, Orcutt VL, Colder BM. *Mycobacterium avium-intracellulare* infection limited to the skin and lymph nodes in patients with AIDS. Rev Infect Dis 1989;11:625–628.
72. Rogers PL, Walker RE, Wayne HC, et al. Disseminated *Mycobacterium haemophilum* infection in two patients with AIDS. Am J Med 1988;84:640–642.
73. Rohatgi PK, Palazzolo JV, Saini NB. Acute miliary tuberculosis of the skin in acquired immunodeficiency syndrome. J Am Acad Dermatol 1992;26:285–287.
74. Boudes P, Sobel A, Deforges L, et al. Disseminated *Mycobacterium bovis* infection from BCG vaccination and HIV infection [letter]. JAMA 1989;262:2386.

75. Roth C, Theodore C, Aitkin C, et al. Presumed disseminated *Mycobacterium tuberculosis* infection presenting with cutaneous lesions in a patient with AIDS [abstract]. In: Abstracts of the 8th International Conference on AIDS, Amsterdam, 1992.
76. Rogers PL, Walker RE, Lane HC, et al. Disseminated *Mycobacterium haemophilum* infection in two patients with AIDS. Am J Med 1988;84:640–642.
77. Piketty C, Lons Danic D, Weiss L, et al. Atypical sporotrichosis-like infection caused by *Mycobacterium avium* in AIDS [abstract]. In: Abstracts of the 8th International Conference on AIDS, Amsterdam, 1992.
78. Quinn TC, Cannon RO, Glasser D, et al. The association of syphilis with risk of human immunodeficiency virus infection in patients attending sexually transmitted disease clinics. Arch Intern Med 1990; 159:1297–1302.
79. Gregory N, Sanchez M, Buchness MR. The spectrum of syphilis in patients with human immunodeficiency virus infection. J Am Acad Dermatol 1990;22:1061–1067.
80. Glover RA, Piaquadio DJ, Kern S, et al. An unusual presentation of secondary syphilis in a patient with human immunodeficiency virus infection: a case report and review of the literature. Arch Dermatol 1992;128:530–534.
81. Ficarra G, Zaragoza AM, Stendardi L, et al. Early oral presentation of lues maligna in a patient with HIV Infection: a case report. Oral Surg Oral Med Oral Pathol 1993;75:728–732.
82. Johns DR, Tierney M, Felsenstein D. Alteration of the natural history of neurosyphilis by concurrent infection with the human immunodeficiency virus. N Engl J Med 1987;316:1569–1572.
83. Sadick N, Kaplan MH, Pahwa SG, et al. Unusual features of scabies complicating human T-lymphotrophic virus type III infection. J Am Acad Dermatol 1986;15:482–486.
84. Hirschmann JV, Chu AC. Skin lesions with disseminated toxoplasmosis in a patient with the acquired immunodeficiency syndrome. Arch Dermatol 1988;124:1446–1447.
85. Insera DW, Bickley LK. Crusted scabies in acquired immunodeficiency syndrome. Int J Dermatol 1990;29:287–289.
86. Raur C, Baird IM. Crusted scabies in a patient with acquired immunodeficiency syndrome [letter]. J Am Acad Dermatol 1986;15:1058–1059.
87. Jucowics P, Ramon ME, Donn PC, et al. Norwegian scabies in an infant with acquired immunodeficiency syndrome. Arch Dermatol 1989;125:1670–1671.
88. Skinner SM, DeVillez RL. Sepsis associated with Norwegian scabies in patients with acquired immunodeficiency syndrome. Arch Dermatol 1992;50:213–216.
89. O'Donnell BF, O'Loughlin S, Powell FC. Management of crusted scabies. Int J Dermatol 1990;29:258–266.
90. Gherman CR, Ward RR, Bassis ML. *Pneumocystis carinii* otitis media and mastoiditis as the initial manifestation of the acquired immunodeficiency syndrome. Am J Med 1991;127:250–252.
91. Hennessey NP, Parro EL, Cockerell CJ. Cutaneous *Pneumocystis carinii* infection in patients with acquired immunodeficiency syndrome. Arch Dermatol 1991;127:1699–1701.
92. Litwin MA, Williams CM. Cutaneous *Pneumocystis carinii* infection mimicking Kaposi's sarcoma. Ann Intern Med 1992;117:48–49.
93. Portnoy BL, Micheletti GA. *Acanthamoeba* infection of skin and sinuses in an AIDS patient: diagnosis and treatment [abstract]. In: Abstracts of the 8th International Conference on AIDS, Amsterdam, 1992.
94. Glezerov V, Masci JR. Disseminated strongyloidiasis and other selected unusual infections in patients with acquired immunodeficiency syndrome. Prog AIDS Pathol 1990;2:137–142.
95. Klein RS, Harris CA, Small CB, et al. Oral candidiasis in high-risk patients as the initial manifestation of the acquired immunodeficiency syndrome. N Engl J Med 1984;311:354–358.
96. Wolf JE, Little JR, Pappagianis D, et al. Disseminated coccidioidomycosis in a patient with the acquired immune deficiency syndrome. Diagn Microbiol Infect Dis 1986;5:331–336.
97. Prichard JG, Sorotzkin RA, James RE III. Cutaneous manifestations of disseminated coccidioidomycosis in the acquired immunodeficiency syndrome. Cutis 1987;39:203–205.
98. Fish DG, Ampel NM, Galgiani JN, et al. Coccidioidomycosis during human immunodeficiency virus infection: a review of 77 patients. Medicine 1990;69:384–391.
99. Manrique P, Mayo J, Alvarez JA, et al. Polymorphous cutaneous cryptococcosis: nodular, herpes-like, and molluscum-like lesions in a patient with the acquired immunodeficiency syndrome. J Am Acad Dermatol 1992;26:122–124.
100. Cusini M, Cagliani P, Grimalt R, et al. Primary cutaneous cryptococcosis in a patient with the acquired immunodeficiency syndrome [letter]. Arch Dermatol 1991;127:1848–1849.
101. Jones C, Orengo I, Rosen T, et al. Cutaneous cryptococcosis simulating Kaposi's sarcoma in the acquired immunodeficiency syndrome. Cutis 1990;45:163–167.
102. Lynch DP, Naftolin LZ. Oral *Cryptococcus neoformans* infection in AIDS. Oral Surg Oral Med Oral Pathol 1987;64:449–453.
103. Rico NJ, Penneys NS. Cutaneous cryptococcosis resembling molluscum contagiosum in a patient with AIDS. Arch Dermatol 1985;121:901–902.
104. Mares M, Sartori MT, Carretta M, et al. Rhinophyma-like cryptococcal infection as an early manifestation of aids in a hemophilia B patient. Acta Haematol 1990;84:101–103.
105. Cohen PR, Grossman ME, Silvers DN. Disseminated histoplasmosis and human immunodeficiency virus infection. Int J Dermatol 1991; 30:614–622.
106. Hazelhurst JA, Vismer JF. Histoplasmosis presenting with unusual skin lesions in acquired immunodeficiency syndrome (AIDS). Br J Dermatol 1985;113:345–348.
107. Kalter DC, Tschen JA, Klima M. Maculopapular rash in a patient with acquired immunodeficiency syndrome. Arch Dermatol 1985;121:1455–1456.
108. Lindgren AM, Fallon JD, Horan RF. Psoriasiform papules in the acquired immunodeficiency syndrome: disseminated histoplasmosis in AIDS. Arch Dermatol 1991;127:722–723, 725–726.
109. Chaker MB, Cockerell CJ. Concomitant psoriasis, seborrheic dermatitis and disseminated cutaneous histoplasmosis in a patient infected with human immunodeficiency virus: J Am Acad Dermatol 1993;29:311–313.
110. Cole MC, Cohen PR, Satra KH, et al. The concurrent presence of systemic disease pathogens and cutaneous Kaposi's sarcoma in the same lesion: *Histoplasma capsulatum* and Kaposi's sarcoma coexisting in a single skin lesion in a patient with AIDS. J Am Acad Dermatol 1992;26:285–287.
111. Lipstein-Kresch E, Isenberg HD, Singer C, et al. Disseminated *Sporothrix schenckii* infection with arthritis in a patient with acquired immunodeficiency syndrome. J Rheumatol 1985;12:805–808.
112. Shaw JC, Levinson W, Montanara A. Sporotrichosis in the acquired immunodeficiency syndrome. J Am Acad Dermatol 1989;21:1145–1147.
113. Fitzpatrick JE, Eubanks S. Acquired immunodeficiency syndrome presenting as disseminated cutaneous sporotrichosis. Int J Dermatol 1988;27:406–407.
114. Bibler MR, Luber HJ, Glueck HI, et al. Disseminated sporotrichosis in a patient with HIV infection after treatment for acquired factor VIII inhibitor. JAMA 1986;256:3125–3126.
115. Fraser VJ, Keath EJ, Powderly WG. Two cases of blastomycosis from a common source: use of DNA restriction analysis to identify strains. J Infect Dis 1991;163:1378–1381.
116. Wood GM, McCormack JG, Muir DB, et al. Clinical features of human infection with *Scedosporium inflatum*. Clin Infect Dis 1992;14:1027–1033.
117. Scherr GR, Evans SG, Kiyabu MT, et al. *Pseudallescheria boydii* in the acquired immunodeficiency syndrome. Arch Pathol Lab Med 1992;116:535–536.

118. Hevia O, Kligman D, Penneys NS. Nonscalp hair infection caused by *Microsporum canis* in a patient with acquired immunodeficiency syndrome. J Am Acad Dermatol 1991;24:789–790.
119. Frazer R, Stoole E, Schmidt J, et al. Head and neck zygomycetes/aspergillus infections in patients with AIDS. Presented at the 9th International Conference on AIDS, Berlin, 1993.
120. Sanders M. Panza-Wilson I. Cutaneous zygomycosis. Presented at the 9th International Conference on AIDS, Berlin, 1993.
121. Sachot LJ, Hadderingh RJ, Devriese PP. Facial palsy and HIV infection [abstract]. In: Abstracts of the 8th International Conference on AIDS, Amsterdam, 1992.
122. Supparatpinyo K, Chiewchanvit S, Hirunsri P, et al. *Penicillium marneffei* in patients infected with HIV [abstract]. In: Abstracts of the 8th International Conference on AIDS, Amsterdam, 1992.
123. Terrell CL, Hughes CE. Antifungal agents used for deep-seated mycotic infections. Mayo Clin Proc 1992;67:69–91.
124. Mathes BM, Douglass MC. Seborrheic dermatitis in patients with acquired immunodeficiency syndrome. J Am Acad Dermatol 1985;13:947–951.
125. Rao BK, Cockerell CJ. Histologic findings in inflammatory dermatoses in a patient with HIV Infection. Presented at the 7th International Conference on AIDS, Florence, Italy, 1991.
126. Duvic M, Johnson TM, Rapini RP, et al. Acquired immunodeficiency syndrome-associated psoriasis and Reiter's syndrome. Arch Dermatol 1987;123:1622–1623.
127. Kaplan MH, Sadik NS, Weider J, et al. Antipsoriatic effects of zidovudine in human immunodeficiency virus–associated psoriasis. J Am Acad Dermatol 1989;20:76–82.
128. Kaye BR. Rheumatologic manifestations of infection with human immunodeficiency virus (HIV). Ann Intern Med 1989;111:158–167.
129. Herman LE, Curbin AK. Eryrthroderma as a manifestation of the AIDS-related complex. J Am Acad Dermatol 1987;17:507.
130. Soeprono FF, Schinella RA. Eosinophilic pustular folliculitis in patients with acquired immunodeficiency syndrome. J Am Acad Dermatol 1986;14:1020–1022.
131. Rosenthal D, LeBoit PE, Klumpp L, et al. Human immunodeficiency virus–associated eosinophilic folliculitis: a unique dermatitis associated with advanced human immunodeficiency virus infection. Arch Dermatol 1991;127:206–209.
132. Buchness MR, Lim HW, Hatcher VA, et al. Eosinophilic pustular folliculitis in the acquired immunodeficiency syndrome. N Engl J Med 1988;318:1183–1186.
133. Sadik NS, McNutt NS. Cutaneous hypersensitivity reactions in patients with AIDS. Int J Dermatol 1993;32:621–627.
134. Miadonna A, Zeger E, Tedeschi A, et al. Enchanced basophil releasability in subjects infected with human immunodeficiency virus. Clin Immunol Immunopathol 1990;54:237–246.
135. Tateno M, Gonzales-Scarano F, Levy JA. Human immunodeficiency virus type 1 can infect CD-4 negative human fibroblastoid cells. Proc Natl Acad Sci U S A 1989;11:4287–4290.
136. Valerie K, Delers A, Bruck C, et al. Activation of human immunodeficiency virus type 1 by DNA damage in human cells. Nature 1988;333:78–81.
137. Meola T, Soter NA, Ostrecher R, et al. The safety of UVB phototherapy in patients with HIV infection. J Am Acad Dermatol 1993;29:216–20.
138. King DA, Ion D, Berger TG, et al. Itraconazole for treatment of HIV-associated eosinophilic folliculitis. Presented at the 9th International Conference on AIDS, Berlin, 1993.
139. Toback AC, Longley J, Cardello AC, et al. Severe chronic photosensitivity in association with acquired immunodeficiency syndrome. Arch Dermatol 1986;15:2056–2057.
140. Tojo N, Yoshimura N, Yoshizawa M, et al. Vitiligo and chronic photosensitivity in human immunodeficiency virus infection. Jpn J Med 1991;30:255–259.
141. Lobato MN, Berger TG. Porphyria cutanea tarda associated with the acquired immunodeficiency syndrome. Arch Dermatol 1988;124:1009–1010.
142. Herranz MT, el Amrani A, Aranegui P, et al. Porphyria cutanea tarda and acquired immunodeficiency syndrome: pathogenetic mechanisms. Arch Dermatol 1991;12:1585–1586.
143. Picard C, Crickx B, Fegueuz S, et al. Porphyria cutanea tarda in HIV infection. Presented at the 7th International Conference on AIDS, Florence, Italy, 1991.
144. Egbert BM, LeBoit PE, McCalmont T, et al. Caterpillar bodies: distinctive, basement membrane-containing structures in blisters of porphyria. Am J Dermatopathol 1993;15:199–202.
145. Reference deleted.
146. Anderson KE, Goeger DE, Carson RW, et al. Erythropoietin for the treatment of porphyria cutanea tarda in a patient on long-term hemodialysis. N Engl J Med 1990;322:315–317.
147. Coopman SA, Johnson RA, et al. Cutaneous disease and drug reactions in HIV infection. N Engl J Med 1993;328:1670–1674.
148. Gordin FM, Simon GL, Wofsy CD, et al. Adverse reactions to trimethoprim–sulfamethoxazole in patients with the acquired immunodeficiency syndrome. Ann Intern Med 1984;100:495–499.
149. Raviglione MC, Dinan WA, Pablo-Mendez A, et al. Fatal toxic epidermal necrolysis during prophylaxis with pyrimethamine and sulfadoxine in a human immunodeficiency virus–infected person. Arch Intern Med 1988;148:2683–2685.
150. Nunn P, Wasunna K, Kwanyah G, et al. Cutaneous hypersensitivity reactions to thiacetazone among HIV-1 seropositive tuberculosis patients in Nairobi. Presented at the 7th International Conference on AIDS, Florence, Italy, 1992.
151. Snyder DE, Graczyk J, Beck E, et al. Supervised six-month treatment of newly diagnosed pulmonary tuberculosis using isoniazid, rifampin and pyrazinamide with and without streptomycin. Am Rev Respir Dis 1984;130:190–194.
152. Battegay M, Opravil M, Wuthrich B, et al. Rash with amoxicillin–clavulanate therapy in HIV-infected patients [letter]. Lancet 1989;2:1100.
153. Donn PC, Fusco F, Fried P, et al. Nail dyschromia associated with zidovudine. Ann Intern Med 1990;112:145–146.
154. Furth PA, Kazakis AM. Nail pigmentation changes associated with azidothymidine (zidovudine). Ann Intern Med 1987;107:350.
155. Greenberg RG, Berger TG. Nail and mucocutaneous hyperpigmentation with azidothymidine therapy. J Am Acad Dermatol 1990;327:330.
156. Merenich JA, Hannen RN, Gentry RH, et al. Azidothymidine-induced hyperpigmentation mimicking primary adrenal insufficiency. Am J Med 1989;86:469–470.
157. Gaglioti D, Ficarra G, Adler-Storthz K, et al. Zidovudine-related oral lichenoid reactions. Presented at the 7th International Conference on AIDS, Florence, Italy, 1991.
158. Bessen LJ, Greene JB, Louis E, et al. Severe polymyositis-like syndrome associated with zidovudine or AIDS or ARC [letter]. N Engl J Med 1988;311:708.
159. Feingold I. Oral desensitization of trimethoprim-sulfamethoxasole in a patient with acquired immunodeficiency syndrome [letter]. J Allergy Clin Immunol 1986;78:905.
160. Leonidas JR. Hair alteration in black patients with acquired immunodeficiency syndrome. Cutis 1987;39:537–538.
161. Casanova JM, Puig T, Rubio M. Hypertrichosis of the eyelashes in acquired immunodeficiency syndrome. Arch Dermatol 1987;123:1599–1601.
162. Foon KA, Dougher G. Increased growth of eyelashes in a patient given leukocyte a interferon [letter]. N Engl J Med 1984;311:1259.
163. Kaplan MH, Sadik NS, Talmor M. Aquired trichomegaly of the eyelashes a cutaneous marker of acquired immunodeficiency syndrome: J Am Acad Dermatol 1991;25:801–804.
164. Casanova JM, Puig T, Rubio M. Hypertrichosis of the eyelashes in acqured immunodeficiency syndrome. Arch Dermatol 1987;123:1599-1601.

165. Schonwetter RS, Nelson EB. Alopecia areata and the acquired immunodeficiency syndrome related complex [letter]. Ann Intern Med 1986;104:287.
166. Sadick NS. Clinical and laboratory evaluation of AIDS trichopathy. Int J Dermatol 1993;32:33–38.
167. Chernosky ME, Findley VK. Yellow-nail syndrome in patients with AIDS. J Am Acad Dermatol 1985;13:731–737.
168. Scher RK. Acquired immunodeficiency syndrome and yellow nails. J Am Acad Dermatol 1988;18:758–759.
169. Yabe Y, Tanimura Y, Sakai A, et al. Molecular characteristics and physical state of human papillomavirus DNA change with progressing malignancy: studies in a patient with epidermodysplasia verruciformis. Int J Cancer 1989;43:1022–1028.
170. Sitz KV, Keppen M. Metastatic basal cell carcinoma in acquired immunodeficiency syndrome–related complex. JAMA 1987;257:340–343.
171. Berger TG, Sawchuk WS, Leonardi C, et al. Epidermodysplasia verruciformis-associated papillomavirus infection complicating human immunodeficiency virus disease. Br J Dermatol 1991;126:79–83.
172. Fink MJ, Fretcher R, Mamand M, et al. Cytology, colposcopy and histology in HIV-positive women. Presented at the 9th International Conference on AIDS, Berlin, 1993.
173. Guinness K, LaGuardia K. Cryotherapy in the management of cervical dysplasia in HIV-infected women. Presented at the 9th International Conference on AIDS, Berlin, 1993.
174. Parker SC, Fenton DA, McGibbon DH. L'homme rouge and the acquired immunodeficiency syndrome. N Engl J Med 1989;321:906–907.
175. Kobayashi M, Yoshimoto S, Fujishita M, et al. HTLV-positive T-cell lymphoma/leukemia in an AIDS patient. Lancet 1984;1:1361–1362.
176. Nagatani T, Miyazawa T, Matsuzaki T, Iemoto G, et al. Adult T-cell leukemia/lymphoma (ATL): clinical, histopathological, immunological and immunohistochemical characteristics. Exp Dermatol 1992;1:248–252.
177. Knowles DM, Chamulak G, Subar M, et al. Clinical pathologic immunophenotypic and molecular genetic analysis of AIDS-associated lymphoid neoplasia: clinical and biologic implications. Pathol Annu 1988;23:33–67.

32

ORAL MANIFESTATIONS OF HIV INFECTION AND AIDS

John S. Greenspan and Deborah Greenspan

EPIDEMIOLOGY

Significance of Oral Manifestations

Oral candidiasis was one of the lesions observed in the initial reports of the condition that became known as acquired immune deficiency syndrome (AIDS) (1). With the discovery of hairy leukoplakia (HL) (2) and the observation of its relationship with human immunodeficiency virus (HIV) infection and the development of AIDS in otherwise asymptomatic individuals in the then-recognized AIDS risk groups (3), we and others postulated that those two lesions, as well as other opportunistic oral infections, were important indicators of HIV infection and of probable progression of disease in patients with that infection. In principle, this finding should not be unexpected because the mouth, even in healthy individuals, houses a varied and energetic flora prone to become aggressive and to cause opportunistic disease in the presence of even slight weakening of local or systemic immune defenses (4). However, this group of lesions also is of specific prognostic significance independent of other available markers of immunosuppression, both direct and surrogate (5). The biologic implication of that relationship is that the oral flora can detect and take advantage of subtle, perhaps local mucosal, detects that are beyond the sensitivity of current assays of immune function. The defects in host ability to resist oncogenic influences, which also include microbiologic agents such as human papillomavirus (HPV) and human herpesvirus 8 (HHV8) and lead to at least some the malignancies seen in AIDS, must be particularly marked in the oral cavity of HIV-infected individuals, because Kaposi's sarcoma (KS) and non–Hodgkin's lymphoma commonly present first in the mouth and oropharynx. Autoimmune disorders, and presumably autoimmune diseases associated with HIV infection, such as aphthous ulcers and salivary gland disease, also cause clinically important oral lesions.

The oral lesions described in this chapter are thus of both theoretic and practical importance in the diagnosis of HIV infection (3, 6–9), in staging schemes for HIV diseases (10–12), in assessing prognosis (13, 14), and in initiating use (15) and judging response to antiretroviral therapy. Both oral candidiasis and oral HL are included in the 1993 expanded AIDS surveillance case definition. In the presence of CD4 counts lower than $200/mm^3$, both lesions are listed as symptomatic conditions in category B3, thus qualifying patients for a diagnosis of AIDS (16). Oral candidiasis and HL feature in the Pan American Health Organization ("Caracas") definition of AIDS (17, 18), and both lesions have been used as entry criteria or as "soft end points" in HIV therapy (19) and vaccine trials.

The published literature on oral HIV-associated diseases and their management, as well as on the broader professional implications of AIDS for oral health care, is extensive and is growing rapidly. This chapter emphasizes the recognition, significance, and management of the oral lesions and cites mostly those papers that describe initial observations or illustrate important issues. For a more complete listing of publications in this field, the reader may refer to other reviews (20–23).

Prevalence and Incidence

Many accounts of the frequency of the oral lesions have been based on clinic populations (24–27). Although providing valuable insight into the range of oral HIV-associated disease, such accounts do not determine how common the conditions are among persons with HIV infection.

A widely held impression is that oral lesions are common features of HIV disease. However, few well-designed population-based studies are available. Published reports include descriptions of otherwise asymptomatic HIV-seropositive individuals (original United States Centers for Disease Control and Prevention [CDC] group II or 1993 CDC category A), those with persistent lymphadenopathy and other manifestations of HIV infection short of full AIDS (original CDC group III and IV A, C2, and E; 1993 CDC category B), and patients with AIDS (original CDC group IV C1 and D; 1993 CDC category C). The presence of oral lesions significantly affects the CDC group category to which cases are assigned in both the original version (10) and the 1993 classification. Examples of the prevalence of oral lesions of any type in such convenience sample–based studies ranged from 15%, in HIV-seropositive women in Nairobi in 1989 (28), through about 50%, in patients in all CDC original-staging group IV categories in Tanzania in 1987 (29) and in England in 1988 (26), to even higher percentages, including 80% of a sample of HIV-positive patients in CDC groups II, III, and IV in Mexico City who were examined in 1989 and 1990 (27) and almost 100% of a sample of hospitalized AIDS patients in Zaire in 1989 (30). HL was found in 29.5% of a mixed population of outpatients at an HIV clinic in Antwerp reported in 1992 (31), but this lesion was less common in some studies from Africa. However, none of those studies represented population-based cohorts. Thus, all the data reflect referral or other selection bias.

At the University of California, San Francisco Oral AIDS Center, we have examined subjects in several cohorts who are enrolled in longitudinal studies of the natural history of HIV infection. These include homosexual or bisexual men, injection drug users, transfusion recipients, hemophiliacs, heterosexual women and men, and children. Our oral examinations of these cohorts began in 1987. The prevalences of the commonest HIV-associated lesions in HIV-infected men who have sex with men (excluding men with AIDS) were approximately 19% for HL, 9% for candidiasis, and 4% for all other oral lesions (32). The prevalence of any oral lesion was almost 30%. These men had acquired their HIV infection at different times, but most were probably infected between 1978 and 1984, generally toward the later date. Because the study was performed from 1987 to 1990, most of the subjects would have been seropositive for 3 to 10 years. The data are therefore probably representative of HIV-positive, non-AIDS patients who have not received significant antiretroviral therapy. Among women with HIV infection resulting from heterosexual transmission or injection drug use, we found a prevalence of oral lesions of 22% (15% candidiasis and 10% HL) (33). The types and frequency of oral lesions were similar to those seen in our studies of men. Among children seen in a pediatric AIDS clinic (34), we found that 72% had oral candidiasis, 47% had parotid enlargement, 24% had herpes simplex, and 2% had HL.

Little evidence is available to suggest major differences in the prevalence or type of oral lesions among risk groups or based on geography, gender, or ethnicity apart from the relative rarity of KS in women (35) and of the rarity of that lesion and of HL in children.

Classification

Few investigators disagree concerning the association between HIV infection and its commonest oral manifestations. However, at least 40 oral lesions have been claimed as features of HIV infection. Detailed classifications have been established under the auspices of the European Union (36, 37) and a U.S. collaborative group (38). However, many of the oral lesions described in the literature have been reported as single cases and may be only coincidentally associated with HIV infection. Table 32.1 lists the oral lesions most frequently seen and clearly associated with HIV infection.

Table 32.1. Oral Lesions of HIV Infection

Neoplastic
  Kaposi's sarcoma
  Lymphoma
Fungal
  Candidiasis
  Histoplasmosis
  Cryptococcosis
  Aspergillosis
  Geotrichosis
  Penicilliosis
Viral
  Herpes simplex
  Herpes zoster
  Hairy leukoplakia (Epstein–Barr virus)
  Cytomegalovirus disease
  Warts
Bacterial
  Gingivitis
  Periodontitis
  Necrotizing stomatitis
  Tuberculosis
  Mycobacterium avium-intracellulare complex infection
Autoimmune/idiopathic
  Recurrent aphthous ulcers
  Immune thrombocytopenic purpura
  Salivary gland disease
  Abnormal pigmentation

NEOPLASMS

Kaposi's Sarcoma

The oral lesions of KS are often the first manifestation of AIDS (37), particularly among men who have sex with men, but also occasionally in women (39), and these lesions were among the first oral features of the epidemic to be identified (40, 41). Investigators now know that KS may be caused by the recently described HHV8 (42, 43); although the route of transmission is not known, herpesviruses in humans often spread through saliva, so an oral route is possible. What, if any, relationship exists between the route of transmission and the location of KS lesions is not clear. However, the frequency of oral lesions is intriguing in that regard. The palate is the commonest location for oral KS (Fig. 32.1), and lesions may also be seen on the gingiva and tongue, in the salivary glands, and within the mandible or cervical lymph nodes (44, 45). Oral KS may present as blue, purple, or red flat or raised patches, nodules, or extensive tumors. Yellow staining of the mucosa adjacent to the lesion may be seen. Occasionally, oral KS may be covered by normal-colored mucosa (20). Large or nodular lesions may ulcerate and may become secondarily infected. The differential diagnosis includes hemangioma, purpura or eccymosis, pyogenic granuloma, and many other benign or malignant oral nodular lesions. Biopsy is required for definitive diagnosis. The histopathologic features are the same as those of KS lesions of skin and viscera (46).

The oral lesions of KS may be painful because of ulceration and secondary infection. They may interfere with mastication and swallowing, and the appearance of visible lesions may be embarrassing to the patient. Small lesions usually respond well to local therapy, for example, surgical or laser excision or intralesional chemotherapy, using agents such as vinblastine (47). Sclerosing agents have also proved useful (48). Larger lesions have responded well to radiation therapy, although mucositis may be a complication (39). Oral lesions should be treated, early if possible, to slow progress and to reduce the morbidity associated with secondary infection that may mimic HIV-related periodontal disease.

Lymphoma

Non–Hodgkin's lymphoma (49, 50) is the other form of malignant disease commonly found in AIDS, and many patients have oral lesions that may precede lesions at other sites. These oral manifestations may be the only lesions and so may be the presenting and diagnostic lesions of AIDS (51). AIDS lymphoma may be found anywhere in the mouth and can present as diffuse swellings, discrete nodules, or ulcers of varied shapes, sizes, and surface characteristics (Fig. 32.2). As with oral lymphomas in other populations, these lesions can resemble other conditions causing mucosal ulceration, and repeated biopsies may be needed for diagnosis. Most lymphomas are of B-cell origin; many harbor Epstein–Barr virus (EBV) DNA, although a few are predominantly T-cell lesions, and in a small number, assigning a phenotype may be difficult. We and others have seen multifocal oral lymphoma (52), as well as oral ulcers that are histologically lymphoma but that spontaneously resolve, only to reappear later elsewhere in the mouth as lymphoma (53). Oral HL predicted the development of lymphoma in one study of more than 1000 patients with advanced HIV disease who were receiving zidovidine (54). No accounts of oral lesions of AIDS-related Hodgkin's disease have been published.

Oral Cancer

Basal cell carcinoma and low-grade squamous cell carcinoma of the skin appear to be associated with HIV infection

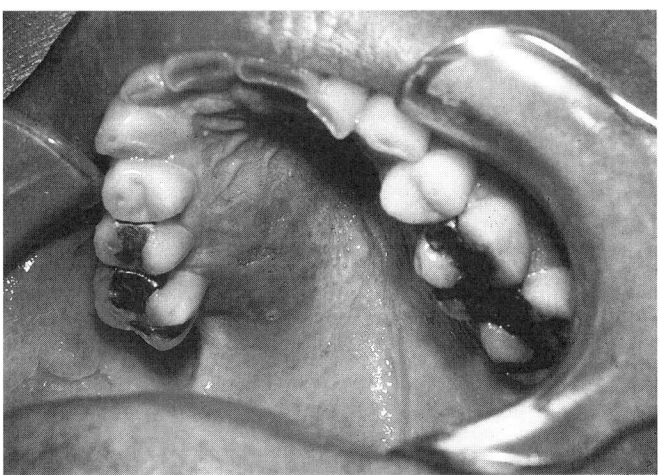

Figure 32.1. Kaposi's sarcoma of the palate. (See color section.)

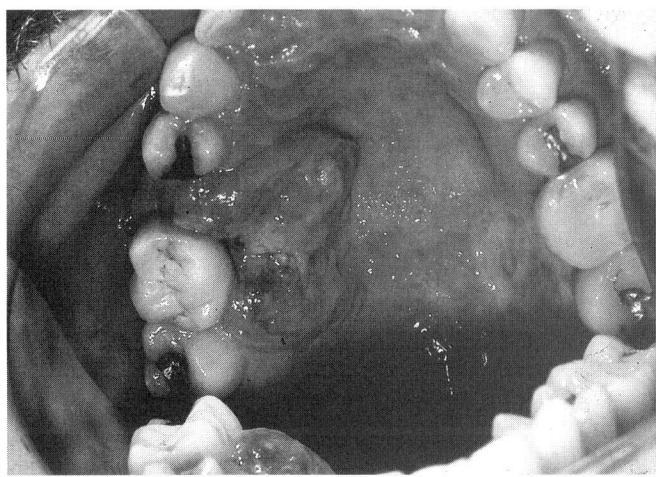

Figure 32.2. Lymphoma of the palate. (See color section.)

(55). However, no convincing evidence indicates an association between oral squamous cell carcinoma and HIV infection, notwithstanding a few, probably coincidental, case reports (56). However, the possibility exists that, as the life expectancy of HIV-infected individuals increases, oral cancer resulting from papillomavirus and prolonged tobacco use may occur. Clear evidence indicates increased incidence of anogenital precancer (57). HL, a lesion caused by the potentially oncogenic organism EBV, does not appear to be premalignant.

FUNGAL LESIONS

Oral Candidiasis

Oral and esophageal candidiasis were among the first opportunistic infections identified in the original description of what was to become known as AIDS (1, 58). Candidiasis of the esophagus was an AIDS-defining condition in CDC group IV category C1 of the 1986 definition. Oral candidiasis was included in group IV category C2 of that definition and is included in category B3 of the 1993 revised definition. Oral candidiasis also occurs as a feature of the acute syndrome that may be associated with primary HIV infection (59, 60). *Candida* and related yeasts can be identified even in the healthy mouth (61). *Candida* counts are higher in persons with asymptomatic HIV infection and increase as the CD4 cells diminish in number (62). Oral candidiasis, also known as candidosis, can be associated with many predisposing factors other than HIV infection and is one of the more common infections seen in oral medicine practice. These other factors include systemic disease such as diabetes and anemia, infancy, old age, and the wearing of dentures. Immunosuppressed patients, including those receiving corticosteroids and other immunosuppressive medications, as well as HIV-infected individuals, are particularly prone to the disease (11, 63). The presence of this lesion is therefore not nearly as indicative of HIV infection as is the presence of HL.

The diagnosis of oral candidiasis can usually be made on clinical appearance, although some simple tests are helpful if available. The best of these tests is the use of a potassium hydroxide, periodic acid–Schiff, or Gram-stained smear from the lesions to demonstrate *Candida* hyphae. A culture can be used to determine the species of fungus, but culture is not helpful in diagnosis. An association between oral candidiasis and esophageal candidiasis was reported in the early stages of the AIDS epidemic (64), but this relation has not been confirmed. Our attempts to find esophageal lesions using endoscopy in patients with both pseudomembranous and erythematous oral candidiasis have been unsuccessful.

Candidiasis, like certain other oral mucosal lesions, is one of the early clinical indicators of progression of HIV infection. Although usually commensal in healthy individuals, *Candida* becomes superficially invasive in many immunosuppressed patients and causes lesions. In HIV-infected women, vaginal candidiasis appears even earlier in the decline of CD4 cells than does oral candidiasis in both men and women infected with the virus (65). With the transition from commensal to invasive disease, the fungus undergoes morphologic and genetic alterations that may be important factors in pathogenesis. Thus, commensal yeastlike forms become hyphal, the form usually isolated from lesions. Concurrently, gene expression is altered, and the repertoire of macromolecules, including surface antigens and potential virulence factors, also changes. Superimposed on these events is a process of phenotypical switching that influences a range of other cell properties (66). Clinically relevant events appear to include the effects of phenotypical switching on drug sensitivity and the expression of virulence associated with a secreted aspartyl protease (67).

Several reports indicate that most individuals carry a single strain of *Candida*, as defined by restriction length polymorphism and other criteria, during the course of HIV infection, both when mucosal lesions are absent and when they are present (68–70). The absence of unique or specifically pathogenic strains (71, 72) is evidence of a primary role for defects in host defense mechanisms in the events initiating the pathogenesis of oral mucosal candidiasis.

In association with HIV infection, candidiasis occurs as three types: erythematous candidiasis, pseudomembranous candidiasis (thrush), and angular cheilitis. Two or even all three may be seen together, and any or all types can occur at the same time as HL. Hyperplastic candidiasis, also known as candidal leukoplakia, is not a feature of oral disease in persons with HIV infection, although HL is sometimes mistakenly diagnosed as that lesion.

ERYTHEMATOUS CANDIDIASIS

Lesions of erythematous candidiasis appear as red areas of the mucosa (Fig. 32.3). The typical location is the palate, but lesions on the dorsal tongue in the form of papillary atrophy are common, and involvement of other oral mucosal sites also occurs. Erythematous candidiasis is usually asymptomatic, although soreness and burning may be reported. No objective evidence suggests that the apparently milder erythematous type precedes the more florid pseudomembranous form. Indeed, our studies show both forms to be equally predictive

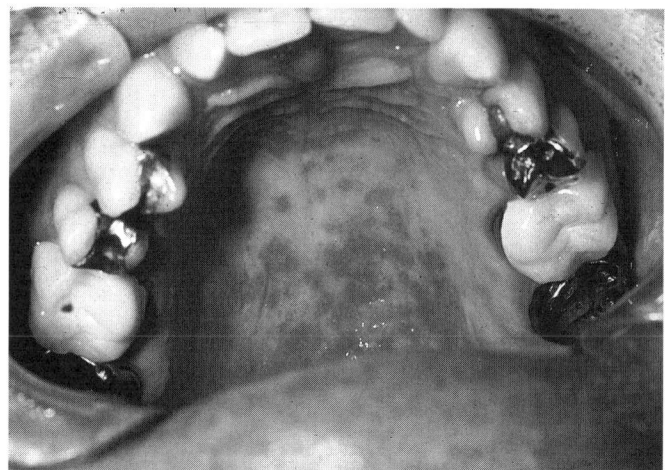

Figure 32.3. Erythematous candidiasis of the palate. (See color section.)

of progression of HIV infection (73). Because of its subtle nature, erythematous candidiasis is frequently overlooked, particularly by personnel lacking special training in the area of diagnosis of oral mucosal disease. Thus, many studies involving oral lesions as predictors of progression of HIV infection omit reference to the erythematous form. This omission is of significance because, as mentioned earlier, erythematous candidiasis is equally predictive of the development of AIDS in those with earlier stage infection as is the more noticeable pseudomembranous variety (73).

PSEUDOMEMBRANOUS CANDIDIASIS

Frequently still known by its ancient name of thrush, pseudomembranous candidiasis presents as white or cream-colored patches. The plaques can be removed, revealing a bleeding surface. Although the palate is again the commonest location, any oral or pharyngeal mucosal surface may be involved, including the gingiva (Fig. 32.4). The adjoining mucosa is often red, resembling erythematous candidiasis, and the patient may complain of pain, soreness, and dysphagia.

ANGULAR CHEILITIS

The angular cheilitis lesion is notable for cracks or fissures at the angles of the mouth and is often due to candidal infection. Therapy for oral candidiasis is indicated to deal with the symptoms, which include pain, burning sensations, soreness, and dysguesia. Such complaints may occur with any of the clinical presentations of oral candidiasis.

Therapy involves the use of topical or systemic antifungal agents. Topical treatment approaches for oral candidiasis include the use of mycostatin, either as vaginal troches (100,000 U, dissolved slowly in the mouth three to four times a day) or as mycostatin oral pastilles (200,000 U; one to two pastilles dissolved in the mouth five times a day). Other preparations include clotrimazole (Mycelex) oral troches (10 mg; one tablet dissolved in the mouth five times a day). With good compliance, any of these remedies usually clears the oral lesions. Unfortunately, compliance can be a problem because of the unpleasant flavor of some of the preparations and the length of time the tablets should be held in the mouth each day. Systemic antifungal therapy has the advantage of once-daily dosage. However, systemic antifungal drugs may interact with other medications prescribed in association with HIV infection.

Ketoconazole should be taken (one 200-mg tablet per day) at the same time as food. Adverse effects of ketoconazole can include changes in liver function, changes in adrenal hormone metabolism, nausea, and skin rash. Furthermore, ketoconazole may not be adequately absorbed in people with HIV infection because they can experience changes in gastric pH, poor absorption, and other gastrointestinal problems associated with HIV infection (74).

Fluconazole is a newer and frequently effective agent. The recommended dose is one 100-mg tablet per day for 9 to 14 days. Fluconazole interacts with certain other drugs, such as rifampin, so the use of fluconazole should be avoided in these cases. Fluconazole inhibits candidal adherence to oral epithelial cells (75). Fluconazole is well absorbed and well tolerated, but its use may be associated with the emergence of resistant strains of the fungus (76).

Although true antifungal resistance, established by laboratory testing, appears to be rare and confined to the use of fluconazole among the agents mentioned, clinical lack of efficacy is seen and probably results from poor compliance or poor absorption of the antifungal drug used. Relapses are common, and once an individual has had two episodes of oral candidiasis, maintenance therapy may be helpful (77), although the introduction of topical amphotericin B offers a powerful new (in fact, rediscovered) topical remedy for oropharyngeal candidiasis. No consensus exists on the effectiveness and value of long-term antifungal prophylaxis for oral candidiasis in HIV-positive individuals who have not yet developed this oral lesion (78).

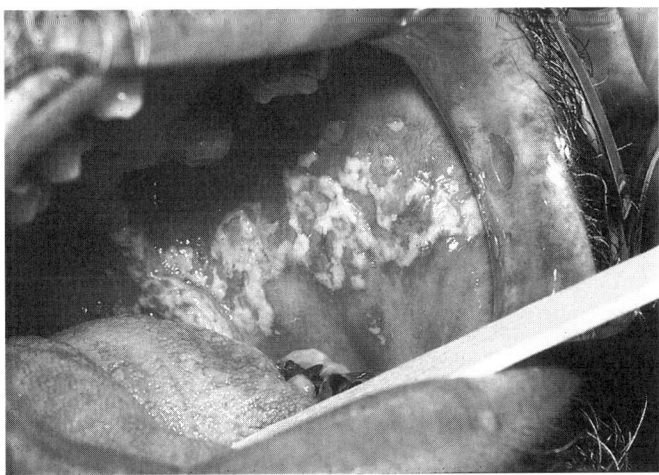

Figure 32.4. Pseudomembranous candidiasis of the cheek. (See color section.)

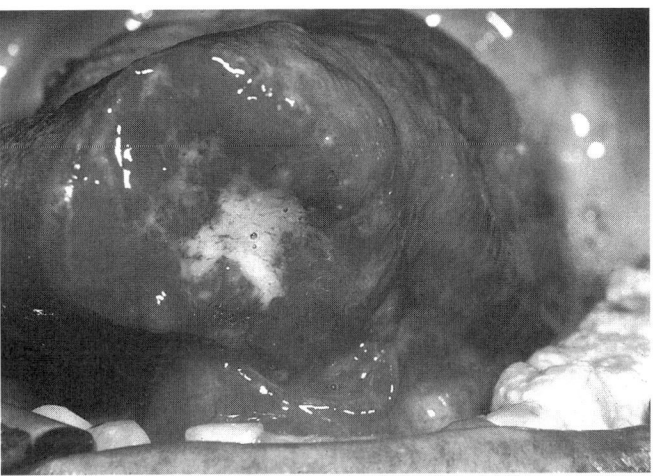

Figure 32.5. Histoplasmosis of the tongue. (See color section.)

Other Oral Fungal Lesions

Occasional examples of oral histoplasmosis (79) (Fig. 32.5), cryptococcosis (80–82), aspergillosis (83), geotrichosis (84), and penicilliosis (85) have been reported. Although most lesions are seen in people with systemic fungal infection, such oral lesions can also be the first-diagnosed or the only lesion of these conditions, leading to prompt diagnosis and care.

VIRAL LESIONS

Herpes Simplex

Orofacial herpes simplex is commonly seen in HIV infection (24). The typical lesions are recurrent intraoral ulcers (Fig. 32.6) or recurrent herpes labialis (25). However, the lesions may be larger and may last much longer than in the immunocompetent individual. They can also be found in unusual oral locations, such as the dorsal tongue. Although herpes simplex virus type 1 (HSV-1) is the predominant type involved, HSV-2 is also occasionally found (86). Acyclovir capsules (200 mg; five to six tablets a day) may be useful in shortening the duration of large herpes labialis lesions and in treating more troublesome intraoral lesions. Acyclovir-resistant oral and perioral herpes caused by HSV-2 is seen increasingly in association with HIV infection (86–88). The lesions respond to foscarnet (trisodium phosphonoformate hexahydrate) (86).

Varicella/Herpes Zoster

The varicella-zoster virus (VZV) is a further human herpes virus that causes oral lesions in patients with HIV infection. Oral lesions of chickenpox have been reported. These lesions responded to high doses of systemic acyclovir (89). Orofacial herpes zoster, caused by reactivation of VZV in patients with failing cell-mediated immunity, is seen in the course of HIV disease. AIDS-defining illness developed in 23% of such patients in 2 years and in 46% in 4 years (90, 91). Herpes

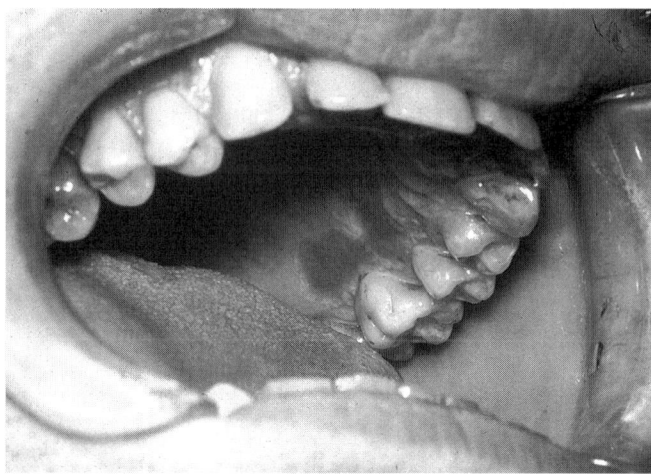

Figure 32.6. Recurrent intraoral herpes simplex of the palate. (See color section.)

zoster produces painful vesicles and ulcers that occur in the distribution of one or more branches of the trigeminal nerve. The lesions usually heal, but treatment with high doses of acyclovir (up to 4 g per day as tablets or even intravenous acyclovir) is indicated to treat or prevent eye lesions. Postherpetic neuralgia after orofacial zoster may be a common and painful complication.

Cytomegalovirus

The herpes-group virus cytomegalovirus (CMV) is common in the healthy population and infects most people who are HIV positive. Oral ulcers that resemble large aphthous ulcers may be seen as features of disseminated CMV disease, as the first clinical sign of such infection, or rarely as isolated lesions in the absence of other features of CMV infection (92, 93). Other presentations include gingival necrosis resembling HIV-associated periodontal disease (94) and ulcers that are coinfected with CMV and HSV (93, 95).

Hairy Leukoplakia

HL was originally observed among homosexual men in San Francisco and was shown to be associated with a human herpes virus (2), soon identified as EBV (96), as well as to presage the development of AIDS (3). This white lesion is found predominantly on the lateral surface of the tongue (Fig. 32.7), although it is seen occasionally elsewhere on the oropharyngeal mucosa (97). The lesion is present in the mouths of a significant proportion of HIV-seropositive patients of all risk groups (31–33, 98). Thus, it is present in approximately 20% of asymptomatic HIV-positive people (30) and becomes more common as the disease progresses. HL is not found in mucosal sites other than the mouth and oropharynx, but it is seen, albeit rarely, in association with non–HIV-induced immunosuppression, notably renal transplant recipients (99, 100), among whom one study found as high a prevalence as among HIV-infected patients (101).

Patients receiving cancer chemotherapy may have HL (102), as may cardiac and bone marrow transplant recipients (103), as well as liver transplant recipients (104). The lesion has been seen occasionally in patients who appear to be immunocompetent (105). HL in the presence of HIV infection is of itself a criterion for group IV category C2 of the original CDC surveillance definition and category B3 of the 1993 definition. Progression to AIDS is significantly more frequent and rapid in HIV-positive patients with HL than in those without the lesion, even after adjustment for CD4 count (32, 106). In our 1987 study (3), approximately 30% of patients with HL developed AIDS within 36 months; in a later study, the probability was 47% by 2 years and 67% by 4 years (107). Other groups have confirmed these observations. We have shown that the rate of progression to AIDS is similar among men with either HL or oral candidiasis (106). However, not all patients with HL progress to AIDS as rapidly, and those who do so are much more likely to have had skin tests negative to *Candida* antigen at diagnosis of HL, a finding indicating significant immunosuppression at that time (107). No relationship exists between the size of the lesion and progression, because we found that patients with small HL lesions were equally prone to develop AIDS as were those with larger lesions (108).

The classic "hairy" or corrugated appearance of the HL lesion on the lateral tongue may represent an exaggeration of the normal structure of that part of the oral mucosa (109). As the lesion extends onto the ventral tongue, it may present a smoother appearance, although lesions of HL on other oral and oropharyngeal surfaces can be of either type (97). On biopsy and histologic examination, the HL lesion shows features of epithelial thickening, including hyperparakeratosis and acanthosis, with a characteristic irregularity to the junction between the parakeratinized surface zone and the underlying prickle cell layer. Enlarged and vacuolated prickle cells resembling koilocytes are present at one or more levels, extending from just above the basal cell layer to the surface parakeratin zone. These cells may be present as a small group

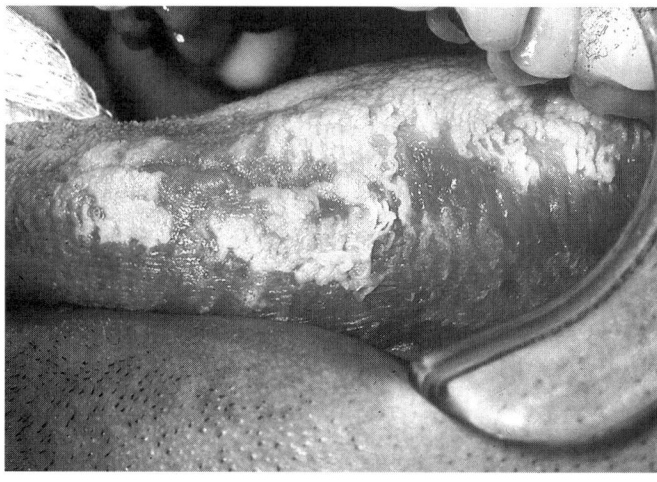

Figure 32.7. Hairy leukoplakia of the tongue. (See color section.)

or as larger clumps, or they may occupy much of the prickle cell layer. Careful examination of routinely stained paraffin sections reveals characteristic changes in nuclear cytology that can be useful for the diagnosis of HL in circumstances in which molecular biology, histochemistry, or electron microscopy techniques are not readily available (110, 111).

Many of the enlarged and vacuolated prickle cells, and also some of the more superficial cells, contain huge numbers of particles of EBV (Fig. 32.8) in fully replicating form (2, 96, 112, 113). Although a presumptive diagnosis of HL can be made on clinical appearance, and histopathologic examination with particular attention to nuclear cytologic features can be useful in strengthening that diagnosis, the presence of EBV is required for the definitive diagnosis of HL (114–117). Cells scraped from the lesion can be used for this purpose in a noninvasive approach using in situ hybridization, histochemistry, or electron microscopy (118). The demonstration of EBV serves to distinguish HL from oral lesions with similar clinical and histologic appearances (119). These include frictional keratosis, smokers' leukoplakia, other forms of leukoplakia resulting from epithelial dysplasia and squamous cell carcinoma, geographic tongue, oral lesions of certain genodermatoses, hyperplastic candidiasis (candidal leukoplakia), and a variant of oral lichen planus (20). EBV appears to be the cause of HL, as indicated by the association between the presence of EBV in HL. When acyclovir or another agent is used to eliminate EBV, the lesion regresses, and clinical recurrence is accompanied by renewed EBV activity (120, 121). However, debate exists about whether EBV is reactivated from a site of latency within the tongue epithelium or whether the virus infects or reinfects that epithelium from the oral cavity or perhaps from circulating B lymphocytes. No viral DNA is found in the basal layers of HL (116, 122–126), suggesting that EBV is not latently cycling, although one report places the viral early gene product BZLF1 at that location (127). EBV small nuclear RNAs are also not expressed (128, 129), an observation consistent with the permissive nature of the EBV infection and the lack of a latent phase.

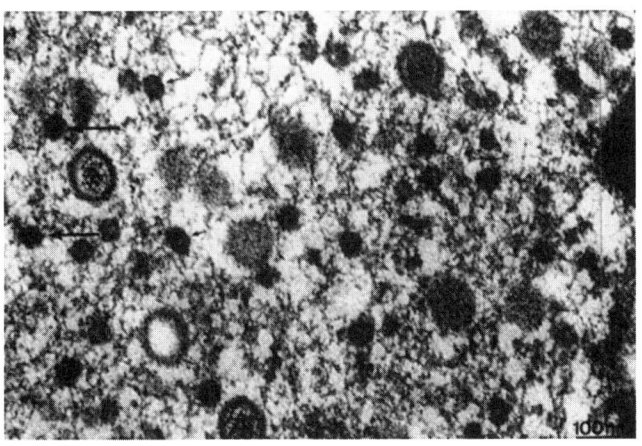

Figure 32.8. Epstein–Barr virus in an epithelial cell of hairy leukoplakia.

Investigators have suggested that some lesions of HL contain defective EBV (130) and perhaps multiple strains of EBV (129, 131–133). However, no oncogenic influences of EBV appear to occur (134), in contrast to the suspected role of that virus in nasopharyngeal carcinoma, certain other upper aerodigestive tract carcinomas, epithelial thymoma, and Burkitt's lymphoma. Carcinoma has not been reported to arise in HL lesions, and the pattern of keratin differentiation in HL does not suggest a premalignant potential (124, 126, 135). Transgenic mice expressing the EBV oncogene BNLF-1, which encodes the latent membrane protein LMP, showed skin thickening and the presence of the hyperproliferation keratin K6 (136). A lesion superficially resembling HL has been described in rhesus macaques bearing simian EBV (137). However, the relationship of these two sets of animal observations with the pathogenesis and significance of human HL is unclear.

The epithelium of the HL lesion contains fewer than normal numbers of Langerhans' cells (138). The function of these and other dendritic cells may be defective in HIV infection (139, 140). Mucosal dendritic cells may be a target, even a site of infection and replication, of HIV. This could permit the infection, or reinfection, of this site by EBV. However, the lack of Langerhans' cells in HL could also be a consequence rather than a cause of the presence of EBV. Reports have linked the location of the HL lesion to the presence of EBV receptors on the lateral margins of the tongue (141), but the specificity of the monoclonal antibodies used is unclear.

Therapy for HL is occasionally indicated because of discomfort or appearance (142). The lesion may change in appearance, waxing and waning in extent. Antifungal therapy should be used to reduce or eliminate superinfection with *Candida,* and systemic acyclovir is occasionally indicated. Although acyclovir is effective, the lesions recur (120). We have found that the antiviral agent desciclovir can be effective in eliminating the clinical lesion and EBV in the tissue (121). Although some case reports suggest that HL may disappear in association with ganciclovir (143) and zidovudine (144) therapy, we have shown that the lesion increases or decreases in size in patients taking the latter drug (145). Podophyllum resin also has been used (146).

Papillomavirus Lesions

In association with HIV infection, oral and labial lesions resulting from HPV take the form of papilliferous and flat warts. Many papilliferous warty lesions contain HPV7, found previously only in skin warts in butchers (102, 147, 148). The oral flat warts found in HIV infection (Fig. 32.9) are identical to the condition known as focal epithelial hyperplasia (Heck's disease). This condition was previously largely confined to the indigenous people of the Americas, Greenland inhabitants, and certain other racial or geographic groups. These lesions are associated with HPV13 and 32, although some unusual, even dysplastic warts associated with new HPV types have occurred (149, 150). If troublesome,

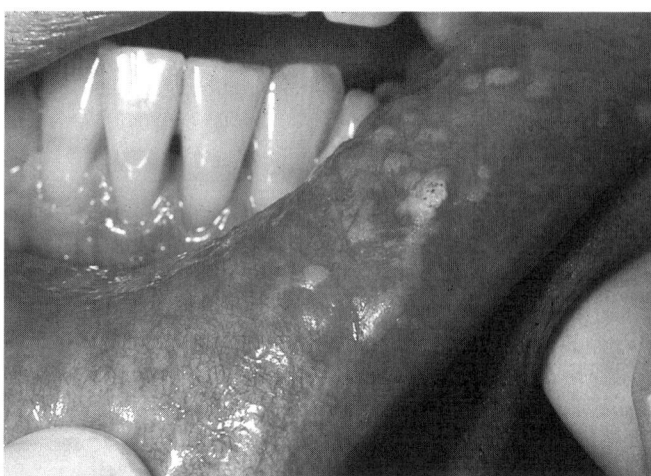

Figure 32.9. Focal epithelial hyperplasia of the lower lip. (See color section.)

oral warts may be excised surgically or by laser, but recurrence is common.

BACTERIAL INFECTIONS

Because defects in cell-mediated immunity are the most prominent immunologic consequence of HIV infection, most opportunistic infections in HIV infection and AIDS are due to viruses, fungi, or protozoa. However, some bacterial infections are also seen. These include tuberculosis and infections caused by other encapsulated bacteria that evoke cell-mediated immune responses. Oral bacterial infections are seen, including those resulting from enterobacteria (151) and mycobacteria (152). Oral lesions of epithelioid (bacillary) angiomatosis have been reported in one or two cases (153). However, the most common and dramatic forms of oral bacterial infection seen in association with HIV infection are the various forms of severe periodontal disease noted in this group of patients.

Periodontal Diseases

The forms of periodontal infection described in HIV infection include gingivitis (linear gingival erythema), necrotizing gingivitis, severe periodontitis (necrotizing ulcerative periodontitis), and the more extensive lesion necrotizing stomatitis. In association with HIV infection, periodontal diseases may have unusual clinical features, including rapid progression to destructive disease and poor response to standard therapy (154). However, HIV-positive individuals are just as prone to conventional periodontal diseases as are the rest of the population, and it has not proved easy to distinguish between HIV-related and conventional forms for studies of epidemiology, etiopathogenesis, and management (155). Although these disorders are widely described and discussed, no general consensus exists concerning their definition or criteria for their diagnosis.

Estimates of the prevalence and incidence of periodontal diseases in the HIV-positive population suggest that the severe forms described here are not a common component of the epidemic (155–157). However, to those who experience these lesions, not to mention the clinicians to whom they offer challenges of diagnosis and management, these diseases can be formidable, causing severe pain and morbidity and presenting the possibility of local or even systemic spread of anaerobic infection (158, 159). Symptoms of severe and rapid periodontal disease may lead patients who are unaware that they are HIV positive to seek care. Another problem is that the effective management of these lesions requires the skills of appropriately trained dental specialists, who are not available in many AIDS care environments.

GINGIVITIS/LINEAR GINGIVAL ERYTHEMA

In the unusual condition originally named HIV gingivitis and now called linear gingival erythema, (160) a thin band of erythema is seen along the gingival margins of one or more groups of teeth. The patient may complain of waking with blood in the mouth because of spontaneous bleeding. Such signs and symptoms may occur in the absence of the plaque and calculus that cause conventional gingivitis. Necrotizing ulcerative gingivitis is also seen, with ulceration of the tips of gingival papillae, marginal inflammation, fetid breath, and fever (161).

HIV-ASSOCIATED PERIODONTITIS/NECROTIZING ULCERATIVE PERIODONTITIS

This condition is distinguished from conventional periodontitis by the rapid and simultaneous loss of both supporting bone and overlying mucosa, leading to exposure of root tissue, tooth mobility, and even tooth loss (154) (Fig. 32.10). Because of the type and rapidity of tissue loss, little periodontal pocketing is seen. These changes are often accompanied by ulceration and necrosis of soft tissue and by complaints of severe pain. Spread to adjoining soft tissue may occur, accompanied by sequestration of portions of alveolar bone (necrotizing stomatitis) (158, 159).

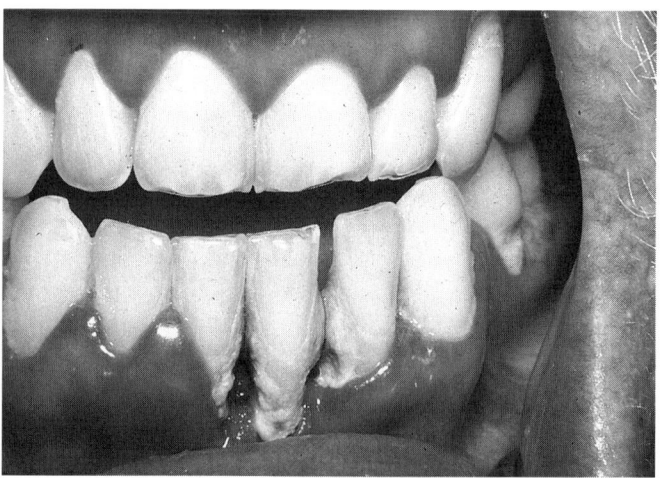

Figure 32.10. HIV-associated periodontal disease. (See color section.)

ETIOLOGY

The causes of this group of lesions are poorly understood. The associated microorganisms appear to be a similar Gram-negative flora to that seen in conventional periodontal disease and include *Bacteroides intermedius, Porphyromonas gingivalis, Actinobacillus actinomycetemcomitans, Fusobacterium nucleatum, Wolinella recta,* and *Eikenella corrodens* (162). *Candida* species are also found, as are spirochetes; however, polymorphonuclear leukocyte defects may also be involved (163).

THERAPY

Treatment for these conditions (164, 165) involves debridement of necrotic tissue including bony sequestra, root planing, and curettage, accompanied by irrigation of the affected areas with 10% povidone–iodine (Betadine) followed by chlorhexidine (Peridex) mouth rinses. Administration of antibiotics such as metronidazole, clindamycin, or amoxicillin is often helpful.

IDIOPATHIC/AUTOIMMUNE LESIONS

Recurrent Aphthous Ulcers

Recurrent oral ulcers without identifiable cause, known as recurrent aphthous ulcers (RAU) or canker sores, are common in the general population. Some evidence suggests a moderate increase in the prevalence of this condition in individuals with HIV infection (32). However, patients with a prior history of RAU experience a dramatic increase in the severity of the lesions (166), with larger and longer-lasting lesions, often after an interruption of many years. RAU of the major form (Fig. 32.11) has become more common than the minor or herpetiform varieties in HIV infection. These are large (1 to 2 cm), painful ulcers that can be either solitary or multiple. They often persist for weeks, sometimes months, and frequently the attendant pain interferes with chewing and swallowing. Their occurrence in HIV infection is associated with diminished CD4 and CD8 lymphocyte numbers than are the other two forms of RAU (166). Minor aphthae present as crops of ulcers about 5 mm in diameter that usually heal more rapidly than the major form, yet they persist much longer than in HIV-negative patients. The least common form of RAU in the general population, called herpetiform because of faint clinical resemblance to herpes simplex, consists of crops of tiny (1- to 2-mm) ulcers that may coalesce. These, too, are proportionally more frequent in persons with HIV infection. The cause of RAU has not been identified, but the association with HIV infection supports the hypotheses of opportunistic infection or defects in immune regulation.

Aphthous ulcers can usually be controlled with topical steroids such as Lidex ointment (0.05% mixed half and half with Orabase and applied to the ulcers five to six times a day). Systemic steroids may be indicated in some cases (167). Thalidomide has been used with some success in Europe and South America (168, 169), whereas the recently completed AIDS Clinical Treatment Group (ACTG) 251 trial indicates good efficacy of this drug in the United States.

Large, painful necrotizing oral ulcers are also seen in HIV infection. Some represent major aphthous ulcers further complicated by bacterial infection, or they may be a form of necrotizing stomatitis. These ulcers may be associated with similar lesions elsewhere in the gastrointestinal tract. They respond to a combination of topical steroids and antibiotics directed against Gram-negative bacteria. The differential diagnosis is extensive and includes lymphoma, squamous cell carcinoma, CMV infection, tuberculosis, cryptococcosis, and various other conditions. The nature and etiology of the oral ulcers seen in association with primary HIV infection (170) have not been investigated.

HIV-Associated Salivary Gland Disease

Both xerostomia (dry mouth) and enlargement of major salivary glands are seen in HIV-infected patients (171, 172) (Fig. 32.12). These conditions can occur together or separately, and salivary flow may be reduced. Appropriate measures to alleviate symptoms and to prevent caries include saliva substitutes, control of sugar intake, fluoride rinses, and fluoride applications.

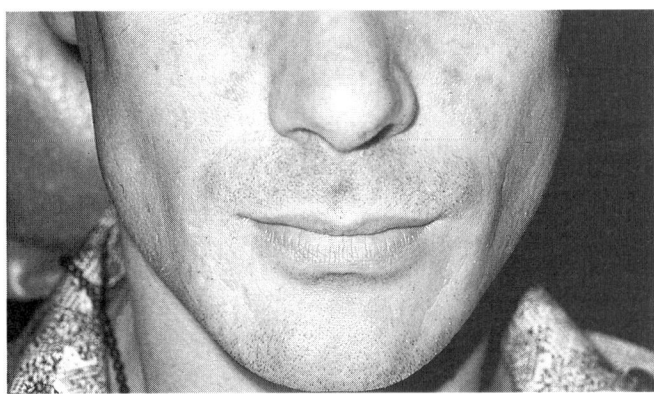

Figure 32.12. Salivary gland enlargement. (See color section.)

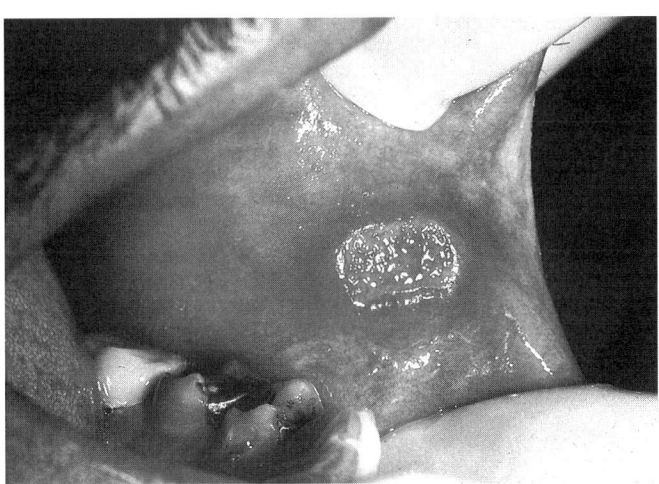

Figure 32.11. Major aphthous ulcer of the cheek. (See color section.)

Initially seen in pediatric AIDS cases (173, 174), salivary gland, notably parotid, enlargement has now been seen in adults of all risk groups (175). The swelling is bilateral, diffuse, and soft, but not fluctuant. Patients may have dry eyes and other features suggestive of Sjögren's syndrome, but significant serologic and immunohistochemical differences distinguish HIV-associated salivary gland disease from Sjögren's syndrome (172). HIV-associated salivary gland disease may include cases described as branchial cleft cysts or lymphoepithelial cysts of salivary glands (176), and all these may be the salivary gland expression of the diffuse infiltrative CD8 lymphocytosis syndrome in HIV infection described by Itescu and colleagues (177, 178). No viral or other microbial causes have been identified, but associations with HLA-DR5 and HLA-B35 have been suggested (179).

Immune Thrombocytopenic Purpura

Oral lesions of immune thrombocytopenic purpura are occasionally seen in patients with HIV infection (180). They consist of small purpuric lesions or large ecchymoses. Spontaneous gingival bleeding can also be caused by this condition, and thus it can be confused with periodontal disease.

Abnormal Pigmentation

Unusual brown pigmentation of the oral mucosa in HIV-infected patients is most commonly associated with zidovudine or ketoconazole therapy (181). In some cases, no obvious predisposing factors other than HIV infection are found, and the lesions take the form of oral melanotic macules (182). Oral hyperpigmentation in association with HIV infection may also be due to adrenal cortical insufficiency (183, 184).

PEDIATRIC HIV INFECTION: ORAL COMPLICATIONS

Oral candidiasis, HIV-associated salivary gland disease (parotid enlargement), and herpes simplex are common features of pediatric HIV infection (34, 185–187). HL is occasionally seen (188), although other oral lesions are uncommon. In a study of 98 children with perinatally acquired HIV infection (34), the cumulative prevalences were 72% for oral candidiasis, 47% for parotid enlargement, and 24% for herpes simplex. The median time from birth to development of an oral lesion was 2.4 years for candidiasis, 4.6 years for parotid enlargement, and 5 years for herpes simplex. The median time from the appearance of oral lesions to death was 3.4 years for candidiasis, 5.4 years for parotid enlargement, and 4.3 years for herpes simplex. In a time-dependent proportional hazards model, oral candidiasis was associated with more rapid progression to death than was parotid enlargement. Caries may be a problem in children with HIV infection because of neglect and the high sugar content of many pediatric medications. Oral hygiene instruction and maintenance are important components of care for this population. Topical fluoride rinses or gels are recommended as means of preventing caries.

OTHER ORAL PROBLEMS ASSOCIATED WITH HIV INFECTION

Although isolated reports of delayed oral wound healing and problems with endodontic therapy have been published, the few careful studies of this issue have failed to support this notion (189, 190). Thus, antibiotic prophylaxis before these and other oral surgical procedures, including periodontal therapy, is not appropriate for HIV-infected patients unless it is indicated for other medical reasons. Countless oral and dental surgical procedures are performed each year in this population without complication.

In conclusion, initial clinical impressions concerning the frequency of oral lesions and their place in the natural history and progression of HIV disease and AIDS have been supported by substantial numbers of studies. These conditions are common, and they present a potentially bewildering array of appearances and possible diagnoses. Thus, agreed and standardized classification schemes, definitions, and diagnostic criteria are essential elements in the recognition of oral HIV disease, to allow their incorporation in staging systems for HIV infection, as well as to permit rational approaches to their control. The ability to recognize the presence of oral lesions and some familiarity with their management are essential features of contemporary AIDS and HIV care, and yet this simple recommendation is far from being universally heeded (191).

Acknowledgments

The work referred to in this chapter was supported by National Institutes of Health–National Institute of Dental Research grant P01-DE-07946.

References

1. Gottlieb MS, Schroff R, Schantez HM. *Pneumocystis carinii* pneumonia and mucosal candidiasis in previously healthy homosexual men: evidence of a new acquired cellular immunodeficiency. N Engl J Med 1981;305:1425–1431.
2. Greenspan D, Greenspan JS, Conant M, et al. Oral "hairy" leucoplakia in male homosexuals: evidence of association with both papillomavirus and a herpes-group virus. Lancet 1984;2:831–834.
3. Greenspan D, Greenspan JS, Hearst NG, et al. Relation of oral hairy leukoplakia to infection with the human immunodeficiency virus and the risk of developing AIDS. J Infect Dis 1987;155:475–481.
4. Peterson DE, Greenspan D, Squier CA. Oral infections in the immunocompromised host: International Association for Dental Research symposium, 19 April 1991, Acapulco, Mexico. J Oral Pathol Med 1992;21:193–198.
5. Greenspan JS. Sentinels and signposts: epidemiology and significance of the oral manifestations of HIV infection. Oral Dis 1997;3(Suppl 1):513–517.
6. Melnick SL, Engel D, Truelove E, et al. Oral mucosal lesions: association with the presence of antibodies to the human immunodeficiency virus. Oral Surg Oral Med Oral Pathol 1989;68:37–43.
7. Schiødt M, Bakilana PB, Hiza JF, et al. Oral candidiasis and hairy leukoplakia correlate with HIV infection in Tanzania. Oral Surg Oral Med Oral Pathol 1990;69:591–596.

8. Colebunders R, Ryder R, Francis H, et al. Seroconversion rate, mortality, and clinical manifestations associated with the receipt of a human immunodeficiency virus–infected blood transfusion in Kinshasa, Zaire. J Infect Dis 1991;164:450–456.
9. Farizo KM, Buehler JW, Chamberland ME, et al. Spectrum of disease in persons with human immunodeficiency virus infection in the United States. JAMA 1992;267:1798–1805.
10. Schulten EAJM, ten Kate RW, van der Waal I. The impact of oral examination on the Centers for Disease Control classification of subjects with human immunodeficiency virus infection. Arch Intern Med 1990;150:1259–1261.
11. Crowe SM, Carlin JB, Stewart KI, et al. Predictive value of CD4 lymphocyte numbers for the development of opportunistic infections and malignancies in HIV-infected persons. J Acquir Immune Defic Syndr 1991;4:770–776.
12. Fleischer AB, Gallagher PN, Van Der Horst C. Mucocutaneous abnormalities predicted by lymphocyte counts in patients infected by the human immmunodeficiency virus. South Med J 1992;85:687–690.
13. Begg MD, Panagreas KS, Mitchell-Lewis D, et al. Oral lesions as markers of severe immunosuppression in HIV-infected homosexual men and injection drug users. Oral Surg Oral Med Oral Pathol 1996;82:276–283.
14. Coates RA, Farewell VT, Raboud J, et al. Using serial observations to identify predictors of progression to AIDS in the Toronto sexual contact study. J Clin Epidemiol 1992;45:245–253.
15. Carpenter CCJ, Fischl Ma, Hammer SM, et al. Antiretroviral therapy for HIV infection in 1996. JAMA 1996;276:146–154.
16. Centers for Disease Control. 1993 revised classification system for HIV infection and expanded surveillance case definition for AIDS among adolescents and adults. MMWR 1993;41:1–19.
17. Gallant JE, Somani J, Chaisson RE, et al. Diagnostic accuracy of three clinical case definitions for advanced HIV disease. AIDS 1992;6:295–299.
18. Weniger BG, Quinhoes EP, Sereno AB, et al. A simplified surveillance case definition of AIDS derived from empirical clinical data. J Acquir Immune Defic Syndr 1992;5:1212–1223.
19. Fischl MA, Richman DD, Hansen N, et al. The safety and efficacy of zidovudine (AZT) in the treatment of subjects with mildly symptomatic human immunodeficiency virus type 1 (HIV) infection. Ann Intern Med 1990;112:727–737.
20. Greenspan D, Greenspan JS, Pindborg JJ, et al. AIDS and the mouth. Copenhagen: Munksgaard, 1990.
21. Greenspan JS, Greenspan D, eds. Oral manifestations of HIV infection: proceedings of the 2nd International Workshop on the Oral Manifestations of HIV Infection, January 31–February 3 1993, San Francisco, California. Carol Stream, IL: Quintessence, 1995.
22. Lifson AR. Oral lesions and the epidemiology of HIV. In: Greenspan JS, Greenspan D, eds. Oral manifestations of HIV infection: proceedings of the 2nd International Workshop on the Oral Manifestations of HIV Infection, January 31–February 3 1993, San Francisco, California. Carol Stream, IL: Quintessence, 1995:38–41.
23. Glick M, ed. Dental management of patients with HIV. Carol Stream, IL: Quintessence, 1994.
24. Silverman S, Migliorati CA, Lozada-Nur F, et al. Oral findings in people with or at risk for AIDS: a study of 375 homosexual males. J Am Dent Assoc 1986;112:187–192.
25. Reichart PA, Gelderblom HR, Becker J, et al. AIDS and the oral cavity: the HIV infection—virology, etiology, origin, immunology, precautions and clinical observations in 110 patients. J Oral Maxillofac Surg 1987;16:129–153.
26. Porter SR, Luker J, Scully C, et al. Orofacial manifestations of a group of British patients infected with HIV-1. J Oral Pathol Med 1989;18:47–48.
27. Ramirez V, Gonzales A, de la Rosa E, et al. Oral lesions in Mexican HIV-infected patients. J Oral Pathol Med 1990;19:482–485.
28. Wanzala P, Manji F, Pindborg JJ, et al. Low prevalence of oral mucosal lesions in HIV-1 seropositive African women. J Oral Pathol Med 1989;18:416–418.
29. Schiodt M, Bygberg I, Bakilana P, et al. Oral manifestations of AIDS in Tanzania. J Dent Res 1988;67:201.
30. Tukutuku K, Muyembe-Tamfum L, Kayembe K, et al. Oral manifestations of AIDS in a heterosexual population in a Zaire hospital. J Oral Pathol Med 1990;19:232–234.
31. Ramael M, Colebunders R, Colpaert C, et al. The prevalence of hairy leukoplakia in HIV seropositive and HIV seronegative immunocompromised patients. Int J STD AIDS 1992;3:251–254.
32. Feigal DW, Katz MH, Greenspan D, et al. The prevalence of oral lesions in HIV-infected homosexual and bisexual men: three San Francisco epidemiological cohorts. AIDS 1991;5:519–525.
33. Shiboski CH, Hilton JF, Greenspan D, et al. HIV-related oral manifestations in two cohorts of women in San Francisco. J Acquir Immune Defic Syndr Hum Retrovirol 1994;7:964–971.
34. Katz MH, Mastrucci MT, Leggott PJ, et al. Prognostic significance of oral lesions in children with perinatally acquired human immunodeficiency virus infection. Am J Dis Child 1993;147:45–48.
35. Dodd CL, Greenspan D, Greenspan JS. Oral Kaposi's sarcoma in a woman as a first indication of infection with the human immunodeficiency virus. J Am Dent Assoc 1991;122:61–63.
36. Pindborg JJ. Classification of oral lesions associated with HIV infection. Oral Surg Oral Med Oral Pathol 1989;67:292–295.
37. EEC Clearinghouse on Oral Problems Related to HIV Infection. An update of the classification and diagnostic criteria of oral lesions in HIV infection. J Oral Pathol Med 1991;20:97–100.
38. Greenspan JS, Barr CE, Sciubba JJ, et al. Oral manifestations of HIV infection: definitions, diagnostic criteria and principles of therapy. Oral Surg Oral Med Oral Pathol 1992;73:142–144.
39. Ficarra G, Person AM, Silverman S, et al. Kaposi's sarcoma of the oral cavity: a study of 134 patients with a review of the pathogenesis, epidemiology, clinical aspects, and treatment. Oral Surg Oral Med Oral Pathol 1988;66:543–550.
40. Lozada F, Silverman S, Conant M. New outbreak of oral tumours, malignancies and infectious disease strikes young male homosexuals. Calif Dent Assoc J 1982;10:39–42.
41. Lozada F, Silverman S, Migliorati CA, et al. Oral manifestations of tumors and opportunistic infections in the acquired immunodeficiency syndrome (AIDS): findings in 53 homosexual men with Kaposi's sarcoma. Oral Surg Oral Med Oral Pathol 1983;56:491–494.
42. Chang Y, Cesarmen E, Pessin M, et al. Identification of herpesvirus-like DNA sequences in AIDS-associated Kaposis's sarcoma. Science 1994;266:1866.
43. Rickinson AB. Changing seroepidemiology of HHV-8. Lancet 1996;348:1110–1111.
44. Yeh CK, Fox PC, Fox CH, et al. Kaposi's sarcoma of the parotid gland in acquired immunodeficiency syndrome. Oral Surg Oral Med Oral Pathol 1989;67:308–312.
45. Langford A, Pohle H-D, Reichart P. Primary intraosseous AIDS-associated Kaposi's sarcoma. Int J Oral Maxillofacial Surg 1991;20:366–368.
46. Regezi JA, MacPhail LA, Daniels TE. Oral Kaposi's sarcoma: a 10-year retrospective histopathologic study. J Oral Pathol Med 1993;22:292–297.
47. Epstein JB, Scully C. Intralesional vinblastine for oral Kaposi's sarcoma in HIV infection. Lancet 1989;2:1100–1101.
48. Lucatoto FM, Sapp JP. Treatment of oral Kaposi's sarcoma with a sclerosing agent in AIDS patients. Oral Surg Oral Med Oral Pathol 1993;75:192–198.
49. Ziegler JL, Drew WL, Miner RC, et al. Outbreak of Burkitt's-like lymphoma in homosexual men. Lancet 1982;2:631–633.
50. Ziegler JL, Beckstead JA, Volberding PA, et al. Non–Hodgkins lymphoma in 90 homosexual men: relation to generalized lymphadenopathy and the acquired immunodeficiency syndrome. N Engl J Med 1984;311:565–570.

51. Kaugars GE, Burns JC. Non–Hodgkin's lymphoma of the oral cavity associated with AIDS. Oral Surg Oral Med Oral Pathol 1989;67:433–436.
52. Dodd CL, Greenspan D, Heinic GS, et al. Multifocal oral non–Hodgkin's lymphoma in an AIDS patient. Br Dent J 1993;175:373–377.
53. Dodd CL, Greenspan D, Schiodt M, et al. Unusual oral presentation of non–Hodgkin's lymphoma in association with HIV infection. Oral Surg Oral Med Oral Pathol 1992;73:603–608.
54. Moore RD, Kessler H, Richman DD, et al. Non–Hodgkin's lymphoma in patients with advanced HIV infection treated with zidovudine. JAMA 1991;265:2208–2211.
55. Lobo DV, Chu P, Grekin RC, Berger TG. Nonmelanoma skin cancers and infection with the human immunodeficiency virus. Arch Dermatol 1992;128:623–627.
56. Epstein JB, Scully C. Neoplastic disease in the head and neck of patients with AIDS. Int J Oral Maxillofacial Surg 1992;21:219–226.
57. Palefsky JM. Human papillomavirus infection among HIV-positive individuals and its implication for development for malignant tumors. Hematol Oncol Clin North Am 1991;5:357–370.
58. Klein RS, Harris CA, Small CR, et al. Oral candidiasis in high-risk patients as the initial manifestation of the acquired immunodeficiency syndrome. N Engl J Med 1984;311:354–358.
59. Tindal B, Hing M, Edwards P, et al. Severe clinical manifestations of primary HIV infection. AIDS 1989;3:747–749.
60. Dull JS, Sen P, Raffanti S, Middleton JR. Oral candidiasis as a marker of acute retroviral illness. South Med J 1991;84:733–9.
61. Arendorf TM, Walker DM. The prevalence and intra-oral distribution of Candida albicans in man. Arch Oral Biol 1980;25:1–10.
62. Hamilton JN, Thompson SH, Scheidt MJ, et al. Correlation of subclinical candidal colonization of the dorsal tongue surface with the Walter Reed staging scheme for patients infected wirh HIV-1. Oral Surg Oral Med Oral Pathol 1992;73:47–51.
63. Lifson AR, Hessol NA, Buchbinder SP, et al The association of clinical conditions and serologic tests with CD4+ lymphocyte counts in HIV-infected subjects without AIDS. AIDS 1992;5:1209–1215.
64. Tavitian A, Raufman JP, Rosenthal LE. Oral candidiasis as a marker for esophageal candidiasis in the acquired immunodeficiency syndrome. Ann Intern Med 1986;104:54–55.
65. Imam N, Carpenter CC, Mayer KH, et al. Hierarchical pattern of mucosal candidiasis infections in HIV-seropositive women. Am J Med 1990;89:142–146.
66. Soll DR. A molecular approach to the role of switching in oral candidiasis. In: Greenspan JS, Greenspan D, eds. Oral manifestations of HIV infection. Chicago: Quintessence, 1995:93–102.
67. Agabian N, Miyasaki SH, Kohler G, et al. Candidiasis and HIV infection: virulence as an adaptive response. In: Greenspan JS, Greenspan D, eds. Oral manifestations of HIV infection. Chicago: Quintessence, 1995:85–92.
68. Schmid J, Odds FC, Wiselka MJ, et al. Genetic similarity and maintenance of *Candida albicans* strains from a group of AIDS patients, demonstrated by DNA fingerprinting. J Clin Microbiol 1992;30:935–941.
69. Powderly WG, Robinson K, Keath EJ. Molecular typing of *Candida albicans* isolated from oral lesions of HIV-infected individuals. AIDS 1992;6:81–84.
70. Miyasaki SH, Hicks JB, Greenspan D, et al. The identification and tracking of *Candida albicans* isolates from oral lesions in HIV-seropositive individuals. J Acquir Immune Defic Syndr 1992;5:1039–1042.
71. Stevens DA, Odds FC, Scherer S. Application of DNA typing methods to *Candida albicans* epidemiology and correlations with phenotype. Rev Infect Dis 1990;12:258–266.
72. Whelan WL, Kirsch DR, Kwon-Chung KJ, et al. *Candida albicans* in patients with the acquired immunodeficiency syndrome: absence of a novel or hypervirulent strain. J Infect Dis 1990;162:513–518.
73. Dodd CL, Greenspan D, Katz MH, et al. Oral candidiasis in HIV infection: pseudomembranous and erythematous candidiasis show similar rates of progression to AIDS. AIDS 1991;5:1339–1343.
74. Lake BG, Tom W, Lake BD, et al. Gastropathy and ketoconazole malabsorption in the acquired immunodeficiency syndrome (AIDS). Ann Intern Med 1988;109:471–473.
75. Darwazeh AMG, Lamey P-J, Lewis MAO, et al. Systemic fluconazole therapy and in vitro adhesion of Candida albicans to human buccal epithelial cells. J Oral Pathol Med 1991;20:17–19.
76. Maenza JR, Keruly JC, Moore RD, et al. Risk factors for fluconazole-resistant candidiasis in human immunodeficiency virus–infected patients. J Infect Dis 1996;173:219–225.
77. Esposito R, Castagna A, Uberti FC. Maintenance therapy of oropharyngeal candidiasis in HIV-infected patients with fluconazole [letter]. AIDS 1990;4:1033–1034.
78. Just-Nubling G, Gentschew G, Meisner K, et al. Fluconazole prophylaxis of recurrent oral candidiasis in HIV-positive patient. Eur J Clin Infect Dis 1991;10:917–921.
79. Heinic G, Greenspan D, MacPhail LA, et al. Oral *Histoplasma capsulatum* in association with HIV infection: a case report. J Oral Pathol Med 1992;21:85–89.
80. Glick M, Cohen SG, Cheney RT, et al. Oral manifestations of disseminated *Cryptococcus neoformans* in a patient with acquired immunodeficiency syndrome. Oral Surg Oral Med Oral Pathol 1987;64:454–459.
81. Kuruvilla A, Humphrey DM, Emko P. Coexistent oral cryptococcosis and Kaposi's sarcoma in acquired immunodeficiency syndrome. Cutis 1992;49:260–264.
82. Tzerbos F, Kabani S, Booth D. Cryptococcosis as an exclusive oral presentation. J Oral Maxillofac Surg 1992;50:759–760.
83. Shannon MT, Sclaroff A, Colm SJ. Invasive aspergillosis of the maxilla in an immunocompromised patient. Oral Surg Oral Med Oral Pathol 1990;70:425–427.
84. Heinic GS, Greenspan D, MacPhail LA, et al. Oral *Geotrichum candidum* infection in association with HIV infection. Oral Surg Oral Med Oral Pathol 1992;73:726–728.
85. Borradori L, Schmit JC, Stetzkowski M, et al. *Penicilliosis marneffei* infection in AIDS. J Am Acad Dermatol 1994;31:843–846.
86. MacPhail LA, Greenspan D, Schiodt M, et al. Acyclovir-resistant, foscarnet-sensitive oral herpes simplex type 2 lesion in a patient with AIDS. Oral Surg Oral Med Oral Pathol 1989;67:427–432.
87. Erlich KS, Mills J, Chatis P, et al. Acyclovir-resistant herpes simplex virus infections in patients with the acquired immunodeficiency syndrome. N Engl J Med 1989;320:293–296.
88. Epstein JB, Scully C. Herpes simplex virus in immunocompromised patients: growing evidence of drug resistance. Oral Surg Oral Med Oral Pathol 1991;72:47–50.
89. Schiodt M, Rindum J, Bygbert I. Chickenpox with oral manifestations in an AIDS patient. Dan Dent J 1987;91:316–319.
90. Melbye M, Grossman RJ, Goedert JJ, et al. Risk of AIDS after herpes zoster. Lancet 1987;1:728–731.
91. Colebunders R, Mann J, Francis H, et al. Herpes zoster in African patients: a clinical predictor of human immunodeficiency virus infection. J Infect Dis 1988;157:314–318.
92. Langford A, Kunze R, Timm H, et al. Cytomegalovirus associated oral ulcerations in HIV-infected patients. J Oral Pathol Med 1990;19:71–76.
93. Jones AC, Freedman PD, Phelan JA, et al. Cytomegalovirus infections of the oral cavity. Oral Surg Oral Med Oral Pathol 1993;75:76–85.
94. Heinic G, Greenspan D, Greenspan JS. Oral CMV lesions and the HIV infected: early recognition can help prevent morbidity. J Am Dent Assoc 1993;124:99–104.
95. Smith KJ, Skelton HG, III, James WD, et al. Concurrent epidermal involvement of cytomegalovirus and herpes simplex virus in two HIV-infected patients. J Am Acad Dermatol 1991;25:500–506.
96. Greenspan JS, Greenspan D, Lennette ET, et al. Replication of Epstein–Barr virus within the epithelial cells of "hairy" leukoplakia, an AIDS-associated lesion. N Engl J Med 1985;313:1564–1571.

97. Kabani S, Greenspan D, de Souza Y, et al. Oral hairy leukoplakia with extensive oral mucosal involvement. Oral Surg Oral Med Oral Pathol 1989;67:411–415.
98. Ficarra G, Barone R, Gaglioti D. Oral hairy leukoplakia among HIV-positive intravenous drug abusers: a clinico-pathologic and ultrastructural study. Oral Surg Oral Med Oral Pathol 1988;65:421–426.
99. Itin P, Rufli I, Rudlinser R, et al. Oral hairy leukoplakia in a HIV-negative renal transplant patient: a marker for immunosuppression. Dermatologica 1988;17:126–128.
100. Greenspan D, Greenspan JS, DeSouza YG, et al. Oral hairy leukoplakia in an HIV-negative renal transplant recipient. J Oral Pathol Med 1989;18:32–34.
101. King GN, Healy CM, Glover MT, et al. Prevalence and risk factors associated with leukoplakia, hairy leukoplakia, erythematous candidiasis, and gingival hyperplasia in renal transplant recipients. Oral Surg Oral Med Oral Pathol 1994;78:18–26.
102. Syrjanen S, von Krogh G, Kellokoski J, et al. Two different human papillomavirus (HPV) types associated with oral mucosal lesions in an HIV-seropositive man. J Oral Pathol Med 1989;18:366–370.
103. Epstein JB, Priddy RW, Sherlock CH. Hairy leukoplakia-like lesions in immunosuppressed patients following bone marrow transplantation. Transplantation 1988;46:462–464.
104. Reggiani M, Paulizzi P. Hairy leukoplakia in liver transplant patients. Acta Derm Venerol (Stockh) 1990;70:87–88.
105. Eisenberg E, Krutchkoff D, Yamaes H. Incidental oral hairy leukoplakia in immunocompetent persons. Oral Surg Oral Med Oral Pathol 1992;74:332–323.
106. Katz MH, Greenspan D, Westenhouse J, et al. Progression to AIDS in HIV-infected homosexual and bisexual men with hairy leukoplakia and oral candidiasis. AIDS 1992;6:95–100.
107. Greenspan D, Greenspan JS, Overby G, et al. Risk factors for rapid progression from hairy leukoplakia to AIDS: a nested case control study. J Acquir Immune Defic Syndr 1991;4:652–658.
108. Schiodt M, Greenspan D, Daniels TE, et al. Clinical and histologic spectrum of oral hairy leukoplakia. Oral Surg Oral Med Oral Pathol 1987;64:716–720.
109. Andersen L, Philipsen HP, Reichart PA. Macro- and microanatomy of the lateral border of the tongue with special reference to oral hairy leukoplakia. J Oral Pathol Med 1990;19:77–80.
110. Fowler CB, Reed KD, Brannon RB. Intranuclear inclusions correlate with the ultrastructural detection of herpes-type virions in oral hairy leukoplakia. Am J Surg Pathol 1989;13:114–119
111. Fernandez JF, Benito MAC, Lizaldez EB, et al. Oral hairy leukoplakia: a histopathologic study of 32 cases. Am J Dermatopathol 1990;12:571–578.
112. Greenspan JS, Rabanus JP, Petersen V, et al. Fine structure of EBV-infected keratinocytes in oral hairy leukoplakia. J Oral Pathol Med 1989;18:565–572.
113. Rabanus JP, Greenspan D, Petersen V, et al. Subcellular distribution and life cycle of Epstein–Barr virus in keratinocytes of oral hairy leukoplakia. Am J Pathol 1991;139:185–197.
114. Loning T, Henke R-P, Reichart P, et al. In situ hybridization to detect Epstein–Barr virus DNA in oral tissues of HIV-infected patients. Virchows Arch A Anat Pathol Histopathol 1987;412:127–133.
115. Greenspan JS, Greenspan D. Oral hairy leukoplakia: diagnosis and management. Oral Surg Oral Med Oral Pathol 1989;67:396–403.
116. DeSouza YG, Greenspan D, Gelton JR, et al. Localization of Epstein–Barr virus DNA in the epithelial cells of oral hairy leukoplakia using in-situ hybridization on tissue sections [letter]. N Engl J Med 1989;320:1559–1560.
117. Greenspan JS, Greenspan D, Palefsky JM. Oral hairy leukoplakia after a decade. Epstein Barr Virus Rep 1995;2:13–218.
118. DeSouza YG, Freese UK, Greenspan D, et al. Diagnosis of Epstein–Barr virus infection in hairy leukoplakia by using nucleic acid hybridization and noninvasive techniques. J Clin Microbiol 1990;28:2775–2778.
119. Green TL, Greenspan JS, Greenspan D, et al. Oral lesions mimicking hairy leukoplakia: a diagnostic dilemma. Oral Surg Oral Med Oral Pathol 1989;67:422–426.
120. Resnick L, Herbst JHS, Ablashi DV, et al. Regression of oral hairy leukoplakia after orally administered acyclovir therapy. JAMA 1988;259:384–388.
121. Greenspan D, DeSouza Y, Conant MA, et al. Efficacy of desciclovir in the treatment of Epstein–Barr virus infection in oral hairy leukoplakia. J Acquir Immune Defic Syndr 1990;3:571–578.
122. Young LS, Lau R, Rowe M, et al. Differentiation-associated expression of the Epstein-Barr virus BZLF1 transactivator protein in oral hairy leukoplakia. J Virol 1991;65:2868–2874.
123. Niedobitek G, Young LW, Lau R, et al. Epstein–Barr virus infection in oral hairy leukoplakia: virus replication in the absence of a detectable latent phase. J Gen Virol 1991;72:3035–3046.
124. Thomas JA, Felix DH, Wray D, et al. Epstein–Barr virus gene expression and epithelial cell differentiation in oral hairy leukoplakia. Am J Pathol 1991;139:1369–1380.
125. Sandvej KS, Krenacs L, Hamilton-Dutoit SJ, et al. Epstein–Barr virus latent and replicative gene expression in oral hairy leukoplakia. Histopathology 1992;20:387–395.
126. Felix DH, Thomas JA, Wray D, et al. Patterns of Epstein–Barr virus gene expression and epithelial cell differentiation in hairy leukoplakia. In: Greenspan JS, Greenspan D, eds. Oral manifestations of HIV infection. Chicago: Quintessence, 1995:184–191.
127. Becker J, Leser U, Marschall M, et al. Expression of proteins encoded by Epstein–Barr virus trans-activator genes depends on the differentiation of epithelial cells in oral hairy leukoplakia. Proc Natl Acad Sci U S A 1991;88:8332–8336.
128. Gilligan K, Rajadurai P, Resnick L, et al. Epstein–Barr virus small nuclear RNAs are not expressed in permissively infected cells in AIDS-associated leukoplakia. Proc Natl Acad Sci U S A 1990;87:8790–8794.
129. Raab-Traub N, Walling DM, Miller W. Epstein–Barr virus strain variation and expression in oral hairy leukoplakia. In: Greenspan JS, Greenspan D, eds. Oral manifestations of HIV infection. Chicago: Quintessence, 1995:159–165.
130. Patton DF, Shirley P, Raab-Traub N, et al. Defective viral DNA in Epstein–Barr virus-associated oral hairy leukoplakia. J Virol 1990;64:397–400.
131. Walling DM, Edmiston SN, Sixbey JW, et al. Coinfection with multiple strains of the Epstein–Barr virus in human immunodeficiency virus-associated hairy leukoplakia. Proc Natl Acad Sci U S A 1992;89:6560–6564.
132. Walling DM, Raab-Traub N. Epstein–Barr virus intrastrain recombination in oral hairy leukoplakia. J Virol 1994;68:7909–17.
133. Walling DM, Perkins AG, Webster-Cyriaque J, et al. The Epstein–Barr virus ENBA-2 gene in oral hairy leukoplakia: strain variation, genetic recombination, and transcriptional expression. J Virol 1994;68:7918–7926.
134. Young LS, Lau R, Rowe M, et al. Differentiation-associated expression of the Epstein-Barr virus BZLF1 transactivator protein in oral hairy leukoplakia. J Virol 1991;65:2868–2874.
135. Williams DM, Leigh IM, Greenspan D, et al. Altered patterns of keratin expression in oral hairy leukoplakia: prognostic implications. J Oral Pathol Med 1991;20:167–171.
136. Wilson JB, Weinberg W, Johnson R, et al. Expression of the BNLF-2 oncogene of Epstein–Barr virus in the skin of transgenic mice induces hyperplasia and aberrant expression of keratin 6. Cell 1990;61:1315–1327.
137. Baskin GB, Roberts ED, Kuebler D, et al. Squamous epithelial proliferative lesions associated with Rhesus Epstein–Barr virus in simian immunodeficiency virus–infected rhesus monkeys. J Infect Dis 1995;172:535–539.
138. Daniels TE, Greenspan D, Greenspan JS, et al. Absence of Langerhans cells in oral hairy leukoplakia, an AIDS-associated lesion. J Invest Dermatol 1987;89:178–182.

139. Riccardi R, Pimpinelli N, Ficarral G, et al. Morphology and membrane antigens of nonlymphoid accessory cells in oral hairy leukoplakia. Hum Pathol 1990;21:897–904.
140. Pimpinelli N, Borgognoni L, Riccardi R, et al. CD36(OKM5)+ dendritic cells in the oraol mucosa of HIV- and HIV+ subjects. J Invest Dermatol 1991;97:537–542.
141. Corso B, Eversole LR, Hutt-Fletcher L. Hairy leukoplakia: Epstein–Barr virus receptors on oral keratinocyte plasma membranes. Oral Surg Oral Med Oral Pathol 1989;67:416–421.
142. Greenspan D, Greenspan JS. The significance of oral hairy leukoplakia. Oral Surg Oral Med Oral Pathol 1992;73:151–154.
143. Newman C, Polk BF. Resolution of hairy leukoplakia during therapy with 9-(1,3-dihydroxy-2-propoxymethyl) guanine (DHPG). Ann Intern Med 1987;107:348–350.
144. Brockmeyer NH, Kreuzfelder E, Mertins L, et al. Zidovudine therapy of asymptomatic HIV-1-infected patients and combined zidovudine-acyclovir therapy of HIV-1-infected patients with oral hairy leukoplakia. J Invest Dermatol 1989;92:647.
145. Katz MH, Greenspan D, Heinic GS, et al. Resolution of hairy leukoplakia: an observational trial of zidovudine versus no treatment [letter]. J Infect Dis 1991;164:1240–1241.
146. Gowdey G, Lee RK, Carpenter WM. Treatment of HIV-related hairy leukoplakia with podophyllum resin 25% solution. Oral Surg Oral Med Oral Pathol 1995;79:64–67.
147. Greenspan D, de Villiers EM, Greenspan JS, et al. Unusual HPV types in the oral warts in association with HIV infection. J Oral Pathol 1988;17:482–487.
148. de Villiers EM. Prevalence of HPV-7 papillomas in the oral mucosa and facial skin of patients with human immunodeficiency virus. Arch Dermatol 1989;125:1590.
149. Volter C, He Y, Roy-Burman A, et al. Novel HPV types present in oral papillomatous lesions from patients with HIV infection. Int J Cancer 1996;66:453–456.
150. Regezi JA, Greenspan D, Greenspan JS, et al. HPV-associated epithelial atypia in oral warts in HIV+ patients. J Cutan Pathol 1994;21:217–223.
151. Schmidt-Westhausen A, Fehrenbach FJ, Reichart PA. Oral enterobacteriaceae in patients with HIV infection. J Oral Pathol 1990;19:229–231.
152. Fowler CB, Nelson JF, Henley DW, et al. Acquired immune deficiency syndrome presenting as a palatal perforation. Oral Surg Oral Med Oral Pathol 1989;67:313–318.
153. Speight PM. Epithelioid angiomatosis affecting the oral cavity as a first sign of HIV infection. Br Dent J 1991;171:367–370.
154. Winkler JR, Murray PA, Grassi M, et al. Diagnosis and management of HIV-associated periodontal lesions. J Am Dent Assoc 1989; 119(Suppl):S25–S34.
155. Lamster I, Grbic J, Fine J, et al. A critical review of periodontal disease as a manifestation of HIV infection. In: Greenspan JS, Greenspan D, eds. Oral manifestations of HIV infection. Chicago: Quintessence, 1995:247–256.
156. Masouredis CM, Katz MH, Greenspan D, et al. Prevalence of HIV-associated periodontitis and gingivitis in HIV-infected patients attending an AIDS clinic. J Acquir Immune Defic Syndr 1992;5:479–483.
157. Winkler JR, Herrera C, Westenhouse J, et al. Periodontal disease in HIV-infected and uninfected homosexual and bisexual men [letter]. AIDS 1992;6:1041–1043.
158. Williams CA, Winkler JR, Grassi M, et al. HIV-associated periodontitis complicated by necrotizing stomatitis. Oral Surg Oral Med Oral Pathol 1990;69:351–355.
159. SanGiacomo TR, Tan PM, Loggi DG, et al. Progressive osseous destruction as a complication of HIV-periodontitis. Oral Surg Oral Med Oral Pathol 1990;70:476–479.
160. Winkler JR, Grassi M, Murray PA. Clinical description and etiology of HIV-associated periodontal diseases. In: Robertson PB, Greenspan JS, eds. Perspectives on oral manifestations of AIDS: diagnosis and management of HIV-associated infections. Littleton, MA: PSG, 1988:49–70.
161. Pindborg JJ, Thorn JJ, Schiodt M, et al. Acute necrotizing gingivitis in an AIDS patient. Dan Dent J 1986;90:450–453.
162. Zambon JJ, Reynolds H, Smutko J, et al. Are unique bacterial pathogens involved in HIV-associated periodontal diseases? In: Greenspan JS, Greenspan D, eds. Oral manifestations of HIV infection. Chicago: Quintessence, 1995:257–262.
163. Ryder MI, Winkler JR, Weintreb RN. Elevated phagocytosis, oxidative burst and F actin formation in PMNs from individuals with intraoral manifestations of HIV infection. J Acquir Immune Defic Syndr 1988;1:346–353.
164. Grassi M, Williams CA, Winkler JR, et al. Management of HIV-associated periodontal diseases. In: Robertson PB, Greenspan JS, eds. Perspectives on oral manifestations of AIDS: diagnosis and management of HIV-associated infections. Littleton, MA: PSG, 1988:119–130.
165. Palmer G. Periodontal therapy for patients with HIV infection. In: Greenspan JS, Greenspan D, eds. Oral manifestations of HIV infection. Chicago: Quintessence, 1995:273–280.
166. MacPhail LA, Greenspan D, Feigal DW, et al. Recurrent aphthous ulcers in association with HIV infection: description of ulcer types and analysis of T-cell subsets. Oral Surg Oral Med Oral Pathol 1991;71:678–683.
167. MacPhail LA, Greenspan D, Greenspan JS. Recurrent aphthous ulcers in association with HIV infection: diagnosis and treatment. Oral Surg Oral Med Oral Pathol 1992;73:283–288.
168. Revuz J, Guillaume J-C, Janier M, et al. Crossover study of thalidomide vs placebo in severe recurrent aphthous stomatitis. Arch Dermatol 1990;126:923–927.
169. Ryan J, Colman J, Pedersen J, et al. Thalidomide to treat esophageal ulcer in AIDS [letter]. N Engl J Med 1992;327:208–209.
170. Rabeneck L, Popovic M, Gartner S, et al. Acute HIV infection presenting with painful swallowing and esophageal ulcers. JAMA 1990;263:2318–2322.
171. Schiodt M, Dodd CL, Greenspan D, et al. Natural history of HIV-associated salivary gland disease. Oral Surg Oral Med Oral Pathol 1992;74:326–331.
172. Schiodt M, Dodd CL, Greenspan D, et al. HIV-associated salivary gland disease. In: Greenspan JS, Greenspan D, eds. Oral manifestations of HIV infection. Chicago: Quintessence, 1995:145–151.
173. Pawha S, Fikrig S, Kaplan M, et al. Expression of HTLV-III infection in a pediatric population. Adv Exp Med Biol 1985;187:45–-51.
174. Soberman N, Leonidas JC, Berdon WE, et al. Parotid enlargement in children seropositive for human immunodeficiency virus: imaging findings. AJR Am J Roentgenol 1991;157:553–556.
175. Bem C, Barucha H, Patil PS. Parotid disease and human immunodeficiency virus infection in Zambia. Br J Surg 1992;79:768–770.
176. Huang RD, Pearlman S, Friedman WH, et al. Benign cystic vs. solid lesions of the parotid gland in HIV patients. Head Neck 1991;13:522–527.
177. Itescu S, Brancato LJ, Winchester R. A sicca syndrome in HIV infection: association with HLA-DR5 and CD8 lymphocytosis [letter]. Lancet 1989:466–468.
178. Itescu S, Dalton J, Zhang HZ, et al. Tissue infiltration in a CD8 lymphocytosis syndrome associated with human immunodeficiency virus-1 infection has the phenotypic appearance of an antigenically driven response. J Clin Invest 1993;91:2216–2225.
179. Itescu S, Mathur-Wagh U, Skovron ML, et al. HLA-B35 is associated with accelerated progression to AIDS. J Acquir Immune Defic Syndr 1991;5:37–45.
180. Greenspan D, Grenspan JS, Pindborg JJ, et al. AIDS and the dental team. Copenhagen: Munksgaard, 1986.
181. Langford A, Pohle HD, Gelderblom H, et al. Oral hyperpigmentation in HIV-infected patients. Oral Surg Oral Med Oral Pathol 1989;67:301–307.

182. Cohen LM, Callen JP. Oral and labial melanotic macules in a patient infected with human immunodeficiency virus. J Am Acad Dermatol 1992;26:653–654.
183. Porter SR, Glover S, Scully C. Oral hyperpigmentation secondary to adrenocortical suppression in a patient with AIDS. Oral Surg Oral Med Oral Pathol 1990;70:59–60.
184. Ficarra G, Shillitoe EJ, Adler-Storthz K, et al. Oral melanotic macules in patients infected with human immunodeficiency virus. Oral Surg Oral Med Oral Pathol 1990;70:748–755.
185. Leggott PJ, Robertson PB, Greenspan D, et al. Oral manifestations of primary and acquired immunodeficiency diseases in children. Pediatr Dent 1987;9:89–104.
186. Moniaci D, Cavallari M, Greco D, et al. Oral lesions in children born to HIV-1 positive women. J Oral Pathol Med 1993;22:8–11.
187. Ramos-Gomez FJ, Hilton JF, Canchola AJ, et al. Risk factors for HIV-related orofacial manifestations in children. Ped Dent 1996;18:121–126.
188. Greenspan JS, Mastrucci T, Leggott P, et al. Hairy leukoplakia in a child. AIDS 1988;2:143.
189. Robinson PG, Cooper H, Hatt J. Healing after dental extractions in men with HIV infection. Oral Surg Oral Med Oral Pathol 1992;74:426–430.
190. Porter SR, Scully C, Luker J. Complications of dental surgery in persons with HIV disease. Oral Surg Oral Med Oral Pathol 1993;75:165–167.
191. Paauw DS, Wenrich MD, Curtis R, et al. Ability of primary care physicians to recognize physical findings associated with HIV infection. JAMA 1995;274:1380–1382.

33

GASTROINTESTINAL MANIFESTATIONS OF HIV DISEASE, INCLUDING THE PERITONEUM AND MESENTERY

Douglas T. Dieterich, Michael A. Poles, Mitchell S. Cappell, and Edward A. Lew

The overwhelming global epidemiologic impact of human immunodeficiency virus (HIV) is amply reviewed elsewhere in this book. The importance of the gastrointestinal system in this grand scheme cannot be underestimated. From mouth to anus, the entire gastrointestinal tract plays an important role in the epidemiology, pathophysiology, and treatment of acquired immunodeficiency syndrome (AIDS). The mucosa of the gastrointestinal tract is many times larger than the skin and is the major surface on which contact between human beings and their environment takes place. Inside the system, only a single layer of gut epithelium separates the "milieu interior" from the hostile external world. Through this single layer of cells, nutrients must be absorbed, and infectious and toxic matter must be defended against and excluded.

The distal colon is likely the portal of entry for HIV infection in patients who acquire the disease through homosexual contact. The virus may enter the circulation through breaks in the rectal mucosa, or it may be shuttled by mucosal antigen-presenting M cells to lymphocytes, which may disseminate throughout the body. The gut-associated lymphoid tissue, which collectively represents the largest lymphoid organ in the body, may also act as a reservoir for HIV-infected lymphocytes. Altered activity of these lymphocytes likely contributes to the functional abnormalities of the gut-associated lymphoid tissue that is partly responsible for the digestive diseases of AIDS patients (1).

The clinical significance of AIDS-related gastrointestinal problems is enormous. Estimates of the prevalence of gastrointestinal complaints in patients with HIV range from 30 to 90%. It seems that, in the United States, more gay men (80%) than intravenous drug users (58%) complain of gastrointestinal problems (2). In Australia, Lane and colleagues reported that 60% of AIDS patients reported gastrointestinal symptoms (3); in Germany, Heise and associates found 49% (4), and in France, 62% were reported (5). Even more disturbing are the statistics from developing countries, where more than 90% of patients have gastrointestinal complaints (6), and most of those patients will die of malnutrition and wasting. The African cases had been called "slim disease" because of the degree of wasting associated with it. Much of the morbidity and mortality of advanced AIDS is due to gastrointestinal disease, and this significantly affects the use of health care resources. The health care costs associated with HIV in the United States alone were $15 billion in 1995 (7).

In the second decade of the study and treatment of HIV, advances in the clinical and basic science have given us grounds for optimism. New antiretroviral drugs and new treatments for many opportunistic infections have led some optimists to proclaim that the scourge of AIDS will soon be behind us. In the first half of 1996, AIDS-related deaths decreased 19% from the same period of the previous year. This change is due, in part, to the use of combination therapy that includes protease inhibitors (highly active antiretroviral therapy [HAART]). These trends have an effect on the gastrointestinal tract as well. Longer life span means more opportunities for development of infections and neoplasms in the gastrointestinal tract. Nonetheless, the reality is that, although we have made advances in controlling the spread of the virus in industrialized countries, spread in the developing world continues unabated. No room exists for complacency. Estimates suggest that more than 30 million people worldwide are HIV infected; by the year 2000, the number will probably grow to 40 million. AIDS has become the third leading cause of death among women in the United States who are 25 to 44 years of age, and it is already the leading cause of death in white men of the same age group.

GENERAL APPROACH

In formulating a general approach to the patient with gastrointestinal problems (Table 33.1), the clinician must first and foremost be suspicious of every conceivable disease. New pathogens in common places and common pathogens in new places are the rule and not the exception. An

Table 33.1. General Approach to the Patient with HIV and Gastrointestinal Complaints

1. Be suspicious of every conceivable disease.
2. Consider new pathogens in common sites and common pathogens in new sites.
3. An aggressive approach to diagnosis leads to more successful and earlier treatment and better outcomes for the patient.
4. It is more common to find more than one pathogen at a time than to find only one.
5. When standard tests are unrevealing, perform endoscopic or percutaneous biopsies.
6. If no gastrointestinal condition is found, look elsewhere.
7. When an infection is found:
   It may not respond to standard therapy.
   Relapse is frequent.
   Permanent maintenance therapy may be required.
8. All problems are not necessarily HIV related; do not overlook the fact that HIV-infected persons also are subject to nonopportunistic, non-HIV–related processes typical for their age and sex.

aggressive approach to diagnosis will lead to more successful and earlier treatment and better outcomes for the patients. No room exists for complacency or therapeutic nihilism in the care of people with AIDS and gastrointestinal problems. It is more common to find more than one pathogen at a time than to find only one. Therefore, if a patient is not responding to therapy, the clinician should continue looking. If no pathogen is found, one should continue looking. For instance, ascribing diarrhea to "AIDS enteropathy" is easy when no obvious pathogens are located. However, microsporidia, *Cyclospora*, and many as yet unidentified pathogens may be playing a role. When standard stool and blood tests are unrevealing, one should perform endoscopic or percutaneous biopsies. Several studies have shown that endoscopic or liver biopsy yields a diagnosis of a potentially treatable condition in more than 50% of cases. If no gastrointestinal condition is identified, one should look elsewhere. *Pneumocystis carinii* pneumonia sometimes presents with diarrhea. Nausea, vomiting, and anorexia are sometimes caused by central nervous system processes such as lymphoma, toxoplasmosis, or cryptococcal meningitis.

When a condition is found and treated, long-term maintenance therapy for life is more frequently required than not. Finally, in one's zeal to find an opportunistic infection, the clinician must not forget that HIV-infected persons are also subject to nonopportunistic, non–HIV-related processes typical for their age and sex. Moreover, some processes that afflict nonimmunosuppressed persons, such as inflammatory bowel disease (8) and peptic ulcer disease (9), may be seen less frequently or in a more benign fashion among patients with AIDS.

HAART has had a profound impact on the care of patients infected with HIV. We are encountering far fewer patients with gastrointestinal complaints resulting from opportunistic infections. Additionally, patients with such infections may experience resolution associated with the immune reconstitution afforded by HAART. Still, not all patients benefit to the same extent, and HAART may only result in expansion of the memory CD4 cell population already present; if the immunologic memory for a given pathogen is lost in advanced AIDS, it may be lost forever, despite HAART. Finally, the agents used in HAART, including protease inhibitors, may cause symptoms and signs, including diarrhea and elevations of liver-associated substances.

ESOPHAGEAL DISEASE

A target of many diseases, the esophagus is an extremely important organ in HIV-infected patients. These patients may suffer from decreased appetite or from severe malnutrition or dehydration as a result of reduced intake despite preserved appetite. At some point in their disease, at least one-third of HIV-infected patients suffer from esophageal disease (10). Further, opportunistic infection of the esophagus is a sign of severely diminished immunologic function and is a predictor of poor survival (10).

The most common symptom described by patients with esophageal disease is odynophagia or painful swallowing. Next is dysphagia, a feeling of food "sticking" in the retrosternal area. Frequently, of course, the two are found together. Two-thirds of patients with esophageal symptoms, more commonly with odynophagia, are diagnosed with a specific infectious or neoplastic disorder (11). Regularly overlooked signs of esophageal disease include singultus or "hiccups," usually caused by esophagitis, and substernal chest pain or gastrointestinal bleeding.

Etiology

Most HIV-infected patients with esophageal symptoms have opportunistic infections that can be identified. The most common esophageal diseases are listed in Table 33.2. *Candida albicans* is by far the most frequently identified etiologic agent, occurring 42 to 79% of the time (12). It usually occurs with oropharyngeal candidiasis, although not necessarily. Symptomatic esophageal candidiasis is an AIDS-defining diagnosis. Two rarely seen fungal pathogens are *Candida glabrata*, *Histoplasma capsulatum* (13, 14), *Aspergillus* species, and *Cryptococcus*.

The most common viral pathogen found in the esophagus is cytomegalovirus (CMV). It has been found in 10 to 40% of endoscopic biopsies of esophageal ulcers (15). CMV infection can appear as either diffuse esophagitis, single or multiple ulcers usually at the middle esophagus or gastroesophageal junction, or giant ulcers involving the whole esophagus. It may be discovered only after treatment of *Candida* because these pathogens coexist in up to 20% of patients (Fig. 33.1) (16). Patients with a diagnosis of CMV esophagitis, whether treated or not, have a poor long-term prognosis; before the expanded use of protease inhibitors, few survived longer than a year. Few data are available on the survival of patients receiving these drugs. Less common viral causes of esophagitis include Epstein–Barr virus, herpes simplex virus (HSV), papovavirus (17), and human herpesvirus type 6 (18). Finally, HIV itself appears to cause both acute and chronic esophageal disease (19).

Bacterial and mycobacterial esophageal disease is rare. *Mycobacterium tuberculosis* causes symptoms, usually from erosion of a contiguous mediastinal lymph node into the esophagus. *Mycobacterium avium* complex (MAC) rarely causes direct esophageal infection. Reports have noted superinfection by *Actinomyces* of CMV esophageal ulcers (20), esophageal bacillary angiomatosis (21), and nocardial esophagitis (22). Extremely rare protozoal causes of esophagitis include *Cryptosporidium parvum* (23), *Pneumocystis* (24), and *Leishmania* (25).

Kaposi's sarcoma (KS) is occasionally found in the esophagus. It is usually submucosal and rarely causes symptoms unless it ulcerates, obstructs the lumen, bleeds, or occurs at a sphincter. More and more lymphomas are also being found in the esophagus as a primary or a secondary site (26).

Aphthous or idiopathic ulceration of the esophagus is a significant problem, typically in patients with severe immunosuppression. Frequently, a solitary ulcer or multiple large ulcers will be identified, and biopsy examination reveals only ulcer with granulation tissue, but no identifiable pathogens (Fig. 33.2). These ulcers may be caused by established pathogens missed by biopsy, they may be caused by HIV itself (19), or they may result from unknown pathogens. The response of

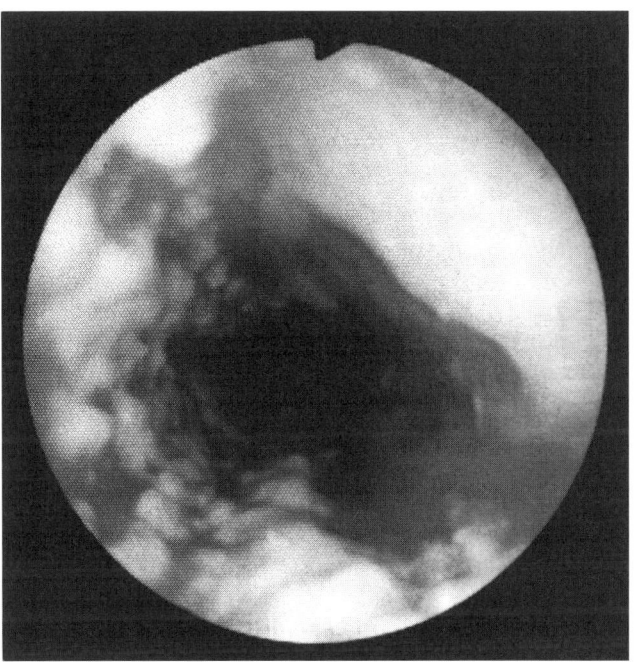

Figure 33.1. Cytomegalovirus ulcer with opposing candidal esophagitis.

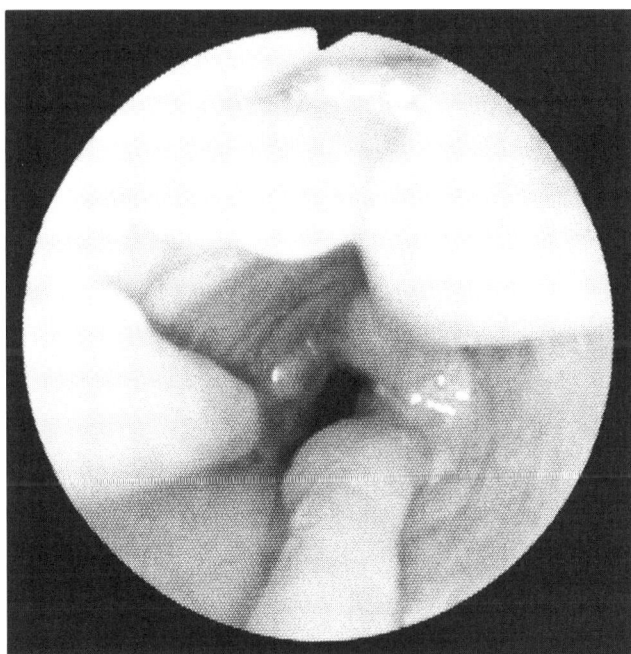

Figure 33.2. Large, nearly circumferential aphthous ulcer at the lower esophageal sphincter.

Table 33.2. Etiology of HIV-Associated Esophageal Disease

Fungal
   Candida albicans
   Candida glabrata
   Histoplasma capsulatum
   Aspergillus sp.
   Cryptococcus neoformans
Viral
   Cytomegalovirus
   Herpes simplex virus
   Epstein–Barr virus
   Papovavirus
   Human herpes virus-6
   HIV
Bacterial
   Mycobacterium tuberculosis
   Mycobacterium avium complex
   Actinomyces
   Bartonella henselae
   Nocardia sp.
Protozoal
   Cryptosporidium parvum
   Pneumocystis carinii
   Leishmania donovani
Neoplastic
   Kaposi's sarcoma
   Lymphoma
Miscellaneous
   Aphthous (idiopathic)
   Acid reflux
   Pill esophagitis

aphthous ulcers to thalidomide, an agent that inhibits cytokine tumor necrosis factor (TNF), suggests that perhaps overexpression of cytokines may play an important role. Regardless of the cause, the end result appears to be induction of apoptosis or programmed cell death (27). Gastroesophageal reflux disease is uncommon among patients with AIDS (10), but these patients may experience pill esophagitis, especially from zidovudine and dideoxycytidine (zalcitabine; ddC). Other offending medications include doxycycline, potassium preparations, and nonsteroidal agents.

Diagnosis

A thorough history and physical examination, including an evaluation for oropharyngeal candidiasis and CMV retinitis, may yield clues to the cause of esophageal disease in the HIV-seropositive patient (Fig. 33.3). Regardless of whether or not oropharyngeal candidiasis is present, empiric antifungal treatment for *Candida* for 7 to 10 days is warranted as the initial part of the diagnostic algorithm. This strategy was shown to be safe, with an associated cost savings of $738 per patient when compared with immediate endoscopy (28). If the complaints resolve as a result of antifungal therapy, then no further testing is required. If the odynophagia or dysphagia does not resolve, endoscopy is usually the next step. Barium esophagography is seldom useful. It can enable one to identify *Candida* esophagitis, but the diagnosis of CMV, HSV, lymphoma, or two simultaneous pathogens is often missed. In one study, radiography produced a correct diagnosis only 25% of the time; when two pathogens were involved, one was missed in 100% of the cases (29). When an ulcer is identified on barium swallow, endoscopy is necessary for biopsy diagnosis. Barium radiography should be used when one suspects a fistula or stricture.

Candidiasis can appear in a range of severity from scattered, small, yellow to tan plaques to larger lesions that coalesce to the point of coating the mucosa or clogging the lumen. Removal of the plaque often reveals an erythematous or eroded base. It commonly obscures concomitant esophageal infections such as CMV. CMV esophagitis may also be focal or may appear as diffuse esophagitis. Rarely, giant (larger than 2 cm) ulcers are present. HSV lesions appear vesicular, as small, discrete "volcano" ulcers, or as a diffuse process. Endoscopic biopsy is required for diagnosis of ulcerative lesions, and specimens should should be taken from the periphery and crater of these lesions. The sensitivity of histopathologic diagnosis may be increased by immunohistochemical staining.

Treatment

In the past, many agents were used to treat candidal esophagitis, including nystatin, clotrimazole, and miconazole as local agents, ketoconazole, fluconazole, itraconazole, and 5-flucytosine as oral agents, and amphotericin B and fluconazole intravenously. The local agents are typically effective against oropharyngeal candidiasis; however, esophageal disease requires systemic therapy.

Fluconazole, 200 mg each day, is the treatment of choice for candidal esophagitis. Ketoconazole had been preferred, but problems related to hepatotoxicity, resistance, interactions with other medications, and poor absorption because of hypochlorhydria put it at a disadvantage (30). Although ketoconazole is one-third as expensive, fluconazole has greater in vivo activity against *Candida* and is better absorbed, even at neutral pH (31). A trial that compared these agents showed an endoscopic cure in 91% of the patients given fluconazole versus 52% in those given ketoconazole, with no difference in adverse events (32). In other comparative studies, itraconazole was found to have an efficacy superior to that of fluconazole and ketoconazole. Patients who develop candidal esophagitis despite fluconazole use may be treated with triple the dose or with intravenous amphotericin. No strong data suggest that maintenance antifungal therapy to prevent relapse is cost effective, and it may induce resistance to an important class of drugs. Instead, secondary prophylaxis should be considered with fluconazole, 100 mg daily, if the patient experiences a relapse.

Two drugs, ganciclovir and foscarnet, have been studied in the treatment of CMV-induced gastrointestinal disease. Each has its own advantages and disadvantages, and the choice of initial therapy should be tailored to the patient. Regardless of the agent used, the patient should be treated with a 2- to 4-week induction period. Ganciclovir was approved first, and in five published studies (33–37), the response to ganciclovir appears to be about 70 to 80%, equivalent to the response rate for CMV retinitis. Ganciclovir is easy to administer intravenously (5 to 10 mg/kg daily), but it frequently induces dose-limiting neutropenia or thrombocytopenia, especially in the presence of zidovudine (38). This complication can be treated successfully with colony-stimulating factors, which are costly. Foscarnet (60 mg/kg three times daily or 90

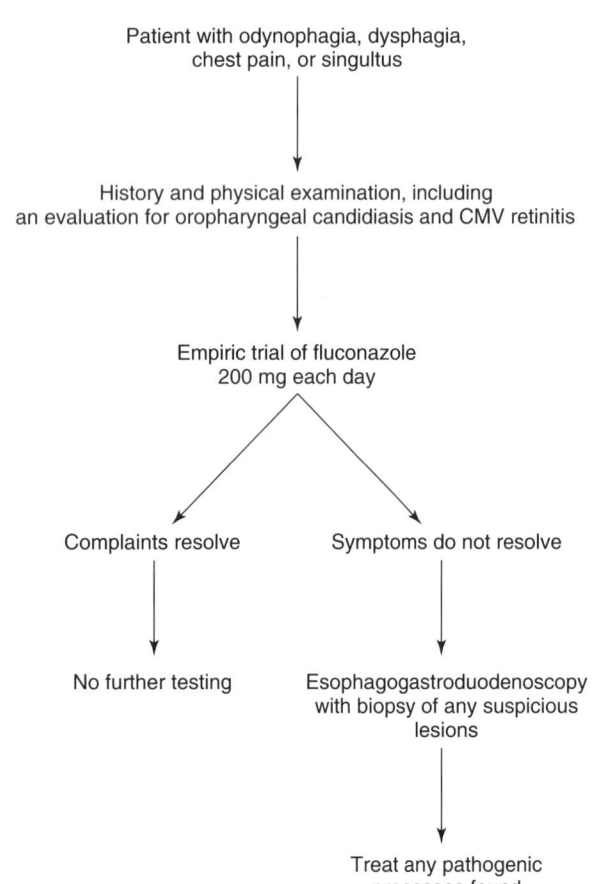

Figure 33.3. Algorithm for approach to the patient with HIV-related esophageal disease.

mg/kg twice daily) is effective in treating both "new" CMV esophageal disease and relapses after treatment with ganciclovir fails (39). The principal side effects of foscarnet are nephrotoxicity and renal wasting of electrolytes. At present, thrice-daily administration is suggested, but a twice-daily schedule appears to be equivalent in efficacy and pharmacokinetics (40). Esophageal strictures have been reported after treatment with both drugs (41), presumably as a result of healing. Now that patients are living longer, the question arises about what to do when a CMV esophageal ulcer recurs after therapy with both ganciclovir and foscarnet. Some evidence suggests that both drugs can be used together successfully in standard doses both in induction and maintenance therapy of CMV (42). Whether maintenance treatment is required after initial therapy is still open to question. Many factors enter into this decision. Most patients achieve long-term remission after standard induction therapy without maintenance. If relapse occurs, retreatment with induction doses of the same drug is reasonable, followed by maintenance therapy. Oral ganciclovir has been approved by the United States Food and Drug Administration (FDA) for maintenance therapy of CMV retinitis, but its role in gastrointestinal disease is yet to be established. Preliminary evidence suggests that maintenance therapy is associated with a trend toward lower remission, but this evidence dates from before the use of protease inhibitors (43). A recent trial describing elevated levels of TNF-α mRNA in the tissue from CMV-associated esophageal ulcers suggests that thalidomide may be used as adjunctive therapy to improve healing of these lesions (44).

Herpes esophagitis should be treated with intravenous acyclovir, at a dose of 15 to 30 mg/kg each day. Foscarnet is effective against acyclovir-resistant HSV.

Treatment of idiopathic or aphthous ulcers is controversial. Symptomatic therapy with acid-blocking agents or sucralfate may help, as does treatment of the underlying HIV disease. Reports have been published of successful treatment with prednisone, at a dose of 40 mg orally each day until symptoms improve, and then tapering 10 mg each week (45). This regimen appears to be safe and effective, with a low relapse rate (46). Reports have also noted a benefit from treatment with thalidomide (47).

Bacterial and mycobacterial infections of the esophagus generally respond to standard antibiotic regimens. Effective therapies exist for both *Mycobacterium tuberculosis* and MAC, and clinicians have every reason to treat these patients. The response of neoplasia in the esophagus to chemotherapy is no different from the response seen at other locations.

GASTRIC DISEASE

The stomach, with a few rare exceptions, is subject to the same disease processes and pathogens as the esophagus, including CMV, HSV, mycobacteria, *Toxoplasma*, lymphoma, and KS (Fig. 33.4). Some overlap with small intestinal disease also exists. *Candida*, perhaps because of sensitivity to acidic pH, is not usually a significant problem. However, patients infected with HIV may exhibit parietal cell

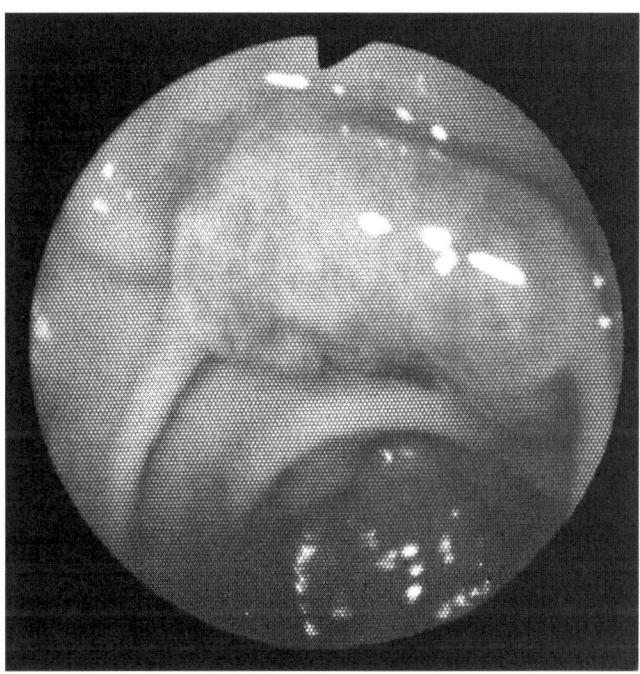

Figure 33.4. Large Kaposi's sarcoma lesion in the antrum.

dysfunction that can lead to a reduction in maximal acid output (48). The resultant hypochlorhydria may lower the "acid barrier" to infection, thus allowing bacterial overgrowth in the small bowel and diarrhea. Hypochlorhydria may also interfere with the absorption of acid-soluble drugs such as ketoconazole.

Helicobacter pylori infection is the primary risk factor for development of peptic ulcer disease worldwide, but most studies have shown that the prevalence of this infection is significantly lower in AIDS patients (49). One study determined that diminished *H. pylori* and peptic ulcer disease prevalence were most marked for patients with fewer than 200 CD4 cells/mm³ (9). For unclear reasons, *H. pylori* is not a significant pathogen in HIV-infected patients. Dyspeptic symptoms and nausea in HIV-infected patients may be due to motility dysfunction related to HIV-associated visceral neuropathy (50).

Treatment of gastric pathogens is the same as that of esophageal or enteric pathogens. Treatment of peptic ulcer disease or gastritis may be different because of the problem of hypochlorhydria. If no acid is present, use of histamine-2 blockers or proton pump inhibitors is unlikely to help. Therefore, mucosal protective agents such as sucralfate may be more effective. Because of the high incidence of diarrhea in AIDS patients, magnesium-containing antacids should be avoided in favor of aluminum- or bismuth-based antacids.

ENTEROCOLITIS AND DIARRHEA

At least half of North American and European patients with HIV will develop diarrhea sometime during their clinical course; those at greater risk include patients with a CD4 cell count lower than 200 to 250 cells/mm³ and male homosexuals (51, 52). This number ranges up to 90% in developing countries (6). A pathogen can be identified in 50 to 85% of HIV-infected patients with diarrhea (53, 54), especially in homosexual men (2), in patients with significant weight loss (52), and in those with prolonged diarrhea (52, 55). The number of pathogens found and treated is continually expanding. Whatever the cause of diarrhea, it is significantly associated with diminished quality of life, and it is an independent predictor of poor prognosis in patients with AIDS (56). In addition to substantial work lost, such patients incur annual health costs that are 50% higher than those of comparable patients without diarrheal symptoms (57).

The intensity of the diagnostic investigation of patients with HIV-related chronic diarrhea remains controversial. The strongest evidence for a minimal evaluation comes from an initial cost-to-benefit analysis published in 1990 (58). The authors of that study concluded that a minimal initial evaluation with stool culture alone was associated with the same diarrhea remission rate as a more extensive evaluation that included stool culture, ova and parasite examination, blood cultures, upper gastrointestinal tract endoscopy, and colonoscopy with biopsies. They also concluded that the minimal approach was cost effective and suggested that endoscopy be reserved for patients who fail to respond to nonspecific antidiarrheals. This early study has been criticized because it assumed that diarrhea would resolve in 67% of patients treated with diphenoxylate regardless of the cause, and it did not take into account many treatable enteropathogens and the effectiveness of new therapies. More recent studies have proved that more extensive workups are more effective, and most experts recommend an intensive approach including endoscopic examination in most patients with advanced HIV disease (52, 59, 60). Still, finding a diarrhea-causing organism does not guarantee its role in the patient's symptoms, nor does it guarantee a response to treatment. Even when an enteropathogen is found and treated, the benefit may not outweigh the cost and discomfort of an extensive evaluation (61). Certainly, further investigations are required.

Regardless of the extent of evaluation, when an HIV-positive patient presents with diarrhea, standard medical practice is the best way to approach the problem (Fig. 33.5). A thorough history and physical examination are first, with particular attention to travel history, medications that can cause diarrhea, and diet (e.g., lactose). In addition, the number and volume of bowel movements can help to point to either a small bowel or large bowel source of diarrhea. Large-volume or relatively infrequent or nocturnal diarrhea points to the small bowel. Frequent bloody bowel movements with abdominal pain and rebound tenderness point to the colon. Stool studies are next and should be tested for all bacterial pathogens, for standard ova and parasites, for *Clostridium difficile* toxin, for *Cryptosporidium* using modified acid-fast stain, direct fluorescent antibody (DFA), and enzyme-linked immunosorbent assay (ELISA), and for microsporidia using chromotrope-based techniques, "Fungi-fluor" stains, or polymerase chain reaction (PCR) that allows speciation (62). If *Giardia* is a consideration, then DFA staining or detection of *Giardia* antigens in the stool by ELISA should be undertaken. Commonly, three sets of stool studies are sent to the laboratory, because shedding of these organisms is episodic, although no data support this concept. If fever accompanies the diarrhea, blood cultures, chest radiography, and urinalysis are also indicated. Sometimes, bacterial pathogens only appear in the blood and not in the stool cultures. If results of stool tests done in a reliable laboratory are negative, then endoscopic biopsy is the next step.

Patients with classic small bowel diarrhea should have upper gastrointestinal tract endoscopy first, with small bowel biopsy from the distal duodenum or proximal jejunum. Aspirates and cytologic brushings as well as biopsy samples placed directly in glutaraldehyde may be performed. A sample can be set aside for electron microscopy should the initial workup be unrevealing. If the history suggests colitis, then endoscopy of the lower gastrointestinal tract should be performed. The choice of lower endoscopic procedure is controversial. Some studies suggest that the yield of flexible sigmoidoscopy is adequate for detection of enteric pathogens, with colonoscopy reserved for patients in whom flexible sigmoidoscopy fails to reveal the cause but in whom colitis is likely (52). Our published data (63) suggest that sigmoidoscopy alone would miss at least 33% of cases of CMV-related colitis. Another study suggested that if flexible sigmoidoscopy had been used rather than colonoscopy, 30% of pathogens, mostly treatable, and 75% of lymphomas would have escaped detection (64). Instead of subjecting a patient to two procedures, one colonoscopy is probably preferable. Multiple random biopsies should be performed for histopathologic examination and possibly for mycobacterial culture, even if the mucosa appears normal, because MAC and CMV can be found in grossly normal-appearing mucosa. Whether investigation of the upper or lower gastrointestinal tract should be performed first is not clear. Both may be performed on the same day; if one is negative, then the alternative procedure should be performed. When all tests are unrevealing, although frustration is a common reaction, it should not be. Symptomatic therapy with nonspecific antidiarrheal agents such as loperamide, diphenoxylate, paregoric, or opium is frequently successful in alleviating symptoms. Empiric therapy with a fluoroquinolone and metronidazole may also be used. Lactose-free low-fat diets can also help. If malnutrition is a problem, then nutritional therapy should be instituted either enterally or parenterally. If diarrhea persists after 6 to 8 weeks, the diagnostic cycle should begin again, with stool tests and then endoscopic biopsies. If this cycle is repeated several times, a pathogen is almost always identified. In some patients, no cause is identified despite intensive investigations. Patients in whom no diagnosis can be established after an extensive workup often have spontaneous resolution of their symptoms and longer survival than patients who have an identified pathogen (52, 65).

Etiology

The list of most common pathogens isolated from the small or large bowel is included in Table 33.3. The frequency and prevalence of each of these pathogens are difficult to judge. They vary geographically, seasonally, and by risk factor. The best approach is to keep an open mind and to search for all pathogens. In addition, other causes of diarrhea must always be included in the differential diagnosis. Almost all patients with HIV are lactose intolerant but may be consuming large quantities of milk or ice cream to gain weight. Most drugs used in the treatment of AIDS, including reverse transcriptase inhibitors, protease inhibitors, and antibiotics, are associated with diarrhea. Other drugs such as dideoxyinosine (ddI), ddC, trimethoprim–sulfamethoxazole (TMP–SMX), and pentamidine can cause pancreatitis, which can lead to maldigestion and steatorrhea. Other proposed mechanisms of cryptogenic diarrhea include altered intestinal permeability, bile acid malabsorption, dysregulation of the enteric immune system, local production of lymphokines, autonomic denervation, and increased HIV in GALT tissue.

CYTOMEGALOVIRUS

This ubiquitous herpesvirus often affects the colon (67% in one series [66]), but it can cause damage throughout the gastrointestinal tract. Infection may result in colitis, only visible microscopically, to deep fibrin-covered ulcers. Most commonly, CMV causes mild, patchy colitis (Fig. 33.6), although mucosal ulceration is not atypical (Fig. 33.7). The

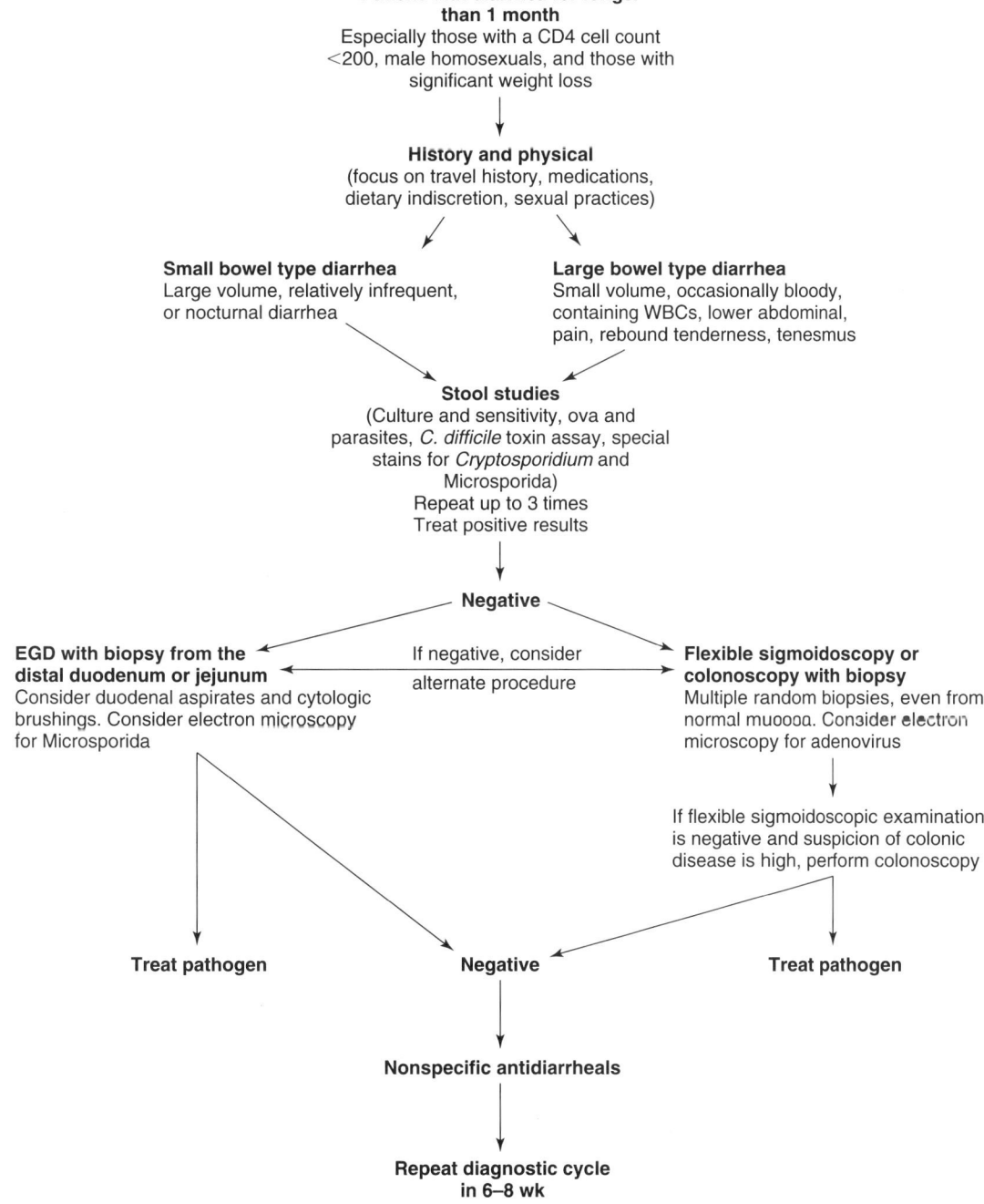

Figure 33.5. Algorithm for approach to the patient with HIV-related diarrheal disease.

Table 33.3. Etiology of HIV-Associated Diarrheal Disease

Small Intestine
   Cytomegalovirus
   Histoplasma capsulatum
   Cryptosporidium parvum
   Microsporidia
   Isospora belli
   Giardia lamblia
   Cyclospora cayetanensis
   Blastocystis hominis?
   Pneumocystis carinii
   Toxoplasma gondii
   Mycobacterium avium complex
   Salmonella species
   Campylobacter species
   Mycobacterium tuberculosis
   HIV
Large Intestine
   Cytomegalovirus
   Adenovirus
   Astroviruses, caliciviruses, and rotavirus
   Herpes simplex virus
   Histoplasma capsulatum
   Candida albicans
   Cryptococcus neoformans
   North American blastomycoses
   Cryptosporidium parvum
   Coccidioides immitis
   Entamoeba histolytica
   Mycobacterium avium complex
   Shigella; group D
   Clostridium difficile
   Campylobacter jejuni
   Enteroadherent *Escherichia coli*
   HIV
Miscellaneous
   Lactose intolerance
   Medication-induced disease
   Pancreatitis

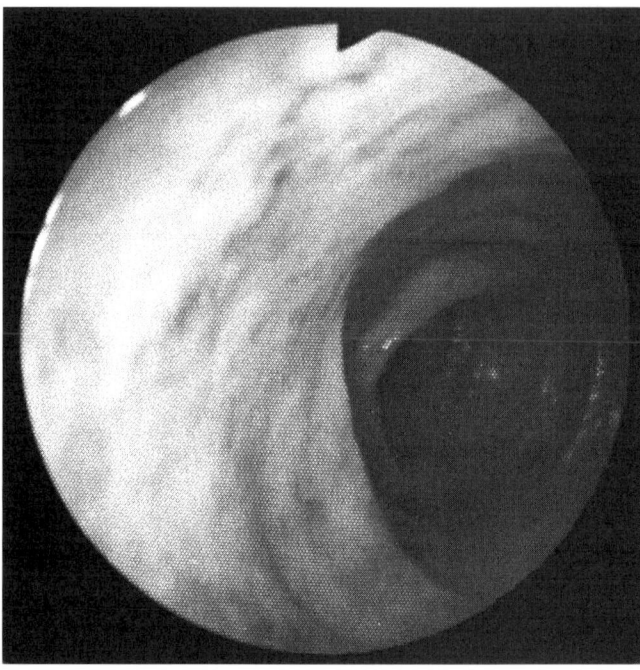

Figure 33.6. Mild cytomegalovirus colitis.

probable mechanism of CMV-induced end-organ damage is vasculitis, leading to thrombosis, occlusion, and ischemia. Clinical CMV disease usually occurs after the CD4 cell count has fallen to below 100 cells/mm^3 and increases linearly below this level (67). Most patients with CMV colitis present with intermittent or persistent diarrhea, crampy lower abdominal pain, tenesmus, and weight loss. The stool may be formed or semiformed and may be positive for blood and fecal leukocytes. Rebound tenderness strongly suggests peritonitis from CMV-induced inflammation or perforation (68). The diagnosis of CMV colitis is made histologically. Multiple biopsy samples should be taken of involved mucosa. CMV may also be found in normal-appearing mucosa, so biopsy specimens should be taken there as well. Histopathologic examination reveals characteristic large mononuclear, epithelial, endothelial, or smooth muscle cells containing intranuclear or cytoplasmic inclusions. The inclusion body may be surrounded by a halo of clear space suggestive of the appearance of a classic "owl's eye." In some cases, the viral inclusions are atypical or sparse, and special staining with immunoperoxidase and DNA in situ hybridization, as well as PCR, may increase the sensitivity and specificity of histologic examination. Despite these measures, sensitivity may still depend on the number of biopsies taken and the diligence of the pathologist (69). The significance of finding CMV inclusions in an area devoid of endoscopic or histologic inflammation is unclear at this time, although many clinicians would treat such a patient.

ADENOVIRUS

Adenovirus has been described as a cause of diarrhea in immunosuppressed adults and normal children (70). It has been identified in colon biopsy samples from AIDS patients with chronic diarrhea in both inflamed and normal-appearing mucosa, as well as in the stool of AIDS patients without diarrhea (71). Thus, its causal role in the pathogenesis of diarrhea is questionable. Patients with CD4 cell counts lower than 200 cells/mm^3 are prone to more prolonged adenovirus infection (72). The histopathologic changes of adenovirus are different from those of CMV, and the sensitivity of light microscopy is improved by immunostains (73).

Additional studies using stringent techniques have led to the discovery of other viral pathogens that may contribute to diarrhea in patients with AIDS, including astroviruses, caliciviruses, coronavirus, and rotavirus (74). As with adenovirus, the significance of these viruses in the pathogenesis of diarrhea is confounded by their presence in many asymptomatic AIDS patients. One study revealed stool virus by electron microscopy in 17% of AIDS patients undergoing endoscopy; coronavirus and adenovirus were more common in patients with diarrhea (75). Coinfection with other enteropathogens was common.

HERPES SIMPLEX VIRUS

HSV infection of the rectum can cause diarrhea or constipation, hematochezia, and tenesmus resulting from painful perianal ulcers. Gastrointestinal symptoms may also be accompanied by dysuria, paresthesias from sacral nerve involvement, and urinary or fecal incontinence. Early infection may appear as small vesicles on the colonic mucosa that may rupture and coalesce to form ulcers. Given the similarity of HSV to CMV infection in endoscopic appearance and symptoms, these pathogens must be distinguished histopathologically. Examination of biopsy specimens reveals the characteristic Cowdry type A intranuclear inclusions in multinucleated cells. Viral culture or immunohistochemistry also help in the diagnosis.

FUNGI

Fungal causes of diarrhea are rare. However, in endemic areas, *Histoplasma capsulatum* is a common cause of gastrointestinal symptoms. Reactivated *Histoplasma* may lead to a chronic infection with dissemination to lymphatic tissue. Any segment of the gastrointestinal tract may be affected, but the terminal ileum with its abundant lymphoid tissue is the most common site. Infection may be asymptomatic, but it is more commonly symptomatic, with diarrhea, weight loss, fever, and abdominal pain. Advanced intestinal disease may result in strictures or perforation. Endoscopically, the mucosa appears inflamed, occasionally with ulcerations or plaques. The organism may be seen on histopathologic examination of Giemsa-stained biopsy material. In many patients, the diagnosis is not made until autopsy. Other fungi, such as *Candida albicans*, *Cryptococcus neoformans*, *Blastomyces dermatitidis* (the agent of North American blastomycosis), and *Coccidiomyces immitis*, have been reported to cause diarrhea in patients with AIDS, although the significance of these pathogens remains unclear.

PROTOZOANS

Cryptosporidium parvum is a coccidian protozoal parasite that may inhabit the microvillous border of intestinal epithelial cells. Transmission of this organism occurs by fecal–oral spread and by contaminated water. Infection occurs in as many as 20% of HIV-infected patients with diarrhea in the United States and in much higher percentages in developing countries. Although infection in immunocompetent hosts is self-limited, with a duration of about 2 weeks, in the immunosuppressed patient the organism may cause debilitating diarrhea. The diarrhea is nonbloody, can be voluminous, frequently occurs at night, and may be associated with nausea, vomiting, severe weight loss, and cramps. Fever is not a common accompaniment of cryptosporidial diarrhea. The infection may resolve spontaneously in patients with more than 180 CD4 cells/mm^3, but in patients with greater degrees of immunosuppression, it becomes a chronic illness with many exacerbations and remissions (76). Patients with fewer than 50 CD4 cells/mm^3 commonly experience fulminant disease, with passage of more than 2 L of stool daily, that is often refractory to therapy. The ileum and jejunum are the predominant sites of infection, but cryptosporidia have been found in the colon 25% of the time and occasionally in other areas of the gastrointestinal tract. The diagnosis is usually made on modified acid-fast stain or ELISA of stool. However, enteric or colonic biopsies may be necessary when results of stool studies are negative. Infection results in cell injury with partial villous atrophy and flattening and variable inflammation of the lamina propria.

Microsporidia are small, obligate spore-producing intracellular protozoa found widely in vertebrate and invertebrate hosts. They are considered a significant cause of chronic diarrhea, malabsorption, and wasting among HIV-infected patients, although one study found no difference in the frequency of microsporidia among HIV-infected patients with and without chronic diarrhea (77). Patients are usually severely immunodeficient, with CD4 cell counts lower than 100 cells/mm^3, and they present with nonbloody watery diarrhea, abdominal discomfort, and occasional nausea, but no fever. The incidence of this disease is still emerging, but it ranges from 15 to 30% of AIDS patients with chronic diarrhea (77, 78). Although several species of microsporidia are recognized, approximately 90% of human infections are due to *Enterocytozoon bieneusi*. A second microsporidian, *Encephalitozoon intestinalis*, is unique in its ability to infect lamina propria macrophages and to disseminate to distant sites (79). Speciation is possible with electron microscopy and PCR techniques. Given the organism's small size and inconsistent staining by hematoxylin and eosin, the best way to make the diagnosis in the past was by electron microscopy of small bowel biopsies. Improved staining methods including modified trichrome stain, fluorescent stains, and immunologic staining of biopsy and stool specimens, as well as PCR

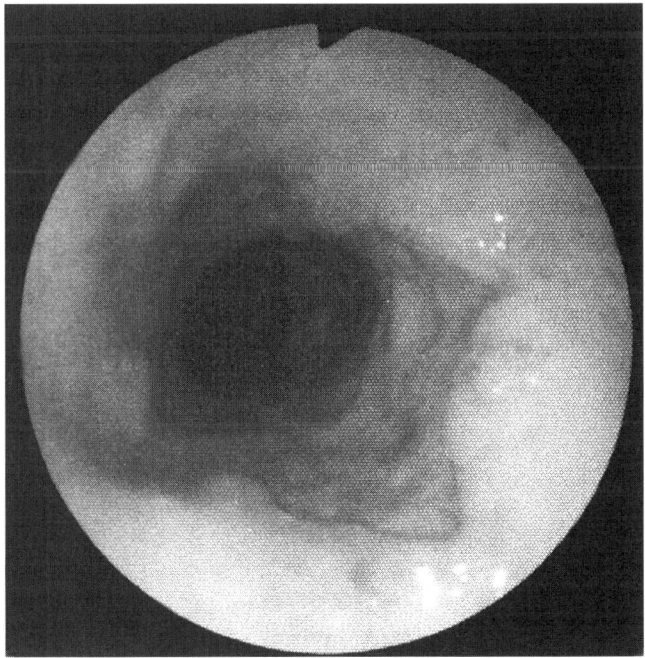

Figure 33.7. Cytomegalovirus ulcer in the ascending colon.

of stool specimens, have allowed for accurate diagnosis by light microscopy. Infection is greatest in the proximal jejunum, in which round to oval plasmodia, sporonts, and mature spores are seen in the supranuclear cytoplasm of infected cells.

Other presumed protozoal pathogens include *Entamoeba histolytica, Giardia lamblia, Isospora belli, Cyclospora cayetanensis,* and *Blastocystis hominis.* The latter is not considered a pathogen in immunocompetent hosts by most scientists; however, debate remains about its role in HIV-related diarrhea. *Entamoeba* is transmitted by fecal–oral spread. Trophozoites invade and ulcerate the colonic mucosa. In its most severe form, amebiasis may present as a fulminant colitis with bloody diarrhea and a high mortality. *Giardia* is transmitted by contaminated drinking water or through person-to-person contact. The organism is released from cysts in the upper small intestine, where it adheres to the brush border, resulting in disrupted crypt architecture. *Isospora* is a rare cause of diarrhea in North America, but it assumes far greater significance in developing countries, occurring in up to 20% of AIDS patients from Haiti or Africa (80). *Cyclospora,* previously described as a blue-green alga, is a coccidian organism that may infect the small bowel and cause watery chronic diarrhea in severely immunosuppressed AIDS patients (81). Like *Cryptosporidium,* it may be discovered on acid-fast staining of the stool, but it is larger. Other protozoal infections, such as *Pneumocystis carinii* (82), and *Toxoplasma gondii* (83), may infect the bowel and should be considered in the differential diagnosis.

BACTERIA

MAC is a ubiquitous organism in the environment, and it is the most common systemic bacterial infection in HIV-infected individuals, especially in patients with CD4 cell counts lower than 50 cells/mm^3. Studies suggest that approximately 10 to 24% of AIDS patients are infected with MAC, and most of these infections occur in the gastrointestinal tract (84, 85). The gastrointestinal tract probably serves as the portal of entry for these bacteria and the site from which dissemination occurs. The diarrheal disease caused by MAC is typically protracted and is associated with abdominal pain, fever, anemia, weight loss, and night sweats. Complications of gastrointestinal MAC infection include obstruction, fistula formation, bleeding, and perforation, occasionally exacerbated by the improved immune response associated with the use of protease inhibitors.

The diagnosis of disseminated MAC infection is readily made by culture of blood or bone marrow, but the diagnosis of gastrointestinal disease may require endoscopy. Endoscopically, MAC may appear as granular white nodules measuring 1 to 4 mm in diameter with a surrounding rim of erythema. The mucosa may appear erythematous, friable, and occasionally ulcerated. In many patients, the mucosa appears normal. Fresh stool samples may contain heavy bacterial loads. Although this finding suggests gastrointestinal infection, it may represent colonization, and the definitive diagnosis of MAC infection is usually made on biopsy of either the small bowel or the colon. The organism is found within foamy macrophages on Ziehl–Neelsen staining. Culture of biopsy samples increases the sensitivity of diagnosis. *Mycobacterium tuberculosis* is a rarer cause of diarrhea in AIDS, but it is clinically similar to MAC.

When a patient has fever, particularly when it is higher than 101°F, bacterial diarrhea is frequently the cause. *Salmonella* species, *Shigella flexneri,* and *Campylobacter jejuni* are the most likely pathogens. *Salmonella* and *Campylobacter* are associated with advanced immunosuppression, but *Shigella* is more commonly diagnosed in the early stages of HIV (86). The febrile diarrheal illness caused by these bacteria may include cramping, bloating, nausea, and possibly tenesmus. It may rarely be associated with toxic megacolon or pseudomembranous colitis. The absence of a normal humoral and cytotoxic immune response may be associated with failure to clear these organisms from the intestine and may lead to a long-term asymptomatic carrier state that often persists despite antibiotic therapy (87). The incidence of *Salmonella* bacteremia is lowered by the use of zidovudine or TMP–SMX prophylaxis (88). Clinicians have noted an increased incidence of enteroadherent *Escherichia coli* associated with diarrhea in AIDS. This organism is typically localized to the right colon (89, 90). Diagnosis is usually made by stool culture, but often only blood cultures are positive. Enteroadherent *E. coli* may be found by light microscopy, in clusters adherent to the small bowel or colonic mucosa brush border.

A frequently overlooked pathogen is *Clostridium difficile.* It is common in HIV-infected patients and may occur with or without the prior use of antibiotics. It typically results in bloody, mucoid diarrhea with abdominal pain and fever. One study reported that *C. difficile* is more virulent in HIV-positive patients (91), but other investigators have refuted this concept (92). The diagnosis and treatment of *C. difficile* enterocolitis are no different from that in immunocompetent patients (Fig. 33.8).

HIV ENTEROPATHY

The prevalence of small intestinal injury and D-xylose malabsorption in patients with HIV is high (93). Moreover, HIV itself can be isolated from enterocytes and colonic cells both in vitro and in vivo (94, 95). A controversial cause of diarrhea is HIV itself, the so-called "HIV or AIDS enteropathy." HIV has been identified in mononuclear cells of the bowel wall in 30 to 39% of patients with AIDS (96). HIV infection of mucosal cells is believed to result in altered enterocyte maturation and function. Kotler and associates showed that HIV p24 antigen expression in the colonic mucosa is associated with an inflammatory disease that appears to be unrelated to other pathogens (97). Therefore, invoking HIV as a cause of diarrhea is tempting when testing is unrevealing; however, it should be carefully considered. Other pathogens are likely to be found if the diagnostic search is repeated. It is much to the patient's advantage to be

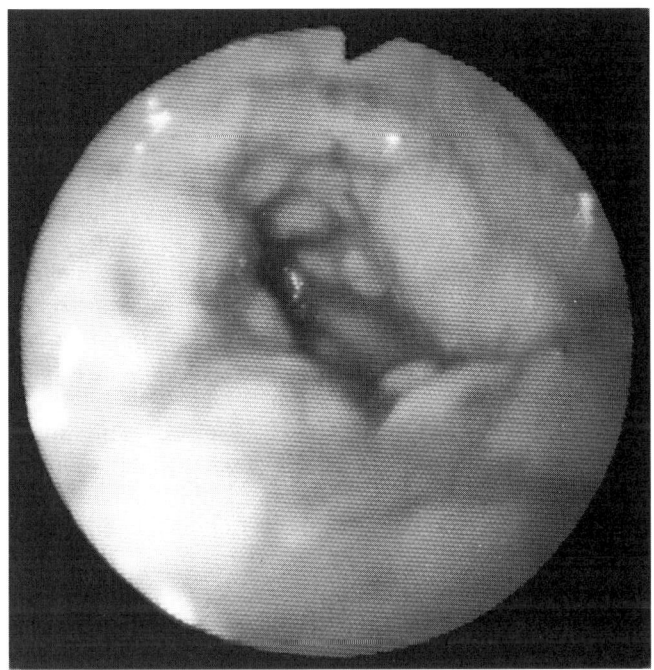

Figure 33.8. Pseudomembranous colitis caused by *Clostridium difficile*.

treated for a specific pathogen than to be treated nonspecifically for diarrhea. Other possible causes of pathogen-negative diarrhea in HIV-infected patients include bacterial overgrowth (98), decreased mucosal immune function (99), and altered enteric neural and endocrine function (100). Undoubtedly, HIV plays a role in the etiology of diarrhea, but more pathogens will probably appear as medical science advances. Currently, no criteria exist on which to base the diagnosis of HIV enteropathy.

The prognosis may actually be better for HIV-infected patients with pathogen-negative diarrhea after an extensive evaluation. In one prospective study, the median survival for patients with pathogen-negative diarrhea (48.7 months) was similar to that of control patients, and it was significantly longer than in those with an enteric pathogen (9.6 months) (65).

Treatment

Few general principles of treatment for diarrhea exist. Drug resistance develops rapidly, recurrences are the rule rather than the exception, more than one disease is common, and maintenance therapy may be required for life.

CYTOMEGALOVIRUS INFECTION

AIDS patients with CMV disease have poor long-term survival, but mortality may be improved with treatment. The usual treatment for CMV infection in the lower gastrointestinal tract is the same as treatment for esophageal disease. Both ganciclovir and foscarnet are beneficial, and a randomized open-label trial comparing them showed similar efficacy (101). More published data support the use of ganciclovir in the colon, so most patients receive it as induction therapy at a dose of 5 to 10 mg per kg twice daily (33–35, 102). Foscarnet, at a dose of 90 mg/kg thrice daily, can be used either as a first-line drug or when treatment with ganciclovir fails (39). Both drugs can also be used in combination after failure of one or both (42). Not enough information is available to support maintenance after induction therapy at this time. In past studies (33, 34), the time to relapse for CMV gastrointestinal disease was 9 weeks versus 3 weeks for CMV retinitis, but some patients had relapse-free intervals for as long as 1 year. The decision to place a patient on maintenance therapy after the initial presentation should be individualized, although it may prolong the duration of remission. However, after one relapse, maintenance therapy should probably be used in all patients. Quantitative PCR for CMV DNA at the end of induction therapy may be useful in monitoring the response to therapy and the risk of relapse (103). Surgical treatment of CMV-induced perforation and peritonitis is imperative. The segment of perforated bowel should be resected, and the proximal bowel should be exteriorized because of the high incidence of anastomotic breakdown if the bowel is reanastomosed. Despite surgical treatment, perforation caused by CMV is often a terminal event.

HERPES SIMPLEX VIRUS INFECTION

The treatment for HSV infection is acyclovir, either intravenously or orally. For these patients, oral therapy is usually effective, and maintenance therapy is appropriate.

CRYPTOSPORIDIOSIS

No completely effective therapy for *Cryptosporidium* infection exists at present, and supportive care and rehydration remain the main interventions. More than 100 drugs have been tried with limited success. Higher CD4 levels are the only obvious answer to the cryptosporidiosis question. Overall, the macrolides, which include azithromycin and clarithromycin, and the poorly absorbed antiamebic paromomycin have shown the most promise. Paramomycin, at high doses of 1500 to 3000 mg per day in divided doses, decreases stool frequency and oocyst shedding and improves intestinal function in patients with cryptosporidiosis, but it has not been uniformly effective (104). Azithromycin, also at high doses of 1500 to 2000 mg per day, may have promise. Antisecretory therapy and oral passive immunization with powdered bovine serum colostrum have been used with mixed success, but no large-scale studies have validated their usefulness. One study did show that use of this agent for cryptosporidial diarrhea is associated with a significant decrease in stool weight, a nonsignificant weight gain, and decreased oocyst shedding (105). No consensus exists regarding the length of therapy necessary, but maintenance therapy is probably necessary in all responders.

MICROSPORIDIOSIS

The therapy for microsporidiosis is not proved. Several medications have been tried, but no randomized placebo-controlled trials have been published to date. The most promising agent is albendazole, which has broad-spectrum anthelmintic activity. In uncontrolled studies (106), albendazole, at a dose of 400 mg twice daily for 28 days, significantly reduced diarrhea and produced weight gain in patients with *Enterocytozoon bieneusi*, although the parasite was not eradicated from repeated small bowel biopsies. Although no known therapy is uniformly effective in the treatment of *E. bieneusi*, investigators have noted marked clinical and parasitologic responses of *Encephalitozoon intestinalis* to albendazole. The parasite disappears from follow-up small bowel biopsies and disseminated sites (107). Placebo-controlled studies are ongoing to confirm the activity of albendazole and other benzimidazole agents. Other agents suggested to provide a benefit against microsporidia species include nitaroxid, furazolidone, and nonspecific agents including thalidomide (108, 109).

Bacterial Infections

The treatment of bacterial enteropathogens in patients with AIDS is similar to that in the immunocompetent patient, and if possible, it should be guided by the sensitivity of the organism to in vitro testing. Maintenance therapy may be required because of the propensity for recurrent infection. When stool workup reveals Gram-negative bacteria, but speciation is not possible, empiric therapy with ciprofloxacin is probably warranted, as a result of the effectiveness of this drug against most common pathogens. *Clostridium difficile* infection should be treated with oral metronidazole (250 mg four times daily) or oral vancomycin (125 to 500 mg four times daily). Cholestyramine may also be used to bind toxin and to help alleviate symptoms.

The incidence of MAC gastrointestinal disease may be reduced by the use of prophylactic rifabutin (300 mg orally once daily) in patients with CD4 cell counts lower than 100 cells/mm^3 (110). Encounters with MAC infection should not evoke therapeutic nihilism because many drugs are effective against it, particularly in combination. The United States Public Health Service Task Force recommends treatment with at least two agents including azithromycin or clarithromycin to which may be added ethambutol (15 mg/kg per day), ciprofloxacin (1500 mg/day), rifabutin (300 mg per day), rifampin (600 mg per day), and amikacin (500 mg intravenously for 6 weeks) (110). Treatment of these patients may result in symptomatic improvement, but sustained clinical response has not been proved.

HIV-RELATED DIARRHEA

Whether or not a cause of diarrhea is established, symptomatic treatment is necessary for the patient's quality of life. Three categories of antidiarrheal agents exist: luminal agents, antimotility agents, and hormones. Luminal agents may be considered, but they are seldom effective enough to be used alone. Fiber, one such agent, seemingly paradoxically, takes up water and builds bulk in the stool when a patient has diarrhea. Another luminal agent, cholestyramine, binds bile acids that can stimulate fluid secretion. Most antimotility agents reduce diarrhea by increasing transit time, thus prolonging contact with the absorptive surface. Loperamide is an over-the-counter drug that is useful as a first-line agent. Lomotil, a combination of diphenoxylate and atropine, can also be helpful. If stronger remedies are required, opiates can be used. Codeine, morphine, methadone, paregoric, and deodorized tincture of opium are all appropriate. Higher doses than are recommended in the package insert may be necessary to control devastating HIV-related diarrhea. If these drugs do not provide adequate relief, then hormonal therapy can be attempted.

Octreotide is the synthetic version of the natural somatostatin. It slows transit time, decreases active secretion, and inhibits all gastrointestinal hormones. In one study (111), it decreased stool frequency and volume significantly compared with placebo. More recent studies have shown this agent to be no more effective than placebo (112). It must be administered subcutaneously and can be associated with certain side effects, but in some patients it appears useful. Finally, patients with diarrhea associated with idiopathic colonic inflammation may respond to prednisone (113).

Equally important is ensuring adequate nutritional status. If only colonic disease is present and diarrhea is manageable, oral supplementation is both possible and effective. Generally speaking, if the patient has an abnormal D-xylose test, enteral nutrition will be less effective and parenteral nutrition should be considered. Dietary counseling is mandatory, however, at any level of disease. Lactose intolerance must be assumed, and a low-fat, low-fiber diet may help improve symptoms. The recent discovery of a high incidence of male hypogonadism has led to the use of testosterone and anabolic steroidal agents in the treatment of HIV wasting (114).

HEPATOBILIARY DISEASE

In HIV, the hepatobiliary system plays a much different role than the rest of the gastrointestinal tract. This system is a reservoir of prior infection with hepatitis viruses, it is a place for primary opportunistic infections and possibly HIV itself, and finally it is a window for diagnosing systemic opportunistic infections. Therefore, we should consider hepatobiliary disease slightly differently. Nearly all HIV-infected patients have abnormal liver tests (aspartate transaminase, alanine transaminase, and alkaline phosphatase) at some point in their course, usually when CD4 counts are lower than 200 cells/mm^3. Mere biochemical abnormality is not sufficient to trigger a major clinical investigation, however, unless it is accompanied by symptoms of pain, fever, jaundice, or hepatic decompensation. When these symptoms do occur, aggressive diagnostic testing including liver biopsy should be carried out because a large proportion of hepatobiliary disease is potentially treatable, and treatment may improve the quality and

Table 33.4. Etiology of HIV-Associated Hepatic Disease

Hepatitis
   Hepatitis B, C, D
   Cytomegalovirus
   Epstein–Barr virus
   Herpes simplex virus
   Adenovirus
   Varicella-zoster virus
   HIV
   Hepatotoxic drugs
   Ethanol
Granulomatous inflammation
   Mycobacterial
      Mycobacterium avium complex
      Mycobacterium tuberculosis
      Other atypical mycobacteria
   Fungal
      Histoplasma capsulatum
      Cryptococcus neoformans
      Coccidioides immitis
      Candida albicans
   Protozoal
      Pneumocystis carinii
      Toxoplasma gondii
      Microsporidian species
      Schistosoma sp.
      Cryptosporidium parvum
Hepatotoxic drugs
Mass lesions
   Kaposi's sarcoma
   Non–Hodgkin's lymphoma
   Other neoplasms
Vascular lesions
   Peliosis hepatis
   Kaposi's sarcoma
Nonspecific findings

quantity of life. Every physician caring for patients with AIDS requires a systematic method of evaluating and treating patients with hepatobiliary disease, to ensure that morbidity, mortality, and medical costs are minimized and that patients' quality of life is optimal.

Etiology

The main causes of hepatic diseases (Table 33.4) are opportunistic infections, viral hepatitis, and neoplasia. Drug-induced and other nonspecific causes should also be considered.

OPPORTUNISTIC INFECTIONS

MAC is by far the most common infection found in the liver of HIV-infected patients, typically in patients with advanced disease. Liver disease is usually part of a disseminated infection. In autopsy studies, it was found in 20 to 50% of patients (115, 116), and it has been identified in 10 to 30% of antemortem liver biopsy samples in patients with AIDS (115, 117–119). Patients characteristically present with nausea, diarrhea, and abdominal pain, and on examination, they may have hepatomegaly or biliary obstruction resulting from enlarged nodes at the porta hepatis. MAC infection has been associated with disproportionally elevated alkaline phosphatase levels, but abnormal transaminases may be the sole liver-associated enzyme abnormality in this disease (120). Liver biopsy commonly reveals diffuse, poorly formed granulomas, composed primarily of foamy histiocytes, with a paucity of other cells and lack of caseation. Acid-fast bacilli are found within and surrounding the granulomas. In the face of severe immunosuppression, granulomas may be absent, and MAC may be isolated within Kupffer cells. Culture occasionally uncovers mycobacteria in the absence of acid-fast organisms on biopsy.

Mycobacterium tuberculosis is a less common cause of liver disease in patients infected with HIV. Extrapulmonary *Mycobacterium tuberculosis* infection is seen in 60% of AIDS patients with lung disease, and in one study, 7.5% of patients with extrapulmonary disease had hepatic infection (121). Patients typically present with fever, night sweats, weight loss, cough with sputum production, anorexia, lymphadenopathy, and hepatomegaly. Laboratory analysis typically reveals an elevated alkaline phosphatase, with mildly elevated bilirubin and aminotransferase levels. Hepatic abscesses resulting from *Mycobacterium tuberculosis* have also been described (122). Infection usually occurs with less immunosuppression than with MAC. Granulomas tend to be more fully formed, with less tissue load of acid-fast bacilli than with MAC. Unfortunately, mycobacterial culture is usually necessary to distinguish the species. Other mycobacteria implicated in hepatic disease include *Mycobacterium xenopi*, *M. genavense*, and *M. kansasii*.

Bacillary peliosis hepatis is caused by *Bartonella quintana* or *B. henselae* and is characterized by dilated vascular lakes in the hepatic parenchyma. Liver involvement is heralded by fever, weight loss, abdominal pain, and hepatosplenomegaly in patients who are generally severely immunosuppressed. These patients may or may not have cutaneous or bone lesions of bacillary angiomatosis. Laboratory analysis may reveal mild to moderate elevations of aminotransferase levels and a moderate to severe elevation of alkaline phosphatase. Abdominal computed tomographic (CT) examination displays multiple, small, low-attenuated lesions throughout the hepatic parenchyma (123). Peliosis hepatis is best diagnosed histologically. Biopsy reveals cystic blood-filled spaces within the liver that are a few millimeters in diameter (Fig. 33.9). These peliotic spaces are often associated with fibromyxoid stroma containing few inflammatory cells and clumps of bacilli (124). The Gram-negative organism can be detected by Warthin–Starry stain or by electron microscopy, both intracellularly in sinusoidal endothelial cells and extracellularly (125). Peliosis hepatis with blood sequestration has been reported to result in transfusion-unresponsive anemia, thrombocytopenia, and consumptive coagulopathy (126). Cultures are usually negative.

CMV is the most common viral opportunistic infection of the liver (115). It involves the liver as part of disseminated disease in patients with advanced immunosuppression. In a study by Bonacini (127), it comprised 14% of combined autopsy and biopsy results. However, in another large series of antemortem liver biopsies (120), it was found in only 1.6% of patients. CMV hepatitis is rarely symptomatic, but it may result in fever, malaise, hepatomegaly, and weight loss; it is much more likely to come to medical attention when affecting the biliary tree. CMV hepatitis is characterized by mild transaminitis and mild cholestasis. Liver biopsy reveals sparse hepatonecrosis with mild portal and periportal inflammation. Viral inclusions are seen in hepatocytes, Kupffer cells, bile duct epithelium, and endothelial cells.

Both herpesvirus and adenovirus have been reported to cause hepatitis in AIDS patients, and both may cause devastating illnesses (120). Other viral agents implicated in HIV-related hepatic disease include human herpesvirus type 6 (128), varicella-zoster virus (129), and Epstein–Barr virus. They all may cause hepatocellular necrosis, rarely leading to death.

Fungal liver disease occurs in patients with advanced immunosuppression and commonly causes a granulomatous response. These granulomas are usually poorly formed and are associated with minimal inflammatory response. Fungal hepatitis is often asymptomatic except for fever and right upper-quadrant pain. Laboratory analysis usually reveals a cholestatic picture and variably elevated bilirubin levels. Cryptococcal liver involvement is found in 19% of patients with extraneural disease (127). Occasionally, cryptococcal infection of the liver may result in abscess formation (Fig. 33.10). *Histoplasma capsulatum* disseminates to the liver in 16% of infected patients (127). Fulminant disease presenting with shock, multisystem organ failure, and disseminated intravascular coagulation has been described (130). Demonstration of characteristic yeast forms or pseudohyphae on Gomori's methamine silver stain of biopsy samples is diagnostic for candidal hepatic infection. Hepatic infection with *Coccidioides immitis*, *Aspergillus* sp., and *Sporothrix schenckii* has also been described in the literature (131).

Pneumocystis carinii is a common infectious organism in HIV-infected patients. One autopsy study reported finding hepatic *Pneumocystis* in 39% of patients receiving aerosolized

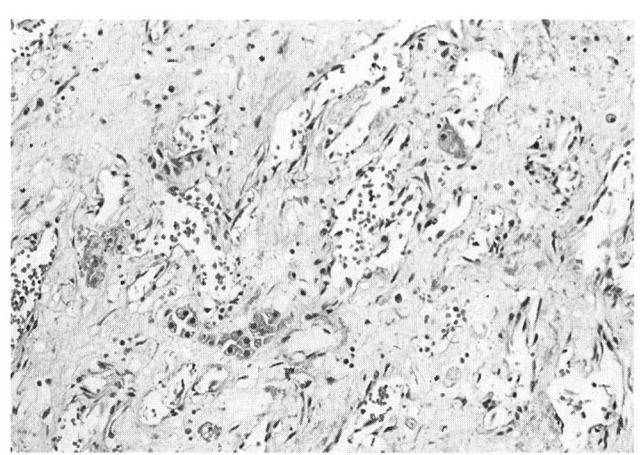

Figure 33.9. Peliosis hepatis.

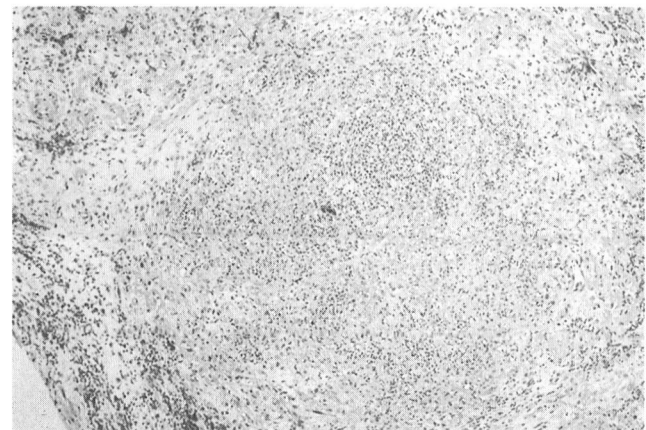

Figure 33.10. Cryptococcal liver abscess.

pentamidine (127). Patients may present with mild abdominal pain associated with variable elevations of transaminases and alkaline phosphatase. Abdominal CT scans, and rarely, plain radiographs, may exhibit diffuse punctate calcifications of the liver (132). Liver biopsy reveals foamy nodules that contain numerous *Pneumocystis* cysts that stain with methenamine silver and are associated with minimal inflammation. *Toxoplasma gondii* may also be hematogeneously disseminated to the liver (133). Although the organism can be seen histologically, PCR analysis of liver biopsy samples has also been used (134). Microsporidial infection of the liver is a rarity, but it has been associated with elevated bilirubin, transaminases, and especially alkaline phosphatase (135). Light microscopy reveals focal granulomatous and suppurative necrosis, mainly in the portal area, accompanied by characteristic spores, sporoblasts, and sporonts. *Entamoeba histolytica* may invade the bowel wall and may spread to the liver and form an abscess. Other rare hepatic protozoal pathogens include *Schistosoma* sp. and *Leishmania donovani* (136).

HEPATITIS VIRUSES

Given the shared epidemiologic risks of sexual contact, intravenous drug use, and, in the past, use of blood products, it is not surprising that up to 95% of patients with AIDS have serologic markers of past hepatitis B virus (HBV) infection (anti-HBs or anti-HBc positive), and 10 to 15% are chronic carriers (HBsAg positive) (116, 119, 137). Immunologic dysfunction induced by HIV may modify the course of HBV infection. HIV seropositivity appears to increase the risk of becoming a chronic HBV carrier (138), and HBV clearance appears to be inversely associated with the degree of immunosuppression. HIV-infected patients who do clear the infection may suffer reactivation of quiescent HBV, a rare occurrence in the immunocompetent patient. Reactivation is believed to be due to the progressive decline in humoral and cellular immunity (139), and it can be fulminant, resulting in death (140). Data also suggest that the natural history of acute hepatitis B infection is influenced by HIV coinfection. In these patients, HBV replicates with greater frequency, as evidenced by higher levels of DNA polymerase levels and increased core and HBeAg titers (138, 141). Although these characteristics predict poor survival in immunocompetent patients, in coinfected patients, liver disease does not appear to histologically worsen, and survival does not appear to be affected (142). The presumed pathogenesis of HBV offers us an explanation of this phenomenon. CD4 lymphocytes play an essential role in the host's immune response to hepatocytes infected with HBV; increased proportions of these cells infiltrate the liver and trigger cytotoxic CD8 cell activity, resulting in hepatocellular necrosis (143). Thus, as cell-mediated immunity wanes with HIV, less immunologic damage to infected hepatocytes may occur, and HBV replication may proceed unopposed. Because hepatic inflammation is minimized, progression to cirrhosis is unusual.

Patients with HIV frequently cannot be vaccinated successfully against HBV (144), but every attempt should be made to vaccinate patients at risk. Although HBV appears capable of increasing the replication of HIV in vitro and in vivo (145), large epidemiologic studies do not suggest that this characteristic affects progression to AIDS, CD4 cells titers, or survival (146, 147).

Hepatitis C virus (HCV) is most commonly transmitted parenterally, either through blood transfusions or by intravenous drug use. Sexual transmission, through both heterosexual and homosexual contact, and transplacental transmission of HCV appear to occur, but less efficiently than through the parenteral route. The incidence of HCV infection is increased in patients with HIV disease, reflecting shared epidemiologic risks. Investigators estimate that 50 to 90% of HIV-seropositive patients who acquired the disease though intravenous drug use or hemophilia are coinfected with HCV (148). The incidence of coinfection is much lower among gay men, approximately the same as in HIV-seronegative homosexuals, a finding supporting exposure to infected blood products as the primary means of transmission (149). Overall, approximately 14% of HIV-seropositive patients are coinfected with HCV, although this number may be an underestimation resulting from the unreliability of our diagnostic abilities (150).

HCV, in contrast to HBV, is believed to be a cytopathic virus, and coinfection with HIV appears to have adverse effects on liver disease caused by HCV. In the setting of HIV-induced immunosuppression, HCV may exhibit uncontrolled replication (151, 152). The HCV viral load measured by RNA PCR appears to increase soon after HIV infection and remains higher than seen in patients without immunodeficiency. Eyster and associates showed a 58-fold increase in HCV RNA levels several years after HIV seroconversion compared with a 3-fold increase in HIV-negative patients with HCV (153). In some studies, the HCV RNA levels appeared to correlated inversely with the decline of CD4 cell counts (153, 154), although other studies noted no such correlation (155). Liver failure in these patients may also be associated with CD4 cell counts lower than 100 cells/µL (156). Increased viral replication and increased viral load probably heightens the virulence of HCV and accelerates the progression to cirrhosis. In a study of 223 patients with hemophilia and HCV, 9% of the HIV-coinfected patients developed liver failure, whereas none of the HIV-seronegative patients developed liver failure (156). In yet another study of 225 hemophiliac patients with HCV, the patients coinfected with HIV had a 21-fold higher risk of hepatic decompensation (157). Still, coinfection with HIV does not appear to increase the risk of chronic HCV infection, and HCV infection is not an independent determinant of mortality in nonhemophiliacs with AIDS (158). Most studies have concluded that HCV infection does not accelerate the progression of HIV as judged by measurement of surrogate markers including CD4 cell counts, p24 antigenemia, or serum β_2-microglobulin (159). Increased replication of HCV under the influence of HIV-induced immunosuppression does appear to increase the risk of sexual and vertical transmission of HCV.

Many diagnostic techniques now exist for the detection of HCV. Screening tests are immunologically based. Present HCV screening usually entails testing with the second-generation ELISA assay and confirmation with a recombinant immunoblot (RIBA) assay to improve specificity. Immunosuppressed patients may have diminished reactivity to HCV antigens, leading to indeterminate RIBA and ELISA results; a single negative assay for antibodies to HCV cannot exclude active infection in HIV-seropositive patients (160). Indeed, PCR may be necessary. Immunologic assays do not allow quantification of the viral load; they only reflect the immune response and cannot determine whether the patient has active viremia. Thus, they are of little value in monitoring the effects of treatment. This problem may be circumvented by using PCR or branched-chain DNA assays to measure or quantify HCV RNA.

Little is known about the direct relationship between HIV and the liver. The liver contains the body's largest population of tissue macrophages, Kupffer cells, whose position within the sinusoids allows for interaction with blood-borne viruses and infected blood cells (161). Kupffer cells may represent a reservoir for HIV during early and latent HIV disease, allowing viral persistence and later dissemination. Immunoreactivity for HIV-1 antigens can be shown in 80% of liver biopsies of patients with AIDS (162). Despite a lack of CD4 receptors on hepatocytes, hepatoma cells lines can be productively infected by HIV-1 in vitro (163), and in vivo testing has revealed HIV-1 RNA in the hepatocytes of patients with AIDS (164). What effect these changes have on liver function, morbidity, or mortality is not clear, but a correlation does not appear to exist between HIV-1 RNA and histologic liver injury (165).

NEOPLASIA

Both Hodgkin's and non–Hodgkin's lymphomas (NHL) may affect the liver of patients with HIV. In patients with AIDS, NHL is associated with a high incidence of extranodal disease, and the liver is the most commonly affected solid organ (Fig. 33.11). The tumor is typically a high-grade

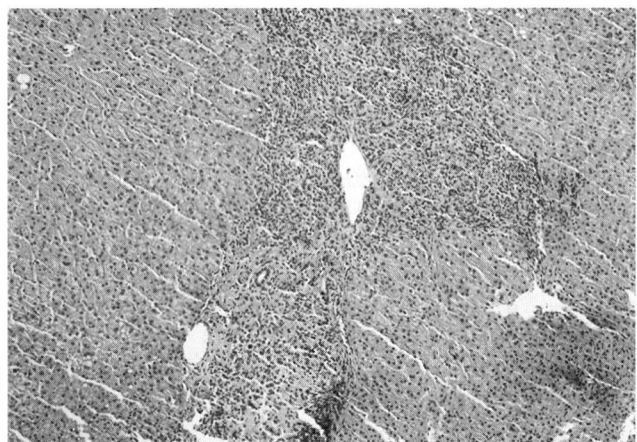

Figure 33.11. Diffuse large cell non–Hodgkin's disease of the liver.

malignancy of the B-cell type. Liver involvement has been reported in 14% of patients with lymphoma elsewhere and 29% of all patients with intra-abdominal involvement (166). Fifteen reports of primary hepatic lymphomas occurring in patients with AIDS have been published (167). Hepatic NHL may remain asymptomatic, but it commonly presents with weight loss, fever, and night sweats, similar to the symptoms of many opportunistic infections. When bulky, lymphoma may cause dull right upper-quadrant pain or hepatomegaly. NHL may be associated with elevated liver associated enzymes, especially alkaline phosphatase. Ultrasound examination may show various-sized solitary or multiple mass lesions larger than those seen in opportunistic infection or KS. They may be low-attenuated and hypoechoic lesions throughout, but occasionally they are cystic with septations or targetoid (168). On CT, masses are usually less dense than the surrounding hepatic parenchyma, and they may be surrounded by a thin, enhancing rim (166). Radiographic examination may yield false-negative results, with subsequent diagnosis made by random liver biopsy or at autopsy. Compression of the extrahepatic bile duct by portal or peripancreatic lymphadenopathy may cause intrahepatic biliary dilatation, and patients may present with painless jaundice. Hodgkin's lymphoma is less common, but it may also involve the liver at an advanced stage.

Despite the presence of hepatic KS in approximately one-third of all patients with cutaneous involvement, this lesion is seldom found on antemortem liver biopsy. This situation is presumed to be the result of sampling error. Hepatic KS is rarely symptomatic and does not appear to shorten life expectancy. Patients occasionally present with abdominal pain and hepatosplenomegaly with an elevated alkaline phosphatase. Ultrasound examination typically reveals only hepatomegaly because the lesions are too small to delineate sonographically. When seen, tumors are represented by multiple, small, hyperechoic nodules. On a noncontrast CT scan, KS lesions are hypoattenuated, but they enhance after a bolus of contrast (169). Liver biopsy is the best tool to diagnose hepatic KS, but given the vascular nature, the safety of liver biopsy has been questioned (170). This worry appears to be unfounded. On macroscopic examination, KS appears as irregular, purple-brown, soft nodules deep to the capsule or in the hilar region. Microscopically, KS appears as areas of vascular endothelial cell proliferation with associated spindle-shaped cells, extravasated erythrocytes, and vascular lakes.

Other neoplastic mass lesions that have been discovered in the livers of AIDS patients include malignant fibrosarcoma (171), chronic lymphocytic leukemia, leiomyoma (172), hepatoma, cholangiocarcinoma, and metastatic disease.

DRUG-INDUCED LIVER DISEASE

The treatment of HIV requires the use of many drugs. Many of these are potentially hepatotoxic and necessitate constant attention to detail. In fact, up to 90% of AIDS patients are treated with at least one drug associated with hepatotoxicity, often necessitating dose reduction or discontinuation (Table 33.5) (173). Medications are the most common cause of jaundice in AIDS patients (174). A hepatocellular pattern of liver-associated enzyme abnormalities is related to the use of amphotericin B (Fungizone), isoniazid (Nydrazid), rifampin (Rifadin; Rimactane), ethionamide (Trecator), pyrazinamide, metronidazole (Flagyl), tetracycline (Achromycin-V), penicillins, ganciclovir (Cytovene), azole antifungals, pentamidine (Pentam 300), phenytoin (Dilantin), sulfa-containing drugs, including TMP–SMX (Bactrim; Septra), and nucleoside analogs, such as zidovudine (Retrovir) and ddI (Videx) and protease inhibitors such as ritonavir (Norvir) and nelfinavir (Viracept). Indinavir (Crixivan) may be associated with a Gilbert-like syndrome that is worse in patients coinfected with viral hepatitis or with other coexistent liver disease (175). Hepatotoxic drugs associated with cholestatic liver-associated enzymes include albendazole, azithromycin (Zithromax), erythromycin (E-mycin; Ery-

Table 33.5. Potentially Hepatotoxic Drugs Used in Patients with AIDS

Hepatocellular	Cholestatic	Mixed
Zidovudine (AZT)	Albendazole	Trimethoprim–sulfamethoxazole
Dideoxyinisine (ddI)	Azithromycin	
Ketoconazole	Erythromycin	Carbamazepine
Isoniazid	Prochlorperazine	Indinavir
Rifampin	Indinavir	
Phenytoin		
Valproic acid		
Pentamidine		
Penicillins		
Amphotericin B		
Ethionamide		
Pyrazinamide		
Metronidazole		
Tetracyclines		
Ganciclovir		
Ritonavir		
Saquinavir		
Nelfinavir		

Tab; Ilosone), TMP–SMX, and prochlorperazine (Compazine). A mixed hepatocellular and cholestatic pattern is often seen, especially with TMP–SMX and carbamazepine (Tegretol). The danger of nucleoside analog therapy is highlighted by the occurrence of severe hepatotoxicity and mortality from fialuridine (FIAU) used to treat HBV (176). All nucleoside analogs, like this one, may be incorporated into mitochondrial DNA, resulting in disturbed protein synthesis and oxidative phosphorylation and a fatal syndrome of lactic acidosis and fulminant or subfulminant liver failure. Although this syndrome is believed to be rare, physicians are advised to monitor carefully patients receiving nucleoside analog therapy who have elevated liver-associated enzymes or hepatomegaly. The widespread use of TMP–SMX as *Pneumocystis carinii* pneumonia prophylaxis makes this the most common cause of drug-related hepatotoxicity in patients with AIDS; its use is associated with abnormalities in liver function serologic studies in half the patients who are treated (164). A large problem is mycobacterial therapy. Nearly all the drugs used have potential hepatotoxicity, but therapeutic changes have to be made in only 5% of patients. The presence of eosinophils on liver biopsy and the absence of organisms on special stains suggest drug-induced liver disease in patients with a compatible history. Clearly, withdrawal of potentially hepatotoxic medication is the first step in the diagnostic workup of any HIV-infected patient with elevated liver enzymes.

BILIARY TRACT DISEASE

The biliary tree, including the gallbladder, is a common site of infection in HIV-infected patients with low CD4 counts. It may be involved in the form of acalculous cholecystitis and AIDS cholangiopathy. The major pathogens responsible, *Cryptosporidium*, microsporidia (177), MAC, and CMV, are most commonly found at CD4 counts lower than 50 cells/mm^3, although in half the patients no organism is found (178). Acalculous cholecystitis, a recognized manifestation of AIDS, most commonly presents with right upper-quadrant or epigastric pain, fever, nausea, vomiting, and commonly diarrhea and weight loss. Jaundice is a rare symptom, but alkaline phosphatase is markedly elevated most of the time. One may see mild elevations of transaminases. Ultrasound may show a thickened, dilated gallbladder, or it may be normal. Gallbladder sludge is often seen. Cholangitis is a common accompaniment; involvement of the biliary tree occurs in more than 50% of cases with acalculous cholecystitis (179).

AIDS cholangiopathy was first described in three patients complaining of right upper-quadrant pain and fever (178). Pathologically, such patients experience periductal inflammation affecting the extrahepatic, and often the intrahepatic, bile ducts with mural thickening, beading, and nodularity. This change results in irregular narrowing along the length of the involved bile duct segment. When the papilla of Vater is involved, common bile duct, and occasionally pancreatic duct, dilatation may result. The presentation of cholangiopathy is essentially the same as that of acalculous cholecystitis: pain and fever, nausea, and vomiting, with an elevated alkaline phosphatase and usually normal bilirubin levels. The most commonly used classification of the endoscopic retrograde cholangiopancreatography (ERCP) changes of AIDS cholangiopathy was proposed by Cello (180). He described four different patterns of disease: type I, combined sclerosing cholangitis and papillary stenosis; type II, papillary stenosis alone; type III, sclerosing cholangitis alone; and type IV, long extrahepatic bile duct strictures. If ERCP is performed, abnormalities are found in 77% (180). Ultrasonography and CT are not as sensitive (75 to 87%) as ERCP (180, 181). Biliary obstruction, resulting from ductal compression by NHL or KS, occurs rarely. Immunosuppression predisposes to superimposed bacterial cholangitis. AIDS cholangiopathy does not appear to affect survival (182).

Diagnosis

When an HIV-positive patient presents with liver disease, a rational diagnostic approach can narrow the broad differential diagnosis, permitting more directed evaluation (Fig. 33.12). Because opportunistic diseases cause liver disease through blood-borne or lymphatic dissemination, thorough history and physical examination as the starting points may reveal extrahepatic clues to the diagnosis. The clinician should pay particular attention to prior opportunistic infections that may have disseminated to the liver, use of potentially hepatotoxic medications or alcohol, recent travel, a history of viral hepatitis, and the patient's risk factors for HIV disease. The absolute CD4 cell count is equally important in the determination of a differential diagnosis. For example, an HIV-infected patient with a normal CD4 cell count is unlikely to have an opportunistic infection of the liver but may have tuberculosis or KS, whereas patients with CD4 cell counts lower than 100 cells/mm^3 become susceptible to MAC or CMV infection. The combination of abnormal liver enzyme tests and fever is common. Hepatomegaly, right upper-quadrant pain, and jaundice are less common. The clinician must bear in mind that when CD4 counts are lower than 50 cells/mm^3, almost all HIV-infected patients have some abnormality of liver enzymes. Many have nonspecific abnormalities on liver biopsy, such as steatosis, which may be caused by malnutrition, total parenteral nutrition, tumor necrosis factor and other cytokines, and possibly alcohol. Biopsy for every patient with abnormal liver enzymes is not practical or rewarding; in fact, it may even be dangerous.

Abnormalities in liver tests can be separated into cholestatic (predominance of alkaline phosphatase) and hepatocellular (predominance of transaminases) abnormalities, but this distinction does not yield specific diagnoses. Patients with elevated alkaline phosphatase levels commonly have granulomatous liver disease. The sensitivity and specificity of a serum alkaline phosphatase level higher than 220 IU/L for granulomas were 81 and 34%, respectively, whereas a level above 300 IU/L has a sensitivity and specificity of 75% for any diagnosis (183). The positive predictive value of an alkaline phosphatase level higher than 200 IU/L for a specific diagnosis was 58 to 74% (120, 184).

Liver biopsy is a controversial element in the evaluation of liver disease in patients with AIDS. Because the liver is commonly involved in systemic disease that has disseminated lymphohematogenously, a diagnosis may often be established through less invasive procedures that produce less morbidity. These procedures involve biopsy and culture of peripheral sites such as the blood, skin, gastrointestinal mucosa, lymph nodes, and bone marrow. Liver biopsy should be reserved for workup when these less invasive procedures and a trial of hepatotoxic medication withdrawal have failed to yield a diagnosis. Studies in immunocompetent patients have shown liver biopsy to be a safe procedure, with a morbidity of 0.1 to 0.6% and a mortality of 0 to 0.12% (185). However, patients with AIDS may have a slightly higher risk of bleeding; in one study, the rate of major hemorrhage was 2% and mortality 1.6% (186, 187). We avoid biopsy in patients with a prothrombin time longer than 3 seconds over control or a platelet count less than 50,000. If biopsy is an emergency in these patients, supplementation with fresh frozen plasma or platelets should be given.

Despite an increased risk associated with liver biopsy, it is the most specific diagnostic technique for parenchymal liver disease in patients seropositive for HIV. Opponents of liver biopsy cite studies that failed to find a correlation between indications for liver biopsy and histopathologic findings (137) and note liver biopsy rarely results in new AIDS-specific diagnoses or improved survival (188, 189). Proponents of liver biopsy highlight studies that revealed a specific diagnosis from biopsy in 30 to 80% of patients with AIDS and note that the finding of opportunistic infections or neoplasms

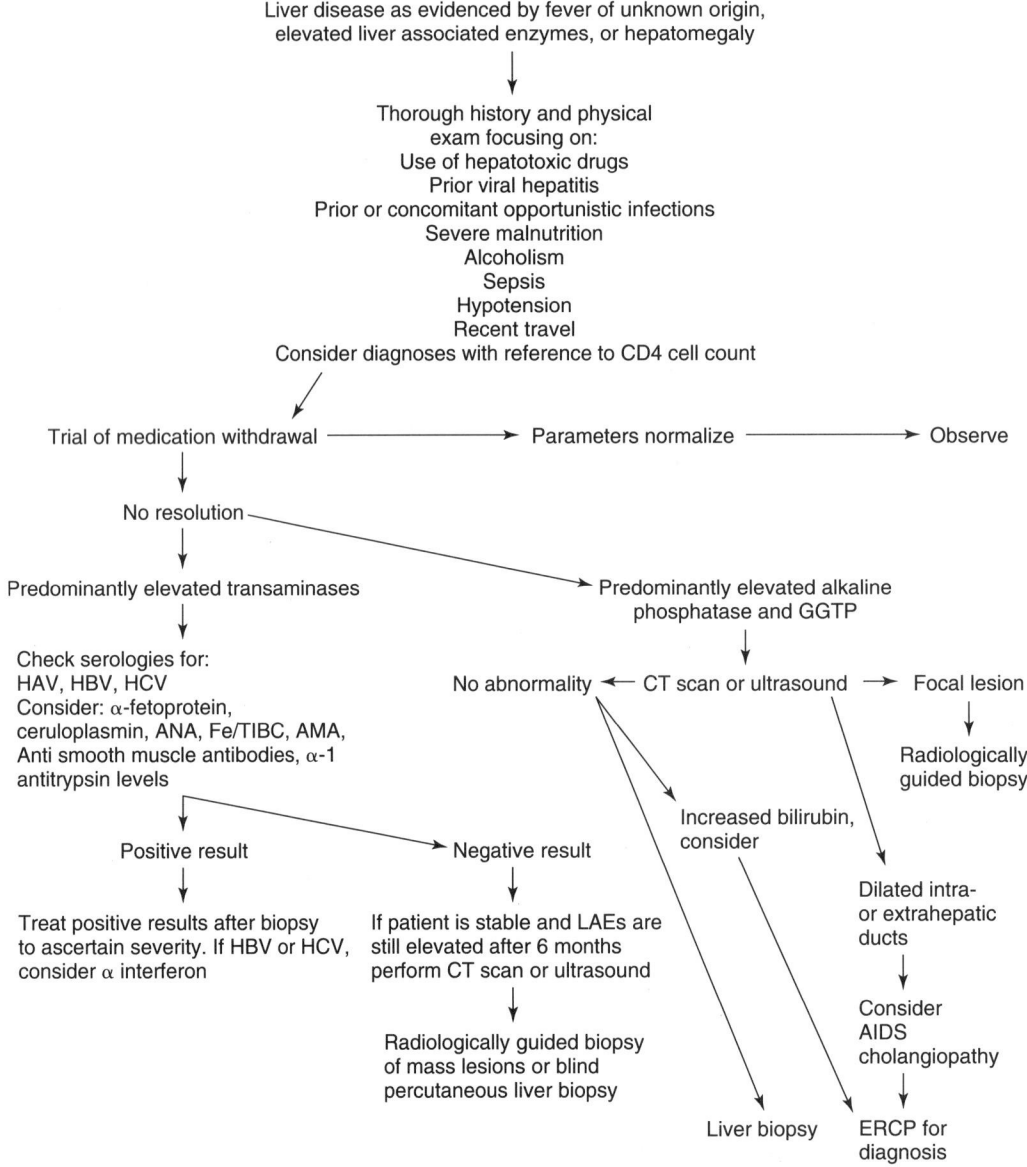

Figure 33.12. Algorithm for approach to the patient with HIV-related hepatic disease.

on liver biopsy may yield important prognostic information (116, 118, 120, 137, 162, 183, 184, 188, 190, 191). A review that compiled autopsy and liver biopsy data from 22 previous studies, composed of 635 patients infected with HIV (127), concluded that 34% of liver biopsies yielded important diagnostic information. In a recent retrospective analysis of 501 liver biopsies performed on AIDS patients with abnormalities of liver chemistry studies, fever, hepatomegaly, or right upper-quadrant pain, we found that 64.3% of liver biopsies yielded a histopathologic diagnosis, 45.7% of which represented potentially treatable disease (120). Further, 58.2% of patients with fever who had already undergone nondiagnostic workup including bone marrow biopsy had a diagnosis diagnosed based on liver biopsy. The yield of liver biopsy may be enhanced when the procedure performed on patients with a longer history of HIV infection, with a history of multiple opportunistic infections before biopsy, or with fever and an alkaline phosphatase or γ-glutamyl transferase level more than 1.5 times the upper limit of normal (183, 192). Laparoscopic biopsy was evaluated in the diagnosis of 54 HIV-infected patients with elevated liver enzymes, hepatomegaly, ascites, fever of unknown origin, and right upper-quadrant pain (193). In 46%, abnormalities were directly visualized on examination, and the use of liver biopsy resulted in diagnoses in 70% of patients with AIDS and in 30% of HIV-seropositive patients without AIDS.

Noninvasive imaging with ultrasound or CT has an important role in the diagnosis of liver disease in HIV-infected patients. Imaging may reveal biliary or gallbladder abnormalities or mass lesions attributable to lymphoma, other neoplasms, infection, or even the peliotic spaces of peliosis hepatis. Unfortunately, the presence of multiple disorders and the high incidence of unsuspected disease on subsequent biopsy make these imaging techniques too nonspecific and insensitive to use alone (194). Patients with AIDS often have asymptomatic thickening of the gallbladder wall that does not require treatment. ERCP is more sensitive than radiologic imaging in the diagnosis of AIDS cholangiopathy, although radiology is usually used before ERCP. One study found that ultrasound was almost perfectly accurate in the prediction of normal or abnormal ERCP examination, with a sensitivity of 97% and a specificity of 100% (195). This finding suggests that ultrasound should be the initial screening procedure, with ERCP reserved for patients in whom abnormalities are discovered. ERCP is better at defining the shagginess and mucosal irregularity that characterizes this disease. ERCP may also be used for therapeutic intervention such as sphincterotomy or stent placement, as well as biopsy of the ampulla and distal common bile duct. Ampullary biopsy specimens should be obtained to examine for parasites, protozoa, fungi, and CMV. Hepatobiliary scintiscans may be useful for establishing the diagnosis of HIV-associated acalculous cholecystitis. These scans reveal delayed or nonvisualization of the gallbladder. Pathologic examination often reveals inflammation and edema of the gallbladder with mucosal ulceration (196).

Treatment

Few differences exist between treatment of hepatobiliary opportunistic infections and of other opportunistic infections. The same treatment is used for infections wherever they exist. The only therapy that is different is the treatment of chronic viral hepatitis B and C.

Treatment of both hepatitis B and C with interferon-α has been approved by the FDA and has a reasonable success rate in immunocompetent patients. The value in patients with HIV is debatable. The responsiveness of interferon in HIV-infected patients with chronic HBV appears to be lower than in immunocompetent patients. Wong and colleagues reported that a response, as defined as loss of HBeAg antigen and HBV DNA, was one-fifth as likely in HIV-infected patients (197). Few studies have evaluated the use of interferon in the treatment of HCV-infected patients who are also HIV infected. Most of these studies concluded that treatment of this population is as efficacious as in the HIV-seronegative population (198, 199). Unfortunately, none of the studies evaluated patient survival. Multiple variables probably play a role in modulating the efficacy of interferon in the coinfected population. A correlation appears to exist between the decline of CD4 cell counts and a lack of responsiveness of patients to interferon therapy. In a study by Soriano, multiple logistic regression analysis showed that a CD4 cell count higher than 500 cells/mm^3 was independently associated with a better response to interferon (199). The response to interferon therapy may also depend on the infecting strain of HCV. A full response to interferon is seen in fewer than 25% of patients who harbor HCV genotype 1b (200, 201). Patients who acquire HCV infection through parenteral drug use are more likely to be infected with multiple HCV strains; this also appears to decrease the likelihood of a positive response to therapy, as well as a greater likelihood of infection with genotype 1b. In addition, responsiveness to interferon may be decreased in patients with high serum viral titers, as is characteristic of HIV-seropositive patients (202). Despite these variables, most studies have shown that treatment with interferon of HIV-positive patients who have not yet progressed to AIDS is beneficial. Combination of interferon with a nucleoside analog ribavirin may well become standard therapy for patients with sustained HCV replication after the use of interferon alone, or as initial therapy in HCV-infected patients. This regimen improved biologic and virologic response rates compared with interferon alone (203).

Despite the high incidence of adverse effects associated with the use of interferon, the incidence of intolerance among the patients who are HIV infected does not seem to be increased. A few studies have noted that use of interferon is associated with a risk of a precipitous fall in the CD4 cell count of HIV-infected patients who are treated (199, 204). Despite this finding, no studies have shown that the incidence of opportunistic infections is increased by interferon. Lamivudine, a nucleoside analog, has activity against both HIV and HBV in coinfected patients and will likely become a key component in the treatment of these patients (205).

Treatment of HIV-related biliary disease is also similar to that for immunocompetent patients. Patients with cholecystitis should undergo cholecystectomy. This procedure alleviates symptoms, although it is unlikely to help patients with coexistent cholangitis. The operative findings are often less remarkable than anticipated from a patient's clinical picture (206). Most cases do reveal an edematous, inflamed, and ulcerated gallbladder mucosa, but no gangrene or necrosis. In one review, open cholecystectomy in 11 AIDS patients with CMV cholecystitis was associated with 9% morbidity, but no mortality (207). Other series have reported mortality as high as 33% (208). Laparoscopic cholecystectomy may lead to decreased morbidity and mortality in this population. After identification of the causative organism, directed antimicrobial therapy should be instituted.

Patients with AIDS cholangiopathy, especially papillary stenosis, may benefit from endoscopic sphincterotomy or stent insertion for focal biliary duct strictures. Sphincterotomy has been shown to reduce long-term pain scores significantly, but laboratory abnormalities commonly remain, perhaps because of progressive intrahepatic disease (209). Secondary bacterial infection of the abnormal biliary tree is a significant factor to be considered and should always be treated with antibiotics even when other pathogens are present. Ursodeoxycholic acid has also been used in the treatment of AIDS-related cholangiopathy (210).

PANCREATIC DISEASE

The pancreas is a frequent site of inflammatory disease in patients with HIV, far more frequent (4 to 22%) (211) than is generally realized; most AIDS-related pancreatic disease remains asymptomatic. Autopsy studies have revealed pancreatic lesions in 50 to 70% of patients with AIDS (212). Serum levels of trypsin and elastase I are elevated in the asymptomatic phase of disease, a finding suggesting that pancreatic damage is common throughout the course of HIV infection (213), although enzyme elevations are more common with increasing immunosuppression (214). Drugs, opportunistic infections, neoplasms, and perhaps HIV itself can involve the pancreas and even may lead to endocrine or exocrine failure (Table 33.6). In addition, patients with AIDS, especially intravenous drug users, have an increased incidence of alcoholism, and they are therefore at risk of acute or chronic alcoholic pancreatitis. Pancreatic disease is also common in patients with concomitant biliary disease (215). Pancreatic disease in patients with AIDS usually takes the form of pancreatitis or mass lesions, although overlap is extensive.

Pancreatic infection most commonly results in pancreatitis. Acute pancreatitis is characterized by abdominal pain, nausea, vomiting, and anorexia, and it is typically diagnosed by hyperamylasemia and hyperlipasemia. When these values are elevated, the patient should have an abdominal roentgenogram and CT scan. Radiology commonly reveals an

Table 33.6. Etiology of HIV-Related Elevations in Pancreatic Enzymes

Opportunistic infections
  Cytomegalovirus
  Toxoplasma gondii
  Candida albicans
  Cryptococcus neoformans
  Herpes simplex virus
  Cryptosporidium parvum
  Mycobacterium tuberculosis
  Mycobacterium avium complex
Neoplasms
  Non–Hodgkin's lymphoma
  Kaposi's sarcoma
Non-HIV causes
  Ethanol use
  Gallstone disease
  Hypercalcemia
  Hypertriglyceridemia
  Salivary gland disease
  Macroamylasemia
  Renal failure
Drug-related causes
  Pentamidine
  Dideoxyinosine
  Dideoxycytidine
  Trimethoprim–sulfamethoxazole
  Octreotide
  Paramomycin

enlarged and edematous pancreas with peripancreatic fluid. Many AIDS-related pancreatic disorders result in pancreatitis. One study reported hyperamylasemia in 46% of AIDS patients in an intensive care unit during their first week of hospitalization (216). Autopsies were performed on eight patients who died, and all had pancreatic disease. CMV was found in two, together with *Toxoplasma gondii* in one, *Candida* in one, and *Cryptococcus* in one. The other four patients had nonspecific steatonecrosis of the pancreas. These investigators concluded that most opportunistic infections involving the pancreas are rarely recognized before death. CMV is the most common infection (66%), followed by *Cryptococcus* (16%) and toxoplasmosis (10%). Other pancreatic diseases that may cause pancreatitis in these patients include HSV, *Cryptosporidium*, NHL, and KS. The infections and neoplasia are usually part of a disseminated process.

Drugs have long been known to cause pancreatitis in persons who are not infected with HIV, and the list of drugs used in HIV-related disease is rapidly expanding. Pentamidine, used for *Pneumocystis* infection, is a lipophilic drug that accumulates in the pancreas, and it may have a cytolytic effect on pancreatic β cells. This effect may manifest as pancreatitis days, weeks, or months after initiation of therapy. Histologically, the pancreas may show spotty acinar necrosis, steatonecrosis, focal hemorrhage, inflammation, and inspissated ductular secretions (217). Typically, it is not seen until the patient has received at least 1 g of pentamidine (218). The first effect is pancreatic injury leading to release of insulin and hypoglycemia. This effect is exacerbated in patients who have renal impairment caused by pentamidine. Later, hypoglycemia occurs in the presence of low serum C-peptide levels. This condition indicates a requirement for insulin and permanent islet cell injury (219). The second drug approved for use to treat HIV was ddI. Many anecdotal reports of pancreatitis are attributed to ddI, and two large studies (211, 220) address the issue. The first, involving 51 patients, reported clinical pancreatitis in 12 (23.5%) and asymptomatic hyperamylasemia in another 10 (20%). The other series reported on 44 patients, 7 of whom (16%) developed clinical pancreatitis. The cumulative dose of ddI appeared to correlate best with the development of pancreatitis, and in some patients rechallenge at a lower dose was tolerated. The onset of pancreatitis is typically between 6 and 24 weeks after initiating therapy (221). The agent ddC also may cause pancreatitis, but much less commonly. TMP–SMX has been reported to cause pancreatitis, presumably as a consequence of its sulfa component. Finally, octreotide, used in the treatment of AIDS-related diarrhea (222), and paromomycin, used for cryptosporidial infection (223), may also result in pancreatitis.

A diagnosis of hyperamylasemia does not equate with a diagnosis of pancreatitis. Another cause of hyperamylasemia is macroamylasemia. Circulating immune complexes that bind amylase may form macroamylase. The presence of macroamylase would obviate the need for diagnostic intervention. AIDS is associated with macroamylasemia, possibly because of circulating immune complexes produced by polyclonally activated B lymphocytes (224). The diagnosis can be ruled out by isoamylase studies or the amylase-to-creatinine ratio. Renal failure may be associated with mild increases in amylase and lipase. The incidence of salivary gland disease is also increased in AIDS patients and may be associated with an elevated amylase level in the face of a normal lipase level. Hypertriglyceridemia, a common problem in HIV-infected patients, has also been associated with pancreatitis in AIDS (225). One approach to the diagnosis of pancreatic disease is seen in Figure 33.13.

Mass lesions in and around the pancreas may be due to intrinsic lesions, peripancreatic lymph nodes, or surrounding organs. Neoplastic lesions in the pancreas commonly are solid on imaging, whereas infections and pseudocysts, associated with pancreatitis, are fluid-filled or are mixed solid and cystic. These processes may be difficult to distinguish, but infections more typically present with fever, night sweats, and other severe systemic complaints. Mass lesions may compress neighboring structures. Masses of the pancreatic head may obstruct the common bile duct and may even compress the duodenum. The most common infectious causes of pancreatic or peripancreatic abscess are *Mycobacteria tuberculosis* and MAC (226). Other infectious mass lesions include CMV, fungal abscesses, and toxoplasmosis. Pancreatic involvement is an uncommon accompaniment to disseminated AIDS-associated neoplasia such as KS and NHL, but when present, mass lesions are common. Evaluation of a pancreatic or peripancreatic mass, discovered on radiologic examination, requires a biopsy diagnosis. This procedure is typically accomplished under CT or ultrasound guidance, but if it is unsuccessful, laparotomy may be required. Endoscopic ultrasound allows for transvisceral biopsy from a few centimeters' distance, and it may become the optimal diagnostic technique for these patients (227). Samples should be sent

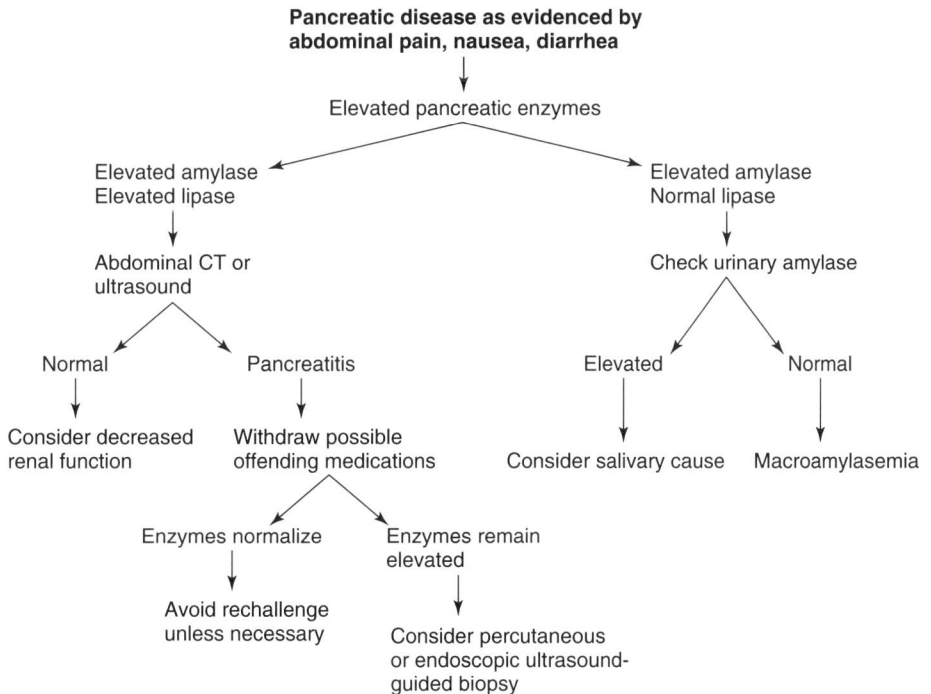

Figure 33.13. Algorithm for approach to the patient with HIV-related pancreatic disease.

Table 33.7. Etiology of HIV-Associated Peritoneal and Mesenteric Disease

Cause	Intrabdominal Process
Malignancy	
Lymphoma	Lymphadenopathy, perforation, bowel obstruction, masses, ascites
Kaposi's sarcoma	Lymphadenopathy, perforation, appendicitis, bowel obstruction, masses
Mycobacteria	
Mycobacterium tuberculosis	Lymphadenopathy, perforation, chronic peritonitis, bowel obstruction, abscess, ascites
Mycobacterium avium complex	Lymphadenopathy, chronic peritonitis, bowel obstruction, abscess, ascites
Atypical mycobacteria	Lymphadenopathy, abscess, ascites
Bacteria	
Nocardia brasiliensis	Lymphadenopathy, cholecystitis, abscess
Campylobacter fetus	Perforation
Fungi	
Coccidioides immitis	Lymphadenopathy, chronic peritonitis, abscess, ascites
Cryptococcus neoformans	Lymphadenopathy, perforation, chronic peritonitis, abscess, ascites
Histoplasma capsulatum	Lymphadenopathy, perforation, chronic peritonitis, abscess, ascites
Candida	Perforation, chronic peritonitis, cholecystitis, abscess, ascites
Aspergillus	Chronic peritonitis, abscess, ascites
Protozoa	
Pneumocystis carinii	Lymphadenopathy, chronic peritonitis, abscess, ascites
Toxoplasma gondii	Lymphadenopathy, chronic peritonitis, abscess, ascites
Microsporidia	Chronic peritonitis, cholecystitis, abscess, ascites
Cryptosporidium parvum	Cholecystitis
Strongyloides stercoralis	Bowel obstruction
Virus	
Cytomegalovirus	Lymphadenopathy, perforation, chronic peritonitis, appendicitis, cholecystitis, bowel obstruction, ascites
?HIV	Chronic peritonitis

for cytologic analysis, histologic examination, and culture for mycobacteria, fungi, and viruses.

The treatment of pancreatitis in the setting of HIV is exactly the same as in patients who are not infected with HIV. Endocrine and exocrine failure requires supplementation with insulin and pancreatic enzymes. Acute pancreatitis is treated with pain medication, fluids, and supportive therapy. Potentially offending drugs should be removed immediately if any elevation of amylase is noted. Rechallenge is usually not warranted, but it may be attempted if absolutely necessary.

PERITONEAL AND MESENTERIC DISEASE

Peritoneal disease in patients with AIDS is usually due to extension of gastrointestinal disease, and, like gastrointestinal disease, it usually involves opportunistic infections and atypical presentations of diseases unrelated to immunosuppression (Table 33.7).

Intraperitoneal Abscess or Masses

Clinical findings associated with intraperitoneal abscesses include fever, night sweats, abdominal pain, malaise, localized tenderness, a palpable mass, and leukocytosis. The diagnosis is usually made by abdominal ultrasound, CT, or, more recently, endoscopic ultrasound. AIDS-related pathogens implicated in intraperitoneal abscesses include *Mycobacterium tuberculosis* and MAC and, less commonly, *Histoplasma capsulatum*, *Aspergillus*, *Candida* (216), microsporidia (228), and *Nocardia*. Biopsy is required for diagnosis, and specimens may be obtained using percutaneous aspiration under roentgenographic guidance, through the use of endoscopic ultrasound, or at laparotomy.

Other abdominal masses include organomegaly, lymphadenopathy, tumor, or pancreatic pseudocyst. Again, radiologic methods often delineate the nature and the origin of the mass. Whenever masses or abscesses undergo biopsy for diagnosis, the samples should be evaluated histologically and should be cultured for bacterial, mycobacterial, fungal, and even viral causes of disease. Given the association between gastrointestinal and intraperitoneal disease, in these patients, stool analysis and endoscopic biopsies may also yield important information.

Ascites

AIDS-related causes of ascites include opportunistic infections, neoplasia, liver disease, renal disease such as HIV-associated or heroin-induced nephropathy, and hypoalbuminemia from malnutrition. Some opportunistic organisms described as causes of ascites include *Mycobacterium tuberculosis*, MAC, peliosis-causing *Bartonella*, fungi such as *Aspergillus*, *Candida*, *Coccidioides immitis*, *Cryptococcus neoformans*, and *Histoplasma capsulatum*, protozoa such as microsporidia, *Pneumocystis carinii*, and *Toxoplasma gondii*, and CMV. Many AIDS patients with NHL and intraabdominal KS present with cytology-positive ascites (229, 230). The workup of ascites should be the same as for the nonimmunocompromised population. Paracentesis is a safe and effective clinical diagnostic tool in the evaluation of these patients, and it may permit diagnosis of AIDS-defining diagnoses in up to 25% of patients (231). Tests that should be routinely performed include cytologic analysis, albumin level, total protein level, cell count, and culture for bacterial, mycobacterial, and fungal organisms inoculated in culture bottles at the bedside.

The diagnosis of tuberculous ascites often requires more than 1 L of fluid for analysis. The fluid is typically turbid with a high lymphocyte count. Histologic stains for acid-fast bacilli and mycobacterial cultures are positive in only half the patients. The ascites caused by *Pneumocystis carinii*, on the other hand, usually contains few leukocytes (232). Cytologic examination may reveal reactive mesothelial cells and foamy eosinophilic material, with cyst forms stained by Gomori's methenamine silver stain. *Toxoplasma gondii* infection of the peritoneum results in a neutrophilic ascites, and diagnosis may be made by culture or staining with Wright–Giemsa stain.

Peritonitis: Acute and Chronic

Symptoms and signs of peritonitis include abdominal pain, fever, tachypnea, hypotension, involuntary abdominal guarding, direct and rebound abdominal tenderness, and abdominal distension. AIDS patients may have delayed, attenuated, or atypical inflammatory responses to peritoneal inflammation that may equate with a decrease in the typical physical and laboratory signs of peritonitis (233). Further, concomitant extra-abdominal opportunistic infection can modify the clinical presentation of peritonitis.

An abdominal roentgenogram with the patient erect may demonstrate pneumoperitoneum from bowel perforation. It may also reveal other signs of significant intra-abdominal disease such as bowel wall thickening, intestinal mucosal thumbprinting, indistinct colonic haustra, intramural intestinal air, air in the portal vein, and signs of obstruction. Patients with an acute abdomen should be evaluated with abdominal CT, and with paracentesis if ascites is present. When evaluating ascites in patients with AIDS, leukocytes may be remarkably absent in the ascites in the face of severe immunosuppression despite peritonitis. Chronic peritoneal infections, including tuberculosis and fungal infections, present with lymphocytic ascites.

Gastrointestinal perforation leads to secondary bacterial contamination of the peritoneum. The most common pathogens encountered include aerobic coliform bacteria, particularly *Escherichia coli*, anaerobic *Bacteroides*, anaerobic and aerobic streptococci, enterococci, and *Clostridium*. AIDS patients may develop chronic peritonitis or spontaneous bacterial peritonitis without bowel perforation. The risk of spontaneous bacterial peritonitis is increased in patients with ascites, especially with low ascites protein, cirrhosis, advanced immunosuppression, and poor medical status. AIDS patients are at increased risk of spontaneous bacterial peritonitis from *Salmonella*, as well as the more typical bacteria, which include *Escherichia coli*, *Klebsiella pneumoniae*, and *Streptococcus*. HIV itself has been postulated as a cause of peritonitis in patients with a negative extensive evaluation (234). AIDS patients with peritonitis should be treated with antibiotics directed against the inciting organism or with broad-spectrum antibiotics in none is found. Surgery should be undertaken if needed.

Laparotomy

About 4% of patients with AIDS require laparotomy (208). The causes of emergency laparotomy in patients with AIDS are similar to those in the nonimmunosuppressed population and include bowel perforation, appendicitis, cholecystitis, bowel obstruction, and intestinal ischemia. What commonly differs in these populations is the etiology behind those causes. The AIDS-related causes of bowel perforation include malignancy such as KS or lymphoma and opportunistic infections such as CMV, *Mycobacterium tuberculosis*, and fungi including *Candida*, *Cryptococcus*, and *Histoplasma*. Appendicitis in AIDS may be caused by CMV or KS, and cholecystitis may be caused by CMV, *Candida*, *Cryptosporidium*, and *Nocardia*. Bowel obstruction in AIDS patients may also be precipitated by AIDS-related opportunistic infections and neoplasms that include CMV, *Mycobacterium tuberculosis*, MAC, *Strongyloides stercoralis*, KS, and lymphoma.

The morbidity and mortality in patients with AIDS who are undergoing laparotomy are increased because of delayed diagnosis resulting from atypical presentations, poor wound healing, malnutrition, protein deficiency, poor medical status, and concurrent infections. Although early reports noted a mortality of up to 60% for emergency laparotomy in AIDS patients, this number has been reduced by greater attention to preoperative hyperalimentation and correction of metabolic disturbances (235, 236). Despite these measures, many AIDS patients undergoing laparotomy experience wound dehiscence.

References

1. Janoff EN, Jackson S, Wahl SM, et al. Intestinal mucosal immunoglobulins during human immunodeficiency virus type 1 infection. J Infect Dis 1994;170:299–307.
2. Antony MA, Brandt LJ, Klein RS, et al. Infectious diarrhea in patients with AIDS. Dig Dis Sci 1988;33:1141–1146.
3. Lane GP, Lucas CR, Smallwood RA. The gastrointestinal and hepatic manifestations of the acquired immune deficiency syndrome. Med J Aust 1989;150:139–143.
4. Heise W, Mostertz P, Arasteh K, et al. Gastrointestinal findings in HIV infection. Dtsch Med Wochenschr 1988;113:1588–1593.
5. Girard PM, Marche C, Maslo C, et al. Digestive manifestations in acquired immunodeficiency disease. Ann Med Interne (Paris) 1987; 138:411–415.
6. Colebunders R, Francis H, Mann JM, B et al. Persistent diarrhea, strongly associated with HIV infection in Kinshasa, Zaire. Am J Gastroenterol 1987;82:859–864.
7. Dieterich DT, Wilcox CM. Diagnosis and treatment of esophageal diseases associated with HIV infection. Am J Gastroenterol 1996;91: 2265–2269.
8. Yoshida EM, Chan NH, Herrick RA, et al. Human immunodeficiency virus infection, the acquired immunodeficiency syndrome, and inflammatory bowel disease. J Clin Gastroenterol 1996;23:24–28.
9. Cacciarelli AG, Marano BJ, Gualtieri NM, et al. Lower *Helicobacter pylori* infection and peptic ulcer disease prevalence in patients with AIDS and suppressed CD4 counts. Am J Gastroenterol 1996;91: 1783–1784.

10. Connolly GM, Hawkins D, Harcourt-Webster JN, et al. Oesophageal symptoms, their causes, treatments and prognosis in patients with the acquired immune deficiency syndrome. Gut 1989;30:1033–1039.
11. Bonacini M, Young T, Laine L. Histopathology of human immunodeficiency virus-associated esophageal disease. Am J Gastroenterol 1993;88:549–551.
12. Wilcox M. Esophageal disease in the acquired immunodeficiency syndrome: etiology, diagnosis and management. Am J Med 1992;92:412–421.
13. Tom W, Aaron JS. Esophageal ulcers caused by *Torulopsis glabrata* in a patient with acquired immunodeficiency syndrome. Am J Gastroenterol 1987;82:766–768.
14. Forsmark CE, Wilcox CM, Darragh TM, et al. Disseminated histoplasmosis in AIDS: an unusual case of esophageal involvement and gastrointestinal bleeding. Gastrointest Endosc 1990;36:604–605.
15. Gould E, Kory WP, Raskin JB, et al. Esophageal biopsy findings in acquired immunodeficiency syndrome: clinicopathological correlation in 20 patients. South Med J 1988;81:1392–1396.
16. Laine L, Bonacini M, Sattler F, et al. Cytomegalovirus and *Candida* esophagitis in patients with AIDS. J Acquir Immune Defic Syndr 1992;5:605–609.
17. Schechter M, Pannain VL, de Oliveira AV. Papovavirus-associated esophageal ulceration in a patient with AIDS. AIDS 1991;5:238.
18. Corbellino M, Lusso P, Gallo RC, et al. Disseminated human herpesvirus 6 infection in AIDS. Lancet 1993;342:1242.
19. Kotler DP, Wilson CS, Haroutiounian G, et al. Detection of human immunodeficiency virus-1 by 35S-RNA in situ hybridization in solitary esophageal ulcers in two patients with the acquired immune deficiency syndrome. Am J Gastroenterol 1989;84:313–317.
20. Poles MA, McMeeking AA, Scholes JV, et al. *Actinomyces* infection of a cytomegalovirus esophageal ulcers in two patients with acquired immunodeficiency syndrome. Am J Gastroenterol 1994;89:1569–1572.
21. Chang AD, Drachenberg CI, James SP. Bacillary angiomatosis associated with extensive esophageal polyposis: a new mucocutaneous manifestation of acquired immunodeficiency disease (AIDS). Am J Gastroenterol 1996;91:2220–2223.
22. Kim J, Minamoto GY, Grieco MH. Nocardial infection as a complication of AIDS: report of six cases and review. Rev Infect Dis 1991;13:624–629.
23. Kazlo PG, Shah K, Bdnkov KJ, et al. Esophageal cryptosporidiosis in a child with AIDS. Gastroenterology 1986;91:1301–1303.
24. Grimes MM, Lapook JD, Bar MH, et al. Disseminated *Pneumocystis carinii* infection in a patient with acquired immunodeficiency syndrome. Hum Pathol 1987;18:307–308.
25. Villanueva JL, Torre-Cisneros J, Jurado R, et al. *Leishmania* esophagitis in an AIDS patient: an unusual form of visceral leishmaniasis. Am J Gastroenterol 1994;89:273–275.
26. Bernal A, del Junco GFW. Endoscopic and pathological features of esophageal lymphoma: a report of four cases in patients with acquired immune deficiency syndrome. Gastrointest Endosc 1986;32:96–99.
27. Houghton JM, Korah RM, Kim KH, et al. A role for apoptosis in the pathogenesis of AIDS-related idiopathic esophageal ulcers. J Infect Dis 1997;175:1216–1219.
28. Wilcox CM, Alexander LN, Clark WS, et al. Fluconazole compared with endoscopy for human immunodeficiency virus-infected patients with esophageal symptoms. Gastroenterology 1996;110:1803–1809.
29. Connolly GM, Forbes A, Gleeson JA, et al. Investigation of upper gastrointestinal symptoms in patients with AIDS. AIDS 1989;3:453–456.
30. Sugar AM, Alsip SG, Galgiani JN, et al. Pharmacology and toxicity of high dose ketoconazole. Antimicrob Agents Chemother 1987;31:1874–1878.
31. Como JA, Dismukes WE. Oral azole drugs as systemic antifungal therapy. N Engl J Med 1994;330:263–270.
32. Laine L, Dretler RH, Conteas CN, et al. Fluconazole compared with ketoconazole for the treatment of *Candida* esophagitis in AIDS: a randomized trial. Ann Intern Med 1992;117:655–660.
33. Chachoua A, Dieterich D, Krasinski K, et al. 9-(1,3-Dihydroxy-2-propoxymethyl)guanine (ganciclovir) in the treatment of cytomegalovirus gastrointestinal disease with the acquired immunodeficiency syndrome. Ann Intern Med 1987;107:133–137.
34. Dieterich DT, Chachoua A, Lefleur F, et al. Ganciclovir treatment of gastrointestinal infections caused by cytomegalovirus in patients with AIDS. Rev Infect Dis 1988;10(Suppl 3):S532–S537.
35. Jacobson M, O'Donnell J, Porteus D, et al. Retinal and gastrointestinal disease due to CMV in patients with AIDS: prevalence, natural history and response to ganciclovir therapy. Q J Med 1988;65:463–486.
36. Wilcox CM, Diehl DL, Cello JP, et al. Cytomegalovirus esophagitis in patients with AIDS. A clinical, endoscopic, and pathologic correlation. Ann Intern Med 1990;113:589–593.
37. Wilcox CM, Straub RF, Schwartz DA. Cytomegalovirus esophagitis in AIDS: a prospective evaluation of clinical response to ganciclovir therapy, relapse rate, and long-term outcome. Am J Med 1995;98:169–176.
38. Hochster H, Dieterich DT, Bozzette S, et al. Toxicity of combined ganciclovir and zidovudine for cytomegalovirus disease associated with AIDS: an AIDS Clinical Trials Group Study. Ann Intern Med 1990;113:111–117.
39. Dieterich DT, Poles MA, Dicker M, et al. Foscarnet treatment of cytomegalovirus gastrointestinal infections in acquired immunodeficiency syndrome patients who have failed ganciclovir induction. Am J Gastroenterol 1993;88:542–548.
40. Dieterich DT, Poles MA, Lew EA, et al. Treatment of gastrointestinal cytomegalovirus infection with twice daily foscarnet: a pilot study with pharmacokinetics in patients with HIV. Antimicrob Agents Chemother 1997;41(6):1226–1230.
41. Goodgame RW, Ross PG, Kim HS, et al. Esophageal stricture after cytomegalovirus ulcer treated with ganciclovir. J Clin Gastroenterol 1991;13:678–681.
42. Dieterich DT, Poles MA, Lew E, et al. Concurrent use of ganciclovir and foscarnet to treat cytomegalovirus infection in AIDS patients. J Infect Dis 1993;167:1184–1188.
43. Reeves-Darby V, Laine L, Rodrigue D, et al. A randomized trial of foscarnet maintenance therapy versus observation for CMV gastrointestinal disease (FOS 29). In: 11th International Conference on AIDS, Vancouver, 1996.
44. Wilcox CM, Harris PR, Redman TK, et al. High mucosal levels of tumor necrosis factor α messenger RNA in AIDS-associated cytomegalovirus-induced esophagitis. Gastroenterology 1998;114:77–82.
45. Kotler D, Reka S, Borcich A, et al. Corticosteroid therapy of idiopathic esophageal ulcers. Gastrointest Endosc 1990;36:191.
46. Wilcox CM, Schwartz DA. Etiology, response to therapy, and long-term outcome of esophageal ulceration in patients with human immunodeficiency virus infection. Ann Intern Med 1995;122:143–149.
47. Paterson DL, Georghiou PR, Allworth AM, et al. Thalidomide as treatment of refractory aphthous ulceration related to human immunodeficiency virus infection. Clin Infect Dis 1995;20:250–254.
48. Lake-Bakaar G, Elsakr M, Hagag N, et al. Changes in parietal cell structure and function in HIV disease. Dig Dis Sci 1996;41:1398–1408.
49. Marano BJ Jr, Smith F, Bonanno CA. *Helicobacter pylori* prevalence in acquired immunodeficiency syndrome. Am J Gastroenterol 1993;88:687–690.
50. Konturek JW, Fischer H, van der Voort IR, et al. Disturbed gastric motor activity in patients with human immunodeficiency virus infection. Scand J Gastroenterol 1997;32:221–225.
51. Rabeneck L, Crane MM, Risser JM, et al. Effect of HIV transmission category and CD4 count on the occurrence of diarrhea in HIV-infected patients. Am J Gastroenterol 1993;88:1720–1723.
52. Wilcox CM, Schwartz DA, Cotsonis G, et al. Chronic unexplained diarrhea in human immunodeficiency virus infection: determination of the best diagnostic approach. Gastroenterology 1996;110:30–37.

53. Smith PD, Lane HC, Gill VJ, et al. Intestinal infections in patients with the acquired immunodeficiency syndrome (AIDS): etiology and response to therapy. Ann Intern Med 1988;108:328–333.
54. Rene E, Marche C, Regnier B, et al. Intestinal infections in patients with acquired immunodeficiency syndrome: a prospective study in 132 patients. Dig Dis Sci 1989;34:773–780.
55. Connolly GM, Shanson D, Hawkins DA, et al. Non-cryptosporidial diarrhoea in human immunodeficiency virus (HIV) infected patients. Gut 1989;30:195–200.
56. Watson A, Samore MH, Wanke CA. Diarrhea and quality of life in ambulatory HIV-infected patients. Dig Dis Sci 1996;41:1794–1800.
57. Lubeck DP, Bennett CL, Mazonson PD, et al. Quality of life and health service use among HIV-infected patients with chronic diarrhea. J Acquir Immune Defic Syndr 1993;6:478–484.
58. Johanson JF, Sonnenberg A. Efficient management of diarrhea in the acquired immunodeficiency syndrome (AIDS): a medical decision analysis. Ann Intern Med 1990;112:942–948.
59. Blanshard C, Francis N, Gazzard BG. Investigation of chronic diarrhoea in acquired immunodeficiency syndrome: a prospective study of 155 patients. Gut 1996;39:824–832.
60. Wilcox CM, Rabeneck L, Friedman S. AGA technical review: malnutrition and cachexia, chronic diarrhea, and hepatobiliary disease in patients with human immunodeficiency virus infection. Gastroenterology 1996;111:1724–1752.
61. Bini EJ, Kornacki S. Electron microscopic examination of small bowel biopsies in HIV-positive patients with chronic diarrhea: is it worth the added cost? Gastroenterology 1997;112:A935.
62. Da Silva AJ, Bornay-Himes FJ, del Aguila de la Puerta C, et al. Diagnosis of *Enterocytozoon bieneusi* (microsporidia) infections by polymerase chain reaction in stool samples using primers based on the region coding for small-subunit ribosomal RNA. Arch Pathol Lab Med 1997;121:874–879.
63. Dieterich DT, Rahmin M. Cytomegalovirus colitis in AIDS: presentation in 44 patients and a review of the literature. J Acquir Immune Defic Syndr 1991;4(Suppl 1):S29–S35.
64. Bini EJ, Weidel EH. Endoscopic evaluation of chronic human immunodeficiency virus–related diarrhea: is colonoscopy superior to flexible sigmoidoscopy? Am J Gastroenterol 1998;93:56–60.
65. Blanshard C, Gazzard BG. Natural history and prognosis of diarrhoea of unknown cause in patients with acquired immunodeficiency syndrome. Gut 1995;36:283–286.
66. Chachoua A, Dieterich DT, Krasinski K, et al. '9-(1,3-Dihydroxy-2-propoxymethyl)guanine (ganciclovir) in the treatment of cytomegalovirus gastrointestinal disease with the acquired immunodeficiency syndrome. Ann Intern Med 1987;107:133.
67. Gallant J, Moore RD, Richman DD, et al. Incidence and natural history of cytomegalovirus disease in patients with advanced human immunodeficiency virus disease treated with zidovudine. J Infect Dis 1992;166:1223.
68. Dieterich DT. Ganciclovir treatment of cytomegalovirus gastrointestinal disease in patients with AIDS. In: Spector S, ed. Ganciclovir therapy for cytomegalovirus infection. New York: Marcel Dekker, 1991:129–144.
69. Goodgame RW, Genta RM, Estrada R, et al. Frequency of positive tests for cytomegalovirus in AIDS patients: endoscopic lesions compared with normal mucosa. Am J Gastroenterol 1993;88:338–343.
70. Smith PD, Saini SS, Orenstein JM. Infections in the immunosuppressed host. In: Phillips SF, Pemberton JH, eds. Large intestine: physiology, pathophysiology, and disease. New York: Raven Press, 1991:121–138.
71. Janoff EN, Orenstein JM, Manischevitz JF, et al. Adenovirus colitis in the acquired immunodeficiency syndrome. Gastroenterology 1991;100:976–979.
72. Laughon BE, Druckman DA, Vernon A, et al. Prevalence of enteric viral pathogens in homosexual men with acquired immunodeficiency syndrome. Gastroenterologt 1988;94:984.
73. Yan Z, Son M, Singh M, et al. Adenovirus colitis in HIV infection: an underdiagnosed entity [abstract 388]. Lab Invest 1996;74:68A.
74. Grohman GS, Glass RI, Pereira HG, et al. Enteric viruses and diarrhea in HIV-infected patients. N Engl J Med 1993;329:12.
75. Schmidt W, Schneider T, Heise W, et al. Stool viruses, coinfections, and diarrhea in HIV-infected patients. J Acquir Immune Defic Syndr Hum Retrovirol 1996;13:33–38.
76. Flanigan T, Whalen C, Turner J, et al. *Cryptosporidium* infection and CD4 counts. Ann Intern Med 1992;116:840–842.
77. Rabeneck L, Gyorkey F, Genta RM, et al. The role of *Microsporidia* in the pathogenesis of HIV-related chronic diarrhea. Ann Intern Med 1993;119:895–899.
78. Kotler DP, Orenstein JM. Prevalence of intestinal microsporidiusis in HIV-infected individuals referred for gastroenterological evaluation. Am J Gastroenterol 1994;89:1998–2002.
79. Orenstein JM, Dieterich DT, Kotler DP. Systemic dissemination by a newly recognized intestinal microsporidia species in AIDS. AIDS 1992;6:1143.
80. Dehovitz JA, Pape JW, Boney M, et al. Clinical manifestations and therapy of *Isospora belli* infections in patients with the acquired immunodeficiency syndrome. N Engl J Med 1986;315:87.
81. Ortega YR, Sterling CR, Gilman RH, et al. *Cyclospora* species: a new protozoal pathogen of humans. N Engl J Med 1993;328:1308.
82. Dieterich DT, Lew EA, Bacon DJ, et al. Gastrointestinal pneumocytstosis in HIV infected patients on aerosolized pentamidine: report of five cases and review of the literature. Am J Gastroenterol 1992;87:1763–1770.
83. Bonacini M, Kanel G, Alamy M. Duodenal and hepatic toxoplasmosis in a patient with HIV infection: review of the literature. Am J Gastroenterol 1996;91:1838–1840.
84. Horsburgh CR. *Mycobacterium avium* complex infection in the acquired immunodeficiency syndrome. N Engl J Med 1991;324:1332.
85. Rotterdam H, Tsang P. Gastrointestinal disease in the immunocompromised patient. Hum Pathol 1994;25:1123.
86. Nelson MR, Shanson DC, Hawkins DA, et al. *Salmonella*, *Campylobacter* and *Shigella* in HIV-seropositive patients. AIDS 1992;6:1495.
87. Blaser MJ, Hale TL, Formal SB. Recurrent shigellosis complicating human immunodeficiency virus infection: failure of pre-existing antibodies to confer protection. Am J Med 1989;86:105.
88. Salmon D, Detruchis P, Leport C, et al. Efficacy of zidovudine in preventing relapses of *Salmonella* bacteremia in AIDS. J Infect Dis 1991;163:415.
89. Mayer HB, Wanke CA. Enteroaggregative *Escherichia coli* as a possible cause of diarrhea in an HIV-infected patient. N Engl J Med 1995;332:273.
90. Orenstein JM, Kotler DP. Diarrheogenic bacterial enteritis in acquired immune deficiency syndrome: a light and electron microscopy study of 52 cases. Hum Pathol 1995;26:481.
91. Cappell MS, Clark P. *Clostridium difficile* infection as a treatable cause of diarrhea in patients with advanced human immunodeficiency virus infection: A study of seven consecutive patients admitted from 1986 to 1992 to a university teaching hospital. Am J Gastroenterol 1993;88:891.
92. Lu SS, Schwartz JM, Simon DM, et al. *Clostridium difficile*-associated diarrhea in patients with HIV positivity and AIDS: a prospective controlled study. Am J Gastroenterol 1994;89:1226.
93. Ehrenpreis ED, Ganger DR, Kodhvar GT, et al. D-Xylose malabsorption: characteristic finding in patients with the AIDS wasting syndrome and chronic diarrhea. J Acquir Immune Defic Syndr 1992;5:1047–1050.
94. Heise C, Dandekar S, Kumar P, et al. Human Immunodeficiency virus infection of enterocytes and mononuclear cells in human jejunal mucosa. Gastrenterology 1991;100:1521–1527.
95. Fleming SC, Kapembwa MS, McDonald TT, et al. Direct in vitro infection of human intestine with HIV-1. AIDS 1992;6:1099–1104.
96. Jarry A, Cortez A, Rene E, et al. Infected cells and immune cells in the gastrointestinal tract of patients with AIDS: an immunoistochemical study of 127 cases. Histopathology 1990;16:133.

97. Kotler DP, Reka S, Clayton F. Intestinal mucosal inflammation associated with human immunodeficiency virus infection. Dig Dis Sci 1993;38:1119.
98. Belitsos PC, Greenson JK, Yardley JH, et al. Association of gastric hypoacidity with opportunistic enteric infections in patients with AIDS. J Infect Dis 1992;166:277–284.
99. Keating J, Bjarnason I, Somasundaram S, et al. Intestinal absorptive capacity, intestinal permeability and jejunal histology in HIV and their relation to diarrhoea. Gut 1995;37:623–629.
100. Sharkey KA, Sutherland LR, Davison JS, et al. Peptides in the gastrointestinal tract in human immunodeficiency virus infection. Gastroenterology 1992;103:18–28.
101. Blanshard C, Benhamou Y, Dohin E, et al. Treatment of AIDS-associated gastrointestinal cytomegalovirus infection with foscarnet and ganciclovir: a randomized comparison. J Infect Dis 1995;72:622–628.
102. Dieterich DT, Kotler DP, Busch DF, et al. Ganciclovir treatment of cytomegalovirus colitis in AIDS: a randomized double-blind, placebo controled multicenter trail. J infect Dis 1993;167:278–282.
103. Cotte L, Drouet E, Bailly F, et al. Cytomegalovirus DNA level on biopsy specimens during treatment of cytomegalovirus gastrointestinal disease. Gastroenterology 1996;111:439–444.
104. White AC, Chappell CL, Hayat CS, et al. Paramomycin for cryptosporidiosis in AIDS: a prospective double-blind trial. J Infect Dis 1994;170:419–424.
105. Greenberg PD, Cello JP. Treatment of severe diarrhea caused by *Cryptosporidium parvum* with oral bovine immunoglobulin concentrate in patients with AIDS. J Acquir Immune Defic Syndr Hum Retrovirol 1996;13:348–354.
106. Dieterich DT, Lew EA, Kotler DP, et al. Treatment with albendazole for intestinal disease due to *Enterocytozoon bieneusi* in patients with AIDS. J Infect Dis 1994;169:178–183.
107. Joste NE, Rich JD, Busam KJ, et al. Autopsy verification of *Encephalitozoon intestinalis* (microsporidiosis) eradication following albendazole therapy. Arch Pathol Lab Med 1996;120:199–203.
108. Dionisio O, Manneschi LI, Di Lullo S, et al. *Enterocytozoon bieneusi* in AIDS: symptomatic relief and parasitic changes after furazolidone. J Clin Pathol 1997;50:472–476.
109. Sharpstone D, Rowbottom A, Francis N, et al. Thalidomide: a novel therapy for microsporidiosis. Gastroenterology 1997;112:1823–1829.
110. Masur H. Recommendations on prophylaxis and therapy for disseminated *Mycobacterium avium* complex disease in patients infected with human immunodeficiency virus. N Engl J Med 1993;329:898–904.
111. Cello JP, Grendell JH, Basuk, et al. Effect of octreotide on refractory AIDS-associated diarrhea. Ann Intern Med 1991;115:705–710.
112. Simon DM, Cello JP, Valenzuela J, et al. Multicenter trial of octreotide in patients with refractory acquired immunodeficiency syndrome–associated diarrhea. Gastroenterology 1995;108:1753–1760.
113. Gopul DV, Hassaram S, Morcon NE, et al. Idiopathic colonic inflammation in AIDS: an open trial of prednisone. Am J Gastroenterol 1997;92:2237–2240.
114. Poles MA, Lin A, Weiss WR, et al. Oxandrolone as a treatment for AIDS-related weight loss and wasting. Gastroenterology 1997;112:A1062.
115. Waisman J, Rotterdam H, Niedt GN, et al. AIDS: an overview of the pathology. Pathol Res Pract 1987;182:729–754.
116. Gordon SC, Reddy KR, Gould EE, et al. The spectrum of liver disease in the acquired immunodeficiency syndrome. J Hepatol 1986;2:475–484.
117. Hawkins CC, Gold JW, Whimbey E, et al. *Mycobacterium avium* complex infections in patients with the acquired immunodeficiency syndrome. Ann Intern Med 1986;105:184–188.
118. Kahn SA, Saltzman BR, Klein RS, et al. Hepatic disorders in the acquired immune deficiency syndrome: a clinical and pathological study. Am J Gastroenterol 1986;81:1145–1148.
119. Lebovics E, Dworkin BM, Heier SK, et al. The hepatobiliary manifestations of human immunodeficiency virus infection. Am J Gastroenterol 1988;3:1–7.
120. Poles MA, Dieterich DT, Schwarz ED, et al. Liver biopsy findings in 501 patients infected with human immunodeficiency virus (HIV). J Acquir Immune Defic Syndr Hum Retrovirol 1996;11:170–177.
121. Chaisson RE, Schecter GF, Theuer CP, et al. Tuberculosis in patients with the acquired immunodeficiency syndrome: clinical features, response of therapy and survival. Am Rev Respir Dis 1987;136:570–574.
122. Weinberg JJ, Cohen P, Malhotra R. Primary tuberculous liver abscess associated with the human immunodeficiency virus. Tubercle 1988;69:145–147.
123. Wyatt SH, Fishman EK. Hepatic bacillary angiomatosis in a patient with AIDS. Abdom Imag 1993;18:336–338.
124. Perkocha LA, Geaghan SM, Yen TS, et al. Clinical and pathological features of bacillary peliosis hepatis in association with human immunodeficiency virus infection. N Engl J Med 1990;323:1581–1586.
125. Leong SS, Cazen RA, Yu GS, et al. Abdominal visceral peliosis associated with bacillary angiomatosis: ultrastructural evidence of endothelial destruction by bacilli. Archiv Pathol Lab Med 1992;116:866–871.
126. Garcia-Tsao G, Panzini L, Yoselevitz M, et al. Bacillary peliosis hepatis as a cause of acute anemia in a patient with the acquired immunodeficiency syndrome. Gastroenterology 1992;102:1065–1070.
127. Bonacini M. Hepatobiliary complications in patients with human immunodeficiency virus infection. Am J Med 1992;92:404–411.
128. Knox KK, Carrigan DR. Disseminated active HHV-6 infections in patients with AIDS. Lancet 1994;343:577–578.
129. Soriano V, Bru F, Gonzalez-Lahoz J. Fatal varicella hepatitis in a patient with AIDS. J Infect 1992;25:107.
130. Wheat LJ, Small CB. Disseminated histoplasmosis in the acquired immune deficiency syndrome. Arch Intern Med 1984;144:2147–2149.
131. Bibler MR, Luber HJ, Glueck HI, et al. Disseminated sporotrichosis in a patient with HIV infection after treatment for acquired factor VIII inhibitor. JAMA 1986;256:3125–3126.
132. Radin DR, Baker EL, Klatt EL, et al. Visceral and nodal calcification in patients with AIDS-related *Pneumocystis carinii* infection. AJR Am J Roentgenol 1990;154:27–31.
133. Oksenhendler E, Matheron S. Toxoplasmosis: new aspects, diagnosis and treatment. Rev Pract 1992;42:155–159.
134. Liesenfeld O, Roth A, Weinke T, et al. A case of disseminated toxoplasmosis: value of PCR for the diagnosis. J Infect Dis 1994;29:133–138.
135. Terada S, Reddy KR, Jeffers LJ, et al. Microsporidan hepatitis in the acquired immunodeficiency syndrome. Ann Intern Med 1987;107:61–62.
136. Federico G, Cauda R, Pizzigallo E, et al. Visceral leishmaniasis in patients with AIDS: description of 2 cases. Pathologica 1989;81:591–600.
137. Lebovics E, Thung SN, Schaffner F, et al. The liver in acquired immunodeficiency syndrome: a clinical and histologic study. Hepatology 1985;5:293–298.
138. Bodsworth NJ, Cooper DA, Donovan B. The influence of human immunodeficiency virus type 1 infection on the development of hepatitis B virus carrier state. J Infect Dis 1991;163:1138–1140.
139. Vandercam B, Cornu C, Gala JL, et al. Reactivation of hepatitis B virus in a previously immune patient with human immunodeficiency virus infection. Eur J Clin Microbiol Infect Dis 1990;9:701–702.
140. Boue F, Goujard C, Lazzizi Y. et al. Fatal fulminant hepatitis linked to HBV reactivation in AIDS patient [abstract PO-B08-1351]. In: Programs and abstracts of the 9th International Conference on AIDS, Berlin, 1993:360.
141. Mills CT, Lee E, Perrillo R. Relationship between histology, aminotransferase levels and viral replication in chronic hepatitis B. Gastroenterology 1990;99:519–524.

142. Housset C, Pol S, Carnot F, et al. Interactions between human immunodeficiency virus-1, hepatitis delta virus and hepatitis B virus infections in 260 chronic carriers of heptatis B virus. Hepatology 1992;15:578–583.
143. Pham BN, Mosnier JF, Walker F, et al. Flow cytometry CD4+/CD8+ ratio of liver-derived lymphocytes correlates with viral replication in chronic hepatitis B. Clin Exp Immunol 1994;97:403–410.
144. Collier AC, Corey L, Murphy VL, et al. Antibody to human immunodeficiency virus (HIV): a suboptimal response to hepatitis B vaccination. Ann Intern Med 1988;109:101–105.
145. Balsano C, Billet O, Bennoun M, et al. Hepatitis B virus X gene product acts as a transactivator in vivo. J Hepatol 1994;21:103–109.
146. Scharschmidt BF, Held MJ, Hollander HH, et al. Hepatitis B in patients with HIV infection: relationship to AIDS and patient survival. Ann Intern Med 1992;117: 837–838.
147. Solomon RE, VanRaden M, Kaslow RA, et al. Association of hepatitis B surface and core antibody with acquisition and manifestations of human immunodeficiency virus type 1 (HIV-1) infection. Am J Public Health 80:1475–1478.
148. Stevens C, Taylor PE, Pindyck J, et al. Epidemiology of hepatitis C virus: a preliminary study in volunteer blood donors. JAMA 1990; 263:49–53.
149. Esteban JI, Esteban R, Viladomiu L, et al. Hepatitis C virus antibodies among risk groups in Spain. Lancet 1989;2:294–297.
150. Hiyashi PH, Flynn N, McCurdy SA, et al. Prevalence of hepatitis C virus antibodies among patients infected with human immunodeficiency virus. J Med Virol 1991;33:177–180.
151. Soriano V, Bravo R, Mas A, G et al. Impact of immunosuppression caused by HIV infection on the replication of hepatitis C virus. Vox Sang 1995;69:259–260.
152. Thomas DL, Shih JW, Alter HJ, et al. Effect of human immunodeficiency virus on hepatitis C virus infection among injecting drug users. J Infect Dis 1996;174:690–695.
153. Eyster ME, Fried MW, Di Bisceglie AM, et al. Increasing hepatitis C virus RNA levels in hemophiliacs: relationship to human immunodeficiency virus infection and liver disease. Multicenter Hemophilia Cohort Study. Blood 1994;84:1020–1023.
154. Matsuda J, Tsukamoto M, Gohchi K, et al. Hepatitis C virus (HCV) RNA and human immunodeficiency virus (HIV) p24 antigen in the cryoglobulin of hemophiliacs with HIV and/or HCV infection. Clin Infect Dis 1994;18:832–833.
155. Telfer PT, Brown D, Devereaux H, et al. HCV RNA levels and HIV infection: evidence for a viral interaction in haemophiliac patients. Br J Haematol 1994;88:397–399.
156. Eyster ME, Diamondstone LS, Lien J-M, et al. Natural history of hepatitis C virus infection in multitransfused hemophiliacs: effect of coinfection with human immunodeficiency virus. J Acquir Immune Defic Syndr 1993;6:602–610.
157. Telfer P, Sabin C, Devereux H, et al. The progression of HCV-associated liver disesae in a cohort of haemophiliac patients. Br J Haematol. 1994;87:555–561.
158. Wright TL, Hollander H, Pu X, et al. Hepatitis C in HIV-infected patients with and without AIDS: prevalence and relationship to patient survival. Hepatology 1994;20:1152–1155.
159. Llibre JM, Garcia E, Aloy A, et al. Hepatitis C virus infection and progression of infection due to human immunodeficiency virus. Clin Infect Dis 1993;16:182.
160. Marcellin P, Martinot-Peignoux M, Elias M, et al. Hepatitis C virus (HCV) viremia in human immunodeficiency virus-seronegative and seropositive patients with indeterminate HCV recombinant immunoblot assay. J Infect Dis 1994;170:433–435.
161. Persidsky Y, Steffan A-M, Gendrault J-L, et al. Permissiveness of Kupffer cells for simian immunodeficiency virus (SIV) and morphological changes in the liver of rhesus monkeys at different periods of SIV infection. Hepatology 1995;21:1215–1225.
162. Hoda SA, White JE, Gerber MA. Immunohistochemical studies of human immunodeficiency virus-1 in liver tissues of patients with AIDS. Mod Pathol 1991;4:578–581.
163. Cao YZ, Friedman-Kien AE, Huang YX, et al. CD4-independent, productive human immunodeficiency virus type 1 infection of hepatoma cell lines in vitro. J Virol 1990;64:2553–2559.
164. Housset C, Lamas E, Courgnaud V, et al. Presence of HIV-1 in human parenchymal and non-parenchymal liver cells in vivo. J Hepatol 1993;19:252–258.
165. Cao YZ, Dieterich D, Thomas PA, et al. Identification and quantification of HIV-1 in the liver of patients with AIDS. AIDS 1992; 6:65–70.
166. Radin DR, Esplin JA, Levine AM, et al. AIDS-related non-Hodgkin's lymphoma: abdominal CT findings in 112 patients. AJR Am J Roentgenol 1993;160:1133–1139.
167. Scerpella EG, Villareal AA, Casanova PF, et al. Primary lymphoma of the liver in AIDS: report of one new case and review of the literature. J Clin Gastroenterol 1996;22:51–53.
168. Soyer P, Van Beers B, Teillet-Thiebaud F, et al. Hodgkin's and non–Hodgkin's hepatic lymphoma: sonographic findings. Abdom Imaging 1993;18:339–343.
169. Luburich P, Bru C, Ayuso MC, et al. Hepatic Kaposi sarcoma in AIDS: US and CT findings. Radiology 1990;175:172–174.
170. Gottesman D, Dyrszka H, Albarran J, et al. AIDS-related hepatic Kaposi's sarcoma: massive bleeding following liver biopsy. Am J Gastroenterol 1993;88:762–764.
171. Ninane J, Moulin D, Latinne D, et al. AIDS in two African children: one with fibrosarcoma of the liver. Eur J Pediatr 1985;144:385–390.
172. Wachsberg RH, Cho KC, Adekosan A. Two leiomyomas of the liver in an adult with AIDS: CT and MR appearance. J Comput Assist Tomogr 1994;18:156–157.
173. Dworkin BM, Stahl RE, Giardina MA, et al. The liver in acquired immune deficiency syndrome: emphasis on patients with intravenous drug abuse. Am J Gastroenterol 1987;82:231–236.
174. Chalasani N, Wilcox CM. Etiology, evaluation, and outcome of jaundice in patients with acquired immunodeficiency syndrome. Hepatology 1996;23:728–733.
175. Lee C, Stein JJ, Kravetz JD, et al. Hepatic complications in HIV-infected individuals treated with indinavir. J Acquir Immune Defic Syndr Hum Retrovirol (in press).
176. McKenzie R, Fried MW, Sallie R, et al. Hepatic failure and lactic acidosis due to fialuridine (FIAU), an investigational nucleoside analogue for chronic hepatitis B. N Engl J Med 1995;333:1099–1105.
177. Wilson R, Harrington R, Stewart B, et al. Human immunodeficiency virus 1-associated necrotizing cholangitis caused by infection with Septata intestinalis. Gastroenterology 1995;108:247–251.
178. Cello JP. Human immunodeficiency virus–associated biliary tract disease. Semin Liver Dis 1992;12:213–218.
179. Robinson G, Wilson SE, Williams RA. Surgery in patients with acquired immunodeficiency syndrome. Arch Surg 1987;122:170–175.
180. Cello JP. Acquired immunodeficiency syndrome cholangiopathy: spectrum of disease. Am J Med 1989;86:539–546.
181. Bouche H, Housset C, Dumont JL, et al. AIDS-related cholangitis: diagnostic features and course in 15 patients. J Hepatol 1993;17: 34–39.
182. Schneiderman DJ, Cello JP, Laing FC. Papillary stenosis and sclerosing cholangitis in the acquired immunodeficiency syndrome. Ann Intern Med 1987;106:546–549.
183. Cappell MS, Schwartz MS, Biempica L. Clinical utility of liver biopsy in patients with serum antibodies to the human immunodeficiency virus. Am J Med 1990;88:123–130.
184. Comer GM, Mukherjee S, Scholes JV, et al. Liver biopsies in the acquired immune deficiency syndrome: influence of endemic disease and drug abuse. Am J Gastroenterol 1989;84:1525–1531.
185. Piccione F, Sagnelli E, Pasquale G, et al. Complications following percutaneous liver biopsy: a multicentre retrospective study on 68,276 biopsies. J Hepatol 1986;2:165–173.
186. Schwarz E, Lew R, Dicker MA, et al. Complications of liver biopsies in patients seropositive for human immunodeficiency virus (HIV). Gastroenterology 1993;4:A777.

187. Churchill DR, Mann D, Coker RJ, et al. Fatal haemorrhage following liver biopsy in patients with HIV infection. Genitourin Med 1996;72: 62–64.
188. Schneiderman DJ, Arenson DM, Cello JP, et al. Hepatic disease in patients with the acquired immune deficiency syndrome (AIDS). Hepatology 1987;7:925–930.
189. Roger PM, Mondain V, Saint Paul MC, et al. Liver biopsy is not useful in the diagnosis of mycobacterial infections in patients who are infected with human immunodeficiency virus. Clin Infect Dis 1996; 23:1302–1304.
190. Boylston AW, Cook HT, Francis ND, et al. Biopsy pathology of acquired immune deficiency syndrome (AIDS). J Clin Pathol 1987; 40:1–8.
191. Orenstein MS, Tavitian A, Yonk B, et al. Granulomatous involvement of the liver in patients with AIDS. Gut 1985;26:1220–1225.
192. Cavicchi M, Pialoux G, Carnot F, et al. Value of liver biopsy for the rapid diagnosis of infection in human immunodeficiency virus-infected patients who have unexplained fever and elevated serum levels of alkaline phosphatase or gamma-glutamyl transferase. Clin Infect Dis 1995;20:606–610,
193. Jeffers LJ, Alzate I, Aguilar H, et al. Laparoscopic and histologic findings in patients with human immunodeficiency virus. Gastrointest Endosc 40:160–164, 1994.
194. Beale TJ, Wetton WN, Crofton . A sonographic-pathological correlation of liver biopsies in patients with the acquired immune deficiency syndrome (AIDS). Clin Radiol 1995;50:761–764.
195. Daly CA, Padley SPG. Sonographic prediction of a normal or abnormal ERCP in suspected AIDS related sclerosing cholangitis. Clin Radiol 1996;51:618–621.
196. Miller FH, Gore RM, Nemcek AA, et al. Pancreaticobiliary manifestations of AIDS. AJR Am J Roentgenol 1996;166:1269–1274.
197. Wong DKH, Yim C, Naylor CD, et al. Interferon alfa treatment of chronic hepatitis B: randominzed trial in a predominately homosexual male population. Gastroenterology 1995;108:165–171.
198. Marriott E. Navas S, del Romero J, et al. Treatment with recombinant alpha-interferon of chronic hepatitis C in anti-HIV-positive patients. J Med Virol 1993;40:107–111.
199. Soriano V, Garcia-Samaniego J, Bravo R, et al. Intereron alpha for the treatment of chronic hepatitis C in patients infected with human immunodeficiency virus. Clin Infect Dis 1996;23:585–91.
200. Takada N, Takase S, Enomoto N, et al. Clinical backgrounds of the patients having diferent types of hepatitis C virus genomes. J Hepatol 1992;14:35–40.
201. Chemello L, Alberti A, Rose K, et al. Hepatitis C serotype and response to interferon therapy [letter]. N Engl J Med 1994;330:143.
202. Tsubota A, Chayama K, Ikeda K, et al. Factors predictive of response to interferon-alpha therapy in hepatitis C virus infection. Hepatology 1994;19:1088–1094.
203. Reichard O, Noftrans G, Fryden A, et al. Randomised, double-blind, placebo-controlled of interferon alpha-2b with and without ribavirin for chronic hepatitis C. Lancet 1998;351:83–87.
204. Vento S, Di Perri G, Cruciani M, et al. Rapid decline of CD4 cells after IFN alpha treatment in HIV-1 infection [letter]. Lancet 1993;341: 958–959.
205. Benharads Y, Kathman G, Lunel F, et al. Effects of lamivudine on replication of hepatitis B virus in HIV-infected men. Ann Intern Med 1996;125:705–712.
206. Wind P, Chevallier JM, Jones D, et al. Cholecystectomy for cholecystitis in patients with acquired immune deficiency syndrome. Am J Surg 1994;168:244–246.
207. Adolph MD, Bass SN, Lee SK, et al. Cytomegaloviral acalculous cholecystitis in acquired immunodeficiency syndrome patients. Am Surg 1993;59:679–684.
208. LaRaja RD, Rothenberg RE, Odom JW, et al. The incidence of intra-abdominal surgery in acquired immunodeficiency syndrome: a statistical review of 904 patients. Surgery 1989;105:175–179.
209. Cello JP, Chan MF. Long-term follow-up of endoscopic retrograde cholangiopancreatography sphincterotomy for patients with acquired immune deficiency syndrome papillary stenosis. Am J Med 1995;99: 600–603.
210. Castiella A, Iribasth JA, Lopez P, et al. Ursodeoxycholic acid in the treatment of AIDS-associated cholangiopathy. Am J Med 1997;103: 170–171.
211. Maxson CJ, Greenfield SM, Turner JL. Acute pancreatitis as a common complication of 2′-,3′,dideoxyinosine therapy in the acquired immunodeficiency syndrome. Am J Gastroenterol 1992;87:708–713.
212. Dowell SF, Moore GW, Hutchins GM. The spectrum of pancreatic pathology in patients with AIDS. Mod Pathol 1990;3:49–53.
213. Pezzilli R, Gullo L, Ricchi E, et al. Serum pancreatic enzymes in HIV-seropositive patients. Dig Dis Sci 1992;37:286–288.
214. Dutta SK, Tiny CD, Lai LL. Study of prevalence, severity, and etiological factors associated with acute pancreatitis in patients infected with human immunodeficiency virus. Am J Gastroenterol 1997;92:2044–2048.
215. Teare JP, Daly CA, Rodgers C, et al. Pancreatic abnormalities and AIDS-related sclerosing cholangitis. Genitourin Med 1997;73: 271–273.
216. Zazzo JF, Pichon F, Regnier B. HIV and the pancreas [letter]. Lancet 1987;2:1212–1213.
217. Klatt EC. Pathology of pentamidine-induced pancreatitis. Arch Pathol Lab Med 1992;116:162–164.
218. O'Neil MG, Selub SE, Hak LJ. Pancreatitis during pentamidine therapy in patient with AIDS. Clin Pharm 1991;10:56–59.
219. Perrone C, Bricaire F, Leport C, et al. Hypoglycemia and diabetes mellitus following parenteral pentamidine mesylate treatment in AIDS patients. Diabetic Med 1990;7:585–589.
220. Seidlin M, Lambert JS, Dolin R, et al. Pancreatitis and pancreatic dysfunction in patients taking dideoxyinosine. AIDS 1992;6: 831–835.
221. Yarchoan R, Mitsuya H, Plunda JM, et al. The National Cancer Institute phase I study of 2-,3-dideoxyinosine (ddI) administration in AIDS or AIDS related complex: analysis of activity and toxicity profiles. Rev Infect Dis 1990;12(Suppl 5):522–533.
222. Brivet F, Coffin B, Bedossa P, et al. Pancreatic lesions in AIDS [letter]. Lancet 1987;2:570–571.
223. Tan WW, Chopick EK, Abter EZ, et al. Paromomycin-associated pancreatitis in HIV-related cryptosporidiosis. Ann Pharmacother 1995;29:22–24.
224. Greenberg RE, Banks S, Singer C. Macroamylasemia in association with the acquired immunodeficiency syndrome. Postgrad Med J 1987;63:677–679.
225. Grunfield C, Kotler DP, Hamadeh R, et al. Hypertriglyceridemia in the acquired immunodeficiency syndrome. Am J Med 1989;86: 677–679.
226. Jaber B, Gleckman R. Tuberculous pancreatic abscess as an intial AIDS-defining disorder in a patient infected with the human immunodeficiency virus: case report and review. Clin Infect Dis 1995;20: 890–894.
227. Poles MA, Procaccino F, Eysselein VE. Endoscopic ultrasound-guided biopsy in the evaluation of retroperitoneal disease in two patients with acquired immunodeficiency syndrome (AIDS). (Submitted)
228. Zender HO, Arrigoni E, Eckert J, et al. A case of *Encephalitozoon cuniculi* peritonitis in a patient with AIDS. Am J Clin Pathol 1989;92:352–356.
229. Lin O, Scholes JV, Lustbader IJ. Chylous acsites resulting from Kaposi's sarcoma in an AIDS patient. Am J Gastroenterol 1994;89: 2252–2253.
230. Green L, Espiritu E, Ladanyi M, et al. Primary lymphomatous effusions in AIDS: a morphologic, immunophenotypic, and molecular study. Mod Pathol 1995;8:39–45.
231. Cappell MS, Shetty V. A multicenter, case-controlled study of the clinical presentation and etiology of ascites and of the safety and clinical

efficacy of diagnostic abdominal paracentesis in HIV seropositive patients. Am J Gastroenterol 1994;89:2172–2177.
232. Mathews WC, Bozzette SA, Hassity S, et al. *Pneumocystis carinii* peritonitis: antemortem confirmation of disseminated pneumocystosis by cytologic examination of body fluids. Arch Intern Med 1992;152: 867–869.
233. Burdette WJ. The role of the surgeon in the management of AIDS. Surg Rounds 1988;11:22–37.
234. Wilcox CM, Forsmark CE, Darraph T, et al. High protein ascites in patients with the acquired immunodeficiency syndrome. Gastroenterology 1991;100:745–748.
235. Ferguson CM. Surgical complications of human immunodeficiency virus infection. Am Surg 1988;54:4–9.
236. Wilson SE, Robinson G, Williams RA, et al. Acquired immune deficiency syndrome (AIDS): indications for abdominal surgery, pathology and outcome. Ann Surg 1989;210:428–433.

34
LIVER DISEASE AND AIDS

Janice Main, Alastair McNair, Robert Goldin, and Howard C. Thomas

The hepatobiliary complications of human immunodeficiency virus (HIV) infection are common but rarely fatal. The liver, a major part of the immune system, is a reservoir for HIV infection and a target organ for many opportunistic infections. Abnormal liver biochemistry is a frequent feature of HIV disease and is usually asymptomatic. Liver biopsy may yield valuable information during an investigation of a patient with wasting or fever of unknown origin, and an opportunistic infection can be identified in 34% of cases by biopsy (1).

In a retrospective study of 501 liver biopsies in HIV-infected patients (2), the main indications for liver biopsy were unexplained abnormal liver biochemistry (89.5%), unexplained fever (71.9%), and hepatomegaly (52%). *Mycobacterium avium* complex infection was the main diagnosis made after liver biopsy, and in patients with unexplained fever and noncontributory bone marrow examinations, the liver biopsy yielded a diagnosis in 58%. In one study in which ultrasound was compared with liver biopsy, the investigators concluded that liver biopsy produced a significantly greater diagnostic yield (3).

Coinfection with hepatotropic viruses is common, and investigators have recognized that HIV itself can infect hepatocytes in addition to Kupffer cells. The average HIV-infected patient receives many antimicrobial agents, and drug toxicity is a common cause of deranged liver function in this group.

PARENCHYMAL DISEASE

Causes of parenchymal disease include infections, neoplasms, and drug toxicity.

Infections

Implicated pathogens include viruses, fungi, protozoa, and bacteria.

VIRUSES

HIV

The liver can be directly infected by the HIV virus. Both hepatic macrophages, including Kupffer cells, and the sinusoidal endothelial cells express CD4, which mediates viral uptake by cells (4). Human hepatoma cell lines that do not express CD4 can also be infected with HIV (5). The p24 gag protein has been demonstrated immunohistochemically in Kupffer cells and endothelial cells in tissue sections (6), as well as in cultured Kupffer cells (7) and endothelial cells (8). The suggestion has been made that Kupffer cells may act as a reservoir for HIV. Viral replication has also been demonstrated within hepatocytes (9).

HIV and the Hepatotropic Viruses

The defect in cell-mediated immunity associated with HIV infection appears to alter the clinical course of many different conditions caused by coinfecting viruses. In addition, coinfection with other viruses may alter the progression of HIV infection. Evidence exists of interaction of HIV and the hepatotropic viruses at the molecular, cellular, and clinical levels.

Hepatitis A Virus Infection. Several outbreaks of hepatitis A virus (HAV) infection have occurred in homosexual men (10) and intravenous drug users (11). However, no evidence indicates that HIV affects the natural history of HAV infection and vice versa. HAV vaccination has been recommended for people in high-risk groups. The antibody response is reduced in the presence of HIV infection (12), but the vaccine appears to be well tolerated by patients (13).

Hepatitis B Virus Infection. Because the routes of transmission and therefore the risk groups for HIV and hepatitis B virus (HBV) infection are similar, coinfection with both viruses is common (Fig. 34.1). About 90% of patients with acquired immunodeficiency syndrome (AIDS) have markers of past or ongoing HBV infection (14).

HBV is transmitted more efficiently than HIV, a finding that presumably reflects the higher levels of HBV in most body fluids (15, 16). One study examined the seroconversion rates for HIV and HBV in a cohort of initially HIV- and HBV-seronegative homosexual men and estimated that HBV was transmitted 8.6 times more efficiently than HIV (17).

Advances in the understanding of the mechanisms regulating the expression of HIV and HBV have provided insight into the ways in which the two viruses may interact. These interactions may occur directly at the molecular level, or indirectly, through affects on cytokine production or cell-mediated immunity.

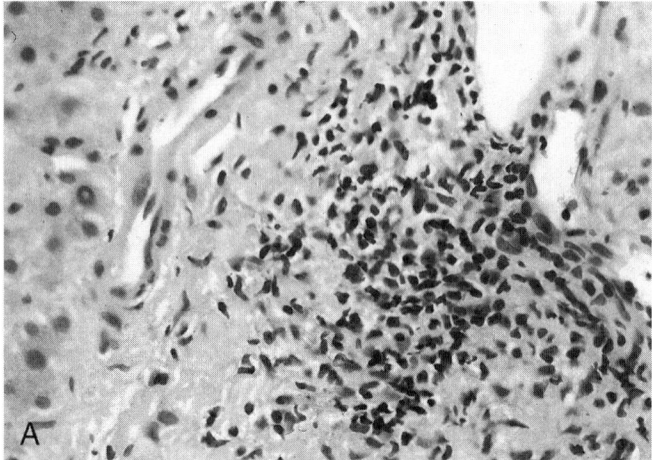
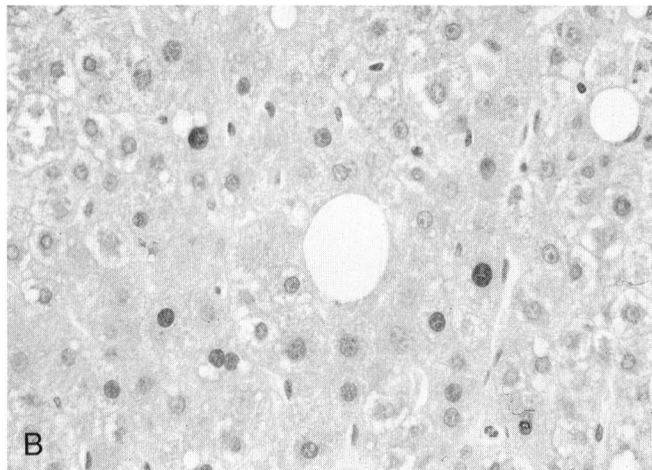

Figure 34.1. A patient with hepatitis B. A. The picture is of mild chronic persistent hepatitis. **B.** Immunohistochemical staining shows large amounts of hepatitis B DNA polymerase indicating active viral replication. (See color section.)

Molecular Interactions of HIV and HBV. A direct interaction between HIV and HBV at the molecular level would require the two viruses to infect the same cells. Although HBV is regarded as predominantly hepatotropic, HBV-related DNA has also been detected in lymphoid cells (18). In a study of 16 HIV-positive men, HBV DNA was detectable in peripheral blood mononuclear cells in all cases by DNA blot hybridization, whereas it was found in only 50% of cases in a control group of HIV-negative patients (19). This finding suggests that HIV may enhance the ability of HBV to infect lymphoid cells, although another study of 29 asymptomatic HIV carriers and 40 HIV-seronegative patients found a similar proportion of HBV DNA in the peripheral blood mononuclear cells of both groups (20). Investigators now know that HIV and HBV can potentially infect the same cell types and therefore may interact directly to influence the level of viral expression. The switch from low- to high-level HIV production in infected CD4+ cells is thought to reflect the activation of transcription factors within the cell that bind to specific elements within the controlling region upstream of the proviral DNA (the long terminal repeat [LTR]), leading to an increase in the rate of transcription of HIV DNA. The HIV LTR contains sequences to which cellular transcription factors can bind, including two sequences recognized by the transcription factors NF-κB and NFAT-1 (21). Both these factors are found in activated T cells and have been linked to the induction of HIV expression after antigen stimulation. The HIV LTR contains two NF-κB sites, deletions of which have been shown to affect the rate of viral replication. Inducers of NF-κB include the cytokine tumor necrosis factor-α (TNF-α), which is known to enhance expression of HIV in chronically infected T lymphocytes and macrophages (22).

Because HIV and HBV can potentially infect the same cell type, proteins produced by HBV have been examined for an effect on HIV expression. The HBV genome contains open-reading frames encoding the DNA polymerase, core and surface antigens, and a transactivation protein, X, which increases the rate of transcription of certain viral and cellular genes (23, 24). Investigators have demonstrated in both hepatocellular and lymphoblastoid cell lines that expression of the X protein is capable of increasing the expression of genes under the control of the HIV LTR (25, 26). This effect is lost if the NF-κB sites in the LTR are disrupted, and because the X protein does not bind directly to DNA, it presumably functions through an interaction with NF-κB or similar transcription factors in HBV-infected cells (27). If this mechanism operates in vivo, the HBV X protein may increase expression of HIV in cells coinfected with both viruses.

The replication of HIV is affected by certain cytokines including TNF-α and interferons (IFNs). Alterations in cytokine production provide HBV with other potential mechanisms of influencing the course of HIV infection. TNF-α increases HIV expression from chronically infected monocytes (28), probably through the induction of NF-κB, and some viruses of the herpes group appear to augment HIV replication by inducing the production of TNF-α (29). Studies of HBV have failed to demonstrate a similar effect. IFN-α has been shown in vitro to have an antiviral effect on HIV-infected T cells and monocytes, although the importance of endogenous IFN production in controlling HIV expression is not clear (30, 31). Some evidence indicates that HBV inhibits both the production and actions of IFNs (32–34), so the expression of HBV proteins in HIV-infected mononuclear cells may oppose the antiviral actions of IFN-α and may allow enhanced HIV replication.

Clinical Course of HBV and HIV Coinfection. Most of the evidence for interactions between HIV and HBV at the molecular level comes from in vitro studies, and, despite the theoretic potential for activation of HIV by HBV, large epidemiologic studies do not suggest that progression to AIDS is more rapid in those coinfected by both viruses. One such study examined a large cohort of homosexual men and concluded that HBV seropositivity is not associated with a more rapid decline in T-helper lymphocyte counts in HIV-positive subjects or with an increased incidence of AIDS at 2.5 years' follow-up (35).

Although evidence of an effect of HBV on the course of HIV infection is limited, considerable clinical and epidemiologic evidence suggests that HIV affects the outcome of HBV infection.

HBV does not appear to be directly cytopathic (36), and the hepatocellular injury of acute and chronic hepatitis B is thought to be mediated by the cellular immune response directed at viral antigens expressed on the hepatocyte surface. Analysis of the lymphocyte infiltrate in liver biopsies from patients with chronic HBV shows the presence of many CD8+ T cells and smaller numbers of CD4+ cells, both of which have specificity for hepatitis B core antigen (HBcAg) but not surface antigen (HBsAg) (37, 38).

Peptides derived from HBcAg are presented at the cell surface in association with major histocompatibility class (MHC) class I antigens allowing recognition by cytotoxic and helper T lymphocytes and elimination of the infected cells (39). Recovery from acute hepatitis B and spontaneous seroconversion in chronic infection results from a clearance of HBV-infected hepatocytes. These events are reflected histologically by a mononuclear cell infiltrate and necrosis of hepatocytes and biochemically by an elevation of liver enzymes. An impairment of the cell-mediated response would be expected to lead to increased replication of HBV and reduced hepatocellular damage. This phenomenon was previously recognized in patients receiving immunosuppressive therapy (40, 41) and has also been reported in association with the impaired cell-mediated immunity caused by HIV infection (42, 43).

HIV may further reduce the elimination of HBV-infected hepatocytes by affecting IFN production. Endogenous and therapeutic IFN is thought to increase the elimination of HBV-infected hepatocytes by enhancing presentation of HBV-related peptides in association with MHC class I antigens at the cell surface (44) and through increased activity of cytotoxic T cells. A direct antiviral action of IFN has also been demonstrated in cultured hepatocytes expressing HBV (45), but the frequent observation of the raised transaminase values during a successful response to IFN-α suggests that IFN immunomodulatory effects are also important. The production of IFN-α by mononuclear cells from patients with AIDS is impaired (46), and this impairment may alter these antiviral actions and allow increased replication of HBV. However, MHC class I antigen expression has been shown to be elevated on peripheral blood mononuclear cells of HBV carriers with coexistent HIV infection (47). Taken together, the evidence suggests that the primary site of the defect of the response to HBV in HIV-infected individuals is in the T-cell response to infected hepatocytes, rather than in IFN production or MHC class I expression.

Many of the epidemiologic data concerning HIV and HBV coinfection have come from trials of IFN therapy and HBV vaccination. The main conclusions from these studies are summarized in Table 34.1. They confirm that HBV replication is increased in HIV coinfection accompanied by an increased risk of developing chronic infection. One such study found that, among a group of HIV-infected men who had not received HBV vaccination, 21% became chronic carriers after HBV infection compared with 7% of those who were HIV seronegative (48). The average duration of HIV infection before HBV was only 8.5 months, and significant immunodeficiency would not be expected at that stage. This trial did not demonstrate a difference between the two groups in liver damage during the acute phase of hepatitis B, with similar peak alanine transaminase (ALT) values and duration of ALT greater than 200 IU/L. However, during follow-up in the 13- to 36-month interval after the onset of infection, those patients with HIV infection and HBV carriage had lower ALT levels than the HIV-negative group. A separate study of chronically HBsAg-positive patients found that subjects who were also HIV positive were more likely to express HBe antigen and HBV DNA in the serum than those who were HIV seronegative (49), although the level of HBeAg and HBV DNA did not correlate with the degree of immune suppression as determined by the CD4 lymphocyte count. In the HBeAg-positive subgroup, concurrent HIV infection was associated with lower serum ALT, the level of which decreased with falling CD4 counts.

A retrospective study from Australia (50) confirmed that HIV-seropositive patients developed chronic HBV infection more frequently than those who were HIV negative (23% versus 4%) and also demonstrated that HIV-positive patients who cleared HBsAg had significantly more circulating CD4+ lymphocytes (mean, 547/mm^3) than those who did not (mean, 352/mm^3). These findings emphasize the importance of an intact cell-mediated immune response for the successful elimination of HBV.

Additional evidence of reduced severity of the liver disease during HIV and HBV coinfection comes from histologic studies. Goldin and colleagues (51) carried out a detailed histologic and immunohistochemical study of 20 HIV-seropositive (non-AIDS) male patients and 30 HIV-negative controls. The histologic activity (using the Knodell histologic activity index) was significantly lower in the HIV-positive group, whereas the expression of HBeAg and HBV polymerase was increased. HBsAg expression was not affected by HIV status.

Therapeutic Implication of HIV and HBV Coinfection. IFN-α therapy in chronic HBV infection is now well established, with an overall response rate of approximately 40% (52) after 3 months of treatment. Early trials of IFN-α

Table 34.1 Summary of the Effects of HIV on the Clinical Course of Hepatitis B

Increased HBV replication, increased HBV DNA
Increased risk of chronic HBV infection after exposure
Reduced liver damage in chronic HBV carriers[a]
Increased risk of reactivation
Reduced response to interferon-α therapy
Reduced response to vaccination

[a]Most studies confirm reduced transaminase levels during chronic infection, at least in HBeAg-positive subjects, and reduced histological disease activity.

found that underlying immunosuppression was associated with a poor response to therapy, and investigators have since shown that treatment with lymphoblastoid or recombinant IFN is unlikely to clear HBV in patients coinfected with HIV (52, 53). Whether impaired cell-mediated immunity alone is responsible for the lack of efficacy of IFN is unclear: other possible factors include the initially heavier HBV load, abnormal cytokine production with high levels of acid-labile IFN (54), downregulation of IFN-α receptors (55), and the presence of anti-IFN antibodies in this group (56). Perrillo and others (57) investigated the effect of pretreatment with a short course of corticosteroids on the response to IFN and found that, although the seroconversion rate was not improved in patients with chronic HBV alone, two of three HIV-seropositive patients cleared HBV. Both had CD4 lymphocyte counts higher than $500/mm^3$, whereas the nonresponder had a much lower CD4 count. However, the use of corticosteroids in this group is unlikely to become routine because of the risks of exacerbating preexisting immunosuppression.

Nucleoside analogs are used in the treatment of HBV infection in HIV-infected patients. HBV DNA polymerase has, like HIV, reverse transcriptase activity. Several reverse transcriptase inhibitors developed as antiretroviral agents also have inhibitory effects on HBV replication in vitro and in vivo.

1. *Zidovudine:* Attempts to improve the seroconversion rate by combining IFN with the reverse-transcriptase inhibitor zidovudine have been disappointing. Zidovudine has inhibitory activity against duck HBV (58), and investigators hoped that similar results would be seen with human HBV. However, in one study of 14 male homosexuals with chronic HBV and symptomatic HIV, zidovudine had no effect on indices of HBV replication (59), and a separate study showed no benefit of combination therapy with IFN-α and zidovudine (60).
2. *Lamivudine,* 3′-thiacytidine, is a deoxynucleoside analog and reverse transcriptase inhibitor routinely used as a component of antiretroviral combination therapy (61). In vitro studies suggested that the drug is active against Hepadnaviridae, and this finding has been confirmed in clinical trials (62). The clearance rates of HBV infection in those who are otherwise healthy have so far been disappointing, but the results of long-term monotherapy studies are awaited. Lamivudine is also being used in the setting of liver transplantation (63) and appears effective as long-term suppressive therapy, although inevitably with long-term monotherapy in the setting of immunosuppression, several reports have noted the development of viral resistance (64, 65). Lamivudine appears well tolerated by both patients with HIV infection and those with hepatitis B liver damage. Inclusion of lamivudine in a combination regimen should therefore be considered for those patients with HIV and HBV infection.
3. *Famciclovir* also has inhibitory effects on HBV replication (66). As with other nucleoside analogs, prolonged monotherapy in an immunosuppressed patient with HIV and HBV infection is unlikely to achieve clearance of chronic HBV, but when one has clinical concerns about HBV-related disease, this drug is a further option to consider.

Protease inhibitors are increasingly used as therapy for HIV infection. An HIV- and HBV-infected patient participated in an early trial of ritonavir monotherapy (67). The reduction in the HIV load and the increase in the CD4 count were accompanied by a flare in the transaminase levels, a reduction in the HBV DNA levels, and a clearance of HBeAg. Investigators postulated that the restoration of immune function that followed effective antiretroviral therapy was followed by immune recognition and lysis of HBV-infected hepatocytes.

Prevention. Because the antibody response to HBsAg is helper T-cell dependent (68), immunosuppressed individuals have a reduced response to HBV vaccination. Approximately 40% of patients undergoing hemodialysis (69) and up to 80% of organ transplant recipients receiving immunosuppressive therapy (70) fail to develop anti-HBs antibodies after vaccination, compared with a nonresponse rate of only 2.5 to 5% in immunocompetent recipients (71). Predictably, therefore, the response rate is poor in HIV-infected individuals. Most trials report low antibody response or nonresponse rates of more than 40% (72–74). One study found that HIV-positive individuals infected with HBV around the time of first HBV vaccination had a high (80%) HBV carriage rate, a finding suggesting that the vaccine may temporarily impair the immune response to HBV in those with HIV coinfection (48).

Reactivation of HBV. Reactivation of HBV replication has been described both spontaneously and during immunosuppressive therapy (75), and several cases have now been reported in patients with HIV infection (76, 77). The reasons underlying the reactivation are unclear. After recovery from acute infection or seroconversion in chronic infection, viral replication can persist for prolonged periods even in the presence of anti-HBs (78). An important factor in reactivation may be the progressive decline in humoral immunity in HIV infection. The levels of anti-HBs decrease with time in HIV-positive individuals with a history of HBV (79) and also after vaccination (74). Reactivation is usually associated with the reappearance of HBsAg and HBV DNA, but HBeAg does not always reappear (80), and anti-HBc antibodies may persist (81). Another unexpected feature of HBV reactivation in this setting is the severity of disease, even in patients with full-blown AIDS and low CD4 lymphocyte counts. Liver damage may be severe, even fatal, and investigators have suggested that mechanisms other than T-cell–mediated cytotoxicity lead to liver cell death. Perhaps, for example, at high levels of viral replication, HBV becomes cytopathic, a situation analogous to the reactivation of HBV seen after liver transplantation. As with patients with high levels of HBV replication after liver transplantation, reports now note the development of fibrosing cholestatic hepatitis in patients with HIV and hepatitis B (82).

Differentiating between reactivation and reinfection is important in these patients, as is continued monitoring of HBV markers. In particular, the absence of HBeAg does not exclude reactivation, and HBV DNA should be sought in an HIV-positive patient with an acute hepatic illness.

Hepatitis C Virus Infection. Hepatitis C virus infection (HCV) appears to be predominantly transmitted by the parenteral route and is commonly found in intravenous drug users and recipients of blood products (83). Sexual transmission probably occurs (84), but it appears rarer than with HBV and HIV, and therefore, coinfection with HIV and HCV is more commonly seen in intravenous drug users and hemophiliacs than in homosexual men.

One group confirmed the low level of sexual transmission in female partners of hemophiliac patients, but noted that the frequency of transmission was five times higher with HIV infection (85). Perhaps HIV and HCV coinfection is associated with higher levels of HCV viremia, and investigators have suggested that this may also explain the higher rates of HCV vertical transmission seen with HIV coinfection (86).

Our understanding of the immunopathogenesis of HCV infection is limited. HCV may have a cytopathic effect on hepatocytes, and more severe disease is reported in patients receiving immunosuppressive therapy (87).

Martin and others (88) described 3 patients with HIV and HCV coinfection who all developed symptomatic cirrhosis within 3 years of the onset of hepatitis, a finding suggesting a more rapidly progressive course than is seen with HCV alone. In one study, the outcome of HCV infection in 44 HIV-negative patients was compared with the outcome in 32 patients with HIV infection (89). Cirrhosis developed within 15 years in 25% of those with HIV and in only 6.5% of those who were HIV negative.

Several reports of patients with hemophilia and HCV have noted more rapidly progressive liver disease in those with HIV infection (90, 91). The same groups have also demonstrated higher levels of HCV RNA in patients with HIV infection (92, 93).

However, not all studies have confirmed these findings. In one study of 512 HIV-infected patients (94), mainly nondrug-using homosexual men, 66 patients with HCV infection were followed-up for a mean of 28 months, and no effect of HCV on HIV or HIV on HCV outcome was demonstrated. In an Italian study (95) of 416 patients with HIV infection, the clinical outcome was compared in those with (214 patients) and without HIV infection. No effect of HCV on HIV outcome, including rate of decline of CD4 count, was demonstrated.

The follow-up period in most of these studies has been short, and few groups have looked at other host and viral factors that are thought to be important in the natural history of HCV infection. Perhaps the relative timing or route of the infections is relevant in determining outcome. Diagnostic difficulties may be encountered when testing HIV-positive patients for HCV infection. Just as with HBV infection, a reduction in the level of antibodies has been described in patients with HIV infection (96), and a high number of indeterminate recombinant immunoblot assays has also been noted (97).

Therapeutic Implications of HIV and HCV Infection. In view of the poor response to IFN therapy seen in HIV-positive patients with chronic HBV, the early HCV trials often excluded patients with HIV infection. In one of the early studies of IFN-α as therapy for HCV in HIV infection, 12 patients were treated, and a biochemical response was noted in 3 (25%) (98). In a larger Spanish study reported by Soriano and others (99), the response to IFN was studied in 88 HIV-positive patients with HCV-associated chronic liver disease and CD4 counts higher than $200/mm^3$. IFN-α was administered for 12 months (5 MU thrice weekly for 3 months and then 3 MU thrice weekly for 9 months). Zidovudine was prescribed for those with CD4 counts of less than $500/mm^3$. The investigators noted that 31 of 72 (43%) patients followed-up for at least 14 weeks achieved complete response. The sustained response rate was higher in those with CD4 counts of more than $500/mm^3$. The risk of subsequent relapse is unknown in this group. Preliminary data suggest a low risk of reactivation (100), but clearly, in a group at risk of subsequent immune suppression, longer term follow-up is important.

Investigators have noted adverse effects of IFN in this setting, with reports of sudden decreases in the CD4 count (101, 102). This phenomenon was studied by Soriano's group in their large study, and three (5.2%) of their HIV-infected patients had a significant decrease in the CD4 count (103).

The combination of ribavirin and IFN appears a promising approach for those patients with chronic HCV who are otherwise healthy (104), and it may be worth considering in those with HIV and severe liver disease related to HCV. However, ribavirin can antagonize the effects of other nucleoside analogs (105) and may therefore limit the antiretroviral choice for the patient.

Hepatitis Delta Virus Infection. Hepatitis delta virus (HDV) is a defective RNA virus that requires HBV as a helper virus either infecting simultaneously with HBV (coinfection) or infecting chronic HBV carriers (superinfection). It leads to more severe liver disease than HBV infection alone.

HDV, like HCV, is thought to be cytopathic, and certainly coinfection with HIV leads to a worsening of liver disease (106). Sexual transmission of HDV is inefficient, so coinfection is uncommon in homosexual men and is mainly found in intravenous drug users and recipients of blood products. In HIV-negative patients, HDV has an inhibitory effect on the replication of HBV (107) with low or undetectable levels of HBV DNA in the serum, although high level expression of both viruses has been described in some patients (108). HIV appears to alter the inhibitory effect of HDV on HBV. One study found that HBV DNA was detectable in 23% of serum samples from patients coinfected HIV and HDV, but it was not detectable in those with HDV alone (109). Another group reported similar findings and also noted that coinfection with HIV decreased the antibody response to HDV and was associated with episodes of reactivation with elevation of transaminase levels (110). In one cross-sectional study (111), 15 patients with HDV and HIV infection were compared with 29 patients with only HDV infection. This study confirmed that HIV reduces the suppressive effect of HDV on HBV replication but found no effect of HIV infection in HDV replication and no increase in the severity of the liver disease. Investigators have also suggested that HDV can suppress HCV replication in patients with HIV infection (112).

The response rate to IFN-α in HIV-negative patients with HDV infection is disappointingly low. Lamivudine, with its inhibitory effects on HBV replication, may be worth incorporating into antiretroviral regimens.

Hepatitis E Virus. The hepatitis E virus (HEV) is an important cause of enterally transmitted non-A, non-B hepatitis, but little information is available concerning the influence of HIV on the outcome of HEV. Reports noted an increased seroprevalence of anti-HEV antibodies in Italian injecting drug users (113) and homosexual men (114), but other reports note false-positive test results in this group (115). Detailed studies suggest that, in homosexual men, foreign travel rather than sexual practice can predispose to HEV infection (116).

HEV carries a mortality of around 20% in pregnant women (117). This mortality is not explained, but if it is related to immunosuppression, more severe episodes of hepatitis E may be anticipated in those with underlying HIV infection.

Hepatitis G Virus Infection. Hepatitis G virus (HGV) infection is commonly detected in patients with a history of exposure to blood products, but as yet little is known about the interactions of HIV and HGV.

Other Viruses

Cytomegalovirus. In both postmortem and liver biopsy series, cytomegalovirus (CMV) is one of the commonest organisms to infect the liver. It may infect the liver parenchyma or more commonly the biliary tree (described later), but usually it is part of a systemic infection (118).

CMV hepatitis is rarely symptomatic in this group, but unusual metastatic-like lesions have been described on computed tomography (119). The histologic features range from classic large, basophilic intranuclear and stippled basophilic intracytoplasmic inclusions to cells with enlarged nuclei in which only a poorly defined inclusion can be seen. When the cells have the former features, one may see an artifactual halo around the nuclear inclusions giving the cell an "owl's eye" appearance (120). In our experience, this is more common in postmortem studies than in biopsy material. The inclusions may be seen in hepatocytes (most often periportal), biliary epithelial cells, Kupffer cells, or endothelial cells. The presence of CMV in the liver can be confirmed immunohistochemically, using antibodies to early antigen, by in situ hybridization or culture (121). The role of these two latter techniques in liver biopsies in which no evidence of CMV is noted on immunohistochemical staining has not been established. The liver usually shows the features of acute hepatitis with evidence of hepatocyte degeneration, necrosis, and regeneration. Collections of neutrophils in the parenchyma have been suggested as useful markers for CMV infection in patients with AIDS, as in transplant recipients. CMV infection may be associated with a lymphocytic infiltrate or with granulomas (122), although the latter is uncommon in patients with AIDS.

The treatment for CMV hepatitis is intravenous ganciclovir or foscarnet.

Herpes Simplex. Herpes simplex virus (HSV) can involve the liver in patients with AIDS as part of a systemic disease (123). HSV produces characteristic gross lesions involving the capsule and the deeper parenchyma. These lesions are composed of multiple soft, hemorrhagic, yellow-orange lesions ranging in size up to several centimeters in diameter (124). Scattered foci of coagulative necrosis are surrounded by hepatocytes that contain "ground glass" and irregular eosinophilic Cowdry type A intranuclear inclusions often surrounded by a halo. The diagnosis can be confirmed immunohistochemically or by culture.

Intravenous acyclovir is the treatment of choice.

Varicella-Zoster Virus. Fatal hepatitis complicating chickenpox was described in one AIDS patient (125) who had no apparent response to intravenous acyclovir.

Adenovirus. Adenovirus infections have been diagnosed rarely ante mortem in patients with AIDS (126). Adenovirus infection is associated with extensive nonzonal hepatocyte necrosis and hemorrhage. Hepatocytes surrounding such areas may contain "smoky" intranuclear inclusions that can also be seen electron microscopically. Immunohistochemical techniques can also be applied to diagnosis.

Epstein–Barr Virus. Epstein–Barr virus has been associated with chronic hepatitis in children with AIDS (127–129). This virus does not appear to be a significant cause of liver disease in adults. As in liver transplant recipients, Epstein–Barr virus infections may be associated with lymphoproliferative disorders and lymphoma (130). Immunohistochemical detection of the virus can now be carried out in both paraffin and frozen sections: in situ hybridization can also be useful.

FUNGI

Cryptococcus neoformans, Histoplasma capsulatum, Candida albicans, Coccidioides immitis, and *Penicillium marneffei* may all involve the liver, usually as part of a systemic disease (131–133). Primary involvement of the liver may occur, but it is rare (131, 134). The inflammatory response associated with these infections may be granulomatous, although the granulomas are often poorly formed and consist of loose aggregates of macrophages surrounding microabscesses (Fig. 34.2). Although the organisms may be visible on hematoxylin and eosin staining, special stains, especially diastase periodic acid–Schiff or methenamine silver, are essential.

Invasive fungal disease with *Aspergillus* sp. is usually reported in the setting of neutropenia or significant neutro-

Pneumocystis carinii

Pneumocystis carinii infection is a major cause of lung disease in AIDS and has now been increasingly recognized as a cause of extrapulmonary disease (136–138). The liver can be involved, and many cases have been associated with the use of nebulized pentamidine prescribed for *Pneumocystis* pneumonia prophylaxis, although cases have also occurred when more systemic agents were prescribed. The histologic features can be similar to those seen in the lung, with a foamy eosinophilic exudate containing cysts that can be demonstrated with methenamine silver staining within the hepatic sinusoids (Fig. 34.3). In some cases, acellular nodules composed of these organisms have been described (139). These lesions are characterized by the lack of inflammatory response.

Diagnosis. In the absence of associated lung disease, this diagnosis may be difficult to make clinically, and a high index of suspicion is required, particularly if the patient is receiving nebulized pentamidine for *Pneumocystis carinii* pneumonia prophylaxis. Respiratory symptoms may be absent, and the patient may present with fever or with impaired liver function. The infection has no particularly characteristic bio-

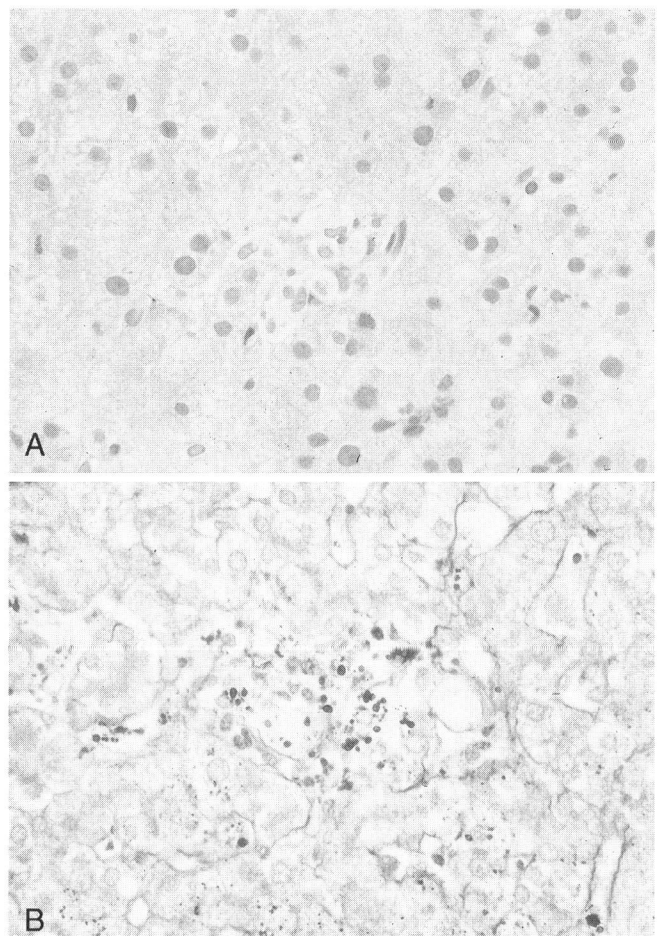

Figure 34.2. **A.** Poorly formed granuloma from an African patient. **B.** The Grocott stain revealed fungi with features consistent with histoplasmosis. (See color section.)

phil dysfunction and is, predictably, not a major feature of HIV-associated immunosuppression. The use of myelotoxic agents including zidovudine, ganciclovir, and cytotoxic regimens can lead to neutropenia, however, and *Aspergillus* abscesses have been reported (135).

Diagnosis

In most systemic fungal disease, the diagnosis is more likely to be made from more accessible sites than the liver. For example, histoplasmosis may be diagnosed after sputum culture, and cryptococcal infection may be ascertained from serum antigen tests or culture of cerebrospinal fluid.

Treatment

Standard antifungal therapy can be prescribed with fluconazole or amphotericin for cryptococcal and *Candida* infection and itraconazole or amphotericin for *Aspergillus* and *Histoplasma* infection. If invasive fungal infection has occurred in the setting of significant neutropenia, then potentially myelotoxic drugs should be dose adjusted, or the use of granulocyte colony-stimulating factor should be considered.

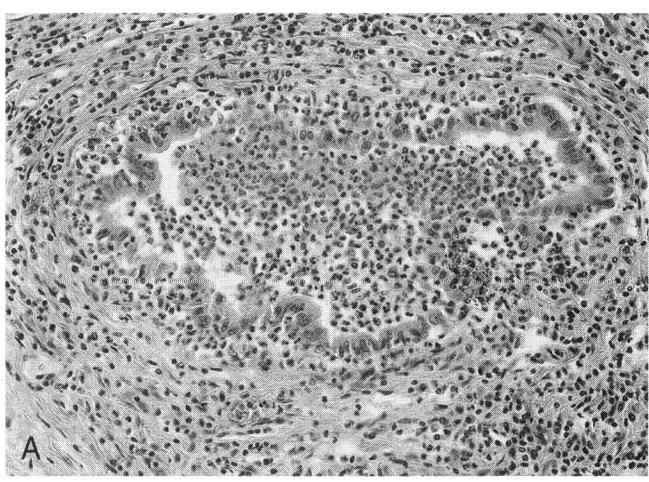

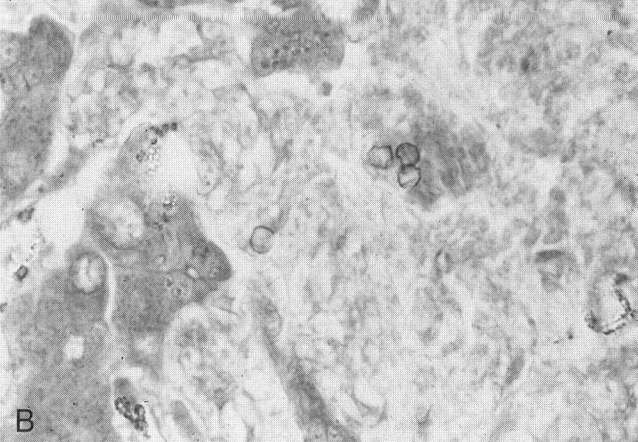

Figure 34.3. **A.** Liver containing a granular exudate. The patient had been receiving pentamidine prophylaxis for *Pneumocystis*. **B.** *P. carinii* cysts are present in the Grocott stain. (See color section.)

chemical features, and the diagnosis therefore relies on the biopsy appearances.

Treatment. Systemic treatment is required with trimethoprim–sulfamethoxazole or second-line agents as required.

PROTOZOA

Toxoplasmosis

Toxoplasmosis can involve the liver as part of systemic disease (140).

Leishmaniasis

Hepatic leishmaniasis has now been frequently reported in HIV-infected patients (Fig. 34.4). Fever is usually the main presenting symptom, and bone marrow involvement is also common. Obtaining a detailed travel history is important in all AIDS patients because such infections can reactivate many years after their initial acquisition. The response to treatment is generally disappointing (141–144), and many drugs such as the antimonials are potentially toxic and do not have activity against all the subtypes. More promising results have been described with liposomal amphotericin and pentamidine.

BACTERIA

Mycobacteria

Mycobacterial infection of the liver is the most common infection diagnosed on liver biopsy in patients with AIDS (145). Enlarged intra-abdominal lymph nodes can cause biliary obstruction.

Mycobacterium tuberculosis, *M. avium-intracellulare*, *M. xenopi*, and *M. kansasii* may all involve the liver (146–149). In one retrospective study of 501 liver biopsies (145), the most common diagnosis was *M. avium* complex, seen in 17.4% of specimens. Reactivation of *M. tuberculosis* is com-

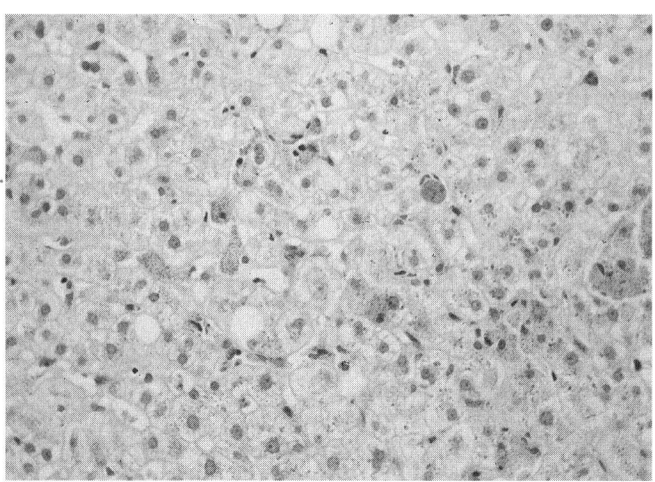

Figure 34.4. Leishmaniasis. This shows Leishman–Donovan bodies in sinusoidal macrophages. (See color section.)

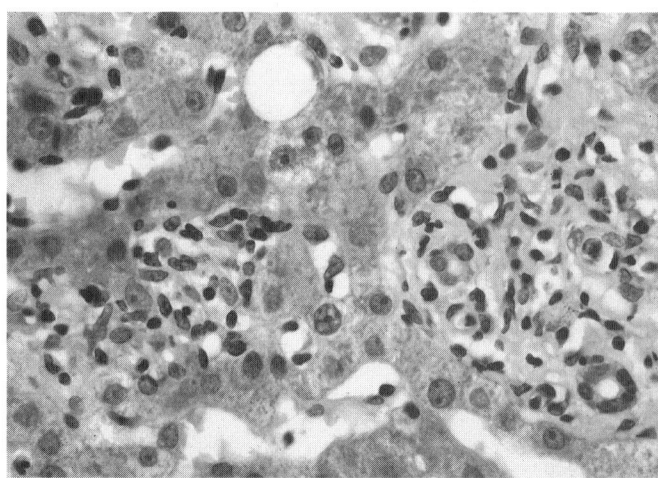

Figure 34.5. Loose aggregate of macrophages from a case in which *Mycobacterium tuberculosis* was cultured. No acid-fast bacilli were seen on special stains. (See color section.)

mon in early disease, and infection with atypical mycobacteria such as *M. avium-intracellulare* is more common after a prolonged period of immunosuppression, such as characterized by a CD4 count lower than $50/mm^3$. The degree of immunosuppression is often reflected in the liver biopsy appearances, with well-formed granulomas and few acid-fast bacilli seen in early disease (usually *M. tuberculosis*) and more poorly formed granulomas and more organisms in later disease (more typical of *M. avium-intracellulare*) (Fig. 34.5). The granulomas may be noncaseating, or one may see poorly defined aggregates of foamy macrophages or even bacilli within single macrophages (131, 134, 146, 149–151). Ziehl–Neelsen and diastase periodic acid–Schiff staining techniques are essential to identify these organisms. Investigators have claimed that histologic examination is more sensitive than culture in detecting mycobacteria in liver biopsies, although culture is necessary to identify the different types of organisms and to establish drug sensitivities (152). Furthermore, culture may detect tuberculosis even in the absence of bacilli or granulomas on biopsy.

Diagnosis. Culture of the liver biopsy specimen in addition to routine histologic examination is important because culture may prove positive in the absence of negative microscopy. In terms of diagnostic yield, bone marrow is usually superior to liver biopsy (1).

The patient with *Mycobacterium tuberculosis* infection may have other clinical features to suggest the diagnosis, with cervical lymphadenopathy or lung disease, particularly affecting the upper lobes. Fever may be the only clue. The classic description of the elevated alkaline phosphatase may be present, but only the transaminases may be elevated, or the results of liver function tests may be completely normal. *M. avium-intracellulare* infection usually occurs in late stage disease, and presentation may be with fever or weight loss.

Treatment. Appropriate antimycobacterial therapy should be prescribed. The pyrexia and other features may some weeks to respond fully to therapy.

Bartonella

Bartonella henselae and *Bartonella quintana* (previously known as *Rochalimaea*) have been identified as the cause of bacillary angiomatosis in patients with AIDS (153, 154). These spiral organisms can be visualized using tinctorial stains (including silver stains such as Warthin–Starry or Steiner's, Brown–Hopps, or Brown–Brenn) and electron microscopy. Bacillary angiomatosis can involve the liver. In the liver, this infection may be associated with peliosis hepatis ("bacillary peliosis") (155), although not all cases of peliosis hepatis can be ascribed to this pathogen. Peliosis hepatis associated with bacillary angiomatosis appears as multiple cystic, blood-filled spaces a few millimeters in diameter. Typically, they are usually associated with fibromyxoid stroma containing a few inflammatory cells, capillaries, and clumps of granular blue material containing the organisms (155).

Diagnosis. The classic skin appearances of bacillary angiomatosis may be present. Peliosis hepatis may be suggested by ultrasound appearances, and the biopsy appearances are also diagnostic.

Treatment. Erythromycin is the treatment of choice, although spontaneous resolution has been reported (156).

Other Bacteria

Acute hepatitis has also been described in the setting of HIV with *Listeria monocytogenes* (157), *Fusobacterium* (158), and spirochetal infection (159).

Neoplasms

The most common neoplasms associated with AIDS are lymphomas, both non–Hodgkin's lymphoma (NHL) and less commonly Hodgkin's disease (HD), and Kaposi's sarcoma (KS) (121). Both lymphoma and KS of the liver are seen as part of systemic disease, although pure hepatic involvement is also possible. KS is the commonest liver neoplasm found at postmortem examination, although it rarely pro-

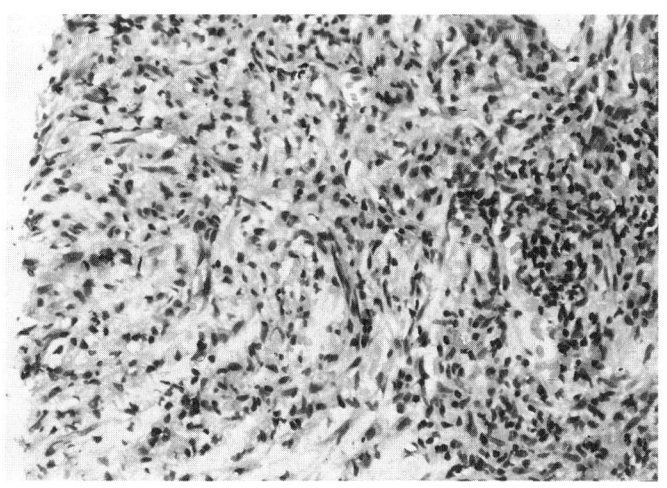

Figure 34.6. This postmortem specimen shows Kaposi's sarcoma involving the portal tract. (See color section.)

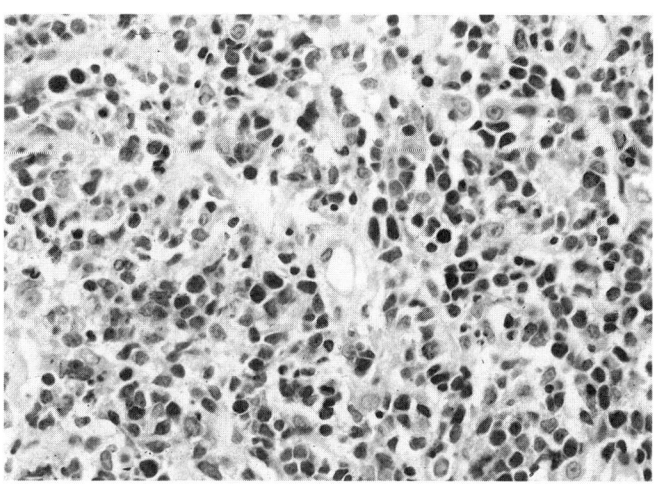

Figure 34.7. Pleomorphic centroblastic B-cell lymphoma in a patient with AIDS. Organ involvement was widespread. (See color section.)

duces clinical problems in life (Fig. 34.6). KS, in patients with AIDS, tends to involve multiple organ systems, and the liver is involved late in the course of disease. Primary involvement of the liver with KS can occur (160). One-third of patients with cutaneous KS have liver involvement (131, 146), and generally involvement of the liver is seen in association with KS in other viscera, especially the intestines and the lungs.

At postmortem examination, KS appears as irregular, purplish brown nodules most frequently seen deep to the capsule or in the hilar region (131). Histologically, multifocal nodules are often hemorrhagic and tend to involve the larger portal tracts and are therefore rarely detected on liver biopsy. They have the typical histologic features of KS seen elsewhere in the body.

LYMPHOMA

Lymphoma, both NHL and HD, may occur in patients with HIV and behaves atypically. NHL in these patients is usually a high-grade lymphoma of B-cell origin, commonly with both widespread disease and extranodal involvement (161, 162) (Fig. 34.7).

Histologically, these tumors are usually small or large cell noncleaved cell lymphomas or immunoblastic lymphomas with plasmacytoid differentiation. T-cell lymphomas, some of which are CD30 (Ki-1) positive, have also been described (163). Although primary involvement of the liver or bile ducts has been reported, it is rare (146, 150, 162, 164, 165).

HD, although less common than NHL, is also a more aggressive tumor, both histologically and clinically, in patients with AIDS (161, 166, 167).

Drugs and Hepatotoxicity

Hepatotoxicity is common with many of the agents used in the management of HIV infection. In one study of 36 HIV-infected patients with jaundice, drug-induced hepatitis was diagnosed in 11 (31%) (168). Moreover, particularly in patients with a history of recreational drug use, hepatitis can be associated with many agents including Ecstacy, and increased alcohol intake is a common way of "coping with HIV."

ANTIRETROVIRAL AGENTS

Acute cholestatic hepatitis has been suggested as an adverse effect of zidovudine. However, in view of the large numbers of patients who have been treated with this agent, the incidence of this complication must be low (169, 170). Massive hepatic steatosis and lactic acidosis have also been reported in patients taking zidovudine (171). Dideoxyinosine (ddI) has been associated with fatal hepatitis with microvesicular and macrovesicular fatty change, hepatocellular necrosis, cholestasis, and fibrosis in patients receiving the drug (172, 173).

Although these toxic reactions are rare, they are similar to the reports of multisystem failure and lactic acidosis reported in patients participating in a trial of fialuridine, another nucleoside analog, for chronic hepatitis B (174). Many of these agents appear to be able to damage host mitochondria (175).

Protease inhibitors can also cause liver toxicity, and mildly deranged liver function tests have been reported with indinavir and ritonavir. Raised serum bilirubin has also been described with protease inhibitors and may be secondary to hepatotoxicity or hemolysis. The protease inhibitors inhibit the hepatic cytochrome P450 system and therefore have many potential interactions with other agents.

ANTIMICROBIAL AGENTS

Granulomas have been ascribed to the use of cotrimoxazole in patients with AIDS (169, 176). Liver disease caused by this drug appears to be more common in patients with AIDS than in others (177), but this finding may reflect the high doses used to treat *Pneumocystis carinii* pneumonia. Antifungal agents and antituberculous drugs are commonly associated with hepatotoxicity, and therapeutic modifications are often necessary (178).

IRON OVERLOAD

The early use of zidovudine was generally at high doses and as monotherapy. Transfusion-dependent anemia was not unusual and led to significant iron overload in some patients (179). Iron is initially deposited in the Kupffer cells and portal tracts, and as more iron accumulates, it is found within hepatocytes. Although this phenomenon may be associated with portal fibrosis, as yet no descriptions of progressive liver disease have been published.

Nonspecific Lesions

As part of the generalized lymphoid depletion that may be seen in patients with AIDS, the portal tracts may contain fewer lymphocytes than normal (180). Histologic findings in the liver for which no specific cause has been found include fatty change, focal hepatocyte necrosis, granulomas, sinusoidal abnormalities, prominent Kupffer cells, portal inflammation, fibrosis, and bile duct proliferation (4, 131, 132, 148, 150, 151, 180–182). Large-droplet fatty change is extremely common. The fat is frequently periportal (resembling the appearances in protein–calorie malnutrition), but it may be perivenular (14, 147). Investigators have suggested that it is caused by associated malnutrition or systemic disease. No study has correlated the severity or the distribution of fatty change with either nutritional status or other disease processes. Although alcoholic liver disease does occur in patients with AIDS, it is uncommon (14, 182). Kupffer cells containing ceroid pigment may be conspicuous (180). They also may contain iron or display erythrophagocytosis, probably resulting from associated viremia.

The presence of iron may not always be associated with a history of blood transfusion. It may result from mobilization of iron storage pools, and it could be secondary to the erythrophagocytosis.

The sinusoidal abnormalities range from sinusoidal dilatation to peliosis hepatis. Sinusoidal dilatation in patients with AIDS is usually focal and does not show a particular zonal distribution. It is often associated with atrophy of the adjacent hepatocytes, and perisinusoidal fibrosis may be present (183).

The frequency of sinusoidal dilatation has varied considerably in different studies. Peliosis hepatis is common in patients with AIDS (4, 131), and, as described previously, it has been linked to bacillary angiomatosis.

Veno-occlusive disease has been described in patients with AIDS (184). Liver involvement has also been reported in patients with the diffuse infiltrative lymphocytosis syndrome (185).

Electron microscopy of the liver in AIDS has also been performed, with interesting results (186). Cytoplasmic collections of membranous rings were found in many hepatocytes. Prominent Ito cells were also noted.

BILIARY TRACT DISEASE

Biliary tract complications of HIV infection include cholangiopathy and alcalculous cholecystitis (187). Involvement by tumors occurs, but it is uncommon. Cholangiopathy is rarely a cause of jaundice in patients with AIDS (188). Drugs are the most common cause of jaundice in this group of patients.

Cholangiopathy

HIV-associated cholangiopathy has many similarities with sclerosing cholangitis. The trigger is thought to be associated opportunistic infection, and patients often have evidence of CMV infection, cryptosporidiosis (189), microsporidiosis, or *Cyclospora* infection (190), but often no pathogen is identified (189).

Microsporidia are the most common pathogens when blood cultures and multiple stool tests are negative (191).

Electron microscopy is necessary to distinguish the two most common species (*Enterocytozoon bieneusi, Encephalitozoon intestinalis*) (190).

DIAGNOSIS

The patient may complain of right hypochondrial discomfort and tenderness. The typical biochemical response, which may predate the symptoms, is a climbing alkaline phosphatase. Jaundice may follow. Conversely, liver function tests may be normal despite biliary tract disease demonstrated by endoscopic retrograde cholangiopancreatography (ERCP) (192). Ultrasound examination usually suggests cholangiopathy, but results may be normal, and ERCP is required to establish the diagnosis. This technique has the advantage that samples can be taken from the biliary tree for diagnosis of infection, and, if necessary, sphincterotomy can be performed. Four distinct ERCP patterns have been described (193):

1. *Papillary stenosis:* dilated common bile duct with appearances of stricture in the distal 2 to 4 mm and retention of contrast medium.
2. *Sclerosing cholangitis:* focal strictures and dilatations in intrahepatic and extrahepatic bile ducts (Fig. 34.8).
3. *Both papillary stenosis and sclerosing cholangitis:* This is the commonest pattern seen in approximately 60% of patients.
4. Long extrahepatic bile duct strictures.

Narrowing of the bile ducts may be associated with pancreatic inflammation or neoplasia (Fig. 34.9). In contrast to sclerosing cholangitis in immunocompetent individuals, the entire common bile duct appears diseased, and marked dilatation of the entire biliary tree is common.

In Cello's description of 40 patients with AIDS cholangiopathy (189), ampullary biopsy demonstrated inflammation only in 22 cases, evidence of CMV infection in 7, cryptosporidiosis in 5, *Mycobacterium avium-intracellulare* in 3, both CMV and cryptosporidiosis in 1 lymphoma in 1, and KS in 1. More recent studies have tended to produce a higher diagnostic yield (194). Liver biopsy has little role to play in the evaluation of this group of patients. Biopsy samples can be taken from the duodenum or biliary tree (after sphincterotomy). Brush cytology and examination of

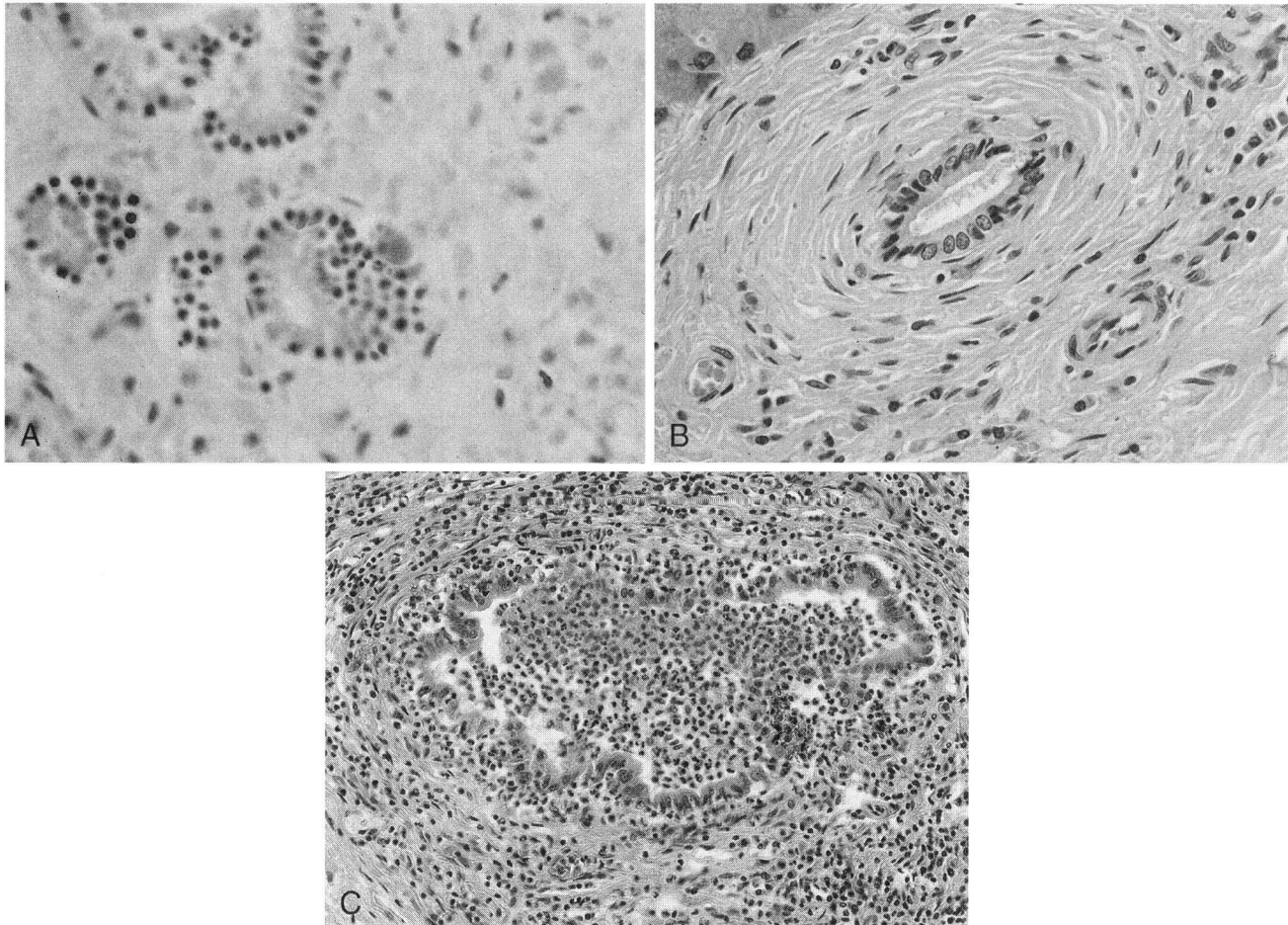

Figure 34.8. Postmortem material from a patient who died after recurrent episodes of cholangitis. A. Cytomegalovirus was present at all levels of the biliary tree. **B.** Some of the bile ducts showed the features of sclerosing cholangitis. **C.** Elsewhere, evidence of suppurative cholangitis was noted. (See color section.)

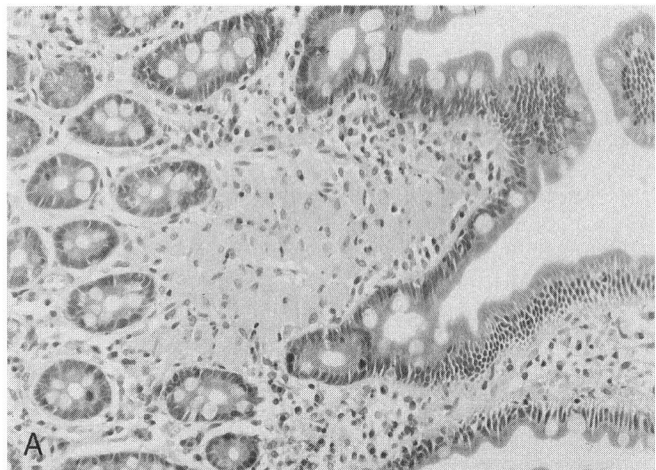
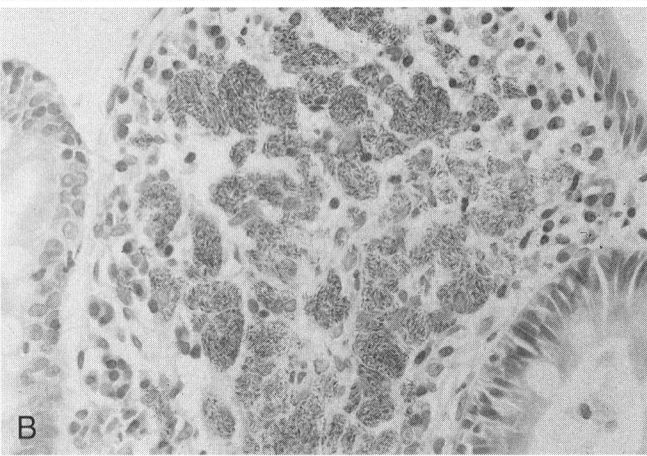

Figure 34.9. A and B. Ampullary biopsy from a patient with bile duct obstruction. Sheets of foamy macrophage containing large numbers of acid-fast bacilli are present. Culture confirmed the presence of Mycobacterium avium-intracellulare. (See color section.)

the biliary fluid are useful in the diagnosis of microsporidiosis and cryptosporidiosis.

TREATMENT

Even when a pathogen is identified, the response to appropriate antimicrobial therapy is disappointing. Successful chemotherapy of lymphoma has been associated with resolution of the condition (195). Some symptomatic benefit often follows sphincterotomy, although alkaline phosphatase levels may continue to rise because of progressive intrahepatic disease (196). The prognosis of patients with AIDS cholangiopathy is poor. The reason is that opportunistic infections of the biliary tree occur in patients with low CD4 counts, but survival is not worse than in matched patients with low CD4 counts and no biliary tract disease (192).

Acalculous Cholecystitis

Acalculous cholecystitis can follow *Campylobacter* or *Salmonella* enteritis. It may also be seen in association with cryptosporidiosis (197), CMV infection (198, 199), microsporidiosis (200), or *Isospora belli* infection (201) and often in association with cholangiopathy. Gallbladder diseases associated with gallstones may, of course, also be seen (202).

The patient typically presents with right hypochrondrial pain and fever. The alkaline phosphatase level is elevated, and ultrasound examination may demonstrate thickening of the gallbladder wall or gallbladder dilatation. The examination may also be normal.

Cases attributed to *Salmonella* or *Campylobacter* may respond to appropriate antimicrobial therapy, but patients with severe cases may require surgical treatment. The gallbladder wall is usually edematous and may be ulcerated. A laparoscopic approach to therapy is generally favored in this group of patients (202).

In conclusion, recognition and treatment of liver disease in HIV infection may improve the quality of life of an AIDS patient. A detailed history is important, particularly regarding previous travel and current medications. The biochemical liver function tests may point to liver disease rather than to a specific diagnosis, but it is usually possible to establish the diagnosis with a combination of ultrasound, liver biopsy, or, when appropriate, computed tomography or ERCP. For investigation of a fever of unknown cause, bone marrow examination may be more successful in yielding the diagnosis.

References

1. Bonacini M. Hepatobiliary complications in patients with human immunodeficiency virus infection. Am J Med 1992;92:404–411.
2. Poles MA, Dieterich DT, Schwarz ED, et al. Liver biopsy findings in 501 patients infected with human immunodeficiency virus (HIV). J Acquir Immune Defic Syndr Hum Retrovirol 1996;11:170–177.
3. Beale TJ, Wetton CW, Crofton ME. A sonographic–pathological correlation of liver biopsies in patients with the acquired immunodeficiency syndrome (AIDS). Clin Radiol 1995;50:761–764.
4. Scoazec JY, Feldmann G. Both macrophages and endothelial cells of the human hepatic sinusoid express the CD4 molecule, a receptor for the human immunodeficiency virus. Hepatology 1990;13:1265.
5. Cao YZ, Friedman KA, Huang YX, et al. CD4-independent, productive human immunodeficiency virus type 1 infection of hepatoma cell lines in vitro. J Virol 1990;64:2553–2559.
6. Housett C, Boucher O, Girard PM, et al. Immunohistochemical evidence for human immunodeficiency-1 infection of Kupffer cells. Hum Pathol 1990;21:404–408.
7. Schmitt MP, Gendrault JL, Schweitzer C, et al. Permissivity of primary cultures of human Kupffer cells for HIV-1. AIDS Res Hum Retroviruses 1990;6:987–991.
8. Steffan AM, Schmitt MP, Gendrault JL, et al. Productive infection of primary cultures of human immunodeficiency virus. Exp Cell Biol 1989;57:118–119.
9. Cao YZ, Dieterich D, Thomas PA, et al. Identification and quantitation of HIV-1 in the liver of patients with AIDS. AIDS 1992;6:65–70.
10. Henning KJ, Bell E, Braun J, et al. A community-wide outbreak of hepatitis A: risk factors for infection among homosexual men and bisexual men. Am J Med 1995;99:132–136.
11. Centers for Disease Control. Hepatitis A among drug users. MMWR Morb Mortal Wkly Rep 1988;37:297–305.
12. Hess G, Clemens R, Bienzle U, et al. Immunogenecity and safety of an inactivated hepatitis A vaccine in anti-HIV positive and negative homosexual men. J Med Virol 1995;46:40–42.
13. Bodsworth NJ, Neilsen GA, Donovan B. The effect of immunization with inactivated hepatitis A vaccine on the clinical course of HIV-1 infection: 1 year follow up. AIDS 1997;11:747–749.

14. Lebovics E, Dworkin B, Heier S, et al. The hepatobiliary manifestations of human immunodeficiency virus infection. Am J Gastroenterol 1988;83:1–7.
15. Stevens CE, Taylor PE, Zang EA, et al. Human T cell lymphotropic virus type III infection in a cohort of homosexual men in New York City. JAMA 1986;255: 2167–2172.
16. Taylor PE, Stevens CE, DeCordoba SR, et al. Hepatitis B virus and human immunodeficiency virus: possible interactions. In: Zuckerman AJ, ed. Viral hepatitis and liver disease. New York: Alan R. Liss, 1988:198–200.
17. Kingsley LA, Rinaldo CR, Lyter DW, et al. Sexual transmission efficiency of hepatitis B virus among homosexual men. JAMA 1990; 264: 230–234.
18. Laure F, Zagury D, Saimot AG, et al. Hepatitis B virus DNA sequences in lymphoid cells from patients with AIDS and AIDS-related complex. Science 1985;229:561–563.
19. Noonan C, Yoffe B, Mansell P, et al. Extrachromosomal sequences of hepatitis B virus DNA in peripheral blood mononuclear cells of acquired immune deficiency syndrome patients. Proc Natl Acad Sci U S A 1986;83:5698–5702.
20. Bartolome F, Moraleda G, Castillo I, et al. Presence of HBV DNA in the peripheral blood mononuclear cells from anti-HIV symptomless carriers. J Hepatol 1990;10:186–190.
21. Sen R, Baltimore D. Multiple nuclear factors interact with the immunuglobulin enhancer sequences. Cell 1986;46:705–716.
22. Israel N, Hazan U, Alcami J, et al. Tumour necrosis factor stimulates transcription of HIV-1 in human T lymphocytes, independently and synergistically with mitogens. J Immunol 1989;143:3956–3960.
23. Colgrove R, Simon G, Ganem D. Transcriptional activation of homologous and heterologous genes by the hepatitis B virus X gene product in cells permissive for viral replication. J Virol 1989;63: 4019–4026.
24. Twu JS, Schloemer RH. Transcriptional trans-activating function of hepatitis B virus. J Virol 1987;61:3488–3453.
25. Seto E, Yen T, Peterlin B, et al. Transactivation of the human immunodeficiency virus long terminal repeat by the hepatitis B virus X protein. Proc Natl Acad Sci U S A 1988;85:8286–8290.
26. Twu JS, Robinson W. Hepatitis B virus X gene can transactivate heterologous viral sequences. Proc Natl Acad Sci U S A 1989;86: 2046–2050.
27. Siddiqui A, Gaynor R, Srinivasan A, et al. *Trans*-activation of viral enhancers including long terminal repeat of the human immunodeficiency virus by the hepatitis B virus X protein. Virology 1989;169: 479–484.
28. Poli G, Kinter AL, Justement JS, et al. Tumor necrosis factor-α functions in an autocrine manner in the induction of HIV expression. Proc Natl Acad Sci U S A 1990;87:782–785.
29. Clouse KA, Robbins PB, Fernie B, et al. Viral antigen stimulation of the production of human monokines capable of regulating HIV1 expression. J Immunol 1989;143:470–475.
30. Kornbluth RS, Oh PS, Munis JR, et al. Interferons and bacterial lipopolysaccharide protect macrophages from productive infection with human immunodeficiency virus in vitro. J Exp Med 1989;169: 1137–1151.
31. Koyanagi Y, O'Brien WA, Zhao JQ, et al. Cytokines alter production of HIV-1 from primary mononuclear phagocytes. Science 1988;241: 1673–1675.
32. Foster G, Ackrill A, Goldin R, et al. Expression of the terminal protein region of hepatitis B virus inhibits cellular responses to interferons α and γ and double-stranded RNA. Proc Natl Acad Sci U S A 1991;88: 2888–2892.
33. Twu JS, Lee CH, Lin PM, et al. Hepatitis B virus suppresses expression of human beta-interferon. Proc Natl Acad Sci U S A 1988;85: 252–256.
34. Whitten TM, Quets AT, Schloemer RH. Identification of the hepatitis B virus factor that inhibits expression of the beta interferon gene. J. Virol 1991;65:4699–4704.
35. Solomon RE, VanRaden M, Kaslow RA, et al. Association of hepatitis B surface and core antibody with acquisition and manifestations of human immunodeficiency virus type 1 (HIV-1) infection. Am J Public Health 1990;80:1475–1478.
36. Dudley F, Fox RA, Sherlock S. Cellular immunity and hepatitis associated Australia antigen liver disease. Lancet 1972;1:723–726.
37. Ferrari C, Penna A, Mondelli MU, et al. Intrahepatic, HBcAg-specific, regulatory T cell networks in chronic active hepatitis B. In: Zuckerman AJ, ed. Viral hepatitis and liver disease. New York: Alan R. Liss, 1988:645–649.
38. Mondelli MU, Botolotti F, Pontisso P, et al. Definition of hepatitis B virus (HBV)-specific target antigens recognized by cytotoxic T cells in acute HBV infection. Clin Exp Immunol 1987;68:242–250.
39. Naumov N, Mondelli M, Alexander G. Relationship between expression of hepatitis B virus antigens in isolated hepatocytes and autologous lymphocyte cytotoxicity in patients with chronic hepatitis B virus infection. Hepatology 1984;4:63–68.
40. Hoofnagle J, Dusheiko G, Schafer, et al. Reactivation of chronic hepatitis B virus infection by cancer chemotherapy. Ann Intern Med 1982;96:447–449.
41. Weller I, Bassendine M, Murray A, et al. Effects of prednisolone/ azathioprine in chronic hepatitis B viral infection. Gut 1982;23: 650–655.
42. Krogsgaard K, Lindhardt BO, Nielsen JO, et al. The influence of HTLVIII infection on the natural history of hepatitis B virus infection in male homosexual HBsAg carriers. Hepatology 1987;7:37–41.
43. Perrillo RP, Regenstein FG, Roodman ST. Chronic hepatitis B in asymptomatic homosexual men with antibody to human immunodeficiency virus. Ann Intern Med 1986;105:382–383.
44. Pignatelli M, Waters J, Brown D, et al. HLA class I antigens on the hepatocyte membrane during recovery from acute hepatitis B virus infection and during interferon therapy in chronic hepatitis B infection. Hepatology 1986;6:349–353.
45. Hayashi Y, Koike K. Interferon inhibits hepatitis B virus replication in a stable expression system of transfected viral DNA. J. Virol 1989;63: 2936–2940.
46. Rossol S, Voth R, Laubenstein HP, et al. Interferon production in patients infected with HIV-1. J Infect Dis 1989;159:815–821.
47. Paul RG, Roodman ST, Paul DA, et al. Elevated HLA class I antigen expression on PBMC of HBV carriers with coexistent HIV infection. In: Zuckerman AJ, ed. Viral hepatitis and liver disease. New York: Alan R. Liss, 1988:688–690.
48. Hadler SC, Judson FN, O'Malley PM, et al. Outcome of hepatitis B virus infection in homosexual men and its relation to prior human immunodeficiency virus infection. J Infect Dis 1991;163:454–459.
49. Bodsworth N, Donovan B, Nightingale B. The effect of concurrent human immunodeficiency virus infection on chronic hepatitis B: a study of 150 homosexual men. J Infect Dis 1989;160:577–582.
50. Bodsworth NJ, Cooper DA, Donovan B. The influence of human immunodeficiency virus type 1 on the development of the hepatitis B virus carrier state. J Infect Dis 1991;163:1138–1140.
51. Goldin RD, Fish DE, Hay A, et al. Histological and immunohistochemical study of hepatitis B virus in human immunodeficiency virus infection. J Clin Pathol 1990;43:203–205.
52. Brook MG, Chan G, Yap I, et al. Randomised controlled trial of lymphoblastoid interferon alfa in Europid men with chronic hepatitis B virus infection. BMJ 1989;299:652–656.
53. McDonald JA, Caruso L, Karayiannis P, et al. Diminished responsiveness of male homosexual chronic hepatitis B virus carriers with HTLV-III antibodies to recombinant alpha-interferon. Hepatology 1987;7:719–723.
54. DeStefano E, Friedman R, Friedmankien A, et al. Acid-labile human leucocyte interferon in homosexual men with Kaposi's sarcoma. J Infect Dis 1982;146:451–459.
55. Lau A, Read S, Williams B. Downregulation of interferon α but not γ receptor expression in vivo in the acquired immunodeficiency syndrome. J Clin Invest 1988;82:1415–1421.

56. Joller-Jemelka HI, Joller PW. Antibodies to endogenous interferon alpha in contols and HIV infected persons in different disease states [abstract ThBP 133]. In: Abstracts of the 5th International Conference on AIDS, Montreal, 1989.
57. Perrillo R, Regenstein R, Peters M, et al. Prednisone withdrawal followed by recombinant alpha interferon in the treatment of chronic type B hepatitis: a randomized controlled trial. Ann Intern Med 1988;109: 95–100.
58. Haritani H, Uchida T, Okuda Y, et al. Effect of 3'-azido-3'-deoxythymidine on replication of duck hepatitis B virus in vivo and in vitro. J Med Virol 1989;29:244–248.
59. Marcellin P, Pialoux G, Girard P-M, et al. Absence of effect of zidovudine on hepatitis B virus replication in homosexual men with symptomatic HIV-1 infection. AIDS 1989;5:217–220.
60. Hess G, Rossol S, Voth R, et al. Treatment of patients with chronic type B hepatitis and concurrent human immunodeficiency virus with a combination of interferon alpha and azidothymidine. Digestion 1989;43:56–59.
61. Eron JJ, Benoit SL, Jemsek J, et al. Treatment with lamivudine, zidovudine, or both in HIV-positive patients with 200 to 500 CD4+ cells per cubic millimeter. N Engl J Med 1995;333:1662–1669.
62. Dienstag JL, Perrillo RP, Schiff ER, et al. A preliminary trial of lamivudine for chronic hepatitis B infection. N Engl J Med 1995;333: 1657–1661.
63. Grellier L, Mutimer D, Ahmed M, et al. Lamivudine prophylaxis against reinfection in liver transplantation for hepatitis B cirrhosis. Lancet 1996;348:1212–1215.
64. Bartholomew MM, Jansen RW, Jeffers LJ, et al. Hepatitis B virus resistance to lamivudine given for recurrent infection after orthotopic liver transplantation. Lancet 1997;349:20–22.
65. Ling R, Mutimer D, Ahmed M, et al. Selection of mutations in the hepatitis B virus polymerase during treatment of transplant recipients with lamivudine. Hepatology 1996;24:711–713.
66. Main J, Brown JL, Howells C, et al. A double blind placebo-controlled study to assess the effect of famciclovir in virus replication in patients with chronic hepatitis B virus infection. J Viral Hepatitis 1996;3: 211–215.
67. Carr A, Cooper DA. Restoration of immunity to chronic hepatitis B infection in HIV-infected patient on protease inhibitor. Lancet 1997; 349:995–996.
68. Milich DR, Louie RE, Chisari FV. Genetic regulation of the immune response to HBsAg T cell proliferation response and cellular interaction. J Immunol 1983;134:1292–1294.
69. Stevens CE, Alter HJ. Hepatitis B vaccine in patients receiving hemodialysis: Immunogenicity and efficacy. N Engl J Med 1984;311: 496–501.
70. Jacobson IM, Jaffers G, Dienstag JL, et al. Immunogenicity of hepatitis B vaccine in renal transplant recipients. Transplantation 1985;39:393–395.
71. Szmuness W, Stevens CE, Harley EJ, et al. Hepatitis B vaccine: demonstration of efficacy in a controlled clinical trial in a high-risk population in the United States. N Engl J Med 1980;303: 833–841.
72. Carne CA, Weller IV, Waite J, et al. Impaired responsiveness of homosexual men with HIV antibodies to plasma derived hepatitis B vaccine. BMJ 1987;294:866–868.
73. Collier AC, Corey L, Murphy VL, et al. Antibody to human immunodeficiency virus (HIV) and suboptimal response to hepatitis B vaccination. Ann Intern Med 1988;109:101–105.
74. Loke R, Murray-Lyon I, Coleman J, et al. Diminished response to recombinant hepatitis B vaccine in homosexual men with HIV antibody: an indicator of poor prognosis. J Med Virol 1990;31: 109–111.
75. Davis GL, Hoofnagle JH. Reactivation of chronic type B hepatitis presenting as a viral hepatitis. Ann Intern Med 1985;102:762–765.
76. Vandercam B, Cornu C, Gala J, et al. Reactivation of hepatitis B virus infection in a previously immune patient with HIV infection. Eur J Clin Microbiol Infect Dis 1990;9:701–702.
77. Vento S, Di Perri G, Luzzati R, et al. Clinical reactivation of hepatitis B in anti-HBs positive patients with AIDS [letter]. Lancet 1989;1: 332–333.
78. Brechot C, Degos F, Lugassi C, et al. Hepatitis B virus DNA in patients with chronic liver disease and negative tests for hepatitis B surface antigen. N Engl J Med 1985;312:270–276.
79. Laukamm-Josten U, Muller O, Benzie U, et al. Decline of naturally acquired antibodies to hepatitis B surface antigen in HIV-1 infected homosexual men with AIDS. AIDS 1988;2:400–401.
80. Levy P, Marcellin P, Martinot PM, et al. Clinical course of spontaneous reactivation of hepatitis B virus infection in patients with chronic hepatitis B. Hepatology 1990;12:570–574.
81. Waite J, Gilson RJC, Weller IVD, et al. Hepatitis B virus reactivation or reinfection associated with HIV-1 infection. AIDS 1988;2: 443–448.
82. Fang JWS, Wright TL, Lau JYN. Fibrosing cholestatic hepatitis in a patient with human immunodeficiency virus and hepatitis B virus coinfection. Lancet 1993;342:1175.
83. Alter HJ, Purcell RH, Shih JW, et al. Detection of antibody to hepatitis C virus in prospectively followed transfusion recipients with acute and chronic non-A and non-B hepatitis. N Engl J Med 1989; 321:1494–1500.
84. Tedder RS, Gilson RJC, Briggs M, et al. Hepatitis C virus: evidence for sexual transmission. BMJ 1991;302:1299–1302.
85. Eyster ME, Alter HJ, Aledort LM, et al. Heterosexual co-transmission of hepatitis C virus (HCV) and human immunodeficiency (HIV). Ann Intern Med 1991;115:764–768.
86. Giovannini M, Tagger A, Ribero ML, et al. Maternal–infant transmission of hepatitis C virus and HIV infections: a possible interaction. Lancet 1990;335:1166.
87. Schoeman MN, Liddle C, Bilous M, et al. Chronic non-A, non-B hepatitis: lack of correlation between biochemical and morphological activity and effects of immunosuppressive therapy on disease. Aust N Z J Med 1990;20:56–62.
88. Martin P, Di Bisceglie AM, Kassianides C, et al. Rapidly progressive non-A, non-B hepatitis in patients with human immunodeficiency virus infection. Gastroenterology 1989;97:1559–1561.
89. Sanchez-Quijano A, Andreu J, Gavilan F, et al. Influence of human immunodefiency virus type 1 infection on the natural course of chronic parenterally acquired hepatitis C. Eur J Clin Microbiol Infect Dis 1995;14:949–953.
90. Eyster ME, Diamondstone LS, Jau-Min L, et al. Natural history of hepatitis C virus infection in multitransfused hemophiliacs: effect of coinfection with human immunodeficiency virus. J Acquir Immune Defic Syndr 1993;6:602–610.
91. Telfer P, Sabin C, Devereux H, et al. The progression of HCV-associated liver disease in a cohort of haemophiliac patients. Br J Haematol 1994;87:555–561.
92. Telfer PT, Brown D, Devereux H, et al. HCV RNA levels and HIV infection: evidence for a viral interaction in haemophiliac patients. Br J Haematol 1994;88:397–399.
93. Eyster ME, Fried MW, Di Bisceglie AM, et al. Increasing hepatitis C virus RNA levels in hemophiliacs: relationship to human immunodeficiency virus infection and liver disease. Blood 1994;84:1020–1023.
94. Wright TL, Hollander H, Pu X, et al. Hepatitis C in HIV-infected patients with and without AIDS: prevalence and relationship to patient survival. Hepatology 1994;20:1152–1155.
95. Dorruci M, Pezzotti P, Phillips AN, et al. Coinfection of hepatitis C virus with human immunodeficiency virus and progression to AIDS: Italian seroconversion study. J Infect Dis 1995;172:1503–1508.
96. Chamot E, Hirchel B, Wintsch J, et al. Loss of antibodies against hepatitis C virus in HIV-seropositive intravenous drug users. AIDS 1990;4:1275–1277.
97. Nubling NN, Von Wangenheim G, Staszewski S, et al. Hepatitis C virus antibody prevalence among human immunodeficiency virus-1 infected individuals: analysis with different test systems. J Med Virol 1994;44:49–53.

98. Boyer N, Marcellin P, Degott C, et al. Recombinant interferon-alpha for chronic hepatitis C in patients positive for antibody to human immunodeficiency virus: Comite des Anti-Viraux. J Infect Dis 1992; 165:723–726.
99. Soriano V, Bravo R, Samaniego JG, et al. CD4 T-lymphocytopenia in HIV infected patients receiving interferon therapy for chronic hepatitis C. AIDS 1994;8:1621–1622.
100. Soriano V, Bravo R, Garcia-Samaniego J, et al. Relapses of chronic hepatitis C in HIV-infected patients who responded to interferon therapy. AIDS 1997;11:400–401.
101. Vento S, Di Perri G, Cruciani M, et al. Rapid decline of CD4+ cells after IFN-α treatment in HIV-1 infection. Lancet 1993;341: 958–959.
102. Pesce A, Taillan B, Rosenthal E, et al. Opportunistic infection and CD4 lymphopenia with interferon treatment in HIV-1 infected patients. Lancet 1993;341:1597.
103. Soriano V, Garcia-Samaniego J, Bravo R, et al. Efficacy and safety of alpha interferon treatment for chronic hepatitis C in HIV infected patients. J Infect 1995;31:9–13.
104. Chemello L, Cavalletto L, Bernardinello E, et al. The effect of interferon alfa and ribavirin combination therapy in naive patients with chronic hepatitis C. J Hepatol 1995:23(Suppl 2):8–12.
105. Vogt MW, Hartshorn KL, Furman PA, et al. Ribavirin antagonises the effect of azidothymidine on HIV replication. Science 1987;235: 1376–1379.
106. Farci P, Croxson TS, Taylor MB, et al. Effect of human immunodeficiency virus on the increased severity of liver disease associated with delta hepatitis [abstract]. Gastroenterology 1988;94:A578.
107. Krogsgaard K, Kryger P, Aldershville J, et al. Delta infection and suppression of hepatitis B virus replication in chronic HBsAg carriers. Hepatology 1987;7:42–45.
108. Saldanha J, Di Blasi F, Blas C, et al. Detection of hepatitis delta virus RNA in chronic liver disease. J Hepatol 1990;9:23–28.
109. Cassidy W, Govindarajan S, Gupta S, et al. Influence of HIV on chronic hepatitis B and D infection [abstract]. Hepatology 1989;10:690.
110. Govindarajan S, Cassidy WM, Valinluck B, et al. Interactions of HDV, HBV and HIV in chronic B and D infections and in reactivation of chronic D infection. Prog Clin Biol Res 1991;364:207–210.
111. Pol S, Wesenfelder L, Dubois F, et al. Influence of human immunodefiency virus infection in hepatitis delta virus superinfection in chronic HBsAg carriers. J Viral Hepatitis 1994;1:131–137.
112. Eyster ME, Sanders JC, Battegay M, et al. Suppression of hepatitis C virus (HCV) replication by hepatitis D virus (HDV) in HIV infected hemophiliacs with chronic hepatitis B and C. Dig Dis Sci 1995;40: 1583–1588.
113. Zannetti AR, Dawson GJ, Sgoh E. Hepatitis type E in Italy: a seroepidemiological survey. J Med Virol 1994;42:318–320.
114. Montella F, Rezza G, Di Sorra F, et al. Association between hepatitis E virus and HIV infection in homosexual men. Lancet 1994; 344:1433.
115. Medrano FJ, Sanchez QA, Torronteras R, et al. Hepatitis E virus and HIV infection in homosexual men. Lancet 1995;345:127.
116. Bissuel F, Houhou N, Leport C, et al. Hepatitis E antibodies and HIV status. Lancet 1996;347:1494.
117. Myint H, Soe MM, Khin T, et al. A clinical and epidemiological study of an epidemic of non-A, non-B hepatitis in Rangoon. Am J Trop Med Hyg 1985;34:1183–1189.
118. Macher AM, Reichert CM, Strauss SE, et al. Death in the AIDS patient: role of cytomegalovirus. N Engl J Med 1983;309:1454.
119. Vieco PT, Rochon L, Lisbona A. Multifocal cytomegalovirus-associated hepatic lesions simulating metastases in AIDS. Radiology 1990;176:123–124.
120. Snover DC, Horowitz CA. Liver disease in cytomegalovirus mononucleosis: a light microscopical and immunoperoxidase study of six cases. Hepatology 1984;4:408–412.
121. Bach N, Theise ND, Schaffner F. Hepatic histopathology in the acquired immunodeficiency syndrome. Semin Liver Dis 1992;12: 205–212.
122. Clarke J, Craig RM, Saffro R, et al. Cytomegalovirus granulomatous hepatitis. Am J Med 1979;66:264–269.
123. Zimmerli W, Bianchi L, Gudat F, et al. Disseminated herpes simplex type 2 and systemic *Candida* infection in a patient with previous asymptomatic HIV infection. J Infect Dis 1988;157:597–598.
124. Goodman ZD, Ishak KG, Sesterhenn IA, et al. Herpes simplex hepatitis in apparently immunocompetent adults. Am J Clin Pathol 1986;85:694–699.
125. Soriano V, Bru F, Gonzalez-Lahoz J. Fatal varicella hepatitis in a patient with AIDS. J Infect 1992;25:107.
126. Krilov LR, Rubin LG, Frogel M, et al. Disseminated adenovirus infection with hepatic necrosis in patients with human immunodeficiency virus infection and other immunodeficiency states. Rev Infect Dis 1990;12:303–307.
127. Duffy LF, Daum F, Kahn E, et al. Hepatitis in children with the acquired immunodeficiency syndrome. Gastroenterology 1986;90: 173–181.
128. Thung SN, Gerber MA, Benkov KJ, et al. Chronic active hepatitis in a hild with HIV infection. Arch Pathol Lab Med 1988;112:914–916.
129. Kamani N, Lightman H, Leiderman I, et al. Pediatric acquired immunodeficiency syndrome related complex: clinical and immunological features. Pediatr Infect Dis J 1988;7:383–388.
130. Beissner RS, Rappaport FS, Diaz JA. Fatal case of Epstein–Barr virus-induced lymphoproliferative disorder associated with a human immunodeficiency virus infection. Arch Pathol Lab Med 1987;11: 250–253.
131. Glasgow BJ, Anders K, Layfield LJ, et al. Clinical and pathological findings of the liver in the acquired immunodeficiency syndrome (AIDS). Am J Clin Pathol 1985;85:582–588.
132. Lebovics E, Thung SN, Schaffner F, et al. The liver in the acquired immunodeficiency syndrome: a clinical and histological study. Hepatology 1985;5:293–298.
133. Duong TA. Infection due to *Penicillium marneffei*, an emerging pathogen: review of 155 reported cases. Clin Infect Dis 1996;23: 125–130.
134. Orenstein MS, Travitan A, Yonk B, et al. Granulomatous involvement of the liver in patients with AIDS. Gut 1985;26:1220–1225.
135. Filice C, Brunetti E, Carnevale G, et al. Ultrasonographic and microbiological diagnosis of mycetic liver abscesses in patients with AIDS. Microbiologica 1989;12:101–104.
136. Sachs JR, Greenfield SM, Sohn M, et al. Disseminated *Pneumocystis carinii* infection in a patient with the acquired immunodeficiency syndrome. Am J Gastroenterol 1991;86:81–85.
137. Grimes MM, La Pook JD, Bar MH, et al. Disseminated *Pneumocystis carinii* infection in a patient with immunodeficiency syndrome. Hum Pathol 1987;18:307–308.
138. Hagopian WA, Huseby IS. *Pneumocystis* hepatitis and choroiditis despite successful aerosolized pentamidine pulmonary prophylaxis. Chest 1989;96:949–951.
139. Problete RB, Rodriguez K, Foust RT, et al. *Pneumocystis carinii* hepatitis in the acquired immunodeficiency syndrome (AIDS). Ann Intern Med 1989;110:737–738.
140. Oksenhendler E, Matheron S. Toxoplasmosis: new aspects, diagnosis and treatment. Rev Prat 1992;42:155–159.
141. Falk S, Helm EB, Hubner K, et al. Disseminated visceral leishmaniasis (kala azar) in acquired immunodeficiency syndrome (AIDS). Pathol Res Pract 1988;183:253–255.
142. Federico G, Cauda R, Pizzigallo E, et al. Visceral leishmaniasis in patients with AIDS: description of 2 cases. Pathologica 1989;81: 591–600.
143. Fenske S, Stellbrink HJ, Albrecht H, et al. Visceral leishmaniasis in an HIV-infected patient: clinical features and response to treatment. Klin Wochenschr 1991;69:793–796.
144. Montalban C, Calleja JL, Erice A, et al. Visceral leishmaniasis in patients infected with human immunodeficiency virus: Co-operative Group for the Study of Leishmaniasis in AIDS. J Infect 1990;21: 261–270.

145. Poles MA, Dieterich DT, Schwarz ED, et al. Liver biopsy findings in 501 patients infected with human immunodeficiency virus (HIV). J Acquir Immun Defic Syndr Hum Retrovirol 1996;11:170–177.
146. Schneiderman DJ, Arensen DM, Cello JP, et al. Hepatic disease in patients with the acquired immune deficiency syndrome (AIDS). Hepatology 1987;5:925–930.
147. Palmer M, Braly LF, Schaffner F. The liver in acquired immunodeficiency disease. Semin Liver Dis 1987;7:192–202.
148. Kahn SA, Saltzman BR, Klein RS, et al. Hepatic disorders in the acquired immunodeficiency syndrome: clinical and pathological features. Am J Gastroenterol 1986;81:1145–1148.
149. Horsburgh CR, Mason UG, Farhi DC, et al. Disseminated infection with *Mycobacterium avium-intracellulare*: a report of 13 cases and a review of the literature. Medicine (Baltimore) 1985;64:36–48.
150. Welch K, Finkbeiner W, Alpers CE, et al. Autopsy findings in the acquired immunodeficiency syndrome. JAMA 1984;252:1152–1159.
151. Gordon SC, Reddy KR, Gould EE, et al. The spectrum of liver disease in the acquired immunodeficiency syndrome. J Hepatol 1986;2:475–484.
152. Prego V, Glatt AE, Roy V, et al. Comparative yield of blood culture for fungi and mycobacteria, liver biopsy, and bone marrow biopsy in the diagnosis of fever of undetermined origin in human immunodeficiency virus-infected patients. Arch Intern Med 1990;150:333–336.
153. Relman DA, Louht JS, Schmidt TM, et al. The agent of bacillary angiomatosis: an approach to the identification of uncultured pathogens. N Engl J Med 1990;323:1573–1580.
154. Slater LN, Welch DF, Hensel D, et al. A newly recognised fastidious Gram-negative pathogen as a cause of fever and bacteremia. N Engl J Med 1990;323:1587–1593.
155. Perkocha LA, Geaghan SM, Yen TS, et al. Clinical and pathological features of bacillary peliosis hepatis in association with human immunodeficiency virus infection. N Engl J Med 1990;323:1581–1586.
156. Radin DR. Spontaneous resolution of peliosis of the liver and spleen in patient with HIV infection. AJR Am J Roentgenol 1992;158.
157. DeVega T, Echevarria S, Crespo J, et al. Acute hepatitis by Listeria monocytogenes in an HIV patients with chronic HBV hepatitis. J Clin Gastroenterol 1992;15:251–255.
158. Scoular A, Corcoran GD, Malin A, et al. Fusobacterium nucleatum bacteraemia with mutiple liver abscesses in an HIV antibody positive man with IgG2 deficiency. J Infect 1992;24:321–325.
159. Kostman JR, Patel M, Catalano E, et al. Invasive colitis and hepatitis due to previously uncharacterized spirochetes in patients with advanced human immunodeficiency virus infection. Clin Infect Dis 1995;21:1159–1165.
160. Hasan FA, Jeffers LJ, Welsh SW, et al. Hepatic involvement as the primary manifestation of Kaposi's sarcoma in the acquired immune deficiency syndrome. Am J Gastroenterol 1989;84:1449–1451.
161. Knowles DM, Chamaluk GA, Subar M, et al. Lymphoid neoplasia associated with the acquired immunodeficiency syndrome (AIDS). Ann Intern Med 1988;5:744–753.
162. Ziegler JL, Beckstead JA, Volberding PR, et al. Non-Hodgkin's lymphoma in 90 homosexual men: relationship to generalised lymphadenopathy and the acquired immunodeficiency syndrome. N Engl J Med 1984;311:565–570.
163. Chadburn A, Cesarman E, Jagirdar J, et al. CD30 (Ki-1) positive anaplastic large cell lymphomas in individuals infected with the human immunodeficiency virus. Cancer 1993;72:3078–3090.
164. Caccamo D, Pervez NK, Marchevsky A. Primary lymphoma of the liver in the acquired immunodeficiency syndrome. Arch Pathol Lab Med 1986;11:553–555.
165. Lisker MM, Pittaluga S, Pluda JM, et al. Primary lymphoma of the liver in a patient with acquired immune deficiency syndrome and chronic hepatitis B. Am J Gastroenterol 1989;84:1445–1448.
166. Ioachim HL, Cooper MC, Hellman GC. Hodgkin's disease and the acquired immunodeficiency syndrome. Ann Intern Med 1985;101:554.
167. Scheib RG, Siegel RS. Atypical Hodgkin's disease and the acquired immunodeficiency syndrome. Ann Intern Med 1985;102:554.
168. Chalasini N, Wilcox CM. Etiology, evaluation and outcome of jaundice in patients with acquired immunodeficiency syndrome. Hepatology 1996;23:728–833.
169. Richman DD, Fischl MA, Grieco MH, et al. The toxicity of azidothymidine (AZT) in the treatment of patients with AIDS and AIDS-related complex. N Engl J Med 1987;317:192–197.
170. Dubin G, Braffman MN. Zidovudine-induced hepatotoxicity. Ann Intern Med 1989;110:85–86.
171. Olano JP, Borucki MJ, Wen JW, et al. Massive hepatic steatosis and lactic acidosis in a patient with AIDS who was receiving zidovudine. Clin Infect Dis 1995;21:973–976.
172. Kew Lai K, Gang DL, Zawacki JK, et al. Fulminant hepatic failure associated with 2'3'-dideoxyinosine (ddI). Ann Intern Med 1991;115:283–284.
173. Bissuel F, Bruneel F, Habersetzer F, et al. Fulminant hepatitis with severe lactate acidosis in HIV infected patients with didanosine therapy. J Intern Med 1994;235:367–371.
174. McKenzie R, Fried MW, Sallie R, et al. Hepatic failure and lactic acidosis due to fialuridine (FIAU), an investigational nucleoside analogue for chronic hepatitis B. N Engl J Med 1995;333:1099–1105.
175. Cui L, Yoon S, Schinazi RF, et al. Cellular and molecular events leading to mitochondrial toxicity of 1- (2-deoxy-2-fluoro-1-β-D-arabinofuranosyl)-5-iodouracil in human liver cells. J Clin Invest 1995;95:555–563.
176. Gordin FM, Simon GL, Wofsky CB, et al. Adverse reactions to trimethoprim–sulphamethoxazole in patients with the acquired immunodeficiency syndrome. Ann Intern Med 1984;100:495–499.
177. Schaffner F. The liver in HIV infection. Prog Liver Dis 1990;9:505–522.
178. Small PM, Schecter GF, Goodman PC, et al. Treatment of tuberculosis in patients with advanced human immunodeficiency virus infection. N Engl J Med 1991;324:289–294.
179. Goldin RD, Wilkins M, Dourakis S, et al. Iron overload in multiply transfused patients who are HIV seropositive. J Clin Pathol 1993;46:1036–1038.
180. Nakanuma Y, Liew CT, Peters RL, et al. Pathologic features of the liver in the acquired immunodeficiency syndrome (AIDS). Liver 1986;6:158–166.
181. Czapar CA, Weldon-Linne M, Moore DM, et al. Peliosis hepatis in the acquired immunodeficiency syndrome: a clinical and pathological study. Arch Pathol Lab Med 1986;110:611–613.
182. Wilkins MJ, Lindley R, Dourakis SP, et al. Surgical pathology of the liver in HIV infection. Histopathology 1991;18:459–464.
183. Scoazec JY, Marche C, Girard PM, et al. Peliosis hepatis and sinusoidal dilation during infection by the human immunodeficiency virus (HIV): an ultrastructural study. Am J Pathol 1988;131:38–47.
184. Buckley JA, Hutchins GM. Association of hepatic veno-occlusive disease with the acquired immunodeficiency syndrome. Mod Pathol 1995;8:398–401.
185. Kazi S, Cohren PR, Williams F, et al. The diffuse lymphocytosis syndrome: clinical and immunogenetic features in 35 patients. AIDS 1996;10:385–391.
186. Sidhu GS, Stahl RE, el-Sadr W, et al. The acquired immunodeficiency syndrome; an ultrastructural study. Hum Pathol 1985;16:377–386.
187. Goldin RD, Hunt J. Biliary tract pathology in patients with AIDS. J Clin Pathol 1993;46:691–693.
188. Chalasini N, Wilcox CM. Etiology, evaluation and outcome of jaundice in patients with acquired immunodeficiency syndrome. Hepatology 1996;23:728–733.
189. Cello JP. Human immunodeficency virus-associated biliary tract disease. Semin Liver Dis 1992;12:213–218.
190. Goodgame RW. Understanding intestinal spore-forming protozoa: cryptosporidia, microsporidia and *Cyclospora*. Ann Intern Med 1996;124:429–441.
191. Pol S, Romana CA, Richard S, et al. Microsporidia infection in patients with the human immunodeficiency virus and unexplained cholangitis. N Engl J Med 1993;328:95–99.

192. Forbes A, Blanshard C, Gazzard B. Natural history of AIDS related sclerosing cholangitis: a study of 20 patients. Gut 1993;34:116–121.
193. Cello JP. Acquired immunodeficiency syndrome cholangiopathy: spectrum of disease. Am J Med 1989;86:539–546.
194. Bouche H, Houssett C, Dumont JL, et al. AIDS-related cholangitis: diagnostic features and course in 15 patients. J Hepatol 1993;17:34–39.
195. Teare JP, Price DA, Foster GR, et al. Reversible AIDS-related sclerosing cholangitis. AIDS 1995;23:20–-211.
196. Cello JP, Chan MF. Long-term follow-up of endoscopic retrograde cholangiopanreatography sphincterotomy for patients with acquired immunodeficiency syndrome papillary stenosis. Am J Med 1995;99:600–603.
197. Pitlik SD, Fainstein V, Rios A, et al. Cryptosporidial cholecystitis. N Engl J Med 1983;308:967.
198. Kavin H, Jonas RB, Chowdhury L, et al. Acalculous cholecystitis and cytomegalovirus infection in the acquired immunodeficiency syndrome. Ann Intern Med 1986;104:53–54.
199. Aaron JS, Wynter CD, Kirton OC, et al. Cytomegalovirus associated with acalculous cholecystitis in a patient with the acquired immunodeficiency syndrome. Am J Gastroenterol 1988;83:879-891.
200. Knapp PE, Saltzman JR, Fairchild P. Acalculous cholecystitis associated with microsporidial infection in a patient with AIDS. Clin Infect Dis 1996;22:195–196.
201. Benator DA, French AL, Beaudet LM, et al. *Isospora belli* infection associated with acalculous cholecystitis in a patient with AIDS. Ann Intern Med 1994;121:663–664.
202. Wind P, Chevallier JM, Jones D, et al. Cholecystectomy for cholecystitis in patients with acquired human immunodeficiency syndrome. Am J Surg 1994;168:244–246.

35
RENAL DISEASE AND AIDS

Jacques J. Bourgoignie, Jorge Diego, and Carmen Ortiz-Butcher

The early descriptions of the clinical manifestations of the acquired immunodeficiency syndrome (AIDS) did not include renal complications. Nevertheless, renal disease is a relatively common complication in patients infected with the human immunodeficiency virus (HIV). Nephrologists were consulted in 6% of 1635 patients with AIDS seen, between 1982 and 1987, at the University of Miami—Jackson Memorial Medical Center (UM/JMMC) (1). Ninety percent of nephrologists' interventions were for azotemia or proteinuria. Some of these events represented intercurrent disease, but others appeared related to the HIV infection and exhibited characteristic clinical and pathologic features. In addition, some consultations were for complicated electrolyte or acid-base disorders resulting from opportunistic infections or drug interactions associated with AIDS or its treatment.

After a brief review of electrolyte and acid-base complications, this chapter focuses on acute and chronic nephropathies encountered in patients with HIV infection, with an emphasis on clinical presentation, pathogenesis, and treatment.

ELECTROLYTE AND ACID-BASE DISORDERS

Single and mixed acid-base disturbances, lactic acidosis, and various electrolyte disorders, most commonly hyponatremia and hyperkalemia, can be observed in patients with AIDS. These disorders are not usually associated with structural lesions in the kidneys unless acute renal failure (ARF) is also present. These complications may develop spontaneously, or they may follow pharmacologic intervention. Certain drugs used in the treatment of patients with AIDS can induce acid-base or electrolyte abnormalities (Table 35.1) from direct renal toxicity (dideoxyinosine [ddI], foscarnet, pentamidine, rifampin, amphotericin B), other organ toxicity (ddI, foscarnet, rifampin), or interference with uric acid metabolism (ddI, pyrazinamide, ethambutol) (2).

Lactic acidosis type A (anaerobic) is expected in patients with advanced AIDS and tissue hypoxia. Lactic acidosis type B (aerobic) can also occur in patients in whom tissue hypoxia is not apparent. In seven patients, no single drug could be incriminated, and an infectious cause was probable. Patients had no symptoms except hyperventilation. They presented on admission with a mean anion gap of 28 mmol/L, mean arterial pH of 7.22, bicarbonate of 7.0 mmol/L, and arterial lactate of 14.3 mmol/L. Four patients rapidly died of cardiovascular collapse secondary to progressive metabolic acidosis as the arterial lactate concentration exceeded 15 mmol/L and arterial pH fell to less than 6.83 (3).

Hyponatremia is the most prevalent electrolyte abnormality, observed in 26 to 56% of patients hospitalized with AIDS (4–8). It is often associated with hypovolemia in patients with gastrointestinal fluid losses. In the absence of an evident source of fluid loss, volume depletion may be related to renal salt wasting as a result of defective tubular reabsorption of sodium from tubulointerstitial disease or hormonal imbalances. Hyporeninemic hypoaldosteronism has been reported (9, 10). Mineralocorticoid deficiency, resulting from pituitary–adrenal dysfunction, may exist but is usually subclinical (11–13). Although the adrenal gland is the endocrine organ most commonly affected by opportunistic infections in AIDS, overt Addison's disease is rare, inasmuch as less than 50% of the gland is typically involved (14). Nevertheless, the possibility that hyponatremia reflects adrenal insufficiency must always be considered. In euvolemic patients, hyponatremia is compatible with inappropriate secretion of antidiuretic hormone in patients with pulmonary or central nervous system disease (6, 7, 15). Determination of urinary sodium concentration (UNa) is helpful for diagnostic purpose. In a series of 103 hospitalized patients with AIDS, hyponatremia (serum sodium concentration less than 130 mmol/L) was due to hypovolemia (UNa, 10 to 18 mmol/L) in 12, adrenal insufficiency (UNa, 43 mmol/L) in 1, and inappropriate secretion of antidiuretic hormone (UNa, 36 to 192 mmol/L) in 23 (7). Hyponatremia in hypervolemic patients is dilutional in origin as a result of excessive free water intake in a context of renal insufficiency (8).

Hypernatremia is much less common and is usually the result of drug-induced nephrogenic diabetes insipidus, particularly after administration of amphotericin B, rifampin, or foscarnet (16, 17).

Hypokalemia can occur in 17% of patients with AIDS as a result of gastrointestinal losses from diarrhea, metabolic alkalosis induced by prolonged vomiting, or urinary losses associated with drug-induced tubular acidosis (amphotericin B, rifampin, cotrimoxazole) (18).

Table 35.1 Fluid and Electrolyte Complications of Drugs Used to Treat Aids

Complication	Drug
Hypernatremia	Foscarnet, rifampin, amphotericin B
Hypokalemia	ddI, rifampin, amphotericin B, foscarnet
Hyperkalemia	Pentamidine, trimethoprim, ketoconazole
Hypercalcemia	Foscarnet
Hypocalcemia	Foscarnet, pentamidine, ddI
Hyperuricemia	ddI, pyrazinamide, ethambutol
Hypomagnesemia	Pentamidine, amphotericin B
Tubular acidosis	Amphotericin B, rifampin, trimoxazole

ddI, dideoxyinosine

Hyperkalemia can develop in 16 to 24% of hospitalized patients (5). It is associated with renal insufficiency in only half the cases (19). In the absence of nephropathy, the cause may be hypoaldosteronism as a result of ketoconazole, adrenal insufficiency, or pentamidine toxicity (19, 20). Many of these patients, however, were receiving trimethoprim–sulfamethoxazole therapy for opportunistic infections. Trimethoprim has now been shown to mimic the action of amiloride and to inhibit sodium reabsorption by decreasing the number of open sodium channels in the luminal membrane of the cortical collecting tubule. The ensuing decrease in sodium reabsorption thereby decreases potassium secretion to produce hyperkalemia (20). In one study, 20% of patients treated with oral trimethoprim–sulfamethoxazole developed hyperkalemia in excess of 5mEq/L (21). The average serum potassium may increase from 0.6 to 1.1 mEq/L with occasional severe hyperkalemia (22). Drug-induced hyperkalemia resolves with removal of the responsible agent. Experimentally, maneuvers that increase sodium delivery in the distal nephron can abrogate the antikaliuretic effects of trimethoprim (23, 24). Pentamidine appears to act by the same mechanism as trimethoprim, by blocking distal potassium secretion.

More rarely, *hypocalcemia* unaccounted for by hypoalbuminemia or *hypercalcemia* has been reported with foscarnet use. Hypocalcemia may result from *hypomagnesemia* caused by urinary losses of magnesium and inhibition of parathyroid hormone secretion (pentamidine, amphotericin B, aminoglycoside antibiotics) (25, 26) or from drug-induced pancreatitis (pentamidine, ddI, foscarnet) (2). *Hypercalcemia* can occur in association with granulomatous disorders, disseminated cytomegalovirus infection, lymphoma, human T-cell leukemia related to human T-cell leukemia/lymphoma virus type 1 (HTLV-1) infection (27), or foscarnet administration. Calciphylaxis has been observed in hypercalcemic or eucalcemic AIDS patients with renal disease and severe hyperparathyroidism (28).

Hypouricemia was described in 22% of 96 patients as a result of an intrinsic tubular defect in urate transport unrelated to drugs (29). It was associated with increased morbidity and mortality but was not a terminal finding. In contrast, *hyperuricemia* usually is the result of drug interference with purine metabolism (ddI) or inhibition of tubular urate secretion (pyrazinamide, ethambutol) (2).

The renal, fluid, and electrolyte complications of drugs used to treat HIV and associated opportunistic infections and dosing guidelines for the use of these drugs in patients with renal insufficiency were reviewed and updated by Berns and colleagues (2, 30). The reader is referred to those extensive reports.

In patients with renal insufficiency, not only should dosages be reduced for nephrotoxic drugs, but also for drugs eliminated or metabolized by the kidney. Accumulation of these drugs or their metabolites in renal insufficiency may have toxic effects at extrarenal sites. For instance, ganciclovir is not nephrotoxic, but it accumulates in patients with renal insufficiency and may then result in nightmares, visual hallucinations, and severe agitation (31). Thus, a definite need exists for regular urinalysis and for measurements of serum electrolytes and renal function during the treatment of patients with AIDS.

ACUTE RENAL FAILURE

ARF is a frequent complication in patients with AIDS. Defining ARF by an increase in serum creatinine of 2 mg/dL, ARF was reported in 20% of hospitalized patients seen at Bellevue Hospital in New York (32). The same incidence was found at L. Sacco Hospital in Milan (33).

The cause of ARF in patients with AIDS is variable, with volume depletion accounting for one-third and drugs used to treat AIDS and associated infections, sepsis, or the diagnostic use of radiocontrast agents accounting for 40 to 50% of the cases (32) (Table 35.2). Other causes of ARF include acute tubulointerstitial nephritides, rapidly progressive glomerulopathies, and obstructive nephropathies. In many patients, the origin of ARF is multifactorial.

Prerenal Azotemia and Acute Tubular Necrosis

Azotemia, often prerenal initially (5, 32–36), occurs in a context of extracellular fluid volume depletion, but it may lead to structural changes of acute tubular necrosis if left unattended or after hemodynamic disturbances or nephrotoxic insults, related to the treatment of sepsis with antimicrobial drugs or the administration of pentamidine, amphotericin B, foscarnet, cidofovir, acyclovir, or ritonavir (32–40). The reported prevalence of acute tubular necrosis in patients dying of AIDS varies from 8 to 30% (5, 38).

Table 35.2 Etiology of Acute Renal Failure

Acute tubular necrosis from hypovolemic, anoxic, septic, or toxic injuries
Allergic interstitial nephritis
Rapidly progressive immune-complex glomerulonephritis
Thrombotic thrombocytopenic purpura and hemolytic-uremic syndrome
Obstructive nephropathy from crystal-induced renal failure, uric acid nephropathy, retroperitoneal fibrosis
Rhabdomyolysis and myoglobinuric renal failure

The clinical presentation, laboratory findings, and course of acute tubular necrosis are not different in patients with AIDS and those in other clinical settings. ARF commonly occurs in patients with AIDS and rarely in patients without AIDS but with HIV infection. Unlike glomerulosclerosis, ARF occurs equally commonly in black and white patients. Preventive correction of the electrolyte and intravascular volume derangements, drug dosage adjustment appropriate to the level of renal function, and identification and withdrawal of the offending agents usually result in recovery of renal function, unless renal failure is a terminal event related to infections, central nervous system lesions, or multiple organ failures. Dialysis may be needed before renal function improves (1, 33, 34).

Acute Tubulointerstitial Nephritis

ARF associated with acute tubulointerstitial nephritis is usually a complication of drugs such as trimethoprim–sulfamethoxazole, rifampin, foscarnet, sulfadiazine, or ciprofloxacin (38, 41). Pathologic features are characterized by the presence of a diffuse interstitial inflammatory infiltrate consisting predominantly of mononuclear cells including eosinophils. The clinical course, prognosis, and treatment are similar to those of acute tubulointerstitial nephritis in HIV-seronegative individuals.

Physicians must remain alert to the possibility of acute tubulointerstitial nephritis because unorthodox drugs may be used in AIDS patients. For instance, germanium-containing compounds, promoted as "immunostimulants," may result in severe and irreversible tubulointerstitial nephritis (42, 43).

Thrombotic Thrombocytopenic Purpura and Hemolytic-Uremic Syndrome

Instances of clinical thrombotic thrombocytopenic purpura (TTP) and hemolytic-uremic syndrome (HUS) are reported with increased frequency in HIV-seropositive patients and in patients with AIDS (44–55). Although few detailed reports of renal histopathology in cases of HIV-related TTP/HUS have been published, the findings generally have been similar to those seen with TTS/HUS unrelated to HIV infection. The anemia associated with TTP/HUS is characterized by red blood cell fragments or helmet cells in the absence of a positive Coombs' test. In some instances, microangiopathic renal disease precedes the development of opportunistic infections, a finding supporting the possibility of a direct viral cytotoxic effect. TTP/HUS may occur as a complication of chemotherapy; no clear association exists with *Escherichia coli* 0157:H7 infection, and an intercurrent infection has been demonstrated in only one-third of patients. HIV-related circulating immune complexes may play a role in immune-mediated thrombocytopenia in HIV-infected patients (56). An elevated plasma tissue-type plasminogen activator has been found in HIV-infected patients with thrombotic microangiopathy (57).

Renal involvement in TTP is frequently minimal, whereas glomerular and vascular renal involvement is more extensive in HUS and can lead to renal cortical necrosis (48, 49). The distinction between the two entities sometimes is tenuous. TTP/HUS can occur at any stage of HIV infection, and the prognosis is poor. As in all HIV-associated renal diseases, tubuloreticular cytoplasmic inclusions (TRIs) are frequently present on electron microscopy. Arteriolar and glomerular capillary thromboses are also seen in septic patients with AIDS. Treatment with plasmapheresis using fresh-frozen replacement plasma should be instituted as soon as a diagnosis of HIV-related TTP/HUS is made (58).

Rapidly Progressive Immune-Complex Glomerulonephritis

ARF rarely results from rapidly progressive proliferative intracapillary, as well as necrotizing crescentic mesangiocapillary glomerulonephritis (GN) (59–61). Specific HIV antigens have not been identified in these acute glomerulopathies. Their clinical presentation, course, and glomerular lesions appear similar to those observed in HIV-seronegative patients with the same type of glomerulopathy (see later).

Acute Intrarenal or Extrarenal Obstruction

Obstructive nephropathy may occur under conditions that favor the tubular precipitation of sulfadiazine (62–65), acyclovir (66), or urate crystals during the chemotherapy of AIDS-related lymphoma (67). Characteristic crystals can be observed in the urine sediment when examined under polarized light. This complication can be prevented by maintaining appropriate hydration and high urine output and by the administration of alkalinizing agents to keep the urine pH higher than 6.0 to 6.5. On the other hand, 4% of patients taking indinavir develop symptoms of clinical nephrolithiasis with collecting-duct crystalluria. The solubility of indinavir is low, at pH 6 (68). Obstruction without hydronephrosis may also develop in patients with lymphoma as a result of lymphomatous ureteropelvic infiltration or retroperitoneal fibrosis (69–72).

Myoglobinuric Acute Renal Failure

Myoglobinuria may follow zidovudine or pentamidine treatment, but it seldom results in acute renal insufficiency (73, 74). Myoglobinuric ARF was reported in a patient with acute HIV infection (75). More often, however, this disorder is the result of illicit drug abuse (76).

Outcome of Severe Acute Renal Failure

Rao and Friedman (77) reported a decade's experience in the management of severe ARF (serum creatinine of at least 6 mg/dL) in 146 patients with HIV disease (132 with AIDS, 14 HIV seropositive) and in 306 contemporaneous HIV-seronegative (non-HIV) patients. The patients with HIV dis-

Table 35.3 Comparison of Severe Acute Renal Failure (ARF) between HIV and Non-HIV Patients

	HIV	Non-HIV	P
Number of patients	146	306	
Men (%)	77	64	NS
Mean age, (y)	38.4	55.2	< .001
Etiology of ARF			
Sepsis (%)	52	24	< .001
Nephrotoxins (%)	23	18	NS
Miscellaneous (%)	25	17	NS
Obstructive uropathy (%)	0	17	< .001
Surgical trauma (%)	0	26	< .001

NS, not significant.

ease were younger, sepsis was more frequent, but obstructive uropathy and surgical or traumatic causes of ARF were less frequent than in the group of non-HIV patients (Table 35.3).

The management and the outcome of ARF in these patients are presented in Table 35.4. In both groups, 83 to 85% of patients requiring only conservative therapy recovered renal function. Among patients requiring dialysis, many more patients with HIV disease (42%) than non-HIV patients (22%) were not offered aggressive replacement therapy and died rapidly. Among dialyzed patients, 56% in the HIV group and 47% in the non-HIV group recovered renal function. Overall mortality was not statistically different between the two groups. Eventually, 29% of HIV patients and 38% of non-HIV patients were discharged home (77).

Chronic Glomerulopathies in HIV-Seropositive Patients

All types of glomerular lesions have been reported in HIV-seropositive patients. Some glomerulopathies are infrequent and may be coincidental. In contrast, others, such as focal or global glomerular sclerosis in adults or diffuse mesangial hyperplasia in children, are frequently associated with HIV infection. Table 35.5 illustrates the way in which specific types of histologically proved chronic glomerulopathies were reported in the literature in 1993 in adults and children with HIV infection. It is now evident, however, that the distribution presented in Table 35.5 is skewed because glomerulosclerosis is essentially observed only in patients of African origin. Thus, the evidence of various types of glomerulopathies differs in different populations and geographic areas. Unlike ARF, chronic glomerulopathies occur in otherwise asymptomatic HIV-seropositive patients as well as in patients with AIDS. The finding by polymerase chain reaction of HIV nucleic acids in kidneys of all HIV-infected patients with or without renal disease emphasizes the role of genetic, immunologic, and other host factors in determining the renal pathologic expression and outcome of HIV-associated glomerulopathies (78, 79).

Focal or Global Glomerulosclerosis

By far, the most common glomerulopathy reported is a rapidly progressive form of glomerulosclerosis that accounts for 60 to 70% of chronic glomerular lesions in adults and for 33% of such lesions in children. The nephropathy has been described in otherwise asymptomatic HIV-seropositive individuals; thus, it is designated in the literature as HIV-associated, rather than AIDS-associated, nephropathy. This term, however, does not imply a direct pathogenic link between HIV and the nephropathy, nor does it exclude the possibility that other glomerular lesions may be mediated by the virus (80). In fact, several HIV-associated nephropathies are now recognized. Therefore, the nomenclature of HIV-associated nephropathies should be amended to include the associated qualifying histologic feature (81). HIV-associated glomerulosclerosis has characteristic clinical manifestations and histologic features (38, 82–86).

Demography and Epidemiology

An increased incidence of focal glomerulosclerosis in AIDS patients was first reported from New York and Miami in 1984 (87–89). Chronic renal disease, however, had been virtually absent in early autopsy series of patients with AIDS. Moreover, subsequent studies in Bethesda, Maryland (90), Dallas (5), and San Francisco (91) failed to confirm this association. Focal glomerulosclerosis can be found in intravenous drug users. Because intravenous drug use is a definite risk factor for AIDS, the possibility was raised that intravenous drug use was responsible for the glomerulosclerosis of AIDS. It became rapidly evident, however, that AIDS-associated glomerulosclerosis also occurred in patients who did not use intravenous drugs (34) and in children with perinatal AIDS (84). These observations, together with characteristic histologic and ultrastructural features of glomerulosclerosis in HIV-infected patients, indicated that the

Table 35.4 Management and Outcome of Severe ARF between HIV and Non-HIV Patients

Management	HIV	Non-HIV	P
Patients conservatively managed	20 (14%)	42 (14%)	NS
Recovered renal function	17/20 (85%)	35/42 (83%)	NS
Patients needing dialysis	126	264	
Dialysis not initiated	53 (42%)	57 (22%)	< .003
Dialyzed	73	207	
Recovered renal function	41/73 (56%)	98/207 (47%)	NS
Outcome			
Immediate mortality	88/146 (60%)	173/306 (56%)	NS
Mortality within 3 mo	103/146 (71%)	191/306 (62%)	NS
Discharged home	43/146 (29%)	115/306 (38%)	NS

NS, not significant.

nephropathy was different from that seen in intravenous drug users.

The conflicting reports about the prevalence of HIV-associated glomerulosclerosis in different areas of the United States reflect geographic differences in the composition of the populations studied (92–94). A demographic examination of the various populations with AIDS indicates a high prevalence of glomerulosclerosis among series in which intravenous drug users and black patients prevail, whereas series with a low prevalence of this disorder include a high proportion of white homosexuals (84). The predilection of the disease for blacks is striking. At UM/JMMC, where the ratio of white to black patients with AIDS was 3 to 1, chronic renal disease was found 10 times more frequently in blacks than in whites (92). Similarly, although the prevalence of HIV-associated glomerulosclerosis in the literature was only about 1% in autopsy studies of 690, predominantly white, patients, our experience at UM/JMMC uncovered a 15% incidence of glomerulosclerosis in 118 consecutive autopsies of patients with AIDS, of whom 70% were black (94). In contrast, reports from Europe in 1992 denied the existence of HIV-associated glomerulosclerosis on the basis of autopsy or biopsy findings in a white population (95). These negative findings support the contention that race, for whatever reason, is an important cofactor in the expression of HIV-associated glomerulosclerosis. The converse argument can be held for the well-known predominance of immunoglobulin A (IgA) nephropathy in whites, whether the disorder be idiopathic or HIV associated (see later). Reports from ethnically mixed populations in San Francisco (96), Rio de Janeiro (97), and Paris (98) confirmed the vulnerability of blacks to HIV-associated glomerulosclerosis. Essentially, all cases of HIV-associated glomerulosclerosis reported from Europe are described in black patients originating from central Africa or the Caribbean basin (98–101), but no European cases have been reported in white patients. An outstanding incidence of collapsing glomerulosclerosis has not yet been reported from tropical Africa, where autopsies and renal biopsies, however, are rarely performed.

Table 35.5 Chronic Glomerulopathies in HIV-Seropositive Patient

Disorder	Adults	Children
Glomerulosclerosis	30 (66%)	20 (33%)
Mesangial hyperplasia	63 (13%)	15 (25%)
Minimal-change GN	29 (5%)	5 (8%)
Other glomerulopathies	81 (16%)	20 (33%)
Proliferative GN	47	16
Membranous GN	5	1
SLE-like GN	10	1
IgA nephropathy	12	2
Sclerosing GN	1	—
Amyloidosis	3	—
Diabetes mellitus	2	—
End-stage renal disease	1	—

[a]GN, glomerulopathy; SLE, systemic lupus erythematosus.

Table 35.6 Distinctive Pathologic Findings in HIV-Associated Glomerulosclerosis

"Collapsed" glomerular capillaries
Visceral glomerular epitheliosis
Microcystic tubules with variegated casts
Focal tubular simplification
Endothelial tubuloreticular inclusions

Pathology

At autopsy, the kidneys in HIV glomerulosclerosis often are grossly enlarged and edematous (84). Histologic examination shows striking abnormalities in glomeruli and tubular interstitium. Although many glomeruli exhibit a global sclerosis (38), glomeruli with early segmental lesions and others with intermediate changes in the progression to global sclerosis are usually identified in the same kidney (102).

The glomerular and tubulointerstitial lesions found in HIV-associated glomerulosclerosis are listed in Table 35.6. At an early stage, glomeruli show only capillary collapse, with large hyperplastic visceral epithelial cells loaded with hyaline protein droplets compressing the capillary loops and filling Bowman's space. In late stages, the collapsed capillaries are progressively compacted into lobular masses. Simultaneously, progressive expansion of the mesangium occurs, with overproduction of matrix, and the lobules are contracted and solidified into sclerosed structures. Frequently, Bowman's space appears dilated and filled with a proteinaceous acidophilic material similar to that observed within the dilated tubules surrounding the glomerulus (80).

The tubulointerstitial changes in HIV-associated glomerulosclerosis are unusually prominent when compared with those present in other types of glomerulosclerosis. Proximal tubular convolutions frequently lack brush borders and show occasional cell desquamation. Nuclei are irregular in distribution, size, and staining. The epithelium is flattened in dilated tubules, which may reach microcystic proportions. Massive tubular casts distend tubules and Bowman's space and contain all types of plasma proteins, but they lack Tamm–Horsfall protein (85). These distended tubules may compress and displace glomeruli, other tubules, and interstitial capillaries. The tubulointerstitial changes likely play an important role in the pathogenesis of the renal insufficiency, thus explaining the pronounced decrease in renal function sometimes observed in patients who exhibit only mild glomerular changes. These changes may be responsible for disturbances in sodium reabsorption or renal tubular acidosis seen particularly in children.

An interstitial, predominantly mononuclear, inflammatory infiltrate is an important component of the nephropathy. Most cells are of the CD8 phenotype, similar to those seen in peripheral blood (38, 80).

Whereas none of the glomerular or tubular changes individually is specific or pathognomonic of HIV-associated glomerulosclerosis, the concomitant presence of these lesions is highly suggestive of this disease. The same lesions of collapsing glomerulosclerosis can be found in HIV-seronegative patients of African extraction (103, 104).

On immunofluorescence examination, findings in glomeruli are nonspecific and are similar in HIV-associated glomerulosclerosis and in idiopathic focal and segmental glomerular sclerosis, consisting largely of IgM and C3 deposited in a segmental and granular pattern in the mesangium and capillaries (38, 84, 85). Mesangial deposits of IgM and C3 are seen in 70 to 90% of patients with HIV-associated nephropathy. Conversely, immunofluorescent deposits of IgM and C3 do also occur in 30% of AIDS patients without renal disease.

Electron microscopy discloses various nuclear and cytoplasmic inclusions in renal endothelial, epithelial, or interstitial cells. No evidence indicates that these ultrastructural inclusions have a role in the pathogenesis of HIV-associated nephropathy. Most characteristic are TRIs in endothelial cells consisting of anastomosing microtubules, 20 to 25 nm in diameter, with a limiting membrane continuous with the endoplasmic reticulum. An abundance of TRIs is virtually diagnostic of HIV infection, provided systemic lupus erythematosus, another condition in which TRIs are abundant, has been excluded (80). TRIs can be induced in normal human leukocytes and cultured endothelial cells exposed to interferon-α; therefore, their presence in patients suffering from renal complications associated with the administration of interferon treatment can be misleading. However, TRIs are not found in the idiopathic variety of collapsing glomerulosclerosis (103).

Pathogenesis

The pathogenesis of HIV-associated glomerulosclerosis remains unknown. An important role cannot be ascribed to the numerous complications that define AIDS, or drugs used to treat AIDS, because the nephropathy also occurs in otherwise asymptomatic HIV-seropositive patients or in patients with only constitutional symptoms (38, 84, 104–106). The lack of immunopathologic features, usually associated with immune-complex glomerulopathies, mitigates against an immune pathogenesis, although complexes of viral antigens and antibodies may be pathogenic in other HIV-associated glomerulopathies such as IgA nephropathy (107) or after primary HIV infection (75, 108–110).

Intraglomerular hemodynamic changes such as those associated with glomerular hypertrophy produced experimentally after partial renal ablation were suggested by Langs and associates (102) because of the striking glomerular capillary wall collapse present in renal biopsy specimens in the absence of widespread glomerulosclerosis. The renal protection afforded by angiotensin-converting enzyme (ACE) inhibitors provides some support for this hypothesis (see later).

Other theories have implicated a mycoplasma (111), immunodeficiency per se (112), tubular necrosis (85), tubular obstruction by paraprotein casts (113, 114), renotropic strains of the retrovirus (115), or the genetic makeup of the affected host as pathogenic factors (78, 79). Whereas some of

Table 35.7 Evidence Suggesting Involvement of HIV in the Kidney

Renal transplantation
HIV replication in glomerular cells
CD4 expression in mesangial cells
P24 HIV antigen in epithelial cells
HIV genome by in situ hybridization in tubular and glomerular epithelial cells
Viral DNA by polymerase chain reaction in renal parenchymal cells
Simian immunodeficiency
Transgenic mouse with noninfectious HIV provirus

these may be important cofactors in the expression of HIV-associated glomerulosclerosis, they are unlikely to serve a primary role in the pathogenesis of the nephropathy.

In 1990, we speculated that infected blood-borne lymphocytes or monocytes/macrophages could disseminate HIV to the kidney or, alternatively, directly infect glomerular or tubular cells bearing the CD4 antigen receptor or subpopulations of resident monocytes/macrophages. Activation of parenchymal renal cells or resident monocytes/macrophages could spread HIV to other cell populations and produce an inflammatory response that would mediate the destruction of renal tissue (35). If HIV were renotropic, the kidney could serve as sanctuary for the virus, as was demonstrated for cytomegalovirus (116).

Accumulating and substantial evidence indicates that HIV can localize in the kidney. A direct relationship, however, between the presence of HIV in renal parenchymal cells and the pathogenesis of HIV-associated glomerulosclerosis has not been established conclusively because of inconsistent observations or demonstration of HIV in renal cells of patients with, as well as without, nephropathy (117). Therefore, the mechanisms whereby HIV may lead eventually to glomerulosclerosis remain unknown. Several arguments provide evidence of HIV localization in the kidney (Table 35.7):

1. Indirect evidence stems from the well-documented patients who have had a renal transplant and became infected with HIV by a cadaver kidney despite extensive ex vivo perfusion of the donor organ (118).
2. T lymphocytes and monocytes/macrophages expressing the CD4 molecule are the primary receptor cells for HIV. In these cells, the CD4 antigen is the membrane receptor for the envelope glycoprotein (gp120). A preliminary report describes the presence of CD4 antigen in mesangial cells of normal human kidney, suggesting that direct HIV infection of glomeruli is possible (119). This finding, however, has not been confirmed (120).
3. Direct evidence of HIV localization in the kidney was provided by Cohen and associates (121). Using a monoclonal antibody, these investigators localized HIV core p24 antigen by immunohistochemistry in the cytoplasm of tubular epithelium. Replication of these findings, however, has been difficult because of problems of specificity with the various immunohistochemical probes used for virus antigen detection (122–124).

4. Using the more sensitive in situ hybridization technique and a cDNA probe for HIV nucleic acid, the same investigators found the HIV genome not only in tubular epithelial cells, but also in glomerular epithelia in 10 of 11 patients with HIV-associated glomerulosclerosis, unlike in kidneys from HIV-seropositive patients with immune-complex GN or HIV-seronegative patients (121). Using alternate DNA probes, however, other investigators have been unable to detect HIV genomic nucleic acid in renal tissue, but only in passenger leukocytes (123, 124).

5. Green and colleagues (125) succeeded in infecting glomerular cells by exposing homogeneous cultures of human glomerular capillary endothelial cells, mesangial cells, and epithelial cells to HIV in vitro. Infection developed fast and consistently, and it was generalized with glomerular endothelial cells, whereas infection was slow, inconsistent, and limited with mesangial cells. Infectivity attempts were unsuccessful with glomerular epithelial cells. Erice and Kim (126) also succeeded in infecting human mesangial cells in culture, whereas Alpers and colleagues (120) could not. The method used by the last researchers, however, may not have been sensitive enough to detect a low level of mesangial infection, because other investigators have found that coculture with normal peripheral blood mononuclear cells after exposure to HIV or detection of HIV DNA by polymerase chain reaction was required (125). Shukla and associates (127) transfected human mesangial cells in culture with a functional HIV gene.

6. Using the polymerase chain reaction technique, Kimmel and colleagues (117) detected HIV DNA in 28 renal biopsies of 29 HIV-infected patients with nephrotic proteinuria of various causes. Moreover, microdissection of glomeruli, tubules, interstitial cells, and infiltrating inflammatory cells identified the HIV genome in all but interstitial cells. The HIV genome was present in renal cells of HIV-infected patients with or without nephropathy, but not of HIV-seronegative patients. Thus, in these studies, the HIV genome appears to be ubiquitous in renal tissue of HIV-seropositive patients regardless of nephropathologic outcome, risk factor, and stage of HIV infection. The studies do not identify which cells within the glomerulus contained the HIV genome. The finding of HIV proviral DNA in renal tissue of HIV-infected patients regardless of nephropathy indicates that the presence of the HIV genome is not sufficient for the development of glomerulosclerosis. Some triggering local mechanism must be crucial for the expression of renal disease. Host factors related to immune or genetic response to HIV must be associated with the induction of the nephropathy.

7. The difficulties of unraveling the pathogenesis of HIV-associated glomerulosclerosis have been compounded by the lack of an animal model. In monkeys, simian immunodeficiency virus may produce a disease similar to AIDS in humans. In the rhesus, *Macaca mulatta*, mesangial hyperplasia as well as a sclerosing glomerulopathy may ensue. No virus, however, was identified in the kidney (128).

8. Another animal model was described by Dickie and colleagues (129). They produced transgenic mice using a noninfectious HIV provirus transgene in which *gag* and *pol* sequences encompassing the coding sequences for p24, p15, protease, reverse transcriptase, and the amino terminus of p34 endonuclease were deleted. The transgenic animals remained healthy and transmitted the transgene to their progeny. Tissue expression and specificity were variable and possibly dependent on host transcriptional proteins. Three lines of mice in which the transgene was present in the kidney were produced from eight transgenic founders. The heterozygous mice were immunocompetent and did not experience opportunistic infections, but they eventually developed renal disease. Renal expression of proviral mRNA was transient and evident in glomeruli, but not in tubules, before the onset of proteinuria. The proteinuria was progressive, leading to a severe nephrotic syndrome, uremia, and death (130). The kidneys of severely proteinuric animals were enlarged (twice normal size) and showed a spectrum of pathologic changes resembling HIV-associated glomerulosclerosis including microcystic dilated tubules filled with proteinaceous casts, simplification of tubular epithelium, mild mononuclear interstitial nephritis, segmental or global glomerulosclerosis with reactive epithelial cells, and marked expansion of mesangial cell matrix with increased deposition of laminin, collagen, and heparin sulfate proteoglycan (130). Some glomeruli showed mesangial hypercellularity. Subcellular ultrastructural particles, such as tubuloreticular inclusions, were absent (129). Renal tubular cells expressed increased amounts of tissue growth factor-β (TGF-β) and normal cell polarization for sodium–potassium–adenosine triphosphatase (131). Because the virus is not replicating in those models, these findings suggest that HIV-1 gene products alone can induce many of the features of HIV-associated glomerulosclerosis and implicate HIV genes directly in its pathogenesis.

Increasing evidence indicates that cytokines and growth factors play an important role in the progression of idiopathic glomerulosclerosis (132). The tubular hyperplasia and dilatation characteristic of HIV-associated glomerulosclerosis suggest a role for cytokines and growth factors in the expression of the nephropathy. Emerging evidence suggests that such factors may contribute importantly to the rapid progression and possibly the pathogenesis of HIV-associated glomerulosclerosis. An increased influx of macrophages, increased production of cytokines, and increased expression of TGF-β have been described in the kidneys of patients with HIV-associated glomerulosclerosis. TGF-β particularly has been implicated in the mesangial expansion and sclerosis evident in HIV-associated glomerulosclerosis (133). TGF-β, but not tumor necrosis factor or platelet-derived growth factor, has also been shown to activate HIV gene expression in human mesangial cells transfected with an HIV provirus (79, 127).

Clinical Course

Patients usually present with proteinuria, a nephrotic syndrome, or renal insufficiency. Their age and male-to-female ratio are not different from values reported for AIDS patients without renal disease (1, 38). As previously indicated, HIV-associated glomerulosclerosis occurs predominantly in blacks or in intravenous drug users (34, 84). Children with HIV-associated glomerulosclerosis had a mean age of 3 years, and 96% were African-American or Haitian. All children became infected perinatally from mothers with HIV infection (61).

Nephrotic-range proteinuria is usually present in HIV-associated glomerulosclerosis (1, 34, 102), with features of the nephrotic syndrome including hypoalbuminemia. Renal insufficiency is often evident, with serum creatinine concentrations in excess of 2 mg/dL at initial presentation (1, 104); 10 to 20% of these patients may have normal renal function (102). The onset of the nephropathy is often abrupt, with massive proteinuria and uremia. These fulminant lesions may present as ARF.

In contrast to other types of nephrotic syndrome, AIDS patients with HIV-associated glomerulosclerosis frequently have minimal peripheral edema (1, 102). Dehydration and low blood pressure as a consequence of constitutional symptoms, chronic diarrhea, or malnutrition or malabsorption may result in intravascular volume depletion and may prevent the accumulation of fluid in the interstitial tissue. The presence of hyperglobulinemia may have the same effect (134). Blood pressure is often normal, even in patients with advanced renal failure (1, 86, 102). Serum albumin is decreased, often without a reciprocal increase in serum cholesterol concentration (34, 102, 104). Functional manifestations of tubulointerstitial involvement such as tubular acidosis and salt wasting have been described.

The diagnosis of HIV-associated glomerulosclerosis is not difficult in patients with AIDS. In the absence of clinical AIDS, the diagnosis should be suspected when risk factors are elicited. Investigations of patients with HIV-associated glomerulosclerosis fail to detect other known causes of nephrotic syndrome. Serum complement proteins are normal. One may see a polyclonal increase in serum immunoglobulins. CD4 cell counts are variable, from normal to low. HIV infection should be confirmed by the finding of circulating HIV antibodies. As awareness of the nephropathy increases, the nephropathy is often diagnosed clinically. However, not all HIV-seropositive patients developing proteinuria and renal insufficiency have HIV-associated glomerulosclerosis. In our opinion, accurate and early histopathologic diagnosis remains essential, particularly if the effects of antiviral agents or other therapy are to be assessed on the course of the nephropathy. Sometimes, a renal biopsy performed in the workup of an idiopathic nephrotic syndrome leads to an unexpected diagnosis of HIV-associated glomerulosclerosis.

In HIV-seropositive individuals with a nephrotic syndrome, the identification of large kidneys (13 to 15 cm) with increased echogenicity supports a diagnosis of HIV-associated glomerulosclerosis (1, 84, 135–137) inasmuch as kidney size is usually decreased in most other types of chronic renal disease in the absence of diabetes mellitus or amyloidosis. Amyloidosis with nephrotic syndrome and large kidneys can occur in HIV-infected patients and should be considered in the differential diagnosis (34, 138, 139). The enlargement of the kidneys does not correlate with the severity of the proteinuria.

The meaning of modest proteinuria (0.5 to 2.0 g per 24 hours) is uncertain in patients with AIDS in the absence of histologic evaluation. Discrete proteinuria was found in 32 of 75 adult outpatients studied consecutively (1) and in 32 of 55 children with perinatal AIDS (140). Clinically "silent" HIV glomerulosclerosis has been described at autopsy of patients with only modest proteinuria and normal renal function (97, 141). In our experience, the glomeruli of patients dying of AIDS who have discrete proteinuria and no clinical manifestation of renal disease usually are normal or show mild mesangial changes at autopsy (84).

The progression of renal insufficiency is rapid, particularly in nephrotic patients and in blacks, with an interval from initial clinical presentation to dialysis of only weeks to a few months, with a median of 11 weeks (34, 102, 104). The rate of progression can vary, however, and appears slower in Hispanics than in blacks (86). In nonnephrotic patients, kidney survival is prolonged. Children with HIV-associated glomerulosclerosis have a more protracted clinical course, with an average interval of 1 year from the time of detection of the nephropathy to end-stage renal failure. In adults and children, survival is dictated by the clinical progression of AIDS and is independent of the renal disease (61, 104). The rapidity with which renal function deteriorates in HIV-associated glomerulosclerosis contrasts with the slower progression of glomerulosclerosis associated with other diseases (34).

Treatment

No prospective randomized treatment trials of HIV-associated glomerulosclerosis have been conducted. One reason has been the concern of treating infected patients with steroids or immunosuppressive agents. The other is that the pharmacokinetics of new antiviral agents are unknown, and their toxicities are not established in patients with renal insufficiency. Current therapies include zidovudine, immunosuppressants (corticosteroid and cyclosporine), and ACE inhibitors.

Isolated reports note clinical improvement with zidovudine, at a dose of 300 to 800 mg per day, consisting of temporary remission of proteinuria or delayed occurrence of renal failure for several months (142–145), including one patient who was able to discontinue maintenance hemodialysis temporarily. Zidovudine, however, was ineffective in nephrotic children (146). We have seen disease progression in patients with HIV-associated glomerulosclerosis despite administration of zidovudine. Nevertheless, our clinical impression is that HIV-associated glomerulosclerosis occurs less frequently in the last few years than it did 5 to 10 years ago, and progression of the renal disease may not be as explosive in patients who receive antiretroviral therapy than in those who do not. Whether this decrease is due to treatment with antiviral agents or to other factors is unknown.

Several reports support a clinical effect of antiviral agents on HIV-associated glomerulosclerosis. One retrospective analysis of six patients with histologically proved HIV-associated glomerulosclerosis indicated no benefit of zidovudine (300 to 800 mg per day) in two patients with advanced renal disease, but it showed an important delay for the need of long-term hemodialysis for up to 33 months in four patients with less advanced renal dysfunction (serum creatinine 1.2 to 5.1 mg/dL) (100).

In another study, 15 patients with minimal renal dysfunction (mean serum creatinine 0.95 mg/dL) were prospectively treated with zidovudine at 400 to 800 mg per day. After 6 to 26 months of follow-up, mean serum creatinine was unchanged for the group, and no patient developed overt nephropathy or progressed to end-stage renal failure. This study included four patients with biopsy-proved HIV-associated glomerulosclerosis in whom azotemia stabilized or decreased, and proteinuria improved after 3 to 24 months of treatment with 400 mg per day zidovudine (147).

In the third study, 43 or 54 patients with 2+ proteinuria received zidovudine, whereas 11 did not. Zidovudine had little effect in patients already azotemic at the time of initiation of therapy; all patients became uremic or developed end-stage renal failure. On the other hand, only 5 of 37 nonazotemic patients who were given zidovudine became azotemic after 2 years of treatment, whereas 4 of 10 nonazotemic patients who remained untreated developed end-stage renal failure (148).

These observations suggest that zidovudine treatment may protect the kidney, at least when used early in proteinuric patients before azotemia develops. Using regression analysis, an improved outcome was shown to be related specifically to antiretroviral therapy (149). Whether the newer antiretroviral drugs or combinations thereof may improve the course of HIV-associated nephropathy, especially if these drugs are used early in the course of renal disease, is unknown.

Cyclosporine has been used in children with HIV-associated glomerulosclerosis, and it induced a remission of the nephrotic syndrome for up to 1 year in three children with perinatal AIDS and normal renal function. At follow-up, two of these children were in remission, and one, who had two renal biopsies, showed no progression of HIV-associated glomerulosclerosis after 12 months (146). No report on the use of cyclosporine in adults with HIV-associated glomerulosclerosis has been published.

Corticosteroids usually have been ineffective in children (61, 140). An isolated report described a remission of the nephrotic syndrome in an HIV-seropositive white man who had a biopsy showing diffuse mesangial hypercellularity but not the classic picture of HIV-associated glomerulosclerosis (150).

One study reported improvement in renal function and proteinuria in 20 HIV-seropositive patients (14 with biopsy-proved glomerulosclerosis, 3 with mesangial hyperplasia and proliferation, and 3 who did undergo biopsy) who were given prednisone at a dose of 60 mg per day for 2 to 1 weeks followed by slow tapering over 2 to 26 weeks (151). Nineteen patients had serum creatinine concentrations greater than 2 mg/dL: 2 progressed to end-stage renal disease within 5 weeks; in 17, mean serum creatinine decreased from 8.1 to 3.0 mg/dL ($P<.001$). Four patients who had been receiving dialysis at the beginning of the study were able to discontinue dialysis. Twelve of 13 patients showed a reduction in 24-hour urinary protein excretion from a mean of 9.1 to 3.2 g per day ($P<.005$). Six of these patients suffered serious, new opportunistic infections during prednisone therapy including cytomegalovirus retinitis, *Mycobacterium avium* infection, or candidemia. Two patients developed steroid-related psychosis. After a follow-up of 2 to 24 months, 7 patients were alive (5 off and 2 on dialysis), 11 patients had complications of AIDS, and 2 were lost to follow-up. Relapses after discontinuation of prednisone may respond to a second course of steroids (151, 152).

Thus, in selected patients undergoing close medical supervision, prednisone may retard the occurrence of end-stage renal failure. In one patient with HIV-associated glomerulosclerosis and superimposed thrombotic microangiopathic changes treated with prednisone, the improvement in renal function correlated with a marked reduction in interstitial inflammation and tubular damage and the resolution of thrombotic microangiopathy (153).

Treatment with ACE inhibitors is beneficial in several proteinuric glomerular diseases. Similarly, ACE inhibitors have been shown to improve renal survival in patients with HIV-associated glomerulosclerosis. Serum ACE levels are elevated in patients with HIV-infection (154). This enzyme may play a pathogenetic role in the development of glomerulosclerosis through modulation of mesangial cell growth and matrix synthesis. A reduction in proteinuria was observed by Burns and colleagues (155) in a patient with biopsy-proved HIV-associated glomerulosclerosis and the nephrotic syndrome treated with fosinopril. In a case-control study, the mean renal survival time from initiation of captopril therapy (6.25 to 25 mg orally three times daily) to initiation of dialysis was 156 days in nine patients with HIV-associated glomerulosclerosis, compared with 37 days in matched control cases not treated with captopril (149). Burns and associates (156) expanded and confirmed their original observation with 10 mg fosinopril orally once daily in 20 patients, all with biopsy-proved HIV-associated glomerulosclerosis and early renal disease (serum creatinine up to 2 g per day, no prior renal disease, and nonintravenous drug users). They compared seven patients with proteinuria less than or equal to 2 g per day treated with fosinopril against four similar patients not given fosinopril. Baseline serum creatinine (1.3 and 1.0 mg/dL) and proteinuria (1.6 and 0.8 g per day) were similar in the two groups of patients. At 24 weeks, serum creatinine in treated and untreated patients was

1.5 and 4.9 mg/dL ($P<.006$), and proteinuria was 1.3 and 8.5 g per day ($P<.005$), respectively.

Similar renal protection was observed in patients with nephrotic-range proteinuria. Baseline serum creatinine and proteinuria averaged 1.7 mg/dL and 5.4 g per day, respectively, in five treated patients and 1.9 mg/dL and 5.2 g per day in four untreated patients. After 12 weeks of follow-up, serum creatinine and proteinuria for patients given 10 mg fosinopril averaged 2.0 mg/dL and 2.8 g per day compared with 9.2 mg/dL ($P<.02$) and 10.5 g per day ($P<.008$) in untreated patients, respectively (156).

These striking results need confirmation. They also emphasize the need for early referral, tissue diagnosis, and treatment in patients with HIV infection and renal disease. The mechanisms whereby ACE inhibition may be protective in HIV-associated glomerulosclerosis are still unclear, but they may include effects on glomerular hemodynamics, expression of growth factors and cytokines stimulated by angiotensin, or even inhibition of protease activity.

Overall, the therapy for HIV-associated glomerulosclerosis remains controversial, but the outlook is certainly brighter than it was a decade ago. Early diagnosis and biopsy documentation of the nephropathy associated with HIV are important. Use of ACE inhibitors early in the disease appears beneficial. The use of immunosuppressive drugs (corticosteroids and cyclosporine) remains experimental in view of their potential harmful side effects. A combination therapy could include, in selected patients who rapidly develop end-stage renal failure, a short course of corticosteroids followed by ACE inhibitor therapy in those patients who respond to steroids.

Renal Replacement Therapy

In the absence of effective treatment, all patients with HIV-associated glomerulosclerosis eventually progress to end-stage renal failure and require renal replacement therapy in the form of dialysis or kidney transplantation. The prognosis of patients with HIV infection who are receiving hemodialysis is related to the stage of the HIV infection. In the 1980s, AIDS patients survived for less than 3 months while receiving dialysis. Patients with constitutional symptoms survived for 276 days, whereas 14 asymptomatic HIV-seropositive patients were alive 488 days after commencing dialysis treatment (157). Three of the last group of initial patients reported in 1988 eventually survived more than 10 years while receiving dialysis (two on hemodialysis, one on peritoneal dialysis).

In comparison with the 1980s, the survival of HIV-infected patients receiving hemodialysis has improved. Ifudu and colleagues (158) identified 34 patients (91% black, 95% with AIDS) who were receiving maintenance hemodialysis in four outpatient facilities in Brooklyn, New York. These patients had been receiving maintenance hemodialysis for a mean of 57 months, with a mean duration of HIV infection of 50.5 months (range, 2 to 144 months). The reasons for this improved outcome of uremia therapy in patients with end-stage renal disease is unclear. It is not due to antiretroviral therapy because only 18% of the foregoing patients were receiving zidovudine or ddI. Rather, it may relate to a combination of factors such as better treatment of opportunistic infections, use of permanent vascular access (only one patient had a temporary access) providing blood flow in excess of 350 mg per minute and allowing for better dialysis, correction of anemia with erythropoietin, use of bicarbonate dialysate, and more biocompatible dialyzers, in addition to changes in the definition of AIDS and possibly the selection of patients. Patients with AIDS may develop a syndrome of unexplained malnutrition and wasting, a "failure to thrive" that is unresponsive to intensive nutritional support (87).

In a separate study, the use of zidovudine in patients undergoing hemodialysis was associated with a significantly longer survival of HIV-infected patients (15.2 versus 6.2 months, $P<.01$) (159). In this study, variables predicting survival in HIV-infected patients receiving maintenance hemodialysis included CD4 counts and blood pressure ($P<.001$); patients with the lowest values had the worst survival. Infection rate and urine protein excretion both had a significant negative correlation with survival ($P<.01$ and $<.02$, respectively).

Long-term peritoneal dialysis is a reasonable option and is equivalent to hemodialysis for patients with HIV infection (160). Outcome is also related to the stage of the HIV infection. The decision to withhold dialysis in individual patients with terminal AIDS must be individualized (161).

Renal transplantation in HIV-infected patients with end-stage renal disease is complex. Experience is not large and is mostly retrospective. HIV can be transmitted by an infected organ. Thus, HIV screening is mandatory for all potential kidney donors. The feasibility, risk, and cost-effectiveness of renal transplantation in HIV-infected patients with end-stage renal disease is controversial. Most centers do not perform renal transplantation in this population (118).

MINIMAL-CHANGE DISEASE AND MESANGIAL HYPERPLASIA

Several instances of minimal-change disease have been reported in proteinuric patients with AIDS, including two who later evolved to glomerulosclerosis. The significance of minimal change glomerulopathy or focal mesangial hyperplasia in the pathogenesis of glomerular sclerosis must await prospective studies that include serial renal biopsies (80).

Diffuse and global mesangial hyperplasia, on the other hand, is readily identified histologically in approximately 25% of children with perinatal AIDS and nephrotic-range proteinuria and in 13% of adults (see Table 35.5). The characteristic tubulointerstitial histologic features and the kidney enlargement of HIV-associated glomerulosclerosis are absent in patients with diffuse mesangial lesions. The kidneys are not enlarged at autopsy (84), a finding supporting the dominant role of the tubulointerstitial lesions in the pathogenesis of the nephromegaly. Clinically, these patients have massive proteinuria with little decrease in renal function.

As with minimal lesions and focal mesangial hyperplasia, the possibility that diffuse mesangial lesions may precede glomerulosclerosis is an attractive hypothesis, suggested by documented, although rare, transitions to HIV-associated glomerulosclerosis (94). The nephrotic syndrome in AIDS patients with minimal glomerular lesions or with diffuse mesangial hyperplasia is variably responsive to steroid treatment (61, 146). The role of antiviral agents or ACE inhibitors on the proteinuria and progression of renal diseases in these patients is unknown.

IMMUNE-COMPLEX GLOMERULONEPHRITIS

Another major form of chronic renal disease in patients infected with HIV is immune-complex GN of various types (79). These disorders occur more often in white and in male patients with HIV infection. Their prevalence is a function of the population studied in different geographic areas. For instance, in an Italian study of 26 HIV-infected subjects (all white adults, with most being intravenous drug abusers), the glomerular lesions included 2 minimal-change disease, 1 mesangial proliferative GN, 6 postinfectious GN, 1 crescentic membranoproliferative GN, 3 membranous GN, 4 IgA nephropathy, 3 mixed membranous and proliferative GN and 3 diffuse proliferative lupus-like GN. No patient had HIV-associated glomerulosclerosis (162). Except for the frequent occurrence of TRIs on electron microscopy, the lesions are similar to those encountered in HIV-seronegative patients with GN. These patients present with proteinuria, azotemia, or microscopic hematuria. They more often have hypertension and hematuria than patients with HIV-associated glomerulosclerosis. The rate of progression to end-stage renal may be rapid (79, 163).

Mesangial Proliferative and Membranoproliferative Glomerulonephritis

The pathogenesis of these glomerulonephritides remains controversial. They may be HIV associated, they may be a manifestation of coinfection (hepatitis C, postinfectious), they may develop coincidentally, or they may be related to treatment with interferon (164–166).

HIV infection may modify and prolong the natural course of postinfectious GN, as demonstrated by Korbet and Schwartz (167) in a patient in whom lingering manifestations of active streptococcal infection remained serologically and histopathologically evident for 7 months. The importance of coinfection in the pathogenesis of immune-complex GN needs emphasis. Stokes and associates (166) identified 12 patients with renal disease (all intravenous drug abusers, African-Americans) who were coinfected with HIV and hepatitis C virus. Eleven patients had immune-complex GN, and 1 had HIV-associated glomerulosclerosis with immune-complex deposits. Renal biopsy showed mesangial proliferative GN in 5 patients, membranoproliferative GN in 5, membranous GN in 1, and "collapsing" glomerulosclerosis with immune-complex deposits in 1. The contribution of hepatitis C virus infection on HIV-associated immune-complex GN is still unraveling.

Membranous Glomerulonephritis

Membranous glomerulopathy has been described in HIV-seropositive individuals and can occur in patients coinfected with hepatitis B (168–170) or hepatitis C (166). Hepatitis B surface and e antigens and hepatitis C virus antigen each were identified in the glomerular deposits of one patient (169). Glomerular membranous lesions have also been shown in a patient with AIDS and secondary syphilis whose nephrotic syndrome cleared with penicillin treatment (171) and in a child with perinatal AIDS and antinuclear and double-stranded DNA antibodies consistent with systemic lupus erythematosus (172).

Systemic Lupus Erythematosus

Clinical and serologic manifestations of systemic lupus erythematosus have been reported in adults and children with AIDS in association with membranous as well as mesangial and intracapillary proliferative glomerular lesions (61, 98, 162, 172). To what extent these lesions represent a manifestation of autoimmunity related to the viral infection has not been elucidated inasmuch as autoimmune processes frequently occur with HIV infection. Low titers of antinuclear antibodies (up to 1:160) without anti-ds DNA antibodies can occur in HIV-infected patients without renal disease (173). Two HIV-infected patients with strong clinical and serologic evidence of systemic lupus and renal disease have been reported to underscore the need for renal biopsy to define the underlying nephropathy. One patient had diffuse proliferative GN compatible with systemic lupus nephritis, whereas the other had collapsing glomerulosclerosis compatible with HIV-associated nephropathy (174).

Immunoglobulin A Nephropathy

More than 20 cases of IgA nephropathy have been reported in HIV-seropositive patients (162, 175, 176). All were white, generally homosexuals (2 intravenous drug abusers) or children with normal or low CD4 cell counts. All presented with microscopic or macroscopic hematuria, minimal or modest renal insufficiency, proteinuria usually less than 1 g per 24 hours (only 4 had nephrotic-range proteinuria), increased serum IgA or IgA/IgG (but normal IgM) concentrations, and increased circulating immune complexes. Progression of renal disease appears slow. Renal histologic examination revealed, in various instances, normal glomeruli, focal or diffuse mesangial proliferation, or crescentic GN (2 patients). All had IgA deposits in the glomerular mesangium, alone or in combination with C3, C1q, IgG, or IgM. Tubuloreticular inclusions were identified when sought.

Selective abnormalities of IgA regulation are frequent in patients with AIDS, and circulating complexes containing

IgA can be found in 57% of patients, as well as polymeric IgA1 rheumatoid factor (177–179). In contrast, intrarenal deposits of IgA are rare at autopsy of AIDS patients (178, 180) or at biopsy of patients with HIV-associated nephropathy (84). The occurrence of IgA nephropathy appears to be HIV related. Indeed, Katz and colleagues (181) demonstrated the presence of circulating anti-HIV IgA in two patients with HIV infection and IgA nephropathy. Kimmel and associates (107) isolated circulating immune complexes composed of idiotypic IgA antibody reactive with anti-HIV IgG or IgM in two patients with IgA nephropathy, and the identical immune complex was eluted from the renal biopsy tissue of one patient studied. These observations support an immune-complex pathogenesis associated with HIV infection, even though the HIV antigen was not present in these complexes.

OTHER RENAL LESIONS

Various other renal lesions can be found in AIDS that often remain clinically silent and are found at autopsy.

Nephrocalcinosis

Foci of calcium deposition can be found in up to 40% of kidneys of AIDS patients examined at autopsy (5, 38). Clinical manifestations are absent. Nephrocalcinosis can occur in association with pulmonary granulomatosis (38), possibly as a result of increased vitamin D production or *Mycobacterium avium-intracellulare* infection (182), or as a manifestation of extrapulmonary *Pneumocystis* infection (183–186). A high incidence of unexplained hypocalcemia has been found in patients with calcium deposits (5). Nephrocalcinosis can be identified by increased echogenicity on ultrasound and increased density in computed tomographic examination.

Opportunistic Infections

Virtually all opportunistic infections seen in AIDS may localize in the renal parenchyma as a manifestation of disseminated disease. The degree of interstitial reaction and tubular damage varies, but it is usually mild, and renal function is usually not compromised.

Acute bacterial pyelonephritis is rare, although genitourinary infections are common. Referrals to urologists have increased in AIDS patients for renal and perirenal abscesses with uncommon organisms (*Candida albicans, Mucor, Aspergillus*). Conservative therapy with percutaneous drainage may be effective (187–189).

Cytomegalovirus infection is the most common opportunistic infection found in the kidney and has been suggested to facilitate the development of HIV-associated glomerulosclerosis. The kidneys of 78 HIV-infected patients, examined for the presence of cytomegalovirus by immunohistochemistry and in situ hybridization, disclosed the virus in 10 patients (12.8%), but in none of 5 with HIV-associated glomerulosclerosis (190). Invasion of the kidney by opportunistic organisms is rarely identified in patients with HIV-associated glomerulosclerosis. Renal infection with mycobacteria is a manifestation of miliary tuberculosis. Disseminated microsporidial infections are increasingly recognized as having clinically significant renal involvement ranging from hematuria to ARF (191, 192). In areas of endemicity, histoplasmosis frequently produces overwhelming systemic infections in part leading to ARF (193).

Neoplasms

Non–Hodgkin's lymphoma and Kaposi's sarcoma are the most frequent renal neoplasms found in AIDS patients, usually as a local manifestation of a disseminated involvement. Lymphomas are reported in 2% of autopsies (5). Renal cell carcinoma may appear in AIDS patients who are younger than serologically negative individuals, although an increased prevalence is not established. An angiocarcinoma has also been reported (80).

References

1. Bourgoignie JJ, Meneses R, Ortiz C, et al. The clinical spectrum of renal disease associated with human immunodeficiency virus. Am J Kidney Dis 1988;12:131–137.
2. Berns JS, Cohen RM, Stumacher RJ, et al. Renal aspects of therapy for human immunodeficiency virus and associated opportunistic infections. J Am Soc Nephrol 1991;1:1061–1080.
3. Chattha G, Arieff AI, Cummings C, et al. Lactic acidosis complicating the acquired immunodeficiency syndrome. Ann Intern Med 1993; 118:37–39.
4. Glassock RJ, Cohen AH, Danovitch G, et al. Human immunodeficiency virus (HIV) infection and the kidney. Ann Intern Med 1990;112:35–49.
5. Seney FD Jr, Burns DK, Silva FG. Acquired immunodeficiency syndrome and the kidney. Am J Kidney Dis 1990;16:1–13.
6. Vitting KE, Gardenswartz MH, Zabetakis PM, et al. Frequency of hyponatremia and nonosmolar vasopressin release in the acquired immunodeficiency syndrome. JAMA 1990;263:973–976.
7. Agarwal A, Soni A, Ciechanowsky M, et al. Hyponatremia in patients with the acquired immunodeficiency syndrome. Nephron 1989;53: 317–321.
8. Tang WW, Kapstein EM, Feinstein EI, et al. Hyponatremia in hospitalized patients with acquired immune deficiency syndrome and the AIDS related complex Am J Med 1993;94:169–174.
9. Greene LW, Cole W, Greene JB, et al. Adrenal insufficiency as a complication of the acquired immunodeficiency syndrome. Ann Intern Med 1984;101:497–498.
10. Kalin G, Torensky L, Seras DS, et al. Hyporeninemic hypoaldosteronism associated with the acquired immunodeficiency syndrome. Am J Med 1987;82:1035–1038.
11. Guenthner EE, Rabinowe SL, Van Niel A, et al. Primary Addison's disease in a patient with the acquired immunodeficiency syndrome. Ann Intern Med 1984;100:847–848.
12. Membreno L, Irony I, Dere W, et al. Adrenocortical function in acquired immunodeficiency syndrome. J Clin Endocrinol Metab 1987;65:482–487.
13. Biglieri EG. Adrenocortical function in the acquired immunodeficiency syndrome (AIDS). West J Med 1988;148:70–73.
14. Glasgow BJ, Steinsapir KD, Anders K, et al. Adrenal pathology in the acquired immunodeficiency syndrome. Am J Clin Pathol 1985;84: 594–597.
15. Santos GI, Garcia PI, del Arco GC, et al. Sindrome de secrecion inapropiada asociado con el sindrome de immunodeficiencia adquirida. Rev Clin Esp 1991;188:120–122.

16. Farese RV Jr, Schambelan M, Hollander H, et al. Nephrogenic diabetes insipidus associated with foscarnet treatment of cytomegalovirus retinitis. Ann Intern Med 1990;112:955–956.
17. Navarro JF, Quereda C, Quereda C, et al. Nephrogenic diabetes insipidus and renal tubular acidosis secondary to foscarnet therapy. Am J Kidney Dis 1996;27:431–434.
18. Peter SA. Electrolyte disorders and renal dysfunction in acquired immunodeficiency syndrome patients. J Natl Med Assoc 1991;83:889–891.
19. Briceland LL, Bailie GR. Pentamidine-associated nephrotoxicity and hyperkalemia in patients with AIDS. Drug Intell Clin Pharmacol 1991;25:1171–1174.
20. Lachaal M, Venuto RC. Nephrotoxicity and hyperkalemia in patients with acquired immunodeficiency syndrome treated with pentamidine. Am J Med 1989;87:260–263.
21. Velasquez H, Perazella MA, Wright FS, et al. Renal mechanism of trimethoprim-induced hyperkalemia. Arch Intern Med 1993;119:296–301.
22. Medina I, Mills J, Leoung G, et al. Oral therapy for *Pneumocystis carinii* pneumonia in the acquired immunodeficiency syndrome: a controlled trial of trimethoprim–sulfamethoxazole versus trimethoprim–dapsone. N Engl J Med 1990;323:776–782.
23. Greenberg S, Reiser IW, Chou SY, et al. Trimethoprim–sulfamethoxazole induces reversible hyperkalemia. Ann Intern Med 1993;119:291–295.
24. Reiser IW, Chou SY, Brown ML, et al. Reversal of trimethoprim-induced antikaliuresis. Kidney Int 1996;50:2063–2069.
25. Shah GM, Alvarado P, Kirrschenbaum MA. Symptomatic hypocalcemia and hypomagnesemia with renal magnesium wasting associated with pentamidine therapy in a patient with AIDS. Am J Med 1990;89:380–382.
26. Mani S. Pentamidine induced renal magnesium wasting [letter]. AIDS 1992;6:594–595.
27. Jacobs MB. The acquired immunodeficiency syndrome and hypercalcemia. West J Med 1986;144:469–471.
28. Cockerell CJ, Dolan ET. Widespread cutaneous and systemic calcification (calciphylaxis) in patients with the acquired immunodeficiency syndrome and renal disease. J Am Acad Dermatol 1992;26:559–562.
29. Maesaka JK, Cusano AJ, Thies HL, et al. Hypouricemia in acquired immunodeficiency syndrome. Am J Kidney Dis 1990;15:252–257.
30. Berns JS, Cohen RM, Rudnick MR, et al. Renal aspects of antimicrobial therapy for HIV infection. In: Renal and urologic aspects of HIV infection. Contemp Issues Nephrol 1996;29:195–235.
31. Chen JL, Brocavich JM, Lin AY. Psychiatric disturbances associated with ganciclovir therapy. Ann Pharmacother 1992;26:193–195.
32. Valeri A, Neusy AJ. Acute and chronic renal disease in hospitalized AIDS patients. Clin Nephrol 1991;35:110–118.
33. Genderini A, Bertoli S, Scorza D, et al. Acute renal failure in patients with acquired immune deficiency syndrome. J Nephrol 1991;1:45–47.
34. Rao TK, Friedman EA. Renal syndromes in the acquired immunodeficiency syndrome (AIDS): lessons learned from analysis over 5 years. Artif Organs 1988;12:206–209.
35. Bourgoignie JJ. Renal complications of human immunodeficiency virus type 1. Kidney Int 1990;37:1571–1584.
36. Cantor ES, Kimmel PL, Bosch JP. Effect of race on expression of acquired immunodeficiency syndrome–associated nephropathy. Arch Intern Med 1991;151:125–128.
37. Comtois R, Pouliot J, Vinet B, et al. Higher pentamidine levels in AIDS patients with hypoglycemia and azotemia during treatment of *Pneumocystis carinii* pneumonia. Am Rev Respir Dis 1992;146:740–744.
38. D'Agati V, Cheng JI, Carbone L, et al. The pathology of HIV-nephropathy: a detailed morphologic and comparative study. Kidney Int 1989;35:1358–1370.
39. Polis MA, Spooner KM, Baird BF, et al. Anticytomegaloviral activity and safety of cidofovir in patients with human immunodeficiency virus infection and cytomegalovirus viruria. Antimicrob Agents Chemother 1995;39:882–886.
40. Seidel EA, Koenig S, Polis MA. A dose escalation study to determine the toxicity and maximally tolerated dose of foscarnet. AIDS 1993;7:941–945.
41. Rashed A, Azadeh B, Abu Romeh SH. Acyclovir-induced acute tubulo-interstitial nephritis. Nephron 1990;56:436–438.
42. Raisin J, Hess B, Blatter M, et al. Toxicity of an organic germanium compound: deleterious consequences of a "natural remedy." Schweiz Med Wochenschr 1992;122:11–13.
43. Hess B, Raisin J, Zimmermann A, et al. Tubulointerstitial nephropathy persisting 20 months after discontinuation of chronic intake of germanium lactate citrate. Am J Kidney Dis 1993;21:548–552.
44. Jokela J, Flynn T, Henry K. Thrombotic thrombocytopenic purpura in a human immunodeficiency virus (HIV)–seropositive homosexual man. Am J Hematol 1987;25:341–343.
45. Nair JMG, Bellevue R, Bertoni M, et al. Thrombotic thrombocytopenic purpura in patients with the acquired immunodeficiency syndrome (AIDS)–related complex: a report of 2 cases. Ann Intern Med 1988;109:209–212.
46. Platanias NC, Paiusco D, Bernstein S, et al. Thrombotic thrombocytopenic purpura as the first manifestation of human immunodeficiency virus infection. Am J Med 1989;87:699–700.
47. Leaf AN, Laubenstein LJ, Raphael B, et al. Thrombotic thrombocytopenic purpura associated with human immunodeficiency virus type 1 infection. Ann Intern Med 1988;109:194–197.
48. Charasse C, Michelet C, Le Tulzo Y, et al. Thrombotic thrombocytopenic purpura in patients with the acquired immunodeficiency syndrome: a pathologically documented case report. Am J Kidney Dis 1991;17:80–82.
49. Boccia RV, Gelmann EP, Baker CC, et al. A hemolytic uremic syndrome with the acquired immunodeficiency syndrome. Ann Intern Med 1984;101:716–717.
50. Esforzado N, Poch E, Almirall J, et al. Hemolytic uremic syndrome associated with HIV infection [letter]. AIDS 1991;5:1041–1042.
51. Segal GH, Tubbs RR, Ratliff NB, et al. Thrombotic thrombocytopenic purpura in a patient with AIDS. Cleveland Clin J Med 1990;57:360–366.
52. Meisenberg BR, Robinson WL, Mosley CA, et al. Thrombotic thrombocytopenic purpura in human immunodeficiency (HIV) seropositive males. Am J Hematol 1988;27:212–215.
53. Rarick MU, Espina B, Mocharnuk R, et al. Thrombotic thrombocytopenic purpura in patients with human immunodeficiency virus infection: a report of three cases and review of the literature. Am J Hematol 1992;40:103–109.
54. Thompson CE, Damon LE, Ries CA, et al. Thrombotic microangiopathies in the 1980s: clinical features, response to treatment, and the impact of the human immunodeficiency virus epidemic. Blood 1992;80:1890–1895.
55. Frem GJ, Rennke HG, Sayegh MH. Late renal allograft failure secondary to thrombotic microangiopathy–human immunodeficiency virus nephropathy. J Am Soc Nephrol 1994;4:1643–1648.
56. Karpatkin S, Nardi M. Autoimmune anti-HIV-1 gp120 antibody with anti-idiotype–like activity in sera and immune complexes of HIV-1-related immunologic thrombocytopenia. J Clin Invest 1992;89:356–364.
57. Peraldi MN, Berrou J, Flahaut A, et al. Elevated plasma tissue type plasminogen activator (tPA) in HIV-infected patients with thrombotic microangiopathy [abstract]. J Am Soc Nephrol 1996;7:1377.
58. Berns JS. Hemolytic uremic syndrome and thrombotic thrombocytopenic purpura associated with HIV infection. Contemp Issues Nephrol 1996;29:111–133.
59. Coleburn NH, Scholes JV, Lowe FC. Renal failure in patients with AIDS-related complex. Urology 1991;37:523–527.
60. Jindal KK, Trillo A, Bishop G, et al. Crescentic IgA nephropathy as a manifestation of human immune deficiency virus infection. Am J Nephrol 1991;11:147–150.

61. Strauss J, Abitbol C, Zilleruelo G, et al. Renal disease in children with the acquired immunodeficiency syndrome. N Engl J Med 1989;321: 625–630.
62. Christin S, Baumelou A, Bahri S, et al. Acute renal failure due to sulfadiazine in patients with AIDS. Nephron 1990;55:233–234.
63. Carbone LG, Bendixen B, Appel GB. Sulfadiazine-associated obstructive nephropathy occurring in a patient with the acquired immunodeficiency syndrome. Am J Kidney Dis 1988;12:72–75.
64. Molina JM, Belenfant X, Doco-Lecompte T, et al. Sulfadiazine-induced crystalluria in AIDS patients with toxoplasma encephalitis. AIDS 1991;5:587–589.
65. Becker K, Jablonowski H, Haussinger D. Sulfadiazine-associated nephrotoxicity in patients with the acquired immunodeficiency syndrome. Medicine (Baltimore) 1996;75:185–194.
66. Sawyer MH, Webb DE, Balow JE, et al. Acyclovir-induced acute renal failure. Clinical course and histology. Am J Med 1988;84:1067–1071.
67. Ogea Garcia JL, Villanueva Marcos JL, Jurado R, et al. Linfoma de Burkitt y AIDS presentacion como hepatomegalia tumoral e insuficiencia renal aguda debida a depositos de uratos [letter]. An Med Interna 1989;6:551–552.
68. Tashima KT, Horowitz JD, Rosen S. Indinavir nephropathy [letter]. N Engl J Med 1997;336:138–139.
69. Mohler JL, Jarow JP, Marshall FF. Unusual urological presentations of acquired immune deficiency syndrome: large cell lymphoma. J Urol 1987;138:627–629.
70. Spector DA, Katz RS, Fuller H, et al. Acute non-dilating obstructive renal failure in a patient with AIDS. Am J Nephrol 1989;9:129–132.
71. Comiter S, Glasser J, Al-Askari S. Ureteral obstruction in a patient with Burkitt's lymphoma. Urology 1992;39:277–289.
72. Kuhlman JE, Browne D, Shermak M, et al. Retroperitoneal and pelvic CT of patients with AIDS: primary and secondary involvement of the genitourinary tract. Radiographics 1991;11:473–483.
73. Gertner E, Thurn JR, Williams DN, et al. Zidovudine-associated myopathy. Am J Med 1989;86:814–817.
74. Sensakovic JW, Suarez M, Perez G, et al. Pentamidine treatment of *Pneumocystis carinii* pneumonia in the acquired immunodeficiency syndrome: association with acute renal failure and myoglobinuria. Arch Intern Med 1985;145:2247.
75. del Rio C, Soffer O, Widell JL, et al. Acute human immunodeficiency virus infection temporarily associated with rhabdomyolysis, acute renal failure, and nephrosis. Rev Infect Dis 1990;12:282–285.
76. Roth D, Alarcon FJ, Fernandez JA, et al. Acute rhabdomyolysis associated with cocaine intoxication. N Engl J Med 1988;319: 673–677.
77. Rao TK, Friedman EA. Outcome of severe acute renal failure in patients with acquired immunodeficiency syndrome. Am J Kidney Dis 1995;25:390–398.
78. Rappaport J, Kopp JB, Klotman PE. Host virus interaction and the molecular regulation of HIV-1. Kidney Int 1994;46:16–27.
79. Kimmel PL, Phillips TM. Immune complex glomerulonephritis associated with HIV infection. Contemp Issues Nephrol 1996;29: 77–110.
80. Pardo V, Wetli, Strauss J, et al. Renal complications of drug abuse and human immunodeficiency virus. In: Tischer C, Brenner BM, eds. Pathology of the kidney. 2nd ed. Philadelphia: JB Lippincott, 1994; 390–418.
81. Bourgoignie J. Glomerulosclerosis associated with HIV infection. Contemp Issues Nephrol 1996;29:59–75.
82. Humphreys MH. Human immunodeficiency virus–associated glomerulosclerosis. Kidney Int 1995;48:311–320.
83. D'Agati V, Appel GB. HIV infection and the kidney. J Am Soc Nephrol 1997;8:138–152.
84. Pardo V, Meneses R, Ossa L, et al. AIDS-related glomerulopathy: occurrence in specific risk groups. Kidney Int 1989;31:1167–1173.
85. Cohen AH, Nast CC. HIV-associated nephropathy: a unique combined glomerular, tubular and interstitial lesion. Mod Pathol 1988;1:87–97.
86. Soni A, Agarwal A, Chander P, et al. Evidence for an HIV-related nephropathy: a clinicopathological study. Clin Nephrol 1989;31: 12–17.
87. Rao TK, Filippone EJ, Nicastri AD, et al. Associated focal and segmental glomerulosclerosis in the acquired immunodeficiency syndrome. N Engl J Med 1984;310:669–673.
88. Pardo V, Aldana M, Colton RM, et al. Glomerular lesions in the acquired immunodeficiency syndrome. Ann Intern Med 1984;101: 429–434.
89. Gardenswartz MH, Lerner CW, Seligson GR, et al. Renal disease in patients with AIDS: a clinicopathologic study. Clin Nephrol 1984;21: 197–204.
90. Balow JE, Macher AM, Rook AH. Paucity of glomerular disease in acquired immunodeficiency syndrome (AIDS) [abstract]. Kidney Int 1986;29:178.
91. Mazbar SA, Schoenfeld PY, Humphreys MH. Renal involvement in patients infected with HIV: experience at San Francisco General Hospital. Kidney Int 1990;37:1325–1332.
92. Bourgoignie JJ, Ortiz-Interian C, Green DF, et al. The epidemiology of human immunodeficiency virus-associated nephropathy. In: Hatano M, ed. Nephrology. vol 1. Tokyo: Springer-Verlag, 1991: 484–492.
93. Humphreys MH. Human immunodeficiency virus-associated nephropathy: east is east and west is west? Arch Intern Med 1990; 150:253–255.
94. Bourgoignie JJ, Pardo V. The nephropathology in human immunodeficiency virus (HIV-1) infection. Kidney Int 1991;35:S19–S23.
95. Brunkhorst R, Brunkhorst U, Eisenbach GM, et al. Lack of clinical evidence for a specific HIV-associated glomerulopathy in 203 patients with HIV infection. Nephrol Dial Transpl 1992;7:87–92.
96. Frassetto L, Schoenfeld PY, Humphreys MH. Increasing incidence of human immunodeficiency virus-associated nephropathy at San Francisco General Hospital. Am J Kidney Dis 1991;18:655–659.
97. Lopes GS, Marques LP, Rioja LS, et al. Glomerular disease and human immunodeficiency virus infection in Brazil. Am J Nephrol 1992;12: 281-287.
98. Nochy D, Gotz D, Dosquet P, et al. Renal disease associated with HIV infection: a multicentric study of 60 patients from Paris hospitals. Nephrol Dial Transplant 1993;8:11–19.
99. van der Reijden HJ, Schipper MEF, Danner SA, et al. Glomerular lesions and opportunistic infections of the kidney in AIDS: an autopsy study of 47 cases. Adv Exp Med Biol 1989;252:181–189.
100. Michel C, Dosquet P, Ronco P, et al. Nephropathy associated with human immunodeficiency virus: a report of 11 cases including 6 treated with zidovudine. Nephron 1992;62:434–440.
101. Esforzado N, Feliz T, Almirall J, et al. Nephropathy in human immunodeficiency virus infection. Med Clin (Barc) 1992;98:764–767.
102. Langs C, Gallo GR, Schacht RG, et al. Rapid renal failure in AIDS-associated focal glomerulosclerosis. Arch Intern Med 1990; 150:287–292.
103. Detwiler RK, Falk RJ, Hogan SL, et al. Collapsing glomerulopathy: a clinically and pathologically distinct variant of focal segmental glomerulosclerosis. Kidney Int 1994;45:1416–1424.
104. Valeri A, Barisoni L, Appel GB, et al. Idiopathic collapsing focal segmental glomerulosclerosis: a clinicopathologic study. Kidney Int 1996;50:1734–1746.
105. Carbone L, D'Agati V, Cheng JT, et al. Course and prognosis of human immunodeficiency virus-associated nephropathy. Am J Med 1989;87:389–395.
106. Rao TK, Friedman EA. AIDS (HIV)-associated nephropathy: does it exist? An in-depth review. Am J Nephrol 1989;9:441–453.
107. Kimmel PL, Phillips TM, Farkas-Szallasi T, et al. Idiotypic IgA nephropathy in patients with HIV infection. N Engl J Med 1992;327: 702–706.
108. Patri B, Doazan H, N'Guyen Phuong T, et al. Hepatite et insuffisance rénale aigues associées a une séroconversion au virus de l'immunodéficience humaine [letter]. Presse Med 1988;17:1094–1095.

109. Lawrenson JJ, Chapman P, Getfen L, et al. Proteinuria and the acute mononucleosis-like illness associated with seroconversion in HIV infection [letter]. S Afr Med J 1991;79:625–626.
110. Schindler JM, Neftel KA. Simultaneous primary infection with HIV and CMV leading to severe pancytopenia, hepatitis, nephritis, perimyocarditis, myositis, and alopecia totalis. Klin Wochenschr 1990;68:237–240.
111. Bauer FA, Wear DJ, Angritt P, et al. *Mycoplasma fermentans* (incognitas strain) infection in the kidneys of patients with acquired immunodeficiency syndrome and associated nephropathy: a light microscopic, immunohistochemical, and ultrastructural study. Hum Pathol 1991;22:63–69.
112. Foster S, Hawkins E, Hanson CG, et al. Pathology of the kidney in childhood immunodeficiency: AIDS-related nephropathy is not unique. Pediatr Pathol 1991;11:63–74.
113. Heriot K, Hallquist AE, Tomar KH. Paraproteinemia in patients with acquired immunodeficiency syndrome. Clin Chem 1985;31:1224–1226.
114. Papadopoulos NM, Lane HC, Costello R, et al. Oligoclonal immunoglobulin in patients with the acquired immunodeficiency syndrome. Clin Immunol Immunopathol 1987;35:43–46.
115. Cheng-Mayer C, Levy LA. Distinct biological and serological properties of human immunodeficiency viruses from the brain. Ann Neurol 1988;23:S58–S61.
116. Heieren MH, Vander Woude JF, Balfour HM. Cytomegalovirus replicates efficiently in human kidney mesangial cells. Proc Natl Acad Sci U S A 1988;85:1642–1646.
117. Kimmel PL, Ferreira-Centeno A, Farkas-Szallasi T, et al. Viral DNA in microdissected renal biopsy tissue from HIV infected patients with nephrotic syndrome. Kidney Int 1993; 43:1347–1352.
118. Feduska NJ. Human immunodeficiency virus, AIDS, and organ transplantation. Transplant Rev 1996;4:93–107.
119. Karlsson-Parra A, Dimeny E, Fellstrom B, et al. HIV receptors (CD4 antigen) in normal human glomerular cells [letter]. N Engl J Med 1989;320:741.
120. Alpers CE, McClure J, Bursten SL. Human mesangial cells are resistant to productive infection by multiple strains of human immunodeficiency virus types 1 and 2. Am J Kidney Dis 1992;19:126–130.
121. Cohen AH, Sun NCJ, Shapshak P, et al. Demonstration of human immunodeficiency virus in renal epithelium in HIV-associated nephropathy. Mod Pathol 1989;2:125–128.
122. Barbiano di Belgiojoso G, Genderini A, Vago L, et al. Absence of HIV antigens in renal tissue from patients with HIV-associated nephropathy. Nephrol Dial Transplantant 1990;5:489–492.
123. Pardo V, Shapshak P, Yoshioka M, et al. HIV associated nephropathy (HIVN). Direct renal invasion or indirect glomerular involvement [abstract]. FASEB J 1991;5:907A.
124. Nadasdy T, Hanson-Painton O, Davis L, et al. Conditions affecting detection of HIV in formalin fixed paraffin embedded sections in kidneys and organs from AIDS patients [abstract]. Lab Invest 1991;64:98A.
125. Green DR, Resnick L, Bourgoignie JJ. HIV infects glomerular endothelial and mesangial cells but not epithelial cells in vitro. Kidney Int 1992;41:956–960.
126. Erice A, Kim Y. In-vitro infection of human renal cells by human immunodeficiency virus: pathogenic implications for HIV-associated nephropathy [abstract]. Clin Res 1991;39:219A.
127. Shukla RR, Kumar A, Kimmel PL. Transforming growth factor beta increases the expression of HIV-1 gene in human mesangial. Kidney Int 1993;44:1022–1029.
128. Alpers CE, Baskin GB. Sclerosing glomerulopathy in rhesus monkeys with simian AIDS [abstract]. Kidney Int 1989;35:339.
129. Dickie P, Felser J, Eckhaus M, et al. HIV-associated nephropathy in transgenic mice expressing HIV-1 genes. Virology 1991;185:109–119.
130. Kopp JB, Klotman ME, Adler SH, et al. Progressive glomerulosclerosis and enhanced renal accumulation of basement membrane components in mice transgenic for human immunodeficiency virus type 1 genes. Proc Natl Acad Sci U S A 1992;89:1577–1581.
131. Kopp JB, McCunie BK, Notkins AL, et al. Increased expression of transforming growth factor beta in HIV-transgenic mouse kidney [abstract]. J Am Soc Nephrol 1991;1:600.
132. Wolthuis A, van Goor H, Weening JJ, et al. Pathobiology of focal sclerosis. Curr Opin Nephrol Hypertens 1993;2:458–464.
133. Bodi I, Abraham AA, Kimmel PL. Macrophages in human immunodeficiency virus-associated kidney disease. Am J Kidney Dis 1994;24:762–767.
134. Guardia J, Ortiz-Butcher C, Bourgoignie J. Contribution of globulins to plasma oncotic pressure and the presence of edema in HIV patients with proteinuria [abstract]. J Am Soc Nephrol 1995;6:419.
135. Hamper UM, Goldblum LE, Hutchins GM, et al. Renal involvement in AIDS: sonographic pathologic correlation. AJR Am J Roentgenol 1988;150:1321–1325.
136. Schaffer RM, Schwartz GE, Becker JA, et al. Renal ultrasound in acquired immune deficiency syndrome. Radiology 1984;153:511–513.
137. Kay CJ. Renal disease in patients with AIDS: sonographic findings. AJR Am J Roentgenol 1992;159:551–554.
138. Baumelou A, Assogba V, Beaufils H, et al. Pathologie rénale associée à l'infection à virus VIH et au syndrome d'immunodéficience acquise. In: Chatelain C, Jacobs C, eds. Séminuro-néphrologie. Paris: Masson, 1989:42–49.
139. Cozzi PJ, Abu-Jawdah GM, Green RM, et al. Amyloidosis in association with human immunodeficiency virus infection. Clin Infect Dis 1992;14:189–191.
140. Strauss J, Zilleruelo G, Abitbol C, et al. Human immunodeficiency virus nephropathy. Pediatr Nephrol 1993;7:220-225.
141. Baquera Heredia J, Angeles Angeles A, Reyes Gutierrez E, et al. Nephropatia asociada al sindrome de inmunodeficiencia adquirida. Rev Invest Clin 1987;39:105–115.
142. Babut-Gay ML, Echard M, Kleinknecht D, et al. Zidovudine and nephropathy with human immunodeficiency virus (HIV) infection [letter]. Ann Intern Med 1989;111:856–857.
143. Cook PP, Appel RG. Prolonged clinical improvement in HIV-associated nephropathy with zidovudine therapy [abstract]. J Am Soc Nephrol 1990;1:842.
144. Lam M, Park MC. HIV-associated nephropathy: beneficial effect of zidovudine therapy [letter]. N Engl J Med 1990;323:1775–1776.
145. Harrer T, Hunzelmann N, Stoll R, et al. Therapy for HIV-1 related nephritis with zidovudine. AIDS 1990;4:815–817.
146. Ingulli E, Tejani A, Fikrig S, et al. Nephrotic syndrome associated with acquired immunodeficiency syndrome in children. J Pediatr 1991;119:710–716.
147. Ifudu O, Rao TK, Tan CC, et al. Zidovudine is beneficial in human immunodeficiency virus associated nephropathy. Am J Nephrol 1995;15:217–221.
148. Ahmed V, Kloser P, Miller MA, et al. Does zidovudine slow the progression of HIV nephropathy [abstract]. J Am Soc Nephrol 1993;6:269.
149. Kimmel PL, Mishkin GJ, Umana WO. Captopril and renal survival in patients with human immunodeficiency virus nephropathy. Am J Kidney Dis 1996;28:202–208.
150. Appel RG, Neill J. A steroid-responsive nephrotic syndrome in a patient with human immunodeficiency virus (HIV) infection. Ann Intern Med 1990;113:892–893.
151. Smith MC, Austen JL, Carey JT, et al. Prednisone improves renal function and proteinuria in human immunodeficiency virus-associated nephropathy. Am J Med 1996;101:41–48.
152. Watterson MK, Detwiler RD, Bolin P Jr. Clinical response to prolonged corticosteroids in a patient with human immunodeficiency virus-associated nephropathy. Am J Kidney Dis 1997;29:624–626.
153. Briggs WA, Tnawattancharoen S, Choi MJ, et al. Clinicopathologic correlates of prednisone treatment of HIV-associated nephropathy. Am J Kidney Dis 1996;28:618-621.

154. Ouelette DR, Kelly JW, Anders JT. Serum angiotensin converting enzyme level is elevated in patients with HIV-infection. Arch Intern Med 1992;152:321–324.
155. Burns GC, Matute R, Onyema D, et al. Response to inhibition of angiotensin-converting enzyme in human immunodeficiency virus-associated nephropathy: a case report. Am J Kidney Dis 1994;23: 441–443.
156. Burns G, Paul SK, Sivak SL, et al. Effect of angiotensin-converting enzyme inhibition in HIV-associated nephropathy. J Am Soc Nephrol 1997;8:1140–1146.
157. Ortiz C, Meneses R, Jaffe D, et al. Outcome of patients with human immunodeficiency virus on maintenance hemodialysis. Kidney Int 1988;34:248–253.
158. Ifudu O, Mayers JD, Matthew JJ, et al. Uremia therapy in patients with end-stage renal disease and human immunodeficiency virus infection: has the outcome changed in the 1990s? Am J Kidney Dis 1997;29: 549–552.
159. Perinbasekar S, Brod-Miller S, Pal S, et al. Predictors of survival in HIV-infected patients on hemodialysis. Am J Nephrol 1996;16: 280–286.
160. Kimmel PL, Umana WO, Simmens SJ, et al. Continuous ambulatory peritoneal dialysis and survival of HIV infected patients with end-stage renal disease. Kidney Int 1993;44:373–378.
161. Pennell JP, Bourgoignie JJ. Should AIDS patients be dialyzed? Trans Am Soc Artif Intern Organs 1988;34:907–911.
162. Casanova S, Mazzucco G, Barbiano di Belgiojoso G, et al. Pattern of glomerular involvement in human immunodeficiency virus-infected patients: an Italian study. Am J Kidney Dis 1995;26:446–453.
163. Rodriguez RA, Johansen KL, Balkovetz DF, et al. Clinical characteristics and renal biopsy findings in human immunodeficiency virus infected outpatients with renal disease [abstract]. J Am Soc Nephrol 1996;7:1342.
164. Kimmel PL, Phillips TM, Ferreira-Centeno A, et al. HIV-associated immune-mediated renal disease. Kidney Int 1993;44:1327–1340.
165. Kimmel PL, Abraham AA, Phillips TM. Membranoproliferative glomerulonephritis in a patient treated with interferon-alpha for human immunodeficiency virus infection. Am J Kidney Dis 1994; 24:858–863.
166. Stokes MB, Chawla H, Brody RI, et al. Immune complex glomerulonephritis in patients co-infected with human immunodeficiency virus and hepatitis C virus. Am J Kidney Dis 1997;29:514–525.
167. Korbet SM, Schwartz MM. Human immunodeficiency virus infection and nephrotic syndrome. Am J Kidney Dis 1992;20:97–103.
168. Guerra IL, Abraham AA, Kimmel PL, et al. Nephrotic syndrome associated with chronic persistent hepatitis B in an HIV antibody positive patient. Am J Kidney Dis 1987;10:385–388.
169. Collins AB, Khan AK, Dienstag H, et al. Hepatitis B immune complex glomerulonephritis: simultaneous glomerular deposits of hepatitis B surface and e antigens. Clin Immunol Immunopathol 1983;28:137–153.
170. Schectman JM, Kimmel PL. Remission of hepatitis B-associated membranous glomerulonephritis in human immunodeficiency virus infection. Am J Kidney Dis 1991;17:716–718.
171. Kusner DJ, Ellner JJ. Syphilis, a reversible cause of nephrotic syndrome in HIV infection [letter]. N Engl J Med 1991;324:341–342.
172. D'Agati V, Seigle R. Coexistence of AIDS and lupus nephritis: a case report. Am J Nephrol 1990;10:243–247.
173. Koppelman RG, Zolla-Pazner S. Association of human immunodeficiency virus infection and autoimmune phenomena. Am J Med 1988;84:82–88.
174. Contreras G, Green DF, Pardo V, et al. Systemic lupus erythematosus in two adults with human immunodefiency virus infection. Am J Kidney Dis 1996:28:292–295.
175. Bourgoignie JJ, Pardo V. Human immunodeficiency virus-associated nephropathies [editorial]. N Engl J Med 1992;327:729–730.
176. Beanfils H. Jouanneau C, Katlama C, et al. HIV-associated IgA nephropathy: a post-mortem study. Nephrol Dial Transplant 1995; 10:35–38.
177. Jackson S, Dawson LM, Kotler DP. IgA 1 is the major immunoglobulin component of immune complexes in the acquired immunodeficiency syndrome. J Clin Immunol 1988;8:64–68.
178. Jackson S, Tarkowski A, Collins JE, et al. Occurrence of polymeric IgA1 rheumatoid factor in the acquired immunodeficiency syndrome. J Clin Immunol 1988;8:390–396.
179. Jackson S. Immunoglobulin: antiimmunoglobulin interactions and immune complexes in IgA nephropathy. Am J Kidney Dis 1988;12: 425–429.
180. Béné MC, Canton P, Amiel C, et al. Absence of mesangial IgA in AIDS: a postmortem study. Nephron 1991;58:240–241.
181. Katz A, Bargman JM, Miller DC, et al. IgA nephritis in HIV-positive patients: a new HIV-associated nephropathy? Clin Nephrol 1992; 38:6–68.
182. Falkoff GE, Rigsby CM, Rosenfield AT. Partial, combined cortical and medullary nephrocalcinosis: US and CT patterns in AIDS-associated MAI infection. Radiology 1987;162:343–344.
183. Bargman JM, Wagner C, Cameron R. Renal cortical nephrocalcinosis: a manifestation of extrapulmonary *Pneumocystis carinii* infection in the acquired immunodeficiency syndrome. Am J Kidney Dis 1991; 17:712–715.
184. Feuerstein IM, Francis P, Raffeld M, et al. Widespread visceral calcifications in disseminated *Pneumocystis carinii* infection: CT characteristics. J Comput Assist Tomogr 1990;14:149–151.
185. Radin DR, Baker EL, Klatt EC, et al. Visceral and nodal calcification in patients with AIDS-related *Pneumocystis carinii* infection. AJR Am J Roentgenol 1990;154:27–31.
186. Ravalli S, Garcia RL, Vincent RA, et al. Disseminated *Pneumocystis carinii* infection in the acquired immunodeficiency syndrome. N Y State J Med 1990;90:155–157.
187. Grateau G, Soffer M, Fritz P, et al. Guerison par drainage externe d'un abcés périrénal au cours du SIDA. Ann Med Interne 1988; 139:403–404.
188. Gelabert Mas A, Arango O, Bielsa O, et al. Drenaje percutaneo de los abscesos renales y perinefriticos. Actas Urol Esp 1992;16:513–516.
189. Valle Gerhold J, Monzón Alebesque F, López López JA. Tratamiento percutaneo de absceso renal micótico por *Aspergillus fumigatus* en un paciente con SIDA. Actas Urol Esp 1992;16:492–494.
190. Nadasdy T, Miller KW, Johnson LD, et al. Is cytomegalovirus associated with renal disease in AIDS patients? Mod Pathol 1992;5: 277–282.
191. Aarons EJ, Woodrow D, Hollister WS, et al. Reversible renal failure caused by a microsporidian infection. AIDS 1994;8:1119–1121.
192. Weber R, Kuster H, Visvesvara GS, et al. Disseminated microsporidiosis due to Encephalitozoon hellem: pulmonary colonization, microhematuria, and mild conjunctivitis in a patient with AIDS. Clin Infect Dis 1993;17:415–419.
193. Clinicopathologic Conference. Fever and acute renal failure in a 31-year-old male with AIDS. Am J Med 1997;102:310–315.

36
CARDIAC INVOLVEMENT IN THE PATIENT WITH AIDS

Melvin D. Cheitlin

It is nearly a decade and a half since the acquired immunodeficiency syndrome (AIDS) was first recognized. By the year 2000, when the pandemic will have finished its second decade, investigators estimate that 30 million people will be infected worldwide (1). During this time, the human immunodeficiency virus (HIV) has been identified, and the mechanism by which the virus invades the host cell and incorporates itself into the host genetic material, its method of replication, and transmission to other cells, ultimately destroying the host immune system, have all been determined. With all these advances, the fear generated in the general population by AIDS has rivaled that seen with earlier pandemics, such as the influenza pandemic of 1918 and the poliomyelitis epidemic, diseases we knew little about at the time they terrorized humankind.

With the understanding of the biology of HIV and the pathogenesis of the disease have come marked advances in developing therapeutic agents to inhibit viral attachment to the host cells and viral replication. Antiviral agents such as zidovudine (formerly known as azidothymidine), dideoxyinosine (ddI), and dideoxycytidine (ddC), which prolong the latency period, the time from infection to the development of clinical disease, have been developed, and, with the development of protease inhibitor drugs such as saquinavir, ritonavir, and indinavir, one can inhibit viral replication and viral binding. In many infected patients, these drugs have diminished or even eliminated the presence of virus in the blood. Nonetheless, the disease has not been eliminated, and most infected patients probably will ultimately die of AIDS.

When the AIDS epidemic first began, investigators noted early that cardiac involvement could occur. As the number of patients with AIDS increased, it became obvious that clinical cardiac involvement was unusual. Cardiac involvement was seen in the following ways:

1. Incidental involvement by opportunistic infections
2. Valvular involvement with marantic endocarditis, infective endocarditis, especially in intravenous (IV) drug abusers, and mitral valve prolapse
3. Involvement with tumor, such as, Kaposi's sarcoma and lymphoma, especially non–Hodgkin's lymphoma
4. Pericarditis
5. Pulmonary hypertension and cor pulmonale
6. Myocarditis
   A. Focal myocarditis
   B. Diffuse myocarditis
      i. Caused by a known pathogen
      ii. Of unknown origin
7. Myocardial dysfunction
   A. Asymptomatic
   B. Cardiomyopathy with congestive heart failure

INCIDENTAL CARDIAC INVOLVEMENT

At autopsy, organisms such as *Toxoplasma*, *Histoplasma*, and *Candida* occasionally are found in the myocardium. Most of these patients had no clinical indication of myocardial disease. Because these organisms may be seen without any cellular reaction surrounding them, they likely were disseminated throughout the body and were found incidentally in the myocardium.

Early in the epidemic, autopsy series were commonly reported. With the maturing of the epidemic and the realization of the danger of infection to the prosectors, the incidence of autopsies has dropped dramatically in patients with AIDS. In autopsy series, the incidence of cardiac involvement varied, depending on how it was defined, from no involvement at all to abnormalities in 70% of the hearts examined (2–11). The major reason for the wide range depends on the institution reporting the autopsy series, whether a facility is for tertiary care or primary care for the treatment of AIDS patients, and whether cellular infiltration without myocardial cell necrosis is counted as cardiac involvement. In the large series of consecutive autopsies from primary care centers, the incidence of cardiac involvement is between 5 and 20%. Most often, even cardiac involvement that is recognized clinically plays little or no role in the patient's outcome. The common causes of death in AIDS patients are respiratory failure and infection (8, 10, 12). Neoplasm, specifically non–Hodgkin's lymphoma, and encephalopathy are also frequent causes of death (13). In a review of 15 series of autopsies in the literature, of 815 patients, only 9 (1%) had a cardiac cause of death. At least half of these cardiac deaths were caused by pathogens such as *Toxoplasma,* which are known to cause cardiac involvement.

VALVULAR INVOLVEMENT

Valvular involvement occurs in three ways: infective endocarditis with the usual purulent pathogens, marantic endocarditis, and mitral valve prolapse.

Infective Endocarditis with the Usual Purulent Pathogens

Infective endocarditis is almost exclusively seen in patients for whom IV drug abuse is their HIV risk factor (14). It is not surprising that in a population such as that of New York City, where IV drug abusers constitute 50% of the patients with AIDS, infective endocarditis is seen frequently. In the San Francisco population, only about 15% of HIV-positive patients admit to a history of IV drug abuse. In patients in San Francisco, I have occasionally seen tricuspid endocarditis, but only in IV drug abusers.

When infective endocarditis occurs, it may have a more virulent course in the immunocompromised patient with AIDS (15). The common pathogens seen in endocarditis in IV drug users with AIDS are *Staphylococcus aureus,* which is present in almost three-fourths of these patients, and *Streptococcus pneumoniae* and *Haemophilus influenzae,* which are seen less commonly (16). Austrian's syndrome, originally described in alcoholics, characterized by *S. pneumoniae*-induced infective endocarditis, pneumonia, and meningitis, has also been seen in IV drug users with AIDS (15). Fungal endocarditis, mostly from infection with *Candida* and *Cryptococcus,* usually the result of systemic fungemia, is infrequent and, again, is seen almost exclusively in IV drug users. No specific differences exist in the diagnosis and therapy of infective endocarditis in patients with and without AIDS. When valve replacement is necessary, it should be performed, although judgment must be used in patients in the late stages of AIDS.

Marantic Endocarditis

Marantic endocarditis is also reported, and at autopsy it may be the most common endocardial involvement (17, 18). Because these vegetations are sterile, the valve leaflets are not destroyed; therefore, valvular insufficiency is not usually created. Marantic endocarditis is found mostly because of the occurrence of embolization with cerebral infarction (19) or other systemic emboli, or it is an incidental finding at autopsy. It occurs most often with cachexia, a frequent occurrence in the late stages of AIDS (4).

Mitral Valve Prolapse

Mitral valve prolapse, at least as seen by echocardiography, has been reported, most often without clinical evidence of mitral valve prolapse such as an ejection click with or without a late systolic murmur. The mitral valve prolapse probably is secondary to cachexia and loss of left ventricular volume. Because the valve and its supporting structures remain the same size and end-diastolic left ventricular volume is reduced, during systole the otherwise normal mitral valve prolapses into the left atrium.

NEOPLASMS

One of the first examples of cardiac involvement reported was the incidental finding of Kaposi's sarcoma involving the myocardium and pericardium (20). Most often, the Kaposi's sarcoma implants are asymptomatic and are found incidentally (3). At present, involvement with lymphoma, especially non–Hodgkin's-type lymphoma, is seen most frequently (21–23). The tumor can cause problems by infiltrating the myocardium, growing into the lumen of the heart, or causing pericardial effusion. Diffuse myocardial infiltration is the most common pattern of involvement, but discrete nodular lesions have been described (5, 8).

Myocardial neoplastic infiltration can be clinically silent, or it may cause symptoms of congestive heart failure, heart block, or atrial or ventricular arrhythmias (24). Pericardial effusion can be silent or may cause tamponade. For patients with an intraluminal tumor, surgical resection may be appropriate to relieve obstruction to blood flow (25). Kelsey and colleagues (26) reported complete remission with combination chemotherapy in an HIV-infected patient with large cell lymphoma.

PERICARDITIS

Pericarditis is the most frequent clinical cardiac involvement seen in the AIDS population. This disorder is reported in autopsy series in as few as 3% of cases, as in the series of Wilkes and associates (6), and in as many as 26.9% of cases, as in the series of Marche and colleagues (27).

Echocardiographic evidence of pericardial effusion, especially in AIDS patients, is not uncommon. The prevalence of pericardial effusion varied from 39 of 102 (38%) patients in the series of Corallo and associates (28) to 21% in the series of Monsuez and colleagues (29). In a prospective series of 151 HIV-positive patients who had echocardiograms reported by Steffen and colleagues (30), 29 patients (19%) had pericardial effusion. In 88 consecutive patients with echocardiograms performed at San Francisco General Hospital (SFGH), 26 (30%) had a pericardial effusion. The patients were referred for echocardiography for clinical reasons and were not simply consecutive AIDS patients. In a review of 17 references in the literature, pericardial effusion was found in 310 of 1506 (20.6%) HIV-infected patients by echocardiography.

Clinical pericardial involvement is most frequently discovered by the onset of chest pain, usually pleuritic, the finding of an enlarged cardiac silhouette on the chest radiograph, and occasionally the development of pericardial tamponade (31,

32). The pericarditis can be due to specific organisms, such as *Mycobacterium tuberculosis* (29, 33, 34) or *M. avium-intracellulare* (35, 36). Pericarditis can be caused by purulent bacterial infection such as with *Streptococcus pneumoniae* or *Staphylococcus aureus* (32, 33). Lymphoma is another well-recognized cause of pericardial involvement. Frequently, no etiologic agent is identified.

In the SFGH experience, my colleagues and I have seen 25 patients with AIDS or persistent generalized lymphadenopathy with pericardial disease (37). In 10 of these patients, we obtained either fluid or tissue or both from pericardiocentesis or surgery. None of these patients had tuberculosis or an infection with any other identifiable organism. The incidence of cardiac tamponade varied depending on the series. Of these 25 patients, 32% presented with tamponade. In the series of Monsuez and colleagues (29), of 18 patients with effusion, 5 (28%) had tamponade.

The cause of the pericarditis is not fully understood. Some cases possibly could be due to HIV infection, but implants from lymphoma, opportunistic infection with coxsackievirus B, and cytomegalovirus may also be possible in the immunocompromised patient. Reynolds and colleagues reported 14 AIDS patients with effusion; 8 (37%) had suggestive evidence of mycobacterial disease (38). Managing these patients is usually not complicated. If the patient is found to have an effusion by enlargement of the cardiac silhouette on the chest radiograph, and if the effusion is large on the echocardiogram, then pericardiocentesis with culture of the fluid and cytologic examination are indicated. If organisms such as *Mycobacterium* are cultured, then treatment appropriate to the organism is indicated. Large effusions can cause symptoms by pericardial tamponade or compression of the lung, in which case pericardiocentesis should be performed to minimize symptoms. Usually, I leave a catheter in the pericardium with vacuum drainage to render the pericardium as dry as possible for 24 hours and then remove the catheter. Patients usually have no recurrence.

If the effusion is small and asymptomatic, I usually do not recommend pericardiocentesis, except when the patient is septic and purulent pericarditis is a possibility. In patients with a symptomatic, relatively small effusion, open drainage, usually through the subxiphoid approach, is indicated; in this way, one obtains not only pericardial fluid to culture and to examine, but also a pericardial biopsy specimen, thus improving the chance of finding the cause of the pericarditis.

The presence of pericardial effusion may have prognostic significance in patients with AIDS (39). At SFGH, Heidenreich and colleagues performed echocardiograms every 4 months on 231 subjects recruited over a 5-year period (39). At the time of entrance into the study, 59 subjects had asymptomatic HIV infection, 62 had AIDS-related complex, 74 had AIDS, 21 were HIV-negative healthy gay men, and 15 subjects had non-HIV end-stage medical illness. The incidence of developing pericardial effusion was 4% per year for all HIV-infected patients and 11% per year for AIDS patients. The AIDS patients with pericardial effusion had a lower survival at 6 months than those without pericardial effusion (36% versus 93%). The relative risk after adjustment for lead time bias in those with compared to those without the development of pericardial effusion was 2.2 (95% confidence interval; 1.2 to 4.0; $P = .01$) (39).

PULMONARY HYPERTENSION

In autopsy series, enlargement of the right ventricle and even right ventricular hypertrophy have been reported. Anderson and colleagues (9) reported right ventricular hypertrophy or right ventricular dilatation in 12 of 71 patients (17%). Lewis, in a large consecutive autopsy series, reported right ventricular hypertrophy or dilatation in 18 of 115 patients (16%) (8).

Reitano and colleagues in 1984 reported echocardiograms on 21 AIDS patients; 6 had right ventricular dilatation (40). Himelman and colleagues in 1989 reported echocardiograms in 51 AIDS patients and 13 HIV-positive patients with chronic lymphadenopathy; 8 had right ventricular dilatation (41). In the series of Steffen and colleagues (30) of 151 HIV positive patients, 2 had right ventricular dilatation. At SFGH, in a consecutive series of 88 autopsied patients, 2 (2.3%) had right ventricular dilatation (10). In 1989, Himelman and colleagues reported 6 patients from the University of California, San Francisco who had right ventricular hypertrophy or right ventricular failure with elevated pulmonary arterial pressure from increased pulmonary vascular resistance (42). Five of the 6 patients had had repeated episodes of *Pneumocystis carinii* pneumonia, and 1 had not had any such infection. The probable explanation is that progressive fibrosis and destruction of the interstitium caused loss of the small vessels in the lung and an increase in pulmonary vascular resistance.

Another possibility has been suggested as a result of finding severe pulmonary hypertension in patients without a history of significant pulmonary infection or IV drug use. Two reports noted seven such patients, and in the four patients who later were studied by autopsy, three had smooth muscle medial hypertrophy of the small pulmonary arteries, and one had plexogenic endothelial proliferation (43, 44). These findings are characteristic of pulmonary vascular disease in patients with primary pulmonary hypertension. A hypothesis was advanced that a growth factor stimulating pulmonary endothelial proliferation may be formed from infected T cells or possibly directly from HIV (45).

MYOCARDITIS

The incidence of focal myocarditis found at autopsy in AIDS patients varies according to whether myocardial necrosis must be present with an inflammatory infiltrate. In a series of 88 consecutive autopsies at SFGH, 20% had focal myocarditis at autopsy with and without evidence of myocardial necrosis (10). Half of these patients had known organisms such as *Histoplasma*, *Toxoplasma*, and *Cryptococcus* found in the myocardium after a diligent search. No case had clinical evidence of myocardial involvement. In other series, the incidence of focal myocarditis is much higher.

In an autopsy series from the Armed Forces Institute of Pathology, 46 of 105 cases (44%) had microscopic foci of myocarditis. Of these, 48% had no organisms found and were called idiopathic (9). Lewis reported 115 consecutive autopsies in AIDS patients, with 10 cases of focal myocarditis (8). The prevalence of focal myocarditis is much higher than the incidence of clinically important myocarditis or cardiomyopathy. Lewis' study of 115 autopsies reported 2 cases of dilated cardiomyopathy, both without interstitial infiltration and interstitial fibrosis (8).

In a review of 9 autopsy series from the literature, "myocarditis" was present in 214 of 656 (33%) patients with AIDS (24). The definition of myocarditis included round cell infiltration with and without myocardial cell necrosis. No specific cause was present in more than 80% of the patients.

The histologic pattern in AIDS-associated HIV myocarditis is a nonspecific, focal round cell infiltrate without myocardial necrosis. Next most frequent is round cell infiltration with myocyte necrosis meeting the Dallas criteria for the histologic diagnosis of myocarditis (46). The least common is myocyte cell necrosis without cellular inflammatory infiltrate.

Although histologic myocarditis is frequent, the cause of the myocarditis is not clear, and the relation of myocarditis to clinical findings or functional abnormalities of the ventricle is not certain. Baroldi and colleagues (7) reported focal lymphocytic myocarditis by the Dallas criteria in 9 (34%) and lymphocytic infiltration in 20 (77%) of 26 autopsy studies of patients who had no clinical cardiac disease before death. Eight of the patients had undergone an echocardiogram; 6 had abnormal left ventricular function, 5 had a globular left ventricle and diffuse hypokinesis, and 3 had left ventricular dilatation. Of the 6 with an abnormal echocardiogram, 4 met Dallas criteria for myocarditis. These investigators speculated that myocarditis could precede the development of cardiomyopathy. However, they concluded that the lymphocytic myocarditis was insufficient to account for the myocardial dysfunction. More recently, Hansen reported Dallas criteria for myocarditis in 25 (42%) of 60 consecutive autopsies of patients with AIDS (11). Hansen concluded that the myocarditis led to fibrosis and ultimately to dilated cardiomyopathy. In 99 consecutive autopsies in patients with AIDS at SFGH, 21% had focal myocarditis, and none had clinical cardiomyopathy (10). In the autopsy study of Lewis, 9% of 115 patients had myocarditis, and only 1 patient had clinical cardiomyopathy (8).

CARDIOMYOPATHY

The first evidence that HIV disease could be associated with clinical cardiomyopathy was reported in 1986 by Cohen and colleagues (47), who reported 3 patients with clinical echocardiographic and morphologic findings of dilated cardiomyopathy. All had decreased ejection fraction, and 2 had clinical findings of congestive heart failure. At autopsy, 2 had findings compatible with myocarditis resulting in cardiomyopathy. Reilly and colleagues (48) reported 58 consecutive autopsies; 7 (12%) had major clinical cardiovascular abnormalities, including 4 with congestive heart failure and others with ventricular tachycardia. All had focal myocarditis with round cell infiltration and myocardial fiber necrosis.

Cardiac involvement with focal myocarditis is common at autopsy, yet death resulting from myocarditis is rare. In 14 autopsy studies reported in the literature, 1009 patients were described. Eight died of cardiac involvement; 1 had cryptococcal myocarditis, 1 had toxoplasmic myocarditis, and 5 of the patients came from a single institution (9). Echocardiography has provided evidence of myocardial functional impairment, most of the time in patients without clinical cardiomyopathy. Himelman and colleagues reported 71 patients with AIDS, 8 of whom had left ventricular dilatation or decreased contractility (41). Four patients had congestive heart failure. In the echocardiographic study of Corallo and colleagues in 102 consecutive AIDS patients, none had congestive heart failure, although 41% had left ventricular hypokinesis (28).

That cardiomyopathy occurs in AIDS patients is not in doubt. The cause of the cardiomyopathy is a matter of considerable controversy. The possible origin of cardiomyopathy in patients with HIV disease can be cataloged as follows: 1) HIV myocarditis leading to cardiomyopathy; 2) opportunistic infection; 3) dilated cardiomyopathy as a postviral disease; 4) impaired immune system; 5) cytokines and cardiomyopathy; 6) nutritional cardiomyopathy; and 7) drug-induced cardiomyopathy.

HIV Myocarditis Leading to Cardiomyopathy

HIV myocarditis with subsequent cardiomyopathy is the most logical explanation. In support of this hypothesis are the occasional reports of HIV organisms cultured from cardiac muscle biopsy. In 1987, Calabrese and colleagues reported culturing the organism from a right ventricular myocardial biopsy sample in a patient with a hypokinetic right ventricle and a normal left ventricle (49). Contamination from the blood, infected macrophages, or endothelial cells could not be excluded.

One argument against HIV infection as a cause of myocarditis is that little evidence indicates that the HIV organism can invade the myocardial cell. The myocardial cell has no CD4 receptors, the major means by which the virus enters the cell. Grody and colleagues reported detecting HIV nucleic acid sequences by in situ hybridization in myocardial tissue from 6 of 22 patients who died of AIDS (50). None had clinical cardiac involvement, and all had normal myocardium by light microscopy. These investigators believed the target to be myocardial cells, but one cannot be certain of this determination by this technique, and the sequences could have been in macrophages, endothelial cells, or the serum. The cells showing positive hybridization signals were sparse. Others investigators have also reported finding HIV DNA either by in situ hybridization or by polymerase chain reaction (51, 52), but one cannot say that the HIV was within the myocardial cell. Most patients have neither clinical nor microscopic evidence of myocardial involvement. Many other reports of patients with cardiomyopathy have not shown evidence of the viral genome in the myocardial cell (52–54). Wu and colleagues used immunocytochemical analysis to identify HIV in the heart of a 35-year-old AIDS patient (55). Confirmed with in situ hybridization studies, HIV was found in the lymphocytic infiltrate and not in the myocardial cells. Given all the patients seen with AIDS and the rarity of clinical cardiomyopathy, it is doubtful whether the HIV organism causes severe myocarditis, at least not often.

The mechanism by which the HIV organism could cause myocardial damage is not clear. The HIV organism could possibly invade the myocardial cell even in the absence of CD4 receptors. If the myocardial cell is injured, entrance of the HIV virion may be facilitated. Epstein–Barr virus has been shown to facilitate entry and replication of HIV into CD4 receptor-negative cells (56). Alternatively, the HIV organism can exact a direct cytolytic effect by means of an "innocent bystander" mechanism that has been postulated as the way in which neurologic cell injury occurs in AIDS-associated encephalitis (57). The latter hypothesis involves the paracrine effect of the release of toxic enzymes or lymphokines by replicating HIV in the myocardial interstitial lymphocytes and macrophages.

Opportunistic Infection

Because AIDS patients are subject to opportunistic bacterial, viral, mycotic, and protozoal infections, perhaps cardiomyopathy is related to these known myocardial pathogens. Epstein–Barr virus and cytomegalovirus are both known to cause cardiomyopathy in AIDS patients (58, 59). Niedt and Schinella (60) detected cytomegalovirus histologically from various organs in 43 (77%) of 56 patients with AIDS at autopsy. These investigators demonstrated inclusion bodies and myocarditis in 4 of the cases with congestive heart failure, arrhythmia, or electrocardiographic changes. Other studies using in situ hybridization techniques demonstrated many infected cells including myocytes, which do not show the characteristic inclusion bodies seen in cytomegalovirus infection (61). The absence of these inclusion bodies has been cited as the reason for diminishing the role of this organism as a cause of myocarditis in HIV-infected patients.

Myocarditis caused by *Cryptococcus neoformans* and *Toxoplasma gondii* is also well known (62–64), and *Aspergillus*-associated endocarditis and myocarditis have been reported (65). *Toxoplasma* is the most common infectious cause of myocarditis in AIDS patients. Early studies revealed a small incidence of cardiac toxoplasmosis: 1 case in 71 (1.4%) in 1 series (9) and 1 case in 24 (4%) in another (7). A report of 18 consecutive AIDS autopsies revealed 4 cases of *T. gondii* myocarditis (66). A study from France reported 21 (12%) cases of myocardial toxoplasmosis in 170 autopsies. Five of these patients had extensive lesions (67). Coxsackievirus B is a well-known cause of myocarditis, and this pathogen also has been reported in AIDS patients (54, 68, 69).

Dilated Cardiomyopathy as a Postviral Disease

Increasing evidence indicates that idiopathic cardiomyopathy in the non-AIDS population results from immunologic reaction to myocardial cellular injury, at least much of the time caused by viral myocarditis (70). This can be a cross-reactivity to viral antigen with some element of the myocardial cell or an immunologic reaction to myocardial antigen that is altered by the viral infection to act as a foreign antigen. The immune reaction, mediated through the binding of complement, results in the myocardial necrosis and inflammatory cell infiltration and fibrosis characteristic of cardiomyopathy (70). The evidence rests on the detection of elevated viral antibody titers and viral-specific RNA sequences found in myocardial biopsies (71–73).

Impaired Immune System

Autoimmune mechanisms may cause cardiomyopathy (64, 69, 74, 75). Herskowitz and colleagues demonstrated cardiac autoantibodies in four of six patients with AIDS and cardiomyopathy (76). No such antibodies were seen in HIV-positive patients without AIDS cardiomyopathy. These investigators were unable to demonstrate by in situ hybridization with genomic probes any evidence of HIV or other viruses in the myocardial cell. By enzyme-linked immunospecific assay, they noted a high titer of immunoglobulin G antibody to myosin, as well as to cardiac mitochondrial adenine nucleotide. One possibility is that the autoantibodies found are an epiphenomenon, that is, the result of myocardial injury rather than its cause.

Another possibility is that the T-lymphocyte abnormalities may affect suppressor cell function, thus resulting in myocardial injury. Fowles and colleagues (77) and Bolte (78) found defective suppressor cell function in patients with idiopathic congestive cardiomyopathy and suggested this as a mechanism for the progression of myocarditis to dilated cardiomyopathy. Patients with AIDS may have an abnormality of T-helper cell function that could result in uncontrolled hypergammaglobulinemia, high serum immune complexes that can cause inflammatory lesions in many organs including the myocardium (64).

Cytokines and Cardiomyopathy

In explaining neuroglial cell dysfunction in AIDS, Ho and colleagues proposed a primary role for cytokines released by nearby HIV-infected monocytes (79). They termed this concept the "innocent bystander mechanism." Cytokines, including tumor necrosis factor (TNF), interleukin-1 and interleukin-2, and interferon-α, are released by immune cells as soluble proteins; these biologically active mediators can affect cells in the immediate vicinity, or they can affect distant cells by an increase in cytokine concentration in the circulation. Certain of these cytokines have been implicated in the production of myocardial depression seen in septic shock (80, 81). The substance depresses myocardial cell function and may be the same as TNF (82, 83).

Reversible depression of myocardial function with depression in stroke volume and decrease in ejection fraction is well documented in patients with endotoxic shock (80, 81). Suffredini and colleagues administered endotoxin-released TNF to volunteers and demonstrated transient depression of left ventricular function independent of left ventricular volume or loading conditions (84).

In support of cytokine involvement in HIV disease, Lähdevirta and colleagues reported increased circulating TNF with advanced HIV-1 infection (85). Other investigators have reported an increased production of cytokine TNF by peripheral monocytes in patients with AIDS (86). Finally, Levine and colleagues demonstrated high levels of circulating TNF in patients with severe clinical congestive heart failure (87). Again, investigators have not been able to demonstrate that cytokines are the cause of the cardiomyopathy rather than the result of the congestive heart failure.

Nutritional Cardiomyopathy

Many AIDS patients who have cardiomyopathy are late in the course of their disease when nutritional problems are severe, resulting in marked cachexia (17, 64). Vitamin deficiency, especially vitamin B_1 deficiency, could cause or contribute to cardiomyopathy (64, 69). Perhaps cachexia itself can result in decreased myocardial function. Left ventricular wall motion abnormalities and decreased stroke volume have been seen by echocardiography in patients with bulimia and anorexia nervosa, as compared with controls (88). Starvation and refeeding experiments in animals have demonstrated decreased left ventricular compliance and decreased peak systolic force in the hearts of these animals as well as cardiac interstitial edema and myofibrillar atrophy (89).

Protein–calorie deficiency in patients can result in cardiac dysfunction with congestive heart failure occurring during refeeding and recovery (90, 91). In patients with severe malnutrition, deficiencies in microelements could result in cardiomyopathy. Selenium deficiency in Keshan disease is one example. Selenium deficiency has been reported, especially in pediatric patients with AIDS (92–94). Supporting this concept, Zazzo and colleagues showed decreased left ventricular fractional shortening by echocardiography in 10 patients with AIDS (95). Six of 8 patients repleted with sodium selenite showed improvement in left ventricular function within 3 weeks (95). Other investigators have also reported improved cardiac function with selenium supplementation (92, 93, 96).

Drug-induced Cardiomyopathy

Patients with AIDS take many drugs, both illicit and therapeutic, that could result in cardiomyopathy. Known cardiotoxic drugs, such as doxorubicin, interleukin-2 (97), and interferon-α_2 (98, 99), have all been reported to cause cardiomyopathy, at times reversible, and congestive heart failure. Brown and colleagues reported an AIDS patient with two episodes of severe congestive heart failure, the second associated with cardiogenic shock and a left ventricular ejection fraction less than 20%, associated with the administration of foscarnet (100). After the foscarnet was stopped, the situation was rapidly and totally reversible on both occasions (100).

The most common drugs used in AIDS are those that inhibit reverse transcriptase enzyme essential to the replication of the HIV organism. Zidovudine was the first of these drugs, and through phase I clinical trials as well as in a study by Richman and colleagues, no cardiac toxicity was reported (101). Dalakas and colleagues, however, demonstrated a toxic mitochondrial skeletal muscle myopathy after 1 year of therapy with zidovudine (102). Whether this effect can involve cardiac muscle as well is not clear.

Herskowitz and colleagues reported improvement in echocardiographic function in AIDS patients when zidovudine was stopped (103). These investigators have recommended a "drug holiday" in patients with decreased left ventricular function shown by echocardiography or frank cardiomyopathy. In contrast to this finding is a study by Lipshultz and colleagues in which pediatric AIDS patients showed no evidence of echocardiographic differences in myocardial function before and after starting zidovudine treatment (104). Compared with healthy children, AIDS patients had progressively increased left ventricular volume and mass, but not sufficient to maintain normal wall stress. No differences were found between the HIV-infected children who received zidovudine and those who did not.

Finally, AIDS patients are simultaneously taking many drugs whose interactions are unknown. Possibly, the interaction of drugs can result in myocardial damage.

Cocaine, a commonly used drug in this population, can cause coronary artery spasm. Myocardial necrosis has been described as causing myocarditis and reversible cardiomyopathy (105).

Frequency of Cardiomyopathy

Several prospective echocardiographic studies have attempted to define by echocardiography the prevalence and incidence of cardiomyopathy or at least decreased left ventricular function in patients with AIDS. Blanchard and colleagues (106) found 7 of 50 (14%) to have abnormal left ventricular function. Three improved, as shown on serial echocardiography. Of the 4 who had persistent left ventricular dysfunction, all died within 1 year of follow-up.

DeCastro and colleagues did a prospective serial echocardiographic study of 136 HIV-positive patients over a mean time of 415 ± 220 days (107). Seven AIDS patients developed clinical and echocardiographic findings of left ventricular dysfunction. Six of the patients died, and 5 underwent autopsy. Three had lymphocytic myocarditis, 1 had cryptococcal myocarditis, and 1 had interstitial fibrosis (107).

At SFGH, 74 outpatients with AIDS were recruited, and serial quantitative Doppler echocardiograms were performed every 4 months (108). Control populations included HIV-positive patients without disease, HIV-positive patients with

AIDS-related complex, and HIV-negative gay men. Over a follow-up time of 16.5 ± 12 months, no significant change in left ventricular function, either systolic or diastolic, was found, and no differences between the AIDS patients and the control group were detected.

In a report by Herskowitz and colleagues, 69 AIDS patients were randomly selected to be followed for a mean of 11 months with serial echocardiograms (109). At entry, 10 (14.5%) had global hypokinesia. Of the 59 patients with initially normal echocardiograms, 11 subsequently developed evidence of global dysfunction during a total of 725 months of follow-up (1.5 per 100 person-months). For the 21 patients combined, 20 were clinically silent, and only 1 was found to have unsuspected congestive heart failure on physical examination. Herskowitz and colleagues, in evaluating 450 HIV-infected patients from 6 echocardiographic series, reported the prevalence of left ventricular hypokinesis in 79 (17.5%); of these, 28 (6.2%) had or developed congestive heart failure. At the Johns Hopkins Hospital in Baltimore, investigators estimated of all the AIDS patients followed, cardiomyopathy was seen in 2.1% of their population (109).

No doubt exists that cardiomyopathy can occur in patients with AIDS. What is clear is that although wall motion abnormalities shown by echocardiography are not uncommon, clinical cardiomyopathy with left ventricular failure occurs in appreciably fewer than 5% of AIDS patients.

The evidence is against direct infection by HIV organism resulting in myocarditis as a cause of cardiomyopathy. The cause of the cardiomyopathy is unclear and may be multifactorial.

CARDIOVASCULAR SURGERY IN AIDS PATIENTS

When patients with AIDS have problems that are usually evaluated by cardiac catheterization and treated by cardiac surgery, the fear of infection of the health care worker creates a lively ethical discussion concerning the care of these patients. A legitimate question, especially in these times of finite resources, is related to the advisability of an expensive procedure that incapacitates the patient for a period of time when the final outcome is not affected. In such AIDS patients, coronary or valvular surgical procedures are not likely to be justified if the goal is to prolong life, inasmuch as 70% of patients with AIDS die within 3 to 4 years of the diagnosis (110), although this prognosis has been changing since the introduction of protease inhibitor drugs and multiple therapy. However, in patients who are receiving maximal medical management and who are still incapacitated by their coronary or valvular disease, surgery to relieve symptoms is justifiable.

The major concern relates to HIV-infected patients who have no defining diagnosis of AIDS. Such patients may have 10 to 15 years before they manifest this ultimately fatal disease. In such patients, cardiac catheterization and surgery should be considered and performed for the usual indications.

The only reason for disagreement with the foregoing recommendation is the health care worker's fear of becoming infected with HIV. As of 1997, 52 health care workers have been reported who seroconverted after workplace exposure. Combining 14 prospective studies of the risk of HIV-1 transmission to health care workers, 2042 parenteral exposures occurred in 1948 subjects (74). The chance of seroconversion was 0.29% per exposure (95% confidence interval; 0.13 to 0.7%), and 668 people with 1051 mucous membrane exposures had no seroconversions (95% confidence interval; upper bound, 0.28% per exposure). Therefore, the risk of HIV seroconversion from work-related exposure was low, approximately 1 infection in 300 documented parenteral exposures to HIV-positive blood (111).

The fear is understandable; however, other occupations regularly expose their practitioners to danger and even death as part of the profession (e.g., firemen, policemen, military personnel). Medicine as a profession and physicians as professionals must do no less.

References

1. World Health Organization, Office of Information. Press release WHO/101. Geneva: December 10, 1993.
2. Silver MA, Macher AM, Reichert CM, et al. Cardiac involvement by Kaposi's sarcoma in acquired immune deficiency syndrome (AIDS). Am J Cardiol 1984;53:983–985.
3. Welch K, Finkbeiner W, Alpers CE, et al. Autopsy findings in the acquired immune deficiency syndrome (AIDS). JAMA 1984;252:1152–1159.
4. Cammarosano C, Lewis W. Cardiac lesions in acquired immune deficiency syndrome (AIDS). J Am Coll Cardiol 1985;5:703–706.
5. Roldan EO, Moskowitz L, Hensley GT. Pathology of the heart in acquired immunodeficiency syndrome. Arch Pathol Lab Med 1987;111:943–946.
6. Wilkes MS, Fortin AH, Felix JC, et al. Value of necropsy in acquired immunodeficiency syndrome. Lancet 1988;2:85–88.
7. Baroldi G, Corallo S, Moroni M, et al. Focal lymphocytic myocarditis in acquired immunodeficiency syndrome (AIDS): a correlative morphologic and clinical study in 26 consecutive fatal cases. J Am Coll Cardiol 1988;12:463–469.
8. Lewis W. AIDS: cardiac findings from 115 autopsies. Prog Cardiovasc Dis 1989;32:207–215.
9. Anderson DW, Virmani R, Reilly JM, et al. Prevalent myocarditis at necropsy in the acquired immunodeficiency syndrome. J Am Coll Cardiol 1988;11:792–799.
10. Magno J, Margaretten W, Cheitlin M. Myocardial involvement in acquired immunodeficiency syndrome: incidence in a large autopsy study [abstract]. Circulation 1988;78(Suppl II):II-459.
11. Hansen BF. Pathology of the heart in AIDS: a study of 60 consecutive autopsies. APMIS 1992;100:273–279.
12. Moskowitz L, Hensley GT, Chan JC, et al. Immediate causes of death in acquired immunodeficiency syndrome. Arch Pathol Lab Med 1985;109:735–738.
13. Murray JF, Garay SM, Hopewell PC, et al. NHLBI workshop summary. Pulmonary complications of the acquired immunodeficiency syndrome: an update. Report of the second National Heart, Lung and Blood Institute workshop. Am Rev Respir Dis 1987;135:504–509.

14. Currie PF, Sutherland GR, Jacob AJ, et al. A review of endocarditis in acquired immunodeficiency syndrome and human immunodeficiency virus infection. Eur Heart J 1995;16(Suppl B):15–18.
15. Francis CK. Cardiac involvement in AIDS. Curr Probl Cardiol 1990;15:569–639.
16. Nahass RG, Weinstein MP, Bartels J, et al. Infective endocarditis in intravenous drug users: a comparison of human immunodeficiency virus type 1–negative and–positive patients. J Infect Dis 1990;162:967–970.
17. Kaul S, Fishbein MC, Siegel RJ. Cardiac manifestations of acquired immune deficiency syndrome: a 1991 update. Am Heart J 1991;122:535–544.
18. Lopez JA, Ross RS, Fishbein MC, et al. Nonbacterial thrombotic endocarditis: a review. Am Heart J 1987;113:773–784.
19. Pinto AN. AIDS and cerebrovascular disease. Stroke 1996;27:538–543.
20. Autran B, Gorin I, Leibowitch M, et al. AIDS in a Haitian woman with cardiac Kaposi's sarcoma and Whipple's disease. Lancet 1983;1:767–768.
21. Goldfarb A, King CL, Rosenzweig BP, et al. Cardiac lymphoma in the acquired immunodeficiency syndrome. Am Heart J 1989;118:1340–1344.
22. Holladay AO, Siegel RJ, Schwartz DA. Cardiac malignant lymphoma in acquired immune deficiency syndrome. Cancer 1992;70:2203–2207.
23. Dalli E, Quesada A, Paya R. Cardiac involvement by non–Hodgkin's lymphoma in acquired immune deficiency syndrome. Int J Cardiol 1990;26:223–225.
24. Michaels AD, Lederman RJ, MacGregor JS, et al. Cardiovascular involvement in AIDS. Curr Probl Cardiol 1997;22:109–148.
25. Horowitz MD, Cox MM, Neibart RM, et al. Resection of right atrial lymphoma in a patient with AIDS. Int J Cardiol 1992;34:139–142.
26. Kelsey RC, Saker A, Morgan M. Cardiac lymphoma in a patient with AIDS. Ann Intern Med 1991;115:370–371.
27. Marche C, Trophilme D, Mayorga R, et al. Cardiac involv[e]ment in AIDS: a pathological study [abstract]. In: International Conference on AIDS, Stockholm, 1988;4:403.
28. Corallo S, Mutinelli MR, Moroni M, et al. Echocardiography detects myocardial damage in AIDS: prospective study in 102 patients. Eur Heart J 1988;9:887–892.
29. Monsuez JJ, Kinney EL, Vittecoq D, et al. Comparison among acquired immune deficiency syndrome patients with and without clinical evidence of cardiac disease. Am J Cardiol 1988;62:1311–1313.
30. Steffen H-M, Müller R, Schrappe-Bächer M, et al. Prevalence of echocardiographic abnormalities in human immunodeficiency virus 1 infection. Am J Noninvas Cardiol 1991;5:280–284.
31. Steigman CK, Anderson DW, Macher AM, et al. Fatal cardiac tamponade in acquired immunodeficiency syndrome with epicardial Kaposi's sarcoma. Am Heart J 1988;116:1105–1107.
32. Karve MM, Murali MR, Shah HM, et al. Rapid evolution of cardiac tamponade due to bacterial pericarditis in two patients with HIV-1 infection. Chest 1992;101:1461–1463.
33. Hsia J, Ross AM. Pericardial effusion and pericardiocentesis in human immunodeficiency virus infection. Am J Cardiol 1994;74:94–96.
34. D'Cruz IA, Sengupta EE, Abrahams C, et al. Cardiac involvement, including tuberculous pericardial effusion, complicating acquired immune deficiency syndrome. Am Heart J 1986;112:1100–1102.
35. Woods GL, Goldsmith JC. Fatal pericarditis due to *Mycobacterium avium-intracellulare* in acquired immunodeficiency syndrome. Chest 1989;95:1355–1357.
36. Choo PS, McCormack JG. *Mycobacterium avium:* a potentially treatable cause of pericardial effusions. J Infect 1995;30:55–58.
37. Galli FC, Cheitlin MD. Pericardial disease in AIDS: frequency of tamponade and therapeutic and diagnostic use of pericardiocentesis [abstract]. J Am Coll Cardiol 1992;19:266A.
38. Reynolds M, Berger M, Hecht S, et al. Large pericardial effusions associated with the acquired immune deficiency syndrome (AIDS) [abstract]. J Am Coll Cardiol 1991;17:221A.
39. Heidenreich PA, Eisenberg MJ, Kee LL, et al. Pericardial effusion in AIDS: incidence and survival. Circulation 1995;92:3229–3234.
40. Reitano J, King M, Cohen H, et al. Cardiac function in patients with acquired immune deficiency syndrome (AIDS) or AIDS prodrome [abstract]. J Am Coll Cardiol 1984;3:525.
41. Himelman RB, Chung WS, Chernoff DN, et al. Cardiac manifestations of human immunodeficiency virus infection: a two-dimensional echocardiographic study. J Am Coll Cardiol 1989;13:1030–1036.
42. Himelman RB, Dohrmann M, Goodman P, et al. Severe pulmonary hypertension and cor pulmonale in the acquired immunodeficiency syndrome. Am J Cardiol 1989;64:1396–1399.
43. Coplan NL, Shimony RY, Ioachim HL, et al. Primary pulmonary hypertension associated with human immunodeficiency viral infection. Am J Med 1990;89:96–99.
44. Mette SA, Palevsky HI, Pietra GG, et al. Primary pulmonary hypertension in association with human immunodeficiency virus infection: a possible viral etiology for some forms of hypertensive pulmonary arteriopathy. Am Rev Respir Dis 1992;145:1196–1200.
45. Nakamura S, Salahuddin SZ, Biberfeld P, et al. Kaposi's sarcoma cells: long-term culture with growth factor from retrovirus-infected $CD4^+$ T cells. Science 1988;242:426–430.
46. Aretz HT. Myocarditis: the Dallas criteria. Hum Pathol 1987;18:619–624.
47. Cohen IS, Anderson DW, Virmani R, et al. Congestive cardiomyopathy in association with the acquired immunodeficiency syndrome. N Engl J Med 1986;315:628–630.
48. Reilly JM, Cunnion RE, Anderson DW, et al. Frequency of myocarditis, left ventricular dysfunction and ventricular tachycardia in the acquired immune deficiency syndrome. Am J Cardiol 1988;62:789–793.
49. Calabrese LH, Proffitt MR, Yen-Lieberman B, et al. Congestive cardiomyopathy and illness related to the acquired immunodeficiency syndrome (AIDS) associated with isolation of retrovirus from myocardium. Ann Intern Med 1987;107:691–692.
50. Grody WW, Cheng L, Lewis W. Infection of the heart by the human immunodeficiency virus. Am J Cardiol 1990;66:203–206.
51. Lipshultz SE, Fox CH, Perez-Atayde AR, et al. Identification of human immunodeficiency virus-1 RNA and DNA in the heart of a child with cardiovascular abnormalities and congenital acquired immune deficiency syndrome. Am J Cardiol 1990;66:246–250.
52. Cenacchi G, Re MC, Furlini G, et al. Human immunodeficiency virus type 1 antigen detection in endomyocardial biopsy: an immunomorphological study. Microbiologica 1990:13:145–149.
53. Henry K, Dexter D, Sannerud K, et al. Recovery of HIV at autopsy [letter]. N Engl J Med 1989;321:1833–1834.
54. Dittrich H, Chow L, Denaro F, et al. Human immunodeficiency virus, coxsackievirus, and cardiomyopathy [letter]. Ann Intern Med 1988;108:308–309.
55. Wu AY, Forouhar F, Cartun RW, et al. Identification of human immunodeficiency virus in the heart of a patient with acquired immunodeficiency syndrome. Mod Pathol 1990;3:625–630.
56. Goldblum N, Daefler S, Llana T, et al. Susceptibility to HIV-1 infection of 2 human B-lymphoblastoid cell line, DG75, transfected with subgenomic DNA fragments of Epstein–Barr virus. Dev Biol Stand 1990;72:309–313.
57. Ho DD, Pomerantz RJ, Kaplan JC. Pathogenesis of infection with human immunodeficiency virus. N Engl J Med 1987;317:278–286.
58. Lafont A, Marche C, Wolff M, et al. Myocarditis in acquired immunodeficiency syndrome (AIDS): etiology and progress [abstract]. J Am Coll Cardiol 1988;11:196A.
59. Stewart JM, Kaul A, Gromisch DS, et al. Symptomatic cardiac dysfunction in children with human immunodeficiency virus infection. Am Heart J 1989;117:140–144.
60. Niedt GW, Schinella RA. Acquired immunodeficiency syndrome: clinicopathologic study of 56 autopsies. Arch Pathol Lab Med 1985;109:727–734.

61. Myerson D, Hackman RC, Nelson JA, et al. Widespread presence of histologically occult cytomegalovirus. Hum Pathol 1984;15:430–439.
62. Kinney EL, Monsuez JJ, Kitzis M, et al. Treatment of AIDS-associated heart disease. Angiology 1989;40:970–976.
63. Grange F, Kinney EL, Monsuez JJ, et al. Successful therapy for *Toxoplasma gondii* myocarditis in acquired immunodeficiency syndrome. Am Heart J 1990;120:443–444.
64. Acierno LJ. Cardiac complications in acquired immunodeficiency syndrome (AIDS): a review. J Am Coll Cardiol 1989;13:1144–1154.
65. Cox JN, di Dió F, Pizzolato GP, et al. *Aspergillus* endocarditis and myocarditis in a patient with the acquired immunodeficiency syndrome (AIDS): a review of the literature. Virchows Arch A Pathol Anat Histopathol 1990;417:255–259.
66. Matturri L, Quattrone P, Varesi C, et al. Cardiac toxoplasmosis in pathology of acquired immunodeficiency syndrome. Panminerva Med 1990;32:194–196.
67. Hofman P, Bernard E, Michiels JF, et al. Extracerebral toxoplasmosis in the acquired immunodeficiency syndrome (AIDS). Pathol Res Pract 1993;189:894–901.
68. Schwimmbeck PL, Schultheiss H-P, Strauer BE. Identification of a main autoimmunogenic epitope of the adenine nucleotide translocator which cross-reacts with coxsackie B3 virus: use in the diagnosis of myocarditis and dilative cardiomyopathy [abstract]. Circulation 1989;80(Suppl II):II-665.
69. Patel RC, Frishman WH. Cardiac involvement in HIV infection. Med Clin North Am 1996;80:1493–1512.
70. Lowry PJ, Thompson RA, Littler WA. Cellular immunity in congestive cardiomyopathy: the normal cellular immune response. Br Heart J 1985;53:394–399.
71. Zee-Cheng CS, Tsai CC, Palmer DC, et al. High incidence of myocarditis by endomyocardial biopsy in patients with idiopathic congestive cardiomyopathy. J Am Coll Cardiol 1984;3:63–70.
72. Parrillo JE, Aretz HT, Palacios I, et al. The results of transvenous endomyocardial biopsy can frequently be used to diagnose myocardial diseases in patients with idiopathic heart failure: endomyocardial biopsies in 100 consecutive patients revealed a substantial incidence of myocarditis. Circulation 1984;69:93–101.
73. Bowles NE, Richardson PJ, Olsen EGJ, et al. Detection of coxsackie-B-virus–specific RNA sequences in myocardial biopsy samples from patients with myocarditis and dilated cardiomyopathy. Lancet 1986;1:1120–1122.
74. Lieberman EB, Herskowitz A, Rose NR, et al. A clinicopathologic description of myocarditis. Clin Immunol Immunopathol 1993;68:191–196.
75. Herskowitz A, Willoughby S, Wu TC, et al. Immunopathogenesis of HIV-1–associated cardiomyopathy. Clin Immunol Immunopathol 1993;68:234–241.
76. Herskowitz A, Ansari AA, Neumann DA, et al. Cardiomyopathy in acquired immuno-deficiency syndrome: evidence for autoimmunity [abstract]. Circulation 1989;80(Suppl II):II-322.
77. Fowles RE, Bieber CP, Stinson EB. Defective in vitro suppressor cell function in idiopathic congestive cardiomyopathy. Circulation 1979;59:483–491.
78. Bolte HD. Immunological defects precursors of myocarditis and dilated cardiomyopathy? J Mol Cell Cardiol 1985;17(Suppl 2):69–71.
79. Ho DD, Pomerantz RJ, Kaplan JC. Pathogenesis of infection with human immunodeficiency virus. N Engl J Med 1987;317:278–286.
80. Parker MM, Shelhamer JH, Bacharach SL, et al. Profound but reversible myocardial depression in patients with septic shock. Ann Intern Med 1984;100:483–490.
81. Natanson C, Fink MP, Ballantyne HK, et al. Gram-negative bacteremia produces both severe systolic and diastolic cardiac dysfunction in a canine model that simulates human septic shock. J Clin Invest 1986;78:259–270.
82. Parrillo JE, Burch C, Shelhamer JH, et al. A circulating myocardial depressant substance in humans with septic shock: septic shock patients with a reduced ejection fraction have a circulating factor that depresses in vitro myocardial cell performance. J Clin Invest 1985;76:1539–1553.
83. Cunnion RE, Parrillo JE. Myocardial dysfunction in sepsis: recent insights [editorial]. Chest 1989;95:941–945.
84. Suffredini AF, Fromm RE, Parker MM, et al. The cardiovascular response of normal humans to the administration of endotoxin. N Engl J Med 1989;321:280–287.
85. Lähdevirta J, Maury CPJ, Teppo AM, et al. Elevated levels of circulating cachectin/tumor necrosis factor in patients with acquired immunodeficiency syndrome. Am J Med 1988;85:289–291.
86. Wright SC, Jewett A, Mitsuyasu R, et al. Spontaneous cytotoxicity and tumor necrosis factor production by peripheral blood monocytes from AIDS patients. J Immunol 1988;141:99–104.
87. Levine B, Kalman J, Mayer L, et al. Elevated circulating levels of tumor necrosis factor in severe chronic heart failure. N Engl J Med 1990;323:236–241.
88. Goldberg SJ, Comerci GD, Feldman L. Cardiac output and regional myocardial contraction in anorexia nervosa. J Adolesc Health Care 1988;9:15–21.
89. Abel RM, Grimes JB, Alonso D, et al. Adverse hemodynamic and ultrastructural changes in dog hearts subjected to protein–calorie malnutrition. Am Heart J 1979;97:733–744.
90. Heymsfield SB, Bethel RA, Ansley JD, et al. Cardiac abnormalities in cachectic patients before and during nutritional repletion. Am Heart J 1978;95:584–594.
91. Schocken DD, Holloway JD, Powers PS. Weight loss and the heart: effects of anorexia nervosa and starvation. Arch Intern Med 1989;149:877–881.
92. Kavanaugh–McHugh A, Rowe S, Benjamin Y, et al. Selenium deficiency and cardiomyopathy in malnourished pediatric AIDS patients [abstract]. In: 5th International Conference on AIDS, Montreal, 1989; section B:329.
93. Dworkin BM, Antonecchia PP, Smith F, et al. Reduced cardiac selenium content in the acquired immunodeficiency syndrome. JPEN J Parenter Enteral Nutr 1989;13:644–647.
94. Kavanaugh–McHugh AL, Ruff A, Perlman E, et al. Selenium deficiency and cardiomyopathy in acquired immunodeficiency syndrome. JPEN J Parenter Enteral Nutr 1991;15:347–349.
95. Zazzo JF, Chalas J, Lafont A, et al. Is nonobstructive cardiomyopathy in AIDS a selenium deficiency-related disease? [letter]. JPEN J Parenter Enteral Nutr 1988;12:537–538.
96. Dworkin BM. Selenium deficiency in HIV infection and the acquired immunodeficiency syndrome (AIDS). Chem Biol Interact 1994;91:181–186.
97. Samlowski WE, Ward JH, Craven CM, et al. Severe myocarditis following high-dose interleukin-2 administration. Arch Pathol Lab Med 1989;113:838–841.
98. Deyton LR, Walker RE, Kovacs JA, et al. Reversible cardiac dysfunction associated with interferon alfa therapy in AIDS patients with Kaposi's sarcoma. N Engl J Med 1989;321:1246–1249.
99. Zimmerman S, Adkins D, Graham M, et al. Irreversible, severe cardiomyopathy occurring in association with interferon alpha therapy. Cancer Biother 1994;9:291–299.
100. Brown DL, Sather S, Cheitlin MD. Reversible cardiac dysfunction associated with foscarnet therapy for cytomegalovirus esophagitis in an AIDS patient. Am Heart J 1993;125:1439–1441.
101. Richman DD, Fischl MA, Grieco MH, et al. The toxicity of azidothymidine (AZT) in the treatment of patients with AIDS and AIDS-related complex: a double-blind, placebo-controlled trial. N Engl J Med 1987;317:192–197.
102. Dalakas MC, Illa I, Pezeshkpour GH, et al. Mitochondrial myopathy caused by long-term zidovudine therapy. N Engl J Med 1990;322:1098–1105.
103. Herskowitz A, Willoughby SB, Baughman KL, et al. Cardiomyopathy associated with antiretroviral therapy in patients with HIV infection: a report of six cases. Ann Intern Med 1992;116:311–313.

104. Lipshultz SE, Orav EJ, Sanders SP, et al. Cardiac structure and function in children with human immunodeficiency virus infection treated with zidovudine. N Engl J Med 1992;327:1260–1265.
105. Chokshi SK, Moore R, Pandian NG, et al. Reversible cardiomyopathy associated with cocaine intoxication. Ann Intern Med 1989;111:1039–1040.
106. Blanchard DG, Hagenhoff C, Clow LC, et al. Reversibility of cardiac abnormalities in human immunodeficiency virus (HIV)–infected individuals: a serial echocardiographic study. J Am Coll Cardiol 1991;17:1270–1276.
107. De Castro S, d'Amati G, Gallo P, et al. Frequency of development of acute global left ventricular dysfunction in human immunodeficiency virus infection. J Am Coll Cardiol 1994;24:1018–1024.
108. Cheitlin MD. Cardiovascular complications of HIV infection. In: Sande MA, Volberding PA, eds. The medical management of AIDS. 4th ed. Philadelphia: WB Saunders, 1995;332–344.
109. Herskowitz A, Vlahov D, Willoughby S, et al. Prevalence and incidence of left ventricular dysfunction in patients with human immunodeficiency virus infection. Am J Cardiol 1993;71:955–958.
110. Centers for Disease Control. Update: acquired immunodeficiency syndrome—United States. MMWR Morb Mortal Wkly Rep 1986;35:17–21.
111. Henderson DK, Fahey BJ, Willy M, et al. Risk for occupational transmission of human immunodeficiency virus type 1 (HIV-1) associated with clinical exposures: a prospective evaluation. Ann Intern Med 1990;113:740–746.

37

HEMATOLOGIC MANIFESTATIONS OF HIV INFECTION

John P. Doweiko

The first human retroviruses were discovered in the late 1970s (1). Type 1 human immunodeficiency virus (HIV-1), previously known as human T-cell lymphotropic virus type III or lymphadenopathy-associated virus, is a member of the Lentivirus group of the family Retroviridae (2, 3). An estimated 1 million people in the United States, and 8 to 10 million worldwide, have been infected with this virus (4).

Despite its relatively simple structure, HIV-1 has a complicated mechanism of replication (5). Its genome is encoded within a single strand of RNA that is enclosed within a "shell" of p24 protein (6). This shell is itself contained within a glycoprotein envelope that is studded with the transmembrane p41 protein to which is attached the gp120 protein (2, 3). The gp120 glycoprotein is necessary for binding to the CD4 protein of the target cells (7).

HIV-1 is genetically more complex than other members of the Retroviridae family (3). HIV-1 has three genes that are characteristic of replicative retroviruses (2, 3): the *Gag* gene that encodes for the core structural proteins of the virus, the *Pol* gene encoding for the viral enzymes (reverse transcriptase, integrase and protease), and the *Env* gene encoding for the surface glycoproteins of the virus. In addition, the genome of HIV-1 also includes six other genes that are currently less well understood (2).

Certain genes of HIV-1 are error prone, particularly those encoding reverse transcriptase and the envelope proteins. Having this propensity to mutate in vivo, progression of the infection within a host is associated with evolution toward a quasispecies composed of viral variants (8–10). This property allows for extensive genomic variation to develop from a single infecting event.

The CD4 protein is contained on T lymphocytes and cells of the monocyte/macrophage line and is a member of the immunoglobulin superfamily (11). This protein is in high concentration on T-helper cells and monocytes, designating these cells as the major targets of the infection (12–15). Although the CD4 antigen may be the sole high-affinity cellular receptor for HIV-1 (12, 13), other cell-surface proteins act as coreceptors and augment entry into the cell by a factor of at least a thousandfold compared with cell membranes that lack these other proteins (11, 16). The chemokine receptors that function as cell-surface binding sites for HIV-1 include, but are not limited to, fusin, now known as CXCR-4 (11). This is a coreceptor for strains of HIV-1 that primarily invade T-cell lines. The β-chemokine receptor CCR5 serves as a coreceptor for strains that infect cells of monocytic lineage (11, 16).

The process of binding of HIV-1 to the CD4 antigen allows the virus to enter the cell. In addition, other important events that result from this binding are inhibition of signal transduction by the T-cell CD3 receptor and secretion of a multitude of cytokines by the infected cell that include interleukin-1β (IL-1β), tumor necrosis factor-α (TNF-α), and granulocyte–monocyte colony-stimulating factor (GM-CSF) (11, 17).

Other cells also express surface CD4 antigen, rendering them vulnerable to infection by HIV-1 (18). These include fibroblasts and related cells such as glial cells, as well as the stromal reticular cells of the bone marrow (12, 13). Cells may be infected by routes other than the CD4 antigen (12, 13), including galactosylceramide on neurons and enterocytes (11). Entry into cells may also occur by Fc receptors when HIV-1 is bound to antibody within immune complexes (11).

Some strains of HIV-1 preferentially infect monocytes, whereas others display selectivity for CD4 lymphocytes (12). This characteristic is important to the evolution of the intricate syndrome that results from this viral infection. The two major sequelae of HIV-1 infection are degradation of cellular immunity and an ultimately detrimental cytokine response. The fundamental morbidity of this infection is degradation of the cellular immune system (19). The clinical manifestations largely result from opportunistic infections and neoplasms, as well as metabolic disturbances from the cytokines produced in response to the infection (20, 21).

The monocyte, as well as the CD4+ lymphocyte, plays an important role in the pathogenesis of HIV infection. In the early phases of infection, monocytotropic strains of HIV-1 predominate over lymphocytotropic strains (19, 22). Although HIV assembles almost exclusively on the plasma membrane of CD4 lymphocytes, it can assemble and accumulate within cytoplasmic vacuoles of monocytes and macrophages, where it remains hidden from the immune system (15). Infection of cells of the monocyte/macrophage line is not lethal for these cells.

Cells of monocytic lineage become important reservoirs of HIV-1 and vectors for spread of the virus throughout the body (4, 23, 24). In nonlymphoid tissues, such as the central nervous system, local infection is predominately sustained by cells of monocytic lineage (22, 25). Derivatives of the monocyte/macrophage cell line such as glial cells of the central nervous system may be infected by and harbor the virus (26). Within these cells, the virus may replicate more rapidly than in other tissues (26).

Cells of monocytic lineage are central to the complex network of growth factors and cytokines that sustains and regulates the hematopoietic and immune systems. Infection of these cells is responsible, in large part, for one of the major sequelae of this viral infection: an ultimately detrimental cytokine response that accelerates HIV infection and promotes tissue injury (24). Levels of inflammatory cytokines in the serum increase as the viral infection progresses (27).

Progression of HIV-1 infection is associated with a shift toward more lymphocytotropic variants of the virus (22). This feature is important to the cellular immune dysfunction characteristic of AIDS (24).

One life cycle for HIV is about 1.2 days in vivo, with about 0.9 days of this cycle being intracellular and the remainder of time representing the half-life of the virion within the tissues or blood (28, 29). Investigators previously thought that after the initial viremia of HIV infection, the virus entered a "latent phase" during which viral replication took place at reduced rate. More recent studies have shown that viral replication persists throughout the course of the HIV infection (30, 31). During the clinical "latent" phase, those infected may be only minimally symptomatic. A large reservoir of HIV-1, however, is sequestered within lymphoid and other tissues wherein viral replication continues (30, 32, 33).

HIV-infected persons produce and destroy about 30% of the total body viral burden daily (28, 29, 34). The clearance of HIV virions is relatively constant during the course of HIV infection, regardless of the CD4+ lymphocyte counts (27, 29). Associated with this brisk viral replication rate is a daily turnover rate of about 5% of the total CD4 lymphocyte pool (27, 29). The decline in the CD4+ lymphocyte count that occurs with progression of HIV infection is due to the destructive capacity of HIV-1 for these cells that eventually exceeds the replicative capacity of the body (28, 29, 32, 34–36). This process results in a progressive deterioration of the cellular immune system (35, 36).

Unlike the viral production rate, which tends to be constant, the CD4 lymphocyte production rate varies from patient to patient (27, 29). This feature may explain, in large part, the variations in disease course among patients. Some patients infected with HIV-1, however, do not succumb to the infection as rapidly as do others (37). In long-term survivors, the viral burden in the plasma and peripheral blood mononuclear cells is less by several orders of magnitude than in less fortunate patients with a similar duration of disease (38, 39). These long-term survivors seem to have a vigorous viral-inhibitory CD8 lymphocyte response and a stronger neutralizing antibody response than is typically seen (38). Genetic alterations in the chemokine receptors may also confer some resistance to HIV-1 and may promote survival (11).

SPECIFIC CYTOPENIAS

Infection with HIV-1 is associated with suppression of hematopoiesis (39–42) (Table 37.1). The hematologic perturbations encountered with HIV-1 infection not only have morbidity of their own, but also hinder therapy directed toward the primary viral infection and the secondary infectious and neoplastic complications (43, 44). The need to reduce doses or to interrupt therapy because of poor hematologic tolerance may cause the emergence of drug-resistant organisms and progression of infections or neoplasms (43, 44).

Anemia

The most common cytopenia associated with HIV-1 infection is anemia. The degree of anemia correlates with the stage of the HIV-1 infection. Although 10 to 20% of patients are anemic at the time of presentation, 70 to 80% eventually become anemic with progression of the infection (45–49). The major cause of anemia in HIV-infected patients is impaired erythropoiesis.

The anemia is typically normochromic and normocytic and is associated with an inappropriately low reticulocyte count (50). Macrocytosis is unusual, and it tends to occur in patients treated with zidovudine (50, 51). Iron stores are almost always normal or elevated, and one typically sees a decrease in serum iron along with a parallel decrease in the total iron binding capacity that is characteristic of the "anemia of chronic disease." Serum ferritin levels are often increased (50), and these levels tend to parallel the severity and duration of the infection with HIV-1 (52–54). Although decreases in serum vitamin B_{12} levels are found in about 20% of HIV-infected patients (50, 55–57), the extent to which these low levels contribute to the cytopenias of HIV is not clear (56, 58–60). Patients usually do not have other manifestations of vitamin B_{12} deficiency, and typically they do not improve markedly with parenteral repletion (50, 57, 58). Conversely, investigators have demonstrated that in the non–HIV-infected population, serum vitamin B_{12} levels may

Table 37.1. Causes of Cytopenias in HIV Infection

Ineffective hematopoiesis
    Effects of HIV-1 on stem cells
    Effects of HIV-1 on marrow stromal cells
    Alterations in growth factors
    Alterations in cytokines
Myelosuppressive medications
Opportunistic infections involving the bone marrow
Tumor involvement of the bone marrow

have poor predictive value (61): Anemia may be absent in patients who are found to be deficient in vitamin B_{12} using assays that rely on vitamin B_{12}-dependent metabolic pathways (61). The low vitamin B_{12} levels that occur with HIV infection seem to be due to altered serum transport of the vitamin (56, 58), but patients may have abnormal absorption with advanced HIV infection (56). Considering the controversy over the exact role of vitamin B_{12} in the anemia associated with HIV infection, some evidence that cobalamins may hinder binding of HIV-1 to the CD4 molecule (57), and the ease of parenteral administration, this therapy should be considered in an anemic HIV-infected patient.

Although some patients have a positive Coombs test, this is usually nonspecific and is not a major contributing factor to the anemia. Sensitive assays show that 2 to 44% of asymptomatic HIV-infected patients are directly Coombs positive, as are 60 to 70% with AIDS-related complex and up to 85% of those with AIDS (44, 50). Although these antibodies may be reactive with specific minor antigens on erythrocytes (44, 46, 50), they are most commonly due to nonspecific binding of antiphospholipid antibodies or deposition of immune complexes on erythrocytes (44, 46, 50). Immune hemolysis is rare (44, 50).

Paraproteinemia may occur in more than half of all HIV-infected patients (50). The peripheral smear may demonstrate rouleaux; dimerization or comigration of these proteins during electrophoresis may result in the appearance of a monoclonal protein (50). However, a polyclonal pattern on electrophoresis is more common, and the paraproteinemia does not cause or contribute to the cytopenias seen with HIV-1 infection (50).

Neutropenia

Granulocytopenia tends to occur concomitantly with anemia (53). Although 10 to 30% of patients with AIDS-related complex may be neutropenic, this number may progress to about three-fourths of those with AIDS (44, 46, 48, 53, 55). Review of the peripheral smear reveals a variable deficiency of neutrophils, lymphocytes, and perhaps monocytes; atypical lymphocytes may be seen. Vacuolization of the monocytes is a typical finding, and hypolobulation of the neutrophils may occur and may imitate a leftward shift (53, 62).

Impaired myelopoiesis is the major cause of the leukopenia associated with HIV-1 infection (53, 63–65). Myelotoxic medications may exacerbate this problem, and concurrent use of these drugs may be synergistic in this regard. Although about one-third of patients have antibodies on the circulating neutrophils, the presence of these antibodies correlates neither with the incidence nor the severity of the neutropenia (50).

Thrombocytopenia

Although anemia and granulocytopenia tend to occur concomitantly, with a severity that parallels the course of the HIV-1 infection, thrombocytopenia can occur independently of other cytopenias and at all stages of HIV infection (45, 48, 53, 66–69). Thrombocytopenia of varying severity may occur in 30 to 60% of HIV-infected patients (43, 45–47, 66, 68–71). Of these thrombocytopenic, HIV-infected patients, 16 to 40% of those with platelet counts below 50,000 cells/mm^3 may have clinically significant bleeding (68, 71). By itself, thrombocytopenia is not prognostic of the HIV infection (72, 73).

The causes of thrombocytopenia in HIV infection include reduced bone marrow production and immune and nonimmune destruction (74). Although immune mechanisms and reduced platelet life span may be more important in the early stages of HIV-associated thrombocytopenia, decreased production may be more important in the later stages of disease (74, 75).

Most HIV-infected patients have antibodies coating the platelets (76–78). Although some of these may be due to nonspecific binding of immune complexes (45, 79), molecular mimicry between gp160/120 antigen of HIV-1 and gpIIb/IIIa of platelets may lead to production of more specific antibodies to the platelet surface (76, 77, 80–82). The presence of antibodies on the surface of the platelets does not, however, correlate well with the platelet count, because of defective reticuloendothelial clearance in HIV-infected patients (83–85). In addition to immune destruction, infections and fevers that occur with HIV infection decrease the life span of circulating platelets. Other causes of nonimmune destruction of circulating platelets are hemolytic-uremia syndrome and thrombotic thrombocytopenia purpura, which occur more commonly in HIV-infected patients (67, 86, 87).

A progressive reduction in the productive capacity of megakaryocytes that occurs with HIV infection leads to a lack of compensatory megakaryocytopoiesis in HIV-infected patients to counter ongoing peripheral destruction (69, 79, 88–90). Megakaryocyte precursors in HIV-1–seropositive patients demonstrate an increase in apoptosis compared with normal controls, and the degree has been shown to correlate inversely with the circulating platelet count (69). HIV-1 may directly suppress platelet production in that megakaryocytes are potential targets of infection by the virus (46, 79, 90, 91), and this process may result in quantitative and morphologic abnormalities of megakaryocytes (74). HIV-1 indirectly suppresses platelet production by exposing or altering antigens on the surface of the megakaryocyte that then renders them targets of antiplatelet antibodies (67, 76). Compounding this situation are the changes in cytokines and growth factors that occur during the HIV infection and that alter platelet production (88, 92).

TREATMENT

No well-controlled, prospectively randomized trials have been conducted to test the various treatment options for HIV-associated thrombocytopenia (50) (Table 37.2). Spontaneous remissions may occur in 10 to 20% of patients (52, 93). A sudden elevation in the platelet count, however, may indicate deterioration in the immune system and may

Table 37.2. Treatment Modalities for HIV-Associated Thrombocytopenia

Modality	Acute Response Rate (% of patients)	Durable Response Rate (% of patients)
Spontaneous remissions	10–20	10
Nucleoside analogs	20–30	10
Dapsone	20–30	10
Corticosteroids	20–30	10
Vincristine	10	10
Anabolic steroids	10–30	10
High-dose ascorbic acid	Case reports to date	
Interferons	Small and uncontrolled studies	
Anti-D (anti-Rh) antibody	70–80	10
Splenectomy	60–90	60
Low-dose splenic irradiation	40–60	40

herald the onset of AIDS (67, 93). In patients who have a sustained decrease in platelet count, therapy is not always necessary, because the incidence of significant bleeding episodes may be low despite low platelet counts (94–96). However, to predict the risk of bleeding based solely on platelet count is difficult (97).

In patients with thrombocytopenia associated with HIV infection, administration of zidovudine may result in elevations of platelet counts in approximately 30% of patients within 12 weeks of initiation of therapy (51, 67, 68, 92, 93). Although some studies have shown a dose response, this effect has not been demonstrated in other studies (51). Other nucleoside reverse transcriptase inhibitors have not, as yet, been shown to have this effect (91). Like zidovudine, dapsone may elevate platelet counts in a few patients within 3 weeks of initiating therapy (78). Although the mechanism of zidovudine is not clear, that of dapsone may be due to a reduction in phagocyte-mediated destruction (78).

Corticosteroids elevate platelet counts in 40 to 80% of those patients with HIV-associated immune thrombocytopenia; long-term remissions occur in only 10 to 20% after such therapy (67). Although long-term, low-dose steroids may be effective in maintaining an acceptable platelet count (84), side effects preclude their use. No controlled trials thus far demonstrate any adverse effects of short-term steroids on HIV infection (84).

Patients in whom the foregoing treatments have failed have been tried on other therapies. Vincristine and anabolic steroids have an overall response rate of about only 10% (98, 99). High-dose ascorbate (2 to 4 g per day) over several months has been shown in small studies to increase platelet counts in patients with HIV-associated immune thrombocytopenia; the mechanism and durability of the response are not entirely clear (67). Interferons (IFNs), particularly IFN-α, have been shown in controlled trials to have some efficacy in patients with zidovudine-resistant, HIV-1–related thrombocytopenia (50, 100). One potential mechanism by which IFN-α restores platelet production may be by increasing levels of IL-6 (101), a cytokine with trophic effects on megakaryocytes.

Infusions of γ-globulins offer the potential for a rapid elevation in platelet counts with an acute response rate of 70 to 90% (67, 102, 103); the median response duration is about 3 weeks. Sustained remissions from a single course of such therapy occur in fewer than 10% of patients (67). A similar response is offered by anti-D (anti-Rh) antibody, which has an acute response rate of 75% (104), with sustained remissions in less than 10%. As with γ-globulin infusions, readministration is effective in elevating the platelet counts in patients who initially responded (67, 105, 106). Unlike with γ-globulin, however, the response may take up to 3 weeks to occur, and it may be associated with some hemolysis; anti-D antibody is not effective in patients who have undergone splenectomy or in those who are Rh negative (104). Both immune globulin infusions and anti-D antibody may work by increasing production of thrombopoietic cytokines from cells of the reticuloendothelial system, such as IL-6, rather than by decreasing platelet destruction (107).

When other therapies fail, splenectomy needs to be considered. This procedure has an acute response rate of 60 to 100%, and durable responses occur in 40 to 60% (67). No studies to date demonstrate any detrimental effects of splenectomy on HIV progression (97, 108, 109). This procedure can, however, result in artificial elevations in CD4 counts from peripheral lymphocytosis (108). Consequently, patients who have undergone splenectomy may develop opportunistic infections at higher levels of CD4 than otherwise expected (108). An alternative to splenectomy is offered by low-dose splenic irradiation (78, 110). Small, uncontrolled studies have demonstrated an acute response rate of 70%, with durable responses occurring in about 40% of patients (110). The total doses are about 900 to 1000 cGy over 1 month. Some degree of splenic function is maintained by low-dose radiation (111).

BONE MARROW ABNORMALITIES

The bone marrow in most patients with HIV infection exhibits morphologic aberrations (40, 42, 112, 113) (Table 37.3). The incidence of these changes increases with progression of HIV infection (55, 114). None of the marrow abnormalities seen with HIV infection, however, are specific for the disease (42, 43, 115, 116).

Hypercellularity of the bone marrow is the most common morphologic demonstration encountered in HIV-1–infected patients (117–119). This change occurs in 50 to 60% of cases

Table 37.3. Typical Features of the Bone Marrow in HIV Infection

Cellularity: Increased in 50–60%; normal in 35–40%; hypocellular in 5%
Dysplasia in one or more cell lines occurs in over 70%
Granulocyte > erythrocyte > megakaryocytic
Lymphoid aggregates occur in 20%
Fibrosis occurs in 20%
Less commonly seen: Eosinophilia, plasma cell infiltrates

and is due to absolute hyperplasia of one or more of the nonlymphoid cell lines (114). One may see mild myeloid hyperplasia, but more often, the myeloid-to-erythroid ratio tends to remain close to normal (116). Because much of the hypercellularity may not represent effective hematopoiesis, the marrow cellularity correlates neither with the peripheral blood counts nor with the stage of HIV infection (50, 116, 118, 119). Hypocellularity of the marrow is rare, occurring in fewer than 5% of cases, and is usually a manifestation of advanced HIV infection (43, 47, 55). In the end stages of HIV infection, atrophy or necrosis of the marrow may occur (116).

Dysplasia of at least one cell line occurs in more than 70% of HIV-infected patients (47, 62, 117). This dysplasia is similar to that of the myelodysplastic syndromes, but it is largely not distinguishable from the latter on morphologic criteria alone (47, 120). Dysplasia of the granulocyte series is the most frequent occurrence, with vacuolization of the granulocyte precursors in the marrow and in the peripheral neutrophils (121). Erythrocytic dysplasia is less common, seen in 50 to 60% of HIV-infected patients, and dysplasia of the megakaryocytes is seen in about one-third of HIV-infected patients (117). In general, the degree and frequency of dysplastic changes in the bone marrow increase with progression of the HIV-1 infection and also with concurrent opportunistic infections (46).

Less common aberrations include lymphoid aggregates and increased numbers of lymphocytes. This situation is encountered in about 20% of patients, and it occurs despite the peripheral lymphopenia that is characteristic of the viral infection (46, 62). A similar proportion of patients with advanced HIV infection have focal or diffuse increases in reticulin deposition in the bone marrow (46, 55). In general, marrow fibrosis increases in incidence and severity with progression of the HIV-1 infection and with marrow involvement by fungal or mycobacterial organisms (50). Other nonspecific morphologic changes that may be seen in the bone marrow include increases in eosinophils and plasma cells and histiocytic erythrophagocytosis (55, 122).

CAUSES OF CYTOPENIAS

The hematologic abnormalities that occur during the course of HIV infection are largely due to ineffective hematopoiesis. A compounding factor is peripheral destruction. In a few patients with significant splenomegaly, sequestration may further compound the problem.

Hematopoiesis is a process that is both constitutive and inducible. Constitutive hematopoiesis is largely under the direction of the CSFs (123), whereas inducible hematopoiesis is more within the realm of action of other cytokines and interleukins that modulate hematopoiesis during situations of altered demand (124, 125). These cytokines are released from marrow fibroblasts, endothelial cells, T cells, and monocytes in response to a multitude of stimuli (123, 124).

The hematologic perturbations that occur in association with HIV infection may be a result of HIV-1 on stem cells and the marrow stromal cells. The alterations in growth factors and cytokines that occur as a result of HIV infection contribute to hematopoietic abnormalities (126). Other factors that merit recognition are opportunistic infections and neoplasms invading the bone marrow and myelosuppressive medications.

Altered Hematopoiesis from Tumor, Infection, or Medications

HIV infection is associated with the development of lymphomas as well as Kaposi's sarcoma and squamous cell carcinomas. The incidence of neoplasms that occur with HIV infection is likely to increase as the infectious complications of AIDS are better controlled. The bone marrow is affected in about one-third of patients with AIDS-related lymphomas (127). The extent of replacement of the bone marrow by these malignant cells does not, however, correlate well with the peripheral blood counts (127). The antineoplastic drugs needed to treat these tumors are myelosuppressive, and the dose reductions that may be needed to preserve hematopoietic function hinder therapy of the tumors.

The medications used to treat HIV infection and the opportunistic infections that occur in AIDS cause disease-stage and dose-dependent suppression of hematopoiesis (29, 50). All the dideoxynucleoside analogs can inhibit hematopoiesis at sufficiently high doses, with zidovudine the major offender (128, 129). Other myelosuppressive drugs include pentamidine, trimethoprim, sulfonamides, ganciclovir, acyclovir, and pyrimethamine (128). Medications that are not typically associated with decreases in hematopoiesis may cause this effect when given to patients with altered hematopoietic potential such as occurs with HIV infection. Furthermore, concurrently administered myelosuppressive medications are synergistic in their potential to cause bone marrow suppression.

Several opportunistic infections that result from HIV-induced immunosuppression may cause or contribute to bone marrow failure. Mycobacterial infections, particularly with *Mycobacterium avium* complex but also with disseminated *M. tuberculosis* and atypical forms, and fungal infections, most common of which are cryptococcosis and histoplasmosis, are important causes of reduced hematopoietic potential. The bone marrow may reveal a disseminated mycobacterial or fungal infection long before other indications of these infections become apparent in an HIV-infected host (120, 130): Special stains and cultures of the marrow for these organisms are helpful and may be positive before peripheral blood cultures turn positive (120, 130). Small studies have shown that bone marrow examination or culture is positive for mycobacteria or fungi in at least 75% of patients who are subsequently found by other diagnostic methods to have these infections (120, 131).

The most common manifestation of the presence of these infections within the bone marrow is diffuse infiltration with loose aggregates and clusters of macrophages (52, 132). The ability to detect involvement of the bone marrow by mycobacteria and fungi correlates with the number of macrophages in the marrow (52). Although these cells may organize into granulomas, the tendency to do so lessens with advancing immunosuppression (50). Pseudo-Gaucher cells may also be seen as a manifestation of such infections (133).

Opportunistic infections of the bone marrow by viruses other than HIV-1 itself are important causes of marrow failure. In this regard, cytomegalovirus and parvovirus have special significance. Hepatitis B and C, however, merit recognition as causes of bone marrow suppression in an HIV-infected patient (134, 135).

Cytomegalovirus may suppress hematopoiesis and may also cause autoimmune destruction of blood cells (50, 136). Neutropenia, anemia that may be hemolytic, and thrombocytopenia either alone or in combination can be seen with cytomegalovirus infection (137). This virus can infect bone marrow progenitor cells, rendering them less responsive to CSFs (136–138). Furthermore, these infected cells may serve as reservoirs of latent cytomegalovirus within the bone marrow, causing further problems with advancing immunosuppression (136). Cytomegalovirus can infect the bone marrow stromal cells, interfering with their hematopoietic supporting functions, largely by decreasing local growth factor production by these cells (136, 139). Despite the hematologic problems that cytomegalovirus may cause, the virus does not cause distinctive histologic changes of the bone marrow, and it is best cultured from the buffy coat of the blood and not from the marrow itself (136).

HIV-positive patients may be infected with parvovirus B19 that may result in marrow suppression. These patients often do not have the manifestations of fifth disease (fevers, rash, and arthralgias) that are seen in immunologically normal patients (140). The major hematopoietic target of parvovirus B19 is the erythroid progenitor (141). This is the only permissive cell of the hematopoietic system for the virus. Morphologically, such an infection results in giant pronormoblasts (140) and erythroblastopenia that can persist in those who are unable to make antibodies to the virus (135, 141). Parvovirus also has an inhibitory effect on myeloid and megakaryocyte progenitors that may result in varying degrees of neutropenia or thrombocytopenia (140–142). Immunosuppressed patients may not be able to make immunoglobulin M (IgM) antibody to parvovirus, and this inability hinders the spontaneous recovery from the infection as well as the value of serologic testing in diagnosis (143). Treatment of parvovirus B19 infection in patients who are unable to make antibodies to the infection includes intravenous γ-globulin, which results in a reduction in serum viral concentrations and recovery of erythropoiesis (140, 143). Simultaneous infection with parvovirus B19 and HIV-1 does not preclude a response to erythropoietin (140).

Human herpesvirus-6 is the etiologic agent of another viral exanthem of childhood, roseola. Infection usually occurs in the first 3 years of life, and then it establishes latency (144). The primary target of this virus is the CD4 lymphocyte, as well as cells of monocytic lineage (144, 145). Immunosuppression may result in loss of latency; subsequent exposure of marrow precursor cells to this virus inhibits their ability to respond to growth factors, and infection of lymphocytes causes further suppression of T-cell function (144, 145).

Colony-Stimulating Factors

A vast cytokine network composed of over 20 hematopoietic and lymphopoietic growth factors has been identified (146). Important components of this array are the CSFs, which include granulocyte CSF (G-CSF), macrophage CSF (M-CSF), GM-CSF, IL-3, stem cell factor, and erythropoietin (124, 147). These glycoproteins regulate passage of hematopoietic cells into the cell cycle and into the processes of terminal maturation (148). The predominant activity of these cytokines and growth factors is to suppress apoptosis (149–151).

The major sources of CSFs are T and B lymphocytes, natural killer (NK) cells, vascular endothelial cells, smooth muscle cells, and fibroblasts (124, 125). Many of these cells are targets of infection by HIV-1 (126), and when they are infected, their ability to make growth factors progressively diminishes (152). The monocyte, an important primary target for infection by HIV-1, is central to the network of cytokines, interleukins, and growth factors that support and regulate hematopoiesis (125, 132, 153). Although infection of cells of monocytic lineage by HIV-1 enhances their secretion of inflammatory cytokines, it simultaneously diminishes their ability to secrete hematopoietic growth factors (154).

Production of G-CSF, GM-CSF, and M-CSF increases during the early phases of HIV infection (41). This increase may partially explain the hypercellularity of the bone marrow that is often seen at this stage of HIV infection (126). This change is largely due to the effects of low concentrations of IL-1 and other inflammatory cytokines, such as IFN-γ and TNF-α, on cells within the bone marrow that produce these growth factors (126, 155, 156).

As HIV infection advances, however, levels of these inflammatory cytokines progress beyond levels that stimulate hematopoiesis to levels that inhibit it (126, 154). Furthermore, with advancing HIV infection, these increasing levels of inflammatory cytokines alter the receptors on target cells to make them less responsive to growth factors (155–159). Other cytokines that inhibit hematopoiesis, such as transforming growth factor-β (TGF-β) are made in increasing amounts with advancing HIV infection (126, 152).

Major stimuli to the production of these negative regulators of hematopoiesis by monocytes within the bone marrow are products of HIV itself such as the Tat protein (41, 160–162). This protein is released from infected monocytes and lymphocytes and may be taken up by other cells and stimulates them to release proinflammatory cytokines that include TNF-α, IL-1α, IL-1β, and IFN-γ (163, 164). HIV-1 Nef protein also may be released from infected cells and induces IL-6 production and release by peripheral blood lymphocytes (165).

The pharmacokinetics of growth factors administered to cytopenic patients depends on the dose, amount of glycosylation, and route of administration. Cytokines may have effects in combination that are not seen with each alone (126, 146). Exogenous administration of growth factors offers the potential of ameliorating some of the adverse effects of HIV infection on hematopoiesis. Dispensing of growth factors permits the administration of myelosuppressive medications without dose reduction or interruption of therapy (44). With the exception of erythropoietin, these potentials of growth factors have been investigated in uncontrolled studies only (166).

GRANULOCYTE COLONY-STIMULATING FACTOR

G-CSF is produced by activated monocytes, stimulated endothelial cells, and fibroblasts. Exogenous administration of G-CSF results in a sustained, dose-dependent rise in the circulating neutrophil counts (63, 123). High doses may result in modest elevations of monocytes and lymphocytes (123). The relative and absolute elevation in neutrophil count is due to an increase in the number of divisions of neutrophil precursors in the marrow and a decrease in their maturation time (167). In vitro, G-CSF augments neutrophil function (63, 168).

GRANULOCYTE–MONOCYTE COLONY-STIMULATING FACTOR

GM-CSF is produced primarily by stimulated fibroblasts and endothelial cells, but also by T cells. Administration of this growth factor, as with G-CSF, results in a dose-dependent elevation in neutrophils. The kinetic basis of the elevation in neutrophils differs from that of G-CSF in that GM-CSF prolongs the circulating half-life of these cells, rather than decreasing the production time as does G-CSF (123, 169). Unlike G-CSF, however, it also results in a significant elevation in eosinophils and monocytes (64, 65, 170, 171).

GM-CSF and G-CSF have different effects on HIV-infected cells (63, 147, 172). Although G-CSF does not seem to alter HIV replication in cells that are targets for the growth factor, GM-CSF can stimulate HIV replication in vitro in infected cells of monocytic lineage (170, 171, 173, 174). Moreover, activation of monocytes by HIV infection induces them to produce GM-CSF and to stimulate T cells, endothelial cells, and fibroblasts to produce this growth factor, and this augments HIV replication in the monocytes (124, 125). When GM-CSF is administered in conjunction with zidovudine, the result is enhanced antiviral effects because of an increase in the concentration of the active drug within monocytes (170, 171, 173, 175). Thus far, this effect has been shown only for zidovudine, and therefore, GM-CSF should be administered concomitantly with zidovudine in HIV-infected patients (172).

ERYTHROPOIETIN

Most HIV-infected patients with anemia have adequate erythropoietic capacity, but they are unable to augment this capacity during times of demand in large part because of inadequate erythropoietin levels (50). Inappropriately low endogenous levels (lower than 500 mU/mL) of serum erythropoietin are seen in 75% of AIDS patients regardless of the medications they are receiving (44, 126, 176). In addition to a production problem, the cytokines produced in response to the HIV infection, such as IL-1 and TNF-α, blunt the normal exponential elevation between the hematocrit and serum erythropoietin levels (126, 177). Proinflammatory cytokines not only decrease erythropoietin production, but also alter the sensitivity of erythroid precursors to this growth factor (155).

Administration of erythropoietin may reverse the suppression of erythropoiesis that occurs in response to proinflammatory cytokines (155, 178). In placebo-controlled trials, exogenous administration of erythropoietin increased the hematocrit and improved the quality of life for patients with AIDS (176, 179). The elevation in erythrocyte counts was dose dependent (43, 44). Initial concerns about stem cell exhaustion or lineage diversion did not occur (44). Erythropoietin neither promoted nor prevented HIV replication (44, 172).

Despite these promising results, not all patients respond to the administration of this growth factor. The benefits are principally seen in those with baseline erythropoietin levels of less than 500 mU/mL (44). About 25% of patients who are receiving zidovudine do not have a significant elevation in hematocrit with concurrent administration of erythropoietin (44). Opportunistic infections render patients resistant to the effects of exogenous erythropoietin (180).

Administration of erythropoietin offers an alternative to transfusions, which have potential morbidity. Transfusions may be immunosuppressive (181, 182); they have been shown to cause decreases in the ratio of CD4 to CD8 lymphocytes and reductions in NK cell number (183). The time to progression to AIDS is shorter in patients who undergo transfusion (44, 50, 183). Furthermore, these patients risk exposure to new infectious agents with transfusions (44) and alloimmunization transfusion reactions despite the immunodeficiency induced by HIV-1 infection (44, 116).

STEM CELL FACTOR

Stem cell factor (S-CSF, kit ligand) is a multipotential growth factor produced by marrow stromal cells (184). It acts on cells of myeloid, lymphoid, and mast cell lineage (184). For optimal stimulatory effects, it acts in synergy with other, more lineage-restricted, CSFs (124, 184–186).

Levels of endogenous stem cell factor decrease as HIV infection advances, and these levels correlate with overall survival (186). The reduction of these levels may be due to progressively defective function of the stromal cells that make S-CSF (186). When administered to HIV-infected patients, S-CSF increases hematopoiesis in a dose-dependent fashion (187). It has not been shown to alter HIV expression (187).

INTERLEUKIN-3

This growth factor is produced by activated T cells and has direct effects on granulocytes, monocytes, and mast cells, as well as indirect stimulatory activities on erythroid production and T lymphocytes (188). Administration results in a dose-dependent increase in circulating granulocytes, erythrocytes, and platelets (188).

The loss of T cells that is characteristic of advancing HIV infection results in reductions in endogenous IL-3 levels (101, 175, 189–191). This change may contribute to the myelosuppression that occurs with HIV infection (175). Combinations of suboptimal concentrations of IL-3 act in synergy with other growth factors to counter the myelosuppression that occurs with HIV-1 infection. The mechanism of this activity involves preventing the apoptosis of hematopoietic progenitor cells that occurs in the presence of HIV and in the absence of growth factors (151).

Although some investigators have found IL-3 to potentiate HIV expression in monocytes in vitro, others have found no consistent effects on viral activity (192). Like GM-CSF, IL-3 may augment the antiviral effects of zidovudine by elevating the intracellular levels of the active form of the drug (12, 115, 175, 193).

Bone Marrow Progenitor Cells

Results of studies on HIV infection of bone marrow progenitor cells have been conflicting (114). Although data indicate that progenitor cells are targets of HIV infection (53, 92), other investigators have revealed that CD34+ bone marrow progenitor cells are infrequently infected with the virus (40, 41, 194–200). Some have shown that progenitor cell numbers in the bone marrow and peripheral blood (118, 201, 202) are decreased with HIV infection (47, 58, 113), whereas others have noted no significant differences in the numbers of these cells in HIV-infected patients when compared with immunologically normal persons (196, 199, 203, 204).

These ostensibly conflicting results are reconciled when consideration is given to several factors. Studies that investigate the effects of HIV-1 on hematopoietic progenitor cells need to consider the different strains of virus that are known to occur and evolve with advancing infection. Monocytotropic strains of HIV-1 may be more prone to alter hematopoiesis than are lymphocytotropic strains (203). The cytopathic capacity of different strains of HIV-1 also differs (197, 199), with some strains known to impair hematopoiesis in a dose-dependent manner (197, 205–207).

Obtaining highly purified populations of CD34 cells from the bone marrow is difficult (200). When this impediment is overcome, however, it becomes apparent that only a few CD34+ progenitor cells are also positive for CD4, and therefore, only an unimportant number of progenitor cells are major targets for HIV-1 (76, 198, 208–211). Direct infection of the hematopoietic cells by HIV-1 does not seem to be a major contribution to the hematopoietic defect that occurs with HIV-1 infection (151, 162, 203, 212).

The presence or absence of accessory cells within the marrow cultures is also important to the myelosuppression that occurs in vitro in the presence of HIV-1. T cells, monocytes, adipocytes, fibroblasts, and vascular endothelial cells are important components of the bone marrow stroma and influence hematopoiesis by production of growth factors (53, 59, 126, 152). These cells, particularly the stromal cells of monocytic lineage, are targets for HIV and may serve as reservoirs of virus within the bone marrow (40, 41, 153, 213). When infected with HIV-1, these cells are less able to make growth factors (53, 59, 154). Because the major function of growth factors may be to prevent apoptosis, the deficiency in local production permits bone marrow progenitor cells to undergo this process (203). Furthermore, these cells may produce inhibitors of hematopoiesis such as TGF-β, platelet factor 4, IFNs, and TNF-α (124, 212, 214–216). In vitro depletion of marrow cultures of these cells increases hematopoiesis (212, 213, 217).

The progenitor cells of HIV-1–infected patients may have defective activity without being directly affected by productive infection by HIV-1 (40, 203). Protein products of HIV-1 can directly inhibit marrow progenitor cells, and this effect does not depend on the presence of active virus (41, 113, 218). The gp120 and gp160 envelope proteins of HIV-1 have been shown to cause a dose-dependent decrease in viable CD34+ cell counts by a process that stimulates apoptosis in these hematopoietic cells (42, 151, 210, 219). Preincubation of HIV-1 with neutralizing anti-gp120 antibody prevents the apoptosis that occurs in hematopoietic cells when envelope gp120 interacts with the low levels of CD4 antigen present on these cells (151, 203). Prevention of apoptosis does not occur if HIV-1 or recombinant gp120 treatment of hematopoietic cells is followed by the addition of the same gp120 antibody (203). This finding implicates the engagement of CD4 antigen present in low levels on progenitor cells as a trigger to programmed cell death in these cells, thus depleting the hematopoietic reserve (203, 211). Anti-CD4 and anti-gp120 antibodies also may induce apoptosis in hematopoietic cells (67, 76, 217, 220). The mechanism that permits anti-CD4 antibodies to do this may be by altering protein kinase C activity and intracellular calcium levels (162, 218).

Indirectly, gp120 can suppress hematopoiesis by inducing other cells to produce cytokines that inhibit hematopoiesis such as TNF-α (41, 42, 156, 212, 221). Protein products of the *Tat* and *Nef* genes suppress hematopoiesis either directly (40, 162) or indirectly by causing other marrow stromal cells to produce inhibitors of hematopoiesis such as TGF-β and TNF-α (41, 42, 212, 221, 222).

Other factors need to be recognized when one looks at studies that investigate the effects of HIV-1 on bone marrow progenitor cells. At least with respect to megakaryocytes, HIV-1 infection induces alterations in surface antigens that render them potential targets of antiplatelet and anti–HIV-1 antibodies (88, 92, 82). The presence of antiretroviral drugs may influence the results of experiments on the presence of HIV-1 in bone marrow progenitors (199, 223).

Taken all together, the data indicate that the effects of HIV-1 on the bone marrow progenitor cells are largely indirect, rather than a result of direct infection of these cells. The summation of these indirect effects on hematopoietic cells is a reduction in the potential of the progenitor cells to differentiate and proliferate (44, 206, 207).

Other Cytokines and Interleukins

INTERLEUKIN-1

IL-1 is one of the primary mediators of the acute-phase response (224). This cytokine is produced largely by cells of monocytic lineage (224–226), but it is also produced by dendritic cells, B and T lymphocytes, NK cells, fibroblasts, and vascular endothelial cells (1). IL-1 causes fever and anorexia and contributes to a catabolic state (225). With respect to hematopoiesis, it induces secretion of CSFs by accessory cells in the bone marrow, particularly G-CSF, M-CSF, and GM-CSF (124, 227), and also IL-6 (224, 227). In this way, it enhances hematopoiesis (124, 224). Prolonged secretion of IL-1, however, induces secretion of TNF-α and other inflammatory cytokines that suppress hematopoietic activity (215, 224, 227). In vivo and in vitro, levels of IL-1 tend to increase with progression of HIV-1 infection (154, 157, 216, 225, 228).

INTERLEUKIN-2

IL-2 is a primary growth factor for T cells (124, 125), and it secondarily stimulates proliferation and differentiation of B cells (147). IL-1 and TNF-α are the major stimuli for production of IL-2 by T cells, and these cytokines also increase IL-2 receptor numbers and binding capacity on the T-cell membrane (124, 125, 147).

IL-2 can indirectly decrease hematopoiesis by its ability to induce synthesis of IFN-γ by other cells (124). More important, production of IL-2 during the chronic inflammatory state of HIV infection augments replication of HIV-1 in infected cells (12, 115, 229, 230). In this way, production of this cytokine directly upregulates HIV-1 production, and it indirectly contributes to the suppression of hematopoiesis that is characteristic of advancing HIV-1 infection.

INTERLEUKIN-6

HIV infection is associated with increased production of IL-6 primarily by monocytes (154). This increase may occur as a result of the interaction of gp160 antigen with the CD4 receptors of these cells (101, 154, 231). IL-6 may also be produced by stimulated B cells, T cells, and fibroblasts (124, 125, 147, 185, 227). Circulating neutrophils and eosinophils as well as vascular endothelial cells have been shown to produce this cytokine in the presence of HIV-1 (231, 232). HIV-1 Tat protein has been shown to upregulate IL-6 expression directly and indirectly (222).

IL-6 can act in synergy with IL-3 to enhance hematopoiesis (83, 95, 124, 233–235). In this regard, the elevated levels of IL-6 that occur with advancing HIV-1 infection (216, 228) would be expected to upregulate hematopoiesis (101, 154). This cytokine, however, also induces hepatocytes to produce acute-phase proteins (101), primarily IL-1, and this directly and indirectly downregulates hematopoietic potential (85, 154, 185, 207, 236). Furthermore, IL-6 can upregulate HIV-1 production by infected cells (13, 115, 229, 236), and it may cause T-cell proliferation, thereby expanding the pool of HIV-infected cells (185).

INTERFERONS

The IFNs are a family of cytokines that are produced by leukocytes (IFN-α), fibroblasts (IFN-β), and cells of lymphocyte and monocytic lineage (IFN-γ) (27). The last may be produced by cytotoxic T lymphocytes on contact with target cells that present HIV antigens (27).

Serum IFN levels tend to increase with progression of HIV infection (195, 237, 238). IFNs in general, and INF-α in particular, inhibit marrow progenitor cells (238–240). This effect may be mediated by inducing secretion of other cytokines such as TNF-α and IL-1 from bone marrow monocytes and T cells (12, 13, 115, 215, 227, 241).

TUMOR NECROSIS FACTOR

TNF-α (cachectin) is produced by stimulated monocytes and macrophages (115, 125, 227), T lymphocytes (27), stimulated B cells (242), and vascular endothelial cells (226). Although it is not produced constitutively by HIV-infected cells, it can be produced in response to diverse stimuli concurrent with the HIV infection (225, 226, 243). The Tat protein of HIV-1 may activate TNF-α genes in vitro (157, 228). Cytotoxic T lymphocytes are capable of producing TNF-α on contact with target cells presenting HIV-1 antigens (27), and monocytes and macrophages are capable of producing TNF-α after contact with gp120 (25, 212). This production does not require the presence of live virus (212).

TNF-α levels are elevated in the sera of HIV-infected patients (212, 225, 228, 244), and they rise progressively with the disease. In vitro, TNF-α can maintain HIV expression in chronically infected cells (13, 115, 226, 245, 246). TNF-α is therefore important to the autocrine and paracrine regulation of HIV infection (169).

TNF-α can act as both a positive and a negative regulator of hematopoiesis (212, 226, 247). TNF-α has indirect suppressive effects on hematopoiesis by inducing the production of IL-1 by monocytes that, in turn, suppress hematopoiesis (124, 215). It can alter the production of growth factors by marrow stromal cells as well as modulate the expression of cell-surface receptors for growth factors on cells that are targets of HIV infection (124, 212, 224, 226, 247).

The concentration of TNF-α is important to the quantitative effect on hematopoiesis (247, 248): Low concentrations stimulate IL-3 and GM-CSF–induced colony formation, but high levels inhibit the actions of these growth factors (124, 215). TNF-α also has different effects on various hematopoietic cell lines: The same concentration of

TNF-α that stimulates growth of committed granulocyte and monocyte progenitor cells inhibits erythroid growth (248). TNF-α has at least two receptors, a 55-kd receptor and a 75-kd receptor, and these seem to use different signaling pathways and result in different effects on hematopoiesis. Although the inhibitory effects of TNF-α on progenitor cells involve p55 and p75, the p55 receptor alone mediates the stimulatory effects on progenitors (247, 248).

TRANSFORMING GROWTH FACTOR-β

TGF-β is a stimulatory agent for some cell lines, fibroblasts in particular, but it is a potent inhibitor of hematopoietic proliferation (42, 214, 249, 250). It has a reversible, suppressive effect on bone marrow progenitors (214). It acts on early cells in hematopoiesis in a multipotential and nonlineage-specific fashion (214). Its mechanism of action may be by downregulation of cell-surface C-kit expression and downmodulation of IL-1 receptors (249).

Levels of TGF-β increase progressively as infection with HIV-1 advances (251). The Tat protein of HIV-1 upregulates production of this cytokine in a direct and an indirect manner (222). Moreover, TGF-β is capable of inducing its own synthesis (251).

In addition to its effects on hematopoiesis, TGF-β is a potent endogenous immunosuppressive factor (251). It downregulates activity of B cells, T cells, monocytes, and macrophages (251). Its overall effect is to augment the immunosuppression and hematosuppression characteristic of HIV-1 infection (251–253). Moreover, TGF-β enhances HIV-1 expression in infected cells (254).

Hematopoietic Microenvironment

The bone marrow stroma consists of cellular and acellular components that provide a structural framework organizing hematopoiesis into a nonrandom distribution confined to the marrow cavities (255–257). Adhesion events among hematopoietic cells, the stromal cells, and the extracellular matrix are important to the regulation of hematopoiesis (258, 259). In addition to providing sites of attachment for hematopoietic cells, the marrow stromal cells produce growth factors and cytokines that regulate hematopoiesis (255, 257–260).

The cytokines released in response to infection with HIV-1, particularly IL-1 and TNF-α, alter the adhesion molecules on the marrow stromal cells (261). These alterations in the attachment events between marrow stromal cells and hematopoietic cells (47, 261) may result in suppression of hematopoiesis (259).

HIV-1 infection of accessory cells within the marrow adversely alters hematopoiesis (262, 263). Monocytes and lymphocytes within the bone marrow are important cellular components of the bone marrow stroma, and they regulate hematopoiesis by their capacity to produce growth factors locally, particularly GM-CSF and IL-3 (264). During the early phases of infection by HIV-1, lymphocytes and monocytes within the bone marrow may increase production of these growth factors; this may partially explain the bone marrow hypercellularity commonly seen during this stage of HIV infection (114, 264).

As the viral infection progresses, however, lymphocytes and monocytes within the marrow begin to produce increasing levels of IL-1 and IL-2 (14, 215, 227, 264) that not only decrease hematopoietic potential (47, 124, 215, 224, 227), but also upregulate HIV replication within these and other cells (115, 215, 226, 227). As noted earlier, these cells may also serve as a reservoir for HIV within the bone marrow (265, 266).

Nonhematopoietic cells within the bone marrow are also important to the structure and function of the bone marrow microenvironment. A major component of the stroma is the reticulum cell (fibroblast). This cell accounts for 60 to 70% of the volume of the marrow framework (189). The marrow reticulum cell is a target of HIV infection (18, 40, 107, 118, 213, 267, 268). When infected with HIV-1, these cells are less able to support hematopoiesis in vitro (265, 266, 268, 269) because of an impaired ability to secrete growth factors (270). Moreover, HIV-infected marrow stromal cells may also secrete factors that inhibit hematopoiesis (162, 200). Medications used to treat the HIV infection, such as zidovudine, have the potential to inhibit the growth and development of these stromal cells in addition to that of the hematopoietic cells themselves (223).

The endothelial cells that line the marrow sinusoids are also important to the structure of the bone marrow. These cells are essential to the homing of circulating hematopoietic cells, and, in addition, they regulate migration of marrow cells into the circulation. They also secrete growth factors. These cells are targets for HIV infection (231, 270). When infected by HIV-1, they undergo alterations in surface receptors, and their ability to secrete growth factors is hindered, thus adversely altering their ability to support hematopoiesis. In addition, these cells may serve as reservoirs of HIV-1 within the bone marrow (270).

COAGULATION ABNORMALITIES

Clotting disorders are not uncommon in HIV infection (271, 272). The most common of these disorders is the "lupus anticoagulant" (273). This is one of several antibodies to acidic phospholipids that can occur as a result of the abnormal immune responses characteristic of HIV infection. These antibodies are found in 20 to 66% of HIV-infected patients (274–278). Titers tend to increase during active opportunistic infections (69, 278).

The antiphospholipid antibodies include the lupus anticoagulant and nonspecific antibodies that may give positive results for the Venereal Disease Research Laboratory test and anticardiolipin antibody assays. These antibodies tend to cause abnormalities of in vitro tests of coagulation (50). Most commonly, one sees elevation of the activated partial thromboplastin time that does not correct with one-to-one mixing of normal and patient plasma. The prothrombin time may be prolonged to a mild degree in about 10% of patients who have antiphospholipid antibodies. Also abnormal are the dilute thromboplastin inhibition assay and the viper venom clotting time. Once thought to be clinically insignificant, the lupus anticoagulant in HIV-infected patients may be associated with major thromboembolic phenomena (273).

Thromboembolic events may also occur as a result of reduced levels of active protein S (272, 279, 280). This peptide is the cofactor for protein C, acting to localize active protein C to the phospholipid surface. Mean total and free protein S levels are statistically lower in HIV-infected patients with or without thromboses than in healthy male controls (272, 279, 280). The levels of free and total protein S do not correlate with CD4 counts, stage of HIV infection, p24 antigen levels, or use of antiretroviral medications (279). Protein S binds to C4b-binding protein, and increases in C4b-binding protein in the chronic inflammatory state encountered with HIV infection result in greater binding of protein S, so less is available to prevent aberrant thrombotic events (279). Another mechanism that may contribute to lower levels of active protein S in HIV-infected patients is the presence of antiprotein S antibodies in these patients. These antibodies bind protein C, thus decreasing the unbound and active forms of the protein (280).

Several of the opportunistic viral infections that result from the immunosuppression induced by HIV-1 may cause or contribute to the prothrombotic state characteristic of HIV infection. Quiescent endothelial cells have control mechanisms that restrict expression of procoagulant phospholipids to areas of vascular injury (281, 282). Cytomegalovirus and herpes simplex types 1 and 2 can convert vascular endothelial cells from a noncoagulative to a procoagulative phenotype (281, 282). The mechanism seems to be alteration in surface phospholipids to forms that are active in the coagulation system (281, 282).

Increases in levels of antigenic von Willebrand factor that correlate with CD4 lymphocyte counts and decreases in plasminogen activator inhibitor levels also occur in patients infected with HIV-1 (280) and may contribute toward a prothrombotic state. Other abnormalities in coagulation that may occur with HIV infection include isolated deficiencies in prothrombin levels (282), and abnormal platelet aggregation (281, 282). Acquired circulating anticoagulations with antifactor V activity also have been reported, as well as deficiencies in heparin cofactor II (278, 283). The hypoalbuminemia that occurs with advancing HIV infection may cause fibrin polymerization and fibrinolytic defects (271, 284).

References

1. Gallo RC. Human retroviruses: a decade of discovery and link with human disease. J Infect Dis 1991;164:235–243.
2. Hirsch MS, Kaplan JC. The biomedical impact of the AIDS epidemic. In: Broder S, Merigan TC, Bolognesi D, eds. Textbook of AIDS medicine. Baltimore: Williams & Wilkins, 1994:3–12.
3. Huff JR. HIV protease: a novel chemotherapeutic target for AIDS. J Med Chem 1991;34:2305–2314.
4. Kessler HA, Bick JA, Pottage JC Jr, et al. AIDS: part I. Dis Mon 1992;38:633–690.
5. Jeffries DJ. Targets for antiviral therapy of human immunodeficiency virus infection. J Infect 1989;1:5–13.
6. Edlin BR, Weinstein RA, Whaling SM, et al. Zidovudine–interferon-α combination therapy in patients with advanced human immunodeficiency virus type 1 infection: biphasic response of p24 antigen and quantitative polymerase chain reaction. J Infect Dis 1992;165: 793–798.
7. Capon DJ, Ward RHR. The CD4–gp120 interaction and AIDS pathogenesis. Annu Rev Immunol 1991;9:649–678.
8. Torbett BE, Healy PA, Shao LE, Mosier DE, Yu J. HIV-1 infection is latent in primary and transformed bone marrow stromal cells [abstract 1904]. Blood 1994;84:480a.
9. O'Brien WA. Viral determinants of cellular tropism. Pathobiology 1992;60:225–229.
10. Ball JK, Holmes EC, Whitwell H, et al. Genomic variation of human immunodeficiency virus type 1 (HIV-1): molecular analyses of HIV-1 in sequential blood samples and various organs obtained at autopsy. J Gen Virol 1994;75:67–79.
11. Levy JA. Infection by human immunodeficiency virus—CD4 is not enough. N Engl J Med 1996;335:1528–1530.
12. Greene WC. The molecular biology of human immunodeficiency virus type 1 infection. N Engl J Med 1991;321:308–317.
13. Merigan TC, Katzenstein DA. Relation of pathogenesis of human immunodeficiency virus infection to various strategies for its control. Rev Infect Dis 1991;13:292–302.
14. Gendelman HE, Baca LM, Turpin JA. Interactions between interferon and the human immunodeficiency virus. J Exp Pathol 1990;5:53–67.
15. Orenstein JM. Ultrastructural pathology of human immunodeficiency virus infection. Ultrastruct Pathol 1992;16:179–210.
16. Langner KD, Niedrig M, Fultz P, et al. Antiviral effects of different CD4-immunoglobulin constructs against HIV-1 and SIV: immunological characterization, pharmacokinetic data and in vivo experiments. Arch Virol 1993;130:157–170.
17. Oyaizu N, McCloskey TW, Coronesi M, et al. Accelerated apoptosis in peripheral blood mononuclear cells (PBMCs) from human immunodeficiency virus type-1 infected patients and in CD4 cross-linked PBMCs from normal individuals. Blood 1993;82:3392–3400.
18. Joling P, Bakker LJ, van Wichen DF, et al. Binding of HIV-1 to human follicular dendritic cells. Adv Exp Med Biol 1993;329:455–460.
19. Albert J, Wahlberg J, Lundeberg J, et al. Persistence of azidothymidine-resistant human immunodeficiency virus type 1 RNA genotypes in posttreatment sera. J Virol 1992;66:5627–5630.
20. Hersh EM, Brewton G, Abrams D, et al. Ditiocarb sodium (diethyldithiocarbamate) therapy in patients with symptomatic HIV infection and AIDS: a randomized, double-blind, placebo-controlled, multicenter study. JAMA 1991;265:1538–1544.
21. Merigan TC, Amato DA, Balsley J, et al. Placebo-controlled trial to evaluate zidovudine in treatment of human immunodeficiency virus infection in asymptomatic patients with hemophilia: NHF-ACTG 036 Study Group. Blood 1991;78:900–906.
22. Poli G, Pantaleo G, Fauci AS. Immunopathogenesis of human immunodeficiency virus infection. Clin Infect Dis 1993;17(Suppl 1): S224–S229.
23. Crowe SM, McGrath MS, Elbeik T, et al. Comparative assessment of antiretrovirals in human monocyte-macrophages and lymphoid cell lines acutely and chronically infected with the human immunodeficiency virus. J Med Virol 1989;29:176–180.
24. Chiodi F, Keys B, Albert J, et al. Human immunodeficiency virus type 1 is present in the cerebrospinal fluid of a majority of infected individuals. J Clin Microbiol 1992;30:1768–1771.
25. Rivas CI, Golde DW, Vera JC, et al. Involvement of the sphingomyeline pathway in autocrine tumor necrosis factor signaling for human immunodeficiency virus production in chronically infected HL-60 cells. Blood 1994;83:2191–2197.
26. Mitsuya H, Yarchoan R. Development of antiretroviral therapy for AIDS and related disorders. In: Broder S, Merigan TC, Bolognesi D, eds.Textbook of AIDS medicine. Baltimore: Williams & Wilkins, 1994:721–742.

27. Jassoy C, Harrer T, Rosenthal T, et al. Human immunodeficiency virus type 1-specific cytotoxic T lymphocytes release gamma interferon, tumor necrosis factor alpha (TNF-α), and TNF-β when they encounter their target antigens. J Virol 1993;67:2844–2852.
28. Kim SY, Byrn R, Groopman J, et al. Temporal aspects of DNA and RNA synthesis during human immunodeficiency virus infection: evidence for differential gene expression. J Virol 1989;63:3708–3713.
29. Wei X, Ghosh SK, Taylor ME, et al. Viral dynamics in human immunodeficiency virus type 1 infection. Nature 1995;373;117–122.
30. Perelson AS, Neumann AU, Markowitz M, et al. HIV-1 dynamics in vivo: virion clearance rate, infected cell life-span, and viral generation time. Science 1996;271:1582–1586.
31. Piatak M Jr, Saag MS, Yang LC, et al. High levels of HIV-1 in plasma during all stages of infection determined by competitive PCR. Science 1993;259:1749–1754.
32. Pantaleo G, Graziosi C, Demarest JF, et al. HIV infection is active and progressive in lymphoid tissue during the clinically latent stage of disease. Nature 1993;362:355–358.
33. Kalams SA, Walker BD. The cytotoxic T-lymphocyte response in HIV-1 infection. Clin Lab Med 1994;14;271–299.
34. Ho DD, Neumann AU, Perelson AS, et al. Rapid turnover of plasma virions and CD4 lymphocytes in HIV-1 infection. Nature 1995;373: 123–126.
35. McLean AR. The balance of power between HIV and the immune system. Trends Microbiol 1993;1:9–13.
36. Baltimore D. Lessons from people with nonprogressive HIV infection. N Engl J Med 1995;332;259–260.
37. Bates P. Chemokine receptors and HIV-1: an attractive pair? Cell 1996;86:1–3.
38. Cao Y, Qin L, Zhang L, et al. Virologic and immunologic characterization of long-term survivors of human immunodeficiency virus type-1 infection. N Engl J Med 1995;322:201–208.
39. Pantaleo G, Menzo S, Vaccarezza M, et al. Studies in subjects with long-term nonprogressive human immunodeficiency virus infection. N Engl J Med 1994;332:209–216.
40. Louache F, Henri A, Bettaieb A, et al. Role of human immunodeficiency virus replication in defective in vitro growth of hematopoietic progenitors. Blood 1992;80:2991–2999.
41. Re MC, Furlini G, Zauli G, et al. Human immunodeficiency virus type 1 (HIV-1) and human hematopoietic progenitor cells. Arch Virol 1994;137:1–23.
42. Zauli G, Davis BR, Re MC, et al. Tat protein stimulates production of transforming growth factor-beta 1 by marrow macrophages: a potential mechanism for human immunodeficiency virus-1–induced hematopoietic suppression. Blood 1992;80:3036–3043.
43. Mir N, Costello C, Luckitt J, et al. HIV-disease and bone marrow changes: a study of 60 cases. Eur J Haematol 1989;42:339–343.
44. Miles SA. Hematopoietic growth factors in HIV infection. Hematopoiet Ther Index Rev 1991;1:1–10.
45. Abrams DI, Kiprov DD, Goedert JJ, et al. Antibodies to human T-lymphotropic virus type III and development of the acquired immunodeficiency syndrome in homosexual men presenting with immune thrombocytopenia. Ann Intern Med 1986;104:47–50.
46. Zon LI, Arkin C, Groopman GE. Hematologic manifestations of the human immunodeficiency virus (HIV). Br J Haematol 1987;66: 251–256.
47. Ganser A. Abnormalities of hematopoiesis in the acquired immunodeficiency syndrome. Blut 1988;56:49–53.
48. Jacobson MA, Peiperl L, Volberding PA, et al. Red cell transfusion therapy for anemia in patients with AIDS and ARC. Transfusion 1990;30:133–137.
49. Spivak JL, Barnes DC, Fuchs E, et al. Serum immunoreactive erythropoietin in HIV infected patients. JAMA 1989;261:3104–3107.
50. Aboulafia DM, Mitsuyasu RT. Hematologic abnormalities in AIDS. Hematol Oncol Clin North Am 1991;5:195–214.
51. Richman DD, Fischl MA, Grieco MH, et al. The toxicity of azidothymidine (AZT) in the treatment of patients with AIDS and AIDS-related complex. N Engl J Med 1987;317:192–197.
52. Castella A, Croxson TS, Mildvan D, et al. The bone marrow in AIDS: a histologic, hematologic and microbiologic study. Am J Clin Pathol 1985;84:425–432.
53. Zon LI, Groopman JE. Hematologic manifestations of the human immune deficiency virus (HIV). Semin Hematol 1988;25:208–218.
54. Gupta S, Inman A, Licorish K. Serum ferritin in acquired immune deficiency syndrome. J Clin Lab Immunol 1986;20:11.
55. Scadden DT, Zon LI, Groopman JE. Pathophysiology and management of HIV-associated hematologic disorders. Blood 1989;74: 1455–1463.
56. Harriman GR, Smith PD, Horne MK, et al. Vitamin B_{12} malabsorption in patients with acquired immunodeficiency syndrome. Arch Intern Med 1989;149:2039–2041.
57. Weinberg JB, Sauls DL, Misukonis MA, et al. Inhibition of productive human immunodeficiency virus-1 infection by cobalamins. Blood 1995;86:1281–1287.
58. Remacha AF, Riera A, Cadafalch J, et al. Vitamin B_{12} abnormalities in HIV-infected patients. Eur J Haematol 1991;47:60–64.
59. Baum MK, Mantero-Atienza E, Shor-Posner, et al. Association of vitamin B_6 status with parameters of immune function in early HIV-1 infection. J Acquir Immune Defic Syndr 1991;4:1122–1132.
60. Falguera M, Perez-Mur J, Puig T, et al. Study of the role of vitamin B_{12} and folinic acid supplementation in preventing hematologic toxicity of zidovudine. Eur J Haematol 1995;55:97–102.
61. Sumner AE, Chin MM, Abrahm JL, et al. Elevated methylmalonic acid and total homocysteine levels show high prevalence of vitamin B_{12} deficiency after gastric surgery. Ann Intern Med 1996;124:469–476.
62. Treacy M, Lai L, Costello C. Peripheral blood and bone marrow abnormalities in patients with human immunodeficiency virus related disease. Br J Haematol 1987;65:289–294.
63. Miles SA, Mitsuyasu RT, Moreno J, et al. Combined therapy with recombinant granulocyte colony-stimulating factor and erythropoietin decreases hematologic oxicity from zidovudine. Blood 1991;77: 2109–2117.
64. Groopman JE, Mitsuyasu RT, DeLeo JM, et al. Effect of recombinant human granulocyte-macrophage colony-stimulating factor on myelopoiesis in the acquired immunodeficiency syndrome. N Engl J Med 1987;317:593–598.
65. Davey RT Jr, Davey VJ, Metcalf JA, et al. A phase I/II trial of zidovudine, interferon-alpha, and granulocyte-macrophage colony-stimulating factor in the treatment of human immunodeficiency virus type I infection. J Infect Dis 1991;164:43–52.
66. Murphy MF, Metcalfe P, Waters AH, et al. Incidence and mechanism of neutropenia and thrombocytopenia in patients with human immunodeficiency virus infection. Br J Haematol 1987;66:337–340.
67. Stricker RB. Hemostatic abnormalities in HIV disease. Hematol Oncol Clin North Am 1991;5:249–265.
68. Marroni M, Gresele P, Vezza R, et al. Thrombocytopenia in HIV infected patients: prevalence and clinical spectrum. Recenti Prog Med 1995;86:103–106.
69. Zauli G, Catani L, Gibellini D, et al. Impaired survival of bone marrow GPIIb/IIIa+ megakaryocytic cells as an additional pathogenetic mechanism of HIV-1-related thrombocytopenia. Br J Haematol 1996;92:711–717.
70. Perkocha LA, Rodgers GM. Hematologic aspects of human immunodeficiency virus infection: laboratory and clinical considerations. Am J Hematol 1988;29:94–105.
71. Sloand EM, Klein HG, Banks SM. Epidemiology of thrombocytopenia in HIV infection. Eur J Haematol 1992;48:168–172.
72. Holzman RS, Walsh CM, Karpatkin S. Risk for the acquired immunodeficiency syndrome among thrombocytopenic and nonthrombocytopenic homosexual men seropositive for the human immunodeficiency virus. Ann Intern Med 1987;106:383–386.
73. Galli M, Musicco M, Gervasoni C, et al. No evidence of a higher risk of progression to AIDS in patients with HIV-1–related severe thrombocytopenia. J Acquir Immune Defic Syndr Hum Retrovirol 1996;2: 268–275.

74. Sullivan PS, McDonald TP. Evaluation of murine leukemia virus infection as a model for thrombocytopenia of HIV/AIDS: mechanism of thrombocytopenia and modulation of thrombocytopenia by thrombopoietin. AIDS Res Hum Retroviruses 1995;11:837–842.
75. Najean Y, Rain JD. The mechanisms of thrombocytopenia in patients with human immunodeficiency virus infection. J Lab Clin Med 1994;123:415–420.
76. Louache F, Bettaieb A, Henri A, et al. Infection of megakaryocytes by human immunodeficiency virus in seropositive patients with immune thrombocytopenic purpura. Blood 1991;78:1697–1705.
77. Bettaieb A, Fromont P, Louache F, et al. Presence of cross-reactive antibody between human immunodeficiency virus (HIV) and platelet glycoproteins in HIV-related immune thrombocytopenic purpura. Blood 1992;80:162–169.
78. Durand JM, Lefevre P, Hovette P, et al. Dapsone for thrombocytopenic purpura related to human immunodeficiency virus infection. Am J Med 1991;90:675–677.
79. Dominguez A, Gamallo G, Garcia R, et al. Pathophysiology of HIV related thrombocytopenia: an analysis of 41 patients. J Clin Pathol 1994;47:999–1003.
80. Dominguez CA, Vazquez Rodriguez JJ. Thrombocytopenia associated with HIV infection. Med Clin (Barc) 1992;98:671–675.
81. Stanworth DR, Solder B, Lewin IV, et al. Related epitopes in HIV viral coat protein and human IgG. Lancet 1989;1:1158–1159.
82. Gonzalez-Conejero R, Rivera J, Rosillo MC, et al. Association of autoantibodies against platelet lycoproteins Ib/IX and IIb/IIIa, and platelet-reactive anti-HIV antibodies in thrombocytopenic narcotic addicts. Br J Haematol 1996;93:464–471.
83. Bender BS, Quinn TC, Spivak JL. Homosexual men with thrombocytopenia have impaired reticuloendothelial system Fc receptor specific clearance. Blood 1987;70:392–395.
84. Karpatkin S. Immunologic thrombocytopenic purpura in HIV-seropositive homosexuals, narcotic addicts and hemophiliacs. Semin Hematol 1988;25:219–229.
85. Baldwin GC, Fleischmann J, Chung Y, et al. Human immunodeficiency virus causes mononuclear phagocyte dysfunction. Proc Natl Acad Sci U S A 1990;87:3933–3937.
86. Leaf AN, Laubenstein LH, Raphael B, et al Thrombotic thromocytopenic purpura asociated with human immunodeficiency virus type 1 (HIV-1) infection. Ann Intern Med 1988;109:194–197.
87. Thompson CE, Damon LE, Ries CA, et al. Thrombotic microangiopathies in the 1980s: clinical features, response to treatment, and the impact of the human immunodeficiency virus epidemic. Blood 1992;80:1890–1895.
88. Zauli G, Re MC, Gugliotta L, et al. Lack of compensatory megakaryocytopoiesis in HIV-1-seropositive thrombocytopenic individuals compared with immune thrombocytopenic purpura patients. AIDS 1991;5:1345–1350.
89. Berstein L, Cappacino A, Cappacino H. Platelet function and bound antibodies in AIDS-ARC patients with thrombocytopenia [abstract]. Blood 1987;70:118a.
90. Davis BR, Zauli G. Effect of human immunodeficiency virus infection on haematopoiesis. Baillieres Clin Haematol 1995;8:113–130.
91. Zucker-Franklin D, Sermetis S, Zeng ZY. Internalization of human immunodeficiency virus type 1 by megakaryocytes and platelets. Blood 1990;77:481–485.
92. Ballem PJ, Belzberg A, Devine DV, et al. Kinetic studies of the mechanisms of thrombocytopenia in patients with human immunodeficiency virus infection. N Engl J Med 1992;327:1779–1784.
93. Walsh C, Kriegel R, Lennette E, et al. Thrombocytopenia in homosexual patients. Ann Intern Med 1985;103:542–545.
94. Takatsuki F, Okano A, Suzuki C, et al. Interleukin-6 perfusion stimulates reconstitution of the immune and hematopoietic systems after 5-fluorouracil treatment. Cancer Res 1990;50:2885–2890.
95. Hill RJ, Warren MK, Levin J. Stimulation of thrombopoiesis in mice by human recombinant interleukin-6. J Clin Invest 1990;85:1242–1247.
96. Luikart S, MacDonald M, Herzan D. Ability of twice daily granulocyte-macrophage colony-stimulating factor (GM-CSF) to support dose escalation of etoposide (VP-l6) and carboplatin (CBDCA) in extensive small cell lung cancer (SCLC) [abstract]. Proc Am Soc Clin Oncol 1991;10:825a.
97. Cazzola M, Ponchio L, Beguin Y, et al. Subcutaneous erythropoietin for treatment of refractory anemia in hematologic disorders: results of a phase I/II clinical trial. Blood 1991;79:29–37.
98. Ahn YS. Efficacy of danazol in hematologic disorders. Acta Haematol 1990;84:122–123.
99. Dhawan S, Weeks BS, Abbasi F, et al. Increased expression of alpha 4 beta 1 and alpha 5 beta 1 integrins on HTLV-1–infected lymphocytes. Virology 1993;197:778–781.
100. Marroni M, Gresele P, Landonio G, et al. Interferon-alpha is effective in the treatment of HIV-1–related, severe, zidovudine-resistant thrombocytopenia: a prospective, placebo-controlled, double-blind trial. Ann Intern Med 1994;121:423–429.
101. Beard J, Savidge GF. High-dose intravenous immunoglobulin and splenectomy for the treatment of HIV-related immune thrombocytopenia in patients with severe haemophilia. Br J Haematol 1988;68:303–306.
102. Zauli G, Re MC, Gugliotta L, et al. The elevation of circulating platelets after IFN-alpha therapy in HIV-1 seropositive thrombocytopenic patients correlates with increased plasma levels of IL-6. Microbiologica 1993;16:27–34.
103. Pollak AN, Jaminis J, Green D. Successful intravenous immune globulin therapy for human immunodeficiency virus–associated thrombocytopenia. Arch Intern Med 1988;148:695–697.
104. Oskenhendler E, Bierling P, Brossard Y, et al. Anti-Rh immunoglobulin therapy for human immunodeficiency virus–related immune thrombocytopenia. Blood 1989;71:1499–1502.
105. Biniek R, Malessa R, Brochmeyer NH, et al. Anti-Rh(D) immunoglobulin for AIDS-related thrombocytopenia. Lancet 1986;2:627–631.
106. Than S, Oyaizu N, Pahwa RN, et al. Effect of human immunodeficiency virus type-1 envelope glycoprotein gp120 on cytokine production from cord-blood T cells. Blood 1994;84:184–188.
107. Louache F, Canque B, Marandin A, et al. HIV-1 infection of human bone marrow stromal cells and hematopoiesis [abstract 1921]. Blood 1994;84:484a.
108. Transfusion Safety Study Group. Splenectomy and HIV-1 progression. [abstract 1922]. Blood 1994;84:484a.
109. Zambello R, Trentin L, Agostini C, et al. Persistent polyclonal lymphocytosis in human immunodeficiency virus-1-infected patients. Blood 81:1993:3015–3021.
110. Calverley DC, Jones GW, Kelton JG. Splenic radiation for corticosteroid-resistant immune thrombocytopenia. Ann Intern Med 1992;116:977–981.
111. Gold E, Chadha M, Culliney B, et al. Failure of splenic irradiation to treat HIV-associated immune thrombocytopenia [abstract 2787]. Blood 1994;84:204.
112. Calenda V, Chermann JC. The effects of HIV on hematopoiesis. Eur J Haematol 1992;48:181–186.
113. Schwartz GN, Kessler SW, Szabo JM, et al. Negative regulators may mediate some of the inhibitory effects of HIV-1 infected stromal cell layers on erythropoiesis and myelopoiesis in human bone marrow long term cultures. J Leukoc Biol 1995;57:948–955.
114. Sugiura K, Oyaizu N, Pahwa R, et al. Effect of human immunodeficiency virus-1 envelope glycoprotein on in vitro hematopoiesis of umbilical cord blood. Blood 1992;80:1463–1469.
115. Rosenberg ZF, Fauci AS. Immunopathogenic mechanisms of HIV infection: cytokine induction of HIV expression. Immunol Today 1990;11:176–180.
116. Perkocha LA, Rodgers GM. Hematologic aspects of human immunodeficiency virus infection. Am J Hematol 1988;29:94–105.
117. Goasguen JE, Bennett JM. Classification and morphologic features of myelodysplastic syndromes. Semin Oncol 1992;19:4–13.

118. Stutte HJ, Muller H, Falk S, et al. Pathophysiological mechanisms of HIV-induced defects in haematopoiesis: pathology of the bone marrow. Res Virol 1990;141:195–200.
119. Karcher DS, Frost AR. The bone marrow in human immunodeficiency virus (HIV)-related disease: morphology and clinical correlation. Am J Clin Pathol 1991;95:63–71.
120. Zarabi CM, Thomas R, Adesokan A. Diagnosis of systemic histoplasmosis in patients with AIDS. South Med J 1992;85:1171–1175.
121. Candido A, Rossi P, Menichella G, et al. Indicative morphological myelodysplastic alterations of bone marrow in overt AIDS. Haematologica 1990;75:327–333.
122. Abrams DI, Chinn EK, Lewis BJ, et al. Hematologic manifestations in homosexual men with Kaposi's sarcoma. Am J Clin Pathol 1984;81:13–18.
123. Lieschke GJ, Burgess AW. Granulocyte colony-stimulating factor and granulocyte-macrophage colony-stimulating factor (first of two parts). N Engl J Med 1992;327:28–35.
124. Brach MA, Herrmann F. Hematopoietic growth factors: interactions and regulation of production. Acta Haematol 1991;86:128–137.
125. Sieff CA. Biological and clinical aspects of the hematopoietic growth factors. Annu Rev Med 1990;41:483–496.
126. Zauli G, Davis BR. Role of HIV infection in the hematologic manifestations of HIV seropositive subjects. Criti Rev Oncol Hematol 1993;15:271–283.
127. Levine AM. Acquired immunodeficiency–related lymphoma. Blood 1992;80:8–20.
128. Pluda JM, Mitsuya H, Yarchoan R. Hematologic effects of AIDS therapies. Hematol Oncol Clin North Am 1991;5:229–248.
129. Bhalla K, Birkhofer M, Li GR, et al. 2′-Deoxycytidine protects normal human bone marrow progenitor cells in vitro against the cytotoxicity of 3′-azido-3′-deoxythymidine with preservation of antiretroviral activity. Blood 1989;74:1923–1928.
130. Poropatich CO, Labriola AM, Tuazon CU. Acid-fast smear and culture of respiratory secretions, bone marrow and stools as predictors of disseminated mycobacterium avium complex infection. J Clin Microbiol 1987;25:929.
131. Neubauer MA, Bodensteiner DC. Disseminated histoplasmosis in patients with AIDS. South Med J 1992;85:1166–1170.
132. Cohen RJ, Samoszuk MK, Busch D, et al. Occult infections with *M. intracellulare* in bone marrow biopsy specimens from patients with AIDS. N Engl J Med 1983;308:1475–1476.
133. Solis OC, Belmonte AH, Ramaswamy G. Pseudo-Gaucher cells in *Mycobacterium avium-intracellulare* infection in the acquired immune deficiency syndrome (AIDS). Am J Clin Pathol 1986;85:233–235.
134. Zeldis JB, Farraye FA, Steinberg HN. In vitro hepatitis B virus suppression of erythropoiesis is dependent on the multiplicity of infection and is reversible with anti-HBs antibodies. Hepatology 1988;8:755–759.
135. Zeldis JB, Boender PJ, Hellings JA, et al. Inhibition of human hemopoiesis by non-A, non-B hepatitis virus. J Med Virol 1989;27:34–38.
136. Maciejewski JP, Bruening EE, Donahue RE, et al. Infection of hematopoietic progenitor cells by human cytomegalovirus. Blood 1992;80:170–178.
137. Lazzarotto T, Furlini G, Re MC, et al. Human cytomegalovirus replication correlates with differentiation in a hematopoietic progenitor cell line and can be modulated by HIV-1. Arch Virol 1994;135:13–28.
138. Movassagh M, Gozlan J, Senechal B, et al. Direct infection of CD34+ progenitor cells by human cytomegalovirus: evidence of inhibition of hematopoiesis and viral replication. Blood 1996;88:1277–1283.
139. Almeida GD, Porada CD, St. Jeor S, et al. Human cytomegalovirus alters interleukin-6 production by endothelial cells. Blood 1994;83:370–376.
140. Frickhofen N, Abkowitz JL, Safford M, et al. Persistent B19 parvovirus infection in patients infected with human immunodeficiency virus type 1 (HIV-1): a treatable cause of anemia in AIDS. Ann Intern Med 1990;113:926–933.
141. Pont J, Puchhammer-Stockl E, et al. Recurrent granulocytic aplasia as clinical presentation of a persistent parvovirus B 19 infection. Br J Haematol 1992;80:160–165.
142. Baurmann H, Schwarz TF, Oertel J, et al. Acute parvovirus B19 infection mimicking myelodysplastic syndrome of the bone marrow. Ann Hematol 1992;64:43–45.
143. Gyllensten K, Sonnerborg A, Jorup-Ronstrom C, et al. Parvovirus B19 infection in HIV-1 infected patients with anemia. Infection 1994;22:356–358.
144. Flamand L, Gosselin J, Stefanescu I, et al. Immunosuppressive effect of human herpesvirus 6 on T-cell functions: suppression of interleukin-2 synthesis and proliferation. Blood 1995;85:1263–1271.
145. Carrigan DR, Knox KK. Human herpesvirus 6 (HHV-6) isolated from bone marrow: HHV-6 bone marrow suppression in bone marrow transplant patients. Blood 1994;84:3307–3310.
146. Hermans P. Clinical use of haematological growth factors in patients with human immunodeficiency virus (HIV-1) infection. Biomed Pharmacother 1994;48:69–72.
147. Ohmann AB, Babink LA, Harland R. Cytokine synergy with viral cytopathic effects and bacterial products during the pathogenesis of respiratory tract infections. Clin Immunol Immunopathol 1991;60:153–170.
148. Gabrilove J. The development of granulocyte colony-stimulating factor in its various clinical applications. Blood 1992;80:1382–1385.
149. Williams GT, Smith CA, Spooncer E, et al. Haemopoietic colony-stimulating factors promote cell survival by suppressing apoptosis. Nature 1990;343:76–79.
150. Yu H, Bauer B, Lipke GK, et al. Apoptosis and hematopoiesis in murine fetal liver. Blood 1993;81:373–384.
151. Zauli G, Vitale M, Re MC, et al. In vitro exposure to human immunodeficiency virus type 1 induces apoptotic cell death of the factor-dependent TF-1 hematopoietic cell line. Blood 1994;83:167–175.
152. Re MC, Zauli G, Furlini G, et al. GM-CSF production by CD4+ T-lymphocytes is selectively impaired during the course of HIV-1 infection: a possible indication of a preferential lesion of a specific subset of peripheral blood CD4+ T-lymphocytes. Microbiologica 1992;15:265–270.
153. Canque B, Marandin A, Rosenzwajg M, et al. Susceptibility of human bone marrow stromal cells to human immunodeficiency virus (HIV). Virology 1995;208:779–783.
154. Esser R, Glienke W, von Briesen H, et al. Differential regulation of proinflammatory and hematopoietic cytokines in human macrophages after infection with human immunodeficiency virus. Blood 1996;88:3474–3481.
155. Faquin WC, Schneider TJ, Goldberg MA. Effect of inflammatory cytokines on hypoxia-induced erythropoietin production. Blood 1992;79:1987–1994.
156. Dinarello CA. Biologic basis for interleukin-1 in disease. Blood 1996;87:2095–2147.
157. Buonaguro L, Barillari G, Chang HK, et al. Effects of the human immunodeficiency virus type 1 Tat protein on the expression of inflammatory cytokines. J Virol 1992;66:7159–7167.
158. Schooley JC, Kullgren B, Allison AC. Inhibition by interleukin-1 of the action of erythropoietin on erythroid precursors and its possible role in the pathogenesis of hypoplastic anaemias. Br J Haemotol 1987;67:11–17.
159. Clibon U, Bonewald L, Caro J, et al. Erythropoietin fails to reverse the anemia in mice continuously exposed to tumor necrosis factor-alpha in vivo. Exp Hematol 1990;18:438–444.
160. Bagnara GP, Zauli G, Giovannini M, et al. Early loss of circulating hematopoietic progenitors in human immunodeficiency virus I infected cells. Exp Hematol 1990;18:426–430.

161. Hooper WC. The role of transforming growth factor-beta in hematopoiesis: a review. Leukemia 1991;15:177–187.
162. Chelucci C, Hassan HJ, Locardi C, et al. In vitro human immunodeficiency virus-1 infection of purified hematopoietic progenitors in single-cell culture. Blood 1995;85:1181–1187.
163. Mann DA, Frankel AD. Endocytosis and targeting of exogenous HIV-1 Tat protein. EMBO J 1991;10:1733.
164. Rautonen N, Rautonen J, Martin NL, et al. HIV-1 Tat induces cytokine synthesis by uninfected mononuclear cells. AIDS 1994;8:1504–1508.
165. Chirmule N, Oyaizu N, Saxinger C, et al. Nef protein of HIV-1 has B-cell stimulatory activity. AIDS 1994;8:733–740.
166. Lieschke GJ, Burgess AW. Granulocyte colony-stimulating factor and granulocyte-macrophage colony-stimulating factor (second of two parts). N Engl J Med 1991;327:99–106.
167. Lord BI, Molineux G, Pojda Z, et al. Myeloid cell kinetics in mice treated with recombinant interleukin-3, granulocyte colony-stimulating factor (CSF), or granulocyte-macrophage CSF in vivo. Blood 1991;77:2154–2159.
168. Lindemann A, Herrmann F, Oster W, et al. Hematologic effects of recombinant human granulocyte colony-stimulating factor in patients with malignancy. Blood 1989;74:2644–2651.
169. Lord BI, Gurney H, Chang J, et al. Haemopoietic cell kinetics in humans treated with rGM-CSF. Int J Cancer 1992;50:26–31.
170. Pluda JM, Yarchoan R, Smith PD, et al. Subcutaneous recombinant granulocyte-macrophage colony-stimulating factor used as a single agent and in an alternating regimen with azidothymidine in leukopenic patients with severe human immunodeficiency virus infection. Blood 1990;76:463–472.
171. Perno CF, Yarchoan R, Cooney DA, et al. Replication of human immunodeficiency virus in monocytes. J Exp Med 1989;169:933–951.
172. Perno CF, Cooney DA, Gao W-Y, et al. Effects of bone marrow stimulatory cytokines on human immunodeficiency virus replication and the antiviral activity of dideoxynucleosides in cultures of monocyte/macrophages. Blood 1992;80:995–1003.
173. Hammer SM, Gillis JM, Pinkston P, et al. Effect of zidovudine and granulocyte-macrophage colony-stimulating factor on human immunodeficiency virus replication in alveolar macrophages. Blood 1990;75:1215–1219.
174. Baldwin GC, Gasson JC, Quan SG, et al. Granulocyte-macrophage colony-stimulating factor enhances neutrophil function in acquired immunodeficiency syndrome patients. Proc Natl Acad Sci U S A 1988;85:2763–2766.
175. Schuitemaker H, Kootstra NA, van Oers MHJ, et al. Induction of monocyte proliferation and HIV expression by IL-3 does not interfere with anti-viral activity of zidovudine. Blood 1990;76:1490–1493.
176. Fischl M, Galpin JE, Levine JD, et al. Recombinant human erythropoietin for patients with AIDS treated with zidovudine. N Engl J Med 1990;322:1488–1493.
177. Erslev A. Erythropoietin. N Engl J Med 1991;324:1339–1344.
178. Means RT Jr, Krantz SB. Inhibition of human erythroid colony-forming units by gamma interferon can be corrected by recombinant human erythropoietin. Blood 1991;78:2564–2567.
179. Lyman SD, Williams DE. Biological activities and potential therapeutic uses of Steel factor: a new growth factor active on multiple hematopoietic lineages. Am J Pediatr Hematol Oncol 1991;14:1–7.
180. Miles SA, Golde DW, Mitsuyasu RT. The use of hematopoietic hormones in HIV infection and AIDS-related malignancies. Hematol Oncol Clin North Am 1991;5:267–280.
181. Blachman MA, Bardosy L, Carmen R, et al. Allogeneic blood transfusion-induced enhancement of tumor growth: two animal models showing amelioration by leukodepletion and passive transfer using spleen cells. Blood 1993;81:1880–1882.
182. Brunson ME, Alexander JW. Mechanisms of transfusions-induced immunosuppression. Transfusion 1990;30:651–654.
183. Blumberg N, Heal MJ. Transfusion and recipient immune function. Arch Pathol Lab Med 1989;113:246–253.
184. McNeice IK, Langley KE, Zsebo KM. Recombinant human stem cell factor synergises with GM-CSF, G-CSF, IL-3 and Epo to stimulate human progenitor cells of the myeloid and erythroid lineages. Exp Hematol 1991;19:226–231.
185. Birx DL, Redfield RR, Tencer K, et al. Induction of interleukin-6 during human immunodeficiency virus infection. Blood 1990;76:2303–2310.
186. Manegold C, Jablonowski H, Armbrecht C, et al. Serum levels of stem cell factor are increased in asymptomatic human immunodeficiency virus-infected patients and are associated with prolonged survival. Blood 1995;86:243–249.
187. Miles SA, Lee K, Hutlin L, et al. Potential use of human stem cell factor as adjunctive therapy for human immunodeficiency virus-related cytopenias. Blood 1991;78:3200–3208.
188. Guba SC, Stella G, Turka LA, et al. Regulation of interleukin 3 gene induction in normal human T cells. J Clin Invest 1989;84:1701–1706.
189. Bruno E, Miller ME, Hoffman R. Interacting cytokines regulate in vitro human megakaryocytopoiesis. Blood 1989;73:671–677.
190. Biddell RA, Bruno E, Cooper RJ, et al. Effect of c-kit ligand on in vitro human megakaryocytopoiesis. Blood 1991;78:2854–2859.
191. Briddell RA, Hoffman R. Cytokine regulation of the human burst-forming unit-megakaryocyte. Blood 1990;76:516–522.
192. Scadden DT, Levine JD, Bresnahan J, et al. In vivo effects of interleukin 3 in HIV type 1-infected patients with cytopenia. AIDS Res Hum Retroviruses 1995;11:731–740.
193. Koyanagi Y, O'Brien WA, Zhao JQ, et al. Cytokines alter production of HIV-1 from primary mononuclear phagocytes. Science 1988;241:1673–1675.
194. Fischl M, Galpin JE, Levine JD, et al. Human recombinant erythropoietin therapy for AIDS patients treated with AZT: a double-blind, placebo-controlled clinical study. N Engl J Med 1990;322:1488.
195. Kornbluth RS, Oh PS, Munis JR, et al. The role of interferons in the control of HIV replication in macrophages. Clin Immunol Pathol 1990;54:200–219.
196. Neal TF, Holland HK, Baum CM, et al. CD34+ progenitor cells from asymptomatic patients are not a major reservoir for human immunodeficiency virus-1. Blood 1995;86:1749–1756.
197. Cen D, Zauli G, Szarnicki R, et al. Effect of different human immunodeficiency virus type-1 (HIV-1) isolates on long-term bone marrow haemopoiesis. Br J Haematol 1993;85:596–602.
198. Louache F, Debili N, Marandin A, et al. Expression of CD4 by human hematopoietic precursors. Blood 1994;84:3344–3355.
199. Molina JM, Scadden DT, Sakaguchi M, et al. Lack of evidence for infection of or effect on growth of hematopoietic progenitor cells after in vivo or in vitro exposure to human immunodeficiency virus. Blood 1990;76:2476–2482.
200. Neal TF, Holland HK, Baum CM, et al. CD34+ progenitor cells from asymptomatic patients are not a major reservoir for human immunodeficiency virus-1. Blood 1995;86:1749–1756.
201. Zauli G, Re MC, Giovannini M, et al. Effect of human immunodeficiency virus type 1 on CD4+ cells. Ann N Y Acad Sci 1991;628:273–278.
202. Brizzi MF, Porcu P, Porteri A, et al. Haematologic abnormalities in the acquired immunodeficiency syndrome. Haematologica 1990;75:454–463.
203. Re MC, Qauli G, Gibellini D, et al. Uninfected haematopoietic progenitor (CD34+) cells purified from the bone marrow of AIDS patients are committed to apoptotic cell death in culture. AIDS 1993;7:1049–1055.
204. Marandin A, Canque B, Coulombel L, et al. In vitro infection of bone marrow-adherent cells by human immunodeficiency virus type 1 (HIV-1) does not alter their ability to support hematopoiesis. Virology 1995;213:245–248.
205. Re MC, Zauli G, Furlini G, et al. The impaired number of circulating granulocyte/macrophage progenitors (CFU-GM) in human immunodeficiency virus-type 1 infected subjects correlates with an active HIV-1 replication. Arch Virol 1993;129:53–64.

206. Steinberg HN, Crumpacker CS, Chatis PA. In vitro suppression of normal human bone marrow progenitor cells by human immunodeficiency virus. J Virol 1991;65:1765–1769.
207. Folks TM, Kessler SW, Orenstein JM, et al. Infection and replication of HIV-l in purified progenitor cells of normal human bone marrow. Science 1988;242:919–922.
208. Zucker-Franklin D, Cao Y. Megakaryocytes of human immunodeficiency virus-infected individuals express viral RNA. Proc Natl Acad Sci U S A 1989;86:5595–5599.
209. Kouri YH, Borkowsky W, Nardi M, et al. Human megakaryocytes have a CD4 molecule capable of binding human immunodeficiency virus-1. Blood 1993:81:2664–2670.
210. Arock M, Dedenon A, Le Goff L, et al. Specific ligation of the HIV-1 viral envelope protein gp120 on human CD34+ bone marrow-derived progenitors. Cell Mol Biol 1994;40:319–323.
211. Louache F, Debili N, Marandin A, et al. Expression of CD4 by human hematopoietic progenitors. Blood 1994;84:3344–3355.
212. Maciejewski JP, Weichold FF, Young NS. HIV-1 suppression of hematopoiesis in vitro mediated by envelope glycoprotein and TNF-alpha. J Immunol 1994;153:4303–4310.
213. Watanabe J, Ringler DJ, Nakamura M, et al. Simian immunodeficiency virus inhibits bone marrow hematopoietic progenitor cell growth. J Virol 1990;64:656–663.
214. Axelrod AA. Some hematopoietic negative regulators. Exp Hematol 1990;18:143–150.
215. Merrill JE, Koyanagi Y, Chen IS. Interleukin-l and tumor necrosis factor alpha can be induced from mononuclear phagocytes by human immunodeficiency virus type l binding to the CD4 receptor. J Virol 1989;63:4404–4408.
216. Berman MA, Zaldivar F Jr, Imfeld KL, et al. HIV-1 infection of macrophages promotes long-term survival and sustained release of interleukins 1 alpha and 6. AIDS Res Hum Retroviruses 1994;10:529–539.
217. Donahue RE, Johnson MM, Zon LI, et al. Suppression of in vitro haematopoiesis following human immunodeficiency virus infection. Nature 1987;326:200–203.
218. Gibellini D, Zauli G, Re MC, et al. CD4 engagement by HIV-1 in TF-1 hematopoietic progenitor cells increases protein kinase C activity and reduces intracellular Ca2+ levels. Microbiologica 1994;17:85–92.
219. Zauli G, Re MC, Furlini G, et al. Human immunodeficiency virus type 1 envelope glycoprotein gp120-mediated killing of human haematopoietic progenitors (CD34+ cells). J Gen Virol 1992;73:417–421.
220. Donahue RE, Johnson MM, Zon LI, et al. Suppression of in vitro haematopoiesis following human immunodeficiency virus infection. Nature 1987;326:200–207.
221. Angel JB, Saget BM, Wang MZ, et al. Interleukin-10 enhances human immunodeficiency virus type 1 expression in a chronically infected promonocytic cell line (U1) by a tumor necrosis factor alpha-independent mechanism. J Interferon Cytokine Res 1995;15:575–584.
222. Gibellini D, Zauli G, Re MC, et al. Recombinant human immunodeficiency virus type-1 (HIV-1) Tat protein sequentially up-regulates IL-6 and TGF-beta 1 mRNA expression and protein synthesis in peripheral blood monocytes. Br J Haematol 1994;88:26,126–26,127.
223. Abraham NG, Chertkov JL, Staudinger R, et al. Long-term bone marrow stromal and hemopoietic toxicity to AZT: protective role of heme and IL-1. Exp Hematol 1993;21:263–268.
224. Fibbe WE, Willems R. The role of interleukin-l in hematopoiesis. Acta Haematol 1991;86:148–154.
225. Molina JM, Scadden DT, Burn R, et al. Production of tumor necrosis factor alpha and interleukin 1 beta by monocytic cells infected with human immunodeficiency virus. J Clin Invest 1989;84:733–737.
226. Valentin A, Albert J, Svenson SB, et al. Blood-derived macrophages produce IL-1, but not TNF-alpha, after infection with HIV-1 isolates from patients at different stages of disease. Cytokine 1992;4:185–191.
227. Reuben JM, Gonik B, Li S, et al. Induction of cytokines in normal placental cells by the human immunodeficiency virus. Lymphokine Cytokine Res 1991;10:195–199.
228. Dolei A, Serra C, Arca MV, et al. Mutual interactions between HIV-1 and cytokines in adherent cells during acute infection. Arch Virol 1994;134:157–168.
229. Tsunetsugy-Yokota Y, Honda M. Effect of cytokines on HIV release and IL-2 receptor alpha expression in monocyte cell lines. J Acquir Immune Defic Syndr 1990;3:511–516.
230. Kovacs JA, Baseler M, Dewar RJ, et al. Increases in CD4 lymphocytes with intermittent courses or interleukin-2 in patients with human immunodeficiency virus infection. N Engl J Med 1995;332:567–575.
231. Heinrich MC, Dooley DC, Freed AC, et al. Constitutive expression of steel factor gene by human stromal cells. Blood 1993;82:771–783.
232. Melani C, Mattia GF, Silvani A, et al. Interleukin-6 expression in human neutrophil and eosinophil peripheral blood granulocytes. Blood 1993;81:2744–2749.
233. Ishibashi T, Kimura H, Uchida T, et al. Human interleukin 6 is a direct promotor of maturation of megakaryocytes in vitro. Proc Natl Acad Sci U S A 1989;86:5953–5958.
234. Williams N, De Giorgio T, Banu N, et al. Recombinant interleukin 6 stimulates immature murine megakaryocytes. Exp Hematol 1990;18:69–72.
235. Kimura H, Ishibashi T, Uchida T, et al. Interleukin 6 is a differentiation factor for human megakaryocytes in vitro. Eur J Immunol 1990;20:1927–1931.
236. Fauci AS. Cytokine regulation of HIV expression. Lymphokine Res 1990;94:527–531.
237. Michaelis B, Levy JA. HIV replication can be blocked by recombinant human interferon beta. AIDS 1989;3:27–31.
238. Francis ML, Meltzer MS, Gendelman HE. Interferons in the persistence, pathogenesis and treatment of HIV infection. AIDS Res Hum Retroviruses 1991;8:199–207.
239. Mansan KF, Zidar B, Shadduck RK. Interferon-induced aplasia: evidence for T-cell mediated suppression of hematopoiesis and recovery after treatment with horse antihuman thymocyte globulin. Am J Hematol 1985;19:401–405.
240. Ganser A, Carlo-Stella C, Greher J, et al. Effect of recombinant interferons alpha and gamma on human bone marrow-derived megakaryocytic progenitor cells. Blood 1987;70:1173–1179.
241. Collart MA, Belin D, Vassalli J-D, et al. Gamma interferon enhances macrophage transcription of the tumor necrosis factor/cachectin, interleukin 1, and urokinase genes, which are controlled by short-lived repressors. J Exp Med 1986;164:2113–2118.
242. Boue F, Wallon C, Goujard C, et al. HIV induces IL-6 production by human B lymphocytes: role of IL-4. J Immunol 1992;148:3761–3767.
243. Shalaby MR, Espevik T, Rice GC, et al. The involvement of human tumor necrosis factors-alpha and -beta in the mixed lymphocyte reaction. J Immunol 1988;141:499–503.
244. Means FT, Krantz SB. Progress in understanding the pathogenesis of the anemia of chronic disease. Blood 1992;80:1639–1647.
245. Mabondzo A, Le Naour R, Raoul H, et al. In vitro infection of macrophages by HIV. Res Virol 1991;142:205–212.
246. Carlo-Stella C, Ganser A, Hoelzer D. Defective in vitro growth of the hematopoietic progenitor cells in the acquired immunodeficiency syndrome. J Clin Invest 1987;80:286–293.
247. Rusten LS, Jacobsen FW, Lesslauer W, et al. Bifunctional effects of tumor necrosis factor alpha (TNF-α) on the growth of mature and primitive human hematopoietic progenitor cells: Involvement of p55 and p75 TNF receptors. Blood 1994;83:3152–3159.
248. Rusten LS, Jacobsen SEW. Tumor necrosis factor (TNF)-α directly inhibits human erythropoiesis in vitro: role of p55 and p75 TNF receptors. Blood 1995;85:989–996.
249. Dubois CM, Ruscetti RW, Stankova J, et al. Transforming growth actor-beta regulates c-kit message stability and cell-surface protein expression in hematopoietic progenitors. Blood 1994;83:3138–3145.
250. Bonewald LF, Dallas SL. Role of active and latent transforming growth factor beta in bone formation. J Cell Biochem 1994;55:350–357.

251. Kekow J, Wachsman W, McCutchan JA, et al. Transforming growth factor beta and noncytopathic mechanisms of immunodeficiency in human immunodeficiency virus infection. Proc Natl Acad Sci U S A 1990;87:8321–8325.
252. Leiderman IZ, Greenberg ML, Adelsberg BR, et al. A glycoprotein inhibitor of in vitro granulopoiesis associated with AIDS. Blood 1987;70:1267–1272.
253. Seddiki N, Ben Younes-Chennoufi A, et al. Membrane glycolipids and human immunodeficiency virus infection of primary macrophages. AIDS Res Hum Retroviruses 1996;12:695–703.
254. Lazdins JK, Klimkait T, Alteri E, et al. TGF-β: upregulator of HIV replication in macrophages. Res Virol 1991;142:239–242.
255. McGinnes K, Quesniaux V, Hitzler J, et al. Human B-lymphopoiesis is supported by bone marrow-derived stromal cells. Exp Hematol 1991;19:294–303.
256. Johnson A, Dorshkind K. Stromal cells in myeloid and lymphoid long term bone marrow cultures can support hematopoiesis and modulate the production of hematopoietic growth factors. Blood 1986;68:1348–1354.
257. Lichtman M. The ultrastructure of the hemopoietic environment: a review. Exp Hematol 1981;9:391–410.
258. Tavassoli M, Hardy CL. Molecular basis of homing of intravenously transplanted stem cells to the marrow. Blood 1990;76:1059–1070.
259. Levesque J-P, Haylock DN, Simmons PJ. Cytokine regulation of proliferation and cell adhesion are correlated events in human CD34+ hemopoietic progenitors. Blood 1996;88:1168–1176.
260. Yang Y-C, Schickwann T, Wong GG, et al. Interleukin-1 regulation of hematopoietic growth factor production by human stromal fibroblasts. J Cell Physiol 1988;134:292–296.
261. Simmons PJ, Masinovsky B, Longenecker BM, et al. Vascular cell adhesion molecule-l expressed by bone marrow stromal cells mediates the binding of hematopoietic progenitor cells. Blood 1992;80:388–395.
262. Bagby GC, Rigas D, Bennett RM, et al. Interaction of lactoferrin, monocytes and T lymphocyte subsets in the regulation of steady state granulopoiesis in vitro. J Clin Invest 1981;68:56–63.
263. Ganser A, Ottmann OG, von Briesen H, et al. Changes in the hematopoietic progenitor cell compartment in the acquired immunodeficiency syndrome. Res Virol 1990;141:185–193.
264. Platzer E. Human hematopoietic growth factors. Eur J Haematol 1989;42:1–15.
265. Scadden DT, Zeira M, Woon A, et al. Human immunodeficiency infection of human bone marrow stromal fibroblasts. Blood 1990;76:317–322.
266. Anonymous. Human immunodeficiency virus infection of human bone marrow stromal fibroblasts [editorial]. Dis Markers 1991;9:57.
267. Neil JC, Onions DE. Feline leukaemia viruses: molecular biology and pathogenesis. Anticancer Res 1985;5:49–64.
268. Linenberger ML, Abkowitz J. Studies in feline long-term marrow culture: hematopoiesis on normal and feline leukemia virus infected stromal cells. Blood 1992;80:651–662.
269. Chehimi J, Prakash K, Shanmugam V, et al. In-vitro infection of peripheral blood dendritic cells with human immunodeficiency virus-1 causes impairment of accessory functions. Adv Exp Med Biol 1993;329:521–526.
270. Moses AV, Williams S, Heneveld ML, et al. Human immunodeficiency virus infection of bone marrow endothelium reduces induction of stromal hematopoietic growth factors. Blood 1996;87:919–925.
271. Toulon P, Blanche P, Bachmeyer D, et al. Thromboembolism and HIV-infection: protein S deficiency and hypoalbuminemia as risk factors for thrombosis. [abstract 1910]. Blood 1994;84:481a.
272. Hassell KL, Kressin DC, Neumann A, et al. Correlation of antiphospholipid antibodies and protein S deficiency with thrombosis in HIV-infected men. Blood Coagul Fibrinolysis 1994;5:455–462.
273. Cappell MS, Simon T, Tiku M. Splenic infarction associated with anticardiolipin antibodies in a patient with acquired immunodeficiency syndrome. Dig Dis Sci 1993;38:1152–1155.
274. Denis A, Baudeau C, Verdy E, et al. Acquired circulating anticoagulant with anti-factor V activity in AIDS: first case report. Nouv Rev Fr Hematol 1995;37:165–169.
275. Gold JE, Haubenstock A, Zalusky R. Lupus anticoagulant and AIDS. N Engl J Med 1986;314:1252–1253.
276. Bloom EJ, Abrams DI, Rodgers GM. Lupus anticoagulant in the acquired immunodeficiency syndrome. JAMA 1986;256:491–493.
277. Cohen H, Mackie IJ, Anagnostopoulos N, et al. Lupus anticoagulant, anticardiolipin antibodies, and human immunodeficiency virus in haemophilia. J Clin Pathol 1989;42:629–633.
278. Cohen AJ, Philips TM, Kessler CM. Circulating coagulant inhibitors in the acquired immunodeficiency syndrome. Ann Intern Med 1986;104:175–180.
279. Stahl CP, Sideman CS, Spira TJ, et al. Protein S deficiency in men with long-term human immunodeficiency virus infection. Blood 1993;81:1801–1807.
280. Lafeuillade A, Sorice M, Griggi T, et al. Role of autoimmunity in protein S deficiency during HIV-1 infection. Infection 1994;22:201–203.
281. Lafeuillade A, Alessi MC, Poizot-Martin I, et al. Endothelial cell dysfunction in HIV infection. J Acquir Immune Defic Syndr 1992;5:127–131.
282. Pryzdial ELG, Wright JF. Prothrombinase assembly on an enveloped virus: evidence that the cytomegalovirus surface contains procoagulant phospholipid. Blood 1994;84:3749–3757.
283. Toulon P, Lamine M, Ledjev I, et al. Heparin cofactor II deficiency in patients infected with the human immunodeficiency virus. Thromb Haemost 1993;70:730–735.
284. Toulon P, Frere E, Bachmeyer C, et al. Fibrin polymerization defect in HIV-infected patients: evidence for a critical role of albumin in the prolongation of thrombin and reptilase clotting times. Thromb Haemost 1995;73:349–355.

38

ENDOCRINE ABNORMALITIES ASSOCIATED WITH HIV INFECTION AND AIDS

Deborah E. Sellmeyer, Carl Grunfeld, and Morris Schambelan

Human immunodeficiency virus (HIV) infection and the acquired immunodeficiency syndrome (AIDS) are associated with many alterations in endocrine function. These changes can be direct consequences of the opportunistic infections and malignancies associated with HIV infection, or they may be complications of medications used in the treatment of these disorders. Moreover, any severe illness can change the rate of hormone secretion or clearance, or both, even in the absence of pathologic involvement of the organs responsible for hormone production or metabolism. In practice, it may prove difficult to determine whether an abnormality in endocrine function is due to the cytopathologic effects of the virus or to intercurrent illnesses or therapies. Additionally, as in other chronic illnesses, the presence of HIV infection and its complications may be associated with alterations in the results of tests of endocrine function without overt clinical manifestations.

This chapter reviews abnormalities in endocrine gland pathology and function that have been reported in association with HIV and AIDS, distinguishing whether alterations are clinically significant, are specific to HIV infection and its treatment, or are representative of a normal response to severe illness.

ADRENAL GLAND

Pathology

Adrenal pathology is common at postmortem examination in patients who have died of AIDS (1–9). In autopsy series, cytomegalovirus (CMV) inclusion bodies have been found in 40 to 88% of adrenal glands studied (1–10). The adrenal pathologic abnormalities associated with CMV infection range from focal inflammation to extensive hemorrhagic necrosis, often affecting the adrenal medulla more than the cortex (3–7, 10). In autopsy series of AIDS patients, the maximum amount of adrenal cortical necrosis found has been 60 to 70% (7, 10); clinical adrenal insufficiency is not thought to occur until 90% of the gland has been destroyed. However, two patients with adrenal insufficiency caused by CMV adrenalitis have been reported; both had extensive adrenal necrosis and CMV inclusion bodies at autopsy (11, 12). Other pathologic processes that involve the adrenal gland in patients with AIDS include hemorrhage, infection with *Toxoplasma, Cryptococcus, Mycobacterium tuberculosis,* and *M. avium* complex, and infiltration with Kaposi's sarcoma and lymphoma (1, 4, 5, 7, 9). However, in these studies, only CMV infection appeared to be associated with significant adrenal destruction.

Evaluation of Adrenal Glucocorticoid Secretion

Cortisol, the major glucocorticoid hormone in humans, is secreted by the inner zone of the adrenal cortex (zona fasciculata) in response to changes in corticotropin (ACTH) secretion by the pituitary, which, in turn, is regulated by the secretion of corticotropin-releasing hormone (CRH) by the hypothalamus. Secretion of ACTH and cortisol is pulsatile, manifests a diurnal circadian rhythm, and is under negative feedback control. Elevations in circulating levels of cortisol and, to a lesser extent, of ACTH are frequently seen during severe illness, including infection (13, 14). These changes are likely produced by cytokines, such as interleukin-1 (IL-1) and tumor necrosis factor (TNF), which have been shown to stimulate cortisol secretion directly (15). Additionally, IL-1, and IL-6 appear to stimulate release of ACTH and CRH directly (15–19).

When cortisol secretion is increased under conditions of severe illness (even when circulating levels may not be frankly elevated), the response to dynamic stimulatory tests of adrenal function (using ACTH, insulin, or metyrapone) may not be normal. Sibbald and colleagues reported that 19% of patients with surgical sepsis had normal basal levels of cortisol but failed to respond to acute ACTH stimulation (20); these patients were subsequently found to have normal adrenal function after recuperation. Recovery from both meningococcal and blastomycosis-induced adrenal insufficiency has also been reported (21, 22). Patients with chronic diseases and severe malnutrition also tend to have subnormal rates of urinary excretion of 17-keto- and 17-hydroxycorticosteroids that respond sluggishly to longer ACTH infusions (23).

Extensive destruction of adrenal tissue leads to decreased levels of cortisol, increased levels of ACTH, and a subnormal response to stimulation by exogenously administered ACTH. However, because adrenal reserve is substantial, loss of more than 90% of adrenal tissue may be required before a clinically significant reduction in cortisol levels occurs. Pathologic involvement of the hypothalamus or pituitary results in decreased levels of both ACTH and cortisol, with a subnormal response to stimulation of the hypothalamic–pituitary axis with insulin-induced hypoglycemia or metyrapone. Additionally, ACTH deficiency leads to atrophy of the adrenal cortex and a subnormal response to a single-dose ACTH stimulation test. Measurement of plasma ACTH levels should distinguish between primary and secondary causes of cortisol deficiency, but samples must be processed appropriately for results to be interpretable. Therefore, single data points (or limited analyses) are not always able to differentiate among the causes of adrenocortical abnormalities.

Adrenocortical Secretion in AIDS

Despite the frequency with which adrenal pathology is noted at postmortem examination, clinically significant impairment of glucocorticoid hormone secretion appears to be uncommon in patients with AIDS. Addison's disease was reported in one HIV-infected patient in an early case report; however, adrenal insufficiency preceded the patient's diagnosis of AIDS by 4 months and occurred at a time when the patient's ratio of helper to suppressor T cells was normal (24). After this report, a prospective study was performed in 20 patients with AIDS who were referred specifically because of symptoms and signs suggestive of adrenal insufficiency (25). A blunted response of plasma cortisol to stimulation with ACTH was noted in 4 patients, 2 of whom had hyperpigmentation and elevated plasma ACTH levels that further suggested the presence of primary glucocorticoid hormone deficiency. However, 3 of these patients had received rifampin and 2 had received ketoconazole, both of which can affect steroidogenesis and may have altered their cortisol responses.

Although these early reports suggested a substantial frequency of adrenal insufficiency in AIDS, larger series have found basal cortisol levels in HIV-infected patients to be normal (26–28) or, more commonly, elevated (29–36). Basal ACTH levels in patients with HIV infection have been found to be elevated, normal, or even decreased. In HIV-infected patients with elevated basal cortisol levels, morning ACTH levels were found to be elevated by Verges and associates (29), but normal by Membreno and colleagues (31). Eight of 25 ambulatory, HIV-infected patients in a longitudinal study had elevated morning ACTH levels at the end of 2 years, although basal cortisol levels remained normal (28). In a study of circadian ACTH secretion, Villette and associates found elevated basal cortisol with decreased ACTH (30), a finding suggesting adrenal cortical stimulation by a nonpituitary factor.

More than 90% of HIV-infected patients studied have had normal responses to ACTH stimulation testing (26–29, 31, 32, 35, 37). Azar and colleagues administered 1 μg/kg intravenous CRH and measured plasma cortisol and ACTH over the following 120 minutes (38). In response to CRH stimulation, 50% of 25 HIV-infected patients with CD4 cell counts under 500 cells/mm^3 but no acute illness and no symptoms of adrenal insufficiency had normal cortisol and ACTH responses, 25% had normal ACTH responses with reduced cortisol responses, and 25% had both reduced cortisol and ACTH responses. All these patients had normal basal ACTH and cortisol levels compared with controls; however, the response to CRH stimulation suggests a loss of reserve at either the pituitary or adrenal level in up to half the HIV-infected patients. Similar results were found by Lortholary and associates in their study of 22 AIDS patients (35). Although all 22 patients had elevated basal cortisol levels and normal ACTH stimulation tests, 14 had reduced responses to CRH stimulation. In contrast, Biglino and associates found delayed or absent ACTH and cortisol responses to CRH stimulation in 8 patients with symptomatic HIV infection but no opportunistic disease (34). However, these patients were all drug users; opiate use may blunt ACTH release (39).

Cortisol secretion has also been found to be normal in pediatric patients with HIV infection. Laue and colleagues studied 9 children with failure to thrive (40); each child had normal adrenal function. In 10 children with HIV infection who were studied by Oberfield and coworkers (41), both baseline and ACTH stimulated cortisol levels were either normal or slightly elevated in comparison with a control population. The response to CRH has not been tested in children with HIV infection.

Although clinically significant glucocorticoid deficiency is relatively infrequent, subclinical abnormalities of adrenal biosynthesis may be common in patients with HIV infection. Membreno and associates measured plasma concentrations of the secretory products of the two major ACTH-dependent steroid biosynthetic pathways in the adrenal zona fasciculata (31): 17-hydroxysteroids (cortisol) and 17-deoxysteroids (corticosterone, deoxycorticosterone, and 18-OH-deoxycorticosterone) in HIV-infected patients. Basal levels of cortisol were significantly higher in patients with AIDS than in controls. In response to ACTH stimulation, the average cortisol level among the AIDS patients was slightly less than among controls, but the plasma concentrations of the products of the 17-deoxysteroid pathway were substantially reduced. When ACTH was administered for 3 consecutive days, cortisol levels increased normally, but levels of the 17-deoxysteroids remained subnormal. A diminished response of 17-deoxysteroids with normal cortisol levels after acute ACTH stimulation testing has also been noted in children with HIV infection (41).

The 17-deoxysteroid products are probably not functionally important at normal plasma concentrations; therefore, these findings cannot be taken as evidence of clinically significant adrenal functional impairment. Whether this biosynthetic pattern could represent a harbinger of subsequent impaired adrenal capacity in patients with AIDS (31) requires further study. Moreover, whether this subtle abnormality of the zona fasciculata is unique to HIV infection or whether it also occurs in other acute and chronic illnesses is not known. Conceivably, this alteration in steroid metabolism could represent a common adaptive mechanism that preserves cortisol secretion at the expense of reduced secretion of steroids that do not appear to have biologic significance.

The concept of shunting of adrenal biosynthetic products toward glucocorticoids is also suggested by studies of adrenal androgens. Villette and colleagues found decreased dehydroepiandrosterone (DHEA) and DHEA sulfate levels with elevated cortisol levels in HIV-infected men undergoing studies of hormonal circadian variation (30). Basal adrenal androgen secretion has been found to be lower in HIV-infected patients compared with controls (42–44), and decreased adrenal androgen response to ATCH stimulation has been found at all stages of HIV infection (28). DHEA levels have been shown to decline with falling CD4 cell counts (44). In two studies, lower DHEA levels predicted progression to AIDS independent of CD4 cell counts (42, 43). Honour and colleagues found that urinary excretion of adrenal androgens was lower in HIV-seronegative patients in intensive care units as well as in HIV-infected outpatients and hospitalized AIDS patients compared with healthy seronegative controls (45). These data suggest that the lower DHEA levels found in HIV-infected patients may be found in other illness states as well. In vitro, DHEA has been shown to be a modest inhibitor of HIV replication (46); an open-label dose-escalation trial of DHEA in HIV-infected patients showed no sustained improvements in CD4 counts or serum p24 antigen levels (47). No randomized, controlled trials of adrenal androgen replacement therapy in AIDS have been reported.

Norbiato and associates reported a syndrome of glucocorticoid resistance in HIV-infected patients (48). These patients exhibited weakness, fatigue, weight loss, and hyperpigmentation with elevated cortisol levels and mildly increased ACTH levels. Mononuclear lymphocytes from these patients were found to have an increased number of receptors and decreased receptor affinity for glucocorticoids (48). In a series of HIV-infected patients, 17% of whom were believed to have glucocorticoid resistance, the abnormal glucocorticoid receptor was accompanied by continual stimulation of interferon-α secretion (49). The prevalence and clinical significance of this syndrome have not been fully elucidated. These patients have a clinical syndrome that includes hyperpigmentation. However, one could speculate that partial glucocorticoid resistance could explain the elevated basal cortisol levels and variability in response to stimulatory testing more commonly found in HIV-infected patients (50).

Several medications used in the treatment of HIV infection and AIDS can affect glucocorticoid metabolism. Ketoconazole inhibits cortisol synthesis and could lead to adrenal insufficiency, particularly in patients with limited adrenal reserve (51). Rifampin enhances hepatic cortisol metabolism and can cause adrenal insufficiency in patients with Addison's disease who are receiving maintenance glucocorticoid therapy (52), and it may lead to adrenal insufficiency in patients with limited adrenal reserve (53). Megestrol acetate, currently used as an appetite stimulant for patients with the AIDS wasting syndrome, can reduce plasma serum cortisol levels, perhaps because of its intrinsic cortisol-like activity at the high doses used for such therapy. Patients with low cortisol levels while taking megestrol have been shown to have low ACTH levels even in response to metyrapone testing (54). The endocrinologic effects of medications used in the treatment of HIV infection are summarized in Table 38.1.

Clinical Approach to Adrenocortical Abnormalities in AIDS

Because most patients with HIV infection have normal or elevated basal cortisol levels and normal response to ACTH stimulation testing, little evidence of widespread adrenal insufficiency exists in patients with AIDS. However, more subtle alterations may occur in the hypothalamic–pituitary–adrenal axis. Given the wide spectrum of changes in this axis that occur with any form of severe illness, mild abnormalities in adrenal function, particularly in the cortisol response to ACTH stimulation, should not be taken as proof of adrenal insufficiency.

Symptoms resembling Addison's disease, particularly fatigue and orthostasis, may be common in patients with advanced stages of AIDS. Patients with symptoms or signs consistent with the diagnosis of adrenal insufficiency should undergo provocative testing. Glucocorticoid maintenance therapy should be considered in patients with AIDS and low baseline cortisol levels who fail to respond to stimulation with ACTH, insulin-induced hypoglycemia, or metyrapone. These patients likely need short-term doses of glucocorticoids under stress. It is more difficult to propose the appropriate treatment for patients with a normal or elevated basal cortisol level who show minimal or no further increase in response to provocative testing. Most of these patients have a normal cortisol response to prolonged ACTH stimulation (31) and probably do not require maintenance therapy. However, glucocorticoids could be considered in these patients at times of stress, provided treatment is limited in duration to prevent adverse effects of exogenous steroid therapy.

Evaluation of Adrenal Mineralocorticoid Hormone Secretion

Aldosterone, the principal mineralocorticoid hormone, is secreted by the outer zone of the adrenal cortex (zona glomerulosa) under the control of the renin–angiotensin system and, to a lesser extent, by potassium and ACTH. Aldosterone plays a critical role in the modulation of sodium, potassium, and acid-base balance and in the regulation of extracellular fluid volume. Aldosterone deficiency results in renal sodium wasting, hypotension, hyperkalemia, metabolic acidosis, and elevated levels of plasma renin activity.

In contrast to the extensive evaluations of the functional capacity of the adrenal zona fasciculata, studies of steroid

Table 38.1. Endocrinologic Effects of Medications Used in the Treatment of HIV Infection and AIDS

Medication	Mechanism of Action	Clinical Effects
Rifampin	Induces hepatic microsomal enzymes leading to increased hormone clearance	Normal subjects: decreased T_4, rT_3, increased T_3, normal TSH Hypothyroidism in patients with impaired thyroid reserve Adrenal insufficiency in patients with limited reserve Decrease 25-hydroxy vitamin D levels; no change in calcium levels
Ketoconazole	Inhibits adrenal and gonadal steroidogenesis	Adrenal insufficiency in patients with limited reserve Reduced 1,25 hydroxy vitamin D levels; decreased total, but not ionized calcium levels Decreased testosterone levels
Megestrol acetate	Intrinsic glucocorticoid-like activity Progesterone activity	Lower serum cortisol levels, decreased response to provocative testing, hyperglycemia Lower testosterone levels
Trimethoprim	Impairs potassium secretion by inhibiting sodium channels in distal nephron	Hyperkalemia, metabolic acidosis
Sulfonamides	Interstitial nephritis	Hyponatremia, salt wasting Hyporeninemic hypoaldosteronism
Pentamidine	Nephrotoxicity Pancreatic toxicity	Hyperkalemia Acutely hypoglycemia Chronically hyperglycemia
Foscarnet	Complexes with ionized calcium; possible renal effects	Hypocalcemia Nephrogenic diabetes insipidus
Amphotericin B	Impairs proximal and distal tubular reabsorption of electrolytes	Renal magnesium and potassium wasting
Protease inhibitors	Unknown	Hyperglycemia

T_3, Triiodothyronine (rT_3, reverse T_3); T_4, thyroxine; TSH, thyroid-stimulating hormone.
(From Sellmeyer DE, Grunfeld C. Endocrine and metabolic disturbances in human immunodeficiency virus infection and the acquired immune deficiency syndrome. Endocr Rev 1996;17:518–532.)

secretion by the zona glomerulosa and of the integrity of the renin–angiotensin system in AIDS are limited. One patient who presented with hyponatremia, hyperkalemia, and normal cortisol levels may have had a primary abnormality of zona glomerulosa function because aldosterone levels were low normal despite hyperreninemia (55). However, cortisol reserve appeared to be subnormal in response to ACTH stimulation in this patient, and the apparent benefit of treatment with a mineralocorticoid (fludrocortisone) may have been due in part to concomitant administration of a glucocorticoid (hydrocortisone).

In four patients with AIDS and unexplained hyperkalemia, the finding of low renin and aldosterone values that failed to increase normally in response to intravenous furosemide and upright posture suggested the diagnosis of hyporeninemic hypoaldosteronism (56). However, these patients were taking trimethoprim–sulfamethoxazole at the time they were studied. Sulfonamides can cause interstitial nephritis (57), a disorder associated with hyporeninemic hypoaldosteronism (58). Alternatively, abnormalities of potassium homeostasis in patients taking trimethoprim–sulfamethoxazole may be due to trimethoprim, which, in the large doses frequently used in the treatment of *Pneumocystis carinii* pneumonia, can block amiloride-sensitive luminal sodium channels and secondarily may limit potassium secretion in distal nephron segments (59). Transient hyperkalemia was also reported during treatment with pentamidine, a finding that was reversed on discontinuation of the agent and that was attributed to nephrotoxicity (60).

In larger series, mineralocorticoid deficiency is uncommon. Verges and colleagues found no abnormalities in circulating renin or aldosterone levels in 63 HIV-infected patients, 23 of whom had AIDS (29). Similarly, Membreno and associates did not find abnormalities in aldosterone or renin levels in 74 patients with AIDS and in 19 with AIDS-related complex (31). Aldosterone levels also increased normally in response to direct stimulation of the zona glomerulosa with an angiotensin II-derived peptide. In a longitudinal study of HIV-infected patients, there was no change in basal plasma aldosterone or plasma renin activity over 2 years (28). There was some degree of impaired aldosterone response to ACTH in up to 26% of CDC class II-III patients and up to 53% of CDC class IV patients at each study interval; however, mean peak aldosterone response did not differ from normal subjects.

Interpretation of even the few published results of renin and aldosterone measurements in patients with AIDS should be done cautiously. Electrolyte abnormalities in HIV-infected patients are more likely to be the result of medication effects or renal disease than mineralocorticoid dysfunction. The endocrinologic effects of medications used in the treatment of HIV infection are summarized in Table 38.1.

HYPOTHALAMIC–PITUITARY AXIS

Pathology

The most frequent findings in postmortem studies that reviewed the pathologic findings in the pituitary glands of

AIDS patients were varying degrees of infarction and necrosis in approximately 10% of glands (61–63). In a series of 49 AIDS patients, direct infectious involvement was noted in 6 adenohypophyses (5 by CMV and 1 by *Pneumocystis carinii*) and 3 neurohypophyses (2 by CMV and 1 by *Toxoplasma gondii*) (63). Pituitary involvement by *Mycobacterium tuberculosis* has also been reported (64). In all instances, these changes were associated with generalized or cerebral infection by these same agents. Noninfectious lesions such as pituitary microadenomas and hyperplastic nodules were also noted, but not in greater prevalence than in age-matched controls. Neither Kaposi's sarcoma nor lymphoma was noted in the pituitary glands directly; however, 3 patients with cerebral lymphoma had peripheral involvement of the gland (63).

Pituitary Function

Generalized pituitary dysfunction appears to be rare in patients with AIDS. One patient in whom panhypopituitarism was attributed to cerebral toxoplasmosis had a large necrotic pituitary at autopsy and *Toxoplasma* demonstrated in cerebral abscesses although not in the pituitary itself (65). One patient with hypothalamic dysfunction attributable to CMV has also been described (66). In contrast to these two reports, studies that have systematically evaluated pituitary functional reserve using gonadotropin- or thyrotropin-releasing hormone (TRH)–stimulating hormones in patients with HIV infection have not found evidence of anterior pituitary dysfunction (26, 27, 37).

Basal and TRH-stimulated prolactin levels in HIV-infected patients have generally been found to be normal (26, 37, 67). In two reports, however, mean prolactin levels were found to be increased in patients with AIDS (68, 69).

Growth failure has been observed in some children with HIV infection, prompting studies of growth hormone (GH) secretion in these patients (40, 70, 71). Overt GH deficiency does not appear to be common. In a study of 22 boys with hemophilia, HIV infection, and lymphadenopathy, 3 were found to have short stature. All 3 had normal peak GH levels, but 2 had subnormal 24-hour mean GH levels and low insulin-like growth factor-1 (IGF-1) levels (70). Schwartz and colleagues found normal GH responses to glucagon in 14 HIV-infected children with failure to thrive (71); however, despite normal GH dynamics, these children had subnormal IGF-1 levels. Among 24 children with perinatally acquired HIV, Matarazzo and associates found reduced IGF-1 levels in 45% of symptomatic children and in 86% of children with advanced infection (72). Subnormal IGF-1 levels, in the face of apparently normal GH levels, are common in malnutrition (73). Although nutritional status may be a contributing factor, many of the children with low IGF-1 levels did not appear to be malnourished and did not have weight loss. In contrast, Laue and associates studied 9 children with AIDS and failure to thrive (40). All the children in this study were below the fifth percentile for weight and were receiving parenteral or enteral supplementation. Eight of the 9 had normal basal IGF-1 levels. All but 1 child had a normal GH response to provocative testing. In adults with HIV infection, 24-hour GH profiles showed normal number, amplitude, length, and interval of secretory rates (74).

Geffner and colleagues compared in vitro hormone sensitivity among asymptomatic HIV-infected children, symptomatic HIV-infected children, and a control group of seronegative children with short stature (75). Basal levels of IGF-1 and height–weight scores were similar among all three groups. However, a quantitative reduction in erythroid progenitor cell colony formation in response to IGF-1, GH, and insulin was noted in symptomatic HIV-infected children compared with asymptomatic children and controls, a finding suggesting that resistance could occur to the growth-promoting actions of these hormones (75). Adult patients with HIV infection also demonstrate blunting of the IGF-1 response to GH stimulation; particularly in patients with weight loss (76–79).

Hyponatremia is a common finding in patients with AIDS, and it raises the possibility of the syndrome of inappropriate antidiuretic hormone secretion (SIADH). Hyponatremia has been reported in 30 to 50% of inpatients (80–83) and 20% of outpatients with AIDS (81). Agarwal and associates observed that, at the time of hospital admission with an opportunistic infection, 36 of 103 patients with AIDS had a serum sodium value less than 130 mEq/L (80). Twenty-three of the hyponatremic patients were believed to be euvolemic on the basis of clinical assessment, and serum sodium levels remained subnormal despite saline administration. When 11 of the patients in the euvolemic subgroup were investigated further, arginine vasopressin levels were noted to be inappropriately high for the serum osmolality, a finding suggesting a diagnosis of SIADH (Fig. 38.1). Nearly all these patients had *Pneumocystis carinii* pneumonia, which, like any pulmonary

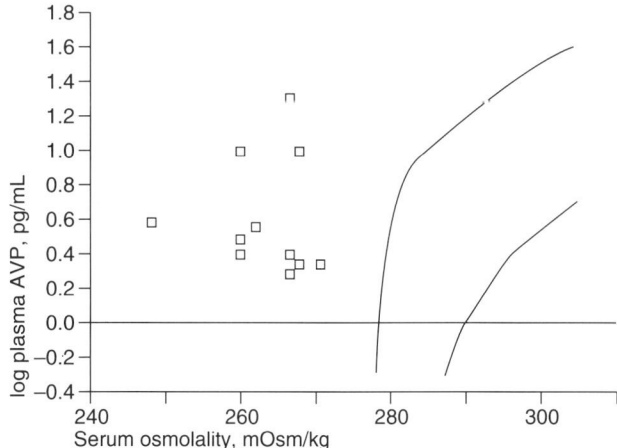

Figure 38.1. Relationship between serum vasopressin levels and osmolality in 11 euvolemic AIDS patients with hyponatremia. The area between the *solid lines* represents the normal range. The levels of vasopressin in the AIDS patients are inappropriately high for the serum osmolality. (From Agarwal A, Soni A, Ciechanowsky M, et al. Hyponatremia in patients with the acquired immunodeficiency syndrome. Nephron 1989;53:317–321.)

infection, could cause SIADH. Additionally, more than half the patients in this group were being treated with trimethoprim, which could have impaired sodium conservation during saline replacement (59). Impaired sodium conservation can lead to volume contraction and nonosmotic stimulation of ADH. Finally, intravenous administration of trimethoprim requires infusion of large volumes of hypotonic solution and may lead to dilutional hyponatremia (84).

Central diabetes insipidus has been reported in one HIV-infected patient with herpetic meningoencephalitis (85). Damage of the posterior pituitary or hypothalamus from any cause could potentially induce diabetes insipidus.

THYROID

Infectious and Tumor Effects

Opportunistic infections such as with *Mycobacterium avium*, *Cryptococcus neoformans*, CMV, and *Pneumocystis carinii* and AIDS-related neoplasms such as Kaposi's sarcoma have been found in the thyroid gland at autopsy in patients dying of AIDS (1). As in the adrenal and pituitary glands, CMV inclusion bodies can be identified in the absence of clinically significant thyroid destruction (86).

In contrast, inflammatory thyroiditis from *Pneumocystis carinii* infection accompanied by alterations in thyroid function has been reported (87–96). Thyroid function testing was performed in 11 of these cases; 7 patients had hypothyroidism (87, 90, 91, 93, 94, 96), 3 had hyperthyroidism (88, 90, 92), and 1 had normal thyroid function (89). Radionuclide scanning, performed in 7 cases, showed nonvisualization of the affected gland (88–90, 92, 94). Hyperthyroidism resolved with treatment for the *Pneumocystis carinii* infection in 2 patients (90, 92). Involvement of the thyroid gland by *Cryptococcus neoformans* (97) and *Aspergillus fumigatus* (98) has been reported in patients with disseminated infection; these patients had normal thyroid function.

Kaposi's sarcoma has also been described in the thyroid glands of two patients (99, 100). In one of these cases, the thyroid was almost completely destroyed by tumor, and the patient had hypothyroidism (99).

Thyroid Hormone Secretion

Regulation of thyroid hormone secretion is initiated by a TRH of hypothalamic origin that stimulates the release of thyrotropin (thyroid-stimulating hormone [TSH]) from the pituitary. TSH, in turn, stimulates the thyroid gland to release two thyroid hormones, thyroxine (T_4) and triiodothyronine (T_3). Although 80% of the secreted thyroid hormone is in the form of T_4, most of this is converted in the periphery to T_3, which is the active form of the hormone, and a small amount to reverse T_3 (rT_3), which is inactive. Homeostatic control is maintained by a feedback effect of T_3 at both hypothalamic and pituitary levels.

Destruction of the thyroid leads to decreases in T_4 and compensatory increases in TSH. T_3 levels may be either frankly low or in the low-normal range. Severe systemic nonthyroidal illness also results in decreased circulating T_3 levels as a consequence of impaired conversion of T_4 to T_3; T_4 levels vary and may occasionally be slightly increased in this setting. These changes in thyroid hormone metabolism are known as the euthyroid sick syndrome (101, 102), and they are usually accompanied by increases in rT_3 levels. Investigators have proposed that the decreases in T_3 limit both protein catabolism and energy expenditure in severe illness (101, 102). During caloric deprivation accompanied by decreased T_3, replacement therapy with T_3 accelerates negative nitrogen balance (103, 104), although this concept has been challenged in another study (105).

As in other acute and chronic illnesses, abnormalities of thyroid function tests occur frequently in patients with AIDS, but frank hypothyroidism is uncommon. Some studies have reported decreased T_3 levels in asymptomatic HIV-infected patients and patients with AIDS (27, 37, 106). These patients all had normal basal and TRH-stimulated TSH levels. Other studies have not found a decrease in T_3 levels in HIV-infected patients (26, 107–109). Because many patients with advanced AIDS do not show decreases in T_3, investigators have questioned whether the failure to decrease T_3 is inappropriate and could contribute to the wasting syndrome. However, patients with AIDS have an appropriate decrease in serum T_3 levels in response to severe illness. Serum T_3 levels are consistently depressed in patients with *Pneumocystis carinii* pneumonia and other infections (110–113). Serum T_3 levels are decreased in proportion to the severity of illness at the time of study, and, indeed, patients who die during hospitalization are likely to have low T_3 levels (37, 112, 113). Although many patients with AIDS show wasting at some time during the disease, their weight is stable for long periods (107, 114). Those patients who have active weight loss, frequently in the setting of secondary infection, show appropriate decreases in T_3 levels (111).

Other changes in thyroid homeostasis may be unique to AIDS, but their significance is not fully understood. In the euthyroid sick syndrome, TSH usually does not increase during illness but may do so in the recovery phase. In patients with AIDS, TSH levels are significantly higher than in controls, although these levels are rarely frankly elevated (108, 111). TSH pulse amplitude is increased (Fig. 38.2), and the TSH response to TRH is exaggerated (108). These data are consistent with a compensated hypothyroid state, particularly in patients with AIDS who are not infected and whose weight is stable (108).

Thyroid-binding globulin is increased in HIV infection and AIDS (106, 108, 109, 111, 112, 115). The clinical significance of the elevated thyroid-binding globulin found in HIV infection is unclear; however, it should be considered when interpreting measurements of total T_3 and T_4.

Levels of rT_3 decrease early in the course of HIV infection and AIDS (111, 112). In most, but not all, nonthyroidal illnesses, when T_3 is reduced because of decreased conversion of T_4, rT_3 usually increases. The decrease in rT_3 in AIDS occurs before T_3 levels decrease. Increases in rT_3 do occur in

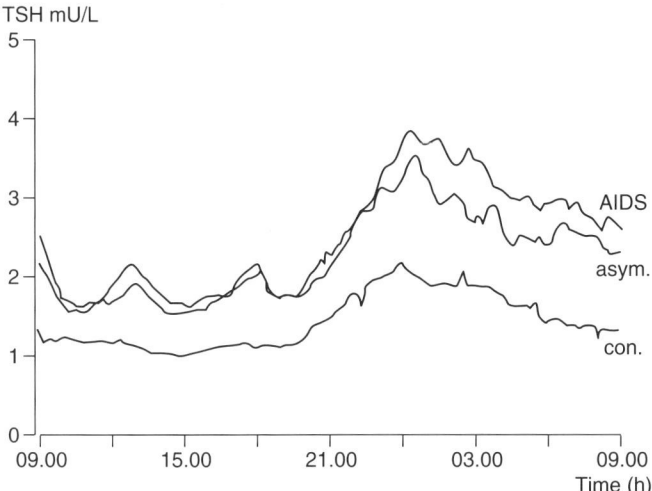

Figure 38.2. Increased 24-hour thyroid-stimulating hormone levels and pulse amplitude in patients with asymptomatic HIV infection and AIDS compared with seronegative controls. (From Hommes MJT, Romijn JA, Endert E, et al. Hypothyroid-like regulation of the pituitary-thyroid axis in stable human immunodeficiency virus infection. Metabolism 1993;42: 556–561.)

Table 38.2. Alterations in Thyroid Function Tests in HIV Infection

Test	HIV Seronegative, Severe Nonthyroidal Illness	HIV Infected, Stable	HIV Infected, Ill
T_3	Decreased	Normal	Decreased
rT_3	Increased	Decreased	Decreased or normal
TBG	Increased	Increased	Increased
T_4	Normal or decreased	Normal	Normal
TSH	Normal, may be increased during recovery	Normal	Normal

T_3, Triiodothyronine (rT_3, reverse T_3); T_4, thyroxine; TBG, thyroxine-binding globulin; TSH, thyroid-stimulating hormone.
(From Sellmeyer DE, Grunfeld C. Endocrine and metabolic disturbances in human immunodeficiency virus infection and the acquired immune deficiency syndrome. Endocr Rev 1996;17:518–532.)

a subset of severely ill AIDS patients, especially those who do not survive (112). The alterations in thyroid function tests found in HIV infection are summarized in Table 38.2.

In addition to its effect on hepatic steroid metabolism, rifampin also increases L-thyroxine clearance by induction of hepatic microsomal enzyme activity, and patients receiving L-thyroxine replacement may require dose adjustment. Rifampin may also cause hypothyroidism in patients with marginal thyroid or pituitary reserve (116). The endocrinologic effects of medications used in the treatment of HIV infection are summarized in Table 38.1.

GONADAL FUNCTION

Pathology

Pathologic destruction of the gonads leads to decreased circulating sex steroids (testosterone, estradiol, or progesterone) and high levels of the pituitary gonadotropins (luteinizing hormone [LH] and follicle-stimulating hormone [FSH]) that regulate gonadal function. Severe illness and malnutrition decrease the production of sex steroids, but they lead to normal or only slightly elevated levels of gonadotropins. Chronic illness and malnutrition can eventually cause atrophy of the gonads with reduced spermatogenesis and disturbances in menstrual function and ovulation (117).

Chabon and associates examined the testes of 32 men with AIDS at autopsy and found that 62% had marked decreases in spermatogenesis, 30% had thickening of the tunica propria, and 53% had a mild-to-moderate interstitial infiltrate that was mononuclear and frequently perivenular (118). Opportunistic infections were present in 25% of cases: 6 patients had CMV, 1 had toxoplasmosis, and 1 had tuberculosis. De Paepe and Waxman found that testes of patients with AIDS had a significantly lower degree of spermatogenesis, more prominent thickening of tubular basement membranes, and interstitial fibrosis (119). Testicular infections were present in 18 of 57 patients with AIDS; CMV was the most common pathogen, followed by *Mycobacterium avium* complex and *Toxoplasma*. Kaposi's sarcoma has also been found in the testes of a patient dying of AIDS (120). Da Silva and colleagues noted peritubular fibrosis in the testes of all 14 patients with AIDS whom they examined, with total tubal sclerosis occurring in 3 cases (121).

Sperm counts were found to be decreased in two of four published studies (122–125). More commonly, sperm looked abnormal and were less motile, and semen was more viscous. Pyosemia may be responsible for some of these changes (125). Further analysis is needed to determine which aspects of HIV infection and its complications contribute to changes in sperm and semen. Additionally, HIV DNA was shown to infect the spermatogonia selectively in the testes in several studies (125, 126). Because of the effects of chronic illness on testicular function, interpreting the significance of the findings of decreased testicular volume and spermatogenesis is difficult; however, the frequency of infiltration and infection of the testes is a striking finding. Changes in ovarian pathology in AIDS have not been studied.

Testicular Function

Changes in gonadal function clearly occur in patients with HIV infection. Dobs and associates found that 28 of 42 patients with AIDS had decreased libido, and 14 were impotent (26). Free testosterone levels were below the normal range in 25% of asymptomatic HIV patients, 29% of patients with AIDS-related complex, and 45% of patients with AIDS (Fig. 38.3). Notably, 75% of these patients with low free testosterone levels did not have elevated LH and FSH levels. Furthermore, 7 of the 8 patients who underwent stimulation with gonadotropin-releasing hormone (GnRH) had a normal response. Thus, most patients with low free testosterone levels appeared to have inappropriately low LH and FSH levels and normal GnRH responsiveness, a finding

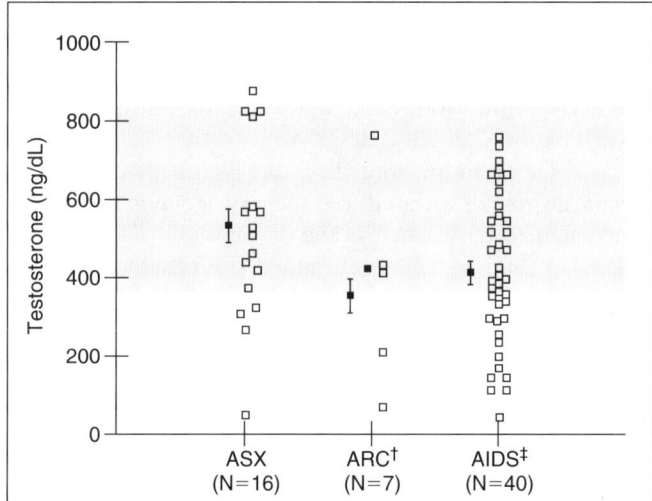

Figure 38.3. Serum testosterone levels in men with asymptomatic HIV infection, AIDS-related complex, and AIDS. *Shaded area* represents the normal range. *Open squares,* individual values; *closed squares,* mean ± SEM. (From Dobs AS, Dempsy MA, Ladenson PW, et al. Endocrine disorders in men infected with the human immunodeficiency virus. Am J Med 1988;84:611–616.)

suggesting a functional disorder of the hypothalamus with respect to GnRH secretion. Raffi and colleagues also found decreased total testosterone levels in 8 of 28 patients with AIDS (27). They also noted that the LH and FSH levels were inappropriately low for the serum testosterone levels and the response to GnRH was normal in all cases. Subnormal testosterone levels in AIDS patients have been demonstrated in several other studies as well (30, 33, 127, 128). Croxson and colleagues also found lower total testosterone levels in patients with AIDS (68), but they did not observe inappropriately low LH or FSH values in their study. Thus, their results implied low testosterone resulting from primary testicular failure rather than from hypogonadotropic hypogonadism. One possible explanation for this disparity is that the latter study excluded intravenous drug users; opiate use itself is known to cause hypogonadotropic hypogonadism (129). Serum bioavailable testosterone levels have been found to be lower in HIV-infected patients with weight loss who subsequently went on to develop wasting (130). Free testosterone levels positively correlated with lean body mass and exercise functional capacity in hypogonadal men with advanced HIV infection and wasting (79).

Testosterone levels have been found to be normal or even elevated early in the course of HIV infection (27, 30, 33, 37, 68). In patients with early HIV infection, Merenich and associates found elevated testosterone levels with higher basal LH and an enhanced LH response to GnRH (37), a finding suggesting an alteration at the pituitary–hypothalamic level.

Most studies have found normal sex hormone–binding globulin levels at all stages of HIV infection (26, 37, 68, 115); however, Martin and associates found sex hormone–binding globulin was increased 46% above controls and had an increased affinity for testosterone (131). Increased concentration or affinity of this serum protein would lead to lower levels of free sex steroids.

Drugs used in the treatment of patients with AIDS may also have an impact on gonadal function. In addition to its effects on adrenal function, ketoconazole is associated with decreased levels of total and free testosterone, leading to oligospermia, azoospermia, and gynecomastia (51). Megestrol acetate, a progestational agent, can result in lower testosterone levels through feedback inhibition on gonadotropin secretion (127). In a therapeutic trial of the treatment of wasting, megestrol significantly reduced testosterone levels (132). The endocrinologic effects of medications used in the treatment of HIV infection are summarized in Table 38.1.

In summary, men with AIDS tend to have an increased incidence of impotence and low testosterone levels. The low testosterone values probably are due to a functional disorder of the hypothalamus, primary testicular failure, or a combination of both. However, which of these potential causes is more important is not clear. The finding of decreased testosterone with normal to slightly increased (inappropriately low) gonadotropin levels suggests the effects of systemic illness. On the other hand, clear-cut primary testicular failure (low testosterone with highly elevated gonadotropin levels) suggests a localized infection. Although infection of the pituitary and hypothalamus occurs, it is exceedingly rare, and secondary hypogonadism should only be considered in the face of other endocrine or central nervous system disorders.

Ovarian Function

Much less information is currently available on gonadal function in women with HIV infection. Amenorrhea was noted in 26% of 308 HIV-infected women in Uganda (133). Among HIV-infected women with CD4 counts higher than 200 cells/mm^3, 92% of asymptomatic and 100% of symptomatic women had regular menstrual cycles (134). Shelton and colleagues also found no menstrual irregularities or changes in hormone levels in HIV-infected women (135). Two cross-sectional studies also found no significant differences in menstrual function between HIV-infected and HIV-seronegative women (136, 137).

PANCREAS

Pathology

The pancreas is frequently abnormal in autopsy series of patients dying of AIDS. Among 82 HIV-infected patients, opportunistic infections and malignancies of the pancreas were found much more commonly in AIDS patients than in patients who were immunocompromised for other reasons (138). Most of these pancreatic lesions do not appear to cause clinically significant pancreatic dysfunction. Clinically significant pancreatic tuberculous abscesses have been described in patients with AIDS; however, these patients presented with febrile illnesses rather than pancreatic dysfunction (139).

Pancreatic Function

Clinically stable HIV-infected men were found to have increased rates of insulin clearance and increased sensitivity of peripheral tissues to insulin during euglycemic clamp studies compared with seronegative controls (140). In contrast, other infections and cytokine administration induce insulin resistance.

Trends exist toward decreased glucose oxidation and increased nonoxidative glucose disposal in HIV infection (76, 140, 141), but these trends were not statistically significant in published reports based on small numbers of subjects. If glucose disposal is increased, the likely cause is increased insulin-mediated glucose disposal (141).

Intravenous pentamidine for *Pneumocystis carinii* infections can rarely cause acute pancreatitis (142, 143). More commonly, it results in β-cell toxicity leading to acute hypoglycemia. Risk factors for the development of hypoglycemia in patients taking pentamidine include longer duration of therapy, higher cumulative doses, and renal insufficiency (144–146). AIDS patients who become hypoglycemic while receiving pentamidine have elevated insulin levels (147). In vitro studies on insulinoma cells showed that pentamidine caused acute insulin release after 30 minutes of exposure followed by subsequent inhibition of insulin release (144). With continued pentamidine exposure cytolysis occurred, and after 3 weeks no cell structure remained.

Patients who develop acute hypoglycemia while taking pentamidine often subsequently develop diabetes mellitus (144–147). C-peptide levels in these patients are low, a finding suggesting significant β-cell destruction (148). Hypoglycemia and diabetes mellitus may also occur during treatment with inhaled pentamidine (149, 150). Despite similar fasting blood glucose values, postprandial glucose, glycosylated hemoglobin, and fasting C-peptide were all found to be higher in HIV-infected patients receiving aerosolized pentamidine therapy compared with AIDS patients who had never received inhaled pentamidine, a finding suggesting frequent, subclinical β-cell toxicity (151).

Megestrol acetate, used in the treatment of anorexia and cachexia in AIDS, has been reported to induce diabetes mellitus (152); however, hyperglycemia has been uncommon in controlled trials (153). Whether this side effect is secondary to increased caloric intake or to a pharmacologic effect of the drug such as its intrinsic cortisol-like activity is not known.

The United States Food and Drug Administration has sent a "Dear Doctor" warning indicating that increasing numbers of new cases of diabetes mellitus or hyperglycemic exacerbations of preexisting cases of diabetes mellitus have been reported in patients taking protease inhibitors for treatment of HIV (154). The incidence of hyperglycemia during therapy with protease inhibitors is currently low. The cases are indistinguishable from classic diabetes mellitus. No known mechanism exists by which protease inhibitors induce hyperglycemia. The endocrinologic effects of medications used in the treatment of HIV infection are summarized in Table 38.1.

BONE AND MINERAL HOMEOSTASIS

Hypercalcemia has been reported in four patients with AIDS-related lymphoma (155). One of these patients had a markedly elevated 1,25-dihydroxy vitamin D level that returned to normal during therapy for lymphoma. Hypercalcemia with elevated 1,25-dihydroxy vitamin D and suppressed parathyroid hormone (PTH) levels has also been reported in an AIDS patient with *Mycobacterium avium* complex (156), which responded to prednisone therapy. These reports of hypercalcemia appear to be due to enhanced conversion of 25-hydroxy vitamin D to 1,25-dihydroxy vitamin D by the lymphoma or granuloma.

Baseline and ethylenediamine tetraacetic acid (EDTA)–stimulated intact PTH levels were found to be lower in AIDS patients compared with healthy controls and severely ill patients with malignancies despite comparable magnesium and vitamin D levels (157). Mean maximal increments in PTH levels were similar among the three groups, but at each calcium level, PTH concentrations were lower in patients with AIDS than in healthy controls (Fig. 38.4).

After tetracycline labeling, iliac crest bone biopsies in AIDS patients showed a decrease in some histomorphometric parameters of bone turnover compared with asymptomatic HIV-infected patients (158). Whether these changes are specific to advanced HIV infection or occur with other types of severe illness is unknown.

Foscarnet, a pyrophosphate analog used in the treatment of CMV retinitis, has been reported to cause hypocalcemia,

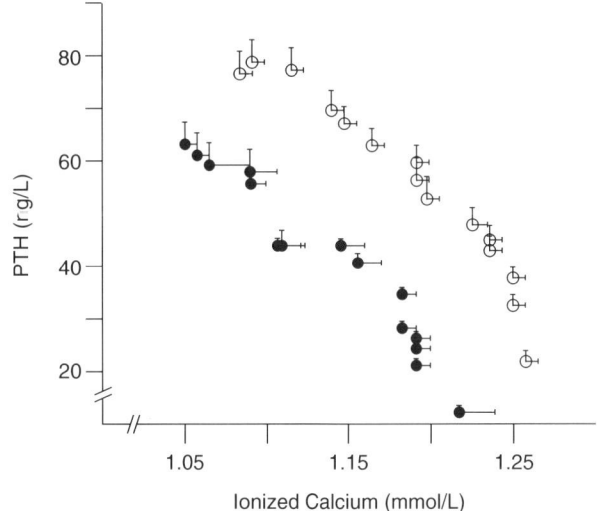

Figure 38.4. The relationship between serum intact parathyroid hormone and ionized calcium concentration during ethylenediamine tetraacetic acid (EDTA) infusion. *Open circles*, seronegative controls; *closed circles*, patients with AIDS (± SEM). At each level of calcium, AIDS patients have lower parathyroid hormone values. (From Jaeger P, Otto S, Speck RF, et al. Altered parathyroid gland function in severely immunocompromised patients infected with human immunodeficiency virus. J Clin Endocrinol Metab 1994;79:1701–1705.)

possibly by forming a complex with ionized calcium (159–161). Hypocalcemia and hypomagnesemia have been reported in association with pentamidine use (162, 163). The hypocalcemia can result in potentially serious clinical sequelae. Fatal hypocalcemia has been reported when foscarnet was given together with parenteral pentamidine (159). Hypomagnesemia, hyperphosphatemia, and hypokalemia can also occur with foscarnet treatment (164), as can nephrogenic diabetes insipidus (165). Amphotericin B, used in the treatment of fungal infections, causes renal magnesium and potassium wasting by impairing proximal and distal tubular reabsorption of electrolytes (166).

Ketoconazole lowered 1,25-dihydroxy vitamin D levels in both normal and hypercalcemic subjects; however, ionized calcium and PTH values were unchanged (167, 168). Similarly, rifampicin induced a 56 to 90% reduction in 1,25 dihydroxy vitamin D levels among eight normal men taking 600 mg per day (169). Calcium and PTH levels remained unchanged throughout the study. The endocrinologic effects of medications used in the treatment of HIV infection are summarized in Table 38.1.

In summary, multiple endocrine abnormalities have been described in association with HIV infection and AIDS. These abnormalities are rarely due to HIV infection itself, and they are rarely due to infection or tumor infiltration of endocrine glands. More commonly, these aberrations result from classic consequences of organ involvement such as SIADH from pulmonary or central nervous system lesions, the effects of systemic illness, or the medications used in the treatment of HIV infection or its complications.

References

1. Welch K, Finkbeiner W, Alpers CE, et al. Autopsy findings in the acquired immune deficiency syndrome. JAMA 1984;252:1152–1159.
2. Klatt EC, Shibata D. Cytomegalovirus infection in the acquired immunodeficiency syndrome. Arch Pathol Lab Med 1988;112:540–544.
3. Guarda LA, Luna MA, Smith L, et al. Acquired immune deficiency syndrome: postmortem findings. Am J Clin Pathol 1984;81:549–557.
4. Bricaire F, Marche C, Zoubi D, et al. Adrenocortical lesions and AIDS. Lancet 1988;1:881.
5. Laulund S, Visfeldt J, Klinken L. Pathoanatomical studies in patients dying of AIDS. Acta Pathol Microbiol Immunol Scand 1986;94:201–221.
6. Pillay D, Lipman MCI, Lee CA, et al. A clinicopathological audit of opportunistic viral infections in HIV-infected patients. AIDS 1993;7:969–974.
7. Glasgow BJ, Steinsapir KD, Anders K, et al. Adrenal pathology in the acquired immunodeficiency syndrome. Am J Clin Pathol 1985;84:594–597.
8. Drew WL. Cytomegalovirus infection in patients with AIDS. J Infect Dis 1988;158:449–456.
9. Tapper ML, Rotterdam HZ, Lerner CW, et al. Adrenal necrosis in the acquired immunodeficiency syndrome. Ann Intern Med 1984;100:239–241.
10. Pulakhandam U, Dincsoy HP. Cytomegaloviral adrenalitis and adrenal insufficiency in AIDS. Am J Clin Pathol 1990;93:651–656.
11. Angulo JC, Lopez JI, Flores N. Lethal cytomegalovirus adrenalitis in a case of AIDS. Scand J Urol Nephrol 1994;28:105–106.
12. Bleiweiss IJ, Pervez NK, Hammer GS, et al. Cytomegalovirus-induced adrenal insufficiency and associated renal cell carcinoma in AIDS. Mt Sinai J Med 1986;53:676–679.
13. Edgehl RH, Meguid MM, Aun F. The importance of the endocrine and metabolic responses to shock and trauma. Crit Care Med 1977;5:257–263.
14. Beisel WR. Metabolic response to infection. New York: Grune & Stratton, 1981.
15. Darling G, Goldstein DS, Stull R, et al. Tumor necrosis factor: immune endocrine interaction. Surgery 1989;106:1155–1160.
16. Rivier C, Chizzonite R, Vale W. In the mouse, the activation of the hypothalamic–pituitary–adrenal axis by a lipopolysaccharide (endotoxin) is mediated through interleukin-1. Endocrinology 1989;125:2800–2805.
17. Rivier C. Role of endotoxin and interleukin-1 in modulating ACTH, LH, and sex steroid secretion. Adv Exp Med Biol 1990;274:295–301.
18. Sapolsky R, Rivier C, Yamamoto G, et al. Interleukin-1 stimulates the secretion of hypothalamic corticotropin-releasing factor. Science 1987;238:522–524.
19. Woloski BM, Smith EM, Meyer WJ, et al. Corticotropin-releasing activity of monokines. Science 1985;230:1035–1037.
20. Sibbald WJ, Short A, Cohen MP, et al. Variations in adrenocortical responsiveness during severe bacterial infections. Ann Surg 1977;186:29–33.
21. Osa SR, Peterson RE, Roberts RB. Recovery of adrenal reserve following treatment of disseminated South American blastomycosis. Am J Med 1981;71:298–301.
22. Bosworth DC. Reversible adrenocortical insufficiency in fulminant meningococcemia. Arch Intern Med 1979;139:823–824.
23. Cooke JNC, James VHT, Landon J, et al. Adrenocortical function in chronic malnutrition. Br Med J 1964;1:662–666.
24. Guenthner EE, Rabinowe SL, Van Niel A, et al. Primary Addison's disease in a patient with the acquired immunodeficiency syndrome. Ann Intern Med 1984;100:847–848.
25. Greene LW, Cole W, Greene JB, et al. Adrenal insufficiency as a complication of the acquired immunodeficiency syndrome. Ann Intern Med 1984;101:497–498.
26. Dobs AS, Dempsy MA, Ladenson PW, et al. Endocrine disorders in men infected with the human immunodeficiency virus. Am J Med 1988;84:611–616.
27. Raffi F, Brisseau JM, Planchon B, et al. Endocrine function in 98 HIV infected patients: a prospective study. AIDS 1991;5:729–733.
28. Findling JW, Buggy BP, Gilson IH, et al. Longitudinal evaluation of adrenocortical function in patients infected with the human immunodeficiency virus. J Clin Endocrinol Metab 1994;79:1091–1096.
29. Verges B, Chavanet P, Desgres J, et al. Adrenal function in HIV infected patients. Acta Endocrinol (Copenh) 1989;121:633–637.
30. Villette JM, Bourin P, Doinel C, et al. Circadian variations in plasma levels of hypophyseal, adrenocortical and testicular hormones in men infected with human immunodeficiency virus. J Clin Endocrinol Metab 1990;70:572–577.
31. Membreno L, Irony I, Dere W, et al. Adrenocortical function in acquired immunodeficiency syndrome. J Clin Endocrinol Metab 1987;65:482–487.
32. Hilton CW, Harrington PT, Prasad C, et al. Adrenal insufficiency in the acquired immunodeficiency syndrome. South Med J 1988;81:1493–1495.
33. Christeff N, Gharakhanian S, Thobie N, et al. Evidence for changes in adrenal and testicular steroids during HIV infection. J Acquir Immune Defic Syndr 1992;5:841–846.
34. Biglino A, Limone P, Forno B, et al. Altered adrenocorticotropin and cortisol response to corticotropin-releasing hormone in HIV-1 infection. Eur J Endocrinol 1995;133:173–179.
35. Lortholary O, Christeff N, Casassus P, et al. Hypothalamo–pituitary–adrenal function in human immunodeficiency virus–infected men. J Clin Endocrinol Metab 1996;81:791–796.
36. Laudat A, Blum L, Guechot J, et al. Changes in systemic gonadal and adrenal steroids in asymptomatic human immunodeficiency virus–infected men: relationship with the CD4 cell counts. Eur J Endocrinol 1995;133:418–424.

37. Merenich JA, McDermott MT, Asp AA, et al. Evidence of endocrine involvement early in the course of human immunodeficiency virus infection. J Clin Endocrinol Metab 1990;70:566–570.
38. Azar ST, Melby JC. Hypothalamic–pituitary–adrenal function in non-AIDS patients with advanced HIV infection. Am J Med Sci 1993;305:321–325.
39. Dackis CA, Gurpegui M, Pottash ALC, et al. Methadone induced hypoadrenalism. Lancet 1982;1:1167.
40. Laue L, Pizzo PA, Butler K, et al. Growth and neuroendocrine dysfunction in children with acquired immunodeficiency syndrome. J Pediatr 1990;117:541–545.
41. Oberfield SE, Cowan L, Levine LS, et al. Altered cortisol response and hippocampal atrophy in pediatric HIV disease. J Acquir Immune Defic Syndr Hum Retrovirol 1994;7:57–62.
42. Jacobson MA, Fusaro RE, Galmarini M, et al. Decreased serum dehydroepiandrosterone is associated with an increased progression of human immunodeficiency virus infection in men with CD4 cell counts of 200–499. J Infect Dis 1991;164:864–868.
43. Mulder JW, Jos Frissen PH, Krijnen P, et al. Dehydroepiandrosterone as predictor for progression to AIDS in asymptomatic human immunodeficiency virus–infected men. J Infect Dis 1992;165:413–418.
44. Wisniewski TL, Hilton CW, Morse EV, et al. The relationship of serum DHEAS and cortisol levels to measures of immune function in human immunodeficiency virus–related illness. Am J Med Sci 1993;305:79–83.
45. Honour J, Schneider MA, Miller RF. Low adrenal androgens in men with HIV infection and the acquired immunodeficiency syndrome. Horm Res 1995;44:35–39.
46. Henderson E, Yang J, Schwartz A. Dehydroepiandrosterone (DHEA) and synthetic DHEA analogs are modest inhibitors of HIV-1 III-B replication. AIDS Res Hum Retroviruses 1992;8:625–631.
47. Dyner TS, Lang W, Geaga J, et al. An open-label dose-escalation trial of oral dehydroepiandrosterone tolerance and pharmacokinetics in patients with HIV disease. J Acquir Immune Defic Syndr 1993;6:459–465.
48. Norbiato G, Bevilacqua M, Bago T, et al. Cortisol resistance in acquired immunodeficiency syndrome. J Clin Endocrinol Metab 1992;74:608–613.
49. Norbiato G, Bevilacqua M, Vago T, et al. Glucocorticoid resistance in the acquired immunodeficiency syndrome: effects on the immunosystem. Presented at the 76th annual meeting of the Endocrine Society, Anaheim, CA, 1994.
50. Sellmeyer DE, Grunfeld C. Endocrine and metabolic disturbances in human immunodeficiency virus infection and the acquired immune deficiency syndrome. Endocr Rev 1996;17:518–532.
51. Pont A, Graybill JR, Craven PC, et al. High-dose ketoconazole therapy and adrenal and testicular function in humans. Arch Intern Med 1984;144:2150–2153.
52. Kyriazopoulou V, Parparousi O, Vagenakis AG. Rifampicin-induced adrenal crisis in addisonian patients receiving corticosteroid replacement. J Clin Endocrinol Metab 1984;59:1204–1206.
53. Ediger SK, Isley WL. Rifampicin-induced adrenal insufficiency in the acquired immunodeficiency syndrome: difficulties in diagnosis and treatment. Postgrad Med J 1988;64:405–406.
54. Loprinzi CL, Jensen MD, N Jiang, et al. Effect of megestrol acetate on the human pituitary–adrenal axis. Mayo Clin Proc 1992;67:1160–1162.
55. Guy RJC, Turber Y, Davidson RN, et al. Mineralocorticoid deficiency in HIV infection. Br Med J 1989;298:496–497.
56. Kalin MF, Poretsky L, Seres DS, et al. Hyporeninemic hypoaldosteronism associated with acquired immune deficiency syndrome. Am J Med 1987;82:1035–1038.
57. Appel GB, Neu HC. The nephrotoxicity of antimicrobial agents (third of three parts). N Engl J Med 1977;296:784–787.
58. Schambelan M, Sebastian A, Biglieri EG. Prevalance, pathogenesis, and functional significance of aldosterone deficiency in hyperkalemic patients with chronic renal insufficiency. Kidney Int 1980;17:89–101.
59. Choi MJ, Fernandez PC, Patnaik A, et al. Brief report: trimethoprim-induced hyperkalemia in a patient with AIDS. N Engl J Med 1993;328:703–706.
60. Lachaal M, Venuto RC. Nephrotoxicity and hyperkalemia in patients with acquired immunodeficiency syndrome treated with pentamidine. Am J Med 1989;87:260–263.
61. Ferreiro J, Vinters HV. Pathology of the pituitary gland in patients with the acquired immune deficiency syndrome (AIDS). Pathology 1988;20:211–215.
62. Mosca L, Costanzi G, Antonacci C, et al. Hypophyseal pathology in AIDS. Histol Histopathol 1992;7:291–300.
63. Sano T, Kovacs K, Scheithauer BW, et al. Pituitary pathology in acquired immunodeficiency syndrome. Arch Pathol Lab Med 1989;113:1066–1070.
64. Sie L, Linssen W. Hypophyseal tuberculosis in a patient with AIDS. Clin Infect Dis 1994;19:550–551.
65. Milligan SA, Katz MS, Craven PC, et al. Toxoplasmosis presenting as panhypopituitarism in a patient with the acquired immune deficiency syndrome. Am J Med 1984;77:760–764.
66. Sullivan WM, Kelley GG, O'Connor PG, et al. Hypopituitarism associated with a hypothalamic CMV infection in a patient with AIDS. Am J Med 1992;92:221–223.
67. Gorman JM, Warne PA, Begg MD, et al. Serum prolactin levels in homosexual and bisexual men with HIV infection. Am J Psychiatry 1992;149:367–370.
68. Croxson RS, Chapman WE, Miller KL, et al. Changes in the hypothalamic–pituitary–gonadal axis in human immunodeficiency virus–infected homosexual men. J Clin Endocrinol Metab 1989;68:317–321.
69. Graef AS, Gonzalez SS, Baca VR, et al. High serum prolactin levels in asymptomatic HIV-infected patients and in patients with acquired immunodeficiency syndrome. Clin Immunol Immunopathol 1994;72:390–393.
70. Kaufman FR, Gomperts ED. Growth failure in boys with hemophilia and HIV infection. Am J Pediatr Hematol Oncol 1989;11:292–294.
71. Schwartz LJ, St Louis Y, Wu R, et al. Endocrine function in children with human immunodeficiency virus infection. Am J Dis Child 1991;145:330–333.
72. Matarazzo P, Palomba E, Lala R, et al. Growth impairment, IGF-1 hyposecretion and thyroid dysfunction in children with perinatal HIV-1 infection. Acta Paediatr Scand 1994;83:1029–1034.
73. Hintz RL, Suskind R, Amatayakul E, et al. Plasma somatomedin and growth hormone values in children with protein–calorie malnutrition. J Pediatr 1978;92:153–156.
74. Heijligenberg R, Sauerwein HP, Brabant G, et al. Circadian growth hormone secretion in asymptomatic human immune deficiency virus infection and acquired immunodeficiency syndrome. J Clin Endocrinol Metab 1996;81:4028–4032.
75. Geffner ME, Yeh DY, Landaw EM, et al. In vitro insulin-like growth factor-1, growth hormone, and insulin resistance occurs in symptomatic human immunodeficiency virus-1–infected children. Pediatr Res 1993;34:66–72.
76. Mulligan K, Grunfeld C, Hellerstein M, et al. Anabolic effects of recombinant human growth hormone in patients with wasting associated with human immunodeficiency virus infection. J Clin Endocrinol Metab 1993;77:956–962.
77. Lieberman SA, Butterfield GE, Harrison D, et al. Anabolic effects of recombinant insulin-like growth factor-I in cachectic patients with the acquired immunodeficiency syndrome. J Clin Endocrinol Metab 1994;78:404–410.
78. Frost RA, Fuhrer J, Steigbigel R, et al. Wasting in the acquired immune deficiency syndrome is associated with multiple defects in the serum insulin-like growth factor system. Clin Endocrinol (Oxf) 1996;44:501–514.
79. Grinspoon S, Corcoran C, Lee K, et al. Loss of lean body and muscle mass correlates with androgen levels in hypogonadal men with acquired immunodeficiency syndrome and wasting. J Clin Endocrinol Metab 1996;81:4051–4058.

80. Agarwal A, Soni A, Ciechanowsky M, et al. Hyponatremia in patients with the acquired immunodeficiency syndrome. Nephron 1989;53:317–321.
81. Cusano AJ, Thies HL, Siegal FP, et al. Hyponatremia in patients with acquired immune deficiency syndrome. J Acquir Immune Defic Syndr 1990;3:949–953.
82. Tang WW, Kaptein EM, Feinstein EI, et al. Hyponatremia in hospitalized patients with the acquired immunodeficiency syndrome (AIDS) and the AIDS-related complex. Am J Med 1993;94:169–174.
83. Vitting KE, Gardenswartz MH, Zabetakis PM, et al. Frequency of hyponatremia and nonosmolar vasopressin release in the acquired immunodeficiency syndrome. JAMA 1990;263:973–978.
84. Ahn Y, Goldman JM. Trimethoprim–sulfamethoxazole and hyponatremia. Ann Intern Med 1989;103:161–162.
85. Madhoun ZT, DuBois DB, Rosenthal J, et al. Central diabetes insipidus: a complication of herpes simples type 2 encephalitis in a patient with AIDS. Am J Med 1991;90:658–659.
86. Frank TS, LiVolsi VA, Connor AM. Cytomegalovirus infection of the thyroid in immunocompromised adults. Yale J Biol Med 1987;60:1–8.
87. Battan R, Mariuz P, Raviglione MC, et al. *Pneumocystis carinii* infection of the thyroid in a hypthyroid patient with AIDS: diagnosis by fine needle aspiration biopsy. J Clin Endocrinol Metab 1991;72:724–726.
88. Drucker D, Bailey D, Rotstein L. Thyroiditis as the presenting manifestation of disseminated extrapulmonary *Pneumocystis carinii* infection. J Clin Endocrinol Metab 1990;71:1663–1665.
89. Gallant J, Enriques R, Cohen KL, et al. *Pneumocystis carinii* thyroiditis. Am J Med 1988;84:303–306.
90. Guttler R, Singer PA. *Pneumocystis carinii* thyroiditis: report of three cases and review of the literature. Arch Intern Med 1993;153:393–396.
91. McCarty M, Coker R, Claydon E. Case report: disseminated *Pneumocystis carinii* infection in a patient with the acquired immune deficiency syndrome causing thyroid gland calcification and hypothyroidism. Clin Radiol 1992;45:209–210.
92. Patel A, Sowden D, Kemp R, et al. *Pneumocystis* thyroiditis. Med J Aust 1992;156:136–137.
93. Ragni MV, Dekker A, DeRubertis FR, et al. *Pneumocystis carinii* infection presenting as necrotizing thyroiditis and hypothyroidism. Am J Clin Pathol 1991;95:489–493.
94. Vijayakumar V, Bekerman C, Blend MJ, et al. Role of Ga-67 citrate imaging in extrapulmonary *Pneumocystis* in HIV positive patients. Clin Nucl Med 1993;18:337–338.
95. Walts AE, Pitchon HE. *Pneumocystis carinii* in FNA of the thyroid. Diagn Cytopathol 1991;7:615–617.
96. Spitzer RD, Chan JC, Marks JB, et al. Case report: hypothyroidism due to *Pneumocystis carinii* thyroiditis in a patient with acquired immunodeficiency syndrome. Am J Med Sci 1991;302:98–100.
97. Machac J, Mejatheim M, Goldsmith SJ. Gallium-67 citrate uptake in cryptococcal thyroiditis in a homosexual male. J Nucl Med Allied Sci 1985;29:283–285.
98. Martinez-Ocana JC, Romen J, Llatjos M, et al. Goiter as a manifestation of disseminated aspergillosis in a patient with AIDS. Clin Infect Dis 1993;17:953–954.
99. Mollison LC, Mijch A, McBride G, et al. Hypothyroidism due to destruction of the thyroid by Kaposi's sarcoma. Rev Infect Dis 1991;13:826–827.
100. Krauth PH, Katz J. Kaposi's sarcoma involving the thyroid in a patient with AIDS. Clin Nucl Med 1987;12:848–849.
101. Cavalieri RR. The effects of nonthyroid disease and drugs on thyroid function tests. Med Clin North Am 1991;75:27–39.
102. Wartofsky L, Burman KD. Alterations in thyroid function in patients with systemic illnesses: the euthyroid sick syndrome. Endocr Rev 1982;3:164–217.
103. Gardner DF, Kaplan MM, Stanley CA, et al. Effect of triiodothyronine replacement on the metabolic and pituitary responses to starvation. N Engl J Med 1979;300:579–584.
104. Burman KD, Wartofsky L, Dinterman RE, et al. The effect of T_3 and reverse T_3 administration on muscle protein catabolism during fasting as measured by 3- methylhistidine excretion. Metabolism 1979;28:805–813.
105. Byerley LO, Heber D. Metabolic effects of triiodothyronine replacement during fasting in obese subjects. J Clin Endocrinol Metab 1996;81:968–976.
106. Bourdoux PR, DeWit SA, Servais GM, et al. Biochemical thyroid profile in patients infected with the human immunodeficiency virus. Thyroid 1991;1:147–149.
107. Hommes MJT, Romijn JA, Godfried MH, et al. Increased resting energy expenditure in human immunodeficiency virus–infected men. Metabolism 1990;39:1186–1190.
108. Hommes MJT, Romijn JA, Endert E, et al. Hypothyroid-like regulation of the pituitary–thyroid axis in stable human immunodeficiency virus infection. Metabolism 1993;42:556–561.
109. Olivieri A, Sorcini M, Fazzini C, et al. Thyroid hypofunction related with the progression of human immunodeficiency virus infection. J Endocrinol Invest 1993;16:407–413.
110. Fried JC, LoPresti JS, Micon M, et al. Serum triiodothyronine values: prognostic indicators of acute mortality due to *Pneumocystis carinii* pneumonia associated with the acquired immunodeficiency syndrome. Arch Intern Med 1990;150:406–409.
111. Grunfeld C, Pang M, Doerrler W, et al. Indices of thyroid function and weight loss in human immunodeficiency virus infection and the acquired immunodeficiency syndrome. Metabolism 1993;42:1270–1276.
112. LoPresti JS, Fried JC, Spencer CA, et al. Unique alterations of thyroid hormone indices in the acquired immunodeficiency syndrome. Ann Intern Med 1989;110:970–975.
113. Tang WW, Kaptein EM. Thyroid hormone levels in the acquired immunodeficiency syndrom (AIDS) or AIDS-related complex. West J Med 1989;151:627–631.
114. Grunfeld C, Pang M, Shimizu L, et al. Resting energy expenditure, caloric intake, and short-term weight change in human immunodeficiency virus infection and the acquired immunodeficiency syndrome. Am J Clin Nutr 1992;55:455–460.
115. Lambert M, Zech F, DeNayer P, et al. Elevation of serum thyroxine binding globulin (but not of cortisol binding globulin and sex hormone–binding globulin) associated with the progression of human immunodeficiency virus infection. Am J Med 1990;89:748–751.
116. Isley WL. Effect of rifampin therapy on thyroid function tests in a hypothyroid patient on replacement L-thyroxine. Ann Intern Med 1987;107:517–518.
117. Russell GFM. Psychological and nutritional factors in disturbances of menstrual function and ovulation. Postgrad Med J 1972;48:10–13.
118. Chabon AB, Stenger RJ, Grabstald H. Histopathology of testis in acquired immune deficiency syndrome. Urology 1987;29:658–663.
119. De Paepe ME, Waxman M. Testicular atrophy in AIDS: a study of 57 autopsy cases. Hum Pathol 1989;20:210–214.
120. Reichert CM, O'Leary TJ, Levens DL, et al. Autopsy pathology in the acquired immune deficiency syndrome. Am J Pathol 1983;112:357–382.
121. da Silva M, Shevchuk MM, Cronin WJ, et al. Detection of HIV related protein in testes and prostates of patients with AIDS. Am J Clin Pathol 1990;93:196–201.
122. Martin PM, Gresenguet G, Herve VM, et al. Decreased number of spermatozoa in HIV-1–infected individuals [letter]. AIDS 1992;6:130.
123. Politch JA, Mayer KH, Abbott AF, et al. The effects of disease progression and zidovudine therapy on semen quality in human immunodeficiency virus type 1 seropositive men. Fertil Steril 1994;61:922–928.
124. Crittenden JA, Handelsman DJ, Stewart GJ. Semen analysis in human immunodeficiency virus infection. Fertil Steril 1992;57:1294–1299.

125. Krieger JN, Coombs RW, Collier AC, et al. Fertility parameters in men infected with human immunodeficiency virus. J Infect Dis 1991;164:464–469.
126. Nuovo GJ, Becker J, Simsir A, et al. HIV-1 nucleic acids localize to the spermatogonia and their progeny: a study by polymerase chain reaction in situ hybridization. Am J Pathol 1994;144:1142–1148.
127. Wagner G, Rabkin JG, Rabkin R. Illness stage, concurrent medications, and other correlates of low testosterone in men with HIV illness. J Acquir Immune Defic Syndr Hum Retrovirol 1995;8:204–207.
128. Lefrere JJ, Laplanche JL, Vittecoq D, et al. Hypogonadism in AIDS. AIDS 1988;2:135–136.
129. Smith CG, Asch RH. Drug abuse and reproduction. Fertil Steril 1987;48:355.
130. Dobs AS, Few WL III, Blackman MR, et al. Serum hormones in men with human immunodeficiency virus–associated wasting. J Clin Endocrinol Metab 1996;81:4108–4112.
131. Martin ME, Benassayag C, Amiel C, et al. Alterations in the concentrations and binding properties of sex steroid binding protein and corticosteroid-binding globulin in HIV+ patients. J Endocrinol Invest 1992;15:597–603.
132. Engelson ES, Pi-Sunyer FX, Kotler DP. Effects of megestrol acetate therapy on body composition and circulating testosterone concentrations in patients with AIDS [letter]. AIDS 1995;9:1107–1108.
133. Widy-Wirski R, Berkely S, Downing R, et al. Evaluation of the WHO clinical case definition of AIDS in Uganda. JAMA 1988;260:3286–3289.
134. Shah PN, Smith JR, Wells C, et al. Menstrual symptoms in women infected by the human immunodeficiency virus. Obstet Gynecol 1994;83:397–400.
135. Shelton M, Adams J, Gugino L, et al. Menstrual cycle hormone patterns in HIV infected women. Presented at the 3rd Conference on Retroviruses and Opportunistic Infections, Washington, DC, 1996.
136. Ellerbrock TV, Wright TC, Bush TJ, et al. Characteristics of menstruation in women infected with human immunodeficiency virus. Obstet Gynecol 1996;87:1030–1034.
137. Chirgwin KD, Feldman J, Muneyyirci-Delale O, et al. Menstrual function in human immunodeficiency virus–infected women without acquired immunodeficiency syndrome. J Acquir Immune Defic Syndr Hum Retrovirol 1996;12:489–494.
138. Dowell SF, Moore GW, Hutchins GM. The spectrum of pancreatic pathology in patients with AIDS. Mod Pathol 1990;3:49–53.
139. Desmond NM, Kingdon E, Beale TJ, et al. Tuberculous pancreatic abscess: an unusual manifestation of HIV infection. J R Soc Med 1995;88:109P–110P.
140. Hommes MJT, Romijn JA, Endert E, et al. Insulin sensitivity and insulin clearance in human immunodeficiency virus–infected men. Metabolism 1991;40:651–656.
141. Heyligenberg R, Romijn JA, Hommes JT, et al. Non–insulin-mediated glucose uptake in human immunodeficiency virus–infected men. Clin Sci 1993;84:209–216.
142. Murphey SA, Josephs AS. Acute pancreatitis associated with pentamidine therapy. Arch Intern Med 1981;141:56–58.
143. Salmeron S, Petitpretz P, Katlama C, et al. Pentamidine and pancreatitis. Ann Intern Med 1986;105:140–141.
144. Osei K, Falko JM, Nelson KP, et al. Diabetogenic effect of pentamidine: in vitro and in vivo studies in a patient with malignant insulinoma. Am J Med 1984;77:41–46.
145. Stahl-Bayliss CM, Kalman CM, Laskin OL. Pentamidine-induced hypoglycemia in patients with the acquired immune deficiency syndrome. Clin Pharmacol Ther 1986;39:271–275.
146. Waskin H, Stehr-Green JK, Helmick CG, et al. Risk factors for hypoglycemia associated with pentamidine therapy for Pneumocystis pneumonia. JAMA 1988;260:345–347.
147. Bouchard PH, Sai P, Reach G, et al. Diabetes mellitus following pentamidine-induced hypoglycemia in humans. Diabetes 1982;31:40–45.
148. Perronne C, Bricaire F, Leport C, et al. Hypoglycemia and diabetes mellitus following parenteral pentamidine mesylate treatment in AIDS patients. Diabetic Med 1990;7:585–587.
149. Karboski JA, Godley PJ. Inhaled pentamidine and hypoglycemia. Ann Intern Med 1988;108:490.
150. Chen JP, Braham RL, Squires KE. Diabetes after aerosolized pentamidine. Ann Intern Med 1991;114:913–914.
151. Uzzan B, Bentata M, Campos J, et al. Effects of aerosolized pentamidine on glucose homeostasis and insulin secretion in HIV-positive patients: a controlled study. AIDS 1995;9:901–907.
152. Henry K, Rathgaber S, Sullivan C, et al. Diabetes mellitus induced by megestrol acetate in a patient with AIDS and cachexia. Ann Intern Med 1992;116:53–54.
153. Von Roenn JH, Armstrong D, Kotler DP, et al. Megestrol acetate in patients with AIDS-related cachexia. Ann Intern Med 1994;121:393–399.
154. Lumpkin MM. Reports of diabetes and hyperglycemia in patients receiving protease inhibitors for the treatment of human immunodeficiency virus. Food and Drug Administration public health advisory. Washington, DC: United States Food and Drug Administration, 1997.
155. Adams JS, Fernandez M, Gacad MA, et al. Vitamin D metabolite–mediated hypercalcemia and hypercalciuria patients with AIDS- and non–AIDS-associated lymphoma. Blood 1989;73:235–239.
156. Delahunt JW, Romeril KE. Hypercalcemia in a patient with the acquired immunodeficiency syndrome and Mycobacterium avium intracellulare infection. J Acquir Immune Defic Syndr Hum Retrovirol 1994;7:871–872.
157. Jaeger P, Otto S, Speck RF, et al. Altered parathyroid gland function in severely immunocompromised patients infected with human immunodeficiency virus. J Clin Endocrinol Metab 1994;79:1701–1705.
158. Serrano S, Marinoso ML, Soriano JC, et al. Bone remodelling in human immunodeficiency virus-1–infected patients: a histomorphometric study. Bone 1995;16:185–191.
159. Youle MS, Clarbour J, Gazzard B, et al. Severe hypocalcaemia in AIDS patients treated with foscarnet and pentamidine. Lancet 1988;1:1455–1456.
160. Jacobson MA, Gambertoglio JG, Aweeka FT, et al. Foscarnet-induced hypocalcemia and effects of foscarnet on calcium metabolism. J Clin Endocrinol Metab 1991;72:1130–1135.
161. Gearhart MO, Sorg TB. Foscarnet-induced severe hypomagnesemia and other electrolyte disorders. Ann Pharmacother 1993;27:285–288.
162. Shah GM, Alvarado P, Kirschenbaum MA. Symptomatic hypocalcemia and hypomagnesemia with renal magnesium wasting associated with pentamidine therapy in a patient with AIDS. Am J Med 1990;89:380–382.
163. Burnett RJ, Reenta SB. Severe hypomagnesemia induced by pentamidine. DICP Ann Pharmacother 1990;24:239–240.
164. Anonymous. Foscarnet. Med Lett Drugs Ther 1992;34:3–4.
165. Farese RV, Schambelan M, Hollander H, et al. Nephrogenic diabetes insipidus associated with foscarnet treatment of cytomegalovirus retinitis. Ann Intern Med 1990;112:955–956.
166. Gallis HA, Drew RH, Pickard WW. Amphotericin B: 30 years of clinical experience. Rev Infect Dis 1990;12:308.
167. Glass AR, Eil C. Ketoconazole-induced reduction in serum 1,25-dihydroxyvitamin D. J Clin Endocrinol Metab 1986;63:766–769.
168. Glass AR, Eil C. Ketoconazole-induced reduction in serum 1, 25-dihydroxyvitamin D and total serum calcium in hypercalcemic patients. J Clin Endocrinol Metab 1988;66:937.
169. Brodie MJ, Boobis AR, Dollery CT, et al. Rifampicin and vitamin D metabolism in man [proceedings]. Br J Clin Pharmacol 1980;9:286P–287P.
170. Fisher DA, Pandian MR, Carlton E. Current clinical concepts: vasopressin (antidiuretic hormone). San Juan Capistrano, CA: Nichols Institute, 1986.

39

THE WASTING SYNDROME: PATHOPHYSIOLOGY AND TREATMENT

Carl Grunfeld and Morris Schambelan

The wasting syndrome and the ensuing debilitation that accompanies it are among the most feared and devastating aspects of acquired immunodeficiency syndrome (AIDS). In Africa, where AIDS-related therapies are limited, AIDS is known as "slim disease" because of the unrelenting syndrome of weight loss that frequently precedes death (1). Even in Western societies, where therapies are increasingly successful in the control of opportunistic infections, malignancies, and human immunodeficiency virus (HIV) itself, the wasting syndrome still contributes substantially to morbidity and mortality in AIDS (2–4). Early in the epidemic, the United States Centers for Disease Control and Prevention (CDC) designated weight loss of more than 10% of body weight associated with more than 30 days of fever or diarrhea and the presence of antibody against HIV as a criterion to establish the diagnosis of AIDS, even in the absence of an AIDS-defining infection or malignancy (5). How the new triple antiretroviral regimens with protease inhibitors will affect the wasting syndrome is not yet clear, but impressive weight gain has not been seen in patients enrolled in controlled studies reported to date (6).

Weight loss is also characteristic of other untreated infections and malignancies. Many different metabolic disturbances are found in malignancies and chronic infections, including infection with HIV. Early reports regarding the mechanism of wasting suggested that weight loss was inexorably driven by these changes in metabolism. These concepts were greatly influenced by the hypermetabolic state of sepsis, in which negative nitrogen balance is so profound that it cannot be influenced by nutritional support such as hyperalimentation (7, 8). These prior theories of cachexia combined with the poor quality of life and grave prognosis of AIDS patients with the wasting syndrome led to initial pessimism about reversing the wasting syndrome in AIDS. However, wasting in AIDS should not be compared with sepsis. Data from animal model systems and, in particular, from clinical studies of AIDS itself indicate the following: 1) wasting is not inevitable in AIDS; 2) the body can compensate for many of the metabolic disturbances seen in AIDS; 3) weight loss may be a marker for secondary disease in HIV infection; 4) weight gain can occur with appropriate treatment of underlying conditions; and 5) a role for nutritional support and/or pharmacologic therapy of the wasting syndrome is being developed. This chapter describes the status of our understanding of the wasting syndrome in AIDS.

WEIGHT LOSS, BODY COMPOSITION, AND SURVIVAL

Death from Weight Loss

Starvation leads to death when weight is reduced to below 66% of ideal body weight, even in the absence of other underlying diseases (9–12). Patients with the wasting syndrome who have AIDS (3) also die when body weight reaches similar levels. These studies suggest that the degree of wasting per se is the cause of death rather than the specifics of an underlying disease. Furthermore, if body weight determines time of death, then, in theory, maintaining weight could prolong life.

Epidemiologic studies have demonstrated that the presence of wasting is a strong predictor of death in patients with AIDS (4, 13, 15). In multivarial analysis, wasting is an independent predictor even when the effects of CD4 count and other AIDS-related illnesses are accounted for (13–15). As could be expected, wasting contributes to decreased function in AIDS (16). Furthermore, the presence of wasting in AIDS patients is an independent risk factor for future hospitalization (17).

Body Composition in Disease

Body composition can be separated into multiple compartments. The simplest division is fat-free mass versus fat. Fat-free mass (also called lean body mass) can be divided into the intracellular cellular component (known as body cell mass) and the extracellular component (including intravascular and extravascular fluid and the mineral content of bone). The predominant constituents of body cell mass are muscle, the vital internal organs, and skin. During simple caloric restriction, the tendency is to maximize loss of fat while attempting to minimize loss of muscle (7, 11, 12, 18). The more body fat present at the beginning of weight loss, the higher the ratio of fat to lean body mass that is lost during starvation (18). However, in anorexia nervosa, in which a loss continues far below ideal body weight, but activity continues, body fat is reduced to a minimum (2).

Early studies indicated that in AIDS patients with the wasting syndrome, body fat is more variable (2, 19). Women with the wasting syndrome show dramatic depletion of body fat similar to that seen in anorexia nervosa (2). Men may have relatively more sparing of fat. Early studies of body composition of patients with AIDS included a high proportion of those who were acutely ill, especially with diarrhea; such persons show more loss of lean body mass (2) than would be predicted from caloric restriction alone (18). However, when AIDS patients are studied during clinically stable periods after having lost weight (20–22), their losses of fat and lean body mass are consistent with those predicted from starvation (18).

In acutely ill patients, in whom body cell mass may be more depleted, body cell mass becomes a more reliable predictor of death than weight in the wasting syndrome of AIDS, with death occurring at 54% of ideal body cell mass (3). Likewise, muscle mass is an excellent predictor of death in cancer with the wasting syndrome (23). Finally, loss of body cell mass best correlates with decreased function in AIDS (16).

In sepsis and some cancers, aggressive alimentation can restore body fat, but it has no effect on maintaining positive nitrogen balance (8, 24). Likewise, hyperalimentation of AIDS patients with inadequately treated secondary infection increases body fat without increasing body cell mass (25). These findings on alimentation, combined with the strong relation between body cell mass and death, suggest that optimal therapy directed at the wasting syndrome should induce positive nitrogen balance and increase body cell mass rather than fat. As discussed in this chapter, the efficacy of alimentation may be better in patients with AIDS and gastrointestinal disease.

MECHANISMS AND MEDIATORS OF WASTING

Energy Balance and Weight Loss

To maintain body weight, energy expenditure must be equal to caloric intake. Energy expenditure includes the needs of metabolism as well as activity. When caloric intake exceeds energy expenditure, the excess energy is stored as body fat or as body cell mass. When caloric intake is less than energy expenditure (because of either a decrease in caloric intake or an increase in energy expenditure), the body converts its tissue components into energy to supply the extra needs. In health, the body preferentially uses fat to provide this energy (7, 9, 11, 12, 18). However, in many diseases (of which sepsis is the most clear-cut), body cell mass is rapidly depleted to provide these energy needs (7, 8).

Caloric intake can be decreased in disease by multiple mechanisms, most of which can be found in AIDS. Anorexia is a common component of illnesses such as infection, cancer, and depression. Fatigue and dementia can prevent patients from obtaining adequate food. Mechanical obstruction can occur when gastrointestinal lesions prevent adequate food intake. Finally, malabsorption may contribute to decreased nutrient availability.

Likewise, many metabolic disturbances are present that could contribute to excess use of energy or wasting of protein (body cell mass). Sepsis and many malignant diseases are characterized by hypermetabolism, in particular, an increase in resting energy expenditure. During infection, the substrates of intermediary metabolism may be involved in substrate cycles (formerly called futile cycles) that waste energy. Substrates may also be inappropriately used by less efficient pathways. Finally, investigators have postulated that the body may specifically increase its breakdown of protein to provide energy during infection. As outlined later in this chapter, it has now become apparent that the body is able to compensate for many of these changes in metabolism, and more than one defect may be necessary for significant wasting to occur.

Cytokines as Mediators of Metabolic Disturbances and Wasting

The degree of metabolic disturbances and the rate of wasting in infection and cancer do not correlate with the amount of infective burden or with tumor size (26). In addition, many of the metabolic disturbances that occur during infection can be reproduced by injection of bacterial fragments (27, 28). Therefore, investigators long have postulated that the disturbances in metabolism and wasting are due to the host response to infection. More recent data indicate that these metabolic changes are mediated by cytokines, the normal mediators of the host immune response (29).

Fat Cell Catabolism and the Cachectin Hypothesis

The search for a cytokine mediator of wasting began with the cachectin hypothesis (30). Noting that infections characterized by weight loss are also accompanied by severe hypertriglyceridemia, Beutler and Cerami found, in an animal parasitic infection, that the hypertriglyceridemia of infection was accompanied by reduced clearance of triglyceride-rich lipoproteins because of a decrease in lipoprotein lipase, the enzyme responsible for clearance of triglycerides (30). These investigators showed that supernatants from activated macrophages induced broad catabolic effects in cultured fat cells, including reductions in lipoprotein lipase activity, decreased synthesis of fatty acids, and increased lipolysis (the breakdown of stored triglyceride). These supernatants also induced weight loss when given daily to rodents. These researchers therefore postulated that a single factor, which they named "cachectin," promoted weight loss by its catabolic effects on adipose tissue. When the cachectin factor was purified based on its ability to inhibit lipoprotein lipase, it was found to be the cytokine tumor necrosis factor (TNF) (30).

The availability of recombinant cytokines allowed further exploration of this catabolic model. Purified TNF was shown to have the same activity as "cachectin" in cultured fat cells, decreasing lipoprotein lipase activity and fatty acid synthesis while promoting lipolysis (29, 31). However, other cytokines, including interleukin-1 (IL-1), IL-6, leukemia-inhibiting factor (LIF), and interferon-α, β, and γ share many or all of these catabolic effects in cultured fat cells (29, 31–35). Thus, if promoting fat cell catabolism is the mechanism by which cachexia occurs, then multiple cytokines could be considered cachectins.

As discussed earlier, adipose tissue depletion is variable in the wasting syndrome, and increased alimentation often leads to effective storage of fat during cachexia (7, 8, 24, 25). When investigators demonstrated that the ability of cytokines to promote fat cell catabolism in vitro could not be reversed by insulin (29, 31), the major hormone promoting fat storage, it became clear that the original cultured fat cell model did not adequately represent the metabolic disturbances that occur in vivo.

Cytokines and In Vivo Lipid Metabolism

Both TNF and IL-1 induce rapid increases in plasma triglycerides when given to rats and mice (36–40). TNF has also been shown to increase plasma triglycerides in monkeys and humans (41–43).

The mechanism of cytokine-induced hypertriglyceridemia has been studied extensively in rodents. In contrast to what was found using cultured fat cells, TNF has little effect on lipoprotein lipase activity in vivo under conditions in which serum triglycerides are increased (28, 44–46). In fact, TNF, IL-1, and IL-6 are not able to induce a decrease in triglyceride clearance (38, 39, 46). Rather, these and other cytokines including LIF, ciliary neurotropic factor, nerve growth factor, and keratinocyte growth factor increase plasma triglycerides by increasing hepatic fatty acid synthesis and production rates of very low density lipoprotein (VLDL), a triglyceride-rich lipoprotein (29, 36, 39, 41). The doses required for TNF and IL-1 to stimulate hepatic fatty acid synthesis are similar to those that induce fever, that is, endogenous pyrogen activity. Indeed, the induction of hypertriglyceridemia is one of the most sensitive host responses to endotoxin, with the median effective dose occurring at 1/500,000 the median lethal dose for endotoxin (47). At these low doses, endotoxin increases serum triglycerides by increasing VLDL production, a finding suggesting that the normal host response to infection would induce an increase in hepatic lipogenesis (47). At least two other cytokines, IL-6 and interferon-α, have also been shown to increase hepatic fatty acid synthesis (48, 49).

Under certain circumstances, hepatic fatty acid synthesis is an example of inappropriate use of substrate, which could theoretically contribute to wasting. The synthesis of fatty acid from glucose (de novo lipogenesis) is a mechanism for converting excess energy from glucose into fatty acid for more efficient storage as triglyceride. On a weight basis, triglyceride stores more energy than glycogen. However, the synthesis of fatty acid from glucose uses 30% of the glucose calories to perform the synthesis, storing only 70% of the calories in the fatty acid and glycerol that are synthesized. In a state such as cachexia, wherein the body should be repleting muscle (body cell mass) or at least attempting to minimize negative nitrogen balance rather than storing fat, increased de novo synthesis of fatty acids in the liver could be inappropriate.

Another TNF-induced change in lipid metabolism could also contribute to energy wasting. TNF acutely mobilizes free fatty acids from peripheral fat stores (50). The fatty acids are returned to the liver where they are reesterified into triglyceride, which, in turn, provides more substrate to increase VLDL production. This VLDL then returns to the periphery, where its triglyceride is broken down by lipoprotein lipase, and the free fatty acids are stored again inside the fat cell as triglyceride. Every time triglyceride is synthesized from fatty acids (whether in the liver or the fat cell), energy is used. In the optimal condition, fatty acid should be stored as triglyceride in adipose tissue and muscle when excess food is eaten, and it should be called out only when its energy is needed. The futile cycle, in which fatty acids derived from lipolysis return to the liver, are reesterified into triglyceride, and are sent back to the fat cell for restorage, wastes energy with each extra cycle. Fatty acid–triglyceride substrate (futile) cycling has also been found in sepsis (51). Such substrate cycling of fatty acid and triglyceride could contribute to wasting by increasing energy expenditure.

TNF-Induced Changes in Lipid Metabolism Do Not Drive Wasting

As noted earlier, crude preparations of cachectin (endotoxin-stimulated macrophage supernatants) induced progressive weight loss when injected on a daily basis into rodents (30, 52). However, when rats were given daily or even twice-daily injections of pure recombinant TNF, the rats initially lost weight but then rapidly regained it (29, 53–61). The TNF-induced weight loss was secondary to decreased food intake, decreased water intake, and increased urine output (60). With the development of tachyphylaxis to these effects of TNF, rodents gained weight. Thus, the syndrome of cachexia first demonstrated with crude cachectin could not be reproduced with injections of pure TNF.

However, rats do not become resistant to all the actions of TNF. A striking finding was that long-term TNF treatment produced persistent hypertriglyceridemia despite weight gain (60). Thus, the TNF-induced disturbances in lipid metabolism that lead to hypertriglyceridemia are not sufficient to cause wasting. This experiment led to the necessity of reexamining whether any specific metabolic disturbance, which could *theoretically* contribute to weight loss, was indeed the cause of the wasting syndrome in AIDS.

Cytokines and Hypertriglyceridemia in AIDS

Like other chronic infections, AIDS is accompanied by significant hypertriglyceridemia (62, 63). Multiple disturbances in triglyceride metabolism contribute to the hypertriglyceridemia of AIDS. First, patients with AIDS show decreased levels of lipoprotein lipase and a striking decrease in triglyceride clearance (62). Second, patients with AIDS and HIV infection show increased hepatic lipogenesis in the fasting state and after feeding (64). Finally, plasma-free fatty acids are elevated, and fatty acid turnover may be increased in AIDS (64, 65), findings that raise the possibility of futile cycling of fatty acid and triglyceride.

Although an initial study reported increased TNF levels in AIDS (66), multiple other laboratories have not found significant elevations of unbound or bioactive serum TNF levels in patients with AIDS (63, 64, 67–70). However, AIDS patients do have high levels of interferon-α in their circulation (63, 64, 69). A significant correlation exists between serum triglyceride levels and serum interferon-α levels in AIDS and HIV infection (63, 69). When the metabolic changes that produce hypertriglyceridemia are studied, one sees even a higher correlation between interferon-α levels and both the decrease in triglyceride clearance and the increase in fasting de novo hepatic fatty acid synthesis (63, 64). When AIDS patients with both elevated triglyceride and interferon-α levels receive new antiretroviral therapy, the levels of interferon-α and triglycerides fall in parallel (71). Some assays that measure total TNF detect small but significant increases in circulating TNF in AIDS (72–74). However, AIDS is also accompanied by an increase in circulating soluble TNF receptors (73–79). Because the level of receptor is several logs higher than that of total TNF (74), circulating TNF is bound and is not bioactive. No correlation exists between levels of triglycerides and levels of TNF or TNF receptors (63, 64, 79).

These studies suggest that circulating interferon-α contributes to hypertriglyceridemia in AIDS, but a direct causal relationship has not yet been established. Interferon-α has been shown to increase hepatic lipogenesis in rodents (48). Treatment with interferon-α induces hypertriglyceridemia in humans with certain diseases such as skin disorders, but not in those with malignant disease (80–83). However, perhaps interferon-α represents a marker for immune activation, and another cytokine is the cause of hypertriglyceridemia.

Disturbances in Triglyceride Metabolism Do Not Predict Weight Loss in AIDS

AIDS is accompanied by disturbances in lipid metabolism that could potentially contribute to wasting. These include decreased storage of triglyceride in fat cells resulting from decreased lipoprotein lipase, inappropriate use of substrate secondary to increased de novo hepatic fatty acid synthesis, and potentially increased fatty acid–triglyceride futile cycling (63–65). Nevertheless, as seen in animal models, no relationship exists between the presence of hypertriglyceridemia and the presence of wasting in AIDS (62). Although half the patients in one study had hypertriglyceridemia and half had wasting as analyzed by body cell mass, no correlation was found between triglycerides and wasting (62). More important, when patients with hypertriglyceridemia were followed-up, they all showed persistent hypertriglyceridemia, but most showed stable weight and body cell mass for several months (62). These data suggest that humans can compensate for infection-induced disturbances in lipid metabolism; hypertriglyceridemia is not invariably associated with wasting.

ENERGY BALANCE AND WASTING IN AIDS

Hypermetabolism in Diseases with Wasting

Hypermetabolism, particularly in the basal state (increased resting energy expenditure), has been found in many diseases with wasting. The most striking hypermetabolism is found in sepsis or burns (8, 9, 84, 85). In some severe cases, negative nitrogen balance and even weight loss continue in the face of aggressive hyperalimentation (8). In contrast, not all malignant diseases are accompanied by hypermetabolism (86–90), and in some of these malignancies decreased food intake is the dominant cause of weight loss, so normal nitrogen balance can be restored with any type of alimentation (91). The range of metabolic disturbances clearly depends on the nature of the infection or the malignancy.

The exact causes of hypermetabolism have not yet been delineated for any disease. Among the potential contributors are futile cycling, inappropriate use of substrates, and uncoupling of enzymatic events from energy formation. Although these processes clearly waste energy and are usually found in diseases associated with hypermetabolism, limited data indicate that the quantitative contribution of a given pathway is small. For example, fatty acid–triglyceride futile cycling contributes less than 15% of the increased resting energy expenditure seen in sepsis (51). The caloric contribution of increased de novo hepatic lipogenesis would be even less (64). In theory, one should be able to compensate for the increased use of energy found in hypermetabolism with increased caloric intake, suggesting that hypermetabolism itself, like the defects in lipid metabolism, would not be sufficient to drive wasting directly. However, the metabolic disturbances underlying hypermetabolism may contribute to disproportionate use of protein or body cell mass to meet these needs.

Hypermetabolism Is Common in AIDS and HIV Infection

Multiple studies have found that resting energy expenditure is elevated in HIV infection and AIDS (65, 68, 92–99). A striking finding was that asymptomatic patients with HIV infection who had normal CD4 lymphocyte counts also showed a significant increase in resting energy expenditure (92). Because many of the underlying metabolic disturbances that contribute to hypermetabolism have been shown to be part of the host response and are not due to the metabolic requirements of the invading pathogen, hypermetabolism early in the course of HIV infection probably is a marker for the host immune response to HIV. Therefore, HIV likely is not latent during this early period, but the hypermetabolism likely reflects the attempt of the body to contain the virus.

Resting energy expenditure is increased early in HIV infection, and this expenditure appears to increase further with the progression to AIDS (94). Resting energy expenditure shows a significant but weak ($r = .4$) correlation with HIV viral load (100). Patients with secondary opportunistic and bacterial infections may have even higher resting energy expenditure (94, 95). Therefore, perhaps undetected secondary infections are responsible for some of the increase in resting energy expenditure seen in AIDS (94, 95).

Despite dramatic increases in resting energy expenditure, most patients with AIDS do not have short-term weight loss. In several studies, the weight of most patients with HIV infection or with AIDS by CDC criteria was stable in the absence of secondary infections despite elevated resting energy expenditure (68, 94, 97). Thus, just as the metabolic disturbances that cause hypertriglyceridemia in animals (60) and in patients with AIDS (62) do not inevitably cause wasting, neither does hypermetabolism, a broad-based indicator of underlying metabolic disturbances.

Not all patients with AIDS show increased resting energy expenditure (96, 99, 101, 102). Indeed, the variance is wider in AIDS (102), so individual patients may have reduced levels (99, 101, 102). Hypometabolism may be more common in subjects with gastrointestinal disease or malabsorption (99, 101), as discussed later.

Role of Secondary Infection and Anorexia in the Weight Loss of AIDS

Although many patients with AIDS and HIV infection have stable weights, weight loss is extremely prominent in patients with AIDS who have active secondary infection. In one study, patients lost an average of 5% of their body weight in 28 days during episodes of secondary infection (94). The link between secondary infection and rapid weight loss in AIDS has been confirmed in a prospective study (103). A cohort of patients was followed prospectively with frequent recording of individual weight. Thirty-three acute episodes of weight loss (defined as more than 4 kg of body weight in less than 4 months) were identified. Of those acute weight loss episodes, 82% were clearly associated with (nongastrointestinal) secondary infections (103). Likewise, weight gain was often associated with recovery from opportunistic infection (103).

An increase in resting energy expenditure could not account for the episodes of weight loss (94, 97). Subjects with AIDS and HIV infection who had stable weight maintained relatively normal caloric intake per kilogram of body weight (68, 94, 97). However, AIDS patients with active secondary infection and rapid weight loss had marked anorexia (94, 97). With successful treatment of secondary infections, patients increased their caloric intake and gained weight (94, 97). As a consequence, weight change in patients with AIDS correlates highly with caloric intake.

The response to decreased caloric intake in normal subjects includes a decrease in resting energy expenditure (7, 11, 12). In patients with AIDS and secondary infection, increased resting energy expenditure continues in the face of striking decreases in caloric intake (94, 97), a phenomenon similar to the maladaption seen when starvation is followed by sepsis (7, 12). Patients with AIDS and weight loss are not truly hypermetabolic in terms of total energy expenditure (97). They show decreased total energy expenditure (97), but their caloric intake is less than that needed to cover their needs (97). Indeed, their caloric intake may be less than even their elevated resting energy expenditure (94, 97), let alone their total needs, which include diet-induced thermogenesis (104) and energy expended in activity (97).

Protein Wasting

In highly catabolic states such as sepsis or burns, protein catabolism is greatly accelerated, a phenomenon that is not driven by decreases in caloric intake (7, 12). In normal subjects, long-term decreases in caloric intake lead to sparing of muscle protein in parallel to the decrease in resting energy expenditure discussed earlier (7, 11, 12). The presence of overwhelming infection or burns clearly overrides these compensatory mechanisms, leading to accelerated protein loss as well as hypermetabolism. On the other hand, in certain malignant diseases, negative nitrogen balance is purely the result of decreased food intake, and aggressive alimentation can return disturbances in protein metabolism to normal (105).

The data on protein metabolism in AIDS are limited and contradictory. In one study of AIDS patients in the absence of secondary infection, tracer studies found that both protein synthesis and protein degradation were nearly equally depressed, a pattern more consistent with chronic starvation than the increased turnover of sepsis (106). However, a decrease in the protein synthetic rate could be harmful in the long run, because it could impede the rebuilding of body cell mass that is lost during secondary infection. In another study, urinary nitrogen loss was not accelerated in HIV infection, in AIDS in the absence of secondary infection, or in AIDS in patients with secondary infection (107). However, given the decreased caloric (and protein) intake during secondary infection, those AIDS patients with secondary infection were in striking net negative nitrogen balance (99, 107). A third study, using a different tracer technique, found increases in both protein synthesis and protein degradation (108). Provision of extra calories, however, induced positive protein balance (108). A fourth study found that provision of increased amino acids to patients with AIDS acutely improved whole-body protein balance by improving synthesis (109). Probably, varying degrees of protein loss occur in AIDS, such that some losses can be reversed by caloric intake, whereas in other states, true accelerated protein turnover may be seen. More studies need to be performed during secondary infections and weight loss.

Weight Loss and Cytokines

The underlying mechanisms behind the weight loss and negative nitrogen balance of infection (or cancer) are not yet understood. Cytokines likely play a role in these processes because the systemic administration of cytokines produces symptoms typical of infection including fever, myalgia, nausea, anorexia, fatigue, and lethargy; higher doses produce hypotension and shock (110). TNF has been shown to decrease gastric motility, causing food retention in the upper gastrointestinal tract (53, 111), a phenomenon that could contribute to anorexia. Other studies have demonstrated that administration of IL-1, interferon-α, interferon-γ, and transforming growth factor-β (TGF-β) can lead to anorexia and weight loss (112–117). The mechanisms by which cytokines induce anorexia are not fully understood. The most studied cytokine, IL-1, induces changes in the feeding control areas of the hypothalamus, such as increasing corticotropin-releasing factor levels, that would promote anorexia (118). IL-1 and other cytokines acutely increase the levels of leptin (119, 120), a hormone synthesized in fat cells that regulates food intake and energy expenditure (121). Inappropriately elevated levels of leptin could falsely signal satiety, causing anorexia. However, leptin levels are not increased in patients with AIDS during secondary infection or weight loss (122, 123).

Animal tumor models have suggested that TNF, interferon-γ, IL-6, or LIF may contribute to the cachexia syndrome (124–129). However, serum TNF levels are not elevated in adult humans with malignant disease (130–133). Administration of a single cytokine often results in rapid tachyphylaxis to its anorectic and cachectic effects (29, 53–61, 114, 115). Antibodies against single cytokines are only partially able to reverse the weight loss seen in tumor animal models (124–127).

These findings with single cytokine administration and anticytokine therapy suggest that no single cytokine is responsible for the complete syndrome of cachexia, and synergy among cytokines is required for significant wasting. This hypothesis is consistent with the concept that the body has mechanisms to compensate for metabolic disturbances such as hypertriglyceridemia and hypermetabolism. When multiple stimuli perturb metabolism by different mechanisms, the body cannot adequately compensate, and wasting ensues.

Models for cytokine synergy have been developed. Doses of TNF and IL-1 that have little effect on their own produce shock when infused together (134). Likewise, the combined infusion of TNF and IL-1 promotes negative nitrogen balance, increased glucose recycling, muscle catabolism, and hypermetabolism (135, 136).

The possibility that synergy among cytokines is responsible for the rapid weight loss in AIDS during secondary infection must be raised, although definitive data are lacking. As discussed earlier, patients with AIDS often have long-term elevation of one cytokine, interferon-α. During secondary infection, monokines such as TNF and IL-1 likely are secreted. However, some, but not all, investigators have found increased circulating TNF levels in AIDS patients with secondary infection (66, 94). Although interferon-α has metabolic properties similar to those of TNF and IL-1, such as stimulating hepatic lipogenesis (48), interferon-α works by a different mechanism than TNF or IL-1. As a consequence, interferon-α is synergistic with TNF and IL-1 in its metabolic effects (137). Thus, the possibility must be raised that when multiple cytokines disturb metabolism, the body cannot develop tachyphylaxis or adequate compensatory changes. More detailed discussions of cytokine synergy in animal models of wasting have been published (29, 138, 139).

Catabolic hormones such as glucocorticoids, glucagon, and especially catecholamines have been shown to play an important role in the hypermetabolism and metabolic disturbances of sepsis (84). However, the available data suggest that catecholamines, glucocorticoids, and glucagon are not above normal in AIDS (68). Small but statistically significant increases in plasma cortisol can occur (see Chap. 38). Likewise, acute sepsis and injury are characterized by insulin resistance (140, 141); however, patients with HIV infection show increased insulin sensitivity (142). During acute illness or caloric deprivation, one mechanism by which the body conserves protein and energy is by decreasing the conversion of thyroxine to triiodothyronine, a phenomenon known as the "euthyroid sick syndrome" (143). Although patients with HIV infection and AIDS who are in stable condition have normal triiodothyronine levels, those with anorexia and weight loss have decreased circulating triiodothyronine (107). However, this decrease in triiodothyronine is not sufficient to block the protein wasting that occurs in AIDS during secondary infection (107).

Gastrointestinal Disease and Weight Loss

Intermittent or chronic diarrhea is common in AIDS. Diarrhea along with weight loss establishes the diagnosis of AIDS in the absence of AIDS-indicating infections or malignancies (5). The gastrointestinal tract is affected by opportunistic infections, malignant diseases, and HIV itself during the course of AIDS. As a consequence, small intestinal or colonic injury may contribute to nutritional abnormalities in AIDS. Diseases affecting the gastrointestinal tract in AIDS are discussed in detail in Chapters 21 and 33.

The mechanisms by which gastrointestinal disease affects nutrition in AIDS are complex. First, gastrointestinal infection, particularly with cytomegalovirus or with *Mycobacterium avium* complex (MAC), may represent a systemic infection that leads to the rapid weight loss syndrome because of a secondary infection (94, 103). However, a second syndrome of wasting has also been described in which weight loss is much slower, that is, more than 4 kg in more than 4 months (103). When those patients with slower weight loss were examined, 65% had gastrointestinal disease, often accompanied by diarrhea (103).

Damage to the intestinal tract may lead to malabsorption or diarrhea, which, in turn, may contribute to this weight loss. Partial villous atrophy has been reported in the gastrointestinal tract of patients with HIV infection and AIDS (144–147). One group reported an association between villous atrophy and malabsorption (146). The presence of villous atrophy has also been reported to correlate with gut protozoal infections (144); however, other investigators have not found such an association (147). Intestinal pathogens associated with these changes include the agents of cryptosporidiosis, isosporiasis, microsporidiosis, and cytomegalovirus infection. MAC leads to a different lesion characterized by infiltration of the lamina propria and intestinal lymphatics with macrophages, producing a physical block to absorption and exudative enteropathy (148). In Africa, most patients dying of AIDS and severe cachexia now have disseminated *Mycobacterium tuberculosis* infection on autopsy (G Griffin, unpublished data).

In one study, 50% of patients with HIV infection and chronic diarrhea had enteric pathogens evident on endoscopy that were undetected by routine stool studies (147). In contrast, fewer than 10% of AIDS patients without diarrhea had intestinal pathogens. The presence of diarrhea and intestinal pathogens indicated a poor prognosis because these patients had greater weight loss and shorter survival than those who had diarrhea and no identified pathogens (147). Diarrhea and small intestinal injury accompanied by no identifiable pathogen has been termed "AIDS enteropathy" (149). HIV itself can infect the gastrointestinal tract (149–153). Whether AIDS enteropathy is due to intestinal infection with HIV or to other not yet identified pathogenic factors is unknown.

Malabsorption

Investigators often presume that the mechanism by which gastrointestinal disease leads to wasting is by malabsorption of nutrients. Villous atrophy and other functional defects of pathogen-damaged cells are often accompanied by nutrient malabsorption (154). One group noted an association between the presence of villous atrophy and significant malabsorption in AIDS (146). Villous atrophy decreases the surface area through which nutrient absorption occurs. This lesion may be accompanied by compensatory crypt hyperplasia with rapid turnover of epithelial cells leading to a functional immaturity of the epithelia. As a consequence, the epithelial cells have decreased levels of the enzymes involved in metabolism of peptides and complex sugars such as lactose and sucrose (155).

Malabsorption, as indicated by abnormal functional tests or stool composition, is commonly found in AIDS, but it has not been definitively linked to identifiable intestinal pathogens (98, 156–162). For example, malabsorption of D-xylose and vitamin B_{12}, abnormal lactose breath tests, steatorrhea, and bile salt deconjugation have been reported in AIDS, but these abnormalities may occur in the absence of significant intestinal disease (98, 156–162). Abnormalities in sugar and fat absorption are found in patients who do not have diarrhea (156, 157). Malabsorption of vitamin B_{12} may occur early in the course of HIV infection, before the development of AIDS-indicating illnesses (156–159).

More important from the viewpoint of the mechanisms underlying wasting, significant malabsorption in terms of abnormal diagnostic tests may occur in the absence of wasting (156, 157). In fact, HIV-infected children with measurable malabsorption are capable of normal growth patterns, a sensitive indicator of adequate nutrition (156). Thus, the body appears to have mechanisms to adapt to malabsorption, just as it can adapt to metabolic disturbances such as hypermetabolism. One potential mechanism for compensatory adaptation to malabsorption has been reported. A cohort of adult patients with malabsorption but stable weight was reported to be hypometabolic (101). Another group of AIDS patients with protozoal infections of the gastrointestinal tract was also found to have lower resting energy expenditure (99). Thus, these patients may be able to maintain weight or to minimize loss by decreasing energy expenditure in a manner similar to that seen in normal subjects in response to decreased nutrient intake (7, 11, 12).

Malabsorption of nutrients itself may not be the major contributor to weight loss. Significant malabsorption leads to diarrhea. In other diseases, weight loss correlates better with the presence of diarrhea than with abnormal malabsorption tests. Patients with significant diarrhea decrease their food intake, perhaps to minimize their symptoms. (An increase in food input over time could compensate for malabsorption.) Diarrhea is prominent in patients with AIDS who have gastrointestinal disease and a slow course of wasting (103). A trend toward decreased food intake was found in AIDS patients with the slow weight loss syndrome (97). A preliminary report suggests that steatorrhea is common in AIDS patients with severe diarrhea or weight loss (162). The relative contributions of decreased food intake, malabsorption, and changes in resting energy expenditure must be more thoroughly evaluated in patients with AIDS and wasting from gastrointestinal disease.

CLINICAL APPROACH AND TREATMENT

Importance of Documenting Weight Trends in the Management of Patients

Data presented here and elsewhere (94, 103) indicate that rapid weight loss (more than 4 kg in less than 4 months) is frequently (82% of episodes) due to secondary infection. Slower weight loss (more than 4 kg in more than 4 months) may result from (65% of cases) gastrointestinal disease manifested by diarrhea and malabsorption (103). As a consequence, investigators have proposed that patients with HIV infection or AIDS should have their weights measured frequently and recorded on a graph kept in their clinical record (163). Graphic presentation of weights should permit accurate assessment of the rate of weight loss and should direct the clinician toward the proper workup for infection or gastrointestinal disease. For children with HIV infection, measuring length or height, a standard in pediatric practice, may be the most sensitive measure of wasting (164). Sophisticated assessment of body composition may provide further sensitivity in detecting the deleterious changes in nutritional status (2, 13, 163).

Nutritional Status Improves with Treatment of Infection

Episodes of weight gain occur frequently in the recovery period after treatment of secondary infection (94, 97, 103). In one study, when patients who received alimentation were excluded, nearly all the weight gain occurred after treatment of infection (103). Patients with cytomegalovirus infection who are treated with ganciclovir show increases in body weight, body cell mass, body fat, and serum albumin, whereas untreated historic controls showed worsening of nutritional status (165). Investigators have suggested that ganciclovir treatment also prolongs the survival of cytomegalovirus-infected patients (166). However, the efficacy of treatment of systemic cytomegalovirus remains controversial (see Chap. 23). Treatment of HIV infection itself with antiretroviral drugs may also lead to weight gain. The institution of zidovudine therapy in HIV-infected patients led to an average weight gain of 3 kg (167). Surprisingly, preliminary data from controlled studies of potent suppression of HIV load with three antiretroviral agents including a protease inhibitor do not show more impressive gains (6), despite anecdotes of large weight gain.

However, existing data suggest that recovery from bouts of weight loss after infection is usually not complete (97, 103, 139). The result is net long-term weight loss over the course of AIDS. As detailed later, a rationale for therapeutic interventions specifically aimed at the wasting syndrome may be indicated even in patients whose wasting is due to intermittent secondary infection.

Treatment of Gastrointestinal Disease

Pathologic lesions of the oral mucosa (see Chap. 32) and of the esophagus (see Chap. 33) can lead to decreased food intake. Dysphagia from invasive candidiasis is amenable to antifungal treatment (see Chap. 22). Early endoscopic examination or presumptive treatment of patients with dysphagia should be considered.

The situation is more complex with regard to small intestinal and colonic pathogens. Trimethoprim–sulfamethoxazole is effective in the treatment of isosporiasis, but long-term suppressive therapy is required. No effective treatment is known for cryptosporidiosis or microsporidiosis. For these two latter diseases and for idiopathic diarrhea, symptomatic antidiarrheal therapy is indicated but not always effective. Multiple trials are in progress to determine the most efficacious treatment of MAC (see Chap. 17). Idiopathic diarrhea may be self-limiting, with weight loss occurring only during severe symptomatic episodes (168, 169).

Successful treatment of gastrointestinal pathogens may take extended periods during which weight loss progresses. As seen with acute secondary infection, the recovery from the slower weight loss that results from gastrointestinal disease may also not be complete (103). Therefore, the use of supplemental alimentation and other therapeutic modalities should be considered during the course of treatment of patients with AIDS and chronic gastrointestinal disease.

Alimentation in Patients with Malignant Disease

Pessimism about the efficacy of aggressive alimentation has been due in part to the results reported in patients with malignant disease. Because of the decrease in nutritional intake seen during cancer chemotherapy, several groups have examined the ability of hyperalimentation during chemotherapy to prolong survival in cancer patients. A meta-analysis suggests that hyperalimentation during chemotherapy decreases long-term survival, perhaps by promoting tumor growth (170). The risk of infection is increased fourfold in cancer patients receiving hyperalimentation during chemotherapy (170). The risk of infection may also be increased in patients with AIDS who receive parenteral hyperalimentation (171, 172), but it can be minimized with careful training (173).

In the absence of chemotherapy, two patterns of response to alimentation occur that are more relevant to the circumstances of AIDS. Although hyperalimentation of patients with lymphoma leads to significant weight gain, this gain represents primarily body fat with no significant increase in muscle mass (24). In contrast, patients with gastric or esophageal carcinoma (conditions associated with significant decreases in food intake) showed improvement in protein balance with any form of vigorous alimentation (105). These studies suggest that, under specific circumstances during malignant disease (i.e., decreased food intake), therapy with enteral or parenteral alimentation is effective in treating cancer-related cachexia.

Studies of Alimentation in AIDS

Only a few studies document the response to alimentation in patients with AIDS. Data available to date suggest some limited efficacy of alimentary therapy. In one study, 8 patients with wasting were given enteral alimentation by percutaneous gastrostomy (174). In this small group, 6 patients had eating or swallowing disorders associated with neurologic disease, and 1 had a deep painful esophageal ulcer. The eighth patient had MAC infection. These patients showed a 3-kg weight gain over 2 months. Increased body cell mass accounted for much of this gain (174). In another study of unselected AIDS patients with the wasting syndrome, enteral alimentation induced fat storage rather than muscle formation (175). In a third study of gastrostomy feeding, only 6 out of 10 subjects tolerated feeding; they gained 0.98 lb per week (176).

The effect of total parenteral nutrition (TPN) on body composition has also been analyzed. In one study, 12 patients with AIDS and the wasting syndrome were treated for a median of 14 weeks (25). Five of those patients had gastrointestinally based alterations in intake or malabsorption as the primary cause of their wasting syndrome; all 5 patients showed increased body cell mass as well as weight. In contrast, the other 7 patients, who had systemic secondary infection as the cause of their wasting syndrome, showed an average decrease in body cell mass over the course of hyperalimentation despite gaining weight, which was primarily fat. Only 2 of the 7 patients with systemic infection showed increases in body cell mass (25). Another study of TPN consisted of patients who had lost more than 10% of body weight and had severe diarrhea or an inability to be fed enterally (177). Sixteen patients were randomized to TPN and 15 to conventional dietary counseling. Weight, lean body mass, and body cell mass improved in the TPN group, but these values declined in the control group. Short-term survival was not affected (177), but a survival difference was found in a limited longer-term follow-up (178).

Thus, enteral or parenteral alimentation appears to be most effective at increasing muscle mass in patients with AIDS wasting who have gastrointestinal disease of a degree sufficient to prevent adequate food intake and who have no secondary systemic infection. This group (in the absence of infection) should be the focus of intensive nutritional intervention.

One study examined supplementary feeding early in the course of HIV infection, before significant weight loss (179). A specialized formula seemed to have better results with regard to maintenance of weight and fewer subsequent hospitalizations. However, the intake of supplement was low, and the reasons for hospitalization were not specified (179).

Drugs That Stimulate Appetite

Dronabinol (Δ-9-tetrahydrocannabinol) was the first drug approved for treatment of the anorexia associated with weight loss in patients with AIDS (180). In a small, open-label study, dronabinol stimulated appetite and increased weight (181). However, three subsequent studies did not find weight gain (182–184). In one double-blind placebo-controlled crossover study, 12 patients were entered, but only 5 completed the study (182). No improvement in weight or appetite score was seen, although fat mass increased during treatment (182). In a longer study, 72 patients were randomized to dronabinol and 67 to placebo, with 50 and 38 patients evaluable at end of study (183). Appetite, mood, and nausea were shown to be statistically improved by use of analog visual scales. However, weight was not significantly improved (183). In a subsequent open-label study (184), patients receiving dronabinol lost an average of 2 kg of weight.

Megestrol acetate has also been approved as an appetite stimulant in AIDS. A pilot open-label study demonstrated that megestrol acetate can increase the weight of patients with AIDS and a history of weight loss (185). Two large randomized, double blind placebo-controlled trials have confirmed that megestrol acetate increases weight, but the weight gain is predominantly fat, with no or small increases in lean body mass (186, 187). In a dose-ranging study, patients with significant wasting (about a 30-lb loss) were randomized to placebo or to 200, 400, or 800 mg of megestrol acetate (186). At 800 mg, patients had a significant gain in weight (7.8 lb) compared with placebo (−1.6 lb) at the last evaluable visit (only 71 to 74% of subjects were evaluable). Patients were dropped from study for secondary infections. Most of the weight gained (5.3 of 7.6 lb) was fat by bioelectrical impedance analysis (186).

Patients were randomized to placebo or to 800 mg megestrol acetate in another study (187). Only 42% completed 12 weeks of study. At that point, treated subjects showed a 4.2-kg weight gain, whereas those receiving placebo lost 0.6 kg. Using bioelectrical impedance, the megestrol-treated subjects were found to have gained 4.5 kg of fat and to have lost 0.3 kg of lean body mass (187). In the latter two studies, patients reported subjective improvements in appetite, well-being, and appearance (186, 187).

Given that lean body mass is a major determinant of both function and survival (3, 12), optimal therapy would restore lean body mass. However, building a fat reserve could theoretically allow preservation of more lean body mass during subsequent periods of wasting (18). In these short, 12-week studies, no survival advantage could be seen with megestrol therapy.

The reason for the failure to gain significant lean body mass in these studies is not clear. Megestrol acetate is a progestational agent and as such reduces serum testosterone (188), a phenomenon that could by itself reduce lean body mass (megestrol acetate also induces impotence). However, replacement of testosterone during megestrol therapy adds only a small amount of gain in lean body mass (189). As discussed in the next section, the symptoms of AIDS may also contribute to the difficulty in building lean body mass. Finally, megestrol acetate therapy may be associated with an increase in deep vein thrombosis and pulmonary embolism (190). The combination of dronabinol and megestrol acetate is no more effective at inducing weight gain than megestrol acetate alone (184).

Role of Symptoms Such as Lethargy and Fatigue

The role of constitutional symptoms, such as lethargy and fatigue, in the process of wasting is increasingly recognized (94, 97, 138, 139). During periods of weight maintenance, total energy expenditure must equal caloric intake. Total energy expenditure is the sum of resting energy expenditure plus dietary thermogenesis plus energy expended in activity. During periods of stable weight, patients with HIV disease and AIDS show increased resting energy expenditure, yet they have normal caloric intake and total energy expenditure (94, 97). Thus, in AIDS and HIV infection, caloric intake is not increased proportionately to the increase in resting energy expenditure. (The other component of energy expenditure, dietary thermogenesis, plays a small role in total energy balance.) Therefore, because weight maintenance requires that total energy expenditure equal caloric intake, patients with AIDS and HIV infection must have a decrease in their energy expended in activity to prevent an increase in their total energy expenditure (97). The symptoms of lethargy and fatigue, which decrease activity, help to maintain weight in the presence of increased resting energy expenditure and normal caloric intake.

Although decreased activity can maintain weight over the short-term, decreased activity is detrimental in the long-term. Muscle mass, the most important component of body cell mass, requires activity for maintenance; inactivity leads to muscle atrophy. Systemic symptoms leading to inactivity also result in a poor ability to regain muscle mass after bouts of wasting. Decreased muscle mass is part of a downward spiral of debilitation, because inadequate strength increases the frequency of fatigue and makes activities such as food preparation and eating even more difficult (139). Finally, inactivity by itself (even in the absence of hormonally stimulated negative nitrogen balance) may contribute to the lack of efficacy of alimentary therapy; in the presence of limited activity, aggressive alimentation produces fat storage in disproportion to muscle mass, as is often seen in malignant disease and AIDS (15, 16, 175, 186, 187, 189).

In a controlled study of exercise, a supervised exercise program was able to increase strength and duration (exercise tolerance) compared with controls who received counseling (191). No deleterious effects of exercise were noted on immune function or disease status. Furthermore, in a preliminary report, progressive resistance training increased lean body mass and fat in AIDS patients who had already lost significant weight (192).

Anabolic Therapies

Newer anabolic therapies have focused on building lean body mass. Growth hormone has been demonstrated to induce protein synthesis and positive nitrogen balance in various states characterized by catabolism or decreased nutrient intake (193). As a consequence, growth hormone and related factors have been tested in AIDS patients with wasting, and growth hormone has received approval for use in the wasting syndrome by the United States Food and Drug Administration. In an early, small, nonplacebo-controlled trial, 12 weeks of therapy with growth hormone increased weight and lean body mass in HIV-infected men (194). Muscle power and endurance also improved (194). In a metabolic ward study of patients with HIV infection who had lost 19% of their body weight, growth hormone induced weight gain and significantly sustained positive nitrogen balance (65). The proportion of positive potassium balance to nitrogen balance was consistent with increases in body cell mass. Treated patients showed decreased protein oxidation and increased fatty acid oxidation (65). Some of the metabolic effects of growth hormone are mediated by insulin-like growth factor I (IGF-I). In a similar metabolic ward study, IGF-I also induced positive nitrogen balance in AIDS patients with previous weight loss; however, the effect was not sustained (195).

Results of several larger studies of low- and high-dose growth hormone therapy, either alone or in combination with IGF-I therapy, have been published. Growth hormone (0.34 mg subcutaneously once daily) plus IGF-I (5 mg subcutaneously twice daily) was given 142 subjects for 12 weeks (196). In the 80 evaluable subjects, weight was increased at 3 weeks (1.5 kg), and fat-free mass was increased at 6 weeks (0.8 kg), but neither was significantly increased at 12 weeks. No significant change was seen in those receiving placebo (196). A subset of these patients underwent more detailed body composition analysis (197). At 6 weeks, increases were seen in weight (1.5 kg), lean body mass (2.1 kg), and body cell mass by total body potassium (2.1 kg), whereas fat decreased. No changes were significant in the patients receiving placebo treatment. By 12 weeks, only the increase in lean body mass (1.6 kg) and the decrease in fat mass remained significant (197).

Another study compared the effects of placebo, a higher dose of growth hormone (1.4 ng per day), IGF-I (5 mg twice daily), and the combination of growth hormone and IGF-I (198). All therapeutic arms showed increases (1 to 3.2 kg) in lean body mass at 6 weeks, but this increase was sustained at 12 weeks only in the group receiving combination therapy. Weight increased significantly only at 6 weeks in either arm of the trial that received growth hormone. IGF-I decreased fat mass. The combination therapy produced improvement in strength and quality of life (198).

Clearer results were obtained when an even higher dose of growth hormone (0.1 mg/kg, average 6 mg) was used (199); the dose was similar to that used in the earlier successful studies (65, 194). Of 178 randomized patients, 140 (80%) were evaluable, and increases in weight (1.6 kg) and lean body mass (3.0 kg) were sustained over 12 weeks of growth hormone therapy, whereas fat decreased (199). No significant changes were found in patients treated with placebo. Analysis of extracellular and intracellular water demonstrated that the lean body mass gained during growth hormone therapy was of the same ratio as normal tissue. Furthermore, growth hormone increased the ability of subjects to perform work on a treadmill. Improvement in work was proportioned to improvement in lean body mass. Quality of life by subjective scales did not change (199). The studies with growth hormone are the first to demonstrate that treatment of the wasting syndrome in AIDS improves function (194, 199); these studies provide a new standard for evaluating future therapies.

Androgens and anabolic steroids are being evaluated, but controlled data are limited, and these agents are not currently approved for the wasting syndrome in AIDS. Testosterone levels are frequently reduced in patients with AIDS, but rarely to the level seen in classic hypogonadism (see Chap. 38).

In an open-label study, HIV-infected men with sexual dysfunction and low testosterone were treated with replacement therapy of 400 mg testosterone cyprinate every other week

(200). Serum testosterone rose from 3.6 to 10.9 ng/mL. These subjects were not underweight at baseline. After 12 weeks of therapy, they showed no significant increase in weight (group difference was +0.9kg). A significant increase was seen in fat-free mass (1.2 kg) and in body cell mass (1.2 kg), whereas fat mass did not change (−0.2 kg) (200). Although these results are encouraging, the failure to use a placebo group or study patients with prior wasting does not allow extrapolation of these results to the clinically relevant group of AIDS patients with wasting.

Open-label studies of anabolic steroids (including stanozolol, nandrolone, and oxymethalone) in patients with AIDS wasting syndrome and weakness have reported weight gain or increases in strength (201–204). In a double-blind randomized study, placebo was compared with 5 or 15 mg of oxandrolone per day. The high dose transiently induced a significant increase in weight that reached 1.8 kg at 14 weeks, whereas placebo treatment resulted in a 0.7-kg loss. By 16 weeks, however, the difference between the groups was not significant. The 5-mg dose led to smaller, more variable changes. Patients receiving 15 mg per day reported subjective increases in appetite and physical activity. No objective changes in strength were found. Body composition was not analyzed.

Further studies on the treatment of the AIDS wasting syndrome with anabolic steroids are clearly warranted. Results of body composition and physical performance will be key in evaluation of their efficacy.

Anticytokine Therapy

Because of the potential role of cytokines in mediating the wasting syndrome (29, 30, 139), therapies that decrease the production of cytokines, in particular TNF, have been tested in the AIDS wasting syndrome. Therapy with fish oil has been shown in healthy subjects to decrease the ability of endotoxin to stimulate release of TNF and IL-1 from circulating white blood cells (205) and to prevent cytokine-induced anorexia in animals (115). In a trial of fish oil therapy in HIV-infected patients with significant weight loss, no significant weight gain occurred on the average (159). Patients who did not develop new AIDS-related complications gained weight, whereas those who did develop complications lost weight (206). Preliminary results from a double-blind placebo-controlled study also found no weight gain or body composition change in the group treated with fish oil, but the placebo group had a 1-kg decrease in lean body mass and a 1.8-kg increase in fat (207).

Ketotifen is an inhibitor of TNF release from peripheral blood mononuclear cells that is available in Europe. In an open-label trial, subjects receiving ketotifen gained 2.7 kg (208). However, in another study in which ketotifen or placebo was added to an open-label therapy with an anabolic steroid, ketotifen induced no increase in weight compared with placebo (203).

Another compound that inhibits TNF production in patients with AIDS is pentoxifylline (209, 210). In three separate trials, pentoxifylline did not prevent weight loss or stimulate weight gain in patients with AIDS (209–211). Indeed, on average, patients lost weight in these studies. Furthermore, concern has been raised that pentoxifylline therapy may increase the susceptibility to infection in patients with AIDS (211). TNF is an important component of the host defense (110). Treatment of macrophages from control and HIV-infected patients with pentoxifylline leads to enhanced growth of MAC (212).

In contrast, a third drug that inhibits TNF production in vitro, thalidomide, has been shown to induce weight gain in AIDS. Thalidomide was given for 14 days to patients undergoing treatment for tuberculosis, of whom 43% were HIV positive (213). All patients received multidrug antituberculosis therapy (213). The weight gain in 21 patients receiving thalidomide (from both open-label and placebo-controlled trials) was 6% of body weight. In contrast, 8 patients receiving placebo gained only 2% of weight. In another randomized double-blind placebo-controlled trial, 39 HIV-positive male patients presenting to Chest and Venereal Disease Clinics in Thailand were randomized to thalidomide or placebo (214). Thirty-two patients completed the study, 16 patients had tuberculosis, and 16 patients did not. Eight patients from each of those groups received thalidomide, and 8 received placebo. In the HIV-positive patients with tuberculosis, weight gain while receiving thalidomide was 8%, whereas those receiving placebo lost 1%. Among patients with HIV infection alone, those receiving thalidomide gained 5% weight, whereas those receiving placebo gained only 2% (214). In another small, randomized, double-blind placebo-controlled trial in 28 patients with advanced HIV disease, weight gain occurred in 8 of 14 patients receiving thalidomide and in only 1 of 14 patients receiving placebo (215). No body composition studies were performed. These data are encouraging, and a large, multicenter, double-blind placebo-controlled trial for AIDS wasting has been completed. Unpublished reports indicate modest weight gain (G Kaplan, unpublished data). A surprising finding in another study in which thalidomide was used to treat aphthous ulcers, however, was an increase in total TNF in serum rather than a decrease (216). Thus, the mechanism by which thalidomide induces weight gain still needs to be explored.

In summary, wasting is not an inevitable component of AIDS, but rather it is a manifestation of underlying secondary disease. Although metabolic disturbances are universally found in AIDS, these disturbances do not necessarily cause rapid wasting. In the absence of secondary diseases, nitrogen balance is not profoundly negative. Slow weight loss may be a sign of gastrointestinal disease and is frequently accompanied by diarrhea. Rapid weight loss accompanied by anorexia is often due to secondary infection. During secondary infection, the cytokines mediating the immune and inflammatory response are likely to produce metabolic disturbances and anorexia that exceed the ability of the body to compensate resulting in rapid weight loss. However, no single cytokine causes sustained wasting in AIDS or in animal models.

Direct therapy of the wasting syndrome is evolving. Administration of alimentation is indicated when decreased nutrient intake is due to treatable gastrointestinal lesions; such therapy can replete body cell mass. In other cases, alimentation or appetite stimulation may induce weight gain, but most gain occurs in fat rather than in body cell mass. Growth hormone therapy promotes positive nitrogen balance, increases weight and body cell mass, and improves function. However, one must still continually reexamine AIDS patients with active wasting for secondary infection, malignant disease, or gastrointestinal diseases that are amenable to treatment.

Acknowledgments

This work was supported in part by grants from the University AIDS Research Program (R90SF211), the National Institutes of Health (DK40990, DK45833, DK49440, DK52610), and the Research Service of the Department of Veterans Affairs.

References

1. Serwadda D, Sewankambo NK, Carswell JW, et al. Slim disease: a new disease in Uganda and its association with HTLV-III infection. Lancet 1985;2:850–852.
2. Kotler DP, Wang J, Pierson R. Studies of body composition in patients with the acquired immunodeficiency syndrome. Am J Clin Nutr 1985;42:1255–1265.
3. Kotler DP, Tierney AR, Francisco A, et al. The magnitude of body cell mass depletion determines the timing of death from wasting in AIDS. Am J Clin Nutr 1989;50:444–447.
4. Chlebowski RT, Grosvenor MB, Bernhard NH, et al. Nutritional status, gastrointestinal dysfunction, and survival in patients with AIDS. Am J Gastroenterol 1989;84:1288–1293.
5. Centers for Disease Control. Revision of the CDC case surveillance definition for acquired immunodeficiency syndrome. MMWR Morb Mortal Wkly Rep 1987;36(Suppl 1S):3S–14S.
6. Teixeira A, Leu JC, Honderlick P, et al. Variation in body weight and plasma viral load in HIV patients treated with tritherapy including a protease inhibitor [abstract]. Nutrition 1997;13:269.
7. Brennan MF. Uncomplicated starvation versus cancer cachexia. Cancer Res 1977;37:2359–2364.
8. Streat SJ, Beddoe AH, Hill GL. Aggressive nutritional support does not prevent protein loss despite fat gain in septic intensive care patients. J Trauma 1987;27:262–266.
9. Brozek J, Wells S, Keys A. Medical aspects of semistarvation in Leningrad (siege 1941–1942). Am Rev Soviet Med 1946;4:70–86.
10. Fliederbaum J. Clinical aspects of hunger disease in adults. In: Winick M, ed. Hunger disease. New York: John Wiley & Sons, 1979:11–43.
11. Keys A, Brozek J, Henschel A, et al. The biology of human starvation. Minneapolis: University of Minnesota Press, 1950.
12. Cahill GF. Starvation in man. N Engl J Med 1970;282:668–675.
13. Guenter P Muurahainen N, Simons G, et al. Relationships among nutritional status, disease progression and survival in HIV infection. J Acquir Immune Defic Syndr 1993;6:1130–1138.
14. Suttman U, Ockenga J, Selberg O, et al. Incidence and prognostic value of malnutrtion and wasting in human immunodeficiency virus–infected outpatients. J Acquir Immune Defic Syndr Hum Retrovirol 1995;8:239–246.
15. Palenicek JG, Graham NMH, He YD, et al. Weight loss prior to clinical AIDS as a predictor of survival. J Acquir Immune Defic Syndr Hum Retrovirol 1995;10:366–373.
16. Turner J, Muurahainen N, Graber TC, et al. Nutritional status and quality of life [abstract]. In: Proceedings of the 10th International Conference on AIDS, Yokohama, Japan, 1994;2:35.
17. Cohan GR, Muurahainen N, Guenter P, et al. HIV-related hospitalization, CD4 percent and nutritional markers [abstract]. In: Proceedings of the 7th International Conference on AIDS, Amsterdam, 1992:67.
18. Forbes GB. Growth, aging, nutrition and activity. In: Human body composition. New York: Springer-Verlag, 1987:209–247.
19. Wang J, Kotler DP, Russell M, et al. Body fat measurement in patients with acquired immunodeficiency syndrome: which method? Am J Clin Nutr 1992;56:963–967.
20. Paton NIJ, Macallan DC, Jebb SA, et al. Longitudinal changes in body composition measured with a variety of methods in patients with AIDS. J Acquir Immune Defic Syndr Hum Retrovirol 1997;14:119–127.
21. Oliver CJ, Rose A, Blagojevic N, et al. Total body protein status of males infected with the human immunodeficiency virus. In: Ellis KJ, Eastman JD, eds. Human body composition. New York: Plenum Press, 1993:197–200.
22. Mulligan K, Tai VW, Schambelan M. Cross-sectional and longitudinal evaluation of changes in body composition in men with HIV infection. J Acquir Immune Defic Syndr Hum Retrovirol 1997;14:43–48.
23. Heymsfield SB, McManus C, Smith J, et al. Anthropometric measurement of muscle mass: revised equations for calculating bone-free arm muscle area. Am J Clin Nutr 1982;36:680–690.
24. Popp MB, Fisher RI, Wesley R, et al. A prospective randomized study of adjuvant parenteral nutrition in the treatment of advanced diffuse lymphoma: influence on survival. Surgery 1981;90:195–202.
25. Kotler DP, Tierney AR, Culpepper-Morgan JA, et al. Effect of home total parenteral nutrition upon body composition in patients with AIDS. JPEN J Parenter Enteral Nutr 1990;14:454–458.
26. Beisel WR. Metabolic response to infection. In: Sanford JB, Luby JP, eds. The science and practice of clinical medicine. New York: Grune & Stratton, 1981:28–35.
27. Kaufmann RL, Matson CG, Beisel WR. Hypertriglyceridemia produced by endotoxin: role of impaired triglyceride disposal mechanisms. J Infect Dis 1976;133:548–555.
28. Lang CH, Bagby GJ, Spitzer JJ. Glucose kinetics and body temperature after lethal and nonlethal doses of endotoxin. Am J Physiol 1985;248:R471–R478.
29. Grunfeld C, Feingold KR. The metabolic effects of tumor necrosis factor and other cytokines. Biotherapy 1991;3:143–158.
30. Beutler B, Cerami A. Cachectin and tumor necrosis factor as two sides of the same biological coin. Nature 1986;320:584–588.
31. Patton JS, Shepard HM, Wilking H, et al. Interferons and tumor necrosis factors have similar catabolic effects on 3T3-L1 cells. Proc Natl Acad Sci U S A 1986;83:8313–8317.
32. Beutler BA, Cerami A. Recombinant interleukin-1 suppresses lipoprotein lipase activity in 3T3-L1 cells. J Immunol 1986;135:3969–3971.
33. Mori M, Yamaguchi K, Abe K. Purification of a lipoprotein lipase inhibiting protein produced by a melanoma cell line associated with cancer cachexia. Biochem Biophys Res Commun 1989;160:1085–1092.
34. Feingold KR, Doerrler W, Dinarello CA, et al. Stimulation of lipolysis in cultured fat cells by TNF, IL-1 and the interferons is blocked by inhibition of prostaglandin synthesis. Endocrinology 1992;130:10–16.
35. Greenberg AS, Nordon RP, McIntosh J, et al. Interleukin-6 reduces lipoprotein lipase activity in adipose tissue of mice in vivo and in 3T3-L1 adipocytes: a possible role for interleukin-6 in cancer cachexia. Cancer Res 1992;52:4113–4116.
36. Feingold KR, Grunfeld C. Tumor necrosis factor alpha stimulates hepatic lipogenesis in the rat in vivo. J Clin Invest 1987;80:184–190.
37. Chajek-Shaul T, Friedman G, Stein I, et al. Mechanisms of the hypertriglyceridemia induced by tumor necrosis factor administration to rats. Biochim Biophys Acta 1989;1001:316–432.

38. Krauss RM, Feingold KR, Grunfeld C. Tumor necrosis factor acutely increases plasma levels of very low density lipoproteins of normal size and composition. Endocrinology 1990;127:1016–1021.
39. Feingold KR, Soued M, Adi S, et al. The effect of interleukin-1 on lipid metabolism in the rat: similarities to and differences from tumor necrosis factor. Arterioscler Thromb 1991;11:495–500.
40. Memon RA, Grunfeld C, Moser AH, et al. Tumor necrosis factor mediates the effects of endotoxin on cholesterol and triglyceride metabolism in mice. Endocrinology 1993;132:2246–2253.
41. Starnes HF Jr, Warren RS, Jeevanandam M, et al. Tumor necrosis factor and the acute metabolic response to tissue injury in man. J Clin Invest 1988;82:1321–1325.
42. Sherman ML, Spriggs DR, Arthur KA, et al. Recombinant human tumor necrosis factor administered as a five day continuous infusion in cancer patients: phase I toxicity and effects on lipid metabolism. J Clin Oncol 1988;6:344–350.
43. Ettinger WH, Miller LD, Albers JJ, et al. Lipopolysaccharide and tumor necrosis factor cause a fall in plasma concentrations of lecithin: cholesterol acyltransferase in cynomolgus monkeys. J Lipid Res 1990;31:1099–1107.
44. Semb H, Peterson J, Tavernier J, et al. Multiple effects of tumor necrosis factor on lipoprotein lipase in vivo. J Biol Chem 1987;62:8390–8394.
45. Grunfeld C, Gulli R, Moser AH, et al. The effect of tumor necrosis factor administration in vivo on lipoprotein lipase activity in various tissues of the rat. J Lipid Res 1989;30:579–585.
46. Feingold KR, Soued M, Staprans I, et al. The effect of TNF on lipid metabolism in the diabetic rat: evidence that inhibition of adipose tissue lipoprotein lipase activity is not required for TNF induced hyperlipidemia. J Clin Invest 1989;83:1116–1121.
47. Feingold KR, Staprans I, Memon R, et al. Endotoxin rapidly induces changes in lipid metabolism that produce hypertriglyceridemia: low doses stimulate hepatic triglyceride production while high doses inhibit clearance. J Lipid Res 1992;33:1765–1776.
48. Feingold KR, Soued M, Serio MK, et al. Multiple cytokines stimulate hepatic lipid synthesis in vivo. Endocrinology 1989;125:267–274.
49. Grunfeld C, Adi S, Soued M, et al. Search for mediators of the lipogenic effects of tumor necrosis factor: potential role for interleukin-6. Cancer Res 1990;50:4233–4238.
50. Feingold KR, Adi S, Staprans I, et al. Diet affects the mechanisms by which TNF stimulates hepatic triglyceride production. Am J Physiol 1990;259:E177–E184.
51. Wolfe RR, Shaw JHF, Durkot MJ. Effect of sepsis on VLDL kinetics: responses in basal state and during glucose infusion. Am J Physiol 1985;248:E732–E740.
52. Cerami A, Ikeda Y, Latrang N, et al. Weight loss associated with an endotoxin induced mediator from peritoneal macrophages: the role of cachectin (tumor necrosis factor). Immunol Lett 1985;11:173–177.
53. Patton JS, Peters PM, McCabe J, et al. Development of partial tolerance to the gastrointestinal effects of high doses of recombinant tumor necrosis factor alpha in rodents. J Clin Invest 1987;80:1587–1596.
54. Tracey KJ, Wei H, Manogue KR. Cachectin/tumor necrosis factor induces cachexia, anemia and inflammation. J Exp Med 1988;167:1211–1227.
55. Socher SH, Friedman A, Martinez D. Recombinant human-tumor necrosis factor induces acute reductions in food-intake and body-weight in mice. J Exp Med 1988;167:1957–1962.
56. Stovroff MC, Fraker DL, Swedenborg JA, et al. Cachectin/tumor necrosis factor, a possible mediator of cancer anorexia in the rat. Cancer Res 1988;48:920–925.
57. Kettelhut IC, Goldberg AL. Tumor necrosis factor can induce fever in rats without activating protein breakdown in muscle or lipolysis in adipose tissue. J Clin Invest 1988;81:1384–1389.
58. Kramer SM, Aggarwal BB, Eessalu TE, et al. Characterization of the in vitro and in vivo species preference of human and murine tumor necrosis factor alpha. Cancer Res 1988;48:920–925.
59. Mahony SM, Tisdale MJ. Induction of weight loss and metabolic alterations by human recombinant tumor necrosis factor. Br J Cancer 1988;58:345–349.
60. Grunfeld C, Wilking H, Neese R, et al. Persistence of the hypertriglyceridemic effect of tumor necrosis factor despite development of tachyphylaxis to its anorectic/cachectic effects in rats. Cancer Res 1989;49:2554–2560.
61. Mullen BJ, Harris RBS, Patton JS, et al. Recombinant tumor necrosis factor-alpha chronically administered in rats: lack of cachectic effect. Proc Soc Exp Biol Med 1990;193:318–325.
62. Grunfeld C, Kotler DP, Hamadeh R, et al. Hypertriglyceridemia in the acquired immunodeficiency syndrome. Am J Med 1989;86:27–31.
63. Grunfeld C, Pang M, Doerrler W, et al. Lipids, lipoproteins, triglyceride clearance and cytokines in human immunodeficiency virus infection and the acquired immunodeficiency syndrome. J Clin Endocrinol Metab 1992;74:1045–1052.
64. Hellerstein MK, Grunfeld C, Wu K, et al. Increased de novo hepatic lipogenesis in HIV-infected humans. J Clin Endocrinol Metab 1993;76:559–565.
65. Mulligan K, Grunfeld C, Hellerstein MK, et al. Anabolic effects of recombinant human growth hormone in patients with wasting associated with human immunodeficiency virus infection. J Clin Endocrinol Metab, 1993;77:956–962.
66. Lahdevirta J, Maury CPJ, Teppo AM, et al. Elevated levels of circulating cachectin/tumor necrosis factor in patients with acquired immunodeficiency syndrome. Am J Med 1988;85:289–291.
67. Reddy MM, Sorrell SJ, Lange M, et al. Tumor necrosis factor and HIV P24 antigen in the serum of HIV-infected population. J Acquir Immune Defic Syndr 1988;1:436–440.
68. Hommes M, Romijn JA, Godfried MH, et al. Increased resting energy expenditure in human immunodeficiency virus–infected men. Metabolism 1990;39:1186–1190.
69. Grunfeld C, Kotler DP, Shigenaga JK, et al. Circulating interferon alpha levels and hypertriglyceridemia in the acquired immunodeficiency syndrome. Am J Med 1991;90:154–162.
70. Dworkin BM, Seaton T, Wormser G. The role of tumor necrosis factor (TNF) and altered metabolic rate in weight loss in AIDS [abstract]. In: Proceedings of the 6th International Conference on AIDS, San Francisco, 1990;1:218.
71. Mildvan D, Machado SG, Wilets II, et al. Endogenous interferon and triglyceride concentrations to assess response to zidovudine in AIDS and advanced AIDS-related complex. Lancet 1992;339:453–456.
72. Hober D, Haque A, Wattre P, et al. Production of tumour necrosis factor-alpha (TNF-α) and interleukin-1 (IL-1) in patients with AIDS: enhanced level of TNF-α is related to a higher cytotoxic activity. Clin Exp Immunol 1989;78:329–333.
73. Aukrust P, Liabakk NB, Muller F, et al. Serum levels of tumor necrosis factor α (TNF-α) and soluble TNF receptors in human immunodeficiency virus type I infection: correlations to clinical, immunologic and virologic parameters. J Infect Dis 1994;169:420–424.
74. Thea DM, Porat R, Nagimbi K, et al. Plasma cytokines, cytokine antagonists, and disease progression in African women infected with HIV-1. Ann Intern Med 1996;124:757–762.
75. Godfried MH, van der Poll T, Jansen J, et al. Soluble receptors for tumor necrosis factor: a putative marker of disease progression in HIV infection. AIDS 1993;7:33–36.
76. Godfried MH, van der Poll T, Weverling GJ, et al. Soluble receptors for tumor necrosis factor as predictors of progression to AIDS in asymptomatic human immunodeficiency virus type I infection. J Infect Dis 1994;169:739–745.
77. Suttmann U, Selberg O, Gallati H, et al. Tumour necrosis factor receptor levels are linked to the acute phase response and malnutrition in human immunodeficiency virus infected patients. Clin Sci 1994;86:462–467.
78. Zangerle R, Gallati H, Sarcletti M, et al. Increased serum concentrations of soluble tumor necrosis factor in HIV infected individuals are associated with immune activation. J Acquir Immune Defic Syndr Hum Retrovirol 1994;7:79–85.

79. Godfried MH, Romijn JA, van der Poll T, et al. Soluble receptors for tumor necrosis factor are markers for clinical course but not for major metabolic changes in human immunodeficiency virus infection. Metabolism 1995;44:1554–1569.
80. Olsen EA, Lichtenstein GR, Wilkinson WE. Changes in serum lipids in patients with condylomata acuminata treated with interferon alpha-n1 (Wellferon). J Am Acad Dermatol 1988;19:286–289.
81. Graessle D, Bonacini M, Chen S. Alpha-interferon and reversible hypertriglyceridemia. Ann Intern Med 1993;118:316–317.
82. Ehnholm C, Aho K, Huttenen JK, et al. Effect of interferon on plasma lipoproteins and on the activity of post-heparin plasma lipases. Arteriosclerosis 1982;2:68–73.
83. Massaro ER, Borden EC, Hawkins MJ, et al. Effects of recombinant interferon-alpha$_2$ treatment upon lipid concentrations and lipoprotein composition. J Interferon Res 1986;6:655–662.
84. Wilmore DW, Long JM, Mason AD, et al. Catecholamines: mediators of the hypermetabolic response to thermal injury. Ann Surg 1974;180:653–669.
85. Long CL, Schaffel N, Geiger JW, et al. Metabolic response to injury and illness: estimation of energy and protein needs from indirect calorimetry and nitrogen balance. JPEN J Parenter Enteral Nutr 1979;3:452–456.
86. Dempsey DT, Feurer ID, Knox LS, et al. Energy expenditure in malnourished gastrointestinal cancer patients. Cancer 1984;53:1265–1273.
87. Hansell DT, Davies JWL, Burns HJG. The relationship between resting energy expenditure and weight loss in benign and malignant diseases. Ann Surg 1986;203:240–245.
88. Nixon DW, Kutner M, Heymsfield S, et al. Resting energy expenditure in lung and colon cancer. Metabolism 1988;37:1059–1064.
89. Fredrix EWHM, Soeters PB, Wouters EFM, et al. Effect of different tumor types on resting energy expenditure. Cancer Res 1991;51:6138–6141.
90. Arbeit JM, Lees DE, Corsey R, et al. Resting energy expenditure in controls and cancer patients with localized and diffuse disease. Ann Surg 1984;199:292–298.
91. Burt ME, Stein TP, Brennan MF. A controlled, randomized trial evaluating the effects of enteral and parenteral nutrition on protein metabolism in cancer-bearing man. J Surg Res 1983;34:303–314.
92. Hommes MJT, Romijn JA, Endert E, et al. Resting energy expenditure and substrate oxidation in human immunodeficiency virus (HIV)–infected asymptomatic men: HIV affects host metabolism in the early asymptomatic stage. Am J Clin Nutr 1991;54:311–315.
93. Melchior JD, Salmon D, Rigaud D, et al. Resting energy expenditure is increased in stable, malnourished HIV-infected patients. Am J Clin Nutr 1991;53:437–441.
94. Grunfeld C, Pang M, Shimizu L, et al. Resting energy expenditure, caloric intake and short-term weight change in human immunodeficiency virus infection and the acquired immunodeficiency syndrome. Am J Clin Nutr 1992;55:455–460.
95. Melchior JC, Raguin G, Boulier A, et al. Resting energy expenditure in human immunodeficiency virus–infected patients: comparison between patients with and without secondary infections. Am J Clin Nutr 1993;57:614–619.
96. Suttmann U, Ockenga J, Hoogestraat L, et al. Resting energy expenditure and weight loss in human immunodeficiency virus–infected patients. Metabolism 1993;42:1173–1179.
97. Macallan DC, Noble C, Baldwin C, et al. Energy expenditure and wasting in human immunodeficiency virus infection. N Engl J Med 1995;333:83–88.
98. Sharpstone DR, Murray CP, Ross HM, et al. Energy balance in asymptomatic HIV infection. AIDS 1996;10:1377–1384.
99. Sharpstone DR, Ross HM, Gazzard BG. The metabolic response to opportunistic infections in AIDS. AIDS 1996;10:1529–1533.
100. Mulligan K, Tai VW, Schambelan M. Energy expenditure in human immunodeficiency virus infection. N Engl J Med 1997;336:70–71.
101. Kotler DP, Tierney AR, Brenner SK, et al. Preservation of short-term energy balance in clinically stable patients with AIDS. Am J Clin Nutr 1990;51:7–13.
102. Schwenk A, Hoffer-Belitz E, Jung B, et al. Resting energy expenditure, weight loss, and altered body composition in HIV infection. Nutrition 1996;12:595–601.
103. Macallan DC, Noble C, Baldwin C, et al. Prospective analysis of patterns of weight change in stage IV HIV infection. Am J Clin Nutr 1993;58:417–424.
104. Poizot-Martin I, Benourine K, Philibert P, et al. Diet-induced thermogenesis in HIV infection. AIDS 1994;8:501–504.
105. Burt ME, Stein TP, Brennan MF. A controlled, randomized trial evaluating the effects of enteral and parenteral nutrition on protein metabolism in cancer-bearing man. J Surg Res 1983;34:303–314.
106. Stein TP, Nutinsky C, Condoluci D, et al. Protein and energy substrate metabolism in AIDS patients. Metabolism 1990;39:876–881.
107. Grunfeld C, Pang M, Doerrler W, et al. Indices of thyroid function and weight loss in human immunodeficiency virus infection and the acquired immunodeficiency syndrome. Metabolism 1993;42:1270–1276.
108. Macallan DC, NcNurlan MA, Milne E, et al. Whole-body protein turnover from leucine kinetics and the response to nutrition in human immunodeficiency virus infection. Am J Clin Nutr 1995;61:818–826.
109. Selberg O, Suttmann U, Melzer A, et al. Effect of increased protein intake and nutritional status on whole-body protein metabolism of AIDS patients with weight loss. Metabolism 1995;44:1159–1165.
110. Grunfeld C, Palladino, MA. Tumor necrosis factor: immunologic, antitumor, metabolic and cardiovascular activities. Adv Intern Med 1990;35:45–72.
111. Feingold KR, Soued M, Serio MK, et al. The effect of diet on tumor necrosis factor stimulation of hepatic lipogenesis. Metabolism 1990;39:623–632.
112. Sherwin SA, Knost JA, Fein S, et al. A multiple-dose phase I trial of recombinant leukocyte A interferon in cancer patients. JAMA 1982;248:2461–2466.
113. Vadhan-Raj S, Al-Katib A, Bhalla R, et al. Phase I trial of recombinant interferon gamma in cancer patients. J Clin Oncol 1986;4:137–146.
114. Fujii T, Sato K, Ozawa M, et al. Effect of interleukin-1 (IL-1) on thyroid hormone metabolism in mice: stimulation by IL-1 of iodothyronine 5′-deiodinating activity (type I) in the liver. Endocrinology 1989;124:167–174.
115. Hellerstein MK, Meydani SN, Meydani M, et al. Interleukin-1 induced anorexia in the rat. J Clin Invest 1989;84:228–235.
116. DiBisceglie AM, Martin P, Kassianides C, et al. Recombinant interferon alpha therapy for chronic hepatitis C: a randomized, double-blind, placebo-controlled trial. N Engl J Med 1989;321:1506–1520.
117. Zugmaier G, Paid S, Wilding G, et al. Transforming growth factor β1 induces cachexia and systemic fibrosis without an antitumor effect in nude mice. Cancer Res 1991;51:3590–3594.
118. Plata Salaman CR. Immunoregulators in the nervous system. Neurosci Biobehav Rev 1991;15:185–215.
119. Grunfeld C, Zhao C, Fuller J, et al. Endotoxin and cytokines induce expression of leptin, the ob gene product, in hamsters: a role for leptin in the anorexia of infection. J Clin Invest 1996;97:2152–2157.
120. Sarraf P, Frederich RC, Turner EM, et al. Multiple cytokines and acute inflammation raise mouse leptin levels: potential role in inflammatory anorexia. J Exp Med 1997;185:171–175.
121. Zhang Y, Proenca R, Maffei M, et al. Positional cloning of the mouse obese gene and its human homologue. Nature 1994;372:425–431.
122. Grunfeld C, Pang M, Shigenaga JK, et al. Serum leptin levels in the acquired immunodeficiency syndrome. J Clin Endocrinol Metab 1996;81:4342–4346.
123. Yarasheski KE, Zachwieja JJ, Horgan MM, et al. Serum leptin concentrations in human immunodeficiency virus–infected men with low adiposity. Metabolism 1997;46:303–305.
124. Sherry BA, Gelin J, Fong Y, et al. Anticachectin/tumor necrosis factor-alpha antibodies attenuate development of cachexia in tumor models. FASEB J 1989;3:1956–1962.

125. Langstein HN, Doherty GM, Fraker DL, et al. The roles of interferon gamma and tumor necrosis alpha in an experimental rat model of cancer cachexia. Cancer Res 1991;51:2302–2306.
126. Matthys P, Heremans H, Opdenakker G, et al. Anti-interferon-gamma antibody treatment, growth of Lewis lung tumours in mice and tumour-associated cachexia. Eur J Cancer 1991;27:182–187.
127. Strassmann G, Fong M, Kenney JS, et al. Evidence for the involvement of interleukin-6 in experimental cancer cachexia. J Clin Invest 1992; 89:1681–1684.
128. Black K, Garrett IR, Mundy GR. Chinese hamster ovarian cells transfected with the murine interleukin-6 gene cause hypercalcemia as well as cachexia, leukocytosis and thrombocytosis in tumor-bearing nude mice. Endocrinology 1991;128:2657–2659.
129. Mori M, Yamaguchi K, Honda S, et al. Cancer cachexia syndrome developed in nude mice bearing melanoma cells producing leukemia inhibitory factor. Cancer Res 1991;51:6656–6659.
130. Waage A, Espevik T, Lamvik J. Detection of tumor necrosis factor–like cytotoxicity in serum from patients with septicaemia but not from untreated cancer patients. Scand J Immunol 1986;24:739–743.
131. Scuderi P, Lam KS, Ryan KJ, et al. Raised serum levels of tumor necrosis factor in parasitic infections. Lancet 1986;2:1364–1365.
132. Socher SH, Martinez D, Craig JB, et al. Tumor necrosis factor not detectable in patients with clinical cancer cachexia. J Leukoc Biol 1988;43:436–444.
133. Saarinen UM, Koskelo E-K, Teppo A-M, et al. Tumor necrosis factor in children with malignancies. Cancer Res 1990;50:592–595.
134. Okusawa S, Gelfand JA, Ikejima T, et al. Interleukin-1 induces a shock-like state in rabbits: synergism with tumor necrosis factor and the effect of cyclooxygenase inhibition. J Clin Invest 1988;81:1162–1172.
135. Tredget EE, Yu YM, Zhong S, et al. Role of interleukin 1 and tumor necrosis factor on energy metabolism in rabbits. Am J Physiol 1988;255:E760–E768.
136. Flores EA, Bistrian BR, Pomposelli JJ, et al. Infusion of tumor necrosis factor/cachectin promotes muscle catabolism in the rat: a synergistic effect with interleukin 1. J Clin Invest 1989;83:1614–1622.
137. Grunfeld C, Soued M, Adi S, et al. Evidence for two classes of cytokines that stimulate hepatic lipogenesis: relationships among tumor necrosis factor, interleukin-1 and interferon-alpha. Endocrinology 1990;127:46–54.
138. Kotler DP, Grunfeld C. Pathophysiology and treatment of the AIDS wasting syndrome. AIDS Clin Rev 1995/1996:229–275.
139. Grunfeld C, Feingold KR. Metabolic disturbances and wasting in the acquired immunodeficiency syndrome. N Engl J Med 1992;327:329–337.
140. Black PR, Brooks DC, Bessey PQ, et al. Mechanisms of insulin resistance following injury. Ann Surg 1982;196:420–435.
141. Yki-Jarvinen H, Sammalkorpi K, Koivisto VA, et al. Severity, duration and mechanisms of insulin resistance during acute infections. J Clin Endocrinol Metab 1989;69:317–323.
142. Hommes MJT, Romijn JA, Endert E, et al. Insulin sensitivity and insulin clearance in human immunodeficiency virus–infected men. Metabolism 1991;40:651–656.
143. Wartofsky L, Burman KD. Alterations in thyroid function in patients with systemic illness: the "euthyroid sick syndrome." Endocr Rev 1982;3:164–217.
144. Kotler DP, Francisco A, Clayton F, et al. Small intestinal injury and parasitic disease in the acquired immunodeficiency syndrome (AIDS). Ann Intern Med 1990;113:444–449.
145. Batman PA, Miller AR, Forster SM, et al. Jejunal enteropathy associated with human immunodeficiency virus infection: quantitative histology. J Clin Pathol 1989;42:275–281.
146. Ullrich R, Zeitz M, Heise M, et al. Small intestinal structure and function in patients infected with human immunodeficiency virus (HIV): evidence for HIV-induced enteropathy. Ann Intern Med 1989;111:15–21.
147. Greenson JK, Belitsos PC, Yardley JH, et al. AIDS enteropathy: occult enteric infections and duodenal mucosal alterations in chronic diarrhea. Ann Intern Med 1991;114:366–372.
148. Roth RI, Owen RL, Keren DF, et al. Intestinal infection with *Mycobacterium avium* in acquired immunodeficiency syndrome (AIDS): histological and clinical comparison with Whipple's disease. Dig Dis Sci 1985;30:497.
149. Kotler DP, Gaetz HP, Lange M, et al. Enteropathy associated with the acquired immunodeficiency syndrome. Ann Intern Med 1984;101:421–428.
150. Nelson JA, Wiley CA, Reynolds-Kohler C, et al. Human immunodeficiency virus detected in bowel epithelium from patients with gastrointestinal symptoms. Lancet 1988;2:259–262.
151. Mathijs JM, Hing M, Grierson J, et al. HIV infection of rectal mucosa. Lancet 1988;1:111.
152. Fox CH, Kotler DP, Tierney AR, et al. Detection of HIV-1 RNA in intestinal lamina propria of patients with AIDS and gastrointestinal disease. J Infect Dis 1989;159:467–471.
153. Rene E, Jarry A, Brousse N, et al. Demonstration of HIV infection of the gut in AIDS patients: relation with symptoms and other digestive infection. Gastroenterology 1988;94:373A.
154. Shiau UF, Kotler DP, Levine GM. Can normal small bowel morphology be equated with normal function? Gastroenterology 1979;76:1246A.
155. Boyle JT, Celano P, Koldovsky O. Demonstration of a difference in expression of maximal lactase and sucrase activity along the villus in the adult rat jejunum. Gastroenterology 1980;79:503–507.
156. Miller TL, Orav EJ, Martin SR, et al. Malnutrition and carbohydrate malabsorption in children with vertically transmitted human immunodeficiency virus 1 infection. Gastroenterology 1991;100:1296–1302.
157. Zeitz M, Ullrich R, Heise W, et al. Malabsorption is found in early stages of HIV infection and independent of secondary infections [abstract]. In: Proceedings of the 7th International Conference on AIDS, Florence, Italy, 1991;2:46.
158. Harriman GR, Smith PD, McDonald KH, et al. Vitamin B_{12} malabsorption in patients with the acquired immunodeficiency syndrome. Arch Intern Med 1989;149:2039–2041.
159. Burkes RL, Cohen E, Kralo M, et al. Low serum cobalamin levels occur frequently in the acquired immunodeficiency syndrome and related disorders. Eur J Hematol 1987;38:141–147.
160. Kotler DP, Haroutiounian G, Greenberg R, et al. Increased bile salt deconjugation in AIDS. Gastroenterology 1985;88:1455A.
161. Kapembwa M, Bridges C, Joseph AE, et al. Ileal and jejunal absorptive function in patients with AIDS and enterococcidial infectin. J Infect 1990;21:43–53.
162. Koch J, Scott MK, Steuerwald MH, et al. Steatorrhea is nearly universal in patients with HIV-associated unexplained weight loss or diarrhea [abstract]. Nutrition 1997;13:268.
163. Grunfeld C, Feingold KR. Body weight as essential data in the management of patients with human immunodeficiency virus infection and the acquired immunodeficiency syndrome. Am J Clin Nutr 1993;58:317–318.
164. Henderson RA, Hutton N, Derusso P, et al. Viral load is associated with nutritional status in HIV-infected children [abstract]. Nutrition 1997;13:269.
165. Kotler DP, Tierney AR, Altilio D, et al. Body mass repletion during ganciclovir therapy of cytomegalovirus infections in patients with acquired immunodeficiency syndrome. Arch Intern Med 1989;149:901–905.
166. Kotler DP, Culpepper-Morgan J, Tierney AR, et al. Treatment of disseminated cytomegalovirus infection with 9-(1,3-dihydroxy-2-propoxymethyl) guanine: evidence of prolonged survival in patients with the acquired immunodeficiency syndrome. AIDS Res 1987;2:299–308.
167. Yarchoan R, Weinhold KJ, Lyerly HK, et al. Administration of 3′-azido-3′-deoxythymidine, an inhibitor of HTLV-III/LAV replica-

tion, to patients with AIDS or AIDS-related complex. Lancet 1986; 1:575–580.
168. Connolly GM, Forbes A, Gazzard BG. Investigation of seemingly pathogen-negative diarrhoea in patients infected with HIV-1. Gut 1990;31:886–889.
169. Wilcox CM, Schwartz DA, Cotsonis G, et al. Chronic unexplained diarrhea in human immunodeficiency virus infection: determination of the best diagnostic approach. Gastroenterology 1996;110:30–37.
170. American College of Physicians. Position paper: parenteral nutrition in patients receiving cancer chemotherapy. Ann Intern Med 1989;110: 734–736.
171. Raviglione MC, Battan R, Pablos-Mendez A, et al. Infections associated with Hickman catheters in patients with acquired immunodeficiency syndrome. Am J Med 1989;86:780–786.
172. Skoutelis AT, Murphy RL, MacDonel KB, et al. Indwelling central venous catheter infections in patients with acquired immune deficiency syndrome. J Acquir Immune Defic Syndr 1990;3:335–342.
173. Sweed M, Guenter P, Lucente K, et al. Long-term central venous catheters in patients with acquired immunodeficiency syndrome. Am J Infect Control 1995;23:194–199.
174. Kotler D, Tierney A, Ferraro R, et al. Effect of enteral alimentation upon body cell mass in patients with the acquired immunodeficiency syndrome. Am J Clin Nutr 1991;53:149–154.
175. Kelson K, Malcolm J, Brantsma A, et al. Percutaneous endoscopic gastrostomy feeding in AIDS [abstract]. In: Proceedings of the 7th International Conference on AIDS, Florence, Italy, 1991;1:285.
176. Garcia-Shelton Y, Keiserman M, Rockey DC, et al. Gastrostomy feeding for severe weight loss in patients with AIDS [abstract]. Nutrition 1997;13:271.
177. Melchior J-C, Chastang C, Gelas P, et al. Efficacy of 2-month total parenteral nutrition in AIDS patients: a controlled randomized prospective trial. AIDS 1996;10:379–384.
178. Melchior JC, Gelas P, Carbonnel F, et al. Improved survival by home total parenteral nutrition in AIDS patients: follow up of a controlled randomized prospective trial [abstract]. Nutrition 1997;13:272.
179. Chlebowski RT, Beall G, Grosvenor M, et al. Long-term effects of early nutritional support with new enterotropic peptide-based formula vs. standard enteral formula in HIV-infected patients: randomized prospective trial. Nutrition 1993;9:507–512.
180. Nightingale SL. Dronabinol approved for use in anorexia associated with weight loss in patients with AIDS. JAMA 1993;269:1361.
181. Gorter R, Seefried M, Volberding P. Dronabinol effects on weight in patients with HIV infection [letter]. AIDS 1992;6:127.
182. Struwe M, Kaempfer SH, Geiger CJ, et al. Effect of dronabinol on nutritional status in HIV infection. Ann Pharmacol 1993;27: 827–831.
183. Beal JE, Olson R, Laubenstein L, et al. Dronabinol as a treatment for anorexia associated with weight loss in patients with AIDS. J Pain Symptom Manage 1995;10:89–97.
184. Timpone JG, Wright DJ, Li N, et al. The safety and pharmacokinetics of single-agent and combination therapy with megestrol acetate and dronabinol for the treatment of HIV wasting syndrome. AIDS Res Human Retroviruses 1997;13:305.
185. Von Roenn JH, Murphy RL, Weber KM, et al. Megestrol acetate for treatment of cachexia associated with human immunodeficiency virus (HIV) infection. Ann Intern Med 1988;109:840–841.
186. Von Roenn JH, Armstrong D, Kotler DP, et al. Megestrol acetate in patients with AIDS-related cachexia. Ann Intern Med 1994;121: 393–399.
187. Oster MH, Enders SR, Samuels SJ, et al. Megastrol acetate in patients with AIDS and cachexia. Ann Intern Med 1994;121:400–408.
188. Engelson ES, Pi-Sunyer FX, Kotler DP. Effects of megestrol acetate therapy on body composition and circulating testosterone concentrations in patients with AIDS. AIDS 1995;9:1107–1108.
189. Strawford A, Hoh R, Neese R, et al. The effects of combination megestrol acetate (MA) and testosterone (T) replacement therapy in AIDS wasting syndrome (AWS) [abstract]. Nutrition 1997;13:276.
190. Gilbert CL, Koller EA, Green L, et al. Thrombotic events with megestrol acetate for AIDS wasting [abstract]. Nutrition 1997;13:271.
191. Rigsby LW, Dishman RK, Jackson WA, et al. Effects of exercise training on men seropositive for the human immunodeficiency virus-1. Med Sci Sports Exerc 1992;24:6–12.
192. Roubenoff R, Suri J, Raymond J, et al. Feasibility of increasing lean body mass in HIV-infected adults using progressive resistance training [abstract]. Nutrition 1997;13:271.
193. Wilmore DW. Catabolic illness: strategies for enhancing recovery. N Engl J Med 1991;325:695–702.
194. Krentz AJ, Koster FT, Crist DM, et al. Anthropometric, metabolic and immunological effects of recombinant human growth hormone in AIDS and AIDS-related complex. J Acquir Immune Defic Syndr 1993;6:245–251.
195. Lieberman SA, Butterfield GE, Harrison D, et al. Anabolic effects of recombinant insulin-like growth factor-I in cachectic patients with the acquired immunodeficiency syndrome. J Clin Endocrinol Metab 1994;78:404–410.
196. Lee PDK, Pivarnik JM, Bukar JG, et al. A randomized, placebo-controlled trial of combined insulin-like growth factor I and low dose growth hormone therapy for wasting associated with human immunodeficiency virus infection. J Clin Endocrinol Metab 1996;81: 2968–2975.
197. Ellis KJ, Lee PDK, Pivarnik JM, et al. Changes in body composition of human immunodeficiency virus–infected males receiving insulin-like growth factor I and growth hormone. J Clin Endocrinol Metab 1996;81:3033–3038.
198. Waters D, Danska J, Hardy K, et al. Recombinant human growth hormone, insulin-like growth factor 1, and combination therapy in AIDS-associated wasting: a randomized, double-blind, placebo-controlled trial. Ann Intern Med 1996;125:865–872.
199. Schambelan M, Mulligan K, Grunfeld C, et al. Recombinant human growth hormone in patients with HIV-associated wasting: a randomized, placebo-controlled trial. Ann Intern Med 1996;125:873–882.
200. Engelson ES, Rabkin JG, Rabkin R, et al. Effects of testosterone upon body composition. J Acquir Immune Defici Syndr Hum Retrovirol 1996;11:510–511.
201. Berger JR, Pall L, Winfield D. Effect of anabolic steroids on HIV related wasting myopathy. South Med J 1993;86:865–866.
202. Gold J, High HA, Li Y, et al. Safety and efficacy of nandrolone decanoate for treatment of wasting in patients with HIV infection. AIDS 1996;10:745–752.
203. Hengge UR, Baumann M, Maleba R, et al. Oxymetholone promotes weight gain in patients with advanced human immunodeficiency virus (HIV-1) infection. Br J Nutr 1996;75:129–138.
204. Berger JR, Pall L, Hall CD, et al. Oxandrolone in AIDS-wasting myopathy. AIDS 1996;10:1657–1662.
205. Endres S, Ghorbani R, Kelley VE, et al. The effect of dietary supplementation with n-3 polyunsaturated fatty acids on the synthesis of interleukin-1 and tumor necrosis factor by mononuclear cells. N Engl J Med 1989;320:265–271.
206. Hellerstein MK, Wu K, McGrath M, et al. Effects of dietary n-3 fatty acid supplementation in men with weight loss associated with the acquired immune deficiency syndrome: relation to indices of cytokine production. J Acquir Immune Defic Syndr Hum Retrovirol 1996;11: 258–270.
207. Jonkers C, Heijligenberg R, Leeuwen RV, et al. Dietary supplementation with fish-oil prevents the loss of lean body mass and attenuates the increase in TNF-α production in AIDS [abstract]. Nutrition 1997;13:273.
208. Ockenga J, Rohde F, Suttmann U, et al. Ketotifen in HIV-infected patients: effects on body weight and release of TNF-α. Eur J Clin Pharmacol 1996;50:167–170.
209. Dezube BJ, Pardee AB, Chapman B, et al. Pentoxifylline decreases tumor necrosis factor expression and serum triglycerides in people with AIDS: NIAID AIDS Clinical Trials Group. J Acquir Immune Defic Syndr 1993;6:787–794.

210. Dezube BJ, Lederman MM, Spritzler JG, et al. High-dose pentoxifylline in patients with AIDS: inhibition of tumor necrosis factor production: National Institute of Allergy and Infectious Diseases AIDS Clinical Trials Group. J Infect Dis 1995;171: 1628–1632.
211. Landman D, Sarai A, Sathe SS. Use of pentoxifylline therapy for patients with AIDS-related wasting: pilot study. Clin Infect Dis 1994;18:97–99.
212. Sathe SS, Sarai A, Tsigler D, et al. Pentoxifylline aggravates impairment in tumor necrosis factor-α secretion and increases mycobacterial load in macrophages from AIDS patients with disseminated *Mycobacterium avium-intracellulare* complex infection. J Infect Dis 1994; 170:484–487.
213. Tramontana JM, Utaipat U, Molloy A, et al. Thalidomide treatment reduces tumor necrosis factor α production and enhances weight gain in patients with pulmonary tuberculosis. Mol Med 1995;1:384–397.
214. Klausner JD, Makonkawkeyoon S, Akarasewi P, et al. The effect of thalidomide on the pathogenesis of human immunodeficiency virus type 1 and *M. tuberculosis* infection. J Acquir Immune Defic Syndr Hum Retrovirol 1996;11:247–257.
215. Reyes-Teran G, Sierra-Madero JG, Martinez del Cerro V, et al. Effects of thalidomide on HIV-associated wasting syndrome: a randomized, double-blind, placebo-controlled clinical trial. AIDS 1996; 10:1501–1507.
216. Jacobson JM, Greenspan JS, Spritzler J, et al. Thalidomide for the treatment of oral apthous ulcers in patients with human immunodeficiency virus infection: National Institute of Allergy and Infectious Diseases AIDS Clinical Trials Group. N Engl J Med 1997;336: 1486–1493.

40

ASSAYS FOR THE DIAGNOSIS OF HIV INFECTION

Denis Henrard and Patricia Reichelderfer

Human immunodeficiency virus (HIV) is endemic in the United States and is one of the leading causes of death among adults aged 25 to 44 years (1). Although men who have sex with men constitute the largest infected population, the number of cases of women, adolescents, and young adults is increasing rapidly (2). The first blood test for the diagnosis of HIV-1 became available in 1985. Today, less than 1 in 10,000 blood donors in the United States is identified as being infected with HIV-1. This finding reflects the extremely low prevalence (0.008%) of HIV-1 infection among blood donors (3). On the other hand, the seroprevalence is much higher among patients in hospitals and other health care settings. For example, anonymous testing of nearly 200,000 consecutive patients admitted to 20 acute care hospitals revealed that almost 5% of them were infected with HIV (4).

The laboratory diagnosis of HIV-1 infection in adults is most often accomplished by analysis of a blood sample. This may include testing for antibody, for p24 antigen, or for culturable virus or gene amplification. Specific serologic assays for the diagnosis of HIV in urine and saliva samples are also available. The diagnosis of infection in infants born to HIV-infected women cannot rely on antibody detection and must use assays to detect the presence of virus.

HIV infection remains largely undiagnosed and is often not detected until late in infection. In 1995, the United States Centers for Disease Control and Prevention (CDC) conducted a survey of 2441 AIDS cases from 11 states and found that 87% of the participants were tested only 2 months to 1 year before being diagnosed with AIDS (5). Most (58%) of these patients were diagnosed while admitted for an illness at an acute care hospital. Fewer than 13% of subjects sought testing at a designated counseling center for high-risk behavior (5). Lack of testing has been attributed to denial of risk, lack of access to or knowledge of available tests, and physicians who do not consider the diagnosis or who are unaware of potential therapeutic interventions.

The testing environment and attitude of clinicians can have a major impact on patient awareness of HIV infection. For example, in the early 1990s, only 15 to 25% of HIV-infected patients admitted to the Johns Hopkins Hospital in Baltimore knew about their serostatus. Today, after several collaborative studies on routine screening (6, 7) and primary infection (8, 9) were conducted, HIV testing is offered to every admitted patient. As a result, more than 75% of infected patients know about their serostatus (T Quinn, unpublished data).

This chapter presents a summary of the types of assays and specimens that can be reliably used for the diagnosis of HIV-1 infection and the clinical context in which these assays are most useful. To understand the underlying principles of the various diagnostic assays presented here, the reader should refer to discussions of basic viral properties (see Chaps. 2 and 3).

Although this summary focuses on HIV-1, another strain of HIV, HIV-2, was identified in West Africa in 1985 (10, 11). HIV-2 has also been identified in the United States, albeit at a low prevalence. Fewer than 60 persons to date have been diagnosed with HIV-2 infection in the United States (see Chap. 57).

DIAGNOSIS OF INFECTION IN BLOOD SPECIMENS FROM ADULTS

Defining the Window of Seroconversion

After the initial contact with an infectious agent, a variable period occurs during which the presence of the microorganism or antibodies directed against the pathogen cannot be detected. For many pathogens, this "incubation" period lasts about 2 weeks (e.g., varicella) and occasionally up to 6 weeks (e.g., Epstein–Barr virus). Early reports of a prolonged seronegative "latent period" in HIV infection have not been substantiated (12, 13). The results were obtained using unvalidated diagnostic methods that were notoriously prone to false-positive reactions resulting from specimen contamination. Subsequent studies using validated tests and conducted under carefully controlled conditions designed to minimize specimen contamination demonstrated that the seronegative window of HIV infection is approximately 3 to 5 weeks (14).

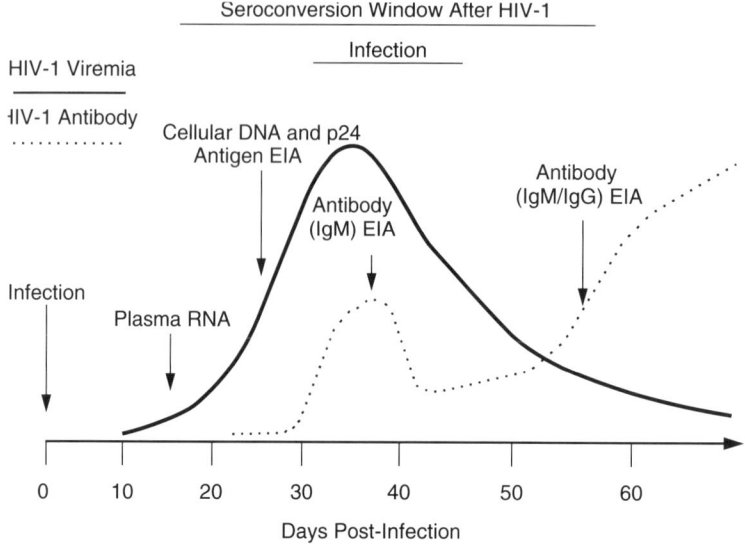

Figure 40.1. Typical seroconversion profile illustrating the timing of appearance of diagnostic markers after infection.

The order in which diagnostic markers of HIV infection appear has also been well defined (15, 16). Retrospective studies of blood donors, plasma donors, and individuals at risk of HIV infection who seroconverted have been particularly useful to determine the sequence and timing of appearance of diagnostic markers. A typical profile of seroconversion is shown in Figure 40.1. Approximately 2 weeks after infection, the presence of viral RNA encapsulated in viral particles can be detected in serum or plasma. A few days later, HIV DNA associated with infected peripheral blood mononuclear cells (PBMC), as well as HIV p24 antigen, become detectable. The first sign of an immune response usually appears about 1 week later in the form of immunoglobulin M (IgM), which quickly reaches a peak and then decreases over the following weeks. Approximately 1 week after IgM antibody detection, IgG antibody levels rise significantly and reach a plateau within a few months. Thus, the immunologic profile of seroconversion to HIV is similar to that of other infectious agents.

The ability to detect diagnostic markers during the early events of HIV infection depends on the sensitivity of the assay used to measure the marker and also on the individual response of the person to the virus. Studies of closely spaced (two to four times per week) sequential serum samples obtained from individuals around the time of seroconversion have always identified IgM before IgG antibodies (15, 17, 18). In contrast, HIV RNA and DNA can be detected in almost all persons before IgM and IgG antibodies become detectable. Similarly, p24 antigen can be detected before HIV antibodies in more than 90% of subjects (15). Before an effective immune response is mounted, the levels of HIV RNA, DNA, and p24 antigen are generally extremely high, corresponding to 10^6 to 10^9 viruses per milliliter of blood, reflecting intense viral replication in the absence of immune containment (19, 20). The specific level of viral replication may be associated with a particular virus strain, or it may be host related.

Antibody Testing

The serologic diagnosis of antibody to HIV in blood specimens takes approximately 1 week. First, pretest counseling is provided, followed by phlebotomy to obtain the specimen. The specimen is then sent to a central hospital laboratory or to an outside testing laboratory. The antibody test is typically completed within 2 to 3 hours. If the sample is nonreactive, the patient can be informed quickly, within a day. However, if the sample is reactive, it is retested in duplicate and then is analyzed further by supplemental tests to confirm HIV infection. This process usually takes several days, after which the results can be disclosed to the tested person by a clinician or special counselor.

The easiest and most widely used test for identification of HIV infection is the enzyme immunoassay (EIA). It is an indirect test that measures the presence of antibody to HIV proteins. Dozens of EIAs for HIV antibody are commercially available. They differ in format and in the nature of the antigens (viral lysate recombinant proteins and peptides) and in the conjugates used for detection (21). Viral proteins or peptides coated on a solid support are used to capture anti-HIV antibodies from serum or plasma. Captured antibodies are then detected using a "conjugate," which is a color-producing enzyme attached to an immunologic component. The nature of the proteins coated on the solid support and that of the conjugate can significantly affect test performance.

Most current EIAs use recombinant proteins, synthetic peptides, or a combination of both, on the solid phase; these are "cleaner" and easier to make than purified viral lysate. However, this increased "cleanliness" can adversely affect performance when testing various HIV strains (22) (see the final section of this chapter). Until 1992, antihuman antibodies were used in the conjugate of EIAs for screening blood donors. These antibody conjugates can only bind to the heavy chain (Fab) of HIV antibody and thus can detect only IgGs. Currently, the conjugates used in assays consist of specific HIV antigens coupled to an enzyme. These antigen conjugates can bind to any type of antibody, including IgM. Thus, the sensitivity of these tests has increased, particularly at the early stage of seroconversion (15). However, the limited number and restricted nature of antigenic sites on these conjugates can also adversely affect test performance when testing divergent HIV strains.

The performance of a test is often defined by its sensitivity (percentage of true positive samples that react with the test) and its specificity (percentage of true negative samples that do not react with the test) (23). Although the sensitivity should always be as close to 100% as possible, the specificity can vary greatly depending on the type of test and the prevalence HIV infection in population studied. For example, in blood donors, about 0.1% (1 in 1000) of the specimens are reactive by EIA, of which approximately 10% (1 in 10,000) are confirmed as positive by Western blot (WB) (3). In contrast, in sexually transmitted disease clinics, 10% (100 in 1000) or more of the specimens may be reactive by EIA, of which about 90% may be confirmed by WB (T Quinn, unpublished data). As a result, the probability that a sample reactive in a sexually transmitted disease clinic is truly positive is much higher (90%) compared with a sample from a blood donor (10%). However, the total number of samples that give a false-positive EIA reaction will also be higher in the sexually transmitted disease clinic ($n=10$) than in the blood donor population ($n=0.9$).

Confirmation of Reactivity

As previously discussed, every diagnostic test has a small but significant rate of false-positive results, mostly caused by nonspecific reactions. Therefore, a single sample positive by a primary screening EIA should be classified as "HIV reactive," *not positive*, and should be confirmed by one or more supplemental tests.

The WB has been the most commonly used supplemental test. Viral proteins are separated by size on a gel, transferred to a nitrocellulose sheet, and cut into individual "strips," which are incubated with serum samples. Antibodies bind to the HIV proteins on the paper and are revealed by antihuman antibodies conjugated to an enzyme that produces a colored reaction. This produces a distinctive pattern of bands corresponding to single HIV antigens. Antibodies can be identified to six major HIV proteins: gp41 and gp120 (envelope), p24 and p17 (core), and p66 and p31 (reverse transcriptase).

Reactivity to a WB strip can also be nonspecific. Therefore, one must use appropriate interpretation criteria. Several organizations, including the CDC (24), the World Health Organization (25), and the Consortium for Retrovirus Serology Standardization (26) have proposed criteria for interpreting WB reactivity. The two most commonly used criteria recommend that reactivity to 1) p24 *and* gp 41 or gp120/160 or 2) p24 or p31 *and* gp41 or gp 120/160 be observed to classify a sample as positive for HIV-1. (For diagnosis of HIV-2, p26 and gp36 antigens correspond to HIV-1 p24 and gp41 antigens, respectively.) Reactivity patterns that do not fit the foregoing criteria are classified as indeterminate.

Nonspecific reactivity by WB is relatively common and sometimes difficult to interpret. In fact, approximately 15 to 30% of EIA-negative samples produce indeterminate results on WB. Among EIA-reactive samples, a significant proportion (4 to 20%) can produce indeterminate WB results (27, 28). The use of an alternative confirmatory commercial test, the Recombinant Immunoblot Assay (RIBA), has reduced the number of indeterminate results by more than 80% (K Sayer, unpublished data). Nonetheless, the continued presence of indeterminate results points to one of the challenges in the identification of persons truly infected or not truly infected by HIV.

Some studies have shown that most people with samples producing indeterminate patterns on HIV WB are not infected by HIV (28–30). However, a small proportion of true infections will produce an indeterminate WB pattern. This can happen at the advanced stage of HIV disease in subjects with declining antibody levels resulting from a severely depressed immune system (31, 32). Such a pattern is also expected at the early stages of seroconversion, before antibody production reaches a sufficient level (33, 34). During that time, lack of confirmation by WB is a particular problem because third-generation EIAs are more sensitive than WB. Therefore, true EIA reactivity during seroconversion often is not confirmed by WB or RIBA. In these cases, p24 antigen and viral RNA detection are useful supplemental tests (33, 35). Some testing laboratories routinely use p24 antigen or RNA detection for specimens reactive by EIA but indeterminate by WB.

Testing for p24 Antigen and HIV RNA

The presence of HIV p24 antigen can be detected about 1 week before HIV antibodies, and therefore, it allows for earlier identification of primary infection. In June, 1996, the p24 antigen test was implemented for blood donor testing in the United States, and it has since identified a few donors who were seroconverting, yet still antibody negative. However, p24 testing is probably most useful in a hospital setting where the number of patients with primary HIV infection is much higher. For example, in a retrospective study of 2120 antibody-negative subjects attending the Johns Hopkins Hospital Emergency Department, 6 (0.28%) had detectable p24 antigen and additional findings indicating primary HIV infection (9). Schacker and associates (36) used a similar testing strategy to identify 46 patients prospectively at the time of primary infection.

Reactivity to p24 antigen EIA, similar to antibody EIA, can be nonspecific. Thus, one must confirm p24 antigen reactivity by supplemental testing. Confirmation can be obtained by a neutralization test. If the sample is truly positive, more than 50% of the reactivity should be neutralized by the addition of exogenous p24. Alternatively, the detection of virion RNA can be used to confirm p24 antigenemia.

The detection of plasma virion RNA by genomic amplification is more sensitive than p24 antigen EIA (37, 38). Furthermore, plasma HIV RNA is always present when p24 antigen is detected during seroconversion (35, 39). Thus, considerable interest exists in using HIV RNA detection for screening in blood banks. Because of its increased sensitivity, virion RNA testing probably will replace the current p24 antigen testing of blood donors. Similarly, clinicians from hospitals could be tempted to use virion RNA tests to diagnose HIV infection. However, although quantitative RNA assays have been developed for prognostic and monitoring purposes, none of the currently available tests are licensed for diagnostic use. Although an RNA test can give additional information during the acute infection stage, critical issues such as false reactivity and confirmation of the results remain.

Testing Algorithms

At the time of seroconversion, up to 93% of subjects infected by HIV have nonspecific symptoms consistent with an acute viral illness (40, 41). These include fever (more than 95%), fatigue (more than 90%), pharyngitis (60 to 70%), myalgia or arthralgia (60 to 70%), swollen lymph nodes (50 to 65%), headache (45 to 55%), nausea (30 to 50%), weight loss (35 to 70%), and rash (30 to 40%) (8, 36). Therefore, subjects presenting to a hospital with such symptoms should be suspected of acute primary HIV infection. The diagnosis in these individuals during the acute stage of infection can lead not only to counseling, but also to early treatment and prevention of HIV transmission (40, 41).

A summary of two testing algorithms for the hospital or clinical setting is given in Table 40.1. The first describes patients who admit to various risk factors or for whom the physician believes a test is warranted. The second algorithm is for patients who present with nonspecific symptoms indicating a possible acute infection. The major difference between these two testing strategies is the request for antibody *and* p24 antigen (or HIV RNA) determination at the time of initial tests for patients with possible acute primary infection.

DIAGNOSIS OF INFECTION IN INFANTS

Considerations for the Diagnosis of Infant Infection

The rapid and accurate diagnosis of HIV-infected infants is essential to initiate therapy as soon as possible. However, diagnosis of HIV-1 infection during the neonatal period cannot simply be based on the presence of IgG antibody, because all babies born to HIV-1 infected mothers are HIV IgG antibody positive for up to 18 months as a result of passive transfer from their mothers (42). HIV-infected infants develop HIV IgA antibody between 3 and 6 months of age. However, studies have shown that the detection of IgA was not sensitive (less than 70%) (43–46). Therefore, the accurate early diagnosis of HIV infection represents a challenge for which several technologies, which primarily identify the virus itself, are useful alone or in combination.

Infants born to HIV-infected mothers may acquire the virus either in utero or in the intrapartum period. The Pediatric AIDS Clinical Trials Group has arbitrarily defined early (in utero) versus late (intrapartum) infection based on the ability to detect HIV-1 during the first 48 hours of life versus during the period from day 7 to day 90 (47). This definition is based on several studies including a meta-analysis of 12 studies that used DNA polymerase chain reaction (PCR) for virus detection. This analysis, which involved 271 HIV-infected children, showed that approximately 38% of children were infected in utero and 62% were infected in the intrapartum period (48). The results of

Table 40.1 Algorithm for Diagnosis of HIV-1 in Blood Specimens from Adults

Patient with Known Risk Factors	Patient with Nonspecific Symptoms and Possible Acute Infection
Pretest counseling and blood draw ↓	Pretest counseling and blood draw ↓
Request for HIV diagnosis by EIA/WB ↓	Request for HIV diagnosis by EIA AND p24 antigen or RNA ↓
If EIA negative, report as negative ↓	If both negative, report as negative ↓
If EIA reactive, test is repeated and WB/p24 antigen used to confirm ↓	If EIA reactive, follow same steps as for column 1 ↓
• If WB/p24 antigen negative, report as negative	• If EIA negative and p24 antigen or RNA positive, confirm by retesting on a second sample
• If WB or p24 antigen positive and confirmed, report as positive	• If positive, report as primary HIV infection; follow-up with EIA/WB 2–4 wk later
• If WB indeterminate and p24 antigen negative, report as negative; may recommend follow-up testing at 1–3 mo	• If negative, report as negative; may recommend follow-up testing in 1–3 mo

EIA, enzyme immunoassay; WB, Western blot.

another study, which used culture for the detection of HIV, also indicated that about 27% of children were infected in utero (49). Therefore, about two-thirds of HIV-positive children do not have virus detected at delivery and appear to become infected at that time.

The arbitrary definition of the route of infection based on a cutoff period of up to 48 hours for in utero infection and at least 7 days for postpartum infection may give the false impression that no infants produce virus between those two time points. This situation is simply not the case because infants can become positive for viral markers at any time between birth and a few months of age. In addition, other factors, such as the relative sensitivity of the assays and the timing of sample collection, also play a role in estimating the time and route of infection (49). Detectable virus and high viral loads at birth have been associated with increased rate of disease progression in some, but not all, studies (50, 51). Children can also become infected by breast-feeding, but this route is unlikely in the United States because of active programs to persuade seropositive mothers not to breast-feed. The intrapartum or postpartum HIV infection resembles the acute primary infection in adults and, similarly, requires repeat sampling and testing to confirm HIV infection.

Several methods are available for the early diagnosis of pediatric infection. Direct detection of HIV in infants has been achieved by viral culture (52), as well as measurements of HIV-1 proviral copy number in infant cells (DNA PCR) (53), p24 antigen (54), and immune-complex–dissociated p24 antigen (55). Most recently, the direct detection of HIV has been achieved by plasma HIV-1 viral RNA (RNA PCR) (56). Additionally, infant-specific immune response to HIV has been detected by in vitro antibody production (57). At present, most routine diagnosis is based on a combination of assays (53).

A summary of the major studies that have assessed the relative sensitivity of various assays for diagnosing infant infection during the first 6 months of life is presented in Table 40.2 (46, 52–59). The relative sensitivity of each assay increases with increasing age. The reason, at least in part, is the window period between intrapartum infection and the detection of viral markers in the infected child, as well as the relative sensitivity of the assays.

The results presented in Table 40.2 have been obtained primarily with specimens from patients who had not been treated or who had received, at most, a short course of zidovudine therapy. However, more recent data show that zidovudine and other antiviral treatments can have an effect on the rate of transmission that, in turn, can affect the relative sensitivity of the assay. For example, in infants tested at more than 30 days of age, the positive predictive value of DNA PCR testing was 95% if the transmission rate was high (25.5%), that is, the mother was untreated, and 83% if the transmission rate was low (8.3%), that is, the mother was treated (60). Zidovudine therapy for 6 months or less does not seem to affect the time at which a definitive *negative* diagnosis can be made, be it by culture or DNA PCR (61).

Table 40.2 Relative Sensitivities of Various Assays for Diagnosing Infant Infection During the First 6 Months of Life

Assay	Time to Detection; Number Positive Over Total Tested (% Positive)			Reference
	1–14 d	1–4 mo	6 mo	
Culture	19/40 (48)	30/40 (75)		54
	6/21 (29)	—	98/111 (88)	53
	7/29 (24)	96/111 (86)	43/49 (88)	46
	10/22 (45)	16/16 (100)	34/38 (90)	58
	10/17 (59)	14/15 (93)	21/21 (100)	59
			23/27 (89)	57
Mean sensitivity	41%	88.5%	91%	
DNA PCR	6/21 (29)	24/26 (92)	27/27 (100)	53
	14/25 (56)	18/19 (95)	42/43 (98)	58
	10/17 (57)	10/12 (83)	18/18 (100)	59
	3/19 (16)	26/35 (49)	10/11 (91)	56
Mean sensitivity	39.5%	79.8%	97%	
p24	7/40 (18)	11/40 (28)	—	54
	9/19 (47)	8/13 (62)	23/45 (51)	58
	7/17 (41)	10/17 (59)	23/26 (88)	57
	0/9 (0)	1/9 (11)	2/11 (18)	57
			18/27 (66)	55
Mean sensitivity	26.5%	40%	55.8%	
Immune complex–dissociated p24	0/9 (0)	9/9 (100)	11/11 (100)	55
	12/19 (63)	15/16 (93)	21/30 (73)	58
Mean sensitivity	31.5%	96.5%	86.5%	
RNA PCR	6/19 (32)	32/35 (91)	11/11 (100)	56
Immunoglobulin A	12/24 (50)	20/23 (87)	49/50 (98)	52
In vitro antibody production	—	—	25/27 (93)	57

PCR, polymerase chain reaction.

However, whether therapy that suppresses viral load sufficiently can delay *positive* diagnosis of infected infants remains to be established.

A final concern for pediatric diagnosis is specificity. Occasionally, HIV has been detected at birth by one or more assays and has not been confirmed by repeat testing. These infants have been reported as "transiently" infected (62). In addition are reports of DNA PCR-positive results from seroreverting infants who were never infected (63, 64). Many of these cases appear to be the result of samples misattributed to the subjects, and no case has had satisfactory documentation that the virus detected was indeed from the corresponding mother (J Mullens, unpublished data). Because each method has been reported to have spurious erroneous results, either false-positive or false-negative, clearly a need exists to repeat testing on a second specimen to verify initial results (65).

Peripheral Blood Mononuclear Cell Culture

In infants, culture of virus from PBMCs is the current standard to which all other assays have been compared. HIV is produced by patient cells that can be activated to express virus in vitro, as well as those that are already expressing virus. Blood specimens from neonates have, in general, extremely high levels of circulating lymphocytes. Therefore, culture can be successfully performed with small volumes of blood. Infection status is generally determined from culturing 1 million lymphocytes (66). In specimens with limited numbers of lymphocytes, a modified protocol can be used without appreciable loss of detectability (66). The lymphocytes are first separated from blood plasma and are cultured in the presence of normal donor PBMCs that have been activated to support viral replication. Current culture technology is based on consensus protocols (66) and takes 14 to 28 days. As described historically (see Table 40.2), the sensitivity increased over time from a mean of 41% at 2 weeks to 91% at 6 months. However, using current culture methods, sensitivity is usually more than 90% for children older than 2 weeks of age (49). More important, for diagnosis in infants, the specificity of culture is greater than 99.6% (52).

Qualitative DNA PCR

Qualitative DNA PCR is probably the most commonly used assay for the diagnosis of infection in infants. DNA PCR measures all integrated proviral DNA in the PBMCs, regardless of the ability of the DNA to make infectious virus. The only test licensed for HIV-1 DNA PCR diagnosis is the Roche Amplicor HIV-1 test (Roche Molecular Systems, Somerville, NJ). A 500-µL aliquot of whole blood collected in ethylenediamine tetraacetic acid (EDTA) or acid–citrate–dextrose is treated to lyse red blood cells, and leukocytes are then separated as a dry cell pellet by centrifugation. Alternatively, cell pellets of 1 million PBMCs can also be obtained using the lymphocyte separation technique developed for culture (66). Lymphocyte pellets may be tested immediately or frozen for batch assay and shipment to a central laboratory. After extraction of DNA from the cells and amplification, detection of DNA PCR products is determined colorimetrically using biotinylated probes. As for antibody EIAs, reactivity greater than the cutoff indicates that a specimen is positive.

The major advantage of DNA PCR over culture is the rapid turnaround time to report results. Most DNA PCR results, even when tested in batch mode, are generally available within 1 week or less, compared with 3 weeks for culture. The major disadvantage of DNA PCR over culture is the possible risk of false-positive results from contamination of the specimen. Methods have been developed to help minimize this possibility (67). False-negative results can also occur if the specimen contains inhibitors for the PCR reaction such as hemoglobulin or heparin (68), or when the assay contains fewer cells than expected. As an internal quality control for the number of available cells, testing of pediatric specimens for HIV DNA should also include concurrent testing for HLA DQα by PCR amplification.

The use of HIV-1 DNA PCR for early infant diagnosis was examined in a meta-analysis of 32 studies (60). The range of sensitivity (31 to 100%) and specificity (50 to 100%) was a function of infant age and transmission rates. As expected, the combined sensitivity was higher in older (more than 30 days) infants (98.2%) than in neonates (93.3%). As with culture, early studies have shown that the sensitivity of the assay increased over time from 40% at 2 weeks to 97% at 6 months (see Table 40.2). At the present time, most untreated infants, or infants treated with zidovudine, will be HIV-1 DNA PCR positive during the first month of life. The occurrence of false-positive reactions results in an average specificity that is lower than that of culture (97%) (53).

The detection of HIV DNA PCR has also been successfully performed on dried blood spots and has been shown to have a sensitivity and specificity similar to those obtained with PBMCs (69). The dried blood spot requires a small volume, typically from a heel stick. These features are particularly advantageous for use in field trials and diagnosis in developing countries.

Plasma HIV-1 RNA Detection

The latest approach to infant diagnosis is by the detection of HIV-1 plasma RNA. Cell-free HIV-1 RNA in the plasma of infected subjects is associated with both infectious and noninfectious virus. Currently, RNA detection assays are quantitative tests that are useful for prognosis and monitoring patients on therapy, but they are not qualitative diagnostic tests. The only licensed RNA assay is the Roche HIV-1 Monitor assay, and, as stated previously, it is not licensed for diagnostic use. Nonetheless, initial investigations into the use of plasma RNA quantification suggests that this may hold promise for the early diagnosis of pediatric infection (56). Studies are needed to define the specificity of the test. In general, one would expect that advantages and disadvantages that apply to DNA PCR will also apply to RNA PCR.

Testing Algorithm for Pediatric Diagnosis

All findings to date point to the need for repeat testing and use of multiple assay formats to diagnose infection in infants. An algorithm for defining pediatric infectious status has been proposed by the Women and Infants Transmission Studies Group (70) based, in part, on guidelines from the CDC (71). Definitive HIV *infection* can be ascertained if one or more HIV diagnostic assay (HIV culture, DNA PCR, immune-complex–dissociated p24 antigen, serum p24 antigen, or anti-HIV IgA) is positive on at least two samples collected at different times. For patients without clinical signs of disease and who have no other positive diagnostic assay results, definitive HIV-1 *uninfected* status can be ascertained by two negative cultures or DNA PCR results, one of which must be obtained when the patient is at least 6 months of age (70). In general, two separate samples, drawn over a 3-month period, and tested by culture and DNA PCR, appear to have a 100% sensitivity and a 95% specificity (53). Thus, either repeat testing by viral culture or DNA PCR or culture combined with DNA PCR allows for the determination of infection status in 100% of children infected by 6 months of age. This 6-month period may be shortened in the future as methods for testing improve. Infection status in children who are at least 18 months old is established as for adults.

In some cases, one cannot obtain two samples over the required time frame to make a definitive diagnosis, and the infant's status is classified as indeterminate. Indeterminate status occurs if 1) a single *positive* test result (culture, PCR, p24 antigen EIA, or ICD p24 antigen EIA) is not confirmed by testing another specimen or 2) a single *negative* result (culture, PCR, p24 antigen EIA, or ICD p24 antigen EIA) is not confirmed by testing a second sample obtained at 6 months of age or older. In each case, the second test can be done by the same or a different method. In a study of 885 infants born to HIV-infected mothers, 56 infants (5%) were found be indeterminate (70). These infants had only one culture determination and were otherwise lost to follow-up for various reasons, including death. The failure to determine infant infection status definitively is therefore a function of appropriate follow-up and sampling and not of test failure.

DIAGNOSIS OF INFECTION IN SPECIMENS OTHER THAN BLOOD

Specific EIAs have been improved or developed to allow the use of samples other than blood, such as urine or saliva, for the diagnosis of HIV infection. Confirmatory WB assays have been similarly modified to detect HIV-1 antibodies in urine and oral fluids. Although tests have been approved by the United States Food and Drug Administration (FDA) for testing fluids other than blood, this approval has so far included the specific warning that these tests are not as accurate as blood tests (72, 73).

Testing Urine Specimens

Several early studies provided conflicting results on the sensitivity of urine testing. Although some investigators found a sensitivity equivalent to that obtained with blood specimens (74, 75), others reported a sensitivity in the range of 70 to 98% (76, 77). These discrepancies may reflect differences in patient populations or in specimen handling, or both.

In 1996, the FDA approved a urine HIV-1 antibody EIA (Calypte Biomedical, Berkeley, CA). During preliminary clinical studies, the EIA used in combination with a specifically designed WB test was found to be 100% sensitive and specific (78). However, it was not approved as a stand-alone diagnostic test. Patients with reactive specimens have to be retested using a blood specimen.

Testing Oral Fluids

The collection of saliva instead of blood can be especially advantageous outside the hospital setting. The procedure is simple and does not require qualified personnel to be present, thereby allowing for sample collection outside of the clinic. It is also applicable to patients from whom drawing blood may be difficult, such as patients with hemophilia.

The low sensitivity observed in early studies (79) on saliva was primarily the result of two independent factors. First, the levels of IgG in saliva are a thousandfold lower than in serum. Second, the presence of bacterially produced proteases that degrade immunoglobins contributes significantly to the reduced sensitivity of the test. Today, the detection of HIV antibody in oral fluid can be as sensitive and specific as in blood specimens. This improvement is primarily due to advances in collection devices that concentrate and stabilize the immunoglobulins in oral fluid, combined with assays designed specifically for testing oral fluids.

One of these collection devices, the OraSure (Epitope, Beaverton, OR), was approved in 1994 by the FDA. The device consists of an absorbent pad attached to a plastic stick that is rubbed gently along the tooth and gum margin and then is allowed to sit to concentrate immunoglobulins that primarily arise from the gingival crevical fluid. The sticks are placed in transport vials containing buffer and antimicrobial agents. The collection device concentrates IgG three- to fourfold and stabilizes the antibody levels for up to 21 days at temperatures ranging from −20 to 37°C.

Modifications of EIA and WB have also increased the sensitivity of antibody detection in oral fluids (80). The Oral Fluid Vironostika HIV-1 Microelisa System (Organon Teknika, Durham, NC) and the OraSure HIV-1 WB kit (Epitope, Beaverton, OR) in combination with the OraSure Collection system correctly identified HIV antibody in 99.9% of 3569 saliva specimens from HIV-infected patients (81). Overall, the diagnosis of HIV antibody in saliva has a sensitivity of 97.2 to 100% and a specificity of 97.7 to 100% (82).

ALTERNATIVE TESTING STRATEGIES

Testing with Rapid Assays

Rapid and simple methods are valuable for testing patients in doctor's offices, outpatient clinics, and other situations without fast and easy access to a testing laboratory. The sensitivity and specificity of rapid, instrument-free assay methods have been compared to enzyme-linked immunosorbent assay and WB for blood, oral, and urine specimens. Several rapid tests are commercially available, but only one, the Simple Use Diagnostic System (SUDS) test (Murex Corp., Norcross, GA) is currently licensed in the United States. Many of these rapid tests are based on agglutination or dot-blot methods.

A comprehensive review of studies evaluating the performance of rapid assays has been previously published (21). One of these studies (83) evaluated the sensitivity and specificity of six rapid assays, including the SUDS assay licensed in the United States, in four distinct specimen types. The format of these assays included solid-phase capture ($n=3$), dot-immunoblot assays ($n=2$), and latex agglutination ($n=1$). The specimens tested included 399 collected from seronegative blood donors and obstetric patients, 202 EIA and WB seropositive specimens, and 99 sera that were reactive by EIA and positive, negative, or indeterminate by WB. The highest mean sensitivity (more than 99%) and specificity (more than 91%) were observed with the solid-phase assays ($n=3$). The SUDS assay had the greatest overall sensitivity, that is, 100%. On the other hand, the GENIE assay (Genetic Systems Corp., Seattle, WA) had no false-positive results, that is, a specificity of 100%. Therefore, although the GENIE assay did not detect all positive specimens, any reactive sample was 100% likely to be a true positive.

The relative sensitivity and specificity of the SUDS and other rapid assays have also been evaluated using various seroconverter panels (84, 85). The ability of the SUDS assay to detect both IgM and IgG antibody makes it particularly useful in diagnosing early infection. Indeed, the SUDS assay had equal or greater sensitivity than the Abbott third-generation EIA (84). However, the assay also reacted with some seronegative and PCR negative specimens, indicating false-positive reactions. Therefore, the authors of these studies recommended the SUDS assay for rapid confirmation of EIA activity.

The results of a 3-month study using the SUDS assay for testing 984 patients in a sexually transmitted disease clinic or an anonymous testing tenter were similar to those of standard testing; that is, 98% of the tests were negative. Negative results by the SUDS assay do not have to be confirmed and can be directly reported to the patient. The effectiveness of same-day testing and counseling was also measured in a poststudy interview in which 88% of patients who had previously been tested said that they preferred the rapid test (86).

Rapid testing may be most desirable in developing countries, where it is often difficult to ensure that patients will return for results and counseling. A judicious combination of conventional EIAs can have 100% sensitivity and specificity (87). Similarly, studies suggest that testing with a combination of rapid tests could be a cheaper and faster alternative to the EIA/WB approach in developing countries (88).

Testing at Home

Over the past decade, the FDA has conducted several hearings on the pros and cons of home testing. Despite an initial negative bias toward home testing, a growing appreciation of the number of individuals at risk who have not been tested by standard procedures prompted renewed interest in home testing. Several assays have been developed that involve private code registration and pretest counseling. The patient is given instructions along with a specimen collection device that uses a lancet to obtain a drop of blood. The specimen is then placed as a dried blood spot on the "specimen card," which is mailed to a central testing service. After testing is completed, the patient is informed of the results by phone and receives posttest counseling.

In May of 1996, the FDA approved the first home HIV testing and counseling service, Confide (Ortho Diagnostics, Raritan, NJ). Surprisingly, in June of 1997, Confide was withdrawn from the market because of lack of consumer demand. In July of 1996, the FDA approved Home Access and Home Access Express (Home Access Health Corporation, Hoffman Estates, IL). This assay is currently available.

A multicenter evaluation compared anonymous HIV testing using the Home Access system with standard venous blood draw (89). The adequacy of specimen collection was assessed by having the Home Access specimens spotted by both a trained phlebotomist and the patients. The study involved 1255 subjects from 5 sites with a low incidence of HIV. Both procedures correctly identified all samples from subjects who completed the study and had 100% concordant specificity and sensitivity.

New home testing systems are being developed both within and outside the United States. The newer generation of tests will allow the patient to perform the diagnostic test at home. However, even with a newer format, it is unclear from the Confide withdrawal whether home-testing will increase or decrease in the next few years.

HIV TESTING AND HIV-1 VARIABILITY

Understanding the HIV Subtypes or Clades

HIV-1 is a simplistic name for a family of diverse strains. Molecular changes in HIV occur frequently in vivo (90), resulting in a phenomenal degree of genetic variation over time (91). Until 1994, the entity called HIV-1 consisted of five specific subtypes or clades designated A to E. Each of those strains have been found in most countries, but to a different extent, depending on the geographic area (92). For example, subtype or clade B is the most common type in the United States, whereas clades A and E are prominent in Africa and Thailand, respectively. More recently, other clades (F, G, H) have been identified in Europe (93).

In 1990, a highly divergent HIV strain (ANT70) was isolated from a person of African origin living in Belgium (94). It was named subtype "O" for outlier. An increasing number of patients with subtype O virus have now been identified in Europe and elsewhere. Although most patients infected with this subtype were originally from Cameroon or were of Cameroonian origin (95), persons infected with O strains have been identified not only in many other African countries (96), but also in Europe (97, 98) and in the United States (99). In recognition of the diversity of the O strains from the other HIV-1 subtypes, the O strains have been classified as group O and the other A to H strains as group M.

Testing HIV Variants

Most of the tests and methods described earlier for diagnosis have been developed using the original isolate of HIV-1 (HIV_{LAI}), which belongs to clade B. This is the most prevalent clade in the United States and in Europe. Initially, many EIAs, including some of the best screening assays, could not always identify individuals infected with group O strains (22, 100, 101). However, newer screening tests have now been modified to include type O-specific antigens and to ensure optimal detection of HIV. Not surprisingly, similar difficulties in detecting group O strains have been experienced for diagnosis by DNA amplification (102). Additionally, DNA amplification may also fail to detect some group M subtypes (103), because most of the primers used for the assay were optimized for detection of subtype B. Appropriate primers should be used to overcome these deficiencies for both group O and group M strains.

If the clinician still suspects that a patient is infected despite the absence of reactive EIA and PCR test, a PBMC culture test would be an appropriate choice. The sensitivity of culture is similar for HIV group M and group O.

Emerging Variants

After the emergence of HIV-2 in 1985, HIV-1 group O represents the second appearance of a genetically highly divergent HIV strain. Given the ever increasing worldwide movement of individuals, HIV-O and other, yet unidentified divergent strains, will continue to spread around the world. This spread illustrates the challenge of diagnosing HIV infection, because infection is not simply related to one virus, but to a multitude of related variants.

Acknowledgments

We would like to thank Drs. Thomas Quinn and Catherine Wilfert for their helpful reviews of the chapter.

References

1. Centers for Disease Control and Prevention. Update: mortality attributable to HIV infection among persons aged 25–44 years: United States, 1994. MMWR Morb Mortal Wkly Rep 1996;45:121–125.
2. Centers for Disease Control and Prevention. First 500,000 AIDS cases: United States, 1995. MMWR Morb Mortal Wkly Rep 1995;44:849–853.
3. Lackritz EM, Statten GA, Aberle-Grasse J, et al. Estimated risk of transmission of the human immunodeficiency virus by screened blood in the United States. N Engl J Med 1995;333:1721–1725.
4. Janssen RS, St. Louis ME, Statten GA, et al. HIV infection among patients in U.S. acute care hospitals: strategies for the counseling and testing of hospital patients. N Engl J Med 1992;327:445–452.
5. Wortley PM, Chu SY, Diaz T, et al. HIV testing patterns: where, why, and when were persons with AIDS tested for HIV? AIDS 1995;9:487–492.
6. Mundy LM, Gopalan R, Quinn TC. More on routine HIV screening. N Engl J Med 1993;328:1716.
7. Kelen GD, Hexter DA, Hansen KN, et al. Trends in human immunodeficiency virus (HIV) infection among a patient population of an inner-city emergency department: implications for emergency department–based screening programs for HIV infection. Clin Infect Dis 1995;21:867–875.
8. Quinn TC. Acute primary HIV infection. JAMA 1997;278:58–62.
9. Clark SJ, Kelen GD, Henrard DR, et al. Unsuspected primary human immunodeficiency virus type 1 infection in seronegative emergency department patients. J Infect Dis 1994;170:194–197.
10. Barin F, M'Boup S, Denis F, et al. Serological evidence for virus related to simian T-lymphotropic retrovirus II in residents of West Africa. Lancet 1985;2:1387–1389.
11. Clavel F. HIV-2, the West African AIDS virus. AIDS 1987;1:135–140.
12. Imagawa DT, Lee MH, Wolinsky SM, et al. Human immunodeficiency virus type 1 infection in homosexual men who remain seronegative for prolonged periods. N Engl J Med 1989;320:1458–1462.
13. Wolinsky SM, Rinaldo CR, Kwok S, et al. Human immundeficiency virus type 1 (HIV-1) infection a median of 18 months before a diagnostic Western blot. Ann Intern Med 1989;111:961–972.
14. Busch MP, Lee LL, Statten GA, et al. Time course of detection of viral and serologic markers preceding human immunodeficiency virus type 1 seroconversion: implications for screening of blood and tissue donors. Transfusion 1995;35:91–97.
15. Gallarda JL, Henrard DR, Liu D, et al. Early detection of antibody to human immunodeficiency virus type 1 by using an antigen conjugate immunoassay correlates with the presence of immunoglobulin M antibody. J Clin Microbiol 1992;30:2379–2384.
16. Busch MP, Schumacher RT, Stramer SL, et al. Assessment of the window period: detection of RNA, p24 antigen, and antibody in early HIV infection [abstract S165]. Transfusion 1996;36(Suppl):42S.
17. Stramer SL, Heller JS, Coombs RW, et al. Markers of HIV infection prior to IgG antibody seropositivity. JAMA 1989;262:64–69.
18. Healey DS, Maskill WJ, Gust ID. Detection of anti-HIV immunoglobulin M by particle agglutination following acute HIV infection. AIDS 1989;3:301–304.
19. Wei X, Ghosh SK, Taylor ME, et al. Viral dynamics in human immunodeficiency virus type 1 infection. Nature 1995;373:117–122.
20. Ho DD, Neumann AU, Perelson AS, et al. Rapid turnover of plasma virions and CD4 lymphocytes in HIV-1 infection. Nature 1995;373:123–126.
21. Constantine NT. Serologic tests for the retroviruses: approaching a decade of evolution. AIDS 1993;7:1–13.
22. Simon F, Ly TD, Baillou-Baufils A, et al. Sensitivity of screening kits for anti-HIV-1 subtype O antibodies. AIDS 1994;8:1628–1629.
23. Mortimer JY. The influence of assay sensitivity and specificity on error rates in three anti-HIV testing strategies. AIDS 1989;3:199–207.
24. Centers for Disease Control and Prevention. Interpretation and use of Western blot assay for serodiagnosis of HIV-1 infection. MMWR Morb Mortal Wkly Rep 1989;38(Suppl S7):1–7.
25. World Health Organization. Proposed WHO criteria for interpreting results from Western blot assays for HIV-1, HIV-2, and HTLV-I/HTLV-II. Wkly Epidemiol Rec 1990;37:281–283.
26. Consortium for Retrovirus Serology. Standardization. Serological diagnosis of human immunodeficiency virus infection by Western blot testing. JAMA 1988;260:674–679.
27. Kleinman S. The significance of HIV-1–indeterminate Western blot results in blood donor populations. Arch Pathol Lab Med 1990;114:298–303.
28. Genesca J, Shih JW-K, Jett BW, et al. What do Western blot indeterminate patterns for human immunodeficiency virus mean in EIA-negative blood donors. Lancet 1989;2:1023–1025.
29. Jackson JB, MacDonald KL, Cadwell J, et al. Absence of HIV infection in blood donors with inderterminate Western blot tests for antibody to HIV-1. N Engl J Med 1990;322:217–222.
30. Jackson JB, Hanson MR, Johnson GM, et al. Long-term follow-up of blood donors with indeterminate human immunodeficiency virus type 1 results on Western blot. Transfusion 1995;35:98–102.
31. Zaaijer HL, Bloemer MH, Lelie PN. Temporary seronegativity in a human immunodeficiency virus type 1–infected man. J Med Virol 1997;51:80–82.
32. Montagnier L, Brenner C, Chamaret S, et al. Human immunodeficiency virus infection and AIDS in a person with negative serology. J Infect Dis 1997;175:955–959.
33. Zaaijer HL, Exel-Oehlers PV, Kraaijeveld T, et al. Early detection of antibodies to HIV-1 by third generation assays. Lancet 1992;340:770–772.
34. Henrard DR, Phillips J, Windsor I, et al. Detection of human immunodeficiency virus type 1 p24 antigen and plasma RNA: relevance to indeterminate serologic tests. Transfusion 1994;34:376–380.
35. Phair JP, Margolick JB, Jacobson LP, et al. Detection of infection with human immunodeficiency virus type 1 before seroconversion: correlation with clinical symptoms and outcome. J Infect Dis 1997;175:959–962

36. Schacker T, Collier AC, Hughes J, et al. Clinical and epidemiologic features of primary HIV infection. Ann Intern Med 1996;4:257–264.
37. Piatak M, Saag MS, Yang LC, et al. High levels of HIV-1 in plasma during all stages of infection determined by competitive PCR. Science 1993;259:1749–1754.
38. De Saussure P, Yerly S, Tullen E, et al. HIV-1 nucleic acids detected before p24 antigenemia in a blood donor. Transfusion 1993;33:164–167.
39. Mulder J, McKinney N, Christopherson C, et al. Rapid and simple PCR assay for quantitation of human immunodeficiency virus type 1 RNA in plasma: application to acute retroviral infection. J Clin Microbiol 1994;32:292–300.
40. Pedersen C, Lindhart BO, Jensen BL, et al. Clinical course of primary HIV infection: consequences for subsequent course of infection. Br Med J 1989;299:154–157.
41. Tindall B, Cooper DA. Primary HIV infection: host responses and intervention strategies. AIDS 1991;5:1–14.
42. European Collaborative Study. Mother-to-child transmission of HIV infection. Lancet 1988;1;1039–42.
43. Weiblen BJ, Lee FK, Cooper ER, et al. Early detection of HIV infection in infants by detection of IgA HIV antibodies. Lancet 1991;335:988–990.
44. Landesman S, Weblen B, Mendez H, et al. Clinical utility of HIV-IgA immunoblot assay in the early diagnosis of perinatal HIV infection. JAMA 1991;266:3443–3446.
45. Quinn TC, Kline R, Halsey N, et al. Early diagnosis of perinatal HIV infection by detection of viral-specific IgA antibodies. JAMA 1991;266:3439–3442.
46. McIntosh K, Comeau AM, Wara D, et al. for the National Institute of Allergy and Infectious Disease and National Institute of Child Health and Human Development Women and Infants' Transmission Study Group. The utility of IgA antibody to human immunodeficiency virus type 1 in early diagnosis of vertically transmitted infection. Arch Pediatr Adolesc Med 1996;150:598–602.
47. Bryson YJ, Luzuriaga K, Sullivan JL, et al. Proposed definitions for in utero versus intrapartum transmission of HIV-1. N Engl J Med 1992;17:1246–1247.
48. Dunn DT, Brandt CD, Krivine A, et al. The sensitivity of HIV-1 DNA polymerase chain reaction in the neonatal period and the relative contributions of intra-uterine and intra-partum transmission. AIDS 1995;9:F7–F11.
49. Kalish LA, Pitt J, Lew J, et al. for the Women and Infants Transmission Study (WITS). Defining the time of fetal or perinatal acquisition of human immunodeficiency virus type 1 infection on the basis of age of first positive culture. J Infect Dis 1997;175:712–715.
50. Papaevangelou V, Pollack H, Rigaud M, et al. The amount of early p24 antigenemia and not the time of first detection of virus predicts the clinical outcome of infants vertically infected with human immunodeficiency virus. J Infect Dis 1996;173:574–578.
51. Shearer WT, Quinn TC, LaRussa P, et al. for the Women and Infants Transmission Study Group. Viral load and disease progression in infants infected with human immunodeficiency virus type 1. N Engl J Med 1997;336:1337–1342.
52. McIntosh K, Pitt J, Brambilla D, et al. for the Women and Infants Transmission Study Group. Blood culture in the first 6 months of life for the diagnosis of vertically transmitted human immunodeficiency virus infection. J Infect Dis 1994;170:996–1000.
53. Bremer JW, Lew JF, Cooper E, et al. for the Women and Infants' Transmission Study Group. Diagnosis of infection with human immunodeficiency viru type 1 by a DNA polymerase chain reaction assay among infants enrolled in the Women and Infants Transmission Study. J Pediatr 1996;129:198–207.
54. Burgard M, Mayaux M-J, Blanche S, et al. The use of culture and p24 antigen testing to diagnose human immunodeficiency virus infection in neonates. N Engl J Med 1992;17:1192–1197.
55. Quinn TC, Kline R, Moss MW, et al. Acid dissociation of immune complexes improves diagnostic utility of p24 antigen detection in perinatally aquired human immunodeficiency virus infection. J Infect Dis 1993;167:1193–1196.
56. Steketee RW, Abrams EJ, Thea DM, et al. Early detection of perinatal human immunodeficiency virus (HIV) type 1 infection using RNA amplification and detection. J Infect Dis 1997;175:707–711.
57. De Rossi AD, Ades AE, Mammano F, et al. Antigen detection, virus culture, polymerase chain reaction, and in vitro antibody production in the diagnosis of vertically transmitted HIV-1 infection. AIDS 1991;5:15–20.
58. Kovacs A, Xu J, Rasheed S, et al. Comparison of a rapid nonisotopic polymerase chain reaction assay with four commonly used methods for the early diagnosis of human immunodeficiency virus type 1 infection in neonates and children. Pediatr Infect Dis J 1995;14:948–954.
59. Borkowsky W, Krasinski K, Pollack H, et al. Early diagnosis of human immunodeficiency virus infection in children <6 months of age: comparison of polymerase chain reaction, culture and plasma antigen capture techniques. J Infect Dis 1992;166:616–619.
60. Owens DK, Holodniy M, McDonald TW, et al. A meta-analytic evaluation of the polymerase chain reaction for the diagnosis of HIV infection in infants. JAMA 1996;275:1342–1348.
61. Chouquet C, Richardson S, Le Chenadec J, et al. Does zidovudine treatment change the timing of HIV-1 transmission from mother to child? [abstract] In: Conference on Global Strategies for the Prevention of HIV Transmission from Mothers to Infants, Washington, DC, 1997:19.
62. Bryson YJ, Pang S, Wei LS, et al. Clearance of HIV infection in a perinatally infected infant. N Engl J Med 1995;332:833–888.
63. Bakshi SS, Tetali S, Abrams EJ, et al. Repeatedly positive human immunodeficiency virus type 1 DNA polymerase chain reaction in human immunodeficiency virus–exposed seroreverting infants. Pediatr Infect Dis 1995;14:658–662.
64. Newell M-L, Dunn D, Maria AD, et al. Detection of virus in vertically exposed HIV-antibody–negative children. Lancet 1996;347:213–215.
65. Long SS, Lischner HW. Early and accurate detection of infection with human immunodeficiency virus type 1 in vertically exposed infants. J Pediatr 1996;129:189–191.
66. Division of AIDS (DAIDS), National Institute of Allergy and Infectious diseases. DAIDS virology manual for HIV laboratories. NIH-97-3828. Bethesda, MD: National Institutes of Health, 1997.
67. Longo MC, Berninger MS, Hartley JL. Use of uracil DNA glycosylase to control carry-over contamination in polymerase chain reaction. Gene 1990;93:125–128.
68. Jackson JB. Detection and quantitation of human immunodeficiency virus type 1 using molecular DNA/RNA technology. Arch Pathol Lab Med 1993;117:473–477.
69. Comeau AM, Pitt J, Hillyer GV, et al. for the Women and Infants Transmission Study Group. Early detection of human immunodeficiency virus on dried blood spot specimens: sensitivity across serial specimens. J Pediatr 1996;129:111–118.
70. Hansen IC, Pitt J, McIntosh K, et al. Standardized assessment of infants with indeterminate (IND) HIV-infection followed in the Women and Infants Transmission Study (WITS) [abstract We.B.3176]. In: 11th International Conference on AIDS, Vancouver, 1996.
71. Centers for Disease Control and Prevention. 1994 revised classification system for human immunodeficiency virus infection in children less than 13 years of age. MMWR Morb Mortal Wkly Rep 1994;43:1–10.
72. Frank AP, Wandell MG, Headings MD, et al. Anonymous testing using home collection and telemedicine counseling. Arch Intern Med 1997;157:309–314.
73. Tessler LF, Walsh JME. Usefulness of oral mucosal transudate for HIV antibody testing [letter]. JAMA 1997;277:1591–1593.
74. Connell JA, Parry JV, Mortimer PP, et al. Novel assay for the detection of immunoglobulin G antihuman immunodeficiency virus in untreated saliva and urine. J Med Virol 1993;41:159–164.
75. Constantine NT, Zhang X, Ling L, et al. Application of a rapid assay for detection of antibodies to human immunodeficiency virus in urine. Am J Clin Pathol 1994;101:157–161.
76. Tribble DR, Rodier GR, Saad MD, et al. Comparative field evaluation of HIV rapid diagnositic assays using serum, urine and oral mucosal transudate specimens. Clin Diagn Virol 1997;7:127–132.

77. Holm-Hansen C, Constantine NT, Haukenes G. Detection of antibodies to HIV in homologous sets of plasma, urine and oral mucosal transudate samples using rapid assays in Tanzania. Clin Diagn Virol 1993;1:207–214.
78. Berrios DC, Avins AL, Haynes-Sanstad K, et al. Screening for human immunodeficiency virus antibody in urine. Arch Pathol Lab Med 1995;119:139–141.
79. Malamud D. Oral diagnostic testing for detecting human immunodeficiency virus-1 antibodies: a technology whose time has come. Am J Med 1997;102(Suppl 4A):9–14.
80. Emmons WW, Paparello SF, Decker CF, et al. A modified ELISA and Western blot accurately determine anti-human immunodeficiency virus type 1 antibodies in oral fluids obtained with a special collecting device. J Infect Dis 1995;171:1406–1410.
81. Gallo D, Richard GJ, Fitchen JH, et al. Evaluation of a system using oral mucosal transudate for HIV-1 antibody screening and confirmatory testing. JAMA 1997;277:254–258.
82. Emmons WW. Accuracy of oral specimen testing for human immunodeficiency virus. Am J Med 1997;102(Suppl 4A):15–20.
83. Malone JD, Smith ES, Sheffield J, et al. Comparative evaluation of six rapid serological tests for HIV-1 antibody. J Acquir Immune Defic Syndr 1993;6:115–119.
84. Samdel HH, Gutigard B-G, Labay D, et al. Comparison of the sensitivity of four rapid assays for detection of antibodies to HIV-1/HIV-2 during seroconversion. Clin Diagn Virol 1996;7:44–61.
85. Constantine NT, Zhang X, Ling L, et al. Application of a rapid assay for detection of antibodies to human immunodeficiency virus in urine. Am J Clin Pathol 1994;101:157–161.
86. Kassler WJ, Dillon BA, Haley C, et al. On-site, rapid HIV testing with same-day results and counseling. AIDS 1997;11:1045–1051.
87. Urassa WK, Bredberg-Raden U, Mbena E, et al. Alternative confirmatory strategies in HIV-1 antibody testing. J AIDS 1992;5:170–176.
88. Sato PA, Maskill WJ, Tamashiro H, et al. Strategies for laboratory HIV testing: an examination of alternative approaches not requiring Western blot. Bull World Health Organ 1994;72:129–134.
89. Frank AP, Wandell MG, Headings MD, et al. Anonymous testing using home collection and telemedicine counseling. Arch Intern Med 1997;157:309–314.
90. Meyerhans A, Cheynier R, Albert J, et al. Temporal fluctuations in HIV quasispecies in vivo are not reflected by sequential HIV isolates. Cell 1989;58:901–910.
91. Wain-Hobson S. The fastest genome evolution ever described:HIV variation in situ. Curr Opin Genet Dev 1993;3:878–883.
92. Sharp PM, Robertson DL, Gao F, et al. Origins and diversity of human immunodeficiency viruses. AIDS 1994;8(Suppl 1):S27–S42.
93. Giacherri C, Yang Y, Wang B, et al. Highly sensitive detection of HIV RNA of diverse geographical origins [abstract S387]. Transfusion 1997;37(Suppl):97S.
94. De Leys R, Vanderborght B, vanden Haesevelde M, et al. Isolation and partial characterization of an unusual human immunodeficiency retrovirus from two persons of West-Central African origin. J Virol 1990;64:1207–1216.
95. Mauclere P, Loussert-Ajaka I, Damond F, et al. Serological and virological characterization of HIV-1 group O infection in Cameroon. AIDS 1997;11:445–453.
96. Peeters M, Gaye A, Mboup S, et al. Presence of HIV-1 group O infection in West Africa. AIDS 1996;10:343–344.
97. Hampl H, Sawitzky D, Stoffler-Meilicke M, et al. First case of HIV-1 subtype O infection in Germany. Infection 1995;23:369–370.
98. Soriano V. First case of HIV-1 group O infection in Spain. Vox Sang 1996;7:66.
99. Britvan L, Gould K, Drvjanski J, et al. Identification of HIV-1 group O infection: Los Angeles county, California 1996. MMWR Morb Mortal Wkly Rep 1996;45:561–565.
100. Loussert-Ajaka I, Ly TD, Chaix ML, et al. HIV-1/HIV-2 seronegativity in HIV-1 subtype O infected patients. Lancet 1994;343:1393–1394.
101. Apetrei C, Loussert-Ajaka I, Descamps D, et al. Lack of screening test sensitivity during HIV-1 non-subtype B seroconversions. AIDS 1996;10:F57–F60.
102. Loussert-Ajaka I, Descamps D, Simon F, et al. Genetic diversity and HIV detection by polymerase chain reaction. AIDS 1994;8:1628–1629.
103. Arnold C, Barlow KL, Kaye S, et al. HIV type 1 sequence G transmission from mother to infant: failure of variant sequence species to amplify in the Roche Amplicor test. AIDS Res Human Retroviruses 1995;11:999–1001.

41
USE OF PLASMA HIV-1 RNA TO ASSESS PROGNOSIS AND MONITOR THERAPY IN HIV-1 INFECTION

Robert W. Coombs and Patricia S. Reichelderfer

Replication of human immunodeficiency virus type 1 (HIV-1) (viral load) can be assessed by many methods such as p24 antigen detection, culture of peripheral blood mononuclear cells (PBMCs), measurement of proviral copy number (DNA polymerase chain reaction [DNA-PCR]), and measurement of viral RNA (see Chap. 3). However, to date, none of these measures of replication has been shown to have the same sensitivity to detect HIV-1 in untreated individuals as assays that measure plasma HIV-1 RNA (1). The increased sensitivities of the assays that detect viral RNA make them suitable for monitoring HIV-infected patients at all stages of disease, even during primary infection.

Commercial assays to detect plasma HIV-1 RNA have been available since 1991. Three of these assay formats are commonly used for measuring plasma HIV-1 RNA. A brief description of the assays is given in Table 41.1. Each of the assays has advantages and disadvantages. To date, only the Roche Monitor assay has been licensed for clinical use and only for prognosis, not for therapeutic monitoring. All the assays are in the process of being modified to increase their sensitivity. Additional assay formats are expected in the near future.

Guidelines have been developed for the use of antiretroviral agents in the treatment of HIV-infected patients (2–8). Viral load as measured by plasma HIV-1 RNA is an integral part of all the guidelines. The use of plasma HIV-1 RNA levels in patient management is based on our increased understanding of virus replication. These guidelines recommend when to measure plasma HIV-1 RNA, when to initiate therapy based on plasma HIV-1 RNA, and when to alter therapy based on changes in plasma HIV-1 RNA. Many of the recommendations put forth in these guidelines are based on experiences with earlier assay formats. For example, the concept of "undetectable viral RNA" is being continually refined for each assay type. The first plasma HIV-1 RNA assay in general use was the Chiron Quantiplex HIV-1 RNA 1.0 branched DNA (bDNA) assay, which had a lower limit of detection of 10,000 copies/mL (9). At present, more sensitive versions of most of the commercially available assays have lower detection limits of less than 100 HIV-1 RNA copies/mL of plasma (10, 11). However, the lower limit of detection is different from the lower limit of quantification. This point is expanded on later in the chapter.

Some of the recommendations for use of plasma HIV-1 RNA put forth in the foregoing guidelines were based solely on the expert opinion of panel members. The authors of the guidelines fully acknowledge this limitation and hence the need for constant reassessment of these recommendations. The intent of this chapter is to reassess the recommendations that pertain to the use of plasma viral RNA in the context of the evolving concept of viral pathogenesis and therapy in both adult and pediatric infection. In addition, to understand the usefulness and limitations of plasma viral RNA measurement in clinical practice, caveats that pertain to the use of plasma HIV-1 RNA as a marker for viral burden and clinical outcome are discussed.

PROGNOSTIC ABILITY OF PLASMA HIV-1 RNA AND ITS USE IN THE THERAPEUTIC MANAGEMENT OF INFECTED ADULTS

Use of Plasma Viral RNA for Prognosis

NATURAL HISTORY

To appreciate the benefits and limitations of using viral RNA as a measure of disease progression, certain critical elements of viral pathogenesis need to be understood. First, cell-free viral RNA in plasma represents a minority population of infectious virus and a majority population of noninfectious virus particles (12). The ratio between these two depends on the replicative efficiency of the virus itself along with other factors such as the levels of HIV-1–specific p24 antibody (13, 14). Second, the level of plasma viral RNA may not reflect the level of cell-associated infectious virus. As such, cell-associated infectious virus can be recovered from

Table 41.1. Descriptive Differences Between Plasma HIV-1 RNA Quantitation Assays

Procedure	RT-PCR[a]	bDNA[b]	NASBA[c]
Anticoagulant[d]	EDTA or ACD	EDTA	EDTA or ACD or heparin
Sample preparation	Sample plus standard is lysed; sample centrifugation before addition of standard and lysis buffer is used to increase sensitivity	Sample is concentrated by centrifugation before detergent disruption	Sample and 3 calibrators are adsorbed onto silica dioxide gel and eluted before lysis
Amplification	Probes 142 bases in *gag;* HIV-1 genome is separated by heating and then reverse transcribed; this process is repeated many times; inclusion of an internal quantitative standard (QS) adjusts for recovery	Probes multiple regions of *pol;* HIV-1 RNA is captured on a 48-well microtiter plate; target and preamplifier probes bind the RNA; branched DNA amplifiers bind the preamplifier probes; no adjustment is made for recovery	Probes approximately 1200 bases in *gag* and *pol;* a series of 3 enzymes is used to make an RNA:DNA HIV-1 target, which is degraded and amplified; the reaction is isothermic and continuous; the sample and the 3 calibrators are amplified simultaneously, thus adjusting for recovery
Detection	The product is attached to a 48-well microtiter plate and biotinylated; an optical density is determined for the sample and the standard, from which a copy number is calculated	Multiple alkaline phosphatase probes amplify the signal, which is detected by measuring light emission from a chemiluminescent substrate; an external standard curve is used for calculating the RNA copy number	The amplicons are captured on beads and detected by means of electrochemiluminescence; calculation of copy number is based on the relative amount of the sample compared with the 3 internal calibrators
Detection level	200 copies/mL (20 copies/mL)[e]	500 copies/mL	80 copies/mL
Quantitation level	400 copies/mL (40 copies/mL)[e]	500 copies/mL	500 copies/mL[f]

[a]RT-PCR, reverse transcription polymerase chain reaction. Information is derived from the Roche Amplicor HIV-1 Monitor Test package insert and the Amplicor HIV-1 Monitor Ultrasensitive specimen preparation protocol (Roche Molecular Systems, Branchburg, NJ).
[b]bDNA, branched DNA. Information derived from the Chiron Quantiplex HIV-1 RNA 2.0 Assay (bDNA) package insert (Chiron Corporation, Emeryville, CA).
[c]NASBA, nucleic acid sequence–based amplification. Information is derived from the Organon Teknika NucliSens HIV-1 RNA Assay package insert (Organon Teknika Corporation, Advanced BioScience Laboratories, Incorporated, Kensington, MD).
[d]EDTA (ethylenediaminetetraacetic acid), purple-top Vacutaner tubes (Becton Dickinson, Franklin Lakes, NJ); ACD (acid citrate dextrose), yellow-top Vacutaner tubes, not to be confused with yellow-top SPS (sodium polyanethol-sulfonate) tubes used for microbiology cultures; heparin, green-top Vacutaner tubes.
[e]The values in parentheses are for the Roche HIV-1 Monitor Ultrasensitive specimen preparation protocol.
[f]The level of detection and quantitation can vary depending on the initial volume extracted.

the majority of patients who have had plasma viral RNA levels suppressed to below the level of detection after prolonged, potent antiretroviral therapy (15, 16). Third, the viral RNA level in plasma may not reflect the level of virus and kinetics of viral replication (17–20) in other sites and compartments such as latently infected cells in the lymph nodes (21), central nervous system (22), and genital tract (23). Fourth, independent of viral RNA level, syncytium-inducing viral phenotype is strongly associated with disease progression (24–28). Finally, patient attributes such as age (29) and immune status (30) may cause substantial variability in the level of viral replication (31). Together, these factors could explain, in part, the differences in disease progression among patients with similar plasma viral RNA levels, and they represent a limitation to the use of plasma viral RNA as the sole marker of therapeutic efficacy and clinical outcome (32–34).

Nonetheless, one of the most important concepts to emerge from our understanding of HIV disease pathogenesis is that the magnitude of HIV replication in infected persons is associated with the rate of disease progression (13, 35, 36). The level of plasma HIV RNA reflects the infected person's ability to contain viral replication such that the replication and clearance of virus reach a quasisteady state (17–20), and thus this level defines, in part, the subsequent rate of disease progression (13, 14, 24, 35, 37–39). This quasisteady state has been referred to as the viral "set-point" and appears to be established in the first 6 to 12 months after primary infection, during which time an HIV-specific humoral and cytotoxic lymphocyte response is established (40–42). The plasma viral RNA level before the establishment of the steady state does not predict subsequent disease progression (43). The viral steady state represents the nadir of viral containment after which time the plasma viral RNA level may increase slowly (40), conferring additional risk for the development of the acquired immunodeficiency syndrome (AIDS). However, some patients may continue to have a decline in plasma viral RNA from the steady state conferring additional clinical benefit (44).

The viral steady state is not absolute, and each plasma viral RNA level describes a range of times to the development of disease progression. To illustrate this point, Ioannidis and coworkers constructed a model to ascertain the predictive value of serum viral RNA in asymptomatic patients with more than 500 CD4 cells/µL, an unknown time since seroconversion, and no prior antiretroviral therapy (31). They found that the minimum and maximum estimated time to progression to AIDS varied at assigned serum viral RNA serum levels. For example, patients with a viral load of 10,000 (10^4) RNA copies/mL of serum could take 2.8 to 19 years to develop AIDS, and those with 30,000 ($10^{4.5}$) RNA copies/mL could take anywhere from 1.9 to 8 years (31).

In general, patients who are more likely to progress to disease rapidly have a higher plasma viral RNA steady state than do those in whom disease progresses more slowly.

However, the predictive value of high plasma viral RNA levels decreases over time, whereas the predictive value of low CD4+ cell count and CD4+ cell function increases over time. Thus, in the later stages of infection, immune deficiency is most predictive of disease progression (44). A monotonic relationship exists between the plasma viral RNA level and the rate of CD4+ cell decline, such that higher plasma viral RNA levels are associated with a greater rate of CD4+ cell decline (38). For example, the Multicenter AIDS Cohort Study of the natural history of HIV-1 infection showed that the mean (95% confidence interval [CI]) decrease in CD4+ cell count per year was −36.3 (−42.3 to −30.4) cells for subjects with fewer than 500 viral RNA copies/mL of plasma compared with −76.5 (−82.9 to −70.5) cells for subjects with more than 30,000 viral RNA copies/mL of plasma (39).

In most untreated subjects, the plasma viral RNA steady-state level lies within a narrow range between 1000 (10^3) and 100,000 (10^5) RNA copies/mL of plasma (13, 24, 35, 44). For example, in the largest cohort study, 74.3% of 1531 untreated patients had plasma viral RNA levels of less than 30,000 RNA copies by the bDNA assay (39). Mellors and coworkers also defined five risk categories for disease progression based on the arbitrary distribution of 1531 subjects into HIV-1 RNA level quintiles (39). Highly significant differences in the proportion of patients who progressed to AIDS within 6 years of diagnosis were seen in these five risk categories: 500 copies/mL or less, 5.4% (95% CI; 0 to 17%); 501 to 3000 copies/mL, 16.6% (12 to 21%); 3001 to 10,000 copies/mL, 31.7% (7 to 43%); 10,001 to 30,000 copies/mL, 55.2% (25 to 84%); and more than 30,000 copies/mL, 80.0% (58 to 100%) (39).

CLINICAL TRIALS

Because a continuous gradient of risk of disease progression is associated with the viral RNA steady-state level, one of the objectives of antiretroviral therapy is to "reset" this plasma viral RNA steady-state level to one with a lower risk of disease progression. Results from HIV-1 therapy trials show that inhibition of HIV-1 replication (as assessed by plasma HIV-1 RNA level) is associated with a delay in clinical disease progression (25–27, 45, 46). Although the relative clinical benefit of any given decline in plasma viral RNA does not depend on the baseline level of plasma viral RNA, the absolute risk of clinical disease progression remains higher in the patient with the higher pretherapy plasma viral RNA level (28). In summarizing the data from 7 large clinical trials involving 1330 subjects who received primarily nucleoside therapies, Marschner and coworkers (28) showed that a 10-fold decrease in plasma viral RNA level from baseline to week 24 yielded a 72% reduction in the risk of progression (95% CI: 61 to 81%, $P < .001$) and that larger reductions in plasma viral RNA level were associated with greater benefit. Any reduction in excess of the natural variability of plasma HIV-1 RNA measurement (approximately 3-fold or 0.5 $\log_{10}$) was associated with a delay in disease progression (28). However, in this study and in others, the prognostic interpretation of any given plasma viral RNA reduction also depended on the treatment response of the CD4+ cell count (28, 47, 48). Although the change in plasma viral RNA is a better predictor of clinical progression than is the CD4+ cell response, together the viral RNA and CD4+ cell count responses more fully characterize the risk of disease progression than does either one alone (28, 47, 49). These clinical trial data strongly suggest that a more complete assessment of a patient's prognosis can be achieved by monitoring the plasma viral RNA level and CD4+ cell count (28, 47, 49).

Use of Plasma Viral RNA to Initiate Therapy

A decision to initiate antiretroviral therapy should be based on both CD4+ cell and plasma viral RNA measurements performed on two occasions 2 to 4 weeks apart (2). These parameters should not be assessed during intercurrent infection or within the first 1 to 2 months after immunization because of concern regarding the limited and transient immune activation of viral replication associated with these events (50, 51). Moreover, the plasma viral RNA measurements should be done using the same commercial assay and preferably in the same testing laboratory, to ensure consistent results (52–54).

As indicated earlier, defining accurate plasma viral RNA levels to use for clinical management is difficult (54). Most of the recommendations for the use of plasma viral RNA levels clinically are based on published data that may have been influenced by several factors (see the section of this chapter on caveats for the clinical use of plasma HIV-1 RNA). For example, these published data were generated using different quantitative viral RNA assays, in the absence of a common viral RNA standard, and viral RNA measurements in either serum or plasma, using different plasma anticoagulants. As such, these factors may have contributed to uncertainty in prescribing absolute plasma viral RNA levels for decision-making strategies (55). Nevertheless, the excellent precision of the current assays and the availability of more sensitive assays that approach the sampling constraints of the Poisson distribution (11) allow one arbitrarily to separate plasma viral RNA levels into one of five categories: *very low* (fewer than 50 copies/mL); *low* (50 to 500 copies/mL); *moderate* (more than 500 to 5000 copies/mL); *high* (more than 5000 to 50,000 copies/mL); and *very high* (more than 50,000 copies/mL). The precise plasma viral RNA copy number within each category may be less important than the assignment to the specific category.

Asymptomatic HIV-1 Infection

The suitability of using CD4+ cell count and clinical stage of disease to initiate antiretroviral therapy is limited, and earlier studies of their use for asymptomatic patients provided inconsistent results. In clinical trials of zidovudine monotherapy, treatment slowed the decline in CD4+ cell count but did not significantly prolong either AIDS-free or overall survival in asymptomatic patients in some (56–58), but not all (59), studies. These studies were limited by their inability to assess the level of viral replication and the less potent antiretroviral drug regimen that was available at the time. As such, we still do not know how to initiate antiretroviral therapy properly in asymptomatic patients with 500 or more CD4+ cells/μL. Moreover, when to initiate antiretroviral therapy in asymptomatic patients based on the plasma viral RNA level remains controversial and without a definitive clinical trial-based answer (3, 4).

The two current clinical approaches to initiating therapy in the asymptomatic patient population are aggressive and conservative (3, 4, 6). Both approaches are based on assessing the risk of disease progression based on the plasma viral RNA level, and to a lesser extent, the CD4+ cell count.

The aggressive approach treats any HIV-1–infected patient who has detectable plasma HIV-1 RNA, regardless of the CD4+ cell count, and preferably before evidence of significant immunosuppression (4, 6). This approach is primarily based on the belief that plasma viral RNA is the ideal laboratory marker to follow, and clinically significant viral resistance will arise in every patient who does not have their plasma viral RNA completely suppressed.

The conservative approach, on the other hand, delays therapy until the patient has evidence of progressive immune dysfunction as defined by a CD4+ cell count less than 500 cells/μL (6, 27, 60). For patients with more than 500 CD4+ cells/μL, therapy is individually tailored to reflect the perceived risk of disease progression based on the plasma viral RNA levels and overall lower short-term risk of disease progression for those with fewer than 10,000 (bDNA) copies/mL (31, 39).

Empirical viral RNA values from the aforementioned Multicenter AIDS Cohort Study suggest that therapy should be started for any patient with more than 5000 to 10,000 RNA copies/mL of plasma (4, 35, 38, 39). Previous studies have shown that the greatest clinical benefit for asymptomatic patients has been observed when antiretroviral therapy was initiated at CD4+ cell counts lower than 500 cells/μL (60). However, some physicians treat anybody with a detectable viral RNA level regardless of either the CD4+ cell count or the patient's clinical condition. The success of either approach depends on the willingness of the patient to begin therapy, the potential risks and benefits of starting therapy, the unvalidated assumptions about the completeness of plasma viral RNA level alone as a surrogate marker for clinical outcome, and the likelihood of adherence with the therapy regimen (6).

SYMPTOMATIC HIV-1 INFECTION

Any patient with symptomatic infection should be treated aggressively with antiretroviral therapy regardless of the plasma viral RNA level (3–6). The therapeutic objective is to suppress viral replication as much as possible, to arrest further immunosuppression, and to achieve an elevation of the CD4+ cell count and partial return of CD4+ cell function (4, 6). In many cases, prior antiretroviral therapy and concomitant drug therapies for prophylaxis or treatment of opportunistic infections limit the choice of antiretroviral therapy and temper both the magnitude and the durability of the viral RNA response. Unfortunately, many of these patients are not able to suppress viral replication to below the limit of detection. Nevertheless, as discussed earlier, any decrease in viral RNA and stabilization or increase in CD4+ cell count translates into clinical benefit (28).

PRIMARY HIV-1 INFECTION

Several theoretic reasons exist for initiating potent antiretroviral therapy in the earliest stages of primary HIV-1 infection. The rationale is based on infectious disease principles for acute infection and an emerging understanding of the pathogenesis of primary HIV-1 infection. Anecdotal cases of "cure" have been reported (61), and evidence also indicates short-term effects of antiretroviral therapy on viral burden and CD4+ cell count in primary HIV infection (62). In one placebo-controlled study of 77 patients with primary infection who were treated with zidovudine monotherapy (63), patients who received zidovudine had an average gain of 8.9 CD4+ cells/μL per month (95% CI; −1.4 to 19.1) after 6 months of therapy compared with patients who received placebo and had an average loss of −12.0 CD4+ cells/μL per month (95% CI; −5.2 to −18.7). Other than this study, only historical controls are available for comparison. Thus, the absence of long-term controlled studies makes it difficult to interpret both short-term and long-term changes in plasma viral RNA when antiretroviral therapy is started early in HIV-1 infection (64). However, the potential risks and lack of evidence demonstrating a long-term clinical benefit (62) have not tempered the enthusiasm among most experts to treat these patients early in the course of primary infection (4).

Many of the assumptions made in support of early treatment intervention may or may not be valid. First, short-term viral suppression can be maintained for a long time. Second, no significant selection of preexisting virus polymorphisms leads to escape mutants later in infection. Third, the tissue levels of the antiretroviral agents are sufficient in different compartments, such as lymph nodes and genital tract, to prevent cell-associated virus replication and selection of resistant virus. Fourth, if intolerance or resistance develops, alternative therapies will be available. Finally, the benefits of early treatment outweigh the risks of deferring therapy (5, 6).

Several complex biologic determinants of primary HIV-1 infection, although poorly understood, argue against performing antiretroviral placebo-controlled clinical studies in this setting. First, although neither the viral RNA level nor the CD4+ cell count in the first 6 months after acute infection is necessarily predictive of clinical outcome (40, 41), preliminary evidence indicates the irreversible depletion of HIV-1–specific helper cells within this period that may be necessary for later viral containment (42). Second, preliminary studies suggest that the depleted HIV-1–specific helper cells may not be restored by the later use of potent antiretroviral therapy

(65). Thus, for the foreseeable future, uncontrolled clinical trials for addressing the benefit of earlier antiretroviral therapy will be, by necessity, empirical. A definitive answer to the question whether to use immediate or deferred antiretroviral therapy in acute HIV-1 infection will be left unresolved.

Before considering antiretroviral therapy in this setting, acute infection must be carefully documented (40, 66). The potential problem with low levels of plasma viral RNA carryover in the reverse transcription (RT)-PCR reaction and lower specificity with the bDNA assay argue strongly for a careful documentation of acute HIV-1 infection before considering any antiretroviral therapy (67–69). If potent antiretroviral therapy is started, then therapy should aim at suppressing viral replication to below the level of plasma viral RNA detection and continuing therapy either for an indefinite period or until the optimal duration is defined by ongoing clinical trials (4, 6).

Use of Plasma Viral RNA to Monitor Therapy

The frequency for monitoring the plasma viral RNA response to therapy is less controversial. In general, nadir responses occur in most patients between 4 and 12 weeks after initiation of potent antiretroviral therapy. With some potent antiretroviral regimens, plasma viral RNA values decrease to less than 500 RNA copies/mL by 16 weeks in 60 to 80% of subjects and to less than 50 viral RNA copies/mL by 24 weeks in approximately 70%. The number of patients in these categories depends on the study population and on these patients' prior antiretroviral experience (46, 70). With a stable response, continued monitoring at 3- to 4-monthly intervals seems warranted, more frequently if a critical plasma viral RNA value is approached (2). The investigator should plot the plasma viral RNA values on a log_{10} scale and should only repeat the plasma viral RNA measurement for values higher than the upper 95% CI bound for the expected variation in plasma viral RNA level (i.e., 0.5 log_{10} above the mean nadir response value), provided such a change will to lead to a change in therapy (71–74).

The target of therapy must be a durable reduction in the plasma viral RNA by at least threefold (0.5 log_{10}) or more from pretherapy levels (2, 73), to below 1000 copies/mL (28), and by current consensus guidelines, preferably to an "undetectable" level (4). Although no published clinical trial data have carefully delineated the decrease in risk of disease progression associated with decreases in the plasma viral RNA to less than 1000 copies/mL (28), a preliminary analysis of 1083 patients from AIDS Clinical Trials Group (ACTG) 320 (46) showed that only 7 (5.6%) of 126 clinical events were associated with a preceding plasma HIV-1 level below 500 copies/mL; for the remaining 119 clinical events, the plasma viral RNA level was above 500 copies/mL (75).

Nevertheless, many investigators believe that the target for therapy should be at least 1 log_{10} value lower than 500 RNA copies/mL of plasma, that is, fewer than 50 RNA copies/mL. The "as-low-as-you-can-go" concept in HIV treatment (76) is appealing, but it has, by virtue of its repetition, been accepted for truth (33). How this concept pertains to a chronic, persistent viral infection such as HIV-1 still requires careful validation by controlled clinical trials, particularly in asymptomatic subjects with more than 500 cells/FL, because the long-term toxicities of the most potent protease inhibitor–containing combinations are unknown but are potentially worrisome (77, 78).

Therapy should also stabilize or increase the CD4+ cell count, at or above the expected level of biologic variation, by more than 30% in the absolute cell number or by more than 3% in the proportion of cells (71, 79). Interpretation of any given plasma HIV-1 RNA reduction depends on the treatment response of the CD4+ lymphocyte count. Because of the interaction between viral RNA and CD4 cell count, changes in both, along with a consideration of the clinical course, are necessary to consider in the definition of therapeutic failure. For example, in an analysis of several clinical studies of primarily nucleoside therapy, those subjects with no reduction in plasma HIV-1 RNA level and a reduction in CD4+ cell count had a 30% greater risk of clinical progression over 2 years compared with those who had an increase in CD4+ cell count above pretherapy levels (28).

Additionally, therapy should provide an improved sense of patient well-being with minimal side effects. In targeting for the lowest plasma viral RNA level, consideration must be given to prior antiretroviral drug exposure, while balancing therapy compliance, tolerability of the regimen, and long-term toxicity of the therapy regimen (3–6).

Use of Plasma Viral RNA to Define Virologic Failure

A precise definition of therapeutic failure based on viral RNA level is wanting. Such a definition should embrace, as a minimum, the clinical status of the patient, the CD4+ cell count, and the viral RNA level. The failure of plasma viral RNA to decline by at least 30-fold (1.5 log_{10}) or more from baseline after 4 to 8 weeks of therapy is generally considered to represent a suboptimal virologic response (4, 6, 28). In addition, many clinicians also consider the inability to achieve undetectable plasma viral RNA by 12 to 24 weeks of therapy as evidence of therapeutic failure (4–6).

The relative benefit of a decline in plasma viral RNA is the same no matter where the pretherapy viral RNA level started, although the pretherapy plasma viral RNA level itself confers an additional, independent risk of disease progression. For example, a decline from 100,000 (5.0 log_{10}) viral RNA copies/mL of plasma to 10,000 (4.0 log_{10}) viral RNA copies/mL of plasma represents the same relative 72% reduction (95% CI: 61 to 81%, $P < .001$ in risk of disease progression as a change from 4.0 to 3.0 log_{10} viral RNA copies/mL (28). However, the two pretherapy plasma viral RNA levels of 5.0 and 4.0 log_{10} copies/mL each confer a different relative hazard of disease progression, after controlling for the baseline CD4+ cell count and therapy assignment (28). The target of reaching undetectable plasma viral RNA after 12 to 24 weeks of therapy is also affected by the pretherapy plasma viral RNA level. Achieving a detectable plasma viral RNA level of less than 3.7 $\log_{10}$ (5000 copies/mL) when starting with 6.0 $\log_{10}$ (1,000,000 copies/mL) confers clinical benefit and may be all that is obtainable, given a patient's prior antiretroviral therapy experience.

Investigators have arbitrarily set that any sustainable 0.5 $\log_{10}$ (threefold) rise in plasma viral RNA above the therapy-induced plasma viral RNA nadir that is not attributable to intercurrent infection, vaccination, incomplete adherence to the antiretroviral therapy regimen, decreased absorption of antiretroviral drugs, altered drug metabolism, drug–drug interactions, or testing method likely represents viral failure resulting from the emergence of drug-resistant HIV variants (2, 5, 6). However, this concept must be viewed cautiously for the reasons discussed in the following sections.

VIRAL RESISTANCE

Genotypic and phenotypic changes associated with drug resistance in vitro are not always synonymous with clinical drug failure (80). For example, in a large clinical study (81), persons who had received prior zidovudine therapy for more than 6 months benefited clinically after switching to didanosine, but the presence of high-grade phenotypic or genotypic zidovudine resistance at baseline independently predicted clinical disease progression and death regardless of therapy assignment (82, 83). Plasma viral RNA level, viral syncytium-inducing phenotype, and CD4+ cell response to therapy were each independently associated with the risk of clinical progression (25–27, 45, 84). Thus, the independent association of zidovudine susceptibility suggests a more complex relationship among zidovudine susceptibility, these three variables, and other unidentified viral and host factors. Moreover, although a movement exists in clinical practice to use genotypic susceptibility patterns to adjust antiretroviral therapy, one clinical trial showed that viral genotype did not predict the subsequent plasma viral RNA response when patients were switched to a susceptible antiretroviral drug (85).

Clearly, the correct interpretation of viral genotype is complicated by the complexity of the primary and secondary mutational patterns observed, the potential for undetected subpopulations of mutant virus, and residual effects of prior antiretroviral therapy (85). Thus, the clinician should approach the clinical management of patients using viral genotypic analysis cautiously until definitive clinical trial data are available.

DISCORDANT VIRAL RNA AND CD4 CELL RESPONSES

A discordant response may exist between a rise in plasma viral RNA and either a sustained or a continued rise in CD4+ cell count (48, 86). This discordance occurs in approximately 14% of patients who receive antiretroviral therapy (28). The discordant response has been associated with a decrease in disease progression and thus questions the wisdom of changing antiretroviral therapy based solely on the plasma viral RNA response (32, 34). Many clinical trials provide study patients with the end-point measurement (i.e., plasma viral RNA level) on a real-time basis. This practice raises serious concerns about the introduction of selection bias and the ability to define a viral RNA-based therapeutic failure.

Thus, in the absence of clinical trials data, if the sustained rise in plasma viral RNA during therapy is to either less than 0.5 $\log_{10}$ above the plasma viral RNA therapy nadir or 5000 (3.7 $\log_{10}$) copies/mL, whichever is less, then it may be prudent to observe the patient carefully for a further deterioration in CD4+ cell count or clinical disease progression before considering a change of therapy. A sustained rise in plasma viral RNA that exceeds these criteria should warrant a reassessment of the antiretroviral regimen for adherence and possible therapy failure. A more aggressive approach would consider any detectable plasma viral RNA worthy of a switch in therapy. Neither approach, however, has received validation by a controlled clinical trial.

Pregnant Women

Monitoring of viral RNA levels in pregnant women is no different than in nonpregnant women or in men (5–7). Surprisingly, the natural history of plasma viral RNA during pregnancy is not well characterized. In two small studies, the maternal viral load did not rise during pregnancy (87, 88). However, in a larger cohort study of 198 HIV-1–infected women, plasma HIV-1 RNA levels were higher at 6 months post partum than during the antepartum period in many of the women (89). Although both the plasma viral RNA level and the CD4+ cell count are independently predictive of vertical transmission risk, the change in plasma viral RNA level only explains at most 50% of the benefit of zidovudine therapy (90). These data strongly suggest a prophylactic benefit from antiretroviral therapy on vertical transmission. Despite the association between vertical transmission and maternal plasma viral RNA level (90, 91), no data support the use of plasma viral RNA levels as a guide to changing antiretroviral therapy to reduce the risk of vertical transmission during pregnancy. Furthermore, because transmission may occur when plasma HIV-1 RNA is not detectable (89, 90), plasma HIV-1 RNA levels should not be the determining factor when deciding when to use antiretroviral prophylaxis (7).

PROGNOSTIC ABILITY OF PLASMA HIV-1 RNA AND ITS USE IN THE THERAPEUTIC MANAGEMENT OF INFECTED CHILDREN

Use of Plasma Viral RNA for Prognosis

NATURAL HISTORY

Infection with HIV-1 in pediatrics is unique. Most infants are diagnosed when they are acutely infected, usually at birth. However, the lack of a mature immune system implies that the immunopathogenesis of the disease varies from acute infection in adults. The natural history of disease progression in children has been extensively studied in many cooperative national and international cohorts. In general, the progression of disease in children is thought to be much more rapid than in adults, with the development of AIDS occurring in the first 5 years for infants compared with 10 to 15 years for adults (92). Although early studies suggested rapid mortality (93, 94), subsequent longitudinal studies suggest that a large proportion of children will survive beyond the 5-year period (95–99). HIV-infected children appear to fall into two categories (95, 100, 101). Infants who are rapid progressors develop AIDS within 5 years, and they usually do so within the first year of life (102). This course is in contrast to that of slow progressors, who may remain asymptomatic for 5 to 8 years (98). Many parameters other than plasma viral RNA have been shown to contribute to disease progression in infants such as birth weight (103) and age of acquisition of infection (104), as well as several maternal virologic, clinical, and immunologic parameters (98, 105, 106). Most of the earlier studies that assessed infant prognosis did not include measures of viral load, and many of the later studies on prognosis did not include either maternal or infant clinical factors that may be important for determining risk of disease progression independent of virologic and immunologic parameters measured from the infant at birth.

The lack of a mature immune system in the pediatric patient less than 30 months of age means that it is important not only to measure viral load, but also to measure the development of immune competency. Because of the natural decline in the number of CD4+ cells in children with age, both absolute CD4+ cell count and the proportion (percentage) of CD4+ cells should be determined (107, 108). As with adult acute infection, plasma HIV-1 RNA levels change with children over time. Two patterns of RNA change are likely to occur. Children may be born with exceedingly high levels of RNA that either gradually decline with age or remain high. Alternatively, within the first few weeks of life, children may have lower plasma viral RNA levels that rise within the first month and then decline (109, 110). The present thinking is that those infants with the higher viral RNA loads within the first 72 hours were infected in utero, whereas those with the lower, or undetectable, viral loads were likely infected in the peripartum period (111).

Because the viral load in infants at birth may vary with time of infection, it is understandable that using viral load for prognosis is not as straightforward as with adults. This situation is further complicated by the immaturity of the neonate's immune system. In adults, the mature immune response to HIV infection results in the development of a quasisteady state within 6 to 12 months. However, for most children, the viral load naturally decreases over time; thus the prognostic ability may vary with age and may never reach an equilibrium (47, 109, 112). Although present data with zidovudine treatment do not suggest any differences in plasma HIV-1 RNA prognostic ability (112), this may not be the case with infants or their mothers who receive more potent antiretroviral therapy.

Few studies have been conducted of plasma HIV-1 RNA determinations of infected children followed from birth without treatment (109, 110, 112, 113). The largest of these studies ($N = 106$) found a wide variation in plasma viral RNA levels at all time points (112). The predominant pattern was a rapid rise in plasma viral RNA followed by a slow decline. In this particular study, unlike some others (110, 111), most of the infants appeared to be infected later, that is, during the peripartum period, rather than earlier, in utero. However, infants who were infected early had higher early peak viral plasma viral RNA levels, defined as detectable plasma viral RNA within the first 2 months of life. Detection of virus within the first week of life has been associated with rapid disease progression (110, 111). The plasma viral RNA values obtained early in the course of infection were not as prognostic as peak or plateau values obtained during the first 12 months (112). This observation was unaffected by the presence of zidovudine treatment (112). However, because of the great individual variation observed, the utility of plasma HIV-1 RNA levels during the first 12 months of life in individual patient management is unclear. No infant with a plasma HIV-1 RNA value below 70,000 to 80,000 copies/mL during the first 4 months of life had rapidly progressing disease (112).

CLINICAL TRIALS

Few published studies have assessed the effect of treatment on the prognostic ability of plasma HIV-1 RNA levels and CD4+ cell count on clinical outcome (8, 47, 114, 115). These studies have come to similar conclusions, namely, a strong interaction appears to exist between the two parameters, plasma viral RNA level and CD4+ cell count. Thus, as with adults, the greatest prognostic ability is achieved by a combination of plasma viral RNA level and CD4+ count, and at the extremes of the disease spectrum, high viral RNA level and low CD4+ cell count. For example, patients with high viral loads (more than 100,000 copies/mL) and low CD4+ cell counts (less than 15%) progressed most rapidly. Patients with both high viral RNA level and high CD4+ cell count or low viral RNA level and low CD4+ cell count progressed similarly, whereas patients with low RNA level and high CD4+ cell count experienced little or no disease progression (47, 115).

Patients younger than 30 months of age appear to have the highest risk if their plasma viral RNA levels are higher than 100,000 copies/mL and their proportion of CD4+ cells is less than 15%. Conversely, the same patients with more than 15% CD4+ cells, in spite of high viral loads, have a much reduced risk of mortality. Patients more than 30 months of age appear to have parameters more like those of adults. Those with plasma viral RNA levels higher than 150,000 copies/mL are at highest risk for disease progression, whereas those children having plasma viral RNA levels between 1000 and 15,000 copies/mL are at lowest risk (47).

Use of Plasma Viral RNA to Initiate Therapy

ASYMPTOMATIC INFECTION

Given the foregoing problems in defining the prognostic capability of plasma viral RNA level for pediatrics, it is difficult to find a consensus for when to initiate treatment. Many pediatricians believe, as is the case for adult patients, that children should be started on triple-combination therapy with protease inhibitors as soon as a diagnosis is made, regardless of the plasma viral RNA level. Others believe, however, that antiretroviral treatment can be deferred for children who are asymptomatic and have low plasma viral RNA levels and high CD4+ cell counts. Because children at greatest risk for disease appear to be those with plasma viral RNA levels higher than 100,000 copies/mL, most clinicians would agree to initiate therapy in those patients (115). A lower plasma viral RNA copy number may be selected for older children.

Clinical trial data have demonstrated both a clinical and immunologic benefit in treating HIV-infected infants (116). In ACTG 152, the clinical benefit of antiretroviral treatment was greatest in those infants younger than 30 months of age (114, 116). This finding suggests that earlier treatment would be preferred over delayed treatment in this random patient population. Similarly, in a small, open-labeled study using combination therapy, the greatest virologic and immunologic benefit was seen in children treated before 4 months of age (117). However, in patients who have lower initial plasma viral RNA levels, no clinical trial data document that early treatment is preferred over later treatment. For infants infected with HIV-1, the availability of pediatric formulations and the issue of adherence to an antiretroviral regimen are of particular importance in deciding when to initiate therapy.

SYMPTOMATIC INFECTION

Studies have shown that approximately 70% of HIV-1–infected children present with clinical signs and symptoms of HIV-1 disease during the first year of life (92, 96). The estimated mean time of survival of these children is approximately 5 years (92). Thus, like adults, children presenting with symptomatic infection should be started on treatment. Similarly, young children with plasma viral RNA levels higher than 100,000 copies/mL and evidence of immunologic dysfunction, as expressed by CD4+ cell counts lower than 15%, should be offered therapy (8). In a clinical trial of antiretrovirally naive symptomatic children less than 3 years old, a greater reduction in plasma viral RNA level was associated with a better clinical outcome than was a lesser reduction (118).

Use of Plasma Viral RNA to Monitor Therapy and Describe Treatment Failure

Deciding when to change therapy and describing treatment failure are much more complex in pediatric patients than in adults because, as stated previously, the plasma viral RNA levels in young infants are extremely high and only slowly decline. With current therapies, it may be unrealistic to expect the high pediatric values to fall to "undetectable" levels. Similarly, because the levels are so high, it may take longer for a virologic effect to be observed. In two studies, which assessed the effect of combination therapy with zidovudine, didanosine, and nevirapine, maximal suppression was seen after 4 weeks. Treatment differences in terms of plasma viral RNA response varied with prior antiretroviral exposure, as in adults. In the treatment of antiretrovirally naive subjects with this triple-combination regimen, 1.5 $\log_{10}$ plasma viral RNA decreases were observed (117), whereas in antiretrovirally experienced patients, only 0.7 $\log_{10}$ decreases were observed (119). Similar studies with protease inhibitors in combination with nucleoside inhibitors are just being performed in children. Preliminary results suggest that changes in plasma viral RNA with these drugs are in the order of −1.0 to 1.5 $\log_{10}$, with a great deal of individual patient variation (118, 120, 121). These responses have generally been sustained, but many children have difficulty in adhering to these regimens, and toxicity is a problem (120).

Little is known about the natural variability in plasma HIV-1 RNA levels in children. One could presume that, with increased exposure to potential immune activating antigens and the multiple vaccinations during this period, as well as the loss of maternal antibody, natural variation in children would be much greater than in adults. In general, sustained increases in plasma viral RNA levels should be greater than 0.3 to 0.5 $\log_{10}$ and could be used to define virologic failure. Most pediatricians, however, also consider the initial level of plasma viral RNA, as well as the CD4+ cell count and clinical course before initiating a change in therapy. This is particularly important in pediatrics, in which the number of available alternative drug strategies is limited.

VIRAL RESISTANCE

Monitoring of pediatric patients for genotypic resistance mutations has not been used routinely as a criterion for switching therapies, as has been proposed by some practitioners for adults. Little is known about the emergence of viral resistance in pediatric patients and clinical outcome. Earlier studies had documented an association of the emergence of resistance to zidovudine with disease progression (122, 123). These studies, however, looked at the association independent of other confounding variables such as viral RNA and biologic phenotype. Studies with nevirapine as monotherapy and in combination therapy have shown that a rebound in plasma viral RNA level was associated with the appearance of nevirapine-resistant mutations (117). Investigators have observed high-level phenotypic resistance to zidovudine, but not to zalcitabine or didanosine, although genotypic mutations were observed (124, 125). Genotypic mutations associated with protease inhibitor resistance have been found in children both before and after therapy; however, they have not been strictly correlated with plasma viral RNA (126).

Earlier reports that the viral phenotype did not correlate with disease progressions in children (127) have not been corroborated (128). In a study that assessed the interaction between resistance genotype and biologic phenotype, zidovudine therapy for a mean of 3.8 years was associated with the emergence of codon 215 mutation in 64% of the treated children. However, this mutation was not associated with increased morbidity or mortality, although it was associated with the presence of the syncytium inducing phenotype (125). The appearance in children of the syncytium-inducing phenotype, which increases with age (129), was prognostic of increased risk for disease progression and death (125), as is the case with adults (25, 83). However, no study to date has addressed clinical failure with all these parameters, that is, plasma viral RNA, biologic phenotype, resistance, and CD4 cell count.

CAVEATS FOR THE CLINICAL USE OF PLASMA HIV-1 RNA

Uncertainty in Plasma HIV-1 RNA Measurement

Physicians, patients, and technologists need to understand the uncertainty in assigning a value to a single plasma viral RNA measurement (54). This uncertainty arises from specimen handling, performance characteristics of the assay, technical variability of the assay, testing of the different specimens by batch or in real time, and the infected person's natural variation in virus level (71, 73). In total, these factors define, with 95% confidence, a variability in the estimated plasma viral RNA copy number of at least fivefold ($0.7 \log_{10}$) for single RNA measurements (71–73). Consequently, a single measurement of plasma viral RNA is associated with a defined range of values above or below the measured value at least 95% of the time (2.5% of the time values may be either greater than or 2.5% of the time less than this fivefold range). For example, a person with a plasma viral RNA value of 5000 copies/mL obtained from a single plasma specimen taken today may have a measured viral RNA value anywhere from 1000 to 25,000 copies/mL, 95% of the time, on repeat testing of another blood draw taken within the next few days to weeks (23).

A rigorous virology quality assurance program has shown that the intra-assay standard deviation for these assays ranges from less than 0.1 to $0.2 \log_{10}$ HIV-1 RNA copies/mL of plasma (52, 54). This precision enables the assays to distinguish reliably 3- to 8-fold changes in plasma viral RNA for batched testing and 4- to 19-fold changes for real-time testing. Obviously, the uncertainty in defining the true plasma viral RNA level contributes important *uncertainty* for changing antiretroviral therapy based on a single plasma viral RNA value. This point is illustrated in Table 41.2.

In addition to the foregoing considerations, variability in interpreting absolute plasma viral RNA levels across different clinical studies arises because of the patient population studied, the use of serum or plasma to assess the viral RNA level, different viral RNA assay methods, different anticoagulants, and storage conditions. For example, viral RNA levels are generally $0.5 \log_{10}$ less for serum than plasma, depending on the assay method used; bDNA values are generally twofold less than those for RT-PCR, and heparin interferes with the detection of viral RNA by both bDNA and RT-PCR assays, but not nucleic acid sequence–based amplification (NASBA) (54, 55).

As such, some patients could have successful therapy regimens inappropriately changed based on estimates of plasma viral RNA levels that are associated with considerable uncertainty in both their measurement and clinical meaning of the plasma viral RNA value, particularly when the plasma viral RNA and CD4+ cell responses are discordant (28). This possibility is of particular concern for aggressive therapy management decisions based on the detectability of viral RNA near the reliable limit of detection for an assay (see Table 41.1). Plasma viral RNA assessments by both the bDNA and RT-PCR assays are usually concordant for most patients below the level of quantitation. However, this value is discordant in approximately 20% of patients, and the decision to either maintain or switch antiviral therapy based on the assay quantitation limit will be affected by the choice of the viral RNA assay used (130).

Adequacy of Plasma HIV-1 RNA Level Alone for Explaining the Clinical Response to Therapy

Much remains to be learned about the way in which the favorable and relatively short-term laboratory responses to potent antiretroviral therapy translate into the long-term survival of the individual infected with HIV-1. Of particular concern is the recovery of infectious virus from the presumably longer-lived resting T lymphocytes after prolonged, potent antiretroviral therapy (15, 16). Nevertheless, with continued suppression of viral replication and failure to demonstrate the development of genotypic resistance to therapeutic drugs, the long-term outlook for many patients is encouraging (15, 16), provided the potent therapies are tolerated.

The use of plasma viral RNA to monitor HIV-1 infection clinically should be based on the following three critical validation points (25). First, plasma viral RNA is detected in most infected persons, and the level of plasma viral RNA is associated with disease progression. Second, a decline in plasma viral RNA with therapy is associated with improved clinical outcome, and a rise in plasma viral RNA is associated

Table 41.2. Uncertainty in Estimating True Plasma HIV-1 RNA Copy Number

Measured HIV-1 RNA Level for a Single Plasma Specimen		95% Confidence Interval[a]	
		Copies/mL ($\log_{10}$)	
200	(2.30)	<200–1,000	(<2.3–3.0)
2,000	(3.30)	400–10,000	(2.6–4.0)
20,000	(4.30)	4,000–100,000	(3.6–5.0)
200,000	(5.30)	40,000–1,000,000	(4.6–6.0)

[a]The 95% confidence interval represents the ±5-fold range (±0.7 $\log_{10}$) within which a repeat plasma viral RNA value, obtained shortly after the first, would lie 95% of the time. However, 5% of the time the repeat value would be outside of this range. Duplicate specimens rather than singleton specimens would decrease further the 95% confidence intervals for the estimated plasma viral RNA to ±3-fold; that is, ±0.5 $\log_{10}$ (23). The uncertainty in estimating the true viral RNA copy number arises from the variation (biologic and assay) associated with obtaining a measurement.

with clinical disease progression. Third, the change in plasma viral RNA level completely explains the clinical benefit of antiretroviral therapy (34).

Clearly, fulfillment of these three validation criteria is necessary to understand completely the limitations of plasma viral RNA as a substitute marker for disease progression in clinical trials (34). The first two criteria for surrogacy have been fulfilled in several clinical studies, and the associations between plasma viral RNA level and disease progression are highly significant statistically (25, 26, 28, 36, 39, 45, 49, 131). On the basis of both natural history and clinical trial studies (mostly from adult-based studies), investigators now widely accept that the lower the plasma viral RNA level, the better the clinical outcome (28, 39).

The third criterion has not been completely fulfilled. Change in plasma viral RNA level only explains a portion of the clinical response to therapy (probably less than half, but the estimates are imprecise at this time); as such, plasma viral RNA is only a partial surrogate marker for clinical outcome (34, 45, 90). Although this may seem paradoxic given fulfillment of the first two validation criteria and the strong association between the change in plasma viral RNA and disease progression, the partial surrogacy of plasma viral RNA for clinical outcome means that other host and virus properties are necessary for a complete understanding of disease progression in the individual patient (132); presumably, such information may eventually help to define better the individual management of patients in clinical practice (133).

In summary, measurements of plasma HIV-1 RNA play an important part in the prognosis and clinical management of both pediatric and adult patients infected with HIV-1. Plasma HIV-1 viral RNA, in combination with measures of the immune status of the patient (CD4+ cell count), give a more complete assessment of therapeutic outcome. Viral biologic phenotype and drug susceptibility phenotype or genotype provide additional information regarding clinical status, although these parameters are usually not assessed at this time.

Plasma HIV-1 RNA is subject to the same constraints as all other clinical laboratory measurements. Laboratory values assigned differ because of both patient and laboratory variations. The validity and utility of the recommendations for use of these values put forth in recent guidelines need, for the most part, to be confirmed by prospective clinical trials. In spite of all the caveats, HIV-1 plasma viral RNA is an excellent additional tool available to the physician for managing the HIV-1-infected patient.

Acknowledgments

We would like to thank Pam Easterling and Lorita Thykkuttathil for manuscript preparation. This work (RWC) is supported by National Institutes of Health grants AI-27664, AI-27757, and AI-30731 and Social and Scientific Systems, Inc., grants 96VC002 and 97PVCL02.

References

1. Reichelderfer PS, Coombs RW. Virologic parameters as surrogate markers for clinical outcome in HIV-1 disease: verification, variation and validation. J Acquir Immune Defic Syndr Hum Retrovirol 1995;10:S19–S24.
2. Saag MS, Holodniy M, Kuritzkes DR, et al. HIV viral load markers in clinical practice. Nature Med 1996;2:625–629.
3. British HIV Association Guidelines Co-ordinating Committee. British HIV Association guidelines for antiretroviral treatment of HIV seropositive individuals. Lancet 1997;349:1086–1092.
4. Carpenter CCJ, Fischl MA, Hammer SM, et al. Antiretroviral therapy for HIV infection in 1997. JAMA 1997;277:1962–1969.
5. Office of AIDS Research of the National Institutes of Health (NIH). Report of the NIH panel to define principles of therapy of HIV infection (www.hivatis.org/guide6.pdf). Washington, DC: United States Public Health Service, 1997.
6. Unites States Department of Health and Human Services and the Henry J. Kaiser Family Foundation Panel on Clinical Practices for Treatment of HIV Infection. Guidelines for the use of antiretroviral agents in HIV-infected adults and adolescents (ww.hivatis.org/guide6.pdf). Washington, DC: United States Department of Health and Human Services, 1997.
7. Centers for Disease Control and Prevention. Public health service task force recommendations for the use of antiretroviral drugs in pregnant women infected with HIV-1 for maternal health and for reducing perinatal HIV-1 transmission in the United States. MMWR Morb Mortal Wkly Rep 1998;47:1–30.
8. Working Group on Antiretroviral Therapy and Medical Management of HIV Infected Children: National Pediatric and Family HIV Resource Center and the Health Resources and Services Administration (HRSA). Guidelines for the use of antiretroviral agents in pediatrtic HIV infection (www.hivatis.org/guidelin.html). Washington, DC: United States Department of Health and Human Services, 1997.
9. Cao Y, Ho D, Todd J, et al. Clinical evaluation of branched DNA signal amplification for quantifying HIV type 1 in human plasma. AIDS Res Hum Retroviruses 1995;11:353–361.
10. Mulder J, Resnick R, Saget B, et al. A rapid and simple method for extracting human immunodeficiency virus type 1 RNA from plasma: enhanced sensitivity. J Clin Microbiol 1997;35:1278–1280.
11. Collins ML, Irvine B, Tyner D, et al. A branched DNA signal amplification assay for quantification of nucleic acid targets below 100 molecules/mL. Nucleic Acids Res 1997;25:2979–2984.
12. Piatak M, Saag M, Yang L, et al. High levels of HIV-1 in plasma during all stages of infection determined by competitive PCR. Science 1993;259:1749–1754.
13. Henrard DR, Phillips JF, Muenz LR, et al. Natural history of cell-free viremia. JAMA 1995;274:554–558.
14. Hogervorst E, Jurriaans S, De Wolf F, et al. Predictors for non and slow progression in human immunodeficiency virus (HIV) type 1 infection: low viral RNA copy numbers in serum and maintenance of high HIV-1 p24 specific but not V3-specific antibody levels. J Infect Dis 1995; 171:811–821.
15. Finzi D, Hermankova M, Pierson T, et al. Identification of a reservoir for HIV-1 in patients on highly active antiretroviral therapy. Science 1997;278:1295–1300.
16. Wong JK, Hezareh M, Günthard HF, et al. Recovery of replication-competent HIV despite prolonged suppression of plasma viremia. Science 1997;278:1291–1295.
17. Ho D, Neumann AU, Perelson AS, et al. Rapid turnover of plasma virions and CD4 lymphocytes in HIV-1 infection. Nature 1995;373: 123–126.
18. Wei X, Ghosh SK, Taylor ME, et al. Viral dynamics in human immunodeficiency virus type 1 infection. Nature 1995;373:117–122.
19. Perelson AS, Neumann AU, Markowitz M, et al. HIV-1 dynamics in vivo: virion clearance rate, infected cell life-span, and viral generation time. Science 1996;217:1582–1586.
20. Perelson AS, Essunger P, Cao Y, et al. Decay characteristics of HIV-1–infected compartments during combination therapy. Nature 1997;387:188–191.

21. Stellbrink H-J, van Lunzen J, Hufert FT, et al. Asymptomatic HIV infection is characterized by rapid turnover of HIV-RNA in plasma and lymph nodes but not of latently infected lymph-node CD4+ T cells. AIDS 1997;11:1103–1110.
22. Peeters MF, Colebunders RL, van den Abbeele K, et al. Comparison of human immunodeficiency virus biological phenotypes isolated from cerebrospinal fluid and peripheral blood. J Med Virol 1995;47:92–96.
23. Coombs RW, Speck CE, Hughes JP, et al. Association between culturable human immunodeficiency virus type-1 (HIV-1) in semen and HIV-1 RNA levels in semen and blood: evidence for compartmentalization of HIV-1 between semen and blood. J Infect Dis 1998;177:320–330.
24. Jurriaans S, van Gemen B, Weverling GJ, et al. The natural history of HIV-1 infection: virus load and virus phenotype independent determinants of clinical course? Virology 1994;204:223–233.
25. Coombs RW, Welles SL, Hooper C, et al. Association of plasma human immunodeficiency virus type 1 RNA level with risk of clinical progression in patients with advanced infection. J Infect Dis 1996; 174:704–712.
26. Welles SL, Jackson JB, Yen-Lieberman B, et al. Prognostic value of plasma HIV-1 RNA levels in patients with advanced HIV-1 disease and with little or no zidovudine therapy. J Infect Dis 1996;174:696–703.
27. Katzenstein DA, Hammer SM, Hughes MD, et al. The relation of virologic and immunologic markers to clinical outcomes after nucleoside therapy in HIV-infected adults with 200 to 500 CD4 cells per cubic millimeter. N Engl J Med 1996;335:1091–1098.
28. Marschner I, Collier AC, Coombs RW, et al. Use of changes in plasma human immunodeficiency virus type 1 RNA to assess the clinical benefit of antiretroviral therapy. J Infect Dis 1998;177:40–47.
29. Rosenberg PS, Goedert JJ, Biggar RJ, et al. Effect of age at seroconversion on the natural AIDS incubation distribution. AIDS 1994;8: 803–810.
30. Kroner BL, Goedert JJ, Blattner WA, et al. Concordance of human leukocyte antigen haplotype-sharing, CD4 decline and AIDS in hemophilic siblings. AIDS 1995;9:275–280.
31. Ioannidis JPA, Cappelleri JC, Lau J, et al. Predictive value of viral load measurements in asymptomatic untreated HIV-1 infection: a mathematical model. AIDS 1996;10:255–262.
32. Fleming TR, DeMets DL. Surrogate endpoints in clinical trials: are we being misled? Ann Intern Med 1996;125:605–613.
33. Fessel WJ. Human immunodeficiency virus (HIV) RNA in plasma as the preferred target for therapy in patients with HIV infection: a critique. Clin Infect Dis 1997;24:116–122.
34. De Gruttola V, Flemming T, Lin DY, et al. Validating surrogate markers: are we being naive? J Infect Dis 1997;175:237–246.
35. Mellors JW, Kingsley LA, Rinaldo CR, et al. Quantitation of HIV-1 RNA in plasma predicts outcome after seroconversion. Ann Intern Med 1995;112:573–579.
36. O'Brien TR, Blattner WA, Waters D, et al. Serum HIV-1 RNA levels and time to development of AIDS in the multicenter hemophilia cohort study. JAMA 1996;276:105–110.
37. Saksela K, Stevens CE, Rubenstein P, et al. HIV-1 messenger RNA in peripheral blood mononuclear cells with an early marker of risk for progression to AIDS. Ann Intern Med 1995;123:641–648.
38. Mellors JW, Rinaldo CRJ, Gupta P, et al. Prognosis in HIV-1 infection predicted by the quantity of virus in plasma. Science 1996;272:1167–1170.
39. Mellors JW, Muñoz A, Giorgi JV, et al. Plasma viral load and CD4+ lymphocytes as prognostic markers of HIV-1 infection. Ann Intern Med 1997;126:946–954.
40. Schacker TW, Hughes JP, Shea T, et al. Biological and virological characteristics of primary HIV infection. Ann Intern Med 1998; 128(8):613–620.
41. Musey L, Hughes J, Schacker T, et al. Cytotoxic-T-cell responses, viral load, and disease progression in early human immunodeficiency virus type 1 infection. N Engl J Med 1997;337:1267–1274.
42. Rosenberg ES, Billingsley JM, Caliendo AM, et al. Vigorous HIV-1–specific CD4+ T cell responses associated with control of viremia. Science 1997;278:1447–1450.
43. Schacker T, Hughes J, Shea T, et al. Viral load in acute and very early HIV infection does not correlate with disease progression [abstract 475]. In: 4th Conference on Retroviruses and Opportunistic Infections. Washington, DC: American Society for Microbiology, 1997:152.
44. de Wolf F, Spijkerman I, Schellekens PT, et al. AIDS prognosis based on HIV-1 RNA, CD4+ T-cell count and function: markers with reciprocal predictive value over time after seroconversion. AIDS 1997;11:1799–1806.
45. O'Brien WA, Hartigan PM, Martin D, et al. Changes in plasma HIV-1 RNA and CD4+ lymphocyte counts and the risk of progression to AIDS. N Engl J Med 1996;334:426–431.
46. Hammer SM, Squires KE, Hughes MD, et al. A controlled trial of two nucleoside analogues plus indinavir in persons with human immunodeficiency virus infection and CD4 counts of 200 per cubic millimeter or less. N Engl J Med 1997;337:725–733.
47. Mofenson LM, Korelitz J, Meyer WA, et al. The relationship between serum human immunodeficiency virus type 1 (HIV-1) RNA level, CD4 lymphocyte percent, and long-term mortality risk in HIV-1–infected children. J Infect Dis 1997;175:1029–1038.
48. Reichelderfer PS, Coombs RW. Cartesian coordinate analysis of viral burden and CD4+ cell count in HIV disease: implications for clinical trial design and analysis. Antiviral Res 1998 29(1):83–86.
49. Hughes MD, Johnson VA, Hirsch MS, et al. Monitoring plasma HIV-1 RNA levels in addition to CD4+ lymphocyte count improves assessment of antiretroviral therapeutic response. Ann Intern Med 1997;126:929–938.
50. Stanley SK, Ostrowski MA, Justement JS, et al. Effect of immunization with a common recall antigen in viral expression in patients infected with human immunodeficiency virus type 1. N Engl J Med 1996;334: 1222–1230.
51. Staprans SI, Hamilton BL, Follansbee SE, et al. Activation of virus replication after vaccination of HIV-1 infected individuals. J Exp Med 1995;182:1727–1737.
52. Lin HJ, Myers LE, Yen-Lieberman B, et al. Multicenter evaluation of methods for the quantitation of plasma HIV-1 RNA. J Infect Dis 1994;170:553–562.
53. Schuurman R, Descamps D, Weverling GJ, et al. Multicenter comparison of three commercial methods for quantification of human immunodeficiency virus type 1 RNA in plasma. J Clin Microbiol 1996;34:3016–3022.
54. Brambilla R, Leung S, Lew J, et al. Absolute copy number and relative change in determinations of human immunodeficiency virus type 1 RNA in plasma: effect of an external standard on kit comparisons. J Clin Microbiol 1998;36:311–314.
55. Lew J, Reichelderfer P, Fowler M, et al. Plasma HIV-1 RNA determinations: reassessment of parameters affecting assay outcome. J Clin Microbiol 1998 (in press).
56. Volberding PA, Lagakos SW, Grimes JM, et al. The duration of zidovudine benefit in persons with asymptomatic HIV infection: prolonged evaluation of protocol 019 of the AIDS Clinical Trials Group [abstract]. JAMA 1994;272:437–442.
57. Volberding PA, Lagakos SW, Grimes JM, et al. A comparison of immediate with deferred zidovudine therapy for asymptomatic HIV-infected adults with CD4 cell counts of 500 or more per cubic millimeter. N Engl J Med 1995;333:401–407.
58. Concorde Coordinating Committee. MRC/ANRS randomised double-blind controlled trial of immediate and deferred zidovudine in symptom-free HIV infection. Lancet 1994;343:871–881.
59. Cooper DA, Gatell JM, Kroon S, et al. Zidovudine in persons with asymptomatic HIV infection and CD4+ cell counts greater than 400 per cubic millimeter. N Engl J Med 1993;329:297–303.
60. Hammer SM, Katzenstein DA, Hughes MD, et al. A trial comparing nucleoside monotherapy with combination therapy in HIV-infected

adults with CD4 cell counts from 200 to 500 per cubic millimeter. N Engl J Med 1996;335:1081–1090.
61. Vila J, Nugier F, Bargues G, et al. Absence of viral rebound after treatment of HIV-infected patients with didanosine and hydroxycarbamide. Lancet 1997;350:635–636.
62. Lafeuillade A, Poggi C, Tamalet C, et al. Effects of a combination of zidovudine, didanosine, and lamivudine on primary human immunodeficiency virus type 1 infection. J Infect Dis 1997;175:1051–1055.
63. Kinloch-De Loës S, Hirschel B, Hoen B, et al. A controlled trial of zidovudine in primary human immunodeficiency virus infection. N Engl J Med 1995;333:408–413.
64. Lafeuillade A, Chollet L, Hittinger G, et al. Residual human immunodeficiency virus type 1 RNA in lymphoid tissue of patients with sustained plasma RNA of <200 copies/mL. J Infect Dis 1998;177: 235–238.
65. Connors M, Kovacs JA, Krevat S, et al. HIV infection induces changes in CD4+ T-cell phenotype and depletions within the CD4+ T-cell repertoire that are not immediately restored by antiviral or immune based therapies. Nature Med 1997;3:533–540.
66. Clark SJ, Kelen GD, Henrard DR, et al. Unsuspected primary human immunodeficiency virus type 1 infection in seronegative emergency department patients. J Infect Dis 1994;170:194–197.
67. Holodiny M, Mole L, Margolis D, et al. Determination of human immunodeficiency virus RNA in plasma and cellular viral DNA genotypic zidovudine resistance and viral load during zidovudine–didanosine combination therapy. J Virol 1995;69:3510–3516.
68. Schwartz DH, Laeyendecker OB, Arango-Jaramillo S, et al. Extensive evaluation of a seronegative participant in an HIV-1 vaccine trial as a result of false-positive PCR. Lancet 1997;350:256–259.
69. Brown AE, Jackson B, Fuller SA, et al. Viral RNA in the resolution of human immunodeficiency virus type 1 diagnostic serology. Transfusion 1998;37:926–929.
70. Gulick RM, Mellors JW, Havlir D, et al. Treatment with indinavir, zidovudine, and lamivudine in adults with human immunodeficiency virus infection and prior antiretroviral therapy. N Engl J Med 1997;337:734–739.
71. Raboud JM, Montaner JSG, Conway B, et al. Variation in plasma RNA levels, CD4 count and p24 antigen levels in clinically stable men with human immunodeficiency virus infection. J Infect Dis 1996; 174:191–194.
72. Raboud JM, Montaner JSG, Rae S, et al. Issues in the design of trials of therapies for subjects with human immunodeficiency virus infection that use plasma RNA level as an outcome. J Infect Dis 1997; 175:576–582.
73. Paxton WB, Coombs RW, McElrath MJ, et al. Longitudinal analysis of quantitative virologic measures in human immunodeficiency virus–infected subjects with ≥400 CD4 lymphocytes: implications for applying measurements to individual patients. J Infect Dis 1997;175: 247–254.
74. Deeks SG, Coleman RL, White R, et al. Variance of plasma HIV-1 RNA levels measured by branched DNA (bDNA) within and between days. J Infect Dis 1997;176:514–517.
75. Demeter L, Hughes M, Fischl M, et al. Predictors of virologic and clinical responses to indinavir (IDV) + ZDV + 3TC or ZDV + 3TC [abstract 509]. In: 5th National Conference on Retroviruses and Opportunistic Infections. Alexandria, VA: ISDA Foundation for Retrovirology and Human Health, 1998:175.
76. Ho DD. Time to hit HIV: early and hard. N Engl J Med 1995;331: 1173–1180.
77. Dube MP, Johnson DL, Currier JS. Protease inhibitor–associated hyperglycemia. Lancet 1997;350:713.
78. Hengel RL, Watts NB, Lennox JL. Benign symmetric lipomatosis associated with protease inhibitors. Lancet 1997;350:1596.
79. Stein DS, Korvick JA, Vermund SH. CD4+ lymphocyte cell enumeration for prediction of clinical course of human immunodeficiency virus disease: a review. J Infect Dis 1992;165:352–363.
80. Kuritzkes DR. clinical significance of drug resistance in HIV-1 infection. AIDS 1996;10(Suppl 5):S27–S31.
81. Kahn JO, Lagakos SW, Richman DD, et al. A controlled trial comparing continued zidovudine with didanosine in human immunodeficiency virus infection. N Engl J Med 1992;327:581–587.
82. Japour AJ, Welles S, D'Aquila RT, et al. Prevalence and clinical significance of zidovudine resistance mutations in human immunodeficiency virus isolated from patients after long-term zidovudine treatment. J Infect Dis 1995;171:1172–1179.
83. D'Aquilla RT, Johnson VA, Welles SL, et al. Zidovudine resistance and HIV-1 disease progression during antiretroviral therapy. Ann Intern Med 1995;122:401–408.
84. Brun-Vézinet F, Boucher C, Loveday C, et al. HIV-1 viral load, phenotype, and resistance in a subset of drug-naive participants from the Delta trial. Lancet 1997;350:983–990.
85. Para MF, Coombs R, Collier A, et al. Relationship of baseline genotype to RNA response in ACTG 333 after switching from long term saquinavir (SQVhc) to inidinavir (IDV) or saquinavir soft gelatin capsule (SQVsgc) [abstract 511]. In: 5th National Conference on Retroviruses and Opportunistic Infections. Alexandria, VA: ISDA Foundation for Retrovirology and Human Health, 1998:175.
86. Reichelderfer PS, Coombs RW. Cartesian coordinate analysis of viral burden and CD4+ cell count in HIV disease: implications for clinical trial design and analysis. Antiviral Res 1996;29:83–86.
87. Weiser B, Nachman S, Tropper P, et al. Quantitation of human immunodeficiency virus type 1 during pregnancy: relationship of viral titer to mother-to-child transmission and stability of viral load. Proc Natl Acad Sci U S A 1994;91:8037–8041.
88. Melvin AJ, Burchett SK, Watts DH, et al. Effect of pregnancy and zidovudine therapy on viral load in HIV-1–infected women. J Acquir Immune Defic Syndr Hum Retrovirol 1997;14:232–236.
89. Cao Y, Krogstad P, Korber BT, et al. Maternal HIV-1 viral load and vertical transmission of infection. Nature Med 1997;3:549–552.
90. Sperling RS, Shapiro DE, Coombs RW, et al. Maternal viral load, zidovudine treatment, and the risk of transmission of human immunodeficiency virus type 1 from mother to infant. N Engl J Med 1996;335:1621–1629.
91. Dickover RE, Garratty EM, Herman SA, et al. Identification of levels of maternal HIV-1 RNA associated with risk of perinatal transmission: effect of maternal zidovudine treatment on viral load. JAMA 1996; 275:599–605.
92. Barnhart HX, Caldwell MB, Thomas P, et al. Natural history of human immunodeficiency virus disease in perinatally infected children: an analysis from the Pediatric Spectrum of Disease Project. Pediatrics 1996;97:710–716.
93. Scott GB, Hutto C, Makuch RW, et al. Survival in children with perinatally acquired human immunodeficiency virus type 1 infection. N Engl J Med 1989;321:1791–1796.
94. Blanche S, Rouzioux C, Moscato ML, et al. A prospective study of infants born to women seropositive for human immunodeficiency virus virus type 1. N Engl J Med 1989;320:1643–1648.
95. Blanche S, Newell M-L, Mayaux M-J, et al. Morbidity and mortality in European children vertically infected by HIV-1. J Acquir Immune Defic Syndr Hum Retrovirol 1997;14:442–450.
96. Tovo PA, de Martino M, Gabiano C, et al. Prognostic factors and survival in children with perinatal HIV-1 infection. Lancet 1992;339: 1249–1253.
97. Grubman S, Gross E, Lerner-Weiss N, et al. Older children and adolescents living with perinatally acquired human immunodeficiency virus infection. Pediatrics 1995;95:657–663.
98. Italian Register for HIV Infection in Children. Features of children perinatally infected with HIV-1 surviving longer than 5 years. Lancet 1994;343:191–195.
99. European Collaborative Study. Natural history of vertically aquired human immunodeficiency virus-1 infection. Pediatrics 1994;94: 815–819.
100. Duliege AM, Messiah A, Balanche S, et al. Natural history of human immunodeficiency virus type 1 infection in children: prognostic value of laboratory tests on the bimodal progression of the disease. Pediatr Infect Dis J 1992;11:630–635.

101. Blanche S, Tardieu M, Duliege A-M, et al. Longitudinal study of 94 symptomatic infants with perinatally acquired human immunodeficiency virus infections. Am J Dis Child 1990;144:1210–1215.
102. Pizzo PA, Wilfert CM, Pediatric AIDS Siena Workshop II. Markers and determinants of disease progression in children with HIV infection. J Acquir Immune Defic Syndr Hum Retrovirol 1995;8:30–44.
103. Galli L, de Martino M, Tovo P-A, et al. Onset of clinical signs in children with HIV-1 perinatal infection. AIDS 1995;9:455–461.
104. Krasinski K, Borkowsky W, Holzman RS. Prognosis of human immunodeficiency virus infection in children and adolescents. Pediatr Infect Dis J 1989;8:216–220.
105. Blanche S, Mayaux MJ, Rouzioux C, et al. Relation of the course of HIV infection in children to the severity of the disease in their mothers at delivery. N Engl J Med 1994;330:308–312.
106. Turner BJ, Denison M, Eppes SC, et al. Survival experience of 789 children with the acquired immunodeficiency syndrome. Pediatr Infect Dis J 1993;12:310–320.
107. Wilfert CM, Gross PA, Kaplan JE, et al. Quality standard for enumeration of CD4+ lymphocytes in infants and children exposed to or infected with human immunodeficiency virus. Clin Infect Dis 1995;21:S134–S135.
108. European Collaborative Study. Age-related standards for T lymphocyte subsets based on uninfected children born to human immunodeficiency virus 1–infected women. Pediatr Infect Dis J 1992;11:1018–1026.
109. McIntosh K, Shevitz A, Zaknun D, et al. Age and time-related changes in extracellular viral load in children vertically infected by human immunodeficiency virus. Pediatr Infect Dis 1996;15:1087–1091.
110. De Rossi A, Masiero S, Giaquinto C, et al. Dynamics of viral replication in infants with vertically acquired human immunodeficiency virus type 1 infection. J Clin Invest 1996;97:323–330.
111. Dickover RE, Dillon M, Gillette SG, et al. Rapid increase in load of human immunodeficiency virus correlate with early progression and loss of CD4 cells in vertically infected infants. J Infect Dis 1994;170:1279–1284.
112. Shearer WT, Quinn TC, LaRussa P, et al. Viral load and disease progression in infants infected with human immunodeficiency virus type 1. N Engl J Med 1997;336:1337–1342.
113. Palumbo PE, Kwok SH, Waters S, et al. Viral measurement by polymerase chain reaction–based assays in human immunodeficiency virus–infected infants. J Pediatr 1995;126:592–595.
114. Palumbo PE, Raskino C, Fiscus S, et al. Correlation of HIV plasma RNA levels with clinical outcome in a large pediatric trial (ACTG 152) [abstract LB14]. In: 4th Conference on Retroviruses and Opportunistic Infections. Washington, DC: American Society of Microbiology, 1997:208.
115. Valentine ME, Jackson CR, Vavaro C, et al. Evaluation of surrogate markers and clinical outcomes in two-year follow-up of eighty-six human immunodeficiency virus–infected pediatric infants. Pediatr Infect Dis J 1998;17:18–23.
116. Englund JA, Baker CJ, Raskino C, et al. Zidovudine, didanosine or both as the initial treatment for symptomatic HIV-infected children. N Engl J Med 1997;336:1704–1712.
117. Luzuriaga K, Bryson Y, Krogstad P, et al. Combination treatment with zidovudine, didanosine, and nevirapine in infants with human immunodeficiency virus type 1 infection. N Engl J Med 1997;336:1343–1349.
118. Jankelevich S, Mueller B, Smith S, et al. Long-term activity of Indivir/ZDV/3TC in HIV-1 infected children: results of a phase I/II study [abstract 231]. In: 5th Conference on Retrovirus and Opportunistic Infections. Alexandria, VA: ISDA Foundation for Retrovirology and Human Health, 1998:122.
119. Burchett SK, Carey V, Yong F, et al. Virologic activity of didanosine (ddI), zidovudine (ZDV) and nevirapine (NVP) combinations in pediatric subjects with advanced HIV disease (ACTG 245) [abstract 271]. In: 5th Conference on Retrovirus and Opportunistic Infections. Alexandria, VA: ISDA Foundation for Retrovirology and Human Health, 1998:130.
120. Kline MW, Fletcher CV, Harris AT, et al. One-year follow-up of HIV-infected children receiving combination therapy with indinavir, stavudine (d4T), and didanosine (ddI) [abstract 232]. In: 5th Conference on Retrovirus and Opportunistic Infections. Alexandria, VA: ISDA Foundation for Retrovirology and Human Health, 1998:122.
121. Pelton SI, Yogev R, Johnson D. Changes in viral load and immunologic markers in children treated with triple therapy including ritonavir [abstract 234]. In: 5th Conference on Retrovirus and Opportunistic Infections. Alexandria, VA: ISDA Foundation for Retrovirology and Human Health, 1998:123.
122. Ogino MT, Danker WM, Spector S. Development and significance of zidovudine-resistance in children infected with human immunodeficiency virus. J Pediatr 1993;123:1–8.
123. Tudor-Williams G, St-Clair MH, McKinney RE, et al. HIV-1 sensitivity to zidovudine and clincal outcome in children. Lancet 1992;339:15–19.
124. Husson RN, Shirakasa T, Buttler K, et al. High-level resistance to zidovudine but not to zalcitabine or didanosine in human immunodeficiency virus from children receiving antiretroviral therapy. J Pediatr 1993;123:9–16.
125. Mellado MJ, Cilleruelo MJ, Ortiz M, et al. Viral phenotype, antiretroviral resistance and clinical evolution in human immunodeficiency virus–infected children. Pediatr Infect Dis J 1997;16:1032–1037.
126. Tamalet C, Poizot Martin I, Lafeuillade A, et al. Viral load and genotypic resistance pattern in HIV-1 infected patients treated by a triple combination therapy including nucleoside and protease inhibitors initiated at primary infection [abstract 592]. In: 4th Conference on Retroviruses and Opportunistic Infections. Washington DC: American Society of Microbiology, 1997:174.
127. Gupta P, Urbach A, Cosentine L, et al. HIV-1 isolates from children with or without AIDS have a similar in vitro biological properties. AIDS 1993;7:1561–1564.
128. Balotta C, Vigano A, Riva C, et al. HIV type 1 phenotype correlates with the stage of infection in vertically infected children. AIDS Res Hum Retrovir 1996;12:1247–1253.
129. Spencer LT, Ogino MT, Danker WM, et al. Clinical significance of human immunodeficiency virus type 1 phenotype in infected children. J Infect Dis 1994;169:491–495.
130. Yerkovich M, Sampoleo R, Dragavon J, et al. Low HIV-1 RNA copy number assessed by bDNA and RT-PCR assays: implications for managing patients above or below the viral RNA quantitation limit [abstract 303]. In: 5th National Conference on Human Retroviruses. Alexandria, VA: ISDA Foundation for Retrovirology and Human Health, 1998:136.
131. O'Brien WA, Hartigan PM, Daar ES, et al. Changes in plasma HIV RNA levels and CD4+ lymphocyte counts predict both response to antiretroviral therapy and therapeutic failure. Ann Intern Med 1997;126:939–945.
132. Fauci AS. Host factors and the pathogenesis of HIV-induced disease. Nature 1996;384:529–534.
133. Merigan TC. Individualization of therapy using viral markers. J Acquir Immune Defic Syndr Hum Retrovirol 1995;10:S41–S46.

Section V
Control and Prevention

42
AIDS Vaccine Development

Barney S. Graham and David T. Karzon

Human immunodeficiency virus type 1 (HIV-1) was identified in 1983, and the quest for a preventive vaccine has engendered the most expensive and determined international research effort ever mounted. New molecular tools in virology and immunology, new adjuvants, new antigen delivery systems, recent discoveries in HIV entry and pathogenesis, and promising studies of candidate vaccines in animal models have provided reasons to hope that developing a safe and effective acquired immunodeficiency syndrome (AIDS) vaccine will be possible. However, some investigators have argued that preventive vaccination for AIDS will not be possible (1), and the complex biology of HIV-1 makes this a daunting task. Certainly, one cannot predict when an effective vaccine will be available. Nevertheless, one can state with assurance that the process of AIDS vaccine development will provide important information about HIV immunity and pathogenesis that will affect the HIV epidemic and also will influence vaccine design against other pathogens.

Strategies for the control of HIV-1 can be organized into four major categories: 1) public health initiatives, education, and behavioral change (see Chaps. 9, 13, and 51); 2) mechanical barriers and microbicides (see Chap. 43); 3) antiretroviral chemotherapy (see Chaps. 47 and 48); and 4) preventive vaccination. It may require a combination of all these approaches to achieve the ultimate goal of preventing HIV infection, but in this chapter we address issues directly related to the development and clinical evaluation of preventive vaccines. Ethical and logistic issues involved in performing domestic and international efficacy trials are discussed in Chapter 46.

Development of a vaccine against HIV-1 is critical for controlling the global AIDS epidemic. The virus and its disease pathogenesis present singular challenges for vaccine development. In this chapter we address 1) the features of other viruses for which vaccine development has met with success or failure, 2) current information on disease pathogenesis and HIV-1 immunity relevant to vaccine design, 3) vaccine concepts being evaluated in preclinical and clinical trials, and 4) issues involved in advancing to efficacy trial testing.

SUCCESSFUL VIRAL VACCINES

Viral vaccines, whether presented as inactivated whole virus, live attenuated virus, or viral subunit protein, have been highly successful in preventing those infections characterized by a cluster of biologic characteristics (Table 42.1). Many important infections fall into this category, including rabies, smallpox, yellow fever, poliomyelitis, measles, mumps, rubella and hepatitis B. Unfortunately, HIV-1 infection demonstrates few of the characteristics that mark such infections.

In diseases amenable to effective immune intervention, a defined sequence of steps can usually be documented during the course of viral infection (2). Poliovirus infection as seen in primates or humans provides a prototype of the *systemic model* (Table 42.2). Typical of the systemic model, exposure of the host to a viral pathogen at the *portal of entry* results in silent mucosal replication, although the mucosa may be bypassed by direct parenteral entry. A low-grade *primary viremia* ensues, which is clinically silent and may be difficult to document, with dissemination to systemic *parenteral sites*, where viral expansion occurs. This produces a high-titered *secondary viremia*, which, in turn, seeds the *target organ*. To this point, despite active viral replication and systemic distribution and sometimes early immune responses, characteristically the patient remains entirely well. This *incubation period* ends and disease is expressed only when and if virus replicates sufficiently in the target organ to induce physiologic damage. Thus, the incubation period is clinically silent, although nonspecific prodromal symptoms and signs, such as malaise, fever, and headache, may accompany the secondary viremia, as in poliomyelitis. Classic poliomyelitis is characterized by lower motor neuron paralysis, which occurs only when a sufficient number of neurons is destroyed. However, the pathogenic sequence may self-terminate at any point, presumed to be associated with neutralizing antibody appearing as early as the second week of infection. Poliovirus, in fact, usually manifests as an inapparent infection, although it may progress to prodromal symptoms or may even infect a few motor neurons without clinical paralysis. Prior vaccination is effective by interrupting the process at any point before significant viral replication and damage to the target organ, that is, the motor neurons.

Table 42.1. Characteristics of Human Viral Infections With Successful Vaccines; Features Not Shared by HIV-1

Successful Viral Vaccines	HIV-1 Infection
Pathogenesis includes an obligatory viremia before infecting target organ.	Target organs including lymphocytes, macrophages, and dendritic cells and directly infected as early events.
Preexisting neutralizing antibody prevents infection in an individual with intact immune system; infectious agent is free virus; passive antibody, even with minimal titers readily protects.	A high-threshold titer of neutralizing antibody may protect against free virus; CTL role is probably significant; HIV may be transferred as cell-borne integrated virus.
Antigenic serotypes are stable and monotypic or limited in number.	Extensive and evolving genetic diversity exists in individual host as well as in the population.
Infection of vaccinated individual is frequently accompanied by limited local replication; rapid secondary response results in inapparent infection, dampened before target injury.	Infection of vaccinee risks early establishment of proviral state or distribution of virus into sites protected from immune clearance.
A useful animal model is generally available, although it may not reproduce human disease with fidelity.	HIV-1 in chimpanzee induces active and persistent infection but no disease; SIV in macaque causes infection and disease but has important differences in genome structure.
Vaccination with dominant surface antigens induces vigorous and durable functional antibody that confers long-term protection (years).	To date, vaccination with dominant surface antigens results in modest and transient neutralizing antibody.
CD8 + CTLs are not required for protection.	CD8 + CTL response may be essential for protection.
Host immune function is not significantly compromised by infection.	Immune system is major target organ.
Virus usually does not persist and is not integrated in cell genome.	Integration and proviral state are inherent in replication, and occur as early events.
After recovery, protection against subsequent disease (although not infection) is complete, often lifelong; infections are typically benign and self-limiting, although in some instances death or residua may occur.	Untreated HIV-1 infection is nearly always fatal.

In immunized individuals, challenge virus can replicate at the portal of entry (oropharynx and alimentary tract with poliovirus) and cause no disease, but it provides antigenic stimulus and time for recruitment and expansion of memory cells. It is important to distinguish between prevention of infection and prevention of disease. Previous work suggests that all current successful vaccines prevent disease, but none prevent initial clinically inapparent infection. On reexposure to virus, typically virus replication is sufficient to induce a readily demonstrable secondary response. In the group of diseases represented by poliomyelitis, neutralizing antibody appears to be the first line of protection against subsequent viral challenge by clearing or reducing viral load (3, 4). Persistent circulating antibody protects against disease recurrence, whether that antibody is acquired by natural disease, by passive administration, transplacentally, or by vaccination. In this model, circulating neutralizing antibody is necessary and sufficient for protection, and, thus, its presence even at low titer can be accepted as a surrogate marker of protection. The singular effectiveness of antibody depends not only on a several-day time window required for immune expansion, but also on an almost invariant antigenic match between virus and antibody; for example, each of the three serotypes of poliovirus is serologically matched worldwide and can be type-specifically prevented by use of a single trivalent live attenuated or inactivated whole virus vaccine. Finally, the protective success of antibody depends on the presence of an intact immune system providing functional B- and T-cell systems.

Unsuccessful Vaccine Efforts

By contrast, infectious diseases demonstrating pathogenic patterns other than the classic systemic model described are often difficult to prevent. For example, for infections limited to mucosal sites (e.g., respiratory syncytial virus [RSV]), those with sequestered or latent states (e.g., herpes simplex virus [HSV]), agents subject to significant antigenic variation (e.g., influenza virus), or those that can spread through cell-to-cell fusion events (e.g., RSV and HSV), vaccine efforts remain partially or completely unsuccessful. Although these infections can be prevented by sufficiently high "threshold" titer of antibody, this level is generally not sustained after natural infection or achieved with vaccination. These agents may also require the presence of other immune elements such as mucosal immunoglobulin A (IgA) production or specific cytotoxic lymphocytes (CTLs) to prevent or clear infection (5).

RSV is a paramyxovirus that causes yearly epidemics of respiratory tract infection. Unlike poliovirus or measles virus, the portal of entry for RSV is also its target organ. Therefore, systemic antibody, which can efficiently inhibit poliovirus or measles virus during the obligate viremia required to reach the target organ, has less opportunity to interfere with the pathogenesis of RSV. Although RSV does not spread systemically or infect cells of the immune system, as does HIV-1, it shares other features in common with HIV-1. RSV enters susceptible cells by fusion from without, by a mechanism similar to HIV-1, having the identical FLGFL hydrophobic sequence found in gp41 at the amino terminus of its endoproteolytically cleaved fusion (F) protein. Attempts to develop a vaccine for RSV have thus far been unsuccessful. A formalin-inactivated, alum-precipitated whole virus vaccine tested in the 1960s not only failed to protect against infection, but also resulted in vaccine-enhanced illness with parallels to atypical measles induced by the Tween-ether inactivated measles vaccine (6). The basis for the vaccine-enhanced illness appears to have been related to induction of the inappropriate CD4+ T-lymphocyte subset resulting in a virus-induced immune response that produced immunopathology and ineffective RSV clearance (7, 8). Live attenuated RSV vaccines have not produced an enhanced illness syndrome, but they have failed because of inadequate immunogenicity or incomplete attenuation of virulence.

HSV establishes persistence and can recur locally despite the presence of circulating antibody and cell-mediated immunity. Efforts to prepare a satisfactory HSV vaccine for human use have, so far, been unsuccessful. A recent study evaluating a purified recombinant protein subunit approach in a novel adjuvant failed to protect despite promising results in animal models (427). However, successful vaccine development has been achieved for herpes varicella-zoster virus using a live attenuated vaccine approach (9).

In the remainder of the text, poliomyelitis is used as the paradigm of a virus-induced disease for which a successful vaccine has been produced, and RSV is the paradigm for a virus that has eluded vaccine development.

PATHOGENESIS OF HIV-1 INFECTION RELEVANT TO IMMUNE INTERVENTION

Early Events

The most frequent portals of entry for HIV-1 are the urogenital and rectal mucosa, although the intravenous and transplacental routes bypass mucosal sites. The infection probably can be transmitted as either free or cell-associated virus (10). Evidence points to infection with a single or minimal number of clones (11, 12). Tissue tropism is determined in part by host cell determinants required for entry. CD4 is the major cell-surface receptor for HIV, and thereby CD4+ T lymphocytes, blood monocytes, tissue macrophages, and dendritic cells (DCs) are targets for HIV infection (13–17). After CD4 binding, the HIV envelope glycoprotein binds a coreceptor to initiate membrane fusion and uncoating (18, 19). The coreceptors are a family of seven-transmembrane domain proteins that normally function as chemokine receptors. Chemokine receptor use determines virus tropism and syncytium-inducing phenotype. Viruses that use CCR5 are nonsyncytium inducing and infect cells of the monocyte lineage as well as activated T lymphocytes (20, 21), whereas viruses that use CXCR4 are syncytium inducing and can infect T-cell lines as well as activated T lymphocytes (22). Alternative coreceptors have been identified (22–27), and the full range of potential coreceptors probably has yet to be defined. Therefore, simply blocking one chemokine receptor may have an unpredictable effect on the outcome of HIV infection.

Rare individuals who are homozygous for a 32-bp deletion in CCR5 are resistant to HIV infection (28), although exceptions have been described (29–31). Persons heterozygous for this mutation have delayed disease progression (32), but they make up a small fraction of long-term nonprogressors. Interference with CCR5 binding using β-chemokines such as regulated-on-activation normal T-cell expressed and secreted (RANTES), macrophage inflammatory protein-1α (MIP-1α), and MIP-1β can prevent HIV entry even though cell attachment still occurs (33). Antibodies have also been

Table 42.2. Schema of Pathogenesis of Poliovirus, HIV-1, and Respiratory Syncytial Virus

	Poliovirus (Systemic Model, Long Incubation Period)	HIV-1	Respiratory Syncytial Virus (Mucosally Restricted Model, Short Incubation Period)
Portal of entry	Oropharynx, alimentary mucosa and regional nodes, local replication	Mucosal, intravenous or transplacental; local replication	Respiratory mucosa, local replication
Primary viremia	Low titer	Free virus or infected dendritic cell, no viremia macrophage, or lymphocyte in cases of intravenous transmission; unlikely in mucosal transmission	
Parenteral site (viral expansion)	Reticuloendothelial system	Seeding of regional and systemic lymphoid sites	None
Secondary viremia (high titer)	Transient febrile illness at 7–10 days	High-titered viremia, prodromal "primary infection" at 1–6 weeks	None
Target organ	Motor neurons, with spread limited to motor pathways	Persistent infection of lymphoid tissues, CNS, low-grade viremia, clinically silent	Respiratory mucosa
Disease expression when threshold level of disease is reached (end of incubation period)	Paralysis at 11–14 days	Destruction of lymphoid elements; immune deficiency syndrome at 3–10+ years	Respiratory disease at 5–10 days with wheezing
Outcome	Recovery after inapparent infection (usual) or residual paralysis	Recovery not known	Recovery without residua (usual) or residual airway hyperreactivity
Reinfection	Serotype-specific protection	Superinfection in the setting of persistent infection leading to recombination events	Reinfection common, but with diminishing disease severity

described that can interfere with viral entry even when they are added after virus adsorption has occurred (34, 35).

Entry through CD4 can also be facilitated when nonneutralizing antibody is bound to HIV, thus allowing interactions between Fc or complement receptors (36–38). Leukocyte adhesion factor-1 (LFA-1) may also enhance HIV replication in cell culture by promoting cell–cell contact and syncytium formation (39, 40). Macrophage tropism is an important characteristic of most transmitted HIV strains whether transmission is sexual, parenteral, or vertical (41–43). This finding suggests that transmitted virus primarily uses the CCR5 receptor, and macrophages or related antigen-processing cells such as Langerhans' cells or DCs in the genital or rectal submucosa may be sites of initial infection, thereby determining which HIV variants subsequently disseminate. Developing vaccine strategies to exploit the new understanding of HIV entry and targeting vaccine-induced immune responses to the subset of transmitted virus at the site of initial infection are high priorities.

In vitro findings also implicate mucosal epithelial cells as potential targets of HIV-infected cells. HIV-infected CD4 cell lines mixed with cultures of transformed human cervical epithelial cell lines yield infectious virus progeny released from both basal and apical surfaces of the epithelial cells (44). In vivo, this process would result in relay of virus to the genital submucosa, where it would gain access to macrophages and lymphocytes. In vitro, HIV can target gut epithelia, including enterochromaffin cells of the rectal mucosa (45, 46) and oral mucosal epithelia (47).

Because CD4 is not expressed on mucosal epithelium, an alternative entry mechanism must exist. Galactocerebroside has been proposed as a potential HIV receptor on CD4(−) cells (48–50), but whether it or members of the chemokine receptor family of molecules can mediate entry in vivo in the absence of CD4 is not known. In rabbit and mouse models, HIV-1 is transported (presumably nonspecifically) by antigen-transporting M cells of intact rectal mucosa. This provides access to underlying T and B lymphocytes, macrophages, and DCs (51, 52). The M cell has been proposed as a potential entry site in the human rectum. However, M cells are not known to be found in oral, vaginal, or cervical epithelial mucosa (53). Another proposed mechanism of entry is transcytosis of virus across epithelial cells through endosome-like structures (54). Definitions of both innate and vaccine-inducible adaptive immune mechanisms to prevent entry through M cells, epithelial transcytosis, DCs, or sites of epithelial trauma are areas of active investigation.

DCs are major histocompatibility class (MHC) class II CD4+ antigen-presenting cells (APCs) found within squamous epithelia of mucous surfaces including the oral, vaginal, and cervical mucosa, but they are not found in rectal mucosa (55–58). The DCs have direct access through dendritic processes to the lumen. As Langerhans' cells from skin (59, 60), mucosally derived DCs support HIV-1 replication in culture (52, 57, 61). The DCs also promote infection of CD4+ lymphocytes through direct cell–cell contact in the vaginal submucosa or in the crypts of the adenoids, or they transport virus to regional lymph nodes where CD4+ cells in the paracortex are infected. The complex of mucosal structures and regional nodes is considered the portal of entry for further discussion (see Table 42.2). Initial seeding of systemic lymphoid tissues, by analogy with patterns of dissemination of other viral infections, probably occurs within days of the initial contact with virus. Studies of macaques challenged with simian immunodeficiency virus (SIV) demonstrated spread to regional lymph nodes by 48 hours, and widespread lymph node involvement was present by day 4 or 5 (62, 63). Important targets of secondary spread include elements of the immune system, CD4+ T cells, monocyte/macrophages, and DCs, as well as microglial cells in brain (53, 64, 65). Access through paracortical spaces and lymphatics to the blood and dissemination to systemic lymphoid tissues (peripheral nodes, spleen, thymus, bone marrow) allow rapid and massive expansion. This spread is similar to the viremia necessary for poliovirus-induced disease, but it is unlike RSV pathogenesis, which is restricted to the respiratory tract.

The development of viremia provides an important point of intervention for vaccine-induced immune responses to affect disease progression. Infection by intravenous and transplacental routes presumably induces direct primary viremia. Symptomatic, high-titered secondary viremia then occurs within 2 to 3 weeks after initial inoculation and further distributes the virus. In the SIV-infected macaque, virus is found in the semen at 8 days, and it occurs in peripheral blood by 14 days (53, 66). These events precede the appearance of humoral immune responses by several weeks. Breaches of mucosa due to trauma or ulcerative infection do not necessarily result in direct access to the systemic circulation, but they may simply increase the efficiency of the local infection and spread to regional lymph nodes (53). An acute clinical syndrome occurs in 20 to 50% of individuals undergoing primary HIV-1 infection, and it appears 1 to 6 weeks or more after the time of known exposure (67–73). It may be the equivalent of the symptomatic prodromal stage defined in poliovirus infection manifested concurrently with secondary viremia. Symptoms of primary HIV-1 infection can mimic those of infectious mononucleosis and include fever, fatigue, adenopathy, and often rash and central nervous system involvement, all of which usually resolve spontaneously within 2 to 3 weeks (72, 73). A transient rash has been seen in macaques 1 to 3 weeks after SIV infection (74). A peak of viremia and antigenemia occurs during this symptomatic period in acute HIV infection in humans (75–77) and in chimpanzees (78) several weeks before the appearance of immune responses. The monocyte/macrophage may play an important role as an immune haven and transport system, for example, to the brain, which serves as an immunologically privileged site. Early appearance of antigen and virus in the cerebrospinal fluid is evidence of early central nervous system infection (79). The concept of a separate compartment in the brain gains support from sequence studies of the third variable domain (V3) of the gp120 envelope protein. Strains derived from brain specimens showed common conserved elements not seen in strains isolated in blood from the same individuals (80). Investigators have suggested that the eye and the male seminal tract (3, 81) may also serve as immunoprivileged sites and may protect virus from immune-mediated clearance.

Chronic Persistence and Progression to Clinical Disease

The high-titer viremia and antigenemia that accompany the prodromal syndrome are rapidly dampened, temporally associated with the appearance of CD8+ cytotoxic T lymphocytes (82–84), with humoral responses occurring later. Rather than complete clearing with termination of viremia, as occurs in acute infections with other viruses, rapidly emerging antigenic variants are selected as escape mutants (85–88). Thereafter, viral replication persists indefinitely, presumably by iterations of antigenic diversification, immune evasion, and compartmentalization in cells or organs resistant to immune-mediated clearance. A dynamic steady state ensues (see Chap. 1), with "set-point" or steady-state level of virus replication measured as HIV genome copies per milliliter of plasma (89, 90). Substantial titers of functional antibodies mediating neutralization, fusion inhibition, antibody-dependent cell-mediated cytotoxicity (ADCC), binding to V3 loop, and blocking of CD4 binding are present. In addition, MHC class I–restricted CD8+ CTL activity can be detected in the circulation without in vitro stimulation (91–93).

The failure of combined antiviral antibody and CD8+ CTLs to clear virus successfully may be explained by the continuous evolution of variant neutralizing and CD8+ CTL recognition sites, on the basis of kinetics or magnitude of viral load, by virus sequestration in organs or cells resistant to CD8+ CTL recognition or lysis, or by viral mechanisms for diminishing antigen presentation such as *nef* inhibition of MHC class I expression (3, 94). Other factors that influence the supply side of new virus production include intrinsic differences in virus strains (95, 96) and extrinsic activation events that increase transcription of provirus, including coinfections (97–99), antigen stimulation (100), various cytokine influences, and intrinsic cellular events (65, 101). During the years of clinical latency, the integrity of the immune system is gradually eroded through a combination of direct HIV-induced cell destruction or dysfunction and indirect HIV-specific immunopathologic features (see Chap. 5).

DCs appear to play a special role in viral persistence. These cells are represented by epidermal and mucosal Langerhans' cells, peripheral blood (veiled) cells, and follicular DCs (FDCs) found in systemic lymphoid sites (102, 103). DCs serve as a target cell for initial HIV-1 entry, as an HIV-1 reservoir, and as APCs. Viral RNA, a marker for replicating virus, has been found as immune complexes associated with FDC dendritic processes "trapped" in lymphoid follicles (104–108). More than 90% of the HIV genome present in lymph nodes is present in the extracellular space (109, 110). Differences in the reported capacity of virus to replicate and to induce cytopathic effect in DCs may depend on the maturational state or tissue setting of the DC subset (52, 111–114). HIV-1 replicates in DC located in lymphoid follicles (115–119) and in cell-fractionated preparations of DCs from peripheral blood in vitro without apparent cytopathic effect. The end result of infection of lymphoid tissue is a progressive depletion of both CD4+ cells and FDCs during the years of asymptomatic infection and an eventual immune deficiency state with appearance of opportunistic infections. The AIDS clinical syndrome emerges only when a threshold level of damage to the target organ, helper T cells, and DCs reaches a point of uncompensated clinical impairment, making it appear as a rapid event. This situation is not unlike the paradigm for target organ injury seen with other viral systems, but with a much longer time frame.

NATURAL IMMUNITY AGAINST HIV-1 INFECTION: POTENTIAL GUIDE FOR VACCINE-INDUCED IMMUNITY

Various settings suggest that natural immunity to HIV-1 infection may occur in some people, including the following: 1) uninfected persons with frequent high-risk sexual encounters; 2) persons with documented occupational exposures to HIV-1 who have resisted infection; 3) long-term nonprogressors; and 4) noninfected infants born to HIV-infected mothers. These unique populations suggest that induction of protective immunity against HIV-1 is possible, and they may offer direct clues to which components of the immune response are most important for immunity.

A small subset of commercial sex workers in the Gambia and in Kenya has been shown to have a diminishing risk of HIV-1 infection, if these workers have remained uninfected after 6 years of high-risk exposures (120, 121). Although these persons have no evidence of virus infection by culture and polymerase chain reaction, and no detectable HIV-specific antibody responses, HIV-specific CD8+ CTL activity has been demonstrated, suggesting that transient infection may have occurred, thus inducing protective immunity mediated by CD8+ CTLs (121). This group is small, but other factors contributing to protection from infection have not been reported. A few other groups characterized by remaining uninfected despite multiple high-risk exposures have been shown to have the 32-bp deletion mutation in CCR5, but in other groups, no correlate of immunity has been identified (28). In persons who remain uninfected despite significant occupational exposure to HIV-1–contaminated material, studies have focused on HIV-specific T-cell responses. Although HIV-specific antibodies cannot be detected, peripheral blood mononuclear cells (PBMCs) show lymphoproliferative activity when stimulated with HIV-specific peptides (122). HIV-specific CTL responses have also been seen in this cohort (123). This finding suggests that transient infection may have occurred and was cleared with natural immune defenses. Another group of individuals who remain HIV-seronegative despite having HIV-seropositive partners also has been shown to have HIV-specific PBMC production of interleukin 2 (IL-2), and evidence of HIV-specific IgA in mucosal secretions (124), findings suggesting that induction of immunity at mucosal sites may be important.

A subset of persons infected with HIV-1 has persistent infection, but these persons do not progress to AIDS for more than 12 years. Some of these individuals are infected with virus isolates that replicate poorly (125, 126). However, others are infected with viruses that have normal replication capacity, but they have maintained strong and broad humoral and cellular HIV-specific immune responses that appear to be responsible for delayed disease progression. A key to the maintenance of effective immunity may be the preservation of HIV-specific lymphoproliferative responses (127). Whether the high levels of HIV-specific lymphoproliferative responses are the cause of low virus loads or the result of small amounts of virus being unable to clonally delete HIV-specific CD4 populations is not known. The specific effector mechanism has not been defined, but preservation of HIV-specific lymphoproliferative response is clearly associated with low virus load and delayed disease progression (127). This is an example of the principle that small influences on the homeostasis between virus replication and virus clearance can make a large impact on disease progression, and it provides some hope that altering this dynamic early after infection through vaccine-induced immune responses may be possible.

Uninfected infants born to HIV-infected mothers represent another group in which natural immunity is evident. In untreated mothers, approximately 25% of children are infected (128). The factors that prevent infection in the other 75% have not been defined. However, examples of uninfected infants with detectable HIV-specific CTL activity suggest that transient infection can occur with clearance mediated by natural immunity (129).

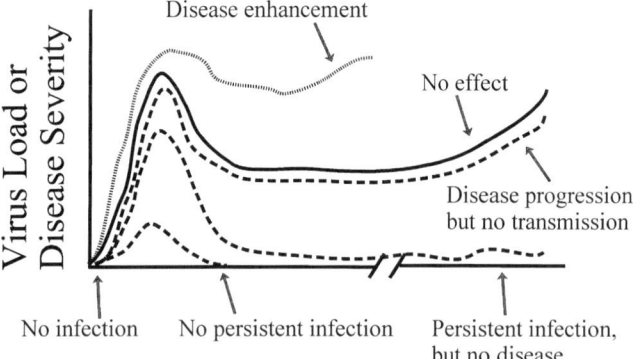

Figure 42.1. Potential outcomes of HIV-1 infection in vaccinated subjects. Some outcomes, expressed as different patterns of viral load, could occur as a consequence of vaccine-induced immunity. These include prevention of infection, which would be unprecedented, prevention of persistent infection (i.e., rapid clearance of virus infected cells), controlled but persistent infection that would not result in clinical disease expression, no effect on virus replication or disease course in the vaccinee but reduced transmissibility of virus to others, no effect, and enhancement of HIV-induced disease.

The parameters of vaccine-induced protective immunity can be defined as 1) the timing or kinetics of the effector response after exposure to the virus, 2) the composition of the vaccine-induced immune response, and 3) the magnitude and duration of the immune response. The possible outcomes of HIV-1 infection acquired in the setting of vaccine-induced immunity are depicted in Figure 42.1. Ideally, infection could be completely prevented, although no precedent exists for this in other successful viral vaccines. Most vaccines work by producing a state of immunity that results in a transient, self-limited infection that does not produce disease. For an HIV vaccine, other acceptable end points could be 1) persistent infection, but no disease progression, and 2) persistent infection and disease progression in the individual, but a reduction in transmissible virus. Unacceptable outcomes would include 1) no effect on virus clearance, on disease progression, or on transmissible virus and 2) enhanced disease. How to assess these end points in vaccine efficacy trials is addressed in Chapter 46.

ANTIGEN TARGETS AND IMMUNOLOGIC EFFECTOR MECHANISMS

Antigenic Diversity

HIV-1 genetic variation represents one of the greatest hurdles to vaccine development. The combination of a high frequency of transcriptional errors and the capacity for recombination has produced a range of variation within and between subtypes that is unprecedented (see Chap. 3). The approaches taken in vaccine development to accommodate this problem include 1) defining the characteristics of naturally transmitted virus, 2) defining conserved epitopes critical for virus survival, 3) production of complex, multicomponent vaccines, 4) development of prototypic vaccine products effective against homologous HIV strains to provide the basis for vaccines against multiple subtypes, and 5) induction of CD8+ CTL response with potential for cross-clade killing activity. Although the genetic diversity of HIV-1 is a daunting challenge for vaccine development, HIV-1 transmission is not efficient. Perhaps a limited number of virions have the ability to be transmitted, and most individuals are infected with a few infectious particles. Therefore, if vaccine-induced immune responses are present before the time of widespread dissemination and expansion of the viral load, they may only need to recognize a small, relatively homogeneous virus swarm to prevent persistent infection. More work is needed to define the characteristics of transmissible virus, and in particular the early events that occur between the time of virus inoculation on a mucosal surface and systemic dissemination. The success of vaccination may hinge on altering events in the early hours after HIV-1 exposure.

Humoral Responses

The envelope glycoprotein gp160 and its cleavage products, transmembrane protein gp41 and surface protein gp120, have up to this point been the principal antigens used for vaccine production. This approach is based on the importance of envelope determinants for neutralizing antibody activity. Several neutralizing epitopes have been defined. The V3 loop and the CD4 attachment domain located within gp120 have long been known to be important neutralizing epitopes (130–132). The V3 loop, known as the principal neutralizing domain, is a continuous region of approximately 35 amino acids linked at its base by a disulfide bond (133–135). The crown of the V3 loop contains an epitope that determines the neutralizing specificity of T-cell line–adapted (TCLA) viruses. The more conserved regions contribute to cell tropism and cytopathogenicity (136–138). V3-specific neutralizing activity in general is type specific, is readily escaped by genetic variants, and does not appear to be a major factor in the neutralization of primary HIV-1 isolates. The CD4 binding site is discontinuous and depends on conformational features (139, 140). Antibodies to the CD4 binding site arising during natural infection can neutralize more broadly than those directed to V3 (140–144). Neutralizing antibodies directed independently to the V3 and CD4 binding sites can act synergistically (145).

Domains in V2 (146–149) and in gp41 (150–152) also are known to be sites for neutralizing antibody binding. Heavy glycosylation and tertiary folding are thought to account for failure to recognize important conserved domains (153–159), and alterations of carbohydrate moieties can modulate specificity and protective efficacy of antibody responses (160). Although structural *gag* and *pol* proteins, as well as regulatory and accessory proteins, induce antibodies measurable in binding assays in infected individuals, they probably do not play an important role in HIV neutralization.

The requirements for neutralizing primary HIV-1 isolates grown in activated PBMCs are different from those needed to neutralize prototype viruses adapted for growth in T-cell lines. TCLA viruses are easy to neutralize in comparison with primary viral isolates (161). Alternative coreceptor usage does not account for the difficulty in neutralizing primary isolates (162, 163). Other factors such as differences in protein folding, glycosylation, and oligomerization are under investigation. Identifying critical gp160 structures that can induce antibodies with neutralizing and fusion inhibiting activity against primary HIV isolates is a major focus of current investigation.

Significant ADCC activity is induced by natural HIV-1 infection (164, 165). The envelope contains the major ADCC targets, including one in the V3 loop and another in the extracellular domain of gp41 (166), and they are accessible on the infected cell surface. ADCC activity is not MHC restricted and thus may uniquely contribute to lysis of virally infected allogeneic donor cells at the time of initial infection. The ADCC mechanism is readily demonstrated using infected cells in vitro and is present in HIV-1 infection, but its role in vivo is yet to be determined.

Cell-Mediated Immune Responses

HIV-1–specific MHC class I–restricted CD8+ CTL activity is readily detected in HIV-infected individuals by direct assay of PBMCs without in vitro expansion (91, 93). With progression to AIDS, CTL activity decreases. CTLs are capable of killing virus-infected cells and are important in the natural termination of many viral infections (5, 167, 168). Multiple CTL epitopes have been mapped, restricted by various MHC class I alleles. CTL epitopes are present in the envelope glycoprotein as well as in internal structural and regulatory proteins. As shown with influenza virus, CTLs directed against sites on relatively conserved internal structural proteins may have broad cross-reactivity (169). However, even gp160-specific CTL responses have been shown to lyse target cells infected with primary HIV-1 isolates from a broad spectrum of HIV-1 subtypes (170, 171). HIV-2 induced CTL responses have also been shown to recognize and lyse HIV-1–infected target cells (172). Therefore, unlike antibody responses, which tend to be type specific with limited activity against primary isolates, CD8+ CTL responses have broad cross-clade killing activity against primary HIV-1 isolates. Nevertheless, within an individual, CTL escape variants have been demonstrated, suggesting that HIV-1 is under immunologic pressure to evade CTL activity (88, 93, 173–175). If a given individual has a limited number of dominant CTL epitope targets, clearing virus early and keeping virus load low will diminish the chance of CTL escape. Whether increasing the number of CTL epitopes in a candidate vaccine will improve immunity is not known. However, because of the documented capacity for genetic variation that allows CTL escape, and other data suggesting that immune responses with a restricted Vβ repertoire can be associated with rapid disease progression (176, 177), vaccines incorporating multiple potential CTL epitopes are favored. Another rationale for incorporating multiple CTL epitopes is that HIV-1 *nef* has been shown to inhibit expression of HLA-A2 and may also diminish expression of other MHC class I proteins. This can lead to a reduction in epitope density and impaired CTL-mediated target cell killing (94). Therefore, increasing the number of potential CTL epitopes in a vaccine may improve the rate of inducing responses not affected by this mechanism.

Vaccine-inducible CD8+ CTLs can kill HIV-infected target cells by classic cell lysis through the perforin–granzyme pathway (178, 179) or through Fas ligand-mediated apoptosis (180). However, CD8+ CTLs can also suppress HIV-1 replication through production of soluble factors that are not related to classic lytic events. An unidentified cell-associated factor (CAF) that inhibits HIV-1 replication at the level of transcription has been described (181, 182). IL-16 has also been shown to inhibit HIV-1 replication (183). Another mechanism involves production of β-chemokines that block entry of viruses dependent on CCR5 for entry (33). The importance of these nonclassic T-cell–mediated virus-suppressing responses for immunity has not yet been defined.

CD4+ T lymphocytes with CTL activity can also be detected in vitro. They recognize processed antigen through MHC class II presentation and are therefore able to respond to a greater number of inductive events than class I–restricted CTLs. CD4+ CTLs can be induced by proteins presented through the MHC class II endocytic pathway, and they have been shown to lyse uninfected CD4+ cells labeled by soluble gp120 (184). They are a vaccine-inducible component of the adaptive immune response (185), but their ability to clear virus-infected cells in vivo has not been as convincingly demonstrated as for CD8+ CTLs, and their potential contribution to immunopathology has not been defined. However, an association exists between maintenance of CD4+ T-cell lymphoproliferative response and delayed disease progression (127). Perhaps the HIV-specific CD4+ T cells provide factors that improve the activity and duration of CD8+ T-cell responses and thereby help in maintaining lower virus titers.

Induction of HIV-specific CD4+ T cells is integral to the initiation and propagation of immune responses because of their ability to provide "help" for other immunologic effector mechanisms. Helper T-cell epitopes are frequent in most viral HIV-1 proteins (186), and they are incorporated as part of all vaccine strategies. As for class I–restricted epitopes, vaccine products will need to be complex and to contain multiple epitopes to encompass the diversity of MHC alleles in the human population. Another consideration besides epitope specificity is the cytokine profile secreted by the vaccine-induced CD4+ T lymphocytes. Progression to AIDS has been linked to a switch from a CD4+ Th1-cell to a Th2-cell preponderance, accompanied by decreased production of IL-2 and interferon-γ (IFN-γ) and an increase in IL-4 and IL-10 levels (187). The cytokines produced by CD4+ T-cell subsets tend to be cross-inhibitory and autostimulatory (188). Vaccine formulations can have a major impact on the composition of subsequent immune responses by expanding one subset out of proportion to another (189). For most other models of virus infection, induction of the type 1 cytokine profile (IL-2, IFN-γ, and tumor necrosis factor-β [TNF-β]) is associated with protection and efficient virus clearance, whereas type 2 cytokines (IL-4, IL-5, IL-10, and IL-13) are associated with poor protection and disease enhancement. This is particularly true for RSV, in which a vaccine-enhanced illness evoked by a formalin-inactivated whole virus vaccine was probably related to induction of type 2 CD4+ lymphocytes that resulted in an immunopathologic response to subsequent RSV infection (7, 190–196).

The need for CD4+ lymphocytes to initiate the adaptive immune response is particularly compelling because these cells are the major target for HIV-1 infection. This situation presents a dilemma for effective induction of protective immunity against HIV-1 without putting vaccine-induced HIV-specific CD4+ at risk of infection. HIV selectively infects and causes the greatest cytopathologic effects in memory or activated CD4+ T cells (197), and as disease progresses, one sees a paucity of naive CD4+ T cells to initiate new immune responses (198). This emphasizes the need for effective immune responses, preexistent at the time of HIV exposure, so virus clearance can be accomplished before expansion of the viral quasispecies, destruction of memory T cells, and depletion of naive T cells.

Mucosal Immunity

Most HIV-1 infections occur across a mucosal barrier. Therefore, to prevent infection of the first cell will require induction of mucosal defenses. IgA can be detected in the mucosal secretions of HIV-1 infected persons, particularly in colostrum. Evidence indicates that IgA can neutralize HIV in vitro, and preliminary studies have suggested that IgA can block HIV transcytosis through the in vitro epithelial cell model (199). Other studies have suggested that IgA could facilitate entry into mucosal macrophages (200). The ability of secretory IgA to neutralize HIV in vivo has not been demonstrated.

Dissemination of SIV to regional nodes occurs within 48 hours after exposure to virus (62, 63). Effective viral clearance requires expansion of resident T-cell memory responses and virus clearance within this time frame. As disease progresses, one sees a disproportionate depletion of mucosal CD4+ T cells relative to the systemic compartment, thus indicating a large viral burden in the gastrointestinal mucosa throughout infection. This finding suggests that immune responses directed to mucosal sites soon after infection may be important for altering the dynamics of virus clearance and replication to avoid persistent infection. As in systemic immune responses, the local CD8+ T lymphocyte is an important mechanism for clearing virus-infected cells. This aspect of mucosal immunity in humans is receiving increased attention (201), but more studies are needed to establish the role of mucosal CTL activity in early HIV infection. Figure 42.2 depicts when and where vaccine-induced adaptive immune responses would have to work to prevent persistent infection.

Potential Disease-Inducing Antigens

Residing in the envelope protein are antigenic sites with the theoretic potential to induce harmful immune responses. No evidence of adverse effects from immunization with *env* products has been reported; however, it is prudent to track potential consequences after HIV-1 immunization. Because most vaccine products are engineered using recombinant DNA technology, options exist to omit such sites in formulating vaccines.

An in vitro antibody-dependent enhancement (ADE) phenomenon was originally observed with dengue virus and was epidemiologically associated with hemorrhagic fever and shock after a second infection with a dengue virus of different serotype (202, 203). ADE has notably been found in infections in which the macrophage is the primary target cell. The dengue ADE mechanism is thought to involve the presence of binding, nonneutralizing antibodies wherein neutralization and ADE activities are induced by distinct epitopes. ADE can be demonstrated in vitro with serum from

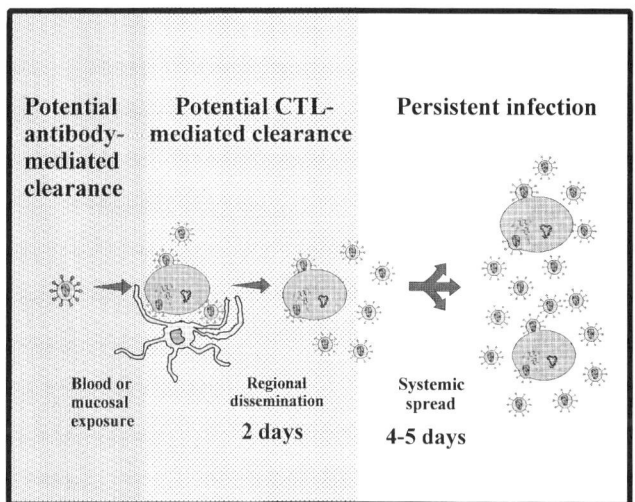

Figure 42.2. *Timing is everything.* Vaccine-induced immunity is a function of preformed antibody reducing inoculum size and expanded populations of memory cells responding to pathogens more rapidly than in primary infection. Early clearance of the pathogen may avoid the consequences of immunopathology resulting from the development of a large antigen load, and it may prevent the establishment of persistent infection. This illustration depicts cell-free virus before infection of the host in the *first shaded portion*. During this time, neutralizing antibody is the only component of the vaccine-inducible adaptive immune response capable of preventing virus infection. In the second phase, HIV-1 is depicted infecting dendritic cells, CD4+ lymphocytes, and macrophages and spreading to regional lymph nodes. Cytolytic T cells are the key component of the vaccine inducible immune response needed to clear virus-infected cells during this time. In the *third panel*, virus infection is shown to be widespread by 4 to 5 days, establishing persistent infection. The immune response probably will not be able to eradicate virus fully at this stage.

HIV-1 infected patients, but no correlation exists with course of infection or illness (204), and the in vitro effect is several orders of magnitude less than that seen with dengue virus infection. In vitro, ADE of HIV-1 has been shown to be mediated by two independent cell-receptor systems, either Fc (205–207) or C' (208). C'-ADE epitopes have been shown to bind to two conserved domains of gp41 (204, 209, 210). An Fc-ADE epitope of HIV-1 was localized to a gp120 conformational site (207).

Molecular mimicry between components of RNA or DNA viruses and host determinants is not uncommon, and antiself antibodies can be demonstrated after infection (211). By and large, these responses seem to be benign and quickly regulated; however, mimicry can cause disease. Autoimmune demyelination associated with Theiler's murine encephalomyelitis virus, mediated by specific cytotoxic T cells, is an example (212). Homology has been identified between several HIV-1 sequences and normal cell constituents. These include thymosin α (p17) (213), neuroleukin (gp120) (214), peptide T or vasoactive polypeptide (CD4 binding site) (215), IL-2 (*env*) (216), and MHC class II HLA β1 domain (gp41) (217, 218). Antibody to the class II domain has been found in 36% of HIV-1–infected patients (217). Anti-idiotypic antibody to CD4 can be detected transiently in some of subjects immunized with *env*-based vaccines (219). The significance of these observations in initiation of autoimmune disease is unknown.

APPROACHES TO VACCINE FORMULATION

Vaccine formulation involves not only the target antigen, but also adjuvants and immunomodulators, delivery vehicle, and route of administration. The antigen determines the specificity of the immune response, but factors such as the composition, kinetics, magnitude, and compartmentalization of immune responses are determined more by other aspects of the vaccine formulation, and they will be critical to vaccine success or failure.

Successful vaccines traditionally have been based on either inactivated whole virus or live attenuated virus preparations (Table 42.3). Considerations of safety have thus far discouraged clinical evaluation of live attenuated or inactivated whole virus HIV-1 preventive vaccines. This section describes approaches to candidate vaccine formulations currently studied or in development. Immunogenicity in nonhuman primates and in clinical trials is described in subsequent sections.

Recombinant Protein Subunits

Initial approaches to produce vaccine antigens have focused on recombinant protein subunit products. This emphasis has been based primarily on safety, but factors including practicality of production, storage, and adaptability have also been considerations. Most products have been based on envelope glycoproteins, either gp120 or gp160, because of their importance for virus attachment and entry. Because subunit proteins are largely limited to presentation through the MHC class II endocytic pathway, their major effect on the adaptive immune response is induction of CD4+ T cells and antibody response. Recombinant subunit gp160 or gp120 has been produced in insect, yeast, and mammalian cells. Mammalian cells allow authentic glycosylation and perhaps more native structure, and they were demonstrated to have immunologic advantages over denatured yeast-derived envelope products (154). Early products studied were prepared from the LAI strain, later replaced with MN or SF-2 strains, all representative of the Western Hemisphere–European B subtype. Newer products are based on non-B clade viruses, and many are derived from non–TCLA primary HIV-1 isolate genes.

The envelope glycoproteins contain the primary epitopes for neutralizing antibody responses, and they will therefore be an important component of any final vaccine strategy. The major challenge for production of the subunit envelope products is to reproduce authentic conformation. This involves considerations not only of amino acid sequence and protein folding, but posttranslational events such as glycosylation patterns, endoproteolytic cleavage, and oligomerization.

Not knowing the correlate of immunity, a perceived need exists for vaccine to induce antibody with "functional"

Table 42.3. Spectrum of Viral Vaccine Development by Category

Live Attenuated	Whole Inactivated	Subunit Protein	Live Vector	Peptides	Virus-like Particle	Nucleic Acid
Licensed Vaccines						
Smallpox	Rabies	Hepatitis B				
Yellow fever	Poliovirus					
Poliovirus	Influenza					
Measles	Hepatitis B					
Mumps	Hepatitis A					
Rubella	Japanese encephalitis					
Adenovirus						
Varicella						
Rotavirus						
Experimental Vaccines in Clinical Trials						
RSV		HIV	HIV	HIV	HIV	HIV
Influenza		Influenza	Rabies			Influenza
		RSV				HSV
		HSV				

HIV, human immunodeficiency virus; HSV, herpes simplex virus; RSV, respiratory syncytial virus.

activity. Although antibody specificity measured in binding assays such as enzyme-linked immunosorbent assay (ELISA) and Western blot may be important, the properties of neutralization, fusion inhibition, inhibition of gp120 binding to CD4 or coreceptor, and ADCC are believed to have greater biologic relevance. In phase I clinical trials, subunit envelope formulations have induced antibody that can neutralize homologous, TCLA HIV-1, but not primary HIV-1 isolates grown in activated PBMCs. Most antibody "functional" activities are directed to conformational epitopes. In addition to the posttranslational events listed previously that affect envelope conformation, some events take place during the process of virus attachment and engagement of selected coreceptor molecules that produce unique conformational determinants in the envelope glycoprotein structure, and they vary depending on HIV tropism and phenotype. Therefore, a CD4-"triggered" or β-chemokine receptor (HIV-coreceptor)-"triggered" envelope glycoprotein may display epitopes that are normally hidden. Antibody responses to these epitopes may be important for neutralization of monocyte tropic, nonsyncytium-inducing, primary isolates. Currently, no subunit envelope products authentically reproduce the oligomeric, glycosylated, and "triggered" structure that gp160 assumes as it mediates HIV-1 entry into cells. This limitation may explain the results in phase I testing to date, which indicate that subunit vaccines induce antibody that is type specific, with limited neutralizing activity against primary HIV-1 isolates.

Not only is the specificity of antibody important, but also the magnitude, duration, and isotype distribution may affect neutralization efficiency. The recombinant subunit vaccines have been formulated with various adjuvants, as listed in Table 42.4, to explore their effects on these parameters.

HIV-1–specific MHC class I-restricted CD8+ CTLs are considered to be a highly desirable effector cell response. Although vehicles have been designed to facilitate antigen delivery to the cytoplasmic compartment to promote MHC class I presentation, initial studies of subunit vaccines in primates and humans suggest that this approach will be much less efficient than recombinant vectors, nucleic acid vaccines, or live attenuated virus for induction of CD8+ CTLs.

The antibody response to immunization with subunit products is in general maximal after the third or fourth injection, it is dose dependent, and it can be attenuated unless a several-month interval exists between injections. Serum antibody titers have a short half-life, and although they can be boosted, the titers generally achieve their peak level after the third or fourth injections. Repeated boosting does not prolong the half-life significantly. Subunit products may find their greatest utility in boosting antibody responses in subjects primed with recombinant vector vaccines (220) or in other strategies that can induce MHC class I–restricted CTL responses.

Synthetic Peptides

Modern biochemical techniques have provided multiple approaches for the formulation of candidate synthetic peptide vaccines. Peptides are attractive because 1) they are safe, 2) large quantities can be prepared inexpensively, 3) they are made synthetically and are therefore free of contaminating host materials, 4) immune responses to precise specificities can be induced, 5) multiple epitopes with desirable immunogenic properties can easily be combined in a single formulation, and 6) theoretically they can be presented through either the MHC class I or II pathways. The major limitations of the peptide vaccine approach are that 1) the breadth of antigenic sites within a given formulation may be too narrow, 2) conformational epitopes are difficult to represent, and 3) historically peptides have not been as immunogenic as more complex antigens.

Several approaches have been taken to produce peptide immunogens as candidate AIDS vaccines. First, peptides based on the V3 loop sequence from one or multiple HIV-1 strains have been covalently linked on an oligolysine back-

Table 42.4. Candidate AIDS Vaccines Evaluated in Clinical Trials

Vaccine Antigen (HIV Strain)	Production Method	Adjuvant or Vehicle	Vaccine Developer	Site of Study or AVEG Protocol Numbers[a]	Reference for Clinical Trial
Envelope Proteins					
Phase I Studies					
rgp160 (LAI)	Baculovirus/insect cells	Aluminum phosphate	MicroGeneSys	National Institutes of Health, Bethesda, MD	373
rgp160 (LAI)	Baculovirus/insect cells	Aluminum phosphate	MicroGeneSys	003, 003A, 003B	356, 374
rgp160 (IIIB)	Vaccinia/vero cells	AL(OH)$_3$ + deoxycholate	IMMUNO-AG	004, 004A, 004B	358, 359
Env 2-3 (SF-2)	Yeast	MF59 ± MTP-PE	Chiron/Biocine	005A, 005B, 005C; Geneva, Switzerland	357, 375
rgp120 (IIIB)	CHO cells	AL(OH)$_3$	Genentech	006	376
rgp120 (MN)					
rgp120 (SF-2)	CHO cells	MF59	Chiron/Biocine	007A, 007B, 007C	377
rgp120 (SF-2)	CHO cells	MF59 ± MTP-PE	Chiron/Biocine		354
rgp120 (MN)	CHO cells	AL(OH)$_3$	Genentech	009	355
rgp120 (IIIB)					
rgp160 (MN)	Vaccinia/vero cells	AL(OH)$_3$ + deoxycholate	IMMUNO-AG	013A	378
rgp160 (MN)	Vaccinia/vero cells	AL(OH)$_3$ + deoxycholate	IMMUNO-AG	013B	Manuscript in preparation[c]
rgp120 (MN)	CHO cells	AL(OH)$_3$	Genentech		
rgp160 (MN/LAI)	Vaccinia/BHK-21 cells	AL(OH)$_3$	Pasteur-Merieux Connaught	Paris, France	379
V3 loop of gp120 (MN)	Synthetic linear peptide	Mineral oil + mannose monooleate (IFA)			
rgp120 (SF-2)	CHO cells	Multiple adjuvants[b]	Chiron/Biocine	015	Manuscript in preparation
rgp120 (MN)	CHO cells	QS-21 and/or AL(OH)$_3$	Genentech	016, 016A, 016B	Manuscript in preparation
rgp120 (SF-2)	CHO cells	MF59	Chiron/Biocine	024	see AVEG 022a
V3 loop of gp120 (15 strains)	Synthetic octameric peptide	AL(OH)$_3$	United Biomedical	017	Manuscript in preparation
V3 loop of gp120 (MN)	Synthetic octameric peptide ± encapsulation	AL(OH)$_3$	United Biomedical	018	Manuscript in preparation
Peptides/Polypeptides					
Ty p17/p24 VLP (LAI)	Yeast transposon	None	British Biotech PLC	England	357
Ty p17/p24 VLP (LAI)	Yeast transposon	None or AL(OH)$_3$	British Biotech PLC	019	Manuscript in preparation
Gag lipopeptide P3C541b	Synthetic linear peptide	Lipid conjugate	United Biomedical	021	Manuscript in preparation
HGP-30 (LAI p17)	Synthetic linear peptide	KLH	Viral Technologies	George Washington University Medical Center, Washington, DC	380–382
V3 loop of gp120 (MN)	Synthetic octameric peptide	AL(OH)$_3$	United Biomedical	011; Yunnan, China; St. Vincent's Hospital, Sydney, Australia; Bangkok, Thailand	383–386
V3 loop of gp120 (MN)	Synthetic linear peptide	PPD	A. Rubinstein	Switzerland	387
V3 loop of gp120 (MN)	Synthetic octameric peptide ± encapsulation	AL(OH)$_3$	United Biomedical	023	Manuscript in preparation
HIV-1 gp120 C4-V3 peptides (MN, EV91, RF, CANO)	Hybrid polyvalent synthetic peptides	Mineral oil + mannose monooleate (IFA)	Wyeth-Lederle Vaccines with Barton Haynes, Duke University	020	In progress
DNA Vaccines					
HIV-1 env/rev	GeneVax DNA plasmid backbone	Bupivacaine ("facilitator")	Apollon	National Institutes of Health, Bethesda, MD	In progress
APL 400-047 HIV-1 core structural proteins (HXB2-gag/pol)	GeneVax DNA plasmid backbone	Bupivacaine ("facilitator")	Apollon	031	In progress

continued

Table 42.4. *(continued)* **Candidate AIDS Vaccines Evaluated in Clinical Trials**

Vaccine Antigen (HIV Strain)	Production Method	Adjuvant or Vehicle	Vaccine Developer	Site of Study or AVEG Protocol Numbers[a]	Reference for Clinical Trial
Poxvirus Recombinants/Combinations					
Vaccinia-gp160 [HIVAC-1e] (LAI)	Recombinant vaccinia		Bristol-Myers Squibb/Onco-gen	Zaire	363
Vaccinia-gp160 [HIVAC-1e] (LAI) rgp160 (LAI)	Recombinant vaccinia Baculovirus/insect cells		Bristol-Myers Squibb/Onco-gen MicroGeneSys	Univ. of Washington-Seattle	364, 365
Vaccinia-gp160 [HIVAC-1e] (LAI) rgp160 (LAI)	Recombinant vaccinia Baculovirus/insect cells	AL(OH)$_3$	Bristol-Myers Squibb/Oncogen MicroGeneSys	002, 002A, 002B	220, 366, 367
Vaccinia-gp160 [HIVAC-1e] (LAI) rgp120 (SF-2) or Env 2-3 (SF-2)	Recombinant vaccinia CHO cells or yeast	MF59	Bristol-Myers Squibb/Oncogen Chiron/Biocine	008	Manuscript in preparation
Vaccinia-gp160 [HIVAC-1e] (LAI) rgp120 (SF-2) or rgp120 (LAI) or rgp160 (MN) or rgp160 (MN)	Recombinant vaccinia CHO cells Vaccinia/vero cells	MF59 AL(OH)$_3$ AL(OH)$_3$ + Deoxycholate	Bristol-Myers Squibb/Oncogen Chiron/Biocine Genentech IMMUNO-AG	010	360
Canarypox-gp160 (MN) (vCP125) rgp160 (MN/LAI)	Recombinant canarypox		Pasteur-Merieux Connaught	Hôpital de l'Institut Pasteur, Paris, France	388, 389
Canarypox-gp160 (MN) (vCP125) rgp120 (SF-2)	Recombinant canarypox CHO cells	MF59	Pasteur-Merieux Connaught Chiron/Biocine	012A, 012B	371
Vaccinia-HIV Env/gag/pol (TBC-3B)	Recombinant vaccinia		Therion Biologics	014A	In progress
Vaccinia-HIV Env/gag/pol (TBC-3B) rgp120 (MN)	Recombinant vaccinia CHO cells	AL(OH)$_3$	Therion Biologics VaxGen	014C	In progress
Canarypox-HIV gp120, TM gp41, gag, protease (MN/LAI) (vCP205) rgp120 (SF-2)	Recombinant canarypox CHO cells	MF-59	Pasteur-Merieux Connaught Chiron/Biocine	022, 022A	Manuscript in preparation
Canarypox-HIV gp120, TM gp41, gag, protease, CTL epitopes in pol and nef (MN/LAI) (vCP300)	Recombinant canarypox		Pasteur-Merieux Connaught	026	Manuscript in preparation
rgp120 (SF-2)	CHO cells	MF59	Chiron/Biocine		

continued

Table 42.4. (continued) Candidate AIDS Vaccines Evaluated in Clinical Trials

Vaccine Antigen (HIV Strain)	Production Method	Adjuvant or Vehicle	Vaccine Developer	Site of Study or AVEG Protocol Numbers[a]	Reference for Clinical Trial
Canarypox-HIV gp120, TM gp41, gag, protease (MN/LAI) (vCP205)[d]	Recombinant canarypox		Pasteur-Merieux Connaught	027	In progress
Canarypox-HIV gp120, TM gp41, gag, protease (MN/LAI) (vCP205)	Recombinant canarypox		Pasteur-Merieux Connaught	029	Manuscript in preparation
rgp120 (SF-2)	CHO cells	MF59	Chiron/Biocine		
Canarypox-HIV gp120, TM gp41, gag, protease (MN/LAI) (vCP205)	Recombinant canarypox	GM-CSF	Pasteur-Merieux Connaught Immunex	033	In progress
Salmonella Typhi Recombinant/Combination					
Salmonella typhi CVD908-HIV-1 LAI rgp120 (VVG 203)	Live attenuated recombinant *Salmonella typhi*		University of Maryland Center for Vaccine Development	028	In progress
rgp120 (MN)	CHO cells	AL(OH)$_3$	VaxGen		
Phase II Studies					
Envelope Proteins					
rgp120 (SF-2)	CHO cells	MF59	Chiron/Biocine	201	Manuscript in preparation
rgp120 (MN)	CHO cells	AL(OH)$_3$	Genentech	201	Manuscript in preparation
Poxvirus Recombinants/Combinations					
Canarypox-HIV gp120, TM gp41, gag, protease (MN/LAI) (vCP205)	Recombinant canarypox		Pasteur-Merieux Connaught	202	In progress
rgp120 (SF-2)	CHO cells	MF59	Chiron/Biocine		

[a]Multiple protocol numbers indicate that significantly different doses, schedules, or administration routes were evaluated. More details about AIDS Vaccine Evaluation Group (AVEG) trial design can be found on the internet at http://www.emmes.com/AVCTN
[b]rgp120(SF-2) administered with one of seven adjuvants (AL(OH)$_3$, Monophosphoryl lipid A [MPL, Ribi ImmunoChem Research], liposome-encapsulated MPL with Alum [Walter Reed Army Institute of Research], MF59 [Chiron Vaccines], MF59 + MTP-PE [Chiron Vaccines], SAF/2 [Chiron Vaccines], SAF/2 with MDP [Chiron Vaccines]) to 15–16 volunteers. The rgp120 (SF-2) + MPL group was not offered an 18-month immunization.
[c]Unpublished studies that have not been performed within the AVEG system may not be listed.
[d]Alternate routes of administration: intramuscular (IM), oral, intranasal, intrarectal, intravaginal, IM + intranasal, IM + intrarectal

bone and formulated with alum for intramuscular injection, or in poly (DL-lactide-coglycolide) microspheres for mucosal administration. The multiple antigen peptide system, on an oligo-lysine backbone (221), improves the immunogenicity of peptide epitopes in animal models and provides a mechanism for bringing helper T-cell and B-cell epitopes together on the same synthetic antigen (221, 222). A second approach has been to synthesize a hybrid linear peptide consisting of helper T-cell, B-cell, and CTL epitopes formulated in incomplete Freund's adjuvant (223, 224). One candidate vaccine based on this strategy has reached the stage of phase I clinical trials, and it combines the V3 loop sequence containing a neutralizing antibody epitope and CTL epitope with a helper T-cell epitope from the C4 domain (223). A third approach involved conjugating a lipid moiety to a peptide from *gag*. In small animal models, the lipid tail augmented the CTL responses induced by the *gag* peptide. Finally, a p17-derived peptide, HGP30, has been of interest because of partial sequence homology with α_1-thymosin. The latter induced antibody reported to neutralize HIV-1$_{BH10}$ in H9 cells (213). Studies using monoclonal antibody subsequently detected a binding site at the p17 amino terminus (225). The mechanism by which antibody specific for an internal protein can neutralize HIV has not been elucidated.

Virus-like Particle Vaccines

One mechanism by which adjuvants augment the immunogenicity of an antigen is through aggregation. Larger particle size facilitates capture by APCs and processing through the endocytic pathway. Another potential advantage is that virus-like particles (VLPs) may allow oligomerization of the surface envelope glycoproteins and may thereby produce conformational structures not available on monomeric subunit immunogens. The first approach takes advantage of HIV-1 assembly events that occur in cells producing *gag*. Cells infected in vitro with recombinant vaccinia expressing *gag* and *envelope* were found to produce noninfectious, genomeless retrovirus-like particles (226, 227). Studies defining the mechanisms of HIV-1 assembly have now shown that *gag* alone is sufficient to yield VLPs (228). Such pseudovirion particles have been produced for evaluation in animal studies (229), but production difficulties have thus far prevented the evaluation of this strategy in clinical trials. Another approach to VLP production has been to take advantage of a self-assembling yeast protein, Ty (230). The recombinant Ty self-assembles into a particle with a diameter of approximately 80 to 100 nm, and when fused with HIV-1 p24 (231) or gp120 V3 (232), it forms a VLP of about 200 nm in diameter. The Ty p24 VLP has been formulated with alum and has been tested in clinical trials both by intramuscular injection and mucosal administration.

Live Recombinant Vectors

Live recombinant viruses as expression vectors for HIV-1 gene products hold several attractions: 1) immunogens are presented in the context of natural infection; that is, oligomeric glycoprotein is expressed on infected cell membranes, with native conformation and glycosylation patterns; 2) antigens are processed by and presented in the context of MHC class I molecules leading to CTL responses; 3) multiple antigens, diverse strain specificities, or immune modifiers may be simultaneously expressed; 4) administration by percutaneous or mucosal routes is simple; and 5) production and delivery are inexpensive. Live bacterial vectors have similar advantages, although posttranslational processing of viral protein differs from that of mammalian processes, and induction of MHC class I–restricted CTLs may be less efficient. An advantage of the bacterial vectors is that the constituents of the vector may provide additional adjuvant properties. Each approach offers unique advantages and disadvantages often related to the tropism and virulence of the parent vector. The diversity of vectors being developed is illustrated by several examples.

Poxvirus vectors have received the most attention thus far. Two parent viruses have been used: vaccinia, the virus used as a vaccine to eradicate smallpox; and canarypox, an avipoxvirus that can enter mammalian cells to express its gene products, but is replication competent only in avian cells. In addition to the general advantages for live virus vectors, they have the following benefits: 1) the genome accommodates the insertion of large sequences of foreign DNA; 2) they are stable and easy to handle; 3) they are able to enter many different cell types; and 4) a precedent exists for using this approach in a successful, large-scale vaccination campaign. Recombinant vaccinia has been produced with the gene encoding HIV-1 envelope interrupting the vaccinia thymidine kinase. This provides a selection mechanism for recombinants, and it also attenuates vaccinia virulence (233–235). The major disadvantage of vaccinia is that after intradermal administration it has a low frequency of side effects caused by spread beyond the site of inoculation or to other individuals (236, 237). To avert this problem, new vaccinia vaccine vectors have been developed with multiple virulence determinants deleted (238–240). However, the balance is delicate because, when replication is attenuated, less recombinant antigen is produced, and immunogenicity may be reduced. Avipoxviruses are fully replication competent in avian cells, but they attain only a single-cycle, nonproductive infection in mammalian cells. Both fowlpox and canarypox parent strains have been used for producing recombinant vaccine vectors. Canarypox vectors have been produced, expressing HIV-1 envelope gene alone or multiple HIV-1 gene products. These vectors have also been constructed to express SIV and HIV-2 gene products for evaluation in animal studies. The major advantage of the avipox approach over vaccinia is the absence of a local pustule or risk of spread from the site of inoculation. However, as with the attenuated vaccinia vectors, one may sacrifice immunogenicity for reduced replication capacity in the vector.

Adenovirus vectors have several desirable features, including feasibility of oral delivery with gut replication, induction of systemic and mucosal immunity after a single oral dose, and a record of safe use for prevention of respiratory disease in the United States military. Adenovirus vectors may be more immunogenic when administered nasally than when given orally, but some reluctance to pursue this route exists because of safety concerns (241).

Other viral vectors that have been investigated include poliovirus (242, 243), influenza virus (244), rhinovirus (245), and hepatitis B virus (246, 247) chimeras. These vectors are of interest because of their ability to induce mucosal immune responses. Their major limitations are the amount of foreign genome that can be accommodated and the virulence properties of the parent vector. A novel approach using the genetic framework of the Venezuelan equine encephalitis (VEE) virus has been described that has unique properties (248). This vector given by a parenteral route not only stimulates systemic immune responses, but also induces mucosal IgA specific for the recombinant antigen (249). This finding suggests that certain mechanisms may be exploited to target inductive sites for mucosal immunity with a parenteral antigen using this or other novel vectors.

Other gene delivery vectors being developed for gene therapy and adapted for use as vaccines are replication incompetent and more closely resemble nucleic acid vaccines than live vaccine vectors. However, adenoassociated virus (AAV) and retrovirus vectors are mentioned in this category because their packaging system is antigenic and may limit the ability to use the vector repeatedly (250, 251).

Attenuated strains of *Salmonella* have been developed as an effective vaccine against typhoid fever (252). Attenuated *Salmonella* parent strains have also been developed as vaccine vehicles to deliver recombinant antigens (253, 254). The advantage of this approach is that it uses the innate strategies that *Salmonella* has developed to reach the inductive sites of the mucosal immune system. The disadvantages of bacterial vectors relative to the viral vector approaches are that the antigens will not be authentically glycosylated and conformational structures may be altered. The other considerations are those of vector virulence and possible transfer to contacts, particularly infants; as with vaccinia, these concerns must be balanced against loss of immunogenicity.

Interest in bacille Calmette-Guérin (BCG) as a live vector stems from its strong adjuvant effect, along with long-lasting infection and antigenic stimulation. BCG is used to immunize infants at birth and has a global record of acceptability (255). Constructs have been developed expressing HIV-1 *gag*, *pol*, and *env* gene products that can induce antibody, helper T-cell, and CTL responses in mice (256, 257), and immunogenicity may be further improved by the coexpression of selected recombinant cytokine genes (258). The molecular biology and immunobiology of this organism are complex, and expression of glycoproteins is often difficult to achieve, making production and adaptability to new genotypic requirements of concern. The potential virulence of this organism is also an issue, as with many of the other live vector approaches.

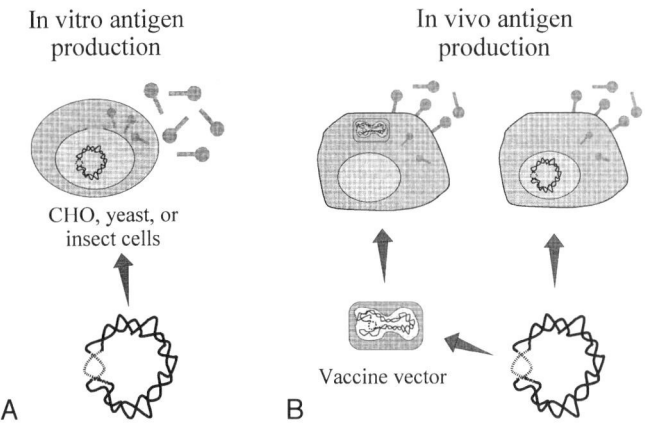

Figure 42.3. Evolution of vaccine antigen production. **A.** Initial approaches relied on vaccine antigen production in vitro for administration of purified recombinant proteins. Current approaches use vectors that allow vaccine antigen production in vivo. **B.** In vivo antigen production leads to the induction of MHC class I–restricted, CD8+ CTL responses and more authentic simulation of antigen presentation events induced by live virus infection. Probably, a combination of vaccine formulations using antigens produced in vivo and in vitro will be needed to achieve optimal immunogenicity.

Other bacterial vectors that have been evaluated as potential vaccine vehicles include *Brucella abortus* (259) and *Listeria monocytogenes* (260). Their development has advanced only to the level of testing in small animal models.

Nucleic Acid Vaccination

Immunization with nucleic acid vectors is a natural progression in the evolution of vaccine concepts based on recombinant DNA technology. Figure 42.3 illustrates the process of recombinant subunit protein production in vitro evolving to in vivo antigen production through an intermediate vaccine vector, to direct inoculation of DNA for expression of genes encoding vaccine antigens. Many of the hurdles in the development of gene therapy turn out to be ideal properties for nucleic acid vectors to deliver vaccine antigens. These include 1) relatively transient expression, 2) lack of integration into host cell genome, and 3) induction of immune responses to the recombinant gene products. Although this immunization technology is still evolving, it promises to be a powerful new weapon. The major considerations in the formulation of nucleic acid vaccines are 1) optimization of the magnitude and duration of gene expression, 2) delivery vehicle and route, 3) methods to combine with adjuvants to promote the desired immune responses, 4) avoidance of sequences that stimulate an immune response to the vector, 5) avoidance of sequences that could lead to integration, and 6) avoidance of genes (such as antibiotic resistance used for in vitro selection) that may alter cell function or provide virulence factors for coexisting pathogens. The ability to produce new specificities quickly and to combine multiple genes in a single vaccine formulation adds to the attractive features of nucleic acid immunization. Other desirable features include

1) induction of antibody and MHC class I–restricted CTL responses, 2) prolonged antigen presentation and durable immune responses, 3) lack of the unnecessary antigens and virulence associated with live recombinant vaccine vectors, and 4) ease of storage and administration. The initial concern about eliciting anti-DNA antibodies has dissipated with new understanding of DNA antigenicity. Palindromic hexamers common in bacterial DNA contain a core CG with two 5′ purine nucleotides and two 3′ pyrimidine nucleotides that have immunostimulatory properties (428). These immunostimulatory motifs induce elements of the innate immune response including IFN-α, IFN-β, and IL-12, and they promote Th1 T-helper differentiation and improved immunogenicity of the recombinant gene product. Antibodies to these bacterial motifs are commonly found in healthy individuals and are distinct from the anti-DNA antibody specificity and isotype profile found in patients with autoimmune diseases such as systemic lupus erythematosus. Learning more about the antigenic properties of DNA, and ways to optimize the formulation and delivery of nucleic acid vaccines, will be a major focus of vaccine development for the next decade.

Another approach to using nucleic acid as a vaccine antigen delivery mechanism is RNA vaccination. For example, by using the replication machinery of Semliki Forest virus, in vitro transcribed RNA has been produced that induced humoral and cellular immune responses in mice after intramuscular injection (261). Unlike plasmid DNA, the RNA vaccine is translated directly in the cytoplasm and does not require transport and processing in the nucleus. Therefore, no risk of integration exists. This approach may be of special importance for recombinant genes from viruses with a cytoplasmic replication program (e.g., RSV) that have not adapted to the nuclear environment. This approach could also be useful for expressing vaccine antigens that have regulatory effects on nuclear transcription factors or that may otherwise adversely affect cell function if production occurs in the nucleus.

Whole Inactivated HIV-1 Vaccines

Whole inactivated virus vaccine formulations have a successful track record against various viral pathogens (see Table 42.3). Techniques including treatment with 1) formaldehyde or glutaraldehyde, 2) β-proprionolactone, and 3) γ-irradiation can be applied to ensure inactivation of the agent used as the basis of the vaccine. The major advantages of this approach are the vast experience available on approaches to vaccine formulation from other systems, the relative ease of vaccine production, and the inclusion of all viral antigens in the product. The limitations of this approach are as follows: 1) the inactivation steps will result in an antigen that will be presented predominantly through the endocytic pathway in the context of MHC class II molecules and will not promote MHC class I–restricted CTLs; 2) in addition to the epitopes important for inducing immunity, undesirable antigens with regulatory properties or regions of molecular mimicry will be included; 3) immunization with whole inactivated measles and RSV vaccines were associated with vaccine-enhanced illness that was unexpected and is still not fully understood, thus indicating that this approach has the potential to induce inappropriate immune responses; 4) it will be difficult to distinguish vacinees from HIV-infected persons using standard antibody-based diagnostic tests; and 5) the fear of incomplete inactivation exists. The use of whole-inactivated SIV in primate models has been informative because of the demonstration that not only could virus-specific antigens mediate protection, but also that cellular proteins incorporated in the virus particles could induce protective immunity (262). This finding has stimulated the investigation of the way in which cellular proteins participate in viral assembly (263), which ones are targets for the protective immune response (264), and whether allogeneic immunization may be a legitimate approach for inducing protective immunity. Studies supporting the validity of this approach include protection of macaques with MHC class II immunization (265), MHC class I immunization (266), or CD4 immunization (267). The discovery of selective HIV-1 coreceptor usage has suggested various new allogeneic antigen candidates to test as vaccine concepts.

Live Attenuated HIV-1 Vaccines

Perhaps the most difficult and important decision to be made in the near future with regard to AIDS vaccine development is the degree of emphasis to put on the development of live attenuated HIV-1 vaccines for clinical trials. Using live attenuated viruses as vaccines has been the most successful and inexpensive approach for preventing viral infections. Thus far, it has been considered an untenable approach for immunizing against HIV in the general population. The reasons for this include the following: 1) a live attenuated lentivirus could integrate into the host genome and potentially could lead to interruption of important host genes; 2) persistent infection with the vaccine virus is needed in animal models to maintain a state of optimal immunity; 3) if persistent infection occurs, the virus will have the opportunity to evolve through genetic variation to become more virulent; 4) persistent infection may lead to disease over a long period, thus limiting the enthusiasm for widespread use until long-term (40 to 50 years) safety experiments have been completed; 5) in some studies, SIV strains attenuated for adult macaques have been lethal for infant macaques (268); 6) if transmission of vaccine virus can occur from mother to infant or between adult partners, the consequences of serial passage in human hosts on HIV virulence must be considered before vaccinating large portions of the population; 7) currently, we have no curative antiviral regimen effective against candidate vaccine viruses that could be used if the vaccine caused illness; and 8) in primate studies, deletion mutants of SIV with attenuated virulence have been repaired in vivo through recombination or gene duplication events leading to restored virulence (269–271).

Nevertheless, in primate studies, the live attenuated virus vaccine approach has shown the most potency in terms of protection against a virulent challenge virus (272). Certain virus constructs have been made and suggested as strategies that deserve further evaluation. Deleting the *nef* gene and a portion of the 3′ long terminal repeat (LTR) leads to attenuated replication in both SIV and HIV (273). Other groups have added genes to provide mechanisms for limiting replication, stimulating early immune responses, and providing a target for antiviral chemotherapy. When IFN-γ is expressed from the SIV genome, it leads to limited replication in macaques, but within a few weeks the gene is excluded from the virus in vivo (274). Adding the herpes simplex thymidine kinase gene to HIV-1 makes it susceptible to ganciclovir in vitro (275) and has been proposed as a strategy to make the live attenuated vaccines "fail safe." Other deletions in HIV-1 accessory genes, such as *vif*, that can add to the attenuation of the vaccine virus may make this approach safer (96).

Based on epidemiologic data from West Africa suggesting that infection with HIV-2 provides some protection against HIV-1 infection (276), other live attenuated virus vaccine approaches are possible. One approach would be to base the live attenuated vaccine strain on the less virulent HIV-2 virus and to add further attenuating mutations, immunomodulatory genes, and genes providing antiviral susceptibility. Another approach could be to use chimeric virus constructs as the basis for the attenuated virus vaccine. SHIV viruses are chimeras produced by replacing the SIV envelope genes with the envelope genes from HIV-1 (277). This procedure allows a virus expressing HIV-1 gp120 to replicate in macaques and to be used as a challenge stock for evaluation of HIV-1 candidate vaccines. Replacement of genes leads to altered rates of replication and virulence that can be restored by serial passage in animals. The chimeric virus approach may allow the expression of envelope glycoproteins of more than one specificity in the same virion to broaden immunity.

Continued development of the live attenuated virus vaccine approach is critical to the process of AIDS vaccine development, because it may be the benchmark for protection in animal models. Whether this approach is safe for use in clinical trials is still debated, but in the meantime, important studies using live attenuated virus vaccines are being performed in primate models to determine the correlates of vaccine-induced immunity. These studies will provide direction for future development of vaccine vectors, nucleic acid vaccines, and recombinant subunit products.

Strategies for Vaccine Adjuvants and Delivery Systems

The adjuvant component of a vaccine can determine the composition, magnitude, and duration of the immune response to the antigenic component of the vaccine formulation. The delivery vehicle for the vaccine antigen will influence which type of APC is responsible for initiating the immune response and which immunologic compartment is activated. The influence of adjuvants is crucial to the immunogenicity of synthetic peptide and recombinant subunit antigens, which alone are poor immunogens. This discussion therefore focuses on adjuvants being evaluated for peptide and recombinant proteins, then briefly mentions a few new approaches to packaging vaccine antigens in new delivery systems. Alum, the term for various aluminum salts, has been the only acceptable adjuvant for more than 40 years and is the adjuvant used for currently licensed vaccines. The primary advantages of alum are its proven track record and safety. The major limitations of alum for use in HIV vaccine development are as follows: 1) the process of alum precipitation is deleterious to the native structure of proteins; 2) the product is only presented through the endocytic antigen-processing pathway in the context of MHC class II molecules; and 3) alum promotes Th2 CD4+ T-cell differentiation and IL-4 production, which may not be as favorable for clearance of intracellular pathogens as Th1 T cells and IFN-γ. These features of alum have led to a major effort to evaluate adjuvants that differ in these fundamental properties. Therefore, the focus has been on oil-based emulsions and products that promote Th1 CD4+ T-cell differentiation or CD8+ T-cell activation. Products that have received the most attention include MF59 ± MTP-PE (Chrion-Biocine, Emeryville, CA), QS21 (Cambridge Biotech, Cambridge, MA), Detox (RIBI ImmunoChem Research, Hamilton, MT), MPL containing liposomes (278), SAF ± MDP (279), and incomplete Freund's adjuvant (280). These products use the following components in various forms: muramyl dipeptides or tripeptides, monophosphoryl lipid A, deoxycholate, saponin, squalene, liposomes, and emulsifier (281, 282) (see Table 42.4).

The discovery and characterization of cytokines, chemokines, cellular adhesion, and costimulatory molecules and their ligands have opened opportunities for the development of vaccines with more targeted aims for immune activation (189). Investigators envision that future vaccine formulations will use a combination of cytokines and costimulatory molecules rather than generic immune modulators. These molecules can be delivered by coadministration or by coexpression in vectors and nucleic acid constructs. Granulocyte–macrophage colony-stimulating factor, in particular, has shown promise as an adjuvant for vaccines against cancer and infectious pathogens in animal models (283). It is thought to work through stimulation of DC activation and enhanced antigen presentation. It tends to induce a cytokine expression pattern of a Th2-like response. In contrast, IL-12 has been shown to have potent adjuvant affects for CD4+ cells that produce IFN-γ. The properties of these and other potential recombinant adjuvants such as IL-2, CD80 and CD86, CD40 ligand, and FLT-3 ligand are still being defined in preclinical studies. Each pathogen probably will require a different combination of molecules for optimal immunity, but the rewards will be a more focused and efficient vaccine-induced immune response with less chance for immunopathologic effects.

The technology of vaccine antigen delivery has also been advancing. Techniques for packaging vaccine antigens in particles, or expressing them from nucleic acid or live recombinant vectors, are described earlier. In addition, time-released delivery by microspheres that incorporate antigens in biodegradable polymers permits targeting to an immune compartment with a desired release interval (284, 285). Cochleates are phospholipid complexes (286) that can package peptides, proteins, or plasmids and can colocalize their delivery to APCs. This approach has shown promise for delivering vaccine antigens to the mucosal immune compartment (287). Other approaches for targeting the induction of mucosal immunity include 1) live vectors with tropism for mucosal sites, 2) coexpression of cytokines with IgA promoting properties (288), and 3) adjuvants or conjugate molecules that target cells involved in mucosal immune induction such as cholera toxin (289, 290).

CONTRIBUTION OF ANIMAL MODELS

Animal Models in Vaccine Development

Historically, animal models have played a key role in the development of vaccines. Defining patterns of virus tropism, replication, and spread, mechanisms of disease, and correlates of immunity in animal models has guided the development of most licensed vaccines. Animal models have also been used in vaccine evaluation including the assessment of vaccine efficacy and safety, such as poliovirus vaccine (291). However, animal models often fall short of duplicating human infection, clinical disease, and pathogenic mechanisms. Models may require exotic challenge routes and manipulation of virulence or tissue tropism, or they may exhibit incomplete disease expression (292–298). Therefore, data obtained from animal model vaccine evaluation must be interpreted with a complete understanding of how virus-induced disease pathogenesis in the model compares to that in humans. Several animal models of lentivirus infection have been developed and applied to HIV-1 vaccine development. After briefly describing the animal models in general, they are discussed with respect to the antigenic properties, virulence, dose, and route of the challenge virus. Although none of the current models reproduce the exact features of HIV-1 transmission and disease pathogenesis in humans, they can be used to rank order the potential efficacy of candidate vaccines, and they are invaluable for gaining insight into mechanisms of disease pathogenesis and defining approaches to achieve vaccine-induced immunity.

HIV-1 INFECTION IN CHIMPANZEES

HIV-1 replicates in the chimpanzee as a chronic persistent infection, with antigenemia and immune responses resembling human infection, but the infection does not progress to clinical immune deficiency in most cases. HIV-1 strains have recently been adapted to cause an AIDS-like disease in chimpanzees (299, 300). The major limitations of the chimpanzee as a model for HIV-1 is its restricted availability and high cost. Critical experiments are typically performed with one or two animals in each experimental group. The small group size does not allow evaluation of less efficient challenge routes (e.g., mucosal), and does not allow a statistical analysis of parameters such as virus load that have an inherent variability. Despite these constraints, the conserved genetics, particularly in CD4 and coreceptor sequences, and the susceptibility to HIV-1 challenge make the chimpanzee a model that may provide unique insights into vaccine behavior.

HIV-2 INFECTION IN BABOONS

Baboons have been used to predict the immunologic behavior of HIV-1 vaccines in humans (154, 301, 302). These animals can be infected with SIV in the wild (303) and are infectable with HIV-2 (304) or SIV (305) experimentally. Some HIV-2 strains lead to persistent infection, CD4 lymphocyte decline, and an AIDS-like disease within 2 years (306).

SIV INFECTION IN MACAQUES

Lentiviruses endemic in African primates (particularly African green and mangabey monkeys) comprise a group of viruses that cause an AIDS-like disease in Asian macaques (92). These viruses, collectively called SIV, are named according to the monkey and site from which they were originally isolated. *Macaca mulatta* (rhesus macaque) is the primary species used for studies of pathogenesis, but *M. fascicularis* (cynomolgus macaque), and *M. nemestrina* (pigtailed macaque) are also used. SIV can cause a disease in macaques that is clinically and pathologically similar to HIV infection in humans. The SIV/macaque model has therefore been of singular importance for our understanding of disease pathogenesis and for demonstrating potential mechanisms of vaccine-induced immunity against lentiviruses. A range of virulence can be seen that is determined by characteristics of the host and the SIV strain used for infection. For example, one SIVsm variant, designated PBj14, can cause a rapidly lethal disease with acute gastrointestinal symptoms (307), whereas SIVmac engineered to have a deletion in *nef* and a portion of the 3′ LTR has attenuated virulence (273). Another example of how host characteristics may affect pathogenesis is that SIV attenuated for adult macaques can be lethal in neonates (268). Typically, SIVmac$_{251}$ infection of *M. mulatta* results in CD4 decline and AIDS in 18 to 36 months (92). This course is more rapid than HIV-1 infection of humans and allows the assessment of rate of disease progression as an end point for vaccine studies if sufficiently large groups are evaluated (308, 309). Therefore, instead of complete virus clearance as a primary end point for a vaccine trial, studies using the SIV/macaque model can ask whether vaccine-induced immunity can alter the dynamics of SIV replication and disease progression in animals infected despite vaccination.

The organization of SIV envelope structural domains is similar to that of HIV-1, and the functional roles may have significant parallels. In particular, the homolog of CCR5 in macaques serves as a coreceptor for SIV entry (310). The SIV/macaque model can therefore be used to evaluate vaccines formulated with SIV antigens to test concepts that may be relevant to HIV-1 vaccine development. It is especially useful for defining immunologic correlates of immunity.

The evaluation of vaccine concepts in the macaque was initially limited by the lack of macaque-specific immunologic reagents and the incomplete definition of the genetics of the major histocompatibility complex. However, the MHC is being defined, and MHC class I and II molecules have now been demonstrated with specificity for epitopes in both SIV *gag* and *envelope* genes (311–317). Moreover, reagents to detect cytokines (318), chemokines (319), costimulatory molecules (320), lymphocyte adhesion molecules (321), other T-cell surface markers (322), and antibody have now been developed. The value of the SIV/macaque model has thus grown in significance, limited now by factors such as cost and facilities available for housing.

Another advance in the development of the macaque model is the production of a chimeric virus, designated SHIV. These viruses contain the replication machinery and *gag* components of SIV with *envelope* and some regulatory genes from HIV-1 (277). SHIV virus adapted for growth in macaques by serial passage can become virulent (323, 324), and thus it serves as a disease-inducing challenge for macaques that can be used to evaluate the efficacy of HIV-1 *envelope* vaccine-induced immunity (325).

Other than the SHIV challenge of macaques, no animal model exists with AIDS-like disease expression in which HIV vaccines can be directly evaluated on a large scale. HIV-2 has a high degree of sequence identity with SIV (326), and it can persistently infect macaques, but it does not lead to disease progression (327). *Macaca nemestrina* is infectable by HIV-1. However, initiation of infection depends on a high input of virus, and disease progression does not occur (328).

NONPRIMATE MODELS

Some small animal models have been developed to investigate vaccine approaches against AIDS, but it is beyond the scope of this chapter to discuss them in detail. Feline immunodeficiency virus (FIV) infection of cats is the most relevant to HIV-1 pathogenesis and vaccine development (329). It has the same advantage of the SIV/macaque model, in that FIV is a lentivirus that can cause an AIDS-like illness in cats. However, FIV is even more distantly related to HIV than SIV, and the lack of sophisticated immunologic reagents is even more profound for cats than for macaques. The severe combined immunodeficiency (SCID) mouse reconstituted with human PBMCs has been a model that has contributed to the evaluation of pharmacologic and passive immunotherapy approaches in HIV-1 infection (330–332). However, too many confounding problems have arisen with antigen presentation mechanisms, compartmentalization of cells and virus, and distribution of relevant cells to use this system for evaluation of immunity induced by active immunization (333). Transgenic mouse models that express human CD4 and CCR5 or CXCR4 (chemokine receptors that serve as coreceptors for HIV-1 entry) are being developed. Having an HIV-susceptible mouse would be a great advantage for immunologic studies because of the wealth of immunologic reagents and the availability of inbred strains that allow lymphocyte transfer experiments to be done. However, whether murine cells can be altered sufficiently to allow the high levels of HIV-1 replication needed to induce AIDS-like disease progression is not known. HIV-1 entry may not be the only factor in murine cells that limits replication rates (334). Attaining high levels of HIV-1 replication does not appear to be a significant problem in rabbit cells (335). Therefore, attempts are also under way to develop transgenic rabbits expressing the human CD4 and chemokine receptor genes. Development of a small animal model of HIV-1 infection would be a significant advance in the ability to evaluate candidate AIDS vaccines.

Immunization and Challenge Studies

Animal models have demonstrated that vaccine-induced immunity can protect against infection with lentiviruses (Table 42.5), and it can also modify the course of disease in animals infected despite vaccination (308). This finding alone justifies the extensive work that has been done in animal model development and the optimism that it will be possible to develop a vaccine that can prevent AIDS in humans. The more difficult questions to ask using animal models are the following: 1) What vaccine formulation is sufficient to protect against infection or disease progression? 2) Which immunologic effector mechanisms are necessary for protection from infection or disease progression? and 3) How can these findings be safely applied in humans to achieve immunity against HIV-1? The answers to these questions remain open and will require careful interpretation of nuances in each of the models. Rather than list the details of all studies performed to date, an approach for interpreting animal model studies is proposed.

The key variable in studies evaluating candidate vaccines in animal models is the virus challenge. The outcome and interpretation of such studies depend on the timing relative to immunization, route, dose, virus properties (replication kinetics, phenotype, tropism, molecular clone or swarm, homology of challenge virus and vaccine antigen), and preparation of challenge stock. Most studies have been performed by giving the virus challenge 2 weeks after the last immunization. This is presumably the peak of immunity, and the timing is designed to provide the greatest chance for protection. Challenge of immunized animals at a time more distant from last immunization is a more critical test of efficacy.

The route of HIV-1 infection is usually across a mucosal surface, and transmission is infrequent. Infection probably is produced by a small number of viruses from the inoculum (11, 41). For practical reasons, animal model studies are designed to produce a high rate of infection, so nearly all the

Table 42.5. Rank Order of Primate Models of Lentivirus Infection by Virulence or Challenge Virus[a]

Virulence of Challenge in Nonvaccinated Animal	Genus	Virus Stock[b]	Level of Protection by Vaccine Approach		Reference
			Virus Load Reduction	Viral Clearance	
Transient infection	Chimpanzee	HIV-1$_{SF2}$		Envelope subunit	390–392
				Adenovirus + subunit	393
				DNA + subunit	394
		HIV-1$_{DH12}$	Envelope subunit	Envelope subunit	391, 395
	Macaca	HIV-2		Whole killed	396
				Envelope subunit	397
				ALVAC + subunit	398, 399
				NYVAC + subunit	399, 400
		SHIV (LAI)		Envelope subunit	Berman, in preparation
				DNA + subunit	401
				SIV live attenuated	402
			RNA		403
Persistent infection without disease	Chimpanzee	HIV-1$_{LAI}$		Envelope subunit	404, 405
		HIV-1$_{LAI}$ (infected cells)		Vaccinia + subunit	406
	Macaca	SIVmac$_{Bk28}$[c]	Env +/– gag subunits		407
		SHIV (DH12)	SIV live attenuated		408
		SHIV (NM-3rN)		SHIV	409
Progressive AIDS-like disease	Macaca	SIVmne$_{E11S}$†	Envelope peptides		410
				Vaccinia + subunit	411, 412
		SIVmac$_{J5}$[c] (rectal)		Envelope subunits	413
		SHIV (LAI$_{KU-1P}$)		SIV Live attenuated or SHIV	414
		HIV-2$_{287}$	HIV-2 live attenuated		Wong-Staal, in preparation
		SHIV (89.6P)	SIV live attenuated		Rud, in preparation
		SIVmac32H (rectal)	NYVAC		Benson, in press
		SIVsm$_{E660}$ (infected cells)	MVA + subunit		415
		SIVsm$_3$	HIV-2 live attenuated		416
		SIVsm$_3$ (rectal)	SHIV (LAI) live attenuated		417
		SIVsm$_3$ (rectal)		HIV-2 live attenuated	418
		SIVsm$_{B670}$	DNA + vaccinia		419
				SIV live attenuated	420
		SIVsm$_{E543}$	Whole inactivated SIV		308
		SIVmac$_{239}$ (vaginal)	SHIV (89.6)		421
		SIVmac$_{251}$ (vaginal)	Adenovirus + subunit		422
		SIVmac$_{251}$	Vaccinia + subunit		423
			ALVAC + subunit		424
				SIV live attenuated	272, 425
Acute, lethal infection	Macaca	SIVsm$_{-PBj14}$	RNA + subunit		426
		SIVsm$_{-PBj14, Clone 6.6}$[c]	SIV live attenuated		Rud, in preparation

[a]Examples of vaccine failures are not listed, but all approaches have failed. Recombinant vectors listed expressed envelope glycoproteins and some co-expressed internal proteins. This table does not account for factors of time between last vaccination and challenge, challenge dose, level of homology between challenge virus and virus from which vaccine was derived, and the species of macaque used. These details can be obtained from the listed references. The purpose of the table is to list the relative potency of a general vaccine approach in context of the relative virulence of a virus challenge in a given animal model system. Other challenge stocks are being prepared for future vaccine challenge studies, particularly SHIV constructs adapted for virulence in macaques.
[b]Inoculum was given IV unless noted. SIV, simian immunodeficiency virus. Additional terms include abbreviation for monkey species from which the virus was originally isolated, and specific strain or clone is listed as subscript; SHIV, chimeric virus with genome encoding internal structural proteins of SIV$_{mac}$ and env from HIV-1. HIV-1 strain is given in parentheses; HIV, human immunodeficiency virus with strain designation given as subscript.
[c]Virus stock was derived from a cloned virus.

control group is infected. Therefore, challenge virus is often administered intravenously at a dose of more than 10 AID$_{50}$ (10-fold higher than the dose needed to infect 50% of animals). One AID$_{50}$ may represent between 1 and 10 tissue culture infective dose (TCID$_{50}$), depending on the cells and conditions used for titrations. This magnitude of virus challenge may represent an artificial and excessive hurdle for vaccine-induced immunity to resist. Efforts to infect uniformly across a mucosal barrier have made some advances, but the amount of virus in the challenge inoculum is even higher for mucosal challenge studies than for intravenous challenges, and the infection rate is variable. Treatment with progesterone is an innovation that improves the rate of infection when inoculating the vagina (336).

The properties that characterize virus involved in transmitting human infection include 1) CCR5 coreceptor usage, 2) nonsyncytium-inducing phenotype, 3) macrophage-tropic phenotype, 4) both cell-free and cell-associated, 5) genotypically a quasispecies, and 6) slow replication rates. In contrast, many challenge stocks contain viruses that use CXCR4, are syncytium inducing and lymphocyte tropic, are cell free and derived from a molecular clone, and have a high replication rate. In addition, the initial test of vaccine-induced immunity is performed with virus that is homologous to that from which the vaccine antigens were derived. Few studies have addressed the breadth of vaccine-induced immunity by challenging with divergent strains. These factors produce a confounding set of variables, with the net effect making vaccine-induced immunity against the experimental challenge either more or less likely than it would be against natural transmission.

The method by which a challenge stock is produced can have a profound effect on vaccine-induced protection. The best examples are early studies showing vaccine-induced protection with whole inactivated SIV (337–339). After extensive analysis, investigators discovered that the best correlate of protection was antibody to human cell constituents (262). When the virus used to produce vaccine was grown in human cells, and the virus challenge stock was grown in the same human cells, allogenic responses to the human proteins incorporated by the virus were the dominant mechanism of protection (262, 264, 340). Studies done with vaccine produced in monkey cells did not show consistent protection.

More than 500 primate studies of active or passive immunization followed by virus challenge have been performed as of early 1998. These studies have been performed by more than 50 research groups from Europe and the United States. Detailed data on specific vaccine formulations and study end points can be found through references compiled in an ongoing survey of primate studies (341–344).

Because of the practical issues that do not permit a virus challenge that accurately reproduces the conditions of a human exposure to HIV-1, one must determine which questions can legitimately be answered in primate models. Animal models can answer questions about pathogenesis, immune correlates of protection from a particular virus challenge, and the potential for a vaccine formulation to resist virus challenge. However, vaccine-induced protection or vaccine failure in animal models is unlikely to correlate directly with efficacy in humans. Nevertheless, by evaluating vaccine approaches in various animal model systems, one can rank order their relative potency against virus challenge of varying stringency (see Table 42.5). In Table 42.5, the primate species and virus challenge stocks are listed in order of ascending disease severity. When vaccine approaches have effectively prevented persistent infection or have delayed disease progression, they are listed in the appropriate column. Caveats are listed in the table footnote. Although one cannot yet know where the threshold of clinical efficacy will be with respect to potency of a vaccine approach in animal model systems, this information will accrue as data from larger-scale human studies become available.

CLINICAL TRIALS FOR SAFETY AND IMMUNOGENICITY

Conduct of Trials

Clinical trials in seronegative volunteers have been performed to evaluate the safety and immunogenicity of candidate AIDS vaccines. Candidate vaccines are rigorously tested in preclinical toxicity and immunogenicity studies in small and large animals. In addition, safety profiles and immunogenic properties must be sufficiently promising to warrant clinical evaluation. The Division of AIDS, National Institute of Allergy and Infectious Diseases, National Institutes of Health, along with industry and university colleagues, is actively engaged in a national program of discovery, development and phase I/II clinical trials in anticipation of defining potential promising vaccine candidates for efficacy trials; similar programs are in effect in other countries. Studies in the United States have been conducted by independent investigators in direct collaboration with industry or by the AIDS Vaccine Evaluation Group (AVEG). The AVEG includes six AIDS Vaccine Evaluation Unit (AVEU) trial sites based at university research centers. An independent AIDS vaccine selection group reviews products of potential interest and makes recommendations concerning their priority for evaluation by the AVEG. The AVEG also includes central immunology laboratories performing most of the immune assays, as well as a data coordinating and analysis center. Each AVEU has an associated community advisory board. A data and safety monitoring board exercises independent oversight, and a reagent program and sample repository have been developed to facilitate assay development and collaboration with outside investigators.

A standardized approach to experimental design, clinical and immunologic assessments, and data analysis permits direct comparison of vaccine approaches. More than 2300 HIV-negative volunteers have been enrolled in double-blind, randomized, placebo-controlled studies in the AVEG program in the United States between 1988 and 1998. Most phase I trials include 25 to 100 individuals. Participating volunteers are healthy seronegative adults who are selected to be at low risk for HIV infection, to minimize potential for confounding HIV infections during trials. Two phase II studies have enrolled 296 and 420 subjects, including some individuals judged to be at high risk of infection. Volunteers are carefully screened, extensively counseled, and informed about potential adverse consequences and implications of vaccine-induced positive serologic results. Recipients are monitored for a broad spectrum of physiologic and immunologic parameters, and repeatedly counseled about maintaining low-risk behavior. Immune responses are assessed by measures of humoral and cell-mediated responses. Assays routinely performed to measure humoral and mucosal responses include detection of HIV-specific antibody by enzyme immunoassay (EIA), Western blot, ELISA using selected protein and peptide antigens as reagents, homologous and heterologous virus neutralization of both TCLA viruses and primary isolates, fusion inhibition, CD4 binding inhibition, and ADCC. Cellular responses are routinely measured by classic CTL and lymphocyte proliferation assays. New approaches to measuring immune responses are also explored in these studies that are responsive to current concepts in HIV immunobiology, and cryopreserved samples allow the evaluation of future assay concepts. Samples include plasma, serum, PBMCs, and mucosal secretions from various sites.

Safety

Vaccine candidates have demonstrated a safety record comparable to that seen with other viral vaccines. Volunteers have experienced mild local reactions, including pain, redness and swelling, and occasional systemic reactions not significantly different from control subjects. Biochemical and hematologic studies have not been abnormal. In particular, CD4 numbers and mitogen responses were unchanged. One adjuvant, MF59/MTP-PE (polysorbate 80/sorbitan triolate emulsifier [MF59] plus muramyl tripeptide [MTP] covalently linked to dipalmitoyl phosphatidylethanolamine [PE]), used with rgp120 (Biocine) (see Table 42.4), caused significant transient local and systemic reactions that appeared to be related to the MTP-PE component. MTP-PE had an equivocal adjuvant effect beyond that of MF59. Low titers of C'-ADE can be found frequently in vaccinees who have developed significant antibody responses, although no adverse effects have been noted (204, 345). No evidence of autoimmune syndromes has been noted, although a few subjects immunized with envelope antigens develop transiently detectable anti-idiotype antibody to CD4 (219).

Breakthrough Infections

During the course of evaluating candidate vaccines, there have been a small number of subjects infected with HIV-1 despite vaccination (346–348). Because the subjects came from various phase I and phase II vaccine protocols containing few placebo recipients, the data cannot be used to make estimates of vaccine efficacy. However, the subjects have been evaluated in detail, to look for evidence of vaccine effects on the infecting virus, immune responses, and pathogenesis of subsequent disease (346–350). Most of the subjects had received purified envelope protein subunit products only, but a few subjects had been immunized with a recombinant vaccinia vector expressing gp160$_{LAI}$ and a baculovirus rgp160 (346, 348).

The characteristics of breakthrough viruses and those recovered from nonvaccinated controls are similar with respect to their syncytium-inducing phenotype, cell tropism, replication kinetics, neutralizability, and genotypes (350). Selected breakthrough viruses have slight sequence changes in epitopes from the V3, C4, and V2 domains of envelope (349), but when compared with contemporary, nonvaccinated subjects with acute HIV-1 infections, the frequency of these changes does not appear significant (348, 350). The biologic significance of minor antigenic changes in the infecting virus compared with the strain from which the vaccine antigen was derived is unknown, but it emphasizes the importance of incorporating antigenic specificities of prevalent strains in vaccine design.

No significant difference in preinfection antibody levels was noted between subjects with breakthrough infections and uninfected matched vaccine recipients (348). No significant alteration occurred in the postinfection antibody response measured by ELISA or in the magnitude or specificity of CD8+ CTL activity in subjects with breakthrough infections compared with nonvaccinated subjected undergoing acute HIV infection (350).

Subjects with breakthrough infection had no evidence of accelerated disease progression or induction of C'-ADE beyond that seen in nonvaccinated subjects with acute HIV infection. The follow-up period has not been sufficient to determine whether long-term impact on disease progression may become apparent, but virus load and CD4+ lymphocyte counts at 1 year after infection in breakthrough subjects are not significantly different from those in nonvaccinated subjects with acute HIV infection (348).

Recombinant Envelope Protein Subunit Vaccines

Certain recombinant envelope products, rgp120 or rgp160, produced in insect, yeast, or mammalian cell substrates formulated with various adjuvants have been evaluated in clinical trials (see Table 42.4). All products evaluated at this time have been derived from sequences of syncytium-inducing, TCLA X4 viruses from clade B. The studies have defined the way in which parameters of dose, schedule, and formulation affect immunogenicity of purified protein subunit preparations as primary immunogens and in combination with other vaccine modalities. The principal findings related to the immunogenicity of purified protein subunits tested to date include the following:

1. Although type-specific neutralization can be induced, particularly to the vaccine antigen, neutralization of primary isolate R5 virus is not induced (351). This problem is considered serious for vaccine development because this type of virus is responsible for most transmission events. Designing vaccine products that can induce neutralizing antibody effective against R5 viruses is an important focus of current research.
2. Antibody is induced that can bind oligomeric, R5 virus presented on the surface of virus-infected cells (352). This finding suggests that the monomeric envelope

products currently being tested can produce antibody that recognizes oligomeric envelope structures, even though the affinity and specificity are not sufficient to result in virus neutralization.

3. Antigens produced in mammalian cells induce higher titer of neutralizing antibody against TCLA virus than those produced in baculovirus or yeast systems (353–356). This phenomenon is thought to be a result of more authentic glycosylation and conformation when the envelope glycoprotein is produced in a mammalian cell line.

4. rgp120 products induce less binding antibody, but more neutralizing antibody, than rgp160 products (353, 354, 357). As noted earlier, the neutralizing activity does not include primary isolate R5 viruses.

5. A four-dose immunization regimen is more effective for antibody induction when a several-month interval occurs between doses (353, 354). Intervals of at least 3 to 4 months between the second, third, and fourth immunization increase the magnitude of response.

6. A rapid (every month) vaccination schedule results in attenuation of antibody responses after the fourth dose (353). Titers of both binding and functional antibody activities are reduced after a monthly immunization schedule using rgp120 in MF59 (353). The attenuating effect of rapid dosing is not as apparent with other adjuvants (358).

7. A fifth dose of rgp120, regardless of interval, does not boost antibody response, but only returns it to previous level.

8. The half-life of vaccine antigen-specific antibody titers is less than 3 months in subjects receiving only purified recombinant protein subunits, regardless of number of doses. The mechanism responsible for brief duration of antibody maintenance is not known.

9. Priming with one subtype and boosting with another demonstrate subtype-specificity in antibody response (359). When a subject is initially immunized with rgp120 derived from a clade B, TCLA X4 HIV strain, subsequent boosting with another clade B strain does not effectively broaden the response significantly, and it does not boost the response to the initial envelope antigen as well as the original rgp120.

10. Envelope subunits can induce CD4+ CTLs, but they rarely induce CD8+ CTLs even when formulated with novel adjuvants (353, 360). This finding is an expected result of obligate processing through the endocytic pathway leading to MHC class II presentation. New adjuvants and delivery systems may improve MHC class I presentation of purified protein antigens, but they are not likely ever to approach the efficiency of antigens produced intracellularly by approaches such as DNA immunization, live recombinant vectors, or live attenuated vaccines.

11. Antigen dose effects on magnitude of antibody production depend on the adjuvant formulation. QS21 appears to allow a reduction in the antigen dose by more than 10- to 100-fold without affecting the magnitude of antibody response (361).

The major focus in the area of recombinant envelope subunits is on devising new immunogens that can induce neutralizing antibody responses to a broad array of primary HIV-1 isolates. This may require more complex oligomeric structures or production of protein from genes derived from primary isolates. It may also require cocktails of products with different antigenic specificities. Even if key structures in the envelope of primary HIV-1 isolates can be made immunogenic, additional steps may be needed to make transmitted virus susceptible to the types of immune responses generated by vaccination.

Peptide Vaccines

Certain peptide vaccine formulations have been evaluated in phase I clinical trials (see Table 42.4). The peptides tested to date have been derived from envelope V3 loop or *gag* sequences of clade B or multiple clades. They have been presented conjugated to an oligolysine backbone, as a lipopeptide conjugate, mixed with adjuvant, or as a fusion protein with the self-assembling yeast protein Ty as a particle. They have been administered intramuscularly in the deltoid or anterior thigh (to target lymph nodes that also drain the rectal mucosa), rectally and orally as Ty-gag VLPs, and orally encapsulated in polylactide copolymers. Preparations tested to date have been weakly immunogenic. Low levels of binding antibody have been detected in most trials, but significant levels of neutralizing antibody even to TCLA viruses have not been achieved. In one study with the Ty-gag-VLP without alum, CD8+ CTL responses were detected in a few subjects (362). Current studies are evaluating a more complex peptide that contains T-helper epitopes from the C4 domain of gp120 and neutralizing antibody and CTL epitopes from the V3 domain. Peptides from four strains of HIV-1 are combined in incomplete Freund's adjuvant and are administered intramuscularly. This approach has been immunogenic in both small animals and primates, but immunogenicity data are not yet available from human trials.

The current experience with peptide vaccines in humans suggests that this approach may not be sufficiently immunogenic to be a primary vaccine. The initial impetus for exploring peptide vaccination was that it appeared to be an approach that could address the problem of genetic variation. However, the problem of genetic variation has been superseded by the challenge of inducing neutralizing antibody against primary HIV-1 isolates, which will probably require a more complex antigenic structure than peptides can provide. Nevertheless, additional work is needed on new formulations and on the role peptides vaccines could serve as mechanisms to either broaden or focus immune responses to particular epitopes when given as a boost after primary vaccination with another preparation.

Live Recombinant Vectors and Nucleic Acid Vaccines

Recombinant vaccinia and canarypox vectors have been evaluated in phase I or II clinical trials, and recombinant *Salmonella* and DNA vaccine constructs are currently being evaluated. These approaches are considered together because their fundamental property is to promote intracellular production of vaccine antigen (see Fig. 42.3). This feature provides many advantages over vaccine approaches that deliver vaccine antigen extracellularly. In particular, intracellular antigens are more likely to be processed and presented like those produced during live virus infection, and they have the capacity to induce MHC class I–restricted CD8+ CTLs.

Initial studies used recombinant vaccinia expressing gp160$_{LAI}$ (220, 360, 363–367). These investigations demonstrated the following:

1. Approaches for secure containment of recombinant vaccinia are possible in the outpatient setting (366).
2. Preexisting immunity to vaccinia diminished immunogenicity of the recombinant antigen (364, 366).
3. Induction of CD8+ CTL responses is possible (365, 368, 369).
4. Delayed induction of humoral responses with vector alone is possible (366).
5. Effective priming for antibody responses elicited by subsequent boosting with purified recombinant envelope subunit formulations occurs (220, 365).
6. Specificity of the antibody response is determined more by the initial antigen expressed by the recombinant vector than by the subsequent purified recombinant subunit antigen given as booster (360, 367), and priming immunization with recombinant vaccinia induces type-specific memory for the recombinant gene product that is not boosted by subsequent immunization with heterologous recombinant subunit envelope proteins (360).

Investigators showed that the dominant antibody response in vaccinees was directed against a gp41 epitope (aa 720-740) that was not a major target for sera from HIV-1$_{LAI}$-infected laboratory workers (370). Like the antibody induced by purified envelope subunit proteins, most neutralizing antibody in vaccinee serum is directed against the V3 loop, is type specific, and is only active against TCLA viruses. A recombinant vaccinia construct that encodes *gag*, *pol*, and *env* genes is currently in phase I trials, but immunogenicity data are not yet available. One of the key questions in the development of vaccinia vectors is how much attenuation of virulence is possible without losing immunogenicity.

Canarypox vectors that express gp160, gp120/*gag*/protease, or gp120/*gag*/protease/*nef* epitopes have been developed and evaluated in phase I (371) and II clinical trials. Canarypox has an abortive replication cycle in mammalian cells, and therefore it does not cause pustular lesions and systemic symptoms, as does vaccinia. The safety profile in trials to date has been excellent, with virtually no local or systemic side effects. Prior vaccinia immunity does not

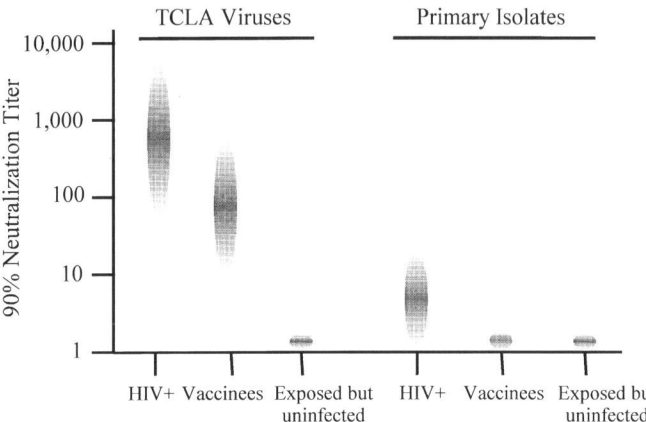

Figure 42.4. Schematic representation of neutralizing antibody data. These data are compiled from HIV-infected persons who remain asymptomatic, vaccine recipients in many different studies (see Table 42.4), and persons repeatedly exposed but uninfected. TCLA, T-cell line adapted.

attenuate responses to the recombinant antigens expressed by canarypox vectors. However, antibody responses to the vector develop after three to four injections, and they attenuate the response to recombinant antigen on subsequent injections. The major findings related to immunogenicity from clinical trials with recombinant canarypox vectors include the following:

1. CD8+ CTL responses to HIV-specific antigens are induced in up to 60% of vaccinated subjects.
2. HIV-specific CD8+ CTLs are detected in 15 to 30% of subjects at any single time.
3. Vectors expressing multiple HIV antigens increase the frequency of CTL induction above that induced by a single recombinant antigen.
4. CD8+ CTL responses are more durable when subsequent boosting with a purified recombinant envelope subunit protein is performed.
5. The HIV-specific antibody response after recombinant canarypox immunization alone is weak, but subsequent boosting with purified recombinant envelope subunit protein induces HIV-specific antibody titers of the same magnitude and quality as three or four inoculations of the purified recombinant envelope subunit protein alone.

Future work with recombinant canarypox vectors will focus on mechanisms to induce mucosal immunity, defining CTL precursor frequencies, defining the pattern of CTL epitope specificity, and determining the role of boosting with purified recombinant subunit proteins on induction and maintenance of the CTL response. In addition, vector construction will be manipulated to improve recombinant gene expression and in vitro replication kinetics. Studies of recombinant *Salmonella* expressing gp160, and DNA vaccines constructed to express *env/rev* or *gag/pol* are in the initial phase of clinical testing; immunogenicity data are not yet available.

Summary of Immunogenicity Data from Clinical Trials

The immunogenicity of candidate AIDS vaccines evaluated in clinical trials is summarized in Figures 42.4 to 42.6. Schematized composite data are shown from all studies, with ranges compared with those reported for HIV-infected patients and for persons who remain uninfected despite multiple exposures. Neutralizing antibody responses against TCLA viruses induced by the most immunogenic formulations are still 5- to 10-fold lower than those produced by HIV-1 infection. The responses are type specific with a short half-life, and they are unable to neutralize primary isolate R5 viruses.

Lymphoproliferative responses have been induced by all vaccine approaches and range in magnitude from stimulation indices of more than 100 for some subjects vaccinated with recombinant vaccinia vectors and boosted with purified recombinant envelope proteins to 5 to 10 for recombinant canarypox-primed subjects. In general, gp160-based formulations have induced higher lymphoproliferative responses than gp120-based formulations. One of the features of HIV-1 infection is that virus-specific lymphoproliferative responses are rapidly lost. Maintenance of HIV-specific lymphoproliferative activity is associated with long-term nonprogression (127). The value of having increased precursor frequencies of HIV-specific CD4+ T lymphocytes before HIV-1 exposure is not known.

HIV-specific CD8+ CTLs can be induced in most subjects receiving recombinant poxvirus vectors, and in a subset, CTL activity is detectable for more than 6 months. Unlike antibody responses, vaccine-induced CTL responses are broadly reactive (170). CTLs induced by recombinant canarypox vectors have been shown to lyse target cells infected with primary HIV-1 isolates from multiple clades (170). Not only is classic MHC class I–restricted cytolytic activity induced, but also vaccine-induced noncytolytic CD8+-mediated sup-

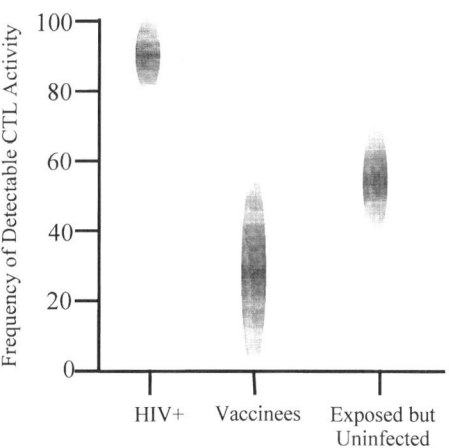

Figure 42.6. Schematic representation of frequency of detecting cytotoxic lymphocyte (CTL) activity in the groups listed in Figure 24.4. Data were derived from the literature for HIV-infected and exposed but uninfected groups and were obtained from the AIDS Vaccine Evaluation Group database for vaccinees. The assay methods varied among groups, with the most significant difference being that the data from HIV-infected subjects is from direct CTL assays and data from the other groups required in vitro stimulation of effector populations.

pression of HIV-1 replication (372) has been demonstrated in recipients of recombinant canarypox vaccines.

CURRENT STATUS OF AIDS VACCINE DEVELOPMENT

HIV-1 is the most complex virus for which vaccine development has ever been attempted. The development effort made to this point is unprecedented and is still far short of the need. To complete the process will require further exploration of fundamental HIV biology and immunopathogenesis, improved approaches to vaccine formulation and design, continued evaluation of new vaccine approaches in both animal models and clinical trials, and performance of large-scale clinical trials in subjects at high risk for HIV-1 infection.

HIV-1 infection presents various handicaps mitigating against successful immune intervention. These include 1) multiple routes of transmission, 2) infection transmitted by cell-free or cell-associated virus, 3) integration of provirus early in infection, 4) biologically significant antigenic diversification and immune escape during persistent infection as well as marked geographic diversity, 5) high frequency of genetic recombination, 6) direct cell–cell fusion, 7) infection of central immune elements including helper T lymphocytes, macrophages, DCs, and thymic and bone marrow precursors, 8) HIV-1–induced immune dysfunction in both infected and bystander cells, 9) rapid systemic dissemination establishing conditions that support persistent viral replication in lymphoid tissue, 10) infection in immunologically sequestered sites, 11) infection of cells that resist virus and immune-mediated lysis, 12) virus-encoded mechanisms to evade immune detection of infected cells, 13) the failure of natural immunity to clear infection in

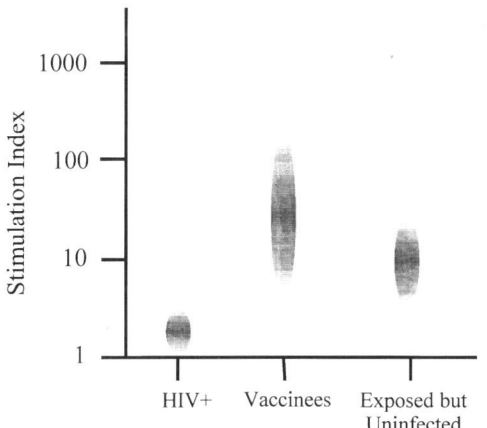

Figure 42.5. Schematic representation of lymphoproliferation data shown as stimulation indices for the same groups listed in Figure 42.4. Antigens used for stimulation were purified recombinant envelope subunit proteins compared with mock preparations from the same cell source.

virtually all cases, and 14) the inability of current vaccine formulations to induce neutralizing antibody responses against primary isolate R5 virus.

Equally compelling factors provide hope that vaccine development will some day be successful. They include the following: 1) HIV-1 transmission is relatively inefficient; 2) transmitted virus may have a restricted set of structural and genotypic features that are susceptible to immune interference; 3) the infectious inoculum may be only a few virions in most cases; 4) HIV-specific immune responses have occurred in some exposed-but-uninfected persons that suggest it may be possible for natural immunity to clear virus infection; 5) examples of vaccine-induced immunity have been reported in primate models; 6) vaccine-induced immune responses include CTL activity against multiple clades of primary HIV-1 isolates; 7) continued gains in our knowledge of antigen presentation, cytokines, chemokines, costimulatory molecules, and their ligands will lead to new vaccine approaches; and 8) new vaccine approaches promise to improve the immunogenicity of vaccine antigens and their delivery into appropriate immunologic compartments.

One of the next major steps in vaccine development will be the performance of larger-scale trials in higher-risk populations. The appropriate timing, vaccine approach, trial design, and trial location for such a study are issues of current controversy and debate. The performance of a phase III clinical trial should be based on 1) its potential for defining a biologic impact of the vaccine on HIV-induced disease based on results from animal model studies and phase I/II trials, 2) its potential for answering questions about correlates of immunity, and 3) the importance of establishing a benchmark against which future vaccine design and development can be measured.

Acknowledgments

We are grateful to Ms. Joyce Keltner for database assistance. Drs. Alan Schultz and Nancy Miller of the Division of AIDS, National Institute of Allergy and Infectious Diseases, National Institutes of Health, Bethesda, MD assisted with development and proofreading of Table 42.5. Ms. Sophia Pallas of the EMMES Corporation assisted with Table 42.4. This work was supported by contract NO1-AI-45210 from the National Institutes of Health.

References

1. Sabin AB. Improbability of effective vaccination against human immunodeficiency virus because of its intracellular transmission and rectal portal of entry. Proc Natl Acad Sci U S A 1992;89:8852–8855.
2. White DO, Fenner F. Pathogenesis and pathology of viral infections. In: Medical virology. 3rd ed. Orlando, FL: Academic Press, 1986:134–143.
3. Ada GL. Prospects for HIV vaccines. J Acquir Immune Defic Syndr 1988;1:295–303.
4. Ada GL. Modern vaccines: the immunological principles of vaccination. Lancet 1990;335:523–526.
5. Cannon MJ, Stott EJ, Taylor G, et al. Clearance of persistent respiratory syncytial virus infections in immunodeficient mice following transfer of primed T cells. Immunology 1987;62:133–138.
6. Graham BS. Pathogenesis of respiratory syncytial virus vaccine–augmented pathology. Am J Respir Crit Care Med 1995;152:S63–S66.
7. Graham BS, Henderson GS, Tang YW, et al. Priming immunization determines T helper cytokine mRNA expression patterns in lungs of mice challenged with respiratory syncytial virus. J Immunol 1993;151:2032–2040.
8. Tang YW, Graham BS. Anti–IL-4 treatment at immunization modulates cytokine expression, reduces illness, and increases cytotoxic T lymphocyte activity in mice challenged with respiratory syncytial virus. J Clin Invest 1994;94:1953–1958.
9. Arvin AM, Gershon AA. Live attenuated varicella vaccine. Annu Rev Microbiol 1996;50:59–100.
10. Anderson DJ, Politch JA, Martinez A, et al. White blood cells and HIV-1 in semen from vasectomised seropositive men. Lancet 1991;338:573–574.
11. Wolinsky SM, Wike CM, Korber BTM, et al. Selective transmission of human immunodeficiency virus type-1 variants from mothers to infants. Science 1992;255:1134–1137.
12. Wolfs TF, Zwart G, Bakker M, et al. HIV-1 genomic RNA diversification following sexual and parenteral virus transmission. Virology 1992;189:103–110.
13. Klatzmann D, Champagne E, Chamaret S, et al. T-lymphocyte T4 molecule behaves as receptor for human retrovirus LAV. Nature 1984;312:767–771.
14. Dalgleish AG, Beverley PC, Clapham PR, et al. The CD4 (T4) antigen is an essential component of the receptor for the AIDS retrovirus. Nature 1984;312:763–767.
15. Gartner S, Markovits P, Markovitz DM, et al. The role of mononuclear phagocytes in HTLV-III/LAV infection. Science 1986;233:215–219.
16. Gendelman HE, Orenstein JM, Baca LM, et al. The macrophage in the persistence and pathogenesis of HIV infection. AIDS 1989;3:475–495.
17. McElrath MJ, Pruett JE, Cohn ZA. Mononuclear phagocytes of blood and bone marrow: comparative roles as viral reservoirs in human immunodeficiency virus type 1 infections. Proc Natl Acad Sci U S A 1989;86:675–679.
18. Alkhatib G, Combadiere C, Broder CC, et al. CC CKR5: a RANTES, MIP-1α, MIP-1β receptor as a fusion co-factor for macrophage-tropic HIV-1. Science 1996;272:1955–1958.
19. Feng Y, Broder CC, Kennedy PE, et al. HIV-1 entry co-factor: functional cDNA cloning of a seven-transmembrane, G protein-coupled receptor. Science 1996;272:872–877.
20. Wu L, Paxton WA, Kassam N, et al. CCR5 levels and expression pattern correlate with infectability by macrophage-tropic HIV-1, in vitro. J Exp Med 1997;185:1681–1691.
21. Dragic T, Litwin V, Allaway GP, et al. HIV-1 entry into CD4+ cells is mediated by the chemokine receptor CC-CKR-5. Nature 1996;381:667–673.
22. Bjorndal A, Deng H, Jansson M, et al. Co-receptor usage of primary human immunodeficiency virus type 1 isolates varies according to biological phenotype. J Virol 1997;71:7478–7487.
23. Dittmar MT, Simmons G, Hibbitts S, et al. Langerhans cell tropism of human immunodeficiency virus type 1 subtype A through F isolates derived from different transmission groups. J Virol 1997;71:8008–8013.
24. Michael NL, Louie LG, Rohrbaugh L, et al. The role of CCR5 and CCR2 polymorphisms in HIV-1 transmission and disease progression. Nature Med 1997;3:1160–1162.
25. Frade JMR, Llorente M, Mellado M, et al. The amino-terminal domain of the CCR2 chemokine receptor acts as co-receptor for HIV-1 infection. J Clin Invest 1997;100:497–502.
26. He J, Chen Y, Farzan M, et al. CCR3 and CCR5 are co-receptors for HIV-1 infection of microglia. Nature 1997;385:645–649.
27. Choe H, Farzan M, Sun Y, et al. The beta-chemokine receptors CCR3 and CCR5 facilitate infection by primary HIV-1 isolates. Cell 1996;85:1135–1148.
28. Liu R, Paxton WA, Choe S, et al. Homozygous defect in HIV-1 co-receptor accounts for resistance of some multiply-exposed individuals to HIV-1 infection. Cell 1996;86:367–377.

29. Balotta C, Bagnarelli P, Violin M, et al. Homozygous delta 32 deletion of the CCR-5 chemokine receptor gene in an HIV-1 infected patient. AIDS 1997;11:F67–F71.
30. O'Brien TR, Winkler C, Dean M, et al. HIV-1 infection in a man homozygous for CCR-5 delta 32. Lancet 1997;349:1219.
31. Theodorou I, Meyer L, Magierowska M, et al. HIV-1 infection in an individual homozygous for CCR5 delta 32: Seroco Study. Lancet 1997;349:1219–1220.
32. Huang Y, Paxton WA, Wolinsky SM, et al. The role of a mutant CCR5 allele in HIV-1 transmission and disease progression. Nature Med 1996;2:1240–1243.
33. Cocchi F, DeVico AL, Garzino-Demo A, et al. Identification of RANTES, MIP-1 alpha, and MIP-1 beta as the major HIV-suppressive factors produced by CD8+ T cells. Science 1995;270:1811–1815.
34. Durda PJ, Bacheler L, Clapham P, et al. HIV-1 neutralizing monoclonal antibodies induced by a synthetic peptide. AIDS Res Hum Retroviruses 1990;6:1115–1123.
35. Graham BS, Rowland JM, Modliszewski A, et al. Antifusion activity in sera from persons infected with human immunodeficiency virus type 1. J Clin Microbiol 1990;28:2608–2611.
36. Homsy J, Meyer M, Levy JA. Serum enhancement of human immunodeficiency virus (HIV) infection correlates with disease in HIV-infected individuals. J Virol 1990;64:1437–1440.
37. Takeda A, Tateno M, Levy JA. Antibody-enhanced infections by HIV-1 via Fc receptor–mediated entry. Science 1988;242:580–583.
38. Robinson WE Jr, Montefiori DC, Mitchell WM. Antibody-dependent enhancement of human immunodeficiency virus type 1 infection. Lancet 1988;1:790–794.
39. Shattock RJ, Griffin GE. Cellular adherence enhances HIV replication in monocytic cells. Res Virol 1994;145:139–145.
40. Hildreth JE, Orentas RJ. Involvement of a leukocyte adhesion receptor (LFA-1) in HIV-induced syncytium formation. Science 1989;244:1075–1078.
41. Zhu T, Mo H, Wang N, et al. Genotypic and phenotypic characterization of HIV-1 in patients with primary infection. Science 1993;261:1179–1181.
42. Van't Wout AB, Kootstra NA, Mulder-Kampinga GA, et al. Macrophage-tropic variants initiate human immunodeficiency virus type 1 infection after sexual, parenteral, and vertical transmission. J Clin Invest 1994;94:2060–2067.
43. Nielsen C, Pedersen C, Lundgren JD, et al. Biological properties of HIV isolates in primary HIV infection: consequences for the subsequent course of infection. AIDS 1993;7:1035–1040.
44. Tan X, Pearce-Pratt R, Phillips DM. Productive infection of a cervical epithelial cell line with human immunodeficiency virus: implications for sexual transmission. J Virol 1993;67:6447–6452.
45. Levy JA, Margaretten W, Nelson J. Detection of HIV in enterochromaffin cells in the rectal mucosa of an AIDS patient. Am J Gastroenterol 1989;84:787–789.
46. Mathijs JM, Hing M, Grierson J, et al. HIV infection of rectal mucosa. Lancet 1988;1:1111.
47. Qureshi MN, Barr CE, Seshamma T, et al. Infection of oral mucosal cells by human immunodeficiency virus type 1 in seropositive individuals. J Infect Dis 1995;171:190–193.
48. Harouse JM, Bhat S, Spitalnik SL, et al. Inhibition of entry of HIV-1 in neural cell lines by antibodies against galactosyl ceramide. Science 1991;253:320–323.
49. Bhat S, Spitalnik SL, Gonzalez-Scarano F, et al. Galactosyl ceramide or a derivative is an essential component of the neural receptor for human immunodeficiency virus type 1 envelope glycoprotein gp120. Proc Natl Acad Sci U S A 1991;88:7131–7134.
50. Yahi N, Baghdiguian S, Moreau H, et al. Galactosyl ceramide (or a closely related molecule) is the receptor for human immunodeficiency virus type 1 on human colon epithelial HT29 cells. J Virol 1992;66:4848–4854.
51. Amerongen HM, Weltzin R, Farnet CM, et al. Transepithelial transport of HIV-1 by intestinal M cells: a mechanism for transmission of AIDS. J Acquir Immune Defic Syndr 1991;4:760–765.
52. Langhoff E, Terwilliger EF, Bos HJ, et al. Replication of human immunodeficiency virus type 1 in primary dendritic cell cultures. Proc Natl Acad Sci U S A 1991;88:7998–8002.
53. Miller CJ, McGhee JR, Gardner MB. Mucosal immunity, HIV transmission, and AIDS. Lab Invest 1993;68:129–145.
54. Bomsel M. Transcytosis of infectious human immunodeficiency virus across a tight human epithelial cell line barrier. Nature Med 1997;3:42–47.
55. Lehner T, Hussain L, Wilson J, et al. Mucosal transmission of HIV. Nature 1991;353:709.
56. Frankel SS, Tenner-Racz K, Racz P, et al. Active replication of HIV-1 at the lymphoepithelial surface of the tonsil. Am J Pathol 1997;151:89–96.
57. Frankel SS, Wenig BM, Mannan P, et al. Replication of HIV-1 in dendritic cell–derived syncytia at the mucosal surface of the adenoid. Science 1996;272:115–117.
58. Hussain LA, Lehner T. Comparative investigation of Langerhans' cells and potential receptors for HIV in oral, genitourinary and rectal epithelia. Immunology 1995;85:475–484.
59. Pope M, Gezelter S, Gallo N, et al. Low levels of HIV-1 infection in cutaneous dendritic cells promote extensive viral replication upon binding to memory CD4+ T cells. J Exp Med 1995;182:2045–2056.
60. Pope M, Betjes MG, Romani N, et al. Conjugates of dendritic cells and memory T lymphocytes from skin facilitate productive infection with HIV-1. Cell 1994;78:389–398.
61. Miller CJ, Kang DW, Marthas M, et al. Genital secretory immune response to chronic simian immunodeficiency virus (SIV) infection: a comparison between intravenously and genitally inoculated rhesus macaques. Clin Exp Immunol 1992;88:520–526.
62. Joag SV, Adany I, Li Z, et al. Animal model of mucosally transmitted human immunodeficiency virus type 1 disease: intravaginal and oral deposition of simian/human immunodeficiency virus in macaques results in systemic infection, elimination of CD4+ T cells, and AIDS. J Virol 1997;71:4016–4023.
63. Spira A, Marx PA, Patterson BK, et al. Cellular targets of infection and route of viral dissemination after an intravaginal inoculation of simian immunodeficiency virus into rhesus macaques. J Exp Med 1996;183:215–225.
64. Terwilliger EF, Sodroski JG, Haseltine WA. Mechanisms of infectivity and replication of HIV-1 and implications for therapy. Ann Emerg Med 1990;19:233–241.
65. Rosenberg ZF, Fauci AS. Immunopathology and pathogenesis of human immunodeficiency virus infection. Pediatr Infect Dis J 1991;10:230–238.
66. Yasutomi Y, Reimann KA, Lord CI, et al. Simian immunodeficiency virus-specific CD8+ lymphocyte response in acutely infected rhesus monkeys. J Virol 1993;67:1707–1711.
67. Cooper DA, Gold J, MacLean P, et al. Acute AIDS retrovirus infection: definition of a clinical illness associated with seroconversion. Lancet 1985;1:537–540.
68. Wantzin GRL, Lindhart BO, Weismann I, et al. Acute HTLV III infection associated with exanthema, diagnosed by seroconversion. Br J Dermatol 1986;115:601–606.
69. Sindrup JA, Lisby G, Weismann K, et al. Skin manifestations in AIDS, HIV infection, and AIDS-related complex. Int J Dermatol 1987;26:267–272.
70. Dewolf F, Lange JMA, Bakker M, et al. Influenza-like syndrome in homosexual men: a prospective diagnostic study. J R Coll Gen Pract 1988;38:443–446.
71. Pantaleo G, Graziosi C, Fauci AS. The immunopathogenesis of human immunodeficiency virus infection. N Engl J Med 1993;328:327–335.
72. McElrath MJ, Schacker T, Graham BS. Primary HIV-1 Infection. In: An update for Mandell, Douglas, and Bennett's principles and practice of infectious diseases. New York: Churchill Livingstone, 1996:1–19.
73. Schacker T, Collier AC, Hughes J, et al. Clinical and epidemiologic features of primary HIV infection. Ann Intern Med 1996;125:257–264.

74. Ringler DA, Murphy GF, King NW. An erythematous maculopapular eruption in macaques infected with an HTLV-III–like virus. J Invest Dermatol 1986;87:674–677.
75. Albert J, Gaines H, Sonnerborg A, et al. Isolation of human immunodeficiency virus (HIV) from plasma during primary HIV infection. J Med Virol 1987;23:67–73.
76. Clark SA, Saag MS, Decker WD, et al. High titers of cytopathic virus in plasma of patients with symptomatic primary HIV-1 infection. N Engl J Med 1991;324:954–960.
77. Daar ES, Moudgil T, Meyer RD, et al. Transient high levels of viremia in patients with primary human immunodeficiency virus type 1 infection. N Engl J Med 1991;324:961–964.
78. Saxinger C, Alter HJ, Eichberg JW, et al. Stages in the progression of HIV infection in chimpanzees. AIDS Res Hum Retroviruses 1987;3:375–385.
79. Goudsmit J, de Wolf F, Paul DA, et al. Expression of human immunodeficiency virus antigen (HIV-Ag) in serum and cerebrospinal fluid during acute and chronic infection. Lancet 1986;2:177–180.
80. Korber B, Wolinsky S, Haynes B, et al. HIV-1 intrapatient sequence diversity in the immunogenic V3 region. AIDS Res Hum Retroviruses 1992;8:1461–1465.
81. Krieger JN, Coombs RW, Collier AC, et al. Recovery of human immunodeficiency virus type 1 from semen: minimal impact of stage of infection and current antiviral chemotherapy. J Infect Dis 1991;163:386–388.
82. Koup RA, Safrit JT, Cao YZ, et al. Temporal association of cellular immune responses with the initial control of viremia in primary human immunodeficiency virus type 1 syndrome. J Virol 1994;68:4650–4655.
83. Borrow P, Lewicki H, Hahn BH, et al. Virus-specific CD8+ cytotoxic T-lymphocyte activity associated with control of viremia in primary human immunodeficiency virus type 1 infection. J Virol 1994;68:6103–6110.
84. Reimann KA, Tenner-Racz K, Racz P, et al. Immunopathogenic events in acute infection of rhesus monkeys with simian immunodeficiency virus of macaques. J Virol 1994;68:2362–2370.
85. Albert J, Abrahamsson B, Nagy K, et al. Rapid development of isolate-specific neutralizing antibodies after primary HIV-1 infection and consequent emergence of virus variants which resist neutralization by autologous sera. AIDS 1990;4:107–112.
86. Nara PL, Smit L, Dunlop N, et al. Emergence of viruses resistant to neutralization by V3-specific antibodies in experimental human immunodeficiency virus type 1 IIIB infection of chimpanzees. J Virol 1990;64:3779–3791.
87. Burns DP, Desrosiers RC. Selection of genetic variants of simian immunodeficiency virus in persistently infected rhesus monkeys. J Virol 1991;65:1843–1854.
88. McMichael AJ, Phillips RE. Escape of human immunodeficiency virus from immune control. Annu Rev Immunol 1997;15:271–296.
89. Mellors JW, Rinaldo CR Jr, Gupta P, et al. Prognosis in HIV-1 infection predicted by the quantity of virus in plasma. Science 1996;272:1167–1170.
90. Mellors JW, Munoz A, Giorgi JV, et al. Plasma viral load and CD4+ lymphocytes as prognostic markers of HIV-1 infection. Ann Intern Med 1997;126:946–954.
91. Walker BD, Flexner C, Paradis TJ, et al. HIV-1 reverse transcriptase is a target for cytotoxic T lymphocytes in infected individuals. Science 1988;240:64–66.
92. Letvin NL, King NW. Immunologic and pathologic manifestations of the infection of rhesus monkeys with simian immunodeficiency virus of macaques. J Acquir Immune Defic Syndr 1990;3:1023–1040.
93. Phillips RE, Rowland-Jones S, Nixon DF, et al. Human immunodeficiency virus genetic variation that can escape cytotoxic T cell recognition. Nature 1991;354:453–459.
94. Collins KL, Chen BK, Kalams SA, et al. HIV-1 nef protein protects infected primary cells against killing by cytotoxic T lymphocytes. Nature 1998;391:397–401.
95. Connor RI, Chen BK, Choe S, et al. Vpr is required for efficient replication of human immunodeficiency virus type-1 in mononuclear phagocytes. Virology 1995;206:935–944.
96. Gibbs JS, Regier DA, Desrosiers RC. Construction and in vitro properties of SIVmac mutants with deletions in "nonessential" genes. AIDS Res Hum Retroviruses 1994;10:607–616.
97. Popik W, Pitha PM. The presence of tat protein or tumor necrosis factor alpha is critical for herpes simplex virus type 1–induced expression of human immunodeficiency virus type 1. J Virol 1994;68:1324–1333.
98. Heng MC, Heng SY, Allen SG. Co-infection and synergy of human immunodeficiency virus-1 and herpes simplex virus-1. Lancet 1994;343:255–258.
99. Blanchard A, Montagnier L, Gougeon ML. Influence of microbial infections on the progression of HIV disease. Trends Microbiol 1997;5:326–331.
100. Glesby MJ, Hoover DR, Farzadegan H, et al. Effect of influenza vaccination on human immunodeficiency virus type 1 load: a randomized, double-blind, placebo-controlled study. J Infect Dis 1996;174:1332–1336.
101. Vicenzi E, Biswas P, Mengozzi M, et al. Role of pro-inflammatory cytokines and beta-chemokines in controlling HIV replication. J Leukocyte Biol 1997;62:34–40.
102. Steinman RM. Dendritic cells: clinical aspects. Res Immunol 1989;140:911–927.
103. Steinman RM, Witmer-Pack M, Inaba K. Dendritic cells: antigen presentation, accessory function and clinical relevance. Adv Exp Med Biol 1993;329:1–9.
104. Fox CH, Cottler-Fox M. The pathobiology of HIV infection. Immunol Today 1992;13:353–356.
105. Fox CH, Tenner-Racz K, Racz P, et al. Lymphoid germinal centers are reservoirs of human immunodeficiency virus type 1 RNA. J Infect Dis 1991;164:1051–1057.
106. Gray D, Skarvall H. B-cell memory is short-lived in the absence of antigen. Science 1988;336:70–73.
107. Szakal AK, Kosco MH, Tew JG. A novel in vivo follicular dendritic cell–dependent icosome-mediated mechanism for delivery of antigen to antigen-processing cells. J Immunol 1988;140:341–353.
108. Burton GF, Kosco MH, Szakal AK, et al. Icosomes and the secondary antibody response. J Immunol 1991;73:271–276.
109. Lafeuillade A, Poggi C, Tamalet C, et al. Human immunodeficiency virus type 1 dynamics in different lymphoid tissue compartments. J Infect Dis 1997;175:804–806.
110. Cavert W, Notermans DW, Staskus K, et al. Kinetics of response in lymphoid tissues to antiretroviral therapy of HIV-1 infection. Science 1997;276:960–964.
111. Cameron PU, Freudenthal PS, Barker JM, et al. Dendritic cells exposed to human immunodeficiency virus type-1 transmit a vigorous cytopathic infection to CD4+ T cells. Science 1992;257:383–387.
112. Tenner-Racz K, Racz P, Bofill M, et al. HTLV-III/LAV viral antigens in lymph nodes of homosexual men with persistent generalized lymphadenopathy and AIDS. Am J Pathol 1986;123:9–15.
113. Macatonia SE, Lau R, Patterson S, et al. Dendritic cell infection, depletion and dysfunction in HIV-infected individuals. Immunology 1990;71:38–45.
114. Cameron PU, Forsum U, Teppler H, et al. During HIV-1 infection most blood dendritic cells are not productively infected and can induce allogeneic CD4+ T cells clonal expansion. Clin Exp Immunol 1992;88:226–236.
115. Spiegel H, Herbst H, Niedobitek G, et al. Follicular dendritic cells are a major reservoir for human immunodeficiency virus type 1 in lymphoid tissues facilitating infection of CD4+ T-helper cells. Am J Pathol 1992;140:15–22.
116. Braathen LR, Ramirez G, Gelderblom H, et al. Langerhans cells as primary target cells for HIV infection. Lancet 1987;87:1094.
117. Braathen LR. Langerhans cells and HIV infection. Biomed Pharmacother 1988;42:305–308.

118. Tschachler E, Groh V, Popovic M, et al. Epidermal Langerhans cells: a target for HTLV-III/LAV infection. J Invest Dermatol 1987;88: 233–237.
119. Rappersberger K, Gartner S, Schenk P, et al. Langerhans' cells are an actual site of HIV-1 replication. Intervirology 1988;29:185–194.
120. Fowke KR, Nagelkerke NJ, Kimani J, et al. Resistance to HIV-1 infection among persistently seronegative prostitutes in Nairobi, Kenya. Lancet 1996;348:1347–1351.
121. Rowland-Jones S, Sutton J, Ariyoshi K, et al. HIV-specific cytotoxic T cells in HIV-exposed but uninfected Gambian women. Nature Med 1995;1:59–64.
122. Clerici M, Levin JM, Kessler HA, et al. HIV-specific T-helper activity in seronegative health care workers exposed to contaminated blood. JAMA 1994;271:42–46.
123. Pinto LA, Sullivan J, Berzofsky JA, et al. ENV-specific cytotoxic T lymphocyte responses in HIV seronegative health care workers occupationally exposed to HIV-contaminated body fluids. J Clin Invest 1995;96:867–876.
124. Mazzoli S, Trabattoni D, Lo Caputo S, et al. HIV-specific mucosal and cellular immunity in HIV-seronegative partners of HIV-seropositive individuals. Nature Med 1997;3:1250–1257.
125. Deacon NJ, Tsykin A, Soloman A, et al. Genomic structure of an attenuated quasi species of HIV-1 from a blood transfusion donor recipients. Science 1995;270:988–991.
126. Kirchhoff F, Greenough TC, Brettler DB, et al. Brief report: absence of intact nef sequences in a long-term survivor with nonprogressive HIV-1 infection. N Engl J Med 1995;332:228–232.
127. Rosenberg ES, Billingsley JM, Caliendo AM, et al. Vigorous HIV-1–specific CD4+ T cell responses associated with control of viremia. Science 1997;278:1447–1450.
128. Connor EM, Sperling RS, Gelber R, et al. Reduction of maternal–infant transmission of human immunodeficiency virus type 1 with zidovudine treatment. N Engl J Med 1994;331:1173–1180.
129. Rowland-Jones SL, Nixon DF, Aldhous MC, et al. HIV-specific cytotoxic T-cell activity in an HIV-exposed but uninfected infant. Lancet 1993;341:860–861.
130. Ivanoff LA, Looney DJ, McDanal C, et al. Alteration of HIV-1 infectivity and neutralization by a single amino acid replacement in the V3 loop domain. AIDS Res Hum Retroviruses 1991;7:595–603.
131. Javaherian K, Langlois AJ, Larosa GJ, et al. Broadly neutralizing antibodies elicited by the hypervariable neutralizing determinant of HIV-1. Science 1990;250:1590–1593.
132. Ho DD, Kaplan JC, Rackauskas IE, et al. Second conserved domain of gp120 is important for HIV infectivity and antibody neutralization. Science 1988;239:1021–1023.
133. Larosa GJ, Davide JP, Weinhold K, et al. Conserved sequence and structural elements in the HIV-1 principal neutralizing determinants. Science 1990;249:932–935.
134. Putney SD, McKeating JA. Antigenic variation in HIV. AIDS 1990; 4(Suppl) 1:S129–S136.
135. Moore JP, Nara PL. The role of the V3 loop of gp120 in HIV infection. AIDS 1991;5(Suppl 2):S21–S33.
136. Hwang SS, Boyle TJ, Lyerly HK, et al. Identification of the envelope V3 loop as the primary determinant of cell tropism in HIV-1. Science 1991;253:71–74.
137. Page KA, Stearns SM, Littman DR. Analysis of mutations in the V3 domain of gp160 that affect fusion and infectivity. J Virol 1992;66: 524–533.
138. Wyatt R, Sullivan N, Thali M, et al. Functional and immunologic characterization of human immunodeficiency virus type 1 envelope glycoproteins containing deletions of the major variable regions. J Virol 1993;67:4557–4565.
139. Ho DD, McKeating JA, Li XL, et al. Conformational epitope on gp120 important in CD4 binding and human immunodeficiency virus type 1 neutralization identified by a human monoclonal antibody. J Virol 1991;65:489–493.
140. Thali M, Olshevsky U, Furman C, et al. Characterization of a discontinuous human immunodeficiency virus type 1 gp120 epitope recognized by a broadly reactive neutralizing human monoclonal antibody. J Virol 1991;65:6188–6193.
141. Skinner MA, Langlois AJ, McDanal CB, et al. Neutralizing antibodies to an immunodominant envelope sequence do not prevent gp120 binding to CD4. J Virol 1988;62:4195–4200.
142. Steimer KS, Scandella CJ, Skiles PV, et al. Neutralization of divergent HIV-1 isolates by conformation-dependent human antibodies to gp120. Science 1991;254:105–108.
143. Thali M, Furman C, Ho DD, et al. Discontinuous, conserved neutralization epitopes overlapping the CD4-binding region of human immunodeficiency virus type 1 gp120 envelope glycoprotein. J Virol 1992;66:5635–5641.
144. Kang CY, Nara P, Chamat S, et al. Anti-idiotype monoclonal antibody elicits broadly neutralizing anti-gp120 antibodies in monkeys. Proc Natl Acad Sci U S A 1992;89:2546–2550.
145. Tilley SA, Honnen WJ, Racho ME, et al. Synergistic neutralization of HIV-1 by human monoclonal antibodies against the V3 loop and the CD4-binding site of gp120. AIDS Res Hum Retroviruses 1992;8: 461–467.
146. Fung MS, Sun CR, Gordon WL, et al. Identification and characterization of a neutralization site within the second variable region of human immunodeficiency virus type 1 gp120. J Virol 1992;66: 848–856.
147. Ho DD, Fung MS, Yoshiyama H, et al. Discontinuous epitopes on gp120 important in HIV-1 neutralization. AIDS Res Hum Retroviruses 1992;8:1337–1339.
148. Sullivan N, Thali M, Furman C, et al. Effect of amino acid changes in the V1/V2 region of the human immunodeficiency virus type 1 gp120 glycoprotein on subunit association, syncytium formation, and recognition by a neutralizing antibody. J Virol 1993;67:3674–3679.
149. McKeating JA, Shotton C, Cordell J, et al. Characterization of neutralizing monoclonal antibodies to linear and conformation-dependent epitopes within the first and second variable domains of human immunodeficiency virus type 1 gp120. J Virol 1993;67:4932–4944.
150. Muster T, Steindl F, Purtscher M, et al. A conserved neutralizing epitope on gp41 of human immunodeficiency virus type 1. J Virol 1993;67:6642–6647.
151. Chanh TC, Dreesman GR, Kanda P, et al. Induction of anti-HIV neutralizing antibodies by synthetic peptides. EMBO J 1986;5: 3065–3071.
152. Ho DD, Sarngadharan MG, Hirsch MS, et al. Human immunodeficiency virus neutralizing antibodies recognize several conserved domains on the envelope glycoproteins. J Virol 1987;61:2124–2128.
153. Botarelli P, Houlden BA, Haigwood NL, et al. N-glycosylation of HIV-gp120 may constrain recognition by T lymphocytes. J Immunol 1991;147:3128–3132.
154. Haigwood NL, Nara PL, Brooks E, et al. Native but not denatured recombinant human immunodeficiency virus type 1 gp120 generates broad-spectrum neutralizing antibodies in baboons. J Virol 1992;66: 172–182.
155. Wyatt R, Thali M, Tilley S, et al. Relationship of the human immunodeficiency virus type 1 gp120 third variable loop to a component of the CD4 binding site in the fourth conserved region. J Virol 1992;66:6997–7004.
156. Thali M, Furman C, Wahren B, et al. Cooperativity of neutralizing antibodies directed against the V3 and CD4 binding regions of the human immunodeficiency virus gp120 envelope glycoprotein. J Acquir Immune Defic Syndr 1992;5:591–599.
157. Lu M, Blacklow SC, Kim PS. A trimeric structural domain of the HIV-1 transmembrane glycoprotein. Nat Struct Biol 1995;2:1075–1082.
158. Lee WR, Syu WJ, Du B, et al. Nonrandom distribution of gp120 N-linked glycosylation sites important for infectivity of human immunodeficiency virus type 1. Proc Natl Acad Sci U S A 1992;89: 2213–2217.
159. Sattentau QJ, Moore JP. Human immunodeficiency virus type 1 neutralization is determined by epitope exposure of the gp120 oligomer. J Exp Med 1995;182:185–196.

160. Benjouad A, Gluckman JC, Rochat H, et al. Influence of carbohydrate moieties on the immunogenicity of human immunodeficiency virus type 1 recombinant gp160. J Virol 1992;66:2473–2483.
161. Moore JP, Cao Y, Qing L, et al. Primary isolates of human immunodeficiency virus type 1 are relatively resistant to neutralization by monoclonal antibodies to gp120, and their neutralization is not predicted by studies with monomeric gp120. J Virol 1995;69:101–109.
162. Montefiori DC, Collman RG, Fouts TR, et al. Evidence that antibody-mediated neutralization of human immunodeficiency virus type 1 by sera from infected individuals is independent of co-receptor usage. J Virol 1998;72:1886–1893.
163. Trkola A, Ketas T, Kewal Ramani VN, et al. Neutralization sensitivity of human immunodeficiency virus type 1 primary isolates to antibodies and CD4-based reagents is independent of co-receptor usage. J Virol 1998;72:1876–1885.
164. Tyler DS, Stanley SD, Nastala CA, et al. Alterations in antibody-dependent cellular cytotoxicity during the course of HIV-1 infection: humoral and cellular defects. J Immunol 1990;144:3375–3384.
165. Baum LL, Cassutt KJ, Knigge K, et al. HIV-1 gp120-specific antibody-dependent cell-mediated cytotoxicity correlates with rate of disease progression. J Immunol 1996;157:2168–2173.
166. Tyler DS, Stanley SD, Zolla-Pazner SB, et al. Identification of sites within gp41 that serve as targets for antibody-dependent cellular cytotoxicity by using human monoclonal antibodies. J Immunol 1990;145:3276–3282.
167. Ada G, Leung KN, Erti H. An analysis of effector T cell generation and function in mice exposed to influenza A or Sendai viruses. Immunol Rev 1981;58:5–24.
168. Zinkernagel RM, Rosenthal KL. Experiments and speculation on antiviral specificity of T and B cells. Immunol Rev 1981;58:131–155.
169. Lu LY, Askonas BA. Cross-reactivity for different type A influenza viruses of a cloned T-killer cell line. Nature 1980;288:164–165.
170. Ferrari G, Humphrey W, McElrath MJ, et al. Clade B-based HIV-1 vaccines elicit cross-clade cytotoxic T lymphocyte reactivities in uninfected volunteers. Proc Natl Acad Sci U S A 1997;94:1396–1401.
171. Cao H, Kanki P, Sankale JL, et al. Cytotoxic T-lymphocyte cross-reactivity among different human immunodeficiency virus type 1 clades: implications for vaccine development. J Virol 1997;71:8615–8623.
172. Bertoletti A, Cham F, McAdam S, et al. Cytotoxic T cells from human immunodeficiency virus type 2–infected patients frequently cross-react with different human immunodeficiency virus type 1 clades. J Virol 1998;72:2439–2448.
173. Borrow P, Lewicki H, Wei X, et al. Antiviral pressure exerted by HIV-1–specific cytotoxic T lymphocytes (CTLs) during primary infection demonstrated by rapid selection of CTL escape virus. Nature Med 1997;3:205–211.
174. Price DA, Goulder PJR, Klenerman P, et al. Positive selection of HIV-1 cytotoxic T lymphocyte escape variants during primary infection. Proc Natl Acad Sci U S A 1997;94:1890–1895.
175. Rowland-Jones SL, Phillips RE, et al. Human immunodeficiency virus variants that escape cytotoxic T-cell recognition. AIDS Res Hum Retroviruses 1992;8:1353–1354.
176. Pantaleo G, Demarest JF, Soudeyns H, et al. Major expansion of CD8+ T cells with a predominant V beta usage during the primary immune response to HIV. Nature 1994;370:463–467.
177. Pantaleo G, Demarest JF, Schacker T, et al. The qualitative nature of the primary immune response to HIV infection is a prognosticator of disease progression independent of the initial level of plasma viremia. Proc Natl Acad Sci U S A 1997;94:254–258.
178. Masson D, Zamai M, Tschopp J. Identification of granzyme A isolated from cytotoxic T-lymphocyte granules as one of the proteases encoded by CTL-specific genes. FEBS Lett 1986;208:84–88.
179. Masson D, Tschopp J. A family of serine esterases in lytic granules of cytolytic T lymphocytes. Cell 1987;49:679–685.
180. Takayama H, Kojima H, Shinohara N. Cytotoxic T lymphocytes: the newly identified Fas (CD95)–mediated killing mechanism and a novel aspect of their biological functions. Adv Immunol 1995;60:289–321.
181. Walker CM, Moody DJ, Stites DP, et al. CD8+ lymphocytes can control HIV infection in vitro by suppressing virus replication. Science 1986;234:1563–1566.
182. Mackewicz CE, Blackbourn DJ, Levy JA. CD8+ T cells suppress human immunodeficiency virus replication by inhibiting viral transcription. Proc Natl Acad Sci U S A 1995;92:2308–2312.
183. Mackewicz CE, Levy JA, Cruikshank WW, et al. Role of IL-16 in HIV replication. Nature 1996;383:488–489.
184. Siliciano RF, Lawton T, Knall C, et al. Analysis of host–virus interactions in AIDS with anti-gp120 T cell clones: effect of HIV sequence variation and a mechanism for CD4+ cell depletion. Cell 1988;54:561–575.
185. Stanhope PE, Liu AY, Pavlat W, et al. An HIV-1 envelope protein vaccine elicits a functionally complex human CD4+ T cell response that includes cytolytic T lymphocytes. J Immunol 1993;150:4672–4686.
186. Cease KB. Peptide component vaccine engineering: targeting the AIDS virus. Int Rev Immunol 1990;7:85–107.
187. Clerici M, Shearer GM. A Th→Th2 switch is a critical step in the etiology of HIV infection. Immunol Today 1993;14:107–111.
188. Street NE, Mosmann TR. Functional diversity of T lymphocytes due to secretion of different cytokine patterns. FASEB J 1991;5:171–177.
189. Tang YW, Graham BS. Potential for directing appropriate responses to vaccines by cytokine manipulation. Clin Immunother 1996;5:327–333.
190. Chin J, Magoffin RL, Shearer LA, et al. Field evaluation of a respiratory syncytial virus vaccine and a trivalent parainfluenza virus vaccine in a pediatric population. Am J Epidemiol 1969;89:449–463.
191. Fulginiti VA, Eller JJ, Sieber OF, et al. Respiratory virus immunization. I. A field trial of two inactivated respiratory virus vaccines: an aqueous trivalent parainfluenza virus vaccine and an alum-precipitated respiratory syncytial virus vaccine. Am J Epidemiol 1969;89:435–448.
192. Kim HW, Canchola JG, Brandt CD, et al. Respiratory syncytial virus disease in infants despite prior administration of antigenic inactivated vaccine. Am J Epidemiol 1969;89:422–434.
193. Kapikian AZ, Mitchell RH, Chanock RM, et al. An epidemiologic study of altered clinical reactivity to respiratory syncytial (RS) virus infection in children previously vaccinated with an inactivated RS virus vaccine. Am J Epidemiol 1969;89:405–421.
194. Waris ME, Tsou C, Erdman DD, et al. Respiratory syncytial virus infection in BALB/c mice previously immunized with formalin-inactivated virus induces enhanced pulmonary inflammatory response with a predominant Th2-like cytokine pattern. J Virol 1996;70:2852–2860.
195. Alwan WH, Kozlowska WJ, Openshaw PJM. Distinct types of lung disease caused by functional subsets of antiviral T cells. J Exp Med 1994;179:81–89.
196. Graham BS. Immunological determinants of disease caused by respiratory syncytial virus. Trends Microbiol 1995;4:290–294.
197. Chun TW, Chadwick K, Margolick J, et al. Differential susceptibility of naive and memory CD4+ T cells to the cytopathic effects of infection with human immunodeficiency virus type 1 strain LAI. J Virol 1997;71:4436–4444.
198. Connors M, Kovacs J, Krevat S, et al. HIV infection induces changes in CD4+ T-cell phenotype and depletions within the CD4+ T-cell repertoire that are not immediately restored by antiviral or immune-based therapies. Nature Med 1997;3:533–540.
199. Hocini H, Belec L, Iscaki S, et al. High-level ability of secretory IgA to block HIV type 1 transcytosis: contrasting secretory IgA and IgG responses to glycoprotein 160. AIDS Res Hum Retroviruses 1997;13:1179–1185.
200. Janoff EN, Wahl SM, Thomas K, et al. Modulation of human immunodeficiency virus type 1 infection of human monocytes by IgA. J Infect Dis 1995;172:855–858.
201. Musey L, Hughes J, Schacker T, et al. Cytotoxic T-cell responses, viral load, and disease progression in early human immunodeficiency virus type 1 infection. N Engl J Med 1997;337:1267–1274.

202. Porterfield JS. Antibody-dependent enhancement of viral infectivity. Adv Virus Res 1986;31:335–355.
203. Halstead SB, O'Rourke EJ. Antibody-enhanced dengue virus infection in primate leukocytes. Nature 1977;265:739–741.
204. Montefiori DC, Lefkowitz LB Jr, Keller RE, et al. Absence of a clinical correlation for complement-mediated, infection-enhancing antibodies in plasma or sera from HIV-1–infected individuals: Multicenter AIDS Cohort Study Group. AIDS 1991;5:513–517.
205. Homsy J, Meyer M, Tateno M, et al. The Fc and not CD4 receptor mediates antibody enhancement of HIV infection in human cells. Science 1989;244:1357–1360.
206. Kliks S. Antibody-enhanced infection of monocytes as the pathogenetic mechanism for severe dengue illness. AIDS Res Hum Retroviruses 1990;6:993–998.
207. Takeda A, Robinson JE, Ho DD, et al. Distinction of human immunodeficiency virus type 1 neutralization and infection enhancement by human monoclonal antibodies to glycoprotein 120. J Clin Invest 1992;89:1952–1957.
208. Robinson WD Jr, Montefiori DC, Mitchell WM. Antibody-dependent enhancement of human immunodeficiency virus type 1 infection. Lancet 1988;1:790–794.
209. Jiang SB, Lin K, Neurath AR. Enhancement of human immunodeficiency virus type 1 infection by antisera to peptides from the envelope glycoproteins gp120/gp41. J Exp Med 1991;174:1557–1563.
210. Robinson WE Jr, Gorny MK, Xu JY, et al. Two immunodominant domains of gp41 bind antibodies which enhance human immunodeficiency virus type 1 infection in vitro. J Virol 1991;65:4169–4176.
211. Oldstone MBA, Notkins AL. Molecular mimicry. In: Notkins AL, Oldstone MBA, eds. Concepts in viral pathogenesis II. New York: Springer Verlag, 1986:195–202.
212. Johnson RT, Griffin DE. Virus-induced autoimmune demyelinating disease of the central nervous system. In: Notkins AL, Oldstone MBA, eds. Concepts in viral pathogenesis II. New York: Springer Verlag, 1986:203–209.
213. Sarin PS, Sun DK, Thornton AH, et al. Neutralization of HTLV-III/LAV replication by antiserum to thymosin alpha 1. Science 1986;232:1135–1137.
214. Lee MR, Ho DD, Gurney ME. Functional interaction and partial homology between human immunodeficiency virus and neuroleukin. Science 1987;237:1047–1051.
215. Ruff MR, Martin BM, Ginns ME, et al. CD4 receptor binding peptides that block HIV infectivity cause human monocyte chemotaxis. FEBS Lett 1987;211:17–22.
216. Reiher WE, Blalock JE, Brunck TK. Sequence homology between acquired immunodeficiency syndrome virus envelope protein and interleukin 2. Proc Natl Acad Sci U S A 1986;83:9188–9192.
217. Golding H, Robey FA, Gates FTI, et al. Identification of homologous regions in human immunodeficiency virus I gp41 and human MHC class II β1 domain. J Exp Med 1988;167:914–923.
218. Golding H, Shearer GM, Hillman K, et al. Common epitope in human immunodeficiency virus (HIV) 1: GP41 and HLA class II elicits immunosuppressive autoantibodies capable of contributing to immune dysfunction in HIV 1–infected individuals. J Clin Invest 1989;83:1430–1435.
219. Keay S, Tacket CO, Murphy JR, et al. Anti-CD4 anti-idiotype antibodies in volunteers immunized with rgp160 of HIV-1 or infected with HIV-1. AIDS Res Hum Retroviruses 1992;8:1091–1098.
220. Graham BS, Matthews TJ, Belshe RB, et al. Augmentation of human immunodeficiency virus type1 neutralizing antibody by priming with gp160 recombinant vaccinia and boosting with rgp160 in vaccinia-naive adults: the NIAID AIDS Vaccine Clinical Trials Network. J Infect Dis 1993;167:533–537.
221. Wang CY, Looney DJ, Li ML, et al. Long-term high-titer neutralizing activity induced by octameric synthetic HIV-1 antigen. Science 1991;254:285–288.
222. Defoort JP, Nardelli B, Huang W, et al. Macromolecular assemblage in the design of a synthetic AIDS vaccine. Proc Natl Acad Sci U S A 1992;89:3879–3883.
223. Palker TJ, Matthews TJ, Langlois A, et al. Polyvalent human immunodeficiency virus synthetic immunogen comprised of envelope gp120 T helper cell sites and B cell neutralization epitopes. J Immunol 1989;142:3612–3619.
224. Ahlers JD, Dunlop N, Pendleton CD, et al. Candidate HIV type 1 multideterminant cluster peptide-P18MN vaccine constructs elicit type 1 helper T cells, cytotoxic T cells, and neutralizing antibody, all using the same adjuvant immunization. AIDS Res Hum Retroviruses 1996;12:259–272.
225. Papsidero LD, Sheu M, Ruscetti FW. Human immunodeficiency virus type 1–neutralizing monoclonal antibodies which react with p17 core protein: characterization and epitope mapping. J Virol 1989;63:267–272.
226. Haffar O, Garrigues J, Travis B, et al. Human immunodeficiency virus-like, nonreplicating, gag-env particles assemble in a recombinant vaccinia virus expression system. J Virol 1990;64:2653–2659.
227. Shioda T, Shibuta H. Production of human immunodeficiency virus (HIV)–like particles from cells infected with recombinant vaccinia viruses carrying the gag gene of HIV. Virology 1990;175:139–148.
228. Spearman P, Wang JJ, Vander Heyden N, et al. Identification of human immunodeficiency virus type 1 Gag protein domains essential to membrane binding and particle assembly. J Virol 1994;68:3232–3242.
229. Daniel MD, Mazzara GP, Simon MA, et al. High-titer immune responses elicited by recombinant vaccinia virus priming and particle boosting are ineffective in preventing virulent SIV infection. AIDS Res Hum Retroviruses 1994;10:839–851.
230. Adams SE, Burns NR, Layton GT, et al. Hybrid Ty virus-like particles. Int Rev Immunol 1994;11:133–141.
231. Mills KH, Kitchin PA, Mahon BP, et al. HIV p24-specific helper T cell clones from immunized primates recognize highly conserved regions of HIV-1. J Immunol 1990;144:1677–1683.
232. Griffiths JC, Berrie EL, Holdsworth LN, et al. Induction of high-titer neutralizing antibodies, using hybrid human immunodeficiency virus V3-Ty viruslike particles in a clinically relevant adjuvant. J Virol 1991;65:450–456.
233. Moss B. Vaccinia virus: a tool for research and vaccine development. Science 1991;252:1662–1667.
234. Panicali D, Paoletti E. Construction of poxvirus as cloning vectors: insertion of the thymidine kinase gene from herpes simplex virus into the DNA of infectious vaccinia virus. Proc Natl Acad Sci U S A 1982;79:4927–4931.
235. Buller RM, Smith GL, Cremer K, et al. Decreased virulence of recombinant vaccinia virus expression vectors is associated with a thymidine kinase–negative phenotype. Nature 1985;317:813–815.
236. Redfield RR, Wright DC, James WD, et al. Disseminated vaccinia in a military recruit with human immunodeficiency virus (HIV) disease. N Engl J Med 1987;316:673–676.
237. Guillaume JC, Saiag P, Wechsler J, et al. Vaccinia from recombinant virus expressing HIV genes. Lancet 1991;337:1034–1035.
238. Tartaglia J, Cox WI, Taylor J, et al. Live vectors as vaccines: highly attenuated poxvirus vectors. AIDS Res Hum Retroviruses 1992;8:1445–1447.
239. Tartaglia J, Perkus ME, Taylor J, et al. NYVAC: a highly attenuated strain of vaccinia virus. Virology 1992;188:217–232.
240. Paoletti E. Applications of pox virus vectors to vaccination: an update. Proc Natl Acad Sci U S A 1996;93:11349–11353.
241. Loker EF Jr, Hodges GR, Kelly DJ. Fatal adenovirus pneumonia in a young adult associated with ADV-7 vaccine administered 15 days earlier. Chest 1974;66:197–199.
242. Porter DC, Wang J, Moldoveanu Z, et al. Immunization of mice with poliovirus replicons expressing the C-fragment of tetanus toxin protects against lethal challenge with tetanus toxin. Vaccine 1997;15:257–264.
243. Porter DC, Ansardi DC, Choi WS, et al. Encapsidation of genetically engineered poliovirus minireplicons which express human immunodeficiency virus type 1 Gag and Pol proteins upon infection. J Virol 1993;67:3712–3719.

244. Muster T, Ferko B, Klima A, et al. Mucosal model of immunization against human immunodeficiency virus type 1 with a chimeric influenza virus. J Virol 1996;69:6678–6686.
245. Arnold GF, Resnick DA, Smith AD, et al. Chimeric rhinoviruses as tools for vaccine development and characterization of protein epitopes. Intervirology 1996;39:72–78.
246. Grene E, Mezule G, Borisova G, et al. Relationship between antigenicity and immunogenicity of chimeric hepatitis B virus core particles carrying HIV type 1 epitopes. AIDS Res Hum Retroviruses 1997;13:41–51.
247. Koletzki D, Zankl A, Gelderblom HR, et al. Mosaic hepatitis B virus core particles allow insertion of extended foreign protein segments. J Gen Virol 1997;78:2049–2053.
248. Caley IJ, Betts MR, Irlbeck DM, et al. Humoral, mucosal, and cellular immunity in response to a human immunodeficiency virus type 1 immunogen expressed by a Venezuelan equine encephalitis virus vaccine vector. J Virol 1997;71:3031–3038.
249. Davis NL, Brown KW, Johnston RE. A viral vaccine vector that expresses foreign genes in lymph nodes and protects against mucosal challenge. J Virol 1996;70:3781–3787.
250. Manning WC, Paliard X, Zhou S, et al. Genetic immunization with adeno-associated virus vectors expressing herpes simplex virus type 2 glycoproteins B and D. J Virol 1997;71:7960–7962.
251. Irwin MJ, Laube LS, Lee V, et al. Direct injection of a recombinant retroviral vector induces human immunodeficiency virus-specific immune responses in mice and nonhuman primates. J Virol 1994;68:5036–5044.
252. Curtiss R, Galan JE, Nakayama K, et al. Stabilization of recombinant a virulent vaccine strains in vivo. Res Microbiol 1990;141:797–805.
253. Cattozzo EM, Stocker BA, Radaelli A, et al. Expression and immunogenicity of V3 loop epitopes of HIV-1, isolates SC and WMJ2, inserted in *Salmonella* flagellin. J Biotechnol 1997;56:191–203.
254. Hone DM, Wu S, Powell RJ, et al. Optimization of live oral *Salmonella*-HIV-1 vaccine vectors for the induction of HIV-specific mucosal and systemic immune responses. J Biotechnol 1996;44:203–207.
255. Colston MJ. Rebirth of a star performer. Nature 1991;351:479–482.
256. Aldovini A, Young RA. Humoral and cell-mediated immune responses to live recombinant BCG–HIV vaccines. Nature 1991;351:479–482.
257. Stover CK, de la Cruz VF, Fuerst TR, et al. New use of BCG for recombinant vaccines. Nature 1991;351:456–460.
258. Murray PJ, Aldovini A, Young RA. Manipulation and potentiation of antimycobacterial immunity using recombinant bacille Calmette-Guérin strains that secrete cytokines. Proc Natl Acad Sci U S A 1996;93:934–939.
259. Lapham C, Golding B, Inman J, et al. Brucella abortus conjugated with a peptide derived from the V3 loop of human immunodeficiency virus (HIV) type 1 induces HIV-specific cytotoxic T-cell responses in normal and in CD4+ cell–depleted BALB/c mice. J Virol 1996;70:3084–3092.
260. Frankel FR, Hegde S, Lieberman J, et al. Induction of cell-mediated immune responses to human immunodeficiency virus type 1 gag protein by using Listeria monocytogenes as a live vaccine vector. J Immunol 1995;155:4775–4782.
261. Atkins GJ, Sheahan BJ, Liljestrom P. Manipulation of the Semliki Forest virus genome and its potential for vaccine construction. Mol Biotechnol 1996;5:33–38.
262. Stott EJ. Anti-cell antibody in macaques. Nature 1991;353:393.
263. Arthur LO, Bess JW Jr, Sowder RC, et al. Cellular proteins bound to immunodeficiency viruses: implications for pathogenesis and vaccines. Science 1992;258:1935–1938.
264. Montefiori DC, Cornell RJ, Zhou JY, et al. Complement control proteins, CD46, CD55, and CD59, as common surface constituents of human and simian immunodeficiency viruses and possible targets for vaccine protection. Virology 1994;205:82–92.
265. Arthur LO, Bess JW, Urban RG, et al. Macaques immunized with HLA-DR are protected from challenge with simian immunodeficiency virus. J Virol 1995;69:3117–3124.
266. Chan WL, Rodgers A, Grief C, et al. Immunization with class I human histocompatibility leukocyte antigen can protect macaques against challenge infection with SIVmac-32H. AIDS 1995;9:223–228.
267. Watanabe M, Chen ZW, Tsubota H, et al. Soluble human CD4 elicits an antibody response in rhesus monkeys that inhibits simian immunodeficiency virus replication. Proc Natl Acad Sci U S A 1991;88:120–124.
268. Ruprecht RM, Baba TW, Liska V. Attenuated HIV vaccine: caveats. Science 1996;271:1790–1791.
269. Wooley DP, Smith RA, Czajak S, et al. Direct demonstration of retroviral recombination in a rhesus monkey. J Virol 1997;71:9650–9653.
270. Whatmore AM, Cook N, Hall GA, et al. Repair and evolution of *nef* in vivo modulates simian immunodeficiency virus virulence. J Virol 1995;69:5117–5123.
271. Stahlhennig C, Dittmer U, Nisslein T, et al. Attenuated SIV imparts immunity to challenge with pathogenic spleen-derived SIV but cannot prevent repair of the nef deletion. Immunol Lett 1996;51:129–135.
272. Daniel MD, Kirchhoff F, Czajak SC, et al. Protective effects of a live attenuated SIV vaccine with a delention in the *nef* gene. Science 1992;258:1938–1941.
273. Desrosiers RC. HIV with multiple gene deletions as a live attenuated vaccine for AIDS. AIDS Res Hum Retroviruses 1992;8:411–421.
274. Giavedoni LD, Yilma T. Construction and characterization of replication-competent simian immunodeficiency virus vectors that express gamma interferon. J Virol 1996;70:2247–2251.
275. Smith SM, Markham RB, Jeang KT. Conditional reduction of human immunodeficiency virus type 1 replication by a gain of herpes simplex virus 1 thymidine kinase function. Proc Natl Acad Sci U S A 1996;93:7955–7960.
276. Travers K, MBoup S, Marlink R, et al. Natural protection against HIV-1 infection provided by HIV-2. Science 1995;268:1612–1615.
277. Li J, Lord CI, Haseltine W, et al. Infection of cynomolgus monkeys with a chimeric HIV-1/SIVmac virus that expresses the HIV-1 envelope glycoproteins. J Acquir Immune Defic Syndr 1992;5:639–646.
278. Alving CR. Lipopolysaccharide, lipid A, and liposomes containing lipid A as immunologic adjuvants. Immunology 1993;187:430–446.
279. Byars NE, Allison AC, Harmon MW, et al. Enhancement of antibody responses to influenza B virus haemagglutinin by use of a new adjuvant formulation. Vaccine 1990;8:49–56.
280. Pye AD, Vandenberg KL, Dyer SL, et al. Selection of an adjuvant for vaccination with the malaria antigen, MSA-2. Vaccine 1997;15:1017–1023.
281. Warren HS, Vogel RF, Chedid LA. Current status of immunological adjuvants. Annu Rev Immunol 1986;4:369–388.
282. Deres K, Schild H, Wiesmuller K, et al. In vivo priming of virus-specific cytotoxic T lymphocytes with synthetic lipopeptide vaccine. Nature 1989;342:561–564.
283. Dranoff G, Jaffe E, Lazenby A, et al. Vaccination with irradiated tumor cells engineered to secrete murine granulocyte–macrophage colony-stimulating factor stimulates potent, specific, and long-lasting anti-tumor immunity. Proc Natl Acad Sci U S A 1993;90:3539–3543.
284. Eldridge JH, Staas JK, Meulbroek JA, et al. Biogradable microspheres as a vaccine delivery system. Mol Immunol 1991;28:287–294.
285. Moldoveanu Z, Novak M, Huang WQ, et al. Oral immunization with influenza virus in biodegradable microspheres. J Infect Dis 1993;167:84–90.
286. Mannino RJ, Gould-Fogerite S. Lipid matrix-based vaccines for mucosal and systemic immunization. Pharmacol Biotech 1995;6:363–387.
287. Gould-Fogerite S, Edghill-Smith Y, Kheiri M, et al. Lipid matrix-based subunit vaccines: a structure-function approach to oral and parenteral immunization. AIDS Res Hum Retroviruses 1994;10(Suppl):S99–S103.
288. Ramsay AJ, Husband AJ, Ramshaw IA, et al. The role of interleukin-6 in mucosal IgA antibody responses in vivo. Science 1994;264:561–563.

289. Gizurarson S, Tamura S, Aizawa C, et al. Simulation of the transepithelial flux of influenza HA vaccine by cholera toxin B subunit. Vaccine 1992;10:101–106.
290. Porgador A, Staats HF, Faiola B, et al. Intranasal immunization with CTL epitope peptides from HIV-1 or ovalbumin and the mucosal adjuvant cholera toxin induces peptide-specific CTLs and protection against tumor development in vivo. J Immunol 1997;158:834–841.
291. World Health Organization. Requirements for poliomyelitis vaccine (oral). WHO Tech Rep Ser 1983;687:107.
292. Gordon JE. The preparation and use of yellow fever vaccine. In: Virus and rickettsial diseases. Cambridge, MA: Harvard University Press, 1948:767–788.
293. Horstmann DM. The use of primates in experimental viral infections: rubella and the rubella syndrome. Ann N Y Acad Sci 1969;162:594–597.
294. Hollinger FB, Dressman GR, Sanchez Y, et al. Experimental hepatitis B polypeptide vaccine in chimpanzees. In: Vyas GN, Cohen SN, Schmid R, eds. Viral hepatitis. Philadelphia: Franklin Institute Press, 1978:557.
295. Hilleman MR, McAleer WJ, Buynak EB, et al. The preparation and safety of hepatitis B vaccine. J Infect Dis 1983;7(Suppl) 1:3–8.
296. La Monica N, Almond JW, Racaniello VR. A mouse model for poliovirus neurovirulence identifies mutations that attenuate the virus for man. J Virol 1987;61:2917–2920.
297. Melnick JL. Live attenuated poliovaccines. In: Plotkin SA, Motimer EA, eds. Vaccines. Philadelphia: WB Saunders, 1988:115–157.
298. Weibel RE. Mumps vaccine. In: Plotkin SA, Motimer EA, eds. Vaccines. Philadelphia: WB Saunders, 1988:223–234.
299. Villinger F, Brar SS, Brice GT, et al. Immune and hematopoietic parameters in HIV-1 infected chimpanzees during clinical progression toward AIDS. J Med Primatol 1997;26:11–18.
300. Novembre FJ, Saucier M, Anderson DC, et al. Development of AIDS in a chimpanzee infected with human immunodeficiency virus type 1. J Virol 1997;71:4086–4091.
301. Anderson KP, Lucas C, Hanson CV, et al. Effect of dose and immunization schedule on immune response of baboons to recombinant glycoprotein 120 of HIV-1. J Infect Dis 1989;160:960–969.
302. Stephens DM, Eichberg JW, Haigwood NL, et al. Antibodies are produced to the variable regions of the external envelope glycoprotein of human immunodeficiency virus type 1 in chimpanzees infected with the virus and baboons immunized with a candidate recombinant vaccine. J Gen Virol 1992;73:1099–1106.
303. Jin MJ, Rogers J, Phillips-Conroy JE, et al. Infection of a yellow baboon with simian immunodeficiency virus from African green monkeys: evidence for cross-species transmission in the wild. J Virol 1994;68:8454–8460.
304. Castro BA, Nepomuceno M, Lerche NW, et al. Persistent infection of baboons and rhesus monkeys with different strains of HIV-2. Virology 1991;184:219–226.
305. Allan JS, Ray P, Broussard S, et al. Infection of baboons with simian human immunodeficiency viruses. J Acquir Immune Defic Syndr Hum Retrovirol 1995;9:429–441.
306. Barnett SW, Murthy KK, Herndier BG, et al. An AIDS-like condition induced in baboons by HIV-2. Science 1994;266:642–646.
307. Fultz PN, McClure HM, Anderson DC, et al. Identification and biologic characterization of an acutely lethal variant of simian immunodeficiency virus from sooty mangabeys (SIV/SMM). AIDS Res Hum Retroviruses 1989;5:397–409.
308. Hirsch VM, Goldstein S, Hynes NA, et al. Prolonged clinical latency and survival of macaques given a whole inactivated simian immunodeficiency virus vaccine. J Infect Dis 1994;170:51–59.
309. Rida W, Meier P, Stevens C. Design and implementation of HIV vaccine efficacy trials: a working group summary. AIDS Res Hum Retroviruses 1993;9:S59–S63.
310. Deng HK, Unutmaz D, Kewal Ramani VN, et al. Expression cloning of new receptors used by simian and human immunodeficiency viruses. Nature 1997;388:296–300.
311. Lekutis C, Letvin NL. HIV-1 envelope-specific CD4+ T helper cells from simian/human immunodeficiency virus-infected rhesus monkeys recognize epitopes restricted by MHC class II DRB1*0406 and DRB*W201 molecules. J Immunol 1997;159:2049–2057.
312. Yasutomi Y, McAdam SN, Boyson JE, et al. A MHC class 1B locus allele-resricted simian immunodeficiency virus envelope CTL epitope in rhesus monkeys. J Immunol 1995;154:2516–2522.
313. Watanabe N, McAdam SN, Boyson JE, et al. A simian immunodeficiency virus envelope V3 cytotoxic T-lymphocyte epitope in rhesus monkeys and its restricting major histocompatibilty complex class I molecule Manu-A*02. J Virol 1994;68:6690–6696.
314. Shen L, Chen ZW, Letvin NL. The repertoire of cytoxic T lymphocytes in the recognition of mutant simian immunodeficiency virus variants. J Immunol 1994;153:5849–5854.
315. Chen ZW, Shen L, Miller MD, et al. Cytotoxic T lymphocytes do not appear to select for mutations in an immunodominant epitope of simian immunodeficiency virus gag. J Immunol 1992;149:4060–4066.
316. Miller MD, Yamamoto H, Hughes AL, et al. Definition of an epitope and MHC class I molecule recognized by gag-specific cytotoxic T lymphocytes in SIVmac-infected rhesus monkeys. J Immunol 1991;147:320–329.
317. Shen L, Chen ZW, Miller MD, et al. Recombinant virus vaccine-induced SIV-specific CD8+ cytotoxic T lymphocytes. Science 1991;252:440–443.
318. Villinger F, Brar SS, Mayne A, et al. Comparative sequence analysis of cytokine genes from human and nonhuman primates. J Virol 1995;155:3946–3954.
319. Zou W, Lackner AA, Simon M, et al. Early cytokine and chemokine gene expression in lymph nodes of macaques infected with simian immunodeficiency virus is predictive of disease outcome and vaccine efficacy. J Virol 1997;71:1227–1236.
320. Zhang D, Johnson RP. Molecular cloning and comparative analysis of the rhesus macaque co-stimulatory molecules CD80 (B7-1) and CD86 (B7-2). Cell Immunol 1997;177:9–17.
321. Stone JD, Heise CC, Canfield DR, et al. Differences in viral distribution and cell adhesion molecule expression in the intestinal tract of rhesus macaques infected with pathogenic and nonpathogenic SIV. J Med Primatol 1995;24:132–140.
322. Matano T, Shibata R, Siemon C, et al. Administration of an anti-CD8 monoclonal antibody interferes with the clearance of chimeric simian/human immunodeficiency virus during primary infections of rhesus macaques. J Virol 1998;72:164–169.
323. Karlsson GB, Halloran M, Li J, et al. Characterization of molecularly cloned simian-human immunodeficiency viruses causing rapid CD4+ lymphocyte depletion in rhesus monkeys. J Virol 1997;71:4218–4225.
324. Joag SV, Li Z, Foresman L, et al. Characterization of the pathogenic KU-SHIV model of acquired immunodeficiency syndrome in macaques. AIDS Res Hum Retroviruses 1997;13:635–645.
325. Lu YC, Salvato MS, Pauza CD, et al. Utility of SHIV for testing HIV-1 vaccine candidates in macaques. J Acquir Immune Defic Syndr Hum Retrovirol 1996;12:99–106.
326. Hirsch VM, Olmsted RA, Murphey-Corb M, et al. An African primate lentivirus (SIVsm) closely related to HIV-2. Nature 1989;339:389–392.
327. Dormont D, Livartowski J, Chamaret S, et al. HIV-2 in rhesus monkeys: serological, virological and clinical results. Intervirol 1989;30(Suppl 1):59–65.
328. Agy MB, Frumkin LR, Corey L, et al. Infection of *Macaca nemestrina* by human immunodeficiency virus type-1. Science 1992;257:103–106.
329. Hoover EA, Mullins JI, Quackenbush SL, et al. Experimental transmission and pathogenesis of immunodeficiency syndrome in cats. Blood 1987;70:1880–1892.
330. Rabin L, Hincenbergs M, Moreno MB, et al. Use of standardized SCID-hu Thy/Liv mouse model for preclinical efficacy testing of

anti-human immunodeficiency virus type 1 compounds. Antimicrob Ag Chemother 1996;40:755–762.
331. Koup RA, Safrit JT, Weir R, et al. Defining antibody protection against HIV-1 transmission in Hu-PBL-SCID mice. Semin Immunol 1996; 8:263–268.
332. Mosier DE, Gulizia RJ, Baird SM, et al. Human immunodeficiency virus infection of human PBL-SCID mice. Science 1991; 251:791–794.
333. McCune JM. Animal models of HIV-1 disease. Science 1997;278: 2141–2142.
334. Wieder KJ, Chatis P, Boltax J, et al. Human immunodeficiency virus type 1 entry into murine cell lines and lymphocytes from transgenic mice expressing a glycoprotein 120–binding mutant mouse CD4. AIDS Res Hum Retroviruses 1996;12:867–876.
335. Yamamura Y, Kotani M, Chowdhury MI, et al. Infection of human CD4+ rabbit cells with HIV-1:the possibility of the rabbit as a model for HIV-1 infection. Intern Med 1991;3:1183–1187.
336. Marx PA, Spira AI, Gettie A, et al. Progesterone implants enhance SIV vaginal transmission and early virus load. Nature Med 1996; 2:1084–1089.
337. Stott EJ, Chan WL, Mills KH, et al. Preliminary report: protection of cynomolgus macaques against simian immunodeficiency virus by fixed infected–cell vaccine. Lancet 1990;336:1538–1541.
338. Murphey-Corb M, Martin LN, Davison-Fairburn B, et al. A formalin-inactivated whole SIV vaccine confers protection in macaques. Science 1989;246:1293–1297.
339. Desrosiers RC, Wyand MS, Kodama T, et al. Vaccine protection against simian immunodeficiency virus infection. Proc Natl Acad Sci U S A 1989;86:6353–6357.
340. Langlois AJ, Weinhold KJ, Matthews TJ, et al. Detection of anti-human cell antibodies in sera from macaques immunized with whole inactivated virus. AIDS Res Hum Retroviruses 1992;8:1641–1652.
341. Warren JT, Dolatshahi M. Worldwide survey of AIDS vaccine challenge studies in nonhuman primates: vaccines associated with active and passive immune protection from live virus challenge. J Med Primatol 1992;21:139–186.
342. Warren JT, Dolatshahi M. First updated and revised survey of worldwide HIV and SIV vaccine challenge studies in nonhuman primates: progress in first and second order studies. J Med Primatol 1993;22:203–235.
343. Warren JT, Dolatshahi M. Annual updated survey of worldwide HIV, SIV, and SHIV challenge studies in vaccinated nonhuman primates. J Med Primatol 1994;23:184–225.
344. Warren JT, Levinson MA. Preclinical AIDS vaccine development: formal survey of global HIV, SIV, and SHIV in vivo challenge studies in vaccinated nonhuman primates. J Med Primatol 1997;26:63–81.
345. Mascola JR, Mathieson BJ, Zack PM, et al. Summary report: workshop on the potential risks of antibody-dependent enhancement in human HIV vaccine trials. AIDS Res Hum Retroviruses 1993;9: 1175–1184.
346. McElrath MJ, Corey L, Greenberg PD, et al. Human immunodeficiency virus type 1 infection despite prior immunization with a recombinant envelope vaccine regimen. Proc Natl Acad Sci U S A 1996;93:3972–3977.
347. Kahn JO, Steimer KS, Baenziger J, et al. Clinical, immunologic, and virologic observations related to human immunodeficiency virus (HIV) type 1 infection in a volunteer in an HIV-1 vaccine clinical trial. J Infect Dis 1995;171:1343–1347.
348. Graham BS, McElrath MJ, Connor RI, et al. Analysis of intercurrent HIV-1 infections in phase I and II trials of candidate AIDS vaccines. J Infect Dis 1998;177:310–319.
349. Berman PW, Gray AM, Wrin T, et al. Genetic and immunologic characterization of viruses infecting MN-rgp120–vaccinated volunteers. J Infect Dis 1997;176:384–397.
350. Connor RI, Korber BTM, Graham BS, et al. Immunological and virological analyses of persons infected by human immunodeficiency virus type 1 while participating in trials of recombinant gp120 subunit vaccines. J Virol 1998;72:1552–1576.

351. Mascola JR, Snyder SW, Weislow OS, et al. Immunization with envelope subunit vaccine products elicits neutralizing antibodies against laboratory-adapted but not primary isolates of human immunodeficiency virus type 1. J Infect Dis 1996;173:340–348.
352. Gorse GJ, Patel GB, Newman FK, et al. Antibody to native human immunodeficiency virus type 1 envelope glycoproteins induced by IIIB and MN recombinant gp120 vaccines. Clin Diagn Lab Immunol 1996;3:378–386.
353. Graham BS, Keefer MC, McElrath MJ, et al. Safety and immunogenicity of a candidate HIV-1 vaccine in healthy adults: recombinant glycoprotein (rgp) 120: a randomized, double-blind trial. Ann Intern Med 1996;125:270–279.
354. Belshe RB, Graham BS, Keefer MC, et al. Neutralizing antibodies to HIV-1 in seronegative volunteers immunized with recombinant gp120 from the MN strain of HIV-1: NIAID AIDS Vaccine Clinical Trials Network. JAMA 1994;272:475–480.
355. Dolin R, Graham BS, Greenberg SB, et al. The safety and immunogenicity of a human immunodeficiency virus type 1 (HIV-1) recombinant gp160 candidate vaccine in humans: NIAID AIDS Vaccine Clinical Trials Network. Ann Intern Med 1991;114:119–127.
356. Keefer MC, Graham BS, McElrath MJ, et al. Safety and immunogenicity of Env 2-3, a human immunodeficiency virus type 1 candidate vaccine, in combination with a novel adjuvant, MTP-PE/MF59. AIDS Res Hum Retroviruses 1996;12:683–693.
357. Belshe RB, Clements ML, Dolin R, et al. Safety and immunogenicity of a fully glycosylated recombinant gp160 human immunodeficiency virus type 1 vaccine in subjects at low risk of infection. J Infect Dis 1993;168:1387–1395.
358. Gorse GJ, Rogers JH, Perry JE, et al. HIV-1 recombinant gp160 vaccine induced antibodies in serum and saliva. Vaccine 1995;13: 209–214.
359. Corey L, McElrath MJ, Weinhold K, et al. Cytotoxic T cell and neutralizing antibody responses to HIV-1 envelope with a combination vaccine regimen. J Infect Dis 1998;177:301–309.
360. Stanhope PE, Clements ML, Siliciano RF. Human CD4+ cytolytic T lymphocyte responses to a human immunodeficiency virus type 1 gp160 subunit vaccine. J Infect Dis 1993;168:92–100.
361. Kallas EF, Evans TG, Gorse G, et al. QS21 is superior to alum as an adjuvant with low dose recombinant MN gp 120 in immunization of HIV-1 uninfected volunteers: cellular and humoral reponses [abstract]. In: 5th Conference on Retroviruses and Opportunistic Infections, Chicago, 1998:88.
362. Martin SJ, Vyakarnam A, Cheingsongpopov R, et al. Immunization of human HIV-seronegative volunteers with recombinant p17/p24:Ty virus-like particles elicits HIV-1 p24–specific cellular and humoral immune responses. AIDS 1993;7:1315–1323.
363. Zagury D, Bernard J, Cheynier R, et al. A group specific anamnestic immune reaction against HIV-1 induced by a candidate vaccine against AIDS. Nature 1988;332:728–731.
364. Cooney EL, Collier AC, Greenberg PD, et al. Safety of and immunological response to a recombinant vaccinia virus vaccine expressing HIV envelope glycoprotein. Lancet 1991;337:567–572.
365. Cooney EL, McElrath MJ, Corey L, et al. Enhanced immunity to human immunodeficiency virus (HIV) envelope elicited by a combined vaccine regimen consisting of priming with a vaccinia recombinant expressing HIV envelope and boosting with gp160 protein. Proc Natl Acad Sci U S A 1993;90:1882–1886.
366. Graham BS, Belshe RB, Clements ML, et al. Vaccination of vaccinia-naive adults with human immunodeficiency virus type 1 gp160 recombinant vaccinia virus in a blinded, controlled, randomized clinical trial: the AIDS Vaccine Clinical Trials Network. J Infect Dis 1992;166:244–252.
367. Graham BS, Gorse GJ, Schwartz DH, et al. Determinants of antibody response after recombinant gp160 boosting in vaccinia-naive volunteers primed with gp160-recombinant vaccinia virus. J Infect Dis 1994;170:782–786.
368. Hammond SA, Bollinger RC, Stanhope PE, et al. Comparative clonal analysis of human immunodeficiency virus type 1 (HIV-1)–specific

CD4+ and CD8+ cytolytic T lymphocytes isolated from seronegative humans immunized with candidate HIV-1 vaccines. J Exp Med 1992;176:1531–1542.
369. El-Daher N, Keefer MC, Reichman RC, et al. Persisting human immunodeficiency virus type 1 gp160-specific human T lymphocyte responses including CD8+ cytotoxic activity after receipt of envelope vaccines. J Infect Dis 1993;168:306–313.
370. Pincus SH, Messer KG, Cole R, et al. Vaccine-specific antibody responses induced by HIV-1 envelope subunit vaccines. J Immunol 1997;158:3511–3520.
371. Clements-Mann ML, Matthews TJ, Weinhold K, et al. HIV-1 immune responses induced by canarypox (ALVAC)–gp160 MN, SF-2 rgp120, or both vaccines in seronegative adults. J Infect Dis (in press).
372. Schwartz DH, Castillo RC, Arango-Jaramillo S, et al. Chemokine-independent in vitro resistance to human immunodeficiency virus (HIV-1) correlating with low viremia in long-term and recently infected HIV-1–positive persons. J Infect Dis 1997;176:1168–1174.
373. Kovacs JA, Vasudevachari MB, Easter M, et al. Induction of humoral and cell-mediated anti-human immunodeficiency virus (HIV) responses in HIV sero-negative volunteers by immunization with recombinant gp160. J Clin Invest 1993;92:919–928.
374. Keefer MC, Graham BS, Belshe RB, et al. Studies of high doses of a human immunodeficiency virus type 1 recombinant glycoprotein 160 candidate vaccine in HIV type 1–seronegative humans. AIDS Res Hum Retroviruses 1994;10:1713–1723.
375. Wintsch J, Chaignat CL, Braun DG, et al. Safety and immunogenicity of a genetically engineered human immunodeficiency virus vaccine. J Infect Dis 1991;163:219–225.
376. Schwartz DH, Gorse G, Clements ML, et al. Induction of HIV-1–neutralising and syncytium-inhibiting antibodies in uninfected recipients of HIV-1IIIB rgp120 subunit vaccine. Lancet 1993;342:69–73.
377. Kahn JO, Sinangil F, Baenziger J, et al. Clinical and immunologic responses to human immunodeficiency virus (HIV) type 1(SF2) gp120 subunit vaccine combined with MF59 adjuvant with or without muramyl tripeptide dipalmitoyl phosphatidylethanolamine in non-HIV-infected human volunteers. J Infect Dis 1994;170:1288–1291.
378. Gorse GJ, McElrath MJ, Matthews TJ, et al. Modulation of immunologic responses to HIV-1 recombinant gp160 vaccine by dose and schedule of administration. Vaccine 1998;16:493–506.
379. Salmon-Ceron D, Excler JL, Sicard D, et al. Safety and immunogenicity of a recombinant HIV type 1 glycoprotein 160 boosted by a V3 synthetic peptide in HIV-negative volunteers. AIDS Res Hum Retroviruses 1995;11:1479–1486.
380. Sarin PS, Mora CA, Naylor PH, et al. HIV-1 p17 synthetic peptide vaccine HGP-30: induction of immune response in human subjects and preliminary evidence of protection against HIV challenge in SCID mice. Cell Mol Biol 1995;41:401–407.
381. Kahn JO, Stites DP, Scillian J, et al. A phase I study of HGP-30, a 30 amino acid subunit of the human immunodeficiency virus (HIV) p17 synthetic peptide analogue sub-unit vaccine in seronegative subjects. AIDS Res Hum Retroviruses 1992;8:1321–1325.
382. Naylor PH, Sztein MB, Wada S, et al. Preclinical and clinical studies on immunogenicity and safety of the HIV-1 p17-based synthetic peptide AIDS vaccine :HGP-30-KLH. Int J Immunopharmacol 1991;13(Suppl 1):117–127.
383. Gorse GJ, Keefer MC, Belshe RB, et al. A dose-ranging study of a prototype synthetic HIV-1 V3 branched peptide vaccine. J Infect Dis 1996;173:330–339.
384. Li D, Forrest BD, Li Z, et al. International clinical trials of HIV vaccines. II. Phase I trial of an HIV-1 synthetic peptide vaccine evaluating an accelerated immunization schedule in Yunnan, China. Asian Pacific J Allergy Immunol 1997;15:105–113.
385. Kelleher AD, Emery S, Cunningham P, et al. Safety and immunogenicity of UBI HIV-1(MN) octameric V3 peptide vaccine administered by subcutaneous injection. AIDS Res Hum Retroviruses 1997;13:29–32.
386. Phanuphak P, Teeratakulpixarn S, Sarangbin S, et al. International clinical trials of HIV vaccines. I. Phase I trial of an HIV-1 synthetic peptide vaccine in Bangkok, Thailand. Asian Pacific J Allergy Immunol 1997;15:41–48.
387. Rubinstein A, Goldstein H, Pettoello-Mantovani M, et al. Safety and immunogenicity of a V3 loop synthetic peptide conjugated to purified protein derivative in HIV-seronegative volunteers. AIDS 1995;9:243–251.
388. Pialoux G, Excler JL, Riviere Y, et al. A prime-boost approach to HIV preventive vaccine using a recombinant canarypox virus expressing glycoprotein 160 (MN) followed by a recombinant glycoprotein 160 (MN/LAI). AIDS Res Hum Retroviruses 1995;11:373–381.
389. Fleury B, Janvier G, Pialoux G, et al. Memory cytotoxic T lymphocyte responses in human immunodeficiency virus type I (HIV-1)–negative volunteers immunized with a recombinant canarypox expressing gp160 of HIV-1 and boosted with a recombinant gp160. J Infect Dis 1996;174:734–738.
390. Berman PW, Murthy KK, Wrin T, et al. Protection of MN-rgp120–immunized chimpanzees from heterologous infection with a primary isolate of human immunodeficiency virus type 1. J Infect Dis 1996;173:52–59.
391. Girard M, vanderRyst E, Barresinoussi F, et al. Challenge of chimpanzees immunized with a recombinant canarypox–HIV-1 virus. Virology 1997;232:98–104.
392. el-Amad Z, Murthy KK, Higgins K, et al. Resistance of chimpanzees immunized with recombinant gp120$_{SF2}$ to challenge by HIV-1$_{SF2}$. AIDS 1995;9:1313–1322.
393. Lubeck MD, Natuk R, Myagkikh M, et al. Long-term protection of chimpanzees against high-dose HIV-1 challenge induced by immunization. Nature Med 1997;3:651–658.
394. Boyer JD, Ugen KE, Wang B, et al. Protection of chimpanzees from high-dose heterologous HIV-1 challenge by DNA vaccination. Nature Med 1997;3:526–532.
395. Shibata R, Seimon C, Cho MW, et al. Resistance of previously infected chimpanzees to successive challenges with a heterologous intraclade B strain of human immunodeficiency virus type 1. J Virol 1996;70:4361–4369.
396. Putkonen P, Nilsson C, Walther L, et al. Efficacy of inactivated whole HIV-2 vaccines with various adjuvants in cynomolgus monkeys. J Med Primatol 1994;23:89–94.
397. Putkonen P, Bjorling E, Akerblom L, et al. Long-standing protection of macaques against cell-free HIV-2 with a HIV-2 iscom vaccine. J Acquir Immune Defic Syndr Hum Retrovirol 1994;7:551–559.
398. Andersson S, Makitalo B, Thorstensson R, et al. Immunogenicity and protective efficacy of a human immunodeficiency virus type 2 recombinant canarypox (ALVAC) vaccine candidate in cynomolgus monkeys. J Infect Dis 1996;174:977–985.
399. Abimiku AG, Franchini G, Tartaglia J, et al. HIV-1 recombinant poxvirus vaccine induces cross-protection against HIV-2 challenge in rhesus macaques. Nature Med 1995;1:321–329.
400. Franchini G, Robert-Guroff M, Tartaglia J, et al. Highly attenuated HIV type 2 recombinant poxviruses, but not HIV-2 recombinant Salmonella vaccines, induce long-lasting protection in rhesus macaques. AIDS Res Hum Retroviruses 1995;11:909–920.
401. Letvin NL, Montefiori DC, Yasutomi Y, et al. Potent, protective anti-HIV immune responses generated by bimodal HIV envelope DNA plus protein vaccination. Proc Natl Acad Sci U S A 1997;94:9378–9383.
402. Bogers WMJM, Niphuis H, ten Haaft P, et al. Protection from HIV-1 envelope-bearing chimeric simian immunodeficiency virus (SHIV) in rhesus macaques infected with attenuated SIV: consequences of challenge. AIDS 1995;9:F13–F18.
403. Berglund P, Quesada-Rolander M, Putkonen P, et al. Outcome of immunization of cynomolgus monkeys with recombinant Semliki Forest virus encoding human immunodeficiency virus type 1 envelope protein and challenge with a high dose of SHIV-4 virus. AIDS Res Hum Retroviruses 1997;13:1487–1495.

404. Berman PW, Gregory TJ, Riddle L, et al. Protection of chimpanzees from infection by HIV-1 after vaccination with recombinant glycoprotein gp120 but not gp160. Nature 1990;345:622–625.
405. Girard M, Kieny MP, Pinter A, et al. Immunization of chimpanzees confers protection against challenge with human immunodeficiency virus. Proc Natl Acad Sci U S A 1991;88:542–546.
406. Fultz PN, Nara P, Barre-Sinoussi F, et al. Vaccine protection of chimpanzees against challenge with HIV-1–infected peripheral blood mononuclear cells. Science 1992;256:1687–1690.
407. Israel ZR, Edmonson PF, Maul DH, et al. Incomplete protection, but suppression of virus burden, elicited by subunit simian immunodeficiency virus vaccines. J Virol 1994;68:1843–1853.
408. Shibata R, Siemon C, Czajak SC, et al. Live, attenuated simian immunodeficiency virus vaccines elicit potent resistance against a challenge with a human immunodeficiency virus type 1 chimeric virus. J Virol 1997;71:8141–8148.
409. Igarashi T, Ami Y, Yamamoto H, et al. Protection of monkeys vaccinated with *vpr*-and/or *nef*-defective simian immunodeficiency virus strain mac human immunodeficiency virus type 1 chimeric viruses: a potential candidate live-attenuated human AIDS vaccine. J Gen Virol 1997;78:985–989.
410. Shafferman A, Lewis MG, McCutchan FE, et al. Prevention of transmission of simian immunodeficiency virus from vaccinated macaques that developed transient virus infection following challenge. Vaccine 1993;11:848–852.
411. Hu S-L, Abrams K, Barber GN, et al. Protection of macaques against SIV infection by subunit vaccines of SIV envelope glycoprotein gp160. Science 1992;255:456–459.
412. Hu SL, Polacino P, Stallard V, et al. Recombinant subunit vaccines as an approach to study correlates of protection against primate lentivirus infection. Immunol Lett 1996;51:115–119.
413. Lehner T, Wang YF, Cranage M, et al. Protective mucosal immunity elicited by targeted iliac lymph node immunization with a subunit SIV envelope and core vaccine in macaques. Nature Med 1996;2:767–775.
414. Stephens EB, Joag SV, Atkinson B, et al. Infected macaques that controlled replication of SIV mac or nonpathogenic SHIV developed sterilizing resistance against pathogenic SHIV (KU-1). Virology 1997;234:328–339.
415. Hirsch VM, Fuerst TR, Sutter G, et al. Patterns of viral replication correlate with outcome in simian immunodeficiency virus (SIV)–infected macaques: effect of prior immunization with a trivalent SIV vaccine in modified vaccinia virus Ankara. J Virol 1996;70:3741–3752.
416. Putkonen P, Walther L, Zhang YJ, et al. Long-term protection against SIV-induced disease in macaques vaccinated with a live attenuated HIV-2 vaccine. Nature Med 1995;1:914–918.
417. Quesada-Rolander M, Makitalo B, Thorstensson R, et al. Protection against mucosal SIVsm challenge in macaques infected with a chimeric SIV that expresses HIV type 1 envelope. AIDS Res Hum Retroviruses 1996;12:993–999.
418. Putkonen P, Makitalo B, Bottiger D, et al. Protection of human immunodeficiency virus type 2–exposed seronegative macaques from mucosal simian immunodeficiency virus transmission. J Virol 1997;71:4981–4984.
419. Fuller DH, Simpson L, Cole KS, et al. Gene gun-based nucleic acid immunization alone or in combination with recombinant vaccinia vectors suppresses viral burden in rhesus macaques challenged with a heterologous SIV. Immunol Cell Biol 1997;75:389–396.
420. Cole KS, Rowles JL, Jagerski BA, et al. Evolution of envelope-specific antibody responses in monkeys experimentally infected or immunized with simian immunodeficiency virus and its association with the development of protective immunity. J Virol 1997;71:5069–5079.
421. Miller CJ, McChesney MB, Lu XS, et al. Rhesus macaques previously infected with simian/human immunodeficiency virus are protected from vaginal challenge with pathogenic SIVmac239. J Virol 1997;71:1911–1921.
422. Buge SL, Richardson E, Alipanah S, et al. An adenovirus-simian immunodeficiency virus env vaccine elicits humoral, cellular, and mucosal immune responses in rhesus macaques and decreases viral burden following vaginal challenge. J Virol 1997;71:8531–8541.
423. Ahmad S, Lohman B, Marthas M, et al. Reduced virus load in rhesus macaques immunized with recombinant gp160 and challenged with simian immunodeficiency virus. AIDS Res Hum Retroviruses 1994;10:195–204.
424. Abimiku AG, Robert-Guroff M, Benson J, et al. Long-term survival of SIVmac251–infected macaques previously immunized with NYVAC–SIV vaccines. J Acquir Immune Defic Syndr Hum Retrovirol 1997;15(Suppl):S78–S85.
425. Wyand MS, Manson KH, Garciamoll M, et al. Vaccine protection by a triple deletion mutant of simian immunodeficiency virus. J Virol 1996;70:3724–3733.
426. Mossman SP, Bex F, Berglund P, et al. Protection against lethal simian immunodeficiency virus SIVsmmPBj14 disease by a recombinant Semliki Forest virus gp160 vaccine and by a gp120 subunit vaccine. J Virol 1996;70:1953–1960.
427. Corey L, Ashley R, Sekulovich R, et al. Lack of efficacy of a vaccine containing recombinant gD2 and gB2 antigens in MF59 adjuvant for the prevention of genital HSV-2 acquisition [abstract]. In: 37th Interscience Conference on Antimicrobial Agents and Chemotherapy, Toronto, 1997:LB-28.
428. Klinman DM, Takeno M, Ichino M, et al. DNA vaccines: safety and efficacy issues. Springer Semin Immunopathol 1997;19:245–256.

43

DEVELOPING HIV VACCINES AND OTHER INTERVENTIONS TO PREVENT AIDS WORLDWIDE

Margaret I. Johnston and Sam Avrett

This chapter reviews the status of the development of biomedical interventions, particularly vaccines, for the prevention of human immunodeficiency virus (HIV) disease worldwide. Nonbiomedical interventions, such as those to encourage condom use and avoidance of risky sexual and drug use behaviors, which are known to reduce the risk of HIV infection, fall beyond the scope of this chapter.

NEED FOR PREVENTION MEASURES

At the end of 1996, the United Nations Joint Programme on HIV/AIDS (UNAIDS) estimated that the number of new infections worldwide was approximately 16,000, including approximately 1600 children, each day. More than 90% of these new infections occur in developing countries. Sub–Saharan Africa is home of 68% or approximately 21 million of the people living with HIV/AIDS worldwide. The epidemic continues to spread on the African continent. For example, in South Africa, the proportion of pregnant women positive for HIV doubled, from about 7.6% in 1994 to about 14.1% in 1996 (1, 2). South Asia and Southeast Asia now represent the area of greatest growth in new infections; the number of HIV-positive individuals now surpasses 6 million. The number of AIDS cases in India is doubling every 14 months. Other areas where the prevalence of HIV has increased dramatically in the past year include Eastern and Central Europe and parts of South America. More detailed information on the impact of HIV infection worldwide can be found in Chapters 7 and 8.

Although significant progress has been made in developing effective therapeutic interventions for those infected with HIV, these advances are not likely to have a significant impact on the worldwide epidemic. The cost of combination chemotherapy is prohibitive for most people in the developing world and for many in industrialized countries. Further, even if drugs could be made available, the technology to ensure continuous and appropriate use, such as viral load measurements and monitoring of resistance, does not exist in most clinics in developing countries. However, success in finding effective antiretroviral agents has demonstrated the degree to which difficult technical problems can be solved when sufficient resources and expertise are applied to the problem.

Three modalities of biomedical interventions to prevent HIV disease are being pursued. These are antibiotic treatment of sexually transmitted diseases (STDs), development of topical microbicides active against HIV (and sometimes other pathogens), and development of preventive vaccines (Table 43.1). If history is any predictor of the future, safe and effective preventive vaccines will be the most effective, practical, long-term solution to halting the spread of HIV.

TREATMENT OF SEXUALLY TRANSMITTED DISEASES

Estimates of the number of new STD cases each year, worldwide, have been as high as 333 million, far greater than the approximately 30 million people infected with HIV (3). Research has shown that STDs increase an individual's risk of becoming infected with HIV. The increase in HIV transmission resulting from STDs may be explained in part by the observation that HIV shedding in the genital tracts of men and women increases as much as seven- to eightfold in the presence of other STDs, particularly genital ulcer disease (4). Recent data have demonstrated that treatment of STDs dramatically reduces the level of virus in the semen of HIV-infected men (5).

Epidemiologic data have demonstrated that STDs have been and continue to be a major public health problem in developing countries and have contributed to the spread of HIV in those countries. For example, about 70% of HIV infections in Africa are found in individuals who also have an STD. In Thailand, the comparable figure is 15 to 30% (6)

Successful management of STDs relies on several components, including education to alter risky sexual behaviors, provision of condoms, promotion of behavior to seek health care, case management of patients with STDs, and early

Table 43.1. Biomedical Interventions That May Help Prevent the Spread of HIV Worldwide

Intervention	Indication
Antibiotics	To treat sexually transmitted diseases

Topical microbicides	To prevent HIV infection:
	  Broad-spectrum agents
	  Inhibitors of HIV entry or replication

Vaccines	To prevent HIV infection or disease:
	  Live-attenuated HIV
	  Whole-killed HIV or synthetic particle approaches
	  Recombinant viral and bacterial vectors
	  Recombinant HIV proteins
	  Synthetic HIV peptides and peptide complexes
	  Host cell proteins alone or complexed with HIV proteins or peptides

detection and treatment of STDs (3). However, this management approach is not easy to implement in developing countries. For example, condom use requires the consent and cooperation of the male partner. Women cannot always negotiate their use, particularly in situations of nonconsensual sex. In addition, for many women, abstinence, the only fail-safe measure against sexual transmission of STDs (and HIV), is not always an option.

Curative therapy is available for many STDs, including infections with *Neisseria gonorrhoeae, Chlamydia trachomatis, Treponema pallidum,* and *Trichomonas vaginalis,* but not for others such as genital herpes and genital human papillomavirus infection. Because treatment of STDs reduces the occurrence and concentration of HIV in genital secretions, prevention strategies have included research on the impact of STD treatment on HIV infections (5).

In Mwanza, Tanzania, a randomized, controlled, community-level study involving more than 8000 volunteers demonstrated that appropriate management of symptomatic STDs resulted in a 42% reduction in HIV incidence in 6 intervention communities compared with 6 control communities over the 2 years of the study (7, 8). The largest impact on HIV incidence was observed in young women ages 15 to 24 years, apparently because young women are more at risk of HIV infection resulting from behavioral or biologic (immature cervix with large area of ectopy) factors. The management strategy used in this trial included training staff, making STD drugs available, providing STD education, and implementing a quality assurance program. The increased cost of these services compared with routine care was estimated to be $0.40 per person per year, a cost that compares favorably with other public health measures in terms of cost per disability-adjusted life-year saved (9).

One potential limitation of STD treatment as an approach to prevent HIV transmission is that persons with asymptomatic infection are difficult to identify and are thus rarely treated (3, 10). This problem is of particular importance to women because their relation of classic symptoms and signs to eventual diagnosis is weak (3). A strong need exists for rapid, reliable, inexpensive, noninvasive diagnostic tests that can be used for widescale screening to detect even asymptomatic STDs.

An alternative approach may be mass treatment of STDs in populations with a high prevalence of HIV and STDs. In the Rakai district of Uganda, a community-based trial involving 30 communities with combined volunteer enrollment of more than 9000 people will determine whether mass treatment of STDs with multiple antibiotics can reduce the spread of HIV (11). Half the volunteers, ages 15 to 58 years, will receive a combination of oral antibiotics every 6 months that should eliminate nonviral, even asymptomatic STDs. The other half will be given vitamins and medications for intestinal parasites. Although those receiving antibiotics have a lower frequency of STDs at the halfway point of the study, it will be 1 to 2 more years before the impact on HIV transmission can be evaluated. Furthermore, the cost effectiveness of this intervention, if successful, will have to be assessed, particularly because two of the antibiotics are costly.

In summary, STD treatment is one possible approach to slow the spread of HIV in communities with high STD rates. However, optimal methods to treat STDs successfully and practically remain under study. In addition, incorporating STD detection and treatment into broader programs of HIV education and prevention, condom promotion, and interventions to reduce risky sexual and drug use behaviors will have to be achieved if these interventions are to have any significant impact on the worldwide epidemic.

TOPICAL MICROBICIDES

Topical microbicides are products administered to genital mucosal surfaces to prevent HIV infection or other STDs. The rationale for developing topical microbicides is that many populations worldwide have a high prevalence of nonconsensual sex or sex without condoms or in the absence of information about the infection status of sexual partners. In addition, reproductive needs and desires may make use of an agent that is also spermicidal unacceptable. Behavioral interventions alone will be unable to halt the spread of HIV, and the first effective HIV vaccines are years away and are unlikely to be 100% effective.

The ideal microbicide will be inexpensive, effective, compatible with barrier methods, portable, safe, and nontoxic even when used multiple times each day, nonirritating to mucosal surfaces, without noticeable or objectionable color, odor, or taste, active against cell-free and cell-associated HIV, available in spermicidal and nonspermicidal formulations so reproductive decisions do not affect the risk of HIV infection, and nondisruptive to the normal mucosal ecology. Ideally, the microbicide will also have physical properties conducive to reproducible and consistent protection, including being biodiffusible, bioadhesive, nonabsorbable, stable at high temperatures, and able to provide efficacy of reasonable duration.

Development of a microbicide with these ideal properties will be technically challenging. Administration of the product will probably be required daily, if not just before each sex act. Furthermore, many high-risk individuals would potentially have to maintain consistent use of the product for years.

Microbicides under consideration or in development fall into two general categories: 1) broad-spectrum microbicides, active against bacteria or viruses; and 2) specific inhibitors of viral replication, including viral entry.

Broad-Spectrum Microbicides

The broad-spectrum microbicides currently in development include surfactants such as nonoxynol-9 (N-9), octoxynol-9 (O-9), C31G, and chorhexidene, acid buffers such as Buffergel, and natural products such as lactobacilli, as well as a synthetic version of fats from human breast milk.

N-9 has been used for more than 30 years as a spermicidal agent and is available over the counter in gels, foams, creams, and films in many countries. N-9 is a detergent-like chemical that is active against gonorrhea, *Chlamydia*, syphilis, *Trichomonas*, herpes, and hepatitis in laboratory experiments and has also been shown to kill HIV in test tube experiments. Vaginally applied spermicides that contain N-9 or O-9 appear to help prevent transmission of two agents of STDs, *Chlamydia trachomatis* and *Neisseria gonorrhoeae*, and thus could also indirectly prevent HIV transmission. A recent meta-analysis of six clinical trials and six observational studies demonstrated that, although spermicides containing N-9 had some protective effect against gonorrhea and chlamydial infection, the data were not sufficient to judge their effect on HIV transmission (12).

Whether vaginal spermicides containing N-9 reduce the rate of HIV infection remains under study. Although N-9 can inactivate HIV at low concentrations in vitro, a contraceptive sponge with 1000 mg N-9 did not protect female sex workers from HIV infection (13). Further, under some conditions of use, N-9 can irritate the vagina (13), raising concern that N-9 could contribute to susceptibility to HIV infection. However, more recent studies of lower-dose (100 to 150 mg) N-9 suppositories suggested that N-9 could protect against HIV infection (14, 15).

Results from a large, 2-year, phase III placebo-controlled study in 941 women in Cameroon showed that an N-9 contraceptive film had no effect on HIV transmission when provided within an overall HIV/STD prevention program (16). The overall infection rate (6.7%) in study participants was lower than that reported previously in this population (10%). However, no difference was noted between the control group who received counseling, STD treatment, condoms, and a placebo film and the treatment group who received the same, except the film contained 70 mg N-9. The N-9 film was reported to have been used in about 83% of all sex acts. The high rate of condom use in this study may have precluded measurement of an effect of the N-9 film alone.

An N-9 gel is in phase III trial in Kenya, and in South Africa, Thailand, the Côte d'Ivoire, and Benin, an N-9 gel for rectal use is in earlier stages of clinical evaluation. Newer N-9 and O-9 formulations are also under study.

A *Lactobacillus* suppository works against HIV through production of lactic acid, which maintains the vagina at low pH. A low pH reduces the risk of bacterial vaginosis, which in theory could diminish the risk of HIV infection. A phase I safety study of this suppository has been completed, and a phase II trial to evaluate dose and potency is under way.

Buffergel also maintains the natural low pH of the vagina and kills sperm and pathogens, including HIV, *Neisseria gonorrhoeae*, *Chlamydia*, and *Treponema pallidum*, in 5 minutes or less. Phase I safety trials are under way in the United States and are planned for Malawi, India, Thailand, and Zimbabwe. In addition, newer formulations with increased buffering capacity are under development.

C31G, a surfactant that disrupts viral and cell membranes, is a broad-spectrum antifungal, antibacterial, anti-HIV agent soon to enter phase I trial. PC213, a component of ice cream, chewing gum, and cosmetics, is a sulfated polysaccharide derived from seaweed that reportedly works by preventing attachment and uptake of HIV. Activity against herpesvirus, *Neisseria gonorrhoeae*, and *Chlamydia* in vitro has also been reported.

HIV-Specific Agents

Drug companies are also exploring new, more specific microbicidal agents that can be applied vaginally or rectally. Products under development include both broad-spectrum antiviral agents and specific inhibitors of HIV replication. Nonspermicidal inhibitors of viral entry that are in or near clinical evaluation include sulfated polysaccharides (dextrin sulfate, PC213), and sulfonated polymers (PRO2000). In earlier stages of development are chemically modified proteins (B69), *N*-docosanol, soluble CD4 and its derivatives, and monoclonal antibodies, which act at the stage of HIV binding to the surface of the target cell. These new products are years and in most cases decades away from the marketplace.

An anti-HIV vaginal gel containing dextrin sulfate, which blocks HIV entry into susceptible cells, was shown to be safe and well tolerated intravaginally at doses up to 0.5 mg in 36 healthy female volunteers (17). Expanded studies are being planned.

PRO2000 is a stable naphthalene sulfonate polymer of approximately 5000 kd of molecular weight that suppresses HIV replication in both T cells and macrophages. The agent has proved to be nontoxic in preclinical studies in animals, including a rabbit vaginal model (18). Absorption into the blood has not been detected after intravaginal administration to small animals. High concentrations show spermicidal activity, but lower concentrations do not. Phase I trials are under way. Preliminary results suggest that PRO2000 gel at the highest concentration tested (4%) is safe and well tolerated when applied once a day for 14 consecutive days. Use of the product did not appear to lead to genital irritation or microscopic inflammation, and it did not affect the normal vaginal pH or microflora.

Other inhibitors of HIV replication include agents that work after binding—agents such as bicyclams that inhibit fusion of HIV with the cell membrane (bicyclams), inhibitors of the HIV reverse transcriptase such as (R)-9-(2-phosphonylmethoxypropyl)adenine (PMPA), lamivudine, and didanosine, and others. PMPA is an acyclic nucleotide reverse transcriptase inhibitor that has been shown to be the most effective agent evaluated to date in preventing simian immunodeficiency virus (SIV) infection in monkeys after systemic administration and intravenous challenge (19). Preclinical studies are under way, and a phase I study of a topical formulation could begin late in 1998.

Oral zidovudine, which has been shown to reduce the transmission of HIV from infected mother to offspring, is being evaluated for its ability to prevent vertical transmission of HIV in several developing countries (11, 20). These trials are designed to determine whether more practical administration doses or schedules are effective in populations for whom the existing regimen is not feasible or affordable.

HIVIG, a polyclonal human plasma–derived anti-HIV immunoglobulin preparation that is administered systemically, is currently under study for its ability to prevent maternal–infant transmission of HIV in a dose-escalating trial in 30 Ugandan women (21). So far, HIVIG appears to be safe and well tolerated, with little change in maternal CD4 and viral RNA levels at the lowest dose evaluated.

Monoclonal antibodies directed against HIV may be able to provide passive protection against the virus. Antiherpes and antispermidical monoclonal antibodies have been studied in small animals without notable safety concerns. Several anti-HIV monoclonal antibodies have been demonstrated to have broad neutralizing activity against HIV, and data demonstrated that a combination of monoclonal antibodies with HIVIG was synergistic or additive in virus-neutralization laboratory assays (22–25). However, neither topical nor systemic studies have been initiated with anti-HIV monoclonal antibodies.

In summary, worldwide attention to the need for topical microbicides has increased, and several products are under study for safety, acceptability, and activity. None of these products have yet to progress to clinical efficacy trials. Development of an ideal microbicide may be as challenging as vaccine development, and the resulting products may have practical limits in their application to different populations.

VACCINE DEVELOPMENT: THE GOAL

Safe and effective HIV vaccines offer the most hope of stopping the spread of HIV disease worldwide. More than 25 candidate preventive vaccines have been evaluated in phase I trials worldwide, although most of these trials have occurred in the United States. Vaccine candidates and clinical trial results are the subject of Chapter 42 and other reviews (26–29).

The ideal vaccine for worldwide use will be inexpensive to manufacture, provide protection against all subtypes of HIV, require minimal if any boost, protect against all methods of spread of HIV for years, and be easily administered, stable to heat, and widely accessible. Developing such a vaccine will require addressing scientific, logistical, ethical, and financial challenges (Table 43.2).

However, the first effective vaccines will likely be less than ideal, and various factors will affect a vaccine's utility in a given population, including safety, stability, route, number of doses required, efficacy, and durability of protection, as well as the population's perceptions of benefit and cost of immunization relative to the success and cost of other available prevention strategies.

Durability of protection may prove particularly important. A partially protective vaccine could provide protection to all recipients but wane over time. The financial cost of sustaining a high level of herd immunity with a vaccine of short duration of protection could be high even if the vaccine is inexpensive because of continuing distribution and follow-up costs. Alternatively, a partially protective vaccine could protect a portion of recipients over their lifetime. Protecting a portion of the population over their lifetime could have a greater impact on the level of herd immunity than protecting all people but only for a few years (30).

Another possibility is that effective vaccines will not block HIV infection completely, but they will either prevent the establishment of a chronic HIV infection or control HIV infection to a level such that neither disease progression nor transmission to others occurs. Use of such a vaccine will require widespread use of technologies that distinguish seroconversion as a result of immunization from true HIV infection. Finally, investigators must establish mechanisms to ensure that effective vaccines are accessible and affordable to those most in need.

This discussion addresses scientific, logistical, ethical, and other challenges to developing vaccines for worldwide testing and use (see Table 43.2). Many of the points made here

Table 43.2. Challenges in Developing Preventive HIV Vaccines for Worldwide Use

Field	Challenge
Scientific	Genetic and immunologic diversity of HIV
	Diversity of HLA subtypes
	Absence of validated correlates of immune protection
	Lack of ideal animal model of HIV disease
Logistical	Complex infrastructure requiring long-term commitment and resources
	Skepticism and mistrust of researchers and foreign governments
	Long-term protection possibly requiring repeated immunizations
Ethical	Difficulties in obtaining informed consent and providing noncoercive incentives
	Linking of trial sites with HIV prevention and health care services
	Ensuring access to successful vaccines
Other	Suboptimal incentives for private sector participation
	Reliance on established models for technology transfer

with respect to vaccine efficacy trials also pertain to the evaluation of other prevention modalities.

SCIENTIFIC CHALLENGES OF HIV DIVERSITY AND VACCINE DESIGN

One of the greatest challenges will be identifying a vaccine or cocktail of vaccines that will protect against all subtypes of HIV. Much is now known about the nine genetic subtypes, or clades, of class M HIV-1 (A thru I) and one class O HIV-1 (see Chap. 3) (31). In addition, recombinants between the genetic clades have been observed in about 10% of the HIV-1 isolates studied (see Chap. 3) (32). For example, A/C, A/D, A/E, A/C/F, B/D, B/F, G/A, H/G, and other recombinants have been reported.

However, although the genetic and phenotypic character of many HIV strains isolated from the blood of HIV-infected individuals has been well characterized, the nature and diversity of HIV genes or gene sequences that need to be incorporated into an HIV vaccine are not known.

First, the diversity of HIV sequences against which the vaccine needs to protect are not fully characterized. For example, HIV sequences found in mucosal secretions of women soon after exposure, which are believed to be responsible for initiating infection, appear to be distinct but related to HIV sequences that exist in blood, but few studies to explore this question have been done (33). In some cases, HIV proviral sequences in secretions were closely related to a minor variant in blood; in another, viruses in both compartments were relatively homogeneous (34).

With respect to phenotype, macrophage-tropic, non–syncytia-forming HIV appears to predominate in mucosal isolates, a finding suggesting that macrophage-tropic, non–syncytia-forming isolates should also serve as the basis for vaccine design (35). However, because syncytia-forming HIV can also cause primary infection, one can rationalize the use of any primary virus isolate, which is one that has undergone minimal passage in peripheral blood mononuclear cells, given that passage in cell lines appears to alter envelope epitopes (36–39).

More important than sequence characterization, however, is the immunologic significance of HIV diversity, which remains undefined. The relevance of genetic subtypes to neutralization serotypes has been explored using different analytic methods, including a mathematical procedure referred to as the neutralization index method and an artificial neural network algorithm (40–42). Investigators generally agree with earlier work that genetic subtype does not predict serotype, except perhaps for the E subtype of HIV in Thailand (22). Serotypes relevant to neutralization of primary isolates of HIV appear to be defined by complex conformational determinants rather than simple linear epitopes (25, 41).

Data obtained with certain antisera and monoclonal antibodies have suggested that candidate vaccines may not have to be based on the genotype of HIV circulating in the trial population. Specifically, rare antisera and monoclonal antibodies neutralize primary HIV across the genetic clades, a finding demonstrating that cross-reactive epitopes do exist on the HIV envelope protein (22, 25). Theoretically, it may be possible to find ways to present these epitopes to induce broadly cross-reactive antibodies that recognize HIV from across the genetic clades. Although attempts to induce such antisera using complexed and oligomeric forms of envelope have shown promise, experimental induction of high-titer broadly cross-neutralizing antibodies has not yet been achieved (43–47). Until broadly neutralizing antisera can be induced reliably in animals, candidate vaccines designed to stimulated antienvelope antibodies in human volunteers should continue to be based on HIV strains that circulate in that target population.

With respect to cellular immunity, one approach to inducing broadly reactive cytotoxic T lymphocytes (CTLs) would be to include diverse T-cell epitopes in the candidate vaccine (48). Unfortunately, although a significant amount of work has led to identification of T-cell epitopes of clade B HIV, which predominates in the United States and Europe, identification of T-cell epitopes of HIV from non–clade B HIV is far from complete. If this approach to CTL induction is going to work for developing countries, the following information will be required: 1) genetic sequences of non–class B HIV proteins, especially gag, pol, and nef; 2) substantially more knowledge of T-cell epitopes in non–clade B HIVs; 3) the major histocompatibility types of people in developing countries, particularly Africa and Asia; and 4) knowledge about the epitopes to which each population, given its specific HLA types, will be likely to respond. Until this information is available, one cannot rationally select T-cell epitopes to include in vaccines designed for testing in and eventual use by a specific population. Novel computer algorithms to help narrow the search for epitopes have begun to be used and are likely to increase the feasibility of this approach to meet worldwide needs (49).

An alternative approach to the induction of broadly reactive CTL responses in a specific population would be to include in the candidate vaccine as many different antigens, particularly conserved antigens, as possible and then empirically to determine the breadth of responses induced in a particular trial population and ascertain whether this breadth is sufficient to provide protection against some or all viruses to which the person becomes exposed. The feasibility of this approach is supported by data that CTLs elicited by a candidate HIV vaccine based on clade B HIV can recognize and kill cells infected by HIV of other clades. More specifically, studies have demonstrated that at least some individuals immunized with a live canarypox vector expressing *env, gag*, and a portion of *pol* have CTL precursors that, after stimulation ex vivo, kill target cells infected with some isolates of HIV from other clades (50). Additional studies along these lines in diverse populations are needed. A phase I trial of this canarypox vaccine will be initiated in Uganda in 1998 to determine whether that population, with its unique range of divergent HLA subtypes, responds with a similar breadth of

CTL responses as vaccine recipients from the United States and Europe. Unfortunately, CTLs arising after ex vivo expansion may or may not reflect the true precursor frequency in vivo (51).

Evidence that CTLs play an important role in controlling HIV infection continues to mount. If CTLs are critical to protection, then induction of cross-clade CTL responses suggests that a broadly protective HIV vaccine can be designed. The ability of CTLs from vaccine recipients to kill cells infected with a breadth of HIVs from different genetic clades should undergo intense examination in the coming years. In addition, the protective effect of such responses will need to be determined in expanded human trials in volunteers who are at risk of HIV infection.

With respect to specific HIV vaccine designs, DNA vaccines have captured the attention of those interested in HIV vaccines suitable for worldwide use (52–54). Although DNA vaccines remain unproved in the field of vaccinology, if DNA vaccines at reasonable doses are shown to be effective in humans, they may prove well suited for the needs of developing countries. DNA vaccines are expected to be relatively inexpensive to produce, readily adaptable to different genotypes and serotypes, and stable. In addition, several developing countries would have the capacity to perform at least the final stage of the vaccine manufacturing or vialing process, a feature that would help to minimize the final cost of the vaccine.

Live-attenuated HIV also deserves specific note with respect to worldwide vaccine development efforts. Live-attenuated HIV is not currently being developed because of uncertainties about long-term safety, concerns that outweigh any potential benefit to populations of relatively low seroincidence (55, 56). However, given the unparalleled protection afforded by live-attenuated lentiviral vaccines in animal models and the growing body of safety information from animal models and persons infected with apparently attenuated strains of HIV, live-attenuated HIV needs to continue to receive judicious consideration by populations in whom HIV spread is most threatening (57–61). Additional preclinical and clinical research to address safety issues and breadth of protection in animal models is needed.

LOGISTICAL CHALLENGES IN CONDUCTING CLINICAL TRIALS IN DEVELOPING COUNTRIES

Clinical testing of candidate vaccines, particularly trials in developing countries, will be a challenge to scientists, communities, and policy makers. Scientific uncertainties about initiating an efficacy trial in the absence of known immune correlates of protection, the costs associated with the conduct of efficacy trials (particularly large trials in lower seroincidence populations), and the potential impact of vaccine "failure" on the willingness of populations to participate in subsequent trials are all factors that will make decisions about efficacy trials particularly difficult. Yet, many factors argue that multiple efficacy trials in developing countries will be required to identify an effective HIV vaccine.

- The first HIV vaccines to enter efficacy trials will probably not prove to be 100% effective, thus necessitating additional trials of improved products.
- The highest rates of new infection occur in developing countries; therefore, the greatest need and the greatest ability to affect the epidemic worldwide rest in finding vaccines effective in those populations.
- Trials in higher-risk populations will require fewer participants to obtain estimates of vaccine efficacy; all else being equal, trials that require fewer participants will proceed more quickly and at lower cost that larger trials.
- A successful vaccine should protect against all subtypes of HIV to which the individual may be exposed; only subtype B currently predominates in industrialized countries, although other subtypes are entering these countries; trials in developing countries will be required to determine whether a vaccine protects against non–subtype B HIV.
- If the vaccine is effective by controlling or clearing HIV replication rather than preventing HIV infection, it may not be possible to conduct efficacy trials in the United States and Europe if the standard of care evolves to include intervention with combination antiretroviral therapy immediately after detection of infection; the dramatic decrease in HIV levels after effective combination therapy is likely to mask any effect of the vaccine on HIV levels and to prohibit measurement of vaccine efficacy.

BENEFITS OF CLINICAL RESEARCH TO DEVELOPING COUNTRIES

Many countries in Africa, Asia, and Latin America have a long history of clinical testing of drugs and vaccines for diseases such as tuberculosis, cholera, and malaria. Clearly, the long-term benefit of clinical trial research to any country is the potential progress in combating disease and improving public health. The eradication of smallpox was achieved with unparalleled international cooperation in research, disease surveillance, and vaccination, and it drew on the commitment of every country in the world. The control of measles, polio, and yellow fever is an additional example of public health benefits derived from vaccine research and development. In the same way, clinical trial research on HIV in both wealthy industrialized countries and the developing world has great potential for controlling the HIV epidemic.

HIV prevention research has been conducted in Africa, Asia, and Latin America for the last 10 years. Already this research has provided some countries with a better understanding of the pattern of HIV transmission in their own country, ways to provide effective education and risk-

Table 43.3. Examples of Successful International HIV Prevention Research Activities

Area of Study	Country (references)
Association STDs with HIV infection	India (68, 98)
Treatment of STDs to reduce HIV levels in semen	Malawi (5)
Treatment of STDs to reduce HIV incidence	Tanzania (8, 9)
Effectiveness of counseling and use of condoms	Thailand (64, 76, 77)
	Zimbabwe (72)
	Cameroon (11)
Reduction perinatal transmission	Malawi (11, 70)
Effect of nonoxynol-9 on HIV transmission	Cameroon (16)

STDs, sexually transmitted diseases.

reduction interventions for populations at high risk, increased diagnostic capabilities, potential approaches for preventing perinatal HIV transmission, and improved control of STDs and other diseases (Table 43.3).

Moreover, in immediate terms, research studies can directly contribute to public health efforts in educating and counseling people about disease prevention and care, supporting medical care and treatment, and involving individuals and entire communities in seeking a solution to the challenges of disease prevention and health care. Although these benefits of research have a far-reaching impact on public health and welfare, they have so far failed to contain the spread of HIV, a finding arguing that HIV vaccine trials should be pursued in developing countries.

ADDRESSING SKEPTICISM, MISTRUST, AND POLITICAL COMMITMENT

Although clinical research in developing countries has been diverse and largely beneficial, examples of ethical transgressions in this research, combined with misinformation and lack of knowledge, have contributed to mistrust of research in many communities worldwide. As recent debates about genetics research and cloning demonstrate, this mistrust is not confined to developing countries. Recruitment and retention of participants require a certain level of understanding of and belief in the process of gaining knowledge through experimentation. A basic understanding of HIV and of the way in which research will help to control its spread is useful. Although trained researchers may seek to conduct HIV-related trials, the surrounding environment may reflect a political and cultural legacy of mistrust, uncomprehending how HIV could be controlled, suspicious of the intentions of researchers coming from or educated elsewhere, and motivated by local economic, political, or social reasons to prevent public participation in or support of clinical research.

The cost of this mistrust is real. Clinical studies can be delayed or prevented, and the resulting benefits of biomedical research—therapies, vaccines, and control of disease—are likewise delayed or lost. For example, the first preventive HIV vaccine trial in Africa has already been significantly delayed because of the need to implement additional unanticipated in-country advisory committees to ensure local support.

The solutions to addressing mistrust lie in engaging critics of research in useful dialogue and informed oversight of the research process. Successful "community education" requires time and resources to go beyond dissemination of information and to bring people into a process in which they can be an informed, useful voice in trial design and implementation. This goal is a challenge, especially when researchers have little experience or understanding of the benefit of community involvement.

Establishing and maintaining a continuity and breadth of political and economic support are other challenges. It is a testimony to the severity of the HIV epidemic that several countries have made the commitment of scarce resources to preparing for HIV vaccine clinical trials. The political will and commitment of a government to identify and allocate scarce expertise and in-kind resources for research over many years are enormous challenges in the context of a multitude of social and public health needs. Funding, trained doctors and health care personnel, drugs, supplies, and educational efforts are extremely limited in many countries, and government leaders may find it difficult to justify continually the comparative value of investing government effort in clinical research and product evaluation.

ECONOMIC RESOURCES AND LOGISTICAL CHALLENGES

Countries deciding to conduct clinical research first need to invest in trial preparation, the activities of which are outlined in detail later. These preparatory activities can have significant impact on the design and thus the cost of eventual vaccine efficacy trials. Specifically, the HIV seroincidence rate and the loss-to-follow-up rate will determine the number of participants to be recruited and the length of the trial (62, 63). Although epidemiologic studies in Africa, Asia, and Latin America may show annual HIV infection rates higher than 10%, infection rates typically drop in the context of counseling and access to condoms and other prevention resources (64).

The costs of designing and implementing clinical research in Africa, Asia, and Latin America are usually provided by a partnership of national governments, international health organizations, and industry. To prepare for HIV vaccine trials and to test other prevention interventions, nine countries currently receive support from the United States National Institutes of Allergy and Infectious Diseases (NIAID), through a network of projects called HIVNET. Several other African and Asian countries have established research sites for large-scale HIV vaccine and prevention studies, through a collaboration of national health agencies, the United Nations and World Health Organization, international pharmaceutical companies, and European and North American partners such as the United States Army, the European Commission, and the Medical Research Councils of the United Kingdom and Canada. For example, preparation for large clinical trials in Thailand through the Thai Ministry of Health, the Royal Thai Army, Chiron Vaccines, Genentech, Pasteur Merieux

Connaught, and the Walter Reed Army Institute of Research has cost more than $3.5 million per year since 1991 (J McNeil, unpublished data).

The human resource and financial costs of conducting a clinical trial in a developing country can also be substantial. Cost to develop local site infrastructure and the capacity to collect and process laboratory specimens and to collect and process data can be significant. Most infrastructure costs extend for as many years as the trial is conducted, and some begin years before even the first phase I trial begins. No phase III efficacy trial of an HIV vaccine has been conducted yet; thus, direct research costs can only be estimated. For example, the estimated cost of a phase III trial in Thailand is approximately $750 per participant per year, or $4.5 million for a 3-year trial involving 2000 volunteers (J McNeil, unpublished data).

BUILDING INFRASTRUCTURE IN DEVELOPING COUNTRIES FOR PREVENTIVE HIV VACCINE EFFICACY TRIALS

As described earlier, large-scale efficacy trials of preventive HIV vaccines will require an infrastructure of trained investigators and staff, space and equipment for study sites, specialized laboratories, and large numbers of participants followed over several years. Infrastructure needs and options can be categorized into 10 areas.

Trained Researchers and Staff

For clinical trials of HIV vaccines to succeed, a team of researchers is needed who have training and experience with the target population and in clinical trial design and implementation, epidemiologic research, laboratory procedures specific to HIV, data collection methods and analysis, informed consent processes and ethical review boards, HIV risk-reduction interventions and services, and clinical care referrals. To assemble a team of investigators with the necessary expertise, collaborations among researchers at local and national universities, researchers from a national Ministry of Health, and researchers from industry, foreign country universities, and governmental organizations may be necessary. For example, preparations for trials in Thailand have been led by a team of investigators from the Royal Thai Ministry of Public Health, the Royal Thai Army Medical Corps, and Chiang Mai University, as well as the Johns Hopkins University and the Walter Reed Army Institute of Research in the United States. Forging new international collaborations such as this, which link different organizations, requires vision and leadership. A basic challenge is that of training new researchers in developing countries. Training new clinical researchers is often sponsored by national governments or by grants and programs, such as those of the Fogarty International Center of the United States National Institutes of Health (65).

Community Preparedness

As discussed earlier, community education and participation are needed to prepare people for large-scale recruitment campaigns for HIV vaccine efficacy trials and to address possible issues of mistrust and political ambivalence. The options for preparing the public for trials vary according to the target audience and the intensity of efforts. Public opinion in many countries is influenced by popular radio and other local media, international media, political leaders, religious leaders, unions, informal communication among community or ethic groups, and prior experience with study-affiliated volunteers, counselors, researchers, and public officials. Although broad-based outreach is not always necessary until the beginning of HIV vaccine trials, it is essential to develop a consistent message about the research plans and goals and to recognize that the formation of public opinion about the trials does not wait until this plan is developed.

Different study sites, depending on their visibility, population of study participants, and readiness for trials, have developed written fact sheets, presentations for radio and news media, community forums and events, or outreach through political, religious, or union networks. Similarly, to varying degrees, study sites have attempted to gather perceptions and advice from study participants and community leaders about reviewing study protocols and study design (66, 67).

Communities need to recognize that vaccine development is a long, incremental process and that requiring assurances of vaccine access before initiation of phase I clinical trials may significantly delay if not completely block initial trials of promising vaccine candidate. However, agreement about the way in which a successful vaccine will be made available to the communities where trials are conducted before initiation of large efficacy trials would help to ensure community support for the trial. Finally, communities need to understand and concur that a trial of even a partially effective vaccine will provide information useful to vaccine development, and a failed trial is only one from which scientific conclusions cannot be derived.

Recruitment of Study Participants

A key infrastructure question is whether a site can quickly recruit a cohort of participants who are eligible for the study, willing and able to be in the study over time, capable of informed consent, and, for phase II and III trials, at a certain level of risk of HIV infection even when participating in a study involving high-quality risk-reduction counseling and services. The level of risk of HIV infection and the ability to follow participants over time are crucial factors in determining the size and length of the trial.

In countries preparing for HIV vaccine efficacy trials, recruitment issues have been addressed in different ways. Some sites have recruited specific professions, such as commercial sex workers or truck drivers, people at specific locations, such as health clinics, workplaces, or particular

Table 43.4. Countries and Populations With Ongoing HIV Vaccine Efficacy Trial Preparations

Country	Population
Brazil	Men who have sex with men, female sex workers
Haiti	Patients with tuberculosis, discordant couples, pregnant HIV-positive women and their infants
India	Patients with STDs, female sex workers
Kenya	Truck drivers, female sex workers
Malawi	Pregnant HIV-positive women and their infants
South Africa	Women at high risk for HIV, perinatal cohorts
Thailand	Military recruits, patients with STDs, female sex workers, injection drug users, discordant couples
Trinidad	Patients with STDs
Uganda	Military personnel, patients with STDs, rural families
United States	Injection drug users, women at high risk for HIV, men who have sex with men
Zambia	Discordant couples, patients with STDs
Zimbabwe	Factory workers (blood donors)

STDs, sexually transmitted diseases.

neighborhoods or villages, or people with specific risk factors for HIV, such as men who have sex with men, intravenous drug users, partners of intravenous drug users, people seeking care for other STDs, or women who are HIV infected and pregnant (Table 43.4) (68–74). Recruitment parameters that are too narrow can impede rapid recruitment. Parameters that are too broad may recruit people who are at low risk or who are unable to join or remain in the study. Recruitment criteria may have to be partially confidential to avoid biasing people's responses to screening questionnaires, to recruit volunteers who do not wish to be identified publicly as being at risk, and to avoid discrimination against those being recruited for the study. When recruiting groups of participants from a small population, recruitment methods must also consider the potential confounding effect that counseling and vaccination of one person may have on the network of participants.

Informed Consent Process and Institutional Review Boards

Each research site must establish protocols and infrastructure to ensure the highest ethical standards of trial design and conduct. In many international collaborative networks of researchers, clinical research protocols are routinely reviewed by an established institutional review boards (IRBs) based at universities or governmental public health institutions (75). Individual informed consent documents also have been developed at many international study sites and often use written educational materials and consent forms, counselor presentations, videos, or peer-to-peer discussion formats (66). However, in preparing for HIV vaccine efficacy trials, many research sites have documented a need to find ways to improve participant comprehension of HIV vaccine trial concepts, including testing a vaccine of unknown efficacy, the meaning of an antibody response, and the meaning of "placebo." International research sites have also noted participant concerns about vaccine side effects and concerns about discrimination by sexual partners, friends, coworkers, and health care providers and insurers. Finally, one of the most difficult aspects of obtaining informed consent in a developing country is assessing the individual's comprehension of the information provided. In some populations, in whom the germ theory of disease is not understood, the challenge of explaining HIV and vaccines can appear insurmountable. In these instances, patience, repetition, analogies from within the individual's culture, and peer explanations have proved helpful.

Laboratory Capacity and Specimen Collection, Transport, Processing, and Analysis

Laboratory infrastructure needs to include the ability to assess the incidence of HIV and other infections, to monitor the magnitude, specificity, and kinetics of antibody, cellular, and other immune responses, and, in breakthrough infections (individuals who become infected after immunization), to monitor viral load and disease progression. Local laboratory capacity is needed to screen trial volunteers and to prepare each vaccine dose. Standardization of laboratory assays and protocols to ensure consistent specimen collection, shipping, and processing is critical for data to be valid, reliable, and comparable across subsites in multicenter trials.

The options regarding which assays can be done locally and which must be done at a central site usually distant from the clinic are changing as technology improves for processing, shipping, and testing specimens and as the capacity of local laboratories to conduct increasingly sophisticated assays is enhanced. In the current state of HIV vaccine trial preparation in developing countries, most local field research laboratories are equipped and trained to carry out HIV enzyme-linked immunosorbent assays and tests for pregnancy, parasitic infections, hepatitis, syphilis, and other diseases. Local research laboratories are also generally equipped to centrifuge and store specimens and to ship samples. Capabilities for performing Western blot antibody tests and viral RNA polymerase chain reaction are less developed, or these tests are unaffordable, in many developing countries. Most neutralization and other antibody assays, CTL assays, and viral load assays to characterize new HIV infections has been done in central laboratories in the United States and Europe, although selected sites in developing countries have these capabilities. Establishing reliable procedures for international shipment of cells, plasma, and other specimens is challenging, and efforts are being made to increase the capacity of in-country laboratories. Building this laboratory capacity is essential. Even in the United States, a limiting factor in initiating a recent phase II HIV vaccine clinical trial was not recruitment of volunteers, but developing laboratory capacity for several of the more sophisticated assays required by the trial protocol.

Data Collection, Processing, and Analysis

To gather valid, reliable information on trial participants at enrollment and throughout the study, research sites require standardized questionnaires, skilled interviewers, and an ability to track visits, immunizations, and test results. Questionnaires need to be designed to obtain information about the participant, including risk factors and incentives and disincentives to participation, in a way that minimizes the inconvenience to the participant and maximizes the usefulness and accuracy of the collected data. Interviewers at each trial site in the United States are trained and directly supervised in interviewing skills. Interviews may be recorded and reviewed later to identify and reduce sources of error and bias. The interview data are compiled, reviewed for completeness and quality, and analyzed to determine whether further revisions are required. At HIV vaccine trial sites in Africa, Asia, Latin America, and the Caribbean, researchers are working to develop data collection procedures that take into account local languages, cultural norms, and unique population characteristics. Data collected to date in the United States and in several developing countries have allowed an accurate assessment of HIV-related risk factors among the populations that could enroll in HIV vaccine efficacy studies.

Counseling

Ethically, research to evaluate methods to prevent HIV infection must also provide what is known to be effective in preventing HIV infection. This means, in theory, that preventive HIV vaccine trials must provide to all participants what is already known to work in HIV prevention education, counseling, and resources. One difficulty is that few HIV prevention methods have been evaluated for efficacy in any population. Only recently have studies begun to address the impact of counseling, education, condom distribution, and needle exchange on behaviors and, most important, on ultimate infection rates (76, 77). Although needle exchange and condom use are associated with lower risk of HIV infection, no consensus exists on behavior change interventions (78). Coordinating several trial sites, which may recruit diverse populations and risk groups, to adopt and adhere to a "standard" high-quality protocol for HIV prevention counseling, when no one method has proved effective for every population, will remain challenging in the foreseeable future.

With this caveat, most international HIV vaccine trial sites have implemented HIV prevention protocols that include an overview of HIV and HIV transmission, an assessment of risk, counseling to reduce that risk and to reinforce safer behaviors, and provision of resources and referrals to support remaining uninfected. Protocols to ensure the quality of this HIV prevention effort generally include counselor training and may include regular supervisory skills assessment, case review, and cross-training.

At many research sites preparing for preventive HIV vaccine efficacy trials, study participant HIV infection rates have declined, and researchers have been able to evaluate changes in behaviors and infection rates. For example, in a vaginal microbicide trial in Cameroon among commercial sex workers, the HIV incidence dropped from 14 to 6% during the study (16). In a vaccine feasibility study among men in the Royal Thai Army, the HIV incidence dropped from as high as 8% per year to less than 1% per year (J McNeil, unpublished data).

Vaccine Administration and Clinical Monitoring

The evaluation of a candidate vaccine in a placebo-controlled trial requires careful dose preparation, randomization, administration of vaccine or placebo such that the participant and clinician do not know which has been given, and careful monitoring of the participant for clinical symptoms or side effects. Clinicians need to be well trained and, to allow comparison of results among all study sites, procedures must be standardized.

Participant Retention

The proportion of participants who remain in the trial and make every appointment within the desired window of time is crucial to the design and outcome of clinical trials. Researchers need to communicate the long-term nature of the study to the participant, to collect correct and reliable locator information from the participant, and to employ outreach workers to locate and communicate with participants who have not come in for visits. International HIV vaccine preparedness trial sites have had success with maintaining cohorts over time, with retention of more than 85% of cohort participants in studies among commercial sex workers in Senegal and Kenya, women from prenatal clinics in Uganda, and men and women from STD clinics in Thailand (W Cates, unpublished data).

Health Services and Service Referrals

Based on the ethical mandate to maximize benefits and to minimize harms, clinical trial sites usually establish standard protocols to go beyond trial-related activities in provision of health services and referrals. However, research sites generally do not establish themselves as the primary sources of health care services. Particularly in poorer populations, this situation is feasible when the trial site is convenient to health care services or transportation to health care sites is available. Research sites that recruit poorer populations who lack access to health care services are faced with enormous challenges in providing a level of health care that is ethical yet not so high that it may be considered coercive.

The services and referrals offered at trial sites depend on the site's capacity and available referral options, but they can include the following: referrals for testing and treatment of many different illnesses and infections; provision of vaccines, antimalarial drugs, obstetric, gynecologic, and perinatal care, drug treatment, and additional counseling; and linkages with providers of food assistance, housing, and health insurance.

WHAT, WHEN, AND WHERE TO CONDUCT VACCINE EFFICACY TRIALS

The selection of specific clinical trial sites to evaluate preventive HIV vaccines depends on the development of adequate infrastructure to conduct the research, the skills and experience of local researchers, the suitability of the candidate vaccine for the trial population, the acceptability of the vaccine design to the trial population, the support of national and local governments, communities, and potential participants for this research, and the likely HIV seroincidence at the trial site in the context of achievable, high-quality counseling and prevention interventions.

Potential risks and benefits must be carefully weighed in decisions about what vaccine strategies a country elects to pursue. This balance will be different for different countries. The dynamics of the spread of HIV in a country or population is of particular relevance in evaluating the potential risks and benefits of proceeding with efficacy trials in that country or population. In countries with high infection rates and insufficient infrastructure for HIV behavior change interventions, even partially effective vaccines may be useful in combating the HIV epidemic. Modeling studies have shown that, with certain assumptions, a vaccine with 50% or less efficacy over a 5-year period could have a significant public health impact in populations with high rates of HIV transmission (30).

Decisions on efficacy trials are particularly difficult given the resources and infrastructure required to conduct such trials successfully. If the correlates of immunity for recovery from or clearance of a viral infection are known, then vaccines that induce that immune response can move quickly into an efficacy trial. Alternatively, if a validated animal model predicts protection in humans, a vaccine that provides protection in that animal model moves quickly through clinical evaluation. In the case of HIV, one has neither documented correlates of immune protection nor a validated animal model of HIV disease. Fortunately, history has aptly demonstrated that effective vaccines can be developed without knowing the correlates of immune protection or having a validated animal model.

Another factor challenging decision makers is that the more "traditional" designs of live-attenuated and whole-killed vaccines have not been actively pursued toward human trials because of perceptions that they are too risky. As a result, the vaccine designs that are currently being evaluated are new biotechnologic approaches to vaccine development and are essentially unproved in the field of vaccinology.

Given this unique combination of challenges, a reasonable approach is to evaluate multiple designs essentially in parallel and continue to move the best designs forward into trials in which efficacy can be determined as long as the vaccines appear to be safe and induce immune responses that may be protective in an acceptable percentage of recipients. Another approach is to conduct more fundamental research until more information about correlates is obtained or until an animal model of HIV disease is developed or some other new knowledge instills wide confidence that a particular vaccine is likely to be effective. The urgency of the AIDS epidemic worldwide argues that fundamental and clinical HIV vaccine research needs to be pursued simultaneously (79, 80).

EFFICACY TRIAL DESIGNS

Phase I trials typically enroll a small number (12 to 100) of healthy individuals at low risk of HIV infection to evaluate safety and immunogenicity of the candidate vaccine. Phase II trials also evaluate safety and immunogenicity in a larger number (50 to 200) of volunteers, including individuals at higher risk of HIV infection. Phase III trials measure vaccine efficacy and require hundreds to thousands of volunteers (600 to 6000), depending on factors such as seroincidence in the trial population, minimum efficacy to be detected, accrual period, desired length of the trial, loss to follow-up and desired statistical parameters (Table 43.5) (62, 81, 82).

Phase III trials typically evaluate the ability of the vaccine to protect individuals who receive the vaccine relative to a control group receiving placebo, with an assumption of equal exposure between two groups. The primary end point could be prevention of infection, prevention of the establishment of chronic infection (e.g., absence of detectable virus at a certain time point after apparent infection), reduction in viral load, or clinical benefit (81).

Clinical benefit is not a practical primary end point in HIV vaccine efficacy trials given the long time between infection and disease. Reduction in viral load may be difficult to accept as a primary end point. Although many data demonstrate that viral load predicts clinical outcome in HIV-infected individuals, a correlation between viral load and clinical outcome has not been demonstrated in individuals who received an experimental vaccine before infection. Given the urgency of the epidemic, however, regulators in some countries may be persuaded to approve a vaccine for higher-seroincidence populations based on a reduction of viral load end point if appropriate follow-up can be accomplished after the trial.

Definitive efficacy trials in populations of lower seroincidence (e.g., 1 to 3%), as found in industrialized countries, would require a large number of volunteers and could be expensive (62). Intermediate-sized or "phase IIb" trials have been designed to estimate whether the vaccine has a minimum efficacy (83). Instead of several thousands of volun-

Table 43.5. Relation of Seroincidence to Efficacy Trial Size[a]

Sample seroincidence (%)	Number of Volunteers
1	8,780
2	4,420
3	2,970
4	2,250

[a]Assumptions: 3-year trial with 90% power to detect 50% efficacy; efficacy achieved over a 6-month immunization period; loss to follow-up 10% per year or less.
(Data from Vermund SH. The efficacy of HIV vaccines: methodological issues in preparing for clinical trials. In: Nicolosi A, ed. HIV epidemiology: models and methods. New York: Raven Press, 1994:187–209.)

teers, each arm of the phase IIb trial would enroll about 1500 volunteers, the exact number depending on seroincidence in that population and other design parameters. Phase IIb trials would not replace phase III trials but would help to guide decisions on whether to move a candidate vaccine into larger trials. Only under the best or worst of circumstances, either low (less than 30%) or high (more than 70%) efficacy, would a phase IIb trial give reasonable proof of the vaccine's ability to protect individuals. Candidate vaccines with observed efficacy in the midrange would have to be evaluated in a larger, definitive trial to obtain a more precise estimate of efficacy. A well-designed and carefully executed phase IIb trial will also provide information on whether neutralizing antibody levels correlate with protection and to some extent whether plasma HIV RNA levels in vaccinated volunteers are reduced compared with controls.

Other alternative trial designs may also be considered, given that the overall public health benefits of a vaccine derive from the combined impact of immunization on the individual and the distribution of the effective vaccine in the population. Community-based trials could be feasible in developing countries. Similar communities would be selected, and a fraction of the communities would receive the candidate vaccine while the control group could receive an unrelated vaccine. All would receive education and counseling. To give a valid measure of vaccine effectiveness, the communities would have to be "closed" to transmission from other communities, changes in behavior could not dramatically differ between communities, and the vaccine's effect would have to be relatively long lasting.

Other designs may also be considered. The indirect or overall public health benefit can be estimated by comparing the impact of an immunization program in different populations with different incident rates. In addition, if information on contacts can be gathered, then the impact of immunization on infectiousness can be evaluated (84).

ETHICAL CHALLENGES IN CONDUCTING VACCINE TRIALS IN DEVELOPING COUNTRIES

Generally, "ethics" is defined as a set of rules or standards governing what is right or wrong. In the context of clinical trials involving human subjects, this issue includes consideration of how research affects trial participants and society at large by the research process and outcomes and how the research trials conform to principles of right and wrong.

The three basic principles of ethics in biomedical and behavioral research, based on definitions in the 1949 Nuremberg Codes and the 1964 World Medical Association Declaration of Helsinki, are the principles of respect for autonomy, beneficence, and justice (85, 86). "Respect for autonomy" establishes the principle that researchers, in their research design and implementation, must support the ability of individual trial participants to make their own informed decisions regarding participation and to be able to act on those decisions. Additional effort and protection must be provided to avoid coercion and to support self-determination when research participants have a restricted ability for independent decision making, such as by imprisonment, military service, or economic or social forces. "Beneficence" essentially means that potential benefits of research should be maximized, and potential harms and risks of harm should be minimized. "Justice" refers to both comparative distribution of risks and benefits and the absolute burden of risks borne by participants and society.

During the past 40 years, these ethical standards and the structures for enforcing them in biomedical research have become increasingly standard throughout the world. IRBs were made mandatory at all research facilities in the United States beginning in 1978, and review and oversight of research to minimize risks of research are also carried out by the United States Food and Drug Administration and by local data safety monitoring boards (87, 88). Moreover, United States companies and universities supporting research in other countries are mandated by law to have foreign IRB approval and project assurance agreements. Several African, Asian, and Latin American countries have established similar structures for ethical oversight of research. The capacity for ethical review in many other countries is sorely lacking. Complicated ethical issues may arise in any research setting, and appropriate institutional review groups and processes are needed in every country where clinical research is conducted (11, 89–92).

ETHICAL ISSUES OF HIV VACCINE RESEARCH

A Just Distribution of Risk and Benefit

Realistically, preventive HIV vaccine trials in many countries probably will involve large numbers of volunteers who are poor, undereducated, and of low social status, simply because these characteristics often correlate with higher risk of HIV infection. A study that enrolls volunteers who are at high risk of HIV infection even with trial-sponsored counseling and intervention will reduce the amount of time, the number of volunteers, and the resources needed for the trial. This factor raises the question about equal distribution of risks and benefits.

In the aftermath of the infamous Tuskegee study on syphilis in the United States, the United States Commission for the Protection of Human Subjects of Biomedical and Behavioral Research stated that "the proposed involvement of . . . disproportionate numbers of racial and ethnic minorities or persons of low socioeconomic status should be justified" (93). Strong scientific justification exists for disproportionate recruitment in HIV vaccine efficacy studies, but consequences are complex for a country or society conducting research disproportionately on people who are disadvantaged socially, politically, or economically. Although immediate benefits of the trial, such as HIV prevention interventions and referral to medical care and treatment, would be directed to populations most in need, assurances must be made that the ultimate benefit of the research, an effective HIV vaccine, be shared by those who bear the risks of the research.

To address the ethical question of distributive justice, international and national agencies have begun efforts to link HIV vaccine trial preparation with HIV prevention campaigns, medical services, and community mobilization. In addition, efforts (discussed later) are being made to ensure international availability to any vaccine that proves efficacious.

Informed Consent and Independent, Noncoerced Participation

The informed consent process should explain the goals of the trial, the reason that the trial would benefit by the participation of the individual, what participation means, the potential risks and benefits of participation to the volunteer and others, alternatives to participation, issues of confidentiality, any compensation for trial participation and for any costs or injuries resulting from trial participation, and the right to end participation at any time. The informed consent process should ensure that the potential participant understands the information and that the person's choice to participate or not is voluntary.

Although informed consent explicitly supports an individual's independent and autonomous decision, decisions in many communities are heavily influenced by peers and a larger social and political context. Furthermore, in less-educated populations, the challenges to gaining fully informed consent from potential research participants is made more difficult when potential volunteers cannot grasp the complex scientific concepts of the research, as described earlier. Finally, the voluntary aspect of informed consent is complicated when potential volunteers seek the medical and HIV prevention services that HIV vaccine efficacy studies, by design, offer and that may not otherwise be available to them.

More specifically, researchers are obliged ethically to provide responsible and achievable HIV behavior change counseling and other prevention interventions, as well as the best possible referrals for clinical diagnosis and care and other health needs. Resolving ethical issues of voluntary consent when trial-related services surpass those outside the trial remain the responsibility of duly appointed international and national ethics review committees.

Maximizing Benefits and Minimizing Risks

The benefits of trial participation have been described above. In addition to maximizing the benefits of participation, researchers ethically attempt to minimize risks to participants, understanding that all risk cannot be eliminated from research studies. The current vaccine candidates that have been tested so far in phase I and phase II human safety and immunogenicity studies have shown little to no major side effects or adverse reactions. Nevertheless, the theoretical risks of participation in an HIV vaccine trial range from minimal inconvenience and short-term side effects, such as a sore arm or dizziness, to an unknown long-term effects of a retrovirus vaccine. In addition to the physical risk and economic cost of participation, research trial volunteers may find themselves stigmatized and at risk of losing income or health care if the research trial is identified as being conducted only among marginalized or high-risk populations. A risk may also arise if the volunteer perceives that the vaccine is protective, or if the vaccine makes the volunteer HIV-antibody positive on routine screening tests.

Most studies provide a guarantee of varying levels of compensation for injuries and inconvenience that result directly from participation in the research study. For HIV vaccine trial participants in developing countries, a question has been raised whether participants will be able to seek compensation through legal means if they are harmed or require medical services resulting from participation in a trial and to which legal systems participants will have access. Possible solutions have been proposed elsewhere (94). One approach would be a treaty between the manufacturer's country and the recipient nation that would waive the legal liability of the pharmaceutical companies in favor of an administrative claims procedure. Claims would be handled by the host country and would be funded by contributions from the governments or foreign or private international relief organizations or by contributions from the pharmaceutical company based on a percentage of the price of each vaccine dose sold.

Researchers can maximize benefits and minimize risks by designing competent trials that use all available preclinical data and knowledge, ensure good use of resources and volunteer time, adequately incorporate good collection of data and specimens, provide good clinical care and referrals, and efficiently answer the research questions.

Building Structures for Ethical Research

In both industrialized and developing countries that are preparing for HIV vaccine trials, the challenge of building institutions that provide independent ethical oversight is complicated by highly political environments, fierce competition for resources, and social and economic inequality that may limit access to information. Researchers and governments can be particularly sensitive to criticism and public debate. However, researchers, government officials, ethics committees, and potential research participants all have a role in encouraging and facilitating a healthy and informed debate about the benefits and costs of HIV vaccine research trials.

These parties can each participate in research oversight mechanisms, including IRBs and data safety monitoring boards, creating appropriate and effective informed consent procedures, setting up services and service referrals for those who opt not to participate in the research, evaluating future means of ensuring access to an effective vaccine, and in a larger sense, weighing the costs of these activities against the potential benefits of improved health and services for the trial community.

PROGRESS TO DATE

Phase I trials of candidate vaccines have taken place predominantly in the United States, European nations including Sweden, Israel, and other industrialized countries (see Chap. 42) (26, 28). A few phase I trials of candidate vaccines have been initiated in less-developed countries, including Thailand, Brazil, and China. Thailand, given it previous vaccine development experience and the dedicated efforts of the United States army in utilizing its infrastructure in northern Thailand, has conducted several trials (Table 43.6). Uganda is slated to initiate a phase I trial of ALVAC vCP215 later in 1998. Other countries are likely to follow in the coming years if additional resources become available to develop products suitable for testing in and use by those populations.

No candidate vaccine has yet to progress beyond phase II trials. In 1994, the NIAID decided to not support expanded trials of rgp120 at that time, but made clear that this decision pertained only to NIAID support of trials in the United States and the dynamics of the epidemic in other countries may yield different decisions. Indeed, the World Health Organization Global Programme on Vaccines declared that trials of rgp120 *could* be undertaken in other countries.

At this time, rgp120, in combination with a recombinant canarypox expressing multiple HIV proteins, is being evaluated in a phase II trial in the United States. This "prime-boost" strategy may progress to larger trials in the United States or Thailand by 1999 to 2000.

NOVEL APPROACHES TO ACCELERATING HIV VACCINE DEVELOPMENT

When HIV was discovered in 1983, investigators predicted that it would take just a few years to develop an HIV vaccine (95). Since then, we have learned that the combination of challenges in developing an HIV vaccine is unique relative to other viruses for which vaccines have been developed successfully. Even though the consensus is that the typical paradigms do not hold for HIV (96), the primary dependence has been on the same technology transfer mechanisms successful for the development of other vaccines and for therapies to treat HIV infection. Specifically, success depends on the full involvement of the private sector to conduct preclinical development, to manufacture vaccine for human trials, and eventually to market and distribute licensed vaccines. To date, almost every HIV vaccine that has entered clinical trial has been prepared by a private company. Few academic investigators have the interest, expertise, capabilities, or resources to translate their vaccine designs into material suitable for even small-scale human trials.

One of the greatest challenges in addressing the HIV/AIDS epidemic on a worldwide scale has been the lack of sufficient incentives to bring the expertise of the private sector fully to bear on the problem (97). Although a public health need exists for safe, effective vaccine and other prevention measures, companies have few incentives to make and test vaccines throughout the world because only a few of those whose lives would benefit from an effective HIV vaccine live in industrialized countries and would be able to purchase the vaccine. In addition to this lack of incentives are many disincentives to companies to become involved in developing HIV vaccines for testing in and use by developing countries, including liability concerns, market size uncertain-

Table 43.6. Outline of Ongoing and Planned HIV Vaccine Trials in non-OECD Countries

Country	Vaccine	Adjuvant	Trial
Brazil	V3 conjugate	Alum	Phase I completed
	vCP205		Phase I under discussion
China	V3-conjugate	Alum	Phase I completed
	Virus-like particles		Phase I under discussion
Cuba	Peptide conjugate		Phase I under way
Haiti	vCP205		Phase I under discussion
Israel	Peptide conjugate		Phase I under discussion
Kenya	Recombinant vaccinia		Phase I under discussion
Thailand	rgp120 (B)	QS21	Phase I completed
	rgp120 (B + E)	QS21	Phase I/II to begin 1999
	rgp120 (B)	MF59	Phase I completed
	rgp120 (B + E)	MF59	Phase II/III to begin 1998–1999
	vCP205		Phase I to begin 1998
	vCP205 + boost		Phase I/II to begin 1998
	ALVAC (E) + boost		Phase I under discussion
	V3-conjugate		Phase I completed
Trinidad	DNA vaccine (E/A)		Phase I under discussion
	vCP205		Phase I under discussion
Uganda	vCP205		Phase I to begin 1998
	DNA vaccine		Phase I under discussion
Zambia	DNA vaccine		Phase I under discussion

ties, patent restrictions, and the absence of public policies about vaccine purchase and distribution.

Incentives that could attract increased involvement of the private sector include direct funding of critical path development activities to decrease costs associated with development and evaluation of candidate HIV vaccines. Such arrangements could include sharing of intellectual property or licenses to facilitate low-cost production and distribution to poorer countries, while allowing companies the freedom to operate in major markets. In addition, efforts to ensure companies some return on their investment should be considered. For example, guaranteed loans to developing countries for the purchase of successful vaccine would provide companies some assurance of market size. Acceptance of multitiered pricing in the United States would encourage United States manufacturers to use this approach to subsidize accessibility by poorer countries. Alternatively, tax breaks, patent extensions, or protection from liability may increase the incentives for companies to be involved in HIV vaccine development.

After several years of international consultations, and with support of several nonprofit organizations, the International AIDS Vaccine Initiative (IAVI) was created in 1996 to ensure development of safe, effective, preventive vaccines for use throughout the world. The strategies currently pursued include the following: advocacy for HIV vaccine development; funding for others to fill critical applied gaps in the vaccine development pipeline, which is now focused on the entry of novel designs into phase I trial and the rapid movement of the most promising candidate vaccines into efficacy trials; and working with others to create incentives for increased investment in vaccine research and development. This novel approach calls on the strengths of the nonprofit sector to complement the activities of publicly supported research programs and privately supported product development, and it represents a new model to address the lack of incentives for full participation by the private sector in product development.

In addition, the international scope of IAVI and its partner, the UNAIDS, will help to focus attention to solving the worldwide problem through development and distribution of safe, effective, preventive HIV vaccines. To this end, IAVI is promoting entry of multiple vaccine designs into human clinical trials in developing countries within the shortest time possible, and it is working with researchers and government officials to determine how developing countries can best contribute to international efforts to identify safe and effective preventive vaccines for worldwide use.

References

1. Pham-Kanter GBT, Steinberg MH, Ballard RC. Sexually transmitted diseases in South Africa. Genitourin Med 1996;72:160–171.
2. Galloway M. Seventh national HIV survey results released. AIDS Bull (Med Res Council S Afr) 1997;1–2:1–4.
3. Adler M. Sexually transmitted diseases control in developing countries. Genitourin Med 1996;72:83–88.
4. St.Louis ME, Wasserheit JN, Gayle HD. Janus consider the HIV pandemic: harnessing recent advances to enhance AIDS prevention [editorial]. Am J Public Health 1997;87:10–12.
5. Cohen MB, Hoffman IF, Royce RA, et al. Reduction of concentration of HIV-1 in semen after treatment of urethritis: implications for prevention of sexually transmitted HIV-1. Lancet 1997;349:1868–1873.
6. Over M, Piot P. HIV infection and sexually transmitted diseases. Washington, DC: World Bank, 1991:HSPR 26.
7. Laga M. STD control for HIV prevention: it works! Lancet 1995;346:518–519.
8. Grosskurth H, Mosha F, Todd J, et al. Impact of improved treatment of sexually transmitted diseases on HIV infection in rural Tanzania: randomised controlled trial. Lancet 1995;346:530–536.
9. Gilson L, Mkanje R, Grosskurth H, et al. Cost-effectiveness of improved treatment services for sexually transmitted diseases in preventing HIV infection in Mwanza region, Tanzania. Lancet 1997;350:1805–1809.
10. Mayaud P, Grosskurth H, Changalucha J, et al. Risk assessment and other screening options for gonorrhea and chlamydial infections in women attending rural Tanzanian antenatal clinics. Bull WHO 1995;73:621–631.
11. Nowak R. Staging ethical AIDS trials in Africa. Science 1995;269:1332–1335.
12. Cook RL, Rosenberg MJ. Sex Transm Dis 1998;25:144–153.
13. Kreiss J, Ngugi E, Holmes K, et al. Efficacy of nonoxynol 9 contraceptive sponge use in preventing heterosexual acquisition of HIV in Nairobi prostitutes. JAMA 1992;268:477–482.
14. Weir SS, Roddy RE, Zekeng L, et al. Nonoxynol-9 use, genital ulcers and HIV infection in a cohort of sex workers. Genitourin Med 1995;71:78–82.
15. Feldblum PJ, Weir SS. The protective effect of nonoxynol-9 against HIV infection. Am J Public Health 1994;84:1032–1034.
16. Roddy RE, Zegeng L, Ryan KA, et al. A randomized controlled trial of the effect of N-9 film use on male-to-female transmission of HIV-1 [abstract]. In: National Conference on Women and HIV, Los Angeles, 1997:135.
17. Stafford M, Cain D, Rosenstein I, et al. A placebo-controlled double-blind prospective study in healthy female volunteers of dextrin sulphate gel. J Acquir Immune Defic Syndr Hum Retrovirol 1997;14:213–218.
18. Sonderfan AJ, Chancellor T, Buckheit R, et al. Safety and in vitro efficacy of a topical microbicide gel for the prevention of HIV-1 transmission [abstract]. In: 4th Conference on Retroviruses and Opportunistic Infections. Washington, DC: American Society for Microbiology, 1997:522.
19. Tsai CC, Follis KE, Sobo A, et al. Prevention of SIV infection in macaques by (R)-9-(2-phosphonylmethoxypropyl) adenine. Science 1995;270:1197–1199.
20. Connor EM, Sperling RS, Gelber R, et al. Reduction of material-infant transmission of human immunodeficiency virus type 1 with zidovudine treatment. N Engl J Med 1994;331:1173–1180.
21. Jackson JB, Guay L, Marum L, et al. Phase I/II trial of HIVIG for prevention of HIV-1 vertical transmission in Uganda [abstract]. In: 4th Conference on Retroviruses and Opportunistic Infections. Washington, DC: American Society for Microbiology, 1997:519.
22. Moore JP, McCutchan FE, Poon S, et al. Exploration of antigenic variation in gp120 from clades A through F of human immunodeficiency virus type 1 by using monoclonal antibodies. J Virol 1994;68:8350–8364.
23. Laal S, Burda S, Gorny MK, et al. Synergistic neutralization of human immunodeficiency virus type 1 by combinations of human monoclonal antibodies. J Virol 1994;68:4001–4008.
24. Mascola JR, Louder MK, Vancott TC, et al. Potent and synergistic neutralization of primary HIV-1 isolates by hyperimmune anti-HIV immunoglobulin (HIVIG) combined with monoclonal antibodies 2F5 and 2G12 [abstract]. In: 4th Conference on Retroviruses and Opportunistic Infections, Washington, DC: American Society for Microbiology, 1997;759.
25. Trkola A, Polamles AB, Yuan H, et al. Cross-clade neutralization of primary isolates of human immunodeficiency virus type 1 by human

monoclonal antibodies and tetrameric CD4-IgG. J Virol 1995;69: 6609–6617.
26. Walker MC, Fast PE. Clinical trials of candidate AIDS vaccines. AIDS 1994;8:S213–S236.
27. Johnston MI. HIV vaccines: problems and prospects. Hosp Pract 1997;32:125–140.
28. Johnston MI. HIV/AIDS vaccine development: challenges, progress and future directions. Rev Med Virol 1996;6:123–140.
29. Clements ML. Clinical trials of human immunodeficiency virus vaccines. In: DeVita VT, Hellman S, Rosenberg SA, eds. AIDS: biology, diagnosis, treatment and prevention. 4th ed. Lippincott–Raven, 1997: 617–626.
30. Anderson RM, Swinton J, Garnett G. Potential impact of low efficacy vaccines in populations with high rates of infection. Proc R Soc Lond [Biol] 1995;261:147–151.
31. Korber BTM, Allen EE, Farmer AD, et al. Heterogeneity of HIV-1 and HIV-2. AIDS 1995;9:S5–S18.
32. Robertson DL, Sharp PM, McCutchan FE, et al. Recombination in HIV-1 [scientific correspondence]. J Virol 1995;374:124-6.
33. Overbaugh J, Anderson RJ, Ndinya-Achola JO, et al. Distinct but related human immunodeficiency virus type 1 variant populations in genital secretions and blood. AIDS Res Hum Retroviruses 1996;12: 107–115.
34. Poss M, Martin HL, Kreiss J, et al. Diversity of virus populations from genital secretions and peripheral blood from women recently infected with human immunodeficiency virus type 1. J Virol 1995;69: 8118–8122.
35. Zhu T, Mo H, Wang N, et al. Genotypic and phenotypic characterization of HIV-1 in patients with primary infection. Science 1994;261: 1179–1181.
36. Moore JP, Cao Y, Qing L, et al. Primary isolates of human immunodeficiency virus type 1 are relatively resistant to neutralization by monoclonal antibodies to gp120, and their neutralization is not predicted by studies with monomeric gp120. J Virol 1995;69:101–109.
37. Sullivan N, Sun Y, Li J, Hofmann W, et al. Replicative function and neutralization sensitivity of envelope glycoproteins from primary and T-cell line–passaged human immunodeficiency virus type 1 isolates. J Virol 1995;69:4413–4422.
38. Moore JP. HIV vaccines: back to primary school. J Virol 1995;376:115.
39. Berman PW, Nakamura GR. Adhesion mediated by intercellular adhesion molecule 1 attenuates the potency of antibodies that block HIV-1 gp160-dependent syncytium formation. AIDS Res Hum Retroviruses 1994;10:585–593.
40. Kostrikis LG, Michalopoulou Z-H, Cao Y, et al. Determining neutralization serotypes of HIV type 1 by neural networks. AIDS Res Hum Retroviruses 1996;12:1667–1669.
41. Kostrikis LG, Cao Y, Ngai H, et al. Quantitative analysis of serum neutralization of human immunodeficiency virus type 1 from subtypes A, B, C, D, E, F, and I: lack of direct correlation between neutralization serotypes and genetic subtypes and evidence for prevalent serum-dependent infectivity enhancement. J Virol 1996;70:445–458.
42. Nyambi PN, Nkengasong J, Lewi P, et al. Multivariant analysis of human immunodeficiency virus type 1 neutralization data. J Virol 1996;70:6235–6243.
43. Devico A, Silver A, Thornton AM, et al. Covalently cross-linked complexes of human immunodeficiency virus type 1 (HIV-1) gp120 and CD4 receptor elicit a neutralizing immune response that includes antibodies selective for primary virus isolates. Virology 1996;218: 258–263.
44. Broder CC, Early P, Long D, et al. Antigenic implications of human immunodeficiency virus type-1 envelope quaternary structure, oligomer-specific and -sensitive monoclonal antibodies. Proc Natl Acad Sci U S A 1996;91:11,699–11,703.
45. Richardson TM, Stryjewski BL, Broder CC, et al. Humoral response to oligomeric human immunodeficiency virus type 1 envelope protein. J Virol 1996;70:753–762.
46. Mascola JR, Vancott TC, Louder M, et al. Neutralizing antibody against primary HIV-1 isolates elicited by immunization with oligomeric, but not monomeric, env glycoprotein [abstract]. In: Conference on Advances in Vaccine Research. Bethesda, MD: National Institutes of Health, 1996.
47. Luke W, Petry H, Dittmer U, et al. Immunization with gp130 oligomers but not gp130 monomers partially protects rhesus macaques against the productive infection with SIVmac32H and disease development [abstract]. In: Conference on Advances in Vaccine Research. Bethesda, MD: National Institutes of Health, 1996.
48. Haynes BF. Scientific and social issues of human immunodeficiency virus vaccine development. Science 1993;260:1279–1286.
49. Roberts CGP, Meister GE, Jesdale BM, et al. Identification of HIV peptide epitopes by a novel algorithm. AIDS Res Hum Retroviruses 1996;12:593–610.
50. Ferrari G, Humphrey W, McElrath MJ, et al. Clade B-based HIV-1 vaccines elicit cross-clade cytotoxic T lymphocyte reactivities in uninfected volunteers. Proc Natl Acad Sci U S A 1997;94:1396–1401.
51. McElrath MJ, Siliciano RF, Weinhold KJ. HIV type 1 vaccine-induced cytotoxic T cell responses in phase I clinical trials: detection, characterization, and quantitation. AIDS Res Hum Retroviruses 1997; 13:211–216.
52. Donnelly JJ, Ulmer JB, Shiver JW, et al. DNA vaccines. Annu Rev Immunol 1997;15:617-48.
53. Weiner DB, Wang B, et al. Induction of humoral and cellular immune responses to the human immunodeficiency type 1 virus in nonhuman primates by in vivo DNA innoculation. Virology 1995;211:102–112.
54. Vogel FR, Sarver N. Nucleic acid vaccines. Clin Microbiol Rev 1995;8:406–410.
55. Baba TW, Jeong YS, Penninck D, et al. Pathogenicity of live attenuated SIV after mucosal infection of neonatal macaques. Science 1995;267: 1820–1825.
56. Bolognesi DP. A live-virus AIDS vaccine? Not yet, it is too early to consider use of a live-attenuated virus vaccine against HIV-1. J NIH Res 1994;6:55–62.
57. Wyand MS, Manson KH, Garcia-Moll M, et al. Vaccine protection by a triple deletion mutant of simian immunodeficiency virus. J Virol 1996;70:3724–3733.
58. Putkonen P, Walther L, Zhang Y, et al. Long-term protection against SIV-induced disease in macaques vaccinated with a live attenuated HIV-2 vaccine. Nature Med 1995;1:914–918.
59. Desrosiers RC. Controversies in Science. Yes, it is time to consider use of a live-attenuated virus vaccine against HIV-1. J NIH Res 1994;6:54–59.
60. Deacon NJ, Tsykin A, Solomon A, et al. Genomic structure of an attenuated quasi species of HIV-1 from a blood transfusion donor and recipients. Science 1995;270:988–991.
61. Kirchhoff F, Greenough TC, Brettler DB, et al. Brief report: absence of intact nef sequences in a long-term survivor with nonprogressive HIV-1 infection. N Engl J Med 1995;332:226–232.
62. Dixon D, Rida W, Fast P, et al. HIV Vaccine trials: some design issues including sample size calculation. J Acquir Immne Defic Syndr 1993; 6:485–496.
63. Halloran ME, Longini IM, Haber M, et al. Exposure efficacy and change in contact rates in evaluating prophylactic HIV vaccines in the field. Stat Med 1994;13:357–377.
64. Nelson K, Celentano D, Eiumtrakul S, et al. Changes in sexual behavior and a decline in HIV infection among young men in northern Thailand. N Engl J Med 1996;335:297–303.
65. Bridbord K. Preparations for AIDS vaccine evaluations: AIDS international training and research program. AIDS Res Hum Retroviruses 1994;10:S227–S229.
66. Esparza J, Mugerwa RD, Ojwok O. Proceedings from the HIV candidate vaccine trial workshop, September 9–11, 1996. Kampala, Uganda: Ugandan Ministry of Health, 1996.
67. Jackson D, Martin H, Bwayo J, et al. Acceptability of HIV vaccine trials in high risk heterosexual cohorts in Mombasa, Kenya. AIDS 1995;9: 1279–1283.
68. Mehendale S, Rodrigues J, Brookmeyer R, et al. Incidence and predictors of HIV-1 seroconversion in patients attending STD clinics in India. J Infect Dis 1995;172:1486–1491.

69. Martin H, Jackson D, Mandaliya K, et al. Preparation for AIDS vaccine evaluation in Mombasa, Kenya: establishment of seronegative cohorts of commercial sex workers and trucking company employees. AIDS Res Hum Retroviruses 1994;10:S235–S237.
70. Miotti P, Canner J, Chiphangwi J, et al. Preparation for AIDS vaccine evaluations: rate of new HIV infection in a cohort of women of childbearing age in Malawi. AIDS Res Hum Retroviruses 1995;10:239–241.
71. Beyrer C, Brookmeyer R, Natpratan C, et al. Measuring HIV-1 incidence in northern Thailand: prospective cohort results and estimates on early diagnostic tests. J Acquir Immune Defic Syndr Hum Retrovirol 1996;12:495–499.
72. Mbizvo M, Machekano R, McFarland W, et al. HIV Seroincidence and correlates of seroconversion in a cohort of male factory workers in Harare, Zimbabwe. AIDS 1996;10:895–901.
73. Fischer R, McNeil J. Preparations for AIDS vaccine evaluations: progress in international cohort development and evaluation. AIDS Res Hum Retroviruses 1994;10:S223–S225.
74. Lawrence D, Hoff R. Progress toward readiness for international trials: conference summary. AIDS Res Hum Retroviruses 1995;11:1291–1295.
75. Nowan R. Staging ethical AIDS trials in Africa. Science 1995;269:1332–1335.
76. Rugpao S, Beyrer C, Tovanabutra S, et al. Multiple condom use and decreased condom breakage and slippage in Thailand. J Acquir Immune Defic Syndr Hum Retrovirol 1997;14:169–173.
77. Kuntolbutra S, Celentano D, Suprasert S, et al. Factors related inconsistent condom use with commercial sex workers in northern Thailand. AIDS 1996;10:556–558.
78. Widom R. Domestic HIVNET risk reduction counseling information and materials. Bethesda, MD: Abt Associates, 1996.
79. Esparza J, Heyward W, Osmanov S. HIV vaccine development: from basic research to human trials. AIDS 1996;10:S123–S132.
80. Anonymous. NIAID strategic plan for HIV vaccine research and development. Bethesda, MD: National Institute of Allergy and Infectious Diseases, 1996.
81. Rida WN, Lawrence DN. Some statistical issues in HIV vaccine trials. Stat Med 1994;13:2155–2177.
82. Vermund SH. The efficacy of HIV vaccines: methodological issues in preparing for clinical trials. In: Nicolosi A, ed. HIV epidemiology: models and methods. New York: Raven Press, 1994:187–209.
83. Rida W, Fast P, Hoff R, et al. Intermediate sized trials for the evaluation of HIV vaccine candidates: a workshop summary. J Acquir Immune Defic Syndr Hum Retrovirol 1997;16:195–203.
84. Rida WN. Asssessing the effect of HIV vaccination on infectiousness. Stat Med 1996;15:2393–2904.
85. Anonymous. Trials of war criminals before the Nuremberg military tribunals under control council law. Washington, DC: US Government Printing Office, 1949;10:181–182.
86. Anonymous. World Medical Association Declaration of Helskinki: Recommendations guiding medical doctors in biomedical research involving human subjects. 1964.
87. The National Commission for the Protection of Human Subjects of Biomedical and Behavioral Research. Institutional review boards: report and recommendations. Washington, DC: US Department of Health, Education and Welfare, 1978:(OS)78-0008.
88. Demets DL, Fleming TR, Whitley RJ. The data safety monitoring board and AIDS clinical trials. Controlled Clin Trials 1997;16:408–421.
89. Foulkes M, Connell C, Fischer R. Ethical and monitoring issues in international trials: conference summary. AIDS Res Hum Retroviruses 1995;11:1313–1314.
90. Lurie P, Bishaw M, Chesney M, et al. Ethical, behavioral, and social aspects of HIV vaccine trials in developing countries. JAMA 1994;271:295–301.
91. Chesney M, Lurie P, Coates T. Strategies for addressing the social and behavioral challenges of prophylactic HIV vaccine trials. J Acquir Immune Defic Syndr Hum Retrovirol 1995;9:30–35.
92. Grady C. The search for an AIDS vaccine: ethical issues in the development and testing of a preventive HIV vaccine. Bloomington: Indiana University Press, 1995.
93. The National Commission for the Protection of Human Subjects of Biomedical and Behavioral Research. The Belmont Report: ethical principles and guidelines for the protection of human subjects of research. Washington, DC: US Department of Health, Education and Welfare, 1978:(OS)78-0012.
94. Wilson JP. Limitation of manufacturer liability for administration of an AIDS vaccine overseas. Int Lawyer 1996;30:783–810.
95. Gallo RC, Sarin PS, Gelmann EP, et al. Isolation of human T-cell leukemia virus in acquired immune deficiency syndrome (AIDS). Science 1983;220:865–867.
96. Fauci AS. An HIV vaccine: breaking the paradigms. Presented at the Clinical Research Meeting of the American Academy of Pediatrics/American Society for Clinical Immunology/American Federation for Clinical Research, May 8, 1995.
97. Anonymous. HIV vaccines: accelerating the development of preventive HIV vaccines for the world. New York: Rockefeller Foundation, 1994.
98. Rodrigues J, Mehendale S, Shepherd M, et al. Risk factors for HIV infection in people attending clinics for sexually transmitted diseases in India. Br Med J 1995;311:283–286.

44

IMMUNE-BASED THERAPIES FOR HIV INFECTION

Michelle Onorato and Richard B. Pollard

As more effective and better tolerated antiretroviral therapy for human immunodeficiency virus (HIV) infection has come into wide clinical use, investigators have increasingly realized that resistance is likely to develop to most pharmaceutical agents, even when these agents are used in combination. This understanding has led to a resurgence of interest in developing alternative therapeutic approaches for HIV infection. Potential strategies for immune-based therapies of HIV infection that are currently being explored include the enhancement of HIV-specific immune responses and stimulation of general immune response. Table 44.1 outlines these approaches. Immunotherapy in patients with early HIV infection could help to modulate the normal responses to infection and lessen the severity of or rate of progression to subsequent immunodeficiency. Investigators also hope that these approaches may be of particular value in the treatment of patients with later stage infection whose high levels of viremia and previous exposure to therapy place them at greatest risk of developing resistance to therapeutic agents and who have the highest risk of opportunistic infection because of severe immunodeficiency. Our early experience has taught us that any such interventions must be carefully juxtaposed with highly active antiretroviral therapy that has significant antiviral and immunologic activity.

THERAPIES TARGETED AT HIV-SPECIFIC IMMUNE RESPONSE

The enhancement of HIV-specific response has been approached by three different mechanisms: the administration of HIV-specific therapeutic and prophylactic vaccines; the administration of passive humoral immunotherapy, by either transfer of pooled immunoglobulin from HIV-infected individuals or monoclonal antibodies to specific viral epitopes; and the passive transfer of specific cell populations in an effort to enhance immune responsiveness to HIV. As the mechanisms of host response to HIV infection have become better understood, particularly cellular immune responses and the development of antibody response (especially neutralizing antibody response), strategies for boosting HIV-specific immune responses have been proposed. However, that enhancement of HIV-specific immune response leads to improved clearance of virus is not yet clear. Several large trials of therapeutic vaccines suggest that, even though immunologic responses to envelope vaccine epitopes are seen, these responses do not necessarily lead to benefit in terms of increased CD4 counts or reductions in HIV viral load.

HIV VACCINES

Interest has been expressed in the development of HIV vaccine not only as a prophylactic measure (for which its potential value is obvious), but also as a therapeutic measure, in hope that the enhanced HIV-specific immunity may add to the efficacy of potent antiretroviral therapy. The first strategy to be used was the development of recombinant glycoprotein vaccines representative of envelope epitopes, similar to the successful hepatitis B surface antigen vaccine. In AIDS Clinical Treatment Group trial 214 (ACTG 214), four vaccines of this type—a IIIB-based gp120 antigen in alum adjuvant, an MN-based gp120 antigen in alum adjuvant, an SF-2 based gp120 antigen in MF-59 adjuvant, and an Env2-3 gp120 antigen in MF-59 adjuvant—were compared to placebo arms of either adjuvant only in a randomized, double-blind trial in HIV-infected patients with CD4 counts higher than 500 cells/mm^3 while receiving no antiretroviral therapy. Primary end points included immunogenicity, as measured by a fivefold increase in immunogen-specific lymphocyte proliferative responses, and toxicity. Secondary end points included change in HIV-1–specific cytotoxic T-lymphocyte (CTL) responses and change in the slope of CD4 count over time. The IIIB-based gp120 vaccine induced immunologic responses in 29% of subjects, and the MN-based gp120 vaccine induced immunologic responses in 24% of subjects; by comparison, the MF-59 conjugated envelope antigens were poorly immunogenic. No effect on CD4 count was noted in any of the treatment arms, and the vaccines were well tolerated, with mild local reactions as the most frequent adverse effect. A companion trial (ACTG 209) examined vaccines in individuals with fewer than 500 CD4 cells/mm^3 at entry. Although some individuals did have evidence of response to the vaccines used, the percentage

Table 44.1. Strategies of Immune-Based Therapy

Enhancement of HIV-specific immunity	Therapeutic vaccine
	Transfer of HIV-specific cell populations
	Transfer of pooled immune sera
	Transfer of monoclonal antibody
General immune enhancement	Inhibition of proinflammatory cytokines
	Administration of immune modulators, i.e., IL-2, IL-12, interferon-α

responding was significantly lower that in those with higher CD4 counts (1, 2). When a gp160 vaccine was studied in patients with earlier HIV infection, investigators found no evidence of a slowing of disease progression as measured by an impact on the decline of T-cell counts (3). A ongoing phase I/II double-blind controlled trial of an MN-based gp160 (Immuno Ag) vaccine versus placebo in HIV-infected patients either with more than 500 CD4 cells/mm^3 or with 200 to 400 CD4 cells/mm^3 who are vaccinated after receiving highly active antiretroviral therapy that has suppressed viral replication not only will address questions regarding the safety and immunogenicity of this vaccine, but also will gather data on viral and immunologic markers. Investigators hope that decreasing the endogenous production of HIV in an infected patient could enhance the ability of a host to develop a heightened immune response to a vaccine epitope.

An alternative approach to vaccine development is the production of peptide vaccines, which have the potential advantage of being less costly than recombinant protein vaccines. In the case of HIV-1, phase I trials of synthetic V3 peptide vaccines have begun using a preparation of 15 peptides in a multiple-antigen presentation system representing 5 different HIV-1 subtypes (4). In a similar vein, a synthetic V3 loop peptide conjugated to purified protein derivative has been shown to induce neutralizing antibodies to a laboratory HIV-MN strain, but not to other clade viruses (5).

Another advance in the development of HIV-1 vaccines has been the interest in DNA vaccines, which have the advantage of being even better adapted to large-scale production than peptide or protein vaccines. A gene encoding the antigen along with a promoter can be inserted into a plasmid, cloned, replicated, and purified; the purified plasmid preparation can then be injected intramuscularly, where the gene can be transcribed, translated, and expressed; this gene product, although expressed in the host cell, is recognized as foreign and provokes an immunogenic response. Potentially, this approach could include multiple genes simultaneously to provoke antigenic response to multiple epitopes. Candidate DNA vaccines using *env* and *rev* genes have reached the stage of phase I trials, and data already are available from primate trials suggesting that vaccination with plasmids expressing HIV-1 or simian immunodeficiency virus type 1 (SIV-1) proteins can induce immunologic responses (6).

An interesting approach capitalizing on the ability to introduce multiple genes has been coinfection with plasmids containing genes for interleukin-12 (IL-12) as well as HIV-1 antigens, in the hope that the enhancement of cell-mediated immunity seen with increased levels of IL-12 translates to a role for IL-12 as an adjuvant in this setting, particularly because decreased levels of IL-12 are among the immune derangements seen in HIV-infected patients. Two groups have independently shown increases in HIV-1–specific cell-mediated immunity in mice who were coimmunized with genes for both HIV-1 antigen and IL-12 compared with HIV antigen alone, findings that spark interest in this cytokine as a potential adjuvant for therapeutic HIV-1 vaccines (7, 8).

Some of the methods described earlier may provide enhanced immune responses to exogenous HIV protein and could stimulate enough of an immune response that antiviral and immunologic improvements will be observed. However, to date no attempts have produced antiviral or generalized immunologic improvement in HIV-infected individuals. Future attempts should be guided by carefully designed initial trials of potential agents.

HIV-SPECIFIC CYTOTOXIC T-CELL RESPONSES

The immunopathogenesis of HIV infection begins with the interaction between HIV-1 and the cellular immune response; so a clearer understanding of this interaction may potentially lead to interventions that can change the natural history of HIV infection. The cellular immune response after primary infection is responsible in part for a several log drop in viral replication after the initial burst of viremia, and so it is an area of intense interest. Primary infection, with its high levels of viremia, is also the time when the virus begins to develop genetic diversity in response to selective pressures exerted by the host immune response. This dynamic interaction at the initial phase of HIV infection sets the stage for the natural history of HIV infection.

Several studies have suggested that the main mechanism responsible for this initial control of viral replication is the cell-mediated immune response, rather than specific neutralizing antibody. Supporting this concept is the observation that HIV-specific CTLs can be found just as high levels of viremia begin to abate and before the rise in neutralizing antibody titers. This finding suggests that the CTL response produces declines in initial viremia (9, 10). In addition, an HIV-1–specific CTL response is demonstrable as early as 21 days after clinical presentation with primary infection and is directed at diverse epitopes within many of the HIV-1 gene products (10–12). Nonhuman primate models of primary infection with SIV show a remarkably parallel sequence of events; within 4 weeks of detecting SIV p27 antigen in blood and SIV RNA in the extrafollicular and sinusoidal areas of lymphoid tissue, p27 antigen is cleared. Increased numbers of CD8+ lymphocytes are detected in the periphery and in lymph nodes, concurrent with this decline in plasma viremia. Humoral and cellular SIV-specific immune responses can be detected within 2 weeks of initial infection. Thus, both human and simian data suggest that the remarkable containment of initial viremia is due in large part to both humoral and cellular immune responses (13, 14). The importance of vigorous response to HIV-1 proliferative responses has been demonstrated by data demonstrating that individuals who have the ability to control HIV infection (long-term nonprogressors) without antiviral therapy have brisk CTL responses and humoral immune responses, in contrast to the undetectable responses usually seen in chronic HIV infection. Furthermore, in three patients presenting with acute seroconversion syndrome who received combination antiretroviral therapy, all demonstrated the development of HIV-1–specific proliferative responses as levels of viremia declined (15).

Further study has shown that, although CTL response during primary infection develops to multiple antigenic determinants, this repertoire is more limited than would be predicted. Perhaps this limitation allows the virus, with its genetic diversity, a chance to escape immune surveillance by mutation of critical epitopes (10, 16). Indeed, in a patient with early HIV infection, serial observations revealed an early CTL response aimed at a highly immunodominant epitope in gp160. However, with mutation that resulted in a single amino acid change, an escape mutant emerged that could not be recognized by epitope-specific CTL. Thus, the CTL response can exert selective pressure that drives the emergence of resistant virus just as is seen with antiretroviral therapy (17). Implications of this finding include vaccine strategies that result in CTL response to multiple codominant epitopes and the importance of concurrent antiretroviral and immune-based approaches to therapy of HIV infection.

Data from natural history studies as well as study of long-term nonprogressors with HIV-1 infection suggest that the immunopathogenesis of HIV infection is affected by the quality of the CTL response. For example, CTL activity is preserved in long-term nonprogressors, in stark contrast to vertically infected children, who generally have little CTL response and rapid progression of clinical disease (18, 19). Furthermore, longitudinal studies of CTL response over time show a steady decline in HIV-1–specific CTL precursor cells, paralleling the decline in the ability of CD8+ cells to suppress HIV replication with progressive infection (20).

Transfer of HIV-Specific Cell Populations

Given the importance of cell-mediated immunity both in primary infection and in asymptomatic nonprogressors, the ex vivo propagation and expansion of lymphocyte populations and reinfusion of expanded cell populations to HIV-infected patients are potential treatment strategies currently being explored. One study examined the ex vivo expansion of unfractionated lymphocytes from an HIV-negative identical twin and infusion of the expanded cell population to the HIV-infected twin. This method appeared to be safe and to result in increases in CD4 counts in the infected twin (21). Another approach is the adoptive transfer of CD8 cells after expansion. Preliminary reports suggest that these reinfused cells have little CTL activity, and most of these cells are rapidly cleared from the circulation. Two other groups are evaluating the administration of CD8 cells expanded ex vivo with IL-2 as potential therapy for Kaposi's sarcoma (22). Another strategy under investigation is the administration of HIV-specific autologous CTL cell lines that have been selected in vitro and expanded for reinfusion; the safety and effects on immunologic parameters of this approach are currently under study. The finding that CD4 can be expanded in vitro in the presence of three antiretroviral drugs holds promise for autologous expanded CD4 cells as therapy as well (23). The limitations of these approaches are the enormous investment in cell culture facilities, careful quality control, and the variable half-life of the reinfused cells requiring repeated administrations.

ENHANCEMENT OF ANTIBODY RESPONSE

The strategy of transfer of pooled antibodies from HIV-infected donors or of monoclonal antibodies directed against HIV is of interest not only as a potential prophylactic measure to prevent infection in exposed seronegative individuals, but also as attempt to enhance antiviral activity in the serum of already infected individuals. This enhancement of antiviral activity could occur not only by neutralization of the virus, but perhaps also by enhancement of antibody-dependent cellular cytotoxicity and increased complement-mediated lysis. The long half-life of antibodies makes this approach particularly attractive, because intermittent therapy at bimonthly intervals may be practical. The drawback of this approach again relates to the genetic diversity of HIV and the potential for development of mutants not recognized by the more specific antibody preparations. In addition, the vast amount of circulating viral antigen could potentially lead to formation of immune complexes, with adverse effects from their deposition in various tissues; however, no adverse events after these infusions that could be related to immune complex deposition have been reported to date.

Trials of Polyclonal Antisera

Two controlled trials have been published that evaluate the effect of HIV immune plasma on disease progression in HIV-positive individuals. In the first trial, 63 volunteers (most of whom had CD4 counts lower than 100 cells/mm^3) were randomized to receive monthly infusions of either HIV immune or HIV antibody–negative plasma. No difference was seen between treatment groups with regard to CD4 counts, frequency of opportunistic infections, or overall survival (24). In a second trial, in which patients received either immune plasma or plasma from negative donors every 2 weeks for a year, investigators noted a significant decrease in the number of opportunistic infections in subjects receiving immune sera (25). Other investigators have reported preliminary results of similar strategies; in one trial, monthly transfusion of pooled hyperimmune plasma to patients with clinical AIDS or AIDS-related complex (ARC) resulted in clinical remissions of 6 to 32 months, with sustained neutralization of HIV viremia. In the patients with ARC, clinical remission lasted beyond the 22-month study period, with both neutralization of HIV viremia as measured by levels of p24 antigenemia and stabilization of CD4 counts (26). This finding is supported by the results of a placebo-controlled study of a sterile, filtered pooled high-titer anti-HIV plasma preparation (treated with β-propiolactone to inactivate any HIV that may be present), administered on a monthly basis to patients with advanced HIV infection. Substantial, although not statistically significant, increases in CD4 count and survival were seen in the group of patients with baseline CD4 counts of more than 50 cells/mm^3 who received the highest doses of immune plasma. However, investigators found no evidence of alteration in virus load because quantitative measurements of HIV RNA by polymerase chain reaction did not differ between the two groups (27).

The role of hyperimmune anti-HIV intravenous immune globulin in preventing perinatal transmission has also been assessed. In a phase I/II double-blind controlled study by the pediatric ACTG, 28 maternal infant pairs were randomized to receive either HIV hyperimmune globulin (HIVIG) or placebo (intravenous immunoglobulin [IVIG]) beginning between 20 and 30 weeks of gestation; all the mothers enrolled were receiving zidovudine. Mothers received infusions every 28 days until delivery; infants received a single infusion within 12 hours of birth. All mothers and infants received zidovudine as per the ACTG 076 protocol. Only mild adverse events were reported, none of which required discontinuation of therapy. Sustained suppression of immune complex–dissociated p24 antigenemia was seen in the treated women, although no change was seen in quantitative HIV RNA. Infants in the treatment group had higher levels of p24 antibody at birth, a finding confirming transplacental transfer of antibody from the HIVIG infusions (28). A recent trial was discontinued early because the rate of vertical transmission had been decreased to such a low level (less than 5%) with antiretroviral agents alone that investigators believed that is was impossible to detect the influence of the immunoglobulin preparation.

Further studies are necessary before the significance of these results and the potential for specific immunoglobulin as therapy are fully understood. Various trials have also examined the efficacy of IVIG without specific anti-HIV activity, and results of these studies consistently show no effect on HIV-related virologic or immunologic parameters, although IVIG may have a role in reducing bacterial infections (29).

Transfer of Monoclonal Antibody

Another approach that has been considered is the administration of specific monoclonal antibodies to various epitopes of HIV. This method has been limited by concerns that the virus would acquire resistance to specific antibodies, although this problem may be overcome by administering combinations that are directed at more than one neutralizing epitope. Another obstacle to clinical trials of specific monoclonal antibodies is the expense of the large-scale production that would be required.

The first step in developing monoclonal antibodies to be tested in clinical trials is to identify epitopes, antibodies to which will result in anti-HIV activity. Most attention to date has focused on antibodies to various surface epitopes of HIV, either to the V3 loop, C4, and gp41 or, in the case of F105, directed against the CD4 binding site. Combinations of these antibodies in vitro show at least additive activity, and against some strains of HIV, they have synergistic activity. The F105 antibody has been evaluated in a dose-escalating phase I/II ACTG trial; although prolonged half-lives of the antibody were seen, no change in HIV titers were observed (30). Chimeric antibodies against the V3 loop and CD4 binding site are also under development, and they have been reported to have initial clinical activity perhaps related to the development of immune responses to the antibody (31). Two other monoclonal antibodies have been examined in vitro and have been accepted as candidates for both adult and pediatric trials that will tentatively begin in 1998. The major limitation of this approach has been the difficulty in obtaining sufficient clinical-grade material to conduct these types of studies.

GENERAL IMMUNE ENHANCEMENT

The availability of cytokine inhibitors, which could potentially counteract the overproduction of cytokines seen in HIV infection, and the availability of general immune stimulators have led to interest in manipulation of the immune system as a therapeutic tool. Theoretically, the general immune stimulation or suppression that may result from these manipulations may, in fact, hasten the rate of HIV progression, particularly because concern exists that stimulation of certain cell populations may enhance HIV replication. Thus, active antiretroviral therapy will have to be administered concurrently with any of these modulators of the immune system.

Inhibition of Proinflammatory Cytokines

The cytokine that has been most extensively studied is tumor necrosis factor-α (TNF-α), both because it is produced at high levels in HIV infection and because it upregulates HIV expression in vitro. Pentoxyphylline, thalidomide, and corticosteroids have all been studied as potential therapies because these agents can inhibit TNF-α production.

With regard to pentoxyphylline, studies of this agent in HIV-infected patients showed that it decreased TNF-α mRNA in the treated patients, and preliminary evidence suggested that some patients do have responses with regard to decreasing viral load. However, in a controlled trial of pentoxyphylline at the highest tolerable dosages, no significant antiviral effect was detected (32). It seems that the benefit is seen mainly in patients who are found to have high pretreatment levels of TNF-α (32, 33). This observation led to the initiation of a placebo-controlled trial of this agent in HIV-infected patients with active pulmonary tuberculosis in Uganda, because patients with concurrent HIV infection and tuberculosis have extremely high levels of circulating TNF-α and have a poorer prognosis than patients with similar stages of disease with HIV infection alone. The patients enrolled in this study had early HIV infection, with a mean CD4 cell count of 380 cells/mm^3, and they did not receive other antiretroviral therapy. Patients in the pentoxyphylline arm of the trial had lower levels of HIV RNA than the control arm, as well as reduced levels of β$_2$-microgloblulin; however, no difference was observed in the two groups with regard to new AIDS-defining illness or survival (34).

Thalidomide is also known to inhibit production of TNF-α and has been shown to inhibit HIV-1 replication in vitro. Multiple uncontrolled observations have been made of its benefit in the treatment of aphthous ulcers in HIV-infected patients, and a placebo-controlled trial has been completed that substantiates this finding and evaluates the effect of thalidomide on HIV replication itself. Patients in the thalidomide arm of the trial appeared to have increases in HIV-1 RNA, a finding underscoring the importance of concurrent antiretroviral therapy; an unexpected finding was that patients in the thalidomide arm actually showed an increase in TNF levels, despite the in vitro evidence to the contrary (35). Another small study is ongoing to examine the safety, tolerability, and antiviral efficacy of thalidomide in patients with CD4 counts higher than 300 cells/mm^3.

The observation that corticosteroids appear to benefit patients with HIV-associated nephropathy has led to interest in this strategy for the interruption of cytokine activity. A placebo-controlled trial of corticosteroid therapy in patients with biopsy-proved typical nephropathy could not be completed because of a lack of eligible patients (36). A small exploratory trial examining the activity of prednisone in a placebo-controlled trial will start shortly (ACTG 349) and will examine the immunologic and virologic activity in patients treated for 8 to 12 weeks with pretreatment CD4 counts lower than 300 cells/mm^3.

Similar to the interest in prednisone, cyclosporine has been proposed as an immunomodulatory agent with potential activity in HIV infection. ACTG 334 is a phase II trial of cyclosporine versus placebo in patients with early HIV infection (CD4 cell count greater than 500 cells/mm^3) that is currently enrolling patients and will explore the role of cyclosporine as an immunosuppressive agent that may decrease some of the enhanced immune functions seen in patients with high CD4 cell counts. End points will include plasma levels of soluble IL-2 receptors, as well as functional assays of immunity and HIV-1 viral load.

Enhancement of Immune Response by Cytokines and Lymphokines

Recent studies of administration of immune modulators have focused mainly on IL-2 and interferon. With regard to interferon, low-dose oral interferon has been studied with and without concurrent antiretroviral administration; it appears to have little benefit with regard to antiviral activity. Subcutaneous administration of interferon in combination with other antiviral agents has also been evaluated. A small study of this agent in combination with zidovudine did not show any benefit with regard to CD4 counts (37). A triple-drug study of interferon with zidovudine and dideoxycytidine suggested a benefit with regard to both CD4 counts and p24 antigens in those patients in the arm of the trial containing interferon, but the sample size was extremely small (38). Data are also available from an uncontrolled trial of interferon and zidovudine in patients with Kaposi's sarcoma, reporting minimal benefit. The most positive data regarding interferon-α to date are for its use in the treatment of HIV-associated thrombocytopenia. Patients in two uncontrolled studies showed benefit with regard to platelet levels at low doses of this agent (39, 40). In general, systemic administration of interferon-α has resulted in unacceptable toxicity and marginal benefit in HIV-infected patients, features that limit its clinical usefulness.

IL-2 has emerged as a potentially exciting agent for immune-based therapy of HIV infection. Results of a small trial of intermittent intravenous IL-2 (5-day continuous infusions every 8 weeks) are encouraging; 60% of patients with baseline CD4 counts higher than 200 cells/mm^3 showed sustained increases in CD4 counts after treatment. This increase in CD4 count was seen over a 14-month follow-up of these patients, although no change was seen in plasma HIV RNA levels or levels of p24 antigenemia. In patients with baseline CD4 counts lower than 100 cells/mm^3, no benefit in terms of CD4 cell count was observed, however, the transient rise in viral load reported in preliminary studies of IL-2 in later stage HIV-infected patients was not seen in this study, presumably because of concurrent antiretroviral therapy (41, 42). A major drawback of this approach is the frequency of continuous intravenous therapy, so trials of subcutaneous or intermittent intravenous IL-2 are planned as well. ACTG 328, a trial of intravenous IL-2 with highly active antiretroviral therapy versus subcutaneous IL-2 with highly active antiretroviral therapy versus highly active antiretroviral therapy alone, will examine the effects on CD4 cell count, HIV-1 viral load, and rates of emergence of resistance to antiretroviral therapy.

IL-12 is currently in phase I clinical trials; it is known to increase natural killer cell and CTL activity in vitro and is known to be deficient in HIV-1 infected patients. Investigators hope that treatment will stimulate development of T-helper type-1 cells, reverting the shift to T-helper type 2 predominance that is seen in HIV infection and that may be a detrimental consequence of the host response to HIV-1 infection (43). ACTG 325, a trial of semiweekly subcutaneous IL-12 in HIV-infected patients with late stage disease (CD4 cell counts less than 50 cells/mm^3) is under way. The end points for this trial include not only safety and tolerability of the agent, but also potential antimycobacterial and immunologic effects. Studies are planned in patients with earlier HIV infection as well.

In summary, both pharmacologic and immunologic approaches to new interventions for HIV infection have yielded some encouraging agents and potential combinations of agents. The challenge will be to sort out which strategies are likely to result in long-term clinical benefit to patients with minimum toxicity. In a rapidly changing environment of new antiretroviral agents, the position of immunologic therapy will have to be understood carefully. Major developments in suppression of HIV with significant improvements in immune function have been reported. However, whether immune function can fully be restored with antiretroviral therapy alone is unclear at present. Immune-based therapies likely will be an important adjuvant to antiretroviral therapy in some patient populations.

References

1. Schooley RT, Spino C, Shiu S, et al. Poor immunogenecity of HIV-1 envelope vaccines with alum or MF59 adjuvant in HIV-1 infected individuals: results of two randomized trials [abstract 756]. In: 4th Conference on Retroviruses and Opportunistic Infections. Washington, DC: American Society for Microbiology, 1997.
2. Kuritzke DR, Spino C, Valentine F, et al. Associations of plasma HIV-1 RNA, CD4 count, and immune response in patients with 50–500 CD4 cells/µl [abstract 757]. In: 4th Conference on Retroviruses and Opportunistic Infections. Washington, DC: American Society for Microbiology, 1997.
3. Birx DL, Davis C, Ruiz, N, et al. Results of a phase II double-blinded multicenter placebo controlled HIV therapeutic vaccine trial [abstract A.275]. In: 11th International Conference on AIDS, Vancouver, 1996.
4. O'Hagen DT, McGee JP, Wang CY, et al. The UBI multicomponent HIV vaccine: the advantages of controlled release microparticles. In: Girard M, Vallete L, Marnes-La-Coquette, eds. Retroviruses of human AIDS and related animal diseases: 8th colloques des "Cent Gardes." Paris: Foundation Marcel Meriux, 1993:309–313.
5. Rubenstein A, Goldstein H, Pettoelle-Mantovani M, et al. Safety and immunogenicity of a V3 loop synthetic peptide conjugated to purified protein derivative in HIV seronegative volunteers. AIDS 1995;9:243–251.
6. Esparza J, Heyward WL, Osmanov S. HIV vaccine development: from basic research to human trials. AIDS 1996;10:S123–132.
7. Kin JJ, Ayyavoo V, Weiner DB, et al. In vivo engineering of a cellular immune response by coadministration of IL-12 expression vector with a DNA immunogen. J Immunol 1997;158:816–826.
8. Tsuji T, Hamajima K, Okuda K, et al. Enhancement of cell mediated immunitiy against HIV-1 induced by co-inoculation of plasmid encoded HIV-1 antigen with plasmid expressing IL-12. J Immunol 1997;158:4002–4013.
9. Koup RA, Safrit JT, Cao Y, et al. Temporal association of cellular immune responses with initial control of viremia in primary HIV-1 syndrome. J Virol 1994;68:4650–4655.
10. Pantaleo G, Demarest JF, Soudeyns H, et al. Major expansion of CD8+ T cells with a predominant Vβ usage during the primary immune response to HIV. Nature 1994;370:463–467.
11. Safrit JT, Andrews CA, Zhu T, et al. Characterization of HIV-1 specific cytotoxic T lymphocyte clones isolated during acute seroconversion: recognition of autologous virus sequences within a conserved immunodominant epitope. J Exp Med 1994;179:463–472.
12. Borrow P, Lewicki H, Hahn BH, et al. Virus specific CD8+ cytotoxic T-lymphocyte activity associated with control of viremia in primary HIV-1 infection. J Virol 1994;68:6103–6110.
13. Reimann KA, Tenner-Racz K, Racz P, et al. Immunopathogenic events in acute infection of rhesus monkeys with SIV of macaques. J Virol 1994;68:2362–2370.
14. Yasutomi Y, Reiman KA, Lord CI, et al. SIV-specific CT8+ lymphocytes response in acutely infected rhesus monkeys. J Virol 1993;67:1701–1711.
15. Rosenberg ES, Billingsley JM, Walker BD, et al. Vigorous HIV-1-specific CD4+ T cell responses associated with control of viremia. Science 1997;278:1447–1450.
16. Coullin I, Culmann–Penciolelli B, Gomard E, et al. Impaired CTL recognition due to genetic variations in the main immunogenic recognition of the HIV-1 nef protein. J Exp Med 1994;180:1129–1134.
17. Borrow P, Lewicki H, Wei X, et al. Antiviral pressure exerted by HIV-1 specific cytotoxic T lymphocytes during primary infection demonstrated by rapid selection of CTL escape virus. Nature Med 1997;3:205–211.
18. Klein MR, Bende RJ, Van Baalen CA, et al. Persistent high gagCTL frequency and low viral load in long term asymptomatic HIV infection [abstract WS-B03-3]. In: 9th International Conference on AIDS/ 4th STD World Congress, Berlin, 1993.
19. Luzuria K, Koup RA, Pikora CA, et al. Deficient HIV-1specific cytotoxic T cell responses in vertically infected children. J Pediatr 1991;119:230–236.
20. Mackewicz CE, Ortega HW, Levy JA. CD8+ cell anti-HIV activity correlates with the clinical status of the infected individual. J Clin Invest 1991;87:1462–1466.
21. Walker R, Larson M, Cartert C, et al. Adoptive immunotherapy using activated expanded synergistic lymphocytes in HIV-infected identical twins [abstract WS-B286]. In: 9th International Conference on AIDS/ 4th STD World Congress, Berlin, 1993.
22. Klimas N, Fletcher M, Walling J, et al. Response of Kaposi's sarcoma to autologous CD8 cells expanded and activated ex vivo and re-infused with rIL-2 [abstract WS-B152]. In: 9th International Conference on AIDS/4th STD World Congress, Berlin, 1993.
23. Wilson CC, Wong JT, Rosenthal TM, et al. Ex vivo expansion of CD4+ T lymphocytes from HIV-1 seropositive persons in the absence of ongoing viral replication [abstract 111]. In: Abstracts of the 1st National Conference on Human Retroviruses. Washington, DC: American Society for Microbiology, 1993.
24. Jacobson JM, Colman N, Ostrow NA, et al. Passive immunotherapy in treatment of advanced HIV infection. J Infect Dis 1993;168:298.
25. Lefrere JJ, Vittecoq D, French Passive Immunotherapy Collaborative Study Group. Passive immunotherapy in AIDS: results of a double blind randomized phase II study [abstract L12]. In: Abstracts of the 1st National Conference on Human Retroviruses. Washington, DC: American Society for Microbiology, 1993.
26. Karpas A, Bainbridge S. Passive Immunization in HIV disease [abstract PO-A28-0659]. In: 9th International Conference on AIDS/4th STD World Congress, Berlin, 1993.
27. Levy J, Youvan T, California Physician Study Group for PHT. Efficacy and safety of passive hyperimmune therapy in HIV disease [abstract PO-B28-2149]. In: 9th International Conference on AIDS/4th STD World Congress, Berlin, 1993.
28. Lambert SJ, Mofenson LM, Fletcher CV, et al. Safety and pharmacokinetics of hyperimmune anti–HIV immunoglobulin administered to HIV-infected pregnant women and their newborns. J Infect Dis 1997;175:283–291.
29. Pollard RB, Forrest BD. Immunologic therapy for HIV-infected individuals, 1993–1994. AIDS 1994;8:S295.
30. Wolfe EJ, Samore MH, Cavacini LA, et al. Pharmacokinetics of F105, a monoclonal antibody, in subjects with HIV infection. Clin Pharmacol Ther 1996;59:662–667.
31. DeZube BJ, Lederman MM, Pardee AB, et al. Pentoxyphyline decreases tumor necrosis factor and may decrease HIV replication in AIDS patients [abstract PO-B28-2142]. In: 9th International Conference on AIDS/4th STD World Congress, Berlin, 1993.
32. Dezube BJ, Lederman ML, Spritzler JG, et al. High-dose pentoxyphylline in patients with AIDS inhibition of tumor necrosis factor production. J Infect Dis 1995;171;1628–1632.
33. Mole L, Margolis D, Holodniy M. A pilot study of pentoxyphylline in HIV-infected patients with CD4+ lymphocytes less than 400 cells/mm^3 [abstract PO-B28-2116]. In: 9th International Conference on AIDS/ 4th STD World Congress, Berlin, 1993.
34. Wallis RS, Nsubuga, Whalen C, et al. Pentoxyphylline therapy in human immunodeficiency virus positive persons with tuberculosis: a randomized, controlled trial. J Infect Dis 1996;174:727–733.

35. Jacobson JM, Greenspan JS, Spritzler J, et al. Thalidomide for the treatment of oral aphthous ulcers in patients with human immunodeficiency virus infection. N Engl J Med 1997;336:1487–1493.
36. Pawar R, Kalayjian R, Graham R, et al. Effect of steroid therapy on progression of HIV-associated nephropathy [abstract PO-B24-1956]. In: 9th International Conference on AIDS/4th STD World Congress, Berlin, 1993.
37. Jablonowski H, Mauss S, Knechten H, et al. Combination therapy with zidovudine and low dose alpha interferon in HIV seropositive patients with rapidly declining CD4+ lymphocyte counts [abstract PO-B28-2148]. In: 9th International Conference on AIDS/4th STD World Congress, Berlin, 1993.
38. Nadler J, Toney J, Holt D, et al. Comparison of Retrovir, HIVID, and Wellferon vs. Retrovir and HIVID in HIV-infected patients without AIDS [abstract 688]. In: 23rd Interscience Conference on Antimicrobial Agents and Chemotherapy, New Orleans, 1993.
39. Vianelli N, Catani L, Gugliotta L, et al. Recombinant alpha interferon 2β in the treatment of HIV-related thrombocytopenia. AIDS 1993;7:823–827.
40. Fabris F, Sgarabotto D, Zanoan E, et al. The effect of a single course of alpha-2β-interferon in patients with HIV-related and chronic idiopathic immune thrombocytopenia. Autoimmunity 1993;14:175–179.
41. Kovacs JA, Baseler M, Lane HC, et al. Increases in CD4 T lymphocytes with intermittent courses of IL-2 in patients with HIV infection. N Engl J Med 1995;332:567.
42. Kovacs JA, Vogel S, Albert JM, et al. Controlled trial of interleukin-2 infusion in patients infected with the human immunodeficiency virus. N Engl J Med 1996;335:1350–1356.
43. Foli A, Saville MW, Baseler MW, et al. Effects of the Th1 and Th2 stimulatory cytokines interleukin-12 and interleukin-4 on HIV replication. Blood 1995;85:2114–2123.

45
DRUG DEVELOPMENT

A. DISCOVERY AND DEVELOPMENT OF ANTIRETROVIRAL THERAPEUTICS FOR HIV INFECTION

Hiroaki Mitsuya and John Erickson

More than a decade has elapsed since the introduction of 3′-azido-2′,3′-dideoxythymidine (formerly known as azidothymidine [AZT] and currently known as zidovudine [ZDV]: Fig. 45A.1, *1*) as the first antiretroviral drug for the therapy of acquired immunodeficiency syndrome (AIDS) and its related diseases. During the mid-1980s, retroviral infection was thought to be inherently untreatable, and indeed, no serious efforts were made to develop antiviral drugs despite the discovery of the first human pathogenic retrovirus, human T-cell leukemia virus type 1 (HTLV-1). However, because treatment of human immunodeficiency virus type 1 (HIV-1) infection proved feasible, some potentially useful strategies for the antiviral therapy of AIDS emerged (1–8). Today, no doubt exists that antiretroviral chemotherapy can bring about reduction of viral load and clinical benefits to individuals infected with HIV-1.

The armamentarium of antiretroviral agents is rapidly growing. Five members of the broad family of antiretroviral 2′,3′-dideoxynucleosides (ddNs)—ZDV, 2′,3′-dideoxyinosine (ddI or didanosine: Fig. 45A.2, *2*), 2′,3′-dideoxycytidine (ddC or zalcitabine: see Fig. 45A.1, *5*), 2′,3′-didehydro-2′,3′-dideoxythymidine (d4T or stavudine: see Fig. 45A.1, *4*), and (−)-2′,3′-dideoxy-3′-thiacytidine (3TC or lamivudine: see Fig. 45A.1, *11*), all targeting the virally coded reverse transcriptase (RT), have been widely used. More nucleoside analogs with the dideoxy-configuration are under clinical or preclinical testing. They include a central nervous system (CNS)–penetrating abacavir (1592U89: see Fig. 45A.2, *10*) and an acid-resistant 2′-β-fluoro-2′,3′-dideoxyadenosine (FddA: see Fig. 45A.2, *7*). Considerable interest also exists in acyclic nucleoside phosphonates, including 9-(2-phosphonylmethoxyethyl)-adenine (PMEA: see Fig. 45A.2, *11*) and its lipophilic prodrug bis-pivaloyloxymethyl-PMEA (bis[POM]PMEA), and a propyl counterpart of PMEA, PMPA (see Fig. 45A.2, *12*). Nonnucleoside RT inhibitors (NNRTIs) have also been available, including nevirapine and delavirdine, and more compounds of this class will emerge in the near future (Fig. 45A.3). In addition, many different therapeutic agents target other stages of the HIV-1 replicative cycle. Among these are inhibitors of the HIV-1 protease, which include saquinavir, ritonavir, indinavir, and nelfinavir (Fig. 45A.4). Several newer protease inhibitors are now in clinical and preclinical development. Efforts to optimize antiretroviral activities of existing compounds have also been made. Investigators have now proved that combinations of multiple classes of antiviral agents, if properly combined, are far more efficacious than monotherapy in patients with HIV infection.

In theory, antiviral drugs exert their effects by interacting with viral structural components, virally encoded enzymes, viral genomes or specific host proteins such as cellular receptors, enzymes, or other factors required for viral replication (1, 2, 6–8). In principle, any virus-specific step in the replicative cycle of HIV-1 that differs from that in normal host cell function can serve as a potential target for the development of antiretroviral therapy. Some selected stages that may be targeted for therapeutic interventions of HIV-1 are illustrated in Table 45A.1. In this chapter, we highlight advances in the antiretroviral therapy against AIDS in terms of their laboratory and preclinical development in the past 10 years. We also discuss some challenges and problems been encountered in the inception of what perhaps we can call the initial success of chemotherapy of HIV-1 infection.

DRUG DISCOVERY, DESIGN, AND DEVELOPMENT

Drug Testing In Vitro

In the long term, it will be possible to design antiviral agents targeting virally encoded components critical for viral replication based on their molecular structures. Structure-based methods including protein crystallography, nuclear magnetic resonance (NMR) spectroscopy, and computational biochemistry are recent additions to the arsenal of drug discovery approaches that have contributed to recent some successes in antiretroviral therapy (9), as discussed later. Nevertheless, the identification of most potential antiviral agents still relies on techniques that permit a large number of test compounds to be screened reliably and rapidly in molecular target-based screen and in cell-based assays using

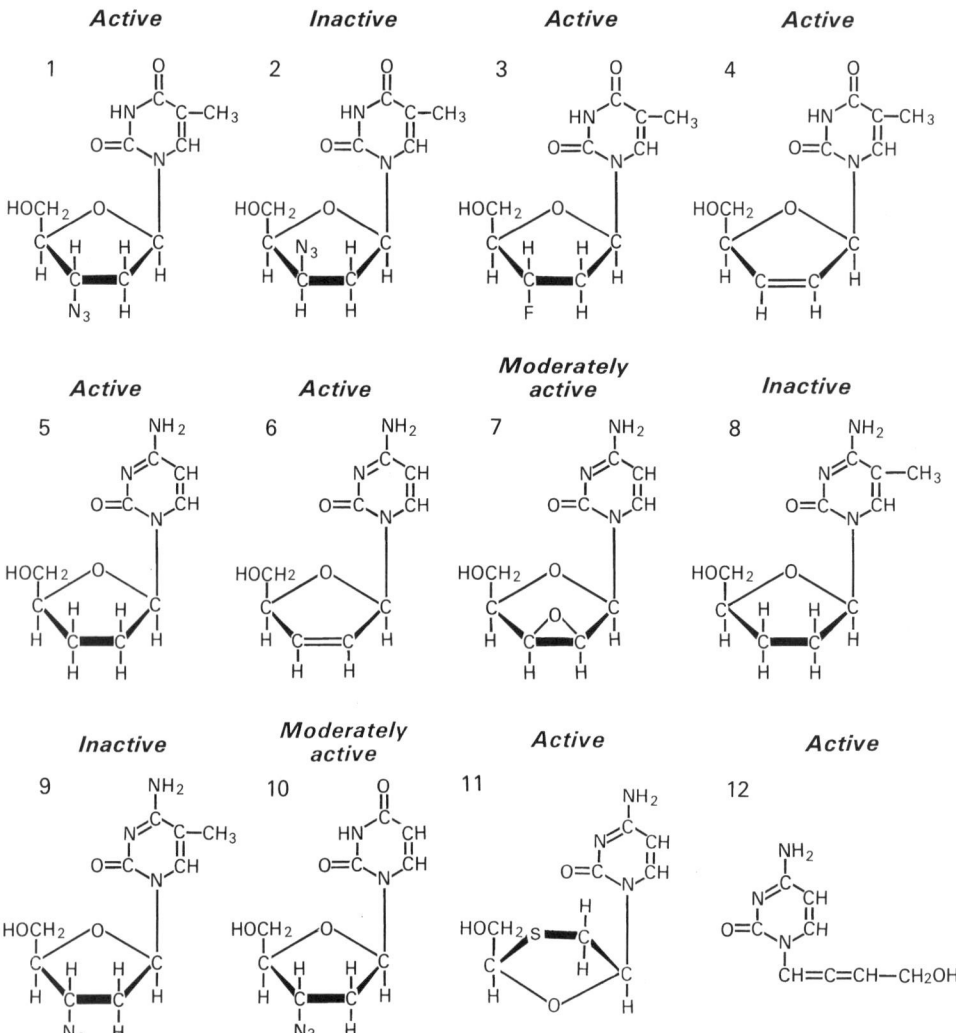

Figure 45A.1. Structures and in vitro antiretroviral activity of 2′,3′-dideoxypyrimidine nucleoside analogs. Antiretroviral activity of each compound was assessed under conditions of high multiplicities of infection (MOI) using ATH8 cells, H9 cells, normal clonal CD4+ T cells, MT-2 cells, or normal unfractionated peripheral blood mononuclear cells, based on the inhibition of the cytopathic effect of HIV, suppression of Gag protein production, or suppression of HIV viral DNA or RNA synthesis (references 2, 8, 10). Compounds that can give a virtually complete inhibition (80 to 100%) of the infectivity and cytopathic effect of HIV at concentrations that do not significantly affect the growth of target cells are defined as active. Compounds that can inhibit the infectivity and replication of HIV-1 by 30 to 80% are defined as moderately active. Compounds that give less than 30% inhibition are defined as inactive. Unless otherwise stated, the in vitro antiviral activity of compounds against HIV-1 defined here was determined by Mitsuya and his coworkers. *1*, 3′-α-azido-2′,3′-dideoxythymidine (AZT or erythro-AZT); *2*, 3′-β-azido-2′,3′-dideoxythymidine (threo-AZT; reference 339); *3*, 3′-α-fluoro-2′,3′-dideoxythymidine; *4*, 2′,3′-didehydro-2′,3′- dideoxythymidine (2′,3′-dideoxythymidinene or d4T); *5*, 2′,3′-dideoxycytidine (ddC); *6*, 2′3′-didehydro-2′,3′-dideoxycytidine (2′,3′-dideoxycytidinene or d4C; reference 340); *7*, 2′,3′-β-epoxy-2′,3′-dideoxycytidine (reference 341); *8*, 5-methyl-2′,3′-dideoxycytidine; *9*, 3′-azido-5-methyl-2′,3′-dideoxycytidine; *10*, 3′-azido-2′,3′-dideoxyuridine (AZddU) (reference 342); *11*, (-)-2′,3′-dideoxy-3′-thiacytidine (3TC); *12*, 1-(4′-hydroxy-1′,2′- butadienyl)cytosine (cytallene; reference 343).

multiple human target cells and HIV-1 strains including clinical HIV-1 isolates (10–14).

The availability of rapid and sensitive assay systems in the mid-1980s facilitated the testing of potential agents for anti–HIV-1 activity and led to the successful development of several ddNs for antiretroviral therapy of HIV-1 infection (10, 15–17). Some in vitro assay systems established in the late 1980s further accelerated the speed of discovering new antiretroviral agents (14, 18). At present, various approaches in assessing drugs for potential usefulness in HIV-related diseases are available. Table 45A.2 shows a set of techniques used in many laboratories. As an initial step of drug testing, one can use various HIV-1 cytopathic effect inhibition assays, using immortalized T-cell lines that are profoundly sensitive to the cytopathic effect of HIV-1 (10, 14–17). Other assay systems can also be used as an initial step of drug testing, depending on end points one would choose.

Certain "conventional" animal models, such as simian immunodeficiency virus (SIV)–infected macaques, have also been available for testing drugs for antiretroviral activity (19, 20). Animal models for HIV-1 infection, such as mice with genetically determined severe combined immunodeficiency

(SCID) engrafted with human hematolymphoid cells from fetal liver, thymus, and lymph node (SCID-hu mice) (21), and SCID mice reconstituted with human peripheral blood leukocytes (hu-PBL-SCID mice) (22) are also useful to expedite the process of drug development.

Rational Drug Design

Random drug screening has met with reasonable success in the development of antibacterial drugs, but random screening efforts for antiviral agents have been disappointing for the most part. The accidental discovery of antiviral drugs is much less likely than is the case for antibacterial screening because the number of viral-specific targets that can be exploited for intervention is much smaller. For example, a virus such as HIV-1 has an average of 15 associated viral proteins, whereas *Escherichia coli* contains approximately 1500 different proteins (23). Advances in the molecular virology of HIV-1 have led to new approaches for designing antiviral agents targeting specific virally encoded functions that are essential in the viral life cycle of HIV-1 (2, 6, 7). This knowledge has profoundly affected the discovery of anti–HIV-1 agents in particular. For example, target-based screens can now be used to identify novel lead compounds for specific targets that would otherwise go unidentified in cell culture–based assays. High-throughput protease assays were responsible for identifying nonpeptidic lead compounds that were subsequently developed into potent protease inhibitors with anti–HIV-1 activity (24), even though the initial lead compounds had no measurable antiviral activity in tissue culture assays. Conversely, a compound that exhibits antiviral activity in a cell culture–based screen can now be subjected to a

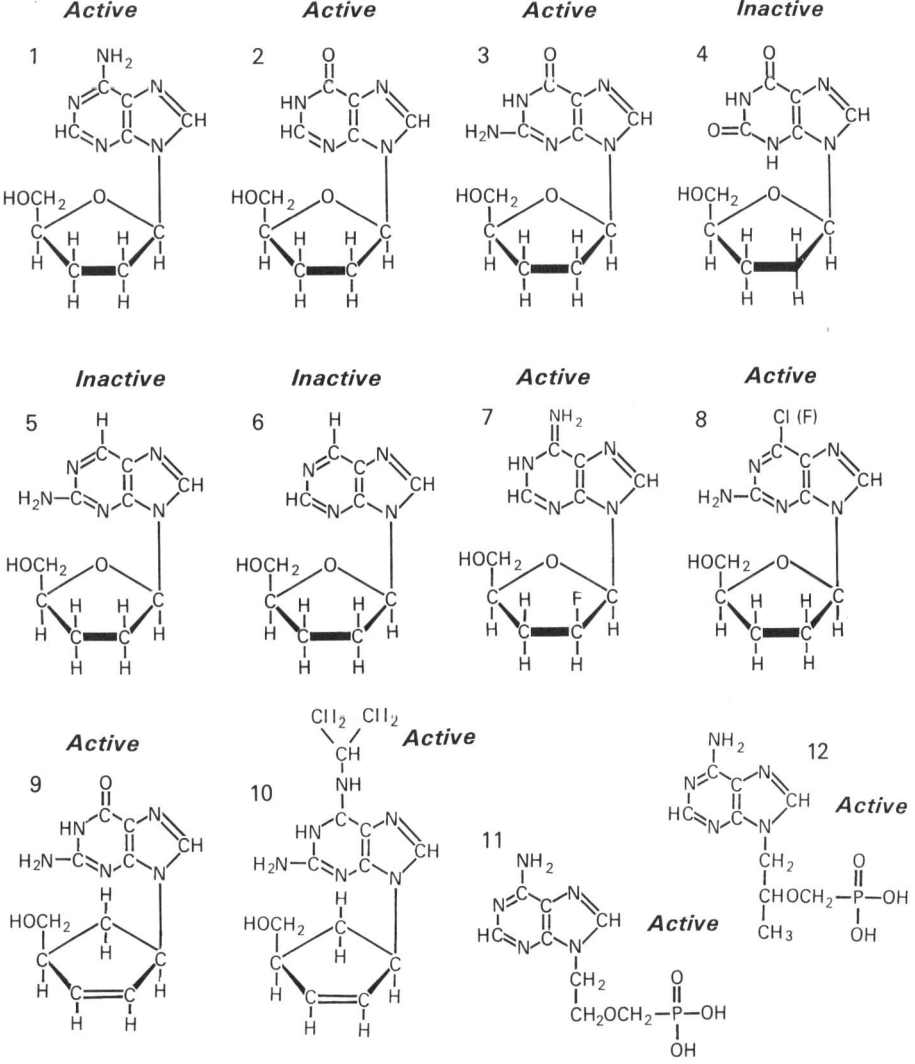

Figure 45A.2. Structures and in vitro antiretroviral activity of 2',3'-dideoxypurine nucleoside analogs. Antiretroviral activity of each compound was assessed as described in the legend to Figure 45A.1. *1*, 2',3'-dideoxyadenosine (ddA); *2*, 2',3'-dideoxyinosine (ddI); *3*, 2',3'-dideoxyguanosine (ddG); *4*, 2',3'-dideoxyxanthosine, *5*, 2-amino-2',3'-dideoxypurine ribofuranoside (reference 339); *6*, 2',3'-dideoxypurine ribofuranoside; *7*, 2'-β-fluoro-2',3'-dideoxyadenosine (FddA); *8*, 2-amino-6-chloro (or -fluoro)-2',3'-dideoxypurine ribofuranoside (references 344, 345); *9*, carbocyclic-2',3'-didehydro-2',3'-dideoxyguanosine (carbovir); *10*, abacavir (1592U89); *11*, phosphonylmethoxyethyladenine (PMEA); *12*, 9-(2-phosphonylmethoxypropyl)-adenine (PMPA).

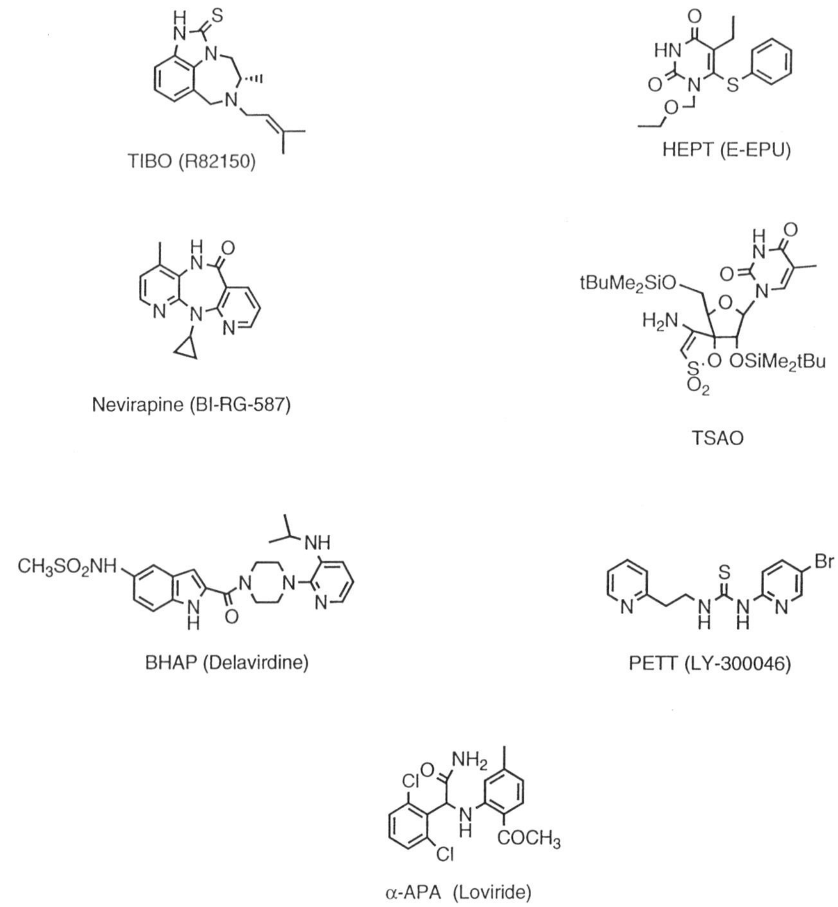

Figure 45A.3. Structures of nonnucleoside reverse transcriptase inhibitors.

battery of mechanism-based tests to profile its mode of action. Such information is important for selecting compounds directed against novel targets as lead compounds for new classes of inhibitors. Perhaps the most important and exciting approach to anti–HIV-1 drug discovery to emanate directly out of basic research on the virus is that of structure-based drug design.

Structure-based drug design approaches were implemented as drug discovery tools over a decade ago and are currently widely used to design safer, more specific, and more effective drugs in cases in which the structure of the molecular target has been determined by x-ray crystallography, NMR, or modeling (9). The first drug design studies with HIV-1 began with HIV protease in the early 1990s (25, 26), and they were made possible by the structure determination of this enzyme in several laboratories. Since then, the x-ray crystallography and NMR structures of certain HIV-1-encoded proteins have been determined including HIV-1 RT inhibitors, RNaseH, integrase, matrix, capsid, nucleocapsid, Tat protein, and, most recently, a domain of gp41. In addition, the envelope-binding domain of soluble CD4 has been determined using x-ray methods (27, 28). Thus far, however, only HIV protease has yielded fruit through structure-guided efforts to design potent and selective antiviral agents. This point perhaps underscores the infancy of the field of drug design. The successful development of HIV protease inhibitors (see later) is arguably the greatest achievement to date for this relatively new method. As structure-based drug design methods improve, investigators have reason to believe that new therapeutic agents will be effectively developed against novel antiviral targets for HIV-1 therapy. The need to continue to search for and to develop such agents should not be underestimated, because the prevalence of new drug-resistant variants of HIV-1 that are insensitive to even the best current regimens of triple and quadruple combination therapy is rising at an alarming rate.

Bringing Anti-HIV Drugs into the Clinic

One of the most important considerations in choosing antiviral agents for further testing is the in vitro therapeutic index, or the ratio of the concentrations at which the drug has activity and toxicity (1, 2, 14). The therapeutic index of a drug is unlikely to be greater in patients than that observed in vitro. Thus, agents for which the toxic concentration is close to the concentration exerting anti–HIV-1 activity have a minimal chance of performing better in patients. For agents with low in vitro therapeutic indices, the possibility exists that what appears to be selective anti–HIV-1 activity is instead simply poor HIV-1 replication resulting from general cellular damage. The potency of the drug and its ability to suppress HIV-1 completely at concentrations that are not toxic also represent important properties of a potential anti–HIV-1 agent. Another critical issue is that candidate antiviral agents should exert their activity against many different HIV-1 strains in various human cells (T cells, monocytes/macrophages, or brain cells). Furthermore, unless the pharmacokinetic profile is highly favorable (see later), the requirement to attain high concentrations of a drug in patients can limit its practicability.

Beyond these central issues, it becomes necessary to weigh various potential benefits and liabilities of each agent. Basic points to consider include the stage of HIV-1 replication at which the agent works, the pharmacokinetic profile (e.g., oral bioavailability, plasma half-life, intracellular half-life), penetration into the CNS, the likely dosing regimens, and the likely toxicity profile (2, 3, 7, 29). As we discuss in greater detail later, another issue that is assuming increasing importance is the potential for inducing resistance and the likelihood of having cross-resistance with available agents. We must also consider the potential for synergistic or antagonistic interactions with the available agents. Moreover, the potential should be considered for developing analogs of a given compound. One may also have a greater interest of bringing a prototype drug of an entirely new class into the clinic.

Identifying a simple algorithm to weigh these various factors is impossible, and indeed, priorities do change as more is learned from experience in the laboratory and clinic. Investigators should consider all available experience in making such decisions, because the time and energy expended in testing a drug in patients are considerable. At the same time, investigators must not become paralyzed by the need to address every possible contingency before moving into the clinic. Indeed, the experience to date would indicate that one often encounters surprises when one tests drugs in

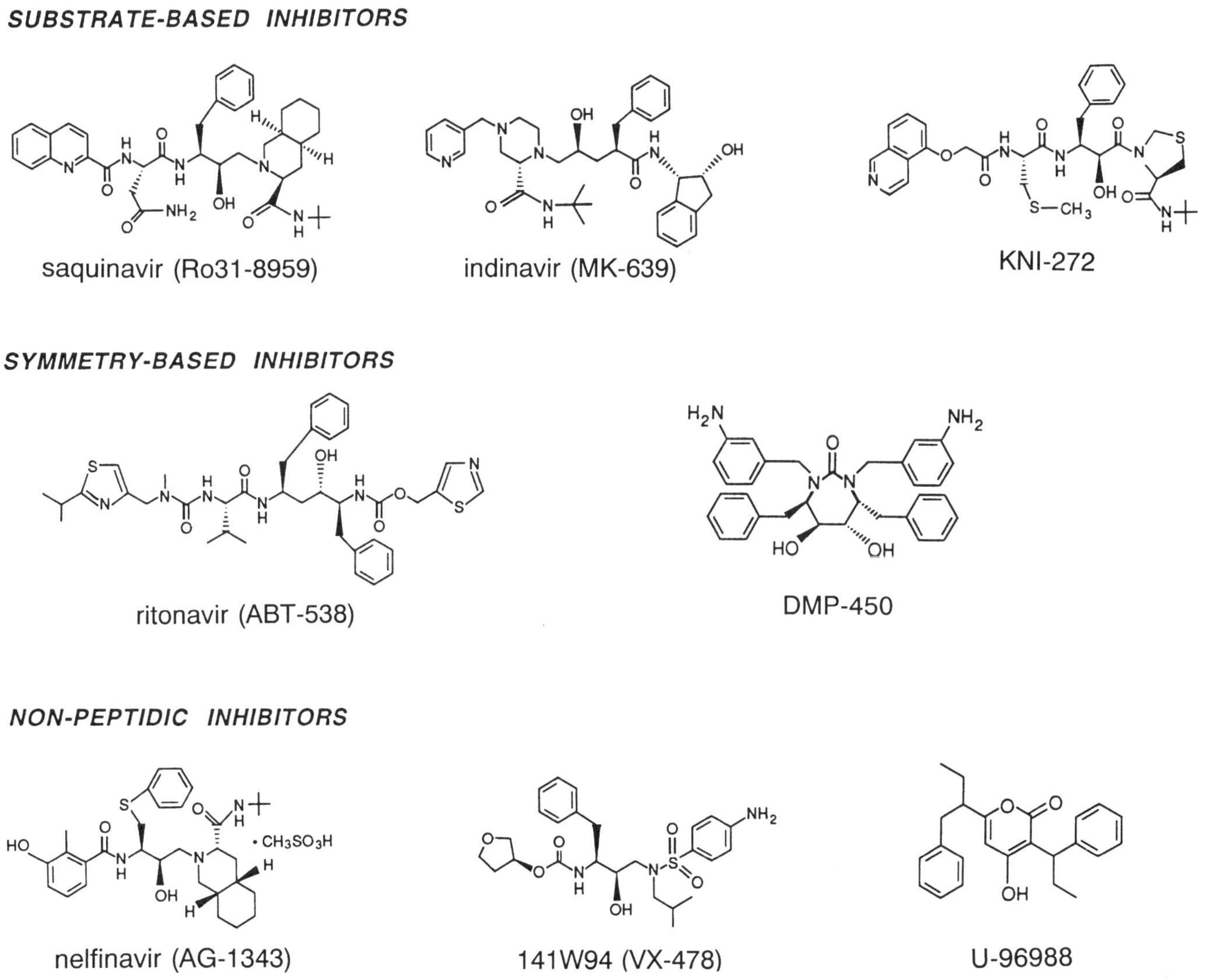

Figure 45A.4. Structures of selected HIV-1 protease inhibitors. Substrate-based inhibitors: saquinavir, indinavir, and KNI-272; symmetry-based inhibitors: ritonavir and DMP-450; and nonpeptidic inhibitors: nelfinavir, 141W94 (VX-478), and U-96988.

patients: some agents, such as ddC, turned out to be much more potent against HIV-1 and more toxic (based on the dose) in patients than anticipated (30, 31), whereas others, such as rCD4, failed to work clinically despite initially observed favorable antiviral and toxicity profiles (32, 33).

Table 45A.1 Stages in the HIV Replicative Cycle that May Serve as Targets for Therapeutic Intervention

Stage	Possible Intervention
Binding to target cell	Antibodies or drugs to block HIV or cellular receptors (CD4, chemokine receptors, etc.)
Fusion to target cell	Antibodies or drugs that block the gp41 fusogenic domain function
Entry, uncoating of RNA, and functional release of HIV RNA	Drugs or antibodies that can block viral entry or uncoating
Reverse transcription	Reverse transcriptase inhibitors (nucleoside and nonnucleoside reverse transcriptase inhibitors)
Accumulation of unintegrated HIV in acute infection	Any intervention described above, which may suppress the cytopathic effect of HIV (if the DNA accumulation of unintegrated HIV DNA relates to premature cell death)
RNA degradation by RNase H activity	Specific inhibitors of HIV RNase H
Migration of viral DNA to nucleus	Agents that block binding of HIV-1 preintegration complexes to karyophilic proteins or agents that inactivate the nuclear localization sequence of matrix antigen
Integration of HIV DNA into host	Agents that inhibit the *pol*-encoded integrase (In protein) function; inhibition of integrase interactor I (Inil 1)
Transcription and translation	Inhibitors of Tat or Rev activity; inhibition of Tat phosphorylation; inhibition of Tat/TAR complex formation, mutant Tat molecules; TAR inhibitors; TAR decoys; HIV mRNA-specific destruction by ribozymes
Enhancement by cellular factors	N-acetyl-cysteine and its analogs
Translation	Antisense constructs against regulatory HIV genes such as the *rev* gene
Ribosomal frameshifting	Ribosomal frameshift inhibitors (as yet unidentified)
Gag-Pol polyprotein cleavage	HIV protease inhibitors
Myristoylation and glycosylation by cellular enzymes	Inhibitors of acyl-coenzyme A synthetase and inhibitors of trimming glucosidase
Dimerization, binding lysine tRNA	Inhibitors of these stages (as yet unidentified)
Assembly/packaging	Zinc-ejecting aromatic compounds; impairment of assembly process (e.g., cyclosporine analogs); antisense constructs against the packaging ψ sequence (as yet unidentified)
Viral budding	Interferons or interferon inducers; antibodies to viral antigens that block viral release
Extracellular processing of Gag-Pol polyproteins	HIV protease inhibitors

Table 45A.2 Selected Basic Methods of Assessing Drugs for Activity Against HIV In Vitro

Protection of target T cells against the cytopathic effect of HIV
Inhibition of viral p24 Gag protein expression
Determination of reverse transcriptase activity produced by target cells
Detection of the synthesis of HIV DNA or RNA in susceptible target cells
Inhibition of HIV-1-caused syncytia formation
Effects on immune reactivities of normal immunocompetent cells

TARGETING REVERSE TRANSCRIPTASE

Inhibitors of RT can be divided into two broad categories. The first group represents nucleoside RT inhibitors (NRTIs) such as ZDV, ddI, and ddC, which, in their triphosphate form, compete with natural substrates and function as chain terminators (1, 16, 34). These compounds are really prodrugs that become phosphorylated by cellular enzymes to the active triphosphate forms. As mentioned earlier, currently five nucleoside analogs are licensed for therapy of HIV-1 infection, but their efficacy has been limited because of toxic side effects and the emergence of drug-resistant viral strains. The second class of RT inhibitors comprises a structurally diverse group of compounds, the NNRTIs, which bind to an allosteric site on the enzyme. NNRTIs are mostly nontoxic, highly potent, and specific for HIV-1 RT, and they can act synergistically with NNRTIs in vitro (35, 36). However, they lead rapidly to the development of drug resistance, usually faster than the nucleoside analogs.

Structure of Reverse Transcriptase

Biochemical and x-ray structural determinations of RT have shown that RT is a heterodimer consisting of two subunits, a catalytically active 66-kd subunit (p66) and an inactive 51-kd subunit (p51). The first 440 amino acids of p66 and p51 are identical, and both subunits contain a polymerase active site. The C-terminal portion of p66 contains the RNase H domain. X-ray crystal structures of RT (37, 38) show that p66 consists of four subdomains, designated fingers, palm, thumb, and connection, as well as the RNase H domain (Fig. 45A.5). The p51 subunit lacks the RNase H domain, and the remaining subdomains are arranged in a different fashion (37–39). Thus, the p66–p51 heterodimer has a highly asymmetric structure, the significance of which is still unclear. The functional polymerase active site is located in the palm subdomain of the p66 subunit and contains the conserved aspartic acids, Asp110, Asp185, and Asp186, which are considered part of the catalytic apparatus of RT. A large cleft of approximately 100 Å between the polymerase active site and the RNase H domain can accommodate an A-form RNA–DNA hybrid. The crystal structure of an RT–DNA–Fab complex shows that the p66 fingers and thumb act as a clamp to position the template primer and that extensive contacts exist between the DNA and the palm, fingers, and thumb subdomains of p66

(37, 38, 40). The subdomains in the p51 subunit are oriented differently such that p51 does not have a DNA-binding cleft. Various crystal structures have shown that RT is a highly flexible molecule (37, 40). The position of the thumb subdomain relative to the palm varies significantly in unliganded, DNA-bound, and inhibitor-bound forms of RT, whereas the basic structural features of the individual subdomains are preserved.

Nucleoside Reverse Transcriptase Inhibitors

In 1977, Sanger and his coworkers established a method for determining nucleotide sequences in DNA by using four 2′,3′-dideoxynucleoside-5′-triphosphates (ddNTPs) as chain-terminating inhibitors (41). These ddNs were synthesized in the 1960s or earlier, and pioneering studies of these ddNs were accomplished over the past 30 years or so (42–49). These agents, after anabolic phosphorylation in target cells, can inhibit HIV RT by DNA chain termination, as discussed later.

In 1985, members of a broad family of nucleosides with a 2′,3′-dideoxyribose moiety were identified to be antiretroviral agents against a divergent range of HIV-1 strains in vitro (1, 16, 34). As a general rule, each drug is unique from the perspective of both its activity and toxicity. The ddN analogs are successively phosphorylated in the cytoplasm of a target cell to ultimately yield ddNTP, although each drug may require a separate metabolic pathway (1–3, 50–52). Several ddNTPs have been extensively studied and are now known to have higher affinities for HIV-1 RT than for cellular DNA polymerase α, although cellular DNA polymerase β and γ appear to be relatively sensitive to ddNTPs (53, 54). These ddNTPs can compete with physiologic nucleotides for RT binding and can also be incorporated into the growing viral DNA chain and bring about termination of the viral DNA because a normal 5′63′ phosphodiester linkage cannot be completed (1, 2, 34). For example, ZDV undergoes anabolic phosphorylation to generate ZDV-TP, which competes with thymidine-TP (50) and functions as a viral DNA-chain terminator (1, 2, 55). In 1986, investigators showed that infected monocytes/macrophages play an important role in the pathogenesis of AIDS, in particular, in the traffic of HIV across the blood–brain barrier and as a reservoir of HIV-1 in vivo (56, 57). Perno and his coworkers subsequently demonstrated that ddN analogs including ZDV also suppress the replication of HIV in monocytes/macrophages in vitro (58, 59).

During the past 10 years, certain ddNs have been identified as potential antiretroviral agents (1–8). Among them are FddA (see Fig. 45A.2, 7), which unlike ddI, is acid stable with retention of antiretroviral activity (60) and 3′-α-fluoro-2′,3′-dideoxythymidine (see Fig. 45A.1, 3) (61, 62), which is slightly more potent against the virus, but also slightly more toxic than ZDV in vitro. Only a moderate level of resistance of HIV-1 against FddA has been seen, and no significant cross-resistance has been documented, at least in vitro (63). FddA is currently undergoing phase I clinical trial. Adefovir (PMEA: see Fig. 45A.2, 11) (64) is an acyclic nucleoside that has a phosphonylmethoxyethyl group instead of the 2′,3′-dideoxyribose, undergoes anabolic diphosphorylation, and serves as a DNA chain terminator on incorporation into the growing viral DNA chain. In this sense, adefovir falls within the DNA chain–terminating nucleoside family. Adefovir is acid resistant, is as potent as ddI/ddA on the basis of molarity, and exerts a broad spectrum of antiviral activity in vitro against several DNA and RNA viruses including HIV (64). Adefovir dipivoxil (GS 840, bis-POM PMEA) is the oral prodrug form of adefovir and is broken down into adefovir within cells with a long half-life, leading to a once-a-day oral dosing regimen. Adefovir dipivoxil is currently undergoing clinical trials in combination with various NRTIs and protease inhibitors. This compound is also being tested for the treatment of hepatitis B infection and as prophylaxis for cytomegalovirus infection.

A 2′,3′-dideoxyguanosine (ddG)–related compound, carbovir (see Fig. 45A.2, 9) (65), has a cyclopentenyl moiety in place of dideoxyribose and exerts potent anti–HIV-1 activity, but it failed as a therapeutic agent because of its limited oral bioavailability and unexpected toxicity in animal studies. However, continued studies to improve the pharmacologic properties of carbovir led to the development of abacavir (see Fig. 45A.2, 10), an N^6-cyclopropylamino derivative, which shows significant advantages over carbovir. Abacavir is phosphorylated by adenosine phosphotransferase (66, 67) but not by the 5′-nucleotidase that monophosphorylates carbovir, ddI, and ddG. Subsequently, abacavir-monophosphate (MP) is converted back to carbovir-MP by a cytosolic deaminase that is ultimately phosphorylated to carbovir-TP, the active moiety, by cellular kinases (67). Thus, abacavir is a prodrug, not of carbovir, but of carbovir-MP. This unique activation pathway appears to enable abacavir to overcome

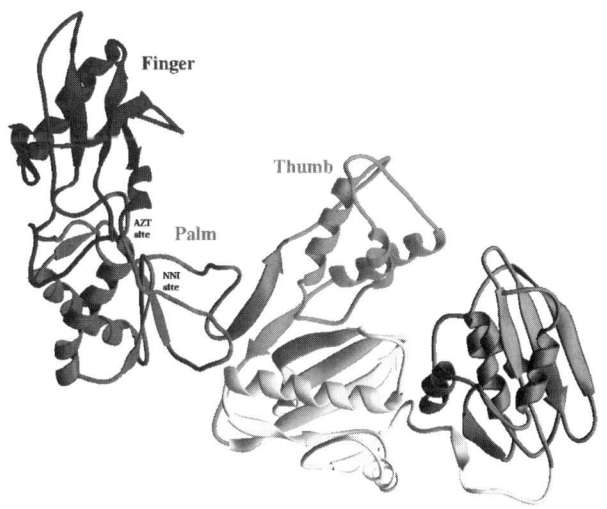

Figure 45A.5. Ribbon diagram of the p66 subunit of HIV-1 reverse transcriptase showing the domain structure. The locations of the nucleoside site (AZT site) and nonnucleoside reverse transcriptase inhibitor binding site (NNI site) are shown. The template primer occupies the groove formed by finger, palm, and thumbs subdomains. (See color section.)

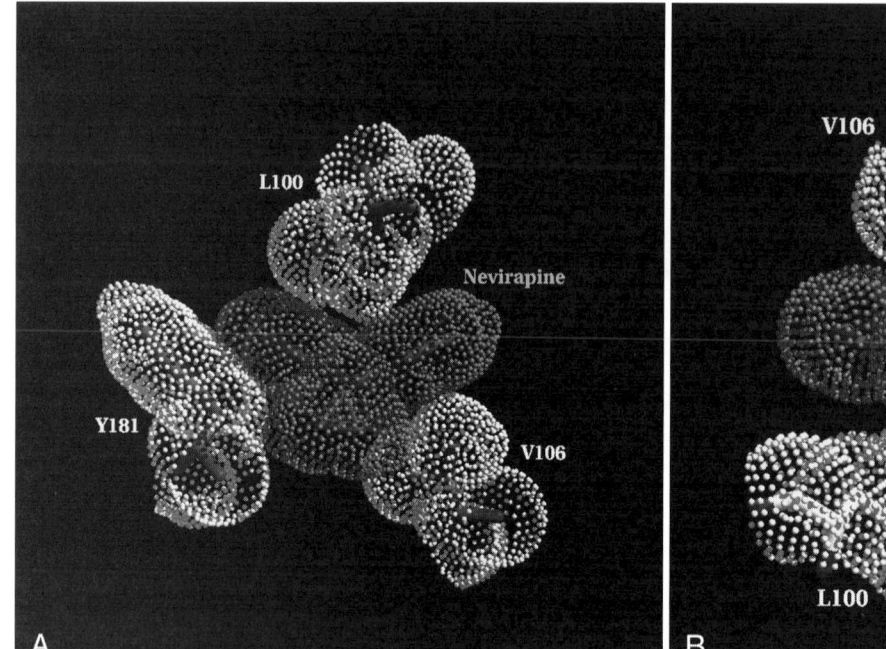

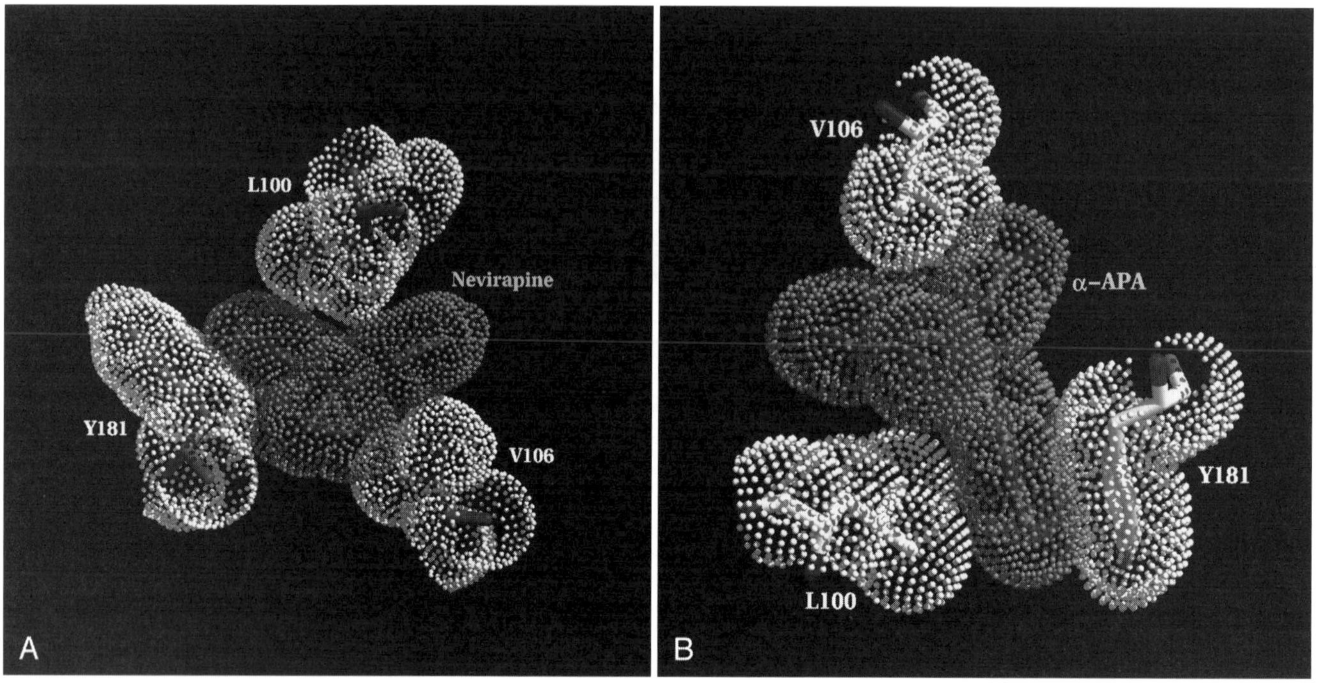

Figure 45A.6. Van der Waals surfaces. These surfaces are depicted for HIV-1 reverse transcriptase *(green)* residing in close contact with the nonnucleoside reverse transcriptase inhibitors *(yellow)*, nevirapine **(A)**, and α-anilinophenylacetamide (α-APA) **(B)** based on the crystallographic coordinates 3HUT and HNI, respectively. (See color section.)

the toxicologic properties of carbovir. Moreover, because of the N^6-cyclopropylamino group, abacavir has a greater lipophilicity than carbovir, which has perhaps enabled abacavir to have greater oral bioavailability and enhanced CNS penetration.

Nonnucleoside Reverse Transcriptase Inhibitors

In 1990 and thereafter, some nonnucleoside compounds that inhibit HIV-1 replication by interfering with RT activity were reported from certain laboratories, mostly affiliated with pharmaceutical companies. These compounds include tetrahydro-imidazo(4,5,1,jk;1,4)-benzodiazepin-2(1H)-one and -thione (TIBO) derivatives (68), dipyridodiazepinone analogs (e.g., BI-RG587 or nevirapine) (69), pyridinone derivatives (e.g., L697,661) (35) and certain bis(heteroaryl)piperazines (BHAP-P compounds) (see Fig. 45A.3) (70). Although these compounds do not appear to be related in structure, they appear to be functionally related in that they are active only against HIV-1 in vitro and inert against other retroviruses such as HIV-2, SIV, and certain animal retroviruses. All these compounds appear to bind to virtually the same, unique site on RT, which is different from the binding site of antiretroviral ddNs (see Fig. 45A.5). A series of nucleoside analogs, 1-([2-hydroxyethoxy]methyl)-6-(phenylthio)-thymine (HEPT) and its derivatives (71, 72), resemble other NNRTIs in that they exert antiviral activity against HIV-1 without phosphorylation, but they are not active against HIV-2 or animal retroviruses (72). HEPT analog, MKC-442, is in a phase Ib clinical trial as a single agent and has shown transient reductions in viral RNA, a finding suggesting the development of resistance (73).

Crystal structures of nevirapine, HEPT, α-anilinophenylacetamide (α-APA), and TIBO complexes with RT reveal that these structurally diverse molecules bind at a common site in the p66 subdomain, although each exhibits slightly different interactions with the enzyme (74). The binding site for NNRTIs is located close to the active site in the p66 subunit (see Fig. 45A.5) and is more of a hydrophobic cavity than a pocket. All inhibitors are able to bind to the pocket in a butterfly shape that appears to be a native structural feature of the molecule or one that the molecule can adopt with little energy penalty (Fig. 45A.6) (75, 76). In the uncomplexed or native crystalline form of the enzyme, the drug-binding cavity does not exist. Thus, the pocket must be created by the flexible motion of the side chains of Trp229, Tyr181, and Tyr188 (see Fig. 45A.6). The mechanism by which NNRTIs inhibit RT is as yet unknown, but several mechanisms have been suggested. One is that inhibitor binding could indirectly affect the conformation of the active site aspartates. A second proposal is that the binding of NNRTIs interferes with the hinge movement between the palm and thumb subdomains. Crystallographic analysis of several complexes of NNRTIs with RT has led to the proposal that NNRTIs block RT function by repositioning the catalytic aspartates. This observation is supported by presteady-state kinetic experiments that show that binding of NNRTIs does not interfere with nucleotide binding itself, but slows down the rate of nucleotide incorporation into the growing viral DNA.

Thus, a functional connection appears to exist between the catalytic site and the NNRTI binding site, although they are spatially distinct (74, 76).

Various NNRTIs exert highly potent and specific activity against HIV-1 in vitro. However, little evidence of favorable antiretroviral activity was seen in patients treated with these NNRTIs in clinical trials. This was subsequently found to be due to the rapid emergence of resistant HIV-1 variants. In several cases, this resulted in termination of clinical trials and near abandonment of NNRTIs, at least as the first-line treatment for HIV infection (77, 78). Indeed, HIV-1 has been shown to develop a high level of resistance even after several passages when it is cultured in the presence of NNRTIs in vitro (79, 80) and in vivo as well. However, magnitude of cross-resistance among NNRTIs varies among compounds, and variants resistant to one NNRTI often can remain susceptible to other NNRTIs in vitro (81, 82). In addition, these NNRTI-resistant HIV-1 variants remain sensitive to NRTIs, and some NNRTIs are synergistic against HIV-1 in vitro when combined with ZDV or other NRTIs (35, 36). Indeed, adding nevirapine to ZDV and ddI was confirmed to improve the long-term immunologic and virologic effects of therapy (83). These results demonstrated the need for continued development of combinations of three or more antiretroviral drugs to increase and prolong HIV-1 suppression.

TARGETING VIRAL PROTEASE

HIV-1 encodes a protease (PR) that is responsible for the posttranslational processing of the viral *gag* and *gag-pol* polyprotein gene products to yield the structural proteins and enzymes of the mature viral particle (84). Processing is required for viral infectivity because either mutation of the active site aspartic acids or chemical inhibition of the enzyme leads to the production of immature, noninfectious viral particles (85–87). Knowledge of the structure and function of HIV-1 protease has led to the successful development of many different potent and chemically diverse inhibitors that have been designed using substrate- and structure-based approaches (84, 88–91).

The possible involvement of protease in the early stages of the retroviral replication was suggested on the basis of observations with equine infectious anemia virus (EIAV) (92) and HIV-1 (93, 94). However, data from several groups demonstrated that protease inhibitors fail to block the synthesis of proviral DNA, its integration into cellular DNA, and transcription, and these investigators concluded that viral protease does not play a role in the early stages of HIV-1 infection (95, 96). Another group has also reached the same conclusion when conditional HIV-1 protease mutants were used as probes (97).

Protease Structure and Substrate-Based Inhibitors

HIV protease is a dimeric aspartic protease that consists of two identical, noncovalently associated subunits of 99 amino acid residues (26). The active site of the enzyme is unusual in that it is formed at the dimer interface and contains two conserved catalytic aspartic acid residues, one from each monomer (Fig. 45A.7). The active site is covered over by two β-hairpin structures, or "flaps," that are highly flexible and

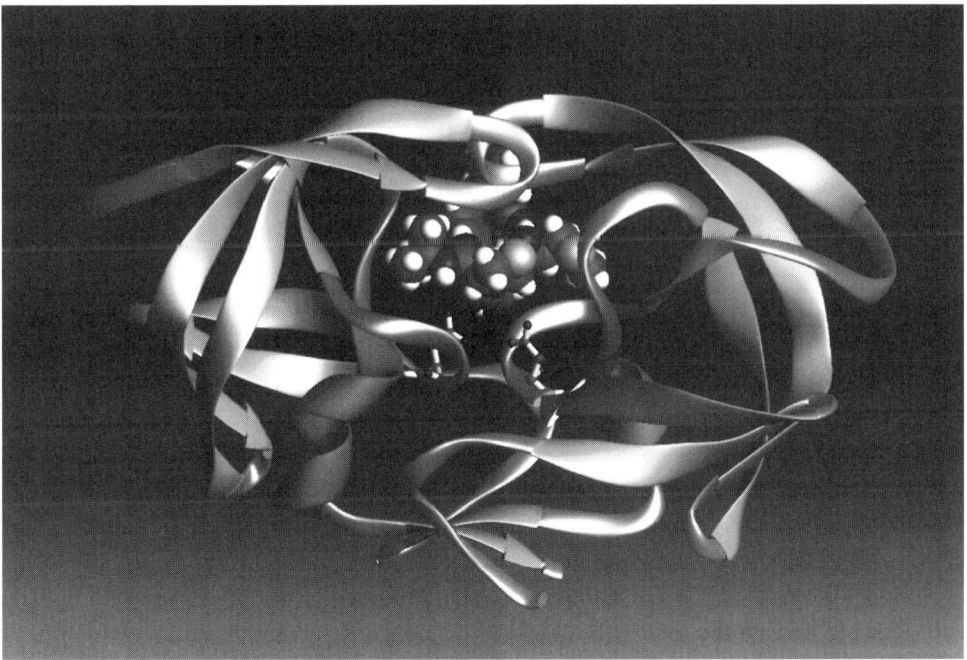

Figure 45A.7. Ribbon diagram of the HIV-1 protease dimer complexed with an inhibitor, KNI-272, showing the catalytic aspartic acid residues (balls and sticks). (See color section.)

760 Section V. Control and Prevention

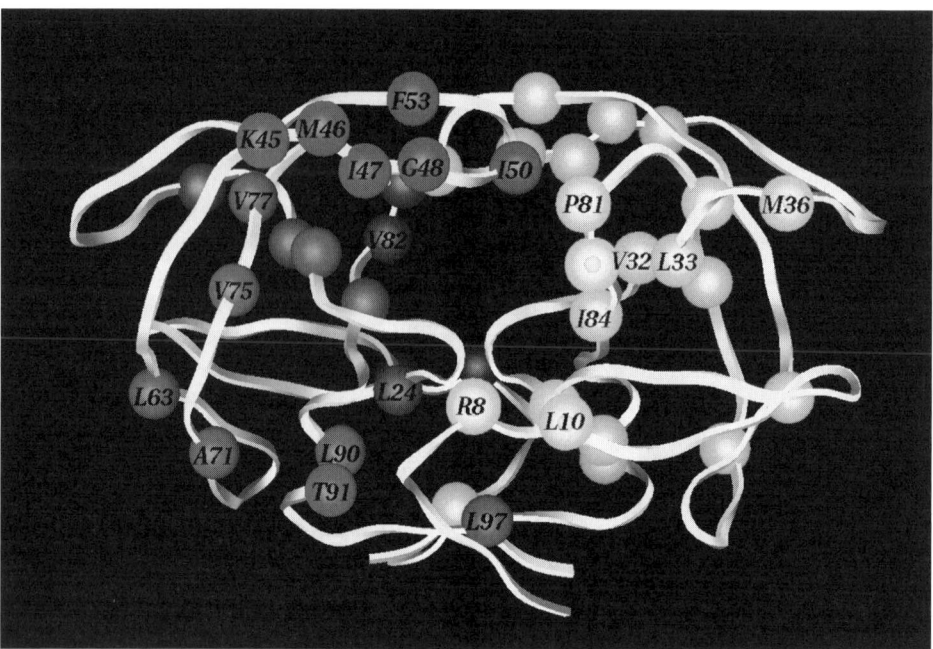

Figure 45A.8. Backbone representations of HIV-1 protease and the locations of amino acid substitutions known to confer resistance against protease inhibitors. The numbering for only one of the two symmetry-related residues of the dimer is given for clarity. (See color section.)

undergo large, localized conformational changes during the binding and release of inhibitors and substrates (98). The close structural and functional relationships between the retroviral and cellular aspartic proteases, together with knowledge of the HIV protease cleavage site sequences on the *gag* and *gag-pol* polyproteins, immediately opened the avenue of peptidomimetic substrate-based approaches that had been developed for designing inhibitors of human renin, an aspartic protease that has long been an important target for the design of antihypertensive agents. Substrate-based inhibitors are essentially peptide substrate analogs in which the scissile peptide bond has been replaced by a noncleavable, transition-state analog or isostere. Examples of this class of inhibitors include saquinavir (Ro-31-8959), KNI-272, and BILA-2011, which are essentially mimics of the Phe-Pro cleavage site sequence (see Fig. 45A.4).

Design of Symmetry-Based Inhibitors

The initial observations that retroviral proteases contain the amino acid triplet, Asp-Thr(Ser)-Gly, and that their proteolytic activity could be inhibited by pepstatin led to the early proposal that these enzymes were related mechanistically to the aspartic protease family of enzymes. The latter are bilobal, single-chain enzymes in which each lobe, or domain, contributes an aspartic acid residue to the active site. The active site itself is formed at the interface of the N- and C-domains and exhibits approximate twofold symmetry at the protein backbone level. With the understanding that the viral enzymes are twofold (C_2) symmetric homodimers in which the active site is formed by the dimer interface and is composed of equivalent contributions of residues from each subunit came the realization that symmetry could be incorporated into the design of inhibitors for the HIV enzyme. Such designs represented a distinct and novel departure from traditional medicinal chemistry approaches to enzyme inhibitor designs, and they constituted the first direct attempts at using the structure of the protein in the design of an antiviral agent for therapy of HIV infection (25, 99). The first symmetry-based inhibitor to enter clinical trials was A-77003 (100). This compound was extremely potent and selective for HIV protease, but it had poor oral bioavailability. Further refinement of A-77003 led to ritonavir (ABT-538; see Fig. 45A.4), which had much better pharmacokinetic properties and is currently approved for clinical use in many countries (101). A second type of symmetry-based inhibitor is represented by the cyclic urea, DMP-450 (see Fig. 45A.4). This class of compound has the added feature that it substitutes a ring carbonyl group for the buried water found in most peptidomimetic inhibitor complexes. In theory, the displacement of the bound water may lead to an increase in binding energetics through favorable entropy (102). Active site symmetry, a feature unique to retroviral proteases, has afforded several novel approaches to inhibitor synthesis and design that would otherwise have been inaccessible to medicinal chemists, and it has led to several clinically useful antiviral agents.

Structure-Based HIV Protease Inhibitors

Well over several hundred crystal structures have been solved for various HIV protease inhibitor complexes, a testimony to the importance placed on structural information in the process of inhibitor design (26, 103–105). Combined with medicinal chemistry and, in some cases, target-based screening efforts, these structural investigations have led to a structurally diverse compendium of inhibitors that include inhibitors, such as nelfinavir (AG-1343), that were derived solely using structure-based design methods and indinavir (MK-639) and amprenavir (141W94, Vx-478), the designs of which were a blend of medicinal chemistry and structural insights. A particularly interesting class of nonpeptidic HIV protease inhibitors is represented by U-96988 (see Fig. 45A.4). The basic 4-hydroxy-2-pyranone ring system was discovered from high-throughput enzyme-based screening by two independent laboratories (106, 107). However, in each case, the potency of the initial lead compounds was too low to possess measurable antiviral activity. Further optimization in both cases was guided by x-ray crystal structure analyses combined with modeling to identify novel binding modes and key positions of the molecules that could be used to incorporate substituents that would fill the enzyme subsites in a preferred manner (107, 108).

Pharmacokinetics of HIV Protease Inhibitors

Unlike the case for the majority of RT inhibitors, most HIV protease inhibitors have serious pharmacokinetic limitations. Poor oral absorption, serum protein binding, liver enzyme metabolism, and other factors can all but eliminate the antiviral benefits of many potent protease inhibitors. Currently approved protease inhibitors need to be ingested often and in large quantities to maintain effective antiviral concentrations in the blood. Furthermore, of the currently available antiviral drugs for HIV-1 infection, protease inhibitors are among the most effective, but they are costly and require complicated treatment regimens. As a result, the failure or dropout rate of patients receiving protease inhibitor therapy tends to be high, the compliance of treatment with protease inhibitors is likely to be poor, and the development of resistance to these highly effective drugs has proved to be a growing problem (109–111) (Fig. 45A.8).

OTHER AGENTS THAT ACT AT EARLY STAGES OF HIV REPLICATION

Inhibitors of Virus Adsorption to Target Cells

Several polyanionic sulfated compounds were found to have anti–HIV-1 activity in vitro (112–114). Suramin, one of the first drugs identified as having anti-HIV activity in vitro (15), also falls into this class. However, these compounds have a high binding avidity for plasma proteins, and their anti–HIV-1 activity is blunted in the presence of high concentrations of serum (as compared with the 10 to 20% serum usually used in tissue culture) (115). Perhaps at least in part because of this property, these compounds failed to exert anti-HIV activity in patients (116, 117). Another possible explanation for this failure is that these agents may be less effective in inhibiting cell-to-cell transmission of HIV-1, in which local concentrations of virus are extremely high.

Soon after the CD4 molecule was identified as the principal receptor for HIV and the CD4 gene was cloned, several groups became interested in the possibility of using CD4 analogs as specific therapy for HIV-1 infection (118–120). The approaches involved the use of recombinant technology to produce soluble forms of CD4 (sCD4), which lacked the cytoplasmic and transmembrane domains (121–125). These preparations were among the first rationally designed therapies for HIV-1 infection, and various versions of sCD4 molecules were shown to exert potent antiviral activity against laboratory HIV-1 strains including macrophage-tropic HIV-1 (126). However, sCD4 and its related agents failed to show significant antiviral activity in patients with HIV-1 infection, perhaps because HIV-1 replicating in patients (clinical strains) have less affinity to CD4 receptors, unlike laboratory strains, which have a high affinity. Moreover, such truncated but large protein molecules may have failed effectively to permeate tissues such as lymphoid organs, where the virus actively replicates.

Inhibitors of HIV-1 by a Chemokine-Related or Chemokine Receptor–Related Strategy

In 1996, Feng and Berger and their group discovered a molecule, designated "fusin," later renamed CXCR-4, a member of the seven-transmembrane segment G-protein–coupled receptor superfamily, as a cofactor for the infection of human CD4+ T cells but not macrophages by HIV-1 (T-cell–tropic HIV-1 strains) (127). In the same year, another molecule, termed CCR-5, which is related to CXCR-4, was found (128, 129) to serve as a coreceptor in the infection of macrophages and CD4+ T cells (macrophage-tropic HIV-1 strains). These findings were led by a preceding discovery that β-chemokines, including regulated-on-activated, normal T-expressed and secreted (RANTES), macrophage inflammatory protein-1α (MIP-1α), and MIP-1β, inhibited the infection of human target cells with HIV-1 in vitro (130). Despite the observed in vitro antiviral activity with a combination of several β-chemokines, it remains to be determined whether chemokines have clinical utility (131–133). Investigators may also be able to exploit chemokine receptors to intervene in the entry of HIV into cells by developing the soluble elements of the chemokine receptors. In this regard, HIV-1 appears to use other receptors as well (e.g., CCR-1, CCR2b, and CCR3), which are different from CD4, CXCR-4, or CCR-5 (128, 134–136). Furthermore, significant variation exists in susceptibility to chemokine inhibition of different strains of HIV-1 (130). Thus, the use of multiple chemokines or multiple soluble chemokine receptors will likely be required if targeting chemokine receptor-mediated viral entry should prove to be clinically relevant.

A series of bicyclams (macrocyclic polyamines) such as AMD3100 (formerly termed JM3100) were reported to inhibit the replication of HIV-1 and HIV-2 in vitro by interacting with a viral uncoating event on the basis of time-of-addition experiments (137, 138). AMD3100 has been shown to bind to CXCR-4 and to inhibit virus fusion and infectivity (139, 140). Clinical trials with AMD3100 have now been planned. In addition, a few small molecules, including ALX40-4C (N-α-acetyl-nona-D-arginine amide) (141) and T22 ([Tyr^{5,12}, Lys^7]-polyphemusin II) (142), inhibit the binding of T- and dual-tropic HIV-1 strains to CXCR-4, thereby inhibiting infection. RANTES interacts with CCR-5 and blocks the infection of peripheral blood mononuclear cells by HIV-1, but only inefficiently. Aminooxypentane (AOP)-RANTES, with the amino terminus of RANTES chemically modified, can, however, achieve full receptor occupancy at nanomolar concentrations and can inhibit infection of diverse cell types including macrophages and lymphocytes by nonsyncytium-inducing, macrophage-tropic HIV-1 strains without inducing chemotaxis (143). This approach, that is, chemical modification of biologic agents, may open a new avenue in developing anti–HIV-1 biologic agents.

OTHER DRUGS THAT ACT AT LATE STAGES

Inhibitors of Nuclear Migration

The double-stranded proviral DNA, synthesized by RT, migrates into the nucleus of a target cell as a large preintegration complex composed of viral nucleic acids and proteins including integrase, viral protein R (Vpr), matrix antigen, and RT (144, 145). The amino acid sequence (residues 26 to 32) is highly conserved among lentiviruses and is homologous to the nuclear localization sequence of SIV and functions as a nuclear targeting signal for HIV-1 preintegration complexes (144, 145). The active importation of the HIV-1 integration complexes occurs when the nuclear localization sequence–containing proteins cross the nuclear pore complex, mediated by karyopherins, the cellular proteins involved in active nuclear import (i.e., karyopherin αβ heterodimers) (146, 147). This active importation of HIV-1 preintegration complexes across the nuclear envelope of nondividing cells obviates the requirement for cell division and allows HIV-1 to infect quiescent cells as well as activated, dividing cells (148). Partial reactions in nuclear import have been reproduced in vitro using a solution binding assay and recombinant karyopherins (149). A compound termed CNI-H0294, which was designed to form Schiff base adducts with contiguous lysines in matrix antigen, has been identified to inhibit the nuclear import of HIV-1 preintegration complexes (150, 151) by inhibiting the binding of HIV-1 preintegration complexes to karyopherins. More recently, investigators have shown that the inhibitory activity of CNI-H0294 apparently requires the presence of RT in the preintegration complexes (151). However, relatively high concentrations of the compound appear to be required for significant levels of viral suppression, and at present, no data have been shown on the oral bioavailability, pharmakokinetics, or stability of CNI-H0294.

Inhibitors of Integrase

Integrase is one of the three virally encoded enzymes essential for the retroviral replication cycle. The initial step in the integration reaction, catalyzed by virally encoded integrase, is an endonucleolytic cleavage event called "processing" that removes the terminal bases from each 3′ end of the linear proviral DNA (152–155). The resulting viral 3′ ends are then joined to target cellular DNA to form the initial recombination intermediate, a polynucleotide transfer or "joining" step. Integrase binds zinc at its N-terminal domain with a stoichiometry of one zinc per integrase monomer, adopts a secondary structure with a high α helical content, and teramizes more readily and acquires more activity than the apoenzyme (156). The mechanism by which host DNA integration sites are selected is unknown, although many regions in the host DNA clearly are accessible to the retroviral integration machinery. This integration of proviral DNA is required for the subsequent generation of new viral particles, and the integrase represents a novel target for intervention of viral replication (157–159). Currently, scores of agents can inhibit HIV-1 integrase activity in cell-free assays, including coumarin analogs (160), hydrazide analogs (161), depsides, and depsidones (159). None of these compounds, however, are free from cytotoxicity, and their anti-HIV activities are marginal or have not been extensively examined.

Analysis of the primary structure of integrase using deletion mutagenesis has shown that full-length integrase (288 residues) contains three structurally important domains (154, 155). Structural work on recombinant HIV-1 integrase was hampered by its inherent biophysical properties because it is highly insoluble and has a tendency to clump. These problems were successfully circumvented by a systematic replacement of the hydrophobic residues in the core domain of HIV-1 integrase and a single amino acid substitution (Phe185Lys and Phe185His), and the crystal structure of the catalytically active core domain of HIV-1 integrase was thus determined (162, 163). The central feature of the structure of integrase is a five-stranded β sheet flanked by helical regions. The overall topology revealed that this domain of integrase belongs to a superfamily of polynucleotidyl transferase (162). A protein, designated Ini1 (integrase interactor 1), has been found to bind to HIV-1 integrase and to stimulate its integrating activity (164). Ini1 is thought to target incoming proviral DNA to active cellular genes, thus ensuring that HIV-1 can quickly replicate in the host cell. To date, advances in the understanding of the structure of integrase have not led to the identification of promising agents. Probably, however, the full elucidation of the structure of integrase should form a basis for designing drugs to block its activity, such as by tailoring agents that inhibit the binding of Ini1 and the integrase or those that bind to and obscure the catalytic sites of integrase.

Inhibitors of Viral Transcription and Translation

HIV-1 contains an essential regulatory gene, designated *tat*. The *tat* gene codes for a diffusible protein that enhances the expression of other viral genes and amplifies the production of new infectious virions at a transcriptional or posttranscriptional step (165). The Tat protein is small (86 amino acids), with a cluster of positively charged amino acids. To exert its effects, the Tat protein, after phosphorylation by the cellular double-stranded RNA-activated kinase (PKR) (166), interacts with a short nucleotide sequence designated TAR (*trans*-acting responsive sequence), which is located within the 5'-long terminal repeat (LTR) and is included in the mRNA transcript of every HIV-1 gene (167). The Tat protein may directly bind to TAR RNA. Cellular RNA binding proteins may also play a role in mediating the *tat*-dependent LTR activation. Although the elucidation of the direct interaction of the Tat protein with TAR requires more research, simple inhibitors that can block the binding of the Tat protein and TAR would efficiently inhibit viral replication. Indeed, a hybrid peptoid–peptide oligomer of 9 residues (CGP64222) has been shown to block the formation of the Tat–TAR complex in vitro at nanomolar concentrations (168). This compound reportedly binds to polypeptides derived from the Tat protein and induces a conformational change in TAR RNA at the Tat-binding site, thus specifically inhibiting the Tat activity and blocking HIV-1 replication in primary human lymphocytes (168). Ro-5-3335, 7-chloro-5-(2-pyrryl)-3H-1,4-benzodiazepine-2-(H)-one, was reported to inhibit the *tat*-dependent LTR-driven gene expression (169) and to inhibit HIV-1 and HIV-2 strains in vitro; however, this agent caused nephrotoxicity and yellow tissue discoloration in early trials. A better tolerated analog, Ro24-7429, was examined in patients with HIV-1 infection only to show no evidence of antiviral activity (170).

Rev protein, a small (116 amino acid) positively charged molecule encoded by the *rev* gene functions as a second essential *trans*-acting factor in viral replication through its binding to a complex RNA stem loop structure, called the Rev-responsive element or RRE, located within the *env* region of HIV-1 (165). In the absence of this second regulatory factor, *gag*- and *env*-encoded protein synthesis is severely diminished. The Rev effector domain has been shown to function as an autonomous nuclear export signal, which causes its rapid nuclear export (171, 172). The Rev protein appears to have evolved to take advantage of a cellular protein export pathway rather than developing a dedicated RNA export pathway, and instead acts as an adaptor that allows the nucleocytoplasmic transport of unspliced viral RNA (171, 172). Although the way in which *rev* works is not understood, the consensus is that this gene is critical for effective viral expression. The *rev* gene therefore is an important target for intervention of HIV-1 replication. The specific interference by drugs or chemicals with the function of the *rev* gene or RRE function could lead to suppression of viral replication in chronically infected cells. In this regard, when an oligonucleotide (RNA decoys) corresponding to the TAR or RRE was expressed at high levels in T cells by using adenoassociated viral vectors, HIV-1 gene expression and replication were transiently inhibited by 70 to 99% (173). Although this finding would not directly lead to gene therapy of HIV infection, it warrants further investigation.

Blocking the expression of retroviral genes by constructing negative-strand (antisense) synthetic oligodeoxynucleotides could be an intriguing strategy for the intervention of viral replication. If an antisense strategy can be developed, such agents should affect the expression of specific viral genes. However, only a few antisense oligomers have been shown to exert such sequence-specific anti-HIV activity. Among them is a nuclease-resistant phosphorothioate oligodeoxynucleotide targeting a highly conserved segment of the *rev* gene, which reduces the level of the genomic viral mRNA transcripts while sparing smaller RNA species (174). Such modified antisense oligodeoxynucleotides may yield important theoretic and clinical insights into the regulation of HIV expression. However, this anti-*rev* construct substantially varies, depending on cell types and HIV-1 strains used in the testing (S Kageyama, H Mitsuya, unpublished data), possibly because of 1) different levels of the target *rev* mRNA expressed in different cell lines, 2) different levels of the oligomer/*rev* mRNA binding, 3) different levels of oligomer penetration into cells, or 4) different patterns of compartmentalization of the oligomer. In any event, this oligomer has been dropped from drug development. A 25-mer phosphorothioate oligomer, termed GEM 91, which is complementary to the *gag* gene initiation site, was initially reported to have sequence-specific antiviral activity (175). However, investigators have had some difficulties in reproducing the initial data, and GEM-91 is no longer considered therapeutic against HIV-1.

Viral Assembly and Maturation

In addition to the protease that processes the viral polyproteins and is required for maturation of the virion, several other viral-specific components are involved in the assembly and maturation of infectious virus particles. Although the structures of such critical components such as capsid (p24) and matrix (p17) proteins have been determined by NMR and x-ray crystallographic methods (176–179), the way in which these proteins assemble into immature virions and the means by which they rearrange to form the mature viral cores remain unclear.

A cyclosporine analog, SDZ-NIM-811, is devoid of immunosuppressive capacity but exhibits potent anti–HIV-1 activity in vitro (180). The viral particles produced by SDZ-NIM-811–treated, chronically infected cells had comparable amounts of capsid proteins, RT activity, and viral RNA, whereas these particles showed a dose-dependent reduction in infectivity, a finding suggesting that SDZ-NIM-811 impairs assembly process (180). Most recently, investigators have shown that SDZ-NIM-811 inhibits the interaction of p24 Gag proteins with cyclophilin A, the intracellular receptor for cyclosporines, causing a significant decrease of cyclophilin incorporation into virions and resulting in reduced infectivity of the newly produced virions (181). Crystallographic analyses of cyclophilin A complexed with a fragment of HIV-1 Gag protein have revealed that this target molecule is likely to function as a chaperone in HIV-1 infectivity (182). Further elucidation of the structure and function of cyclophilin A may lead to discovery of a more potent and selective HIV-1 inhibitor.

NUCLEOCAPSID p7 PROTEIN

The highly basic HIV nucleocapsid protein (p7) preferentially binds to single-stranded RNA, strongly potentiates its dimerization, and has been implicated in both the nucleation and condensation phases of virion assembly (183). Both p7 and a specific site on the viral RNA, designated the psi site, have been identified as being important for proper recognition and specific packaging of genomic RNA into new particles and are also necessary for correct virion assembly and maturation. However, p7 has little demonstrable sequence specificity for binding RNA or DNA in vitro. In this regard, findings of a high-affinity RNA binding site for p7 (184) and the determination of the structure of a complex between p7 and the psi site of genomic RNA (346) may afford new insights into the design of specific inhibitors of this interaction. Certain mutations introduced in p7 affect HIV-1 replication more drastically than RNA incorporation (185), a finding providing a hypothesis that p7 may be involved in other steps of the HIV replication cycle in addition to RNA packaging.

The p7 protein contains two highly conserved and apparently mutationally intolerant retroviral zinc fingers, each with the signature sequence Cys-X2-Cys-X4-His-X4-Cys. The first finger is apparently responsible for RNA packaging, and the second is required for stabilization of viral particles (186). Many different agents cause zinc ejection from either finger and exert antiviral activity in vitro including azocarbonamide and disulfide-containing compounds (187–191). These compounds are thought to react chemically with the zinc chelation complex and display flat structure–activity relationships (192). ^{1}H-NMR studies have revealed that these compounds readily eject zinc from synthetic peptides with sequences corresponding to the zinc fingers, as well as from the intact HIV-1 nucleocapsid protein (191). However, reduced forms of disulfiram and diethyl dithiocarbamate were found to be ineffective at zinc ejection (191). Furthermore, the relative levels of antiviral activity by various disulfide benzamides and benzisothiazolones (108, 190) generally correlate with their kinetic rates of zinc ejection; some disulfide benzamides with zinc ejection have failed to suppress HIV-1 replication (193). Because these zinc-ejecting compounds are in general low-molecular-weight oxidizing agents, issues related to selectivity, toxicity, and stability in the reducing environments of blood and cells must be addressed before the approach of oxidizing retroviral zinc fingers can be developed into a practical therapeutic strategy. On the other hand, the ability of these agents to inactive free HIV particles irreversibly may lead to important prophylactic or vaccine applications.

CAPSID (p24) AND MATRIX (p17) PROTEINS

Two HIV *gag* gene products, capsid (p24) and matrix (p17) proteins, assemble the shell that houses the nucleoprotein complex. Capsid-binding compounds have been developed as antiviral agents for the human rhinoviruses, which are major causative agents of the common cold in humans (194, 195). However, the three-dimensional structure of HIV-1 p24 is entirely different from the β-barrel fold of the icosahedral coat proteins of picornaviruses. The function of HIV-1 p17 protein is even less clear, although it is localized between the envelope and the capsid and must be N-myristoylated for proper assembly and particle budding (see later) to occur at the cellular membrane. For Gag myristoylation, two reactions are involved: 1) conversion of intracellular myristate to myristoyl-coenzyme A (CoA) mediated by acyl-CoA synthetase; and 2) transfer of the myristoyl residue to the N-terminal glycine of Pr55, the precursor of Gag proteins, by N-myristoyl transferase (196). Inhibitors of N-myristoylation, including heteroatom-substituted analogs of myristic acid, analogs of N-myristoyl glycine, and acyl-CoA synthetase inhibitors (see later), have been shown to exhibit antiviral effects (197–199), but so far these compounds have shown only poor clinical utility. Targeting capsid p24 and matrix p17 proteins seems to require more research. However, the unique properties of their structures may afford new approaches to the design of agents that can ultimately inhibit HIV-1 infection.

Inhibitors of Budding

Finally, HIV virion particles are released by a process of viral budding, an as yet poorly understood mechanism. However, myristoylation of Pr55 apparently is essential for virus particle budding, because nonmyristoylated Pr55 obtained by amino acid substitutions fails to bud from the cell surface (200). An inhibitor of acyl-CoA synthetase, termed triacsin C, isolated from *Streptomyces* (197), blocks Gag myristoylation in a dose-dependent manner (0 to 48 μmol/L), but viral particle release was blocked only at a high-concentration 48 μmol/L, as examined using the recombinant baculovirus system (201). These data suggest that small amounts of myristoylated Gag proteins are sufficient for viral budding and that complete inhibition of myristoylation is required for blocking viral budding, findings implying that continuous complete inhibition of myristoylation in therapy of HIV-1 infection may lead to significant cellular damage or side effects.

Interferon-α (IFN-α) appears to have a broad spectrum of activity in the setting of HIV-1 infection. It causes regression of Kaposi's sarcoma with response rates of more than 45%, an increase in CD4 cell counts, and a decrease in the rate of opportunistic infections in a certain patient population (202). It also demonstrates efficacy in hepatitis B and hepatitis C in patients with HIV-1 infection (202). In particular, IFN-α is known to affect the stage of retroviral release from the cell membrane and several other early events in the replicative cycle of HIV-1 (203). Whatever the mechanism, IFN-α has apparent anti–HIV-1 activity both in vitro and in vivo. Although the magnitude of anti–HIV-1 activity is low or moderate as compared with other currently available antiviral therapeutics, reasonable in vitro synergistic antiviral activity with other antiviral agents has been reported (204). When the agent was combined with interleukin 2, a transient increase in CD4+ T-cell percentages, spontaneous lymphocyte blast transformation, and a decrease in HIV-1 titers were observed (205), although the clinical relevance of these transient changes is not known. Combination therapy with ddI and IFN-α was reported to be safely administered to patients with HIV-1 infection (206). In these trials, however, the significance of clinical efficacy of IFN-α itself was not clarified.

EMERGENCE OF DRUG-RESISTANT HIV VARIANTS

The ability to provide effective long-term antiretroviral therapy using single agents for HIV-1 infection became a complex issue when HIV-1 variants were isolated that were less susceptible to ZDV from AIDS patients who had received ZDV therapy for more than 6 months (207). Wainberg and his coworkers also reported in the same year that ZDV-resistant HIV-1 variants were isolated from several patients receiving long-term ZDV therapy when the virions were isolated in the presence of ZDV (208). Sequentially, nucleotide sequence analysis of the RT-encoding region from pairs of ZDV-sensitive and ZDV-insensitive HIV-1 isolates revealed several mutations that result in amino acid substitutions in RT (209, 210). Shortly after HIV protease inhibitors became available for therapy of HIV-1 infection, various amino acid substitutions were reported to occur in the viral protease of HIV-1 isolated from patients receiving such drugs for as short a time as a few months (211, 212). These mutations were confirmed to confer drug resistance to HIV protease inhibitors (213–215).

Mutant viruses appear to emerge in the presence of antiviral agents whenever the balance of mutant virus replication is favorable; that is, the mutant provides a selective advantage to the virus in the presence of drug. The problem is further exacerbated by the infection process for HIV-1, which is chronic, persistent, and characterized by high rates of replication. Pharmacodynamic studies using potent HIV protease inhibitors indicate that the estimated half-life of virus in plasma and virus-producing cells in the body is in the order of 2 days, with new virus being produced at a rate of 10^8 to 10^9 virions per day (216, 217). These conditions, coupled with the high error rate of HIV-1 RT, 1 to 10 nucleotides per replication cycle (218–221), favor rapid mutation and selection of drug-resistant virus (222). Structural implications and mechanisms of resistance to HIV protease inhibitors have been reviewed (223).

The development of viral resistance to antiretroviral agents appears to be a significant factor in the incomplete efficacy of antiviral therapy in patients with HIV-1 infection (224). Indeed, emergence of HIV-1 isolates with decreased susceptibility to ZDV has been linked to deterioration in clinical status in HIV-1–infected individuals being treated with ZDV (225–228). Furthermore, transmission of a drug-resistant HIV-1 variant has been reported (229), and this problem will likely increase in the future.

The isolation of drug-resistant HIV variants and the identification of various drug-related mutations have increased interest in using multiple agents in combination for HIV-1 therapy, as described later. However, the behavior of HIV-1 at the genetic or phenotypic level on exposure to multiple antiretroviral agents varies and remains poorly understood. In patients after long-term therapy with ZDV and ddC or ddI, a high level of resistance to ZDV is easily detected, although only low levels (up to a 10-fold increase in inhibitory concentration of 50% [IC_{50}] values) of resistance to ddI and ddC are found (230–233). These data suggest that the decreased sensitivity to ddC and ddI may be modest as compared with the magnitude of ZDV resistance (230). The alternating combination therapy of ZDV and ddC failed to prevent the emergence of high-level ZDV resistance (230, 231). In contrast, the addition of the ddI-related Leu74Val substitution to ZDV-resistant HIV variants carrying the ZDV-related Thr215Tyr mutation reverses those variants to a more ZDV-sensitive phenotype (234). This observation and other reports of in vitro synergistic activity with combined use of different antiviral agents (235–238) have further warranted combination chemotherapy.

Genetic recombination contributes to the genomic heterogeneity of HIV-1. Indeed, HIV-1 has been shown to develop resistance to two classes of anti–HIV-1 drugs through genetic recombination involving large segments of the viral genome in vitro (239, 240). Perhaps HIV-1 that is insensitive to multiple classes of antiviral agents emerges in patients receiving combination chemotherapy through the same mechanism.

Viral Resistance to Reverse Transcriptase Inhibitors

Drug resistance to NRTIs develops after prolonged treatment, and drug-resistant HIV-1 variants have been identified for all currently known NRTIs. Resistance to ZDV is associated with mutations of Met41Leu, Asp67Asn, Lys70Arg, Thr215Phe, and Lys219Gln (209, 210). Cross-resistance is common among NRTIs. For example, Leu74Val and Val75Thr confer resistance to both ddI and ddC, and Met184Val results in cross-resistance to ddI, ddC, and 3TC (241). The Val75Thr mutation observed with d4T is also cross-resistant to ddI, ddC, d4C, and (-)-2′,3′-dideoxy-5-fluoro-3′-thiacytidine (FTC). With the exception of the Leu74 and Met184 mutations, the mutation pattern seen for each nucleoside analog is unique. The Met184Val mutation can lead to resistance of greater than 100-fold to 3TC and FTC, but it leads to much smaller, although still significant, levels of resistance to ddI and ddC. The substitution of Ile50Thr causes a significant (approximately 30-fold) increase in resistance to d4T.

Unlike NNRTIs, in which the location of drug-resistant mutations can be directly correlated to their effects on binding to and inhibition of RT, the structural mechanisms of resistance to NRTIs are less clear (242). This is primarily because no high-resolution structure of HIV-1 RT is available that contains both a template primer and a nucleoside analog or is dNTP bound. Modeling studies have revealed that most of the resistance mutations observed with the nucleoside analogs do not map to the vicinity of the putative dNTP binding site but are dispersed over the entire finger subdomain (242). Analyses of the crystal structure of HIV RT complexed with double-stranded DNA have revealed that several mutations are in positions that may interact with the template primer (37, 39). Studies on the dependence of ddITP (not ddATP) resistance on the length of the template extension suggest that resistance results from the influence of the mutant side chain on the position or conformation of template primer that alters the ability of the enzyme to select or reject an incoming dNTP (243). Moreover, some mutations, such as Ile135Thr, are found in the p51 subunit at the heterodimer interface. Because this mutation is specific for ddI, it is implied that resistance may, in this case, be mediated through the p51 subunit. A detailed understanding of the resistance pattern for nucleoside analogs awaits further experimental investigations.

A particularly puzzling aspect of nucleoside resistance relates to the phenomenon that a resistance mutation for one compound can suppress a resistance mutation to a second inhibitor. For example, as mentioned earlier, the Leu74Val mutation observed with ddI can reverse the ZDV-resistant effect of the Thr215Tyr mutation (234). The Met184Val and Met184Ile mutations observed with 3TC both can suppress the effects of ZDV-resistant mutations, and the Gln161Leu and His208Tyr mutations observed with foscarnet can increase susceptibility to ZDV, nevirapine, and TIBO by 20- to 90-fold (244). The structural mechanisms for suppression are only poorly understood, but they may be due to compensatory effects of certain combinations of mutations on template-primer binding. These results underscore the need for structural data on ternary complexes of RT with nucleotide analogs and viral DNAs.

A set of five mutations (Ala62Val, Val75Ieu, Phe77Leu, Phe116Tyr, and Gln151Met) in the polymerase domain of RT, which confers on the virus a reduced sensitivity to multiple ddNs (multidideoxynucleoside resistance, MDR), has been identified (245–249). The analysis of the locations of these five mutations revealed that three of the five mutation sites (Val75, Phe77, and Gln151) are located close to the first template base and form part of the "template grip" (247), and a fourth (Phe116) is located close to the proposed dNTP-binding site (250). The locations of these mutations may allow RT to discriminate various ddNTPs from normal dNTPs (247). RT with the five mutations has proved highly resistant to ZDVTP, ddCTP, ddATP, and d4TTP, compared with wild-type RT (RT_{wt}) (251). Steady-state kinetic studies have revealed comparable catalytic efficiency (k_{cat}/K_m) between RTs carrying combined mutations and RT_{wt}, although a marked difference was noted in inhibition constants (K_i) (252). Thus, unlike the cases of ZDV resistance, the alteration of RT's substrate recognition, caused by these mutations, appears to account for the observed multi-ddN-resistance of HIV-1. These HIV-1 variants appear to develop multi-ddN-resistance stepwise through adding one or more mutations, which, however, sacrifice replicative capability; then HIV-1 finally acquires optimal replication competence by further additional mutations (i.e., the fifth Ala62Val mutation) (253).

Although the development of HIV-1 variants with resistance to RT inhibitors is most likely related to clinical deterioration in patients receiving RT inhibitors (225–228), clinical benefits of continuous use of RT inhibitors should still be considered possible because such mutations may impair RT structure or functions, resulting in the production of less replication-competent HIV-1 (222). In this regard, Wainberg and associates reported that RT carrying the 3TC-associated M184V substitution had a greater fidelity of nucleotide insertion than RT_{wt} (254). However, whether the enhanced fidelity observed in such misinsertion fidelity assays has a significant impact on the pathogenesis of HIV-1 diseases remains to be examined. Indeed, HIV-1 carrying M184V appears to acquire other drug-related mutations readily during 3TC-containing therapy (248). In the RT conveying the MDR-conferring five mutations described earlier, no significant changes in the fidelity of the enzyme activity have been detected (255). Nevertheless, it is interesting to examine the fidelity of RTs with various combined mutations that may have substantial constraints because of multiple amino acid substitutions. Other factors constituting the catalytic activity of RT, that is, its RNase H activity, also remain to be analyzed.

Viral Resistance to Nonnucleoside Reverse Transcriptase Inhibitors

The pattern of drug resistance observed for the various NNRTIs can be understood in light of the crystallographic data, and the mutation pattern also confirms the different binding modes of the various NNRTIs to RT. Most of the resistance mutations against NNRTIs occur for those residues that are in direct contact with the inhibitor (see Fig. 45A.6). Leu100, Lys103, Val106, Tyr181, and Gly190 are within van der Waals contact distance with nevirapine, and all these residues exhibit drug-resistance mutations. Tyr181 is not in close contact with nevirapine in the 3.5-Å crystal structure determined in the Steitz laboratory (37), but it does appear to be in close contact in a more recent 2.9-Å structure (256), in agreement with a modeling analysis of NNRTI binding site (257). In the crystal structure of the α-APA–RT complex, Tyr181 is also in contact with α-APA, consistent with mutation data (258). A surface area contact analysis using the published crystal structures of nevirapine and α-APA shows that the residues in the nevirapine complex that make the most contact are Tyr188, Leu100, and Val106. In the α-APA structure, both Tyr181 and Tyr188 make the most contact, followed by Leu100 and Val106. The amount of surface area in contact with the inhibitor correlates well with the observed mutational data. Indeed, a Tyr188 mutation has not yet been reported for α-APA. Examination of the van der Waals contacts between the enzyme and α-APA or nevirapine suggests that mutations of the contact residues will alter the tight packing between the inhibitor and enzyme and will result in altered binding affinity. Residues that make close contact but show no mutations are Leu234 and Trp229. These residues may have a functional role such that any mutations may be detrimental to enzyme function. Experimental evidence shows that the mutation of Trp229Ala results in a noninfective viral mutant (259). The identification and targeting of essential residues in the NNRTI binding site may provide a promising avenue for the design of agents to overcome resistance.

The finding that different classes of NNRTIs bind to the same pocket, although in slightly different fashion, would suggest that cross-resistance would be found among different NNRTIs. Although no crystal structures of mutant RT–drug complexes have been reported, effects of mutations on drug binding can be predicted by modeling mutations into the corresponding wild-type enzyme complex. The mutated amino acids that seem to confer resistance to the largest number of different inhibitors are Leu100, Val106, Tyr181, Val106, and Tyr188 (7, 260, 261). Tyr181 and Tyr188 interact through their aromatic rings with the aromatic rings of the inhibitors. The change from Tyr to Cys is not only a reduction in side chain size, but also in side chain character. The Val106Ala mutation results in loss of favorable hydrophobic side chain interactions with the γ methyl group of Val. Leu100Ile also does not interact with the inhibitors in the same matter because of different side chain rotamer preferences for the two amino acids. The Leu100Ile mutation causes greater than a 100-fold reduction in potency in the case of a TIBO derivative (262). For other, more flexible inhibitors, such as the pyridinones and HEPT, this same mutation results in an increase in resistance by a factor of 2 to 5 (81, 260). Many mutations result in resistance that is limited to one, two, or three classes of molecules, and this opens up the possibility of a combination therapy approach using drugs that exhibit mutually exclusive resistance profiles.

The degree of resistance may be related to conformational rigidity for particular structural classes of NNRTIs (263–265). Rigid compounds, such as TIBO and nevirapine, usually exhibit higher resistance levels than some of the more flexible compounds, such as HEPT and α APA. In addition, resistance can be associated with small structural changes in derivatives of the same class of compounds. In the bis(heteroaryl)piperazine (BHAP) series, Pro236Leu is observed for the U-90152 derivative, whereas Tyr181Cys, Lys103Asn, and Val106Ala are observed with the U-87201 and U-88204 compounds (241, 266). On the other hand, the Gly138Lys mutation seen with TIBO produces only resistance to TSAO and not any other NNRTI (81, 267).

Viral Resistance to Protease Inhibitors

EMERGENCE OF DRUG RESISTANCE TO PROTEASE INHIBITORS

Various drug resistance mechanisms are at play with the protease inhibitors (268). The most important ones, from a purely drug-binding standpoint, are mutations in the active site of the enzyme that lead to loss of anti–HIV-1 activity for the inhibitor. Such mutations are necessary but not sufficient for the emergence of high-level resistance in the clinical setting. The reason for this appears to be that active site mutations alone result in suboptimal virus. This conclusion is consistent with biochemical studies on drug-resistant mutant proteases in vitro (269–271). The structures of protease inhibitor complexes allow us to attempt to rationalize the structural effects of drug-resistance–conferring mutations on the interactions between the enzyme and inhibitor. The inhibitor and enzyme make a pattern of complementary hydrogen bonds between their respective backbone atoms. In some instances, these hydrogen bonds are mediated by bridging water molecules (272). The enzyme also contains well-defined pockets, or subsites, in its active site region into which inhibitor side chains protrude, resulting in tight binding interactions between enzyme and inhibitor. Because a similar pattern of hydrogen bonds is believed to be made for both substrates and peptidomimetic inhibitors, the specificity is believed to reside in the pattern of largely nonpolar subsite interactions between inhibitor and enzyme side chains atoms. Mutations of specificity-determining residues that would directly interfere with inhibitor binding constitute an obvious mechanism for resistance to HIV protease inhibitors. Other resistance pathways could include nonactive site mutations that indirectly interfere with inhibitor binding by long-range structural perturbations of the active site, mutations that result in an enzyme with enhanced catalysis of stability, cleavage site mutations that lead to enhanced processing by mutant enzymes, and "regulatory" mutations elsewhere in the genome that lead to improved viral replication in the presence of protease inhibitors. Combinations of different mutations may lead to additive, synergistic, or even compensatory effects.

Mutations have been observed in at least nearly half of all possible positions in the 99-residue monomer in response to drug-selection pressure (211, 273–281). Many of these mutations may presage the emergence of mutants in the clinical setting in vivo (270, 282, 283). They can be classified as either active site or nonactive site mutations, according to whether they occur inside or outside the inhibitor binding subsites and directly contact inhibitor, as discussed later.

ACTIVE SITE MUTANTS

The first described resistance mutation for HIV protease was a Val82Ala mutation that was selected using a symmetric diol inhibitor (273). Since then, resistance mutations have been observed in each of the unique specificity pockets, S3, S2, S1, and, by symmetry, S1′, S2′ and S3′. However, only a subset of all residues that constitute a particular subsite mutates in response to a particular drug. The structural effects of mutations on drug binding have been modeled using the crystal structures of the appropriate wild-type enzyme inhibitor complexes, and they have been used to rationalize the effects of specific mutations on drug-binding affinities (215, 273–275, 278). For example, KNI-272, a peptidomimetic inhibitor of HIV protease (284–286), contains a norstatine insert as the transition state analog. Two resistance mutations selected in vitro using KNI-272 were found to map to the active site region: Val32Ile and Ile84Val (277). The Ki for the Ile84Val recombinant enzyme is about 30-fold higher than that for the wild-type enzyme (271). Based on a crystal structure obtained for the wild-type enzyme complex, the Ile84Val mutation was modeled into the protease (272). The side chain of Ile84 contacts both the P1 and P2′ groups (and by symmetry, the P1′ and P2 groups) of the inhibitor. The Ile84Val mutation affects both sides of the enzyme active site because of the symmetry of the enzyme. Because the inhibitor is asymmetric, the two mutations were predicted to have different effects, but the net result was a loss of interaction in moving from the bulky isobutyl side chain of Ile to the smaller isopropyl side chain of Val.

Most of the subsite mutations, like Ile84Val and Val82Ala (Ile or Phe), affect hydrophobic and van der Waals' interactions and can be considered to be "packing" mutants, analogous to hydrophobic mutations in a protein core (215, 272, 278). Crystallographic analyses of HIV protease inhibitor complexes show that most of the surface of an inhibitor and its immediate protein environment are solvent inaccessible. Some mutations, such as Val82Ile, are more effective when combined with a second active site mutation, such as Val32Ile, owing to synergistic effects on enzyme activity (274). Other mutations can affect electrostatic contacts. The effect of the Arg8Glu mutation on binding to A-77003 was shown to be due to loss of a charge-induced dipole interaction between the guanidinium side chain of the enzyme and the pyridine ring of the inhibitor (275). Although this mutation resulted in a dramatic loss of inhibition, it also produced a virus with severely impaired replication kinetics. A possible explanation for this defect is the symmetric loss of the intersubunit salt bridge between Arg8 and Asp129 that may decrease the stability of the enzyme. Despite the demonstration of strong cross-resistance of the Arg8Glu protease to ritonavir (ABT-538), indinavir (MK-539), and saquinavir (271), this mutation is infrequently observed in patients. Thus, the design of inhibitors that selectively interact with Arg8 may be a useful strategy for the development of "resistance-repellant" drugs (268).

Although numerous crystal structures of wild-type HIV protease inhibitor complexes have been published, crystal structures of mutant HIV protease inhibitor complexes are only now beginning to emerge in the literature. The structure determination of a Val82Ala mutant of HIV protease complexed to the C_2 symmetry-based inhibitor, A-77003, reveals backbone changes that resulted in the repacking of enzyme and inhibitor atoms in the S1/S1′ and S3/S3′ subsites (215). The structure of the Val82Ile mutant with DMP-323, a cyclic urea-based inhibitor, exhibited a loss of interaction between the γ methyl group of valine and the inhibitor, despite the larger bulk of the mutant isoleucine side chain (287). The reason was that the energetically favored side chain rotamer for isoleucine resulted in a repositioning of the CD1 methyl away from the P1 group of the inhibitor. These changes were unexpected based on modeling studies.

However, Val82 resides in a structurally flexible loop that can exhibit many different conformations in response to different conditions (288). This flexibility is consistent with the finding that Val82 can be replaced by both larger (Ile and Phe) and smaller (Ala) residues in viable mutant enzymes. These studies point out the dangers inherent in reliance on pure modeling approaches and underscore the need for continued experimental studies of inhibitors complexed with resistant mutants of HIV protease.

NONACTIVE SITE MUTANTS

Although the precise structural mechanism of drug resistance can often be pinpointed for active site mutations that directly affect inhibitor binding, the evaluation of nonactive site mutants is more challenging, and several different mechanisms may be at work. Some mutations may act in concert with active site mutations by compensating for a functional deficit caused by the latter. For example, the defective Arg8Glu mutation is found almost exclusively in combination with one or more mutations outside the active site region, such as Met46Ile (275). Mutations of Met46 to Ile, Leu, or Phe are often found in the presence or absence of other active site mutations, such as Val82Ile, Ala or Phe, and Ile84Val. Met46 is in the flap of HIV protease, and molecular dynamics simulations on flap movement have shown that the Met46Ile mutant exhibits different dynamic behavior than the wild-type enzyme (98), and presumably it alters enzyme kinetics. However, a role for Met46 in polyprotein substrate recognition is also possible.

Other nonactive site mutants may indirectly alter the structure of the active site region. Many of these nonactive site mutations are found in multiple combinations with one or more active site mutants. Modeling studies of a hextuple mutant selected using KNI-272 (BD Anderson, H Mitsuya, unpublished data) reveal that mutations far from the active site, such as Ala71Val, may influence inhibitor or substrate binding by a concerted "domino" effect. A similar mechanism may be operative for the saquinavir-resistant Leu90Met mutation. The side chain of residue 90 can affect the conformation of the active site loop that contains the catalytic aspartic acids. Most of these mutations result in a larger hydrophobic side chain that perturbs packing interactions within the enzyme core. This perturbation may be transferred to the active site, where the internal strain energy on the protein may be relieved through alterations in the interaction energy with the inhibitor. In some cases, the introduction of nonactive site mutations alone does not lead to a marked or even measurable reduction in inhibitor binding, in contrast to the case for all known active site mutations (271). However, the observation of certain mutants only in the presence of drug means that they must by definition provide the virus with some selective replication advantage. At least one engineered HIV protease mutant, Gly48Tyr, exhibited greater catalytic efficiency than the wild-type enzyme toward artificial peptide substrates (289). However, this mutant has not been observed either in vitro or in vivo in the presence or absence of inhibitors.

CLEAVAGE SITE MUTANTS

Because active site mutations may be expected to alter the rate of one or more cleavages that must occur during viral maturation, one may imagine that compensating mutations in the cleavage sites on the Gag or Gag-Pol polyproteins could render them better substrates for particular mutant enzymes. Studies have identified a mutation in the p1/p6 gag polyprotein cleavage site (Leu449Phe) substitution that can synergize with the Ile84Val mutant to produce a virus with 350-1,500-fold decreased sensitivity to substrate-based protease inhibitors BILA 1906 BS and BILA 2185 BS (290). The mutation altered the p1/p6 cleavage site from Phe-Leu to Phe-Phe. A synthetic peptide containing the Phe-Phe cleavage site was cleaved at higher catalytic efficiency by the Ile84Val HIV protease mutant than the corresponding peptide with the wild-type sequence (291). When HIV-1 was passaged in the presence of KNI-272 (284, 285) and was selected to develop a high degree of resistance against KNI-272, the same substitution at the p1/p6 gag polyprotein cleavage site (Leu449Phe) was observed (BD Anderson, H Mitsuya, unpublished data). More recently, cleavage site mutations at the p7/p1 cleavage site have been found in breakthrough virus isolated from patients receiving indinavir therapy (292). This finding is important because it confirms the possibility of this mechanism in drug resistance in vivo.

COMBINATION THERAPY

Incomplete virus suppression by inappropriate therapeutic regimens and poor compliance permit HIV-1 to continue to replicate and consequently to develop resistance to the therapeutics (109, 110). Inconvenient and complicated dosing schedules, a great number of pills to be taken, and various inherent side effects all play a major role in the development of drug resistance (109–111). Moreover, the more completely the suppression of viral replication attained, the slower the development of drug resistance. Nevertheless, HIV-1 probably ultimately develops resistance even to the most potent regimens.

Rationale

With the relatively low therapeutic index of most anti-HIV drugs and the propensity of HIV to develop resistance by mutation, the optimal therapy for this disorder probably will involve a combination of drugs and approaches (5, 6, 8, 293–295). In this regard, HIV infection is similar to various tumors or other chronic infectious diseases, such as infection with *Mycobacterium tuberculosis* (296, 297). Combination therapy of AIDS has potential advantages. One is the potential for reducing overall toxicity by combining drugs with different toxicity profiles. This was the initial rationale for testing alternating regimens of ZDV (which primarily causes bone marrow toxicity) and ddC (which primarily causes peripheral neuropathy) (30, 298–300). Pilot studies of such an approach have suggested that a sustained anti-HIV effect can be attained with decreased toxicity from each drug.

Indeed, the potential for combining drugs in this manner is one rationale for developing new drugs with different toxicity profiles than the drugs already in use.

Another reason for combining various drugs is the potential for drug synergy. One would predict that anti-HIV drugs that act at different stages of the HIV life cycle would often be synergistic together, and indeed, this has been observed in vitro with some such combinations (5, 235, 237, 238). Indeed, this is one reason for the interest in targeting different steps. Under certain circumstances, drugs that act at the same step may also be synergistic. For example, two NNRTIs (e.g., ZDV and ddC or ZDV and ddI) can exert antiviral activity either synergistically or additively when tested together (10, 301–303). However, certain drugs can also interfere with each other's activity. For example, ZDV, in part through an effect on thymidylate kinase, reduces the phosphorylation of and activity of d4T (50). In addition, ribavirin reduces the anti-HIV activity of ZDV in vitro by inhibiting its intracellular phosphorylation (304). On the other hand, ribavirin can potentiate the antiviral activity of ddI, ddA, and FddA in vitro, by serving as an inhibitor of inosine-5'-monophosphate dehydrogenase, which is a donor for the phosphorylation of ddI by 5'-nucleotidase (305–308). These examples are reminders that complex interactions can occur among anti-HIV drugs, particularly agents that undergo intercellular activation, and this possibility should be explored before these drugs are used together in clinical trials.

Another potential advantage of using drugs together is that they may target different cell populations. Anti–HIV-1 dideoxynucleoside analogs (ddNs) can be classified into two groups based on the phosphorylation profiles: 1) cell-activation–dependent ddNs, including ZDV and d4T, that are preferentially phosphorylated and yield higher ratios of ddNTP to dNTP in activated cells than in resting cells; and 2) cell-activation–independent ddNs including ddI, ddC, FddA, and PMEA that produce higher ratios of ddNTP to dNTP in resting cells (Table 45A.3) (309–311). As expected, protease inhibitors such as KNI-272, which do not require intracellular activation or anabolic phosphorylation for exhibiting anti–HIV-1 activity, have been confirmed to demonstrate comparable antiviral activity against HIV-1 in both activated cells and resting cells (312). Cellular activation also affects the antiviral activity of NRTIs in monocyte/macrophages (59, 313). Thus, the potential for effective combination chemotherapy is likely to be enhanced when drugs from each of the two categories are combined (e.g., ZDV plus 3TC, ZDV plus ddC, or d4T plus ddI), although the pharmacokinetics of each drug and the emergence of drug-resistant HIV-1 variants also have to be considered as critical factors in designing effective combination antiretroviral chemotherapy.

Interest has been expressed in combining NRTIs with certain inhibitors that may potentiate the antiviral activity of NRTIs by modifying the cellular nucleotide pools. Hydroxyurea, an inhibitor of ribonucleotide reductase, can enhance the anti–HIV-1 activity of ddI, ZDV, and ddC in vitro with

Table 45A.3 Antiviral Activity of Dideoxynucleosides in Resting and Activated Peripheral Blood Mononuclear Cells (PBMs)

	Zidovudine	Stavudine	Didanosine	PMEA	Zalcitabine
Resting PBMs	48.8 µmol/L	45.7	0.2 (×40)	0.19 (×22)	0.008 (×38)
Phytohemagglutin-activated PBMs	0.041 (×1190)	0.41 (×111)	7.9	4.2	0.3

PMEA, 9-(2-phosphonylmethoxyethyl)-adenine.
PBMs were preincubated with various concentrations of each drug for 16 hours, exposed to HIV-1, stimulated with or without PHA, and further cultured in the presence of 5 µmol/L zidovudine for 4 weeks. The amounts of p24 in the supernatants were determined to define IC_{90} values. All experiments were performed in quadruplicate. (reference 346)
(From Shirasaka T, Chokekijchai S, Yamada A, et al. Comparative analysis of anti-human immunodeficiency virus type 1 activities of dideoxynucleoside analogs in resting and activated peripheral blood mononuclear cells. Antimicrob Agents Chemother 1995;39:2555–2559.)

the order of the potentiation being ddI > ZDV ~ ddC at relatively nontoxic concentrations (i.e., 0.1 to 0.4 µmol/L) (314). The greater degree of potentiation by hydroxyurea of ddI than of other ddNs is due to the effective inhibition of dATP synthesis by hydroxyurea in comparison with other dNTPs (dGTP, dTTP, dCTP) (315). In open-label pilot studies, the combination of ddI and hydroxyurea has demonstrated favorable virologic effects against HIV-1 in vivo (316–319). A small, anecdotal study showed that, in several patients who received ddI plus hydroxyurea and stopped the therapy, HIV-1 replication did not resume (320). However, in another study, no such advantages were seen in patients receiving that combination as compared with those receiving ddI monotherapy (321). A possibility existed that the low intracellular dNTP concentrations caused by hydroxyurea could lead to general suppression of HIV-1 without regard to particular drug resistance; however, ddI combined with hydroxyurea apparently did not block or delay the emergence of ddI therapy-related mutations as compared with ddI monotherapy (322). Determination of the utility of the addition of hydroxyurea to currently available therapy with NRTIs requires further clinical evaluation; however, the use of any inhibitors of cellular enzymes such as hydroxyurea may cause intolerable toxicities during long-term antiviral therapy.

Interest also exists in combining anti-HIV agents with drugs that affect the production or activity of stimulatory cytokines. Tumor necrosis factor-α (TNF-α), for example, has been observed to increase HIV replication in vitro (323, 324). The drug pentoxifylline can inhibit the production of TNF-α in vitro, and clinical trials are under way to determine whether it could be of value in advanced HIV infection in combination with ZDV or other anti-HIV agents (325). In addition, the activation of HIV replication induced by TNF-α is associated with a reduction in intracellular glutathione levels, which, in turn, are believed to affect the activity of TNF-α. Cysteine precursors such as N-acetyl-L-cysteine (NAC) are reported to increase intracellular glutathione levels and thus to reduce HIV activation (326). However, because of its inherent toxicity at such high concentrations of NAC reported to be effective against HIV-1 in vitro, reproducing the original reports has been difficult (H Mitsuya, et al., unpublished data).

Finally, some evidence suggests that certain opportunistic infections may hasten the progression of HIV-1–related diseases by various mechanisms. For example, investigators have proposed that *Mycoplasma* infections may potentiate HIV-1–induced apoptosis (327). In addition, regulatory proteins produced by certain herpesviruses can transactivate HIV-1, and infection of CD8-bearing T lymphocytes by human herpesvirus 6 has been shown to induce expression of CD4 on such cells (and thus render them more susceptible to HIV-1 infection) (328, 329). Thus, the administration of drugs against such infections conceivably could secondarily affect the course of HIV-1 infection. This possibility was one of the rationales for using acyclovir in patients with advanced HIV-1 infection (1, 330–332); however, no association between the addition of acyclovir and survival of patients with advanced HIV-1 disease receiving ZDV has been documented (333, 334).

Approaches to Combat Resistance

A key issue in combating resistance is to define the most important resistance mutations for a particular inhibitor, although one has no guarantee that in vitro selection studies will accurately mirror in vivo results. Results of one study, using a panel of over a dozen recombinant protease mutants, suggest that those mutations selected in vivo displayed the highest enzyme "vitality," defined as the ratio of $(K_i \times k_{cat}/K_m)_{mutant}/(K_i \times k_{cat}/K_m)_{wild\ type}$, for a given inhibitor (271). Some studies indicate that cross-resistance is a problem for most clinically useful protease inhibitors (269–271). This observation should not be a surprise because all the inhibitors were highly optimized to bind wild-type enzyme. Mutations have been found in every subsite of HIV protease; however, not every subsite residue has been found to mutate for a particular drug. Further, only a few of the total possible single-step mutations that could occur have actually been found at each variant position. These results suggest that certain constraints limit the potentially available resistance pathways. Beside the usual factors that limit viable mutations in enzymes, such as proper folding, stability, and catalytic function, HIV protease has several unusual constraints because of its structural and functional uniqueness. The homodimeric nature of the enzyme means that every mutation at the genetic level will result in a double mutant at the enzyme level (unless heterodimer formation occurs in vivo). The requirement for recognition and cleavage of 9 or 10 specific cleavage sites on the polyproteins should limit mutations to ones that will not diminish processing below some tolerable threshold. Studies using recombinant HIV protease mutants suggest that this threshold may be below 10% of wild-type enzyme activity (271). Finally, the finding that some subsite amino acids, such as Arg8, also participate in the dimer interface suggests that some subsite mutants may adversely affect dimer stability. Many of the resistance mutations in HIV-1 protease are present in the wild-type sequences of HIV-2 (335) or other retroviral proteases at structurally equivalent locations. EIAV protease behaves like an extreme case of a drug-resistant mutant of HIV-1 protease because it is not susceptible to inhibition by many different HIV-1 protease inhibitors (336). Thus, one may see a limited number of solutions to the protease sequence and substrate specificity combinatorial puzzle for retroviruses, and mutational strategies for resistance tend to evolve toward one or more of them.

Given the unusual constraints on HIV protease and our understanding of inhibitor binding and resistance at an atomic level of detail, investigators should be able to redesign inhibitors that target different mutants. These inhibitors could then be used together in multidrug combination therapy approaches. It may even be possible to design inhibitors that target multiple mutants simultaneously. In certain instances, these second-line drugs could prompt the selection of wild-type revertants, which can then be treated with the original drug. One can thus envision a type of structure-directed oscillation therapy, whereby one treats with a drug designed simultaneously to target the mutant enzyme and to provide selection pressure to mutate back to wild-type or forward toward another treatable variant (268). This proposed strategy differs fundamentally from classic sequential therapy approaches, which have not been successful in controlling infectious diseases, in that it applies specific, structure-guided selection pressure to influence the outcome of therapy.

The situation with HIV RT inhibitors differs from that of HIV protease in several important ways that affect the usefulness of structure-based approaches to combat resistance. Crystallographic studies reveal that NNRTIs bind to a site on HIV-1 RT that is not conserved and evidently is not involved in catalytic function (256). This finding suggests that mutations at this site should be present at a high frequency in the wild-type population. The rapid rise of NNRTI-resistant virus in drug-treated patients supports this assumption. Our understanding of the structural basis of resistance to NRTIs has been hampered by the lack of structural data for an RT–dNTP–DNA inhibitor complex. To make matters worse, for example, resistance to ZDV has been difficult even to speculate about mechanistically, because only slight changes are seen in the sensitivity to ZDVTP of RT with the Thr215Tyr mutation, and RT with the Asp67Asn/Lys70Arg/Thr215Tyr/Lys219Glu mutations accounts only partly for the significantly reduced sensitivity of the virus carrying such mutations to ZDV (252, 337, 338). Thus, perhaps the cross-resistance profile of certain mutant RTs to ddNTPs may not be directly linked to the cross-resistance profile of the virus carrying the same RT.

In conclusion, substantial progress has been made in the therapy of AIDS since HIV was defined as its etiologic agent. More than 10 drugs have been shown to have clinical efficacy, and several others are in various stages of clinical and preclinical development. However, it has become apparent that with the drugs tested so far, only partial immunologic reconstitution is attained in patients with advanced HIV-1 infection. We are at a new forefront in antiviral research that promises to lead to new approaches to deal with various problems in the therapy of HIV-1 infection. In particular, the problem of viral drug resistance poses different challenges than we faced in the design of the first-line drugs because it forces us to think about selection pressure mechanisms in addition to the usual issues of potency, pharmacology, safety, and mechanism of drug action. Unfortunately, those very features that contribute to the specificity and efficacy of RT and protease inhibitors also provide the virus with a strategy to mount resistance. The rapid replication rate of HIV-1 in vivo, coupled with the long duration of viral infection, favors the emergence of resistant mutants to virtually any targeted antiviral agent. Computer simulation studies show that a mutant virus with a selective advantage of only 5% (i.e., a replication rate $1.05 \times$ wild-type virus) will propagate to become the dominant genotype, within approximately 100 virus generations (222). These same considerations imply that those viral mutants that only arise under drug pressure must by definition be less robust than their wild-type progenitors. Our understanding of structural mechanisms of resistance in the case of NNRTIs and protease inhibitors is detailed but still semiquantitative and subject to current methodologic limitations of modeling accuracy. The improvement attained has generally been transient, none of the available therapies are curative, and the need for drug development in AIDS is as urgent as ever. Improved approaches to structure-based drug design and the development of quantitative methods of modeling and binding affinity prediction take on added significance. Meanwhile, one should continue to search for combinations of drugs with complementary resistance profiles and less severe side effects and to explore new treatment modalities such as structure-based approaches that can be used to exert specific selection pressures on HIV-1 in the hopes that at least a stalemate, if not an end-game, strategy can be found to control the progression of AIDS.

References

1. Mitsuya H, Broder S. Strategies for antiviral therapy in AIDS. Nature 1987;325:773–778.
2. Mitsuya H, Yarchoan R, Broder S. Molecular targets for AIDS therapy. Science 1990;249:1533–1544.
3. Yarchoan R, Pluda JM, Perno CF, et al. Anti-retroviral therapy of HIV infection: current strategies and challenges for the future. Blood 1991;78:859–884.
4. Hirsch MS, Kaplan JC. Treatment of human immunodeficiency virus infections. Antimicrob Agents Chemother 1987;31:839–843.
5. Johnson MI, Hoth DF. Present status and future prospects for HIV therapies. Science 1993;260:1286–1293.
6. De Clercq E. Antiviral therapy for human immunodeficiency virus infections. Clin Microbiol Rev 1995;8:200–239.

7. De Clercq E. In search of a selective antiviral chemotherapy. Clin Microbiol Rev 1997;10:674–693.
8. Mitsuya H, ed. Anti-HIV nucleosides: past, present and future. Austin, TX: RG Landes, 1997.
9. Erickson JW, Fesik SW. Macromolecular x-ray crystallography and NMR as tools for structure-based drug design. Annu Rep Med Chem 1992;27:271–289.
10. Mitsuya H, Matsukura M, Broder S. Rapid in vitro systems for assessing activity of agents against HTLV-III/LAV. In: Broder S, ed. AIDS: modern concepts and therapeutic challenges. New York: Marcel Dekker, 1987:303–333.
11. Harada S, Koyanagi Y, Yamamoto N. Infection of HTLV-III/LAV in HTLV-I–carrying cells MT2 and MT4 and application in a plaque assay. Science 1985, 229:563–566.
12. Chesebro B, Wehrly K. Development of a sensitive quantitative focal assay for human immunodeficiency virus infectivity. J Virol 1988;62: 3779–3788.
13. Weislow OS, Kiser R, Fine DL, et al. New soluble-formazan assay for HIV-1 cytopathic effects: application to high flux screening of synthetic and natural products for AIDS-antiviral activity. J. Natl Cancer Inst 1989;81:577–586.
14. Richman DD, Johnson VA, Mayers DL, et al. In vitro evaluation of experimental agents for anti-HIV activity. In: Coligan JE, Kruisbeek AM, Margulies DH, et al., eds. Current protocols in immunology. Unit 12.9. New York, John Wiley & Sons, 1993:12.9.1–12.9.21.
15. Mitsuya H, Popovic M, Yarchoan R, et al. Suramin protection of T cells in vitro against infectivity and cytopathic effect of HTLV-III. Science 1984;226:172–174.
16. Mitsuya H, Weinhold KJ, Furman PA, et al. 3′-Azido-3′-deoxythymidine (BW A509U): an antiviral agent that inhibits the infectivity and cytopathic effect of human T-lymphotropic virus type III/lymphadenopathy-associated virus in vitro. Proc Natl Acad Sci U S A 1985;82:7096–7100.
17. Harada S, Koyanagi Y, Yamamoto N. Infection of HTLV-III/LAV in HTLV-1 carrying cells MT-2 and MT-4 and application in a plaque assay. Science 1985;229:563–566.
18. Pauwels R, Balzarini J, Baba M, et al. Rapid and automated tetrazolium-based colorimetric assay for the detection of anti-HIV compounds. J Acquir Immune Defic Syndr 1988;20:309–321.
19. Ruprecht RM, O'Brien LG, Rossoni LD, et al. Suppression of mouse viraemia and retroviral disease by 3′-azido-3′-deoxythymidine. Nature 1986;323:467–469.
20. Daniel MD, Letvin NL, King NW. Isolation of T-cell tropic HTLV-III–like retrovirus from macaques. Science 1985;228:1201–1204.
21. McCune JM, Namikawa R, Shih C-C, et al. Suppression of HIV infection in AZT-treated SCID-hu mice. Science 1990;247:564–566.
22. Mosier DE, Gulizia RJ, Baird SM, et al. Human immunodeficiency virus infection of human-PBL-SICD mice. Science 1991;251:791–794.
23. Robins RK. Synthetic antiviral agents. Chem Eng News January 27, 1986:28–40.
24. Tummino PJ, Prasad JVNV, Ferguson D, et al. Discovery and optimization of nonpeptide HIV-1 protease inhibitors. Bioorg Med Chem Lett 1996;4:1401–1410.
25. Erickson J, Neidhart DJ, VanDri J, et al. Design, activity, and 2.8 Å crystal structure of a C_2 symmetric inhibitor complexed to HIV-1 protease. Science 1990;249:527–533.
26. Wlodawer A, Erickson JW. Structure-based inhibitors of HIV-1 protease. Annu Rev Biochem 1993;62:543–585.
27. Wu H, Myszka DG, Tendian SW, et al. Kinetic and structural analysis of mutant CD4 receptors that are defective in HIV gp120 binding. Proc Natl Acad Sci U S A 1996;93:15030–15035.
28. Weissenhorn W, Dessen A, Harrison SC, et al. Atomic structure of the ectodomain from HIV-1 gp41. Nature 1997;387:426–430.
29. De Clercq E. Toward improved anti-HIV chemotherapy: therapeutic strategies for intervention with HIV infections. J Med Chem 1995; 38:2491–2517.
30. Yarchoan R, Perno CF, Thomas RV, et al. Phase I studies of 2′,3′-dideoxycytidine in severe human immunodeficiency virus infection as a single agent and alternating with zidovudine (AZT). Lancet 1988;1:76–81.
31. Merigan TC, Skowron G, Bozzette SA, et al. Circulating p24 antigen levels and responses to dideoxycytidine in human immunodeficiency virus (HIV) infections. Ann Intern Med 1989;110:189–194.
32. Kahn JO, Allan JD, Hodges TL, et al. The safety and pharmacokinetics of recombinant soluble CD4 (rCD4) in subjects with the acquired immunodeficiency syndrome (AIDS) and AIDS-related complex: a phase I study. Ann Intern Med 1990;112:254–261.
33. Schooley RT, Merigan TC, Gaut P, et al. Recombinant soluble CD4 therapy in patients with the acquired immunodeficiency syndrome (AIDS) and AIDS-related complex: a phase I-II escalating dosage trial. Ann Intern Med 1990;112:247–253.
34. Mitsuya H, Broder S. Inhibition of the in vitro infectivity and cytopathic effect of human T-lymphotropic virus type III/lymphadenopathy virus-associated virus (HTLV-III/LAV) by 2′,3′-dideoxynucleosides. Proc Natl Acad Sci U S A 1986;83:1911–1915.
35. Goldman ME, Nunberg JH, O'Brien JA, et al. Pyridinone derivatives: specific human immunodeficiency virus type 1 reverse transcriptase inhibitors with antiviral activity. Proc Natl Acad Sci U S A 1991;88: 6863–6867.
36. Vasudevachari MB, Battista C, Lane HC, et al. Prevention of the spread of HIV-1 infection with nonnucleoside reverse transcriptase inhibitors. J Virol 1992;190:269–277.
37. Kohlstaedt LA, Wang J, Friedman JM, et al. Crystal structure at 3.5 Å resolution of HIV-1 reverse transcriptase complexed with an inhibitor. Science 1992;256:1783–1790.
38. Arnold E, Jacob-Monila A, Nanni RG, et al. Structure of HIV1 reverse transcriptase/DNA complex at 7Å resolution showing active site locations. Nature 1992;357:85–89.
39. Jacobo-Molina A, Ding J, Nanni RG, et al. Crystal structure of human immunodeficiency virus type 1 reverse transcriptase complexed with double-stranded DNA at 3.0 Å resolution shows bent DNA. Proc Natl Acad Sci U S A 1993;90:6320–6324.
40. Clark AD Jr, Jacobo-Molina A, Clark P, et al. Crystallization of human immunodeficiency virus type 1 reverse transcriptase with and without nucleic acid substrates, inhibitors, and an antibody Fab fragment. Methods Enzymol 1995;262:171–185.
41. Sanger F, Nicklen S, Coulson AR. DNA sequencing with chain-terminating inhibitors. Proc Natl Acad Sci U S A 1977;75:5463–5467.
42. Horwitz JP, Chua J, Noel M. Nucleosides. V. The monomesylates of 1-(2′-deoxy-β-D-lyxofuranosyl)thymidine. J Organ Chem 1964;29: 2076–2078.
43. Robins MJ, Robins RK. The synthesis of 2′,3′-dideoxyadenosine from 2′-deoxyadenosine. J Am Chem Soc 1964;86:3585–3586.
44. Horwitz JP, Chua J, Noel M, et al. Nucleosides. XI. 2′,3′-Dideoxycytidine. J Organ Chem 1966;32:817–818.
45. Horwitz JR, Chua J, Da Rooge MA, et al. Nucleosides. IX. The formation of 2′,2′-unsaturated pyrimidine nucleosides via a novel β-elimination reaction. J Organ Chem 1966;31:205–211.
46. Toji L, Cohen SS. Termination of deoxyribonucleic acid in *Eschericia coli* by 2′,3′-dideoxyadenosine. J Bacteriol 1970;103:323–328.
47. Ostertag W, Roesler G, Krieg CJ, et al. Induction of endogenous virus and of thymidine kinase by bromodeoxyuridine in cell cultures transformed by Friend virus. Proc Natl Acad Sci U S A 1974;71: 4948–4985.
48. Waqar MA, Evans MJ, Manly KF, et al. Effects of 2′,3′-dideoxynucleosides on mammalian cells and viruses. J Cell Physiol 1984;121:402–408.
49. Furmanski P, Bourguignon GJ, Bolles CS, et al. Inhibition by 2′,3′-dideoxythymidine of retroviral infection of mouse and human cells. Cancer Lett 1980;8:307–315.
50. Furman PA, Fyfe JA, St Clair M, et al. Phosphorylation of 3′-azido-3′-deoxythymidine and selective interaction of the 5′-triphosphate

50. with human immunodeficiency virus reverse transcriptase. Proc Natl Acad Sci U S A 1986;83:8333–8337.
51. Yarchoan R, Mitsuya H, Myers CE, et al. Clinical pharmacology of 3′-azido-2′,3′-dideoxythymidine (zidovudine) and related dideoxynucleosides. N Engl J Med 1989;321:726–738.
52. Johns DG. Pharmacology of antiretroviral nucleoside analogs. In: Mitsuya H, ed. Anti-HIV nucleosides: past, present, and future. Austin, TX: RG Landes, 1997.: 23–50.
53. Starnes MC, Cheng Y-C. Cellular metabolism of 2′,3′-dideoxycytidine, a compound active against human immunodeficiency virus in vitro. J Biol Chem 1987;262:988–991.
54. Cheng Y-C, Dutschman GE, Bastow KF, et al. Human immunodeficiency virus reverse transcriptase: general properties and its interaction with nucleoside triphosphate analogs. J Biol Chem 1987;262:2187–2189.
55. Huang P, Farquhar D, Plunkett W. Selective action of 3′-azido-3′-deoxythymidine 5′-triphosphate on viral reverse transcriptase and human DNA polymerase. J Biol Chem 1990;265:11914–11918.
56. Koenig S, Gendelman HE, Orenstein JM, et al. Detection of AIDS virus in macrophages in brain tissue from AIDS patients with encephalopathy. Science 1986;233:1089–1093.
57. Ho DD, Rota TR, Hirsch MS. Infection of monocyte/macrophages by human T lymphotropic virus type III. J Clin Invest 1986;77:1712–1715.
58. Perno CF, Yarchoan R, Cooney DA, et al. Inhibition of human immunodeficiency virus (HIV-1/HTLV-III$_{Ba-L}$) replication in fresh and cultured human peripheral blood monocytes/macrophages by azidothymidine and related 2′,3′-dideoxynucleosides. J Exp Med 1988;168:1111–1125.
59. Perno C-F, Yarchoan R, Cooney DA, et al. Replication of human immunodeficiency virus in monocytes: granulocyte/macrophage colony-stimulating factor (GM-CSF) potentiates viral production yet enhances the antiviral effect mediated by 3′-azido-2′3′-dideoxythymidine (AZT) and other dideoxynucleoside congeners of thymidine. J Exp Med 1989;169:933–951.
60. Marquez VE, Tseng CK-H, Driscoll JS, et al. 2′,3′-Dideoxy-2′-fluoro-ara-A: an acid-stable purine nucleoside active against human immunodeficiency virus (HIV). Biochem Pharmacol 1987;36:2719–2722.
61. Matthes E, Lehmann C, Drescher B, et al. 3′-Deoxy-3′-fluorothymidinetriphosphate: inhibitor and terminator of DNA synthesis catalysed by DNA polymerase beta, terminal deoxynucleotidyl transferase and DNA polymerase I. Biomed Biochim Acta 1985;44:63–73.
62. Martin JA, Bushnell DJ, Duncan IB, et al. Synthesis and antiviral activity of monofluoro and difluoro analogues of pyrimidine deoxyribonucleosides against human immunodeficiency virus (HIV-1). J Med Chem 1990;33:2137–2145.
63. Tanaka M, Srinivas RV, Ueno T, et al. In vitro induction of human immunodeficiency virus type 1 (HIV-1) variants resistant to 2′-β-fluoro-2′,3′-dideoxyadenosine (F-ddA). Antimicrob Agents Chemother 1997;41:1313–1318.
64. Pauwels R, Balzarini J, Schols D, De Clercq E. Phosphonylmethoxyethyl purine derivatives, a new class of anti-human immunodeficiency virus (HIV) in vitro. Antimicrobial Agents Chemother 1988;32:1025–1030.
65. Vince R, Hua M, Brownell J, et al. Potent and selective activity of a new carbocyclic nucleoside analog (carbovir: NSC 614846) against human immunodeficiency virus in vitro. Biochem Biophys Res Commun 1988;156:1046–1053.
66. Garvey EP, Krenitsky TA. A novel human phosphotransferase highly specific for adenosine. Arch Biochem Biophys 1992;296:161–169.
67. Faletto MB, Miller WH, Garvey EP, et al. Unique intracellular activation of the potent anti-human immunodeficiency virus agent 1592U89. Antimicrob Agents Chemother 1997;41:1099–1107.
68. Pauwels R, Andries K, Desmyter J, et al. Potent and selective inhibition of HIV-1 replication in vitro by a novel series of TIBO derivatives. Nature 1990;343:470–474.
69. Merluzzi VJ, Hargrave KD, Labadia M, et al. Inhibition of HIV-1 replication by a nonnucleoside reverse transcriptase inhibitor. Science 1990;250:1411–1413.
70. Romero DL, Busso M, Tan C-K, et al. Nonnucleoside reverse transcriptase inhibitors that potently and specifically block human immunodeficiency virus type 1 replication. Proc Natl Acad Sci U S A 1991;88:8806–8810.
71. Miyasaka T, Tanaka H, Baba M, et al. A novel lead for specific anti-HIV-1 agents: 1-([2-hydroxyethoxy]methyl)-6-(phenylthio) thymine. J Med Chem 1989;32:2507–2509.
72. Tanaka H, Baba M, Saito S, et al. Specific anti-HIV-1 "acyclonucleosides" which cannot be phosphorylated: synthesis of some deoxy analogues of 1-([2-hydroxyethoxy]methyl)-6-(phneylthio)thymine. J Med Chem 1991;34:1508–1511.
73. Moxham CP, Borroto-Esoda K, Noel D, et al. Preliminary efficacy and safety of repeated multiple doses of MKC-442 in HIV-infected volunteers [abstract 206]. In: 4th Conference on Retrovirology and Opportunistic Infections. Washington, DC, American Society for Microbiology, 1997.
74. Kroeger Smith MB, Rouzer CA, Taneyhill LA, et al. Molecular modeling studies of HIV-1 reverse transcriptase nonnucleoside inhibitors: total energy of complexation as a predictor of drug placement and activity. Protein Sci 1995;4:2203–2222.
75. Ding J, Das K, Moereels H, et al. Structure of HIV-1 RT/TIBO R 86183 complex reveals similarity in the binding of diverse nonnucleoside inhibitors. Nat Struct Biol 1995;2:407–415.
76. Arnold E, Ding J, Hughes SH, et al. Structures of DNA and RNA polymerases and their interactions with nucleic acid substrates. Curr Opin Struct Biol 1995;5:27–38.
77. Pialoux G, Youle M, Dupont B, et al. Pharmacokinetics of R 82913 in patients with AIDS or AIDS-related complex. Lancet 1991;338:140–143.
78. Saag MS, Douglas JI, DeLoach LJ, et al. Safety and relative antiretroviral activity of L697,661 versus zidovudine in HIV-1 infected patients [abstract WeB 1013]. In: 8th International Conference on AIDS, Amsterdam, 1992.
79. Nunberg JH, Schleif WA, Boots EJ, et al. Viral resistance to human immunodeficiency virus type 1-specific pyridinone reverse transcriptase inhibitors. J Virol 1991;65:4887–4892.
80. Richman DD, Shih C-K, Lowy I, et al. Human immunodeficiency virus type 1 mutants resistant to nonnucleoside inhibitors of reverse transcriptase arise in tissue culture. Proc Natl Acad Sci U S A 1991;88:11,241–11,245.
81. Balzarini J, Karlsson A, Perez-Perez M-J, et al. HIV-1–specific reverse transcriptase inhibitors show differential activity against HIV mutant strains containing different amino acid substitutions in the reverse transcriptase. Virology 1993;192:246–253.
82. Goldman ME, O'Brien JA, Ruffing TL, et al. A nonnucleoside reverse transcriptase inhibitor active on human immunodeficiency virus type 1 isolates resistant to related inhibitors. Antimicrob Agents Chemother 1993;37:947–949.
83. D'Aquila RT, Hughes MD, Johnson VA, et al. Nevirapine, zidovudine, and didanosine compared with zidovudine and didanosine in patients with HIV-1 infection: a randomized, double-blind, placebo-controlled trial. National Institute of Allergy and Infectious Diseases AIDS Clinical Trials Group Protocol 241 Investigators. Ann Intern Med 1996;124:1019–1030.
84. Debouck C. The HIV-1 protease as a therapeutic target for AIDS. AIDS Res Hum Retroviruses 1992;8:153–164.
85. Kohl NE, Emini EA, Schleif WA, et al. Active human immunodeficiency virus protease is required for viral infectivity. Proc Natl Acad Sci U S A 1988;85:4686–4690.
86. Seelmeier S, Schmidt H, Turk V, et al. Human immunodeficiency virus has an aspartic-type protease that can be inhibited by pepstatin A. Proc Natl Acad Sci U S A 1988;85:6612–6616.
87. McQuade TJ, Tomasselli AG, Liu L, et al. A synthetic HIV-1 protease inhibitor with antiviral activity arrests HIV-like particle maturation. Science 1990;247:454–456.

88. Tomasselli AG, Howe WJ, Sawyer TK, et al. The complexities of AIDS: an assessment of the HIV protease as a therapeutic target. Chim Oggi 1991;9:6–27.
89. Huff JR. HIV protease: a novel chemotherapeutic target for AIDS. J Med Chem 1991;34:2305–2314.
90. Meek TD. Inhibitors of HIV-1 protease. J Enzym Inhib 1992;6:65–98.
91. Darke PL, Huff JR. HIV protease as an inhibitor target for the treatment of AIDS. Adv Pharmacol 1994;25:399–455.
92. Roberts M, Oroszlan S. The preparation and biochemical characterization of intact capsids of equine infectious anemia virus. Biochim Biophys Res Commun 1989;160:486–494.
93. Baboonian C, Dalgleish A, Bountiff L, et al. HIV-1 proteinase is required for synthesis of proviral DNA. Biochem Biophys Res Commun 1991;179:17–24.
94. Nagy K, Young M, Baboonian C, et al. Antiviral activity of human immunodeficiency virus type 1 protease inhibitors in a single cycle of infection: evidence for a role of protease in the early phase. J Virol 1994;68:757–765.
95. Jacobsen H, Ahlborn L, Gugel R, et al. Progression of early steps of human immunodeficiency virus type 1 replication in the presence of an inhibitor of viral protease. J Virol 1992;66:5087–5091.
96. Uchida H, Maeda Y, Mitsuya H. HIV-1 protease does not play a critical role in the early steps of HIV-1 infection. Antiviral Res 36:107–113, 1997.
97. Kaplan A, Manchester M, Smith T, et al. Conditional human immunodeficiency virus type 1 protease mutants show no role for the viral protease early in virus replication. J Virol 1996;70:5840–5844.
98. Collins JR, Burt SK, Erickson JW. Flap opening in HIV-1 protease simulated by "activated" molecular dynamics. Struct Biol 1995;2:334–338.
99. Kempf D, Norbeck D, Codacovi L, et al. Structure-based, C_2 symmetric inhibitors of HIV protease. J Med Chem 1990;33:2687–2689.
100. Kempf D, Marsh K, Paul D, et al. Antiviral and pharmacokinetic properties of C_2 symmetric inhibitors of the human immunodeficiency virus type 1 protease. Antimicrob Agents Chemother 1991;35:2209–2214.
101. Kempf DJ, Marsh KC, Denissen JF, et al. ABT-538 is a potent inhibitor of human immunodeficiency virus protease with high oral bioavailability in humans. Proc Natl Acad Sci U S A 1995;92:2484–2488.
102. Lam PYS, Jadhav PK, Eyermann CJ, et al. Rational design of potent, bioavailable, nonpeptide cyclic ureas as HIV protease inhibitors. Science 1994;263:380–384.
103. Appelt K. Crystal structures of HIV-1 protease-inhibitor complexes. Perspect Drug Discov Des 1993;1:23–48.
104. Fitzgerald PMD, Springer JP. Structure and function of retroviral proteases. Annu Rev Biophys Biophys Chem 1991;20:299–320.
105. Abdel-Meguid SS. Inhibitors of aspartyl proteinases. Med Res Rev 1993;13:731–778.
106. Prasad JVNV, Para KS, Lunney EA, et al. Novel series of achiral, low molecular weight, and potent HIV-1 protease inhibitors. J Am Chem Soc 1994;116:6989–6990.
107. Thaisrivongs S, Tomich PK, Watenpaugh KD, et al. Structure-based design of HIV protease inhibitors: 4-hydroxycoumarins and 4-hydroxy-2-pyrones as non-peptidic inhibitors. J Med Chem 1994;37:3200–3204.
108. Tummino PJ, Scholten JD, Harvey PJ, et al. The in vitro ejection of zinc from human immunodeficiency virus type 1 nucleocapsid protein by disulfide benzamides with cellular anti-HIV activity. Proc Natl Acad Sci U S A 1996;93:969–973.
109. Carpenter CC, Fischl MA, Hammer SM, et al. Antiretroviral therapy for HIV infection in 1997: updated recommendations of the International AIDS Society—USA panel. JAMA 1997;277:1962–1969.
110. BHIVA Guidelines Co-ordinating Committee. British HIV Association guidelines for antiretroviral treatment of HIV seropositive individuals: BHIVA Guidelines Co-ordinating Committee. Lancet 1997;349:1086–1092.
111. Deeks SG, Smith M, Holodniy M, et al. HIV-1 protease inhibitors: a review for clinicians. JAMA 1997;277:145–153.
112. Ueno R, Kuno S. Dextran sulfate, a potent anti-HIV agent in vitro having synergism with zidovudine. Lancet 1987;1:1379.
113. Mitsuya H, Looney DJ, Kuno S, et al. Dextran sulfate suppression of viruses in the HIV family: inhibition of virion binding to CD4+ cells. Science 1988;240:646–649.
114. Baba M, Snoeck R, Pauwels R, et al. Sulfated polysaccharides are potent and selective inhibitors of various enveloped viruses, including herpes simplex virus, cytomegalovirus, vesicular stomatitis virus, and human immunodeficiency virus. Antimicrob Agents Chemother 1988;32:1742–1745.
115. Hartman NR, Johns DG, Mitsuya H. Pharmacokinetic analysis of dextran sulfate in rats as pertains to its clinical usefulness for therapy of HIV infection. AIDS Res Hum Retroviruses 1990;6:805–812.
116. Broder S, Yarchoan R, Collins JM, et al. Effects of suramin on HTLV-III/LAV infection presenting as Kaposi's sarcoma or AIDS-related complex: clinical pharmacology and suppression of viral replication in vitro. Lancet 1985;2:627–630.
117. Flexner C, Barditch-Crovo PA, Kornhauser DM, et al. Pharmacokinetics, toxicity, and activity of intravenous dextran sulfate in human immunodeficeincy virus infection. Antimicrob Agents Chemother 1991;35:2544–2550.
118. Klatzmann D, Champagne E, Chamaret S, et al. T-lymphocyte T4 molecule behaves as the receptor for human retrovirus LAV. Nature 1984;312:767–768.
119. Dalgleish AG, Beverley PCL, Clapham PR, et al. The CD4 (T4) antigen is an essential component of the receptor for the AIDS retrovirus. Nature 1984;312:763–767.
120. Maddon PJ, Molineaux SM, Maddon DE, et al. Structure and expression of human and mouse T4 genes. Proc Natl Acad Sci U S A 1987;84:9155–9159.
121. Smith DH, Byrn RA, Marsters SA, et al. Blocking of HIV-1 infectivity by a soluble, secreted form of the CD4 antigen. Science 1987;238:1704–1707.
122. Deen KC, McDougal JS, Inacker R, et al. A soluble form of CD4 (T4) protein inhibits AIDS virus infection. Nature 1988;331:82–84.
123. Fisher RA, Bertonis JM, Meier W, et al. HIV infection is blocked in vitro by recombinant soluble CD4. Nature 1988;331:76–78.
124. Hussey RE, Richardson NE, Kowalski M, et al. A soluble CD4 protein selectively inhibits HIV replication. Nature 1988;331:78–81.
125. Traunecker A, Luke W, Karjalainen K. Soluble CD4 molecules neutralize human immunodeficiency virus type I. Nature 1988;331:84–86.
126. Capon DJ, Chamow SM, Mordenti J, et al. Designing CD4 immunoadhesins for AIDS therapy. Nature 1989;337:525–531.
127. Feng Y, Broder CC, Kennedy PE, et al. HIV-1 entry cofactor: functional cDNA cloning of a seven-transmembrane, G protein-coupled receptor. Science 1996;272:872–877.
128. Dragic T, Litwin V, Allaway GP, et al. HIV-1 entry into CD4+ cells is mediated by the chemokine receptor CC-CKR-5. Nature 1996;381:667–673.
129. Deng HK, Unutmaz D, Kewal Ramani VN, et al. Expression cloning of new receptors used by simian and human immunodeficiency viruses. Nature 1997;388:296–300.
130. Cocchi F, DeVico AL, Garzino-Demo A, et al. Identification of RANTES, MIP-1 alpha, and MIP-1 beta as the major HIV-suppressive factors produced by CD8+ T cells. Science 1995;270:1811–1815.
131. Mackewicz CE, Barker E, Greco G, et al. Do beta-chemokines have clinical relevance in HIV infection? J Clin Invest 1997;100:921–930.
132. Mackewicz CE, Barker E, Levy JA. Role of beta-chemokines in suppressing HIV replication. Science 1996;274:1393–1395.
133. Levy JA, Blackbourn DJ, Barker E, et al. HIV variability and host control in HIV pathogenesis [abstract 15]. In: 11th International Conference on AIDS, Vancouver, 1996.
134. Doranz BJ, Rucker J, Yi Y, et al. A dual-tropic primary HIV-1 isolate that uses fusin and the beta-chemokine receptors CKR-5, CKR-3, and CKR-2b as fusion cofactors. Cell 1996;85:1149–1158.

135. Choe H, Farzan M, Sun Y, et al. The beta-chemokine receptors CCR3 and CCR5 facilitate infection by primary HIV-1 isolates. Cell 1996; 85:1135–1148.
136. Cohen OJ, Vaccarezza M, Lam GK, et al. Heterozygosity for a defective gene for CC chemokine receptor 5 is not the sole determinant for the immunologic and virologic phenotype of HIV-infected long-term nonprogressors. J Clin Invest 1997;100:1581–1589.
137. De Clercq E, Yamamoto N, Pauwels R, et al. Potent and selective inhibition of human immunodeficiency virus (HIV)-1 and HIV-2 replication by a class of bicyclams interacting with a viral uncoating event. Proc Natl Acad Sci U S A 1992;89:5286–5290.
138. De Clercq E, Yamamoto N, Pauwels R, et al. Highly potent and selective inhibition of human immunodeficiency virus by the bicyclam derivative JM3100. Antimicrob Agents Chemother 1994;38: 668–674.
139. Schols D, Struyf S, Van Damme J, et al. Inhibition of T-tropic HIV strains by selective antagonization of the chemokine receptor CXCR4. J Exp Med 1997;186:1383–1388.
140. Schols D, Este JA, Henson G, et al. Bicyclams, a class of potent anti-HIV agents, are targeted at the HIV coreceptor fusin/CXCR-4. Antiviral Res 1997;35:147–156.
141. Doranz BJ, Grovit-Ferbas K, Sharron MP, et al. A small-molecule inhibitor directed against the chemokine receptor CXCR4 prevents its use as an HIV-1 coreceptor. J Exp Med 1997;186:1395–1400.
142. Murakami T, Nakajima T, Koyanagi Y, et al. A small molecule CXCR4 inhibitor that blocks T cell line–tropic HIV-1 infection. J Exp Med 1997;186:1389–1393.
143. Simmons G, Clapham PR, Picard L, et al. Potent inhibition of HIV-1 infectivity in macrophages and lymphocytes by a novel CCR5 antagonist. Science 1997;276:276–279.
144. Bukrinsky MI, Haggerty S, Dempsey MP, et al. A nuclear localization signal within HIV-1 matrix protein that governs infection of non-dividing cells. Nature 1993;365:666–669.
145. Bukrinsky MI, Sharova N, McDonald TL, et al. Association of integrase, matrix, and reverse transcriptase antigens of human immunodeficiency virus type 1 with viral nucleic acids following acute infection. Proc Natl Acad Sci U S A 1993;90:6125–6129.
146. Radu A, Blobel G, Moore MS. Identification of a protein complex that is required for nuclear protein import and mediates docking of import substrate to distinct nucleoporins. Proc Natl Acad Sci U S A 1995; 92:1769–1773.
147. Imamoto N, Shimamoto T, Kose S, et al. The nuclear pore-targeting complex binds to nuclear pores after association with a karyophile. FEBS Lett 1995;368:415–419.
148. Lewis P, Hensel M, Emerman M. Human immunodeficiency virus infection of cells arrested in the cell cycle. EMBO J 1992;11:3053–3058.
149. Rexach M, Blobel G. Protein import into nuclei: association and dissociation reactions involving transport substrate, transport factors, and nucleoporins. Cell 1995;83:683–692.
150. Dubrovsky L, Ulrich P, Nuovo GJ, et al. Nuclear localization signal of HIV-1 as a novel target for therapeutic intervention. Mol Med 1995;1:217–230.
151. Popov S, Dubrovsky L, Lee MA, et al. Critical role of reverse transcriptase in the inhibitory mechanism of CNI-H0294 on HIV-1 nuclear translocation. Proc Natl Acad Sci U S A 1996;93:11859–11864.
152. Fujiwara T, Mizuuchi K. Retroviral DNA integration: structure of an integration intermediate. Cell 1988;54:497–504.
153. Bushman FD, Fujiwara T, Craigie R. Retroviral DNA integration directed by HIV integration protein in vitro. Science 1990;249: 1555–1558.
154. Katz RA, Skalka AM. The retroviral enzymes. Annu Rev Biochem 1994;63:133–173.
155. Andrake MD, Skalka AM. Retroviral integrase, putting the pieces together. J Biol Chem 1996;271:19,633–19,636.
156. Zheng R, Jenkins TM, Craigie R. Zinc folds the N-terminal domain of HIV-1 integrase, promotes multimerization, and enhances catalytic activity. Proc Natl Acad Sci U S A 1996;93:13,659–13,664.
157. Mazumder A, Neamati N, Sunder S, et al. Curcumin analogs with altered potencies against HIV-1 integrase as probes for biochemical mechanisms of drug action. J Med Chem 1997;40:3057–3063.
158. Zhao H, Neamati N, Mazumder A, et al. Arylamide inhibitors of HIV-1 integrase. J Med Chem 1997;40:1186–1194.
159. Neamati N, Hong H, Mazumder A, et al. Depsides and depsidones as inhibitors of HIV-1 integrase: discovery of novel inhibitors through 3D database searching. J Med Chem 1997;40:942–951.
160. Zhao H, Neamati N, Hong H, et al. Coumarin-based inhibitors of HIV integrase. J Med Chem 1997;40:242–249.
161. Zhao H, Neamati N, Sunder S, et al. Hydrazide-containing inhibitors of HIV-1 integrase. J Med Chem 1997;40:937–941.
162. Dyda F, Hickman AB, Jenkins TM, et al. Crystal structure of the catalytic domain of HIV-1 integrase: similarity to other polynucleotidyl transferases. Science 1994;266:1981–1986.
163. Bujacz G, Alexandratos J, Qing ZL, et al. The catalytic domain of human immunodeficiency virus integrase: ordered active site in the F185H mutant. FEBS Lett 1996;398:175–178.
164. Kalpana GV, Marmon S, Wang W, et al. Binding and stimulation of HIV-1 integrase by a human homolog of yeast transcription factor SNF5. Science 1994;266:2002–2006.
165. Rosen CA, Pavlakis GN. Tat and Rev: positive regulations of HIV gene expression. AIDS 1990;4:499–509.
166. Brand SR, Kobayashi R, Matthews MB. The Tat protein of human immunodeficiency virus type 1 is a substrate and inhibitor of the interferon-induced, virally activated protein kinase, PKR. J Biol Chem 1997;272:8388–8395.
167. Rosen CA, Sodroski JG, Haseltine WA. The location of cis-acting regulatory sequences in the human T cell lymphotropic virus type III (HTLV-III/LAV) long terminal repeat. Cell 1985;41:813–823.
168. Hamy F, Felder ER, Heizmann G, et al. An inhibitor of the Tat/TAR RNA interaction that effectively suppresses HIV-1 replication. Proc Natl Acad Sci U S A 1997;94:3548–3553.
169. Hsu M-C, Schutt AD, Holly M, et al. Inhibition of HIV replication in acute and chronic infections in vitro by a Tat antagonist. Science 1991;254:1799–1802.
170. Haubrich RH, Flexner C, Lederman MM, et al. A randomized trial of the activity and safety of Ro 24-7429 (Tat antagonist) versus nucleoside for human immunodeficiency virus infection. The AIDS Clinical Trials Group 213 Team. J Infect Dis 1995;172:1246–1252.
171. Fritz CC, Green MR. HIV Rev uses a conserved cellular protein export pathway for the nucleocytoplasmic transport of viral RNAs. Curr Biol 1996;6:848–854.
172. Fridell RA, Bogerd HP, Cullen BR. Nuclear export of late HIV-1 mRNAs occurs via a cellular protein export pathway. Proc Natl Acad Sci U S A 1996;93:4421–4424.
173. Smith C, Lee SW, Wong E, et al. Transient protection of human T-cells from human immunodeficiency virus type 1 infection by transduction with adeno-associated viral vectors which express RNA decoys. Antiviral Res 1996;32:99–115.
174. Matsukura M, Zon G, Shinozuka K, et al. Regulation of viral expression of human immunodeficiency virus in vitro by an antisense phosphorothioate oligodeoxynucleotide against rev (art.trs) in chronically infected cells. Proc Natl Acad Sci U S A 1989;86:4244–4248.
175. Lisziewicz J, Sun D, Klotman M, et al. Specific inhibition of human immunodeficiency virus type 1 replication by antisense oligonucleotides: an in vitro model for treatment. Proc Natl Acad Sci U S A 1992;89:11,209–11,213.
176. Momany C, Kovari LC, Prongay AJ, et al. Crystal structure of dimeric HIV-1 capsid protein. Nat Struct Biol 1996;3:763–770.
177. Gitti RK, Lee BM, Walker J, et al. Structure of the amino-terminal core domain of the HIV-1 capsid protein. Science 1996;273:231–235.
178. Khan R, Chang HO, Kaluarachchi K, et al. Interaction of retroviral nucleocapsid proteins with transfer RNAPhe: a lead ribozyme and ^{1}H NMR study. Nucleic Acids Res 1996;24:3568–3575.

179. Jelinek R, Terry TD, Gesell JJ, et al. NMR structure of the principal neutralizing determinant of HIV-1 displayed in filamentous bacteriophage coat protein. J Mol Biol 1997;266:649–655.
180. Steinkasserer A, Harrison R, Billich A, et al. Mode of action of SDZ NIM 811, a nonimmunosuppressive Cyclosporin A analog with activity against human immunodeficiency virus type 1 (HIV-1): interference with early and late events in HIV-1 replication. J Virol 1995;69:814–824.
181. Mlynar E, Bevec D, Billich A, et al. The non-immunosuppressive Cyclosporin A analogue SDZ NIM 811 inhibits cyclophilin A incorporation into virions and virus replication in human immunodeficiency virus type 1 infected primary and growth-arrested T cells. J Gen Virol 1997;78:825–835.
182. Zhao Y, Chen Y, Schutkowski M, et al. Cyclophilin A complexed with a fragment of HIV-1 gag protein: insights into HIV-1 infectious activity. Structure 1997;5:139–146.
183. Muriaux D, Rocquingny H, Roques BP, et al. NCp7 activates HIV-1Lai RNA dimerization by converting a transient loop–loop complex into a stable dimer. J Biol Chem 1996;271:33686–33692.
184. Fisher RJ, Reth A, Fivash M, et al. Sequence-specific binding of human immunodeficiency virus type 1 nucleocapsid protein to short oligonucleotides. J Virol 1998;82:1902–1909.
185. Poon DT, Wu J, Aldovoni A. Charged amino acid residues of human immunodeficiency virus type 1 nucleocapsid p7 protein involved in RNA packaging and infectivity. J Virol 1996;70:6607–6616.
186. Mizuno A, Ido E, Goto T, et al. Mutational analysis of two zinc finger motifs in HIV type 1 nucleocapsid proteins: effects on proteolytic processing of Gag precursors and particle formation. AIDS Res Hum Retroviruses 1996;12:793–800.
187. Rice W, Schaeffer C, Harten B, et al. Inhibition of HIV-1 infectivity by zinc-ejecting aromatic C-nitroso compounds. Nature 1993;361:473–475.
188. Rice W, Supko J, Malspeis L, et al. Inhibition of HIV nucleocapsid protein zinc fingers as candidates for the treatment of AIDS. Science 1995;270:1194–1197.
189. Rice WG, Turpin JA, Huang M, et al. Azodicarbonamide inhibits HIV-1 replication by targeting the nucleocapsid protein. Nature Med 1997;3:341–345.
190. Rice WG, Baker DC, Schaeffer CA, et al. Inhibition of multiple phases of human immunodeficiency virus type 1 replication by a dithiane compound that attacks the conserved zinc fingers of retroviral nucleocapsid proteins. Antimicrob Agents Chemother 1997;41:419–426.
191. McDonnell NB, De Guzman RN, Rice WG, et al. Zinc ejection as a new rationale for the use of cystamine and related disulfide-containing antiviral agents in the treatment of AIDS. J Med Chem 1997;40:1969–1976.
192. Loo JA, Holler TP, Sanchez J, et al. Biophysical characterization of zinc ejection from HIV nucleocapsid protein by anti-HIV 2,2'-dithiobis(benzamides) and benzisothiazolones. J Med Chem 1996;39:4313–4320.
193. Tummino PJ, Harvey PJ, McQuade T, et al. The human immunodeficiency virus type 1 (HIV-1) nucleocapsid protein zinc ejection activity of disulfide benzamides and benzisothiazolones: correlation with anti-HIV and virucidal activities. Antimicrob Agents Chemother 1997;41:394–400.
194. Hadfield AT, Lee W, Zhao R, et al. The refined structure of human rhinovirus 16 at 2.15 Å resolution: implications for the viral life cycle. Structure 1997;5:427–441.
195. Zhao R, Pevear DC, Kremer MJ, et al. Human rhinovirus 3 at 3.0 Å resolution. Structure 1996;4:1205–1220.
196. Veronese FD, Copeland TD, Oroszlan S, et al. Biochemical and immunological analysis of human immunodeficiency virus gag gene products p17 and p24. J Virol 1988;62:795–801.
197. Omura S, Tomoda H, Xu QM, et al. Triacsins, new inhibitors of acyl-CoA synthetase produced by Streptomyces sp. J Antibiot (Tokyo) 1986;39:1211–1218.
198. Tashiro A, Shoji S, Kubota Y. Antimyristoylation of the gag proteins in the human immunodeficiency virus-infected cells with N-myristoyl glycinal diethylacetal resulted in inhibition of virus production. Biochem Biophys Res Commun 1989;165:1145–1154.
199. Bryant M, Ratner L. Myristoylation-dependent replication and assembly of human immunodeficiency virus 1. Proc Natl Acad Sci U S A 1990;87:523–527.
200. Gheysen D, Jacobs E, de Foresta F, et al. Assembly and release of HIV-1 precursor Pr55gag virus-like particles from recombinant baculovirus-infected insect cells. Cell 1989;59:103–112.
201. Morikawa Y, Hinata S, Tomoda H, et al. Complete inhibition of human immunodeficiency virus Gag myristoylation is necessary for inhibition of particle budding. J Biol Chem 1996;271:2868–2873.
202. Lane HC. Interferons in HIV and related diseases. AIDS 1994;8(Suppl 3):S19–23.
203. Poli G, Orenstein JM, Kinter A, et al. Interferon-α but not AZT supresses HIV expression in chronically infected cell lines. Science 1989;244:575–577.
204. Hartshorn KL, Vogt MW, Chou T-C, et al. Synergistic inhibition of human immunodeficiency virus in vitro by azidothymidine and recombinant alpha A interferon. Antimicrob Agents Chemother 1987;31:168–172.
205. Schnittman SM, Vogel S, Baseler M, et al. A phase I study of interferon-alpha 2b in combination with interleukin-2 in patients with human immunodeficiency virus infection. J Infect Dis 1994;169:981–989.
206. Kovacs JA, Bechtel C, Davey RT Jr, et al. Combination therapy with didanosine and interferon-alpha in human immunodeficiency virus–infected patients: results of a phase I/II trial. J Infect Dis 1996;173:840–848.
207. Larder BA, Darby G, Richman DD. HIV with reduced sensitivity to zidovudine (AZT) isolated during prolonged therapy. Science 1989;243:1731–1734.
208. Rooke R, Tremblay M, Soudeyns H, et al. Isolation of drug-resistant variants of HIV-1 from patients on long-term zidovudine therapy. AIDS 1989;3:411–415.
209. Larder BA, Kemp SD. Multiple mutations in HIV-1 reverse transcriptase confer high-level resistance to zidovudine (AZT). Science 1989;246:1155–1158.
210. Kellam P, Boucher CA, Larder BA. Fifth mutation in human immunodeficiency virus type 1 reverse transcriptase contributes to the development of high-level resistance to zidovudine. Proc Natl Acad Sci U S A 1992;89:1934–1938.
211. Molla A, Korneyeva M, Gao Q, et al. Ordered accumulation of mutations in HIV protease confers resistance to ritonavir. Nature Med 1996;2:760–766.
212. Hammer SM, Kessler HA, Saag MS. Issues in combination antiretroviral therapy: a review. J Acquir Immune Defic Syndr Hum Retrovirol 1994;7(Suppl 2):S24–35.
213. Swanstrom R. Characterization of HIV-1 protease mutants: random, directed, selected. Curr Opin Biotechnol 1994;5:409–413.
214. Borman AM, Paulous S, Clavel F. Resistance of human immunodeficiency virus type 1 to protease inhibitors: selection of resistance mutations in the presence and absence of the drug. J Gen Virol 1996;77:419–426.
215. Baldwin ET, Bhat TN, Liu B, et al. Structural basis of drug resistance for the V82A mutant of HIV-1 protease: backbone flexibility and subsite repacking. Nat Struct Biol 1995;2:244–249.
216. Ho DD, Neumann AU, Perelson AS, et al. Rapid turnover of plasma virions and CD4 lymphocytes in HIV-1 infection. Nature 1995;373:123–126.
217. Wei X, Ghosh SK, Taylor ME, et al. Viral dynamics in human immunodeficiency virus type 1 infection. Nature 1995;373:117–122.
218. Preston BD, Poiesz BJ, Loeb LA. Fidelity of HIV-1 reverse transcriptase. Science 1988;242:1168–1171.
219. Roberts JD, Bebenek K, Kunkel TA. The accuracy of reverse transcriptase from HIV-1. Science 1988;242:1171–1173.
220. Bebenek K, Abbotts J, Roberts JD, et al. Specificity and mechanisms of error-prone replication by human immunodeficiency virus-1 reverse transcriptase. J Biol Chem 1989;262:16948–16956.

221. Mansky LM, Temin HM. Lower in vivo mutation rate of human immunodeficiency virus type 1 than that predicted from the fidelity of purified reverse transcriptase. J Virol 1995;69:5087–5094.
222. Coffin JM. HIV population dynamics in vivo: implications for genetic variation, pathogenesis and therapy. Science 1995;267:483–489.
223. Erickson JW, Burt SK. Structural mechanisms of HIV drug resistance. Annu Rev Pharmacol Toxicol 1996;36:545–571.
224. Gu Z, Wainberg MA. Emergence of HIV-1 variants with resistance to antiretroviral nucleosides. In: Mitsuya H, ed. Anti-HIV nucleosides: past, present, and future. Austin, TX: RG Landes, 1997:101–131.
225. Tudor-Williams G, St Clair M, McKinney R, et al. HIV-1 sensitivity to zidocudine and clinical outcome in children. Lancet 1992;339:15–19.
226. Boucher CAB, Lange JMA, Miedema FF, et al. HIV-1 biological phenotype and the development of zidovudine resistance in relation to disease progression in asymptomatic individuals during treatment. AIDS 1992;6:1259–1264.
227. Kozal MJ, Shafer RW, Winters MA, et al. A mutation in human immunodeficiency virus reverse transcriptase and decline in CD4 lymphocyte numbers in long-term zidovudine recipients. J Infect Dis 1993;167:526–532.
228. D'Aquila RT, Johnson VA, Welles SL, et al. Zidovudine resistance and HIV-1 disease progression during antiretroviral therapy. Ann Intern Med 1995;122:401–408.
229. Erice A, Mayer, DL, Strike DG, et al. Primary infection with zidovudine-resistant human immunodeficiency virus type 1. N Engl J Med 1993;328:1163–1193.
230. Shirasaka T, Yarchoan R, O'Brien M, et al. Changes in drug-sensitivity of human immunodeficiency virus type 1 during therapy with azidothymidine, dideoxycytidine, and dideoxyinosine: as in vitro comparative study. Proc Natl Acad Sci U S A 1993;90:562–566.
231. Husson RN, Shirasaka T, Butler KM, et al. High level resistance to zidovudine but not to zalcitabine or didanosine in human immunodeficiency virus from children receiving antiretroviral therapy. J. Pediatr 1993;123:9–16.
232. Reichman RC, Tejani N, Lambert JL, et al. Didanosine (ddI) and zidovudine (ZDV) susceptibilities of human immunodeficiency virus (HIV) isolates from long-term recipients of ddI. Antiviral Res 1993;20:267–277.
233. Mayers DL, Japour AJ, Arduino JM, et al. Dideoxynucleoside resistance emerges with prolonged zidovudine monotherapy: the RV43 Study Group. Antimicrob Agents Chemother 1994;38:307–314.
234. St Clair MH, Martin JL, Tudor-Williams G, et al. Resistance to ddI and sensitivity to AZT induced by a mutation in HIV-1 reverse transcriptase. Science 1991;253:1557–1559.
235. Kageyama S, Weinstein JN, Shirasaka T, et al. In vitro inhibition of human immunodeficiency virus (HIV) type 1 replication by C_2 symmetry-based HIV protease inhibitors as single agents or in combinations. Antimicrob Agents Chemother 1992;36:926–933.
236. Johnson VA, Barlow MA, Chou T-C, et al. Synergistic inhibition of human immunodeficiency virus type 1 (HIV 1) replication in vitro by recombinant soluble CD4 and 3′-azido-3′-deoxythymidine. J Infect Dis 1989;159:837–844.
237. Johnson VA, Hirsch MS. New developments in combination chemotherapy of anti-human immunodeficiency virus drugs. Ann N Y Acad Sci 1990;616:318–327.
238. Hayashi S, Fine RL, Chou T-C, et al. In vitro inhibition of the infectivity and replication of human immunodeficiency virus type 1 by combination of antiretroviral 2′,3′-dideoxynucleosides and virus-binding inhibitors. Antimicrob Agents Chemother 1990;34:82–88.
239. Moutouh L, Corbeil J, Richman DD. Recombination leads to the rapid emergence of HIV-1 dually resistant mutations under selective drug pressure. Proc Natl Acad Sci U S A 1996;93:6106–6111.
240. Yusa K, Kavlick MF, Kosalaraksa P, et al. HIV-1 acquires resistance to two classes of antiviral drugs through homologous recombination. Antiviral Res 1997;36:179–189.
241. Mellors JW, Larder BA, Schinazi RF. Mutations in HIV-1 reverse transcriptase and protease associated with drug resistance. Intern Antiviral News 1995;3:8–13.
242. Arnold E, Das K, Ding J, et al. Targeting HIV reverse transcriptase for anti-AIDS drug design: structural and biological considerations for chemotherapeutic strategies. Drug Des Discov 1996;13:29–47.
243. Boyer PL, Tantillo C, Jacobo-Molina A, et al. Sensitivity of wild-type human immunodeficiency virus type 1 reverse transcriptase to dideoxynucleotides depends on template length: the sensitivity of drug-resistant mutants does not. Proc Natl Acad Sci U S A 1994;91:4882–4886.
244. Mellors JW, Bazmi HZ, Schinazi RF, et al. Novel mutations in reverse transcriptase of human immunodeficiency virus type 1 reduce susceptibility to foscarnet in laboratory and clinical isolates. Antimicrob Agents Chemother 1995;39:1087–1092.
245. Shirasaka T, Yarchoan R, O'Brien M, et al. Changes in drug-sensitivity of human immunodeficiency virus type 1 during therapy with azidothymidine, dideoxycytidine, and dideoxyinosine: as in vitro comparative study. Proc Natl Acad Sci U S A 1993;90:562–566.
246. Shafer RW, Kozal MJ, Winters MA, et al. Combination therapy with zidovudine and didanosine selects for drug-resistant human immunodeficiency virus type 1 strains with unique patterns of pol gene mutations. J Infect Dis 1994;169:722–729.
247. Shirasaka T, Kavlick MF, Ueno T, et al. Emergence of human immunodeficiency virus type 1 variants with resistance to multiple dideoxynucleosides in patients receiving therapy with dideoxynucleosides. Proc Natl Acad Sci U S A 1995;92:2398–2402.
248. Schmit J-C, Cogniaux J, Hermans P, et al. Multiple drug resistance to nucleoside analogues and nonnucleoside reverse transcriptase inhibitors in an efficiently replicating human immunodeficiency virus type 1 patient strain. J Infect Dis 1996;174:962–968.
249. Kavlick MF, Wyvell K, Yarchoan R, et al. Emergence of multidideoxynucleoside resistant HIV-1 variants, viral sequence variation, and disease progression in patients receiving antiretroviral chemotherapy. J Infect Dis 1998 (in press).
250. Tantillo C, Ding J, Jacobo-Molina A, et al. Locations of anti-AIDS drug binding sites and resistance mutations in the three-dimentional structure of HIV-1 reverse transcriptase: implications for mechanisms of drug inhibition and resistance. J Mol Biol 1994;243:369–387.
251. Ueno T, Shirasaka T, Mitsuya H. Enzymatic characterization of human immunodeficiency virus type 1 reverse transcriptase resistant to multiple 2′,3′-dideoxynucleoside 5′-triphosphates. J Biol Chem 1995;270:23,605–23,611.
252. Ueno T, Mitsuya H. Comparative enzymatic study of HIV-1 reverse transcriptase resistant to 2′,3′-dideoxynucleotide analogs using the single-nucleotide incorporation assay. Biochemistry 1997;36:1092–1099.
253. Maeda Y, Venzon DJ, Mitsuya H. Altered drug sensitivity and fitness of HIV-1 with pol gene mutations conferring multi-dideoxynucleoside resistance. J Infect Dis 1998 (in press).
254. Wainberg MA, Drosopoulos WC, Salomon H, et al. Enhanced fidelity of 3TC-selected mutant HIV-1 reverse transcriptase. Science 1996;271:1282–1285.
255. Rezende LF, Curr K, Ueno T, et al. The impact of nucleoside analog resistance mutations in human immunodeficiency virus type 1 reverse transcriptase on mutation rates and error specificity. J Virol 1998;72:2890–2895.
256. Smerdon SJ, Jager J, Wang J, et al. Structure of the binding site for nonnucleoside inhibitors of the reverse transcriptase of human immunodeficiency virus type 1. Proc Natl Acad Sci U S A 1994;91:3911–3915.
257. Gussio R, Pattabiraman N, Zaharevitz D, et al. All atom models for the non-nucleoside binding site of HIV-1 reverse transcriptase complexed with inhibitors: a 3-D QSAR approach. J Med Chem 1996;39:1645–1650.
258. Ding J, Das K, Tantillo C, et al. Structure of HIV-1 reverse transcriptase in a complex with the non-nucleoside inhibitor alpha-APA R 95845 at 2.8 A resolution. Structure 1995;3:365–379.
259. Jacques PS, Wohrl BM, Howard KJ, et al. Modulation of HIV-1 reverse transcriptase function in "selectively deleted" p66/p51 heterodimers. J Biol Chem 1994;269:1388–1393.

260. Byrnes VW, Sardana VV, Schleif WA, et al. Comprehensive mutant enzyme and viral variant assessment of human immunodeficiency virus type 1 reverse transcriptase resistance to nonnucleoside inhibitors. Antimicrob Agents Chemother 1993;37:1576–1579.
261. Buckheit RW Jr, Fliakas-Boltz V, Yeagy-Bargo S, et al. Resistance to 1-([2-hydroxyethoxy]methyl)-6-(phenylthio)thymine derivatives is generated by mutations at multiple sites in the HIV-1 reverse transcriptase. Virology 1995;210:186–193.
262. Mellors JW, Im GJ, Tramontano E, et al. A single conservative amino aicd substitution in the reverse transcriptase of human immunodeficiency virus-1 confers resistance to (+)-(5S)-4,5,6,7-tetrahydro-5-methyl-6-(3-methyl-2-butenyl)imidazo(4,5,1-jk)(1,4)benzodiazepin-2(1H)-thione (TIBO R82150). Mol Pharmacol 1993;43:11–16.
263. Boyer PL, Currens MJ, McMahon JB, et al. Analysis of nonnucleoside drug-resistant variants of human immunodeficiency virus type 1 reverse transcriptase. J Virol 1993;67:2412–2420.
264. Boyer PL, Ding J, Arnold E, et al. Subunit specificity of mutations that confer resistance to nonnucleoside inhibitors in human immunodeficiency virus type 1 reverse transcriptase. Antimicrob Agents Chemother 1994;38:1909–1914.
265. Boyer PL, Hughes SH. Site-directed mutagenic analysis of viral polymerases and related proteins. Methods Enzymol 1996;275:538–555.
266. Dueweke TJ, Pushkarskaya T, Poppe SM, et al. A mutation in reverse transcriptase of bis(heteroaryl)piperazine-resistant human immunodeficiency virus type 1 that confers increased sensitivity to other non-nucleoside inhibitors. Proc Natl Acad Sci U S A 1993;90:4713–4717.
267. Balzarini J, Velazquez S, San-Felix A, et al. Human immunodeficiency virus type 1-specific (2′,5′-bis-O-(tert-butyldimethylsilyl)-beta-D-ribofuranosyl)-3′-spiro-5′-(4′-amino-1′,2′-oxathiole-2′,2′-dioxide)-purine analogues show a resistance spectrum that is different from that of the human immunodeficiency virus type 1-specific non-nucleoside analogues. Mol Pharmacol 1993;43:109–114.
268. Erickson JW. The not-so-great escape. Nat Struct Biol 1995;2:523–529.
269. Sardana VV, Schlabach AJ, Graham P, et al. Human immunodeficiency virus type 1 protease inhibitors: evaluation of resistance engendered by amino acid substitutions in the enzyme's substrate binding site. Biochemistry 1994;33:2004–2010.
270. Condra JH, Schleif WA, Blahy OM, et al. In vivo emergence of HIV-1 variants resistant to multiple protease inhibitors. Nature 1995;374:569–571.
271. Gulnik SV, Suvorov LI, Liu B, et al. Kinetic characterization and cross-resistance patterns of HIV-1 protease mutants selected under drug pressure. Biochemistry 1995;34:9282–9287.
272. Baldwin ET, Bhat TN, Gulnik S, et al. Structure of HIV-1 protease with KNI-272, a tight-binding transition-state analog containing allophenylnorstatine. Structure 1995;3:581–590.
273. Otto MJ, Garber S, Winslow DL, et al. In vitro isolation and identification of human immunodeficiency virus (HIV) variants with reduced sensitivity to C-2 symmetrical inhibitors of HIV type 1 protease. Proc Natl Acad Sci U S A 1993;90:7543–7547.
274. Kaplan AH, Michael SF, Wehbie RS, et al. Selection of multiple human immunodeficiency virus type 1 variants that encode viral proteases with decreased sensitivity to an inhibitor of the viral protease. Proc Natl Acad Sci U S A 1994;91:5597–5601.
275. Ho DD, Toyoshima T, Mo H, et al. Characterization of human immunodeficiency virus type 1 variants with increased resistance to a C_2-symmetric protease inhibitor. J Virol 1994;68:2016–2020.
276. El-Farrash MA, Kuroda MJ, Kitazaki T, et al. Generation and characterization of a human immunodeficiency virus type 1 (HIV-1) mutant resistant to an HIV-1 protease inhibitor. J Virol 1994;68:233–239.
277. Anderson B, Kageyama S, Ueno T, et al. In vitro induction of HIV-1 with reduced sensitivity to HIV protease inhibitors, KNI-227 and KNI-272 [abstract 516B]. In: 10th International Conference on AIDS and STD, Yokohama, Japan, 1994.
278. Markowitz M, Mo H, Kempf DJ, et al. Selection and analysis of human immunodeficiency virus type 1 variants with increased resistance to ABT-538, a novel protease inhibitor. J Virol 1995;69:701–706.
279. Jacobsen H, Yasargil K, Winslow DL, et al. Characterization of human immunodeficiency virus type 1 mutants with decreased sensitivity to proteinase inhibitor Ro 31-8959. Virology 1995;206:527–534.
280. Patick AK, Rose R, Greytok J, et al. Characterization of a human immunodeficiency virus type 1 variant with reduced sensitivity to an aminodiol protease inhibitor. J Virol 1995;69:2148–2152.
281. Shao W, Everitt L, Manchester M, et al. Sequence requirements of the HIV-1 protease flap region determined by saturation mutagenesis and kinetic analysis of flap mutants. Proc Natl Acad Sci U S A 1997;94:2243–2248.
282. Mous J, Brun-Vezinet F, Duncan IB, et al. Characterisation of in vivo selected HIV-1 variants with reduced sensitivity to proteinase inhibitor saquinavir [abstract 515B]. In: 10th International Conference on AIDS and STD, Yokohama, Japan, 1994.
283. Emini E, Schleif WA, Graham DA, et al. Protease inhibitors: cross resistance and in vivo observations [abstract 15]. In: Proceedings of the 3rd International Workshop on HIV Drug Resistance, Kauai, Hawaii, 1994.
284. Mimoto T, Imai J, Kisanuki S, et al. Kynostatin (KNI)-227 and -272, highly potent anti-HIV agents: conformationally constrained tripeptide inhibitors of HIV protease containing allophenylnorstatine. Chem Pharm Bull (Tokyo) 1992;40:2251–2253.
285. Kageyama S, Mimoto T, Murakawa Y, et al. In vitro anti-human immunodeficiency virus (HIV) activities of transition state mimetic HIV protease inhibitors containing allophenylnorstatine. Antimicrob Agents Chemother 1993;37:810–817.
286. Kageyama S, Anderson BD, Hoesterey BL, et al. Protein binding of human immunodeficiency virus protease inhibitor KNI-272 and alteration of its in vitro antiretroviral activity in the presence of high concentrations of proteins. Antimicrob Agents Chemother 1994;38:1107–1111.
287. Chang C-H, DeLoskey RL, Lam P, et al. Structures of cyclic ureas complexed with native and V82I mutant HIV-1 protease [abstract 110A]. In: 10th International Conference on AIDS and STD, Yokohama, Japan, 1994.
288. Erickson JW. Design and structure of symmetry-based inhibitors of HIV-1 protease. Perspect Drug Discov Des 1993;1:109–128.
289. Lin Y, Lin X, Hong L, et al. Effect of point mutations on the kinetics and the inhibition of human immunodeficiency virus type 1 protease: relationship to drug resistance. Biochemistry 1995;34:1143–1152.
290. Doyon L, Croteau G, Thibeault D, et al. Second locus involved in human immunodeficiency virus type 1 resistance to protease inhibitors. J Virol 1996;70:3763–3769.
291. Lamarre D, Croteau G, Pilote L, et al. Molecular characterization of HIV-1 variants resistant to specific viral protease inhibitors [abstract 10]. In: Proceedings of the 3rd International Workshop on HIV Drug Resistance, Kauai, Hawaii, 1994.
292. Zhang YM, Imamichi H, Imamichi T, et al. Drug resistance during indinavir therapy is caused by mutations in the protease gene and in its Gag substrate cleavage sites. J Virol 1997;71:6662–6670.
293. Boucher CA, Reedijk M. Viral resistance: a major challenge in managing HIV disease. J Biol Regul Homeost Agents 1995;9:91–94.
294. Welles L, Yarchoan R. Therapy of HIV-1 infection with antiretroviral nucleosides. In: Mitsuya H, ed. Anti-HIV nucleosides: past, present, and future. Austin, TX: RG Landes, 1997:51–99.
295. Shafer RW, Merigan TC. Combination therapy of HIV-1 infection with nucleoside analog reverse transcriptase inhibitors. In: Mitsuya H, ed. Anti-HIV nucleosides: past, present, and future. Austin, TX: RG Landes, 1997:134–173.
296. DeVita VT, Serpick AA, Carbone PP. Combination therapy in the treatment of advanced Hodgkin's disease. Ann Intern Med 1970;73:891–895.
297. Fox W. The chemotherapy of pulmonary tuberculosis: a review. Chest 1979, 76S:785–796.
298. Skowron G, Merigan TC. Alternating and intermittent regimens of zidovudine (3′-azido-3′-deoxythymidine) and dideoxycytidine (2′,3′-

dideoxycytidine) in the treatment of patients with acquired immunodeficiency syndrome (AIDS) and AIDS-related complex. Am J Med 1990;88(Suppl 5B):20S–23S.
299. Bozzette SA, Richman DD. Salvage therapy for zidovudine-intolerant HIV-infected patients with alternating and intermittent regimens of zidovudine and dideoxycytidine. Am J Med 1990;88:24S–26S.
300. Meng T-C, Fischl MA, Boota AM, et al. A phase I/II study of combination therapy with zidovudine and dideoxycytidine in subjects with advanced human immunodeficiency virus (HIV) disease. Ann Intern Med 1992;116:13–20.
301. Dornsife RE, St Clair MH, Huang AT, et al. Anti-human immunodeficiency virus synergism by zidovudine (3'-azidothymidine) and didanosine (dideoxyinosine) contrasts with their additive inhibition of normal human marrow progenitor cells. Antimicrob Agents Chemother 1991;35:322–328.
302. Eron JJ Jr, Johnson VA, Merrill DP, et al. Synergistic inhibition of replication of human immunodeficiency virus type 1, including that of a zidovudineresistant isolate, by zidovudine and 2',3'-dideoxycytidine in vitro. Antimicrob Agents Chemother 1992;36:1559–1562.
303. Cox SW, Albert J, Wahlberg J, et al. Loss of synergistic response to combinations containing AZT in AZT-resistant HIV-1. AIDS Res Hum Retrovirol 1992;8:1229–1234.
304. Vogt MW, Hartshorn KL, Furman PA, et al. Ribavirin antagonizes the effect of azidothymidine on HIV replication. Science 1987;235:1376–1379.
305. Balzarini J, Lee CK, Herdewijn P, et al. Mechanism of the potentiating effect of ribavirin on the activity of 2',3'-dideoxyinosine against human immunodeficiency virus. J Biol Chem 1991;266:21509–21514.
306. Bondoc LL Jr, Ahluwalia GS, Hartman NR, et al. Potentiation of the antiretroviral activity and anabolism of purine-2',3'-dideoxynucleoside analoge by inhibitors of IMP dehydrogenase. J Cell Biochem 1992;78(Suppl):16E.
307. Ahluwalia GS, Cooney DA, Shirasaka T, et al. Enhancement by 2'-deoxycoformycin of the 5'-phosphorylation and anti-human immunodeficiency virus activity of 2',3'-dideoxyadenosine and 2'-a-fluoro-2',3'-dideoxyadenosine. Mol Pharmacol 1994;46:1002–1008.
308. Johns DG, Ahluwalia GS, Cooney DA, et al. Enhanced stimulation by ribavirin of the 5'-phosphorylation and anti-human immunodeficiency virus activity of purine 2'-a-fluoro-2',3'-dideoxynucleosides. Mol Pharmacol 1993;44:5195–5223.
309. Gao W-Y, Shirasaka T, Johns DG, et al. Differential phosphorylation of azidothymidine, dideoxycytidine, and dideoxyinosine in resting and activated peripheral blood mononuclear cells. J Clin Invest 1993;91:2326–2333.
310. Gao WY, Agbaria R, Driscoll JS, et al. Divergent anti-human immunodeficiency virus activity and anabolic phosphorylation of 2',3'-dideoxynucleoside analogs in resting and activated human cells. J Biol Chem 1994;269:12,633–12,638.
311. Shirasaka T, Chokekijchai S, Yamada A, et al. Comparative analysis of anti-human immunodeficiency virus type 1 activities of dideoxynucleoside analogs in resting and activated peripheral blood mononuclear cells. Antimicrob Agents Chemother 1995;39:2555–2559.
312. Chokekijchai S, Shirasaka T, Weinstein JN, et al. In vitro anti-HIV-1 activity of HIV protease inhibitor KNI-272 in resting and activated cells: implications for its combined use with AZT or ddI. Antiviral Res 1995;28:25–38.
313. Perno C-F, Cooney DA, Gao W-Y, et al. Effects of bone marrow stimulatory cytokines on human immunodeficiency virus replication and the antiviral activity of dideoxynucleosides in cultures of monocyte/macrophages. Blood 1992;80:995–1003.
314. Gao WY, Johns DG, Mitsuya H. Anti-human immunodeficiency virus type 1 activity of hydroxyurea in combination with 2',3'-dideoxynucleosides. Mol Pharmacol 1994;46:767–772.
315. Gao WY, Johns DG, Chokekuchai S, et al. Disparate actions of hydroxyurea in potentiation of purine and pyrimidine 2',3'-dideoxynucleoside activities against replication of human immunodeficiency virus. Proc Natl Acad Sci U S A 1995;92:8333–8337.
316. Biron F, Lucht F, Peyramond D, et al. Anti-HIV activity of the combination of didanosine and hydroxyurea in HIV-1–infected individuals. J Acquir Immune Defic Syndr Hum Retrovirol 1995;10:36–40.
317. Biron F, Lucht F, Peyramond D, et al. Pilot clinical trial of the combination of hydroxyurea and didanosine in HIV-1 infected individuals. Antiviral Res 1996;29:111–113.
318. Vila J, Biron F, Nugier F, et al. 1-year follow-up of the use of hydroxycarbamide and didanosine in HIV infection. Lancet 1996;348:203–204.
319. Montaner JS, Zala C, Conway B, et al. A pilot study of hydroxyurea among patients with advanced human immunodeficiency virus (HIV) disease receiving chronic didanosine therapy: Canadian HIV trials network protocol 080. J Infect Dis 1997;175:801–806.
320. Vila J, Nugier F, Bargues G, et al. Absence of viral rebound after treatment of HIV-infected patients with didanosine and hydroxycarbamide. Lancet 1997;350:635–636.
321. Simonelli C, Comar M, Zanussi S, et al. No therapeutic advantage from didanosine (ddI) and hydroxyurea versus ddI alone in patients with HIV infection. AIDS 1997;11:1299–1300.
322. De Antoni A, Foli A, Lisziewicz J, et al. Mutations in the pol gene of human immunodeficiency virus type 1 in infected patients receiving didanosine and hydroxyurea combination therapy. J Infect Dis 1997;176:899–903.
323. Ito M, Baba M, Mori S, et al. Tumor necrosis factor antagonizes inhibitory effect of azidothymidine on human immunodeficiency virus (HIV) replication in vitro. Biochem Biophys Res Commun 1990;166:1095–1101.
324. Poli G, Kinter A, Justement JS, et al. Tumor necrosis factor alfa functions in an autocrine manner in the induction of human immunodeficiency virus expression. Proc Natl Acad Sci U S A 1990;87:782–785.
325. Fazely F, Dezube BJ, Allen RJ, et al. Pentoxifylline (Trental) decreases the replication of the human immunodeficiency virus type 1 in human peripheral blood mononuclear cells and in cultured T cells. Blood 1991;77:1653–1656.
326. Staal FJT, Roederer M, Herzenberg LA, et al. Intracellular thiols regulate activation of nuclear factor kB and transcription of human immunodeficiency virus. Proc Natl Acad Sci U S A 1990;87:9943–9947.
327. Lo S-C, Tsai S, Benish JR, et al. Enhancement of HIV-1 cytocidal effects in CD4+ lymphocytes by the AIDS-associated mycoplasma. Science 1991;251:1074–1076.
328. Nabel GJ, Rice SA, Knipe DM, et al. Alternative mechanisms for activation of human immunodeficiency virus enhancer in T cells. Science 1988;239:1299–1302.
329. Lusso P, De MA, Malnati M, et al. Induction of CD4 and susceptibility to HIV-1 infection in human CD8+ T lymphocytes by human herpesvirus 6. Nature 1991;349:533–535.
330. Surbone A, Yarchoan R, McAtee N, et al. Treatment of acquired immunodeficiency syndrome (AIDS) and AIDS-related complex with a regimen of 3'-azido-2',3'-dideoxythymidine (azidothymidine or zidovudine) and acyclovir. Ann Intern Med 1988;108:534–540.
331. Hollander H, Lifson AR, Maha M, et al. Phase I study of low-dose zidovudine and acyclovir in asymptomatic human immunodeficiency virus seropositive individuals. Am J Med 1989;87:628–632.
332. Collier AC, Bozzette S, Coombs RW, et al. A pilot study of low-dose zidovudine in human immunodeficiency virus infection. N Engl J Med 1990;323:1015–1021.
333. Gallant JE, Moore RD, Keruly J, et al. Lack of association between acyclovir use and survival in patients with advanced human immunodeficiency virus disease treated with zidovudine: Zidovudine Epidemiology Study Group (see comments). J Infect Dis 1995;172:346–352.
334. Stein DS, Graham NM, Park LP, et al. Acyclovir in human immunodeficiency virus patients. J Infect Dis 1996;173:504–507.
335. Gustchina A, Weber IT. Comparative analysis of the sequences and structures of HIV-1 and HIV-2 proteases. Proteins 1991;10:325–339.

336. Powell DJ, Bur D, Wlodawer A, et al. Expression, characterisation and mutagenesis of the aspartic proteinase from equine infectious anaemia virus. Eur J Biochem 1996;241:664–674.
337. Lacey SF, Reardon JE, Furfine ES, et al. Biochemical studies on the reverse transcriptase and RNase H activities from human immunodeficiency virus strains resistant to 3′-azido-3′-deoxythymidine. J Biol Chem 1992;267:15,789–15,794.
338. Lacey SF, Larder BA. Novel mutation (V75T) in human immunodeficiency virus type 1 reverse transcriptase confers resistance to 2′,3′-didehydro-2′,3′-dideoxythymidine in cell culture. Antimicrob Agents Chemother 1994;38:1428–1432.
339. Mitsuya H, Yarchoan R, Kageyama S, et al. Targeted therapy of human immunodeficiency virus–related disease. FASEB J 1991;5:2369–2381.
340. Balzarini J, Pauwels R, Herdewijn P, et al. Potent and selective anti-HTLV-III/LAV activity of 2′,3′-dideoxycytidinene, the 2′,3′-unsaturated derivative of 2′,3′-dideoxycytidine. Biochem Biophys Res Commun 1986;140:735–742.
341. Webb TR, Mitsuya H, Broder S. 1-(2,3,-Anhydro-β-D-lyxofuranosyl) cytosine derivatives as potential inhibitors of the human immunodeficiency virus. J Med Chem 1988;31:1475–1479.
342. Schinazi RF, Chu CK, Ahn MK, et al. Selective in vitro inhibition of human immunodeficiency virus (HIV) replication by 3′-azido-2′,3′-dideoxyuridine (CS-87). J Cell Biochem 1987;1(Suppl D):74.
343. Hayashi S, Phadtare S, Zemlicka J, et al. Adenallene and cytallene: acyclic nucleoside analogues that inhibit replication and cytopathic effect of human immunodeficiency virus in vitro. Proc Natl Acad Sci U S A 1988;85:6127–6131.
344. Shirasaka T, Murakami K, Ford H Jr, et al. Lipophilic halogenated congeners of 2′,3′-dideoxypurine nucleosides active against HIV in vitro: a new class of lipophilic prodrugs. Proc Natl Acad Sci U S A 1990;87:9426–9430.
345. Murakami K, Shirasaka T, Yoshioka H, et al. *Escherichia coli*–mediated biosynthesis and in vitro anti-HIV activity of lipophilic 6-halo-2′,3′-dideoxypurine nucleosides. J Med Chem 1991;34:1606–1612.
346. DeGuzman RN, Wu ZR, Stalling CC, et al. Structure of the HIV-1 nucleocapsid protein bound to the SL3 χ-RNA recignition element. Science 1998;287:384–388.

B. Antiretroviral Treatment for HIV Infection

Leslie K. Serchuck, Lauri Welles, and Robert Yarchoan

The therapy of human immunodeficiency virus (HIV) infection has undergone rapid evolution beginning in 1985 with the observation that certain dideoxynucleoside reverse transcriptase inhibitors (RTIs) inhibit viral replication in vitro (1, 2). Shortly after these agents were identified in the laboratory, clinical trials were begun that were able to demonstrate activity in vivo in some cases for prolonged periods (3–9). In the past 10 years, therapeutic strategies have expanded dramatically from treatment with a single medication to combination therapy with two different classes of antiretrovirals. Today, treatment regimens being explored include combinations with as many as three different classes of antiretroviral agents, and ongoing studies are exploring the addition of biologic response modifiers to standard treatment.

The first class of drugs to undergo testing was that of the dideoxynucleoside RTIs, five of which, zidovudine (ZDV, formerly known as azidothymidine or AZT), didanosine (ddI), zalcitabine (ddC), stavudine (d4T), and lamivudine (3TC), have received approval from the United States Food and Drug Administration (FDA). Although the RTIs were originally studied for use as single agents, investigators soon became interested in exploring their use in combination, and early results suggested that, in certain cases, they had synergistic anti-HIV activity (4, 10–14). This finding was subsequently supported by several large, multicenter, international trials (15, 16). During this time, nonnucleoside RTIs (NNRTIs), as well as a new class of antiretroviral agents, HIV protease inhibitors, were commencing evaluation in the clinic. The latter target a different stage of HIV replication than the RTIs and, in particular, inhibit the viral enzyme responsible for the crucial secondary processing of specific viral proteins. Several early small-scale trials demonstrated that these agents had activity by themselves, and subsequent studies provided evidence of substantial immunologic, clinical, and virologic improvements in patients treated with a combination of one or two approved dideoxynucleoside RTIs and a protease inhibitor (17–21). In part, on the basis of these studies, three members of this class of drugs, saquinavir, ritonavir, and indinavir, received rapid FDA approval. In early March, 1997, a fourth protease inhibitor, nelfinavir, also received accelerated approval. The strategy of combination therapy using drugs from two different classes of antiretroviral agents has now entered widespread clinical practice and represents the current standard of treatment for many patients with HIV infection.

A growing understanding of viral replication, kinetics, and host immune response and knowledge regarding enzyme structure and sequencing have contributed to an increasingly rational approach to drug design and therapy (22–24). Looking toward the future, certain stages of HIV replication are actual or potential targets for specific antiretroviral therapy (Table 45B.1). Host factors that may confer innate resistance to primary HIV infection or may slow disease progression are actively being investigated (25, 26). The availability of advanced molecular techniques has improved our ability to monitor HIV disease progression and to make adjustments in antiretroviral therapy. This chapter describes current therapeutic drugs and approaches and provides a basis for understanding potential future strategies elucidated.

A full description of the known elements of the HIV life cycle is beyond the scope of this chapter. Nevertheless, a brief description of those that are known may provide a framework for understanding the physiologic basis of current and future antiretroviral therapies. Infection of CD4 lymphocytes by HIV-1 is initiated by the binding of the viral envelope protein gp120 to the CD4 receptor of its cellular target. The gp120 protein then undergoes a conformational change in each, giving the envelope additional points of attachment (27). The surface protein gp41 then fuses with a second cellular coreceptor. Two proteins that serve this function, CXCR4 (previously called fusin) and CCR5 (previously known as CKR5), have been described (28–31). Both CXCR4 and CCR5 are members of the seven-transmembrane guanosine triphosphate (GTP)–binding protein (G-protein)–coupled family of chemokine receptors. CXCR4, an α-chemokine receptor, is a heterotrimeric G-protein found on resting naive T cells that comediates the binding of T-cell–tropic, syncytium-inducing HIV isolates. CCR5, in contrast, is a β-chemokine receptor expressed on activated or memory T cells for macrophage-tropic, nonsyncytium-inducing HIV strains. Sexually transmitted strains of HIV-1 appear to be primarily M tropic (32). Other cell-surface proteins that can serve as alternate second receptors have been described, and additional research will likely discern further complexities (33). The recognition of these and other coreceptor sites as necessary means of viral entry suggests an exciting potential area for therapeutic intervention.

Once inside the cell, the virus is uncoated and releases the viral RNA genome as a nucleoprotein complex. Replication of the viral genome begins with reverse transcriptase (RT) initiating transcription of a complementary strand of genomic DNA. The RNA template of this RNA–DNA hybrid is degraded by ribonuclease H (RNase H), and RT then catalyzes transcription of the second (positive) DNA strand. This double-stranded DNA form of the HIV genome, known as the provirus, migrates to the cellular nucleus. Within the nucleus, the provirus is incorporated into the cellular DNA. This step is mediated by another *pol* product, integrase. After a variable latency period, which may depend on both host and viral factors, proviral DNA is transcribed to mRNA by host polymerases. A complex interplay of cellular and viral elements, including the *tat* and *rev* genes of HIV, is necessary for the efficient transcription and translation of the virus. Viral mRNA is translated as polyprotein precursors that are cleaved by the HIV protease and cellular enzymes. In the absence of such cleavage, mature virions cannot be produced, and particles that are produced are not infectious. Viral proteins also undergo other changes such as myristoylation and glycosylation (mediated by cellular enzymes), and they are then assembled into infectious, fully processed virions at the cell surface. Finally, these mature virions are released into the extracellular environment by budding through the cellular membrane, and they go on to infect other target cells of the HIV virus.

To suppress HIV viral replication successfully without disruption of normal cellular function, one must target specific components unique to the virus. Theoretically, antiretrovirals that target initial stages of the replicative cycle (prior to provirus formation) should prevent primary infection of cells, yet be ineffective in cells that have already integrated virus. By contrast, drugs that inhibit steps after viral integration can block new virus production by virally infected cells. Our currently approved antiretroviral armamentarium includes RTIs (both nucleoside and nonnucleoside), which act at the early stage of replication, and inhibitors of viral protease, which work in the later stage after viral integration. In the future, viable targets for retroviral therapy may broaden to include ribonuclease H, integrase, envelope glycoprotein, and any one or combination of the six unique HIV genes currently identified. The discussion that follows describes the antiretrovirals currently in use or under study and gives glimpses into the future of therapy for HIV infection.

Table 45B.1 Stages of HIV Replication as Potential Targets for Intervention

Stage	Possible or Actual Intervention
Binding to host cell	Inhibition of CD4 binding to receptors or coreceptors (CCR5, CXCR4, CCR2) by antibodies, modified receptors, or modified ligands
Fusion of virus with host cell	Gp41 inhibitors (pentafuside, plant lectins)
Entry and uncoating of RNA	Inhibitors such as bicyclams and hypericin
Transcription of RNA to DNA by reverse transcriptase	Nucleoside and nonnucleoside reverse transcriptase inhibitors
RNA degradation by RNase H	Inhibitor of RNase (e.g., N-ethylmalemide)
Migration of viral DNA to nucleus	Target or intervention not yet identified
Integration (mediated by integrase)	Integrase inhibitors (e.g., zintevir)
Transcription and translation	Inhibitors of *tat* or *rev*; TAR inhibitors; antisense oligonucleotides
Enhancement by cellular factors	Inhibitors of tumor necrosis factor or other cytokine production (e.g., thalidomide, pentoxyphylline, rolipram)
Ribosomal frameshifting	Ribosomal frameshift inhibitors (not yet identified)
Gag-Pol polyprotein cleavage by protease	Protease inhibitors
Myristoylation and glycosylation	Castanospermine and other glycosylation inhibitors
Assembly and packaging	Zinc finger inhibitors
Viral budding, release	Interferon or interferon inducers

NUCLEOSIDE REVERSE TRANSCRIPTASE INHIBITORS

The first antiretroviral agents to be developed were members of the family of nucleoside analogs called dideoxynucleosides (Table 45B.2). In 1985, Mitsuya and Broder and their colleagues found that certain dideoxynucleosides were potent inhibitors of HIV replication (1, 2). These compounds differ from their naturally occurring counterparts in that the hydroxy (-OH) group in the 3′ position of the sugar ring is replaced by a hydrogen atom or another group that is unable to form phosphodiester linkages. Dideoxynucleosides can enter cells by passive diffusion (34). Their antiviral activity depends on intracellular conversion by serial phosphorylation, using host cellular kinases, to their

Table 45B.2 Antiretroviral Agents Approved by the United States Food and Drug Administration

Drug	Oral Dosage (Adults)	Comments
Nucleoside Reverse Transcriptase Inhibitors		
Didanosine (ddI, dideoxyinosine Videx)	< 60 kg: 125 mg BID (tablet) : 167 mg BID (sachet) ≥ 60 kg: 200 mg BID (tablet) : 250 mg BID (sachet)	More active in resting cells; requires buffering agent; food decreases absorption 50%
Lamivudine (3TC, Epivir)	150 mg BID	More active in resting cells; requires reduced dose in renal impairment
Stavudine (d4T, Zerit)	<60 kg: 30 mg BID ≥60 kg: 40 mg BID	More active in replicating cells; bioavailability: > 80%; CNS penetration: 16–72%; contraindicated with zidovudine
Zalcitabine (ddC, dideoxycytidine, HIVID)	0.75 mg TID	More active in resting cells; bioavailability: 70–80%
Zidovudine (ZDV, formerly azidothymidine [AZT], Retrovir)	200 mg TID (300 mg BID)	More active in replicating cells; 60% CNS penetration; drug of choice for HIV CNS disease

5′-triphosphate (TP) form (35–39). The kinases responsible for this phosphorylation vary among the nucleoside analogs, but they are always cellular in origin because HIV does not encode for any kinases. This property accounts for some of the differences in the activity and toxicity profiles of the different nucleosides. The 5′-TP forms of these compounds are competitive inhibitors of endogenous nucleoside 5′-TPs. In addition, they can act as chain terminators; once they are added to the 3′ end of the growing viral chain of DNA, early chain termination is induced, and replication of the viral genome is halted (38, 40, 41). Dideoxynucleosides have been found to be active in monocyte/macrophages as well as in T cells (42).

Currently, viral resistance is the principal limiting factor for long-term treatment of HIV-infected patients. Resistance to dideoxynucleosides is associated with mutations in the *pol* gene that codes for RT (43). RT is relatively error prone, with mutations occurring at a rate of approximately 1 in 10,000 to 30,000 base pairs (44–46). Data have suggested that the total number of virions produced and released into the extracellular fluid each day is large, on the order of 10 billion particles (47). The entire genome size is 10,000 base pairs, and thus RT averages 1 mutation approximately every 1 to 3 viral replication cycles (48). As a result, constant genetic drift occurs in patients infected with HIV with the accumulation of an increasing number of "quasispecies," some of which may already be resistant to particular anti-HIV drugs. Under selective pressure of nucleoside agents, resistance may rapidly emerge, especially in patients with advanced HIV disease, who characteristically have high viral loads and replication rates (49).

In the face of the evolutionary pressure exerted by therapy with nucleosides, HIV mutations generally accumulate in an ordered, stepwise fashion. Incremental reductions in susceptibility are genetically associated with the acquisition of additional mutations in the *pol* gene. In the case of ZDV, for example, one or two mutations can confer partial resistance to ZDV, whereas high-level resistance is generally seen in strains with three or more of the five most common *pol* substitutions: M41L, D67N, K70R, T215F or T215Y, and K219Q. In the nomenclature used here, M41L denotes a substitution of leucine for methionine at codon 41 (50, 51). Of these mutations, the mutation at codon 215 appears to be the most important (50). The degree of resistance does not strictly depend on the number of mutations, because specific patterns of mutations can have differential effects on HIV replication and may affect one another. For example, strains with M41L and T215Y mutations induce considerably more resistance than either of the mutations when found alone. By contrast, strains that have K70R and T215Y mutations induce less resistance to ZDV than is seen when only one of the mutations is present (44, 52). Phenotypic resistance is usually seen with viruses containing mutations M41L and T215/F or D67N, K70R, and T215Y/F (53).

The observation that specific sets of mutations can be mutually antagonistic provides a rational basis for therapy with certain combinations of nucleosides. The agent ddI generally induces a specific mutation, L74V, that produces partial ddI resistance while restoring sensitivity to ZDV in previously ZDV-resistant strains (54). Thus, for HIV to develop simultaneous resistance to both ZDV and ddI is difficult, and this provides a rationale for using these drugs together. Monotherapy with 3TC, for as little as 4 to 8 weeks, can induce a mutation at codon 184 (M184I or M184V) that rapidly confers high-level resistance to the drug in wild-type HIV strains and correlates clinically with a swift and substantial loss of drug efficacy (51, 55). More interesting, perhaps, is that this mutation also restores ZDV sensitivity in previously resistant strains (51, 56). Largely because of this interaction, the combination of ZDV and 3TC has been found to be active in the clinic (57, 58).

Certain mutations can induce cross-resistance among dideoxynucleosides. One example is a mutation at codon 65 (K65R) of HIV-1 RT that confers resistance to 3TC, ddI, ddC, and 9-(2-phosphonylmethoxyethyl)adenine (PMEA), an acyclic nucleotide (59–63). An even more worrisome finding is that a novel set of five mutations in the polymerase domain of RT (at codons 62, 75, 77, 116, and 151) that can develop in patients receiving combination therapy with ZDV and ddC or ZDV and ddI can confer multidideoxynucleoside resistance to ZDV, ddC, and ddI, as well as to other nucleoside analogs to which the patients have never been exposed (64–66).

Zidovudine

The first dideoxynucleoside to be developed as an anti-HIV drug was ZDV. Originally synthesized as a potential anticancer agent by Jerome Horwitz and colleagues, ZDV was subsequently found to have activity against a broad range of retroviruses, including HIV-1, HIV-2, human T-lymphotropic virus type 1 (HTLV-1), and murine retroviruses (2, 41, 67). ZDV is a thymidine analog, with a 3′-azido (N_3) group replacing the 3′-hydroxyl group. This substitution prevents the triphosphate form, AZT-5′-TP (AZT-TP), from forming 5′ to 3′ phosphodiester linkages, and on incorporation into a growing chain of DNA, it causes chain termination. AZT-TP is also a competitive inhibitor of endogenous thymidine-5′-TP. The compound has greater activity in replicating than in resting cells, because the first step in its phosphorylation is catalyzed by cellular thymidine kinase, an enzyme that is upregulated in dividing cells (68, 69).

Initial phase I studies of ZDV conducted in 1985 at the National Cancer Institute and Duke University provided evidence of the drug's anti-HIV potential and elucidated its pharmacokinetics (3, 70–72). The drug is well absorbed from the gut, with an average bioavailability of 60%. High-fat meals may reduce its bioavailability (73). It is approximately 35% bound to plasma proteins. Although the serum half-life of ZDV is 1.1 hours, the intracellular half-life of AZT-TP is approximately 2 hours longer, allowing for activity with thrice-daily dosing (3, 38, 70, 74). ZDV is excreted in both saliva and semen (75, 76). It penetrates the cerebrospinal fluid and achieves concentrations of approximately 60% of simultaneous serum concentrations 1 hour after intravenous administration (3, 70, 77). ZDV's activity in the central nervous system has been demonstrated by improvement in neurocognitive scores in both adults and children (78–81).

ZDV is metabolized in the liver, primarily by glucuronidation, to an inactive compound (GZDV) and is then excreted by the kidneys (74). GZDV is a dialyzable compound. Approximately 20% of unmetabolized drug is directly excreted by the kidneys and can, if necessary, be cleared by hemodialysis (82). Advanced hepatic disease or renal failure may reduce ZDV clearance, and patients with either of these conditions should be followed closely for signs of toxicity.

In 1986, Yarchoan and associates reported that 15 of 19 patients with acquired immunodeficiency syndrome (AIDS) or AIDS-related complex (ARC) treated in the initial phase I trial of ZDV had increases in their CD4 cell counts (3). A placebo-controlled, randomized, double-blind trial subsequently showed that the drug reduced morbidity and prolonged survival in patients with advanced HIV infection (CD4 counts lower than 200 cells/mm^3) (83, 84). The results of AIDS Clinical Trials Group (ACTG) 019 subsequently showed that ZDV could prolong the short-term progression to AIDS in patients treated early in the course of infection (85). However, different conclusions were reached by the French–British Concorde trial, a double-blind, placebo-controlled study of 1749 asymptomatic HIV-infected patients with CD4 counts of more than 200 cells/mm^3 (42% had CD4 counts higher than 500 cells/mm^3 at entry) (86). Clinical end points (reached by 347 patients during the period of observation) were disease progression to AIDS or death. Patients were given 500 mg of ZDV twice daily or placebo. Early analysis (at 55 weeks) revealed fewer progressions to AIDS in treated patients, but these results were not sustained at the 3-year analysis. In addition, no survival benefit was noted between the patients treated early and those who received ZDV only on disease progression. This lack of benefit at 3 years may have reflected the development of drug resistance. Thus, although the early large-scale studies of previously untreated patients suggested a survival advantage with ZDV monotherapy in patients with CD4 cell counts lower than 200 cells/mm^3 and a decreased rate of disease progression among asymptomatic patients with CD4 cell counts of 200 to 500 cells/mm^3, the benefits of early ZDV monotherapy were generally not sustained in patients with these higher CD4 counts (200 to 500 cells/mm^3).

ZDV has been shown to decrease HIV-related thrombocytopenia, and clinical trial 076 of the ACTG showed that the drug significantly reduces perinatal HIV-1 transmission from 25% in untreated women to approximately 8% in those receiving ZDV during pregnancy and the intrapartum period (infants also received 6 weeks of therapy) (87, 88). The usefulness of ZDV as a single agent is limited, however, both by drug toxicity and the emergence of resistant viral strains.

More recent studies have shown that ZDV in combination with other RTIs can yield superior clinical results, as well as a survival advantage, compared with ZDV monotherapy in patients with moderate immunosuppression. As noted earlier, antagonistic patterns of resistance provided a rationale for testing ZDV with ddI (54). In addition, the drugs selectively work on different cell populations: where ZDV is most active in replicating cells, ddI has preferential activity in resting cells (68, 89). Three small studies in the early 1990s reported relatively large and prolonged CD4 cell count increases when ZDV was administered in combination with ddI (12–14).

On the basis of this information, two large, multicenter trials were initiated: ACTG 175, an American trial, and Delta, an international, European–Australian trial (15, 16). ACTG 175 compared monotherapy with ZDV or ddI to treatment with a combination of ZDV and either ddI or ddC in 2467 patients with CD4 cell counts of 200 to 500 cells/mm^3 (90). Of these patients, 57% were ZDV experienced, and the study duration was 34 months. A significant difference was noted between the time to disease progression observed in patients who were treated with either combination regimen or with ddI monotherapy and the group receiving ZDV treatment alone (16, 90). Both the ZDV and ddI and ddI monotherapy groups demonstrated a 40 to 50% reduced risk of death in the overall population, including both treatment-naive and antiretrovirally experienced patients, as well as in the subgroup with prior antiretroviral therapy (90).

The Delta trial compared monotherapy with ZDV to combination therapy with ZDV and either ddI or ddC in individuals with fewer than 350 cells/mm^3 (15). The study duration was 18 months, and the trial was stratified into two groups: Delta 1 studied 2124 patients who were ZDV naive, and Delta 2 studied 1083 patients who were ZDV experienced. Significantly increased survival was observed among ZDV-naive patients on either combination regimen as compared with ZDV monotherapy (91, 92). Among patients with prior ZDV therapy, a significant increase in survival was observed only in those administered the ZDV and ddI combination (15).

Yet not all studies have shown such clear-cut advantages to combination RTI therapy. The results of one large study of 1100 patients that compared ZDV monotherapy with combination ZDV and ddI or ZDV and ddC in patients with an AIDS-defining condition or CD4 cell counts lower than 200 cells/mm^3 were more equivocal (93). Approximately three-quarters of patients studied were ZDV experienced (median 12 months) at enrollment, and the patients generally had advanced AIDS. In these patients, combination therapy showed no significant advantage over monotherapy and was associated with more side effects and subsequent cessation of study drugs. The authors of this study hypothesized that the reason was, in part, that these patients' advanced HIV disease rendered them more sensitive to the toxic effects of the drugs. In a subset analysis of individuals with less than 12 months of prior ZDV treatment, a small survival advantage and slowed disease progression could be demonstrated in the cohort that received combination therapy.

Thus, the optimal use of ZDV is now believed to be in combination with other agents, and, in fact, ZDV is no longer generally recommended as monotherapy. As noted earlier, ZDV is preferentially phosphorylated in replicating cells, and this provides a rationale for its use with drugs such as ddI, ddC, and 3TC, which are more active in resting cells (42, 94, 95). In addition, the antagonistic resistance patterns observed with ddI and 3TC provide yet another rationale to favor their use with ZDV (51, 54, 56).

As noted earlier, dideoxynucleosides must be phosphorylated within target cells. AZT-5'-monophosphate, the product of the initial step in the phosphorylation of ZDV, blocks the activity of thymidylate kinase, the same enzyme required for the phosphorylation of d4T (38). Such biochemical consideration suggested that ZDV and d4T could be antagonistic when used together, and, in fact, evidence for this suggestion has come from a clinical trial. ACTG 290 was a study in which ZDV-experienced (more than 24 weeks) patients with CD4 cell counts of 300 to 600 cells/mm^3 were enrolled into one of four treatment groups: ZDV and ddI; ZDV and d4T; ddI monotherapy; or d4T monotherapy. An interim analysis of this trial revealed that patients with prior ZDV experience, who received the ZDV and d4T combination, had a dramatic decrease in CD4 cell count ranging from

Table 45B.3 Principal Drug Toxicities of Approved Reverse Transcriptase Inhibitors

Drug	Clinical Toxicities	Laboratory Toxicities
Didanosine	Pancreatitis	Amylasemia
	Peripheral neuropathy	Transaminitis
	Retinal depigmentation	Hyperuricemia
	Diarrhea	
	Headache	
Lamivudine (3TC)	Peripheral neuropathy	Neutropenia
	Pancreatitis (in children)	Amylasemia
Stavudine (d4T)	Peripheral neuropathy	Transaminitis
Zalcitabine (ddC)	Peripheral neuropathy	Amylasemia
	Stomatitis	Transaminitis
	Rash	
	Esophageal ulceration	
	Pancreatitis (rare)	
Zidovudine (ZDV)	Headache	Neutropenia
	Nausea	Anemia
	Myopathy/myositis	Lactic Acidosis
	Hepatic steatosis	Elevated creatine phosphokinase
Delaviridine	Rash (pruritus)	Transaminitis
	Headache	Bilirubinemia
Nevaripine	Rash (Stevens–Johnson)	Transaminitis

approximately 20 cells/mm^3 after 4 weeks of treatment to a decrease of 82 cells/mm^3 after 36 weeks of treatment. Based on these results, the National Institute of Allergy and Infectious Disease issued an advisory to physicians and recommended close monitoring of CD4 cell counts in patients taking this combination (96).

The recommended dosage of ZDV, administered either in combination or as monotherapy, is 600 mg daily, most commonly given in divided doses of 200 mg every 8 hours. In case of toxicity, the dose may be reduced to 100 mg every 8 hours. A newer formulation of 300-mg tablets that can be given twice a day has received approval. The drug is available in three formulations: capsules, an intravenous formulation, and as a raspberry-flavored syrup.

The most common dose-limiting toxicity of ZDV is myelosuppression, most frequently manifested as a macrocytic anemia or granulocytopenia (3, 85, 97–99) (Table 45B.3). Patients with low pretreatment hemoglobin or neutrophil levels, as well as those with low vitamin B$_{12}$ or serum folate, may be at greater risk. Both toxicities are, to some extent, dose dependent and can be mitigated by dose reduction or by the use of hematopoietic growth factors such as erythropoietin for anemia and filgrastim for neutropenia (98, 100–102).

HIV-1 RT is 200 times more sensitive to AZT-TP than is DNA polymerase α, and this principle is the basis for its selective antiviral activity. Other forms of mammalian DNA polymerase such as DNA polymerase γ (found in mitochondria) and β, can however, be inhibited by the compound (38, 41, 103, 104). The long-term use of ZDV has been reported to cause a reversible myopathy that is believed to be due to this effect in the mitochondria of myocytes (105, 106). The myopathy may be difficult to distinguish from that caused by

HIV itself and is characterized by insidious onset of proximal muscle weakness, exercise-induced myalgias, and elevated serum creatinine phosphokinase levels. Muscle biopsy may show mild to moderate myonecrosis. Damage to mitochondria in hepatocytes is thought to be the cause of a rare, sometimes lethal condition similar to Reye's syndrome that has been described predominantly in female patients with good nutritional status (107–109). It consists of lactic acidosis (in the absence of hypoxemia), severe hepatomegaly, and microvesicular hepatic steatosis.

Other reported toxicities of ZDV include headache, which may be severe, and nausea (84). Hyperpigmentation (with a bluish hue) of the nails, seen predominantly in black patients, and excessive eyelash growth also may occur (110). In addition are reports of esophageal ulceration, cardiomyopathy, seizures, orthostatic hypotension, macular edema, and a rare, fatal syndrome resembling Wernicke's encephalopathy (111–113).

ZDV undergoes hepatic glucuronidation and is then secreted by the kidneys. Drugs that interfere with the hepatic metabolism or renal clearance of ZDV, such as probenecid, should be administered with caution in patients receiving this drug (114–116). Although data are insufficient to recommend dose adjustment in patients with impaired liver function, such individuals should be followed closely. In patients with end-stage renal disease, recommended dosing of ZDV is 100 mg every 6 or 8 hours.

Laboratory evidence also indicates that certain drugs may inhibit the antiretroviral activity of ZDV. Ribavirin, for example, may inhibit the phosphorylation of ZDV, so these drugs should probably not be administered concurrently outside the setting of a clinical trial (117, 118). Patients requiring other drugs with similar toxicity profiles similar to that of ZDV should also be monitored closely.

Didanosine

This purine dideoxynucleoside inhibits HIV-1 and HIV-2 replication in human lymphocytes and macrophages (1, 42, 119). As with other dideoxynucleoside analogs, on being phosphorylated to an active moiety, it induces early termination of the growing viral chain and competitively inhibits HIV RT (35). ddI undergoes stepwise intracellular phosphorylation to 2′,3′-dideoxyadenosine-5′-TP (ddATP), the active form, by a pathway involving 5′-nucleotidase. It is effectively phosphorylated to its active moiety in resting cells, a property that it shares with ddC and 3TC (4, 42, 68, 94). By contrast, ZDV, d4T, and other nucleosides that are phosphorylated by a pathway involving thymidine kinase are preferentially phosphorylated in actively replicating cells. These differences provide an additional rationale for a judicious combination of drugs from each of these two groups.

Another notable contrast between ZDV and ddI is that the in vitro activity of ddI is not reversed by its physiologic 2′-deoxynucleoside counterparts, 2′-deoxyinosine or 2′-deoxyadenosine (10). Investigators have reported that the in vitro anti-HIV activity of ddI is potentiated by agents such as hydroxyurea that deplete intracellular pools of dATP, the physiologic nucleotide that directly competes with ddATP for RT and incorporation into proviral DNA (94, 120).

This drug is acid labile, a property that renders it unstable in the acidic gastric environment and reduces its absorption (121). Therefore, it must be formulated with a buffer. Currently available formulations of buffered ddI have an oral bioavailability of about 30 to 40% (121–123). The pharmacokinetics of ddI were first elucidated in a phase I trial at the National Cancer Institute initiated in 1988 (6, 121, 124). The plasma half-life was found to be relatively short, 0.5 to 1.5 hours (121, 123). However, the intracellular half-life of the active form, ddATP, is much longer, lasting 12 to 24 hours or more (125). This relatively long half-life allows for once- or twice-daily dosing of the drug. The drug can be removed by hemodialysis (126). ddI can cross the placental barrier and has been found to penetrate the cerebrospinal fluid, although to a lesser degree than does ZDV (121, 127). Cerebrospinal fluid levels after a dose of ddI were found to be 21% of concurrent plasma levels (121).

Early studies showed that ddI could induce virologic, immunologic and clinical improvement in adult patients with HIV disease (6–8, 121, 124, 128). A follow-up of the 1988 phase I study of ddI showed that the anti-HIV activity of the drug could be sustained for up to 5 years (9). As noted earlier, several lines of evidence suggested that the combination of ZDV and ddI would be particularly active, and initial trials of this combination regimen demonstrated a substantial and prolonged beneficial effect in some patients (12–14, 129). On the basis of these results, the large-scale, multicenter ACTG 175 and Delta trials summarized earlier were initiated. As previously noted, ddI alone or in combination with ZDV was found both to confer a significant survival advantage and to slow disease progression in antiretrovirally naive or experienced patients with CD4 cell counts between 200 and 500 cells/mm^3, whereas lesser benefits were seen in those patients with CD4 cell counts less than 200 cells/mm^3 who were treated with the combination (but not ddI alone) (15, 16).

Currently available commercially as chewable buffered tablets, a buffered powder, or as an oral solution, ddI is given in the following adult doses: in tablet form, 200 mg twice a day for adults weighing more than 60 kg and 125 mg twice daily for those weighing less than 60 kg. The powder (sachet) form is not absorbed as well as the tablets, and dosing is 250 mg twice daily for adults weighing more than 60 kg and 167 mg twice daily for those with lower weights.

The most common dose-limiting toxicities of ddI are painful peripheral neuropathy and pancreatitis (6, 8, 124, 130). The neuropathy presents most commonly in the distal lower extremities and is generally reversible. The pancreatitis is less frequent, but, in some patients, it can be life-threatening (131). Hematologic toxicity is not generally seen with ddI (132). Other reported side effects of ddI include hepatitis, nervousness, insomnia, hyperuricemia, rash, esophageal ulceration, hypoglycemia, and cardiomyopathy

(6–8, 133, 134). Retinal lesions have been noted in children receiving high doses of the drug as well as in some adults (135). Patients receiving the powdered formulation of the drug may experience diarrhea, which can cause hypokalemia. The diarrhea is largely attributable to the citrate–phosphate vehicle rather than the ddI itself.

Coadministration of other drugs known to cause peripheral neuropathy or pancreatitis may increase the risk of these complications. Simultaneous administration of systemic pentamidine, which can cause pancreatitis, should generally be avoided. H_2 blockers such as cimetidine and ranitidine have been reported to induce pancreatitis in their own right and may increase the absorption of ddI (135). Agents that require an acidic gastric environment for absorption, such as ketoconazole and dapsone, are best administered at least 2 hours before ddI to avoid having their absorption decreased by the buffered preparations in the ddI (136).

Zalcitabine

This drug is a dideoxynucleoside analog of 2'-deoxycytidine in which the 3'-hydroxy group of the sugar ring is replaced with a hydrogen atom (1, 119). It undergoes intracellular phosphorylation to its active form, ddC-5'-TP (36). In 1985, ddC was found to have even greater in vitro anti-HIV activity on a molar basis than ZDV (1, 119). In addition, in contrast to ZDV, ddC in high concentrations in vitro was found to completely inhibit viral replication over 21 days in culture (119). This degree of activity was the basis for rapidly initiating clinical trials of the drug.

After oral administration, ddC is well absorbed from the gut with an average bioavailability of approximately 70 to 80% (4, 137). Peak plasma concentrations are generally observed within 0.5 to 2 hours (137, 138). The agent ddC penetrates the cerebrospinal fluid less well than does ZDV. The cerebrospinal fluid concentration ranges from 9 to 37% that of serum concentrations after an intravenous dose (4). The plasma half-life of ddC in HIV-infected adults averages 1.2 to 2 hours, whereas the in vitro intracellular half-life of ddC-5'-TP, the active moiety of ddC, is approximately 2.6 hours (4, 103, 137, 139). Seventy-five percent of the dose of ddC is cleared by the kidney and renal impairment may prolong its elimination half-life (137, 138).

Early phase I studies initiated in 1986 demonstrated that ddC could induce decreases in serum HIV p24 antigen at doses as low as 0.01 mg/kg every 8 hours (4, 5). Increases in CD4 cells were observed at slightly higher doses (0.03 mg/kg every 4 to 8 hours). Large-scale, multicenter trials were subsequently initiated to study monotherapy with ddC. In ACTG 114, ddC was found to be inferior to ZDV in antiretrovirally naive patients (140). However, in ACTG 119, which included only ZDV-experienced patients, no difference was found in survival or progression to clinical end points, although patients receiving ddC had slower rates of decline in CD4 cell counts than those receiving AZT (141). A subsequent trial evaluated the comparative benefits of ddC to ddI in 467 patients with advanced AIDS. Patients enrolled either were intolerant of ZDV monotherapy or this treatment had failed (142). In this trial, after adjustment for differences in entry CD4 cell counts, a slight but statistically significant survival advantage was seen among those patients receiving ddC. In part, on the basis of these results, the FDA approved ddC monotherapy in 1993, at a dose of 0.75 mg every 8 hours in patients with advanced HIV disease in whom ZDV treatment has failed or who are intolerant of ZDV.

ZDV and ddC have different toxicity profiles (see later), and trials using the two drugs in combination began early (4). Indeed, these were among the first trials of combination therapy in HIV infection. Starting in 1987, both pediatric and adult studies of alternating therapy with ZDV and ddC demonstrated that a sustained anti-HIV effect could be observed and suggested that the cumulative tolerable dose of each of the drugs given on an alternating schedule was greater than that of either of the drugs given continuously alone (this effect was more striking in the case of ddC toxicity) (4, 143, 144). Subsequently, combination regimens in which the two drugs were given simultaneously demonstrated substantial increases in CD4 counts that were sustained for up to 1 year (109). ACTG 155, a study designed to assess ZDV and ddC therapy as compared with either ZDV or ddC monotherapy in ZDV-experienced patients with CD4 cell counts less then 300 cells/mm^3 showed no overall advantage to the combination regimen. A subset analysis of this study, however, suggested that ZDV-experienced patients with more than 150 CD4 cells/mm^3 had less disease progression and potential clinical benefit from the ddC and ZDV combination than from ZDV ddC alone (109, 145).

On the basis of these and other observations, the large-scale, multicenter Delta and ACTG 175 trials discussed earlier were undertaken (15, 16). These studies demonstrated a significant reduction in disease progression in patients with CD4 counts below 500 cells/mm^3 who were administered combination therapy with either ZDV and ddC, ZDV and ddI, or ddI monotherapy, as compared with patients receiving ZDV monotherapy. Treatment-naive patients receiving the combination of ZDV and ddC (or the combination of ZDV and ddI) had a significant survival advantage compared with those receiving ZDV monotherapy (15, 16). ddC is currently labeled by the FDA for use in combination with ZDV for the management of HIV infections in adults and children 13 years or older who have had less then 3 months' prior exposure to ZDV.

The recommended dose of ddC is 0.75 mg given orally every 8 hours. Food may decrease the rate and extent of oral absorption. Antacids such as magnesium and aluminum decrease bioavailability of ddC by approximately 25%, and although the clinical importance of this is not known, concomitant administration of antacids and ddC should probably be avoided.

Several mutations have been reported to be associated with ddC resistance, including T69D, K65R, and M186V (60, 146). The latter two mutations are also associated with cross-reactive resistance to 3TC, ddI, and (in the case of K65R) PMEA, an investigational adenine nucleoside analog

(59, 61, 147). However, the resistance associated with these mutations is only partial.

The principal dose-limiting toxicity of ddC is a painful glove-and-stocking peripheral neuropathy, similar to that seen with ddI and hypothesized to be due to the effects of ddC-5′-TP on DNA polymerase γ (4, 5, 148–150). Most patients report gradual symptomatic improvement after discontinuation of the drug, but the condition can worsen during the initial 2 to 4 weeks after therapy has been discontinued. Other toxicities include oral ulcers, aphthous stomatitis, pancreatitis (which occurs infrequently, but can be life-threatening), skin rash, fever, and esophageal ulceration (4, 5, 151). The rash can be self-limiting, even with continued drug administration at a constant dose, and can take diverse forms, ranging from an erythematous morbilliform eruption to papulovesicular lesions (4). Cardiomyopathy has been reported in patients receiving ddC (112).

Caution should be used in administering ddC concomitantly with other drugs capable of causing peripheral neuropathies or pancreatitis, such as ddI or pentamidine. Similarly, drugs that could decrease renal clearance of ddC, such as amphotericin, foscarnet, and aminoglycosides, should also be used with care, because decreased clearance could lead to elevated serum levels of ddC and an increase in adverse events.

Stavudine

This thymidine analog has a mechanism of antiretroviral activity similar to that of the other nucleosides described earlier (152–154). Like ZDV, it is preferentially phosphorylated and exerts more potent anti-HIV activity in activated cells than in resting cells (4, 42, 152–154). However, unlike ZDV (in which the monophosphate inhibits thymidylate kinase), neither d4T nor any of its metabolites inhibits the enzymes responsible for its own phosphorylation (155). As a result of the lack of effect on cellular kinases, less perturbation of cellular nucleotide pools has been observed with d4T than with ZDV, a feature that may, in part, explain its relative lack of bone marrow toxicity.

This drug has greater than 80% bioavailability (156). Maximum drug concentrations are generally attained within 0.5 to 1.5 hours and then rapidly decline. The plasma half-life is 1.22 ± 0.09 hours (range, 0.7 to 2.2 hours) (157). Clinical trials in patients with AIDS or ARC and CD4 cell counts of less than 500 cells/mm^3 (most patients had CD4 cell counts lower than 200 cells/mm^3) who were administered d4T as a single agent in a range of doses have demonstrated improvements in CD4 cell counts and decreases in HIV antigenemia with doses as low as 1.0 mg/kg daily (157, 158). In some studies, these effects were more pronounced at doses of 2.0 mg/kg daily and were sustained for more than 6 months in some patients. Although in phase I trials the maximum tolerated dose of d4T (for short-term use) was determined to be 2.0 mg/kg daily, a multicenter, randomized phase II trial of d4T in 152 HIV-infected individuals with CD4 cell counts of less than 600 cells/mm^3 found that the optimal dose (considering both activity and toxicity) was 0.5 mg/kg daily (159). Preliminary results have become available of an ongoing, randomized, blinded, phase III trial that compared continued treatment with ZDV to treatment with d4T at doses of 40 mg twice a day in 822 ZDV-experienced patients with CD4 cell counts between 50 and 500 cells/mm^3 (160). Significant increases in CD4 cell counts and decreases in p24 antigen and HIV titers were seen in the d4T-treated group, but not in the continued ZDV-treated group. Values returned to baseline approximately 6 months after entry. In part on the basis of these results, d4T received FDA approval for the management of HIV infections in adults who have received prolonged prior ZDV therapy.

Dosage of d4T is based on the patient's weight. The recommended dose for patients weighing 60 kg or more is 40 mg every 12 hours, whereas patients weighing less should take 30 mg every 12 hours. d4T may be taken without regard to meals. The drug dosage should be reduced in patients with renal impairment.

The principal dose-limiting toxicity of d4T is peripheral sensory neuropathy (157–159, 161). Neuropathy appears to be dose related and can resolve with discontinuation of the drug. Some patients with mild neuropathy are able to continue treatment at reduced dose levels without a progression of symptoms. Patients administered combination therapy with d4T and ddC or ddI, either of which can also cause peripheral neuropathy, should be closely followed for signs of toxicity. Laboratory abnormalities seen with use of d4T include asymptomatic elevation of hepatic transaminases (157, 158). Hematologic toxicity does not appear to be a significant adverse effect of treatment with d4T, although one phase I study reported a 14% incidence of anemia (157). However, a phase II multicenter study reported general improvements in hematologic parameters, with significant improvements in platelet counts (159). As noted earlier, ZDV can reduce the phosphorylation of d4T, and these drugs should generally not be used together (162).

Lamivudine

3TC is the (−) enantiomer of 2′-dideoxy-3′-thiacytidine and is structurally related to ddC. The original compound was synthesized as a racemic mixture of both (+) and (−) enantiomers. This mixture was found to be active against HIV (163). The (−) enantiomer (in which the sugar ring is flipped compared to physiologic nucleoside), was found to be more potent than its (+) racemate (164, 165). Perhaps more important, the (−) enantiomer also was found to have relatively less activity against DNA polymerase γ and less cellular (mitochondrial) toxicity in vitro than the (+) racemate. For these reasons, the (−) enantiomer was taken into clinical development. Like ddI and ddC, 3TC is preferentially phosphorylated to its active moiety, the 5′-TP form, in resting cells (94).

3TC is absorbed rapidly after oral administration, with a mean time of maximum concentration (t_{max}) of 1 hour and 82% oral bioavailability. Most the drug is excreted unchanged in the urine (166). Concurrent ingestion of food results in reduced maximum concentration (c_{max}) and delayed t_{max}; however the area under the time-concentration curve (AUC) does not differ in the fasted or fed state. The mean elimination half-life of 3TC is 2.5 hours.

Transient virologic and immunologic improvements have been observed with administration of 3TC as a single agent, particularly at doses of 8.0 mg/kg daily or more, but these improvements were generally not sustained (166, 167). In vitro and in vivo studies have demonstrated the rapid emergence of resistance to 3TC, associated with a mutation at codon 184 (M184I or M184V) of the HIV-1 RT (51, 55). Other RT mutations have also been described, including a lysine-to-arginine substitution at codon 65 (K65R), which confers resistance to 3TC, ddC, ddI, and PMEA (59–62). As mentioned earlier, the 184 mutation induced by exposure to 3TC restores viral sensitivity to ZDV in those strains that are ZDV resistant on the basis of a mutation at codon 215 (51, 56). This finding, as well as the differential phosphorylation of the two drugs in different target cell populations, provides a rationale for administering these two agents together. Investigators have reported that HIV strains with the 184 mutation may have increased RT fidelity (i.e., a decreased ability to mutate) (63). Although investigators have hypothesized that 3TC administration may thus delay the ability of HIV to mutate under the pressure of other RTIs or patients' immunologic responses, this has yet to be proven, and the clinical significance of this find is unknown at present.

In clinical trials, significantly greater increases in CD4 cell counts and greater decreases in HIV-1 RNA polymerase chain reaction (PCR) have been observed with the combination of ZDV and 3TC than with either one administered as a single agent. In one multicenter study, the increase in CD4 cells obtained with use of the combination at 52 weeks was approximately 100 cells/mm^3 (58). Based in part, on an early analysis of this study, the combination of ZDV and 3TC was approved by the FDA in 1995 as front-line therapy for HIV infection in patients with clinical or immunologic evidence of disease progression. The antagonistic resistance pattern observed with ZDV and 3TC has not been demonstrated to occur with other nucleoside combinations involving 3TC, and additional studies will be needed to clarify the role of each combination (51, 56).

At the dose of 3TC recommended for administration (150 mg twice daily), the toxicity profile compares favorably with that of other nucleoside agents. Reported toxicities are peripheral neuropathy, as well as mild and transient episodes of headache, insomnia, fatigue, and abdominal symptoms, with a general downward trend of neutrophil counts seen at higher doses (166). Evidence suggests that 3TC can cause pancreatitis in children (168).

Investigational Nucleoside Reverse Transcriptase Inhibitors

Adefovir dipivoxil (bis-POM-PMEA) is an orally bioavailable prodrug of PMEA, a monophosphated acyclic adenine nucleoside analog that has activity against a broad spectrum of retroviruses and herpesviruses, including cytomegalovirus and HIV types 1 and 2, and is also active against hepatitis B virus (169–172). Its active intracellular metabolite, PMEA diphosphate (PMEApp) is a potent inhibitor of retroviral RT. PMEA has less activity in vitro in lymphocytes than ZDV, but it has more activity in monocytes and macrophages. After prolonged in vitro exposure of HIV to PMEA, mutations in codon 65 or 70 of HIV RT conferring low-level resistance have been described, but whether this change occurs in patients is unclear (59, 173). A phase II randomized, placebo-controlled clinical trial has compared 125 and 250 mg of adefovir dipivoxil daily to placebo in 72 HIV-positive individuals with median CD4 cell counts of 340 cells/mm^3 and HIV plasma RNA levels of 4.9 log copies/mL (174). The initial 6 weeks of treatment were blinded, and the subsequent 6 weeks were with open-label drug. Twelve-week data showed a 0.5 and 0.4 $\log_{10}$ reduction in plasma HIV RNA by PCR in the treatment arms, respectively, with no significant change seen in patients who received placebo. CD4 cell counts increased 57 and 27 cells/mm^3 in the 125- and 250-mg group, respectively (174). Adefovir dipivoxil is currently being tested in phase III clinical trials. In a primate model, an analog of PMEA, PMPA, was shown to block initial infection by the HIV analog, simian immunodeficiency virus (SIV) (175). PMPA is currently in phase I/II trials. A concern with this drug is high rates of Franconi syndrome as a major side effect of treatment using 120 mg/day for several months.

Another RTI currently in development is 2′-β-fluoro-2′,3′-dideoxyadenosine (FddA), a nucleoside RTI with an in vitro activity profile similar to that of ddI (176, 177). FddA, however, contains a fluorine in the 2′-"up" position of purine, making it resistant to acid degradation (177). Therefore, unlike ddI, it does not require administration with buffers. Because of this property, the drug may be better orally absorbed than ddI and may avoid the diarrhea caused by the vehicle of ddI. An even more interesting feature of FddA is that, in vitro, it has been found to have activity in strains of HIV that have ZDV or ddI resistance. Moreover, it is active in strains that have developed multidrug resistance in association with a mutation at codon 151 (178). This characteristic may result in substantial benefit to patients who have multinucleoside-resistant strains of HIV. Phase I trials of FddA in adults and children are now under way at the National Cancer Institute, and additional studies are anticipated.

Another investigational nucleoside RTI is 1592U89 succinate, a potent carbocyclic guanosine nucleoside analog that is not metabolized by the liver (179). It is well absorbed orally and has 18% cerebrospinal fluid penetration. This agent has shown in vitro synergy with other antiretroviral agents and is active against ZDV-resistant strains of HIV (179). The human DNA polymerases α, β, and γ are at least 2 orders of magnitude less sensitive to the active TP metabolite than is RT. Viral resistance to the compound has been associated with the *pol* gene mutations at codons M184V, L74V, and K65R (180, 181). Given the association of resistance with M184V, investigators will be interested in determining whether this drug has activity in patients who have previously received 3TC. A 12-week dose range–finding phase I/II clinical study showed a decrease in HIV RNA of 1.4 logs after the 4-week monotherapy portion of the trial. Half the patients then received a combination of 1592U89 and ZDV, whereas the other half remained on 1592U89 monotherapy for the remaining 8 weeks of the trial. Viral suppression continued even on the monotherapy arm of the trial (179).

Additional promising nucleoside RTIs are in development and offer the potential to expand the range of therapeutic options available to HIV-infected individuals. Indeed, because of the substantial potential of HIV to develop resistance, increasing the number of active drugs likely will optimize the possibility for long-term control of the disease. Moreover, because of the propensity of protease inhibitors to develop resistance when used alone, the development of that class of drugs has actually renewed interest in new nucleoside RTIs.

NONNUCLEOSIDE REVERSE TRANSCRIPTASE INHIBITORS

In the early 1990s, some structurally unrelated non-nucleoside compounds were discovered to be noncompetitive inhibitors of the HIV RT (NNRTIs). They included tetrahydroimidazo(4,5,1,jk;1,4)-benzodiazepin-2(1H)-one and -thrione (TIBO) derivatives, depyridodiazepinone analogs, pyridinone derivatives, and bis(heteroaryl)piperazines (BHAP compounds) (182–184). These agents share the property of having substantial and specific activity for HIV-1, but little activity against HIV-2, SIV, and other retroviruses (183, 185, 186). Unlike the dideoxynucleoside RTIs, which require intracellular phosphorylation to become active and then cause premature chain termination, NNRTIs inhibit viral RNA- and DNA-dependent DNA polymerase activities by disrupting the catalytic site of the enzyme. They bind to the p66 subunit of the enzyme, which lies in a deep pocket close to the presumed primer terminus (187). Nevirapine and delavirdine are two such agents that have gained FDA approval.

Nevirapine

Nevirapine, a dipyridodiazepinone analog, binds to heterodimeric HIV-1 RT and acts as a specific, noncompetitive inhibitor (188). The initial phase I/II dose-escalating trials of nevirapine monotherapy (ACTG 164) showed transient virologic effects. Development of resistance in vitro and in vivo occurred quickly, with most clinical isolates developing a 181 mutation by week 8, and many as early as week 4 (188, 189). Mutations have been observed at amino acid positions 103, 106, 108, 181, 188, and 190, with the 181 mutation being most common. High-level resistance has been seen with concurrent mutations at codons 181 and 106. In a study involving 24 patients, 100% of patient isolates were found to have a more than a 100-fold decreased susceptibility to nevirapine in vitro after 8 weeks of nevirapine monotherapy, and 80% of patient isolates had the 181 mutation (189). Mutations associated with resistance to nevirapine can also confer cross-resistance to other NNRTIs (186).

Modest sustained antiretroviral activity has been attributable to nevirapine administered in combination with nucleoside agents. ACTG 241, a randomized, double-blind trial of 398 antivirally experienced HIV-infected individuals with a median CD4 cell count of 138 cells/mm^3, compared a three-drug regimen of ZDV, ddI, and nevirapine to a combination of ZDV and ddI. Patients in the three-drug arm were found to have an 18% higher mean absolute CD4 cell count and 0.25 log$_{10}$ lower mean HIV-1 RNA plasma level at the end of 48 weeks of therapy than did patients on the two drug combination (190).

In part on the basis of these results, nevirapine was approved for use in combination with nucleosides. Nevirapine should not be used as monotherapy. Although in vitro studies suggested that the nevirapine-initiated RT mutation at codon 181 could counteract ZDV resistance caused by a mutation at codon 215, subsequent in vivo trials have shown that combination therapy with nevirapine and ZDV does not substantially delay the emergence of resistance to nevirapine, even though the RT mutation pattern differs from that seen with nevirapine monotherapy (191, 192). As described later, evidence shows that the development of HIV resistance can be slowed in patients if profound suppression of viral replication is attained (193). Perhaps such a strategy may be found to increase the period that nevirapine can be active in patients.

Nevirapine has a bioavailability of more than 90% that is not affected by coadministration with food or nucleoside RTIs. It is an inducer of the hepatic P450 cytochrome system, with metabolites excreted primarily by the kidney. Nevirapine appears to induce its own metabolism, which results in a fall in the serum half-life from 43 hours at the beginning of therapy to 23 hours 2 weeks later (194). This finding probably explains the reduced rate of adverse events reported when nevirapine dosing is initiated at a lower dose of 200 mg daily for the first 2 weeks of therapy and then increased to twice-daily dosing of 200 mg (400 mg daily) for the balance of therapy (195).

The most common toxicity associated with nevirapine therapy is a morbilliform rash. Headache, somnolence, mouth ulcers, and fever have been reported (196). Laboratory abnormalities include elevated hepatic transaminases, particularly γ-glutamyl transpeptidase and alkaline phosphatase (197). The abnormal transaminases are usually asymptomatic, but they have been associated with clinical hepatitis. The rash induced by nevirapine can be severe in up to 8% of patients, with 0.5% progressing to Stevens–Johnson syndrome (197). One death due to this syndrome has been reported. The rash usually occurs within the first 4 weeks of treatment, but it may occur up to week 8.

Delavirdine

In April, 1997, delavirdine, a BHAP drug, received accelerated approval from the FDA for use in combination with other antiretroviral agents. Like nevirapine, it has activity against HIV-1 alone and binds noncompetitively to the same site located in a pocket next to the RT active site, causing conformational change in the enzyme and reduced activity (198). As with other NNRTIs, resistance to BHAP compounds develops quickly in vitro, and in vivo, exposure for as little as 4 to 8 weeks of monotherapy can lead to a 50- to 500-fold loss of sensitivity (199). This resistance is associated with mutations at codons 103, 181, and 190 of RT (198, 200). Delavirdine also appears to have a unique resistance mutation because of a single amino acid substitution at codon 236 (201). This mutation has been reported to make RT more sensitive to other NNRTIs (202).

Delavirdine is metabolized by the cytochrome P450 CYP3A hepatic enzyme system (198). Unlike nevirapine, however, it acts as an inhibitor of the enzyme system and may also inhibit its own metabolism. Clinical efficacy data are limited. ACTG 261 has enrolled 549 patients with CD4 counts between 100 and 350 cells/mm^3 into one of four groups: ZDV and delavirdine; ddI and delavirdine; ZDV and ddI; or ZDV and ddI and delavirdine. A 48-week analysis has shown no statistically significant CD4 cell count differences among any of the arms of the trial (203).

The current dosing recommendation is 400 mg three times a day. The bioavailability of this agent is not affected by food intake. Antacids decrease its absorption, and therefore, when delavirdine is used in conjunction with ddI, the two should be given at least 1 hour apart. Because of delavirdine's inhibition of cytochrome P450, drug interactions may occur when used concurrently. Plasma levels of sedative hypnotics, of cisapride, and of calcium channel blockers may be increased. Rifampin and rifabutin may decrease the level of delavirdine. Delavirdine increases the AUC of saquinavir fivefold and increases the bioavailability of indinavir (204, 205). This property may make delavirdine an attractive option for use with protease inhibitors in the future. The most frequently reported toxicities include skin rash in which pruritus (but not urticaria) is common, mild to moderate headache, nausea, diarrhea, and fatigue (198). Reversible elevations in liver enzymes and bilirubin have been seen, and rare cases of anemia and neutropenia have been reported.

PROTEASE INHIBITORS

The second step in the HIV life cycle to be successfully targeted is the cleavage of polyprotein by the viral protease (see Table 45B.1). This crucial enzyme is an aspartic endopeptidase that is responsible for the cleavage of viral *gag* and *gag-pol* polyproteins (p55 and p160) to form the structural proteins of the virion core, p17, p24, p9, and p7, as well as the integral viral enzymes RT, integrase, RNase, and protease itself (206–208). This processing occurs during the latter stage of HIV replication and is essential to the production of mature, infectious virions. When protease is inhibited, newly produced virions are not infectious. Unlike the RTIs, this class of antiretroviral agents has the distinct advantage of blocking HIV-1 infection in both acutely and, perhaps more important, chronically infected cells. HIV-infected patients possess long-lived cells chronically infected with HIV. This property allows for the targeting of a viral reservoir not well suppressed by RTIs.

In 1988, the HIV-1 protease enzyme was crystallized, and its three-dimensional structure was elucidated (209–211). Computer modeling then allowed for the consideration of new compounds that specifically fit into the substrate-binding pocket of the protease, thus inhibiting its activity. This information, as well as previous studies elucidating the sequence cleaved by the protease, permitted the rational development of peptidomimetic drugs that were able to compete effectively with substrate for binding sites (212–215). HIV protease is a twofold (C_2)-symmetric homodimer with a single active site composed of a hydrophobic substrate binding pocket located along the central axis at the dimer interface (215). Each 99-amino acid monomer contributes to the formation of eight enzyme subsites that make up the substrate-binding pocket. Two highly conserved aspartic acid residues are found at the active site, each supplied by one of the component monomers. In addition are two flexible "flaps," β-hairpin structures, that cover the active site and undergo conformational change during the binding and release of protease substrates. Identification of these structures has proved critical to the design of protease inhibitors.

Despite the potential of protease as a unique antiretroviral target, several obstacles to the development of clinically useful HIV protease inhibitors were met (213, 214). Many of the original candidate compounds were hydrophobic peptides with poor bioavailability. They possessed a short plasma half-life resulting from rapid degradation, hepatic metabolism, and biliary excretion. Finally, because most of these compounds are complex in structure, they are difficult (and expensive) to synthesize. Nonetheless, by the end of 1996, three HIV protease inhibitors, saquinavir, ritonavir, and indinavir, had entered the clinic and had received FDA approval. In March, 1997, a fourth protease inhibitor, nelfinavir, received accelerated approval. In early-phase clinical trials, significant reductions in viral loads were demonstrated in patients who were administered these antiretrovirals as single agents. However, as monotherapeutic agents, viral resistance is known to emerge rapidly, and optimal use of these medications clearly will be in combination regimens.

Protease genes from drug-resistant strains have been found to contain mutations to residues coding for subsites critical for substrate recognition and binding (216, 217). Thus, mutations tend to follow characteristic patterns. Several key mutations induced by the approved protease inhibitors have been identified. These include mutations at codons M46I and V82A/P induced by ritonavir and indinavir, a mutation at codon L90M induced by saquinavir, and a unique mutation at D30N induced by nelfinavir (216–221). However, one of these mutations is not, in itself, sufficient to confer high-level resistance on a viral strain. Instead, resistance emerges as several mutations accumulate. Cross-resistance among protease inhibitors is frequently found (216, 217). However, because resistance to these drugs is generally associated with the development of several mutations, the issue of cross-resistance among agents is complex. Mutations to protease inhibitors do not confer cross-resistance to nucleoside antiretroviral agents, nor do viral strains with resistance to the nucleosides have decreased susceptibility to the protease inhibitors.

The factors influencing the emergence of resistant virus include the activity of the drug at the doses used, the degree of resistance provided by one or more mutations, and the degree of active viral replication (viral load). The greater the rate of replication and consequent viral titer, the higher the likelihood that mutations will occur. However, the number of potential mutations does not appear to be infinite, and certain mutations possibly may reduce the ability of a viral strain to replicate (222, 223). Resistance can develop rapidly under pressure from certain active agents. In general, the greater the number of mutations required to induce phenotypic resistance, the slower the process. Similarly, the development of drug resistance can be slowed by combinations of antiretroviral agents that yield substantial reductions in viral loads (193). Recent enthusiasm for the administration of triple-drug combination therapy shown to reduce the viral burden to below detectable levels is based in part on this effect (17, 18, 224, 225). However, suboptimal dosing of protease inhibitors with incomplete inhibition of viral replication may lead to the rapid evolution of resistance. This situation may occur if drugs have partial activity at recommended doses, if patients take the drugs at less than the recommended dosages, or if patients take these drugs irregularly. However, abrupt cessation of drug dosing does not enhance the de novo emergence of resistance because no selective, drug-induced pressure occurs.

The protease inhibitors developed to date fall into broad structural categories. Saquinavir contains transition state inserts in place of the dipeptidic cleavage sites of the natural substrates (226, 227). Indinavir, an isosteric transition state substrate analog of the protease cleavage site, contains a hydroxylaminepentanamide moiety (228, 229). The design of C_2- symmetric inhibitors, such as ritonavir, is based on the three-dimensional symmetry of the protease active site (230). Nelfinavir is a nonpeptidic inhibitor of the protease enzyme. Other novel, nonpeptidic protease inhibitors have also been formulated (231). All are reversible competitive inhibitors that are highly selective for viral protease, unlike the nucleoside RTIs. Intracellular conversion of the parent compound is not required for activity of any of the protease inhibitors.

The protease inhibitors have been associated with various adverse effects ranging from gastrointestinal disturbances to nephrolithiasis and hepatitis (Table 45B.4). Increased episodes of bleeding in hemophiliac patients and diabetes mellitus have also been reported with use of protease inhibitors (232).

Saquinavir

The first protease inhibitor to become widely available was saquinavir (Invirase), which received FDA approval in late 1995 for administration in thrice-daily dosing of 600 mg (1800 mg daily total) in combination with a nucleoside analog. The drug is a transition-stage analog of the HIV Phe-Pro protease cleavage site and contains a hydroxyethylamine moiety, making it a highly specific inhibitor of both HIV-1 and HIV-2 (226, 227). It received accelerated FDA approval under an expedited process on the basis of three double-blind studies that demonstrated improvement in surrogate markers of HIV infection.

The pharmacokinetics of saquinavir has been studied in healthy volunteers and in patients with HIV infection (233–236). Saquinavir is poorly absorbed and undergoes extensive first-pass metabolism. Bioavailability of the drug is approximately 4% in the fed state and lower when fasting (234). The steady-state AUC is 2.5 times higher on thrice-daily dosing than after a single daily dose, and the optimal time of dosing is within 2 hours of a high-calorie, high-fat meal (237). Saquinavir has a large volume of distribution yet is 98% bound to plasma proteins, which may limit tissue penetration. Penetration into cerebrospinal fluid is negligible at the approved dose of 1800 mg daily and has not been studied at higher doses. More than 90% of the drug is metabolized by the isoenzyme CYP3A4 of the hepatic P450 cytochrome system, and therefore, care should be taken when it is administered with other drugs similarly metabolized. The metabolites are inactive monohydroxylated and dihydroxylated compounds. After oral administration, 13% of the circulating moiety is attributable to the parent compound and 87% to the inactive metabolites. Excretion in feces and urine is 88% and 17%, respectively (238). A soft gel capsule formulation of saquinavir was approved in 1998 for use with the recommended dose of 1200 mg thrice daily. This formulation (Fortovase) consists of drug dissolved in a liquid consisting of monoglycerides and diglycerides of medium-chain fatty acids. This form is proposed to have threefold greater bioavailability than the hard gel capsules (239).

Saquinavir monotherapy has been studied in doses ranging from 25 mg to 7200 mg daily, with the greatest and most

Table 45B.4 Toxicities Associated With Approved Protease Inhibitors[a]

Drug	Major Toxicities	Laboratory Abnormalities
Indinavir sulfate	Nephrolithiasis	Indirect bilirubinemia
	Nausea	Hematuria
	Abdominal pain	Sterile pyuria
Nelfinavir mesylate	Diarrhea	Neutropenia
	Nausea	Increased creatine phosphokinase
Ritonavir	Nausea	Transaminitis
	Diarrhea	Elevated triglycerides
	Taste perversion	Thrombocytopenia
	Circumoral paresthesias	Granulocytopenia
Saquinavir mesylate	Diarrhea	Neutropenia
	Nausea	Hemolytic anemia
	Abdominal pain	Transaminitis
	Ataxia	

[a]Diabetes mellitus and bleeding episodes in hemophiliac patients have been reported with this class of agents.

sustained improvements in viral load and CD4 cell counts seen at the highest dose (20). At 3600 and 7200 mg daily, patients had maximal viral load reductions of 1.1 and 1.5 logs and sustained reductions at 24 weeks of 0.5 and 0.9 logs, respectively. In one study, CD4 cell count increases were sustained for 24 weeks and were 31 and 100 cells/mm^3 above baseline on the 3600- and 7200-mg daily arms of the trial, respectively (236). By contrast, substantially smaller improvements in surrogate markers of HIV infection were seen at the approved dose of 1800 mg daily, and no clear benefit was observed in patients administered saquinavir monotherapy at daily doses of less than 1800 mg.

At the approved dose of 1800 mg daily, greater improvements in surrogate markers were observed when saquinavir was administered with one or more antiretroviral nucleoside analogs than when any of these agents were administered as monotherapy (20, 236). In one study, a cohort of ZDV-naive patients with CD4 cell counts under 300 cells/mm^3 administered 1800 mg of saquinavir daily, in combination with 600 mg daily of ZDV (both taken on thrice-daily dosing schedules), were observed to have median reductions in viral loads of 0.5 log and median increases in CD4 cell counts of 40 cells/mm^3 at 16 weeks (20). Patients on either monotherapy arm of the trial had median CD4 cell count increases of approximately 10 cells/mm^3 and less notable viral load reductions at 16 weeks. In ACTG 229, ZDV-experienced patients (at least 4 months) with CD4 cell counts under 300 cells/mm^3 were randomized to receive one of the following: triple-drug therapy with saquinavir (1800 mg daily), ZDV, and ddC; combination therapy with the ZDV and ddC; or saquinavir and ZDV (21). Greater improvements in surrogate markers were seen at 24 weeks in patients given the triple combination than in those receiving the two nucleosides without saquinavir. At week 48, a significant number of patients receiving the triple combination were observed to have stable CD4 cell counts above baseline, in contrast to either double-combination therapy arm, in whom CD4 cell count decreases of approximately 20 cells/mm^3 were observed.

Trials are ongoing to evaluate the safety, toxicity, and effect on surrogate markers with combinations of saquinavir and ritonavir. Ritonavir, a powerful inhibitor of cytochrome P450 CYP3A, has been shown to increase the AUC of saquinavir as much as 100-fold (240). In one study of the combination of saquinavir and ritonavir, patients with CD4 cell counts between 100 and 500 cell/mm^3 who were protease inhibitor-naive and who were receiving no other antiretroviral agents were randomized to one of four groups that differed by dose (400 or 600 mg of each agent) and schedule (twice or thrice daily) (241). At 24 weeks, 89% of all patients had undetectable viral loads. Other clinical studies are ongoing.

A 10-fold resistance to saquinavir has been observed with mutations at positions G48V or L90M (242). Less frequently, double mutations occur, leading to reductions in sensitivity up to 100-fold (243). In a group of 85 patients treated with 1800 mg saquinavir daily for 24 weeks, 45% of patients receiving monotherapy and 31% of patients receiving combination therapy with a nucleoside antiretroviral agent developed mutations conferring resistance predominantly at codon 90 (236). By contrast, when saquinavir was used at 7200 mg daily, resistance developed less frequently, a finding suggesting that potent inhibition of viral replication may be able to reduce the development of resistance (236). Cross-resistance to indinavir or ritonavir has not generally been observed in patients, although mutations at sites conferring resistance to the structurally similar nelfinavir have been reported (216, 218, 219). However, more studies are needed to clarify the patterns and frequencies of cross-resistance that may develop with different dosing strategies.

The principal side effects of saquinavir are diarrhea, nausea, and abdominal discomfort (237). Mild decreases in neutrophil numbers and increases in liver function tests have been reported in patients who were receiving concomitant medications. Other serious adverse effects reported with the use of saquinavir include rare occurrences of confusion, ataxia, acute myeloblastic leukemia, hemolytic anemia, seizures, cutaneous reactions, and clinical hepatitis (20, 236).

As noted earlier, saquinavir weakly inhibits and is metabolized by the hepatic CYP3A4 system, and concomitant administration of drugs that induce these enzymes, such as phenobarbital, phenytoin, dexamethasone, or carbamazepine, may reduce plasma concentrations of saquinavir (238). Concentrations of drugs that are potent inhibitors of this system, such as astemizole, ketoconazole, or itraconazole, as well as substrates of related isozymes, such as calcium channel blockers, dapsone, clindamycin, quinidine, and triazolam, may be elevated. All patients receiving both saquinavir and these agents should be closely monitored for toxicity.

Ritonavir

Ritonavir is a C_2-symmetric peptide, the structure of which was designed to optimize antiretroviral activity and bioavailability (207, 211, 230, 244). It has specific activity against HIV-1 and, to a lesser extent, HIV-2. Like saquinavir, the drug has low affinity for human aspartic endopeptidases that have similar structures to the HIV protease (such as pepsin, renin, gastricin, and cathepsins D and E). The median effective concentration (EC_{50}) of the drug in vitro ranges from 3.8 to 153 nmol, with an average of 22 nmol observed for low passage clinical isolates (244).

Ritonavir has a calculated oral bioavailability of approximately 75%, with peak plasma concentrations attained within 2 to 4 hours and a plasma half-life of 3 to 5 hours (244–247). The drug is commercially available in both capsule and liquid formulations. In clinical trials, trough plasma concentrations of ritonavir in patients treated with 600 mg every 12 hours in either dosage form (the recommended dose) were found to exceed the inhibitory concentration of 90% (IC_{90}) of the virus, and the two formulations are considered bioequivalent (244).

Ritonavir is metabolized by the liver (248). The microsomal P450 CYP3A isozymes account for the major portion of metabolism, with CYP2D6 playing a smaller role. Ritonavir is excreted primarily in the stool, both as unchanged drug and metabolites. After oral administration of 600 mg of the oral solution, 86.4% is excreted in stool (33.8% as unchanged drug), whereas 11.3% is excreted in the urine (3.5% as unchanged drug) (247).

Similar patterns of resistance mutations have been observed both in vitro and in vivo (216–219). Protease mutations associated with decreased viral susceptibility to ritonavir in vitro include M46I, I54V, A71V, V82F, and I84V (217). In viral isolates from patients treated with ritonavir, mutations at codons 24 and 36, as well as those previously described, have been observed. At least two mutations are required for the development of high-level resistance to ritonavir, with mutations at both positions 82 and 84 conferring an 8- to 10-fold reduction in drug susceptibility (217). Such mutations may also confer cross-resistance to indinavir and other protease inhibitors, although cross resistance to saquinavir has not been described (217, 223).

Ritonavir has been studied as monotherapy and in combination with nucleosides. Initial phase II studies of monotherapy demonstrated substantial reductions in viral load that frequently returned to baseline within 16 to 20 weeks (246, 247). The use of ritonavir in combination with various regimens of nucleosides in patients with more advanced AIDS has also been studied (19, 249). An international randomized, controlled phase III double-blind trial of 1090 antiretrovirally experienced patients, with fewer than 100 CD4 cells/mm^3 and a median HIV-RNA level of 5.3 copies/mL randomized to receive either ritonavir or placebo in addition to their antiretroviral regimen, has been completed. The primary end point was progression to AIDS or death. After a median duration of 7 months, a significant reduction in both disease progression and mortality was observed among patients in the ritonavir arm of the trial (15.7%) as compared with the placebo arm (33.1%) (241).

As described previously, ritonavir has been shown to increase the plasma concentrations of saquinavir profoundly by inhibition of the hepatic P450 cytochrome isoenzymes when the two drugs are administered in combination. Saquinavir appears to have little effect on the plasma concentrations of ritonavir (250, 251). Studies exploring the combination of ritonavir and nelfinavir are ongoing. Preliminary results indicate that substantial decreases in HIV viral load are attainable with this regimen.

The most frequent adverse effects associated with ritonavir monotherapy have been gastrointestinal. In one clinical study (ABT-245), 23% of patients experienced nausea, 13% emesis, 13% diarrhea, 10% taste perversion, and 3% abdominal pain (252). In studies combining ritonavir with dideoxynucleosides, the incidence of gastrointestinal complaints has often been even greater, with nausea occurring in almost 46% of patients, emesis in 23%, and diarrhea in approximately 22% (252). The incidence of gastrointestinal complaints is lessened when the drug is given with a fat-containing meal. In addition, many reported gastrointestinal complaints are transient and ease by week 4 to 5. Other common complaints include asthenia and anorexia.

The most frequently reported laboratory abnormalities have been elevations in hepatic transaminases, triglycerides, creatine phosphokinase, and uric acid (246, 247, 252). Serum bilirubin is affected less frequently. Anemia, ecchymosis, hemorrhage, leukopenia, lymphocytosis, and thrombocytopenia have been reported in fewer than 2% of patients taking ritonavir. Reports in Europe have noted spontaneous bleeding episodes in patients with hemophilia who were taking protease inhibitors including ritonavir (232). Of the 15 initial cases, 11 presented as hematomas and 5 as hemarthrosis. All cases occurred in patients with advanced disease and who were taking numerous concomitant medications, and therefore a causal relationship could not directly be attributed to the use of protease inhibitors. At this time, no clear evidence suggests that protease inhibitor treatment should be avoided in this population; however, the FDA has recommended that physicians closely monitor patients who are taking protease inhibitors and who have hemophilia for spontaneous bleeding episodes.

Clinically significant drug interactions may occur when ritonavir is administered concomitantly with other agents metabolized by the cytochrome P450 system (Table 45B.5), especially those metabolized by CYP3A, CYP2D6, CYP2C9, and CYP2C19, as well as, to a lesser extent, CYP2A6, CYP1A2, and CYP2E1 (252). Increased plasma concentrations of either drug may occur, and consequent clinical abnormalities may be seen. Special attention should be given to drugs with narrow therapeutic margins, such as oral anticoagulants or immunosuppressants. Agents that may be contraindicated or may require dosage modification include the following: drugs used to treat cardiovascular abnormalities such as arrhythmias or hypercholesterolemia; sedatives, anticonvulsants, narcotic analgesics, the tricyclic antidepressant desipramine, and other drugs that act on the central nervous system; antihistamines; antiemetics; antidiarrheal compounds; hormones or hormone analogs; and select

Table 45B.5 Important Medications That Interact With HIV Protease Inhibitors

Analgesics (meperidine, piroxicam)	Cardiac drugs (amiodarone, amlodipine, diltiazem, flecainide, nifedipine, imodipine, propafenone, quinidine, verapamil)
Antibiotics (clarithromycin, erythromycin, metronidazole)	Corticosteroids
Anticoagulants (warfarin)	Ergot alkaloids (dihydroergotamine, ergotamine)
Anticonvulsants (phenytoin, phenobarbital)	Estrogens
Antifungals (fluconazole, itraconazole, ketoconazole)	Gastrointestinal agents (cimetidine, cisapride)
Antihistamines (astemizole, terfenadine)	Antimalarial agents (quinine)
Antihyperlidemics (clofibrate)	Opioid agonists (alfentanil, fentanyl, methadone)
Antimycobacterials (isoniazid, rifabutin, rifampin)	Psychotropic agents (clozapine, desipramine, sertraline)
Antineoplastics (anthracyclines, tamoxifen)	Sedative/hypnotics (alprazolam, clorazepate, diazepam, estazolam, flurazepam, midazolam, triazolam, zolpidem)

antimicrobial agents (253, 254). Disulfiram-like reactions may occur with the concomitant use of metronidazole because formulations of ritonavir contain alcohol. Given that many patients receiving protease inhibitors also require antimycobacterial prophylaxis, coadministration of ritonavir and rifabutin is specifically contraindicated because it can lead to a 25-fold increase in the C_{max} of rifabutin and substantial hepatic toxicity. Rifampin, on the other hand, increases the activity of P450 CYP3A isoenzymes and thus increases the clearance of ritonavir. However, no specific recommendations regarding dosage adjustments of either rifampin or ritonavir have been suggested by the manufacturers. The C_{max} of clarithromycin is increased by 31% when coadministered with ritonavir, and therefore this agent may be used as prophylaxis against mycobacteria in these patients (255). A list of potential drug interactions is provided by the manufacturer of ritonavir in the prescribing information and should be consulted before initiating therapy (252).

Indinavir

Indinavir sulfate is an isosteric transition state substrate analog of the HIV protease cleavage site that is active against both HIV-1 and HIV-2 (228, 229). Indinavir contains a hydroxylaminepentanamide moiety, which contributes in its being a highly selective, potent inhibitor of the HIV protease. It also contains a basic amide incorporated into the hydroxyethylene backbone, which increases the drug's aqueous solubility and bioavailability.

In the fasting state, indinavir is rapidly absorbed, with the time to peak plasma concentration ranging from 0.5 to 1.1 hours (256). Consumption of a high-fat, high-protein meal reduced peak plasma concentrations by 84% and the AUC by 77%, whereas consumption of a light meal, such as dry toast and coffee, has little to no effect on the oral pharmacokinetics (228, 229). Indinavir is approximately 60% bound to plasma proteins (256).

Indinavir is metabolized by the CYP3A4 isozyme of the hepatic P450 cytochrome system and therefore may interact with drugs metabolized by these isozymes (see Table 45B.5) (251, 257). Less than 20% of the drug is excreted unchanged in the urine, and the elimination half-life is approximately 1.8 hours (228, 229, 258). Patients with hepatic insufficiency who were administered 50% of the standard dose of indinavir were found to have a 60% increase in the mean AUC, as compared with those with normal liver function, and an increase in the elimination half-life to approximately 2.8 hours (256). Such patients should be dosed with caution.

Indinavir has been extensively evaluated in clinical trials involving more than 10,000 patients, and additional trials are under way (17, 18, 224, 225, 259–263). In one randomized, double-blind phase II study of ZDV-experienced adults (median 30.7 months) with mean baseline CD4 counts of 175 cells/mm^3 and HIV-1 RNA levels of approximately 38,400 copies/mL, patients were given indinavir monotherapy, a 2-drug regimen of ZDV and 3TC, or a triple-drug combination of indinavir, ZDV, and 3TC (225). At both 12 and 24 weeks, a greater reduction in HIV-1 RNA level was observed among those patients administered the 3-drug regimen than among those patients in either other arm of the trial. At 24 weeks, serum HIV-1 RNA levels were below the level of detection in 91% of those receiving the triple-drug combination, in 35% of those receiving indinavir monotherapy, and in none of those receiving the combination of the two nucleoside agents.

Resistance to indinavir has been observed both in vitro and in vivo (216, 218, 219). Combinations of mutations in viral strains with decreased in vitro susceptibility to indinavir include the following: M46L and V 82A; V32I, M46L, and V82A (3-fold decrease); and V32I, M46L, A71V, and V82A (14-fold decrease) (216). Resistance-conferring mutations in isolates from patients treated with the drug include L10R/I, M46I, L63P/L, V82A/F/T, and L90M (219). Generally, at least two mutations are needed for the development of high-level resistance to indinavir, and this may also confer resistance to other protease inhibitors, particularly ritonavir (217).

The most serious adverse effect reported to date is nephrolithiasis, which is due to crystallization of the drug. This complication was seen in 5 to 6% of patients in phase II clinical trials and was more likely to occur at doses higher than 2.4 g per day (262, 264). Nephrolithiasis typically presents with flank pain with or without hematuria and responds to drug cessation and vigorous hydration; its incidence may be reduced by hydration with 1 to 2 L of water daily. Sterile pyuria has also been reported (264). Laboratory abnormalities include asymptomatic indirect hyperbilirubinemia, which is seen in more than 10% of patients. This is usually not associated with elevations in hepatic transaminases and does not generally require cessation of drug (263). However, patients with a history of nephrolithiasis, hepatic or renal insufficiency, or hyperbilirubinemia should be monitored closely during therapy with indinavir. Other adverse effects reported in two trials of indinavir therapy include nausea (12% of patients), abdominal pain (9%), headache (6%), diarrhea (5%), and malaise (4%) (256). The gastrointestinal symptoms may be mitigated by the administration of indinavir with a light snack, such as dry toast and apple juice or coffee. Some patients receiving indinavir have had a redistribution of body fat to the abdominal region, causing a noticeable increase in abdominal girth.

Significant drug interactions may occur if patients are treated concurrently with indinavir and other drugs metabolized by the CYP3A4 isozyme, although fewer interactions have been reported than in the case of ritonavir (256). In pharmacokinetic studies, significant drug interactions were observed with ketoconazole, rifabutin, and rifampin. Concomitant administration of indinavir (800 mg every 8 hours) and rifabutin (300 mg daily) led to a 32% decrease in AUC of indinavir and a 204% increase in the AUC of rifabutin. The manufacturer recommends that the dosage of rifabutin be decreased by 50% if it is used in conjunction with indinavir

(265). Other drugs that could potentially interact with indinavir include terfenadine, astemizole, cisapride, triazolam, and midazolam.

The antiretroviral nucleoside ddI contains a buffer that may impair the absorption of indinavir. Patients taking a combination regimen that contains both agents should take indinavir 1 hour before or 1 hour after ddI. Clinicians generally recommend that indinavir be taken in a fasting or near-fasting state, at least 1 hour before or 1.5 hours after meals, at doses of 800 mg three times daily. Indinavir should not be taken with grapefruit juice, because administration of a single 400-mg oral dose with 240 mL of grapefruit juice resulted in a 26% decrease in AUC of the drug.

Nelfinavir

Nelfinavir mesylate is the most recent inhibitor of the HIV aspartyl protease enzyme to receive FDA approval. It is a selective, nonpeptidic inhibitor that received accelerated approval in March, 1997 for the treatment of HIV-1 infection when antiretroviral therapy is warranted. This indication was based on surrogate marker changes in patients who received nelfinavir alone or in combination with nucleoside analogs for 24 weeks (266).

Oral bioavailability ranges from 20 to 80% in animals (267). Maximum plasma concentration and area under the plasma concentration-time curve (AUC) were shown to be two-to threefold higher in the presence of food compared with that of the fasting state. Nelfinavir is 98% protein bound in serum, and less than 2% is excreted in the urine (267). It reaches a peak plasma concentration in 2 to 4 hours and has a half-life of 3.5 to 5 hours. It is commercially available as a tablet or powder for oral solution. The recommended dosage is 750 mg in the tablet form (or 3¾ level teaspoons of oral powder mixed with water or milk) three times a day.

In vitro, mutations observed with nelfinavir have been seen at codons D30N, M46I, and A71V (221). In vivo mutations have been reported to occur at codons D30N, M36I, M46I, A71V, V77I, and N88D. A unique mutation at codon 30 in which an aspartic acid is substituted for an asparagine has been identified. HIV variants with a high-level resistance to nelfinavir are generally susceptible to indinavir, saquinavir, ritonavir, and VX-478 in vitro. In vivo isolates with multiple mutations also occur, and those with substitutions at codons D30N and A71V have a 7-fold decrease in susceptibility, whereas those with mutations at M46I, L63P, A71V, and I84V/A exhibit a 30-fold decrease in susceptibility (221).

At present, no results from controlled trials evaluating the efficacy of therapy with nelfinavir on clinical progression to AIDS or survival are available. A randomized trial of nelfinavir monotherapy (AG 1343-503B), administered at 500, 750, or 1000 mg three times daily over 28 days, involved 30 patients with baseline CD4 cell counts of at least 200 cells/mm^3 and HIV RNA measurements of more than 20,000 copies/mL. At 4 months, patients in all dose groups had a significant increase of approximately 50 CD4 cells/mm^3, whereas viral burden was decreased by 0.6, 1.2, and 1.5 log$_{10}$. A more significant decrease in viral burden of 1.5, 2.4, and 1.8 log$_{10}$, respectively, was observed at 28 days of monotherapy (268).

AG-511 involved 297 treatment-naive patients with baseline CD4 counts of 280 cells/mm^3 and HIV RNA levels of 153,000 copies/mL (269). Patients were randomized to receive nelfinavir (500 or 750 mg thrice daily), ZDV and 3TC, or ZDV and 3TC. At 24 weeks, patients in triple-combination arms of the trial showed an increase of 125 CD4 cells/mm^3 from baseline and a decrease in viral burden of 2.4 log$_{10}$. Of the patients in the high-dose nelfinavir combination arm (750 mg three times daily), 82% had RNA levels below the detectable limits of the assay (500 copies). Patients receiving ZDV and 3TC had an increase of 100 CD4 cells/mm^3 from baseline and a 1.4 log$_{10}$ decrease in HIV RNA copy number. Twenty percent of patients in this arm of the trial had viral loads below detectable limits (269). A 40-week follow-up report of these patients was presented (270). The triple-combination arms continued to show high increases of CD4 cells (approximately 175 cells/mm^3) with reductions in plasma RNA levels of 2 and 1.8 log$_{10}$, respectively. Importantly, 83% of the high-dose nelfinavir group continued to remain below the assays limit of detection as compared with 60% of the low-dose group. An ongoing study is combining nelfinavir (750 mg thrice daily) with the protease inhibitor saquinavir (800 mg thrice daily) (271).

Mild to moderate diarrhea develops in approximately 10% of patients receiving nelfinavir. This can often be controlled with antidiarrheals (267–269). Nausea and vomiting have also been reported when nelfinavir was given in combination with ZDV.

Nelfinavir, like other protease inhibitors, is metabolized by the cytochrome P450 system (specifically the CYP3A isoform). It is a mild inhibitor of the cytochrome P450 isoforms with potential to cause drug interactions. The antimycobacterial drug rifabutin decreases the nelfinavir plasma concentration 32%, whereas its own concentration is increased 207% by nelfinavir. The manufacturers recommend a reduction of 50% the rifabutin dose when these agents are administered concurrently (267). Concomitant use of rifampin, on the other hand, decreases the AUC of nelfinavir 82% and is therefore not recommended. The manufacturer's insert should be consulted before prescribing this agent.

Investigational Protease Inhibitors

Two new protease inhibitors currently being studied in the clinic are worth mentioning. 141W94/VX-478 is a nonpeptide-based protease inhibitor that, in laboratory rats, appeared to cross well into the central nervous system and was found in higher concentrations in lymph tissues than in plasma. A 4-week multiple oral dose, open-labeled dose-escalating study of 4 weeks of monotherapy in 42 protease inhibitor-naive patients has been conducted. The lowest-dose group (300 mg twice a day) had a median CD4 cell increase of 64 cells, whereas the highest group (1200 mg twice a day) experienced a gain of 110 CD4 cells/mm^3. Viral load reductions were −0.58 to −1.95 $\log_{10}$, respectively (272). A phase II 24-week double-blind placebo-controlled combination trial with 141W94/VX478, ZDV, and 3TC is currently enrolling patients.

ABT-378 is a second-generation C_2-symmetry–based peptidomimetic inhibitor that is structurally related to, and is currently being developed for, coadministration with ritonavir. In vitro, it has 10-fold greater activity than ritonavir against HIV-1 (273). In rats, ritonavir inhibited the in vivo hepatic metabolism of ABT-378 and thus increased its bioavailability, causing persistently high levels of ABT-378 to remain in the plasma for as long as 9 to 12 hours (274). Preliminary data indicate that it retains activity against ritonavir-resistant strains (275). ABT-378 is currently in phase I/II testing.

TREATMENT STRATEGIES AND CONTROVERSIES

Over the past 10 years, advances in understanding the biology of HIV infection and substantial experience with a broadening range of antiretroviral agents have evolved hand in hand with techniques for monitoring disease progression and response to therapy. The results of large randomized trials with clinical end points such as time to progression to AIDS and survival data have provided guidance in the use of nucleoside analogs. However, few long-term clinical trials have been conducted to guide the clinician in the use of the newer drugs, particularly protease inhibitors. However, data from trials using surrogate markers (virologic and immunologic) as initial end points, combined with increased understanding of the pathogenesis of HIV, provide optimism that combination therapy using protease inhibitors and nucleoside analogs can sustain viral suppression and clinical benefit to many patients. Using insights gained into the relationship between viral load and disease progression, both national and international panels are attempting to formulate guidelines about how best to use these newer therapies.

In an attempt to interpret the more complete clinical, immunologic, and virologic data that are becoming available, several guidelines for the use and monitoring of antiretroviral therapy in HIV-1 positive patients have been formulated. The clinician must remain alert for new sets of recommendations as more information based on clinical studies is obtained. One set of recommendations was developed by members of the International AIDS Society–USA panel in July, 1996 (276). In September, 1996, the British HIV Association convened to develop its own recommendations (277). In November, 1996, the National Institutes of Health (NIH) Office of AIDS Research met to develop Principles of Therapy and to update treatment guidelines (278). The International AIDS Society–USA panel has updated its recommendations (279). Each panel addressed four central questions: when to initiate therapy; which drugs to use; when to change therapeutic strategies; and which agents to use when a change of therapy is indicated. Recommendations were based on the results of controlled clinical trials when available, but they were also made on the basis of ongoing clinical trials with virologic and immunologic end points, as well as current understanding of the pathophysiology of HIV infection. None of the various panels' recommendations are meant to render a precise algorithm for specific clinical situations, but rather to provide a basis for making rational decisions about therapeutic strategies.

Many data have demonstrated that the rate of disease progression can be predicted by the magnitude of viral burden (active HIV replication) (280, 281). CD4 cell counts, on the other hand, indicate the extent of immune system damage that has already occurred and help to determine, in an individual patient, the current risk of developing an opportunistic infection. The use of both viral load and CD4 cell counts in conjunction enhances the accuracy with which risk of disease progression and death can be predicted (282).

Many studies over the past several years have shown the utility of HIV-1 RNA PCR, and such assays are being used with increasing frequency to make decisions about when to initiate or to adjust antiretroviral regimens (283, 284). This value is only a reflection of circulating virus and is not a comprehensive measurement of infected cells throughout the body. Much of viral replication occurs in fixed lymphoid tissue. Although current data suggest some relationship between the amount of virus measured in the periphery and that in the extravascular compartment, such as fixed lymphoid tissues, the total amount of virus in the body cannot be calculated precisely from the plasma viral RNA level (276). A biologic variability of approximately 0.3 log in plasma HIV RNA levels is observed. Plasma HIV RNA levels of less than 5000 to 10,000 copies/mL are believed to represent low viral loads, whereas levels higher than 30,000 to 50,000 copies/mL are considered evidence of more active HIV infection (285).

The NIH panel set forth certain principles of therapy for HIV-infected individuals (278). First, HIV infection is always harmful, and in the presence of continued high-level replication, true long-term survival free of clinically significant immune dysfunction is exceptional. Treatment decisions should be individualized by level of risk indicated by RNA PCR levels and CD4 cell counts. Decisions about when to begin therapy should be based on risk of disease progression and degree of immunodeficiency. The goal of therapy, once initiated, should be to suppress the level of active HIV replication to below detectable limits. Available antiretroviral medications should be used in combination when evidence indicates additivity or synergy and preferably when the agents possess nonoverlapping toxicities. Ideally, the combination used should delay the emergence of drug-resistant variants. The combination of drugs used should be started simultaneously and should not added sequentially. If one is changing treatment because of drug failure, the new drugs chosen should ideally not be cross-resistant or share similar mutation patterns. If the regimen is failing, then more than one component of it should be changed. Perhaps the most important tenet is that patient education must be extensive (278).

No universal agreement has been reached on when to initiate therapy. All guidelines to date recommend treatment for symptomatic patients regardless of CD4 cell counts or viral load. (Symptoms may include hairy leukoplakia, recurrent thrush, night sweats, weight loss, or unexplained fevers.) The decision to initiate therapy in asymptomatic patients should be based on an assessment of the risk of disease progression as indicated by plasma HIV RNA level and CD4 cell counts, and it should ideally be initiated before irreversible immune system damage occurs. The Department of Health and Human Services panel recommended therapy for all asymptomatic patients with CD4 cell counts lower than 500 cells/mm^3, regardless of viral load. The panel acknowledged controversy among experts regarding treatment of asymptomatic patients whose CD4 counts are between 350 and 500 cells/mm^3 and whose HIV RNA levels are lower than 20,000 copies/mL, but suggested that treatment should be offered to this group of patients. The strength of the recommendations is based on prognosis for disease-free survival and the willingness of the patient to accept therapy. Treatment is believed to be indicated in all patients if their RNA levels are greater than 10,000 copies/mL (bDNA) or 20,000 copies/mL RNA PCR. Patients with CD4 cell counts higher than 500 cells/mm^3 and plasma RNA levels lower than 10,000–20,000 copies/mL can be observed according to the DHHS panel. The International AIDS Society panel recommendations were similar to those of the DHHS panel, except for recommending therapy for patients with CD4 cell counts between 350 and 500 cells/mm^3 and for all patients with plasma HIV RNA concentrations greater than 5000 to 10,000 copies/mL regardless of CD4 cell count (279). The panel suggested that current data do not permit an absolute plasma HIV RNA threshold for initiation of therapy.

The varied panels agree substantially in terms of the goals of treatment and changing therapy, and we present here a consensus view, highlighting differences when appropriate. The goal of treatment, once initiated, should be to suppress the level of active viral replication to below the limits of detection (278). Virologic and immunologic data suggest that durable suppression is best seen when using combination therapy with two nucleoside analog RTIs and a potent protease inhibitor (17, 18, 224, 225, 279). Ideally, medication combinations should be chosen based on evidence, when available, of additivity or synergy and on evidence that the drugs possess nonoverlapping toxicities and that the drugs lack antagonistic pharmacokinetic or antiretroviral properties.

Decisions about the choice of initial therapy may be further guided by emerging data on cross-resistance between agents, toxicity profiles, and an individual patient's clinical status and history (276). Indeed, the most important considerations may be how best to avoid the simultaneous development of resistance and how to avoid unacceptable toxicity. Regimens to which resistance develops slowly are preferred, because a limited number of resistance-conferring mutations appears to be induced by nucleosides and protease inhibitors and because cross-resistance can develop within each class of drug. In this regard, data suggest that the emergence of resistance may be slowed by the use of strategies that substantially suppress HIV, preferably to undetectable levels (236). In addition, resistance mutations are only selected under pressure from active agents. As noted earlier, a common misconception is that once protease inhibitors are started, they cannot be stopped or resistance will develop. Actually, once these drugs are discontinued altogether, no evolutionary pressure exists for resistance to develop. By contrast, reducing or skipping doses of drug can create conditions of partial suppression that permit more rapid emergence of resistance. Thus, while these agents are used, one should maintain continuous dosing at the optimal dose level with all drugs, and particularly with the protease inhibitors. If toxicity develops with one of these agents, it is generally better to discontinue the drug than to reduce the dose (276). At that time, one or more alternative drugs may be substituted. Moreover, in selecting a regimen, one should consider the impact of the associated resistance mutations on possible future regimens.

Once a therapeutic regimen is initiated, alterations in therapy may be considered for three main reasons (276). The first is evidence of treatment failure, as demonstrated by clinical disease progression, immunologic data, or virologic data. The 1997 DHHS panel went so far as to recommend that virologic end points of failure include the following: a less than 10-fold (1 $\log_{10}$) decrease in viral burden as measured by plasma HIV RNA level by 4 weeks after initiation of therapy; failure to drop to below detectable limits of detection of the assay within 4 months after initiation of therapy; repeated detection of virus as measured by plasma HIV RNA levels after suppression to below detectable limits; and any reproducible viral load increase at least 10-fold or 1 $\log_{10}$ from viral load nadir without evidence of intercurrent infection or vaccination (278). The International Committee believes that patients who achieve an initial reduction in plasma HIV concentration as great as 1.5 to 2.0 $\log_{10}$, but whose concentration of virus fails to fall below the limits of detection of the assay may continue current therapy with close observation until a confirmed substantial rise above the nadir is noted (279). Other indications to change treatment are the development of toxicity and a patient's inability to tolerate or to comply with a therapeutic regimen. Based on the best available current data, use of a suboptimal treatment regimen would also necessitate a treatment alteration. For example, investigators now know that ZDV monotherapy is suboptimal, and the treatment strategy should be reevaluated for any patient on that regimen. Choices of alternative regimens depend on the prior regimen as well as the reason for changing it. Problems of toxicity should guide the clinician to a regimen with a different toxicity profile. If evidence suggests treatment failure or if a patient's current therapy is suboptimal, a regimen with greater potency, different mechanisms of activity, and non–cross-resistant patterns of resistance should be sought. For patients in whom therapy fails, at least two antiretroviral agents should be changed.

Although multidrug regimens are expensive and may yield considerable cumulative toxicity, substantial evidence recommends their use in patients with HIV infection. However, the long-term durability of such benefits has yet to be determined, and many patients likely will require modifications of therapy in the course of their disease. Thus, although 11 approved antiretroviral agents are available, the number of sequential 3-drug regimens a given patient can take without reusing drugs is limited. For this reason, considerable thought should be given to the regimen chosen, and a continuing need exists for the development of additional therapeutic agents.

FUTURE DIRECTIONS

The development of new RT and protease inhibitors remains an active area of investigation, and some such agents are already in the pipeline. In addition, entirely novel approaches to antiretroviral therapy are currently being investigated. As noted earlier (see Table 45B.1), the process of HIV replication offers multiple potential targets for novel drug therapies.

An example of an alternative strategy for inhibiting HIV replication under investigation is the use of agents such as thalidomide, pentoxifylline, or rolipram that, directly or indirectly, inhibit tumor necrosis factor-α (TNF-α) (286–288). TNF-α activates proviral HIV and promotes the later steps of HIV replication. Thus, although such inhibition would not likely completely inhibit HIV by itself, these agents may be useful in combination with other treatment modalities in a long-term strategy for therapy of HIV disease.

The HIV-1 nucleocapsid protein zinc fingers are among the more novel targets for antiretroviral therapy. These are structural components necessary for both acute infection and virion assembly that are of particular interest because they are highly conserved and thus may be mutationally intolerant (289). In vitro studies of several disulfide-substituted benzamides, which are inhibitors of the HIV-1 nucleocapsid zinc fingers, have demonstrated significant anti-HIV activity, with inhibition of both acute and chronic infection (290).

An intriguing development is the possibility that we may be able to exploit other host factors, such as CCR5, the HIV coreceptor for monocytotropic strains (28–31). The finding that the initial infection with HIV may be prevented by mutation of the gene that encodes this receptor and that individuals with this mutation may be naturally resistant to HIV makes CCR5 an attractive target for antiretroviral therapy. Potential strategies exploiting this discovery may involve the techniques of gene manipulation, the construction of antisense oligoclonal nucleotides, modification or inhibition of the chemokines or other ligands that bind to this receptor, or allogeneic bone marrow transplantation from donors who have a homozygous CCR5 deletion that makes them naturally resistant to infection by monocytotropic HIV strains.

As more is learned about the disease process initiated by infection with HIV, other approaches to therapy probably will emerge. The advances seen during the past few years, however, are substantial. Available strategies have clearly reduced the morbidity of the disease and have prolonged survival. They also offer the potential to customize therapy based on a particular patient's disease status, history of drug toxicity, and viral resistance patterns. Thus, not only have some patients' lives been extended, but also the quality of their lives has improved, and we have begun to see the transformation of HIV infection from an acute process into a chronic disease. Perhaps most heartening is that these therapeutic advances were based on the practical application of rational drug design. Indeed, the success of this approach to the development of new treatments may be the greatest cause for optimism about the future of antiretroviral therapy.

References

1. Mitsuya H, Broder S. Inhibition of the in vitro infectivity and cytopathic effect of human T-lymphotropic virus type III/lymphadenopathy virus-associated virus (HTLV-III/LAV) by 2′,3′-dideoxynucleosides. Proc Natl Acad Sci U S A 1986;83:1911–1915.
2. Mitsuya H, Weinhold KJ, Furman PA, et al. 3′-Azido-3′-deoxythymidine (BW A509U): an antiviral agent that inhibits the infectivity and cytopathic effect of human T-lymphotropic virus type III/lymphadenopathy-associated virus in vitro. Proc Natl Acad Sci U S A 1985;82:7096–7100.
3. Yarchoan R, Klecker RW, Weinhold KJ, et al. Administration of 3′-azido-3′-deoxythymidine, an inhibitor of HTLV-III/LAV replication, to patients with AIDS or AIDS-related complex. Lancet 1986; 1:575–580.
4. Yarchoan R, Perno CF, Thomas RV, et al. Phase I studies of 2′,3′-dideoxycytidine in severe human immunodeficiency virus infection as a single agent and alternating with zidovudine (AZT). Lancet 1988;1:76–81.
5. Merigan TC, Skowron G, Bozzette SA, et al. Circulating p24 antigen levels and responses to dideoxycytidine in human immunodeficiency virus (HIV) infections. Ann Intern Med 1989;110:189–194.
6. Yarchoan R, Mitsuya H, Thomas RV, et al. In vivo activity against HIV and favorable toxicity profile of 2′,3′-dideoxyinosine. Science 1989; 245:412–415.
7. Cooley TP, Kunches LM, Saunders CA, et al. Once-daily administration of 2′,3′-dideoxyinosine (ddI) in patients with the acquired immunodeficiency syndrome or AIDS-related complex. N Engl J Med 1990;322:1340–1345.
8. Lambert JS, Seidlin M, Reichman RC, et al. 2′,3′-Dideoxyinosine (ddI) in patients with the acquired immunodeficiency syndrome or the AIDS-related complex: a phase I trial. N Engl J Med 1990;322:1333–1340.
9. Nguyen B-Y, Yarchoan R, Wyvill KM, et al. Five-year follow-up of a phase I study of didanosine in patients with advanced human immunodeficiency virus infection. J Infect Dis 1995;171:1180–1189.
10. Mitsuya H, Matsukura M, Broder S. Rapid in vitro systems for assessing activity of agents against HTLV-III/LAV. In: Broder S, ed. AIDS: modern concepts and therapeutic challenges. New York: Marcel Dekker, 1987:303–333.
11. Johnson VA, Hirsch MS. New developments in combination chemotherapy of anti-human immunodeficiency virus drugs. Ann N Y Acad Sci 1990;616:318–327.
12. Collier AC, Coombs RW, Fischl MA, et al. Combination therapy with zidovudine and didanosine compared with zidovudine alone in HIV-1 infection. Ann Intern Med 1993;119:786–793.
13. Yarchoan R, Lietzau JA, Nguyen B-Y, et al. A randomized pilot study of alternating or simultaneous zidovudine and didanosine therapy in patients with symptomatic immunodeficiency virus infection. J Infect Dis 1994;169:9–17.

14. Ragni M, Dafni R, Amato DA, et al. Combination zidovudine and dideoxyinosine in asymptomatic HIV(+) patients [abstract Mo15]. In: 8th International Conference on AIDS/3rd STD World Congress, Amsterdam, 1992.
15. Breckenridge A, Seligmann M, Warrell D, et al. DELTA: a randomized double-blind controlled trial comparing combinations of zidovudine plus didanosine or ddC with zidovudine monotherapy in individuals with HIV infection. Lancet 1996;348:293–291.
16. Katzenstein D, Hammer S, Hughes M. The relation of virologic and immunologic markers to clinical outcomes after nucleoside therapy in HIV-infected adults with 200–500 CD4 cells per cubic millimeter. N Engl J Med 1996;335:1091–1098.
17. Suleiman J, Lewi D, Motti E, et al. Antiretroviral activity and safety of indinavir alone and in combination with zidovudine in zidovudine-naive patients with CD4 cell counts of 50–250 cells/mm^3 [abstract]. In: 11th International Conference on AIDS, Vancouver, 1996.
18. Gulick R, Mellors J, Havlir D, et al. Potent and sustained antiretroviral activity of indinavir (IDV) in combination with zidovudine (ZDV) and lamivudine (3TC) [abstract LB7]. In: 3rd Conference on Retroviruses and Opportunistic Infections. Washington, DC: Infectious Disease Society of America for the Foundation for Retrovirology and Human Health, 1996:40.
19. Cameron B, Heath-Chiozzi M, Kravcik S, et al. Prolongation of life and prevention of AIDS in advanced HIV immunodeficiency with ritonavir [abstract LB6a]. In: 3rd Conference on Retroviruses and Opportunistic Infections. Washington, DC: Infectious Disease Society of America for the Foundation for Retrovirology and Human Health, 1996:40.
20. Vella S. Clinical experience with saquinavir. AIDS 1995;9(Suppl 2):S21–S25.
21. Collier AC, Coombs RW, Schoenfeld DA, et al. Treatment of human immunodeficiency virus infection with saquinavir, zidovudine, and zalcitabine. N Engl J Med 1996;334:1011–1017.
22. Ho D, Neumann A, Perelson A, et al. Rapid turnover of plasma virions and CD4 lymphocytes in HIV-1 infection. Nature 1995;373:123–126.
23. Wei X, Ghosh S, Taylor M. Viral dynamics in human immunodeficiency virus type 1 infection. Nature 1995;373:123–126.
24. Havlir D, Richman D. Viral dynamics of HIV: implications for drug development and therapeutic strategies. Ann Intern Med 1996;124:984–994.
25. Fowke K, Nagelkerke N, Kimani J, et al. Resistance to HIV-1 infection among persistently seronegative prostitutes in Nairobi, Kenya. Lancet 1996;348:1347–1351.
26. Samson M, Libert F, Doranz B, et al. Resistance to HIV-1 infection in Caucasian individuals bearing mutant alleles of the CCR-5 chemokine receptor gene. Nature 1996;382:722–725.
27. Mitsuya H, Yarchoan R, Broder S. Molecular targets for AIDS therapy. Science 1990;249:1533–1544.
28. Deng H, Liu R, Ellmeier W, et al. Identification of a major co-receptor for primary isolates of HIV-1. Nature 1996;381:661–666.
29. Dean M, Carrington M, O'Brien S. Genetic restriction of HIV-1 infection and progression to AIDS by a deletion allele of the CKR5 structural gene. Science 1996;273:1856–1862.
30. Premack B, Schall T. Chemokine receptors: gateways to inflammation and infection. Nature Med 1996;2:1174–1118.
31. Weiss R, Clapham P. Hot fusion of HIV. Nature 1996;381:647–648.
32. Moore JP. Coreceptors: implications for HIV pathogenesis and treatment. Science 1997;276:51–52.
33. Smith M, Dean M, Carrington M, et al. Contrasting genetic influence of CCR2 and CCR5 variants on HIV-1 infection and disease progression. Science 1997;277:959–965.
34. Zimmerman TP, Mahony WB, Prus KL. 3'-Azido-3'-deoxythymidine: an unusual nucleoside analogue that permeates the membrane of human erythrocytes and lymphocytes by nonfacilitated diffusion. J Biol Chem 1987;262:5748–5754.
35. Ahluwalia G, Cooney DA, Mitsuya H, et al. Initial studies on the cellular pharmacology of 2',3'-dideoxyinosine, an inhibitor of HIV infectivity. Biochem Pharmacol 1987;36:3797–3800.
36. Cooney DA, Dalal M, Mitsuya H, et al. Initial studies on the cellular pharmacology of 2',3'-dideoxycytidine, an inhibitor of HTLV-III infectivity. Biochem Pharmacol 1986;35:2065–2068.
37. Cooney DA, Ahluwalia G, Mitsuya H, et al. Initial studies on the cellular pharmacology of 2',3'-dideoxyadenosine, an inhibitor of HTLV-III infectivity. Biochem Pharmacol 1987;36:1765–1768.
38. Furman PA, Fyfe JA, St Clair M, et al. Phosphorylation of 3'-azido-3'-deoxythymidine and selective interaction of the 5'-triphosphate with human immunodeficiency virus reverse transcriptase. Proc Natl Acad Sci U S A 1986;83:8333–8337.
39. Hao Z, Cooney DA, Hartmen NR, et al. Factors determining the activity of 2',3'-dideoxynucleosides in suppressing human immunodeficiency virus in vitro. Mol Pharmacol 1988;34:431–435.
40. Cheng Y-C, Dutschman GE, Bastow KF, et al. Human immunodeficiency virus reverse transcriptase: general properties and its interaction with nucleoside triphosphate analogs. J Biol Chem 1987;262:2187–2189.
41. Mitsuya H, Dahlberg JE, Spigelman Z, et al. 2',3'-Dideoxynucleosides: broad spectrum antiretroviral activity and mechanism of action. In: Bolognesi D, ed. Human retroviruses, cancer, and AIDS: approaches to prevention and therapy. New York: Alan R. Liss, 1988:407–421.
42. Perno CF, Yarchoan R, Cooney DA, et al. Inhibition of human immunodeficiency virus (HIV-1/HTLV-III$_{Ba-L}$) replication in fresh and cultured human peripheral blood monocytes/macrophages by azidothymidine and related 2',3'-dideoxynucleosides. J Exp Med 1988;168:1111–1125.
43. Larder BA, Darby G, Richman DD. HIV with reduced sensitivity to zidovudine (AZT) isolated during prolonged therapy. Science 1989;243:1731–1734.
44. Kellam P, Boucher C, Tunagel T, et al. Zidovudine treatment results in the selection of human immunodeficiency virus type 1 variants whose genotypes confer increasing levels of drug resistance. J Gen Virol 1994;75:341–351.
45. Preston BD, Poiesz BJ, Loeb LA. Fidelity of HIV-1 reverse transcriptase. Science 1988;242:1168–1171.
46. Japour J. Antiretroviral drug resistance. AIDS Clin Care 1995;7:63–67.
47. Perelson A, Neumann A, Markowitz M, et al. HIV-1 dynamics in vivo: virion clearance rate, infected cell life-span, and viral generation time. Science 1996;271:1582–1586.
48. Coffin J. HIV population dynamics in vivo: implications for genetic variation, pathogenesis, and therapy. Science 1995;267:483–489.
49. Richman DD, Grimes J, Lagakos S. Effect of stage of disease and drug dose on zidovudine susceptibilities of isolates of human immunodeficiency virus. J Acquir Immune Defic Syndr 1990;3:743–746.
50. Richman DD. Resistance of clinical isolates of human immunodeficiency virus to antiretroviral agents. Antimicrob Agents Chemother 1993;37:1207–1213.
51. Tisdale M, Kemp SD, Parry NR, et al. Rapid in vitro selection of human immunodeficiency virus type 1 resistant to 3'-thiacytidine inhibitors due to a mutation in the YMDD region of reverse transcriptase. Proc Natl Acad Sci U S A 1993;90:5653–5656.
52. Kellam P, Boucher CAB, Larder BA. Fifth mutation in human immunodeficiency virus type 1 reverse transcriptase contributes to the development of high-level resistance to zidovudine. Proc Natl Acad Sci U S A 1992;89:1934–1938.
53. Mayers D. Rational approaches to resistance: nucleoside analogues. AIDS 1996;10(Suppl 1):S9–S13.
54. St Clair MH, Martin JL, Tudor-Williams G, et al. Resistance to ddI and sensitivity to AZT induced by a mutation in HIV-1 reverse transcriptase. Science 1991;253:1557–1559.
55. Schuurman R, Nijhuis M, van Leeuwen R, et al. Rapid changes in human immunodeficiency virus type 1 RNA load and appearance of

drug-resistant virus populations in persons treated with lamivudine (3TC). J Infect Dis 1995;171:1411–1419.
56. Boucher CA, Cammack N, Schipper P, et al. High-level resistance to (2)enantiomeric 2′-deoxy-3′-thiacytidine in vitro is due to one amino acid substitution in the catalytic site of human immunodeficiency virus type 1 reverse transcriptase. Antimicrob Agents Chemother 1993;37:2231–2234.
57. Antunes F, Atkinson M, Clark A, et al. Randomised trial of addition of lamivudine or lamivudine plus loviride to zidovudine-containing regimens for patients with HIV-1 infection: the CAESAR trial. Lancet 1997;349:1413–1421.
58. Eron J, Benoit S, Jemsek J, et al. Treatment with lamivudine, zidovudine, or both in HIV-positive patients with 200 to 500 CD4 cells per cubic millimeter. N Engl J Med 1995;333:1662–1669.
59. Foli A, Sogocio K, Anderson B, et al. In vitro selection and molecular characterization of human immunodeficiency virus type 1 with reduced sensitivity to 9-[2-(phosphonomethoxy)ethyl]adenine (PMEA). Antiviral Res 1996;32:91–98.
60. Gu Z, Gao Q, Fang H, et al. Identification of a mutation at codon 65 in the IKKK motif of reverse transcriptase that encodes human immunodeficiency virus resistance to 2′,3′-dideoxycytidine and 2′,3′-dideoxy-3′-thiacytidine. Antimicrob Agents Chemother 1994;38:275–281.
61. Gu Z, Salomon H, Cherrington JM, et al. K65R mutation of human immunodeficiency virus type 1 reverse transcriptase encodes cross-resistance to 9-(2-phosphonylmethoxyethyl)adenine. Antimicrob Agents Chemother 1995;39:1888–1891.
62. Gu Z, Arts EJ, Parniak MA, et al. Mutated K65R recombinant reverse transcriptase of human immunodeficiency virus type 1 shows diminished chain termination in the presence of 2′,3′-dideoxycytidine 5′-triphosphate and other drugs. Proc Natl Acad Sci U S A 1995;92:2760–2764.
63. Wainberg M, Drosopoulos W, Prasad V. Enhanced fidelity of 3TC-selected mutant HIV-1 reverse transcriptase. Science 1996;271:1282–1285.
64. Iversen A, Shafer R, Wehrly K, et al. Multidrug-resistant human immunodeficiency virus type 1 strains resulting from combination antiretroviral therapy. J Virol 1996;70:1086–1090.
65. Shafer R, Iversen A, Winters M, et al. Drug resistance and heterogeneous long-term virologic responses of human immunodeficiency virus type 1–infected subjects to zidovudine and didanosine combination therapy. J Infect Dis 1995;172:70–78.
66. Shirasaka T, Kavlick MF, Ueno T, et al. Emergence of human immunodeficiency virus type 1 variants with resistance to multiple dideoxynucleosides in patients receiving therapy with dideoxynucleosides. Proc Natl Acad Sci U S A 1995;92:2398–2402.
67. Horwitz JP, Chua J, Noel M. Nucleosides. V. The monomesylates of 1-(2′-deoxy-β-D-lyxofuranosyl)thymidine. J Org Chem 1964;29:2076–2078.
68. Gao W-Y, Shirasaka T, Johns DG, et al. Differential phosphorylation of azidothymidine, dideoxycytidine, and dideoxyinosine in resting and activated peripheral blood mononuclear cells. J Clin Invest 1993;91:2326–2333.
69. Perno C-F, Cooney DA, Gao W-Y, et al. Effects of bone marrow stimulatory cytokines on human immunodeficiency virus replication and the antiviral activity of dideoxynucleosides in cultures of monocyte/macrophages. Blood 1992;80:995–1003.
70. Klecker RW Jr, Collins JM, Yarchoan R, et al. Plasma and cerebrospinal fluid pharmacokinetics of 3′-azido-3′-deoxythymidine: a novel pyrimidine analog with potential application for the treatment of patients with AIDS and related diseases. Clin Pharmacol Ther 1987;41:407–412.
71. Langtry HD, Campoli-Richards DM. Zidovudine: a review of its pharmacodynamic and pharmacokinetic properties and therapeutic efficacy. Drugs 1989;37:408–450.
72. Yarchoan R, Broder S. Strategies for the pharmacological intervention against HTLV-III/LAV. In: Broder S, ed. AIDS: modern concepts and therapeutic challenges. New York: Marcel Dekker, 1987:335–360.
73. Unadkat JD, Collier AC, Crosby SS, et al. Pharmacokinetics of oral zidovudine (azidothymidine) in patients with AIDS when administered with and without a high-fat meal. AIDS 1990;4:229–232.
74. Blum MR, Liao SH, Good SS, et al. Pharmacokinetics and bioavailability of zidovudine in humans. Am J Med 1988;85(Suppl 2A):189–194.
75. Henry K, Chinnock BJ, Quinn RP, et al. Concurrent zidovudine levels in semen and serum determined by radioimmunoassay in patients with AIDS or AIDS-related complex. JAMA 1988;259:3023–3026.
76. Rolinski B, Wintergerst U, Matuschke A, et al. Evaluation of saliva as a specimen for monitoring therapy in HIV-infected patients. AIDS 1991;5:858–888.
77. Yarchoan R, Broder S. Development of antiretroviral therapy for the acquired immunodeficiency syndrome and related disorders: a progress report. N Engl J Med 1987;316:557–564.
78. Brouwers P, Moss H, Wolters P, et al. Effect of continuous-infusion zidovudine therapy on neuropsychologic functioning in children with symptomatic human immunodeficiency virus infection. J Pediatr 1990;117:980–985.
79. Pizzo PA, Eddy J, Falloon J, et al. Effect of continuous intravenous infusion zidovudine (AZT) in children with symptomatic HIV infection. N Engl J Med 1988;319:889–896.
80. Schmitt FA, Bigley JW, McKinnis R, et al. Neuropsychological outcome of zidovudine (AZT) treatment of patients with AIDS and AIDS-related complex. N Engl J Med 1988;319:1573–1578.
81. Yarchoan R, Berg G, Brouwers P, et al. Response of human-immunodeficiency-virus-associated neurological disease to 3′-azido-3′-deoxythymidine. Lancet 1987;1:132–135.
82. Singlas E, Pioger J-C, Taburet A-M, et al. Zidovudine disposition in patients with severe renal impairment: influence of hemodialysis. Clin Pharmacol Ther 1989;46:190–197.
83. Fischl MA, Richman DD, Grieco MH, et al. The efficacy of azidothymidine (AZT) in the treatment of patients with AIDS and AIDS-related complex: a double-blind, placebo-controlled trial. N Engl J Med 1987;317:185–191.
84. Richman DD, Fischl MA, Grieco MH, et al. The toxicity of azidothymidine (AZT) in the treatment of patients with AIDS and AIDS-related complex: a double-blind, placebo-controlled trial. N Engl J Med 1987;317:192–197.
85. Volberding PA, Lagakos SW, Koch MA, et al. Zidovudine in asymptomatic human immunodeficiency virus infection: a controlled trial in persons with fewer than 500 CD4–positive cells per cubic millimeter. N Engl J Med 1990;322:941–949.
86. Seligmann M, Warrell D, Darbyshire J, et al. Concorde: MRC/ANRS randomised double-blind controlled trial of immediate and deferred zidovudine in symptom-free HIV infection. Lancet 1994;343:871–881.
87. Connor E, Mofenson L. Zidovudine for the reduction of perinatal human immunodeficiency virus transmission: Pediatric AIDS Clinical Trials Group Protocol 076—results and treatment recommendations. Pediatr Infect Dis J 1995;14:536–541.
88. Rarick MU, Espina B, Montgomery T, et al. The long-term use of zidovudine in patients with severe immune-mediated thrombocytopenia secondary to infection with HIV. AIDS 1991;5:1357–1361.
89. Perno CF, Yarchoan R, Cooney DA, et al. Replication of human immunodeficiency virus in monocytes: granulocyte/macrophage colony-stimulating factor (GM-CSF) potentiates viral production yet enhances the antiviral effect mediated by 3′-azido-2′3′-dideoxythymidine (AZT) and other dideoxynucleoside congeners of thymidine. J Exp Med 1989;169:933–951.
90. Hammer S, Katzenstein D, Hughes M, et al. A trial comparing nucleoside monotherapy with combination therapy in HIV-infected adults with CD4 cell counts from 200 to 500 per cubic millimeter. N Engl J Med 1996;335:1091–1098.
91. Choo V. Combination superior to zidovudine in Delta trial. Lancet 1995;346:895.

92. Gazzard B. Further results from European/Australian Delta trial. In: 3rd Conference on Retroviruses and Opportunistic Infections. Washington, DC: Infectious Disease Society of America for the Foundation for Retrovirology and Human Health, 1996:43.
93. Saravolatz L, Winslow D, Abrams D, et al. Zidovudine alone or in combination with didanosine or zalcitabine in HIV-infected patients with the acquired immunodeficiency syndrome or fewer then 200 CD4 cells per cubic millimeter. N Engl J Med 1996;335:1099–1106.
94. Gao W, Agbaria R, Driscoll JS, et al. Divergent anti-human immunodeficiency virus activity and anabolic phosphorylation of 2′,3′-dideoxynucleoside analogs in resting and activated human cells. J Biol Chem 1994;269:12,633–12,638.
95. Shirasaka T, Yarchoan R, O'Brien MC, et al. Changes in drug-sensitivity of human immunodeficiency virus type 1 during therapy with azidothymidine, dideoxycytidine, or dideoxyinosine: an in vitro comparative study. Proc Natl Acad Sci U S A 1993;90:562–566.
96. Anonymous. A note to physicians: important information on the combination of zidovudine (ZDV) and stavudine (d4T) in ZDV-experienced HIV-infected patients. Bethesda, MD: National Institute of Allergy and Infectious Diseases, 1996.
97. Dournon E, Matheron S, Rozenbaum W, et al. Effects of zidovudine in 365 consecutive patients with AIDS or AIDS-related complex. Lancet 1988;2:1297–1302.
98. Fischl M, Parker C, Pettinelli C, et al. A randomized controlled trial of a reduced daily dose of zidovudine in patients with acquired immunodeficiency syndrome. N Engl J Med 1990;323:1009–1014.
99. Fischl M, Richman DD, Hansen N, et al. The safety and efficacy of zidovudine (AZT) in the treatment of subjects with mildly symptomatic human immunodeficiency virus type I (HIV) infection: a double-blind, placebo controlled trial. Ann Intern Med 1990;112:727–737.
100. Fischl M, Galpin JE, Levine JD, et al. Recombinant human erythropoietin for patients with AIDS treated with zidovudine. N Engl J Med 1990;322:1488–1493.
101. Levine JD, Allan JD, Tessitore JH, et al. Recombinant human granulocyte-macrophage colony-stimulating factor ameliorates zidovudine-induced neutropenia in patients with acquired immunodeficiency syndrome (AIDS)/AIDS-related complex. Blood 1991;78:3148–3154.
102. Pluda JM, Yarchoan R, Smith PD, et al. Subcutaneous recombinant granulocyte-macrophage colony-stimulating factor used as a single agent and in an alternating regimen with azidothymidine in leukopenic patients with severe human immunodeficiency virus infection. Blood 1990;76:463–472.
103. Starnes MC, Cheng Y-C. Cellular metabolism of 2′,3′-dideoxycytidine, a compound active against human immunodeficiency virus in vitro. J Biol Chem 1987;262:988–991.
104. Waqar MA, Evans MJ, Manly KF, et al. Effects of 2′,3′-dideoxynucleosides on mammalian cells and viruses. J Cell Physiol 1984;121:402–408.
105. Dalakas MC, Illa I, Pezeshkpour GH, et al. Mitochondrial myopathy caused by long-term zidovudine therapy. N Engl J Med 1990;322:1098–1105.
106. Mhiri C, Baudrimont M, Bonne G, et al. Zidovudine myopathy: a distinctive disorder associated with mitochondrial dysfunction. Ann Neurol 1991;29:606–614.
107. Chattha G, Arieff AI, Cummings C, et al. Lactic acidosis complicating the acquired immunodeficiency syndrome. Ann Intern Med 1993;118:37–39.
108. Freiman JP, Helfert KE, Hamrell MR, et al. Hepatomegaly with severe steatosis in HIV-seropositive patients. AIDS 1993;7:379–385.
109. Meng T-C, Fischl MA, Boota AM, et al. A phase I/II study of combination therapy with zidovudine and dideoxycytidine in subjects with advanced human immunodeficiency virus (HIV) disease. Ann Intern Med 1992;116:13–20.
110. Groak SP, Hood AF, Nelson K. Nail pigmentation associated with zidovudine. J Am Acad Dermatol 1989;21:1032–1033.
111. Edwards P, Turner J, Gold J, et al. Esophageal ulceration induced by zidovudine. Ann Intern Med 1990;112:65–66.
112. Herskowitz A, Willoughby SB, Baughman KL, et al. Cardiomyopathy associated with antiretroviral therapy in patients with HIV infection: a report of six cases. Ann Intern Med 1992;116:3111–3113.
113. Lalonde RG, Dechenes JG, Seamone C. Zidovudine-induced macular edema. Ann Intern Med 1991;114:297–298.
114. de Miranda P, Good SS, Yarchoan R, et al. Alteration of zidovudine pharmacokinetics by probenecid in patients with AIDS or AIDS-related complex. Clin Pharmacol Ther 1989;46:494–500.
115. Kornhauser DM, Petty BG, Hendrix CW, et al. Probenecid and zidovudine metabolism. Lancet 1989;2:473–475.
116. Hedaya MA, Elmquist WF, Sawchuk RJ. Probenecid inhibits the metabolic and renal clearances of zidovudine (AZT) in human volunteers. Pharmacol Res 1990;7:411–417.
117. Baba M, Snoeck R, Pauwels R, et al. Sulfated polysaccharides are potent and selective inhibitors of various enveloped viruses, including herpes simplex virus, cytomegalovirus, vesicular stomatitis virus, and human immunodeficiency virus. Antimicrob Agents Chemother 1988;32:1742–1745.
118. Vogt MW, Hartshorn KL, Furman PA, et al. Ribavirin antagonizes the effect of azidothymidine on HIV replication. Science 1987;235:1376–1379.
119. Mitsuya H, Jarrett RF, Matsukura M, et al. Long-term inhibition of human T-lymphotropic virus type III/lymphadenopathy-associated virus (human immunodeficiency virus) DNA synthesis and RNA expression in T cells protected by 2′,3′-dideoxynucleosides in vitro. Proc Natl Acad Sci U S A 1987;84:2033–2037.
120. Lori F, Malykh A, Cara A, et al. Hydroxyurea as an inhibitor of human immunodeficiency virus-type 1 replication. Science 1994;266:801–805.
121. Hartman NR, Yarchoan R, Pluda JM, et al. Pharmacokinetics of 2′,3′-dideoxyadenosine and 2′,3′-dideoxyinosine in patients with severe HIV infection. Clin Pharmacol Ther 1990;47:647–654.
122. Balis FM, Pizzo RA, Butler KM, et al. Clinical pharmacology of 2′,3′-dideoxyinosine in human immunodeficiency virus-infected children. J Infect Dis 1992;165:99–104.
123. Knupp CA, Shyu WC, Dolin R, et al. Pharmacokinetics of didanosine in patients with acquired immunodeficiency syndrome or acquired immunodeficiency syndrome-related complex. Clin Pharmacol Ther 1991;49:523–535.
124. Yarchoan R, Mitsuya H, Pluda J, et al. The National Cancer Institute phase I study of ddI administration in adults with AIDS or AIDS-related complex: analysis of activity and toxicity profiles. Rev Infect Dis 1990;12(Suppl 5):S522–S533.
125. Ahluwalia G, Johnson MA, Fridland A, et al. Cellular pharmacology of the anti-HIV agent 2′,3′-dideoxyadenosine. In: Proceedings of the American Association for Cancer Research meeting, New Orleans, 1988:345.
126. Singlas E, Taburet AM, Borsa LF, et al. Didanosine pharmacokinetics in patients with normal and impaired renal function: influence of hemodialysis. Antimicrob Agents Chemother 1992;36:1519–24.
127. Pons JC, Boubon MC, Taburet AM, et al. Fetoplacental passage of 2′,3′-dideoxyinosine. Lancet 1991;337:732.
128. Connolly KJ, Allan JD, Fitch H, et al. Phase I study of 2′,3′-dideoxyinosine (ddI) administered orally twice daily to patients with AIDS or AIDS-related complex and hematologic intolerance to zidovudine. Am J Med 1991;91:471–478.
129. Ragni M, Amato D, LoFaro M, et al. Randomized study of didanosine monotherapy and combination therapy with zidovudine in hemophilic and nonhemophilic subjects with asymptomatic human immunodeficiency virus-1 infection. Blood 1995;85:2337–2346.
130. Lambert JS, Seidlin M, Valentine FT, et al. Didanosine: long term follow-up of patients in a phase I study. Clin Infect Dis 1993;16:S40–S44.
131. Dolin R, Amato D, Fischl M, et al. Efficacy of didanosine (ddI) versus zidovudine (ZDV) in patients with no or < 16 weeks of prior ZVD therapy. In: 9th International Conference on AIDS, Berlin, 1993:67.

132. Kahn JO, Lagakos SW, Richman DD, et al. A controlled trial comparing continued zidovudine with didanosine in human immunodeficiency virus infection. N Engl J Med 1992;327:581–587.
133. Yarchoan R, Pluda JM, Thomas RV, et al. Long-term toxicity/activity profile of 2′,3′-dideoxyinosine in AIDS or AIDS-related complex. Lancet 1990;2:526–529.
134. Yarchoan R, Thomas RV, Mitsuya H, et al. Initial clinical studies of 2′,3′-dideoxyadenosine (ddA) and 2′,3′-dideoxyinosine (ddI) in patients with AIDS or AIDS-related complex (ARC). J Cell Biochem 1989;313(Suppl 13B):313–316.
135. Whitcup SM, Butler KM, Caruso R, et al. Retinal toxicity in human immunodeficiency virus-infected children treated with 2′,3′-dideoxyinosine. Am J Ophthalmol 1992;113:1–7.
136. Metroka CE, McMechan MF, Andrada R, et al. Failure of prophylaxis with dapsone in patients taking dideoxyinosine [letter]. Lancet 1991;325:737.
137. Klecker RW Jr, Collins JM, Yarchoan R, et al. Pharmacokinetics of 2′,3′-dideoxycytidine in patients with AIDS and related disorders. J Clin Pharmacol 1988;28:837–842.
138. Whittington R, Brogden RN. Zalcitabine: a review of its pharmacology and clinical potential in acquired immunodeficiency syndrome. Drugs 1992;44:656–683.
139. Gustavson LE, Fukuda EK, Rubio FA, et al. A pilot study of the bioavailability and pharmacokinetics of 2′,3′-dideoxycytidine in patients with AIDS or AIDS-related complex. J Acquir Immune Defic Syndr 1990;3:28–31.
140. Bozzette S, Kanouse D, Berry S, et al. Health status and function with zidovudine or zalcitabine as initial therapy for AIDS: a randomized controlled trial. Roche 3300/ACTG 114 Study Group. JAMA 1995;273:295–301.
141. Fischl MA, Olson RM, Follansbee SE, et al. Zalcitabine compared with zidovudine in patients with advanced HIV-1 infection who received previous zidovudine therapy. Ann Intern Med 1993;118:762–769.
142. Abrams DI, Goldman AI, Launer C, et al. A comparative trial of didanosine or zalcitabine after treatment with zidovudine in patients with human immunodeficiency virus infection. N Engl J Med 1994;330:657–662.
143. Pizzo PA, Butler K, Balis F, et al. Dideoxycytidine alone and in an alternating schedule with zidovudine (AZT) in children with symptomatic human immunodeficiency virus infection. J Pediatr 1990;117:799–808.
144. Skowron G, Bozzette SA, Lim L, et al. Alternating and intermittent regimens of zidovudine and dideoxycytidine in patients with AIDS or AIDS-related complex. Ann Intern Med 1993;118:321–330.
145. Murphy R. Clinical aspects of human immunodeficiency virus disease: clinical rationale for treatment. J Infect Dis 1995;171(Suppl 2):S81–7.
146. Fitzgibbon JE, Howell RM, Haberzettl CA, et al. Human immunodeficiency virus type 1 pol gene mutations which cause decreased susceptibility to 2′,3′-dideoxycytidine. Antimicrob Agents Chemother 1992;36:153–157.
147. Sogocio KM, Foli A, Anderson B, et al. HIV-1 develops reduced sensitivity to 9-(2-phosphonylmethoxyethyl) adenine (PMEA) in vitro through acquisition of K65R. In: Bolognesi D, ed. AIDS research and human retroviruses. Bethesda, MD: Mary Ann Liebert, 1995:S164.
148. Broder S. Pharmacodynamics of 2′,3′-dideoxycytidine: an inhibitor of human immunodeficiency virus. Am J Med 1990;88(Suppl 5B):2S–7S.
149. Dubinsky RM, Yarchoan R, Dalakas M, et al. Reversible axonal neuropathy from the treatment of AIDS and related disorders with 2′,3′-dideoxycytidine (ddC). Muscle Nerve 1989;12:856–860.
150. Yarchoan R, Mitsuya H, Myers CE, et al. Clinical pharmacology of 3′-azido-2′,3′-dideoxythymidine (zidovudine) and related dideoxynucleosides. N Engl J Med 1989;321:726–738.
151. Indorf AS, Pegram PS. Esophageal ulceration related to zalcitabine (ddC). Ann Intern Med 1992;117:133–134.
152. Balzarini J, Kang G-J, Dalal M, et al. The anti-HTLVIII (anti-HIV) and cytotoxic activity of 2′,3′-didehydro-2′,3′-dideoxynucleosides: a comparison with their partental 2′,3′-dideoxynucleosides. Mol Pharmacol 1987;32:162–167.
153. Hamamoto Y, Nakashima H, Matsui T, et al. Inhibitory effect of 2′,3′-didehydro-2′,3′-dideoxynucleosides on infectivity, cytopathic effects, and replication of human immunodeficiency virus. Antimicrob Agents Chemother 1987;31:907–910.
154. Lin TS, Schinazi RF, Prusoff WH. Potent and selective in vitro activity of 3′-deoxythymidin-2′-ene (3′-deoxy-2′,3′-didehydrothymidine) against human immunodeficiency virus. Biochem Pharmacol 1987;36:2713–2718.
155. Ho HT, Hitchcock MJ. Cellular pharmacology of 2′,3′-dideoxy-2′,3′-didehydrothymidine, a nucleoside analog active against human immunodeficiency virus. Antimicrob Agents Chemother 1989;33:844–849.
156. Lea AP, Faulds D. Stavudine: a review of its pharmacodynamic and pharmacokinetic properties and clinical potential in HIV infection. Drugs 1996;51:846–864.
157. Browne MJ, Mayer KH, Chafee SBD, et al. 2′,3′-Didehydro-3′-deoxythymidine (d4T) in patients with AIDS or AIDS-related complex: a phase I trial. J Infect Dis 1993;167:21–29.
158. Murray HW, Squires KE, Weiss W, et al. Stavudine in patients with AIDS and AIDS-related complex: AIDS clinical trials group 089. J Infect Dis 1995;171(Suppl 2):S123–S130.
159. Petersen EA, Ramirez-Ronda CH, Hardy WD, et al. Dose-related activity of stavudine in patients infected with human immunodeficiency virus. J Infect Dis 1995;171(Suppl 2):S131–S139.
160. Riddler SA, Anderson RE, Mellors JW. Antiretroviral activity of stavudine (2′,3′-didehydro-3′-deoxythymidine, d4T). Antiviral Res 1995;27:189–203.
161. Simpson DM, Tagliati M. Nucleoside analogue-associated peripheral neuropathy in human immunodeficiency virus infection. J Acquir Immune Defic Syndr Hum Retrovirol 1995;9:153–161.
162. Hoggard P, Kewn S, Barry M, et al. Effects of drugs on 2′,3′-dideoxy-2′,3′-didehydrothymidine phosphorylation in vitro. Antimicrob Agents Chemother 1997;41:1231–1236.
163. Soudeyns H, Yao X-J, Gao Q, et al. Anti-human immunodeficiency type 1 activity and in vitro toxicity of 2′-deoxy-3′-thiacytidine (BCH-189), a novel heterocyclic nucleoside analog. Antimicrob Agents Chemother 1991;35:1386–1390.
164. Coates JA, Cammack N, Jenkinson HJ, et al. The separated enantiomers of 2′-deoxy-3′-thiacytidine (BCH 189) both inhibit human immunodeficiency virus replication in vitro. Antimicrob Agents Chemother 1992;36:202–205.
165. Schinazi RF, Chu CK, Peck A, et al. Activities of four optical isomers of 2′,3′-dideoxy-3′-thiacytidine (BCH-189) against human immunodeficiency virus type 1 in human lymphocytes. Antimicrob Agents Chemother 1992;36:672–676.
166. van Leeuwen R, Lange JMA, Hussey EK, et al. The safety and pharmacokinetics of a reverse transcriptase inhibitor, 3TC, in patients with HIV infection: a phase I study. AIDS 1992;6:1471–1475.
167. Pluda J, Cooley T, Montaner J, et al. A phase I/II study of 2′-dioxy-3′-thiacytidine (lamivudine) in patients with advanced human immunodeficiency virus infection. J Infect Dis 1995;171:1438–1447.
168. Lewis L, Venzon D, Church J, et al. Phase I/II study of lamivudine in children. J Infect Dis 1996;174:16–25.
169. Balzarini J, Naesens L, Slachmuylders J, et al. 9-(2-Phosphonylmethoxyethyl)adenine (PMEA) effectively inhibits retrovirus replication in vitro and simian immunodeficiency virus infection in rhesus monkeys. AIDS 1991;5:21–28.
170. De Clercq E. Broad-spectrum anti-DNA virus and anti-retrovirus activity of phosphonylmethoxyalkylpurines and pyrimidines. Biochem Pharmacol 1991;42:963–972.
171. Foster SA, Cerny J, Cheng Y. Herpes simplex virus-specified DNA polymerase is the target for the antiviral action of 9-(2-phosphonylmethoxyethyl)adenine. J Biol Chem 1991;266:238–244.

172. De Clercq E, Yamamoto N, Pauwels R. Marked in vivo antiretrovirus activity of 9-(2-phosphonylmethoxy-ethyl)adenine, a selective anti-human immunodeficiency virus agent. Proc Natl Acad Sci U S A 1989;86:332–336.
173. Cherrington J, Mulato A, Fuller M, et al. Novel mutation (K70E) in human immunodeficiency virus type 1 reverse transcriptase confers decreased susceptibility to 9-[2-(phosphonomethoxy) ethyl] adenine in vitro. Antimicrob Agents Chemother 1996;40:2212–2216.
174. Deeks S, Collier A, Lalezari J, et al. A randomized, double-blind, placebo-controlled study of bis-POM-PMEA in HIV-infected patients [abstract 407]. In: 3rd Conference on Retroviruses and Opportunistic Infections. Washington, DC: Infectious Disease Society of America for the Foundation for Retrovirology and Human Health, 1996:129.
175. Tsai CC, Follis KE, Sabo A, et al. Prevention of SIV infection in macaques by (R)-9-(2-phosphonylmethoxypropyl)adenine. Science 1995;270:1197–1199.
176. Johns DG, Driscoll J. 2-β-fluoro-2′,3′-dideoxyadenosine (F-DDA): a new anti-HIV clinical drug candidate [abstract]. In: 11th International Conference on AIDS, Vancouver, 1996:68.
177. Marquez VE, Tseng CK-H, Driscoll JS, et al. 2′,3′-Dideoxy-2′-fluoro-ara-A: an acid-stable purine nucleoside active against human immunodeficiency virus (HIV). Biochem Pharmacol 1987;36:2719–2722.
178. Tanaka MSR, Ueno T, Kavlick MF, et al. In vitro induction of human immunodeficiency virus type 1 variants resistant to 2′-beta-fluoro-2′,3′-dideoxyadenosine. Antimicrob Agents Chemother 1997;41:1313–1318.
179. Saag M. Preliminary data on the safety and antiviral effect of 1592U89, alone and in combination with zidovudine [abstract]. In: 11th International Conference on AIDS, Vancouver, 1996:225.
180. Tisdale M, Parry N, Cousens D, et al. Anti-HIV activity of (1S,4R)-4 [2-amino-6-(cyclopropylamino)-9H-purin-9-yl]-2-cyclopentene-1-methanol (159U89). In: 34th Interscience Conference on Antimicrobial Agents and Chemotherapy, Orlando, FL, 1994.
181. Harrigan R, Stone C, Griffin P, et al. Antiretroviral activity and resistance profile of the carbocyclic nucleoside HIV reverse transcriptase inhibitor 1592U89 [abstract 15]. In: 4th Conference on Retroviruses and Opportunistic Infections. Washington, DC: Infectious Disease Society of America for the Foundation for Retrovirology and Human Health, 1997.
182. Goldman ME, Nunberg JH, O'Brien JA, et al. Pyridinone derivatives: Specific human immunodeficiency virus type 1 reverse transcriptase inhibitors with antiviral activity. Proc Natl Acad Sci U S A 1991;88:6863–6867.
183. Merluzzi VJ, Hargrave KD, Labadia M, et al. Inhibition of HIV-1 replication by a nonnucleoside reverse transcriptase inhibitor. Science 1990;250:1411–1413.
184. Pauwels R, Andries K, Desmyter J, et al. Potent and selective inhibition of HIV-1 replication in vitro by a novel series of TIBO derivatives. Nature 1990;343:470–474.
185. De Clercq E. Basic approaches to anti-retroviral treatment. J Acquir Immune Defic Syndr 1991;4:207–218.
186. De Clercq E. Non-nucleoside reverse transcriptase inhibitors (NNRTIs) for the treatment of human immunodeficiency virus type 1 (HIV-1) infections: strategies to overcome drug resistance development. Med Res Rev 1996;16:125–157.
187. Kohlstaedt LA, Wang J, Friedman JM, et al. Crystal structure at 3.5 Å resolution of HIV-1 reverse transcriptase complexed with an inhibitor. Science 1992;256:1783–1790.
188. Richman D, Shih C-K, Lowy I, et al. Human immunodeficiency virus type 1 mutants resistant to nonnucleoside inhibitors reverse transcriptase arise in tissue culture. Proc Natl Acad Sci U S A 1991;88:11,241–11,245.
189. Myers M, et al. Combination antiretroviral therapy with Viramune (nevirapine). In: Proceedings of the 22nd AIDS Clinical Trials Groups Meeting, Washington, DC, 1996.
190. D'Aquila R, Hughes M, Hirsch M. Nevirapine, zidovudine, and didanosine compared with zidovudine and didanosine in patients with HIV-1 infection. Ann Intern Med 1996;124:1019–1030.
191. Richman D, Havlir D, Corbeil J. Nevirapine resistance mutations of HIV selected during therapy. J Virol 1994;68:1660–1666.
192. Larder B. 3′-Azido-3′ deoxythymidine resistance suppressed by a mutation conferring human immunodeficiency virus type 1 resistance to nonnucleoside reverse transcriptase inhibitors. Antimicrob Agents Chemother 1992;36:2664–2669.
193. Condra J, Holder D, Emini E. Bi-directional inhibition of HIV-1 drug resistance selection by combination therapy with indinavir and reverse transcriptase inhibitors [abstract]. In: 11th International Conference on AIDS, Vancouver, 1996.
194. Erickson D. Induction of drug-metabolizing enzymes in rat liver by BI-RG-587. In: Pharmaceuticals B-I, ed. Nevirapine investigator's brochure. Ridgefield, CT: Roxane Laboratories, 1994:24–31.
195. Cheeseman SH, Hattox SE, McLaughlin MM, et al. Pharmacokinetics of nevirapine: initial single-rising-dose study in humans. Antimicrob Agents Chemother 1993;37:178–182.
196. Viramune (nevirapine) package insert. Ridgefield, CT, Roxane Laboratories, 1996.
197. Murphy R, Montaner J. Nevirapine: a review of its development, pharmacological profile and potential for clinical use. Exp Opin Invest Drugs 1996;5:1183–1199.
198. Freimuth W. Delavirdine mesylate, a potent non-nucleoside HIV-1 reverse transcriptase inhibitor. Adv Exp Med Biol 1996;394:279–289.
199. Demeter L, Shafer R, Para M, et al. Delavirdine (DLV) susceptibility of HIV-1 isolates obtained from patients (pts) receiving DLV monotherapy (ACTG 260) [abstract]. In: 3rd Conference on Retroviruses and Opportunistic Infections. Washington, DC: Infectious Disease Society of America for the Foundation for Retrovirology and Human Health, 1996:43.
200. Kleim J, Bender R, Kirsch R, et al. Mutational analysis of residue 190 of human immunodeficiency virus type 1 reverse transcriptase. Virology 1994;200:696–701.
201. Sardana VV, Emini EA, Gotlib L, et al. Functional analysis of HIV-1 reverse transcriptase amino acids involved in resistance to multiple nonnucleoside inhibitors. J Biol Chem 1992;267:17,526–17,530.
202. Dueweke T. A mutation in reverse transcriptase of bis(heteroaryl) piperazine-resistant human immunodeficiency virus type 1 that confers increased sensitivity to other nonnucleoside inhibitors. Proc Natl Acad Sci U S A 1993;90:4713–4717.
203. Freimuth W, Chuang-Stein C, Greenwald C, et al. Delavirdine combined with zidovudine or didanosine produces sustained reduction in viral burden and increases in CD4 count in early and advanced HIV-1 infection [abstract]. In: 3rd Conference on Retroviruses and Opportunistic Infections. Washington, DC: Infectious Disease Society of America for the Foundation for Retrovirology and Human Health, 1996:43.
204. Cox S, Batts D, Steward F, et al. Evaluation of the pharmacokinetic (PK) interaction between saquinavir (SQV) and delavirdine (DLV) in healthy volunteers [abstract]. In: 4th Conference on Retroviruses and Opportunistic Infections. Washington, DC: Infectious Disease Society of America for the Foundation for Retrovirology and Human Health, 1997.
205. Ferry J, Herman B, Cox S, et al. Delavirdine and indinavir: a pharmacokinetic drug–drug interaction study in healthy adult volunteers [abstract]. In: 4th Conference on Retroviruses and Opportunistic Infections. Washington, DC: Infectious Disease Society of America for the Foundation for Retrovirology and Human Health, 1997.
206. Kramer RA, Schaber MD, Skalka AM, et al. HTLV-III gag protein is processed in yeast cells by the virus pol-protease. Science 1986;231:1580–1584.
207. Erickson J, Neidhart DJ, VanDrie J, et al. Design, activity, and 2.8 Å crystal structure of a C_2 symmetric inhibitor complexed to HIV-1 protease. Science 1990;249:527–533.

208. Meek TD, Lambert DM, Dreyer GB, et al. Inhibition of HIV-1 protease in infected T-lymphocytes by synthetic peptide analogues. Nature 1990;343:90–92.
209. Navia M, Fitzgerald P, McKever B, et al. Three dimensional structure of aspartyl protease from HIV-1. Nature 1989;377:615–620.
210. Weber I, Miller M, Jaskolski M, et al. Molecular modeling of the HIV-1 protease and its substrate binding site. Science 1989;243:928–931.
211. Wlodawer A, Miller M, Jaskolski M, et al. Conserved folding in retroviral proteases: crystal structure of a synthetic HIV-1 protease. Science 1989;245:616–621.
212. Lam PYS, Jadhav PK, Eyermann CJ, et al. Rational design of potent, bioavailable, non-peptide cyclic ureas as HIV protease inhibitors. Science 1994;263:380–384.
213. Thaisrivongs S, Watenpaugh K, Howe W, et al. Structure-based design of novel HIV protease inhibitors: carboxamide-containing 4-hydroxycoumarins and 4-hydroxy-2-pyrones as potent nonpeptidic inhibitors. J Med Chem 1995;38:3624–3637.
214. Thaisrivongs S, Janakiraman M, Chong K, et al. Structure-based design of novel HIV protease inhibitors: sulfonamide-containing 4-hydroxycoumarins and 4-hydroxy-2-pyrones as potent non-peptidic inhibitors. J Med Chem 1996;39:1400–1410.
215. Debouck C. The HIV-1 protease as a therapeutic target for AIDS. AIDS Res Hum Retroviruses 1992;8:153–164.
216. Tisdale M, Myers R, Maschera B. Cross-resistance analysis of HIV-1 variants individually selected for resistance to five different protease inhibitors. Antimicrob Agents Chemother 1995;39:1704–1710.
217. Molla A, Korneyeva M, Kempf D. Ordered accumulation of mutations in HIV protease confers resistance to ritonavir. Nature Med 1996;2:760–766.
218. Chen Z, Li Y, Schock H. Three-dimensional structure of a HIV protease displaying resistance to all protease inhibitors in clinical trials. J Biol Chem 1995;270:21,433–21,436.
219. Condra JH, Schleif WA, Blahy OM, et al. In vivo emergence of HIV-1 variants resistant to multiple protease inhibitors. Nature 1995;374:569–571.
220. Jacobsen H, Hanggi M, Ott M, et al. In vivo resistance to a human immunodeficiency virus type 1 proteinase inhibitor: mutations, kinetics, and frequencies. J Infect Dis 1996;173:1379–1387.
221. Patick A, Mo H, Markowitz M, et al. Antiviral and resistance studies of AG1343, an orally bioavailable inhibitor of human immunodeficiency virus protease. Antimicrob Agents Chemother 1996;40:292–297.
222. Gulnik S, Suvorov L, Lie B, et al. Kinetic characterization and cross-resistance patterns of HIV-1 protease mutants selected under drug pressure. Biochemistry 1995;34:9282–9287.
223. Ridky T, Leis J. Development of drug resistance to HIV-1 protease inhibitors. J Biol Chem 1995;270:29,621–29,623.
224. Berry P, Kahn J, Cooper R, et al. Antiretroviral activity and safety of indinavir alone and in combination with zidovudine in zidovudine-naive patients with CD4 cell counts of 50–250 cells/mm³ [abstract]. In: 11th International Conference on AIDS, Vancouver, 1996.
225. Stein D, Fish D, Bilello J, et al. 24-week open-label phase I/II evaluation of the HIV protease inhibitor MK-639 (indinavir). AIDS 1996;10:485–492.
226. Craig J, Duncan I, Hockley D, et al. Antiviral properties of Ro 31-8959, an inhibitor of HIV proteinase. Antiviral Res 1991;16:295–305.
227. Roberts NA, Martin JA, Kinchington D, et al. Rational design of peptide-based HIV proteinase inhibitors. Science 1990;248:358–361.
228. Dorsey B, Levin R, McDaniel S. L-735,524: the design of a potent and orally bioavailable HIV protease inhibitor. J Med Chem 1994;37:3443–3451.
229. Vacca J, Dorsey B, Schleif W. L-735,524: an orally bioavailable HIV-1 protease inhibitor. Proc Natl Acad Sci U S A 1994;91:4096–4100.
230. Kempf D, Norbeck D, Codacovi L. Structure-based C_2 symmetric inhibitors of HIV protease. J Med Chem 1990;33:2687–2689.
231. Chong U, McGee L, Erickson J. Discovery of potent, orally bioavailable, non-peptidic, cyclic sulfones as HIV protease inhibitors [abstract MoA 1075]. In: 11th International Conference on AIDS, Vancouver, 1996.
232. Ginsburg C, Salmon-Ceron S, Vassilief D, et al. Unusual occurrence of spontaneous haematomas in three asymptomatic HIV-infected haemophilia patients a few days after the onset of ritonavir treatment. AIDS 1997;11:388–389.
233. Delfraissy J, Sereni D, Brun-Vezinet F, et al. A phase I-II dose ranging study of the safety and activity of Ro 31-8959 on previously zidovudine-treated HIV-infected individuals. In: 9th International Conference on AIDS, Berlin, 1993.
234. Kitchen V, Skinner C, Ariyoshi K, et al. Safety and activity of saquinavir in HIV infection. Lancet 1995;345:952–955.
235. Muirhead G, Shaw T, Williams P. Pharmacokinetics of the HIV-proteinase inhibitor Ro 31-8959 after single and multiple oral doses in healthy volunteers. Br J Clin Pharmacol 1992;34:170–171.
236. Schapiro J, Winters M, Stewart F, et al. The effect of high-dose saquinavir on viral load and CD4 T-cell counts in HIV-infected patients. Ann Intern Med 1996;124:1039–1050.
237. Invirase (saquinavir mesylate), capsules: package insert. Nutley, NJ: Roche Laboratories, 1997.
238. Williams P, Madigan M, Mitchel A. A single dose, randomized cross-over study of the absolute and relative bioavailability of Ro 31-8959 in healthy volunteers. In: Roche Research Report. Nutley, NJ: Roche Laboratories, 1992.
239. Lewis JS, II, Terriff CM, Coulston DR, et al. Protease inhibitors: a therapeutic breakthrough for the treatment of patients with human immunodeficiency virus. Clin Ther 1997;19:187–214.
240. Granneman GR, Hsu A, Sun E, et al. Pharmacokinetics/pharmacodynamics of ritonavir-saquinavir combination therapy [abstract 609]. In: 4th Conference on Retroviruses and Opportunistic Infections. Washington DC: Infectious Disease Society of America for the Foundation for Retrovirology and Human Health, 1997.
241. Cameron W, Sun E, Leonard P. Combination use of ritonavir and saquinavir In HIV-infected patients: preliminary safety and activity data [abstract ThB 934]. In: 11th International Conference on AIDS, Vancouver, 1996.
242. Jacobsen H, Yasargil K, Duncan I. Characterizaton of HIV-1 mutants with decreased sensitivity to proteinase inhibitor Ro 31-8959. Virology 1995;206:527–534.
243. Moyle GJ. Use of viral resistance patterns to antiretroviral drugs in optimising selection of drug combinations and sequences. Drugs 1996;52:168–185.
244. Kempf D, Marsh K, Denissen J. ABT-538 is a potent inhibitor of human immunodeficiency virus protease and has high oral bioavailability in humans. Proc Natl Acad Sci U S A 1995;92:2484–2488.
245. Cato A, Hsu A, Granneman R. Assessment of the pharmacokinetic interaction between the HIV-1 protease inhibitor ABT-538 and zidovudine. In: Proceedings of the Interscience Conference on Antimicrobial Agents and Chemotherapy, San Francisco, 1995.
246. Danner S, Carr A, Leonatd J. A short-term study of the safety, pharmacokinetics and efficacy of ritonavir, an inhibitor of HIV-1 protease. N Engl J Med 1995;333:1528–1533.
247. Markowitz M, Saag M, Powderly W. A preliminary study of ritonavir, an inhibitor of HIV-1 protease. N Engl J Med 1995;333:1534–1539.
248. Kumar G, Rodriguez A, Buko A. Cytochrome P450–mediated metabolism of the HIV-1 protease inhibitor ritonavir (ABT-538) in human liver microsomes. J Pharmacol Exp Ther 1996;227:423–431.
249. Mathez D, De Truchis P, Gorin I, et al. Ritonavir, AZT, ddC as a triple combination in AIDS patients. In: 3rd Conference on Retroviruses and Opportunistic Infections. Washington, DC: Infectious Disease Society of America for the Foundation for Retrovirology and Human Health, 1996.

250. Hsu A, Granneman G, Leonard J. Assessment of single- and multiple-dose interactions between ritonavir and saquinavir [abstract LbB 6041]. In: 11th International Conference on AIDS, Vancouver, 1996:30.
251. Kempf D, Marsh K, Denissen J, et al. Coadministration with ritonavir enhances the plasma levels of HIV protease inhibitors by inhibition of cytochrome P450. In: 3rd Conference on Retroviruses and Opportunistic Infections. Washington, DC: Infectious Disease Society of America for the Foundation for Retrovirology and Human Health, 1996:79.
252. Norvir (ritonavir) capsules and oral solution prescribing information: package insert. N. Chicago, IL: Abbott Laboratories, 1997.
253. Bertz R, Cao G, Leonard J. Effect of ritonavir on the pharmacokinetics of desipramine [abstract]. In: 11th International Conference on AIDS, Vancouver, 1996:89.
254. Bertz R, Cao G, Leonard J. Effect of ritonavir on the pharmacokinetics of trimethoprim/sulfanethoxazole [abstract]. In: 11th International Conference on AIDS, Vancouver, 1996:88.
255. Cato A, Cavanaugh J, Leonard J. Assessment of multiple doses of ritonavir on the pharmacokinetics of rifabutin [abstract]. In: 11th International Conference on AIDS, Vancouver, 1996:89.
256. Crixivan (indinavir sulfate) capsules: prescribing information. West Point, PA: Merck, 1997.
257. Anonymous. New drugs for HIV infection. Med Lett Drugs Ther 1996;38:35–38.
258. Balani S, Arison B, Mathai L. Metabolites of L-735,524, a potent HIV-1 protease inhibitor, in human urine. Drug Metab Dispos 1995;23:266–270.
259. Chodakewitz J, Leavitt R, Rockhold F. Crixivan: summary of 24-week experience with Crixivan at 2.4 g/d in phase II trials [abstract MoB 1144]. In: 11th International Conference on AIDS, Vancouver, 1996:79.
260. Emini E, Condra J, Chodakewitz J. Maintenance of long-term virus suppression in patients treated with the HIV-1 protease inhibitor Crixivan (indinavir) [abstract MoB 170]. In: 11th International Conference on AIDS, Vancouver, 1996:18.
261. Massari F, Conant M, Mellors J, et al. A phase II open-label, randomized study of the triple combination of indinavir, zidovudine (ZDV) and didanosine (ddI) versus indinavir alone and zidovudine/didanosine in antiretroviral naive patients. In: 3rd Conference on Retroviruses and Opportunistic Infections. Washington, DC: Infectious Disease Society of America for the Foundation for Retrovirology and Human Health, 1996:90.
262. Steigbigel R, Berry P, Mellors J. Efficacy and safety of the HIV protease inhibitor indinavir sulfate at escalating dose. In: 3rd Conference on Retroviruses and Opportunistic Infections. Washington, DC: Infectious Disease Society of America for the Foundation for Retrovirology and Human Health, 1996:80.
263. Stein D, Fish D, Chodakewitz J. Followup data from an open label phase I evaluation of the HIV protease inhibitor MK-639. In: 3rd Conference on Retroviruses and Opportunistic Infections. Washington, DC: Infectious Disease Society of America for the Foundation for Retrovirology and Human Health, 1996:80.
264. Kopp J, Miller K, Mican J, et al. Crystalluria and urinary tract abnormalities associated with indinavir. Ann Intern Med 1997;127:119–125.
265. McCrea J. Indinavir (MK 639) drug interaction studies [abstract Mo.B. 174]. In: 11th International Conference on AIDS, Vancover, 1996.
266. Powderly W, Sension M, Conant M, et al. Pharmaceuticals VCSGA: the efficacy of VIRACEPT (nelfinavir mesylate) in pivotal phase II/III double-blind randomized controlled trial as monotherapy and in combination with d4T or AZT/3TC [abstract 240]. In: 4th Conference on Retrovirus and Opportunistic Infections. Washington, DC: Infectious Disease Society of America for the Foundation for Retrovirology and Human Health, 1997.
267. Viracept (nelfinavir mesylate) tablets and oral powder prescribing information: package insert. La Jolla, CA: Agouron Pharmaceuticals, 1997.
268. Conant M, Markowitz, M, Hurley A, et al. A randomized phase II dose range-finding study of the HIV protease inhibitor Viracept as monotherapy in HIV positive patients [abstract Tu.B.2129]. In: 11th International Conference on AIDS, Vancover, 1996.
269. Henry K, Lamarca A, Myers R, et al. The safety of Viracept (nelfinavir mesylate) in pivotal phase II/III double-blind randomized controlled trials as monotherapy and in combination with d4T or AZT/3TC. In: 4th Conference on Retroviruses and Opportunistic Infections. Washington, DC: Infectious Disease Society of America for the Foundation for Retrovirology and Human Health, 1997.
270. Chapman S. Update on nelfinavir mesylate phase II/III trial (AG 511). In: 10th International Conference on Antiviral Research, Atlanta, 1997.
271. Kravick S, Sahai J, Kerr B, et al. Nelfinavir mesylate (NFV) increases saquinavir-soft gel capsule (SQV-SGC) exposure in HIV+ patients [abstract 371]. In: 4th Conference on Retroviruses and Opportunistic Infections, Washington, DC: Infectious Disease Society of America for the Foundation for Retrovirology and Human Health, 1997.
272. Tisdale M, Myers RE, Harrigan PR, et al. Analyses of HIV genotype and phenotype during 4 weeks dose-escalating monotherapy with the HIV protease inhibitor 141W94 in HIV-infected patients with CD4 counts 150–400/mm^3. In: 4th Conference on Retroviruses and Opportunistic Infections. Washington, DC: Infectious Disease Society of America for the Foundation for Retrovirology and Human Health, 1997.
273. Marsh K, McDonald E, Sham H, et al. Enhancement of ABT-378 pharmacokinetics when administered in combination with ritonavir. In: 4th Conference on Retrovirus and Opportunistic Infections. Washington, DC: Infectious Disease Society of America for the Foundation for Retrovirology and Human Health, 1997.
274. Kumar G, Jaynati V, Johnson M, et al. Increased bioavailability and plasma levels of the HIV-1 protease inhibitor ABT-378 in rats due to inhibition of the in vivo metabolism by ritonavir. In: 4th Conference on Retrovirus and Opportunistic Infections. Washington, DC: Infectious Disease Society of America for the Foundation for Retrovirology and Human Health, 1997.
275. Sham H, Kempf D, Molla A, et al. Design, synthesis and biological properties of ABT-378, a highly potent HIV protease inhibitor. In: 4th Conference on Retrovirus and Opportunistic Infections. Washington, DC: Infectious Disease Society of America for the Foundation for Retrovirology and Human Health, 1997.
276. Carpenter C, Fischl M, Hammer S, et al. Antiretroviral therapy for HIV infection in 1996: recommendations of an international panel. JAMA 1996;276:146–154.
277. Gazzard B, Moyle G, Weber J, et al. British HIV Association guidelines for antiretroviral treatment of HIV seropositive individuals. Lancet 1997;349:1086–1092.
278. Panel on Clinical Practices for Treatment of HIV Infection. Guidelines for the use of antiretroviral agents in adults and adolescents. Morb Mort Weekly Reports 1998;47 RR–5:43–82.
279. Carpenter C, Fischl M, Hammer S, et al. Antiretroviral therapy for HIV infection in 1997: updated recommendations of the International AIDS Society–USA Panel. JAMA 1997;277:1962–1969.
280. O'Brien W, Hartigan P, Martin D, et al. Changes in plasma HIV-1 RNA and CD4+ lymphocyte count relative to treatment and progression to AIDS. N Engl J Med 1996;334:426–431.
281. Mellors J, Rinaldo C, Phalguni G, et al. Prognosis of HIV-1 infection predicted by the quantity of virus in plasma. Science 1996;272:1167–1170.
282. Mellors JW, Munoz A, Giorgi J, et al. Plasma viral load and CD4 positive lymphocytes as prognostic markers of HIV-1 infection. Ann Intern Med 1997;126:983–985.

283. Mellors J, Munoz A, Giorgi J, et al. Plasma viral load and CD4+ lymphocytes as prognostic markers of HIV-1 infection. Ann Intern Med 1997;126:946–954.
284. Hughes M, Johnson V, Hirsch M, et al. Monitoring plasma HIV-1 RNA levels in addition to CD4+ lymphocyte count improves assessment of antiretroviral therapeutic response. Ann Intern Med 1997; 126:929–938.
285. Saag M, Holodnet M, Kuritzkes D, et al. HIV viral load markers in clinical practice. Nature Med 1996;2:625–629.
286. Angel JB, Saget BM, Walsh SP, et al. Rolipram, a specific type IV phosphodiesterase inhibitor, is a potent inhibitor of HIV-1 replication. AIDS 1995;9:1137–1144.
287. Makonkawkeyoon S, Limson-Pobre RN, Moreira AL, et al. Thalidomide inhibits the replication of human immunodeficiency virus type 1. Proc Natl Acad Sci U S A 1993;90:5974–5978.
288. Moreira AL, Weiguo Y, Shen Z, et al. Thalidomide reduces HIV-1 production in acutely infected human monocytes in vitro. In: 3rd Conference on Retroviruses and Opportunistic Infections. Washington, DC: Infectious Disease Society of America for the Foundation for Retrovirology and Human Health, 1996:111.
289. Rice WG, Schaeffer CA, Harten B, et al. Inhibition of HIV-1 infectivity by zinc-ejecting aromatic C-nitroso compounds. Nature 1993;361:473–475.
290. Rice WG, Supko JG, Malspeis L, et al. Inhibitors of HIV nucleocapsid protein zinc fingers as candidates for the treatment of AIDS. Science 1995;270:1194–1197.

46

BIOSTATISTICAL CONSIDERATIONS IN THE DESIGN AND ANALYSIS OF AIDS CLINICAL TRIALS

Kenneth Stanley and Stephen W. Lagakos

The emerging epidemic of human immunodeficiency virus (HIV) disease is unique in modern medicine. It is the first time that a major infectious disease has emerged rapidly and early in the United States. Based on current knowledge, the HIV epidemic is likely to continue to spread, with a potential for becoming one of the most lethal diseases in history. HIV has also emerged at a time when certain effective clinical and laboratory research tools, developed initially for other diseases, can be rapidly adapted to deal with the problem.

Virtually everything about HIV can be described as rapidly progressing: the spread of infection, the infusion of public and private funds into research, the number of researchers entering the field, the understanding of the disease, the identification of effective new therapies, and the public's expectation of progress. To speed the pace of research, many established mechanisms for drug development are being modified. The United States Food and Drug Administration (FDA) is under considerable pressure to approve drugs for the acquired immunodeficiency syndrome (AIDS) rapidly. This pressure translates into the relaxing of some FDA requirements and the initiation of an accelerated approval process, which can tentatively approve a drug based on early findings on surrogate markers, rather than waiting for definitive clinical information. Often, the major therapeutic questions that clinicians want answered are not envisaged when a study is designed. Sometimes planned studies are obsolete before the first patient is ever entered, and practitioners learn how to evaluate a therapy effectively midway through a study.

The purpose of this chapter is to discuss several biostatistical aspects of study design, monitoring, and evaluation as they relate to clinical trials in HIV disease. We do not intend this chapter to be a comprehensive discussion of clinical trial methods. Rather, we focus on several topics that are specifically relevant to HIV clinical trials. Readers not familiar with the general approach and methods for clinical trials may want to refer to some of the published literature on AIDS (1–5) and other diseases such as cancer and cardiovascular disease (6–13).

STUDY DESIGN

Overall Research Strategy

A clinical trial is a prospective experiment involving human subjects in whom therapy is initiated for the purpose of evaluation. Classically, clinical trials are categorized by phase: phase I, II, or III (Table 46.1).

It is becoming common for phase I HIV studies not to define optimal dose as the maximal tolerated dose, as has been done for years in phase I cancer trials, but rather to use various laboratory and clinical measurements to determine the most effective dose or dosing strategy. Phase II studies for primary HIV disease are designed to look for antiviral activity, commonly measured by HIV RNA levels or CD4 cell counts. Such studies are often randomized to ensure balance among the treatment groups. With the initiation of FDA-expedited approval of dideoxyinosine (didanosine or ddI) and zalcitabine (dideoxycytosine or ddC), primarily based on CD4 trends, some phase II studies are even being used as "pivotal" in the drug-licensing process.

Phase III studies are key in the determination of optimal therapeutic strategies worldwide. For primary HIV disease, each study often involves 500 to 2000 patients, costs $2 to 10 million, and requires the cooperative effort of more than 20 institutions. The impact of these studies is equally large, because some of them determine the therapeutic strategy for millions of current and future patients.

Some basic phase III designs are depicted in Figure 46.1. At the beginning of the HIV epidemic, key studies were randomized comparisons of placebo versus azidothymidine (now known as zidovudine or ZDV). Once ZDV was established as standard therapy, studies began that compared ZDV with drugs such as ddI and ddC. Other studies

Table 46.1. Clinical Trials: Types and Objectives

Type	Objective
Phase I	To determine optimal dose and dosing strategies
Phase II	To determine whether the therapy is active against the disease
Phase III	To compare the experimental therapy with the current standard therapy (or no treatment—placebo)

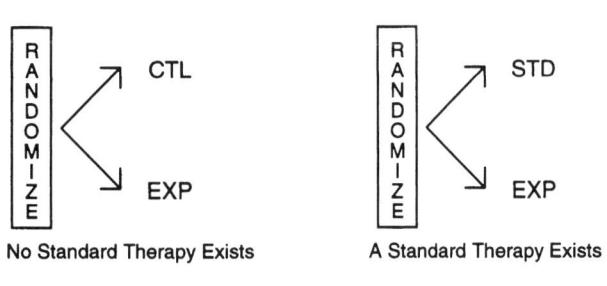

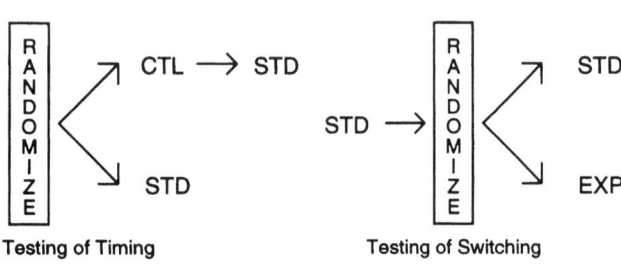

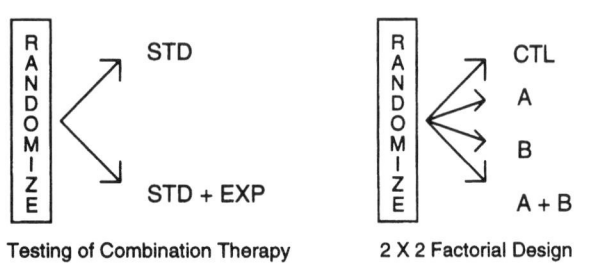

Figure 46.1. Basic phase III designs. *STD*, standard therapy, if it exists; *EXP*, experimental therapy; *CTL*, no therapy or placebo (control); *A + B*, any two therapies.

investigated the timing of the initiation of ZDV (usually depending on CD4 count) and the optimal time of switching (e.g., after 6 months of ZDV). More recent studies are investigating the role of the combinations ZDV plus ddC and ZDV plus ddI, relative to ZDV alone.

The original intention of the phase I, II, III designation was that experimental therapies would progress through phase I, II, and III sequentially, sometimes with more than one study at each phase level, including various patient populations. However, an HIV study typically takes 9 to 12 months or more from concept approval to entry of the first patient. Therefore, hybrid phase I/II and II/III studies are becoming common, as investigators attempt to speed the research process. Although such shortcuts have been viewed by some workers as a step forward, these measures sometimes slow the overall process by forcing investigators to go back and conduct some earlier studies properly. In addition, the medical community may be left with an unresolvable situation if a surrogate marker is used to approve a new compound tentatively and the patients withdraw from the main randomized phase III studies before definitive clinical conclusions are established. Because of the increasing trend for patients to withdraw early because of surrogate marker information and the availability of other new therapies, phase III studies should be designed to follow a larger number of patients for a shorter time rather than fewer patients for a longer time.

Currently, more than 10 anti-HIV drugs have been approved or are in development. It is unlikely that one single drug or combination will suffice for a patient's lifetime. The number of possible combinations and sequences is enormous, and investigators can only test a few. Further, with the availability of real-time RNA, patients and clinicians want to change therapy based on current RNA and CD4 values, a concept we call "switching." Various untested switching strategies are available, and even when the therapeutic strategy is the same, therapy is essentially customized for each patient. The classic phase III clinical trial with clinical progression as an end point is often no longer feasible or interpretable.

This shift has caused a reevaluation of methods of future study design. The key therapeutic questions are as follows: 1) when should therapy start? 2) what classes of drugs should be used at the beginning of therapy? 3) when should one switch therapy? 4) to which classes of drugs should one switch? and 5) when should one stop effective therapy? The concepts of "shorter-term" designs, "longer-term" designs, and "induction trials" have been developed.

Shorter-term designs use RNA and other virologic and immunologic end points and focus on determining the optimal therapy up to a switchpoint and the optimal therapy between switchpoints. For example, a randomized study could compare three different combination therapies as initial therapy, using the proportion of patients reaching an undetectable level of RNA as the primary end point. A second example would be a randomized study of two different combination therapies for patients in whom treatment with a protease inhibitor has failed, with the proportion of patients reaching at least a 2-log drop in RNA serving as the end point.

Longer-term designs use clinical disease progression as an end point and focus on comparing switching criteria or adding a drug from a new class. For example, a randomized study could compare an aggressive versus a conservative RNA-based switching strategy for patients receiving their initial therapy, the former arm of the study switching therapy when RNA returned to a detectable level and the second arm switching therapy when RNA exceeded 10,000 copies/mL. Clinical progression and resistance would be the major measures of therapeutic effectiveness. A second example would be a flexible background trial in which either a drug from a new class or a placebo would be added in a randomized fashion to existing current therapy.

The concepts behind "induction trials" are that viral load (RNA) is believed to be the key to control of HIV, the main objective should be to drive viral load to undetectable levels and keep it there, and a reduction of viral load, but not to undetectable levels, may not be good. Such trials test various levels of aggressive therapeutic approaches and switching strategies. For example, one aggressive approach would be to switch therapy after 12 weeks if the patient has not reached an undetectable level of RNA.

Until recently, trials of antiviral therapies and trials for the prophylaxis of opportunistic infections have proceeded largely independently of each other. However, the efficiency of the clinical research can be improved considerably by using a factorial study design (see Fig. 46.1). If A were an antiviral agent and B were an opportunistic infection prophylaxis agent, a factorial design could test both therapies at the same time. Even if the two therapeutic dimensions are not independent, the precision of the comparisons will improve because of the control of possibly confounding concomitant therapies. Higher-level factorial designs are also feasible.

Selecting the End Points

In phase III trials of many life-threatening diseases, death is the primary study end point for evaluating the benefits of new therapies. However, because of the long latency period of HIV and the rapidly changing standards for medical care of persons infected with HIV, mortality is often not feasible as an end point. In selecting the end points for a phase III HIV trial, several factors must be considered, including the rate of occurrence of the end points in the patient population being considered, the relevance of a treatment effect on the end point, and the reliability in measuring the end point. For a full discussion of these issues, see Amato and Lagakos (14).

Another consideration is the designation of some end points as "primary" end points for the trial and others as "secondary." This important decision should be made before the study is initiated and explicitly described in the protocol. Ideally, a study should have two to three primary end points at most. These should be clinically or biologically important, occur frequently enough for the study to have adequate statistical power, and not be highly correlated with one another. Secondary end points should include those that are potentially important for overall interpretation of the data and those that are clinically relevant yet have limited power because of low event rates.

Selecting the Treatments and Blinding

Three features must be considered in the selection of specific treatments to be used in a trial. First, if successful, is the intervention likely to be implemented in clinical practice? Most AIDS patients in the United States are treated by nonresearchers who are not associated with a unit dedicated to the treatment of the disease. Worldwide, fewer specialized centers are available than in the United States. Second, is the intervention "strong" enough to have a chance of producing a detectable effect? If a new therapy is a cautious, rather than a bold, step forward, the extent of potential additional benefit may be so small as to require the study of extremely large numbers of patients to detect such a minor improvement. Third, will changes in patient management render the results of a trial obsolete before they are available?

Once the treatment arms of the study are selected, one must decide whether these are to be unblinded, blinded to the patient (single blind), or blinded to both the patient and care giver (double blind). In some settings, blinding may cause some difficulties (e.g., the placebo may have side effects). In general, however, it is preferable to conduct a double-blind study than either an unblinded or single-blind study (1). The opportunity for bias in a double-blind study is substantially reduced.

Role of Randomization and Ethical Issues

The basic principle in comparing treatments is that the treatment groups must be alike in all important aspects and must differ only in the treatment each patient receives. Randomization is the treatment allocation mechanism in which each patient has the same chance of receiving any of the treatments under study. In this way, neither the patient nor the physician knows in advance which therapy will be assigned. Some advantages and disadvantages of randomization are presented in Table 46.2. In addition to averaging out the conscious biases of patients and physicians, randomization also attempts to average out the unconscious biases resulting from referral patterns and a myriad of other factors, known and unknown. This averaging out process makes randomization not only vital for phase III trials, but also desirable for phase I and II trials. Random assignment of treatments applied to a relatively homogeneous stream of patients entering a study helps to improve the likelihood that any observed results will be due more likely to the treatments administered than to differences among the groups. Investigators have argued that even phase I studies should be

Table 46.2. Randomization

Advantages
    Eliminates conscious bias caused by physician or patient selection
    Averages out unconscious bias caused by unknown factors
    Groups are "alike on average"
    Necessary for some statistical tests
Disadvantages
    Poses ethical issues concerning equipoise
    Interferes with doctor-patient relationship
    Adds administrative complexity
    "Alike on average" does not guarantee balanced groups

randomized, when possible, to distribute the risks and benefits of the varying dose levels equally from the patient's perspective.

Stratified randomization seeks to improve the balance within treatment groups beyond what can be achieved by randomization alone. Stratification is the mechanism by which separate randomizations are conducted for each of several strata. When the resulting treatment groups are combined, they are more likely to be balanced with respect to these risk factors.

Some patients and physicians may not desire to participate in a randomized trial. They may find it difficult to believe in the reality of equipoise, which is the ethical requirement of randomized trials that both treatments are equally desirable and that no evidence indicates that any other therapy should be preferred. Others firmly believe that a randomized trial interferes with the bond of trust between doctor and patient, the principle that a patient should put full confidence in the doctor's choice of treatment and the doctor should always be seen as knowing what is best for the patient. The idea that a physician would have to admit not knowing which therapy is best and would determine how the patient should be treated by tossing a coin (randomization) is not acceptable to some people.

Increasing concern also has been expressed about the idea that physicians or hospitals sometimes receive academic or monetary compensation for entering patients onto a clinical trial, a practice that possibly hinders the doctor's judgment of what is truly in the best interests of a patient in entering a specific trial. Others argue that, in general, participation in a clinical trial improves the level of care given a patient because of the extra effort to develop optimal patient management guidelines and the external review of the care given. Little doubt exists that randomized double-blind trials are the best available method for determining optimal therapeutic management.

Statistical Power Considerations

The power of a clinical trial is evaluated in the design phase to ensure that the study will have enough patients and follow-up to be definitive. An example is a trial comparing two treatments (A and B) with respect to the proportion of successes observed. This success rate could be the proportion of patients (P) surviving more than 2 years, or it could be the proportion of patients whose CD4 counts remain within 20% of their baseline values or higher after 6 months of therapy. In a randomized phase III trial comparing these two treatments, we are testing the null hypothesis, $H_o: P_A - P_B = O$, that the two treatments produce equivalent results, versus the alternative hypothesis, $H_a: P_A - P_B \neq O$, that the treatments produce different results.

The test of this hypothesis is to conduct a clinical trial and to determine an estimate of $P_A - P_B$. If this estimate is sufficiently different from zero, then we reject the null hypothesis of equivalent treatments and conclude that a treatment difference exists. The question is how far from zero do we need to be before we have sufficient evidence to say the treatments are different?

This statistical problem is usually formulated as follows: Let α be the probability of concluding that the treatments are different when in fact they are really equivalent (reject the H_o given that the H_o is true: a type I error). Let β be the probability of concluding that the treatments are not different when in fact they are different (accept the H_o given that the H_o is false: a type II error). The power of the test is then $1 - \beta$. Further, let Δ be the minimal difference, $P_A - P_B$, considered to be medically significant and biologically plausible.

With the foregoing formulation, the three parameters α, β, and Δ can then be used to determine the appropriate sample size for a particular study design. Most often, α is set at .05, β is set at 0.1 or 0.2, and Δ is the result of a discussion between the study chair and statistician. Frequently, Δ is selected to correspond to a 25 to 50% difference between the treatments; smaller Δs often lead to requirements for unrealistically large studies. The reader is directed to specific references describing sample size determinations for binary end points (15) and "time to event" end points (10, 16–18).

The P value for the evaluation of the primary end point of a trial is the likelihood of the observed result or a more extreme result, assuming no difference between the therapies. If the P value is small, such as $P < .05$, then either we have observed a rare event (which is unlikely) or a difference exists between the treatments. We therefore conclude that a statistically significant difference exists between the therapies. A P value is a function of both the size of the difference between the therapies and the number of patients. Thus, if thousands of patients are studied, a significant P value may indicate a difference of statistical significance, but not necessarily of medical significance.

When the primary end point of a study is survival, time to an AIDS-defining event, time to a 50% decline in CD4 count, or some other "time to event" measure, the statistical power of a study is a function of the number of failures (e.g., deaths or AIDS-defining events) and not the number of patients. For example, the AIDS Clinical Trials Group Study 155 had a target of 400 clinical end points (AIDS-defining events or deaths) to reach the power as designed. The power of the study would be the same if it had observed 400 failures by entering 500 patients and following them for a long time or by entering 2000 patients and following them for a short time.

A common misinterpretation of the results of a clinical trial occurs when a study reports a nonsignificant P value for its primary end point comparison. Usually, it is not appropriate to conclude in this instance that the treatments are equivalent. One can only say that evidence is insufficient to conclude that a difference exists. If the objective of a study is to show the equivalence of two therapies (equivalent to within a prespecified tolerance), then the study is called an equivalence trial, and the power calculation method described previously is inappropriate.

Determining How Many Data Should Be Collected

A mistake often made by beginning investigators is to collect too many data. Clinicians are trained to collect extensive information regarding aspects of patient management. However, little patient management information ever is reported in a published paper. The major data items reported relate to baseline patient characteristics, primary and secondary end points, and severe complications of therapy. Some reporting of the treatment administered and of the necessary modifications occurs, but this is usually brief. The recommended strategy for investigators planning a study is first to draft the abstracts and the key supporting tables and figures of the future articles reporting the major possible conclusions they expect. They should then list the data items needed to produce these tables and figures and design the data collection forms to collect this information directly. Collection of substantial additional data should be discouraged.

INTERIM MONITORING

It is standard and appropriate that some form of interim monitoring of an ongoing clinical trial be carried out. In general, the broad goals are to improve the likelihood that the trial will give meaningful results, to allow for the possibility of early termination of the trial, and to ensure the best interests of the subjects participating in the trial. For a comparative phase III trial, specific areas of concern include the following: 1) quality assurance and logistical issues, including the quality of the data collected, and inconsistencies in the logic or definitions in the protocol; 2) assumptions underlying the duration and sample size of the trial, including the accrual, response, and dropout rates; and 3) the safety and efficacy results of the trial. A brief description of some of these points is presented in the following sections. For a detailed discussion, see DeMets (19) and Pocock (20).

Assessing Definitions, Logic, and Data Quality

Despite the amount of time spent in planning a study and in documenting all aspects in the protocol document, inconsistencies and vagaries invariably arise, usually discovered when the subject evaluation and data collection aspects of the study are carried out for a few patients. Often these problems are associated with the extent of information collected or the timing of the collection; sometimes the actual definitions of key events, such as clinical end points, are unclear. The importance of rectifying these problems early cannot be overstated.

The first interim examination of the data often focuses exclusively on issues of definition, logic, and data quality, with no formal comparative efficacy analysis. Problems in the collection, review, and correction of the database are discussed, with a goal of streamlining the data flow and ensuring that various quality control checks are in place.

Safety and Efficacy Assessment

In most trials, certain adverse events related to the protocol therapies are expected. Thus, the purposes of interim safety analyses are primarily to assess whether the observed rates are consistent with those expected and to determine whether any unexpected and intolerable toxicities are occurring.

Interim monitoring of a clinical trial for efficacy has received much attention in the literature. The main reasons are that the efficacy of a new treatment is usually of great scientific concern, and the type I error rate increases as the data are repeatedly examined. For example, if the data in a trial are examined five times, with a nominal $P=.05$ significance level used in each analysis, the overall type I error may be as large as $P=.18$. In other words, the more times the data are examined, the more likely it is that a false-positive result will occur unless some account is taken of the multiple "looks" at the data.

Many criteria and guidelines exist for how often and when to conduct interim efficacy analyses. For most situations, three to four interim analyses work best, with the analyses timed to occur each time 20 to 25% of the ultimate information in the trial becomes available. For example, in a trial in which the efficacy end point is survival time and four analyses are planned (three interim and one final analysis), the interim analyses should take place when approximately 25%, 50%, and 75% of the total deaths (that are expected at the time of the final analysis) have occurred.

With respect to the issue of multiple looks and inflated false-positive rates, the idea is to "spread" the total desired type I error rate (often 5%) across the interim and final analyses. Currently, the most popular way of doing this is to use what are often referred to as "O'Brien–Fleming" boundaries. These essentially require strong evidence to stop a trial early, but, in turn, they require minor correction from the nominal analyses should the trial not be terminated early. For a full discussion of these issues, see Pocock (20); for a more technical discussion, see Kim and Tsiatis (21).

ANALYZING AND INTERPRETING THE DATA

The literature on statistical methods used to analyze data arising from clinical trials is vast. For researchers with a clinical perspective, the texts by Miké and Stanley (8) and Pocock (20) offer a comprehensive and practical discussion of many of the issues and methods. See also the articles by Byar and colleagues (1) and Ellenberg and associates (2). Rather than attempt to summarize these issues here, we focus on several topics relevant to the interpretation of many AIDS clinical trials. These topics are intent to treat analyses, the effects of noncompliance to study medication, losses to follow-up, and surrogate markers.

Intent to Treat Analyses

"Intent to treat" refers to a philosophy for the analysis of data from randomized clinical trials. Generally speaking, the philosophy states that comparisons among treatment groups should be based on grouping subjects according to how they were intended to be treated (i.e., how they were randomized) rather than actually treated. Thus, all subjects randomized to receive drug A would be analyzed in one comparison group, even if they 1) never initiated treatment with drug A, or 2) immediately began treatment B either through choice, some administrative error, or misunderstanding. The philosophy also extends to the amount of follow-up included in analyses. In particular, for comparisons of groups with respect to time-dependent events (e.g., time until progression of disease or time until death), all of a subject's follow-up information should be included in the analysis; the patient's information should not be censored if he or she discontinued treatment for any reason.

To some investigators, the notion of intent to treat also includes the provision that everyone randomized into the study should be analyzed, regardless of whether they meet the study eligibility requirements. Investigators conducting clinical trials are less unified on this point, however, and some practitioners think it appropriate that ineligible subjects (especially those with gross violations of eligibility criteria) be excluded from the analysis, provided this is specified in advance.

The rationale for the intent to treat approach is twofold. First, the ultimate efficacy of a drug in standard medical practice depends on the magnitude of its effect and the length of time it can be tolerated. A certain proportion of subjects may never begin taking the drug, and others may discontinue its use earlier than prescribed. The intent to treat approach for analysis would tend to reflect the outcomes seen in routine medical practice because of its inclusion of such information. The second rationale for using an intent to treat analysis is that the alternatives proposed are subject to serious bias. For example, if the analysis of trials is based on comparing those subjects who actually received drug A with those who actually received drug B, regardless of which treatment these subjects were assigned at randomization, then a serious selectivity bias could result. Similarly, if time to failure analyses censored information at the time subjects discontinued their initial therapy, a bias could result if the reasons for termination had anything to do with the subject's prognosis (22).

One implication of this philosophy is that follow-up of subjects should continue until they reach a study end point; follow-up should not cease once these patients discontinue their assigned therapy. Unfortunately, this important feature is not adhered to in many clinical trials, thereby clouding interpretation when treatment discontinuation rates are not extremely low.

Effects of Noncompliance

Consider a clinical trial in which subjects are assigned to receive either placebo or some drug, and the data are to be analyzed using an intent to treat philosophy. Assume further that the end point of the trial is time until progression of HIV infection, and follow-up of subjects for disease progression is continued even if treatment is discontinued. In such a case, one can show that discontinuation of protocol treatment for nonmandated reasons (e.g., by a patient's voluntary withdrawal from treatment) can have the effect of attenuating the true drug–placebo difference. This means the study will have less power to detect a real treatment difference than it would have had if subjects had continued to receive their assigned treatments. For example, suppose that in the group assigned to receive the drug, 20% of subjects never take the drug. The power of the study to detect a treatment difference would be about the same as a study having two-thirds the number of subjects in which compliance was complete (23).

Such information is useful when interpreting the results of a trial. For example, if a trial shows no significant difference between the treatment groups, yet evidence indicates substantial noncompliance, then it is not clear whether the drug has no benefit or whether the size of the trial and rate of noncompliance made the power of the study inadequate to detect a real difference. For these reasons, one must assess the extent of noncompliance in clinical trials and use this information when interpreting the results.

Losses to Follow-up

In some trials, follow-up of subjects for the efficacy end points (e.g., clinical progression of their disease or death) is incomplete simply because the data are analyzed before the subject happens to have disease progression. This form of "end of study" censoring poses no problems in the analysis of the data because the standard statistical methods (e.g., Kaplan–Meier curves, logrank tests, Cox proportional hazards model) can account for it. On the other hand, the follow-up of subjects sometimes ends for reasons that could be related to their prognosis. For example, the attending physician may remove a patient from study in the belief that this patient's condition is worsening, or a patient may withdraw from follow-up because he or she believes that the treatment is no longer effective. Another example is CD4 trends over time; if some patients with rapidly declining CD4 counts withdraw from the study after just a few weeks, the average CD4 level of the remaining patients would be artificially high. In these circumstances, the standard methods of statistical analysis could be severely biased because of the informative nature in which the data are censored. Furthermore, no alternative methods of analysis can reliably account for this form of censoring. Thus, losses to follow-up must be minimized in a clinical trial. This goal can be accomplished by rigorous follow-up of subjects as well as by designing trials that allow treatment changes when an indication exists that the current therapy is no longer effective.

Surrogate Markers

Traditionally, phase III comparative trials had as their primary efficacy measure a clinical event such as development of AIDS or death. In the past few years, however, investigators have shown increased interest and use of surrogate end points in comparative clinical trials. This interest was heightened by the 1991 approval by the FDA of ddI, based largely on results indicating that this agent slowed the decline of CD4 cells in patients with AIDS or AIDS-related complex (24). Although this decision was based on other considerations as well, it caused renewed interest in the issue of whether surrogate markers such as CD4 cell count can be used reliably as the primary efficacy end point in a comparative clinical trial.

Much has been written about this subject as it applies to AIDS (25–27), and the issues are complex. As noted by Lagakos and Hoth (28), one can consider the surrogate marker issue from the perspective of regulation of new drugs, with regard to management of individual patients, or as an efficacy end point in a phase III comparative trial. The focus in this chapter is the last of these possibilities. The key question is whether a difference between treatments with respect to the surrogate marker implies and is implied by a treatment difference with respect to the more medically important clinical end point. If not, the use of a surrogate marker could lead to the approval of ineffective drugs or to the abandonment of effective drugs. Thus, one must understand the reliability of CD4, RNA, or some other marker as a surrogate for clinical progression.

Unfortunately, little is known about the value of most markers. CD4 cell count has been the most extensively studied marker (25, 29), and it has been shown to explain some, but not all, of the beneficial clinical effect of ZDV in patients with advanced or early HIV disease. These findings mean that even though an increase or delay in the decline of CD4 cell counts is a good prognostic sign, the ultimate effect of ZDV on clinical progression is partly due to factors not reflected in its effect on CD4 cell count. The implication is that a clinical trial that bases efficacy on a surrogate marker such as CD4 count carries uncertainty about whether any resulting treatment differences, or lack of differences, can reliably be interpreted to indicate corresponding differences in clinical parameters. The value of RNA as a surrogate marker, by itself or in combination with other markers, is just beginning to be investigated (30).

EVALUATING THE LITERATURE

The basic attitude one should take when reviewing the medical literature on any topic is that of the skeptic. Although many patients have the disease, relative to other diseases such as cardiovascular disease and cancer, even HIV specialists have not treated and monitored many patients for any length of time. Many clinicians report their experiences and views based on a few cases. Although these clinicians are accurately reporting what they have seen, one must remember the natural variation or "noise" in the population of patients with HIV disease.

Table 46.3 provides a list of items that should be considered when reviewing the report of a clinical study in the literature. The first item refers to the observation that some clinical studies are primarily "fishing expeditions"; although

Table 46.3. Reviewing the Literature: Features Indicating a High-Quality Study

1. Clear research objective, study design, and evaluation; no evidence of data dredging
2. Use of randomization and stratification
3. Use of placebos and double-blind designs, if feasible
4. Use of standardized criteria and clearly defined end points and response criteria, identified a priori
5. Clear statement of the patient population and accounting of all patients entered
6. Report of extent of follow-up and any resulting limitations on the findings
7. Statement of idealized therapy and actual therapy administered (compliance)
8. Standardization, or at least reporting, of any significant concomitant medications
9. Assessment of end points by an independent or blinded investigator
10. Use of an independent data and safety monitoring board and statement of the number of previous interim analyses for randomized phase III studies
11. Report of the intent to treat analysis of the primary and secondary end points, if the study was randomized
12. Lack of potential bias or conflict of interest of the investigators
13. Statement of statistical power of the study conclusion, if negative
14. Conservative statement of the conclusions; no inferences in the absence of statistical significance

the therapies and case management may be the best available, the research does not appear to have a clear objective. The report of the results of such a study may fail to mention that the specific end points and analyses reported were just a few of many such evaluations conducted and were the only ones that turned out to be interesting. This data evaluation strategy, often referred to as "data dredging," can be misleading because one should expect by chance alone that 1 in 20 analyses should have $P < .05$. One can often pick up clues that such dredging was done by noting variations in the manner of reporting. For example, if the investigators only report the P value for 1 of 6 end points and 1 of 8 subgroups they have described elsewhere in the article, one can be reasonably assured that the P value reported is the smallest of the P values for the 48 (6×8) possible end point subgroup combination analyses. By chance alone, at least 2 of such P values should be less than .05.

A study that produces a definitive result—positive or negative—should be considered a successful clinical trial. However, only a proportion of reported clinical trials can be considered successful. The reasons for failures are many, but they frequently involve the inability to enter the number of patients necessary to produce a definitive study or the selection of therapies and study design in which patients and investigators are unwilling to participate. Others reasons involve studies that are rushed to initiation prematurely, sometimes before the appropriate earlier studies (determining optimal dose or toxicity management) have been completed or before the scientific basis for defining suitable end-point criteria has been established. Whatever the reason, most of these studies eventually are published in the literature.

References

1. Byar DP, Schoenfeld DA, Green SB, et al. Design considerations for AIDS trials. N Engl J Med 1990;323:1343–1348.
2. Ellenberg SS, Finkelstein DM, Schoenfeld DA. Statistical issues arising in AIDS clinical trials. J Am Stat Assoc 1992;87:562–569.
3. Fleming TR. Evaluation of active control trials in AIDS. J Acquir Immune Defic Syndr 1990;3(Suppl 2):S82–S87.
4. Green SB, Ellenberg SS, Finkelstein D, et al. Issues in the design of drug trials for AIDS. Controlled Clin Trials 1990;11:80–87.
5. Volberding PA. Rationale for variations in clinical trial design in different HIV disease stages. J Acquir Immune Defic Syndr 1990;3(Suppl 2):S40–S44.
6. Gelber RD, Zelen M. Planning and reporting of clinical trials. In: Calabresi P, Rosenberg SA, Schein P, eds. Medical oncology: basic principles and clinical management of cancer. New York: MacMillan, 1985:406–425.
7. Meinert CL, Tonascia S. Clinical trials: design conduct and analysis. New York: Oxford University Press, 1986.
8. Miké V, Stanley KE, eds. Statistics in medical research: methods and issues, with applications in cancer research. New York: John Wiley and Sons, 1982.
9. Peto R, Pike MC, Armitage P, et al. Design and analysis of randomised clinical trials requiring prolonged observation of each patient. I. Introduction and design. Br J Cancer 1976;34:585–612.
10. Peto R, Pike MC, Armitage P, et al. Design and analysis of randomised clinical trials requiring prolonged observation of each patient. II. Analysis and examples. Br J Cancer 1977;35:1–39.
11. Schwartz D, Flamant R, Lellouch J. Clinical trials. London: Academic Press, 1980.
12. Weiner JM. Issues in the design and evaluation of medical trials. Boston: G.K. Hall Medical Publishers, 1979.
13. Zelen M. Guidelines for publishing papers on cancer clinical trials: responsibilities of editors and authors. J Clin Oncol 1983;1:164–169.
14. Amato DA, Lagakos SW. Design of clinical trials: endpoints. Consideration in the selection of endpoints for AIDS clinical trials. J Acquir Immune Defic Syndr 1990;3(Suppl 2):S64–S68.
15. Fleiss JL. Statistical methods for rates and proportions. New York: John Wiley and Sons, 1981.
16. Bernstein D, Lagakos SW. Sample size and power determination for stratified clinical trials. J Stat Comput Simulation 1978;8:65–73.
17. Freedman LS. Tables of the number of patients required in clinical trials using the logrank test. Stat Med 1982;1:121–129.
18. Schoenfeld DA, Richter JR. Nomograms for calculating the number of patients needed for a clinical trials with survival as an endpoint. Biometrics 1982;38:163–170.
19. DeMets DL. Data monitoring and sequential analysis: an academic perspective. J Acquir Immune Defic Syndr 1990;3(Suppl 2):S124–S133.
20. Pocock SJ. Clinical trials: a practical approach. New York: John Wiley and Sons, 1983.
21. Kim K, Tsiatis AA. Study duration for clinical trials with survival response and early stopping rule. Biometrics 1990;46:81–92.
22. Lagakos SW, Lim LL-Y, Robins JM. Adjusting for early treatment termination in comparative clinical trials. Stat Med 1990;9:1417–1424.
23. Lagakos SW. Statistical analysis of survival data: applications to the AIDS epidemic. In: Proceedings of the Conference on Health Services Research Methodology: A Focus on AIDS, Tucson, Arizona, June 1988. Rockville, MD: National Center for Health Sciences Research, 1988.
24. Khan JO, Lagakos SL, Richman DD, et al. A controlled trial comparing continued zidovudine with didanosine in human immunodeficiency virus infection. N Engl J Med 1992;327:581–587.
25. De Gruttola V, Wulfsohn M, Tsiatis A, et al. Modeling the relationship between survival and CD4-lymphocytes in patients with AIDS and AIDS-related complex. J Acquir Immune Defic Syndr 1993;6:359–365.
26. Tsiatis A, Dafni U, DeGruttola V, et al. The relationship of CD4 counts over time to survival in patients with AIDS: is CD4 a good surrogate marker? In: Jewell NP, Dietz K, Farewell VT, eds. AIDS epidemiology: methodological issues. Boston: Birkhauser, 1992.
27. Machado SG, Gail MH, Ellenberg S. On the use of laboratory markers in the evaluation of treatment for HIV infection. J Acquir Immune Defic Syndr 1990;3:1065–1073.
28. Lagakos SW, Hoth DF. Surrogate markers in AIDS: where are we? Where are we going? Ann Intern Med 1992;116:599–601.
29. Choi S, Lagakos SW, Schooley R, et al. CD4+ lymphocytes are an incomplete surrogate marker for clinical progression in persons with asymptomatic HIV infection taking zidovudine. Ann Intern Med 1993;118:674–680.
30. Hughes MD, DeGruttola V, Welles SI. Evaluating surrogate markers. J Acquir Immune Defic Syndr Hum Retrovirol 1995;10(Suppl 2):S1–S8.

47

BIOCHEMICAL PHARMACOLOGY

A. NUCLEOSIDE AND NONNUCLEOSIDE REVERSE TRANSCRIPTASE INHIBITORS ACTIVE AGAINST HIV

Jan Balzarini and Erik De Clercq

The formation of the nucleotides that are required for the synthesis of DNA and RNA may be accomplished through two different pathways: the de novo pathway and the salvage pathway (Fig. 47A.1).

In the de novo pathway, ribose, amino acids (i.e., glycine in purine nucleotide metabolism and aspartic acid in pyrimidine metabolism), parts of amino acids (i.e., the NH_2 groups of glutamine and aspartic acid), carbon dioxide (derived from bicarbonate), and formyl, methenyl, and methylene groups derived from formyl-, methenyl-, and methylenetetrahydrofolate (THF) derivatives are combined together and eventually lead to the formation of purine and pyrimidine nucleotides. Starting from inosine monophosphate (IMP), adenine ribonucleotides (i.e., adenosine monophosphate [AMP], adenosine diphosphate [ADP], adenosine triphosphate [ATP]) and guanine ribonucleotides (i.e., guanosine monophosphate [GMP], guanosine diphosphate [GDP], guanosine triphosphate [GTP]) are formed (Fig. 47A.2). Starting from uridine monophosphate (UMP), uridine diphosphate (UDP) and uridine triphosphate (UTP) are formed (Fig. 47A.3). Cytidine triphosphate (CTP) results from the irreversible amination of UTP. All four ribonucleoside 5′-triphosphates (i.e., ATP, GTP, UTP, and CTP) participate in RNA synthesis. The ribonucleoside 5′-diphosphates are reduced to their corresponding 2′-deoxyribonucleoside 5′-diphosphates, which are further converted to thymidine triphosphate (dTTP), dATP, dCTP, and dGTP to participate in DNA synthesis (see Figs. 47A.2 and 47A.3).

In the salvage pathways, free purine and pyrimidine bases and their corresponding nucleosides, derived from breakdown of nucleic acids and nucleotides, are reused to synthesize the corresponding nucleotides. The building blocks of the salvage pathways can be derived from the intracellular as well as the extracellular environment. Bases can be converted to nucleosides by the action of phosphorylases and to nucleotides by the action of phosphoribosyl transferases (PRT). Nucleosides are converted by nucleoside kinases to their 5′-monophosphate derivatives. In addition, 5′-nucleotidase can, under some circumstances, also convert nucleosides to nucleoside 5′-monophosphates. Once the bases and nucleosides have been converted to their corresponding 5′-monophosphate derivatives, they may enter the de novo nucleotide pool and may be converted to their 5′-triphosphate derivatives. The interrelationship between the de novo and the salvage pathways is shown in Figure 47A.1.

PYRIMIDINE 2′-DEOXYRIBONUCLEOTIDE METABOLISM

All 2′-deoxyribonucleotides formed by the de novo pathway are derived from ribonucleotides that are reduced at the level of their 5′-diphosphate derivatives (Fig. 47A.4). The responsible enzyme is ribonucleotide reductase, and it represents an irreversible step in 2′-deoxyribonucleotide synthesis. dUDP and dCDP are subsequently converted to their corresponding 5′-triphosphates dUDP and dCDP, respectively, by nucleoside 5′-diphosphate kinases (NDP kinase) and to their 5′-monophosphate dUMP and dCMP by dTMP (dUMP) kinase and CMP/UMP/dCMP kinase, respectively. Although dCTP can serve as a building block for DNA synthesis, dUTP is converted to dUMP by a specific dUTPase, to avoid erroneous incorporation of dUMP instead of dTMP into cellular DNA. Thymidylate synthase is a key enzyme in dTTP synthesis, and it catalyzes the irreversible conversion of dUMP to dTMP. Thymidylate (dTMP) will then be converted by a dTMP-specific kinase (thymidylate kinase) to dTDP, that is further converted to dTTP by NDP kinase. Besides ribonucleotide reductase and thymidylate synthase, yet another important enzyme in the de novo synthesis of 2′-deoxynucleotides, dCMP deaminase, catalyzes the irreversible conversion of dCMP to dUMP. This enzyme represents the only pathway to convert 2′-deoxycytidine 2′-dCyd) nucleotides into 2′-deoxyuridine (2′-dUrd) nucleotides (see Fig. 47A.4).

As mentioned before, the pyrimidine salvage pathway consists of a limited number of enzymes that play an important role in the activation (phosphorylation) of many antiviral and antitumor compounds. Three different pyrimidine kinases exist: a cytosolic thymidine kinase (TK), which converts dUrd and deoxythymidine (dThd), a mitochondrial

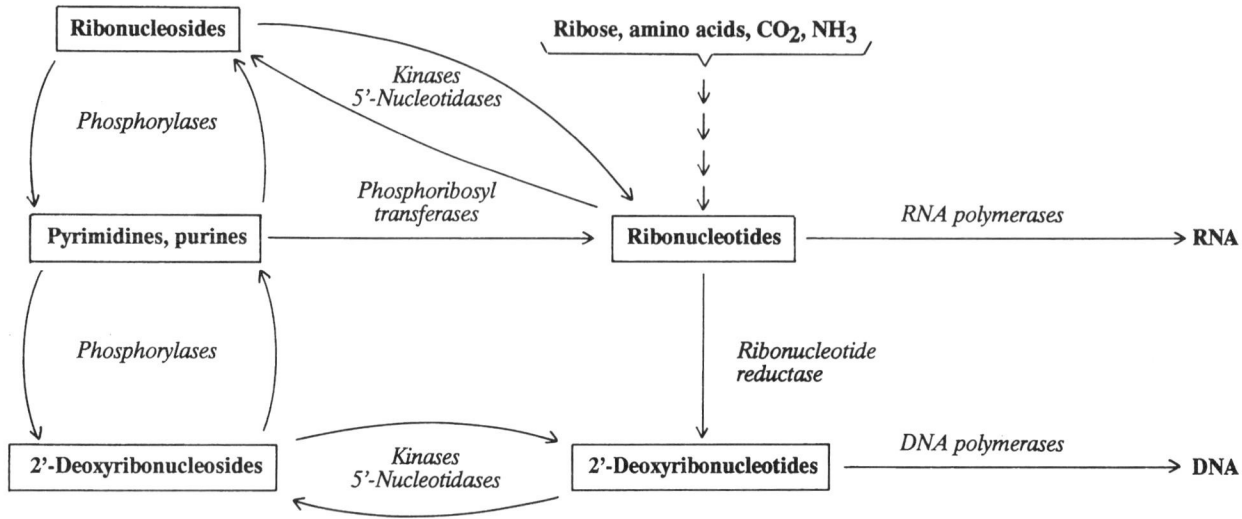

Figure 47A.1. Interrelationship between the salvage and de novo pathways for the biosynthesis of nucleotides.

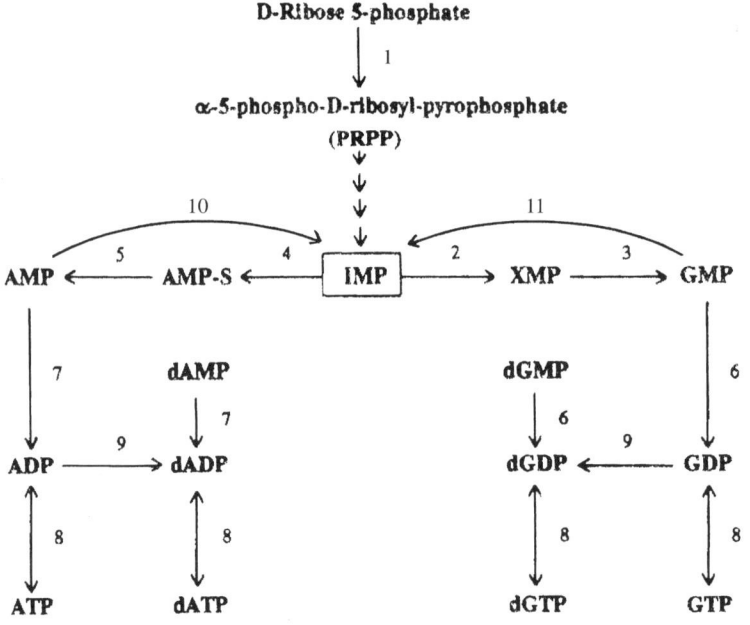

Figure 47A.2. De novo biosynthesis of purine ribo- and 2'-deoxyribonucleotides. Enzymes: *(1)* 5-phosphoribosyl-1-pyrophosphate *(PRPP)* synthetase: *(2)* inosine monophosphate *(IMP)* dehydrogenase; *(3)* guanosine monophosphate *(GMP)* synthetase; *(4)* adenylosuccinate synthetase; *(5)* adenosine monophosphate *(AMP)* lyase; *(6)* guanosine monophosphate *(GMP)* kinase; *(7)* adenosine monophosphate *(AMP)* kinase (myokinase); *(8)* 5'-diphosphate *(DNP)* kinase; *(9)* ribonucleotide reductase; *(10)* adenosine monophosphate *(AMP)* deaminase; *(11)* guanosine monophosphate *(GMP)* reductase.

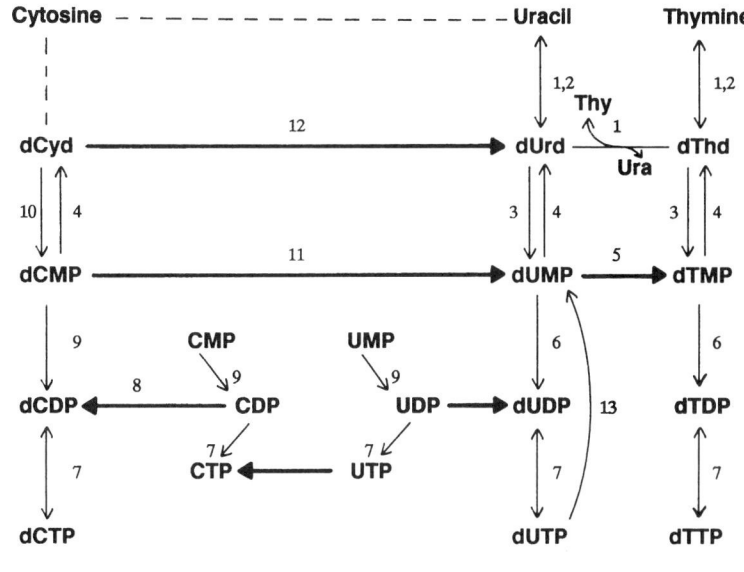

Figure 47A.3. De novo and salvage biosynthesis of pyrimidine ribonucleotides. Enzymes: *(1)* deoxythymidine *(dThd)* phosphorylase; *(2)* uridine/deoxyuridine *(Urd/dUrd)* phosphorylase; *(3)* deoxythymidine *(dThd)* kinase; *(4)* 5'-nucleotidase; *(5)* (2'-deoxy)thymidylate *(dTMP)* synthase; *(6)* (2'-deoxy)thymidylate *(dTMP)* kinase; *(7)* nucleoside 5'-diphosphate *(NDP)* kinase; *(8)* ribonucleotide reductase; *(9)* uridine monophosphate/cytidine monophosphate *(UMP/CMP)* kinase; *(10)* deoxycytidine *(dCyd)* kinase; *(11)* deoxycytidine monophosphate *(dCMP)* deaminase; *(12)* cytidine/deoxycytidine *(Cyd/dCyd)* deaminase; *(13)* deoxyuridine triphosphatase *(dUTPase)*. Thick arrows represent irreversible reactions; thin arrows are reversible reactions; and dashed lines indicate that these do not exist in mammalian cells.

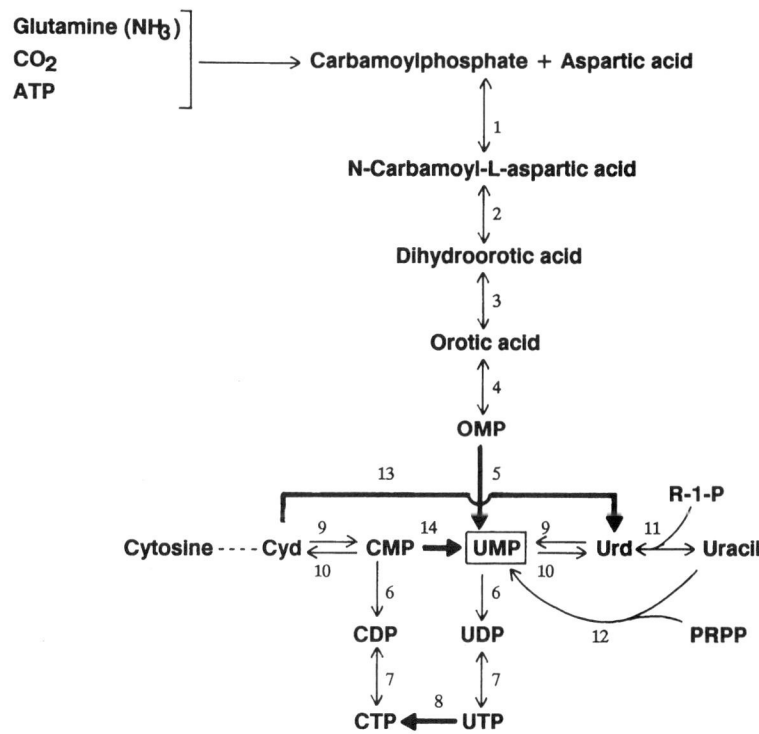

Figure 47A.4. De novo and salvage biosynthesis of pyrimidine 2'-deoxyribonucleotides. Enzymes: *(1)* aspartate carbamoyl transferase *(ATCase)*; *(2)* dihydroorotase; *(3)* dihydroorotate dehydrogenase; *(4)* orotate phosphoribosyl transferase *(ORT)* uridine monophosphate *(UMP)* synthetase; *(5)* orotate monophosphate *(OMP)* decarboxylase; *(6)* uridine monophosphate/cytidine monophosphate *(UMP/CMP)* kinase; *(7)* nucleoside 5'-diphosphate *(NDP)* kinase; *(8)* cytidine triphosphate *(CTP)* synthetase; *(9)* uridine/cytidine *(Urd/Cyd)* kinase; *(10)* 5'-nucleotidase; *(11)* uridine/deoxyuridine *(Urd/dUrd)* phosphorylase; *(12)* uracil phosphoribosyl transferase *(UPRT)*; *(13)* cytidine/deoxycytidine *(Cyd/dCyd)* deaminase; *(14)* cytidine monophosphate/deoxycytidine monophosphate *(CMP/dCMP)* deaminase. Thick arrows represent irreversible reactions; thin arrows are reversible reactions; and dashed lines indicate that these do not exist in mammalian cells.

TK (often called TK-2), which converts dUrd, dThd, and cytosolic dCyd kinase, which converts dCyd to their 5'-monophosphates. These enzymes, as discussed later, have a broad substrate spectrum in that they recognize a series of dUrd and dCyd analogs containing minor changes in the pyrimidine base or deoxyribose moiety and even some purine nucleotides, as in the case of dCyd kinase. The pyrimidine bases uracil and thymine, but not cytosine, can be interconverted to the corresponding nucleosides dUrd and dThd by dThd phosphorylase or uridine (Urd)/dUrd phosphorylase

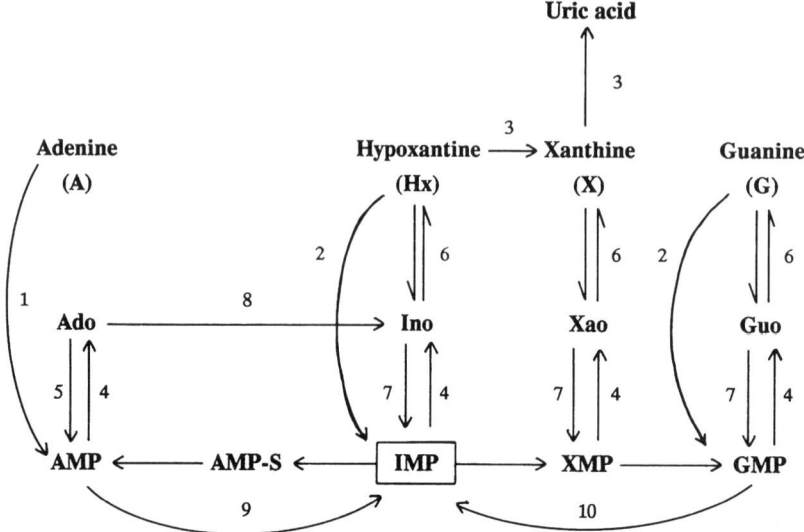

Figure 47A.5. Salvage biosynthesis of purine ribonucleotides. Enzymes: *(1)*, adenine phosphoribosyl transferase *(APRT)*; *(2)* hypoxanthine guanine phosphoribosyl transferase *(HxGPRT)*; *(3)* xanthine oxidase; *(4)* 5′-nucleotidase; *(5)* adenosine kinase; *(6)* purine nucleoside phosphorylase; *(7)* inosine kinase; *(8)* xanthosine kinase; *(9)* adenylate deaminase; and *(10)* guanosine monophosphate *(GMP)* reductase.

in a reversible reaction. In addition, dUrd and dThd can be interconverted by dThd phosphorylase in the presence of the alternative base (see Fig. 47A.4). In this reaction, ribosyl transfer takes place from one nucleoside to the other base and vice versa. The phosphorolytic enzymes basically have a catalytic function and are often responsible for the inactivation of biologically active dThd analogs (i.e., the antiherpetic agent bromovinyldeoxyuridine). A cytidine (Cyd) phosphorylase does not exist in mammalian cells. Finally, many (but not all) cell types contain Cyd/dCyd deaminase activity to convert dCyd (and Cyd) to dUrd (and Urd). This enzyme often plays an "inactivating" role for certain cytosine analogs for which the corresponding uracil nucleoside has no (or diminished) biologic activity (i.e., the antileukemic agent cytosine arabinoside [araC]). A cytosine deaminase does not exist in mammalian cells.

PURINE NUCLEOTIDE METABOLISM

Purine nucleotide metabolism is more complicated, and it consists of more enzymes and more complex feedback regulatory mechanisms than pyrimidine nucleotide metabolism. De novo synthesis of purine nucleotides starts from D-ribose-5-phosphate, which is converted to 5-phosphoribosyl-1-pyrophosphate (PRPP) in an ATP-requiring process catalyzed by PRPP synthetase. This enzyme should be considered as a key enzyme in de novo nucleotide synthesis, both in purine (IMP) and pyrimidine (UMP) nucleotide synthesis.

Starting from PRPP, the purine skeleton is constructed on the activated ribose 5′-phosphate part through 10 enzymatic steps to afford inosinate (IMP). During these anabolic synthetic processes starting from PRPP, at least 4 ATP molecules are consumed, glycine is built into the purine skeleton (thus providing C-4, C-5 and N-7), glutamine and aspartic acid serve as the NH_2-donors for N-9 and N-3, and N-1, respectively), whereas bicarbonate, formyl and methenyl provide the C-6, and C-2 and C-8, respectively. Inosinate (IMP) represents an important branch-point in the de novo purine nucleotide metabolism. On the one hand, it can be converted into GMP through xanthosine monophosphate (XMP) on two subsequent irreversible enzymatic reactions: IMP dehydrogenase and GMP synthetase (see Fig. 47A.2). ATP is the energy source for the synthesis of GMP from XMP. On the other hand, IMP can be converted into succinyl-AMP by adenylosuccinate synthetase, which is then (with GTP as the energy source) converted by adenylosuccinate lyase to AMP. AMP can be converted again to IMP in a one-step reaction, catalyzed by AMP deaminase, whereas GMP can be converted again to IMP by GMP reductase. From AMP and GMP, the corresponding 5′-diphosphate and 5′-triphosphate derivatives are formed. As already mentioned for the pyrimidine 2′-deoxyribonucleotides, the purine 2′-deoxyribonucleotides are formed from ADP and GDP in a reductive irreversible process catalyzed by ribonucleotide reductase.

The salvage pathway for purine ribonucleotide synthesis contains certain important enzymes (Fig. 47A.5). The free bases adenine, hypoxanthine, xanthine, and guanine can be converted directly to their corresponding 5′-monophosphate derivatives by the action of adenine phosphoribosyl transferase (APRT) or hypoxanthine/guanine phosphoribosyl transferase (HGPRT). Physiologically, these phosphoribosyl transferases represent the most active pathways in the salvage of preformed purine bases to the corresponding nucleotide 5′-monophosphates. Only adenosine is efficiently converted to its 5′-monophosphate by adenosine kinase. The other purine nucleosides (i.e., Ino, Xao, and Guo) may be converted to their corresponding nucleotides by the action of 5′-nucleotidases, which normally act in the opposite way (conversion of purine nucleotide 5′-monophosphates to purine nucleosides).

Adenosine deaminase converts Ado into Ino. This substance is ubiquitous in tissues and plasma. Ado deaminase is reponsible for the inactivation of biologically active nucleosides (such as the antiherpetic compound adenine arabinoside [araA]).

Catabolism of purine nucleosides often starts by purine nucleoside phosphorylase (PNPase) that converts Ino to Hx, which is subsequently converted to xanthine and uric acid by xanthine oxidase. However, PNPase may also be considered as an anabolic enzyme, as it can convert Hx and G to Ino and Guo, respectively. Nucleoside kinases are then required to convert the latter to IMP and GMP. However, the two-step nucleoside phosphorylase–nucleoside kinase pathway does not appear to be active, if it exists at all, in most tissues and is generally overtaken by the one-step PRT pathway.

METABOLISM OF 2′,3′-DIDEOXYNUCLEOSIDES

Unlike herpesviruses, human immunodeficiency virus (HIV) and other retroviruses do not encode specific enzymes required for the metabolism of the purine or pyrimidine nucleosides to their corresponding 5′-triphosphates. Moreover, no differences have been observed in the metabolism of the 2′,3′-dideoxynucleosides and acyclic nucleoside phosphonates (ANPs) in virus-infected versus uninfected cells. Thus, HIV replication seems not to have a significant impact on the intracellular pool levels of the 2′,3′-dideoxynucleotides, ANPs, or natural nucleotides. It is inferred, therefore, that 2′,3′-dideoxynucleosides and ANPs must be phosphorylated by host cellular kinases. Because different animal species (or even different cell types within one animal species) may differ in the efficiency of phosphorylation of these drugs, one should be particularly cautious in extrapolating results on the metabolism and antiviral activity of the compounds from one cell type to another, and even more so from one animal species to another, or to humans.

3′-Azido-2′,3′-Dideoxythymidine

The formula for 3′-azido-2′,3′-dideoxythymidine (zidovudine [ZDV], AzddThd, AZT, Retrovir) is shown in Figure 47A.6. Zimmerman and coworkers (1) demonstrated that ZDV permeates the cell membrane chiefly by nonfacilitated diffusion and not through a nucleoside transporter. The initial velocity of ZDV influx proceeds linearly in function of the nucleoside concentration (up to 10 mmol/L), is insensitive to nucleoside transport inhibitors (i.e., dipyridamole, nitrobenzylthioinosine), is insensitive to an excess of other closely related nucleosides (i.e., dThd, Urd), and is almost completely independent of temperature. The unusual ability of ZDV to penetrate cells without the use of a nucleoside transporter may be attributed to the considerable lipophilicity of this compound (1, 2), although other, more polar 2′,3′-dideoxynucleosides (i.e., 2′,3′-dideoxyadenosine [ddAdo], 2′,3′-didehydro-2′,3′-dideoxythymidine [d4T]) may penetrate the cells by a similar mechanism of passive diffusion.

ZDV is metabolized to its 5′-monophosphate, 5′-diphosphate, and 5′-triphosphate in a similar fashion in uninfected and HIV-infected H9 cells (3, 4) (Fig. 47A.7). The cytosol TK (EC 2.7.1.21) is responsible for the phosphorylation of ZDV to its monophosphate (3, 5, 6). TK purified from human lymphocyte H9 cells catalyzes the phosphorylation of dThd and ZDV with apparent Michaelis

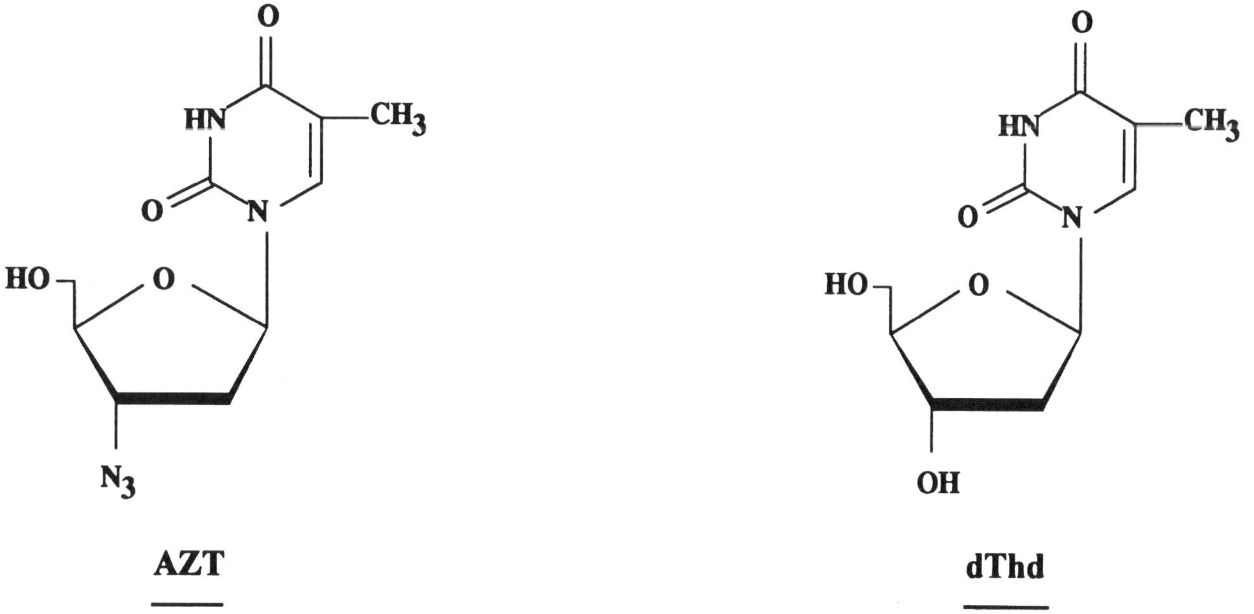

Figure 47A.6. Formulas of 3′-azido-2′,3′-dideoxythymidine *(AzddThd, AZT)*, currently known as zidovudine, and 2′-deoxythymidine *(dThd)*.

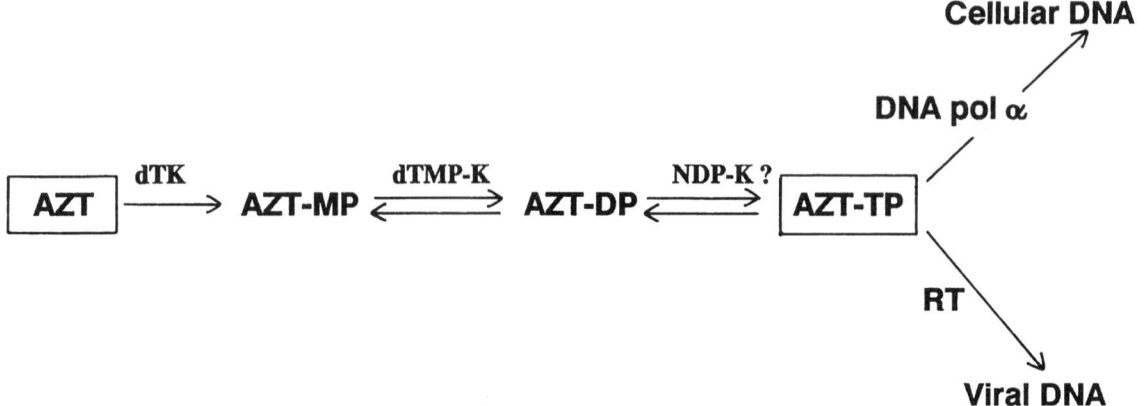

Figure 47A.7. Metabolic conversion of 3′-azido-2′,3′-dideoxythymidine (AZT), currently known as zidovudine, to its 5′-triphosphate derivative. Enzymes: *dTK*, (2′-deoxy)thymidine kinase; *dTMP-K*, (2′-deoxy)thymidylate kinase; *NDP-K*, nucleoside 5′-diphosphate kinase; *DNA pol α*, DNA polymerase α; *RT*, reverse transcriptase.

constant (K_m) values of 2.9 and 3.0 μmol/L, respectively. This means that both compounds have comparable (strong) substrate affinities for TK. The maximal rate of phosphorylation of ZDV is equal to 60% of the rate of dThd.

Furman and associates (3) demonstrated that phosphorylation of ZDV-MP to ZDV-DP is catalyzed by cellular thymidylate (dTMP) kinase (EC 2.7.4.9). The apparent K_m value for ZDV-MP is twofold greater than the K_m for dTMP (8.6 μmol/L versus 4.1 μmol/L), but the maximal phosphorylation rate is only 0.3% of the dTMP rate. ZDV-MP should therefore be considered substrate inhibitor of thymidylate kinase, and this conclusion is compatible with the observation that human T-lymphocytes incubated with ZDV accumulate ZDV-MP, whereas only low levels of the 5′-diphosphate and 5′-triphosphate are achieved. Incubation of H9 cells with 50 μmol/L ZDV resulted in intracellular pool levels of ZDV-MP as high as 790 μmol/L, whereas ZDV-DP and ZDV-TP pool concentrations were only 4.2 and 1.8 μmol/L, respectively (3).

Thus, the intracellular pool levels achieved by ZDV-MP in H9 cells are much higher than those of ZDV-DP and ZDV-TP. This phenomenon has also been observed in other human cell lines: ATH8, Molt/4F, MT-4, CEM, and human bone marrow cells (6–9). It may be generalized to human T-lymphoblast or T-lymphocyte cell lines, and, possibly, to other human cell types as well (i.e., cervix carcinoma HeLa and hepatoblastoma Hep G2.2.2.15 cells) (J Balzarini, B Degrève, E De Clercq, unpublished data). Obviously, ZDV-MP blocks its own phosphorylation to the 5′-diphosphate and 5′-triphosphate (4,6). The higher the initial concentrations of ZDV exposed to the cells (i.e., MT-4), the more ZDV-MP, but not ZDV-DP or ZDV-TP, is formed intracellularly (6). When the initial concentration of ZDV was increased from 0.5 to 50 μmol/L, ZDV-MP pool levels in MT-4 cells increased 50-fold, whereas the ZDV-TP pool levels increased only 3-fold (6). Avramis and coworkers (8) observed only a 5-fold increase of the intracellular ZDV-TP concentration when the input ZDV concentration was increased from 1 to 50 μmol/LEM cell cultures. Lavie and associates revealed the crystal structure of yeast TMP kinase complexed with ZDV-MP (10, 11). They found a 0.5-Å dislocation of the ATP-binding P-loop in the ZDV-MP containing enzyme compared with the dTMP-complexed enzyme, and they correlated this dislocation with the decreased maximum velocity (V_{max}) value of ZDV-MP, relative to dTMP, for dTMP kinase. If the foregoing data can be extrapolated to the in vivo situation, it means that increasing the dose of ZDV will not result in a proportional increase in the intracellular pool levels of ZDV-TP. This, in turn, suggests that high-dose ZDV treatment may not result in comparably higher antiretroviral activity in vivo. Based on this premise, the ZDV dose initially given to patients with acquired immunodeficiency syndrome (AIDS) has been cut down so as to maintain antiviral efficacy while decreasing toxicity.

The accumulation of ZDV-MP, relative to ZDV-DP and ZDV-TP, has not been observed in murine leukemia L1210 cells, in which high pool levels of the monophosphate, diphosphate, and triphosphate of ZDV are achieved (12–14). The efficient conversion of ZDV to ZDV-TP in murine cells may explain the pronounced inhibitory effect of ZDV on Moloney murine sarcoma virus (MSV)–induced transformation of murine C3H/3T3 cells in vitro (14), MSV-induced tumor development in newborn mice (14, 15) and Rauscher murine leukemia virus (RLV)–induced splenomegaly and viremia in Balb/c mice (16).

After ZDV-MP has been converted to ZDV-DP, cellular NDP kinase as well as various other enzymes may be responsible for its further conversion to ZDV-TP. In fact, Véron and collaborators studied the kinetics of ZDV-DP with NDP kinase and revealed the crystal structure of human NDP kinase complexed with ZDV-DP (17, 18). They found that ZDV-DP is a poor substrate for NDP kinase (V_{max} approximately 0.1% of that of dTDP), and this observation is in agreement with the structural data obtained from the ZDV-DP–bound NDP kinase crystals. Intracellular ZDV-TP pool levels decline rapidly after removal of the nucleoside from the culture medium. In H9 cells, ZDV-TP levels decrease by sevenfold within 4 hours after removal of ZDV (50 µmol/L) from the medium (3). Whether and to what extent ZDV-TP is subject to enzymatic hydrolysis and converted back to the 5′-monophosphate or nucleoside form remain to be elucidated.

ZDV-TP competes with dTTP for binding to HIV-1 reverse transcriptase (RT) (3, 19, 20). With poly(A).oligo $(dT)_{12-18}$ as the template/primer, K_m (dTTP) and inhibitory constant (K_i) (ZDV-TP) values are 2.8 and 0.04 µmol/L, respectively. With activated calf thymus DNA as the template, these values are 1.2 and 0.3 µmol/L, respectively (21). For DNA polymerase α, K_m (dTTP) and K_i (ZDV-TP) are as high as 2.4 and 230 µmol/L, respectively; and for DNA polymerase β, they are 6.0 and 73 µmol/L, respectively. Moreover, to DNA polymerase γ, ZDV-TP is much less inhibitory than the closely related 2′,3′-dideoxynucleoside ddTTP (inhibitory concentration of 50% [IC_{50}], 11 and 0.1 µmol/L, respectively) (22). ZDV-TP also functions as an alternative substrate for RT (4, 21). The resulting incorporation of ZDV-TP (as ZDV-MP) into poly (rA).oligo $(dT)_{12-18}$ causes DNA chain termination and premature deceleration of the reaction (Fig. 47A.8). Sommadossi and coworkers (9, 23) demonstrated a specific incorporation of ZDV-MP into human bone marrow cell DNA. The amount of ZDV-MP incorporated into DNA was correlated with the initial extracellular ZDV concentration, and it also correlated with the inhibition of clonal peripheral blood mononuclear cell (PBMC) growth. These observations indicate at least one mechanism responsible for ZDV-induced bone marrow toxicity (see earlier).

Several laboratories have reported on the effect of ZDV on intracellular deoxynucleotide (dNTP) pools. Furman and colleagues (3) observed a four- to fivefold drop of dTTP, a threefold decrease of dGTP, and a twofold increase of dATP levels on incubation of H9 cells with 50 µmol/L ZDV. In addition, a drop of dCTP levels was erroneously reported (3), but it was corrected later by Harrington and associates (24), Frick and Nelson (25), and Frick and

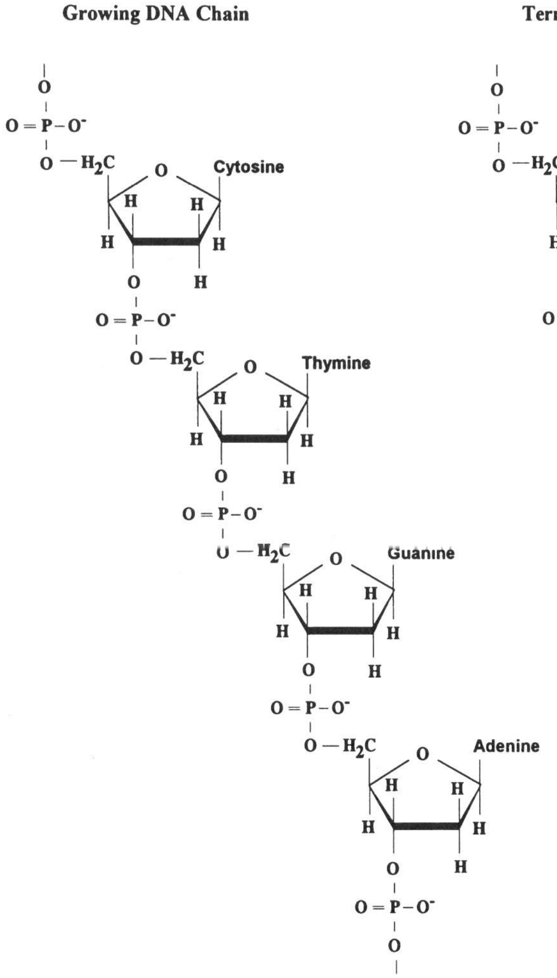

Figure 47A.8. DNA chain termination by 3′-azido-2′,3′-dideoxythymidine (currently known as zidovudine) triphosphate (AZT-TP). A. Growing DNA chain. B. Terminated DNA chain. The azido group at the 3′-end position of the DNA chain prevents incorporation of a new nucleotide and results in DNA chain termination.

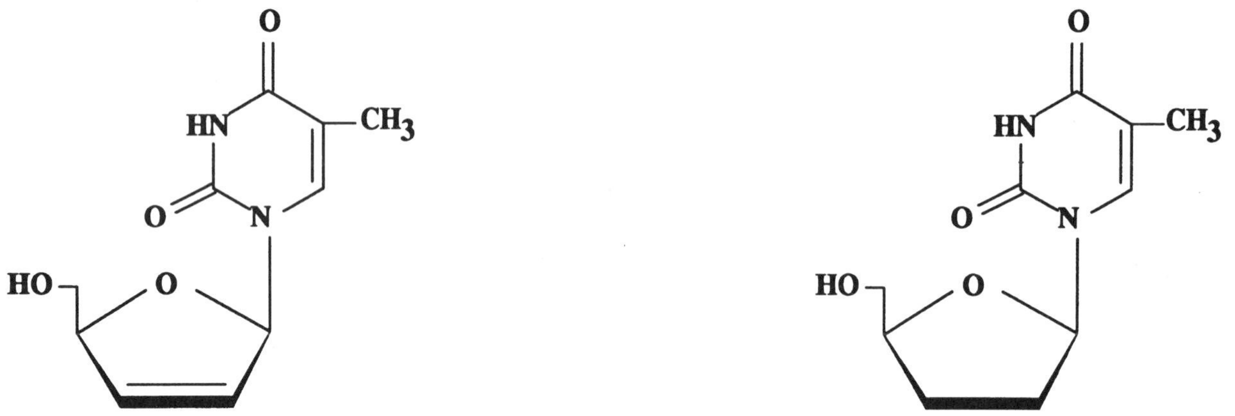

Figure 47A.9. Formulas of 2',3'-didehydro-2',3'-dideoxythymidine *(D4T)* and 2',3'-dideoxythymidine *(ddThd)*.

colleagues (26). Hao and coworkers (27) did not observe consistent changes in endogenous dNTP levels, except for an increase in dCTP after exposure of H9, Molt-4, CEM, and ATH8 cells to 50 µmol/L ZDV during 24 hours. However, in short-term incubations (i.e., 3.5 hours), Frick and Nelson (25) observed a two- to fourfold accumulation of dTMP in ZDV (10 µmol/L)–treated HL-60, H9, and K-562 cells and a concomitant drop of dTTP levels by 10%, 18%, and 56%, respectively. These data are consistent with the inhibitory effect of ZDV on the conversion of radio-labeled dThd to [^{3}H]dTDP and [^{3}H]dTTP in MT-4 and H9 cells and a concomitant increase in intracellular [^{3}H]dTMP pools (6, 28, 29).

All data taken together, the magnitude of the effect of ZDV on intracellular dNTP pools varies from one particular cell line to another. The physiologic relevance of the effects of ZDV on dNTP pools with regard to its cellular toxicity is unclear. Investigators initially suggested that bone marrow toxicity may be due to perturbation of dTTP pools by ZDV. However, arguments against dTTP starvation in human bone marrow cells by ZDV have been provided by Somma-dossi and coworkers (9). These investigators reported that depletion of dTTP pools in human bone marrow cells is minimal, transient, and rapidly reversible: the deoxyribo-nucleotide pools were unaltered after a 24- or 48-hour exposure to 10 µmol/L ZDV.

To explain the cause of anemia and neutropenia in ZDV-treated AIDS patients, Weidner and associates (30) and Weidner and Sommadossi (31) examined the potential mechanism of ZDV-induced anemia by studying the effect of ZDV on hemoglobin synthesis in butyric acid-induced differentiating human K-562 leukemia cells. Unlike other 2',3'-dideoxynucleosides (i.e., 2',3'-dideoxycytidine [ddC], d4T, 3'-fluoro-2',3'-dideoxythymidine [FLT]), exposure of these cells to 25 to 250 µmol/L ZDV for 72 hours resulted in a selective inhibition of hemoglobin synthesis. ZDV reduced the steady-state level of globin mRNA, but not of actin mRNA. The reduction in globin mRNA levels was associated with decreased globin transcription in vitro. The finding that ZDV specifically inhibits globin gene expression may reflect, at least in part, its cytotoxicity for the erythroid cell line.

Another observation made by the same research group (30, 31) is the formation of 3'-amino-ddThd (3'-AmddThd) from ZDV in some cells. 3'-AmddThd can be regarded as a reduction product from ZDV, and it is known to be toxic. However, the potential role of this metabolite in the eventual toxicity of ZDV remains to be demonstrated.

2',3'-Didehydro-2',3'-Dideoxythymidine

The formula for d4T is shown in Figure 47A.9. The metabolism of d4T has been investigated in comparison with that of ZDV. Experiments with H9, MT-4, or CEM cells have revealed that, besides the nucleoside, the 5'-phosphorylated metabolites of d4T (i.e., d4T-MP, d4T-DP, and d4T-TP) rapidly appear intracellularly (32–36). In short-term incubation experiments, the release of free thymine, or formation of [^{3}H]thymidine or [^{3}H]-2',3'-dideoxythymidine, was not observed (6, 32). These observations are in agreement with the findings of Balzarini and associates (33) that d4T is resistant to hydrolytic attack by dThd phosphorylase and thus are not rapidly degraded. Unlike ZDV, d4T does not accumulate as its 5'-monophosphate (d4T-MP), a finding indicating important differences in the kinetic properties of d4T and ZDV for the enzymes involved in their phosphorylation (6, 32, 34, 36).

The agent d4T is much less efficiently phosphorylated to its 5'-monophosphate by MT-4 cell extracts than ZDV (K_m, 142 and 14 µmol/L, respectively; V_{max} d4T, 5% of V_{max} ZDV) (6) (Fig. 47A.10). In addition, Ho and Hitchcock

(34) found with d4T a K_i value of 4600 µmol/L for CEM cells TK compared with a K_m of 6.6 µmol/L with dThd. Marongiu and coworkers (35) reported with d4T a K_m value of 138 µmol/L (versus 1.9 µmol/L for dThd) for purified H9 cytosolic TK, and with dThd a K_i of 1.37 for the same enzyme. The V_{max} for d4T was 9- to 10-fold lower than for dThd. The phosphorylation of d4T by MT-4 cell-free extracts is sensitive to inhibition by dThd (6, 34, 35). Moreover, dTTP, an allosteric inhibitor of TK, inhibits the phosphorylation of d4T by MT-4 cell extracts (6).

At first glance, this finding may suggest that TK is responsible for the phosphorylation of d4T. Thus, Ho and Hitchcock (34) and Marongiu and coworkers (35) demonstrated that [^{3}H]d4T is phosphorylated by purified CEM, Vero, and H9 cell TK. However, Balzarini and colleagues (6) found that the phosphorylation pattern of d4T, unlike that of ZDV, is almost identical in human B-lymphoblast Raji/0 and the TK-deficient Raji/TK – cells. This finding argues against the role of TK in the intracellular activation of d4T, at least in Raji cells. TK may be the principal enzyme responsible for d4T phosphorylation in a number of human T cell lines, but not in human B (Raji) cells.

The observation that d4T, unlike ZDV, does not accumulate in the cells as its 5'-monophosphate form suggests that d4T-MP does not behave as a substrate inhibitor of dTMP kinase. This concept remains to be confirmed in a cell-free dTMP kinase assay. However, the apparent lack of inhibition of dTMP kinase by d4T-MP has been indirectly shown by Balzarini and coworkers (6) and Mansuri and associates (29). Although ZDV has a marked inhibitory effect on the conversion of [^{3}H]thymidine to [^{3}H]dTDP and [^{3}H]dTTP in MT4 and H9 cells and results in an increase in intracellular [^{3}H]dTMP pools, d4T does not cause such perturbation in the intracellular pools of [^{3}H]dTMP, [^{3}H]dTDP, or [^{3}H]dTTP. If dTTP starvation is an important factor in the toxicity of ZDV (see earlier), d4T should have a definite advantage over ZDV, because it does not lead to such dTTP starvation.

The different kinetic behavior of d4T and ZDV at both the dThd kinase level and the dTMP kinase level also affects the formation of their respective 5'-triphosphates. The formation of d4T-TP in MT-4 cells is inferior to ZDV-TP formation if the initial (input) concentration of d4T or ZDV is 1 µmol/L or less. However, if the initial concentration of ZDV and d4T is increased to 10 µmol/L, anabolism of d4T to d4T-TP is facilitated relative to the formation of ZDV-TP from ZDV (6). Obviously, the reason is that, in contrast to ZDV-MP, d4T-MP does not inhibit its further conversion to the 5'-diphosphate and 5'-triphosphate. This phenomenon has also been observed by Ho and Hitchcock (34) in CEM cells. These findings may have a pronounced impact on treatment modalities of HIV-infected individuals with d4T. In contrast to ZDV, higher doses of which do not necessarily result in higher levels of the active metabolite ZDV-TP, higher doses of d4T may result in concomitantly higher levels of the active metabolite d4T-TP. This finding suggests that d4T may have greater efficacy than ZDV at higher drug doses.

Although maximum intracellular pool levels of d4T-MP and d4T-TP are reached within 6 hours after incubation of H9 cells with d4T, these initial levels subsequently decline and then remain constant for up to 72 hours (32). Moreover, in MT-4 cells, sustained d4T-TP levels were observed for 48 hours; they started to decline only at 72 hours (6). In addition, Ho and Hitchcock (34) and Zhu and colleagues (36) found that, after removal of d4T from the (CEM and PBL) cell culture medium, the concentration of d4T-TP diminished with a long half-life (200 to 210 minutes). Thus, inside the cells, the 5'-triphosphate of d4T persists for a long time, a property that must be important for d4T in accomplishing its antiretrovirus activity.

Experiments with [^{3}H]d4T have revealed that the compound is incorporated into both low and high polymeric DNA. The appearance of radioactivity in low polymeric DNA suggests that [^{3}H]d4T is terminally incorporated, thus resulting in the formation of truncated DNA strands (32).

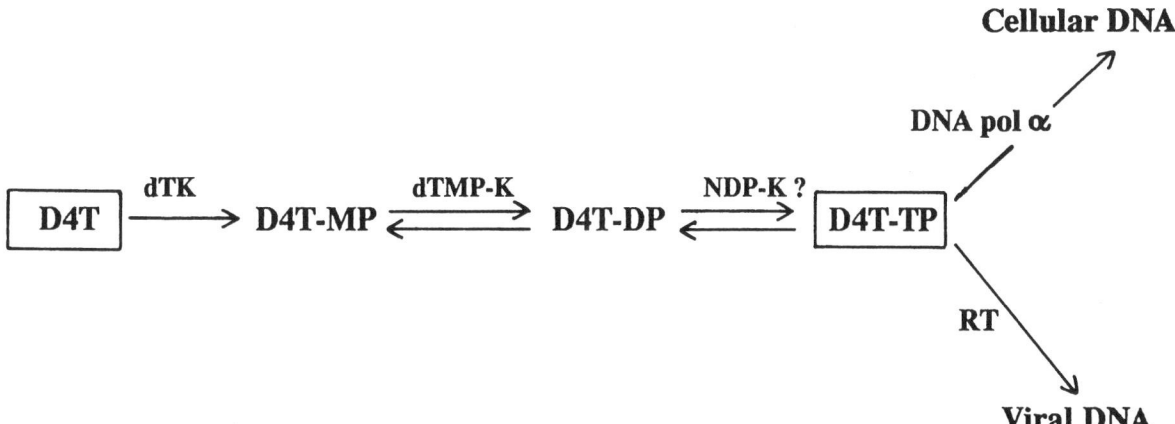

Figure 47A.10. Metabolic conversion of 2',3'-didehydro-2',3'-dideoxythymidine *(D4T)* to its 5'-triphosphate derivative. Enzymes: see legend to Figure 47A.7.

Whether and to what extent the incorporation of d4T in cellular DNA contributes to its cytotoxicity remain to be elucidated.

3′-Azido-2′,3′-Dideoxyuridine

The formula for 3′-azido-2′,3′-dideoxyuridine (AzddUrd) is shown in Figure 47A.11. When exposed to PBMCs and human bone marrow cells, [^{3}H]AzddUrd accumulates as its AzddUMP, representing up to 55 to 65% of the total intracellular radioactivity (37) (Fig. 47A.12). Levels of AzddUDP and AzddUTP are at least 10- to 100-fold lower than that of AzddUMP. In this respect, the metabolism of AzddUrd mimics the metabolism of ZDV in that the 5′-monophosphate metabolite accumulates intracellularly and prevents its further conversion to the 5′-triphosphate derivative. AzddUTP has only been detected in human PBMCs, but not in bone marrow cells (37), a finding that may explain the relatively low toxicity of AzddUrd to bone marrow cells.

Unlike ZDV, AzddUrd gives rise to two novel metabolites. Through the aid of UDP-glucose pyrophosphorylase and in the presence of α-D-glucose-1-phosphate or α-D-N-acetylglucosamine-1-phosphate, AzddUTP is converted to AzddUDP-glucose and AzddUDP-N-acetylglucosamine. In contrast to AzddUTP, which is eliminated by a biphasic process (initial half-life, 1 to 2 hours; terminal half-life, 13 to 30 hours), the AzddUDP-hexose derivatives decay as a monophasic process (half-life, 24 hours) (37). Whether the AzddUDP-hexose metabolites can be converted to AzddUDP or AzddUMP is unclear. If so, they may represent intracellular depot forms of AzddUrd that may eventually be converted to the 5′-triphosphate derivative. AzddUMP is not converted to ZDV-MP by thymidylate synthase, a finding that is in agreement with the absence of any [^{3}H]ZDV derivative found in [^{3}H]AzddUrd-treated bone marrow cells or PBMCs (37).

The pharmacokinetics of AzddUrd in mice has been compared with that of ZDV (34). The half-life, total body clearance (Cl_t), and distribution volume (V_D) proved similar for both compounds at each dose tested (50 and 250 mg/kg). This may be related to the similar chemical structures of both compounds. The decreased Cl_t and V_D at the higher dose indicates a dose dependency for both AzddUrd and ZDV. Possibly, saturation of the hepatic metabolism and renal elimination of unchanged drug are potential causes for the decrease in clearance (38). Brain-to-serum concentration ratios for AzddUrd were 9 4-fold higher than for ZDV at 50 mg/kg (0.23 versus 0.06, respectively).

3′-Fluoro-2′,3′-Dideoxythymidine

Of the 2′,3′-dideoxynucleoside analogs, FLT (FddThd) (Fig. 47A.13) is the most efficiently converted intracellularly to its 5′-triphosphate, as shown in different cell lines (i.e., MT-4, CEM, H9) (Fig. 47A.14). The phosphorylation of FLT to the 5′-monophosphate, 5′-diphosphate, and 5′-triphosphate is similar in uninfected and HIV-infected cells (11, 39, 40).

FLT is a good, although slightly less efficient, substrate for TK than ZDV. Using Molt/4F and MT-4 cell extracts, K_i/K_m values of 3.4 and 0.7 have been found with FLT and ZDV, respectively (5). Phosphorylation of FLT-MP to FLT-DP and FLT-TP proceeds much more efficiently than phosphorylation of ZDV-MP to ZDV-DP and ZDV-TP. FLT only slightly accumulates as its 5′-monophosphate;

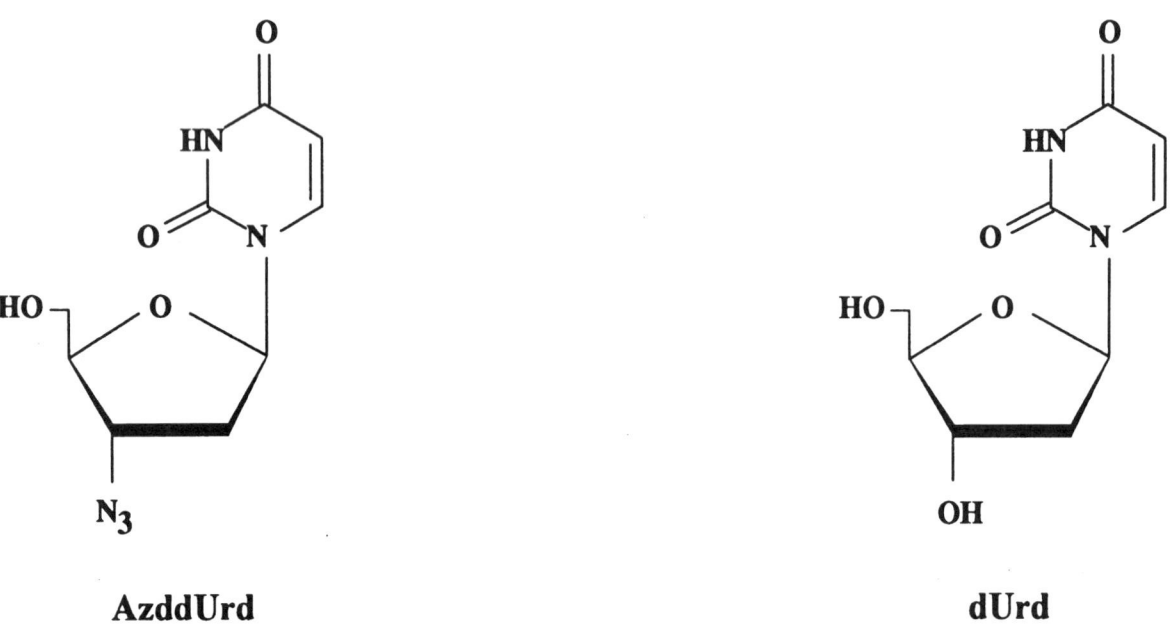

Figure 47A.11. Formulas of 3′-azido-2′,3′-dideoxyuridine *(AzddUrd)* and 2′-deoxyuridine *(dUrd)*.

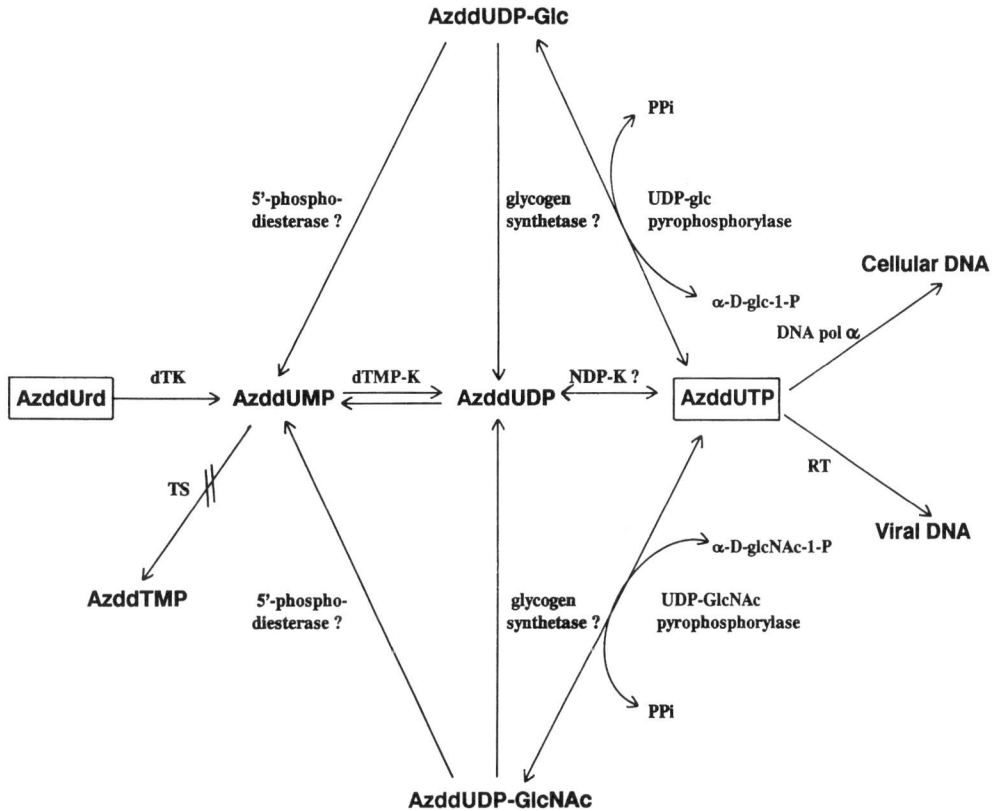

Figure 47A.12. Metabolic conversion of AzddUrd to its 5′-triphosphate derivative. Enzymes: *DNA pol α*, DNA polymerase α; *dTK*, (2′-deoxy)thymidine kinase; *dTMP-K*, (2′-deoxy)thymidylate kinase; *NDP-K*, nucleoside 5′-diphosphate kinase; *PPi*, pyrophosphate; *RT*, reverse transcriptase; *TK*, (deoxy)thymidine kinase; *TS*, (2′-deoxy)thymidylate synthase; *UDP*, uridine 5′-diphosphate.

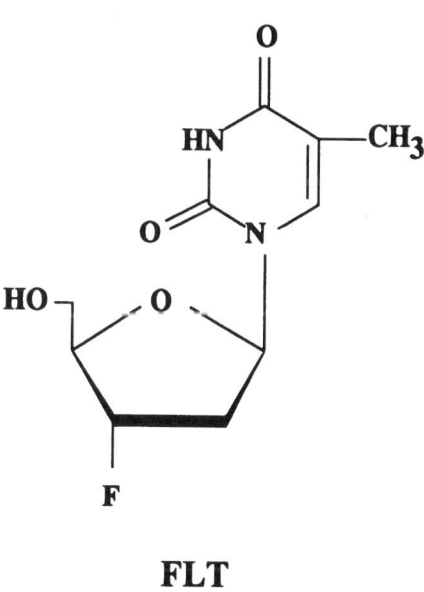

Figure 47A.13. Formulas of 3′-fluoro-2′,3′-dideoxythymidine *(FddThd, FLT)*.

FLT-MP levels are lower than ZDV-MP levels under comparable experimental conditions. Consequently, six- to eight-fold higher levels of FLT-TP than of ZDV-TP are observed when the 2′,3′-dideoxynucleosides (1 μmol/L) are incubated with MT-4 or H9 cells for 24 hours (13). In addition,

FLT-TP, like d4T-TP, persists for a long time after removal of the drug from the H9 cell culture medium (half-life, 4½ hours). In comparison, the half-life for dTTP is much less than 3 hours. As has also been observed for ZDV, FLT is more efficiently phosphorylated in rodent cells than in human cells. Matthes and associates (39) demonstrated that FLT is 2.5- to 3-fold better phosphorylated to FLT-TP in rat NRK-49F and murine 3T3 cells than in MT-4 cells. However, the differences found between the eventual FLT-TP levels in human and rodent cell lines were much less pronounced than for ZDV-TP.

Like ZDV-TP, FLT-TP is a potent inhibitor of HIV RT. The K_i value is 0.08 μmol/L (K_m of the natural substrate, 11.4 μmol/L) when poly(A).oligo(dT)$_{20}$ is used as the template primer. Sterzycki and associates (41) and Mansuri and colleagues (29) also reported for FLT-TP a K_i of 0.26 μmol/L with RNA as template, and 84 μmol/L with DNA as template. In contrast to its high affinity for HIV RT, FLT-TP has only poor affinity for DNA polymerase α (IC_{50}, 200 μmol/L), and moderate affinity for DNA polymerase β (IC_{50}, 3 μmol/L). FLT is endowed with a higher toxicity for human progenitor erythrocyte burst-forming units than ZDV (IC_{50}, 1.0 and 6.7 μmol/L, respectively), but it is much less inhibitory to granulocyte–macrophage colony formation (IC_{50}, 10 and 1 μmol/L, respectively). In this respect, both ZDV and FLT are more toxic to CFU-GM and BFU-E cells than is d4T (IC_{50}, 100 and 10 μmol/L, respectively) (29).

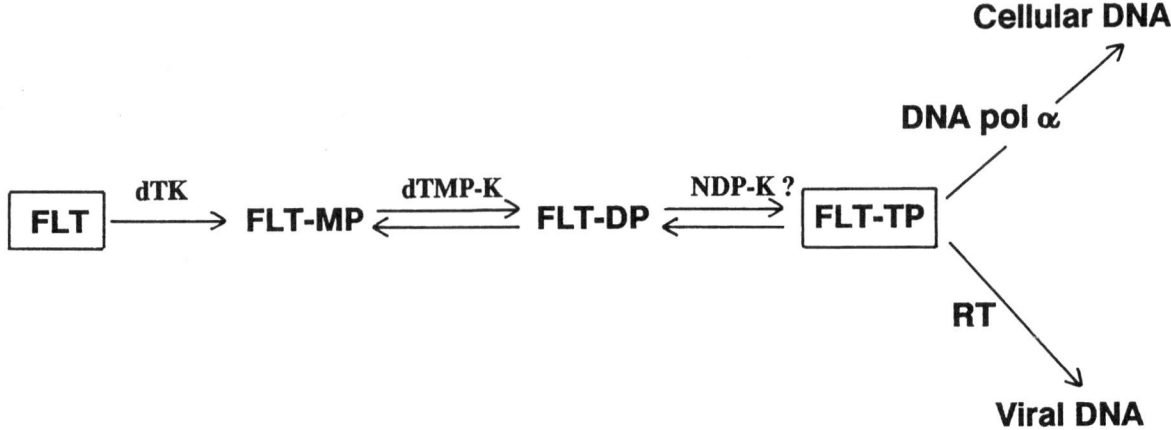

Figure 47A.14. Metabolic conversion of 3′-fluoro-2′,3′-dideoxythymidine *(FLT)* to its 5′-triphosphate derivative. Enzymes: see legend to Figure 47A.7.

2′,3′-Dideoxycytidine

In contrast to ZDV, d4T, and FLT, ddC (ddCyd) is a cytosine derivative (Fig. 47A.15). Therefore, it may be expected to be metabolized in a different way and by different enzymes than the dThd analogs. Cooney and colleagues (42) found no differences in the metabolism of ddC between HIV-infected and uninfected ATH8 cells. Uptake studies (42) revealed that ddC transport depends, at least in part, on the nucleoside carrier. Ullman and coworkers (43) found an 80% diminished rate of [^{3}H]ddC influx in two nucleoside transport–deficient CEM lines and partial resistance of these cell lines to the cytostatic effect of ddC. Phosphorylation of ddC proceeded rapidly to its 5′-triphosphate of ddCTP (Fig. 47A.16). Besides ddCMP, ddCDP, and ddCTP, a ddCDP-choline and a ddCDP-ethanolamine adduct were formed to a significant extent (42, 44).

No deaminated (i.e., ddUrd) metabolites were observed in ATH8 cells exposed to ddC. In fact, Kelley and coworkers (45) determined the rate of deamination of Cyd and ddC by partially purified murine, monkey, and human kidney cell extracts and found that the ratios of Cyd deamination to ddC deamination were 1220, 198, and 1618, respectively. Thus, in contrast to many Cyd analogs, such as Cyd, 2′-dCyd, and araC, which are subject to extensive intracellular deamination by Cyd deaminase or dCMP deaminase, ddC (and its phosphorylated products) are not markedly deaminated to the corresponding ddUrd metabolites in cell cultures.

The findings that 1) the antiretroviral and cytostatic effects of ddC are significantly reversed by dCyd, 2) phosphorylated products of ddC could not be detected in a dCyd kinase (dCK)–deficient murine leukemia (L1210/araC) cell line, and 3) ddC lacks any cytostatic effect against the araC-resistant L1210 cell line point to the pivotal role of cytosol dCK in the activation (phosphorylation) of ddC (46). In addition, Ullman and coworkers (43) demonstrated that a dCK-deficient CEM (ARAC-8D) cell line is completely resistant to growth inhibition by ddC and fails to phosphorylate [^{3}H]ddC. However, ddC is a weak substrate for dCK (10, 46–48). K_m values of ddC for cytosol dCK derived from Molt/4F, thymus, and peripheral chronic lymphocytic leukemia cells are 200, 140, and 180 μmol/L, respectively, as compared with 3, 16, and 3 μmol/L for the natural substrate dCyd. Moreover, the V_{max} for ddC phosphorylation is significantly lower than the V_{max} for dCyd. Nevertheless, ddC phosphorylation is sufficiently fast to yield the necessary intracellular levels of ddCMP, ddCDP, and ddCTP. Whereas dCK is required for the conversion of ddC to ddCMP, further conversion of ddCMP and ddCDP would be most likely accomplished by CMP/dCMP kinase and NDP kinase, respectively.

Cheng and colleagues (49) and Hao and associates (50) reported the competitive inhibitory effect of ddCTP with respect to dCTP against HIV-1 RT. The K_i of ddCTP for HIV-1 RT with poly(I).oligo(dC)$_{18}$ was 0.26 μmol/L (50). The K_i/K_m ratio was 0.04, a finding indicating that ddCTP has a much stronger affinity for HIV-1 RT than the natural substrate dCTP. Mitsuya and coworkers (51) also showed that ddCTP inhibits DNA chain elongation mediated by purified HIV-1 RT, using an M13-based template and an M13 universal oligonucleotide primer in a Sanger sequencing reaction. In addition, Starnes and Cheng (48) demonstrated incorporation of ddC into the DNA of Molt/4 cells. However, the contribution of incorporation of ddC into cellular DNA to the cytotoxicity of ddC has not been ascertained. ddCTP competitively inhibits DNA polymerase α, β, and γ with K_i values of 110, 2.6, and 0.016 μmol/L, respectively (48). Thus, mitochondrial DNA polymerase γ is exquisitely sensitive to the inhibitory effect of ddCTP. Investigators have speculated that inhibition of mitochondrial DNA synthesis by ddC could account for the peripheral neuropathy observed in AIDS patients treated with relatively low doses of ddC (52, 53). However, whether a direct link exists between DNA polymerase γ inhibition by ddCTP and the neuropathy caused by ddC in patients is not clear. In fact, the relationship between ddCTP, ddCDP-choline, ddCDP-ethanolamine, or any other ddC metabolites and the marked neurotoxicity seen with ddC remains to be explored. Observations from Cook and Spence (54) revealed no specific

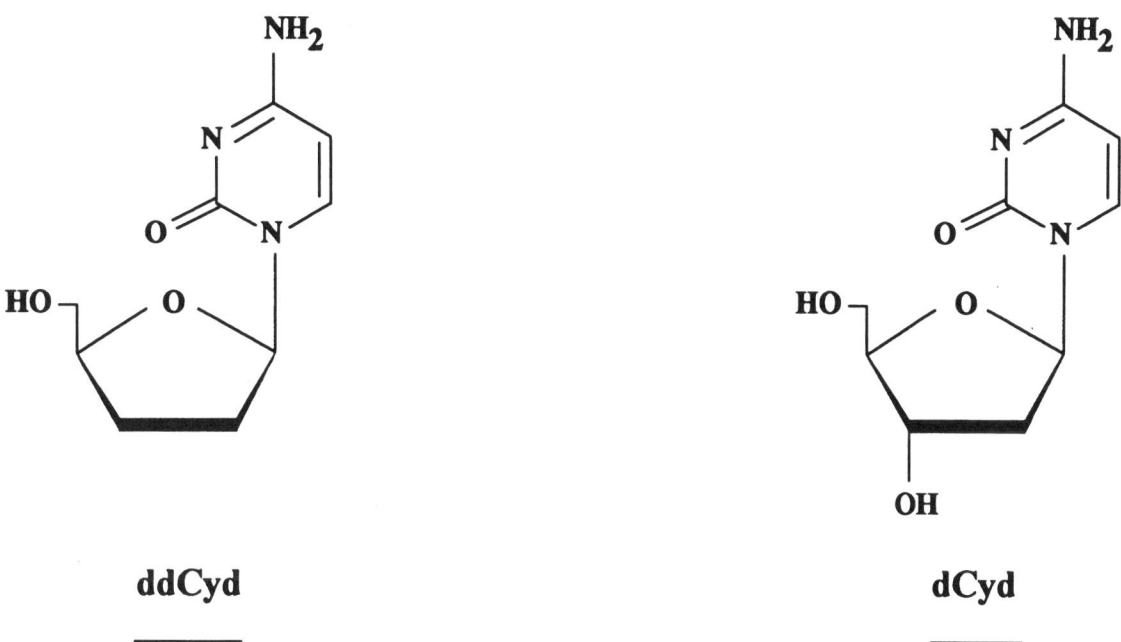

Figure 47A.15. Formulas of 2',3'-dideoxycytidine *(ddCyd, DDC)* and 2'-deoxycytidine *(dCyd)*.

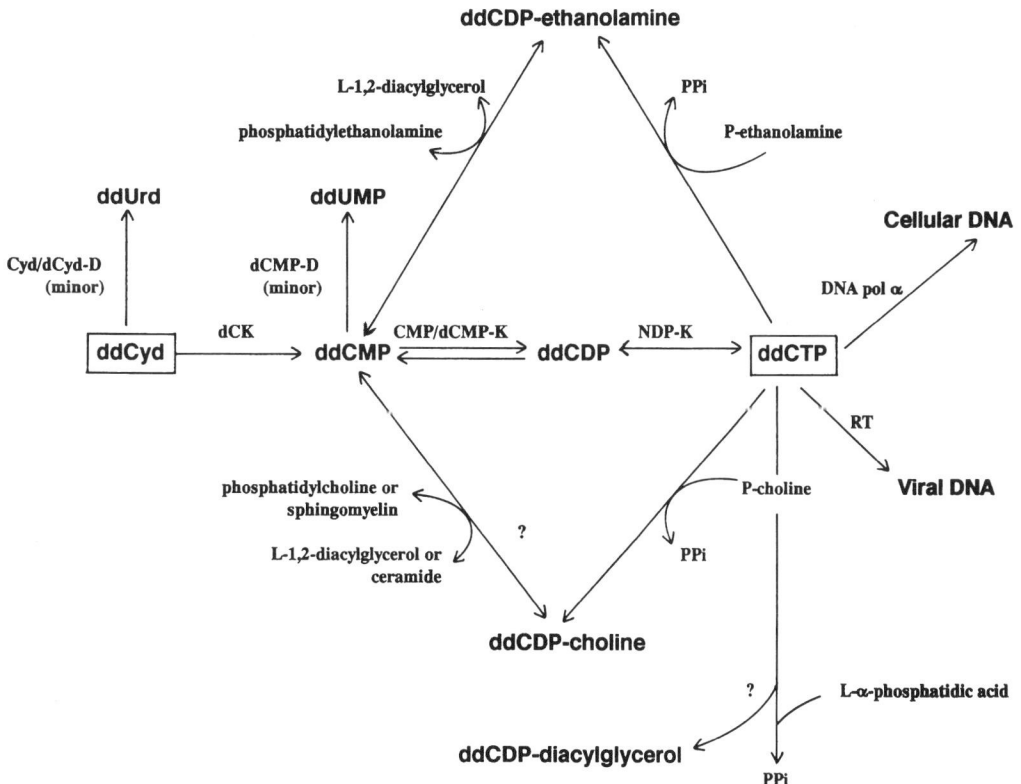

Figure 47A.16. Metabolic conversion of 2',3'-dideoxycytidine *(ddCyd)* to its 5'-triphosphate derivative. Enzymes:*CMP/dCMP-K*, cytidylate/2'-deoxycytidylate kinase;*Cyd/dCyd-D*, cytidine/2'-deoxycytidine deaminase; *dCK*, 2'-deoxycytidine kinase; *dCMP-D*, 2'-deoxycytidylate deaminase; *ddCDP*, 2',3'-dideoxycytidine 5'-diphosphate; *ddCMP*, 2',3'-dideoxycytidine 5'-monophosphate; *ddCTP*, 2',3'-dideoxycytidine 5'-triphosphate; *ddUrd*, 2',3'-dideoxyuridine; *DNA pol α*, DNA polymerase α; *NDP-K*, nucleoside 5'-diphosphate kinase; *PPi*, pyrophosphate; *RT*, reverse transcriptase.

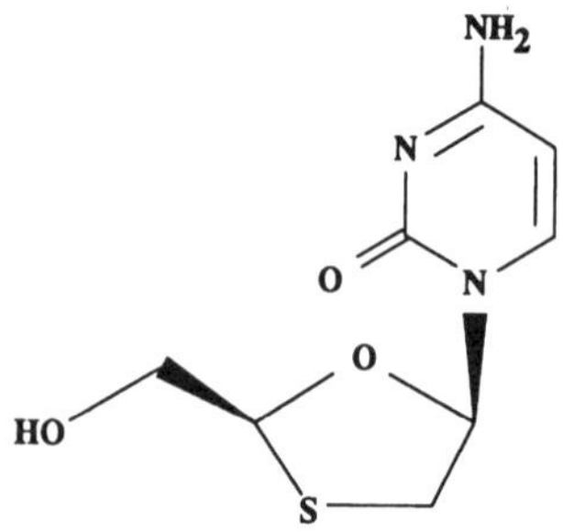

Figure 47A.17. Formulas of 2'-deoxy-3'-thiacytidine *(3TC)* and 2',3'-dideoxy-5-fluoro-3'-thiacytidine *(FTC)*.

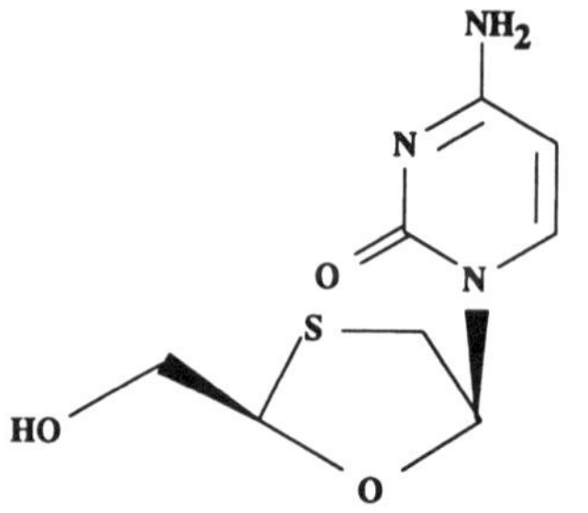

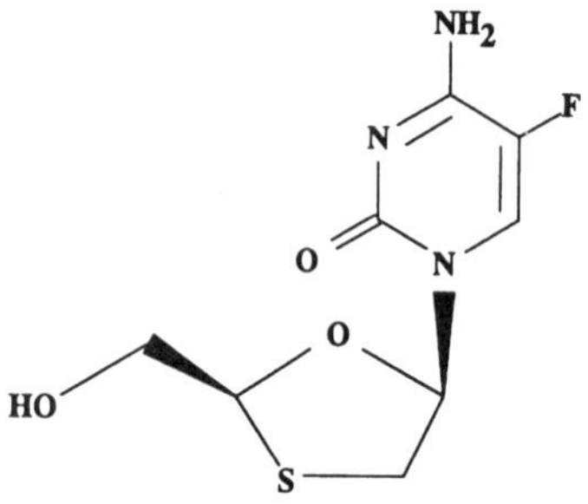

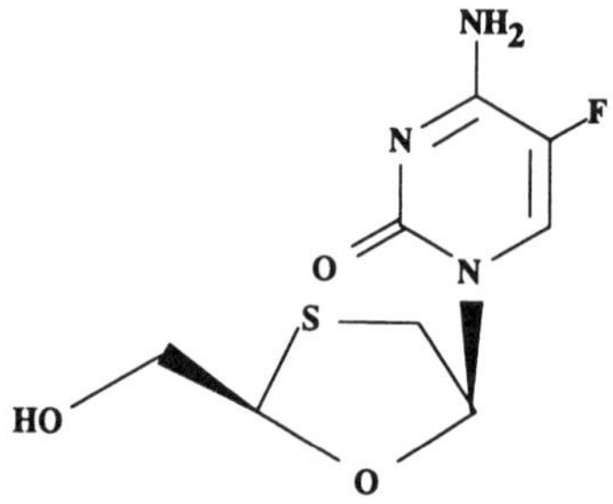

inhibitory effect of ddC on phosphatidylcholine metabolism in neuroblastoma and glioma cells. Balzarini and colleagues (46) found that the metabolism of ddC could be influenced by natural pyrimidine nucleosides and inhibitors of pyrimidine nucleotide biosynthesis. In contrast to dCyd and Cyd, which decreased the phosphorylation rate of ddC, dThd stimulated the formation of phosphorylated ddC products. The degree of this stimulation depended on the preincubation time with dThd and the initial concentration of dThd, and it seemed to correlate with the decrease of the intracellular dCTP pools (resulting from the inhibition of CDP reductase by dTTP). 3-Deazauridine (an inhibitor of CTP synthetase) and hydroxyurea (an inhibitor of ribonucleotide reductase) proved equally effective as dThd in stimulating ddC phosphorylation. However, whether the combination of ddC with any of these compounds (including dThd) is therapeutically advantageous (i.e., leads to an increased therapeutic index in vivo) over the use of ddC as a single drug is unclear.

2'-Deoxy-3'-Thiacytidine and (−)-2',3'-Dideoxy-5-Fluoro-3'-Thiacytidine

The formulas for 2'-deoxy-3'-thiacytidine (3TC, BCH-189) and (−)-2',3'-dideoxy-5-fluoro-3'-thiacytidine [(−)-(FTC)] are shown in Figure 47A.17. A novel nucleoside analog, 3TC, in which the 3'-carbon in the β-ribose ring of 2',3'-dideoxycytidine has been replaced by a sulfur atom (1,3-oxathiolane), was found to be endowed with potent and selective anti-HIV activity in vitro (55, 56). Because 3TC consists of a racemic mixture of the β-D-(+)- and β-L-(−)-enantiomers, both enantiomers were resolved and were found to be equipotent in antiviral activity against HIV-1 and HIV-2 (57). The α-L-(+)- and α-D-(−)-enantiomers proved less antivirally effective than the corresponding β-isomers (58). The (−)-β-enantiomer (3TC) is considerably less toxic than the (+)-β-enantiomer to human lymphocytic cell lines in vitro (57). Sommadossi and coworkers (59) also reported that the (+)-isomer was more toxic to human myeloid and erythroid colony-forming cells—the IC_{50} for granulocyte–macrophage colony-forming units (CFU-GM) and erythroid burst-forming units (BFU-E) were 9 2 μmol/L—than the (−)-isomer (IC_{50} for CFU-GM and BFU-E, 34 and 170 μmol/L, respectively). Both the (−)-enantiomer and the racemic mixture of 3TC are less toxic to T lymphocytes than ZDV (57, 60).

The metabolism of the (−)-enantiomer (3TC) was examined in HIV-1–infected and mock-infected human peripheral blood lymphocytes (PBLs) and U937 cells (61, 62) (Fig.

47A.18). 3TC is metabolized in PBLs to its 5′-monophosphate, 5′-diphosphate, and 5′-triphosphate derivatives. The intracellular concentration of 3TC-TP in phytohemagglutinin (PHA)-stimulated PBLs shows a linear dependence on the extracellular concentration of 3TC up to an extracellular 3TC concentration of 10 μmol/L. This concentration results in intracellular 3TC-TP levels of 5 μmol/L (62). No evidence indicates that 3TC would be deaminated to its Urd counterpart by Cyd/dCyd deaminase or dCMP/CMP deaminase. Nor does evidence suggest the phosphorolysis of 3TC to the free cytosine base by dThd phosphorylase or Urd/dUrd phosphorylase (61). However, incubation of the (+)-enantiomer of 3TC with a platelet-rich suspension revealed deamination to the corresponding 2′-deoxy-3′-thiauridine analog, whereas no free base (uracil) was detected. These observations suggest that, in contrast to the (−)-enantiomer (3TC), the (+)-enantiomer is deaminated but not phosphorolyzed.

The 5′-triphosphate derivative of the 3TC (−)-enantiomer (3TC-TP) consistently represents approximately 40% of the total intracellular metabolites after incubation of PBLs (whether infected with HIV-1 or not) with [³H]3TC for 4 hours; and after a 20-hour incubation, it still represents approximately 20%. The rate of decay (half-life) of 3TC-TP in PBLs was found to be 10.5 to 15.5 hours. The 5′-triphosphate derivative of the (+)-enantiomer has a fivefold greater activity against purified HIV-1 RT (K_i, 8 to 18 μmol/L) than 3TC-TP (61), but it also has a much shorter half-life than that of 3TC-TP (approximately 3.5 to 7 hours) (61). These data may explain the comparable antiviral potency of both enantiomers. 3TC concentrations up to 200 μmol/L did not markedly affect intracellular dNTP pools, whereas ZDV, under identical experimental conditions, increased dCTP and decreased dGTP pool levels.

Because the 3TC concentration producing 90% inhibition of HIV replication in PBL has been reported to be 76 nM, an intracellular 3TC-TP concentration equivalent to the K_i value against HIV-1 RT is attained only when the extracellular 3TC concentration is 2 orders of magnitude higher than the antiviral (90% inhibitory) concentration. However, the apparent discrepancy is explained by the ability of 3TC-TP to act as a substrate (DNA chain terminator) for RT. The IC_{50} values of 3TC-TP for DNA polymerases α, β, and γ and HIV-1 RT at dCTP concentrations equal to the K_m were 10 to 12 μmol/L, 175 μmol/L, 25 μmol/L, and 43 μmol/L, respectively (63). The K_i values for HIV-1 RT and for DNA polymerases β and γ were 10 to 12 μmol/L, 19 μmol/L, and 16 μmol/L, respectively (63). The absence of marked mitochondrial toxicity of 3TC is most likely due to the 3′-5′ exonuclease activity of DNA polymerase γ (62).

Schinazi and coworkers (64) reported on the anti–HIV-1 activity of (−)-2′,3′-dideoxy-5-fluoro-3′-thiacytidine, designated (−)-FTC. This compound differs from 3TC by a substitution of a fluorine at the 5-position of the cytosine ring

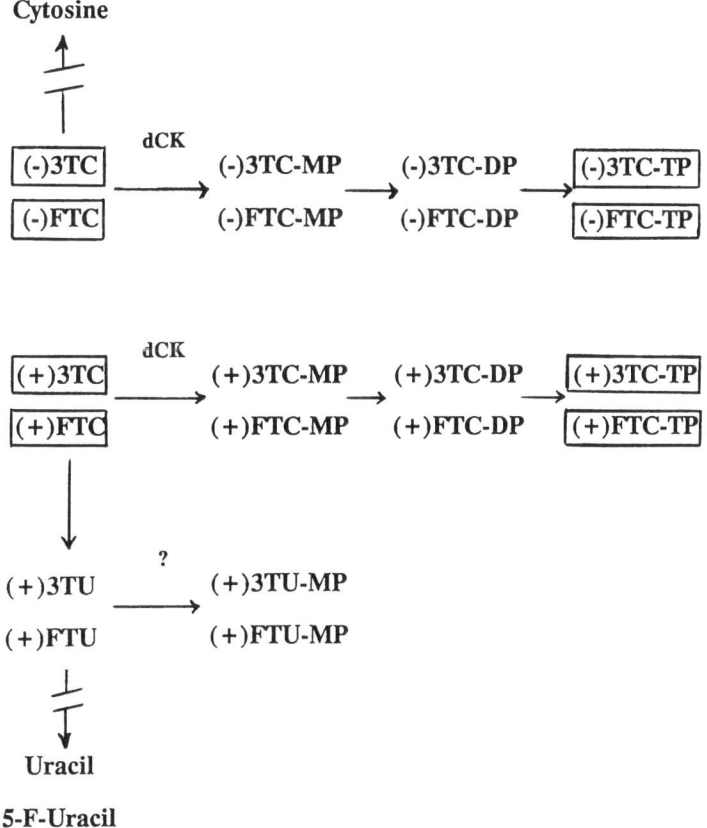

Figure 47A.18. Metabolic conversion of 2′-deoxy-3′-thiacytidine *(3TC)* and the (+)-enantiomer of 3TC.

(see Fig. 47A.18). (−)-FTC has proved to be a potent and selective inhibitor of HIV, simian immunodeficiency virus (SIV), and feline immunodeficiency virus (FIV) in certain cell culture systems, including human monocytes (64). The (−)-enantiomer of FTC was found to be 20-fold more potent against HIV-1 than the (+)-enantiomer. In analogy with the (−)-enantiomeric 3TC, (−)-FTC is less toxic to human bone marrow cells (IC_{50}, more than 30 µmol/L for both CFU-GM and BFU-E) than (+)-FTC (IC_{50}, 7.5 and 53 µmol/L for CFU-GM and BFU-E, respectively) (64). (−)-FTC would be phosphorylated by dCK (64). (−)-FTC-TP has proved to be a potent inhibitor of the HIV-1 RT, with a K_i of 2.9 µmol/L in the presence of poly(I).oligo(dC), whereas (+)-FTC-TP had a two- to threefold decreased affinity for HIV-1 RT. Both compounds act as potent DNA chain terminators in the HIV-1 RT reaction. Furman and coworkers (65) reported that (+)-FTC is a good substrate for Cyd/2′-dCyd deaminase, whereas (−)-FTC is not. Pharmacokinetic and metabolism studies with racemic FTC in rhesus monkeys revealed the presence of the deaminated FTC product (FTU) in serum and urine. However, no 5-fluorouracil was detected in serum or urine (66). This finding is consistent with the observations found for 3TC.

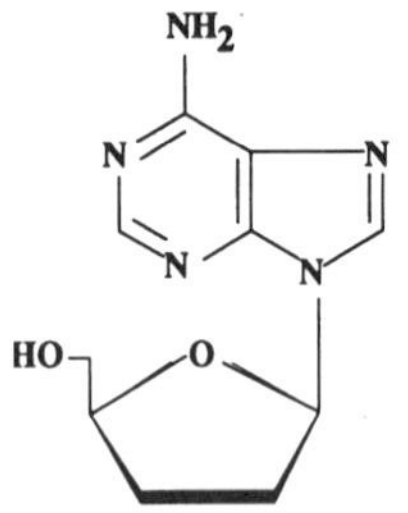

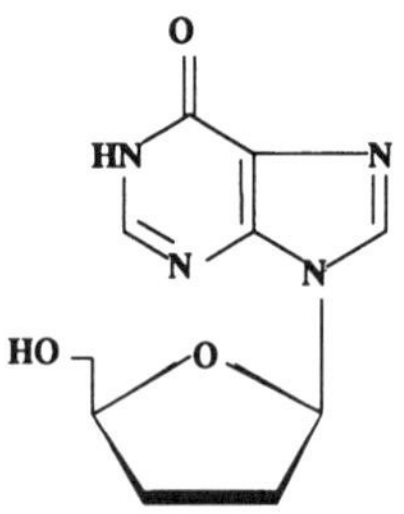

Both 3TC and (−)-FTC have been combined with ZDV and d4T in HIV-infected cell cultures and have been found to inhibit HIV replication synergistically (67). However, the inhibitors 2′,3′-dideoxyinosine (ddI) and ddC were only additive when coadministered with 3TC or (−)-FTC. None of the (−)-nucleoside analogs had additive toxicity in cell culture. They could protect against delayed mitochondrial toxicity associated with ZDV, d4T, ddC, and ddI in drug-treated cells (67).

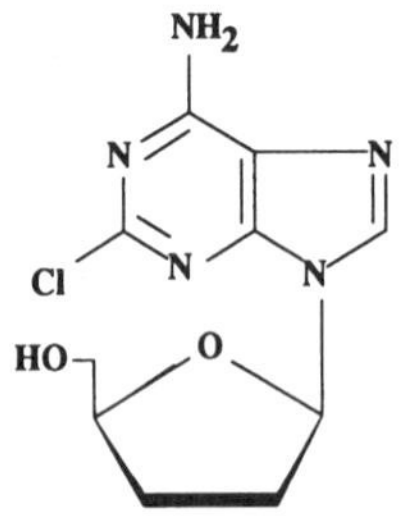

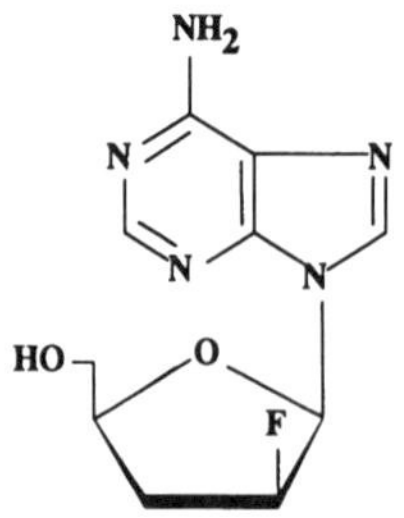

2′,3′-Dideoxyadenosine and 2′,3′-Dideoxyinosine

The formulas for ddAdo and ddI (ddIno) are shown in Figure 47A.19. Because ddAdo uptake by human erythrocytes is not saturated yet at 1 mM and is not inhibited by dipyridamole or nitrobenzylthioinosine, investigators have inferred that ddAdo permeation is not mediated by a nucleoside transporter. In this respect, the cellular uptake of ddAdo resembles that of ZDV (1) (see earlier).

Initial studies on the metabolism of ddAdo and ddI were conducted by Cooney and colleagues (68) and Ahluwahlia and associates (69). In marked contrast to the pyrimidine 2′,3′-dideoxynucleosides (i.e., ZDV, d4T, and ddC), the purine 2′,3′-dideoxynucleosides ddAdo and ddI are extensively catabolized (Fig. 47A.20). Starting from ddAdo, only extremely low intracellular levels of ddATP are generated, and the predominant metabolites are ADP and ATP. These observations are in accord with the finding that ddAdo is readily converted by adenosine deaminase (70) to ddI, whereafter ddI is hydrolyzed to hypoxanthine by PNPase. Eventually, hypoxanthine is anabolized by hypoxanthine–guanine phosphoribosyl transferase to IMP. From IMP, AMP and GMP and the corresponding 5′-diphosphate and 5′-triphosphates are formed through the classic purine nucleotide biosynthetic pathways (see earlier). No evidence has been provided for the formation of ddIDP or ddITP, a finding indicating that deamination of ddAdo to ddI is not followed by anabolic conversion of the latter compound to ddITP. Inhibition of adenosine deaminase by 2′-deoxycoformycin (10 µmol/L) resulted in only slightly higher ddATP levels, whereas catabolism of ddAdo to ddI and reuse of the purine base for the synthesis of the natural purine nucleotides remained the major way to dispose of ddAdo and ddI.

Studies with radiolabeled [^{3}H]ddI have confirmed that ddI anabolites other than ddIMP do not arise intracellularly (69). Moreover, it also appeared that ddI, like ddAdo, acts as a precursor of ddATP. Ahluwahlia and colleagues (69) demonstrated that ddI, on phosphorylation to its ddIMP form, reenters the ddAdo anabolic pathway at the 5′-monophosphate level (i.e., ddIMP ddAMP). Evidence for this reaction stemmed from studies with L-alanosine, a potent inhibitor of adenylosuccinate synthetase. L-Alanosine blocks formation of ddATP from ddI and concomitantly increases ddIMP pool levels. Moreover, L-alanosine suppressed the formation of ddATP starting from [^{3}H]ddAdo, indicating the quantitative predominance of the indirect route (i.e.,

Figure 47A.19. Formulas of 2′,3′-dideoxyadenosine *(ddAdo)*, 2′,3′-dideoxyinosine *(ddIno, ddI)*, 2′,3′-dideoxy-2-chloroadenosine *(ddClAdo)*, and 2′,3′-dideoxy-2′-fluoro-9-β-D-arabinofuranosyladenine *(FddaraA)*.

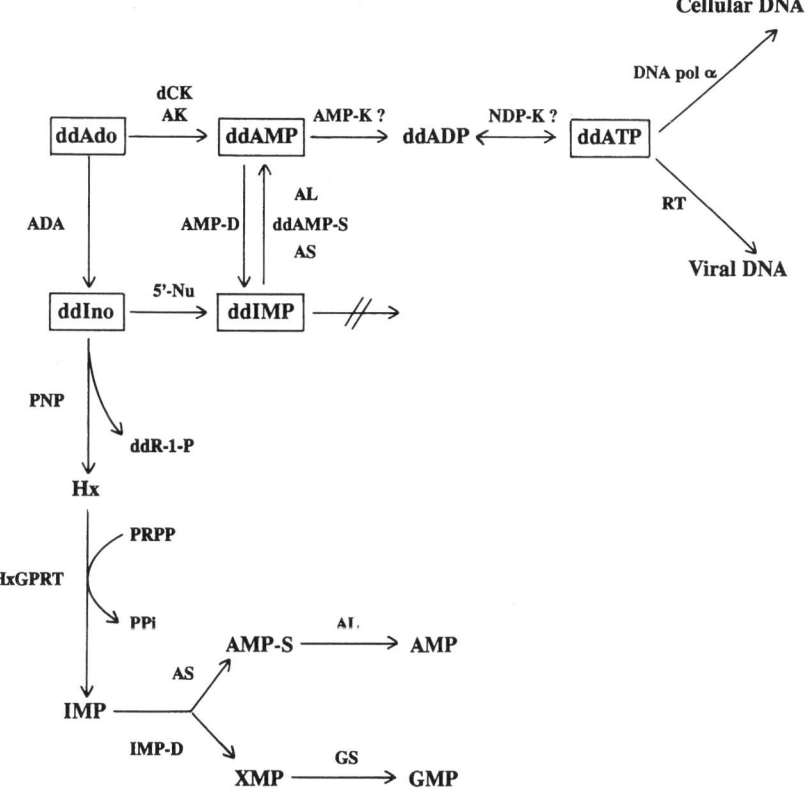

Figure 47A.20. Metabolic conversion of 2′,3′-dideoxyadenosine (*ddAdo*) and 2′,3′-dideoxyinosine (*ddIno*) to their 5′-triphosphate derivatives. Enzymes: *ADA*, adenosine deaminase; *AK*, adenosine kinase; *AL*, adenylosuccinate lyase; *AMP-D*, adenylate deaminase; *AMP-K*, adenylate kinase; *AS*, adenylosuccinate synthetase; *dCK*, 2′-deoxycytidine kinase; *ddR-1-P*, 2′,3′-dideoxyribose-1-phosphate; *DNA pol α*, DNA polymerase α; *GMP*, guanosine-5′-monophosphate; *GS*, guanylate synthetase; *HxGPRT*, hypoxanthine/guanine phosphoribosyl transferase; *IMP-D*, inosinate dehydrogenase; *NDP-K*, nucleoside 5′-diphosphate kinase; *5′-Nu*, 5′-nucleotidase; *PNP*, purine nucleoside phosphorylase; *PPi*, pyrophosphate; *PRPP*, 5-phosphoribosyl-1-pyrophosphate; *RT*, reverse transcriptase; *XMP*, xanthosine-5′-monophosphate.

through ddI) in the conversion of ddAdo to ddAMP, relative to the direct phosphorylation route. Investigators have therefore proposed that ddI, like ddAdo, exerts its antiretroviral activity by virtue of its ability to generate ddATP. Thus, ddAdo can give rise to ddATP by two different routes: directly, through the 5′-phosphorylation of ddAdo, and indirectly, through the intermediary formation of ddI and ddIMP. This dual mechanism of activation of ddAdo has also been confirmed by Johnson and colleagues (71, 72).

Multiple enzymes are involved in the phosphorylation of ddAdo and ddI to their 5′-monophosphates. Cooney and associates (68) provided evidence that ddAdo is phosphorylated by both dCyd kinase and adenosine kinase (K_m values for the partially purified human thymus enzymes, 160 and 50 μmol/L, respectively). The phosphorylation efficiency (V_{max}/K_m) with adenosine kinase was about 10% that of dCyd kinase. Johnson and associates (71, 72) reported that ddAdo was about 500-fold less efficiently phosphorylated by human thymocyte dCyd kinase than dCyd (V_{max}/K_m, 0.004 for ddAdo relative to 1.9 for dCyd). Moreover, Carson and associates (73) confirmed these findings, and they further ascertained that ddAdo in human T cells is phosphorylated predominantly by dCyd kinase. Thus, ddAdo activation in human T lymphocytes may occur by these metabolic pathways: 1) directly, by phosphorylation of ddAdo to ddAMP by dCyd kinase or adenosine kinase; and 2) indirectly, through deamination of ddAdo to ddI and subsequent phosphorylation of ddI to ddIMP, followed by amination of ddIMP to ddAMP by adenylosuccinate synthetase/lyase (72). Neither dCyd kinase nor adenosine kinase seems to be involved in the phosphorylation of ddI. However, Johnson and Fridland (71) found that ddI is phosphorylated by human erythrocytes and thymus extracts that contain 5′-nucleotidase, which acts preferentially with IMP and GMP, but not UMP or TMP. K_m values for ddI and Ino phosphorylation by this enzyme preparation were (in the presence of 10 mM ATP) 4.1 and 2.1 mM, respectively, and (in the absence of ATP) 23.6 and 6.04 mM, respectively. Although the substrate affinity of ddI for 5′-nucleotidase is poor, this enzyme likely is responsible for the conversion of ddI to ddIMP in human lymphoid cells.

The compound ddATP is a potent inhibitor of HIV-1 RT. Its K_m value is 0.22 μmol/L, and the K_i/K_m is 0.02 (50). In this respect, its inhibitory activity against HIV-1 RT is comparable to that of ddCTP and ZDV-TP. In contrast, ddITP is less inhibitory to HIV-1 RT than ddATP. Its K_i is 2.47 μmol/L with poly(C).oligo(dG)$_{12-18}$ as the template primer. In addition, the K_i/K_m value of ddITP is almost

10-fold higher than that of ddATP. The differences in affinity of ddATP and ddITP for the avian myeloblastosis virus (AMV) RT are even more pronounced (K_i: 0.17 and 29.9, respectively) (50). Because no ddITP can be detected in cells exposed to either ddAdo or ddI, and given that ddI serves as a prodrug for ddATP, the lower affinity of ddITP for RT should not be taken into consideration when assessing the chemotherapeutic potential of ddI.

Both ddAdo and ddI are less toxic in cell culture than the pyrimidine 2′,3′-dideoxynucleosides discussed earlier. Their 50% cytotoxic concentration (CC_{50}) values are definitely higher than 500 µmol/L. Moreover, no marked antimetabolic effects have been reported for ddI and ddAdo in vitro. A common property of purine 2′,3′-dideoxynucleosides is their high instability in acidic conditions (low pH). These properties may hamper the oral bioavailability of this type of compounds. Currently, ddI is given orally to HIV-infected individuals together with antacids, to neutralize stomach acidity temporarily and to protect ddI from hydrolysis to hypoxanthine. In addition, to circumvent the problem of instability and thus to overcome the rapid catabolism of ddAdo or ddI, certain 2-halogeno-substituted ddAdo derivatives have been synthesized. These compounds proved stable in acidic conditions and also were resistant to deamination by adenosine deaminase (74).

Haertle and coworkers (74) demonstrated that in CEM cells the 2-chloro-substituted derivative of ddAdo (ddClAdo) is converted intracellularly to its 5′-monophosphate, 5′-diphosphate, and 5′-triphosphate metabolite. dCyd kinase is responsible for the phosphorylation of ddClAdo to ddClAMP. In contrast to ddAdo, ddClAdo is probably not a substrate for adenosine kinase because ddClAdo completely loses its anti–HIV-1 activity in CEM/dCyd kinase⁻ cells that contain normal levels of adenosine kinase (74). CEM cells do not deaminate [³H]ddClAdo, although they convert [³H]ddAdo to [³H]ddI for 98% within 4 hours. In CEM cells, ddClAdo 5′-triphosphate is formed with a similar efficiency, as is ddATP (starting from ddAdo or ddI). Because the 2-halogeno-substituted ddAdo derivatives are much more cytostatic to MT-2 and CEM cells than ddAdo and ddI, they are not advantageous over ddAdo and ddI.

2′-FddaraA, the 2′-fluoro-substituted derivative of ddAdo (with the fluorine in the "up" position) possesses preclinical anti-HIV activity both in vitro (75, 76) and in vivo (77, 78). Unlike ddClAdo, it is devoid of any cytostatic activity in vitro at 500 µmol/L. It is resistant to hydrolytic cleavage in acidic conditions (75, 79, 80). Attempts have been undertaken to study its intracellular metabolism and to compare its kinetic and pharmacologic properties with those of ddAdo and ddI (79). Studies with pyrimidine nucleoside kinase–deficient CEM cell lines indicate that 2′-FddaraA also follows a more direct anabolic pathway toward formation of 2′-FddaraATP than ddAdo. 2′-FddaraA is initially converted to its 5′-monophosphate 2′-FddaraAMP by dCyd kinase (Fig. 47A.21). In Molt/4 cells, 2′-FddaraADP and 2′-FddaraATP levels are 20- and 5-fold higher than the levels of ddADP and ddATP. This observation is in agreement with the findings that 2′-FddaraA is deaminated 10 times less rapidly than ddAdo, and the resulting deaminated product is resistant to hydrolysis by PNPase. Like ddAdo (81), 2′-FddaraA is transported by passive diffusion and does not seem to enter the cells through the purine nucleoside transport carrier (79). The rate of cellular uptake of 2′-FddaraA is about half that of ddAdo. Thus, 2′-FddaraA differs from ddAdo and ddI with regard to its transport into the cells and its subsequent disposition by activating (phosphorylating) and catabolyzing (deaminating) enzymes. Whether these differences translate into any therapeutic benefit over ddI is unclear. 2′-FddaraA has proved effective against ZDV and ddI-resistant HIV-1 strains, and it inhibits all HIV clades A to E in PHA-stimulated PBMCs, although at a lower potency and with a higher variability than ZDV (82).

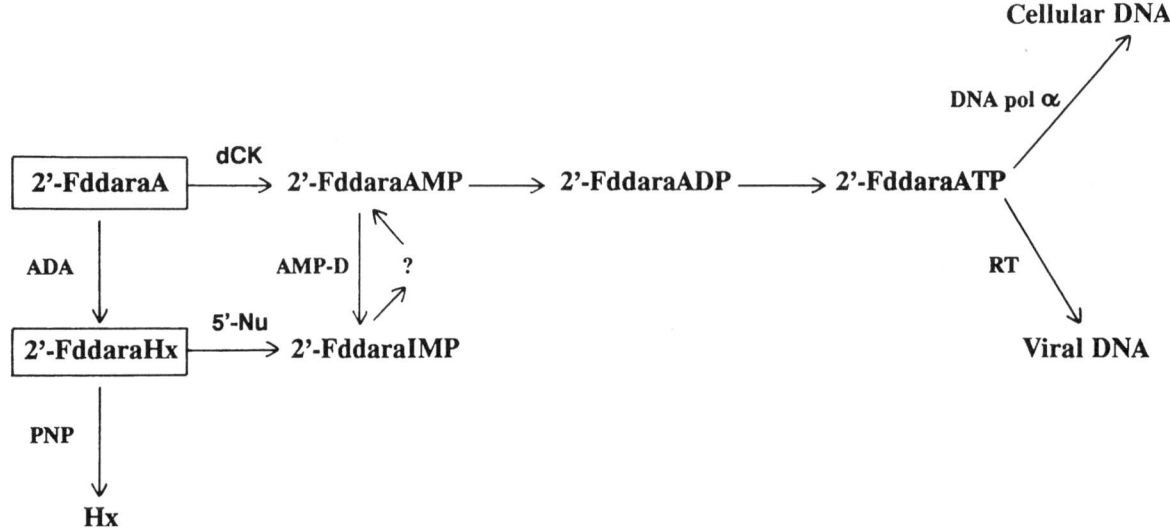

Figure 47A.21. Metabolic conversion of 2′,3′-dideoxy-2′-fluoro-9-β-D-arabinofuranosyladenine *(2′-FddaraA)* to its 5′-triphosphate derivatives. Enzymes: see legend to Figure 47A.20.

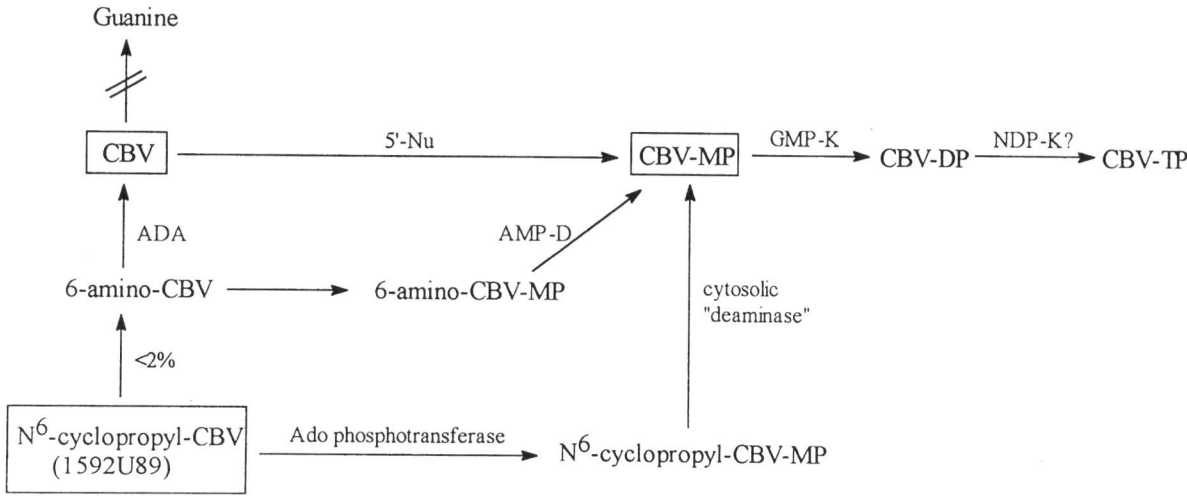

Figure 47A.22. Formulas of carbovir and 1592U89.

Figure 47A.23. Metabolic conversion of carbovir and 1592U89 to carbovir-5′-triphosphate. Enzymes: *ADA,* adenosine deaminase; *Ado phosphotransferase,* adenosine phosphotransferase; *AMP-D,* adenylate deaminase; *CBV-DP,* carbovir diphosphate; *CBV-MP,* carbovir monophosphate; *CBV-TP,* carbovir triphosphate; *GMP-K,* guanylate kinase; *NDP-K,* nucleoside diphosphate kinase; *5′-Nu,* 5′-nucleotidase.

Carbovir and Abacavir (1592U89)

In contrast to many nucleoside analogs, carbocyclic nucleosides lack the labile glycosidic linkage between the heterocycle and the sugar part. They are resistant to phosphorolytic cleavage (hydrolysis of the glycosidic bond) by purine and pyrimidine nucleoside phosphorylases. Unlike the carbocyclic derivatives of ddA, ddI, ddC, ddT, and ddG (83), the carbocyclic analogs 2′,3′-didehydro-ddA, and in particular of 2′,3′-didehydro-ddG, are endowed with a marked anti-HIV activity in cell culture (22, 84). Among the two carbocyclic enantiomers of carbovir (CBV), the (−)-enantiomer is superior to the (+)-enantiomer. The formulas for CBV and 1592U89 are shown in Figure 47A.22.

5′-Nucleotidase (inosine phosphotransferase, 5′-Nu) efficiently converts (±)-CBV to its 5′-monophosphate (±)-CBV-MP (71, 85). The next step catalyzed by GMP kinase is highly stereoselective, and it preferentialy converts (−)-CBV-MP, but not its (+)-enantiomer, to (−)-CBV-DP, with a substrate efficiency (V_{max}/K_m) of 38% of that of GMP. (−)-CBV-DP is eventually converted to its active metabolite (−)-CBV-TP, presumably by NDP kinase, and it specifically inhibits HIV RT (86, 87).

The N^6-cyclopropyl derivative of (−)-CBV (1592U89) (88, 89) shows an entirely different metabolic conversion pathway to CBV-TP (Fig. 47A.23). First, 5′-Nu, which only recognizes the (−)-enantiomer of 1592U89 but not its (+)-enantiomer, is endowed with a low phosphorylation capacity for 1592U89 (approximately 1% of the rate with inosine). Moreover, N^6-cyclopropyl-CBV-MP is an inefficient substrate for the phosphorylation by GMP-K, with a K_m greater than 20-fold higher than for GMP and a V_{max} only 0.1% of that for GMP (relative substrate efficiency, 0.005%).

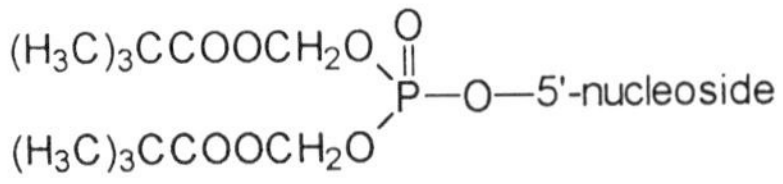

bis(POM)prodrug

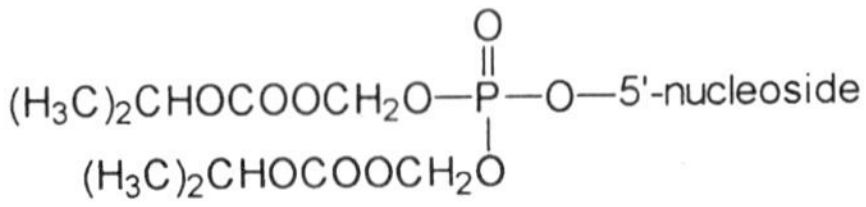

bis(POC)prodrug

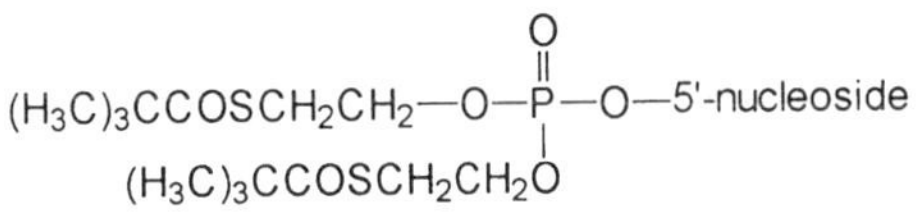

bis(t-Bu-SATE)prodrug

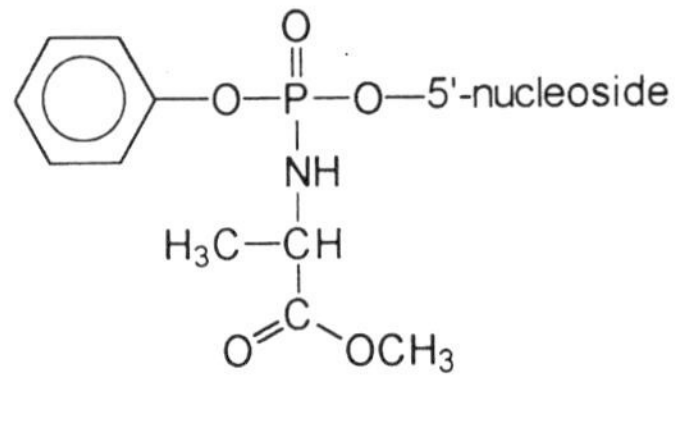

APA prodrug

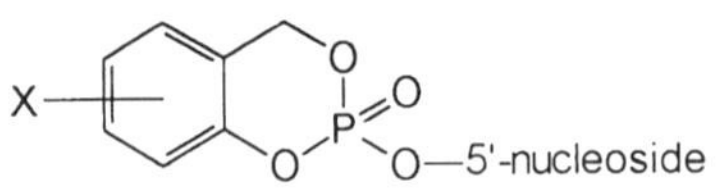

cyclosaligenyl prodrug

Figure 47A.24. General formulas of bis(piareloyloxymethyl) [bis(POM)]-, bis(isopropyloxycarboxymethyl [bis(POC)]-, and bis(tort-butyl) [bis(t-Bu-SATE])-, arylphosphoramidate (APA)-, and cyclosaligenyl prodrugs.

The lack of the capacity of other nucleotide kinases to recognize N^6-cyclopropyl-CBV-MP is in agreement with the lack of observable 5′-diphosphate and 5′-triphosphate metabolites in CEM cell cultures incubated with abacavir. Moreover, abacavir and its 5′-monophosphate derivatives are poor substrates of adenosine deaminase (0.08% of the deamination rate of Ado) and adenylate deaminase (AMP-D) (0.07% of the deamination rate of AMP), respectively. However, adenosine phosphotransferase present in rat liver was identified to anabolize abacavir to its 5′-monophosphate (90). This enzyme could be purified more than 1000-fold from human placenta. It differed from other nucleoside phosphotransferases in its substrate specificity. AMP (K_m, approximately 3 mM) (and also dAMP) can act as an efficient phosphate donor. Ado (K_m, 0.2 mM), but also dAdo and ddAdo, can act as phosphate acceptors. The normal physiologic role of this enzyme is not understood. In addition, a cytosolic deaminase activity, distinct from AMP-D (but still sensitive to the inhibitory effect of 2′-deoxycoformycin) deaminates the N^6-cyclopropyl CBV-MP to CBV-MP. The nucleoside phosphotransferase and cytosolic deaminase participate in the eventual conversion of N^6-cyclopropyl CBV to CBV-TP, the active metabolite of N^6-cyclopropyl CBV (and CBV). Although the active metabolite of CBV and N^6-cyclopropyl-CBV are identical (i.e., CBV-TP), metabolism studies revealed that the formation of 6-amino-CBV and 6-amino-CBV-MP on the one hand and of CBV on the other from N^6-cyclopropyl CBV plays a minor role (if any) in the eventual antiviral activity. Formation of CBV-MP through two successive steps from N^6-cyclopropyl CBV represents a unique pathway of activation of this compound, one clearly distinct from the activation pathway of CBV.

PRODRUGS OF NUCLEOTIDE ANALOGS THAT DELIVER THE NUCLEOSIDE-5′-MONOPHOSPHATES DIRECTLY INTO INTACT CELLS

To overcome the often poor affinity of 2′,3′-dideoxynucleosides for their activating (nucleoside kinase, 5′-nucleotidase) enzymes, several attempts have been made to synthesize prodrugs of the nucleoside 5′-monophosphates and (acyclic) nucleoside phosphonates that neutralize the charges of the phosphate and phosphonate moiety, which ameliorate the uptake (passive diffusion) of the masked phosphates and phosphonates into the cells. Several successful and structurally different approaches have been followed, including the bis(pivaloyloxymethyl) (bis[POM]), bis(isopropyloxycarbonyloxymethyl) (bis[POC]), bis(S-acyl-2-thioethyl) (bis[SATE]), aryloxyphosphoramidate (APA), and CycloSALigenyl approaches (Fig. 47A.24).

The bis(POM) approach was one of the first examples showing that nucleoside monophosphates can be effectively delivered into intact cells (91). Indeed, investigators showed that—in contrast to ddU—bis(POM)-ddUMP was able to inhibit HIV-1 replication in wild-type and TK-deficient CEM cells at 2.5 to 5 μmol/L. Consistent with these observations, substantial amounts of ddUTP (up to approximately 10 μmol/L) were formed intracellularly within 1 hour after the cells had been exposed to 20 μmol/L of the prodrug. This was not the case when ddU was administered to the cells. The lack of biologic activity of ddU is presumably due to the virtual lack of substrate activity of ddU for TK (50). Studies on the bis(POM) derivative of FdUMP, an anticancer agent, revealed that bis(POM) derivatives are stable in the low pH range of 1 to 4 (half-life, more than 100 hours), fairly stable at pH 7.4 (half-life, approximately 40 hours), but rapidly degraded under alkaline conditions (92, 93). Investigators have also shown that mono(POM)-FdUMP is a poor substrate for carboxylate esterases, and both bis- and mono(POM)-FdUMP are resistant to alkaline phosphatase, 5′-nucleotidase, and spleen phosphodiesterases. The bis(POM) (94–97) and, more recently, bis(POC) (98, 99) approaches have also been used successfully to synthesize masked lipophilic prodrugs of the ANPs 9-(2-phosphonylmethoxyethyl)adenine (PMEA) and (R)-9-(2-phosphonylmethoxypropyl)adenine (PMPA) to improve their oral bioavailability. The antiviral efficacy of bis(POM)-PMEA and bis(POC)-PMPA against HIV-1 increased from a median effective concentration (EC_{50}) of 16 to 0.5 μmol/L and from an EC_{50} of 11 to 0.5 μmol/L, respectively.

However, the cytotoxicity of the prodrugs is also increased, presumably because of the higher levels of the relatively (toxic) diphosphate metabolites. Indeed, investigators estimated that the cellular uptake of bis(POM)-PMEA was increased by more than 100-fold, resulting in a concomitant increased formation of the active diphosphorylated metabolites. The finding that the bis(POM) derivatives are chemically unstable and are highly susceptible to serum-mediated hydrolysis limits their potential utility for direct intracellular drug delivery. Thus, the main advantage of bis(POM)-PMEA is a marked increase of the oral bioavailability of PMEA, rather than an increased antiviral potency.

The same conclusion could be drawn for bis(POC)-PMPA, which is chemically stable in buffer but not in biologic media. Bis(POC)-PMPA confers an oral bioavailability of PMPA of 30% in dogs and 21% in mice, and it is effective in suppressing MSV-induced tumor formation in severe combined immunodeficiency (SCID) mice. The reaction mechanisms of the conversion of bis(POM)-dUMP to free PMEA and bis(POC)-PMPA to free PMPA are depicted in Figures 47A.25 and 47A.26.

The bis(SATE) approach has also been applied to ddUMP, in addition to various other ddNMPs (100–104). After being taken up by the cells, the bis(SATE)ddUMP is converted by carboxyesterase activation to a transient thioethanol phosphotriester (releasing acetic acid) that spontaneously decomposes to the corresponding mono(SATE)ddUMP with release of cyclic ethylenesulfide (Fig. 47A.27). The mono(SATE)ddUMP derivative is then further enzymatically converted to free ddUMP. Cell culture studies have shown that the anti-HIV-1 activity of bis(SATE)ddUMP was 5 μmol/L (EC_{50}), which was more than 100-fold better than the parental ddU nucleoside. The compound fully kept its antiviral potency against the TK-deficient CEM/TK–cells, further corroborating the assumed cytosolic ddUMP delivery, because under similar experimental conditions, ddU and ddUMP were devoid of any appreciable antiviral activity. Particularly striking were the findings that bis(SATE)ddAMP proved at least 1000-fold more efficient than an anti-HIV agent in CEM, MT-4, PBMC, and macrophage cell cultures than its corresponding ddA nucleoside. These observations imply that the bis(SATE) approach can be successfully applied to various nucleoside analogs that are endowed with anti-HIV activity.

Nucleoside-5′-monophosphate derivatives can also be delivered into intact cells on introduction on the phosphate of an aryl group and an amino acid ester linked to the

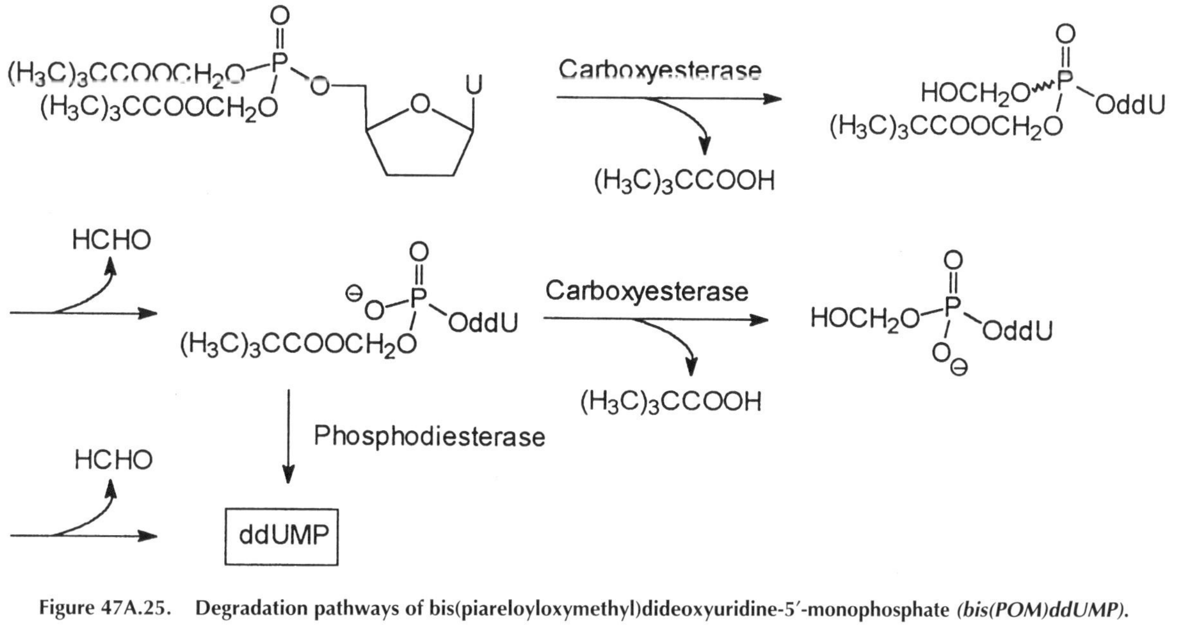

Figure 47A.25. Degradation pathways of bis(piareloyloxymethyl)dideoxyuridine-5′-monophosphate *(bis(POM)ddUMP)*.

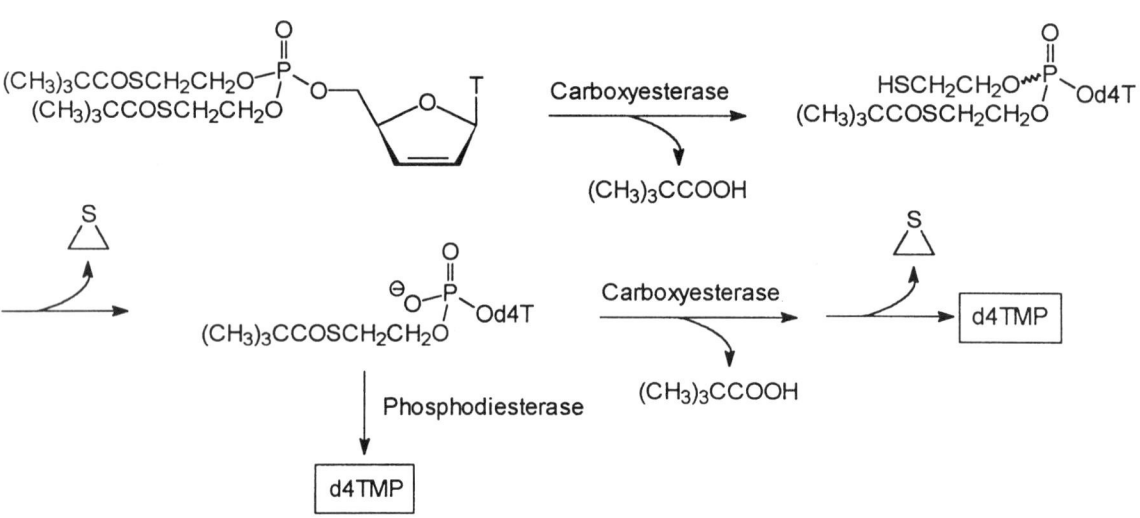

Figure 47A.26. Degradation pathways of bis(POC)9-(2-phosphonylmethoxypropyl)adenine *(PMPA)*.

Figure 47A.27. Degradation pathway of *bis(t-Bu-SATE)d4TMP*.

phosphate through a phosphoramidate bond (Fig. 47A.28). The prototype compound that has been extensively studied is d4T-MP, substituted at its phosphate moiety by a phenyl group and the methyl ester of alanine (designated So 324) (105–111). Investigations with radiolabeled prodrug revealed that 5′-monophosphate, 5′-diphosphate, and 5′-triphosphates of d4T are found in both CEM and CEM/TK– cells to a comparable extent (106). These findings indicate that the d4T-MP is effectively released into the intact cells, which would then explain the pronounced antiviral activity of the prodrug found in HIV-infected CEM/TK– cells. An alaninyl d4T-MP intermediate extensively accumulates in the d4T-MP prodrug-exposed cells. This accumulation can amount up to 100-fold the d4T-TP levels in the cell. The alaninyl d4T-MP may act as an intracellular depot form of d4T or d4T-MP. No evidence of cytostatic activity or toxicity has been found that may be associated with the higher levels of alaninyl d4T-MP. Investigators have also shown that formation of alaninyl d4T-MP and eventually d4T-TP was highly dependent on cell type (107).

Another approach, referred to as the "cyclosaligenyl nucleoside monophosphate approach," has also been reported (112–115). This concept was successfully introduced with d4T-MP and ddAMP as the target nucleotides. The delivery mechanism was originally designed selectively to release the nucleoside 5′-monophosphate and the masking group by a chemically controlled hydrolysis involving a successive, coupled cleavage of the phenyl and benzyl esters of the cyclosal-phosphotriester through a tandem mechanism (Fig. 47A.29). The speed of the first hydrolysis reaction can be influenced by the nature of the substituents present on the cyclosaligenyl moiety. For example, a 5-nitro substituent results in a compound half-life of 0.15 hours at pH 7.3, whereas the presence of a 3-methyl group increases the half-life of the molecule to 10.2 hours. The second hydrolysis step occurs quickly and spontaneously, and it is assumed not to be rate limiting in the eventual conversion of the prodrugs to their respective nucleotides. Thus, this approach may theoretically enable a time-dependent modulation release of the nucleoside 5′-monophosphate into the cells and, consequently, the eventual biologic activity. However, the susceptibility of the prodrugs to cellular enzymes has not been thoroughly studied so far, and one may assume that enzymes will interfere with the chemical hydrolysis process, resulting in complex hydrolysis kinetics of the prodrugs in the intact cell system.

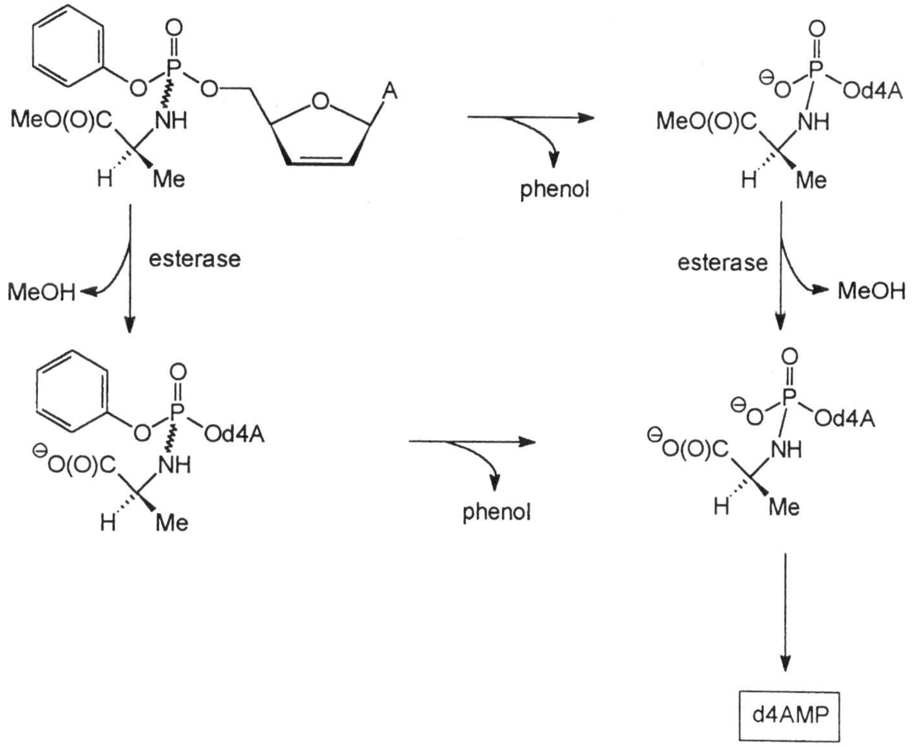

Figure 47A.28. Degradation pathway of the methylester of L-alanine d4A phenylphosphoramidate *(APA)*.

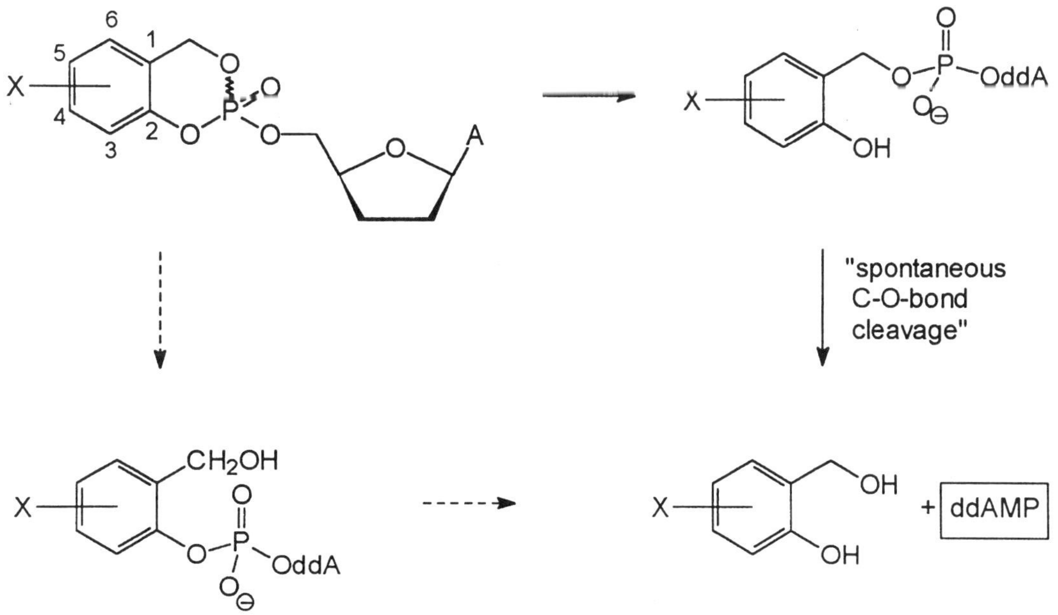

Figure 47A.29. Degradation pathway of cyclosaligenyl dideoxyadenosine-5′-monophosphate *(cycloSALddAMP)*.

Figure 47A.30. Formulas of 9-(2-phosphonylmethoxyethyl)adenine *(PMEA)*, 9-(2-phosphonylmethoxypropyl)adenine *(PMPA)*, and dideoxyadenosine monophosphate *(ddAMP)*.

ACYCLIC NUCLEOSIDE PHOSPHONATES: 9-(2-PHOSPHONYLMETHOXYETHYL)ADENINE AND 9-(2-PHOSPHONYLMETHOXYPROPYL)ADENINE

In 1986, the ANPs were described as a new class of potent antiviral compounds (116). These compounds are now represented by PMEA and PMPA as the prototype compounds endowed with potent antiretroviral activity (116–120) (Fig. 47A.30). PMEA is active against all types of retroviruses that have been investigated: HIV-1, HIV-2, SIV, FIV, feline leukemia virus (FeLV), MSV, Friend murine leukemia virus (FLV), RLV, LP-BM-5 (murine AIDS virus), simian AIDS-related virus (SRV), and visna/maedi virus (117–128). The IC$_{50}$ of PMEA for HIV-1, HIV-2, SIV, FIV, and MSV ranges from 1 to 10 µmol/L. PMEA has also been found effective in inhibiting MSV, RLV, FLV, FIV, FeLV, and SIV replication in animals. PMPA, the (*R*)-enantiomer, differs from PMEA in that PMPA is solely active against retroviruses, whereas PMEA has also additional activity against several herpesviruses (97). Both PMPA and PMEA are active against hepatitis B virus (HBV). The in vivo antiretroviral efficacy of PMEA has been extensively explored against MSV in mice. It was found to be exquisitely active in this model at doses that are at least 10-fold lower than those required for ZDV to give a comparable antiviral efficacy. Moreover, in contrast with ZDV and other antiretroviral agents, PMEA and PMPA are efficacious when administered according to an infrequent dosing schedule (i.e., once or twice a week), which increases the therapeutic index in vivo (97, 128).

The mechanism of cellular uptake of [³H]PMEA has been studied in H9 cells by Palù and colleagues (129) (Fig. 47A.31). Uptake was not sensitive to inhibition by the nucleoside carrier inhibitors nitrobenzylmercaptopurine riboside and dipyridamole. Thus, PMEA does not enter the cells by nucleoside carrier–mediated transport. The observations that uptake of PMEA is virtually abolished at low temperature and that PMEA competes with the cellular uptake of extracellular DNA, but not the natural nucleosides, point to an endocytosis-like process of uptake (129).

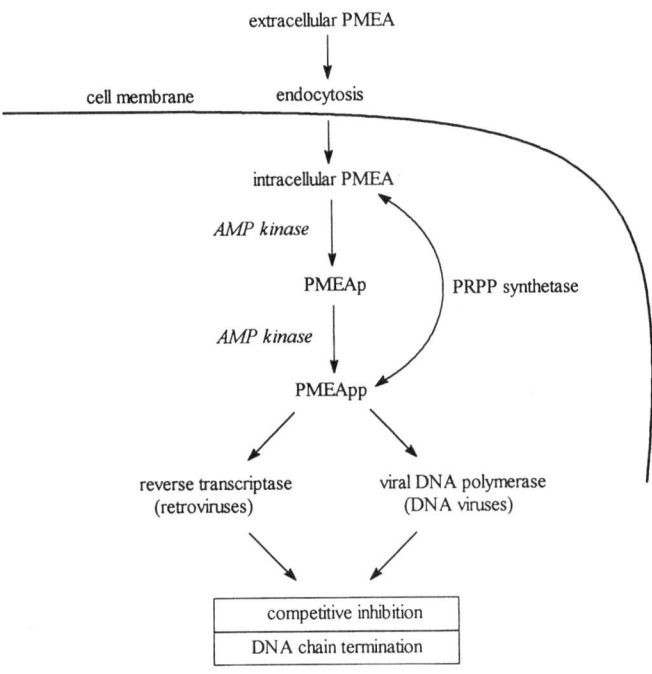

Figure 47A.31. Uptake and metabolism of 9-(2-phosphonylmethoxyethyl)adenine *(PMEA)*. *AMP,* adenosine monophosphate; *PRPP,* 5-phosphoribosyl-1-pyrophosphate.

Metabolism of [³H]PMEA has been studied in MT-4 cells (130). Only the parent compound PMEA and its monophosphorylated (PMEAp) and diphosphorylated (PMEApp) derivatives could be detected by high-performance liquid chromatography (HPLC) analysis. As a rule, intracellular PMEAp and PMEApp levels were invariably 10- to 20-fold lower than the intracellular PMEA levels, irrespective of the initial concentration of PMEA. Moreover, the appearance of phosphorylated derivatives of PMEA proceeded linearly with increasing input concentrations (from 0.5 to 300 µmol/L), a finding suggesting that the uptake process and the phosphorylating enzymes are not saturated at the PMEA concentrations used. Relatively low amounts of PMEApp were detected inside the cells. At equimolar extracellular concentrations (i.e., 10 µmol/L), ZDV and d4T reach 5′-

triphosphate levels that are 10-fold higher than those of PMEApp. However, at equivalent antivirally effective concentrations of ZDV (0.006 µmol/L), d4T (0.2 µmol/L), and PMEA (5 µmol/L) in MT-4 cells, the d4T-TP and PMEApp levels attained within 24 hours are comparable (0.06 and 0.07 nmol/10^9 cells, respectively), whereas ZDV-TP levels are lower (0.01 nmol/10^9 cells). No deaminated metabolites (i.e., PMEHx, PMEAHxp, or PMEAHxpp) were detected in the cells exposed to PMEA. These observations are in agreement with the finding that PMEA is not deaminated by porcine muscle adenylate deaminase.

The diphosphorylated derivative of PMEA (PMEApp) is a potent competitive inhibitor of HIV RT with respect to dATP (130–133). Its K_i for HIV-1 RT is 0.09 µmol/L in the presence of poly(U).oligo(dA) as the template primer and [^{3}H]dATP as the substrate (K_i/K_m, 0.01). In contrast, the K_i/K_m of PMEApp for calf thymus DNA polymerase α is 0.6. Thus, PMEApp is 60-fold less inhibitory to the cellular DNA polymerase than to the retroviral RT, and this property may explain its antiretroviral selectivity. Votruba and associates (133) and Holý and colleagues (132) reported K_i/K_m values of PMEApp of 0.011 and 0.42 for AMV RT and HeLa cell DNA polymerase α, respectively.

Investigators have also demonstrated that PMEApp is incorporated (as PMEA) into the growing DNA chain and thus results in DNA chain termination, in an HIV-1 RT-catalyzed DNA polymerization reaction (130, 132, 133). In this respect, PMEApp proved as effective as ddATP in terminating the DNA chain polymerization at the dAMP sites. DNA chain termination by PMEApp may seem essential for PMEA to exert its antiretroviral action. Simple inhibition of HIV RT by competition with the natural substrate (i.e., dATP) does not suffice to confer antiretroviral activity (our unpublished observations).

PMEApp has a long intracellular half-life (16 to 18 hours), which may explain, at least in part, its long-lasting antiretroviral activity on infrequent dosing. The long half-life of PMEApp may be due to the relatively slow breakdown of PMEApp by ATPase and NDP kinase (130), rather than by the continuous conversion of PMEA to its diphosphorylated form.

The nature of the enzymes responsible for the metabolic conversion of PMEA to PMEAp and PMEApp has been investigated. Several investigators found that AMP kinase from rabbit muscle and several other kinases (e.g., GMP kinase, nucleoside 5′-monophosphate kinase, and pyruvate kinase) cannot catalyze this reaction. However, Merta and associates (134) purified from murine leukemia L1210 cells a PMEA phosphorylating enzyme that also phosphorylated AMP, dAMP, and ADP (134). Phosphorylation of PMEA proceeded with a 1400-fold lower rate than the phosphorylation of AMP. Thus, these investigators concluded that the enzyme responsible for the phosphorylation of PMEA was AMP(dAMP) kinase. However, the PMEA-phosphorylating AMP kinase would be composed of two subunits (MW 40,000 and 29,000), a characteristic different from the known AMP kinases that occur generally as monomers with a molecular weight of 23,000 to 32,000. The role of AMP kinase in the phosphorylation of PMEA was also established by Robbins and colleagues (135, 136) in human CEM cells. The major PMEA phosphorylating activity was found to be associated with the mitochondria and a PMEA-resistant cell variant showed a twofold decrease in mitochondrial adenylate kinase activity. Thus, these observations point to the mitochondrial AMP kinase as the main enzymatic pathway for PMEA phosphorylation.

We have reported that PRPP synthetase is able to convert PMEA directly to PMEApp with a K_m of 1.47 mM and a V_{max} 150-fold lower than the V_{max} for AMP (137, 138). This study was originally performed for PMEA with PRPP synthetase from *Escherichia coli* (130, 137, 138), and it was confirmed for PMEA and PMPA with the rat liver and human erythrocyte enzymes (139). Whether PRPP synthetase plays a significant role in the metabolism of PMEA and PMPA in intact cells, HIV-infected or not, remains to be clarified. A metabolite scheme of PMEA is depicted in Figure 47A.31.

Extensive phosphorylating studies on PMPA have not been performed, but investigators assume that PMPA is metabolized by the same enzymes to its diphosphorylated form as PMEA. However, a striking difference was noted in the sensitivity of PMPApp and PMEApp to its target enzymes (97, 140–142). Indeed, whereas both diphosphorylated derivatives did not significantly differ in inhibitory potential against HIV-1 RT (K_i, 0.98 and 1.55 µmol/L against the DNA-dependent DNA polymerase activity and K_i, 0.012 and 0.022 µmol/L against the RNA-dependent DNA polymerase activity), PMEApp was slightly more inhibitory than PMPApp against DNA polymerases α (K_i, 1.18 µmol/L versus 5.2 µmol/L) and β (K_i, 70.4 µmol/L versus 81.7 µmol/L), and much more inhibitory than PMPApp against DNA polymerase α (K_i, 0.97 µmol/L versus 59.5 µmol/L, respectively). The latter property of PMPApp may explain why PMPA is less toxic (while equally effective) than PMEA.

NONNUCLEOSIDE REVERSE TRANSCRIPTASE INHIBITORS: ANTIVIRAL ACTIVITY, MECHANISM OF ACTION, AND RESISTANCE

Almost 10 years ago, the first leads of highly specific and potent inhibitors of HIV-1 were identified and were designated HEPT (1-[(2-hydroxyethoxy)methyl]-6-(phenylthio)thymine) (143), followed by the TIBO derivatives (tetrahydroimidazo-[4,5,l-jk][1,4]-benzodiazepin-2(1H)-one and -thione) (144). Later, numerous other structural classes of HIV-1-specific compounds were described. Several of them are (or have been) subject of clinical trials: the 9-chloro (R-82913) and 8-chloro-TIBO (R86183) derivatives (144, 145), the dipyridodiazepinone nevirapine (BI-RG-587) (146), the pyridinone derivative L-697,661 (147), the BHAP [bis(heteroaryl)piperazine] derivatives U-87201E (148) and U-90152 (delavirdine) (149), the α-APA (α-anilinophenylacetamide) derivative R-89439 (loviride) (150), the quinoxaline HBY 097 (151), the PETT (phenethylthiazolethiourea) (trovirdine) derivative LY300046.HCl (152), and the (−)6-chloro-4-

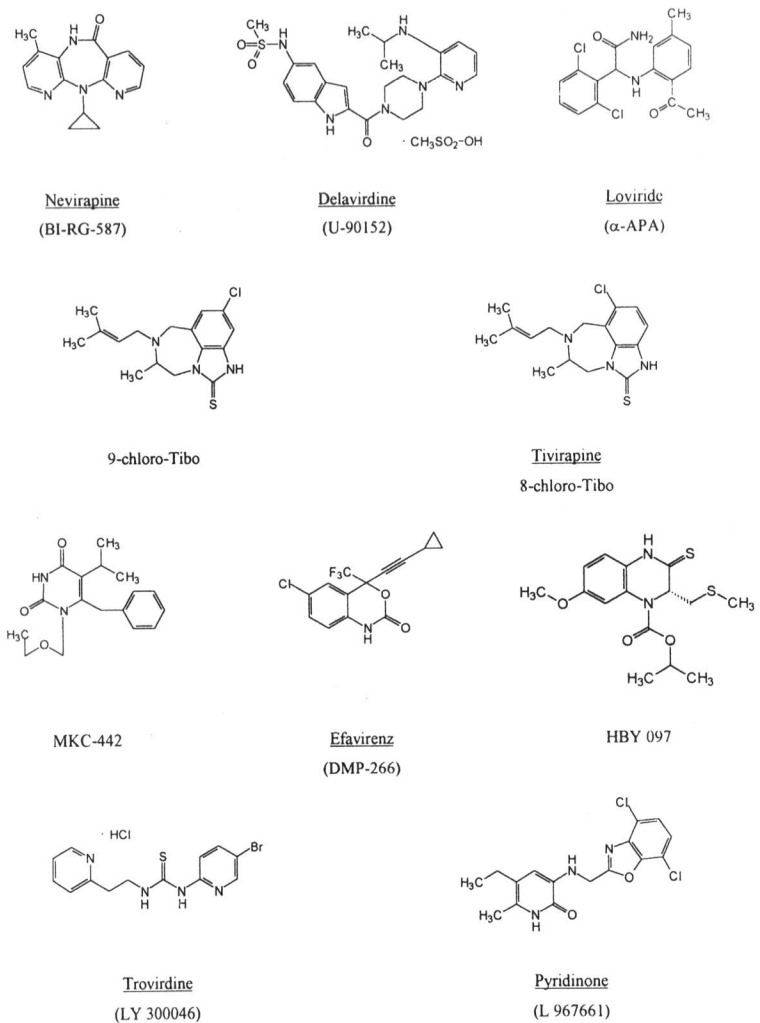

Figure 47A.32. Formulas of nonnucleoside reverse transcriptase inhibitors (NNRTIs).

cyclopropylethynyl-4-trifluoromethyl-1,4-dihydro-2H-3,1-benzoxazin-2-one L 743,726 or DPM 266 (efavirenz) (153) (Fig. 47A.32). Numerous other HIV-1-specific inhibitors—TSAO (1-[2′,5′-bis-O-(*tert*-butyldimethylsilyl)-β-D-ribofuranosyl-3′-spiro-5″-(4″-amino-1″,2″-oxathiole-2″,2″-dioxide)thymine) (154–157), and oxathiin thiocarboxanilides (158–160)—have also been reported but have not yet undergone clinical trials. The HIV-1–specific inhibitors, together with the HIV protease inhibitors, rank among the most potent and selective anti-HIV agents described so far.

Mechanism of Antiviral Action of Nonnucleoside Reverse Transcriptase Inhibitors Compared With Nucleoside Reverse Transcriptase Inhibitors

The nonnucleoside RT inhibitors (NNRTIs) have the propensity solely to inhibit HIV-1 strains, but not HIV-2 strains or other retroviruses. This characteristic is due to a highly specific interaction of the test compounds with the HIV-1 RT (161–165) and a marginal cytotoxicity in cell culture (143–160). The structure and the interaction site of these compounds on HIV-1 RT differ from those of nucleoside analogs. Therefore, these agents have been referred to as "nonnucleoside RT inhibitors," whereas the nucleoside analogs are referred to as "nucleoside RT inhibitors" (NRTIs). Although both NNRTIs and NRTIs act at RT, marked differences exist between NNRTIs and NRTIs. Indeed, both 2′,3′-dideoxynucleoside analogs (i.e., ZDV, ddI) and ANP derivatives (i.e., PMEA, PMPA) interact at the substrate binding site of the RT. In their 5′-triphosphate forms, they compete with the natural substrates (i.e., 2′-deoxynucleoside 5′-triphosphates) of the RT reaction (21, 130, 166, 167). They do not discriminate between HIV-1 and HIV-2 RT. Lineweaver–Burk kinetic plots of the reciprocal of substrate versus the reciprocal of velocity show competitive inhibition for NRTIs with respect to the natural substrate. The 2′,3′-dideoxynucleoside triphosphates and ANP diphosphates inhibit the RT reaction not only by competing with the natural substrates, but also and more importantly by terminating the DNA polymerization process on their incorporation into the growing viral DNA chain. However, as outlined earlier, to inhibit RT, the 2′,3′-dideoxynucleoside and ANP derivatives need first to be metabolically converted (phosphorylated) by cellular enzymes. In contrast, NNRTIs are active on their own right, which means that they do not have to be metabolized to an active derivative. They interact with the RT at a nonsubstrate binding site (162–165), and, as a consequence, they need not compete with endogenous dNTP pools to inhibit the enzyme. Lineweaver–Burk kinetic plots usually show a noncompetitive inhibition of the enzyme against dNTPs and also a noncompetitive or uncompetitive inhibition of the enzyme against homopolymeric templates. The most pronounced inhibition of HIV-1 RT by the NNRTIs has generally been observed in the presence of poly(rC).oligo(dG) as the template primer and dGTP as the substrate, but varying degrees of inhibition were also found in the presence of other artificial homopolymeric template primers such as poly(rA).oligo(dT) and poly(rI).oligo(dC). In contrast to the 2′,3′-dideoxynucleoside triphosphates and ANP diphosphates, NNRTIs do not act as DNA chain terminators.

Emergence of Drug-Resistant Mutant HIV-1 Strains

One of the common properties of NNRTIs is the rapid emergence of resistant virus strains in the presence of the test compounds. This phenomenon has been initially observed in pyridinone- and nevirapine-treated HIV-1–infected cell cultures as well as in nevirapine-treated patients (168–170). The fast emergence of resistance is probably the most important disadvantage of NNRTIs and, it is believed to be the major potential drawback of this category of compounds to afford long-term clinical efficacy and emphasizes the importance of combination therapy.

The resistance of HIV-1 against NNRTIs can be explained by the presence of point mutations in the RT gene of the mutant virus strains. Indeed, investigators have shown that virus strains that have become resistant to one of the NNRTIs show at least one, if not more, amino acid changes in the RT. The degree of resistance and the spectrum of resistance with respect to the different classes of HIV-1–specific RT inhibitors depend on the nature and location of the amino acid change in the RT (168–172). For example, TSAO compounds predominantly select for mutant HIV-1 strains that contain the 138-Glu → Lys mutation in their RT. These virus strains virtually keep full sensitivity to other NNRTIs such as nevirapine, BHAP, and quinoxaline; conversely, virus strains that have emerged in the presence of BHAP or TIBO derivatives and contain a 100-Leu → Ile change in their RT keep marked sensitivity to the inhibitory effects of TSAO or quinoxaline derivatives (171). However, several mutations in the RT severely affect most, if not all, different classes of NNRTIs. For example, a 181-Tyr → Cys mutation in the RT of HIV-1 decreases the inhibitory effects of many NNRTIs such as TIBO, nevirapine, pyridinone, HEPT, and TSAO derivatives. However, several NNRTIs have been identified that are able to suppress 181-Cys–mutant HIV-1 strains at nanomolar concentrations: quinoxaline HBY 097 (173); 5-chloro-3-(phenylsulfonyl)indole-2-carboxamide L-737,126 (174); and several oxathiin thiocarboxanilides (e.g., UC-781) (175). The most common mutation emerging in the HIV-1 RT in NNRTI-treated patients is the 103-Lys → Asn mutation. This mutation causes a pronounced resistance against virtually all NNRTIs in cell culture (176). Another mutation conferring virtually complete resistance to most NNRTIs is the 190-Gly → Glu mutation, arising in the presence of quinoxalines (151, 177). The mutant enzyme has only 5% wild-type catalytic activity. The mutation has not yet been found in HIV-1-infected patients treated with NNRTIs, including quinoxaline HBY 097.

Clustering of the NNRTI-Resistance Mutations in HIV-1 RT and Role of the p66 and p51 RT Subunits in Resistance Development

In general, the amino acid mutations that play a role in the resistance of HIV-1 to NNRTIs can be located in two regions of the RT enzyme: 1) a region that covers the amino acids at positions 98, 100, 101, 103, 106, and 108; and 2) a region that covers the amino acids at positions 179, 181, 188, and 190, as described in the literature (176, 178–181). In addition, the amino acid mutations 236-Pro → Leu, 227-Phe → Leu and 225-Pro → His, which are selected in the presence of BHAP, quinoxaline, or thiocarboxanilides (182–184), and the amino acid mutation 138-Glu → Lys, which emerges in the presence of TSAO, have also been observed in cell culture. However, when the three-dimensional structure of HIV-1 RT is considered, the 98-108, 179-190, and 225, 227, and 236 amino acid sequences are part of a pocket on the p66 subunit of the RT enzyme that is close but distinct from the substrate active site containing the 110-, 185- and 186-aspartic acid triade catalytic center. Indeed, when the p66 subunit of the HIV-1 RT is anatomically compared with a right hand, containing a finger, palm, and thumb subdomain (178, 179), the NNRTI-specific mutations are all clustered in the p66 palm domain at a so-called NNRTI pocket, except the TSAO-specific glutamic acid 138, which is located in a loop at the top of the finger domain of p66 (178–181). However, careful analysis of the x-ray–derived p66/p51 RT heterodimer structure revealed that the location of the amino acid 138-Glu in the p51 subunit of the p66/p51 RT heterodimer enters the p66 NNRTI pocket through the p66/p51 interface (185, 186). This observation reveals a previously unrecognized and important functional and structural role of the p51 subunit in the sensitivity and resistance spectrum of NNRTIs. This role has been proved experimentally for TSAO and some thiocarboxanilide derivatives by constructing p66/p51 RT heterodimers that contain the 138-Lys mutation either in the p51 or in the p66 subunits (159, 185, 186). Indeed, investigators showed that when the TSAO-specific 138-Lys mutation was introduced only in the p51 subunit or in both the p51 and p66 subunits of the HIV-1 RT heterodimer, the enzyme proved fully resistant to TSAO. In contrast, when the 138-Lys mutation was only introduced in the p66 subunit but not in the p51 subunit, the enzyme proved equally sensitive to the inhibitory effects of TSAO as the wild-type RT.

Treatment of HIV-1 with High (Knockout) NNRTI Drug Concentrations

Because one of the characteristics of NNRTIs is their poor toxicity in cell culture and patients, high drug concentrations can be administered to HIV-1–infected cell cultures. At sufficiently high NNRTI concentrations, in the lower micromolar or higher nanomolar concentration range, emergence of drug-resistant virus could be successfully suppressed in long-term HIV-infected cell cultures (187, 188). In these cell cultures, no proviral DNA could be detected by conventional PCR techniques, and when the compounds were withdrawn from the cell cultures after approximately the tenth subcultivation, the cell cultures proved cleared of HIV. The knockout concentrations required to prevent the spread of the HIV-1 infection in cell cultures can be easily achieved in plasma with some of the NNRTIs. Multiple-drug combination of NNRTIs with other HIV inhibitors such as nucleoside analogs or HIV-specific protease inhibitors are currently envisioned in the clinical setting to suppress virus replication completely and to prevent the emergence of drug resistance. In this respect, 3TC-containing combination treatment regimens with NNRTIs have proved particularly attractive (189–192), and they should be further pursued in the treatment of HIV infections.

In conclusion, based on the foregoing observations and the unique properties of NNRTs, these particular compounds represent powerful HIV-1 RT inhibitors that will play a key role in future chemotherapy of HIV-1 infections. A rational drug combination regimen, including NRTIs and NNRTIs, at doses sufficiently high to suppress virus replication completely, should become the cornerstone of our attempts to keep HIV infection under control and to prevent the emergence of resistant mutant virus strains in patients. This treatment regimen should be instituted as soon as possible after HIV-1 infection, based on the observations of Ho and coworkers (193), Wei and associates (194), Perelson and colleagues (195), and Mellors and coworkers (196) that HIV-1 replication starts early after the initial infection and can be suppressed by adequate therapeutic means.

Acknowledgments

Our research has been supported by the Biomedical and Human Capital and Mobility Research Programmes of the European Commission (nos. ERB CHRXCT930258, BMHI-CT93-1691, BMH4-CT-95-1634, and BMHI-CT96-2161) and by a NATO Collaborative Research Grant (no. CRG 920777).

References

1. Zimmerman TP, Mahoney WB, Prus KL. 3′-Azido-3′-deoxythymidine: an unusual nucleoside analog that permeates the membrane of human erythrocytes and lymphocytes by nonfacilitated diffusion. J Biol Chem 1987;262:5748–5754.
2. Balzarini J, Cools M, De Clercq E. Estimation of the lipophilicity of anti-HIV nucleoside analogues by determination of the partition coefficient and retention time on a lichrospher 60 RP-8 HPLC column. Biochem Biophys Res Commun 1989;158:413–422.
3. Furman PA, Fyfe JA, St Clair MH, et al. Phosphorylation of 3′-azido-3′-deoxythymidine and selective interaction of the 5′-triphosphate with human immunodeficiency virus reverse transcriptase. Proc Natl Acad Sci U S A 1986;83:8333–8337.
4. Furman PA, Barry DW. Spectrum and antiviral activity and mechanism of action of zidovudine. Am J Med 1990;85(Suppl 2A):176–181.
5. Balzarini J, Baba M, Pauwels R, et al. Anti-retrovirus activity of 3′-fluoro- and 3′-azido-substituted pyrimidine 2′,3′-dideoxynucleoside analogues. Biochem Pharmacol 1988;37:2847–2856.
6. Balzarini J, Herdewijn P, De Clercq E. Differential patterns of intracellular metabolism of 2′,3′-didehydro-2′,3′-dideoxythymidine (d4T) and 3′-azido-2′,3′-dideoxythymidine (AZT), two potent anti-HIV compounds. J Biol Chem 1989;264:6127–6133.
7. Balzarini J, Van Aerschot A, Pauwels R, et al. 5-Halogeno-3′-fluoro-2′,3′-dideoxyuridines as inhibitors of human immunodeficiency virus (HIV): potent and selective anti-HIV activity of 3′-fluoro-2′,3′-dideoxy-5-chlorouridine. Mol Pharmacol 1989;35:571–577.
8. Avramis VI, Markson W, Jackson RL, et al. Biochemical pharmacology of zidovudine in human T-lymphoblastoid cells (CEM). AIDS 1989;3:417–422.
9. Sommadossi J-P, Carlisle R, Zhou Z. Cellular pharmacology of 3′-azido-3′-deoxythymidine with evidence of incorporation into DNA of human bone marrow cells. Mol Pharmacol 1989;36:9–14.
10. Lavie A, Schlichting I, Vetter IR, et al. The bottleneck in AZT activation. Nature Med 1997;3:922–924.
11. Lavie A, Vetter IR, Konrad M, et al. Structure of thymidylate kinase reveals the cause behind the limiting step in AZT activation. Nature Struct Biol 1997;4:601–604.
12. Balzarini J, Broder S. Principles of antiretroviral therapy for AIDS and related diseases. In: De Clercq E, ed. Clinical use of antiviral drugs. Dordrecht: Martinus Nijhoff, 1988:361–385.
13. Balzarini J, Matthes E, Meeus P, et al. The antiretroviral and cytostatic activity, and metabolism of 3′-azido-2′,3′-dideoxythymidine, 3′-fluoro-2′,3′-dideoxythymidine and 2′,3′-dideoxycytidine are highly cell type-dependent. In: Mikanagi K, Nishioka K, Kelley WN, eds. Purine and pyrimidine metabolism in man. vol. 6, part B. New York: Plenum Press, 1989:407–413.
14. Balzarini J, Pauwels R, Baba M, et al. The in vitro and in vivo anti-retrovirus activity, and intracellular metabolism of 3′-azido-2′,3′-dideoxythymidine and 2′,3′-dideoxycytidine are highly dependent on the cell species. Biochem Pharmacol 1988;37:897–903.
15. Balzarini J, Naesens L, Herdewijn P, et al. Marked in vivo antiretrovirus activity of 9-(2-phosphonylmethoxyethyl)adenine, a selective anti-human immunodeficiency virus agent. Proc Natl Acad Sci U S A 1989;86:332–336.
16. Ruprecht RM., O'Brien LG, Rossoni LD, et al. Suppression of mouse viraemia and retroviral disease by 3′-azido-3′-deoxythymidine. Nature 1986;323:467–469.
17. Bourdais J, Biondi R, Sarfati S, et al. Cellular phosphorylation of anti-HIV nucleosides: role of nucleoside diphosphate kinase. J Biol Chem 1996;271:7887–7890.
18. Morera S, Lebras G, Lascu I, et al. Refined x-ray structure of dictyostelium discoideum nucleoside diphosphate kinase at 1.8 Å resolution. J Mol Biol 1994;243:873–890.
19. Vrang L, Bazin H, Remaud G, et al. Inhibition of the reverse transcriptase from HIV by 3′-azido-3′-deoxythymidine triphosphate and its threo analogue. Antiviral Res 1987;7:139–149.
20. Vrang L, Öberg B, Löwer J, et al. Reverse transcriptases from human immunodeficiency virus type 1 (HIV-1), HIV-2, and simian immunodeficiency virus (SIV_{MAC}) are susceptible to inhibition by foscarnet and 3′-azido-3′-deoxythymidine triphosphate. Antimicrob Agents Chemother 1988;32:1733–1734.
21. St Clair MH, Richards CA, Spector T, et al. 3′-Azido-3′-deoxythymidine triphosphate as an inhibitor and substrate of purified human immunodeficiency virus reverse transcriptase. Antimicrob Agents Chemother 1987;31:1972–1977.
22. White EL, Parker WB, Macy LJ, et al. Comparison of the effect of carbovir, AZT, and dideoxynucleoside triphosphates on the activity of

human immunodeficiency virus reverse transcriptase and selected human polymerases. Biochem Biophys Res Commun 1989;161:393–398.
23. Sommadossi J-P, Carlisle R. Toxicity of 3′-azido-3′-deoxythymidine and 9-(1,3-dihydroxy-2-propoxymethyl)guanine for normal human hematopoietic progenitor cells in vitro. Antimicrob Agents Chemother 1987;31:452–454.
24. Harrington JA, Miller WH, Spector T. Effector studies of 3′-azidothymidine nucleotides with human ribonucleotide reductase. Biochem Pharmacol 1987;36:3757–3761.
25. Frick LW, Nelson DJ. Effects of 3′-azido-3′-deoxythymidine on the deoxynucleoside triphosphate pools of cultured human cells. Adv Exp Med Biol 1989;253B:389–394.
26. Frick LW, Nelson DJ, St Clair MH, et al. Effects of 3′-azido-3′-deoxythymidine on the deoxynucleotide triphosphate pools of cultured human cells. Biochem Biophys Res Commun 1988;154:124–129.
27. Hao Z, Cooney DA, Hartman NR, et al. Factors determining the activity of 2′,3′-dideoxynucleosides in suppressing human immunodeficiency virus in vitro. Mol Pharmacol 1988;34:431–435.
28. Mansuri MM, Starrett JE Jr, Ghazzouli I, et al. 1-(2,3-Dideoxy-β-D-glycero-pent-2-enofuranosyl)thymine (d4T): a highly potent and selective anti-HIV agent. J Med Chem 1989;32:461–466.
29. Mansuri MM, Hitchcock MJM, Buroker RA, et al. Comparison of in vitro biological properties and mouse toxicities of three thymidine analogs active against human immunodeficiency virus. Antimicrob Agents Chemother 1990;34:637–641.
30. Weidner DA, Bridges EG, Sommadossi J-P. 3′-Azido-3′-deoxythymidine (AZT) selectively inhibits globin gene transcription in human K-562 leukemia cells. In: Advances in molecular biology and targeted treatments for AIDS: abstracts of the 3rd annual meeting of the National Institutes of Health National Cooperative Drug Discovery Groups for the Treatment of AIDS, Washington, DC, 1990:129.
31. Weidner DA, Sommadossi JP. 3′-Azido-3′-deoxythymidine (AZT) inhibits globin gene transcription in human K-562 leukemia cells. Proc Am Assoc Cancer Res 1990;31:422, no. 2503.
32. August EM, Marongiu ME, Lin TS, et al. Initial studies on the cellular pharmacology of 3′-deoxythymidin-2′-ene (d4T): a potent and selective inhibitor of human immunodeficiency virus. Biochem Pharmacol 1988;37:4419–4422.
33. Balzarini J, Kang G-J, Dalal M, et al. The anti-HTLV-III (anti-HIV) and cytotoxic activity of 2′,3′-didehydro-2′,3′-dideoxyribonucleosides: a comparison with their parental 2′,3′-dideoxyribonucleosides. Mol Pharmacol 1987;32:162–167.
34. Ho HT, Hitchcock MJM. Cellular pharmacology of 2′,3′-dideoxy-2′,3′-didehydrothymidine, a nucleoside analog active inhibits against human immunodeficiency virus. Antimicrob Agents Chemother 1989;33:844–849.
35. Marongui ME, August EM, Prusoff WH. Effect of 3′-deoxythymidin-2′-ene (d4T) on nucleoside metabolism in H9 cells. Biochem Pharmacol 1990;39:1523–1528.
36. Zhu Z, Ho HT, Hitchcock MJM, et al. Cellular pharmacology of 2′,3′-didehydro-2′,3′-dideoxythymidine (d4T) in human peripheral blood mononuclear cells. Biochem Pharmacol 1990;39:R14–R19.
37. Zhu Z, Schinazi RF, Chu CK, et al. Cellular metabolism of 3′-azido-2′,3′-dideoxyuridine (AzdU) with formation of 5′-O-diphosphohexose derivatives by previously unrecognized metabolic pathways for 2′-deoxyuridine analogs. In: Advances in molecular biology and targeted treatments for AIDS: abstracts of the 3rd annual meeting of the National Institutes of Health National Cooperative Drug Discovery Groups for the Treatment of AIDS, Washington, DC, 1990:130.
38. Doshi KJ, Gallo JM, Boudinot FD, et al. Comparative pharmacokinetics of 3′-azido-3′-deoxythymidine (AZT) and 3′-azido-2′,3′-dideoxyuridine (AzddU) in mice. Drug Metab Dispos Biol Fate Chem 1989;17:590–594.
39. Matthes E, Lehmann C, Scholz D, et al. Phosphorylation, anti-HIV activity and cytotoxicity of 3′-fluorothymidine. Biochem Biophys Res Commun 1988;153:825–831.
40. Matthes E, Lehmann C, Von Janta-Lipinski M, et al. Inhibition of HIV-replication by 3′-fluoro-modified nucleosides with low cytotoxicity. Biochem Biophys Res Commun 1989;165:488–495.
41. Sterzycki R, Mansuri M, Brankovan V, et al. 1-(2,3-dideoxy-3-fluoro-β-D-ribofuranosyl)thymine (FDDT): improved preparation and evaluation as a potential anti-AIDS agent. Nucleosides Nucleotides 1989;8:1115–1117.
42. Cooney DA, Dalal M, Mitsuya H, et al. Initial studies on the cellular pharmacology of 2′,3′-dideoxycytidine, an inhibitor of HTLV-III infectivity. Biochem Pharmacol 1986;35:2065–2068.
43. Ullman B, Coons T, Rockwell S, et al. Genetic analysis of 2′,3′-dideoxycytidine incorporation into cultured human T lymphoblasts. J Biol Chem 1988;263:12,391–12,396.
44. Magnani M, Brandi G, Casabianca A, et al. 2′,3′-Dideoxycytidine metabolism in a new drug-resistant cell line. Biochem J 1995;312:115–123.
45. Kelley JA, Litterst CL, Roth JS, et al. The disposition and metabolism of 2′,3′-dideoxycytidine, an in vitro inhibitor of human T-lymphotrophic virus type III infectivity, in mice and monkeys. Drug Metab Dispos Biol Fate Chem 1987;15:595–601.
46. Balzarini J, Cooney DA, Dalal M, et al. 2′,3′-Dideoxycytidine: regulation of its metabolism and anti-retroviral potency by natural pyrimidine nucleosides and by inhibitors of pyrimidine nucleotide synthesis. Mol Pharmacol 1987;32:798–806.
47. Johnson MA, Johns DG, Fridland A. 2′,3′-Dideoxynucleoside phosphorylation by deoxycytidine kinase from normal human thymus extracts: activation of potential drugs for AIDS therapy. Biochem Biophys Res Commun 1987;148:1252–1258.
48. Starnes MC, Cheng Y-C. Cellular metabolism of 2′,3′-dideoxycytidine, a compound active against human immunodeficiency virus in vitro. J Biol Chem 1987;262:988–991.
49. Cheng Y-C, Dutschman GE, Bastow KF, et al. Human immunodeficiency virus reverse transcriptase: general properties and its interactions with nucleoside triphosphate analogs. J Biol Chem 1987;262:2187–2189.
50. Hao Z, Cooney DA, Farquhar D, et al. Potent DNA chain termination activity and selective inhibition of human immunodeficiency virus reverse transcriptase by 2′,3′-dideoxyuridine-5′-triphosphate (ddUTP). Mol Pharmacol 1990;37:157–163.
51. Mitsuya H, Jarrett RF, Matsukura M, et al. Long-term inhibition of human T-lymptropic virus type III/lymphadenopathy-associated virus (human immunodeficiency virus) DNA synthesis and RNA expression in T cells protected by 2′,3′-dideoxynucleosides in vitro. Proc Natl Acad Sci U S A 1987;84:2033–2037.
52. Yarchoan R, Perno CF, Thomas RV, et al. Phase I studies of 2′,3′-dideoxycytidine in severe human immunodeficiency virus infection as a single agent and alternating with zidovudine (AZT). Lancet 1988;1:76–80.
53. Yarchoan R, Mitsuya H, Myers CE, et al. Clinical pharmacology of 3′-azido-2′,3′-dideoxythymidine (zidovudine) and related dideoxynucleosides. N Engl J Med 1989;321:726–738.
54. Cook HW, Spence MW. Dideoxycytidine, an anti-HIV drug, selectively inhibits growth but not phosphatidylcholine metabolism in neuroblastoma in glioma cells. Neurochem Res 1989;14:279–284.
55. Belleau D, Dixit D, Nguyen-Ba N, et al. Design and activity of a novel class of nucleoside analogues effective against HIV-1 [abstract TC01]. In: Abstracts of the 5th International Conference on AIDS, Montreal, 1989:515.
56. Soudeyns H, Yao X-J, Gao Q, et al. Anti-human immunodeficiency virus type 1 activity and in vitro toxicity of 2′-deoxy-3′-thiacytidine (BCH-189), a novel heterocyclic nucleoside analog. Antimicrob Agents Chemother 1991;35:1386–1390.
57. Coates JAV, Cammack N, Jenkinson HJ, et al. The separated enantiomers of 2′-deoxy-3′-thiacytidine (BCH 189) both inhibit human immunodeficiency virus replication in vitro. Antimicrob Agents Chemother 1992;36:202–205.
58. Schinazi RF, Chu CK, Peck A, et al. Activities of the four optical isomers of 2′,3′-dideoxy-3′-thiacytidine (BCH-189) against human

immunodeficiency virus type 1 in human lymphocytes. Antimicrob Agents Chemother 1992;36:672–676.
59. Sommadossi JP, Schinazi RF, Chu CK, et al. Comparison of cytotoxicity of the (−)- and (+)-enantiomer of 2′,3′-dideoxy-3′-thiacytidine in normal human bone marrow progenitor cells. Biochem Pharmacol 1992;44:1921–1925.
60. Lisignoli G, Facchini A, Cattini L, et al. In vitro toxicity of 2′,3′-dideoxy-3′-thiacytidine (BCH 189/3TC), a new synthetic anti-HIV-1 nucleoside. Antiviral Chem Chemother 1992;3:299–303.
61. Cammack N, Rouse P, Marr CLP, et al. Cellular metabolism of (−)enantiomeric 2′-deoxy-3′-thiacytidine. Biochem Pharmacol 1992; 43:2059–2064.
62. Gray NM, Marr CLP, Penn CR, et al. The intracellular phosphorylation of (−)-2′-deoxy-3′-thiacytidine (3TC) and the incorporation of 3TC 5′-monophosphate into DNA by HIV-1 reverse transcriptase and human DNA polymerase . Biochem Pharmacol 1995;50:1043–1051.
63. Hart GJ, Orr DC, Penn CR, et al. Effects of (−)-2′-deoxy-3′-thiacytidine (3TC) 5′-triphosphate on human immunodeficiency virus reverse transcriptase and mammalian DNA polymerases alpha, beta, and gamma. Antimicrob Agents Chemother 1992;36:1688–1694.
64. Schinazi RF, McMillan A, Cannon D, et al. Selective inhibition of human immunodeficiency viruses by racemates and enantiomers of cis-5-fluoro-1-[2-(hydroxymethyl)-1,3-oxathiolan-5-yl]cytosine. Antimicrob Agents Chemother 1992;36:2423–2431.
65. Furman PA, Davis M, Liotta DC, et al. The anti-hepatitis B virus activities, cytotoxicities, and anabolic profiles of the (−) and (+) enantiomers of cis-5-fluoro-1-[2-(hydroxymethyl)-1,3-oxathiolan-5-yl]cytosine. Antimicrob Agents Chemother 1992;36:2686–2692.
66. Schinazi RF, Boudinot FD, Ibrahim SS, et al. Pharmacokinetics and metabolism of racemic 2′,3′-dideoxy-5-fluoro-3′-thiacytidine in rhesus monkeys. Antimicrob Agents Chemother 1992;36:2432–2438.
67. Bridges EG, Dutschman GE, Gullen EA, et al. Favorable interaction of -L(−) nucleoside analogues with clinically approved anti-HIV nucleoside analogues for the treatment of human immunodeficiency virus. Biochem Pharmacol 1996;51:731–736.
68. Cooney DA, Ahluwahlia G, Mitsuya H, et al. Initial studies on the cellular pharmacology of 2′,3′-dideoxyadenosine, an inhibitor of HTLV-III infectivity. Biochem Pharmacol 1987;36:1765–1768.
69. Ahluwahlia G, Cooney DA, Mitsuya H, et al. Initial studies on the cellular pharmacology of 2′,3′-dideoxyinosine, an inhibitor of HIV infectivity. Biochem Pharmacol 1987;36:3797–3800.
70. Plunkett W, Cohen SS. Two approaches that increase the activity of analogs of adenine nucleosides in animal cells. Cancer Res 1975;35:1547–1554.
71. Johnson MA, Fridland A. Phosphorylation of 2′,3′-dideoxyinosine by cytosolic 5′-nucleotidase of human lymphoid cells. Mol Pharmacol 1989;36:291–295.
72. Johnson MA, Ahluwahlia G, Connelly MC, et al. Metabolic pathways for the activation of the antiretroviral agent 2′,3′-dideoxyadenosine in human lymphoid cells. J Biol Chem 1988;263:15,354–15,357.
73. Carson DA, Haertle T, Wasson DB, et al. Biochemical genetic analysis of 2′,3′-dideoxyadenosine metabolism in human T lymphocytes. Biochem Biophys Res Commun 1988;151:788–793.
74. Haertle T, Carrera CJ, Wasson DB, et al. Metabolism of anti-human immunodeficiency virus-1 activity of 2-halo-2′,3′-dideoxyadenosine derivatives. J Biol Chem 1988;263:5870–5875.
75. Marquez VE, Tseng CK-H, Kelley JA, et al. 2′,3′-Dideoxy-2′-fluoro-ara-A: an acid-stable purine nucleoside active against human immunodeficiency virus (HIV). Biochem Pharmacol 1987;36:2719–2722.
76. Marquez VE, Tseng CK-H, Mitsuya H, et al. Acid-stable 2′-fluoro purine dideoxynucleosides as active agents against HIV. J Med Chem 1990;33:978–985.
77. Boyle MJ, Flanigan ME, Ford H, et al. The Hu-HIV/PBL-SCID mouse: a modified Hu-PBL-SCID model for the study of HIV pathogenesis and therapy. J Immunol 1995;154:6212–6223.
78. Ruxrungtham K, Boone E, Ford H, et al. Potent activity of 2′-fluoro-2′,3′-dideoxyadenosine against human immunodeficiency virus type 1 infection in hu-PBL-SCID mice. Antimicrob Agents Chemother 1996;40:2369–2374.
79. Masood RW, Ahluwahlia GS, Cooney DA, et al. 2′-Fluoro-2′,3′-dideoxyarabinosyladenine: a metabolically stable analogue of the antiretroviral agent 2′,3′-dideoxyadenosine. Mol Pharmacol 1990;37:590–596.
80. Hitchcock MJM, Woods K, De Boeck K, et al. Biochemical pharmacology of 2′-fluoro-2′,3′-dideoxyarabinosyladenine, an inhibitor of HIV with improved metabolic and chemical stability over 2′,3′-dideoxyadenosine. Antiviral Chem Chemother 1990;1:319–327.
81. Plagemann PGW, Woffendin C. Permeation and salvage of dideoxyadenosine in mammalian cells. Mol Pharmacol 1989;36:185–182.
82. Driscoll JS, Mayers DL, Bader JP, et al. 2′-Fluoro-2′,3′-dideoxyarabinosyladenine (F-ddA): activity against drug-resistant human immunodeficiency virus strains and clades A-E. Antiviral Chem Chemother 1997;8:107–111.
83. Mitsuya H, Matsukura M, Broder S. Rapid in vitro systems for assessing activity of agents against HTLV-III/LAV. In: Broder S, ed. AIDS: modern concepts and therapeutic challenges. New York: Marcel Dekker, 1987:309–321.
84. Vince R, Hua M, Brownell J, et al. Potent and selective activity of a new carbocyclic nucleoside analog (carbovir: NSC 614846) against human immunodeficiency virus in vitro. Biochem Biophys Res Commun 1988;156:868–871.
85. Bondoc LL Jr, Shannon WM, Secrist JA III, et al. Metabolism of the carbocyclic nucleoside analogue carbovir, an inhibitor of human immunodeficiency virus, in human lymphoid cells. Biochemistry 1990;29:9839–9843.
86. Parker WB, White EL, Shaddix SC, et al. Mechanism of inhibition of human immunodeficiency virus type 1 reverse transcriptase and human DNA polymerases α, β, and γ by the 5′-triphosphates of carbovir, 3′-azido-3′-deoxythymidine, 2′,3′-dideoxyguanosine, and 3′-deoxythymidine. J Biol Chem 1991;266:1754–1762.
87. Parker WB, Shaddix SC, Bowdon BJ, et al. Metabolism of carbovir, a potent inhibitor of human immunodeficiency virus type 1, and its effect on cellular metabolism. Antimicrob Agents Chemother 1993;37:1004–1009.
88. Daluge SM, Good SS, Faletto MB, et al. 1592U89, a novel carbocyclic nucleoside analog with potent, selective anti–human immunodeficiency virus activity. Antimicrob Agents Chemother 1997;41:1082–1093.
89. Faletto MB, Miller WH, Garvey EP, et al. Unique intracellular activation of the potent anti–human immunodeficiency virus agent 1592U89. Antimicrob Agents Chemother 1997;41:1099–1107.
90. Garvey E, Krenitsky TA. A novel human phosphotransferase highly specific for adenosine. Arch Biochem Biophys 1992;296:161–169.
91. Sastry JK, Nehete PN, Khan S, et al. Membrane-permeable dideoxyuridine 5′-monophosphate analogue inhibits human immunodeficiency virus infection. Mol Pharmacol 1992;41:441–445.
92. Farquhar D, Khan S, Srivastva DN, et al. Synthesis and antitumor evaluation of bis[(pivaloyloxy)methyl]-2′-deoxy-5-fluorouridine 5′-monophosphate (FdUMP): a strategy to introduce nucleotides into cells. J Med Chem 1994;37:3902–3909.
93. Farquhar D, Chen R, Khan S. 5′-[4-(Pivaloyloxy)-1,3,2-dioxaphosphorinan-2-yl]-2′-deoxy-5-fluorouridine: a membrane-permeating prodrug of 5-fluoro-2′-deoxyuridylic acid (FdUMP). J Med Chem 1995;38:488–495.
94. Srinivas RV, Robbins BL, Connelly MC, et al. Metabolism and in vitro antiretroviral activities of bis(pivaloyloxymethyl)prodrugs of acyclic nucleoside phosphonates. Antimicrob Agents Chemother 1993;37:2247–2250.
95. Srinivas RV, Robbins BL, Connelly MC, et al. Pivaloyloxymethyl esters of acyclic nucleoside phosphonates. Int Antiviral News 1994;2:53–55.
96. McGee LR, Shaw J-P, Burman D, et al. Abstract OP11. In: 12th International Roundtable on Nucleosides, Nucleotides, and Their Biological Application, La Jolla, CA, 1996.

97. Naesens L, Snoeck R, Andrei G, et al. HPMPC (cidofovir), PMEA (adefovir) and related acyclic nucleoside phosphonate analogues: a review of their pharmacology and clinical potential in the treatment of viral infections. Antiviral Chem Chemother 1997;8:1–23.
98. Fridland A, Robbins BL, Srinivas RV, et al. Antiretroviral activity and metabolism of bis(POC)PMPA, an oral bioavailable prodrug of PMPA: work presented at the 10th International Conference on Antiviral Research, April 6–11, 1997, Atlanta, Georgia, U S A. Antiviral Res 1997;34:A49, 27.
99. Naesens L, Bischofberger N, Arimilli M, et al. Anti-retrovirus activity and pharmacokinetics in mice of bis(POC)-PMPA, the bis(isopropyloxycarbonyloxymethyl) oral prodrug of PMPA: work presented at the 10th International Conference on Antiviral Research, April 6–11, 1997, Atlanta, Georgia, USA. Antiviral Res 1997;34:A50, 28.
100. Puech F, Gosselin G, Lefebvre I, et al. Intracellular delivery of nucleoside monophosphates through a reductase-mediated activation process. Antiviral Res 1993;22:155–174.
101. Valette G, Pompon A, Girardet J-L, et al. Decomposition pathways and in vitro HIV inhibitory effects of IsoddA pronucleotides: toward a rational approach for intracellular delivery of nucleoside 5′-monophosphates. J Med Chem 1996;39:1981–1990.
102. Girardet J-L, Perigaud C, Aubertin A-M, et al. Increase of the anti-HIV activity of d4T in human T-cell culture by the use of the SATE pronucleotide approach. Bioorg Med Chem Lett 1995;5:2981–2984.
103. Benzaria S, Pelicano H, Johnson R, et al. Synthesis, in vitro antiviral evaluation, and stability studies of bis(S-acyl-2-thioethyl) ester derivatives of 9[2-phosphonomethoxy)ethyl]adenine (PMEA) as potential PMEA prodrugs with improved oral bioavailability. J Med Chem 1996;39:4958–4965.
104. Pompon A, Lefebvre I, Imbach J-L, et al. Decomposition pathways of the mono- and bis(pivaloyloxymethyl) esters of azidothymidine 5′-monophosphate in cell extract and in tissue culture medium: an application of the "on line ISRP-cleaning" HPLC technique. Antiviral Chem Chemother 1994;5:91–98.
105. McGuigan C, Cahard D, Sheeka HM, et al. Aryl phosphoramidate derivatives of d4T have improved anti-HIV efficacy in tissue culture and may act by the generation of a novel intracellular metabolite. J Med Chem 1996;39:1748–1753.
106. Balzarini J, Karlsson A, Aquaro S, et al. Mechanism of anti-HIV action of masked alaninyl d4TMP derivatives. Proc Natl Acad Sci U S A 1996;93:7295–7299.
107. Balzarini J, Egberink H, Hartmann K, et al. Antiretrovirus specificity and intracellular metabolism of 2′,3′-didehydro-2′,3′-dideoxythymidine (stavudine) and its 5′-monophosphate triester prodrug So324. Mol Pharmacol 1996;50:1207–1213.
108. McGuigan C, Wedgwood OM, De Clercq E, et al. Phosphoramidate derivatives of 2′,3′-didehydro-2′,3′-dideoxyadenosine (d4A) have markedly improved anti-HIV potency and selectivity. Bioorg Med Chem Lett 1996;6:2359–2362.
109. Balzarini J, Kruining J, Wedgwood O, et al. Conversion of 2′,3′-dideoxyadenosine (ddA) and 2′,3′-didehydro-2′,3′-dideoxyadenosine (d4A) to their corresponding aryloxyphosphoramidate derivatives markedly potentiates their activity against human immunodeficiency virus and hepatitis B virus. FEBS Lett 1997;410:324–328.
110. McGuigan C, Cahard D, Salgado A, et al. Phosphoramidates as potent prodrugs of anti-HIV nucleotides: studies in the amino region. Antiviral Chem Chemother 1996;7:31–36.
111. McGuigan C, Tsang H-W, Cahard D, et al. Phosphoramidate derivatives of d4T as inhibitors of HIV: the effect of amino acid variation. Antiviral Res 1997;35:195–204.
112. Meier C, Lorey M, De Clercq E, et al. Cyclic saligenyl phosphotriesters of 2′,3′-dideoxy-2′,3′-didehydrothymidine (d4T): a new pronucleotide approach. Bioorg Med Chem Lett 1997;7:99–104.
113. Meier C, Lorey M, De Clercq E, et al. Cyclosaligenyl-3′-azido-2′,3′-dideoxythymidine monophosphate (cycloSal-AZTMP): a new pronucleotide approach? Nucleosides Nucleotides 1997;16:793–796.
114. Meier C, Knispel T, De Clercq E, et al. ADA-bypass by lipophilic cycloSal-ddAMP pronucleotides: a second example of the efficiency of the cycloSal-concept. Bioorg Med Chem Lett 1997;7:1577–1582.
115. Meier C, Lorey M, De Clercq E, et al. CycloSal-2′,3′-dideoxy-2′,3′-didehydrothymidine monophosphate (cycloSal-d4TMP): synthesis and antiviral evaluation of a new d4TMP delivery system. J Med Chem 1998;41(9):1417–1427.
116. De Clercq E, Holý A, Rosenberg I, et al. A novel selective broad-spectrum anti-DNA virus agent. Nature 1986;323:464–467.
117. De Clercq E. Broad-spectrum anti-DNA virus and anti-retrovirus activity of phosphonylmethoxyalkylpurines and -pyrimidines. Biochem Pharmacol 1991;42:963–972.
118. Pauwels R, Balzarini J, Schols D, et al. Phosphonylmethoxyethylpurine derivatives, a new class of anti-human immunodeficiency virus agents. Antimicrob Agents Chemother 1988;32:1025–1030.
119. Balzarini J, Holý A, Jindrich J, et al. Differential antiherpesvirus and antiretrovirus effects of the (S) and (R) enantiomers of acyclic nucleoside phosphonates: potent and selective in vitro and in vivo antiretrovirus activities of (R)-9-(2-phosphonomethoxypropyl)-2,6-diaminopurine. Antimicrob Agents Chemother 1993;37:332–338.
120. Balzarini J, Aquaro S, Perno C-F, et al. Activity of the (R)-enantiomers of 9-(2-phosphonylmethoxypropyl)adenine and 9-(2-phosphonylmethoxypropyl)-2,6-diaminopurine against human immunodeficiency virus in different human cell systems. Biochem Biophys Res Commun 1996;219:337–341.
121. Balzarini J, Naesens L, Herdewijn P, et al. Marked in vivo antiretrovirus activity of 9-(2-phosphonylmethoxyethyl)adenine, a selective anti-human immunodeficiency virus agent. Proc Natl Acad Sci U S A 1989;86:332–336.
122. Balzarini J, Naesens L, Slachmuylders J, et al. 9-(2-Phosphonylmethoxyethyl)adenine (PMEA) effectively inhibits retrovirus replication in vitro and simian immunodeficiency virus infection in rhesus monkeys. AIDS 1991;5:21–28.
123. Gangemi JD, Cozens RM, De Clercq E, et al. 9-(2-Phosphonylmethoxyethyl)adenine in the treatment of murine acquired immunodeficiency disease and opportunistic herpes simplex virus infections. Antimicrob Agents Chemother 1989;33:1864–1868.
124. Hartmann K, Donath A, Beer B, et al. Use of two virustatica (AZT, PMEA) in the treatment of FIV and of FeLV seropositive cats with clinical symptoms. Vet Immunol Immunopathol 1993;35:167–175.
125. Naesens L, Neyts J, Balzarini J, et al. Efficacy of oral 9-(2-phosphonylmethoxyethyl)-2,6-diaminopurine (PMEDAP) in the treatment of retrovirus and cytomegalovirus infections in mice. J Med Virol 1993;39:167–172
126. Hartmann K, Kuffer M, Balzarini J, et al. Efficacy of the acyclic nucleoside phosphonates (S)-9-(3-fluoro-2-phosphonylmethoxypropyl)adenine (FPMPA) and 9-(2-phosphonylmethoxyethyl)adenine (PMEA) against feline immunodeficiency virus. J Acquir Immune Defic Syndr Hum Retrovirol 1998;17:120–128.
127. Thormar H, Georgsson G, Pálsson P, et al. Inhibitory effect of 9-(2-phosphonylmethoxyethyl)adenine on visna virus infection in lambs: a model for in vivo testing of candidate anti-human immunodeficiency virus drugs. Proc Natl Acad Sci U S A 1995;92:3283–3287.
128. Naesens L, Balzarini J, De Clercq E. Single-dose administration of 9-(2-phosphonylmethoxyethyl)adenine (PMEA) and 9-(2-phosphonylmethoxyethyl)-2,6-diaminopurine (PMEDAP) in the prophylaxis of retrovirus infection in vivo. Antiviral Res 1991;16:53–64.
129. Palú G, Stefanelli S, Rassu M, et al. Cellular uptake of phosphonylmethoxyalkylpurine derivatives. Antiviral Res 1991;16:115–119.
130. Balzarini J, Hao Z, Herdewijn P, et al. Intracellular metabolism and mechanism of anti-retrovirus action of 9-(2-phosphonylmethoxyethyl)adenine, a potent anti–human immunodeficiency virus compound. Proc Natl Acad Sci U S A 1991;88:1499–1503.
131. Bronson JJ, Ho H-T, De Boeck H, et al. Biochemical pharmacology of acyclic nucleotide analogues. Ann N Y Acad Sci 1990;616:398–407.

132. Holý A, Votruba I, Merta A, et al. Acyclic nucleotide analogues: synthesis, antiviral activity and inhibitory effects on some cellular and virus-encoded enzymes in vitro. Antiviral Res 1990;13:295–312.
133. Votruba I, Travnicek M, Rosenberg I, et al. Inhibition of avian myeloblastosis virus reverse transcriptase by diphosphates of acyclic phosphonylmethyl nucleotide analogues. Antiviral Res 1990;13:287–293.
134. Merta A, Votruba I, Jindrich J, et al. Phosphorylation of 9-(2-phosphonomethoxyethyl)adenine and 9-(S)-(3-hydroxy-2-phosphonomethoxypropyl)-adenine by AMP(dAMP) kinase from L1210 cells. Biochem Pharmacol 1992;44:2067–2078.
135. Robbins BL, Greenhaw J, Connelly MC, et al. Metabolic pathways for activation of the antiviral agent 9-(2-phosphonylmethoxyethyl) adenine in human lymphoid cells. Antimicrob Agents Chemother 1995;39:2304–2308.
136. Robbins BL, Connelly MC, Marshall DR, et al. A human T lymphoid cell variant resistant to the acyclic nucleoside phosphonate 9-(2-phosphonylmethoxyethyl)adenine shows a unique combination of a phosphorylation defect and increased efflux of the agent. Mol Pharmacol 1995;47:391–397.
137. Balzarini J, De Clercq E. 5-Phosphoribosyl 1-pyrophosphate synthetase converts the acyclic nucleoside phosphonates 9-(3-hydroxy-2-phosphonylmethoxypropyl)adenine and 9-(2-phosphonylmethoxyethyl)adenine directly to their antivirally active diphosphate derivatives. J Biol Chem 1991;266:8686–8689.
138. Balzarini J, De Clercq E. Conversion of acyclic nucleoside phosphonates to their diphosphate derivatives by 5-phosphoribosyl-1-pyrophosphate (PRPP) synthetase. In: Harkness RA, Elion GB, Zöllner N, et al., eds. Purine and pyrimidine metabolism in man. vol. 7, part A. New York: Plenum Press, 1991:29–32.
139. Balzarini J, Nave J-F, Becker MA, et al. Kinetic properties of adenine nucleotide analogues against purified 5-phosphoribosyl-1-pyrophosphate synthetases from E. coli, rat liver and human erythrocytes. Nucleosides Nucleotides 1995;14:1861–1871.
140. Merta A, Votruba I, Rosenberg I, et al. Inhibition of herpes simplex virus DNA polymerase by diphosphates of acyclic phosphonylmethoxyalkyl nucleotide analogues. Antiviral Res 1990;13:209–218.
141. Kramata P, Votruba I, Otová B, et al. Different inhibitory potencies of acyclic phosphonomethoxyalkyl nucleotide analogs toward DNA polymerases α, β, and γ. Mol Pharmacol 1996;49:1005–1011.
142. Cherrington JM, Allen SJW, Bischofberger N, et al. Kinetic interaction of the diphosphates of 9-(2-phosphonylmethoxyethyl)adenine and other anti-HIV active purine congeners with HIV reverse transcriptase and human polymerases α, β, and γ. Antiviral Chem Chemother 1995;6:217–221.
143. Baba M, Tanaka H, De Clercq E, et al. Highly specific inhibition of human immunodeficiency virus type 1 by a novel 6-substituted acyclouridine derivative. Biochem Biophys Res Commun 1989;165:1375–1381.
144. Pauwels R, Andries K, Desmyter J, et al. Potent and selective inhibition of HIV-1 replication in vitro by a novel series of TIBO derivatives. Nature 1990;343:470–474.
145. Pauwels R, Andries K, Debyser Z, et al. New tetrahydroimidazo[4,5-1-jk][1,4]-benzodiazepin-2(1H)-one and -thione derivatives are potent inhibitors of human immunodeficiency virus type 1 replication and are synergistic with 2′,3′-dideoxynucleoside analogs. Antimicrob Agents Chemother 1994;38:2863–2870.
146. Merluzzi VJ, Hargrave KD, Labadia M, et al. Inhibition of HIV-1 replication by a nonnucleoside reverse transcriptase inhibitor. Science 1990;250:1411–1413.
147. Goldman ME, Nunberg JH, O'Brien JA, et al. Pyridinone derivatives: specific human immunodeficiency virus type 1 reverse transcriptase inhibitors with antiviral activity. Proc Natl Acad Sci U S A 1991;88:6863–6867.
148. Romero DL, Busso M, Tan C-K, et al. Nonnucleoside reverse transcriptase inhibitors that potently and specifically block human immunodeficiency virus type 1 replication. Proc Natl Acad Sci U S A 1991;88:8806–8810.
149. Dueweke TJ, Poppe SM, Romero DL, et al. U-90152, a potent inhibitor of human immunodeficiency virus type 1 replication. Antimicrob Agents Chemother 1993;37:1127–1131.
150. Pauwels R, Andries K, Debyser Z, et al. Potent and highly selective HIV-1 inhibition by a new series of -anilinophenyl acetamide (-APA) derivatives targeted at HIV-1 reverse transcriptase. Proc Natl Acad Sci U S A 1993;90:1711–1715.
151. Kleim J-P, Bender R, Billhardt U-M, et al. Activity of a novel quinoxaline derivative against human immunodeficiency virus type 1 reverse transcriptase and viral replication. Antimicrob Agents Chemother 1993;37:1659–1664.
152. Ahgren C, Backro K, Bell FW, et al. The PETT series, a new class of potent non-nucleoside inhibitors of human immmunodeficiency virus type 1 reverse transcriptase. Antimicrob Agents Chemother 1995;39:1329–1335.
153. Young SD, Britcher SF, Tran LO, et al. L-743,726 (DMP-266): a novel, highly potent nonnucleoside inhibitor of the human immunodeficiency virus type 1 reverse transcriptase. Antimicrob Agents Chemother 1995;39:2602–2605.
154. Camarasa M-J, Perez-Perez M-J, San-Felix A, et al. 3′-Spiro nucleosides, a new class of specific human immunodeficiency virus type 1 inhibitors: synthesis and antiviral activity of [2′,5′-bis-O-(tert-butyldimethylsilyl)-β-D-xylo- and -ribofuranose]-3′-spiro-5″-[4″-amino-1″,2″-oxathiole-2″,2″-dioxide] (TSAO) pyrimidine nucleosides. J Med Chem 1992;35:2721–2727.
155. Perez-Perez M-J, San-Felix A, Balzarini J, et al. TSAO analogues: stereospecific synthesis and anti–HIV-1 activity of 1-[2′,5′-bis-O-(tert-butyldimethylsilyl)-β-D-ribofuranosyl]-3′-spiro-5″-(4″-amino-1″,2″-oxathiole-2″,2″-dioxide) pyrimidine and pyrimidine-modified nucleosides. J Med Chem 1992;35:2988–2995.
156. Perez-Perez M-J, San-Felix A, Camarasa M-J, et al. Synthesis of [1-[2′,5′-bis-O-(t-butyldimethylsilyl)–β-D-xylo-and β-D-ribofuranosyl]thymine-3′-spiro-5″-[4″-amino-1″,2″-oxathiole-2″,2″-dioxide] (TSAO): a novel type of specific anti-HIV agents. Tetrahedron Lett 1992;33:3029–3032.
157. Balzarini J, Perez-Perez M-J, San-Felix A, et al. 2′,5′-Bis-O-(tert-butyldimethylsilyl)-3′-spiro-5″-(4″-amino-1″,2″-oxathiole-2″,2″-dioxide)pyrimidine (TSAO) nucleoside analogues: highly selective inhibitors of human immunodeficiency virus type 1 that are targeted at the viral reverse transcriptase. Proc Natl Acad Sci U S A 1992;89:4392–9396.
158. Bader JP, McMahan JB, Schultz RJ, et al. Oxathiin carboxanilide, a potent inhibitor of human immunodeficiency virus reproduction. Proc Natl Acad Sci U S A 1992;88:6740–6744.
159. Balzarini J, Jonckheere H, Harrison WA, et al. Oxathiin carboxanilide derivatives: a class of non-nucleoside HIV-1 specific reverse transcriptase inhibitors (NNRTIs) that are active against mutant HIV-1 strains resistant to other NNRTIs. Antiviral Chem Chemother 1995;6:169–178.
160. Balzarini J, Brouwer WG, Felauer EE, et al. Activity of various thiocarboxanilide derivatives against wild-type and several mutant human immunodeficiency virus type 1 strains. Antiviral Res 1995;27:219–236.
161. Frank KB, Noll GJ, Connell EV, et al. Kinetic interaction of human immunodeficiency virus type 1 reverse transcriptase with the antiviral tetrahydroimidazo[4,5,1-jk]-[1,4]-benzodiazepine-2-(1H)-thione compound, R82150. J Biol Chem 1991;266:14,232–14,236.
162. Cohen KA, Hopkins J, Ingraham RH, et al. Characterization of the binding site for nevirapine (BI-RG-587), a nonnucleoside inhibitor of human immunodeficiency virus type-1 reverse transcriptase. J Biol Chem 1991;266:14,670–14,674.
163. Dueweke TJ, Kezdy FJ, Waszak GA, et al. The binding of a novel bis(heteroaryl)piperazine mediates inhibition of human immunodeficiency virus type 1 reverse transcriptase. J Biol Chem 1992;267:27–30.

164. White EL, Buckheit RW Jr, Ross LJ, et al. A TIBO derivative, R82913, is a potent inhibitor of HIV-1 reverse transcriptase with heteropolymer templates. Antiviral Res 1991;16:257–266.
165. Balzarini J, Perez-Perez M-J, San-Felix A, et al. Kinetics of inhibition of human immunodeficiency virus type 1 (HIV-1) reverse transcriptase by the novel HIV-1–specific nucleoside analogue 1-[2′,5′-bis-O-(*tert*-butyldimethylsilyl)-β-D-ribofuranosyl]-3′-spiro-5″-[4″-amino-1″,2″-oxathiole-2″,2″-dioxide]-thymine (TSAO-T). J Biol Chem 1992;267:11,831–11,838.
166. Balzarini J, De Clercq E. Kinetic and inhibitory properties of nucleoside and non-nucleoside reverse transcriptase inhibitors. Methods Enzymol 1996;275:472–502.
167. Balzarini J, Holý A, Jindrich J, et al. 9-[(2*RS*)-3-fluoro-2-phosphonylmethoxypropyl] derivatives of purine: a class of highly selective antiretroviral agents in vitro and in vivo. Proc Natl Acad Sci U S A 1991;88:4961–4965.
168. Nunberg JH, Schlief WA, Boots EJ, et al. Viral resistance to human immunodeficiency virus type 1–specific pyridinone reverse transcriptase inhibitors. J Virol 1991;65:4887–4892.
169. Richman D, Shih C-K, Lowy I, et al. Human immunodeficiency virus type 1 mutants resistant to nonnucleoside inhibitors of reverse transcriptase arise in tissue culture. Proc Natl Acad Sci U S A 1991;88:11241–11245.
170. Mellors JW, Dutschman GE, Im G-J, et al. In vitro selection and molecular characterization of human immunodeficiency virus-1 resistant to non-nucleoside inhibitors of reverse transcriptase. Mol Pharmacol 1992;41:446–451.
171. Balzarini J, Karlsson A, Vandamme A-M, et al. Human immunodeficiency virus type 1 (HIV-1) strains selected for resistance against the novel class of HIV-1–specific TSAO nucleoside analogues retain sensitivity to HIV-1–specific non-nucleoside inhibitors. Proc Natl Acad Sci U S A 1993;90:6952–6956.
172. Balzarini J, Karlsson A, Perez-Perez M-J, et al. HIV-1–specific reverse transcriptase inhibitors show differential activity against HIV-1 mutant strains containing different amino acid substitutions in the reverse transcriptase. Virology 1993;192:246–253.
173. Balzarini J, Karlsson A, Meichsner C, et al. Resistance pattern of HIV-1 reverse transcriptase to quinoxaline S-2720. J Virol 1994; 68:7986–7992.
174. Williams TM, Ciccarone TM, MacTough SC, et al. 5-Chloro-3-(phenylsulfonyl)indole-2-carboxamide: a novel, non-nucleoside inhibitor of HIV-1 reverse transcriptase. J Med Chem 1993;26:1291–1294.
175. Balzarini J, Pelemans H, Aquaro S, et al. Highly favorable antiviral activity and resistance profile of the novel thiocarboxanilide pentenyloxy ether derivatives UC-781 and UC-82 as inhibitors of human immunodeficiency virus type 1 replication. Mol Pharmacol 1996;50: 394–401.
176. Schinazi RF, Larder BA, Mellors JW, et al. Mutations in retroviral genes associated with drug resistance. Int Antiviral News 1997;5: 129–142.
177. Kleim J-P, Bender R, Kirsch R, et al. Mutational analysis of residue 190 of human immunodeficiency virus type 1 reverse transcriptase. Virology 1994;200:696–701.
178. Kohlstaedt LA, Wang J, Friedman JM, et al. Crystal structure at 3.5 Å resolution of HIV-1 reverse transcriptase complexed with an inhibitor. Science 1992;256:1783–1790.
179. Jacobo-Molina A, Ding J, Nanni RG, et al. Crystal structure of human immunodeficiency virus type 1 reverse transcriptase complexed with double-stranded DNA at 3.0 Å resolution shows bent DNA. Proc Natl Acad Sci U S A 1993;90:6320–6324.
180. Nanni RG, Ding J, Jacobo-Molina A, et al. Review of HIV-1 reverse transcriptase three-dimensional structure: implications for drug design. Perspect Drug Discov Des 1993;1:129–150.
181. Tantillo C, Ding J, Jacobo-Molina A, et al. Locations of anti-AIDS drug binding sites and resistance mutations in the three-dimensional structure of HIV-1 reverse transcriptase: implications for mechanisms of drug inhibition and resistance. J Mol Biol 1994;243:369–387.
182. Dueweke TJ, Pushkarskaya T, Poppe SM, et al. A novel mutation in bisheteroarylpiperazine-resistant HIV-1 reverse transcriptase confers increased sensitivity to other nonnucleoside inhibitors. Proc Natl Acad Sci U S A 1993;90:4713–4717.
183. Balzarini J, Pelemans H, Esnouf R, et al. A novel mutation (F227L) arises in the reverse transcriptase (RT) of human immunodeficiency virus type 1 (HIV-1) upon dose–escalating treatment of HIV-1–infected cell cultures with the non-nucleoside RT inhibitor thiocarboxanilide UC-781. AIDS Res Hum Retroviruses 1997;14: 255–260.
184. Pelemans H, Esnouf R, Dunkler A, et al. Characteristics of the Pro225His mutation in human immunodeficiency virus type 1 reverse transcriptase that appears under selective pressure of dose-escalating quinoxaline treatment of HIV-1. J Virol 1997;71:8195–8203.
185. Jonckheere H, Taymans J-M, Balzarini J, et al. Resistance of HIV-1 reverse transcriptase against [2′,5′-bis-O-(*tert*-butyldimethylsilyl)-3′-spiro-5″-(4″-amino-1″,2″-oxathiole-2″,2″-dioxide)] (TSAO) derivatives is determined by the mutation Glu^{138}6 Lys on the p51 subunit. J Biol Chem 1994;269:25,255–25,258.
186. Boyer PL, Ding J, Arnold E, et al. Subunit specificity of mutations that confer resistance to nonnucleoside inhibitors in human immunodeficiency virus type 1 reverse transcriptase. Antimicrob Agents Chemother 1994;38:1909–1914.
187. Vasudevachari MB, Battista C, Lane HC, et al. Prevention of the spread of HIV-1 infection with nonnucleoside reverse transcriptase inhibitors. Virology 1992;190:269–277.
188. Balzarini J, Karlsson A, Perez-Perez M-J, et al. Knocking-out concentrations of HIV-1–specific inhibitors completely suppress HIV-1 infection and prevent the emergence of drug-resistant virus. Virology 1993;196:576–585.
189. Balzarini J, Pelemans H, Perez-Perez M-J, et al. Marked inhibitory activity of non-nucleoside reverse transcriptase inhibitors against human immunodeficiency virus type 1 when combined with (−)2′,3′-dideoxy-3′-thiacytidine. Mol Pharmacol 1996;49:882–890.
190. Balzarini J, Pelemans H, Karlsson A, et al. Concomitant combination therapy for HIV infection preferable over sequential therapy with 3TC and non-nucleoside reverse transcriptase inhibitors. Proc Natl Acad Sci U S A 1996;93:13,152–13,157.
191. Balzarini J, Pelemans H, De Clercq E, et al. Reverse transcriptase fidelity and HIV-1 variation. Science 1997;275:229–230.
192. Keulen W, Nijhuis M, Schuurman R, et al. Reverse transcriptase fidelity and HIV-1 variation. Science 1997;275:229.
193. Ho DD, Neumann AU, Perelson AS, et al. Rapid turnover of plasma virions and CD4 lymphocytes in HIV-1 infection. Nature 1995;373: 123–126.
194. Wei X, Ghosh SK, Taylor ME, et al. Viral dynamics in human immunodeficiency virus type 1 infection. Nature 1995;373:117–122.
195. Perelson AS, Neumann AU, Markowitz M, et al. HIV-1 dynamics in vivo: virion clearance rate, infected cell life-span, and viral generation time. Science 1996;271:1582–1586.
196. Mellors JW, Rinaldo CR Jr, Gupta P, et al. Prognosis in HIV-1 infection predicted by the quantity of virus in plasma. Science 1996;272:1167–1170.

B. Protease Inhibitors

Emilio A. Emini and Jon H. Condra

The advent of protease inhibitor therapy for the treatment of human immunodeficiency virus type 1 (HIV-1) infection has, in a remarkably short time, fundamentally altered the practice and goals of HIV-1 disease management. Before the availability of the more potent protease inhibitors, investigators assumed that the antiviral effects mediated by anti–HIV-1 therapy would always be transient, limited by rapid selection for resistant viral variants. Given the high turnover rate of HIV-1 in vivo (1, 2), the selection for such resistance occurs in a matter of weeks for those therapies that incompletely suppress ongoing cycles of virus replication. As a result, the clinical benefits obtained from the initial antiviral therapeutic effects are also rapidly diminished subsequent to the development of resistance. However, early clinical trials with the more active protease inhibitors demonstrated that this consequence of antiretroviral therapy is not inevitable, but rather, long-term HIV-1 suppression in patients can indeed be achieved along with associated clinical benefits. The development of viral resistance to protease inhibitors can and does occur. However, the probability of avoiding rapid resistance selection can be enhanced through the appropriate selection, initiation, and maintenance of protease inhibitor–containing therapy.

This chapter reviews our current understanding of the characteristics of the available protease inhibitors, of the genetic basis of HIV-1 resistance and cross-resistance to the inhibitors, and of the principles that should guide optimal use of these highly active antiretroviral agents. The pace of HIV-1 basic and clinical research has been particularly striking over the past several years and continues to be so. As a result, much of what is written here is subject to revision as our state of understanding continues to evolve. The reader is advised to use the information presented here as a fundamental background that should be supplemented with the newest information from updated sources.

MECHANISM OF ACTION

As with other retroviruses, the final steps of HIV-1 replication in cells involve the formation and budding of a nascent viral particle from the plasma membrane of the infected cell. In addition to the viral genetic information, the nascent particle contains multiple copies of various viral proteins that are required for the proper initiation of subsequent viral replication cycles. However, immediately after budding, these proteins exist as immature polyprotein precursors that require cleavage into active forms. The cleavage reactions are mediated by the viral protease enzyme, resulting in the structural and functional maturation of the fully infectious virion. Kohl and associates (3) first demonstrated that genetic inhibition of protease activity exclusively yields immature particles that are incapable of initiating new replication cycles. This observation spurred a decade of subsequent research that eventually culminated in the discovery and licensure for therapeutic use of the currently available protease inhibitors.

The HIV-1 enzyme belongs to the aspartyl protease class of mammalian enzymes (4, 5). Unlike the cellular proteases, the viral enzyme is composed of two identical subunits that associate together to form the protease active site. The successful discovery and development of the viral inhibitors relied on a large body of earlier work with cellular aspartyl proteases such as renin and on a detailed knowledge of the enzyme's three-dimensional crystal structure (6, 7). Most of the interactions between the enzyme and the polyprotein substrates are formed by hydrogen bonds and by hydrophobic associations. These interactions can occur over a length of substrate that can span seven amino acid residues (8). Accordingly, many of the inhibitors that were initially developed proved to be pharmaceutically unacceptable because of their large molecular structures and hydrophobic characteristics, properties that yielded poor bioavailability and rapid metabolism.

As a result, although many hundreds of protease inhibitors have been synthesized and studied in the laboratory, at present only four such inhibitors have been approved for use in humans. The molecular structures of these compounds are presented in Figure 47B.1. Each is described in the following sections, and their summary characteristics are given in Table 47B.1.

SAQUINAVIR

Saquinavir (Invirase, Ro 31-8959, SQV) was the first of the protease inhibitors to be licensed (9, 10). This compound proved to be a potent inhibitor of HIV-1 replication in cell culture, by exhibiting 95% inhibition of viral replication at concentrations of approximately 25 nmol/L. Unfortunately, in spite of its high in vitro potency, the antiviral activity mediated by the compound in infected patients is modest at best, largely because of its relatively low oral bioavailability of only 4%. At the recommended dose of 600 mg, delivered three times per day, saquinavir monotherapy mediated small and transient circulating viral RNA (vRNA) declines. The maximum vRNA drop seen in a representative clinical study was approximately 80% from baseline (11). This was accompanied by similarly modest maximum CD4 cell count recoveries of about 50 cells/mm^3. After 16 weeks of therapy, both vRNA and CD4 cell levels had returned to baseline values. This pattern is similar to that seen with the earlier, relatively weak antiretroviral therapies and is likely the result of resistant virus selection subsequent to incomplete suppression of virus replication (12, 13).

As with all anti–HIV-1 agents, saquinavir's activity is improved when used in a combination therapy regimen (14). The most extensively studied of these agents involved

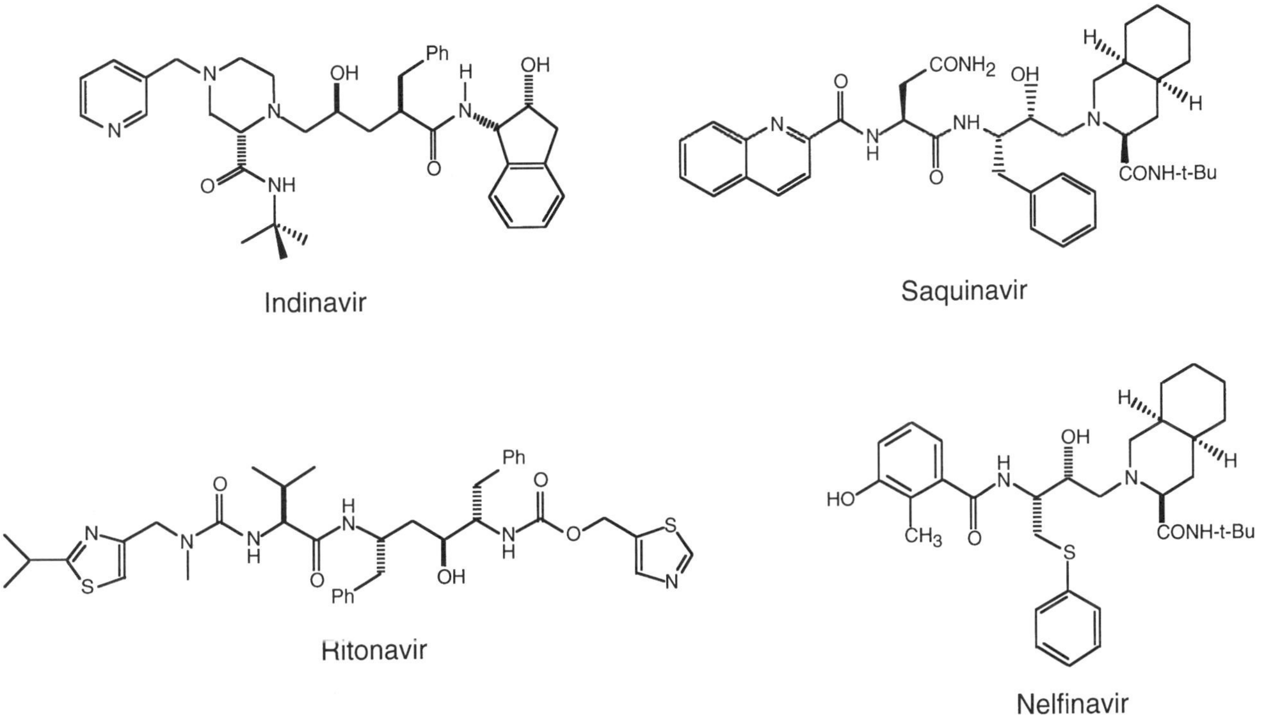

Figure 47B.1. Molecular structures of the licensed HIV-1 protease inhibitors.

saquinavir in combination with the nucleoside analogs zidovudine (ZDV, formerly known as azidothymidine or AZT) and zalcitabine (ddC) (15). The combination therapy mediated greater declines in vRNA levels and larger increases in CD4 levels than did the combination of ZDV and ddC alone. However, the antiviral responses remained transient. In a phase III clinical evaluation, the combination of saquinavir and ddC proved significantly more effective than either saquinavir alone or ddC alone in hindering progression to acquired immunodeficiency syndrome (AIDS)–defining events or death (16). This study did not involve a comparison to standard of care.

In spite of this clinical benefit, saquinavir's weak in vivo antiviral activity limits its usefulness compared with that of the more potent inhibitors. A probe clinical trial that used high doses of saquinavir, up to 7200 mg per day in six divided doses, demonstrated a greater degree and duration of virus suppression and CD4 cell count elevation than those seen at the standard dose (17). This finding demonstrated that the inhibitor's clinical potential could be improved if higher systemic levels of the compound were achieved. To this end, saquinavir has been coadministered with the protease inhibitor ritonavir to take advantage of metabolic interactions that increase saquinavir's plasma concentrations (see later). In addition, a new formulation of the compound, Fortovase, with enhanced oral bioavailability has been developed. Fortovase has been approved in the United States at a dose of 1200 mg, delivered three times daily. Clinical data are not yet available that significantly distinguish the antiviral activities mediated by Fortovase from those of the original formulation of saquinavir (Invirase). Preliminary data from ongoing studies suggest that Fortovase exhibits enhanced antiretroviral activity in patients (18, 19). This formulation of saquinavir has consequently been included in the preferred category (in combination with nucleoside analogues) for initial therapy according to DHHS guidelines for antiretroviral therapy of adults (19a). The availability of Fortovase has made Invirase an antiquated formulation of saquinavir that should be used only in combination with ritonavir.

Saquinavir is delivered as the mesylate salt of the compound. It must be administered with a high-fat meal for adequate oral absorption. In its original and enhanced formulations, saquinavir exhibits toxicities that can include abdominal discomfort, nausea, and diarrhea. No laboratory abnormalities of note have been reported.

RITONAVIR

Ritonavir (Norvir, ABT-538, RTV) was licensed in the United States shortly after saquinavir. This compound is also a potent inhibitor of the HIV-1 protease and exhibits noted anti–HIV-1 activity in cell culture (20). However, unlike saquinavir, ritonavir achieves high plasma concentrations, resulting in profound in vivo antiretroviral activity.

At the recommended dose of 600 mg every 12 hours, ritonavir monotherapy was shown to mediate a mean decline of circulating vRNA levels of almost 2.0 $\log_{10}$ over the initial 32 weeks of therapy. This change was accompanied by a mean increase in CD4 cell count of more than 200 cells/mm^3 (21, 22). Again, ritonavir's antiviral effects were substantially enhanced when used in combination therapy. In one study, the combination of ritonavir, ZDV, and ddC reduced plasma virus loads to less than 500 vRNA copies/mL

Table 47B.1. Characteristics of Protease Inhibitors

Generic Name	Indinavir	Ritonavir	Saquinavir	Nelfinavir
Trade Name	Crixivan	Norvir	Invirase, Fortovase	Viracept
Form	200-, 400-mg caps	100-mg caps; 600-mg/7.5 mL oral solution	200-mg caps	250-mg tablets; 50 mg/g oral powder
Dosing recommendations	800 mg q8h Take 1 hr before or 2 hr after meals; may take with skim milk or low-fat meal	600 mg q12h[a] Take with food if possible	600 mg TID[a] (Invirase) 1200 mg TID (Fortovase) Take with large meal	750 mg TID Take with food (meal or light snack)
Oral bioavailability	65%	Not determined	Hard gel capsule: 4% (Invirase), erratic	20–80%
Serum half-life	1.5–2 h	3–5 h	1–2 h	3.5–5 h
Route of metabolism	P450 cytochrome 3A4	P450 cytochrome 3A4, >2D6	P450 cytochrome 3A4	P450 cytochrome 3A4
Storage	Room temperature	Refrigerate; single dose may be at room temperature for 12 h	Room temperature	Room temperature
Adverse effects	Nephrolithiasis; gastrointestinal intolerance, nausea; laboratory: increase indirect bilirubinemia (inconsequential); headache, asthenia, blurred vision, dizziness, rash, metallic taste, thrombocytopenia	Gastrointestinal intolerance, nausea, vomiting, diarrhea; paresthesia: circumoral and extremities; asthenia; hepatitis; taste perversion; laboratory: triglycerides increase >200%, transaminase elevation, elevated CPK and uric acid	Gastrointestinal intolerance, nausea, and diarrhea; headache; elevated transaminase enzymes	Diarrhea
Drug interactions	Inhibits cytochrome P450 (less than ritonavir); not recommended for concurrent use: rifampin, terfenadine, astemizole, cisapride, triazolam, midazolam, or ergot alkaloids; indinavir levels increased by ketoconazole[c] and delavirdine; indinavir levels reduced by rifampin, rifabutin, nevirapine, and grapefruit juice; didanosine: reduces indinavir absorption unless taken >2 h apart	Inhibits cytochrome P450 (potent inhibitor); ritonavir increases levels of multiple drugs that are not recommended for concurrent use[b] Didanosine: reduced absorption of both drugs: take ≥2 h apart; ritonavir decreases levels of ethinyl estradiol, theophylline, sulfamethoxazole, and zidovudine; ritonavir increases levels of clarithromycin and desipramine	Inhibits cytochrome P450; saquinavir levels increased by ritonavir, ketoconazole, grapefruit juice, nelfinavir, delavirdine; saquinavir levels reduced by rifampin, rifabutin and (?) phenobarbital, phenytoin, dexamethasone and carbamezepine, and nevirapine; not recommended for concurrent use: terfenadine, astemizole, cisapride or ergot alkaloids	Inhibits cytochrome P450 (less than ritonavir); nelfinavir levels reduced by rifampin and rifabutin; not recommended for concurrent use: rifampin, triazolam, midazolam, ergot alkaloids, terfenadine, astemizole, or cisapride; nelfinavir decreases levels of ethinyl estradiol and norethindrone; nelfinavir increases levels of rifabutin, saquinavir, and indinavir

[a]Dose escalation for Ritonavir: Day 1–2: 300 mg bid; Day 3–5: 400 mg bid; Day 6–13: 500 mg bid; Day 14: 600 mg bid
Combination treatment regimen with Saquinavir (400–600 mg po bid) plus Ritonavir (400–600 mg po bid)
[b]Drugs contraindicated for concurrent use with Ritonavir: amioderone (Cordonrone), astemizole (Hismanal), hepridil (Vascar), bupropion (Wellbutin), cisapride (Propulsid), clorazepate (Tranxene), clozapine (Clozaril), diazepam (Valium), ecainide (Enkaid), estazolam (ProSom), flecainide (Tambocor) flurazepam (Dalmane), mepiridine (Demerol), midazolam (Versed), piroxicam (Feldene), propoxyphene (Darvon), propafenone (Rythmol), quinidine, terfenadine (Seldane), triazolam (Halcion), zolpidem (Ambien), ergot alkaloids.
[c]Decrease indinavir to 600 mg q8h.
(From United States Public Health Service.)

in approximately 50% of patients after 52 weeks (23). Ritonavir-containing therapy was also found to reduce the amount of vRNA present in patient lymphoid tissue (24).

Therapy with ritonavir has also demonstrated clinical benefit. In this evaluation, the inhibitor was added to existing background therapy in patients with advanced HIV-1 disease. Compared with placebo, the addition of ritonavir resulted in significantly delayed disease progression and fewer deaths. This clinical benefit continued to be noted through 9 months of observation (25).

The ability to sustain the antiviral response, and apparently to prevent the selection of resistant viral variants, is a function of the therapy's potency and its ability to impose a high genetic barrier to resistance selection (26). An analysis of the genetic basis of HIV-1 resistance to ritonavir showed that high-level resistance is accompanied by the accumulation of multiple coexpressed amino acid substitutions within the protease enzyme (27). Thus, viral variants exhibiting high-level resistance to ritonavir are unlikely to preexist in untreated patients. If complete suppression of new viral replication cycles can be achieved by potent antiretroviral therapy, the required mutations would not be permitted to accumulate, thereby resulting in long-term virus suppression. The identical situation has been described with the protease inhibitor indinavir (see later).

The high plasma concentrations achieved by ritonavir are critical to its antiviral activity. However, these concentrations reflect the ability of the compound to inhibit its own metabolism by the liver cytochrome P450 metabolic pathways. The P450 isozymes predominantly responsible for the inhibitor's metabolism, CYP3A, CYP2D6, and CYP2C9, are also essential for the metabolism of numerous other pharmaceutical agents. As a result, ritonavir interacts strongly with many other drugs, and these interactions must be taken into account when the inhibitor is used. In addition, of all the available protease inhibitors, ritonavir is the least tolerated by patients, with major toxicities that include abdominal pain, nausea, vomiting, diarrhea, and circumoral paresthesia. Due to GI intolerance, ritonavir is generally used in combination with other protease inhibitors to exploit drug interactions via the p450 metabolic pathway; this permits lower doses of ritonavir. Laboratory abnormalities include elevated plasma levels of liver transaminases, triglycerides, and creatinine kinase.

INDINAVIR

Indinavir (Crixivan, L-735,524, MK-639, IDV), licensed at approximately the same time as ritonavir, is the most extensively studied of the HIV-1 protease inhibitors. Many of the current treatment concepts for HIV-1 disease were devised based on data derived from indinavir clinical trials. As with the other inhibitors, indinavir exhibits potent antiviral activity in cell culture (with 95% inhibitory concentrations for virus replication of about 100 nmol/L) and is highly selective for the viral enzyme (28). Moreover, indinavir is unique among the clinically available inhibitors in that it is weakly bound to plasma proteins, thereby enhancing its availability to the infected cell in vivo.

In early clinical trials of indinavir monotherapy, investigators found that the degree and duration of viral suppression were clearly dose related (29). Patients who initiated therapy at the higher doses were not only more likely to exhibit a more profound initial antiviral response, but were also more likely to sustain that response. Patients who started therapy at suboptimal doses and subsequently increased the dose did not achieve the same degree of sustained viral suppression. These observations led to the conclusion that initiating therapy at the appropriate dose is essential, and, more important, a correlation exists between the degree of virus suppression and the ability to maintain the suppression.

Given this finding, the probability of achieving long-term virus suppression, without resistant virus selection in the presence of indinavir, is a function of the starting therapeutic regimen's antiviral potency and the requirement for multiple resistance mutations (the genetic barrier) for indinavir resistance (26, 30, 31). Indinavir monotherapy at the recommended dose of 800 mg every 8 hours mediates a sustained decline of circulating vRNA levels to below 500 copies/mL in about one-third of patients (32). However, remarkable as this appears, indinavir monotherapy is not recommended because its long-term efficacy is greatly enhanced when it is combined with other potent antiretroviral drugs.

In one study of ZDV-experienced patients, the combination of indinavir, ZDV, and lamivudine (3TC) resulted in a drop of circulating vRNA levels to below 500 copies/mL in over 80% of treated subjects for as long as 48 weeks (32). Approximately 75% experienced sustained declines to less than 50 copies/mL. The increase in CD4 cell count at 48 weeks was about 200 cells/mm^3. The drop in circulating vRNA levels was accompanied by an equivalent decline in lymph node cell-associated vRNA (33). Continued observation of these patients has found the antiviral response and CD4 cell count recovery to be sustained for at least 100 weeks (34). In this trials, more than 80% of the patients had carried viruses with mutations associated with ZDV resistance on entry into the study.

Indinavir was also studied in a combination therapy regimen with the nonnucleoside reverse transcriptase inhibitor efavirenz (Sustiva, DMP-266). At 48 weeks, 89% of the treated patients had sustained declines in circulating vRNA levels to less than 500 copies/mL, with an associated mean CD4 cell count increase of 240 cells/mm^3 (35). The apparent potency of such a two-drug combination holds much promise for the development of simplified, yet highly potent, combination therapy regimens.

In a phase III clinical trial in patients with advanced HIV-1 disease (CD4 cell count of 200 cells/mm^3 or lower), indinavir given with ZDV or stavudine (d4T) and 3TC resulted in a 50% decline in disease progression or death compared with the use of the nucleoside analogs alone (36).

Because of the large numbers of patients from various indinavir clinical studies who achieved a substantial decline in circulating vRNA levels, long-term follow-up analyses to ascertain the durability of the viral suppression are possible. In the first of these analyses, investigators determined that, of patients who initiated indinavir-containing therapy and who experienced a drop of plasma vRNA levels to less than 500 copies/mL for at least 12 weeks, about 80% sustained the response without selection for resistant virus for at least 68 weeks (37). In addition, circulating vRNA, obtained from 11 patients treated with the combination of indinavir, ZDV, and 3TC who exhibited a sustained drop in vRNA levels, was analyzed for the appearance of new resistance-associated mutations at various times after the initiation of therapy. Ten of these patients yielded vRNA that was genetically identical (within the protease and reverse transcriptase genes) to the vRNA present at the start of therapy, a finding suggesting the complete suppression of new virus replication cycles (38). Equivalent genetic results have been obtained from patients in the same clinical study using lymphocyte-associated viral DNA obtained up to 96 weeks after therapy initiation (39).

Indinavir is administered as a sulfate salt. The currently approved dose is 800 mg every 8 hours, although more recent investigations have shown that the inhibitor's in vivo antiviral activity may be similar when delivered at 1200 mg every 12 hours (40). Indinavir must be taken 1 hour before or 2 hours after meals or with a low-fat, low-protein meal. The clinically significant major toxicities associated with the inhibitor are abdominal pain and nephrolithiasis. The latter toxicity has been noted in about 5% of patients in clinical trials and has rarely resulted in permanent discontinuation of therapy. However, to lessen the probability of nephrolithiasis, indinavir-treated patients should drink at least 1.5 L of fluid per day. The most commonly observed laboratory abnormality is a moderate elevation of indirect bilirubin levels that is not associated with liver damage.

NELFINAVIR

Nelfinavir (Viracept, AG1343, NFV) is the latest of the HIV-1 protease inhibitors to be licensed and, accordingly, has been the least studied to date. As with the other inhibitors, nelfinavir has potent anti–HIV-1 activity in cell culture and is a selective, competitive inhibitor of the viral protease (41, 42).

Nelfinavir's in vivo antiviral activity appears to be similar to, or slightly less than, that of ritonavir or indinavir. However, this characteristic is difficult to judge in a controlled way because of a relative lack of monotherapy data. Nelfinavir has been primarily studied in combination therapy regimens. In the most significant reported trial, nelfinavir in combination with ZDV and 3TC mediated the decline of circulating vRNA levels to less than 500 copies/mL in about 80% of therapy-naive, treated patients at 24 weeks (43). The mean increase in CD4 cell count was approximately 150 cells/mm^3. The antiviral response was sustained to at least 52 weeks (44). The clinical efficacy of nelfinavir has not been formally established, but the inhibitor is likely to have a beneficial influence on disease progression, given its anti–HIV-1 activity in patients.

Nelfinavir has been reported to select a resistance mutation that is not generally seen with other protease inhibitors (41). However, the clinical relevance of this observation is debated and is discussed in greater detail later. This inhibitor is delivered as a mesylate salt at a recommended dose of 750 mg, three times per day, given with food. As with indinavir, recently reported observations suggest that nelfinavir's antiviral activity may be equivalent when delivered at 1250 mg twice per day (45). The major clinical toxicities are diarrhea and loose stools. No significant laboratory abnormalities have been reported.

RARE ADVERSE EXPERIENCES

Two rare adverse experiences have been associated with the use of the HIV-1 protease inhibitors. The first involves spontaneous bleeding in a small number of HIV-1–positive patients with hemophilia who were treated with protease inhibitors. The second involves the development or aggravation of diabetes, also in a small number of patients treated with the inhibitors. Prolonged highly active antiretroviral therapy, generally including protease inhibitors, has also been associated with evidence of fat redistribution in some patients. This change has involved a thinning of the extremities and buttocks and abdominal deposition of fat. The functional and mechanistic connections between these clinical experiences and the protease inhibitors have not been established; nonetheless, careful observation of patients initiating therapy is advised.

DRUG INTERACTIONS

The potential for metabolic drug interactions must be understood and taken into account when designing combination therapy regimens, particularly for patients who may also be undergoing additional prophylactic or treatment therapies. All four of the available protease inhibitors are metabolized by the liver cytochrome P450 system. The CYP3A isozyme is predominantly involved. As a result, extensive pharmacokinetic interaction studies have been, and continue to be, performed formally to assess the nature of possibly significant interactions. Much of this information is not yet published; however, the following are currently recommended:

- Astemizole, terfenadine, midazolam, triazolam, cisapride, and ergot derivatives should not be coadministered with the protease inhibitors. These drugs all have narrow therapeutic windows, and their plasma concentrations may be inappropriately elevated because of competition for CYP3A by the protease inhibitor.
- Rifampin should not be coadministered with HIV-1 protease inhibitors. This drug is a potent inducer of CYP3A, and coadministration results in plasma protease inhibitor levels that are too low for all four protease inhibitors.
- Protease inhibitors increase plasma concentrations of rifabutin, and rifabutin decreases plasma concentrations of protease inhibitors. Prescribing information for each inhibitor should be consulted.
- Similar caution should be used with all drugs known to be inducers of CYP3A. These include phenobarbital, phenytoin, carbamazepine, and dexamethasone.
- Certain interactions are specific to the individual protease inhibitors. As noted previously, ritonavir inhibits CYP3A, CYP2D6, and CYP2C9, and therefore it can alter the metabolism of numerous drugs. Prescribing information for each inhibitor should be carefully consulted.
- No drug interactions have been reported between the protease inhibitors and the nucleoside analog reverse transcriptase inhibitors. However, interactions with the nonnucleoside reverse transcriptase inhibitors occur and may require dose adjustment depending on the specific combination.
- As expected, each protease inhibitor influences the metabolism of each of the other compounds in the class. The latest information from clinical interaction studies must be consulted before selecting the appropriate doses for combination protease inhibitor therapy.

COMBINATION PROTEASE INHIBITORS

The clinical potential of combination therapy with protease inhibitors is undergoing extensive evaluation. These are potent antiviral agents whose efficacy may be enhanced through combined use. In some cases, drug interactions between pairs of inhibitors may be exploited to increase the overall plasma concentrations of one or both compounds.

The most intensively studied combination to date involves the coadministration of saquinavir with ritonavir. This combination was designed to exploit CYP3A inhibition by ritonavir, thereby leading to high saquinavir plasma concentrations. Various dosing regimens have been studied. Limited data suggest that substantial and sustained antiviral responses can be achieved using 400 mg of saquinavir delivered twice daily with either 400 mg or 600 mg of ritonavir also given twice daily (46). However, the use of this combination is limited in some patients by the poor tolerability of ritonavir at these doses.

Other protease inhibitor combinations actively studied include saquinavir and nelfinavir, indinavir and ritonavir, and indinavir and nelfinavir. Such combinations may prove particularly important in the treatment of patients who already harbor HIV-1 variants that are resistant to the reverse transcriptase inhibitors.

PROTEASE INHIBITOR RESISTANCE

This important topic warrants in-depth discussion. The potential for HIV-1 cross-resistance among the protease inhibitors continues to be debated. This idea is significant because of the need to attempt "salvage" therapy for those patients in whom the initial protease inhibitor–containing therapeutic regimen fails because of resistant virus selection. The design of such salvage therapy is often based on perceptions of the likelihood of cross-resistance.

Genetic Basis of Resistance to HIV-1 Protease Inhibitors

The emergence of resistance to the HIV-1 protease inhibitors is primarily associated with amino acid substitution mutations in the viral protease gene. Unfortunately, assessing the genetic basis of viral resistance to the protease inhibitor class has been difficult because of a substantial imbalance in the amount and quality of available resistance information for the licensed inhibitors. This issue has proved especially problematic when considering the potential for cross-resistance. Nonetheless, as information continues to evolve, common genetic patterns of resistance among the protease inhibitors are becoming apparent, and the clinical significance of these common patterns is also beginning to be appreciated.

In the following discussion of resistance to each protease inhibitor, protease amino acid substitutions are shown using the common convention (e.g., L90M). The number refers to the amino acid residue position in the protease. The first letter designates (by single-letter code) the amino acid present at that position in the North American/European (clade B) consensus viral sequence. The second letter designates the amino acid found in the variant virus.

RESISTANCE TO INDINAVIR

Among the four currently licensed HIV-1 protease inhibitors, the basis of viral resistance to indinavir has been the most extensively studied. Much of our current understanding of the genetic basis of indinavir resistance has come from early phase I and II clinical trials of monotherapy that had used, in retrospect, suboptimal therapeutic doses of the drug.

Clinical resistance to indinavir is accompanied by a rebound in circulating HIV-1 vRNA levels toward pretherapy baseline values, generally during the first 12 to 24 weeks of therapy. Coincident with this rebound, multiple and highly variable combinations of amino acid substitutions were noted in the viral protease (30, 31). These substitutions appeared in no consistent order, suggesting that no particular preexisting single mutation conferred an overriding replicative advantage over the others in the presence of indinavir. The number and combination of the observed substitutions were so variable that no "canonical" pattern of resistance substitutions could be defined among the many patterns observed. In fact, no single amino acid substitution appears to be either necessary or sufficient for resistance to indinavir. However, despite this complexity, some amino acid substitutions have been observed more frequently than others, notably V82 (to A, F, or T), M46 (to I or L), L10 (to I, V, or R), and L63 (usually to P, but often to many others). To date, at least 11 protease residues (L10, K20, L24, M46, I54, L63, I64, A71, V82, I84, and L90) have been implicated in phenotypically measurable resistance to indinavir (31). Substitutions at other positions have also been observed in some patients during therapy, but the potential associations with phenotypic resistance have not yet been verified.

Despite the many amino acid residues that can contribute to indinavir resistance, neither individual substitutions nor any pair of substitutions ever observed exerts a measurable (fourfold or more) loss of viral susceptibility. Certain combinations of three or more substitutions can give rise to measurable resistance, however. For example, the combination M46I/L63P/V82T yields a virus that is fourfold less susceptible to indinavir. By site-directed mutagenesis, the loss of any one of these three substitutions abolishes this resistance (30). Thus, all three substitutions must be present simultaneously for the virus to manifest indinavir resistance.

This result has several implications. First, resistance to indinavir is the cumulative effect of multiple amino acid substitutions whose individual contributions to resistance appear negligible. This finding implies that the effects exerted by these substitutions are critically dependent on the specific ways in which they are combined. Thus, many combinations of the 11 substitutions known to correlate with indinavir resistance appear to have no effect on the level of viral resistance. Other specific combinations, however, have a demonstrable effect. Because of this complexity, it is not yet possible to predict the degree of viral indinavir resistance by knowing the sequence of the protease.

Second, when substitutions are appropriately combined, an association can be demonstrated between the number of substitutions and the level of resistance observed (31). Thus, multiple substitutions that arise during viral replication have a cumulative effect on resistance.

Third, correlates of resistance to indinavir map both within and away from the enzyme's active site. In the previous example, only the V82T substitution affects indinavir binding to the protease. The remaining two, M46I and L63P, do not impinge on the active site and do not affect the inhibitor's binding. Rather, they appear to exert their effects by increasing the catalytic efficiency of the enzyme in a drug-independent manner (47).

Other substitutions selected during indinavir therapy have been shown to occur outside the protease gene altogether. The appearance of protease amino acid substitutions in some indinavir-treated patients has been accompanied by amino acid substitutions in two of the substrate cleavage sites of the protease, within the *gag* gene (48). Thus, viral resistance to indinavir as well as to other investigational protease inhibitors (49) can be accomplished by genetic changes both in the protease and in its substrates.

Finally, many known correlates of resistance to multiple protease inhibitors exist as natural polymorphisms in some untreated patients (31, 50). These include substitutions of L10 (in fewer than 10% of untreated patients), K20 (less than 1%), L63 (approximately 60%), I64 (approximately 10%), and A71 (less than 5%). No evidence, however, indicates that any of these polymorphisms, existing alone, has any effect on resistance to any protease inhibitor. The most common of these is an L63P substitution, which has been observed in over 60% of drug-naive patients. Yet, if not already present, this substitution is usually selected if resistance develops during therapy (30, 31). Moreover, when combined appropriately with additional substitutions (such as M46I, V82T, and I84V), L63P makes a clear contribution to resistance to indinavir, saquinavir, and other agents (30). Thus, genetic polymorphisms can, and do, contribute to resistance to protease inhibitors, but their effects are mediated through complex interactions with other substitutions in the enzyme.

The genetic basis of HIV-1 resistance to indinavir is obviously complex. However, the very complexity and subtlety of these interacting substitutions permit a clear prediction: that viruses carrying the many specific combinations of amino acid substitutions necessary for indinavir resistance are unlikely to preexist in protease inhibitor-naive patients. Therefore, the only way to acquire and select these substitutions is through viral replication in the presence of indinavir (or, as discussed later, other protease inhibitors as well). Thus, a formidable "genetic barrier" exists to the development of indinavir resistance, and when the inhibitor is combined with other effective antiviral agents such as ZDV–ddI or ZDV–3TC, the evolution of resistance to indinavir and to the reverse transcriptase inhibitors can be dramatically reduced or prevented (32, 33, 38, 51).

RESISTANCE TO RITONAVIR

Although the genetic correlates of ritonavir resistance have been less extensively characterized, clinical resistance to ritonavir is associated with the appearance of multiple amino acid substitutions in the protease that, in aggregate, are nearly identical to those seen with indinavir. Thus, resistance to ritonavir is associated with multiple substitutions at residues L10, K20, M46, I54, L63, A71, V82, I84, L90, and others (27).

Unlike indinavir resistance, however, the evolution of resistance to ritonavir appears to be more predictable. In patients whose viruses develop resistance, the first substitution observed in the prevailing viral population is at residue V82, to A, F, T or S (27). After the appearance of this substitution, however, the order of appearance of subsequent substitutions varies widely among patients. That the first substitution observed tends to be at residue 82 suggests that, among the many single mutants that are likely to exist before therapy, V82 substitutions confer the greatest replicative advantage in the presence of ritonavir and are thus the first selected by the drug. This concept is supported by the observation that a single V82S substitution confers a sixfold loss of susceptibility to ritonavir in cell culture (27).

Despite this initial path of least resistance to ritonavir resistance, however, high-level ritonavir resistance appears to require the accumulation of multiple amino acid substitutions in the protease. The initial V82 substitution is insufficient to negate the antiviral effects of ritonavir in vivo, and other substitutions are selected subsequently. This finding is evidence that ritonavir also imposes a high genetic barrier to resistance, reflecting both its high potency and the low impact of individual mutations on resistance.

RESISTANCE TO SAQUINAVIR

Two protease amino acid substitutions have been most frequently associated with resistance to saquinavir, either in vitro or in a clinical setting: G48V and L90M (12, 52). Alone, each substitution confers a 3- to 10-fold loss of susceptibility to the inhibitor, and together, 50- to 100-fold (52). The G48V substitution appears unique to saquinavir, since it is not generally selected by other protease inhibitors in clinical use. However, among patients receiving the recommended dosage of the original (hard gel) formulation of saquinavir, this substitution has been seen less frequently than has L90M.

Based on apparent differences between the resistance pattern of saquinavir and the other protease inhibitors, it was suggested that it might be possible to "sequence" protease inhibitors and derive full clinical benefit from another protease inhibitor following saquinavir failure. As will be discussed below, recent clinical studies have shown this optimistic assumption to be incorrect.

An examination of the available virologic data from saquinavir clinical studies shows the basis of viral resistance to this inhibitor to be more complex than originally thought. Among 21 primary viral isolates in which genotypic and phenotypic resistance to saquinavir were compared, the level of phenotypic resistance observed could not be fully explained by the presence or absence of G48V or L90M alone. Additional substitutions in the protease were found to be correlated with clinical saquinavir resistance, notably L10(I,V), M46I, L63(P and others), A71(V,T), and I84V (12). All these are also associated with resistance to indinavir (30, 31), ritonavir (27), and nelfinavir (41).

Among patients receiving prolonged therapy with saquinavir, "genotypic resistance" (based on detection of G48V or L90M) has been reported to be infrequent, even in monotherapy (ranging from 12 to 63% after approximately 1 year) (12). However, in these studies, viruses carrying resistance substitutions were often seen in mixed populations with wild-type viruses. Because genetic analysis is limited in its ability to detect minor components of mixtures, it is likely that many resistant viruses could not have been detected with the methods used. This cocirculation of wild-type and mutant viruses, however, implies that limited selective pressure is exerted by (current formulation) saquinavir in vivo; otherwise, wild-type virus replication should have been suppressed by the inhibitor. As evidenced by their selection in vitro and in vivo, both G48V and L90M mutants are more fit than wild-type viruses in the presence of suppressive concentrations of saquinavir. Moreover, L90M mutants have been shown to be as fit as wild-type viruses in the absence of drug (52, 53). The limited bioavailability and rapid metabolism of the original formulation of saquinavir result in low (and often undetectable) plasma levels of drug in many patients, as well as a correspondingly weak antiviral effect. However, under conditions of equivalent selective pressure, saquinavir has been found to select for combinations of protease substitutions nearly identical to those observed for indinavir and ritonavir (54, 55). Thus, the apparent lack of resistance selection in many saquinavir-treated patients can likely be explained by low in vivo drug exposure.

As noted, increased exposure to saquinavir in patients has resulted in slightly different patterns of observed resistance to the drug. At higher doses of the current formulation of saquinavir (up to 7.2 g per day) or with the newer, more bioavailable formulation of saquinavir, an increased incidence of G48V substitutions, often associated with V82A substitutions, has been observed (56, 57). Although these results are preliminary, it appears likely that, if in vivo drug exposure of saquinavir can be increased, its clinical resistance pattern may more closely resemble that of the other protease inhibitors.

RESISTANCE TO NELFINAVIR

Because nelfinavir is the most recently approved HIV-1 protease inhibitor, the basis of resistance to this agent has been the least thoroughly studied. Thus, only limited information about nelfinavir resistance is currently available from virologic and clinical studies.

Low-level resistance to nelfinavir (five- to sevenfold) can result from any of several single amino acid substitutions, D30N, I84V, or L90M (41). Among these, D30N appears to confer the greatest replicative advantage in the presence of the drug, and it is thus the most frequently observed single substitution in nelfinavir-resistant viral populations. However, as with the other protease inhibitors, resistance to nelfinavir can evolve along multiple parallel genetic pathways, involving multiple amino acid substitutions in the viral protease.

D30N mutants have not generally been associated with resistance to other protease inhibitors, nor does this single mutation confer measurable (less than fourfold) resistance to indinavir, ritonavir, or saquinavir in vitro (58). Accordingly (as had been proposed for saquinavir), investigators have suggested that initial clinical resistance to nelfinavir could still allow the future use of other protease inhibitors. However, neither virologic findings nor early clinical observations have provided conclusive support for this prediction.

Nelfinavir has been shown to select variants in vitro that exhibited cross-resistance to other protease inhibitors (59). These viruses were found to exist as mixed populations, carrying amino acid substitutions M46I, L63P, A71V, and I84V (41, 59), all of which are associated with resistance to indinavir, ritonavir, and saquinavir (12, 27, 30, 31). Surprisingly, the D30N substitution was not observed among these cross-resistant viruses. Thus, nelfinavir can select for cross-resistance to other protease inhibitors, and it can arise independently of the D30N substitution.

Viruses isolated from five nelfinavir-treated patients, all carrying D30N, were found to be phenotypically susceptible (less than fourfold resistant) to other protease inhibitors in vitro (58). Nonetheless, viral protease sequences obtained from nelfinavir-treated patients have revealed numerous additional substitutions implicated in resistance to the other protease inhibitors. These include L10I, K20(I,R), L24F, D30N, M36I, M46(I,V), L63P, A71(V,T), N88(D,S), I84V, and L90(M,S) (58, 60). As had been observed in vitro (41), nelfinavir-resistant viruses often occur in patients as mixed populations composed of genetically distinct viral variants. Thus, despite the lack of association of the D30N substitution with resistance to other protease inhibitors, the selection by nelfinavir of these additional substitutions would be expected to hasten the development of resistance to subsequently used protease inhibitors.

CROSS-RESISTANCE AMONG HIV-1 PROTEASE INHIBITORS

Each of the available HIV-1 protease inhibitors has been shown to select viral variants that are cross-resistant to other structurally unrelated protease inhibitors. This finding has raised the serious concern that if resistance to any protease inhibitor is allowed to develop in a given patient, the future benefit of this entire class of drugs may be permanently lost for that patient.

Cross-resistance among multiple HIV protease inhibitors was first described in studies of patients receiving indinavir monotherapy (30, 31). Viral isolates from multiple individuals exhibited divergent patterns of amino acid substitutions in the viral protease, and although cross-resistance was infrequent in early isolates that showed only low-level indinavir resistance, the acquisition of additional amino acid substitutions and higher levels of indinavir resistance led to increased cross-resistance to other inhibitors.

This important observation has possible clinical consequences. The apparently restricted cross-resistance and

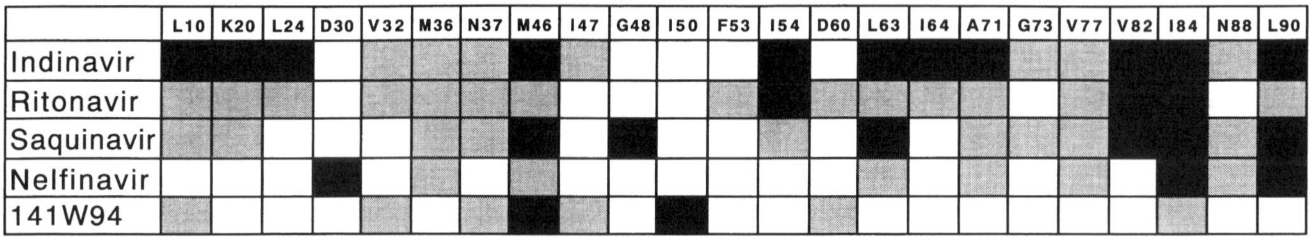

	L10	K20	L24	D30	V32	M36	N37	M46	I47	G48	I50	F53	I54	D60	L63	I64	A71	G73	V77	V82	I84	N88	L90
Indinavir																							
Ritonavir																							
Saquinavir																							
Nelfinavir																							
141W94																							

	L10	K20	L24	D30	V32	M36	N37	M46	I47	G48	I50	F53	I54	D60	L63	I64	A71	G73	V77	V82	I84	N88	L90
Indinavir	30, 31	30, 31	30, 31		30, 31	30, 31	30, 31	30, 31	30, 31				30, 31		30, 31	30, 31	30, 31	31	31	30, 31	30, 31	31	30, 31
Ritonavir	27, 62	27	27, 54		62	27	27, 62	27, 54, 62				27	27, 54, 62	27	27, 54, 62	27	27, 62		27	27, 54, 62	27, 54, 62		27, 62
Saquinavir	12, 54	72				12	72	12, 30		12, 54, 69, 71			17, 54		12, 30, 54, 71		12, 54, 71		54	54	12, 30, 54	12, 30, 54, 71	72	12, 30, 54, 71
Nelfinavir				41, 58, 59	41		58, 59	41, 58, 59							41, 59		41, 58, 59		59	41	41, 59	58, 59	41, 58, 59
141W94	69, 70				69		69	30, 69, 70	70		70			70	30					70			

Figure 47B.2. Amino acid residues in the HIV-1 protease implicated in resistance to the five HIV-1 protease inhibitors currently in clinical use or advanced clinical study (141W94). *Shaded squares* represent amino acids at which substitutions are implicated in resistance, based on in vitro or clinical studies. *Light shaded squares* represent sites at which substitutions have been reported selected by a given drug, but for which no evidence, from controlled virologic studies, indicates that they confer measurable effects on viral phenotypic resistance. In many cases, the relevant experiments have not yet been done. *Dark shaded boxes* represent sites for which direct evidence indicates that substitutions affect viral phenotypic resistance. Often, these effects depend on genetic context. *Unshaded boxes* represent residues that are currently not implicated in resistance with available data. Information was current as of November, 1997. However, this is a work in progress, and as new information is gathered from additional virologic studies, particularly with respect to the less thoroughly studied inhibitors, more correlates of resistance will likely be found. References are indicated in the *lower table*. Referenced boxes *without shading* represent sites at which phenotypic effects have been observed in controlled site-directed mutagenesis experiments, but which, to date, have not been observed to be selected by drug.

lower-level resistance generally manifested by viral isolates early during protease inhibitor resistance selection suggest that switching or intensification of therapy should occur as soon as possible after the loss of virus suppression. The increase in relative resistance and cross-resistance that occurs on continued exposure to the initial failing therapy decreases the likelihood that the second therapeutic regimen will be successful. However, the genetic complexity of viral resistance to the protease inhibitors is such that the generality of this observation is currently unclear.

Cross-resistance manifested during the original indinavir trials was not the result of any unique pattern of amino acid substitutions. Rather, it resulted from the appearance of many alternate combinations of substitutions that are shared among different protease inhibitors. Thus, not only was resistance to indinavir complex, but also it became equally clear that resistance to the other inhibitors could also occur through many unanticipated, and complex, genetic pathways.

Subsequently, other protease inhibitors were also shown to select for viral variants that are cross-resistant to the remaining inhibitors. These included several investigational compounds, such as 141W94 (VX-478) (61), as well as the approved protease inhibitors ritonavir (62), saquinavir (61, 63, 64), and nelfinavir (59). Thus, to the extent that this area has been investigated, the ability to select for cross-resistance appears to be a universal property of HIV-1 protease inhibitors.

From a comparison of sequence specificity, one can understand why cross-resistance is selected by diverse protease inhibitors. Figure 47B.2 shows the amino acid substitutions implicated in resistance to the five HIV-1 protease inhibitors currently in clinical use or in advanced clinical trials. Although some differences exist among the collections of amino acid substitutions selected by the various inhibitors, the observed similarities outweigh the differences. Many of the differences that are apparent between the drugs in Figure 47B.2 are artificial, in that they reflect the incomplete state of knowledge about the newer drugs. Fewer known correlates of resistance would be expected of drugs about which the least is known (e.g., nelfinavir and 141W94) than for the more thoroughly characterized drugs (indinavir and ritonavir).

A growing body of clinical evidence has begun to confirm the virologic observations of in-class cross-resistance among the protease inhibitors. Although only limited studies have been performed to date, several clinical trials have demonstrated that the development of resistance to one protease inhibitor substantially reduces the potential therapeutic benefit of another. Because both saquinavir and nelfinavir were originally proposed to have limited ability to engender cross-resistance to other protease inhibitors, most current studies have addressed the consequences of initial therapy with these compounds. In both cases, the available data suggest that, as expected for indinavir and ritonavir, prior therapy with either saquinavir (65) or nelfinavir (60, 66) also generally compromises the later efficacy of other protease inhibitors, including the use of combinations of protease inhibitors as salvage therapy. In these studies, some individual patients appeared to be successfully treated with the second therapeutic regimen; however, as a whole, protease inhibitor–experienced patients were less likely to manifest sustained viral suppression while receiving these salvage regimens.

The genetic analysis of viral variants expressing multiple protease inhibitor resistance, as a result of sequential protease inhibitor therapy, has demonstrated that the genetic pathway for resistance selection is strongly influenced by the first agent used. For instance, patients initially treated with saquinavir in whom subsequent treatment with indinavir or nelfinavir fails typically yield mutant viruses that predominantly express the L90M substitution along with additional mutations (67, 68). Although both indinavir and nelfinavir can select for L90M, the most commonly observed substitutions in patients in whom initial therapy with these agents fails are usually V82A and D30N, respectively (see earlier). In many of the studied patients, the L90M substitution was not apparent after the period of saquinavir treatment, but it only became apparent after the second protease treatment period (65, 67, 68). These observations have important clinical implications. They emphasize the inadequacy of genetic analysis for assessing the probability of resistance selection on change in therapy. This probability is primarily a function of the genetic changes that occur, under selective pressure, in the "background" viral genetic pool. Most of the available genetic analysis techniques are only capable of providing data on the major circulating virus population and are incapable of analyzing the genetic alterations in the highly diverse genetic pool of minor cocirculating viral variants. However, "new" variants are selected from this pool on a change of therapy. In the clinical examples provided earlier, saquinavir pretreatment apparently enhances the likelihood of resistant virus selection to indinavir by enriching minor variants within this pool, although the major circulating viral population that is detected exhibits no genetic evidence of indinavir resistance.

This discussion shows that the complexities of HIV-1 genetics in vivo and the complexities of protease inhibitor resistance make it impossible accurately to assess the likelihood of cross-resistant virus selection in any single treated patient. Nonetheless, in general, the selection of resistant virus to one inhibitor seems certain to lessen the probability of maintaining an appropriate genetic barrier against resistant virus selection to a second inhibitor. However, the quantification of this lessened probability will be patient specific and will depend on genetic selections that occur in both the major virus population and in the minor viral variant pool. The results of ongoing and planned clinical trials are likely to provide added data and insight.

In conclusion, the discovery and licensure of the more clinically potent HIV-1 protease inhibitors has, over the past 2 years, permitted the development of new concepts to guide the treatment of patients with HIV-1 disease. Investigators now appreciate that long-term virus suppression can be achieved. Moreover, the probability of achieving this goal is a function of the design and institution of the therapy. Successful therapeutic regimens should use combinations of agents that together achieve potent suppression of viral replication and also impose a high genetic barrier to resistance selection. In other words, viral resistance to the therapy should require a combination of coexpressed mutations that are not likely to be present in a patient's pretherapy virus population. In this circumstance, resistance can only be expressed through the accumulation of multiple mutations subsequent to continued virus replication. Therefore, successful therapy should also exhibit a high degree of antiviral potency, to prevent any new viral replication cycles. The 100-week follow-up data have demonstrated that, with at least certain therapeutic combinations, one can indeed forestall resistant virus selection in a high proportion of treated patients.

All the drugs in a combination regimen should be started simultaneously, and the therapy must be maintained. Whether it may eventually be possible to lessen the therapeutic rigor in those patients whose circulating virus levels are rendered below assay limits for extended periods is unclear. Unfortunately, if resistant virus selection is allowed to occur, future therapeutic options will be limited. Although each protease inhibitor may differ from the others with respect to the mutations observed most frequently during therapy, ample evidence indicates common genetic pathways to resistance for all the studied protease inhibitors. Therefore, selection of resistant viral variants to any known protease inhibitor will increase the likelihood of developing resistance to the remaining inhibitors. Given this situation, careful thought must be given to the appropriate clinical use of these compounds so their potential for long-term HIV-1 control in a patient is not irretrievably lost.

References

1. Ho DD, Neumann AU, Perelson AS, et al. Rapid turnover of plasma virions and CD4 lymphocytes in HIV-1 infection. Nature 1995;373: 123–126.
2. Wei XP, Ghosh SK, Taylor ME, et al. Viral dynamics in human immunodeficiency virus type-1 infection. Nature 1995;373:117–122.
3. Kohl NE, Emini EA, Schleif WA, et al. Active human immunodeficiency virus protease is required for viral infectivity. Proc Natl Acad Sci U S A 1988;85:4686–4690.
4. Toh H, Ono M, Saigo K, et al. Retroviral protease-like sequence in the yeast transposon Ty 1. Nature 1985;315:691–692.
5. Pearl LH, Taylor WR. A structural model for the retroviral proteases. Nature 1987;329:351–354.
6. Navia MA, Fitzgerald PMG, McKeever BM, et al. Three-dimensional structure of aspartyl protease from human immunodeficiency virus HIV-1. Nature 1989;337:615–620.
7. Wlodawer A, Miller M, Jaskolski M, et al. Conserved folding in retroviral proteases: crystal-structure of a synthetic HIV-1 protease. Science 1989;245:616–621.
8. Darke PL, Nutt RF, Brady SF, et al. HIV-1 protease specificity of peptide cleavage is sufficient for processing of gag and pol polyproteins. Biochem Biophys Res Commun 1988;156:297–303.
9. Roberts NA, Martin JA, Kinchington D, et al. Rational design of peptide-based HIV proteinase inhibitors. Science 1990;248:358–361.

10. Galpin S, Roberts NA, O'Connor T, et al. Antiviral properties of the HIV-1 proteinase-inhibitor Ro 31-8959. Antiviral Chem Chemother 1994;5:43–45.
11. Kitchen VS, Skinner C, Ariyoshi K, et al. Safety and activity of saquinavir in HIV infection. Lancet 1995;345:952–955.
12. Jacobsen H, Hanggi M, Ott M, et al. In vivo resistance to a human immunodeficiency virus type 1 proteinase inhibitor: mutations, kinetics, and frequencies. J Infect Dis 1996;173:1379–1387.
13. Ives KJ, Jacobsen H, Galpin SA, et al. Emergence of resistant variants of HIV in vivo during monotherapy with the proteinase inhibitor saquinavir. J Antimicrob Chemother 1997;39:771–779.
14. Vella S, Lazzarin A, Carosi G, et al. A randomized controlled trial of a protease inhibitor (saquinavir) in combination with zidovudine in previously untreated patients with advanced HIV infection. Antiviral Ther 1996;1:129–140.
15. Collier AC, Coombs RW, Schoenfeld DA, et al. Treatment of human immunodeficiency virus infection with saquinavir, zidovudine, and zalcitabine. N Engl J Med 1996;334:1011–1017.
16. Lalezari J, Haubrich R, Burger HU, et al. Improved survival and decreased progression of HIV in patients treated with saquinavir (Invirase, SQV) plus HIVID (zalcitabine, ddC) [abstract LB.B.6033]. In: 11th International Conference on AIDS, Vancouver, 1996.
17. Schapiro JM, Winters MA, Stewart F, et al. The effect of high-dose saquinavir on viral load and CD4(+) T-cell counts in HIV-infected patients. Ann Intern Med 1996;124:1039–1050.
18. Slater L. Activity of a new formulation of saquinavir in combination with two nucleosides in treatment-naive patients [abstract 368]. In: 5th Conference on Retroviruses and Opportunistic Infections, Chicago, 1998.
19. Sension M, Farthing C, Pattison TP, et al. Fortovase (saquinavir soft gel capsule; SQV-SGC) in combination with AZT and 3TC in antiretroviral-naive HIV-1 infected patients [abstract 369]. In: 5th Conference on Retroviruses and Opportunistic Infections, Chicago, 1998.
19a. Report of the Panel on Use of Antiretroviral Agents in HIV-infected Adults and Adolescents MMWR 1998 43(RR–5):43–83.
20. Kempf DJ, Marsh KC, Denissen JF, et al. ABT-538 is a potent inhibitor of human immunodeficiency virus protease and has high oral bioavailability in humans. Proc Natl Acad Sci U S A 1995;92:2484–2488.
21. Danner SA, Carr A, Leonard JM, et al. A short-term study of the safety, pharmacokinetics, and efficacy of ritonavir, an inhibitor of HIV-1 protease. N Engl J Med 1995;333:1528–1533.
22. Markowitz M, Saag M, Powderly WG, et al. A preliminary study of ritonavir, an inhibitor of HIV-1 protease, to treat HIV-1 infection. N Engl J Med 1995;333:1534–1539.
23. Mathez D, Bagnarelli P, Gorin I, et al. Reductions in viral load and increases in T lymphocyte numbers in treatment-naive patients with advanced HIV-1 infection treated with ritonavir, zidovudine and zalcitabine triple therapy. Antiviral Ther 1997;2:175–183.
24. Cavert W, Notermans DW, Staskus K, et al. Kinetics of response in lymphoid tissues to antiretroviral therapy of HIV-1 infection. Science 1997;276:960–964.
25. Cameron DW, Heath-Chiozzi M, Kravick S, et al. Prolongation of life and prevention of AIDS complications in advanced HIV immunodeficiency with ritonavir: update. [abstract Mo.B.411]. In: 11th International Conference on AIDS, Vancouver, 1996:24.
26. Condra JH, Emini EA. Preventing HIV-1 drug resistance. Sci Med 1997;4:14–23.
27. Molla A, Korneyeva M, Gao Q, et al. Ordered accumulation of mutations in HIV protease confers resistance to ritonavir. Nature Med 1996;2:760–766.
28. Vacca JP, Dorsey BD, Schleif WA, et al. L-735,524: an orally bioavailable human immunodeficiency virus type-1 protease inhibitor. Proc Natl Acad Sci U S A 1994;91:4096–4100.
29. Mellors J, Steigbigel R, Gulick R, et al. Antiretroviral activity of the oral protease inhibitor, MK-639, in p24 antigenemic, HIV-1 infected patients with <500 CD4/mm^3 [abstract I-172]. In: 35th Interscience Conference on Antimicrobial Agents and Chemotherapy, San Francisco, 1995.
30. Condra JH, Schleif WA, Blahy OM, et al. In vivo emergence of HIV-1 variants resistant to multiple protease inhibitors. Nature 1995;374:569–571.
31. Condra JH, Holder DJ, Schleif WA, et al. Genetic correlates of in vivo viral resistance to indinavir, a human immunodeficiency virus type-1 protease inhibitor. J Virol 1996;70:8270–8276.
32. Gulick RM, Mellors JW, Havlir D, et al. Treatment with indinavir, zidovudine, and lamivudine in adults with human immunodeficiency virus infection and prior antiretroviral therapy. N Engl J Med 1997;337:734–739.
33. Wong JK, Gunthard HF, Havlir DV, et al. Reduction of HIV-1 in blood and lymph nodes following potent antiretroviral therapy and the virologic correlates of treatment failure. Proc Natl Acad Sci U S A 1997;95:12,574–12,579.
34. Gulick R, Mellors J, Havlir D, et al. Indinavir (IDV), zidovudine (ZDV) and lamivudine (3TC): concurrent or sequential therapy in ZDV-experienced patients [abstract I-89]. In: 37th Interscience Conference on Antimicrobial Agents and Chemotherapy, Toronto, 1997.
35. Riddler S, Stein D, Mayers D, et al. Durable clinical anti-HIV-1 activity (48 weeks) and tolerability (24 weeks) for DMP-266 in combination with indinavir (IDV) [abstract]. In: Infectious Disease Society of America 35th annual meeting, San Francisco, 1997.
36. Hammer SM, Squires KE, Hughes MD, et al. A controlled trial of 2 nucleoside analogs plus indinavir in persons with human immunodeficiency virus infection and CD4 cell counts of 200 per cubic millimeter or less. N Engl J Med 1997;337:725–733.
37. Holder DJ, Shivaprakash M, Danovich RM, et al. Duration of HIV-1 load suppression in patients treated with indinavir who experience virus load declines to <500 vRNA copies/mL [abstract 129]. In: International Workshop on HIV Drug Resistance, Treatment Strategies and Eradication, St. Petersburg, FL, 1997:86.
38. Emini EA, Holder DJ, Schleif WA, et al. Evidence for the prevention of new HIV-1 infection cycles in patients treated with indinavir plus zidovudine and lamivudine [abstract 128]. In: International Workshop on HIV Drug Resistance, Treatment Strategies and Eradication, St. Petersburg, FL, 1997:85.
39. Wong JK, Hazarch M, Gunthard HF, et al. Recovery of replication competent HIV from patients despite suppression of plasma viremia for two years. Science 1997;278:1291–1295.
40. Nguyen B-Y, Haas DW, Ramirez-Ronda C, et al. A pilot, multicenter, open-label, randomized study to compare the safety and activity of indinavir sulfate (IDV) administered every 8 hours (h) versus every 12 h in combination with zidovudine (ZDV) and lamivudine (3TC) [abstract I091]. In: 37th Interscience Conference on Antimicrobial Agents and Chemotherapy, Toronto, 1997.
41. Patick AK, Markowitz M, Appelt K, et al. Antiviral and resistance studies of AG1343, an orally bioavailable inhibitor of human immunodeficiency virus protease. Antimicrob Agents Chemother 1996;40:292–297.
42. Kaldor SW, Kalish VJ, Davies JF II, et al. Viracept (nelfinavir mesylate, AG1343): a potent orally bioavailable inhibitor of HIV-1 protease. J Med Chem 1997;40:3979–3985.
43. Henry K, Lamarca A, Myers R, et al. The safety of Viracept (nelfinavir mesylate) in pivotal phase II/III double-blind randomized controlled trials as monotherapy and in combination with d4T or AZT/3TC [abstract 240]. In: 4th Conference on Retroviruses and Opportunistic Infections, Washington, DC, 1997.
44. Saag M, Gersten M, Chang Y, et al. Long-term virological and immunological effect of the HIV protease inhibitor Viracept (nelfinavir mesylate, NFV) in combination with zidovudine (AZT) and lamivudine (3TC) [abstract]. In: Infectious Disease Society of America 35th annual meeting, San Francisco, 1997.
45. Johnson M, Petersen A, Winslade J, et al. Comparison of BID and TID dosing of Viracept (nelfinavor, NFV) in combination with stavudine (d4T) and lamivudine (3TC). In: 5th Conference on Retroviruses and Opportunistic Infections, Chicago, 1998.
46. Cohen C, Sun E, Cameron W, et al. Ritonavir (RTV) in combination with saquinavir (SQV) represents a rational therapeutic regimen for HIV infection based on pharmacokinetic synergy and non-overlapping

resistance [abstract LB7b]. In: 36th Interscience Conference on Antimicrobial Agents and Chemotherapy, New Orleans, 1996.
47. Schock HB, Garsky VM, Kuo LC. Mutational anatomy of an HIV-1 protease variant conferring cross-resistance to protease inhibitors in clinical trials: compensatory modulations of binding and activity. J Biol Chem 1996;271:31,957–31,963.
48. Zhang YM, Imamichi H, Imamichi T, et al. Drug resistance during indinavir therapy is caused by mutations in the protease gene and in its gag substrate cleavage sites. J Virol 1997;71:6662–6670.
49. Doyon L, Croteau G, Thibeault D, et al. Second locus involved in human immunodeficiency virus type 1 resistance to protease inhibitors. J Virol 1996;70:3763–3769.
50. Kozal MJ, Shah N, Shen NP, et al. Extensive polymorphisms observed in HIV-1 clade-B protease gene using high-density oligonucleotide arrays. Nature Med 1996;2:753–759.
51. Condra JH, Holder DJ, Schleif WA, et al. Bi-directional inhibition of HIV-1 drug resistance selection by combination therapy with indinavir and reverse transcriptase inhibitors [abstract Th.B.932]. In: 11th International Conference on AIDS, Vancouver, 1996;(Suppl):19.
52. Jacobsen H, Yasargil K, Winslow DL, et al. Characterization of human immunodeficiency virus type-1 mutants with decreased sensitivity to proteinase-inhibitor Ro 31-8959. Virology 1995;206:527–534.
53. Maschera B, Tisdale M, Darby G, et al. In vitro growth characteristics of HIV-1 variants with reduced sensitivity to saquinavir explain the appearance of L90M escape mutants in vivo [abstract]. Antiviral Ther 1996;1(Suppl 1):53.
54. Smith T, Swanstrom R. Selection for high-level resistance to HIV-1 protease inhibitors used in pairs [abstract]. Antiviral Ther 1996; 1(Suppl 1):12–13.
55. Smith T, Swanstrom R. Biological cross-resistance to HIV-1 protease inhibitors [abstract 15]. In: International Workshop on HIV Drug Resistance, Treatment Strategies and Eradication, St. Petersburg, FL, 1997:10.
56. Schapiro J, Winters M, Lawrence J, et al. Clinical and genotypic cross-resistance between the protease inhibitors saquinavir and indinavir [abstract 87]. In: International Workshop on HIV Drug Resistance, Treatment Strategies, and Eradication, St. Petersburg, FL, 1997:57.
57. Craig C, Race E, Sheldon J, et al. Key amino acid substitutions in HIV proteinase remain unaltered during increased exposure to saquinavir, (SQV-SGC): results from preliminary clinical trials [abstract 243]. In: 6th European Conference on Clinical Aspects and Treatment of HIV-Infection, Hamburg, Germany, 1997:30.
58. Patick AK, Duran M, Cao Y, et al. Genotypic analysis of HIV-1 variants isolated from patients treated with the protease inhibitor nelfinavir, alone or in combination with d4T [abstract 10]. In: 4th Conference on Retroviruses and Opportunistic Infections, Washington, DC, 1997.
59. Patick AK, Duran M, Cao Y, et al. Genotypic and phenotypic characterization of HIV-1 variants isolated from in vitro selection studies and from patients treated with the protease inhibitor, nelfinavir [abstract]. Antiviral Ther 1996;1(Suppl 1):17–18.
60. Henry K, Kane E, Melroe H, et al. Experience with a ritonavir/saquinavir based regimen for the treatment of HIV-infection in subjects developing increased viral loads while receiving nelfinavir [abstract I-204]. In: 37th Interscience Conference on Antimicrobial Agents and Chemotherapy, Toronto, 1997.
61. Tisdale M, Myers RE, Maschera B, et al. Cross-resistance analysis of human immunodeficiency virus type 1 variants individually selected for resistance to five different protease inhibitors. Antimicrob Agents Chemother 1995;39:1704–1710.
62. Schmit JC, Ruiz L, Clotet B, et al. Resistance-related mutations in the HIV-1 protease gene of patients treated for 1 year with the protease inhibitor ritonavir (ABT-538). AIDS 1996;10:995–999.
63. Boucher C. Rational approaches to resistance: using saquinavir. AIDS 1996;10:19.
64. Craig JC, Duncan IB, Gilbert S, et al. Treatment with saquinavir (InviraseJ) should leave the majority of patients the option to use other HIV proteinase inhibitors [abstract]. Antiviral Ther 1996; 1(Suppl 1):19.
65. Rachlis AR, Palmer RH, Bast M, et al. Predictors of decreases in plasma HIV-1 RNA in patients treated with indinavir [abstract A-17]. In: 37th Interscience Conference on Antimicrobial Agents and Chemotherapy, Toronto, 1997.
66. Sampson MS, Barr MR, Torres RA, et al. Viral load changes in nelfinavir treated patients switched to a second protease inhibitor after loss of viral suppression [abstract LB-5]. In: 37th Interscience Conference on Antimicrobial Agents and Chemotherapy, Toronto, 1997.
67. Dulioust A, Paulous S, Guillemot L, et al. Selection of saquinavir-resistant mutants by indinavir following a switch from saquinavir [abstract 16]. International Workshop on HIV Drug Resistance, Treatment Strategies and Eradication, St. Petersburg, FL, 1997:11.
68. Lawrence J, Schapiro J, Pesano R, et al. Clinical response and genotypic resistance patterns of sequential therapy with nelfinavir followed by indinavir plus nevirapine in saquinavir/reverse transcriptase inhibitor-experienced patients [abstract 64]. In: International Workshop on HIV Drug Resistance, Treatment Strategies and Eradication, St. Petersburg, FL, 1997:42.
69. Condra JH, et al. Unpublished data.
70. Partaledis JA, Yamaguchi K, Tisdale M, et al. In vitro selection and characterization of human immunodeficiency virus type 1 (HIV-1) isolates with reduced sensitivity to hydroxyethylamino sulfonamide inhibitors of HIV-1 aspartyl protease. J Virol 1995;69:5228–5235.
71. Vaillancourt M, Irlbeck D, Swanstrom R. Sequence analysis of viral RNA from patients on AZT–saquinavir double therapy (ACTG 229) [abstract]. In: 4th International Workshop on HIV Drug Resistance, Sardinia, Italy, 1995:74.
72. Race E, Sheldon JG, Kaye S, et al. Mutations associated with reduced sensitivity to saquinavir occur in a minority of patients treated in combination with ddC: Results from a phase III clinical trial (NV14256) [abstract 600]. In: 4th Conference on Retroviruses and Opportunistic Infections, Washington, DC, 1997.

48

STRATEGIES FOR ANTIRETROVIRAL THERAPY IN ADULT HIV DISEASE

A. STARTING AND SHIFTING OF ANTIRETROVIRAL THERAPY

Paul A. Volberding

The complexities of devising and applying treatment for human immunodeficiency virus (HIV) infection present a challenge. Progress in HIV therapy has been rapid as the basic biology and pathogenesis have become better understood. Clinical trials have yielded results showing new promise on several therapeutic fronts. As treatment options are expanding, newer laboratory tests permit better monitoring of the disease.

This chapter presents a brief review of the natural history and pathogenesis of HIV disease as they relate to treatment of the disease in adults. Individual agents that have become important in treating HIV disease are discussed, with particular focus on the results of selected clinical trials. Recommendations are presented for therapeutic strategies based largely on recently published treatment guidelines (1, 2) and drawing on clinical experience. Immune-based therapies and experimental treatments that have not yet entered human trials are beyond the scope of this chapter and are reviewed in Chapter 44.

LIFE CYCLE

In the short time since HIV was identified as the cause of the acquired immunodeficiency syndrome (AIDS), basic investigations have revealed many details of the life cycle of this virus within infected cells. In fact, more is known about the replicative cycle of HIV than about that of any other human pathogen, and this knowledge will likely be instrumental in determining the sites for applying antiretroviral therapy. The more each unique point in the life cycle of the virus is identified, the more likely that therapy could be specifically directed at that target, with minimal toxicity to the normal cellular functions of the host. Single-agent therapy for the complex intracellular viral infection, with integration between the viral and the host DNA, is of limited value, and more effective antiviral control requires multiple-agent therapy. Such therapy, because of increased potency, decreases the development of drug resistance.

Attachment

The life cycle of HIV begins with the attachment of the virus to a susceptible cell. Investigators generally believe that the external envelope glycoprotein gp120 (or gp160 when combined with the transmembrane glycoprotein gp41) links with one or more cell-surface receptors. The predominant receptor identified for HIV is the CD4 surface antigen (3). Recently, HIV has been shown to use other cell-surface proteins for attachment along with CD4. The first of these to be described are the receptors for chemokines: CCR5, primarily on the macrophage, and CXCR4, primarily on the T-lymphocyte (4–6). One obvious approach for HIV therapy would be to block either of the cell-surface receptors. This was attempted with soluble CD4, but this approach yielded no evidence of in vivo activity. Strategies to block binding to the chemokine receptors are only now being devised (7).

Fusion of Viral and Cell Membranes

HIV is coated by a cell-derived membrane. For the virus to infect the cell, HIV must fuse its membrane with that of the host. This active process may involve those portions of the envelope that also enable some HIV isolates to fuse cells in culture. Fusion of the virus with the cell membrane may be mediated through interactions among the virus, CD4, and the chemokine receptor. As with attachment, this process may be susceptible to blocking compounds.

Reverse Transcription

The transcription of the RNA genome to a DNA copy is a key early step in the life cycle of HIV (8). Retroviruses, a family of RNA viruses, were given their name because of this step. This phenomenon is the reverse of the normal process whereby RNA is transcribed from DNA. Reverse transcription is catalyzed by RNA-dependent DNA polymerase, or reverse transcriptase. Because this process is unique to retroviruses, it should be possible to block it, with relatively little toxicity to normal host cells. However, this approach does not affect cells that are chronically infected. Once integration between the viral genes and the host DNA has occurred, reverse transcription is no longer necessary, and blockage does not prevent virus-induced cell death.

Numerous approaches to identifying drugs that can block reverse transcription have been explored. The first of these involves using nucleoside analogs, which act, at least in part, as DNA chain terminators. The second approach has arisen from empirical screening of large numbers of compounds against reverse transcriptase systems in vitro, an approach that has resulted in development of several nonnucleoside reverse transcriptase inhibitors (9).

Reverse transcriptase inhibitors can be toxic if they are not selective and block DNA polymerases essential for normal cellular function. Further, because the reverse transcriptase genome is prone to mutation, development of drug resistance is a limitation of these agents in the clinical setting.

Integration

A key step in the early to middle life cycle of HIV is the integration of the host DNA with the DNA copy of the HIV RNA genome. After reverse transcription, the DNA copy, now in a double-strand, circularized form, enters the nucleus and is inserted into the host DNA, facilitated by the enzyme integrase. This enzyme is incompletely characterized but offers another attractive site for the development of inhibitory compounds. HIV can, at this point, become latent, not expressing viral gene products within the infected cell, or it may immediately begin a productive infection. Once integration occurs, eradication of HIV from the host is unlikely.

HIV Genome Activation

At some point, either immediately or after a delay, the HIV proviral genome is activated and transcribes RNA. HIV contains both regulatory and structural genes; the regulatory genes are activated first, followed by those that code structural proteins of the progeny virions (8). Division of the infected cell probably facilitates activation of the HIV genome, but numerous pathways of HIV activation may exist.

HIV Gene Product Translation

After the HIV genome is activated, the cell produces regulatory and structural gene products of HIV. HIV regulatory genes that may increase (e.g., *tat, rev*) or decrease the net level of viral replication may influence the rate of this process (8). Current research is active in this area; as the regulatory control of HIV replication is better understood, inhibitors or stimulators of these genes could be potent therapeutically. Such agents would also be expected to be active in all infected cells and not just in those that are becoming infected.

HIV Protein Processing

In the cytoplasm and after the virus buds from the cell, HIV-related proteins require processing to form infectious virions. Retroviral proteins require cleavage by HIV-specific proteases in a manner analogous to that with insulin or renin (10–12). HIV protease is an aspartyl enzyme that has a high specificity for HIV proteins, making the development of HIV protease inhibitors especially attractive because they can be targeted at viral, as opposed to cellular, enzymes.

Viral Assembly and Budding

During processing, HIV progeny viruses are assembled in the cytoplasm. The mechanisms and controls of this active process have been poorly characterized. HIV progeny particles bud from the surface of the cell, taking a portion of the host cell membrane as the new viral envelope. HIV antigens, particularly gp160, and also some portions of internal proteins are expressed through the membrane.

PATHOGENESIS OF HIV INFECTION

In HIV disease, initial infection is followed quickly by a burst in HIV replication that is reflected in high-titer viremia (13–15). Often, this feature is followed by a drop in viral titer coincident with the appearance of markers of humoral and cellular immune response (16). Active viral replication continues, however, in lymphatic tissue, including that in the spleen, lymph nodes, and tonsils (17). Although true virologic latency is uncommon, prolonged clinical latency is typical. Therapy could be valuable either in the initial burst of HIV replication or in the early asymptomatic phase; these possibilities are the focus of several clinical trials. After a variable period, which may be shorter in infants (18) and in the elderly (19), symptoms develop and clinical disease appears. Eventually, opportunistic diseases that result from progressive immune deficiency develop. The median time to development of advanced disease in adults is 10 to 11 years (20, 21). One laboratory correlate of the disease process is the gradual depletion of CD4-bearing (CD4+) cells in the peripheral blood; thus, the CD4+ cell count is widely used as a means of staging HIV disease (22, 23). However, the immune pathogenesis of HIV disease is more complex, and many other cell populations and aspects of the immune response are affected.

Determining HIV burden is a crucial element in understanding the pathogenesis of HIV disease and in monitoring response to therapy. A higher viral load is associated with more rapid disease progression and with an impaired treatment response. Measurement of viral load is central to improving therapeutic outcome to antiretroviral treatment.

The techniques for quantitating HIV include the bDNA assay (Chiron) (24) and the reverse transcriptase–polymerase chain reaction (RT-PCR) method (Roche Laboratories) (25). Both methods are rapid and accurate, although the actual number of HIV RNA copies reported with the RT-PCR method is approximately twice that with bDNA. The HIV RNA copy number is transiently elevated by vaccinations and after intercurrent infections, and this assay should be avoided at such times. The assay requires prompt specimen handling and the use of appropriate anticoagulants.

Guidelines for clinical application of HIV quantitation have been published regarding these issues (1, 2) and the test's use in antiretroviral therapy (26). Briefly, quantitation should be performed before therapy is initiated as part of disease staging, and in approximately 4 weeks of beginning or altering treatment to determine the activity of the drug combination. Then, the assay should be repeated every 3 to 4 months to monitor continuing response or drug failure.

DRUGS USED IN THE TREATMENT OF HIV DISEASE

The current status of HIV drug therapy difficult to review because it is changing so rapidly. This review focuses on those drugs, by their site of action in the HIV life cycle, now in use (Table 48A.1). Certain drugs that have been found ineffective are discussed as well because of lessons that can be learned from them.

Attachment

An early approach to treat HIV infection was to attempt to block viral binding to the CD4 receptor by neutralizing the virus with small, soluble CD4 components. Even at extremely high doses, however, soluble CD4 had no effect (27, 28). The apparent clinical failure of this drug reflects important differences between HIV directly isolated from patients and that established in the laboratory after repeated passages in T-cell lines. The latter isolates appear to have been conditioned to use CD4 as the viral receptor, although the interaction of primary clinical isolates with CD4 is not as strictly required. This experience should be recalled as efforts increase to develop agents that attempt to block the "second receptor" of HIV, the chemokine receptor.

Reverse Transcriptase Inhibitors

Reverse transcriptase inhibitors were the first successful antiretroviral agents and remain an important component of most combination therapies. Some of these are nucleoside analogs; others have unique chemical structures. Development of drugs in this class continues with at least one nucleoside agent, abacavir, or 1592, which is near approval, and adefovir, a nucleotide. Several new nonnucleoside reverse transcriptase inhibitors are in clinical trials.

NUCLEOSIDE ANALOGS

Nucleoside analogs are, as the name indicates, biochemical variations of endogenous nucleosides. They require phosphorylation by intracellular enzymes to the active triphosphate forms. The active forms of these agents compete with the proviral DNA substrates for binding sites on reverse transcriptase and act as DNA synthesis terminators. The nucleoside analogs approved for the treatment of HIV disease are specific to reverse transcriptase inhibition, with little inhibition of other DNA polymerases. Some of their toxic effects, however, may be due to the inhibition of γ DNA polymerase, particularly in mitochondria. The approved drugs in this class are orally bioavailable. Their serum half-lives tend to be short, although the intracellular half-lives of the active compounds are longer.

With continuous therapy, HIV commonly develops resistance to nucleoside analogs through one or more mutations in the reverse transcriptase genome (29, 30). The rate and degree of the resistance elicited by the drugs in this class vary. Cross-resistance can occur, and resistance mutations to one drug may conversely increase the viral sensitivity to another drug in this class.

Strategies for using the nucleoside analogs continue to evolve. Monotherapy is no longer recommended (1). Com-

Table 48A.1. Antiretroviral Drugs

Drug	Trade Name	Manufacturer	Dosing	Comments/Toxicities
Nucleoside Reverse Transcriptase Inhibitors				
Zidovudine (ZDV)	Retrovir	Glaxo Wellcome	300 mg BID	First drug approved for HIV; can cause anemia, neutropenia, nausea, lethargy/confusion/agitation, and myositis
Didanosine (ddI)	Videx	Bristol-Myers Squibb	200 mg BID	Requires neutral gastric pH; toxicities include peripheral neuropathy and pancreatitis
Zalcitabine (ddC)	Hivid	Roche	0.75 mg TID	Peripheral neuropathy most common toxicity; also pancreatitis
Lamivudine (3TC)	Epivir	Glaxo Wellcome	150 mg BID	Minimal toxicity; rapid resistance; no serious toxicities
Stavudine (d4T)	Zerit	Bristol-Myers Squibb	40 mg BID	Can cause peripheral neuropathy
Nonnucleoside Reverse Transcriptase Inhibitors				
Nevirapine	Viramune	Boehringher/Roxane	200 mg BID	Rapid resistance; good tissue penetration; rash is common
Delavirdine	Rescriptor	Pharmacia/Upjohn	400 mg TID	Less experience; raises level of some protease inhibitors; rash less common than with nevirapine
Protease Inhibitors				
Saquinavir	Inverase	Roche	800 mg TID	Well tolerated but poor bioavailability; mild gastrointestinal disturbances common
Ritonavir	Norvir	Abbott	600 mg BID	Gastrointestinal side effects common
Indinavir	Crixivan	Merck	800 mg TID	Potent; TID dosing; neprolithiasis common; can be reduced with overhydration
Nelfinavir	Viracept	Agouron	750 mg TID	Causes diarrhea; may have less cross-resistance

bination therapy with two drugs from this class can prolong survival, but increasingly these agents are used in conjunction with a third drug to obtain even greater antiviral effect.

Five nucleoside analogs are available, as described in the following sections.

Zidovudine

Zidovudine (3′azido-3′deoxythymidine or ZDV), formerly known as azidothymidine (AZT), was the first agent approved for the treatment of HIV disease (31). It is a structural analog of thymidine. It undergoes intracellular phosphorylation to its active triphosphate form. ZDV is well absorbed after oral administration; the average availability is about 63%. Its serum half-life is approximately 1.1 hours, and the intracellular half-life of its active triphosphate is estimated to be 3 to 4 hours, which permits twice-daily dosing. More frequent dosing, initially recommended because of the short serum half-life, is no longer considered necessary. ZDV is well distributed; in the cerebrospinal fluid, levels reach about 75 ng/mL, or approximately 60% of the serum level after 3 to 4 hours after dosing. ZDV is currently given in doses of 300 mg twice daily, almost always in combination with at least one additional drug.

Zidovudine Resistance Mutations at one or more sites on the reverse transcriptase gene decrease the sensitivity of the enzyme to inhibition by ZDV (32). Mutations at these sites develop only after prolonged treatment unless the patient becomes infected with HIV that is already ZDV resistant. Certain sites tend to mutate before others. Some may be transient; others rarely revert to the wild type in the continued presence of ZDV. The degree of resistance associated with some mutations is greater than with others. High-level resistance requires the accumulation of two or more mutant codons (32). When the selective pressure of ZDV is removed from the resistant virus—that is, when ZDV therapy is discontinued—the dominant HIV population gradually reverts to the wild type (33, 34). The rate of this reversion is poorly defined. How this information can be used in clinical treatment is uncertain.

The correlation between resistance and drug failure is becoming clear: disease progression accelerates with high-level resistance. HIV that is resistant to ZDV remains sensitive to the other nucleoside analogs, although the antiviral effect may be diminished if prior therapy included ZDV.

Clinical Experience Large controlled clinical trials have shown that ZDV has clinical efficacy across a broad range of HIV disease stages. Early trials with ZDV monotherapy in advanced disease showed that it slowed progression to AIDS and decreased mortality (31). Subsequent trials of ZDV monotherapy demonstrated clinical benefit in early, asymptomatic HIV disease (35), although not in one large trial when the CD4 count was greater than 500/mL (36). The consensus now is that ZDV should be considered a component of combination therapy for any patient in whom antiretroviral therapy is indicated.

Toxic Effects Several side effects, both objective and subjective, of ZDV therapy have been reported (37–39). The nature and severity of these side effects vary among patients and tend to be more pronounced in those with more advanced HIV disease. Managing these adverse effects thus requires individualization, with a primary goal of maintaining the patient on a reasonable ZDV dose for as long as the drug is considered effective and as long as the side effects do not outweigh the perceived benefits of this therapy. Anemia is the most frequent objective toxic effect of ZDV that requires dose adjustment or drug discontinuation (40, 41). This side effect is much more common in the advanced stage of HIV disease. Severe anemia developed in 24% of patients with AIDS or advanced AIDS-related complex in the initial licensing trial (31). In a later trial, severe anemia developed in only 1.1% of asymptomatic subjects given ZDV at 500 mg per day, even after 55 weeks of therapy (35). Anemia tends to occur within the first 6 months, but it can appear at any time during the treatment. Therefore, routine monitoring of the hemoglobin level is mandatory in all patients. Anemia may diminish with a reduced dose (300 mg per day), but lower doses may be less effective. If dose reduction is unsuccessful, the addition of recombinant erythropoietin may be considered (42–44). This addition should yield reduced transfusion requirements, but some degree of anemia usually persists. Many clinicians change to an alternative drug such as stavudine (d4T) if anemia severely limits continued use of ZDV. ZDV can cause severe neutropenia, but neutropenia is also a common feature of advanced HIV disease itself (45). As with anemia, dose reduction should be attempted. If this is not successful, coadministration of granulocyte colony-stimulating factor can also raise the neutrophil count (43, 46). A more common and cost-effective strategy, however, is to replace ZDV with another agent. Nausea is the most common subjective side effect of ZDV and is less related to the dose or the disease stage than are the hematotoxic effects. ZDV-induced nausea is usually not well controlled with antiemetics. Patients treated with ZDV report various central nervous system symptoms, including agitation, confusion, lethargy, and headaches. Although some of these symptoms are seen in the absence of ZDV, a relationship with the drug may be established in some cases. Little is known about the pathogenesis of these adverse effects, but reduced dosing can be attempted. With all subjective toxic effects, an important part of management involves appropriate patient education. Patients, particularly those who are asymptomatic when ZDV therapy is initiated, can find even mild to moderate subjective drug side effects intolerable, especially if they have not been apprised of them in advance.

Didanosine

Didanosine (ddI) is an analog of inosine (see Chapter 47A) (47). Like ZDV, ddI undergoes intracellular phosphorylation to the active triphosphate form. The agent ddI is less bioavailable than ZDV and, because it is acid labile, it degrades within several minutes at pH levels of less than 3 (48). The serum half-life of ddI is 1.4 hours, but the intracellular half-life approaches 12 hours, which permits

Table 48A.2. Comparison of Nucleoside Analogs

Drug	Dosage (Total Daily)	Frequency	Side Effects	Indications
Zidovudine (ZDV)	200 mg (500–600 mg)	TID	Anemia Neutropenia Nausea CNS effects	HIV infection, CD4 ≤500 cells/mm^3, thrombocytopenia, dementia
Didanosine (ddI)	200 mg (400 mg)	BID	Pancreatitis Neuropathy Diarrhea Nausea	HIV infection, advanced stage after prior ZDV; ZDV intolerant
Zalcitabine (ddC)	0.75 mg (2.25 mg)	TID	Neuropathy Rash Mouth ulcer Pancreatitis	HIV infection, advanced stage in combination with ZDV

twice-daily dosing. Once-daily dosing is under clinical investigation. The acid lability of ddI requires concurrent gastric acid neutralization, which is accomplished by combining the drug with antacids. The drug should be taken on an empty stomach. The cerebrospinal fluid penetration of ddI, 30 to 50 ng/mL (about 20% of the serum level), is less than that of ZDV (49). Whether this effect decreases efficacy in HIV dementia is, however, not clear, one trial in pediatric HIV disease showed a good response. The recommended dose of ddI is 200 mg twice daily in patients who weigh more than 50 kg. For patients who weigh less, the adult dose is 125 mg twice daily.

Clinical Experience Developed sometime after ZDV, ddI has been tested in a narrower portion of the HIV disease spectrum (50, 51). Shortly after the phenomenon of ZDV resistance became known, clinical trials to explore the clinical significance of this laboratory observation that included ddI were designed. One trial (AIDS Clinical Trials Group [ACTG] 117) enrolled patients who were expected to be ZDV resistant because they had received at least 12 months of prior ZDV therapy (52). A companion study (ACTG 116) randomized patients with either no or less than 12 months of prior ZDV therapy to ZDV or ddI at the same doses (53). In both trials, the primary study end points were clinical progression to AIDS or death. The results of these trials showed that end points were reduced in the antiretrovirally naive patients who were randomized to ZDV. Prior ZDV therapy for 2 months or longer was associated with a clear benefit of ddI over ZDV. In both trials, ddI was associated with a higher frequency of hyperamylasemia and pancreatitis and ZDV with a higher rate of anemia and neutropenia. Overall, however, the rates of severe toxic effects with both drugs were low (Table 48A.2). These results are interesting yet confusing. ZDV emerges as the more effective drug for initial therapy in previously untreated patients with moderate to advanced HIV disease. Yet, after only about 2 to 4 months of ZDV therapy, and long before high-level ZDV resistance is expected, ddI is more effective. These unexpected results imply either that ZDV resistance is clinically important and occurs much more rapidly than expected or that some other mechanism is involved.

Toxic Effects The toxic effects of ddI include pancreatitis, peripheral neuropathy, and diarrhea (54, 55). The neuropathy associated with ddI was recognized early in the development of the drug, and it may be due to the inhibition of γ DNA polymerase in nerve cell mitochondria. This effect depends on the dose administered and the duration of treatment, and it is reversible with dose reduction or drug discontinuation. When therapy is withdrawn, the neuropathy may progress before it declines. It often begins with symmetric dysesthesia or paresthesia of the feet, and if not recognized, it can progress to cause a severe painful ascending axonal neuropathy. Patients must self-monitor for this side effect so the dose can be adjusted accordingly. Generally, ddI therapy is reinstated at half the previous dose after the neuropathy has resolved. This toxicity is more common in patients who are also taking other neurotoxic medications. The toxic effect of greatest concern is pancreatitis. Although rare, cases of fatal, fulminant pancreatitis have been reported (56). It most often, but not exclusively, occurs in patients with a history of pancreatitis or use of drugs also toxic to the pancreas, including alcohol. Pancreatitis associated with ddI is often heralded by a rise in the serum amylase level, but can occur early in drug therapy without warning. Nevertheless, routine monitoring of the serum amylase level is recommended. Asymptomatic elevations of serum amylase should prompt fractionation, as they could be due to salivary sources that may not necessitate dose adjustment.

Zalcitabine

Zalcitabine (ddC) was developed at about the same time as ddI (47). It is a structural analog of cytidine that is well absorbed after oral administration (about 80% bioavailability); absorption is reduced when it is administered with food. Because it is not degraded in a low pH, it can be taken without a buffer. The effective serum half-life of ddC is 1.2 hours, and the estimated intracellular half-life is 2.6 hours; therefore, an 8-hour interval is recommended between doses. The level of drug in the cerebrospinal fluid 2 to 3 hours after administration is 6 to 11 ng/mL, about 20% of that in the plasma. The recommended dose is 0.75 mg three times daily.

Clinical Experience The efficacy of ddC is comparable to that of ddI. The former is often used in similar combinations as the latter, although the two drugs are not combined with each other because of overlapping toxicities. The efficacy of ddC as monotherapy is not impressive, but several trials have shown that ddC in combination with ZDV can delay onset to AIDS and can reduce mortality, particularly in previously antiretrovirally naive populations (57, 58). It is less effective in those with extensive prior therapy (59–61). Combined with the protease inhibitor saquinavir, ddC again prolongs survival and decreases clinical disease progression (62).

Toxic Effects The toxicity of ddC is well understood from phase I trials, later controlled trials, and expanded-access distribution (63). Its principal toxic effect is peripheral neuropathy similar to that associated with ddI (64). This side effect is more common with ddC, but its symptoms and management are the same. The agent ddC also causes mouth ulcers and a rash, effects not seen with other nucleoside analogs. Generally, these effects are uncommon and are not severe enough to require dose interruptions. Pancreatitis has been reported, but it is rare and may reflect underlying pancreatic inflammation caused by HIV infection, cytomegalovirus infection, or other opportunistic diseases; ddC does not cause anemia, neutropenia, or thrombocytopenia. HIV resistant to ZDV remains susceptible to ddC, although, again, prior therapy of any type may decrease the clinical benefits of ddC. The mechanism of this effect is poorly understood.

Lamivudine

Lamivudine (3TC) has several unique features (65). It has the highest short-term potency of any currently approved nucleoside analog. This efficacy is short-lived after the onset of genotypic resistance, which occurs promptly when 3TC is used as monotherapy. The common resistance mutation to 3TC, however, increases sensitivity of previously resistant HIV to ZDV (66).

Some concern has been raised recently, however, that 3TC resistance at the 184 locus may blunt response to subsequent ddI or ddC or even to protease inhibitors. For these reasons, guidelines suggest that 3TC be used in potent three-drug regimens that can prevent resistance selection. 3TC is taken as a 150-mg twice-daily regimen, without dietary restrictions.

Clinical Experience 3TC has had extensive clinical application, including a large expanded-access use. It is particularly popular as a component of combination therapy. 3TC was used in early trials with ZDV because of reports showing that when the HIV genome developed 3TC resistance mutations at the common 184 site, sensitivity to ZDV increased despite previous ZDV resistance (66). Whether this effect is specific to ZDV is not clear, but this characteristic has made the ZDV–3TC drug combination especially common. Use of ZDV along with 3TC results in a clear antiviral benefit (approximately a 1.0 log HIV RNA suppression versus 0.5 log with either drug used alone). Both drugs are used twice daily, and 3TC adds no toxicity; thus, barriers to this combination were low even before clinical end-point data established an improvement in disease progression and survival. End-point data show a nearly 50% reduction in mortality in ZDV–3TC-treated patients (67). 3TC has also been combined with d4T, with antiretroviral potency comparable to that with ZDV (68). Thus, two twice-daily nucleoside reverse transcriptase 3TC-containing regimens are in common use.

Toxic Effects 3TC is unique among current antiretroviral drugs in that it has essentially no common subjective or objective toxicities.

Stavudine

This agent (2′,3′didehydro-3′deoxythymidine; d4T) (69), is well absorbed after oral administration (bioavailability 3%). The drug achieves a high cerebrospinal fluid concentration: 56 ng/mL, or 40% of the serum level (49). The standard dosing regimen of d4T is 40 mg twice daily, without dosing restrictions.

Clinical Experience This agent is widely used in place of ZDV in drug combinations, and it was of modest benefit when used as a single agent in patients switching to d4T from previous ZDV monotherapy (70, 71). It is now used only in combination with other antiretroviral drugs. In one trial, the combination of d4T with 3TC resulted in a 1.66 log reduction in HIV RNA in antiretrovirally naive persons, compared with only a 0.55 log reduction in those who had previous therapy with ZDV, ddI, or ddC (68). Another trial revealed that the combination of d4T with ddI has antiviral potency comparable to that of other nucleoside combinations, without excess peripheral neuropathy (72). However, both trials were small, and have had only a modest duration of follow-up. Use of d4T as an element of three-drug combinations with another nucleoside reverse transcriptase inhibitor and a protease inhibitor is only now being investigated, but we have no reason to believe that these combinations will prove ineffective. Such therapy is already in common clinical use.

Toxic Effects This agent is generally well tolerated (69). Peripheral neuropathy and elevations in transaminase levels are the most common toxic effects (64). The rate of neuropathy is less than reported with either ddI or ddC. Pancreatitis is rarely if ever seen. The agent d4T has been reported to have pharmacologic antagonism with ZDV that may limit its use in combination with that drug.

NONNUCLEOSIDE REVERSE TRANSCRIPTASE INHIBITORS

After extensive laboratory screening, several agents have been identified that inhibit the action of reverse transcriptase but are not nucleosides. The compounds act at a site on the reverse transcriptase enzyme differently from nucleoside analogs. All nonnucleoside reverse transcriptase inhibitors act on the same site, however. They tend to share an exquisite sensitivity for HIV reverse transcriptase, with essentially no activity against the reverse transcriptases from other retroviruses, including HIV-2. In vitro studies of the nonnucleoside reverse transcriptase inhibitors have elucidated their clinical potential and limitations. Several agents, for example, have no cytotoxicity at concentrations in vitro that are several logs greater than their effective antiviral concentration. This finding implies a lower probability of clinical toxicity, as borne out in phase I clinical trials. The specificity of the nonnucleoside reverse transcriptase inhibitors for HIV-1 suggests a great potential for drug resistance. Resistance has developed rapidly in several of these drugs in vitro (after several passages) and in vivo (after several weeks of treatment). In one clinical trial, nonnucleoside reverse transcriptase inhibitor therapy was followed by a rapid fall in HIV p24 antigen levels; but shortly thereafter, this marker rose to baseline levels or greater, and the rise was correlated with the onset of drug resistance (73). Several strategies for use of the nonnucleoside reverse transcriptase inhibitors continue to be explored. First, escalated doses of the drugs appear to make it possible to overcome resistance without excessive toxicity. Second, combining one of these agents with a nucleoside analog may increase efficacy. A third approach being studied in clinical trials is combining a nonnucleoside reverse transcriptase inhibitor with two nucleoside analogs. Several nonnucleoside analogs, including newer chemical variants that are hoped to be less prone to drug resistance, are being developed or are in various stages of laboratory or clinical evaluation.

Nevirapine

Nevirapine was the first nonnucleoside reverse transcriptase inhibitor to be approved. It can be used in a twice-daily (or even once-daily) regimen. Resistance is rapid and is quickly followed by a return in HIV RNA titer to pretreatment levels, but this can be delayed or prevented by using nevirapine in potent three-drug combinations, usually with two nucleoside reverse transcriptase inhibitors (74–76). Nevirapine is being tested in combinations with protease inhibitors as well, but caution is required because nevirapine acts as an inducer of the cytochrome P450 system and thus can reduce serum concentrations of other drugs, perhaps to less effective levels. The usual dose is 200 mg twice daily. Therapy does not entail dietary restrictions.

Clinical Experience The rate of failure from monotherapy with nevirapine was evident early in development, and this agent has usually been tested in combinations with nucleoside reverse transcriptase inhibitors. The primary clinical trial combined nevirapine with ZDV and ddI (77). This trial showed a substantial antiretroviral potency, with nearly 60% of subjects achieving and sustaining suppression of HIV RNA titer below the 500-copy/mL limit of detection. Patients who discontinued therapy had a prompt viral return, but the virus was not nevirapine resistant; this finding suggests that essentially complete suppression had been achieved. Although this effect is significant, it is probably less feasible with a three-drug regimen that includes a protease inhibitor. Therefore, the optimal role of nevirapine in treatment remains unclear.

Toxic Effects Nevirapine is usually well tolerated, although a rash is common (78). This is typically mild but may be limiting in 6% of patients. It is usually erythematous and can be associated with fever. Mucosal involvement is rare and should prompt immediate drug discontinuation.

Delavirdine

Delavirdine, the second approved nonnucleoside reverse transcriptase inhibitor, is as well tolerated as nevirapine and has the same propensity to select for resistant HIV forms rapidly. Delavirdine is used in a thrice-daily regimen and has no dietary restrictions. In contrast to nevirapine, delavirdine is a modest cytochrome P450 inhibitor. Thus, it may raise the serum concentration of other drugs metabolized by that enzyme system, including HIV protease inhibitors. This characteristic may permit more effective or convenient combinations. The dose of delavirdine is 400 mg orally three times daily.

Clinical Experience Little clinical experience has been gained with delavirdine because its development was slowed by problems of resistance and the concomitant development of the potent protease inhibitors. It clearly has some antiretroviral activity and is appropriate to consider in drug combinations (79). This agent generally should not be used as monotherapy. Whether it is as potent as nevirapine is not clear.

Toxic Effects Delavirdine has a toxicity profile comparable to that of nevirapine, but the incidence and severity of rash may be less than with nevirapine.

HIV Protein Processing: Protease Inhibitors

HIV proteins require proteolytic cleavage for final assembly of viable virions, and this process is facilitated by a protease specific to HIV. Several HIV protease inhibitors have been developed (80). These drugs are active in vitro, and clinical application has resulted in impressive gains in clinical improvement in the outcome of HIV disease.

SAQUINAVIR

Saquinavir, the first protease inhibitor developed, has clinical benefits with less toxicity than any other current member of this drug class (80). However, the bioavailability of the compound, especially in its initial formulation, limited antiretroviral potency compared with more recently developed drugs. The resistance mutations selected for by saquinavir may be less common with other protease inhibitors, but this issue is controversial and under active investigation (75). Saquinavir is used in an 800-mg thrice-daily schedule and is taken with a fatty meal to maximize absorption.

Clinical Experience

Saquinavir rapidly selects for resistant HIV mutations when used as a single agent, a feature shared by the other members of this drug class (75, 81). Therefore, it is always used in combination. This agent is metabolized primarily by the cytochrome P450 system, and levels are thus raised by the concomitant use of inhibitors of that enzyme (82). In one trial, saquinavir combined with ddC significantly decreased mortality and disease progression (83). Common practice is to combine this drug with two nucleoside reverse transcriptase inhibitors to gain even more potency. In another study, the combination of saquinavir and another protease inhibitor, ritonavir (a potent cytochrome P450 inhibitor), showed impressive antiretroviral effects (84). Similar, although preliminary, results have been seen with another protease inhibitor, nelfinavir, in combination with saquinavir (85). Each of these dual protease trials raises saquinavir concentrations, thus overcoming the issue of the drug's bioavailability.

Toxic Effects Saquinavir results in some gastrointestinal disturbance in many patients. Bloating, gas, and diarrhea are common. These symptoms are typically mild, however, and do not require drug interruption.

RITONAVIR

Ritonavir, the second approved protease inhibitor, is more bioavailable and hence is more potent in vivo than saquinavir (86). It may be taken with food. It requires refrigeration, however, and commonly causes gastrointestinal symptoms, which may be severe. Ritonavir is used in a 600-mg twice-daily schedule; during dual protease inhibitor therapy, the dose is reduced to 400 mg twice daily.

Clinical Experience

In an early trial, ritonavir was added as a single agent to the current antiretroviral regimen of patients with advanced disease (87). This 1100-person trial showed a nearly 50% reduction in disease progression and mortality with ritonavir treatment. Although it was later appreciated that the potent cytochrome P450 inhibition caused by ritonavir may lead to severe drug interactions (82), few interactions of clinical consequence were seen in this trial. Since it was approved, ritonavir has been used in various combinations and, when tolerated, it has shown clear clinical benefit. Dual protease inhibitor therapy with ritonavir and saquinavir has been explored (82). This has resulted in effective antiviral effects even without the simultaneous use of other drugs, although in clinical practice, most clinicians use dual protease inhibitors along with two nucleoside reverse transcriptase inhibitors.

Toxic Effects

Ritonavir has gastrointestinal symptoms similar to, but often much worse than, those caused by saquinavir (80, 86). Patients also report altered taste and circumoral paresthesias. Starting at a lower dose may reduce side effects, increasing to a full dose over the first week of treatment. Many patients report that side effects are transient, decreasing over the first 4 to 6 weeks of therapy. In the dual protease inhibitor regimen, the reduced ritonavir dose of 400 mg twice daily causes substantially lower toxicity.

INDINAVIR

Indinavir is a potent protease inhibitor with less subjective toxicity than typical with the other drugs in this class (88). It has had the widest application in clinical trials and the broadest clinical experience. Indinavir requires dosing every 8 hours after fasting, and patients must consume substantially more water than normal to reduce the risk of renal stones formed by precipitation of drug in the urine. Indinavir selects for certain genetic mutations, overlapping extensively with ritonavir and potentially other members of this class as well. Indinavir is given as a dose of 800 mg three times daily.

Clinical Experience

Indinavir has been tested in key protocols that, more than any drug in this class, have changed expectations about antiretroviral therapy. Although monotherapy is quickly followed by resistance selection (81), indinavir in combination with two reverse transcriptase inhibitors can suppress HIV RNA to nondetectable levels in most patients, preventing or delaying resistance. Combined with ZDV and 3TC, for example, indinavir rendered 90% of ZDV-experienced patients HIV RNA-nondetectable (89). In a related trial, the combination resulted in a 50% mortality reduction compared with patients receiving ZDV and 3TC (90). Although this agent has been tested less extensively with other nucleoside reverse transcriptase inhibitor pairs, we have no reason to believe that the clinical benefits of this "triple therapy" would not occur with these combinations.

Toxic Effects

Indinavir can cause some gastrointestinal distress (80), but this is uncommon and rarely severe. Asymptomatic hyperbilirubinemia is common, and renal stones are seen in 5 to 10% of patients. This effect is indinavir's primary toxicity, and it can be reduced by encouraging the consumption of additional water, especially for those living in warm climates. The nephrolithiasis is often self-limited, but it may recur and may require discontinuation of drug.

NELFINAVIR

The most recently approved protease inhibitor, nelfinavir is potent and relatively well tolerated. It is used in a thrice-daily schedule, and its resistance pattern may be less cross-resistant to other protease inhibitors. It is a modest cytochrome P450 inhibitor. Combination therapy with nelfinavir and saquinavir is being explored in a way comparable to the ritonavir plus saquinavir combination described earlier (91). Nelfinavir is given at dose of 750 mg three times daily.

Clinical Experience

Nelfinavir is still relatively early in wide-scale use, but it has been tested in combination with two nucleoside reverse transcriptase inhibitors, especially ZDV and 3TC. Again, in clinical use it is being combined with various nucleoside pairs, with apparently good results. In the primary trial to date, use of nelfinavir along with ZDV and 3TC in an antiretrovirally naive group yielded an 80% nondetectable HIV RNA titer, comparable to that seen with indinavir (92).

Toxic Effects

The primary side effect of nelfinavir is gastrointestinal disturbance, especially diarrhea. This effect is usually mild and is controlled with symptomatic remedies.

STRATEGIES FOR HIV TREATMENT

Much attention has been focused on the specific activity of each new antiretroviral agent or combination. Clinically, it seems more important to develop a program of multiple drug administration that provides potent retroviral inhibition that persists for the years; this will be required in most patients. Certainly, several questions dominate the management of antiretroviral therapy. These and certain unique clinical situations are briefly presented herein. Although several guidelines have been published (1, 2), this review primarily reflects my personal opinions. *When should therapy begin?* Given that the immune deficiency of HIV disease is progressive, largely irreversible, and early in onset, it seems reasonable to begin antiretroviral treatment before the disease reaches advanced symptomatic stages, certainly before the CD4 cell count falls below 500 cells/mL; many clinicians initiate therapy earlier. This approach is especially appropriate if the HIV RNA titer is elevated, such as above 20,000 to 50,000 copies/mL. Such a recommendation is based on growing evidence that the response to therapy is augmented in those with lower HIV RNA titers and that resistance selection may be prevented by an aggressive approach. *What should initial therapy include?* Triple-drug therapy yields the strongest evidence of antiretroviral effect. Triple therapy usually includes two nucleoside reverse transcriptase inhibitors and either a protease inhibitor or a nonnucleoside reverse transcriptase inhibitor. A protease inhibitor is usually preferable, especially in patients with higher HIV RNA titers. Saquinavir may be less potent than the other protease inhibitors, but it may be combined with them for greater potency. Monotherapy of any kind is discouraged, and dual therapy is reserved only for those unwilling to accept more aggressive therapy or for occasional patients with extremely low HIV RNA titers, such as below 5000 copies/mL. *Is any single preferred initial combination preferred?* Several nucleoside reverse transcriptase inhibitor combinations have comparable balances between efficacy and ease of use, including ZDV and 3TC, d4T and 3TC, d4T and ddI, ZDV and ddI, and ZDV and ddC. Some of these combinations have more clinical trial supporting data than others, some have better established clinical end-point data, some have less subjective toxicity, and some have theoretic advantages regarding resistance selection. Whether these findings result in a clear first choice is still debated and, in fact, a definitive study will probably never be performed. The clinician and patient must consider issues of tolerability and the strength of data in choosing initial therapy. The choice of protease inhibitor may be similarly challenging. Some agents appear more potent but may be more toxic or inconvenient, and the ultimate degree of benefit in populations of patients may hinge as importantly on ease of use as on biologic efficacy if nonadherence leads to drug resistance and failure. That said, guidelines tend to favor the initial use of the most potent protease inhibitors as first-line therapy. Still, this leaves open the option of considering dual protease inhibitor therapy as an initial approach, which may prove as potent and well tolerated as many other options. When more data are available regarding the degree of clinical cross-resistance within the protease inhibitors, the choice of first-line therapy may be easier because one drug may prove easier to "rescue" after failure than others, an important consideration in prolonging treatment benefit. *How should therapy be monitored?* HIV RNA and CD4 counts should be measured in all patients as therapy is initiated and again after and during therapy to assess response. HIV RNA titer should be obtained about 4 weeks after beginning therapy. The titer should be at least 0.5 logs below baseline and ideally 2.0 logs below. If the titer has not fallen by at least 0.5 logs, a more effective combination should be considered, assuming the patient is compliant with medications. After 4 weeks, the HIV RNA should be followed at 3- to 4-month intervals. Ideally, the titer will become nondetectable by 4 to 6 months after initiating treatment. If so, therapy should be continued. If the titer is reduced from baseline but still detectable, the decision of optimal management must be individualized. Some may continue therapy, especially if CD4+ increases or clinical improvement is evident. Others may wish to intensify the regimen in an attempt to gain virologic control. *What should be done for the patient who becomes intolerant to one of the prescribed medications?* If severe side effects are seen with one drug, one of comparable potency but with a different toxicity profile should replace that agent. The other agents should be continued without interruption. *What should be done if the HIV RNA titer begins to rise after a period of effective suppression?* This situation is increasingly common and complex. The possibility of nonadherence should be assessed, and drug levels should be checked for malabsorption. Resistance genotyping or even phenotyping may help in treatment planning, although how such tests would help in specific cases is often uncertain. If therapy must be altered, at least two, if not all three, drugs should be changed. This approach prevents the sequential monotherapy effect achieved by adding one drug to a failing combination that can no longer control replication. *Should acute HIV infection be treated?* Yes. Most clinicians treat acute infection with an aggressive regimen for at least 6 months. *How should postexposure prophylaxis be approached?* Exposure to HIV, whether through a needlestick occupational injury or through an unprotected sexual act, carries a risk of actual infection. This risk is low in most situations, on the order of 1 in 200 to 1 in

400, per exposure. Use of ZDV monotherapy has been shown effective for occupational exposures, with about a 75% risk reduction. Recent guidelines recommend dual nucleoside therapy or, in the case of more substantial injuries, inclusion of a protease inhibitor in a triple-therapy regimen. One has no reason to believe that similar postexposure therapy would not be effective in those with nonoccupational, primarily sexual, exposures, although substantial difficulties exist in conducting actual clinical trials in this setting. In addition is the real possibility that the postexposure use of antiretroviral therapy could lead some to decrease vigilance regarding safe behavior threatening an actual increase in transmission. Pilot trials of sexual postexposure prophylaxis may be appropriate; in the meantime, such therapy should be considered on a case-by-case basis.

FUTURE DIRECTIONS

Investigators hope that one or more of the newly developed (but not yet available) classes of antiretroviral drugs, perhaps integrase inhibitors or chemokine receptor antagonists, will prove beneficial in combination with the existing agents. Significantly more work must be completed to determine the optimal time to initiate therapy and the individual drugs of choice to be answered. Trials using virologic end points, which address questions of strategy, will expand our insight over the next several years, particularly regarding issues of drug resistance and cross-resistance. Although experience with immune-based or gene therapy has so far been disappointing, this field may become a therapeutic direction. Substantial and, at times, dramatic progress continues in the effort to achieve control over HIV replication, and this effort should offer new optimism in the treatment of patients infected with HIV.

References

1. Carpenter CCJ, Fischl MA, Hammer SM, et al. Antiretroviral therapy for HIV infection in 1997: updated recommendations of the International AIDS Society–USA Panel. JAMA 1997;277:1962–1969.
2. Fauci AS, Bartlett JG, Goosby EP, et al. Draft federal guidelines for the use of antiretroviral agents in HIV infected adults and adolescents. Federal Register June 19, 1997.
3. Habeshaw JA, Dalgleish AG. The relevance of HIV env/CD4 interactions to the pathogenesis of acquired immune deficiency syndrome. J Acquir Immune Defic Syndr 1989;2:457–468.
4. Moore JP. Coreceptors: implications for HIV pathogenesis and therapy. Science 1997;276:51–52.
5. Alkhatib G, Combadiere C, Broder CC, et al. CC CKR5: A RANTES, MIP-1α, MIP-1β receptor as a fusion cofactor for macrophage-tropic HIV-1. Science 1996;272:1955–1958.
6. Feng Y, Broder CC, Kennedy PE, et al. HIV-1 entry cofactor: functional cDNA cloning of a seven-transmembrane, G protein-coupled receptor. Science 1996;272:872–877.
7. Simmons G, Clapham PR, Picard L, et al. Potent inhibition of HIV-1 infectivity in macrophages and lymphocytes by a novel CCR5 antagonist. Science 1997;276:276–279.
8. Greene WC. The molecular biology of human immunodeficiency virus type 1 infection. N Engl J Med 1991;324:308–317.
9. Hirsch MS, D'Aquila RT. Therapy for human immunodeficiency virus infection. N Engl J Med 1993;328:1686–1695.
10. Meek TD, Dreyer GB. HIV-1 protease as a potential target for anti-AIDS therapy. Ann N Y Acad Sci 1990;616:41–53.
11. Robins T, Plattner J. HIV protease inhibitors: their anti-HIV activity and potential role in treatment. J Acquir Immune Defic Syndr 1993;6:162–170.
12. Debouck C. The HIV-1 protease as a therapeutic target for AIDS. AIDS Res Hum Retroviruses 1992;8:153–164.
13. Mellors JW, Kingsley LA, Rinaldo CR Jr, et al. Quantitation of HIV-1 RNA in plasma predicts outcome after seroconversion. Ann Intern Med 1995;122:573–579.
14. Henrard DR, Daar E, Farzadegan H, et al. Virologic and immunologic characterization of symptomatic and asymptomatic primary HIV-1 infection. J Acquir Immune Syndr Hum Retrovirol 1995;9:305–310.
15. Katzenstein TL, Pedersen C, Nielsen C, et al. Longitudinal serum HIV RNA quantification: correlation to viral phenotype at seroconversion and clinical outcome. AIDS 1996;10:167–173.
16. Borrow P, Lewicki H, Hahn BH, et al. Virus-specific CD8+ cytotoxic T-lymphocyte activity associated with control of viremia in primary human immunodeficiency virus type-1 infection. J Virol 1994;68:6103–6110.
17. Haase AT, Henry K, Zupancic M, et al. Quantitative image analysis of HIV-1 infection in lymphoid tissue. Science 1996;274:985–989.
18. Shearer WT, Quinn TC, LaRussa P, et al. Viral load and disease progression in infants infected with human immunodeficiency virus type 1. N Engl J Med 1997;336:1337–1342.
19. Darby SC, Ewart DW, Giangrande PLF, et al. Importance of age at infection with HIV-1 for survival and development of AIDS in UK haemophilia population. Lancet 1996;347:1573–1579.
20. Osmond D, Charlebois E, Lang W, et al. Changes in AIDS survival time in two San Francisco cohorts of homosexual men, 1983 to 1993. JAMA 1994;271:1083–1087.
21. Moss AR, Bacchetti P. Natural history of HIV infection [editorial review]. AIDS 1989;3:55–61.
22. Yust I, Vardinon N, Skornick Y, et al. Reduction of circulating HIV antigens in seropositive patients after treatment with AL-721. Isr J Med Sci 1990;26:20–26.
23. Stites DP, Moss AR, Bacchetti P, et al. Lymphocyte subset analysis to predict progression to AIDS in a cohort of homosexual men in San Francisco. Clin Immunol Immunopathol 1989;52:96–103.
24. Dewar RL, Highbarger HC, Sarmiento MD, et al. Application of branched DNA signal amplification to monitor human immunodeficiency virus type 1 burden in human plasma. J Infect Dis 1994;170:1172–1179.
25. Shafer RW, Merigan TC. New virologic tools for the design and analysis of clinical trials [editorial]. J Infect Dis 1995;171:1325–1328.
26. Saag MS, Holodniy M, Kuritzkes DR, et al. HIV viral load markers in clinical practice. Nature Med 1996;2:625–629.
27. Kahn JO, Allan JD, Hodges TL, et al. The safety and pharmacokinetics of recombinant soluble CD4 (rCD4) in subjects with the acquired immunodeficiency syndrome (AIDS) and AIDS-related complex. Ann Intern Med 1990;112:254–261.
28. Schooley RT, Merigan TC, Gaut P, et al. Recombinant soluble CD4 therapy in patients with the acquired immunodeficiency syndrome (AIDS) and AIDS-related complex. Ann Intern Med 1990;112:247–253.
29. Mellors JW, Larder BA, Schinazi RF. Mutations in HIV-1 reverse transcriptase and protease associated with drug resistance. Int Antiviral News 1996;3:8–13.
30. Strair RK, Mellors JW. Resistance of human immunodeficiency virus-1 to antiretroviral drugs. AIDS Updates 1993;6:1–14.
31. Fischl MA, Richman DD, Griego MH, et al. The efficacy of azidothymidine (AZT) in the treatment of patients with AIDS and AIDS-related complex. N Engl J Med 1987;317:185–191.
32. Larder BA, Kemp SD. Multiple mutations in HIV-1 reverse transcriptase confer high-level resistance to zidovudine (AZT). Science 1989;246:1155–1158.
33. Smith MS, Koerber KL, Pagano JS. Long-term persistence of zidovudine resistance mutations in plasma isolates of human immunodefi-

ciency virus type 1 of dideoxyinosine-treated patients removed from zidovudine therapy. J Infect Dis 1994;169:184–188.
34. Land S, McGavin K, Birch C, et al. Reversion from zidovudine resistance to sensitivity on cessation of treatment. Lancet 1991;338: 830–831.
35. Volberding PA, Lagakos SW, Koch MA, et al. Zidovudine in asymptomatic human immunodeficiency virus infection. N Engl J Med 1990;322:941–949.
36. Concorde Coordinating Committee. Concorde: MRC/ANRS randomised double-blind controlled trial of immediate and deferred zidovudine in symptom-free HIV infection. Lancet 1994;343: 871–881.
37. Koch MA, Volberding PA, Lagakos SW, et al. Toxic effects of zidovudine in asymptomatic human immunodeficiency virus-infected individuals with CD4+ cell counts of 0.50×10^9/L or less. Arch Intern Med 1992;152:2286–2292.
38. Stambuk D, Youle M, Hawkins D, et al. The efficacy and toxicity of azidothymidine (AZT) in the treatment of patients with AIDS and AIDS-related complex (ARC): an open uncontrolled treatment study. Q J Med 1989;70:161–174.
39. Helbert M, Fletcher T, Peddle B, et al. Zidovudine-associated myopathy. Lancet 1988;2:689–690.
40. Pluda JM, Mitsuya H, Yarchoan R. Hematologic effects of AIDS therapies. Hematol Oncol Clin North Am 1991;5:229–248.
41. Gelmon K, Montaner JSG, Fanning M, et al. Nature, time course and dose dependence of zidovudine-related side effects: results from the Multicenter Canadian Azidothymidine Trial. AIDS 1989;3:555–561.
42. Henry DH, Beall GN, Benson CA, et al. Recombinant human erythropoietin in the treatment of anemia associated with human immunodeficiency virus (HIV) infection and zidovudine therapy. Ann Intern Med 1992;117:739–748.
43. Miles SA, Mitsuyasu RT, Moreno J, et al. Combined therapy with recombinant granulocyte colony-stimulating factor and erythropoietin decreases hematologic toxicity from zidovudine. Blood 1991;10: 2109–2117.
44. Fischl MA, Galpin JE, Levine JD, et al. Recombinant human erythropoietin for patients with AIDS treated with zidovudine. N Engl J Med 1990;322:1488–1493.
45. Shaunak S, Bartlett JA. Zidovudine-induced neutropenia: are we too cautious? Lancet 1989;2:91–92.
46. Levine JD, Allan JD, Tessitore JH, et al. Recombinant human granulocyte-macrophage colony-stimulating factor ameliorates zidovudine-induced neutropenia in patients with acquired immunodeficiency syndrome (AIDS)/AIDS-related complex. Blood 1991;78: 3148–3154.
47. Lipsky JJ. Zalcitabine and didanosine. Lancet 1993;341:30–32.
48. Knupp CA, Shyu WC, Dolin R, et al. Pharmacokinetics of didanosine in patients with acquired immunodeficiency syndrome or acquired immunodeficiency syndrome-related complex. Clin Pharmacol Ther 1991; 49:523–535.
49. Foudraine N, de Wolf F, Hoetelmans R, et al. CSF and serum HIV-RNA levels during AZT/3TC and d4T/3TC treatment [abstract]. 1997;1:49.
50. Cooley TP, Kunches LM, Saunders CA, et al. Once-daily administration of 2′,3′-dideoxyinosine (ddI) in patients with the acquired immunodeficiency syndrome or AIDS-related complex. N Engl J Med 1990; 322:1340–1345.
51. Collier AC, Coombs RW, Fischl MA, et al. Combination therapy with zidovudine and didanosine compared with zidovudine alone in HIV-1 infection. Ann Intern Med 1993;119:786–793.
52. Kahn JO, Lagakos SW, Richman DD, et al. A controlled trial comparing continued zidovudine with didanosine in human immunodeficiency virus infection. N Engl J Med 1992;327:581–587.
53. Dolin R, Amato DA, Fischl MA, et al. Zidovudine compared with didanosine in patients with advanced HIV type 1 infection and little or no previous experience with zidovudine. Arch Intern Med 1995;155: 961–974.
54. Kieburtz KD, Seidlin M, Lambert JS, et al. Extended follow-up of peripheral neuropathy in patients with AIDS and AIDS-related complex treated with dideoxyinosine. J Acquir Immune Defic Syndr 1992;5:60–64.
55. Schindzielorz A, Pike I, Daniels M, et al. Rates and risk factors for adverse events associated with didanosine in the expanded access program. Clin Infect Dis 1994;19:1076–1083.
56. Grasela TH, Walawander CA, Beltangady M, et al. Analysis of potential risk factors associated with the development of pancreatitis in phase I patients with AIDS or AIDS-related complex receiving didanosine. J Infect Dis 1994;169:1250–1255.
57. Delta Coordinating Committee. Delta: a randomized double-blind controlled trial comparing combinations of zidovudine plus didanosine or zalcitabine with zidovudine alone in HIV-infected individuals. Lancet 1996;348:283–291.
58. Hammer SM, Katzenstein DA, Hughes MD, et al. Trial comparing nucleoside monotherapy with combination therapy in HIV-infected adults with CD4 cell counts from 200 to 500 per cubic millimeter. N Engl J Med 1996;335:1081–1090.
59. Fischl MA, Stanley K, Collier AC, et al. Combination and monotherapy with zidovudine and zalcitabine in patients with advanced HIV disease. Ann Intern Med 1995;122:24–32.
60. Abrams DI, Goldman AI, Launer C, et al. A comparative trial of didanosine or zalcitabine after treatment with zidovudine in patients with human immunodeficiency virus infection. N Engl J Med 1994; 330:657–662.
61. Fischl MA, Olson RM, Follansbee SE, et al. Zalcitabine compared with zidovudine in patients with advanced HIV-1 infection who received previous zidovudine therapy. Ann Intern Med 1993;118:762–769.
62. Collier AC, Coombs RW, Schoenfeld DA, et al. Treatment of human immunodeficiency virus infection with saquinavir, zidovudine, and zalcitabine. N Engl J Med 1996;334:1011–1017.
63. Merigan TC, Skowron G, ddC Study Group of the AIDS Clinical Trials Group of the NIAID. Safety and tolerance of dideoxycytidine as a single agent. Am J Med 1990;88:5B-11S–5B-15S.
64. Simpson DM, Tagliati M. Nucleoside analogue-associated peripheral neuropathy in human immunodeficiency virus infection. J Acquir Immune Syndr Hum Retrovirol 1995;9:153–161.
65. van Leeuwen R, Katlama C, Kitchen V, et al. Evaluation of safety and efficacy of 3TC (lamivudine) in patients with asymptomatic or mildly symptomatic human immunodeficiency virus infection: a phase I/II study. J Infect Dis 1995;171:1166–1171.
66. Larder BA, Kemp SD, Harrigan PR. Potential mechanism for sustained antiretroviral efficacy of AZT–3TC combination therapy. Science 1995; 269:696–699.
67. CAESAR Coordinating Committee. Randomised trial of addition of lamivudine or lamivudine plus loviride to zidovudine-containing regimens for patients with HIV-1 infection: the CAESAR trial. Lancet 1997;349:1413–1421.
68. Katlama C, Valantin MA, Calvez V, et al. ALTIS: A pilot open study of d4T/3TC in antiretroviral naive and experienced patients [abstract]. 1997;1:49.
69. Skowron G. Biologic effects and safety of stavudine: overview of phase I and II clinical trials. J Infect Dis 1995;171:S113–S117.
70. Katlama C, Molina JM, Rozenbaum W, et al. Stravudine in HIV infected patients with CD4 > 350/mm^3: results of a double-blind randomized placebo controlled study [abstract]. In: Program and Abstracts of the 3rd Conference on Retroviruses and Opportunistic Infections. Washington, DC: American Society for Microbiology 1996:14.
71. Spruance SL, Pavia AT, Mellors JW, et al. Clinical efficacy of monotherapy with stavudine compared with zidovudine in HIV-infected, zidovudine-experienced patients. Ann Intern Med 1997;126:355–363.
72. Pollard R, Peterson D, Hardy D, et al. Antiviral effect and safety of stavudine and didanosine combination therapy in HIV-infected subjects in an ongoing pilot randomized double-blinded trial [abstract]. In:

73. Saag MS, Emini EA, Laskin OL, et al. A short-term clinical evaluation of L-697,661, a non-nucleoside inhibitor of HIV-1 reverse transcriptase. N Engl J Med 1993;329:1065–1072.
74. Havlir D, McLaughlin MM, Richman DD. A pilot study to evaluate the development of resistance to nevirapine in asymptomatic human immunodeficiency virus-infected patients with CD4 cell counts of >500/mm^3: AIDS clinical trials group protocol 208. J Infect Dis 1995;172:1379–1383.
75. Moyle GJ. Resistance to antiretroviral compounds: implications for the clinical management of HIV infection. Immunol Infect Dis 1996;5: 170–182.
76. Richman DD, Havlir D, Corbeil J, et al. Nevirapine resistance mutations of human immunodeficiency virus type 1 selected during therapy. J Virol 1994;68:1660–1666.
77. D'Aquila RT, Hughes MD, Johnson VA, et al. Nevirapine, zidovudine, and didanosine compared with zidovudine and didanosine in patients with HIV-1 infection. Ann Intern Med 1996;124:1019–1030.
78. Cheeseman SH, Havlir D, McLaughlin MM, et al. Phase I/II evaluation of nevirapine alone and in combination with zidovudine for infection with human immunodeficiency virus. J Acquir Immune Syndr Hum Retrovirol 1994;8:141–151.
79. Freimuth WW, Wathen LK, Cox SR, et al. Delavirdine in combination with zidovudine causes sustained antiviral and immunological effects in HIV-1 infected individuals [abstract]. In: Program and Abstracts of the 3rd Conference on Retroviruses and Opportunistic Infections. Washington, DC: American Society for Microbiology, 1996:40–41.
80. Deeks SG, Smith M, Holodniy M, et al. HIV-1 protease inhibitors, a review for clinicians. JAMA 1997;277:145–153.
81. Ridky T, Leis J. Development of drug resistance to HIV-1 protease inhibitors. J Biol Chem 1995;270:29,621–29,623.
82. Kempf D, Marsh K, Denissen J, et al. Coadministration with ritonavir enhances the plasma levels of HIV protease inhibitors by inhibition of cytochrome P450 [abstract]. In: Program and Abstracts of the 3rd Conference on Retroviruses and Opportunistic Infections. Washington, DC: American Society for Microbiology, 1996:79.
83. Collier AC, Coombs RW, Schoenfeld DA, et al. Treatment of Human Immunodeficiency virus infection with saquinavir, zidovudine, and zalcitabine. N Engl J Med 1996;334:1011–1017.
84. Merry C, Barry MG, Mulcahy F, et al. Saquinavir pharmacokinetics alone and in combination with ritonavir in HIV-infected patients. AIDS 1997;11:F29–F33.
85. Kravcik S, Sahai J, Kerr B, et al. Nelfinavir Mesylate (NFV) increases Saquinavir soft gel capsule (SQV-SGC) exposure in HIV+ patients 4th Conf. Retro and Opportun Infect [abstract]. 1997;1:132.
86. Lea AP, Faulds D. Ritonavir. Drugs 1996;52:541–546.
87. Cameron B, Heath-Chiozzi M, Kravci S, et al. Prolongation of life and prevention of AIDS in advanced HIV immunodeficiency with ritonavir [abstract]. In: Program and Abstracts of the 3rd Conference on Retroviruses and Opportunistic Infections. Washington, DC: American Society for Microbiology, 1996:40.
88. Emini EA. Protease inhibitors [abstract]. In: Program and Abstracts from the 3rd Conference on Retroviruses and Opportunistic Infections. Washington, DC: American Society for Microbiology, 1996:1.
89. Gulick R, Mellors J, Havlir D, et al. Potent and sustained antiretroviral activity of indinavir in combination with zidovudine and lamivudine [abstract]. In: Program and Abstracts of the 3rd Conference on Retroviruses and Opportunistic Infections. Washington, DC: American Society for Microbiology, 1996:40.
90. Hammer S. Executive summary: AIDS Clinical Trials Group (ACTG) Trial 320, 1997.
91. Webber S, Shetty B, Wu E, et al. In vitro and in vivo metabolism and cytochrome P450 induction studies with the HIV-1 protease inhibitor, VIRACEPT (AG1343) [abstract]. In: Program and Abstracts of the 3rd Conference on Retroviruses and Opportunistic Infections. Washington, DC: American Society for Microbiology, 1996:79.
92. Agouron Pharmaceuticals Trials S11. Nelfinavir package insert, 1997.

B. Strategy and Use of Antiretroviral Agents in Combination

Scott Hammer

The rapid progress in the field of antiretroviral therapy evident in the past few years has imbued patients and physicians with a new sense of optimism that effective, long-term control of human immunodeficiency virus type 1 (HIV-1) disease can be achieved. This optimism is based on an improved understanding of the nature of the disease process, the availability of viral load monitoring, the advent of the protease inhibitor (PI) era, and clinical trial results that have all contributed to greater disease-free intervals and longer survival for affected persons (1–29). This optimism, however, now presents an enormous challenge because, despite the exploding knowledge base, physicians and patients still must infer from the available data which is the optimal regimen to use initially and how best to sequence drug combinations to maximize their benefit over time. In the current context of therapy, in which the goal is to lower plasma HIV-1 RNA concentrations to below the limits of quantification of the available assays, the choice of a particular regimen is likely to have a cascade effect on the efficacy of future regimens. The concept that a patient's viral strain is irrevocably committed to an evolutionary pathway by a particular therapeutic choice contributes to the growing sense that early choices in a patient's treatment history are the most crucial if long-term success is to be achieved (30). Thus, it is appropriate to approach antiretroviral agent management in a strategic fashion rather than as simply a sequence of independent, unlinked regimens.

The development of a long-term strategic approach must start, of course, with initial choices, and several factors must be taken into account. These include the following: the patient's disease stage as assessed by clinical status, CD4 cell count, and plasma HIV-1 RNA level; prior treatment history, if any; underlying medical conditions; the patient's commitment to treatment and predicted drug adherence; concomitant medications that may contribute to an adverse drug interaction; the available agents and access to them; in vitro data, if available, concerning synergy or antagonism of the agents considered for use in combination; clinical trial results; potency of the regimen; potential for cross-resistance to previously administered or future agents; toxicity profile; cost; the potential effect on the patient's quality of life; and the philosophy of treatment and its goal (Table 48B.1).

The availability of highly potent regimens, most typically but not exclusively represented by three-drug combinations that include a PI, now provides a choice in the overarching goal of therapy: to attempt, if possible, to reduce HIV replication in vivo completely or partially (31–33). It is becoming increasingly clear that, in well-defined circumstances, the suppression of plasma HIV-1 RNA below the limit of quantification of routinely available assays (e.g., lower than 500 copies/mL) actually results in suppression below 50 copies/mL and is associated with marked reductions in HIV RNA expression in lymphoid tissue and genital secretions (9, 28, 34). Such suppression appears to prevent the emergence of resistance that, under other circumstances, would predictably develop in most patients (35). When viewed in these terms, the philosophic choice seems obvious, and quite reasonably, this should dictate the approach to therapy. However, three cautionary notes need to be mentioned: First, "maximal" suppression is not achievable in everyone. This phenomenon is most notable in heavily pretreated patients in whom incremental therapy over the years has resulted in the accumulation of drug resistance mutations. Disease stage, individual variability in bioavailability and drug metabolism, potential sanctuary sites, and other unknown factors all may contribute to the failure to achieve the desired goal. Second, drug adherence is crucial to success. The level of commitment required of an individual who is asked to take numerous pills daily on a rigid schedule cannot be underestimated. This problem is confounded by the potential considerations of the timing of medications in relation to meals, the required vigilance for interactions with other drugs, side effects that need to be tolerated, the uncertainty of whether long-term toxicities will become manifest (e.g., diabetes mellitus in recipients of PIs), and cost. Further, as the field continues to move to recommend therapy in patients with early, asymptomatic disease, these complex regimens carry an additional psychologic burden because a physician is essentially asking a patient to commit to multidrug, around-the-clock adherence for 15 to 20 years or longer (assuming that viral eradication will not be achieved).

Table 48B.1. Factors Involved in the Selection of an Antiretroviral Agent Combination

- Patient's disease stage as assessed by clinical status, CD4 cell count, and plasma HIV-1 RNA level
- Prior treatment history, if any
- Underlying medical conditions
- Patient's commitment to treatment and predicted drug adherence
- Concomitant medications that may contribute to drug interactions with agents being introduced
- Available agents and access to them
- In vitro data, if available, concerning synergy or antagonism of agents being considered for use in combination
- Clinical trial results
- Potency of regimen
- Potential for cross-resistance to previously administered or future agents
- Toxicity profile of agents under consideration
- Potential effect on patient's quality of life
- Philosophy of treatment and its goal
- Cost

The goal of suppression below the limits of HIV-1 RNA detection is laudable, but drug adherence in this circumstance cannot be uniformly assumed. Third, modestly potent regimens still confer a clinical benefit. Investigators have consistently reported that declines of plasma HIV-1 RNA levels in the weeks or months after initiation of treatment are associated with a clinical benefit as measured by a reduction in the incidence of acquired immunodeficiency syndrome (AIDS)–defining illnesses and death (10, 12–15, 17, 18, 36, 37). For example, reductions in the risk of disease progression of 27 to 80% are seen with modest early plasma HIV-1 RNA declines of 0.3 to 1.0 $\log_{10}$ (12–14, 17, 36, 37). Consequently, when complex regimens that include a PI are preferably deferred for whatever reason, therapy with less potent regimens should predictably provide a clinical benefit over time. However, such regimens must be chosen carefully so future options are only minimally compromised.

The evolving standard of care, which is reflected in the recently issued antiretroviral therapy guidelines of the United States Public Health Service and the International AIDS Society–USA (31–33), is to initiate therapy with as potent a regimen as possible within the constraints and considerations just outlined. In the current context, such a regimen is represented by a three-drug combination that includes a potent in vivo PI and two nucleoside analog reverse transcriptase inhibitors (NRTIs). This approach is supported by a wealth of clinical trial data, but although it has become synonymous with the term "triple-drug therapy," the inherent potency of a particular regimen is important irrespective of the number of agents. For example, the term "triple therapy" can also apply to regimens that include a nonnucleoside (HIV-1 specific) reverse transcriptase inhibitor (NNRTI) with two NRTIs or three NRTIs in combination, but whether these regimens will result in the same degree of viral suppression and durability of response is uncertain at this time. Alternatively, dual PI regimens have shown promising activity (38), but how they will compare to the "standard" of a PI combined with two NRTIs is also uncertain. Only direct comparisons within the context of clinical trials will answer this question. Finally, despite the progress and promise inherent in PI–dual NRTI combinations, the response rate is not 100%, particularly in more advanced disease populations (27). Thus, although the development of new agents and classes of agents is awaited, combinations of the currently available PIs, NRTIs, and NNRTIs in three- and four-drug regimens as well as other combinations are currently being evaluated. Table 48B.2 lists the currently approved agents and selected investigational agents of clinical interest.

CONSIDERATIONS IN THE CHOICE OF ANTIRETROVIRAL COMBINATIONS

Baseline Clinical and Laboratory Evaluation

A major component of any therapeutic strategy is the establishment of an accurate baseline because these parameters provide important prognostic information and form the basis for evaluating future treatment responses. This evalua-

Table 48B.2. Approved and Selected Investigational Antiretroviral Agents of the HIV Reverse Transcriptase Inhibitor and Protease Inhibitors Classes

Nucleoside analog reverse transcriptase inhibitors
    Zidovudine (ZDV, AZT, Retrovir)
    Didanosine (ddI, Videx)
    Dideoxycytidine (ddC, HIVID)
    Stavudine (d4T, Zerit)
    Lamivudine (3TC, Epivir)
    Abacavir (ABV, 1592U89)
    Lodenosine (FddA)
Nonnucleoside (HIV-1–specific) reverse transcriptase inhibitors
    Nevirapine (NVP, Virammune)
    Delavirdine (DLV, Rescriptor)
    Efavireuz (EFV, DMP-266, Sustiva)
    Loviride
    HBY-097
    MKC-442
Acyclic nucleoside phosphonate reverse transcriptase inhibitor
    Adefovir dipivoxil (ADV, Preveon)
Protease inhibitors
    Saquinavir (SQV, Invirase)
    Ritonavir (RTV, Norvir)
    Indinavir (IDV, Crixivan)
    Nelfinavir (NFV, Viracept)
    Amprenavir (AMP, 141W94, VX-478)
    ABT-378

tion, of course, needs to encompass both clinical and laboratory parameters because together these define the patient's stage of disease. This may, in turn, influence the nature of the initial regimen chosen as well as the robustness of the antiviral response. Because of assay variability and biologic variation, investigators recommend that two CD4 cell counts and plasma HIV-1 RNA levels be obtained to establish a secure baseline (17, 39). These values should be obtained during a period when no intercurrent illnesses or vaccinations have occurred because these may influence the plasma HIV-1 concentration (40).

Once the baseline status of a patient is established, two questions immediately arise: should the patient be treated with antiretroviral agents, and, if so, with what? Clinical trial and cohort study data suggest that all symptomatic subjects, all subjects with CD4 cell counts lower than 500/mm^3, and all subjects with plasma HIV-1 RNA concentrations higher than 5000 to 10,000 copies/mL should be treated (19, 23, 31–33). Asymptomatic subjects with CD4 cell counts higher than 500/mm^3 and plasma HIV-1 RNA levels lower than 5000 to 10,000 copies/mL are at low risk for near-term disease progression, but most of these subjects still ultimately have disease progression (19). Thus, one should consider instituting treatment in this group as well, particularly because achieving viral suppression should be easier than in patients with advanced disease and high viral loads. The predictably slow progression rate in this group does provide the option of close observation without therapy should one have concerns about the appropriate regimen to start and the patient's commitment to therapy.

Antiretroviral Resistance

Resistance of HIV-1 to the available antiretroviral agents is an important consideration in the selection of an initial regimen from various perspectives. In an antiretrovirally naive subject, the considerations are as follows. First, resistance mutations in the reverse transcriptase or protease gene may exist in the predominant quasispecies as a result of having acquired a resistant strain at the time of infection. Surveillance data suggest that 6 to 8% of new infections in areas of the world with a high penetrance of antiretroviral agent use are with strains harboring zidovudine (ZDV) resistance mutations, and this proportion is increasing with time (41). Plans have been made to expand this surveillance to monitor the acquisition of primary resistance to other reverse transcriptase inhibitors and PIs, but these data do not exist at the present time. Second, the ability of the virus to produce a mutation at every base pair on a daily basis because of the inherent error rate of the reverse transcriptase enzyme and the prolific viral turnover implies that incomplete viral suppression will facilitate the rapid emergence of resistance strains (5). Third, viral strains may exhibit varied patterns of resistance under the influence of the same regimen in different individuals. For example, the reason that the Q151M multidideoxynucleoside genotype complex emerges in approximately 10 to 15% of patients treated with dual nucleoside combinations and whether the baseline polymorphisms in the protease gene affect the pattern of PI resistance are unclear (42, 43). Fourth, agents within a class may differ with respect to their relative ability to induce cross-resistance to other agents within the same class. Table 48B.3 details the mutational resistance pattern among members of the NRTI, NNRTI, and PI classes of agents. This issue is complex, however, because subtle expressions of cross-resistance may exist that are not explicable on a known mutational basis. For example, among the NRTIs, ZDV resistance conferred by the typical ZDV-associated resistance mutations may confer some level of diminished didanosine (ddI) susceptibility not explained by any direct mutational influence (44, 45), and prior experience with with ZDV, ddI, or zalcitabine (ddC) may diminish responsiveness to the dual combination of stavudine (d4T) and lamivudine (3TC) (46). It thus appears that prior drug experience can diminish the response to a new regimen both by direct mutational interactions and by mechanisms not yet fully understood. Finally, although reversion to a more susceptible strain may occur after cessation of selective drug pressure, resistant subspecies persist in the host and can reemerge quickly on reexposure (47).

Evaluation of Response

After the initiation of therapy, the first question to answer is: What is success? Clearly, the expectations for any regimen have risen in the past few years as a result of the availability of new, more potent agents and combinations, the ability to measure responses with plasma HIV-1 RNA quantification more precisely, and the confirmation that peripheral blood markers, HIV-1 expression in lymphoid tissue, prevention of

Table 48B.3. Amino Acid Substitutions Associated with Diminished Susceptibility to Antiretroviral Agents of the HIV Reverse Transcriptase and Protease Inhibitor Classes

A. Nucleoside and Acyclic Nucleoside Phosphonate Reverse Transcriptase Inhibitors

Agent	M41	K65	A62	D67	T69	K70	L74	V75	F77	Y115	F116	Q151	M184	T215	K219	L210
ZDV	L			N		R								Y or F	Q	W
ddI		R			D		V	T					V			
ddC		R					V	T					V	C		
d4T								T								
3TC													V or I			
ABV		R					V						V			
Multi-ddN (ZDV, ddI, ddC, d4T)			V						L	F	Y	M				
ADV		R				E							V			

ABV, abacavir; ADV, adefovir dipivoxil; ddC, dideoxycytidine; dd , didanosine; ddN, dideoxynucleoside; d4T, stavudine; 3TC, lamivudine; ZDV, zidovudine.

B. HIV-1–Specific (Nonnucleoside) Reverse Transcriptase Inhibitors

Agent	L74	V75	A98	L100	K103	V106	V108	E138	V179	Y181	Y188	V189	G190	P236
NVP					N	A	I			C/I	C		A	
DLV				I	N/T					C				L
EFV			G		N					C	L			
Loviride									D					
HBY-097										C	H/L		A	
MKC-442	V/I	L/I			N/R		I	K			I		E/Q/T	

DLV, delavirdine; EFV, efavirenz; NVP, nevirapine.

C. Protease Inhibitors

Agent	L10	K20	L24	D30	V32	L33	M36	M46	I47	G48	I50	I54	L63	A71	V77	V82	I84	N88	L90
SQV	I									V			P	V			V		M
RTV	I/R/V	R				F	I					V		V		A/F/T/S	V		M
IDV		M/R	I		I		I	I				V	P	T/V		A/F/T	V		M
NFV				N										V			V	D	M
AMP	F							I/L	V		V	V	P	V	I				

AMP, amprenavir; IDV, indinavir; NFV, nelfinavir; RTV, ritonavir; SQV, saquinavir.

drug resistance, and clinical outcome parallel one another with more potent therapies (9, 27, 28, 34, 35). Thus, when a patient tolerates a regimen well, is able to maintain a high level of drug adherence, and has an excellent response (defined as reducing the plasma HIV-1 RNA level to below the limits of quantification and raising CD4 cell counts $100/mm^3$ or more), one has little difficulty being comfortable with the therapeutic choice. It is becoming more difficult, however, to declare success when a significant drop in the plasma HIV-1 RNA level is seen, but suppression below the limit of quantification at 16 to 24 weeks does not occur. This difficulty results from the concern that ongoing rounds of virus replication will inevitably lead to the selection of drug-resistant variants. However, is a switch in therapy indicated in someone who has a substantial decrease in viral load (1.5 to 2.0 $\log_{10}$) given that even modest decreases in plasma HV-1 RNA, on the order of 0.5 $\log_{10}$, are associated with a decrease in the risk of disease progression (12, 13)? Given the evolving paradigm of treatment, any detectable virus in the plasma is a concern, and one could justifiably either adjust one component of the regimen or add a fourth drug to try to achieve maximal suppression. Alternatively, and the approach perhaps most commonly taken because of practical concerns, is to continue the same regimen as long as the plasma HIV-1 RNA remains low, even if detectable (e.g., in the range of 400 to 2000 copies/mL) and to change the regimen when a clear rise in plasma HIV-1 RNA is apparent. Given the importance of trying to achieve success with an initial regimen, a strong argument can be made to be aggressive in this circumstance.

The mirror of the difficulty in defining virologic success is that of defining virologic failure. By the strictest definition, any detectable level of virus replication is considered virologic failure, but even this definition is subject to interpretation and is in evolution. For example, in the plasma compartment, increasingly sensitive HIV-1 RNA assays are being developed and applied in clinical trials and will likely move into clinical practice in the near future. Consequently, "detectable" limits of plasma HV-1 RNA will inevitably decline from 400 to 500 copies/mL to 20 to 50 copies/mL. Further, detection of plasma HIV-1 RNA in plasma, which primarily is a reflection of replication in the lymphoid tissue (1–9), is not the only compartment of interest. The central nervous system and genital tract have been termed potential "sanctuary sites." Concentrations of HIV-1 RNA in these anatomic sites cannot be assumed to be direct reflections of the plasma level, although, when antiretroviral therapy is initiated, declines in the HIV-1 RNA concentrations in the cerebrospinal fluid and genital secretions occur in parallel with those seen in plasma (48–51). In the face of "undetectable" plasma HIV-1 RNA concentrations, substantial elevations can be found in these two body compartments, particularly in patients with local infectious or inflammatory conditions (52–55). Sampling of these sites, of course, is not part of routine clinical practice and is not likely to become one. However, one hopes that correlates of virologic success in these compartments will be defined in the context of clinical trials and in this way will become useful tools for the practice setting. For the purposes of this discussion, virologic success is defined as driving the plasma HIV-1 RNA concentration to below the limits of quantification of currently available standard assays (i.e., 400 to 500 copies/mL), with the recognition that this threshold will predictably decrease as more sensitive plasma HIV-1 RNA assays are validated.

INITIAL TREATMENT APPROACHES

From a practical perspective, the choice of a therapeutic strategy involves a regimen that will achieve an acceptable and predictable initial response that is durable, with the simultaneous realization that treatment failure or intolerance is an ever-present possibility. Thus, second and even third alternative regimens need to be thought out in advance. This section attempts to outline several such approaches in an effort to emphasize options without being overly prescriptive, because individualization of therapy is an important basic principle. These approaches are derivative in the sense that specific clinical trials designed to prove the efficacy of a particular strategic approach over the long term have not been done. Results of clinical trials do form the essential database for making recommendations, but one must then link the information from the array of traditional trial designs, which directly compare two or more regimens in a defined population, with cohort studies, knowledge of pathogenesis, and in vitro studies to devise a rational approach to therapy.

Initial Approach No. 1: Protease Inhibitor Plus Two Nucleoside Analog Reverse Transcriptase Inhibitors

This approach has rapidly become the preferential choice for initial therapy. When it is successful, one can expect responses, defined as a dropping plasma HIV-1 RNA copy number below 500 copies/mL, in 70 to 90% of patients. The choice of the dual nucleoside and the PI components should be made on the basis of activity, ease of administration, and the predicted tolerability of the known regimen. Of the approved agents currently available (see Table 48B.2), the dual nucleoside component should be chosen from among ZDV–3TC, d4T–3TC, ZDV–ddI, d4T–ddI, and ZDV–ddC. Of these choices, ZDV–ddI, ZDV–ddC, and ZDV–3TC are supported by clinical and marker end-point data, and d4T–3TC and d4T–ddI are supported by impressive marker response data (23, 24, 46, 56–63). As stand-alone regimens, these five dual nucleoside regimens result in plasma HIV-1 RNA reductions and CD cell count increases of 1.0 to 2.0 $\log_{10}$ copies/mL and 50 to 100 cells/mm^3, respectively. The regimens containing ddI have excellent activity, and extensive data support the clinical benefit of ddI, but intolerance to this agent, the need to take it on an empty stomach, and the presence of the buffer increase the complexity of the regimen and have the potential to affect compliance adversely. Once-daily ddI regimens were studied in the past and are being reinvestigated to reduce the complexity of combination regimens (64, 65). ZDV–3TC and d4T–3TC are the most frequently chosen, based on their activity and tolerability (46, 58–63). Of the available PIs, indinavir (IDV), nelfinavir (NFV), and ritonavir (RTV) offer comparable in vivo activity and thus are preferred as part of initial regimens. Of these three agents, the concern over PI cross-resistance has led to an increasing interest in using NFV in initial regimens because the D30N mutation, generally the first to appear with NFV therapy, does not engender cross-resistance to the other approved PIs (66). The hard gelatin capsule of saquinavir (SQV), because of its low bioavailability, is less ideal, but the development of the soft gelatin capsule may elevate SQV to comparability with the other PIs in the near future (67).

With a potent PI–dual NRTI combination, one should expect an early decline in the plasma HIV-1 RNA concentration within 2 to 4 weeks of initiation of therapy, and it is reasonable to determine that a response has occurred at that time. However, the maximal response to these regimens may not be seen for 16 to 24 weeks because of the "second phase" of HIV-1 RNA decline, presumably reflecting the half-life of longer-lived cell populations, such as monocyte/macrophages (6, 28). Once virologic suppression has occurred, durability for 52 weeks or longer can be attained. Thus, a cautious approach should be taken so potentially efficacious regimens are not prematurely abandoned.

Initial Approach No. 2: Nonnucleoside Reverse Transcriptase Inhibitor Plus Two Nucleoside Analog Reverse Transcriptase Inhibitors

The initiation of treatment with a three-drug regimen consisting of an NNRTI and two NRTIs offers a reasonable alternative to using a PI in drug-naive patients. This choice has been given validity by the preliminary reporting of the INCAS and ISS 047 trials (68, 69). In the INCAS trial, antiretrovirally naive subjects with CD4 cell counts 200 to 600/mm^3 were randomized to one of three arms: ZDV–ddI, ZDV–NVP, or ZDV–ddI–NVP. The proportion of subjects in the ZDV–ddI–NVP arm who achieved a plasma HIV-1 RNA concentration lower than 20 copies/mL at 52 weeks was 51%, a proportion lower than could be expected with a PI regimen (68). Further, in a limited number of subjects studied, NVP resistance was prevented, a finding akin to the prevention of 3TC resistance noted in PI combinations. This finding illustrates that antiretroviral resistance can be prevented by potent virus suppression. In the ISS 047 trial, antiretrovirally naive subjects with less than 200 CD4 cells/mm^3 were randomized to NVP in combination with ZDV–ddI or ZDV–ddI alone. At 24 weeks, most subjects in the three-drug arm had plasma HIV-1 RNA concentrations below 400 copies/mL (69). Although a reasonable alternative, an NNRTI-based three-drug regimen that includes two NRTIs is probably less potent than one that contains a PI, but when the clinician deems it appropriate to defer a PI, this approach is a reasonable alternative that has been endorsed in recently published consensus recommendations (31–33).

Reasons to defer a PI include patient preference and the concern that, should PI resistance develop, the most important class of agents may be compromised. The population for whom this option seems most appropriate is one at a less advanced stage of disease with a moderate plasma HIV-1 RNA level (e.g., fewer than 50,000 copies/mL). For patients with more advanced disease or marked elevations of plasma HIV-1 RNA, a PI-containing regimen is preferred.

Initial Approach No. 3: Two Nucleoside Analog Reverse Transcriptase Inhibitors

The option of treating with a dual NRTI regimen chosen from among ZDV, ddI, ddC, d4T, and 3TC has moved from a primary treatment option to one that is now considered inferior. This evolution in thinking has occurred primarily because these regimens, although conferring benefit, are less potent than three-drug regimens containing either a PI or an NNRTI (27, 28, 68–70). As a consequence, viral suppression is less complete, resistant viral variants can emerge, and the utility of these drugs in future regimens can be compromised. Data indicate, however, that some patients with modest viral loads (e.g., fewer than 10,000 copies/mL) have persistent drops in plasma HIV-1 RNA concentrations below 400 copies/mL (71). However, what proportion of these subjects are highly virally suppressed (i.e., plasma HIV-1 RNA levels lower than 20 to 50 copies/mL), have comparable suppression in lymphoid tissues, and will exhibit durable responses is uncertain. Further, the argument can be made that patients with modest viral loads predictably and durably exhibit virologic suppression on a three-drug regimen, assuming that the caveats inherent in starting a more complex and demanding regimen are considered. Thus, dual NRTI regimens should be reserved for patients who should start treatment but, for whatever reason, who cannot start with a three-drug regimen. In this circumstance, careful thought should be given to which dual NRTI regimen to start. For example, although ZDV–3TC and d4T–3TC are generally well tolerated, easy to administer twice-daily regimens, these regimens inevitably lead to the evolution of the M184V 3TC-associated resistance mutation and potentially severely limit the usefulness of 3TC as a component of a PI-containing regimen in the future. Therefore, should this option be chosen, ZDV–ddI, ZDV–ddC, or d4T–ddI combinations are considered preferable because they will likely preserve 3TC's future usefulness given that the M184V mutation is rarely selected under the selective pressure of ddC or ddI therapy (72, 73).

Initial Approach No. 4: Two Protease Inhibitors

The approach of using two PIs together is based on the additive potency provided by such regimens, the exploitation of pharmacokinetic interactions, and, for some combinations, potentially nonoverlapping or minimally overlapping resistance profiles (38). Most prominent in this regard has been the combination of RTV and SQV. RTV, one of the most powerful CYP3A4 inhibitors, can raise SQV levels 20-fold, and the combination is synergistic in vitro (74). A clinical trial of 4 different dosing regimens of RTV–SQV in nucleoside experienced, protease naive subjects has shown reductions in plasma HIV-1 RNA concentrations on the order of 2.5 $\log_{10}$ with greater than 80% of subjects achieving levels below the quantifiable limit through 48 weeks of follow-up (38). Of the four dosing regimens studied, all were comparably potent, but 400 mg twice daily of both RTV and SQV proved to be the best tolerated. Other dual PI combinations are under evaluation and will likely prove comparably potent in PI-naive patients (Table 48B.4). Data on proper dosing, durability, tolerability, and genotypic resistance patterns that emerge on these regimens will be important to compare their relative merit properly. For example, whether viral variants that breakthrough a dual PI regimen will exhibit broader cross-resistance profiles that will constrain future treatment options is unknown.

Initial Approach No. 5: Protease Inhibitor Plus Nonnucleoside Reverse Transcriptase Inhibitor Plus Nucleoside Analog Reverse Transcriptase Inhibitors

Investigators have shown increasing interest in combining PIs with NNRTIs, given the inherent potency of both classes of agents. Combinations using these two classes have been delayed in their development because of the concerns about drug interactions; both classes of drugs are metabolized by the CYP3A4 P450 hepatic enzyme system, and appropriate drug interaction studies were not available at the time of approval of these agents. This situation, however, is quickly changing as data emerge. Each PI–NNRTI combination needs to be individually studied to derive the correct dosing regimen because the interactions vary with the relative degrees of hepatic enzyme induction, inhibition, or competition for metabolism for which the agents in these classes are responsible. Examples of this complexity are the reduction in PI levels generally noted with NVP and efavirenz (EFV) and the elevation caused by delavirdine.

Most prominent among the PI–NNRTI combinations is IDV–EFV because 88% of subjects have been reported to exhibit plasma HIV-1 RNA levels below 400 copies/mL through 48 weeks of follow-up (75). Despite these impressive and encouraging results, most investigators recommend that, with our currently available agents, a single PI–NNRTI combination be supplemented with NRTIs to try to protect the regimen from virologic breakthrough. This approach is being formally studied in AIDS Clinical Trials Group (ACTG) Study 368, in which the placebo-controlled addition of abacavir (1592U89) to IDV–EFV is being studied in nucleoside-experienced subjects. Numerous other combinations involving NVP, delavirdine, and EFV with various PIs are being studied. Although PI–NNRTI–NRTIs regimens probably will prove efficacious in naive subjects as an initial regimen, data are insufficient to recommend these regimens formally. The risk of such a regimen is that, should viral breakthrough occur, resistance to the three available classes of agents could evolve and compromise many future options.

Initial Approach No. 6: Three Nucleoside Analog Reverse Transcriptase Inhibitors

Data are limited concerning the efficacy of triple NRTI combinations, but modest interest has been shown in pursuing this approach as initial therapy as a way to defer both PI and NNRTI usage. The regimens studied thus far have been predominantly ZDV–ddI–3TC and ZDV–ddC–3TC (76, 77). In patients with primary infection, these combinations have been associated with substantial plasma HIV-1 RNA declines and reductions in lymphoid tissue HIV-1 RNA expression (77). A triple NRTI regimen of particular interest is ZDV–3TC–abacavir, which is currently under study.

MANAGEMENT OF FAILURE OR TOXICITY ON INITIAL REGIMEN

The management of treatment failure is one of the greatest challenges facing patients and clinicians because few data from clinical trials are available to guide decision making. Thus, one must deduce practical information from certain guiding principles. These include the concept that ongoing rounds of viral replication in the face of a failing regimen will lead to increasing degrees of resistance, that the potential for cross-resistance may limit the effectiveness of future options, that antiretrovirally experienced patients, in general, demonstrate smaller degrees of marker responses than antiretrovirally naive subjects that may not always be directly explicable on the basis of known mutations conferring cross-resistance, and that, despite the availability of 11 approved agents with more on the horizon, the options for alternative regimens are limited. These considerations lead to the conclusion, now accepted as a standard of clinical practice, that a minimum of two, and when possible all drugs, in a failing regimen should be changed. This precept may be mitigated in the future to some extent if genotypic resistance testing matures to a state at which greater selectivity in choice may be appropriate, particularly if a change is made at a relatively low plasma HIV-1 RNA concentration. Table 48B.5 lists generic alternatives in the setting of treatment failure after various initial regimens.

Currently, the greatest concern with respect to the management of treatment failure surrounds the issue of managing

Table 48B.4. Dual Protease Inhibitor Combinations Under Consideration for Clinical Use

	Saquinavir	Ritonavir	Indinavir	Nelfinavir	141W94
Saquinavir		X		X	X
Ritonavir	X		X	X	X
Indinavir		X		X	X
Nelfinavir	X	X	X		X
Amprenavir	X	X	X	X	

Table 48B.5. Initial Antiretroviral Agent Combinations and Examples of Alternative Regimens in the Case of Treatment Failure

Initial Regimen[a]	Alternative after Treatment Failure[b]
$NRTI_1/NRTI_2/PI_1$ →	$NRTI_3/NRTI_4/PI_2$
	$NRTI_3/NRTI_4/PI_2/NNRTI$
	$PI_2/PI_3 \pm NRTI_3/NRTI_4 \pm NNRTI$
$NRTI_1/NRTI_2/NNRTI$ →	$NRTI_3/NRTI_4/PI_1$
	$PI_1/PI_2 \pm NRTI_3/NRTI_4$
$NRTI_1/NRTI_2$[c] →	$NRTI_3/NRTI_4/PI_1$
	$PI_1/PI_2 \pm NRTI_3/NRTI_4 \pm NNRTI$
PI_1/PI_2 →	$NRTI_1/NRTI_2/PI_3/NNRTI$
	$NRTI_1/NRTI_2/PI_3/PI_4/NNRTI$
$NRTI_1/NNRTI/PI_1$ →	$NRTI_2/NRTI_3/PI_2/PI_3$
$NRTI_1/NRTI_2/NRTI_3$ →	$PI_1/PI_2 \pm NRTI_4 \pm NNRTI$

NNRTI, nonnucleoside reverse transcriptase inhibitor; NRTI, nucleoside analog reverse transcriptase inhibitor; PI, protease inhibitor.

[a,b]The role of adefovir dipivoxil as part of initial or alternative combination regimens is not yet defined, but its potency suggests that its place will be as a supplement to some of the combination regimens listed.

[a]The first two regimens listed reflect recommendations of currently published guidelines (31–33). See footnote c regarding dual NRTI regimens. The last three options are currently being evaluated and have shown promise, but data are still limited.

[b]In the setting of treatment failure, dual PI regimens should be supplemented with NRTIs or NNRTIs to try to maximize the potency of the alternative regimen given the increasingly limited options, particularly after treatment failure with an initial PI-containing regimen. NNRTIs are not listed as part of alternative regimens after treatment failure with an initial NNRTI-containing regimen because of probable cross-resistance. However, some NNRTIs may be useful in this circumstance, depending on the number and the nature of the NNRTI-associated resistance mutations that have been acquired (e.g., efavirenz retains activity against isolates with the Y181C mutation).

[c]Dual nucleoside analog regimens are now considered suboptimal as initial regimens, but they are included for completeness (see text).

failure with PI-containing regimens, given the degree of cross-resistance that exists among the available agents in this class. The available database is incomplete to guide clinicians fully, but some information is beginning to emerge. Preliminary reports suggest that the response to either IDV or NFV after long-term SQV exposure is blunted (78, 79), and the utility of RTV–SQV in the setting of prior PI failure is variable. Although one report suggests short-term success with this dual PI combination, others suggest that the response rate in this situation is suboptimal (80, 81). Operationally, this situation leaves clinicians in the position of making an empiric choice that typically involves a combination of one or two new PIs with two new NRTIs and possibly an NNRTI. The efficacy of currently approved as well as experimental agents in the management of PI failure is currently being evaluated in numerous studies, and these controlled trial data are urgently needed.

Certain evolving principles in the management of drug toxicity derive from the changing environment created by the era of potent antiretroviral chemotherapy and the desire to avoid extended periods of partially suppressive therapy that could lead to the evolution of resistance. Practically, this translates into avoiding dose reductions whenever possible and, when medication interruption is mandated for more than a brief period by the clinical situation, temporarily stopping the entire regimen rather than one component. If a regimen has been successful and toxicity can be ascribed to one component of a combination, then substitution of that single agent with another drug of comparable potency is appropriate.

STRATEGIC APPROACHES

Several potential strategic approaches to the long-term therapy of HIV disease exist, most of which are being evaluated in the clinical trial setting (Table 48B.6). These approaches are described in the following sections.

Current "Standard"

In the context of this discussion, the current "standard" refers to the approach of initiating therapy with a potent regimen and maintaining as potent a regimen as possible with routine clinical, plasma HIV-1 RNA, and CD4 cell count monitoring. Until data emerge, this can be considered the most conservative approach that is supported by the available information.

Induction and Maintenance

A potentially important strategic approach to the management of HIV disease involves initiating treatment with a potent combination regimen designed to drive viral replication to below quantifiable limits and, after an extended period of viral suppression, reducing the regimen to one that is simpler such that toxicity is minimized and adherence is maximized over the long term. The rationale behind this approach derives from the recently developed views of pathogenesis in which both short- and longer-lived cell pools are theoretically reduced in the face of complete viral suppression (6). If such is indeed the case, then the smaller, suppressed viral population can be held in check by a less potent, simpler maintenance regimen. This approach can

Table 48B.6. Strategic Antiretroviral Therapeutic Approaches

Current standard
  Initiate therapy with a potent combination regimen designed to reduce plasma HIV-1 RNA level below limit of quantification and maintain as long as therapeutic goal is achieved and regimen is tolerated; alternative regimens introduced for treatment failure or toxicity
Induction and Maintenance
  Initiate therapy with a potent combination regimen and, after a period of virus suppression, reduce the regimen to one that is simpler and easier to maintain, to maximize drug adherence
Intensification
  Initiate therapy with a potent combination regimen and intensify regimen with addition of a new agent or agents if a submaximal but acceptable virologic response has been achieved
  For those whose plasma HIV-1 RNA levels are already suppressed below the limits of quantification, add a supplemental agent to try to prolong period of virologic suppression
Eradication
  Currently a hypothetic goal of therapy with numerous challenges, including the integrated nature of retroviral genomes, long-lived cell populations that may harbor replication competent virus, and potential sanctuary sites such as the central nervous system and genital tract

only be recommended after it is proved effective in an appropriate clinical trial setting. This view is supported by the negative results of two clinical trials that were recently reported (82, 83). In these studies (Trilege and ACTG 343), viewed in summary fashion, randomization to simplified regimens (ZDV–3TC, ZDV–IDV, IDV) after 3 to 6 months of induction therapy with ZDV–3TC–IDV was virologically inferior to continuing the three-drug regimen. These studies do not undercut the principle behind the strategy of induction–maintenance, but rather, they suggest that longer induction periods or more potent maintenance regimens will be necessary to achieve durable virologic suppression. Other simplified maintenance protocols are being planned, but a suggestion that this approach is feasible has come from the INCAS trial (68). In this study, as detailed earlier, impressive results were obtained in the ZDV plus ddI plus NVP arm, with 51% of subjects achieving plasma HIV-1 RNA concentrations lower than 20 copies/mL at 52 weeks. Although the ZDV plus NVP arm of the trial performed inferiorly as an initial treatment, five subjects in the three-drug arm who had achieved viral suppression but who discontinued the ddI component were able to maintain virologic suppression (68). Despite this hint of "proof of principle" of the induction–maintenance strategy, obvious questions and risks must be considered. For example, even if the pool of infected cells is reduced during the induction phase, a maintenance regimen of reduced potency may still permit viral escape. If this occurs, the degree of antiretroviral resistance that develops may limit the potential to reintroduce the induction regimen and may compromise other agents because of cross-resistance. The key to this strategy, therefore, relies on the correctness of the underlying pathogenetic principles and the potency of the induction and maintenance regimens. Future regimens that exploit improved pharmacokinetic profiles of newer agents will likely permit maintenance regimens to achieve high degrees of potency, equivalent to our most potent current induction regimens, and simplicity simultaneously.

Intensification

One of the important questions in strategic management is whether the durability of a successful regimen can be prolonged by intensification of treatment. This term refers to the addition of one or more agents to a current combination that has resulted in virologic success, defined as suppression of plasma HIV-1 RNA to below the limit of quantification. The rationale behind this approach is that waiting for virologic failure before making a change in therapy may, in some circumstances, be too late because substantial resistance may have already arisen and alternative regimens may be compromised. Agents that can develop substantial single-step resistance are at most risk (e.g., 3TC and the NNRTIs), but even agents that require multiple mutations to demonstrate a decrease in phenotypic susceptibility (e.g., PIs) may be compromised by the insertion of a "critical" mutation (e.g., V82A/F/T for RTV or IDV; see Table 48B.3) (84–87). Proponents of intensification would argue that the best strategy would be to try to prevent the development of any resistance mutations by preempting the potential for viral escape. For an agent to be useful in this setting, it must be potent, well tolerated, and simple to administer such that adherence to the overall regimen is not adversely affected. Candidate compounds for this role include the NNRTI agents and the experimental nucleoside analog, abacavir, among others. Of course, problems and potential risks associated with pursuing intensification raise certain questions. These include the following: Which drugs to use? When is the proper time to supplement successful therapy? Is the risk of significant drug interactions being introduced? What is the risk to the underlying regimen should a toxicity supervene? The answers to these questions, of course, are only speculative at this stage, and the only way to be able to assess this approach is through appropriately conducted clinical trials. One such study, the placebo-controlled addition of abacavir to subjects with plasma HIV-1 RNA concentrations persistently suppressed below 500 copies/mL with IDV plus ZDV (or d4T) plus 3TC is currently being conducted by the ACTG (ACTG 372A).

Another potential role for intensification is during the initial phase of antiretroviral treatment should the response not be as complete as desired. As noted earlier, the maximum antiviral response achieved with potent regimens may not be evident for 16 to 24 weeks after initiation because of the second phase decay of longer-lived infected cell populations (6, 28). If a regimen demonstrates a good but incomplete response (e.g., a plasma HIV-1 RNA level that declines by 1.5 $\log_{10}$ but does not fall below quantifiable limits), the addition of agents to that regimen may achieve the desired response. This approach has been preliminarily validated in the trial of RTV–SQV in which 13 subjects whose plasma HIV-1 RNA level did not fall below the assay limit of quantification had d4T–3TC added. In 12 of 13 subjects, HIV-1 RNA suppression to below the assay limit was achieved and remained durable through 48 weeks of follow-up (38).

Eradication

In strict terms, eradication of the virus is not a strategy at this time and should only be considered a hypothesis for clinical research. In a certain sense, eradication represents an extension of the rationale behind the induction–maintenance approach in that it depends on maintaining viral suppression long enough to permit latently infected cell populations in all compartments to die. The calculated half-lives of longer-lived infected cell populations had suggested that this could theoretically be accomplished in approximately 3 years, but more recent experimental data suggest that the persistence of infected, resting, memory CD4 lymphocytes will extend this estimate, if not undermine the hypothesis entirely (6, 8, 88).

FUTURE CONSIDERATIONS

The progress made in the monitoring and treatment of patients with HIV infection in the past 2 to 3 years has simultaneously highlighted what is achievable and what further issues need to be addressed. Some of these issues are described in the next sections.

Nonresponders

Clearly, the response to three-drug therapy including a potent PI is not uniform. The proportion of patients who do not respond or do not maintain a response varies from 10 to 50%, depending on the potency of the regimen, the stage of disease, the prior antiretroviral exposure history, the drug susceptibility profile, interpatient variability in drug absorption and metabolism, and drug adherence. For patients with more advanced disease and greater degrees of antiretroviral exposure, more intensive regimens than those represented by a PI and two nucleoside analogs are likely to be required if response rates higher than 90% are to be achieved.

Pharmacologic Considerations

The PI and NNRTI classes of agents have brought into sharp focus the importance of the pharmacologic characteristics of the agents used in multidrug regimens. The influence of food on absorption, the drug interactions among antiretroviral agents and between these agents and the other drugs (both HIV-related and unrelated), the interpatient variability in drug handling, and the differential reporting of the correlation of drug concentrations with either plasma HIV-1 RNA response or the lower potential for the emergence of genotypic resistance have created challenges for clinicians (84, 89). Simultaneously, however, new avenues for investigation, drug development, and patient monitoring have been opened. Drug formulations that maximize bioavailability and extend half-lives will become increasingly important in therapy. For simplicity and safety, it will be desirable to minimize the array of drug interactions now seen with some of the approved agents, but as the field grows more sophisticated, these interactions will be exploited to try to maximize benefit, as has been seen with dual PI combinations (38). Finally, the question whether therapeutic drug level monitoring has value in the routine monitoring of patients needs to be addressed. For this approach to be of value, however, more data will be needed to determine the agents for which these data correlate with response, to decide whether the information truly assists clinicians, and to ascertain whether the cost of the assays can be justified.

Other Modalities

This review has concentrated on the chemotherapeutic aspects of treatment, but interest is keen in other modalities that target the immune system directly. Although the availability of potent combination regimens has resulted in CD4 cell rises not heretofore seen with previously available therapies, immune reconstitution is not complete. Reports to date indicate that, although both memory and naive CD4 cells and functional immune improvement can be restored after PI treatment, restoration to normal levels does not appear to occur (90). Should this observation be confirmed in future studies of current and newer regimens, concomitant immunomodulatory treatment may become an important component of combination regimens for selected individuals. The impressive quantitative results reported thus far with interleukin-2 make this the most prominent such treatment to test (91). For example, although it is not efficacious in patients with CD4 cell counts lower than $200/mm^3$ in the early experience, interleukin-2 may be potentially beneficial when integrated with potent regimens in patients with more advanced disease. In those with earlier stage disease, more complete immune restoration may be accomplishable with immune modulation. Interleukin-2 may also be of interest to study in combination with PIs in the situations in which the CD4 cell rise appears to be "capped" or in those individuals who achieve only a limited or no CD4 cell rise. These situations may provide new pathogenetic insights into CD4 cell regeneration.

Patient Monitoring

As the treatments for HIV infection improve and as disease progression rates continue to decline, an increasing priority will be placed on refining the laboratory aspects of patient monitoring to characterize patients initiating therapy more precisely and to monitor patient responses on treatment more carefully. These developing aspects of more precise patient monitoring include several components. First is the use of *more sensitive HIV-1 RNA assays*. As interest grows in suppressing viral replication as completely as possible and in the ability to assess this goal in the clinical situation, the latest generation of HIV-1 quantification assays likely will increasingly move into routine testing. The ability to assess whether suppression of plasma HIV-1 RNA to levels below 20 to 50 copies/mL occurs rather than the threshold of 400 to 500 copies/mL may have important implications for the reflection of HIV-1 expression in lymphoid tissue and consequently the prevention of viral escape and resistance. The second component is *resistance testing*. Increasing interest has been shown in whether antiretroviral resistance assays (genotypic or phenotypic) will be valuable in patient management. Although such assays are becoming commercially available, the validation that these assays will be useful in routine patient monitoring is awaited. ZDV is the only agent for which phenotypic and genotypic resistance has been associated with clinical disease progression, but loss of plasma HIV-1 RNA or CD4 cell count responses has been associated with genotypic resistance to other NRTIs and members of the NNRTI and PI classes of agents (45, 84–86, 92–95). Therefore, one may logically conclude that assessing drug susceptibilities will be useful in patient management. However, many questions have yet to be answered. These include the type of assay that will prove most useful, the problems inherent in deducing phenotypic susceptibility from a genotypic profile, the possibility that population sequencing may not detect important subpopulations that could quickly emerge as a dominant species when brought under the appropriate selective pressure, and the ability to justify the cost of these assays. Third is *therapeutic drug level monitoring*, which is discussed earlier. The final component is *CD4 subset monitoring*. Although now reserved for research purposes, the monitoring of CD4 cell subpopulation (i.e., memory and naive cell) changes may well enter clinical practice as a means of assessing the degree of immune reconstitution achieved.

Improved Access

Although access to the best current therapies has improved in developed countries as the proof of their benefit has become irrefutable, these same countries have underserved populations for whom greater efforts at outreach need to be made so the benefits of early diagnosis and aggressive treatment can be more widely realized. Perhaps even more pressing is the dilemma this progress has created for governments, nongovernmental organizations, and pharmaceutical firms with respect to the developing world, where most infected persons live and where the greatest numbers of new infections are occurring. Although this access may seem an unlikely and wishful prospect at this stage, only through an imaginative and persistent effort by all interested parties will this gradually emerging moral imperative be addressed.

The developments witnessed in the field of antiretroviral therapy over the past decade have formed the foundation for a well-founded hope that the long-term control of HIV disease can be achieved. An even more intense basic and clinical research effort will be needed over the next decade to secure this progress and to make this hope a reality.

References

1. Wei X, Ghosh SK, Taylor ME, et al. Viral dynamics in human immunodeficiency virus type 1 infection. Nature 1995;373:117–122.
2. Ho DD, Neumann AU, Perelson AS, et al. Rapid turnover of plasma virions and CD4 lymphocytes in HIV-1 infection. Nature 1995;373:123–126.
3. Fauci AS. Host factors and the pathogenesis of HIV-induced disease. Nature 1996;384:529–534.
4. Havlir D, Richman D. Viral dynamics of HIV: implications for drug development and therapeutic strategies. Ann Intern Med 1996;124:984–994.
5. Perelson AS, Neumann AU, Markowitz M, et al. HIV-1 dynamics in vivo: virion clearance rate, infected cell life-span, and viral generation time. Science 1996;271:1582–1586.
6. Perelson AS, Essunger P, Cao Y, et al. Decay characteristics of HIV-1–infected compartments during combination therapy. Nature 1997;387:188–191.
7. Haase AT, Henry K, Zupancic M, et al. Quantitative image analysis of HIV-1 infection in lymphoid tissue. Science 1996;274:985–989.
8. Chun TW, Carruth L, Finzl D, et al. Quantification of latent tissue reservoirs and total body viral load in HIV-1 infection. Nature 1997;387:183–188.
9. Cavert W, Notermans DW, Staskus K, et al. Kinetics of response in lymphoid tissues to antiretroviral therapy of HIV-1 infection. Science 1997;276:960–964.
10. Saag MS, Holodniy M, Kuritzkes DR, et al. HIV viral load markers in clinical practice. Nature Med 1996;2:625–629.
11. Mellors JW, Rinaldo CR Jr, Gupta P, et al. Prognosis in HIV-1 infection predicted by the quantity of virus in plasma. Science 1996;272:1167–1170.
12. Coombs RW, Welles SL, Hooper MD, et al. Association of plasma human immunodeficiency virus type-1 RNA level with risk of clinical progression in patients with advanced infection. J Infect Dis 1996;174:704–712.
13. Welles SL, Jackson JB, Yen-Lieberman B, et al. Prognostic value of plasma HIV-1 RNA levels in patients with advanced HIV-1 disease and with little or no zidovudine therapy. J Infect Dis 1996;174:696–703.
14. Katzenstein D, Hammer S, Hughes M, et al. The relation of virologic and immunologic markers to clinical outcomes after nucleoside therapy in HIV-infected adults with 200 to 500 CD4 cells per cubic millimeter. N Engl J Med 1996;335:1091–1098.
15. Phillips AN, Eron JJ, Bartlett JA, et al. HIV-1 RNA levels and the development of clinical disease. AIDS 1996;10:859–865.
16. Paxton WB, Coombs RW, McElrath MJ, et al. Longitudinal analysis of quantitative virologic measures in human immunodeficiency virus–infected subjects with ≥400 CD4 lymphocytes: implications for applying measurements to individual patients. J Infect Dis 1997;175:247–254.
17. Hughes MD, Johnson VA, Hirsch MS, et al. Monitoring plasma HIV-1 RNA levels in addition to CD4+ lymphocyte count improved assessment of antiretroviral therapeutic response. Ann Intern Med 1997;126:929–938.
18. O'Brien WA, Hartigan PM, Daar ES, et al. Changes in plasma HIV RNA levels and CD4+ lymphocyte counts predict both response to antiretroviral therapy and therapeutic failure. Ann Intern Med 1997;126:939–945.
19. Mellors JW, Munoz A, Giorgi JV, et al. Plasma viral load and CD4+ lymphocytes as prognostic markers of HIV-1 infection. Ann Intern Med 1997;126:946–954.
20. Brun-Vezinet F, Boucher C, Loveday C, et al. HIV-1 viral load, phenotype, and resistance in a subset of drug-naive participants from the Delta trial. Lancet 1997;350:983–990.
21. Hammer SM. Advances in antiretroviral therapy and viral load monitoring. AIDS 1996;10(Suppl 3):S1–S11.
22. Deeks SG, Smith M, Holodniy M, et al. HIV-1 protease inhibitors: a review for clinicians. JAMA 1997;277:145–153.
23. Hammer SM, Katzenstein D, Hughes M, et al. A trial comparing nucleoside monotherapy with combination therapy in HIV-infected adults with CD4 cell counts between 200 and 500 per cubic millimeter. N Engl J Med 1996;335:1081–1090.
24. Delta Coordinating Committee. Delta: A randomised double-blind controlled trial comparing combinations of zidovudine plus didanosine or zalcitabine with zidovudine alone in HIV-infected individuals. Lancet 1996;348:283–291.
25. Cameron DW, Heath-Chiozzi M, Kravcik S, et al. Prolongation of life and prevention of AIDS complications in advanced HIV immunodeficiency with ritonavir: update [abstract Mo.B.411]. In: Abstracts of the 11th International Conference on AIDS, Vancouver, 1996;1:24.
26. Salgo M, Beattie D, Bragman K, et al. Saquinavir (Invirase, SQV) vs. HIVID (zalcitabine, ddC) vs. combination as treatment for advanced HIV infection in patients discontinuing/unable to take Retrovir (zidovudine ZDV) [abstract Mo.B.410]. In: Abstracts of the 11th International Conference on AIDS, Vancouver, 1996;1:24.
27. Hammer SM, Squires KE, Hughes MD, et al. A controlled trial of two nucleoside analogues plus indinavir in persons with human immunodeficiency virus infection and CD4 cell counts of 200 per cubic millimeter or less. N Engl J Med 1997;337:725–733.
28. Gulick RM, Mellors JW, Havlir D, et al. Treatment with indinavir, zidovudine, and lamivudine in adults with human immunodeficiency virus infection and prior antiretroviral therapy. N Engl J Med 1997;337:734–739.
29. Centers for Disease Control and Prevention. Update: trends in AIDS incidence—United States, 1996. MMWR Morb Mortal Wkly Rep 1997;46:861–887.

30. Joep MA, Richman DD. The first blow is half the battle. Antiviral Ther 1997;2:132–133.
31. Carpenter CCJ, Fischl MA, Hammer SM, et al. Antiretroviral therapy for HIV infection in 1997: updated recommendations of the International AIDS Society–USA panel. JAMA 1997;26:1962–1969.
32. Centers for Disease Control and Prevention. Guidelines for the use of antiretroviral agents in HIV-infected adults and adolescents. MMWR Morb Mortal Wkly Rep 1998 (in press).
33. Centers for Disease Control and Prevention. Report of the NIH panel to define principles of therapy of HIV infection. MMWR Morb Mortal Wkly Rep 1998 (in press).
34. Wong JK, Gunthard HF, Havlir DV, et al. Reduction of HIV in blood and lymph nodes after potent antiretroviral therapy [abstract LB10]. In: Program and Abstracts of the 4th Conference on Retroviruses and Opportunistic Infections. Washington, DC: American Society for Microbiology, 1997:207.
35. Gunthard H, Wong J, Ignacio C, et al. Emergence of drug resistance in different tissue compartments in 10 patients using population-based sequencing after 1 year of potent antiretroviral therapy [abstract 66]. In: Abstracts of the International Workshop on HIV Drug Resistance, Treatment Strategies, and Eradication, St. Petersburg, FL, 1997.
36. Freimuth WW, Wathen LK, Cox SR, et al. Delavirdine in combination with zidovudine causes sustained antiviral and immunological effects in HIV-1 infected individuals [abstract LB8a]. In: Abstracts of the 3rd Conference on Retroviruses and Opportunistic Infections. Washington, DC: American Society for Microbiology, 1996.
37. Freimuth WW, Chuang-Stein CJ, Greenwald CA, et al. Delavirdine + didanosine combination therapy has sustained surrogate marker response in advanced HIV-1 population [abstract LB8b]. In: Abstracts of the 3rd Conference on Retroviruses and Opportunistic Infections. Washington, DC: American Society for Microbiology, 1996.
38. Granneman GR, Hsu A, Sun E, et al. Pharmacokinetics/pharmacodynamics of ritonavir–saquinavir combination therapy [abstract 609]. In: Program and Abstracts of the 4th Conference on Retroviruses and Opportunistic Infections. Washington, DC: American Society for Microbiology, 1997:177.
39. Saag MS. Use of HIV viral load in clinical practice: back to the future. Ann Intern Med 1997;126:983–985.
40. Stanley SK, Ostrowski MA, Justement JS, et al. Effect of immunization with a common recall antigen on viral expression in patients infected with human immunodeficiency virus type 1. N Engl J Med 1996;334:1222–1230.
41. Yerly S, Rakik A, Kinloch-de-Loes S, et al. Prevalence of transmission of zidovudine-resistant viruses in Switzerland: l'Etude suisse de cohorte VIH. Schweiz Med Wochenschr 1996;126:1845–1848.
42. Shirasaka T, Kavlick MF, Ueno T, et al. Emergence of human immunodeficiency virus type 1 variants with resistance to multiple dideoxynucleosides in patients receiving therapy with dideoxynucleosides. Proc Natl Acad Sci U S A 1995;92:2398–2402.
43. Iversen AK, Shafer RW, Wehrly K, et al. Multidrug-resistant human immunodeficiency virus type 1 strains resulting from combination antiretroviral therapy. J Virol 1996;70:1086–1090.
44. Mayers DL, Japour AJ, Arduino JM, et al. Dideoxynucleoside resistance emerges with prolonged zidovudine monotherapy: the RV43 Study Group. Antimicrob Agents Chemother 1994;38:307–314.
45. D'Aquila RT, Johnson VA, Welles SL, et al. Zidovudine resistance and HIV-1 disease progression during antiretroviral therapy: AIDS Clinical Trials Group Protocol 116B/117 Team and the Virology Committee Resistance Working Group. Ann Intern Med 1995;122:401–408.
46. Katlama C, Valantin MA, Calvez V, et al. ALTIS: A pilot open study of d4T/3TC in antiretroviral naive and experienced patients [abstract LB4]. In: Program and Abstracts of the 4th Conference on Retroviruses and Opportunistic Infections. Washington, DC: American Society for Microbiology, 1997:206.
47. Boucher CA, van Leeuwen R, Kellman P, et al. Effects of discontinuation of zidovudine treatment on zidovudine sensitivity of human immunodeficiency virus type 1 isolates. Antimicrob Agents Chemother 1993;37:1525–1530.
48. Gisslen M, Norkrans G, Svennerholm B, et al. The effect on human immunodeficiency virus type 1 RNA levels in cerebrospinal fluid after initiation of zidovudine or didanosine. J Infect Dis 1997;175:434–437.
49. Vernazza PL, Gilliam BL, Flepp M, et al. Effect of antiviral treatment on the shedding of HIV-1 in semen. AIDS 1997;11:1249–1254.
50. Gupta P, Mellors J, Kingsley L, et al. High viral load in semen of human immunodeficiency virus type 1–infected men at all stages of disease and its reduction by therapy with protease and nonnucleoside reverse transcriptase inhibitors. J Virol 1997;71:6271–6275.
51. Cohen MS, Hoffman IF, Royce RA, et al. Reduction of concentration of HIV-1 in semen after treatment of urethritis: implications for prevention of sexual transmission of HIV-1. AIDSCAP Malawi Research Group. Lancet 1997;349:1868–1873.
52. Lafeuillade A, Poggi C, Pelligrino P, et al. HIV-1 replication in the plasma and cerebrospinal fluid. Infection 1996;24:367–371.
53. Brew BJ, Pemberton L, Cunningham P, et al. Levels of human immunodeficiency virus type 1 RNA in cerebrospinal fluid correlate with AIDS dementia stage. J Infect Dis 1997;175:963–966.
54. Liuzzi G, Chirianni A, Clementi M, et al. Analysis of HIV-1 load in blood, semen, and saliva: evidence for different viral compartments in a cross-sectional and longitudinal study. AIDS 1996;10:F51–F56.
55. Zhu T, Wang N, Carr A, et al. Genetic characterization of human immunodeficiency virus type 1 in blood and genital secretions: evidence for viral compartmentalization and selection during sexual transmission. J Virol 1996;70:3098–3107.
56. Saravolatz L, Winslow DL, Collins G, et al. Zidovudine alone or in combination with didanosine or zalcitabine in HIV-infected patients with the acquired immunodeficiency syndrome or fewer than 200 CD4 cells per cubic millimeter. N Engl J Med 1996;335:1099–1106.
57. CAESAR Coordinating Committee. Randomised trial of addition of lamivudine or lamivudine plus loviride to zidovudine-containing regimens for patients with HIV-1 infection: the CAESAR trial. Lancet 1997;349:1413–1421.
58. Eron JJ, Benoit SL, Jemsek J, et al. Treatment with lamivudine, zidovudine, or both in HIV-positive patients with 200 to 500 CD4+ cells per cubic millimeter: North American HIV Working Party. N Engl J Med 1995;333:1662–1669.
59. Katlama C, Ingrand D, Loveday C, et al. Safety and efficacy of lamivudine–zidovudine combination therapy in antiretroviral-naive patients: a randomized controlled comparison with zidovudine monotherapy. JAMA 1996;276:118–125.
60. Bartlett J, Benoit S, Johnson VA, et al. Lamivudine plus zidovudine compared with zalcitabine plus zidovudine in patients with HIV infection: a randomized, double-blind, placebo-controlled trial. North American HIV Working Party. Ann Intern Med 1996;125:161–172.
61. Staszewski S, Loveday C, Picazo JJ, et al. Safety and efficacy of lamivudine zidovudine combination therapy in zidovudine-experienced patients: a randomized controlled comparison with zidovudine monotherapy. JAMA 1996;276:111–117.
62. Kuritzkes DR, for the ACTG 306 Study Team. ACTG 306 week 24 final analysis: executive summary, 1997.
63. Pollard R, Peterson D, Hardy D, et al. Stavudine (d4T) and didanosine (ddI) combination therapy in HIV-infected subjects: antiviral effect and safety in an ongoing pilot randomized double-blinded trial [abstract Th.B.293]. In: Abstracts of the 11th International Conference on AIDS, Vancouver, 1996:225.
64. Cooley TP, Kunches LM, Saunders CA, et al. Once-daily administration of 2′,3′-dideoxyinosine (ddI) in patients with acquired immunodeficiency syndrome or AIDS-related complex: results of a phase I trial. N Engl J Med 1990;322:1340–1345.
65. Reynes J, Denisi R, Bicart-See A, et al. Stadi pilot study: once daily administration of didanosine in combination with stavudine in antiretroviral naive patients [abstract 128A]. In: 37th Interscience Conference on Antimicrobial Agents and Chemotherapy, Toronto, 1997.
66. Patick AK, Kuritzkes D, Johnson VA, et al. Genotypic and phenotypic analyses of HIV-1 variants isolated from patients treated with nelfinavir and other HIV-1 protease inhibitors [abstract 18]. In: Abstracts of the

International Workshop on HIV Drug Resistance, Treatment Strategies, and Eradication, St. Petersburg, FL, 1997.
67. Borleffs JC, Boucher CA, Bravenboer B, et al. Saquinavir-soft gelatine capsules versus indinavir as part of AZT and 3TC containing triple therapy [abstract 192]. In: 37th Interscience Conference on Antimicrobial Agents and Chemotherapy, Toronto, 1997.
68. Harris M, Rachlis A, Schillington A, et al. Long-term suppression of HIV in plasma with a combination of two nucleosides and nevirapine [abstract I-86]. In: 37th Interscience Conference on Antimicrobial Agents and Chemotherapy, Toronto, 1997.
69. Vella S, Floridia M, Tomino C, et al. A triple combination of reverse transcriptase inhibitors (2 NRTI + 1 NNRTI) induced pronounced and sustained effects on RNA and CD4 in antiretroviral-naive patients with very advanced disease [abstract LB-7]. In: 37th Interscience Conference on Antimicrobial Agents and Chemotherapy, Toronto, 1997.
70. Powderly W, Sension M, Conant M, et al. The efficacy of viracept (nelfinavir mesylate, NFV) in pivotal phase II/III double-blind randomized controlled trials as monotherapy and combination with d4T or AZT/3TC [abstract 370]. In: Program and Abstracts of the 4th Conference on Retroviruses and Opportunistic Infections. Washington, DC: American Society for Microbiology, 1997:132.
71. Opravil M, Demasi R, Hill A, et al. Baseline HIV RNA determines the durability of RNA suppression during AZT/3TC treatment [abstract I-130]. In: 37th Interscience Conference on Antimicrobial Agents and Chemotherapy, Toronto, 1997.
72. Larder BA, Kohli A, Bloor S, et al. Human immunodeficiency virus type 1 drug susceptibility during zidovudine (AZT) monotherapy compared with AZT plus 2′,3′-dideoxyinosine or AZT plus 2′,3′-dideoxycytidine combination therapy: the protocol 34,225-02 Collaborative Group. J Virol 1996;70:5922–5929.
73. Winters MA, Shafer RW, Jellinger RA, et al. Human immunodeficiency virus type 1 reverse transcriptase genotype and drug susceptibility changes in infected individuals receiving dideoxyinosine monotherapy for 1 to 2 years. Antimicrob Agents Chemother 1997;41:757–762.
74. Merry C, Barry MG, Mulcahy F, et al. Saquinavir pharmacokinetics alone and in combination with ritonavir in HIV-infected patients. AIDS 1997;11:F29–F33.
75. Riddler S, Stein D, Mayers D, et al. Durable clinical anti–HIV-1 activity (48 weeks) and tolerability (24 weeks) for DMP 266 in combination with indinavir [abstract 770]. In: 35th annual meeting of the Infectious Disease Society of America, San Francisco, 1997.
76. Ruiz L, Romeu J, Martinez-Picado J, et al. Efficacy of triple combination therapy with zidovudine (ZDV) plus zalcitabine (ddC) plus lamivudine (3TC) versus double (ZDV + 3TC) combination therapy in patients previously treated with ZDV + ddC. AIDS 1996;10:F61–F66.
77. Lafeuillade A, Poggi C, Tamalet C, et al. Effects of a combination of zidovudine, didanosine, and lamivudine on primary human immunodeficiency virus type 1 infection. J Infect Dis 1997;175:1051–1055.
78. Para MF, Collier A, Coombs R, et al. ACTG 333: antiviral effects of switching from saquinavir hard capsule to saquinavir soft gelatin capsule vs. switching to indinavir after prior saquinavir [abstract 21]. In: 35th annual meeting of the Infectious Disease Society of America, San Francisco, 1997.
79. Lawrence J, Schapiro J, Pesano R, et al. Clinical response and genotypic resistance patterns of sequential therapy with nelfinavir followed by indinavir plus nevirapine in saquinavir/reverse transcriptase inhibitor–experienced patients [abstract 64]. In: Abstracts of the International Workshop on HIV Drug Resistance, Treatment Strategies, and Eradication. St. Petersburg, FL, 1997.
80. Henry K, Kane E, Melroe H, et al. Experience with a ritonavir/saquinavir based regimen for the treatment of HIV-infection in subjects developing increased viral loads while receiving nelfinavir [abstract I-204]. In: 37th Interscience Conference on Antimicrobial Agents and Chemotherapy, Toronto, 1997.
81. Sampson MS, Barr MR, Torres RA, et al. Viral load changes in nelfinavir treated patients switched to a second protease inhibitor after loss of viral suppression [abstract LB-5]. In: 37th Interscience Conference on Antimicrobial Agents and Chemotherapy, Toronto, 1997.
82. Raffi F, Pialoux G, Brun-Vezinet F, et al. Results of Trilege trial, a comparison of three maintenance regimens for HIV-infected adults receiving induction therapy with zidovudine (ZDV), lamivudine (3TC), and indinavir (IDV) [abstract LB15]. In: 5th Conference on Retroviruses and Opportunistic Infections, Chicago, 1998:225.
83. Havlir DV, Hirsch M, Collier A, et al. Randomized trial of indinavir (IDV) vs. Zidovudine (ZDV)/lamivudine (3TC) vs. IDV/ZDV/3TC maintenance therapy after induction IDV/ZDV/3TC therapy [abstract LB16]. In: 5th Conference on Retroviruses and Opportunistic Infections, Chicago, 1998:225.
84. Molla A, Korneyeva M, Gao Q, et al. Ordered accumulation of mutations in HIV protease confers resistance to ritonavir. Nature Med 1996;2:760–766.
85. Condra JH, Schleif WA, Blahy OM, et al. In vitro emergence of HIV-1 variants resistant to multiple protease inhibitors. Nature 1995;374:569–571.
86. Condra JH, Holder DJ, Schleif WA, et al. Genetic correlates of in vivo viral resistance to indinavir, a human immunodeficiency virus type 1 protease inhibitor. J Virol 1996;70:8270–8276.
87. Zhang YM, Imamichi H, Imamichi T, et al. Drug resistance during indinavir therapy is caused by mutations in the protease gene and in its Gag substrate cleavage sites. J Virol 1997;71:6662–6670.
88. Finzi D, Siliciano RF. Analysis of steady state levels and decay rates of latent viral reservoirs in HIV-infected individuals [abstract 91]. In: Abstracts of the International Workshop on HIV Drug Resistance, Treatment Strategies, and Eradication, St. Petersburg, FL, 1997.
89. Lorenzi P, Yerly S, Abderrakim K, et al. Toxicity, efficacy, plasma drug concentrations and protease mutations in patients with advanced HIV infection treated with ritonavir plus saquinavir. AIDS 1997;11:F95–F99.
90. Autran B, Carcelain G, Li TS, et al. Positive effects of combined antiviral therapy on CD4+ T cell homeostasis and function in advanced HIV disease. Science 1997;277:112–116.
91. Kovacs JA, Vogel S, Albert JM, et al. Controlled trial of interleukin-2 infusions in patients infected with the human immunodeficiency virus. N Engl J Med 1996;335:1350–1356.
92. Japour AJ, Welles S, D'Aquila RT, et al. Prevalence and clinical significance of zidovudine resistance mutations in human immunodeficiency virus isolated from patients after long-term zidovudine treatment. J Infect Dis 1995;171:1172–1179.
93. Kozal MJ, Kroodsma K, Winters MA. Didanosine resistance in HIV-infected patients switched from zidovudine to didanosine monotherapy. Ann Intern Med 1994;121:263–268.
94. Schuurman R, Nijhuis M, van Leeuwen R, et al. Rapid changes in human immunodeficiency virus type 1 RNA load and appearance of drug-resistant virus populations in persons treated with lamivudine (3TC). J Infect Dis 1995;171:1411–1419.
95. Richman DD, Havlir D, Corbeil J, et al. Nevirapine resistance mutations of human immunodeficiency virus type 1 selected drug therapy. J Virol 1994;68:1660–1666.

C. Mechanisms Underlying Combination Antiretroviral Therapies

Douglas J. Manion and Martin S. Hirsch

The goal of therapy of human immunodeficiency virus type 1 (HIV-1) infection is to minimize viral replication (1). Because no antiretroviral drug has been able to produce prolonged and profound suppression of HIV replication when it is used alone in large numbers of patients, the use of antiretroviral agents in combination has become the mainstay of anti–HIV-1 therapeutics (2). Antiretroviral drug combinations offer the potential advantages of increased efficacy, broadened access to cellular and tissue reservoirs, widened spectrum of activity against preexisting viral quasispecies, and delayed appearance of drug resistance (3–6). The search is ongoing for antiretroviral combinations that will maximally and durably suppress viral replication not only in the blood but also in sanctuaries such as lymph nodes, the central nervous system, and the genital tract. The prospect of complete long-term viral suppression and eventual senescence of all virus-infected cells raises the possibility of actual eradication of HIV-1 infection (7). Total viral suppression in all body compartments may not currently be achievable, and so breakthrough virus replication may be unavoidable. Thus, the merits of any given multidrug combination in terms of duration of effect will depend on the interplay of residual viral replication and the ability of the virus to mutate to a multidrug-resistant and replication-competent phenotype. In the context of the agents currently available, one must seek out even subtle differences in terms of the efficacy of drugs used in combination. The rapid increase in the number of antiretroviral agents available to treat HIV infection poses the challenge of how best to administer these compounds. Effective use, in turn, depends on an understanding of how drugs interact with one another and with HIV replicative mechanisms leading to the induction of resistance. Although such knowledge is still rudimentary, we have learned enough to favor certain combinations and avoid others. This chapter summarizes some of the knowledge gained regarding mechanisms underlying combination antiretroviral therapy. Details concerning the clinical use of combination regimens are covered Chapter 48B.

ANTIRETROVIRAL COMBINATIONS IN VITRO

Much of what we know regarding the interactions of antiretroviral agents used in combination derives from in vitro combination drug susceptibility assays. Various techniques exist to determine whether drugs in combination act synergistically, additively, or antagonistically (8). Most methods involve tissue culture–based laboratory assays in which a fixed inoculum of virus is added to a given cell type, and viral replication is measured in the presence or absence of drugs. The experimental results are then compared with expected effects, and the interaction is quantified in some manner. A commonly used system is that of Chou and Talalay (9). It models virus–drug interaction according to the law of mass action, estimates the expected additive effect of agents in combination according to Loewe's additivity hypothesis, and quantifies the experimentally obtained interactive effect as a combination index (10). The technique has as its major advantages relative simplicity, ability to be carried out with a finite and manageable number of data points, applicability to the study of combinations of two or more drugs, and adaptability to different cell lines, cell activation status, or viral isolates. It has limitations such as 1) lack of consensus on issues such as inoculum size, drug ratios, and the importance of changes in interactions across varying inhibitory concentrations, 2) arbitrary interpretation of the interaction output measurement, 3) an inability to infer mechanisms, and 4) inherent oversimplification of the system regarding the complexity of in vivo conditions. Newer techniques attempt to address some of these limitations (11, 12), although in the absence of an established standard, debate regarding the optimal method to determine in vitro drug interactions likely will continue. Despite these caveats, the in vitro study of antiviral drug combinations has proved a cornerstone in the evolution of our conceptual approach to HIV pharmacotherapeutics (4, 13).

An expanding body of knowledge has emerged concerning the in vitro interactions of many approved and experimental antiretroviral agents in two-drug and multidrug combinations against HIV-1 isolates of varying drug-resistance profiles (14–33). In vitro combination drug studies have shown that, given favorable interactions among individual drugs, two antiretroviral agents are superior to one (18), three are better than two (15), and four are better than three (20, 21). These studies have also demonstrated the benefit of concomitant over sequential therapy (21). The enumeration of all these studies is beyond the scope of this chapter, but some of these interactions are shown in Table 48C.1. The primary objective of these studies is to identify those combinations with interactions that are either synergistic or antagonistic. Perhaps most important is identification of combinations demonstrating marked antagonism for which added care is warranted should clinical trials of those regimens be undertaken.

The first antiretroviral combination to demonstrate in vitro antagonism was that of ribavirin and zidovudine against wild-type HIV-1 (25). This effect occurred in various cell types (peripheral blood mononuclear cells, T-lymphoblastoid cell lines, monocytes) and under various conditions of inoculation. The underlying mechanism is thought to be reduced active zidovudine triphosphate secondary to negative feedback on the involved thymidine kinase conferred by ribavirin. Zidovudine and stavudine have also been shown to demonstrate marked in vitro antagonism when tested against zidovudine-resistant (23)

Table 48C.1. In Vitro Drug Interactions Among Currently Approved Antiretrovirals

	ZDV	ddI	ddC	d4T	3TC	NVP	DLV	SQV	IDV	RTV	NFV
ZDV	X	+	+	−	+	+	+	+	+		
ddI	+	X		+			+	+	+		
ddC	+		X				+	+			
d4T	−	+		X	+	+		+			
3TC	+			+	X	+		+			
NVP	+			+	+	X					
DLV	+	+	+				X			+	
SQV	+	+	+	+	+			X	−		
IDV	+	+						−	X		
RTV							+			X	
NFV											X

ZDV, zidovudine; ddI, didanosine; ddC, zalcitabine; d4T, stavudine; 3TC, lamivudine; NVP, nevirapine; DLV, delavirdine; SQV, saquinavir; IDV, indinavir; RTV, ritonavir; NFV, nelfinavir; +, additive to synergistic interaction; −, antagonistic interaction.

and multidrug-resistant viruses (34). The mechanism is thought to be competition between zidovudine and stavudine for the same phosphorylation enzymes resulting in lower intracellular concentrations of activated stavudine, the impact of which is magnified by the higher zidovudine drug concentrations needed against resistant isolates (35). This finding underscores the importance of including clinically relevant resistant viral isolates in such in vitro studies. Clinical trials of this drug combination lend support to these in vitro findings. In a phase III study comparing various drug regimens in zidovudine-experienced HIV-seropositive individuals, those subjects randomized to zidovudine and stavudine fared less well in terms of CD4 cell end points, thus prompting the discontinuation of that arm of the trial after interim analysis (36). The contribution of drug antagonism to the clinical failure of combined stavudine and zidovudine is under study, but similar results have been observed by other investigators in open trials (37). Competition at the level of phosphorylation has also been described in vitro for lamivudine and zalcitabine (38), although antagonism between these agents has not been described. In vitro studies of the combination of saquinavir and indinavir have demonstrated low-level antagonism against both zidovudine-sensitive and zidovudine-resistant isolates (39), although the clinical relevance of low-level in vitro antagonism has yet to be determined.

PHARMACOKINETIC CONSIDERATIONS

All the pharmacologic issues considered in use of monotherapies—absorption, distribution, metabolism, and excretion—are also applicable to the use of combinations. In addition, certain additional aspects require attention, including intracellular alterations induced by one drug that affect another drug's metabolism, overlapping toxicities of individual drugs, and the effects that certain agent's requirements for absorption (e.g., use with meals or while fasting) may have on the use of other agents. Finally, an appreciation of the effect of polypharmacy on patient compliance and ultimate effectiveness of complex multidrug antiretroviral regimens is critical to the satisfactory use of this approach.

Much attention has focused on the cytochrome P450 enzyme system, which is involved in the hepatic metabolism and clearance of both protease inhibitors and certain other agents such as the nonnucleoside reverse transcriptase inhibitors (NNRTIs). Some antiretroviral agents induce the cytochrome P450 system, whereas others inhibit this system (Table 48C.2). As a result, the metabolism of antiretroviral agents used concomitantly may be altered significantly. All the protease inhibitors currently approved are metabolized by the CYP3A isoenzyme, for which ritonavir has the highest affinity (40). The greatest impact of ritonavir coadministration is seen with saquinavir, in which increased saquinavir levels of 100-fold were reported in rats (41) and 40-fold in humans (42, 43) without concomitant increases in saquinavir-related toxicities. This phenomenon is being exploited in clinical trials of this combination with encouraging preliminary results in terms of viral load decreases (44, 45).

Other protease inhibitor combinations result in similar interactions, although generally to lesser degrees. The addition of indinavir to saquinavir results in 4- to 7-fold increases in the area under the curve (AUC) for saquinavir (46). Similar increases are seen with the combination of nelfinavir and saquinavir (47). Combining indinavir with nelfinavir results in up to an 80% increase in AUC for each drug (48, 49). Ritonavir increases the AUC for nelfinavir by 150% when administered concomitantly (49). Finally, ritonavir has been shown to increase concentrations of the experimental agent ABT-378 in rats (50, 51), with potential increases of 47-to 770-fold in humans based on in vitro enzymatic studies (52).

Table 48C.2. Interactions Between Antiretroviral Agents and the Hepatic Cytochrome P450 Enzyme (CYP) System

Inducers of CYP	Inhibitors of CYP	Degree of Inhibition
Nevirapine	Delavirdine	+
	Ritonavir	+++
	Saquinavir	+
	Indinavir	+
	Nelfinavir	+

The NNRTI nevirapine increases the metabolism and thus decreases the AUC of saquinavir (27%), indinavir (28%), and ritonavir (11%, not statistically significant) (53, 54). The clinical significance of these findings is not known, although in a small clinical trial nevirapine was not shown to decrease the effect of indinavir on viral load (55). Preliminary results regarding the effect of the NNRTI delavirdine in healthy, HIV-seronegative individuals indicate a more than fivefold increase in the AUC for saquinavir (56) and a 50 to 100% increase in that for indinavir (57). No similar effect was noted with the combination of delavirdine and ritonavir, but studies using the full dose of ritonavir have yet to be reported.

To date, no evidence exists of altered absorption conferred by the addition of one agent to another. This issue has been studied most extensively for the use of concomitant didanosine with other nucleoside analog reverse transcriptase inhibitors (NRTIs). Didanosine's property of acid lability requires administration in the fasting state with the coadministration of a buffered carrier. Indinavir and delavirdine require an acidic environment for good dissolution in the gastrointestinal tract and thus should not be taken within an hour of didanosine administration (58, 59).

The distribution of antiretroviral compounds to pertinent body compartments other than blood is gaining importance as total body clearance of virus becomes a therapeutic goal. Individual drug penetration to sites such as the central nervous system and the genital tract is under active study (60–63).

More is known regarding the correlation of cell type and activation status with conversion of the prodrug NRTIs to their active triphosphate moieties. For example, analyses of zidovudine intracellular metabolism have demonstrated that active triphosphate concentrations are independent of extracellular prodrug concentrations (64), that concentrations of the active forms are lower in monocyte/macrophage cell lines than in activated T-lymphocyte cell lines (65), and that phytohemagglutinin stimulation of peripheral blood mononuclear cells collected from HIV-seropositive patients conferred up to a 150-fold increase in triphosphate concentrations (66). Similar studies have shown preferential activation of the other nucleoside analogs depending on cell type and activation status (67). Active anabolites of stavudine are not found in resting cells (68). Zalcitabine's antiviral activity is independent of the state of activation of the cell. The clinical relevance of these data has not been ascertained. More recent work has focused on the interaction of drugs at the level of intracellular metabolism. Zidovudine is not known to interact with zalcitabine or lamivudine in this respect. However, zidovudine has been shown to decrease the intracellular concentrations of the active form of stavudine because of the higher affinity of the former for thymidine kinase as compared with the latter (35). The intracellular concentrations of active forms of didanosine are increased by ribavirin (69). Hydroxyurea increases the intracellular concentrations of the active forms of zidovudine, lamivudine (70), and particularly didanosine (71).

The biologic basis for the toxic effects of antiretroviral agents has not been fully elucidated. It is not currently possible, based on structure alone, to predict a drug's toxicity profile accurately. Studies of the potentially toxic interactions of drugs are infrequently undertaken before initiating phase II and III clinical trials of drug combinations. Inferences can be drawn when drugs used in combination have overlapping toxicity profiles, such as the neuropathy caused by didanosine, zalcitabine, and stavudine, and greater care is placed on the detection of additive toxicities in the development of clinical trials when these drugs are used together.

RESISTANCE CONSIDERATIONS

Our deepening understanding of the kinetics of emergence of drug-resistant isolates under antiretroviral selective pressures (72) allows for the incorporation of such information in the design of combination drug regimens. Viral breakthrough replication has been the rule in past monotherapy and multidrug clinical trials and is often, but not always, a result of increased viral resistance to the agents used (73). Although newer combinations, such as three-drug regimens using potent protease inhibitors and reverse transcriptase inhibitors, achieve greater suppression of viral replication than ever before, investigators have yet to show that the degree of inhibition of growth will be sufficient to prevent the ultimate emergence of isolates resistant to the drugs in any given combination. In fact, the number of multidrug-resistant isolates emanating from the clinical use of combinations is mounting, with some isolates demonstrating cross-resistance to compounds to which the patient has yet to be exposed (74). The prospect of selecting for pan-resistant isolates mandates continued vigilance lest we repeat the failures seen in past therapeutic efforts, such as in the therapy of tuberculosis, in which incomplete suppression resulted in outbreaks related to multidrug-resistant organisms (75).

The long-term benefit of any antiretroviral drug regimen depends ultimately on the interplay between residual viral replication and the propensity for emergence of an isolate resistant to that regimen. Much is known regarding the specific point mutations that confer resistance to any given compound (72). Clinical trial data support the notion that the duration of drug efficacy when used in monotherapy often correlates with the development of point mutations required for significant resistance. The best example of this phenomenon is the limited utility of the NNRTI nevirapine because of rapid emergence of isolates exhibiting the single point mutation required for high-level resistance (76). This contrasts with the more prolonged time to emergence of resistant isolates in subjects treated with zidovudine or indinavir for which multiple point mutations are required (77–79). One can postulate that, for any given level of suppression of viral replication, the number of drugs used matters less than the ease with which resistant viruses can emerge to evade the antiviral effect. In the presence of high virus titers and relatively low virus inhibitory drug concentrations, resistant viruses may emerge readily. In contrast, with limited virus replication, resistance may be delayed, and with no virus replication, resistance may be prevented altogether. Thus, less complex regimens, such as those used in the context of maintenance therapy, may be sufficient in patients who have had significant decreases in viral load through more aggressive induction therapy.

A growing concern is the emergence of viruses with multidrug-resistant phenotypes in patients receiving combination nucleosides. Several HIV-infected individuals treated with zidovudine and didanosine have developed virus resistance characterized not only by insusceptibility to these agents but to other nucleosides as well (74). For example, an isolate derived from a subject treated with zidovudine and didanosine as part of the AIDS Clinical Trials Group (ACTG) 143 protocol was resistant not only to those compounds but also to stavudine with intermediate resistance to lamivudine (80). Further in vitro passage of this isolate in the presence of lamivudine or nevirapine resulted in successfully selecting for isolates also resistant to these drugs (81). An HIV-1 isolate demonstrating cross-resistance among several members of the protease inhibitor drug class has been described in a subject having received indinavir monotherapy (78), and many more isolates with broad resistance to multiple protease inhibitors have been observed. Given unavoidable issues of patient compliance as well as biologic variation of any regimen's efficacy, one can predict that complex multidrug-resistant isolates will emerge from combinations of currently available antiretroviral agents (82, 83).

A better understanding of viral drug resistance genetics could lead to therapeutic regimens that capitalize on interactive effects of resistance mutations selected for by each component of a combination. This is exemplified by the effects of lamivudine-induced mutations at codon 184 of the HIV-1 reverse transcriptase gene, which confer lamivudine resistance but simultaneously suppress the effects of zidovudine resistance mutations (84). The net effect is prolonged clinical utility of zidovudine and lamivudine when these drugs are used in combination (85).

The advent of rapid, commercially available HIV-1 gene sequencing performed on peripheral blood specimens may allow genotype-based therapeutic decision making. However, measuring the viral genotypes in blood at any one time may not adequately reflect the complete viral complement present in an individual with a complex previous antiretroviral history. Thus, the practicality of initiating clinical trials to address therapeutic questions for all relevant resistance genotypes and phenotypes is questionable. In the absence of sound, prospective clinical data, strategies for treating individuals harboring resistant isolates is empirical. Probably, for the foreseeable future, decisions regarding switching of therapeutic regimen will require the consideration of antiretroviral drug interactions in terms of antiviral activity, pharmacokinetics, pharmacodynamics, and drug resistance. Continued advances in all these areas will be critical to future progress in antiretroviral combination therapy.

Acknowledgment

I acknowledge the support, as a Research Fellow, of the Medical Research Council of Canada.

References

1. Lange J. Combination antiretroviral therapy: back to the future. Drugs 1995;49:32–37.
2. Carpenter CCJ, Fischl MA, Hammer SM, et al. Antiretroviral therapy for HIV infection in 1997: updated recommendations of the International AIDS Society–USA panel. JAMA 1997;277:1962–1969.
3. Hirsch MS, D'Aquila RT. Therapy for human immunodeficiency virus infection. N Engl J Med 1993;328:1686–1695.
4. Caliendo AM, Hirsch MS. Combination therapy for infection due to human immunodeficiency virus type 1. Clin Infect Dis 1994;18: 516–524.
5. Manion DJ, Hirsch MS. Combination chemotherapy for human immunodeficiency virus type 1. Am J Med 1997;102:S76–S80.
6. Hammer SM, Kessler HA, Saag MS. Issues in combination antiretroviral therapy: a review. J Acquir Immune Defic Syndr Hum Retrovirol 1994;7:S24–S35.
7. Markowitz M, Cao Y, Hurley A, et al. Triple therapy with AZT, 3TC, and ritonavir in 12 subjects newly infected with HIV-1 [abstract Th.B.933]. In: Program and abstracts of the 11th International Conference on AIDS, Vancouver, 1996.
8. Prichard MN, Shipman CJ. Analysis of combinations of antiviral drugs and design of effective multidrug therapies. Antiviral Ther 1996;1:9–20.
9. Chou T-C, Talalay P. Quantitative analysis of dose-effect relationships: the combined effects of multiple drugs or enzyme inhibitors. Adv Enzyme Regul 1984;22:27–55.
10. Chou TC. The median-effect principle and the combination index for quantitation of synergism and antagonism in chemotherapy. In: Chou TC, Rideout DC, eds. Synergism and antagonism in chemotherapy. New York: Academic Press, 1991:61–102.
11. Prichard MN, Prichard LE, Shipman CJ. Strategic design and three-dimensional analysis of antiviral drug combinations. Antimicrob Agents Chemother 1993;37:540–545.
12. Belen'kii MS, Schinazi RF. Multiple drug effect analysis with confidence interval. Antiviral Res 1994;25:1–11.
13. Wilson CC, Hirsch MS. Combination antiretroviral therapy for the treatment of human immunodeficiency virus type-1 infection. Proc Assoc Am Physicians 1995;107:19–27.
14. Johnson VA, Walker BD, Barlow MA, et al. Synergistic inhibition of human immunodeficiency virus type 1 and type 2 replication in vitro by castanospermine and 3'-azido-3'-deoxythymidine. Antimicrob Agents Chemother 1989;33:53–57.
15. Johnson VA, Barlow MA, Merrill DP, et al. Three-drug synergistic inhibition of HIV-1 replication in vitro by zidovudine, recombinant soluble CD4, and recombinant interferon-alpha A. J Infect Dis 1990; 161:1059–1067.
16. Johnson VA. Evaluation of candidate anti-HIV agents in vitro. In: Walker BD, Aldovini A, eds. Techniques in HIV research. New York: Stockton Press, 1990:225–237.
17. Johnson VA, Hirsch MS. New developments in antiretroviral drug therapy for human immunodeficiency virus infections. AIDS Clin Rev 1990:235–272.
18. Johnson VA, Merrill DP, Videler JA, et al. Two-drug combinations of zidovudine, didanosine, and recombinant interferon-alpha A inhibit replication of zidovudine-resistant human immunodeficiency virus type 1 synergistically in vitro. J Infect Dis 1991;164:646–655.
19. Johnson VA, Merrill DP, Chou TC, et al. Human immunodeficiency virus type 1 (HIV-1) inhibitory interactions between protease inhibitor Ro 31-8959 and zidovudine, 2',3'-dideoxycytidine, or recombinant interferon-alpha A against zidovudine-sensitive or -resistant HIV-1 in vitro. J Infect Dis 1992;166:1143–1146.
20. Rusconi S, Merrill DP, Hirsch MS. Inhibition of human immunodeficiency virus type 1 replication in cytokine-stimulated monocytes/

macrophages by combination therapy. J Infect Dis 1994;170:1361–1366.
21. Mazzulli T, Rusconi S, Merrill DP, et al. Alternating versus continuous drug regimens in combination chemotherapy of human immunodeficiency virus type 1 infection in vitro. Antimicrob Agents Chemother 1994;38:656–661.
22. Chow YK, Hirsch MS, Merrill DP, et al. Use of evolutionary limitations of HIV-1 multidrug resistance to optimize therapy. Nature 1993;361:650–654.
23. Merrill DP, Moonis M, Chou TC, et al. Lamivudine or stavudine in two- and three-drug combinations against human immunodeficiency virus type 1 replication in vitro. J Infect Dis 1996;173:355–364.
24. St. Clair MH, Millard J, Rooney J, et al. In vitro antiviral activity of 141W94 (VX-478) in combination with other antiretroviral agents. Antiviral Res 1996;29:53–56.
25. Vogt MW, Hartshorn KL, Furman PA, et al. Ribavirin antagonizes the effect of azidothymidine on HIV replication. Science 1987;235:1376–1379.
26. Vogt MW, Durno AG, Chou T-C, et al. Synergistic interaction of 2′,3′-dideoxycytidine and recombinant interferon-alpha-A on replication of human immunodeficiency virus type 1. J Infect Dis 1988;158:378–385.
27. Koshida R, Vrang L, Gilljam G, et al. Inhibition of human immunodeficiency virus in vitro by combinations of 3′-azido-3′-deoxythymidine and foscarnet. Antimicrob Agents Chemother 1989;33:778–780.
28. Craig JC, Duncan IB, Whittaker L, et al. Antiviral synergy between inhibitors of HIV protease and reverse transcriptase. Antiviral Chem Chemother 1993;4:161–166.
29. Craig JC, Whittaker LN, Duncan IB, et al. In vitro anti-HIV and cytotoxicological evaluation of the triple combination: AZT and ddC with HIV protease inhibitor saquinavir (Ro 31-8959). Antiviral Chem Chemother 1994;5:380–386.
30. Daluge SM, Good SS, Faletto MB, et al. 1592U89, a novel carbocyclic nucleoside analog with potent, selective anti-human immunodeficiency viurs activity. Antimicrob Agents Chemother 1997;41:1082–1093.
31. Pagano PJ, Chong K-T. In vitro inhibition of human immunodeficiency virus type 1 by a combination of delavirdine (U-90152) with protease inhibitor U-75875 or interferon-alpha. J Infect Dis 1995;171:61–67.
32. Chong KT, Pagano PJ, Hinshaw RR. A novel BHAP, U-90152, is synergistic with 3′-azido-2′,3′-dideoxythymidine (AZT) and 2′,3′-dideoxycytidine (ddC) against HIV-1 replication in vitro [abstract PO-A25-0606]. In: 9th International Conference on AIDS, Berlin, 1993.
33. Vacca JP, Dorsey BD, Schleif WA, et al. L-735,524: an orally bioavailable human immunodeficiency virus type 1 protease inhibitor. Proc Natl Acad Sci U S A 1994;91:4096–4100.
34. Manion DJ, Merrill DP, Hirsch MS. Combination drug regimens against multi-drug resistant HIV 1 in vitro [abstract 11]. In: 4th Conference on Retroviruses and Opportunistic Infections. Washington DC: American Society for Microbiology, 1997.
35. Hoggard P, Khoo S, Barry M, et al. Intracellular metabolism of zidovudine and stavudine in combination. J Infect Dis 1996;174:671–672.
36. AIDS Clinical Trials Group (ACTG) 290 Protocol Team. A phase II randomized study of the virologic and immunologic effects of d4T versus ddI versus zidovudine plus d4T versus zidovudine plus ddI in HIV infected patients with CD4 cell counts between 300–600/mm^3 and greater than 12 weeks zidovudine experience: ACTG 290 interim review results, 1996.
37. Villalba N, Soriano V, Gomez-Cano M, et al. Short-term efficacy and safety of stavudine (d4T) in pre-treated HIV-infected patients. Antiviral Ther (in press).
38. Veal GJ, Hoggard PG, Barry MG, et al. Interaction between 3TC (lamivudine) and other nucleoside analogues for intracellular phosphorylation. AIDS 1996;10:546–548.
39. Merrill DP, Manion DJ, Chou T-C, et al. Antagonism between human immunodeficiency virus type 1 protease inhibitors indinavir and saquinavir in vitro. J Infect Dis 1997;176:265–268.
40. Kumar GN, Rodrigues AD, Buko AM, et al. Cytochrome P450–mediated metabolism of the HIV-1 protease inhibitor ritonavir (ABT-538) in human liver microsomes. J Pharmacol Exp Ther 1996;277:423–431.
41. Norbeck D, Kumar G, Marsh K, et al. Ritonavir and saquinavir: potential for two-dimensional synergy between HIV protease inhibitors [abstract LB7]. In: 35th Interscience Conference on Antimicrobial Agents and Chemotherapy, San Francisco, 1995.
42. Hsu A, Granneman GR, Sun E, et al. Assessment of single and multiple dose interactions between ritonavir and saquinavir [abstract LB.B.6041]. In: Program and abstracts of the 11th International Conference on AIDS, Vancouver, 1996.
43. Kempf D, Marsh K, Kumar G, et al. Pharmacokinetic enhancement of inhibitors of the human immunodeficiency virus protease by coadministration with ritonavir. Antimicrob Agents Chemother 1996;41:654–660.
44. Granneman GR, Hsu A, Sun E, et al. Pharmacokinetics/pharmacodynamics of ritonavir–saquinavir combination therapy [abstract 609]. In: 4th Conference on Retroviruses and Opportunistic Infections. Washington DC: American Society for Microbiology, 1997.
45. Cameron W, Sun E, Markowitz M, et al. Combination use of ritonavir and saquinavir in HIV-infected patients: preliminary safety and efficacy data [abstract Th.B.934]. In: Program and abstracts of the 11th International Conference on AIDS, Vancouver, 1996.
46. McCrea J, Buss N, Sone J, et al. Indinavir–saquinavir single dose pharmacokinetic study [abstract 608]. In: 4th Conference on Retroviruses and Opportunistic Infections. Washington DC: American Society for Microbiology, 1997.
47. Kravcik S, Sahai J, Kerr B, et al. Nelfinavir mesylate increases saquinavir soft gel capsule exposure in HIV+ patients [abstract 371]. In: 4th Conference on Retroviruses and Opportunistic Infections. Washington DC: American Society for Microbiology, 1997.
48. Yuen G, Anderson R, Daniels R, et al. Investigations of nelfinavir mesylate pharmacokinetic interactions with indinavir and ritonavir [abstract]. In: 4th Conference on Retroviruses and Opportunistic Infections. Washington DC: American Society for Microbiology, 1997.
49. Kerr B, Yuen G, Lee C, et al. Overview of in vitro and in vivo drug interaction studies with nelfinavir mesylate, a new HIV-1 protease inhibitor [abstract 373]. In: 4th Conference on Retroviruses and Opportunistic Infections. Washington DC: American Society for Microbiology, 1997.
50. Kumar GN, Jayanti V, Johnson MK, et al. Increased bioavailability and plasma levels of the HIV-1 protease inhibitor ABT-378 in rats due to inhibition of the in vitro metabolism by ritonavir [abstract 207]. In: 4th Conference on Retroviruses and Opportunistic Infections. Washington DC: American Society for Microbiology, 1997.
51. Marsh K, McDonald E, Sham H, et al. Enhancement of ABT-378 pharmacokinetics when administered in combination with ritonavir [abstract 210]. In: 4th Conference on Retroviruses and Opportunistic Infections. Washington DC: American Society for Microbiology, 1997.
52. Kumar GN, Dykstra J, Jayanti V, et al. Potent inhibition of the in vitro human liver microsomal metabolism of the HIV-1 protease inhibitor ABT-378 by ritonavir- potential for a positive drug interaction [abstract 211]. In: 4th Conference on Retroviruses and Opportunistic Infections. Washington DC: American Society for Microbiology, 1997.
53. Murphy R, Gagnier P, Lamson M, et al. Effect of nevirapine on pharmacokinetics of indinavir and ritonavir in HIV-1 infected patients [abstract 374]. In: 4th Conference on Retroviruses and Opportunistic Infections. Washington DC: American Society for Microbiology, 1997.
54. Sahai J, Cameron W, Salgo M, et al. Drug interaction study between saquinavir and nevirapine [abstract 614]. In: 4th Conference on Retroviruses and Opportunistic Infections. Washington DC: American Society for Microbiology, 1997.
55. Harris M, Durakovic C, Conway B, et al. A pilot study of indinavir, nevirapine, and 3TC in patients with advanced HIV disease [abstract 234]. In: 4th Conference on Retroviruses and Opportunistic Infections. Washington DC: American Society for Microbiology, 1997.

56. Cox SR, Ferry JJ, Batts DH, et al. Delavirdine and marketed protease inhibitors pharmacokinetic interaction studies in healthy volunteers [abstract 372]. In: 4th Conference on Retroviruses and Opportunistic Infections. Washington DC: American Society for Microbiology, 1997.
57. Ferry JJ, Herman BD, Cox SR, et al. Delavirdine and indinavir: a pharmacokinetic drug–drug interaction study in healthy adult volunteers [abstract 121]. In: 4th Conference on Retroviruses and Opportunistic Infections. Washington DC: American Society for Microbiology, 1997.
58. Committee of Proprietary Medicinal Products. European public assessment report (EPAR): crixivan, 1996.
59. Morse GD, Fischl MA, Shelton MJ, et al. Single-dose pharmocokinetics of delavirdine mesylate and didanosine in patients with human immunodeficiency virus infection. Antimicrob Agents Chemother 1997;41:169–174.
60. Blaney SM, Daniel MJ, Harker AJ, et al. Pharmacokinetics of lamivudine and BCH-189 in plasma and cerebrospinal fluid of nonhuman primates. Antimicrob Agents Chemother 1995;39:2779–2782.
61. Portegies P. HIV-1, the brain, and combination therapy. Lancet 1995;346:1244–1245.
62. Hawkins ME, Mitsuya H, McCully CM, et al. Pharmacokinetics of dideoxypurine nucleoside analogs in plasma and cerebrospinal fluid of rhesus monkeys. Antimicrob Agents Chemother 1995;39:1259–1264.
63. Krieger JN, Coombs RW, Collier AC, et al. Seminal shedding of human immunodeficiency virus type 1 and human cytomegalovirus: evidence for different immunologic controls. J Infect Dis 1995;171:1018–1022.
64. Fletcher CV, Kawle SP, Page LM, et al. Intracellular triphosphate concentrations of antiretroviral nucleosides as a determinant of clinical response in HIV-infected patients [abstract 13]. In: 4th Conference on Retroviruses and Opportunistic Infections. Washington DC: American Society for Microbiology, 1997.
65. Perno CF, Yarchoan R, Cooney DA, et al. Inhibition of human immunodeficiency virus (HIV-1/HTLV-III/Ba-L) replication in fresh and cultured human peripheral blood monocytes/macrophages by azidothymidine and related 2′,3′-dideoxynucleosides. J Exp Med 1988;168:1111–1125.
66. Gao WY, Shirasaka T, Johns DG, et al. Differential phosphorylation of azidothymidine, dideoxycytidine and dideoxyinosine in resting and activated peripheral blood mononuclear cells. J Clin Invest 1993;91:2326–2333.
67. Cooney DA, Dalal M, Mitsuya H, et al. Initial studies on the cellular pharmacology of 2′,3′-dideoxycytidine, an inhibitor of HTLV-III infectivity. Biochem Pharmacol 1986;35:2065–2068.
68. Zhu Z, Ho HT, Hitchcock MJ, et al. Cellular pharmacology of 2′,3′-didehydro-2′,3′-dideoxythymidine (d4T) in human peripheral blood mononuclear cells. Biochem Pharmacol 1990;39:R15–19.
69. Balzarini J, Lee CK, Schols D, et al. 1-beta-D-ribofuranosyl-1,2,4-triazole-3-carboxamide (ribavirin) and 5-ethynyl-1-beta-D-ribofuranosylimidazole-4-carboxamide (EICAR) markedly potentiate the inhibitory effect of 2′,2′-dideoxyinosine on human immunodeficiency virus in peripheral blood lymphocytes. Biochem Biophys Res Commun 1991;178:563–569.
70. Palmer S, Cox S. Increased activation fo the combination of 3′-azido-3′-deoxythymidine and 2′-deoxy-3′-thiacytidine in the presence of hydroxyurea. Antimicrob Agents Chemother 1997;41:460–464.
71. Gao WY, Agbaria R, Driscoll JS, et al. Divergent anti-human immunodeficiency virus activity and anabolic phosphorylation of 2′,3′-dideoxynucleoside analogs in resting and activated human cells. J Biol Chem 1994;269:12,633–12,638.
72. Moyle GJ. Use of viral resistance patterns to antiretroviral drugs in optimising selection of drug combinations and sequences. Drugs 1996;52:168–185.
73. Richman DD. The implications of drug resistance for strategies of combination antiviral chemotherapy. Antiviral Res 1996;29:31–33.
74. Shafer RW, Kozal MJ, Winters MA, et al. Combination therapy with zidovudine and didanosine selects for drug-resistant human immunodeficiency virus type 1 strains with unique patterns of pol gene mutations. J Infect Dis 1994;169:722–729.
75. Jacobs RF. Multi-drug–resistant tuberculosis. Clin Infect Dis 1996;19:1–8.
76. de Jong MD, Vella S, Carr A, et al. High-dose nevirapine in previously untreated human immunodeficiency virus type 1–infected persons does not result in sustained suppression of viral replication. J Infect Dis 1997;175:966–970.
77. Loveday C, Kaye S, Tenant-Flowers M, et al. HIV-1 RNA serum-load and resistant viral genotypes during early zidovudine therapy. Lancet 1995;345:820–824.
78. Condra JH, Schleif WA, Blahy OM, et al. In vivo emergence of HIV-1 variants resistant to multiple protease inhibitors. Nature 1995;374:569–571.
79. Vasudevachari MB, Zhang Y-M, Imamichi H, et al. Emergence of protease inhibitor resistance mutations in human immunodeficiency virus type 1 isolates from patients and rapid screening procedure for their detection. Antimicrob Agents Chemother 1996;40:2535–2541.
80. Shafer RW, Iversen AK, Winters MA, et al. Drug resistance and heterogeneous long-term virologic responses of human immunodeficiency virus type 1–infected subjects to zidovudine and didanosine combination therapy: the AIDS Clinical Trials Group 143 Virology Team. J Infect Dis 1995;172:70–78.
81. Shafer RW, Winters MA, Iversen AKN, et al. Genotypic and phenotypic changes during culture of a multinucleoside-resistant human immunodeficiency virus type 1 strain in the presence and absence of additional reverse transcriptase inhibitors. Antimicrob Agents Chemother 1996;40:2887–2890.
82. Kew Y, Salomon H, Olsen LR, et al. The nucleoside analog–resistant E89G mutant of human immunodeficiency virus type 1 reverse transcriptase displays a broader cross-resistance that extends to nonnucleoside inhibitors. Antimicrob Agents Chemother 1996;40:1711–1714.
83. Schmit J-C, Cogniaux J, Hermans P, et al. Multiple drug resistance to nucleoside analogues and nonnucleoside reverse transcriptase inhibitors in an efficiently replicating human immunodeficiency virus type 1 patient strain. J Infect Dis 1996;174:962–968.
84. Larder BA, Kemp SD, Harrigan PR. Potential mechanism for sustained antiretroviral efficacy of AZT-3TC combination therapy. Science 1995;269:696–699.
85. Eron JJ, Benoit SL, Jemsek J, et al. Treatment with lamivudine, zidovudine, or both in HIV-positive patients with 200 to 500 CD4+ cells per cubic millimeter: North American HIV Working Party. N Engl J Med 1995;333:1662–1669.

49
VIRAL RESISTANCE TO ANTIVIRAL DRUGS

Douglas D. Richman

The virus population in an individual infected with an RNA virus has been termed a quasispecies (1). This term describes the existence of many, genetically distinct viral variants that evolve from the initial virus inoculum. These genetic variants are generated because the DNA proofreading mechanisms that have evolved to preserve the genetic composition of organisms with double-stranded DNA genomes do not exist for RNA viruses. As a result, as RNA viruses replicate, each newly copied genome differs from the parental virus on average by a single nucleotide (2, 3). This phenomenon applies not only to HIV, but to hepatitis C virus, influenza virus, poliovirus, and numerous other examples.

These nucleotide differences (termed mutations) may be "neutral," having little impact on viral replication capacity (fitness). As a result, viral polymorphisms (genetic variants with apparently equivalent fitness) are commonly seen among virus populations in infected individuals. These mutations, in contrast, may be lethal or crippling, resulting in variants that cannot replicate and thus are infrequently represented in the viral quasispecies. Other variants may confer a replicative advantage (greater fitness) in the presence of changing selective pressures such as host immune responses or drug treatments. These possibilities illustrate the survival strategy of organisms with high mutation rates, which is to generate large numbers of progeny, each of which has varying prospects for survival, but that collectively provide a large pool of genetic variants with the capacity to adapt to changing selective pressures (4, 5).

Ten billion (10^{10}) virions of HIV have been estimated to be produced daily in an infected individual (6). If each of these contains on average one mutation in a genome of 10,000 (10^4) nucleotides, then replication-competent viruses with every possible single drug-resistance mutation are likely to be generated daily. Double mutants are also likely to be generated, but the probability of generating virus with 3 or more drug-resistance mutations in the same genome is low.

These theoretic estimates are supported by observations from HIV-infected individuals. Viruses or HIV RNA having single but not multiple drug-resistance mutations have been isolated from patients who were infected before the availability of antiretroviral agents and who never received therapy (7–11). Mathematic modeling of the rate of emergence of resistant virus after treatment with nevirapine in previously untreated individuals has permitted estimates of the prevalence in plasma of HIV variants with specific mutations conferring nevirapine resistance. Approximately 1 in 1000 copies of HIV RNA per milliliter of plasma contained the tyrosine to cysteine mutation at amino acid residue 181 of the reverse transcriptase that confers nevirapine resistance (12). These findings confirm that virus-encoding drug-resistance mutations exists in viral quasispecies of HIV-infected individuals before treatment is started.

When the selective pressure of an antiviral drug is applied in an infected individual, the preexisting minor viral species that are resistant to that drug rapidly become the predominant replicating species. These resistant viruses are selected for in the sense of classic Darwinian evolution as the more fit species. For some antiretroviral drugs such as lamivudine (3TC) and nonnucleoside reverse transcriptase inhibitors (NNRTIs; e.g., nevirapine), a single mutation can confer high-level resistance (13–17). When these drugs are administered either as monotherapy or in combinations that only partially suppress virus replication, drug-resistant mutants became predominant within weeks (12, 18–20).

For some other drugs, such as zidovudine (ZDV) and protease inhibitors, high-level resistance requires the accumulation of three or more drug-resistance mutations in a single viral genome (21–23). These highly resistant variants emerge less quickly, requiring months to predominate (22, 24–26). This observation argues against the preexistence of genetic variants with multiple mutations in untreated patients. Rather, development of high-level resistance to these drugs requires persistent viral replication in the presence of the selective pressure of drug treatment. Persistent viral replication permits the evolution of virus with high-level drug resistance by cumulative acquisition of multiple mutations.

What do we know about the development of HIV drug resistance with potent combination therapy? First, the higher the trough plasma concentrations of a protease inhibitor (ritonavir), the more slowly drug-resistance mutations emerge (24). Second, the lower the nadir of plasma HIV RNA, the longer it takes for failure with drug-resistant virus to occur (27). These observations argue that lower rates of virus replication delay the emergence of resistance of drug-resistance mutations.

In patients with suppression below 50 copies HIV RNA/mL of plasma for 1 year, even though HIV RNA and DNA are detectable in lymph nodes, no drug-resistance mutations or other evidence of virus evolution can be discerned (28). In contrast, patients with detectable plasma levels of HIV RNA have indicators of ongoing virus replication including evidence of virus evolution, unlike those patients with fewer than 50 copies/mL. Recent observations documenting the presence of latently infected but replication-competent CD4+ cells in patients with sustained suppression of HIV RNA below detectable levels indicate that the virus isolates from the patients, even after 2 years of treatment, have not evolved and have not acquired drug-resistance mutations since the initiation of treatment (29, 30).

Several practical inferences can be derived from these biologic principles. First, drugs for which only a single mutation is required for high-level resistance, such as 3TC and NNRTIs, should be reserved for combination regimens designed to suppress virus replication completely. Their use in less suppressive regimens is guaranteed to select for high-level resistance. Second, combination regimens should be designed to confer the combined potency and "genetic barrier" necessary to suppress completely the preexisting populations of genetic variants. Such a regimen must suppress all minor populations with one or two mutations that could emerge with any of the individual components of the regimen ("genetic barrier") and could prevent ongoing replication which would permit the cumulative acquisition of mutations. This demanding requirement becomes more formidable in previously treated patients because the duration and complexity of drug treatment add to the deposition of drug resistance in the "genetic archive" sequestered in the patient.

A catalog of resistance mutations that have emerged after selection in vitro and in vivo with antiretroviral drugs has been published (31). This list is large and expanding. An updated version can be accessed on the internet (http://www.viral-resistance.com). Rather than comprehensively review all the drugs, their associated mutations, and the implications, the readers is referred to the relevant chapters in a text devoted to antiviral drug resistance (32) and to the aforementioned website. This chapter provides an overview of resistance with each of the classes of antiretroviral agents, summarizes the assays to detect resistance, and provides some general principles for clinical management to help contend with the problem of drug resistance.

ANTIVIRAL DRUGS

Nucleoside Reverse Transcriptase Inhibitors

ZIDOVUDINE

Isolates from subjects not treated with ZDV (formerly known as azidothymidine or AZT) display a narrow range of susceptibilities to this drug, with the 50% inhibitory concentrations (IC_{50}) ranging from 0.001 to 0.04 µmol/L (25, 26, 33–35). This narrow range of susceptibilities is seen with isolates from subjects of all ages and at all stages of HIV infection, from asymptomatic through advanced AIDS. Isolates of HIV from patients who are administered ZDV chronically display progressive reductions of susceptibility to ZDV over periods of months to years (Fig. 49.1). Isolates with greater than 100-fold increases in the IC_{50} values of ZDV may emerge. In addition to isolates from peripheral blood mononuclear cells, resistant isolates have been documented in plasma (36, 37), cerebrospinal fluid, genital secretions (38), and pulmonary alveolar macrophages (D Richman and R Kornbluth, unpublished data). Diminished susceptibility to ZDV of an isolate of HIV-2 from a patient receiving prolonged therapy has also been reported (39).

The rate of change in susceptibility is correlated with stage of disease. In one study of 55 isolates from 31 patients receiving ZDV (26), patients with late stage HIV infection (AIDS or symptoms with fewer than 200 CD4 lymphocytes/µL) developed resistance significantly sooner than those with early stage disease ($P=.002$) (Fig. 49.2). By 12 months after initiation of ZDV therapy, an estimated 89% (95% confidence interval, 64 to 99%) of persons with late stage HIV infection had developed resistance, compared with 31% (95% confidence interval, 16 to 56%) of those with more than 200 CD4 lymphocytes and minimal or no symptoms.

The clinical significance of resistance is a function of the degree of drug susceptibility. Patients who develop highly resistant virus experience a threefold faster rate of progression to AIDS or death independent of other risk factors (40). This

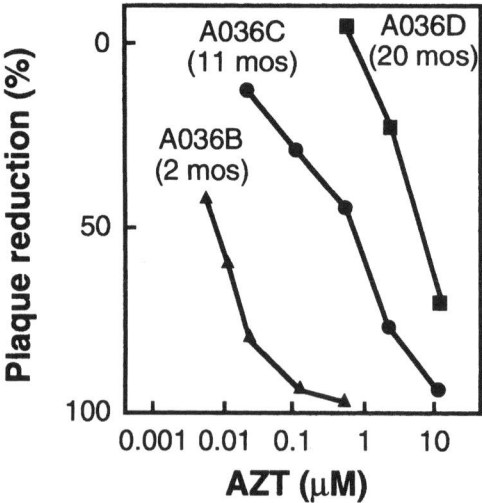

Figure 49.1. Zidovudine *(AZT)* susceptibilities of sequential isolates of HIV-1 from a patient receiving the drug. Isolates from a patient receiving the drug on the original phase II study were assayed in the CD4 expressing HeLa (HT4-6C) cells using syncytial focus (plaque) reduction (25, 92). The percentage of plaque reduction is determined using the number of plaques in the control wells of each isolate assayed without drug. In this assay, the drug is examined at 0.5 $\log_{10}$ (3.16-fold) dilutions. Susceptibility curves are displayed for three isolates obtained from patient A0362 *(triangles)* 11 *(circles)*, and 20 *(squares)* months after the initiation of AZT therapy. (Adapted from Larder BA, Darby G, Richman DD. HIV with reduced sensitivity to zidovudine (AZT) isolated during prolonged therapy. Science 1989;243:1731–1734.)

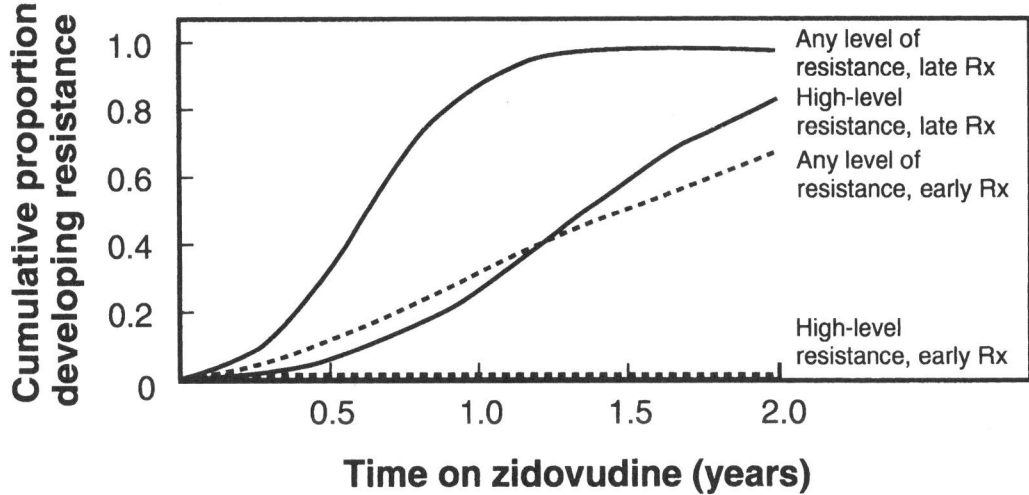

Figure 49.2. Estimated cumulative proportion of patients developing resistant isolates as a function of time since initiation of zidovudine by stage of HIV infection. Patients with late stage infection have fewer than 200 CD4 lymphocytes and HIV-related symptoms. Patients with early stage disease have 200 to 500 CD4 lymphocytes and mild or no symptoms. Any-level resistance is defined as an IC_{10} of at least 0.05 µM. High-level resistance is defined as an IC_{50} of at least 1.0 µM. No high-level resistance was seen in the patients with early stage disease during this interval, but it has been observed in the third and fourth years of therapy (50; D Richman, unpublished data). (Adapted from Richman DD, Grimes JM, Lagakos SW. Effects of stage of disease and drug dose on zidovudine susceptibilities of isolates of human immunodeficiency virus. J Acquir Immune Defic Syndr 1990;3:743–746.)

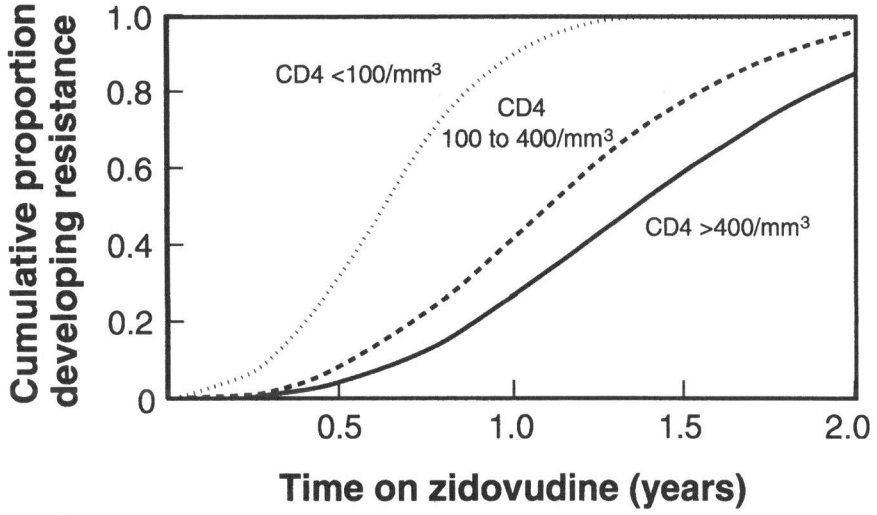

Figure 49.3. Estimated cumulative proportion of isolates developing resistance as a function of time since initiation of zidovudine by CD4 lymphocyte count at the initiation of therapy. Resistance is defined as an IC_{50} of at least 0.05 µmol/L. (Adapted from Richman DD, Grimes JM, Lagakos SW. Effects of stage of disease and drug dose on zidovudine susceptibilities of isolates of human immunodeficiency virus. J Acquir Immune Defic Syndr 1990;3:743–746.)

phenotype correlates with the presence of both the M41L and T215Y or F mutations associated with high-level ZDV resistance (41).

Lower initial CD4 lymphocyte counts were also predictive of increased likelihood of the emergence of resistant isolates ($P=.004$) (26) (Fig. 49.3). The estimated rates of resistance at 1 year were 89%, 41%, and 27% for baseline CD4 cell counts lower than 100, from 100 to 400, and higher than 400 CD4 cells/mm³ (95% confidence intervals, 63 to 99%, 18 to 75%, and 11 to 59%, respectively). These observations are consistent with the observations in cross-sectional analyses of populations that HIV infection is an active persistent process in which levels of virus replication ("virus load") are progressively increasing as CD4 cell counts are diminishing (42–45). The likelihood of the emergence of mutations under the selective pressure of drug therapy should be a product of a relatively constant mutation rate and the number of replicative events.

Development of resistance occurred sooner among individuals assigned to higher daily doses of ZDV (1200 to 1500 mg) than among those assigned to lower doses (500 to 600 mg) (26), although this difference did not attain statistical significance ($P=.18$ without controlling for stage and $P=.06$ after controlling for stage). Higher concentrations of drug may exert greater selective pressure in the face of reduced but persistent virus replication, thus permitting the emergence of resistant isolates.

Isolates resistant to ZDV display diminished susceptibility to other nucleosides containing a 3′-azido moiety, including 3′-azido-2′,3′-dideoxyuridine, 3′-azido-2′,3′-dideoxyguanosine, and 3′-azido-2′,3′-dideoxyadenosine (25, 46) (D Richman, unpublished data). Cross-resistance to other nucleosides, including several thymidine analogs, or to drugs of other classes has not been convincingly documented (25, 46–48).

The antiviral effect of ZDV is conferred by the triphosphate that is generated by anabolic phosphorylation by host cell thymidine kinase and other enzymes (49). ZDV triphosphate inhibits the reverse transcriptase of HIV in cell-free enzyme assays and also acts as a terminator of DNA chain elongation because the 3′-azido group prevents the formation of 3′,5′-phosphodiester bonds. It was not surprising therefore when mutations in the gene for the reverse transcriptase of the resistant virus were documented. What remains puzzling, however, has been the difficulty in demonstrating an enzymologic difference between the mutant and wild-type reverse transcriptases (25). Using enzyme extracted either from ZDV-sensitive and ZDV-resistant virions or prepared from enzyme expressed in *Escherichia coli* after molecular cloning from these viruses, no differences in inhibition by ZDV triphosphate have been demonstrated in cell-free enzyme assays. Because the genetics are definitive, these observations would suggest that cell-free enzyme assays do not reflect the mechanism of inhibition of ZDV triphosphate on the transcription complex in the cell.

Sequencing the reverse transcriptase gene of five pairs of isolates that displayed more than 100-fold reductions in susceptibility during the course of therapy documented multiple mutations, four of which appeared common (21). When these four mutations at amino acid residues 67, 70, 215, and 219 were inserted by site-directed mutagenesis into the susceptible infectious molecular clone pHXB2, a greater than 100-fold reduction in ZDV susceptibility resulted. Sequential isolates from the same individual that displayed progressive, stepwise increments in resistance were associated with the sequential cumulative acquisition of these four mutations (21). Cumulative mutations thus contribute additively or synergistically to stepwise reductions in susceptibility (21, 50).

A fifth mutation at residue 41 (methionine to leucine) also contributes to significant reductions in susceptibility to ZDV (41, 51). The only definitive method to confirm that a mutation in this highly variable virus actually contributes to reduced susceptibility is to quantitate the reduction in susceptibility of a virus with a defined susceptibility and genetic background after introducing the mutation by site-directed mutagenesis (Table 49.1). By assessing the impact on ZDV susceptibility of these mutations singly or in various combinations, these mutations vary quantitatively in their impact, and some combinations appear to result in additive, synergistic, or even antagonistic quantitative changes in drug

Table 49.1. Zidovudine Susceptibility of HIV Variants with Defined Mutations in Reverse Transcriptase[a]

HIV Variant	Mutations Introduced	Zidovudine IC$_{50}$ (µmol)	Change in Susceptibility
HXB2-D		0.01	1
HXB 41L	M41L	0.04	4
HIVRTMF	T215Y	0.16	16
HXB 41L/215Y	M41L, T215Y	0.60	60
HIVRTMC/F	D67N, K70R, T215Y	0.31	31
RTMC/F 41L	M41L, D67N, K70R, T215Y	1.79	179
HIVRTMCY	D67N, K70R, T215Y, K219Q	1.21	121
HIVRTMC	D67N, K70R, T215F, K219Q	1.47	147

[a]The genotypes of HIV variants constructed by site-directed mutagenesis are shown. The codes for the mutations introduced are wild-type amino acid, RT residue number, and mutant amino acid; for example, methionine at 41 to leucine (M41L). Amino acid abbreviations: A, alanine; C, cysteine; D, aspartic acid; E, glutamic acid; F, phenylalanine; G, glycine; H, histidine, I, isoleucine; K, lysine; L, leucine; M, methionine; N, asparagine; Q, glutamine; R, arginine; T, threonine; V, valine; Y, tyrosine.
(Modified from Kellam P, Boucher CA, Larder BA. Fifth mutation in human immunodeficiency virus type 1 reverse transcriptase contributes to the development of high-level resistance to zidovudine. Proc Natl Acad Sci U S A 1992;89:1934–1938.)

susceptibility (51) (see Table 49.1). These effects appear to correlate with the changes in susceptibilities in sequential isolates obtained from patients receiving ZDV therapy and with the patterns of the appearance and even disappearance of some mutations (52).

DIDANOSINE

Four- to 10-fold reductions in susceptibility of sequential isolates from patients receiving prolonged therapy with ddI have been reported (53, 54). Isolates resistant to ZDV at the initiation of ddI therapy may develop increases in ZDV susceptibility in conjunction with reductions in ddI susceptibility (53, 54). St. Clair and associates (53) documented a leucine to valine mutation at residue 74 of the reverse transcriptase in association with these phenotypic changes. Site-directed mutagenesis of an infectious provirus indicated that this mutation could account for both the diminished susceptibility to ddI (and to zalcitabine [ddC]) and the increased susceptibility to ZDV (53). This mutation that produced partial reversal of ZDV resistance had no appreciable effect on the ZDV susceptibility of wild-type (sensitive) virus. In vivo, a consequence of this effect is the delayed emergence of the codon 74 mutation in patients treated with ddI in combination with ZDV (55). The L74V mutation has been associated with diminished antiviral activity of ddI.

ZALCITABINE

A mutation conferring a reduction of ddC susceptibility of approximately fivefold has been identified and confirmed by site-directed mutagenesis at residues 65 and 69 (threonine to aspartic acid) (56, 57). The mutation associated with 3TC treatment, methionine to valine at residue 184, also results in a small quantitative reduction of susceptibility to ddI (58,

59); however, this mutation rarely arises in patients receiving ddI or ddC. In fact, patients receiving regimens containing ddC rarely display diminished susceptibility to ddC (60).

STAVUDINE

Diminished susceptibility rarely emerges to d4T therapy. In vitro selection and site-directed mutagenesis documented a five- to sevenfold diminution of susceptibility of the laboratory strain HXB2 to d4T attributable to a valine to threonine mutation at residue 75 of the reverse transcriptase (61). Nevertheless, this mutation, other characteristic mutations, and phenotypic resistance rarely emerge with d4T therapy (62). Poor responses to d4T therapy have been associated both with "cellular resistance" attributable to impaired anabolic phosphorylation as a consequence of prolonged ZDV therapy and to the multiple nucleoside resistance complex (see later).

LAMIVUDINE

One of two point mutations in residue 184 of the reverse transcriptase confers high-level resistance (more than 1000-fold) to 3TC and its related congener FTC (15–17). The mutations result in a methionine to isoleucine or valine change in the highly conserved YMDD motif in the catalytic site of the polymerase. These mutations rapidly emerge in vivo as well, the isoleucine emerging first (20). This mutant has diminished replication competence (63), however, and is replaced within several weeks by the valine mutant, which becomes predominant in virtually all patients treated with 3TC and who fail to suppress virus replication fully (20). Patients treated with 3TC in a potent protease-containing regimen in whom plasma HIV RNA levels are suppressed below the level of detection maintain the wild-type sequence in PBMC DNA and lymphoid nucleic acid compartments for years (28, 29, 64).

The M184V mutation reverses the reduced susceptibility conferred by ZDV resistance mutations (65), and this effect may account for some of the benefit of the combination regimen in patients harboring ZDV-resistant virus. Nevertheless, 3TC confers at least as much incremental activity for d4T as for ZDV, according to the AIDS Clinical Trial Group (ACTG 306). Moreover, highly dual-resistant virus to ZDV and 3TC emerges over the course of therapy with these two drugs (66), adding to the rationale for the use of 3TC in fully virus-suppressive regimens.

ABACAVIR (1592)

Selection for abacavir-resistant virus has resulted in the sequential accumulation of three mutations (K65R, L74V, M184V) resulting in the progressive reduction in susceptibility by 5- to 20-fold (67). Clinical studies are only preliminary; however, these mutations, as well as preexisting ZDV-resistance mutations, appear to dampen the antiretroviral activity of abacavir.

Multiple Nucleoside Resistance

Shirasaka and associates first described a distinctive pattern of high-level, multiple nucleoside resistance (68). Typically, a patient treated with ZDV and didanosine (ddI) either sequentially or in combination develops virus exhibiting more than 100-fold reductions in susceptibility not only to ZDV and ddI, but to ddC, d4T, 3TC), and abacavir as well. Virus from these patients first acquires a glutamine to methionine mutation at residue 151, and then it acquires additional mutations at residues 62, 75, 77, and 116 (55, 69–71). Patients who first acquire a typical ZDV-resistance mutation, usually at residue 70, do not develop the 151-resistance complex. Conversely, patients with the 151-resistance complex do not appear to acquire ZDV-resistance mutations.

This complex confers high-level resistance to all six of the previously listed nucleosides in clinical use. Still to be precisely defined are the true proportion of patients receiving ZDV–ddI who develop this mutational complex (estimates range widely around 5%) and whether these mutations arise with other nucleoside regimens.

Nonnucleoside Reverse Transcriptase Inhibitors

Some structurally divergent compounds share remarkable similarities (48, 72–76). These compounds do not require cellular metabolism to be active, they are potent inhibitors of HIV-1 replication but are relatively nontoxic in vitro, they inhibit reverse transcriptase activity and replication of HIV-1 but not of HIV-2 or animal lentiviruses, and they are equally effective against ZDV-sensitive and ZDV-resistant isolates (47, 48). This specificity may indicate a potential Achilles heel of these otherwise promising compounds in that lentiviral reverse transcriptase sequences can clearly be fully functional without being susceptible to these compounds. In fact, resistance readily emerges during virus replication in the presence of selective pressure of drug treatment in vitro and in vivo (13, 14, 76, 77)

The reason resistance emerges so readily is, as with 3TC, a single mutation can confer high-level resistance to this class of drugs. Drug-resistant mutants exist as minor subpopulations, as has been shown with the Y181C mutation for nevirapine (12). Treatment with regimens that do not completely suppress viral replication then permit these resistant variants to replicate (78–80). As with 3TC as well, if a regimen is sufficiently potent to suppress virus replication below the levels of detection, resistant virus does not emerge (81).

A 3.5-Å–resolution electron density map of the HIV-1 reverse transcriptase was made possible by complexing the reverse transcriptase heterodimer with nevirapine (82). The p66 subunit of the heterodimer appears to catalyze the multiple activities of the enzyme, making a DNA copy from the genomic RNA, degrading this RNA template (ribonuclease H activity), and making a complementary copy of this new DNA strand to yield the double-stranded viral DNA. The structure of the p66 subunit has been likened to a right hand (Fig. 49.4). This structure maintains remarkable similarity to the structure of the Klenow fragment of the *Escherichia coli* DNA polymerase and other known polymerases (82). The nucleotide binding site is located in the palm. The binding site of nevirapine and the other NNRTIs binds in a pocket in the palm of the p66 subunit (Fig. 49.5). This binding pocket for nevirapine is formed by two β strands composed of amino acid residues 100 to 110 and 180 to 190 (see Fig. 49.5). Mutations in these residues identified for isolates from patients who were administered nevirapine correspond precisely with the amino acid residues that form the binding pocket of the drug. Each of the NNRTIs selects for a subset of the mutations identified in the residues. Thus, in general, resistance to one member of the class selects for partial or complete cross-resistance to other members associated with NNRTI resistance (31, 76).

Resistance Interactions of Reverse Transcriptase Mutations

Cross-resistance of ZDV-resistant isolates has been observed to 3′-azido–containing nucleoside analogs (25, 46). The ddI-resistance mutation at residue 74 confers cross-resistance to ddC and a compensatory reduction of ZDV resistance conferred by residue 215 (53). NNRTIs display cross-resistance, although quantitative differences in the effects of various mutations indicate that the different compounds do not interact with the reverse transcriptase molecule identically (13, 14, 83–85). Additional complexities are being identified. Mutations conferring ZDV resistance can be antagonistic, additive, or synergistic (51). As shown in Table 49.1, the methionine to leucine mutation at amino acid residue 41 (meth 41 leu) is at least additive, if not synergistic with the threonine 215 tyrosine mutation. In contrast, the lysine 70 arginine mutation appears to antagonize the degree of resistance conferred by the 215 mutation. This latter observation may explain the observation that although the 70 mutation often appears first during ZDV therapy (52), it

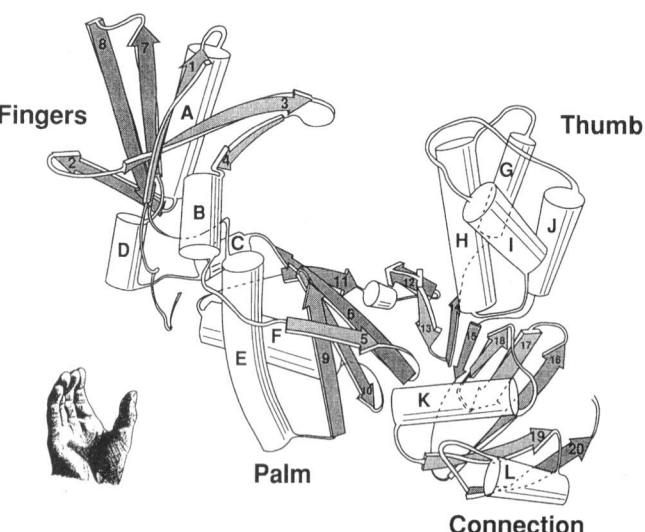

Figure 49.4. The folding structure of the p66 subunit of HIV-1 reverse transcriptase. This subunit has been likened to a right hand with fingers, a palm, and a thumb. Helical regions are represented as *lettered tubes* and β-strands as *numbered arrows*. This subunit is the target of both antiviral nucleoside triphosphates and nonnucleoside transcriptase inhibitors such as nevirapine. (From Kohlstaedt LA, Wang J, Friedman JM, et al. Crystal structure at 3.5-Å resolution of HIV-1 reverse transcriptase complexed with an inhibitor. Science 1992;256:1783–1790, as modified by J NIH Res 1992;4:81.) (See color section.)

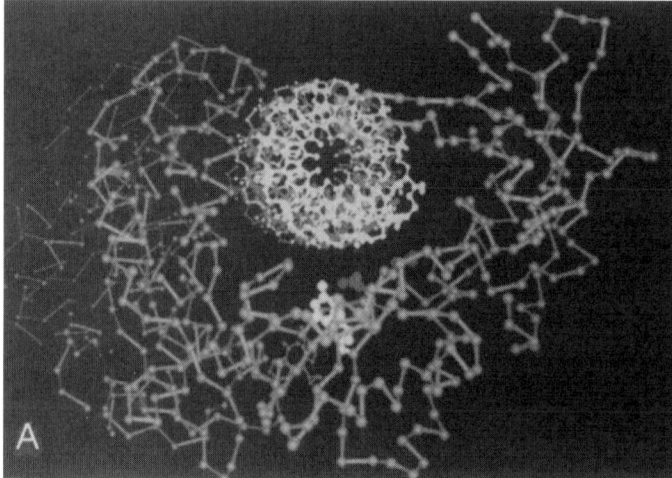
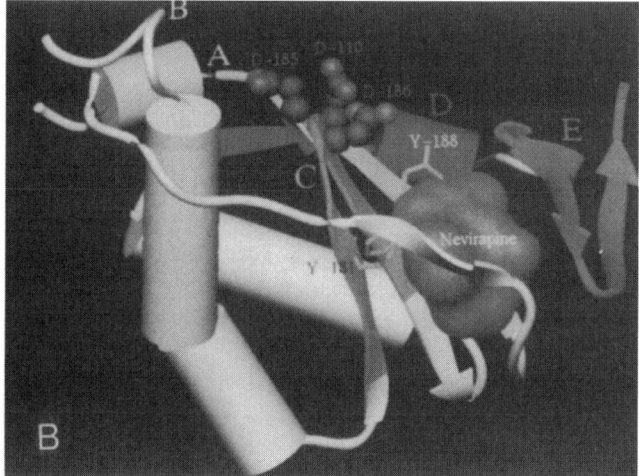

Figure 49.5. The position of nevirapine bound to the p66 subunit of reverse transcriptase. A. α-Carbon backbone *(purple)* of the p66 subunit with model built DNA *(blue and yellow)* showing the aspartic acids *(red)* at amino acid residues 185 and 186 at the presumed catalytic site nearby. Nevirapine *(green)* binds near the tyrosines *(white)* at residues 181 and 188. The view is from the "back" of Figure 49.4, so the "fingers" are on the right and the "thumbs" are on the left. **B.** The palm domain of p66 with nevirapine *(orange)* superimposed. The aspartic acids at residues 110, 185, and 186 presumably participate in the catalytic site. Nevirapine fits into a pocket found by β-strands composed of residues 100 to 110 and 180 to 190. Mutations in these regions including the tyrosines at 181 and 188 to which nevirapine binds result in resistance to nevirapine and the other nonnucleoside reverse transcriptase inhibitors that bind in this pocket. (From Kohlstaedt LA, Wang J, Friedman JM, et al. Crystal structure at 3.5-D resolution of HIV-1 reverse transcriptase complexed with an inhibitor. Science 1992;256:1783–1790.) (See color section.)

Table 49.2. Major Mutations Conferring Resistance to Protease Inhibitors

Drug	Protease Mutation[a]	Reference
Saquinavir	L10I, G48V, L90M	98, 99
Ritonavir	V32I, M46I, I54V, V82A/F/T/S, I84V, L90M	100
Indinavir	L10I/V/R, M46I/L, I54V, 82A/F/T I84V, L90M	22, 90
Nelfinavir	D30N, M46I, I84V, N88D, L90M	101
Aprenavir	M46I, I47V, I50V, I84V	102

[a]See Table 49.1 for abbreviations.

often disappears from the population of mutants when the more potent 215 mutation emerges.

As already described, the leucine 74 valine ddI-resistance mutation both confers cross-resistance to ddC and reduces the degree of resistance to ZDV in those viruses containing the 215 mutation (53). It does not reduce the susceptibility to ZDV of wild-type virus. The Y181C mutation selected by nevirapine and many other NNRTIs reverses the ZDV resistance conferred by mutations at residue 215 (86). Clinically, this interaction results in the emergence of Y181C as the predominant mutation with ZDV monotherapy; however, the coadministration of ZDV forces the virus to follow an alternate evolutionary pathway, and several mutations other than Y181C emerge (79). Several of the piperazine compounds select for a mutation at residue 236 that reverses resistance to nevirapine conferred by Y181C (85). This effect cannot be exploited clinically, however, because certain viral mutants, like those with Y181C itself, confer cross-resistance to both inhibitors.

PROTEASE INHIBITORS

The HIV protease is a homodimer composed of two 99 amino acid subunits. Drugs that inhibit the enzyme compete with substrate for binding at the catalytic site. At least 25 of the amino acid residues have been shown to mutate in association with the selection of drug-resistant virus (31, 87). Some of these mutations clearly reduce the binding affinity (K_i) of the inhibitor for the enzyme and result in a less susceptible virus. Other mutations do not affect drug susceptibility directly but appear to compensate for impairments in fitness, sometimes measurable by catalytic activity of the enzyme or replicative capacity of the virus. This phenomenon is analogous to the phenomenon with the Q151M mutation in reverse transcriptase resistance (see earlier). Recently, mutations in gag cleavage sites have been associated with inhibitor resistance (88, 89). Presumably, these mutant cleavage sequences provide better substrates for the drug-resistant protease, thus improving the replication competence of the resistant virus.

Each protease inhibitor can be shown to select for 8 to 14 different mutations in all; however, in any individual patient or with selection in vitro, various combinations of a subset of these possible mutations emerge, so few patients with resistance to a given protease inhibitor have the same constellation of mutations (23, 90). Table 49.2 lists the most important of the mutations for the protease inhibitors in clinical use.

As resistance emerges, mutations accumulate sequentially, each mutation conferring fitness by improving resistance or replication capacity. Often, the first mutation or several mutations will not confer cross-resistance to other protease inhibitors (22, 90); however, as high-level resistance with multiple mutations emerges, cross-resistance is the rule.

Because high-level protease resistance requires the accumulation of multiple mutations, high-level protease resistant mutants do not preexist. Their emergence requires the persisting replication of virus in the presence of selective pressures (23). For this reason, resistance takes months to emerge in the presence of monotherapy, and combination regimens that can suppress preexisting single and double mutants can prevent the outgrowth of drug-resistant virus (28, 64, 91).

ASSAYS OF DRUG SUSCEPTIBILITY

Phenotypic Assays

Investigators have a widespread desire and need for a dependable, standardized assay of drug susceptibility. The most commonly used assays for antiviral drugs have measured the inhibition of cytopathology, p24 production, or reverse transcriptase production of a laboratory strain of HIV in a lymphoblastoid cell line. Such assays cannot be readily applied to clinical isolates of HIV. The two most commonly used assays of drug susceptibility of clinical isolates have been the syncytial focus assay in CD4-HeLa cells and inhibition of p24 production in primary peripheral blood mononuclear cells (92).

The former assay has a distinct advantage in that it generates a monotonic sigmoid curve that is highly reproducible when the focus number is plotted against the log of the concentration of drug. The assay thus permits reproducible results, quantitative susceptibilities, easy detection of spurious single values, and the detection of phenotypical mixtures (46, 50). A disadvantage of the assay, however, is that it works well with virus stocks that exhibit the syncytium-inducing phenotype that in practice can only be obtained from a few specimens from seropositive individuals. It also works poorly with the drugs that act on posttranslational processing and glycosidase and protease inhibitors (D Richman, unpublished data). The assay in peripheral blood mononuclear cells generates less precise quantitation and is expensive, but it has the advantage of permitting assay for most clinical isolates.

Recent refinements of recombinant assays (93) in which the *pol* gene is amplified by polymerase chain reaction from plasma RNA and is inserted into recombinant constructs that permit the assessment of drug susceptibility, often using robotic methods, promise to transform drug susceptibility testing (94, 95). These assays can be performed from plasma RNA, they are relatively precise, they do not depend on

Table 49.3. Practical Implications of the Biology of HIV Drug Resistance

- Genetic variants of virus with any single and probably many double mutations preexist in all patients before treatment is started; thus, monotherapy and partially suppressive regimens containing lamivudine or nonnucleoside reverse transcriptase inhibitors rapidly fail because of breakthrough replication of resistant variants.
- Genetic variants with three or more drug-resistance mutations probably exist rarely, if at all, in untreated HIV-infected patients; thus, potent combination regimens that require many drug-resistance mutations for viral escape are recommended.
- The prevention of the cumulative acquisition of drug-resistance mutations requires the administration of potent combination regimens that suppress virus replication below the levels of detection.
- Complex mixtures of genetic variants exist in all patients; assays for drug resistance, both genotypic and phenotypic, thus provide information only on the predominant circulating variants.
- Prior treatment may select for drug-resistant mutants that persist in lymphoid tissues but are no longer predominant or even detectable in the absence of drug selection; retreatment with the same drug may not be effective because of the rapid selection of the prior resistant mutants; thus, assays for drug resistance, both phenotypic and genotypic, must be interpreted in the context of the history of drug treatment:
    Assays should be obtained before the patient discontinues the drug. A "sensitive" result may be misleading in a patient with a past history of antiretroviral drug use.

growth characteristics conferred by the viral envelope of each patient's virus, and, in the case of at least one assay, they can be conducted in 8 to 10 days (95). Such assays are being assessed for their clinical utility.

Genotypic Assays

Various technologies have been developed to detect mutations associated with drug resistance. They all require amplification of HIV RNA from plasma or virus isolates. Mutations are then detected by using probes to discriminate wild-type from mutant sequence (e.g., the Line Probe Assay [96]), to use Sanger methods to obtain the nucleotide sequence or, in the case of gene-chip technology, a combination of the two that uses probes to interrogate the nucleotide sequence of the majority of *pol* (97). Each method has its strengths and limitations, and technical improvements are being applied rapidly. One can only infer resistance from genotypic results, an inference that is probably dependable in the case of 41 plus 215 for ZDV, or 184 for 3TC, or 181 for nevirapine, or 151 for multiple nucleoside. On the other hand, inferring cross-resistance patterns for protease inhibitors can often be difficult.

DRUG-RESISTANCE TESTING IN PATIENT MANAGEMENT

Several important considerations must always be kept in mind for all drug-resistance testing, either phenotypic or genotypic (Table 49.3). First, complex mixtures of genetic variants exist in all patients. Assays for drug resistance thus provide information only on the predominant circulating variants. Second, prior treatment may select for drug-resistant mutants that persist in lymphoid tissues but are no longer predominant or even detectable in the absence of drug selection. Retreatment with the same or related drugs may not be effective because of the rapid outgrowth of these resistant mutants. Thus, assays for drug resistance, both phenotypic and genotypic, must be interpreted in the context of the patient's history of drug treatment. Assays should be obtained before the patient discontinues a drug. A result indicating "sensitive" or "wild-type" may be misleading in a patient with a past history of antiretroviral drug use.

Acknowledgments

This work is supported by grants AI 27670, AI 38858, University of California San Diego Center for AIDS Research (AI 36214), AI 29164, the National Institutes of Health, and the Research Center for AIDS and HIV Infection of the San Diego Department of Veterans Affairs.

References

1. Eigen M. Viral quasispecies. Sci Am 1993;269:42–49.
2. Drake JW. Rates of spontaneous mutation among RNA viruses. Proc Natl Acad Sci U S A 1993;90:4171–4175.
3. Lori F, Hall L, Lusso P, et al. Effect of reciprocal complementation of two defective human immunodeficiency virus type 1 (HIV-1) molecular clones on HIV-1 cell tropism and virulence. J Virol 1992;66:5553–5560.
4. Coffin JM. HIV population dynamics in vivo: implications for genetic variation, pathogenesis and therapy. Science 1995;267:483–489.
5. Leigh Brown AJ, Richman DD. HIV-1: Gambling on the evolution of drug resistance? Nature Med 1997;3:268–271.
6. Perelson AS, Neumann AU, Markowitz M, et al. HIV-1 dynamics in vivo: virion clearance rate, infected cell lifetime, and viral generation time. Science 1996;271:1582–1586.
7. Zhang L-Q, Simmonds P, Ludlam CA, et al. Detection, quantitation and sequencing of HIV-1 from plasma of seropositive individuals and from factor VIII concentrate. AIDS 1991;5:675–681.
8. Nájera I, Richman DD, Olivares I, et al. Natural occurrence of drug resistance mutations in the reverse transcriptase of human immunodeficiency virus type 1 isolates. AIDS Res Hum Retroviruses 1994; 10:1479–1488.
9. Nájera I, Holguín A, Quiñones-Mateu ME, et al. *pol* gene quasispecies of human immunodeficiency virus: mutations associated with drug resistance in virus from patients undergoing no drug therapy. J Virol 1995;69:23–31.
10. Wong JK, Ignacio CC, Torriani F, et al. In vivo compartmentalization of HIV: evidence from the examination of *pol* sequences from autopsy tissues. J Virol 1997;70:2059–2071.
11. de Jong MD, Schuurman R, Lange JMA, et al. Replication of a pre-existing resistant HIV-1 subpopulation in vivo after introduction of a strong selective drug pressure. Antiviral Ther 1996;1:34–42.
12. Havlir DV, Gamst A, Eastman S, et al. Nevirapine-resistant human immunodeficiency virus: kinetics of replication and estimated prevalence in untreated patients. J Virol 1996;70:7894–7899.
13. Nunberg JH, Schleif WA, Boots EJ, et al. Viral resistance to human immunodeficiency virus type 1–specific pyridinone reverse transcriptase inhibitors. J Virol 1991;65:4887–4892.
14. Richman DD, Shih C-K, Lowy I, et al. HIV-1 mutants resistant to non-nucleoside inhibitors of reverse transcriptase arise in tissue culture. Proc Natl Acad Sci U S A 1991;88:11,241–11,245.
15. Schinazi RF, Lloyd RM Jr, Nguyen M-H, et al. Characterization of human immunodeficiency viruses resistant to oxathiolane-cytosine nucleosides. Antimicrob Agents Chemother 1993;37:875–881.
16. Tisdale M, Kemp SD, Parry NR, et al. Rapid in vitro selection of human immunodeficiency virus type 1 resistant to 3′-thiacytidine

inhibitors due to a mutation in the YMDD region of reverse transcriptase. Proc Natl Acad Sci U S A 1993;90:5653–5656.
17. Boucher CAB, Cammack N, Schipper P, et al. High-level resistance to (−) enantiomeric 2′-deoxy-3′-thiacytidine in vitro is due to one amino acid substitution in the catalytic site of human immunodeficiency virus type 1 reverse transcriptase. Antimicrob Agents Chemother 1993;37:2231–2234.
18. Wei X, Ghosh SK, Taylor ME, et al. Viral dynamics in human immunodeficiency virus type 1 infection. Nature 1995;373:117–122.
19. van Leeuwen R, Katlama C, Kitchen V, et al. Evaluation of safety and efficacy of 3TC (lamivudine) in patients with asymptomatic or mildly symptomatic human immunodeficiency virus infection: a phase I/II study. J Infect Dis 1995;171:1166–1171.
20. Schuurman R, Nijhuis M, van Leeuwen R, et al. Rapid changes in human immunodeficiency virus type 1 RNA load and appearance of drug-resistant virus populations in persons treated with lamivudine. J Infect Dis 1995;171:1431–1437.
21. Larder BA, Kemp SD. Multiple mutations in HIV-1 reverse transcriptase confer high-level resistance to zidovudine (AZT). Science 1989;246:1155–1158.
22. Condra JH, Schleif WA, Blahy OM, et al. In vivo emergence of HIV-1 variants resistant to multiple protease inhibitors. Nature 1995;374:569–571.
23. Molla A, Korneyeva M, Gao Q, et al. Ordered accumulation of mutations in HIV protease confers resistance to ritonavir. Nature Med 1996;2:760–766.
24. Katzenstein DA, Hammer SM, Hughes MD, et al. The relation of virologic and immunologic markers to clinical outcomes after nucleoside therapy in HIV-infected adults with 200 to 500 CD4 cells per cubic millimeter. N Engl J Med 1996;335:1091–1098.
25. Larder BA, Darby G, Richman DD. HIV with reduced sensitivity to zidovudine (AZT) isolated during prolonged therapy. Science 1989;243:1731–1734.
26. Richman DD, Grimes JM, Lagakos SW. Effect of stage of disease and drug dose on zidovudine susceptibilities of isolates of human immunodeficiency virus. J Acquir Immune Defic Syndr 1990;3:743–746.
27. Kempf D, Rode R, Xu Y, et al. The durability of response to protease inhibitor therapy is predicted by viral load: International Workshop on HIV Drug Resistance, Treatment Strategies and Eradication, St Petersberg, FL [abstract]. Antiviral Ther 1997;2(Suppl).
28. Günthard HF, Wong JK, Ignacio CC, et al. HIV replication and genotypic resistance in blood and lymph nodes after one year of potent antiretroviral therapy. J Virol 1998;72:2422–2428.
29. Wong JK, Hezareh M, Günthard H, et al. Recovery of replication-competent HIV despite prolonged suppression of plasma viremia. Science 1997;278:1291–1294.
30. Finzi D, Hermankova M, Pierson T, et al. Identification of a reservoir for HIV-1 in patients on highly active antiretroviral therapy. Science 1997;278:1295–1300.
31. Schinazi RF, Larder BA, Mellors JW. Mutations in HIV-1 reverse transcriptase and protease associated with drug resistance. Int Antiviral News 1997;5:129–134.
32. Richman DD, ed. Antiviral drug resistance. Chichester: John Wiley & Sons, 1996.
33. Rooke R, Tremblay M, Soudeyns H, et al. Isolation of drug-resistant variants of HIV-1 from patients on long-term zidovudine therapy. AIDS 1989;3:411–415.
34. Land S, Treloar T, McPhee D, et al. Decreased in vitro susceptibility to zidovudine of HIV isolates obtained from patients with AIDS. J Infect Dis 161:326–329, 1990.
35. Tudor-Williams G, St Clair MH, McKinney RE, et al. HIV-1 sensitivity to zidovudine and clinical outcome in children. Lancet 1992;339:15–19.
36. Nielsen C, Gotzsche PC, Nielsen CM, et al. Development of resistance to zidovudine in HIV strains isolated from CD4+ lymphocytes and plasma during therapy. Antiviral Res 1992;18:303–316.
37. Albert J, Wahlberg J, Lundeberg J, et al. Persistence of azidothymidine-resistant human immunodeficiency virus type 1 RNA genotypes in posttreatment sera. J Virol 1992;66:5627–5630.
38. Wainberg MA, Beaulieu R, Tsoukas C, et al. Detection of zidovudine-resistant variants of HIV-1 in genital fluids. AIDS 1993;7:433–434.
39. Pepin J-M, Simon F, Goshi K, et al. HIV-2 resistant in vitro to zidovudine (AZT) isolated during prolonged AZT therapy [abstract PoA 2440]. In: 8th International Conference on AIDS, Amsterdam, 1992.
40. D'Aquila RT, Johnson VA, Welles SL, et al. Zidovudine resistance and HIV-1 disease progression during antiretroviral therapy. Ann Intern Med 1995;122:401–408.
41. Japour AJ, Welles SL, D'Aquila RT, et al. Prevalence and clinical significance of zidovudine resistance mutations in human immunodeficiency virus isolated from patients following long-term zidovudine treatment. J Infect Dis 1995;171:1172–1179.
42. Ho DD, Moudgil T, Alam M. Quantitation of human immunodeficiency virus type 1 in the blood of infected persons. N Engl J Med 1989;321:1621–1625.
43. Coombs RW, Collier AC, Allain J-P, et al. Plasma viremia in human immunodeficiency virus infection. N Engl J Med 1989;321:1626–1631.
44. Saag MS, Crain MJ, Decker DW, et al. High level viremia in adults and children infected with human immunodeficiency virus: relation to disease stage and CD4+ lymphocyte levels. J Infect Dis 1991;164:72–80.
45. Mellors JW, Rinaldo CR Jr, Gupta P, et al. Prognosis in HIV-1 infection predicted by the quantity of virus in plasma. Science 1996;272:1167–1170.
46. Larder BA, Chesebro B, Richman DD. Susceptibilities of zidovudine-susceptible and -resistant human immunodeficiency virus isolates to antiviral agents determined by using a quantitative plaque reduction assay. Antimicrob Agents Chemother 1990;34:436–441.
47. Richman DD, Rosenthal AS, Skoog M, et al. BI-RG-587 is active against zidovudine-resistant human immunodeficiency virus type 1 and synergistic with zidovudine. Antimicrob Agents Chemother 1991;35:305–308.
48. Goldman ME, Nunberg JH, O'Brien JA, et al. Pyridinone derivatives: specific human immunodeficiency virus type 1 reverse transcriptase with antiviral activity. Proc Natl Acad Sci U S A 1991;88:6863–6867.
49. Furman PH, Fyfe JA, St Clair MH, et al. Phosphorylation of 3′-azido-3′-deoxythymidine and selective interaction of the 5′-triphosphate with human immunodeficiency virus reverse transcriptase. Proc Natl Acad Sci U S A 1986;83:8333–8337.
50. Richman DD, Guatelli JC, Grimes J, et al. Detection of mutations associated with zidovudine resistance in human immunodeficiency virus utilizing the polymerase chain reaction. J Infect Dis 1991;164:1075–1081.
51. Kellam P, Boucher CA, Larder BA. Fifth mutation in human immunodeficiency virus type 1 reverse transcriptase contributes to the development of high-level resistance to zidovudine. Proc Natl Acad Sci U S A 1992;89:1934–1938.
52. Boucher CAB, O'Sullivan E, Mulder JW, et al. Ordered appearance of zidovudine resistance mutations during treatment of 18 human immunodeficiency virus–positive subjects. J Infect Dis 1992;165:105–110.
53. St Clair MH, Martin JL, Tudor-Williams G, et al. Resistance to ddI and sensitivity to AZT induced by a mutation in HIV-1 reverse transcriptase. Science 1991;253:1557–1559.
54. McLeod GX, McGrath JM, Ladd EA, et al. Didanosine and zidovudine resistance patterns in clinical isolates of human immunodeficiency virus type 1 as determined by a replication endpoint concentration assay. Antimicrob Agents Chemother 1992;36:920–925.
55. Shafer RW, Kozal MJ, Winters MA, et al. Combination therapy with zidovudine and didanosine selects for drug-resistant human immunodeficiency virus type 1 strains with unique patterns of *pol* gene mutations. J Infect Dis 1994;169:722–729.
56. Fitzgibbon JE, Howell RM, Haberzettl CA, et al. Human immunodeficiency virus type 1 *pol* gene mutations which cause decreased

susceptibility to 2',3'-dideoxycytidine. Antimicrob Agents Chemother 1992;36:153–157.
57. Zhang D, Caliendo AM, Eron JJ, et al. Resistance to 2',3'-dideoxycytidine conferred by a mutation in codon 65 of the human immunodeficiency virus type 1 reverse transcriptase. Antimicrob Agents Chemother 1994;38:282–287.
58. Gao Q, Gu Z, Parniak MA, et al. In vitro selection of variants of human immunodeficiency virus type 1 resistant to 3'-azido-3'-deoxythymidine and 2',3'-dideoxyinosine. J Virol 1992;66:12–19.
59. Gu Z, Gao Q, Li X, et al. Novel mutation in the human immunodeficiency virus type 1 reverse transcriptase gene that encodes cross-resistance to 2',3'-dideoxyinosine and 2',3'-dideoxycytidine. J Virol 1992;66:7128–7135.
60. Richman DD, Meng T-C, Spector SA, et al. Resistance to AZT and ddC during long-term combination therapy in patients with advanced infection with human immunodeficiency virus. J Acquir Immune Defic Syndr Hum Retrovirol 1994;7:135–138.
61. Lacey SF, Larder BA. Novel mutation (V75T) in human immunodeficiency virus type 1 reverse transcriptase confers resistance to 2',3'-didehydro-2',3'-dideoxythymidine in cell culture. Antimicrob Agents Chemother 1994;38:1428–1432.
62. Lin P-F, Samanta H, Rose RE, et al. Genotypic and phenotypic analysis of HIV-1 isolates from patients on stavudine therapy. J Infect Dis 1994;170:1157–1164.
63. Back NK, Nijhuis M, Keulen W, et al. Reduced replication of 3TC-resistant HIV-1 variants in primary cells due to a processivity defect of the reverse transcriptase enzyme. EMBO J 1996;15:4040–4049.
64. Wong JK, Gunthard H, Havlir DV, et al. Reduction of HIV-1 in blood and lymph nodes following potent anti-retroviral therapy and the virologic correlates of treatment failure. Proc Natl Acad Sci U S A 1997;94:12,574–12,579.
65. Larder BA, Kemp SD, Harrigan PR. Potential mechanism for sustained antiretroviral efficacy of AZT–3TC combination therapy. Science 1995;269:696–699.
66. Nijhuis M, Schuurman R, de Jong D, et al. Lamivudine-resistant human immunodeficiency virus type 1 variants (184V) require multiple amino acid changes to become co-resistant to zidovudine in vivo. J Infect Dis 1997;176:398–405.
67. Tisdale M, Alnadaf T, Cousens D. Combination of mutations in human immunodeficiency virus type 1 reverse transcriptase required for resistance to the carbocyclic nucleoside 1592U89. Antimicrob Agents Chemother 1997;41:1094–1098.
68. Shirasaka T, Yarchoan R, O'Brien MC, et al. Changes in drug sensitivity of human immunodeficiency virus type 1 during therapy with azidothymidine, dideoxycytidine, and dideoxyinosine: an in vitro comparative study. Proc Natl Acad Sci U S A 1993;90:562–566.
69. Shirasaka T, Kavlick MF, Ueno T, et al. Emergence of human immunodeficiency virus type 1 variants with resistance to multiple dideoxynucleosides in patients receiving therapy with dideoxynucleosides. Proc Natl Acad Sci U S A 1995;92:2398–2402.
70. Iversen AKN, Shafer RW, Wehrly K, et al. Multidrug-resistant human immunodeficiency virus type 1 strains resulting from combination antiretroviral therapy. J Virol 1996;70:1086–1090.
71. Schmit JC, Cogniaux J, Hermans P, et al. Multiple drug resistance to nucleoside analogues and nonnucleoside reverse transcriptase inhibitors in an efficiently replicating human immunodeficiency virus type 1 patient strain. J Infect Dis 1996;174:962–968.
72. Pauwels R, Andires K, Desmyter J, et al. Potent and selective inhibtion of HIV-1 replication in vitro by a novel series of TIBO derivatives. Nature 1990;343:470–474.
73. Merluzzi VJ, Hargrave KD, Labadia M, et al. Inhibition of HIV-1 replication by a non-nucleoside reverse transcriptase inhibitor. Science 1990;250:1411–1413.
74. Baba M, De Clercq E, Tanaka H, et al. Potent and selective inhibition of human immunodeficiency virus type 1 (HIV-1) by 5-ethyl-6-phenylthiouracil derivatives through its interaction with the HIV-1 reverse transcriptase. Proc Natl Acad Sci U S A 1991;88:2356–2360.
75. Romero DL, Busso M, Tan C-K, et al. Nonnucleoside reverse transcriptase inhibitors that potently and specifically block human immunodeficiency virus type 1 replication. Proc Natl Acad Sci U S A 1991;88:8806–8810.
76. Emini EA. Non-nucleoside reverse transcriptase inhibitors-mechanisms. In: Richman DD, ed. Antiviral drug resistance. Chichester: John Wiley & Sons, 1996:225–240.
77. Havlir D, Richman DD. Non-nucleoside reverse transcriptase inhibitors-clinical aspects. In: Richman DD, ed. Antiviral drug resistance. Chichester: John Wiley & Sons, 1996:241–260.
78. Saag MS, Emini EA, Laskin OL, et al. The L-697 6W: a short-term clinical evaluation of L-697,661, a non-nucleoside inhibitor of HIV-1 reverse transcriptase. N Engl J Med 1993;329:1065–1072.
79. Richman DD, Havlir D, Corbeil J, et al. Nevirapine resistance mutations of human immunodeficiency virus type 1 selected during therapy. J Virol 1994;68:1660–1666.
80. D'Aquila RT, Hughes MD, Johnson VA, et al. Nevirapine, zidovudine, and didanosine compared with zidovudine and didanosine in patients with HIV-1 infection: a randomized, double-blind, placebo-controlled trial. Ann Intern Med 1996;124:1019–1030.
81. Myers MW, Montaner JSG, Incas Study Group. A randomized, double-blinded comparative trial of the effects of zidovudine, didanosine, and nevirapine combinations in antiviral naive, AIDS-free, HIV-infected patients with CD4 counts 200–600 mm^3 [abstract Mo.B.294]. In: 11th International Conference on AIDS, Vancouver, 1996.
82. Kohlstaedt LA, Wang J, Friedman JM, et al. Crystal structure at 3.5 Å resolution of HIV-1 reverse transcriptase complexed with an inhibitor. Science 1992;256:1783–1790.
83. Balzarini J, Karlsson A, Perez-Perez M-J, et al. HIV-1-specific reverse transcriptase inhibitors show differential activity against HIV-1 mutant strains containing different amino acid substitutions in the reverse transcriptase. Virology 1993;192:246–253.
84. Sardana VV, Emini E, Gotlib L, et al. Functional analysis of HIV-1 reverse transcriptase amino acids involved in resistance to multiple nonnucleoside inhibitors. J Biol Chem 1992;267:17,526–17,530.
85. Dueweke TJ, Pushkarskaya T, Poppe SM, et al. A novel mutation in bisheteroarylpiperazine-resistant HIV-1 reverse transcriptase confers increased sensitivity to other nonnucleoside inhibitors. Proc Natl Acad Sci U S A 1993;90:4713–4717.
86. Larder BA. 3'-Azido-3'-deoxythymidine resistance suppressed by a mutation conferring human immunodeficiency virus type 1 resistance to nonnucleoside reverse transcriptase inhibitors. Antimicrob Agents Chemother 1992;36:2664–2669.
87. Markowitz M, Ho DD. Protease inhibitors-mechanisms and clinical aspects. In: Richman DD, ed. Antiviral drug resistance. Chichester: John Wiley & Sons, 1996:261–278.
88. Doyon L, Croteau G, Thibeault D, et al. Second locus involved in human immunodeficiency virus type 1 resistance to protease inhibitors. J Virol 1996;70:3763–3769.
89. Zhang Y-M, Imamichi H, Imamichi T, et al. Drug resistance during indinavir therapy is caused by mutations in the protease gene and in its gag substrate cleavage sites. J Virol 1997;71:6662–6670.
90. Condra JH, Holder DJ, Schleif WA, et al. Genetic correlates of in vivo viral resistance to indinavir, a human immunodeficiency virus type 1 protease inhibitor. J Virol 1996;70:8270–8276.
91. Gulick RM, Mellors JW, Havlir D, et al. Treatment with indinavir, zidovudine, and lamivudine in adults with human immunodeficiency virus infection and prior antiretroviral therapy. N Engl J Med 1997;337:734–739.
92. Richman DD, Johnson VA, Mayers DL, et al. In vitro evaluation of experimental agents for anti-HIV activity. In: Coligan JE, Kruisbeck AM, Margulies DH, et al., eds. Current protocol in immunology. Brooklyn, NY: John Wiley & Sons, 1993:12.9.1–12.9.21.
93. Kellam P, Larder BA. Recombinant virus assay: a rapid, phenotypic assay for assessment of drug susceptibility of human immunodeficiency virus type 1 isolates. Antimicrob Agents Chemother 1994;38:23–30.

94. Hertogs K, Conant M, Schel P, et al. The RT-Antivirogram: a rapid and accurate method to determine phenotypic (multi)-drug resistance in plasma of patients treated with various HIV-1 RT inhibitors [abstract]. In: 5th International HIV Drug Resistance Workshop, Whistler, Canada, 1996.
95. Parkin N, Whitcomb J, Smith D, et al. The use of a rapid phenotypic HIV-1 drug resistance and susceptibility assay in analyzing the emergence of drug-resistant virus during triple combination therapy [abstract]. In: 37th Interscience Conference on Antimicrobial Agents and Chemotherapy, Toronto, 1997.
96. Stuyver L, Wyseur A, Rombout A, et al. Line probe assay (LiPA) for the detection of antiretroviral drug-selected mutations in the HIV-1 reverse transcriptase gene [abstract]. In: 5th International HIV Drug Resistance Workshop, Whistler, Canada, 1996.
97. Kozal MJ, Shah N, Shen N, et al. Extensive polymorphisms observed in HIV-1 clade B protease gene using high-density oligonucleotide arrays. Nature Medicine 1996;2:753–759.
98. Jacobsen H, Hänggi M, Ott M, et al. In vivo resistance to a human immunodeficiency virus type 1 proteinase inhibitor: mutations, kinetics, and frequencies. J Infect Dis 1996;173:1379–1387.
99. Schapiro JM, Winters MA, Stewart F, et al. The effect of high-dose saquinavir on viral load and CD4+ T-cell counts in HIV-infected patients. Ann Intern Med 1996;124:1039–1050.
100. Schmit JC, Ruiz L, Clotet B, et al. Resistance-related mutations in the HIV-1 protease gene of patients treated for 1 year with the protease inhibitor ritonavir (ABT-538). AIDS 1996;10:995–999.
101. Patick AK, Mo H, Markowitz M, et al. Antiviral and resistance studies of AG1343, an orally bioavailable inhibitor of human immunodeficiency virus protease. Antimicrob Agents Chemother 1996;40:292–297.
102. Tisdale M, Myers RE, Maschera B, et al. Cross-resistance analysis of human immunodeficiency virus type 1 variants individually selected for resistance to five different protease inhibitors. Antimicrob Agents Chemother 1995;39:1704–1710.

50

ALTERNATIVE, UNCONVENTIONAL, AND UNPROVEN THERAPIES

J. Allen McCutchan

Despite considerable progress in treating human immunodeficiency virus (HIV) infection and its complications, many patients seek unproven, unconventional, complementary, or alternative therapies. These treatments may be viewed by patients as "alternatives" to scientifically based medical care and thus may represent rejection of or withdrawal from "conventional" providers. In other instances, these patients are seeking complementary therapy, but they remain involved with their scientifically based provider. *Unproven therapy* includes experimental therapy (usually drugs or vaccines) that will be scientifically evaluated in future clinical trials.

Unconventional or unorthodox therapies may be operationally defined as interventions not advocated, taught, practiced, or likely to be tested by scientifically oriented physicians. More fundamentally, many of these diagnostic and therapeutic systems are based on unscientific theories of disease, or, if plausibly based, they have not undergone adequate scientific testing for efficacy. They include such practices as *manipulation* (massage, acupuncture, chiropractic, and reflexology), *altered mental states* (biofeedback, hypnosis, meditation, and visualization), and *unorthodox pharmacotherapy* (herbalism, homeopathy, megavitamins, ozone treatments, and some purportedly antiretroviral or immune-enhancing drugs or vaccines). Specific therapies such as biofeedback or acupuncture may be accepted by conventional practitioners as useful for some conditions, but not for others.

Over the first decade and a half of the acquired immunodeficiency syndrome (AIDS) epidemic, announcements of "research breakthroughs" in the news media or "underground" publications have ranged in credibility from the bizarre to the improbable to the premature. These announcements set off hopeful speculation and questioning among patients and are difficult to address without rigorously acquired and clinically relevant data. An example of the bizarre is the denial that AIDS is caused by HIV (1, 2), whereas an example of the premature is reporting of results of in vitro studies of innovative approaches to treatment (e.g., gene therapy or xenotransplantation) (3). Thus, questions about unconventional or unproven theories and therapies continually confront physicians who care for AIDS patients. Clinicians' willingness to address these questions skillfully and nonjudgmentally can contribute to trust and open communication. This chapter provides background and practical advice for dealing with these issues.

PATTERNS OF USE OF UNCONVENTIONAL THERAPY

Many aspects of unconventional therapy for AIDS have precedents in other debilitating, incurable, or painful conditions such as cancer, arthritis, allergies, or affective disorders (4). Americans are estimated to spend over 13 billion dollars annually on many different treatments for these and less serious disorders such as backache, headache, obesity, and insomnia (5). A large, national telephone survey found that one-third of respondents had used unconventional therapy within the last year (1990). Of those using an unconventional provider, the mean number of visits was 19 annually. Two-thirds of users also saw a physician for the same problem, and of these patients, only one-fourth informed their physician. Consumers of unconventional therapy were more likely to be white, young (25 to 49 years), college educated, and living in the western United States. The broad definition of unconventional therapies used in this survey included commercial weight-loss programs, relaxation techniques, and massage therapy, and the criteria may have influenced these demographics. A similar survey in Australia came to similar conclusions about the extent and demographics of use of unconventional therapy (6).

In contrast to the developed nations, in many parts of the world traditional healers whose practices are not based in scientific medicine provide most health care. Because HIV is epidemic in underdeveloped areas of Africa, Asia, and South America, millions of HIV-infected patients are cared for by traditional medical providers. Traditional medical practices are also available within immigrant communities living in developed countries, and these practices may be used by both immigrants and native-born patients. For example, non-

Western medical practices such as acupuncture, herbal remedies, and meditation have become widely available in the United States.

USE OF UNCONVENTIONAL THERAPY BY PATIENTS WITH HIV INFECTION

Whether AIDS patients use unconventional therapy more commonly than others with life-threatening diseases is unclear. In a survey of 144 patients in Chicago, 9 of 50 (18%) AIDS patients compared with 2 of 30 (7%) cancer patients used unorthodox treatment (7). In more extensive surveys, about 30% of patients attending the AIDS clinics of the San Francisco General Hospital and the Pittsburgh Veteran's Affairs Medical Centers had used unconventional treatments (8, 9). These rates compare with 39% of 69 pediatric cancer patients attending the M.D. Anderson Cancer Center in Houston in the mid-1970s (10).

In a study from San Francisco conducted in 1989, the major factor predicting the number of unorthodox drugs used for HIV infection was a higher level of educational attainment (8). In contrast, income and number and duration of symptoms, but not educational level, were associated with the number of orthodox drugs used. However, a second, smaller study of patients attending the HIV clinic of the Pittsburgh Veteran's Affairs Medical Center found no correlation of use of "nontraditional" therapy with race, education, risk group, stage of disease, Karnofsky performance score, or duration of infection, but this study did find more use in patients older than 35 years (9). A third, larger study (*n*=184) from Philadelphia found that risk group (gay more than intravenous drug user), gender (men more than women) and duration of known infection (diagnosed for more than 2 years more than diagnosed for less than 2 years) were associated with use of alternative therapy, but age, race, income, religion, or stage of disease were not (11). Ten percent of these patients expected their alternative therapy to cure them, and 36% expected a delay in onset of symptoms. The recent advent of more potent antiretroviral drugs and tests for monitoring the effects of these drugs on plasma viremia may change the profile of users of unconventional therapy, but this remains to be seen. Thus, American users of unconventional therapy for AIDS, as for other diseases, are often well educated and have access to conventional treatment, but this pattern may change as therapy improves.

SOCIAL FACTORS INFLUENCING ATTITUDES AND ACCESS TO UNCONVENTIONAL THERAPY

The HIV epidemic has had several features that have promoted unprecedented levels of patient activism. AIDS struck urban gay American men who had preexisting social and political networks that mobilized money, information, and political pressure (12). Their influence on governmental drug regulators and research administrators and on private drug manufacturers has been powerful (13). Because healthy,

Table 50.1. Sources of Information about Experimental and Unconventional Therapy

Publication	Publisher
AIDS Treatment News	John S. James P.O. Box 411256 San Francisco, CA 94141
Treatment Issues	Gay Men's Health Crisis Center New York City Medical Information 129 West 20th Street New York, NY 10001
PWA Health Group Newsletter	PWA Coalition 31 West 26th Street New York, NY 10010
The Body (Website)	www.thebody.com American Foundation for AIDS Research 733 Third Avenue, 12th floor 1515 Broadway, Suite 3601 New York, NY 10017 212-682-7440

PWA, persons with AIDS.

HIV-infected persons at risk of developing AIDS have been diagnosed in large numbers, activists groups have benefited from highly motivated workers and leaders. These groups created sophisticated newsletters covering both unconventional and scientifically based treatments (Table 50.1) and convinced the United States Food and Drug Administration to change regulations concerning importation and premarketing distribution of unproven drugs (14, 15).

Relaxation of restrictions on the importation of unlicensed drugs for "personal use" by terminally ill AIDS patients legitimized a formerly clandestine activity. "Buyers clubs" in many cities provide many different unproven antiretroviral, anti-infective, and "immune-enhancing" drugs. The rationale, safe dose, and potential toxicities of these agents may be unknown or unavailable through conventional sources of medical information. Informational newsletters circulated among patients, but not available in medical libraries, are often the only source of information about unconventional treatments independent of the provider or distributors.

Access to promising experimental drugs through clinical trials or premarketing distribution became a major goal of AIDS activists. Initially, lack of understanding of the complexities of therapeutic research and lack of access to the decision-making process led to fears that indifference, ignorance, or corruption was delaying the search for treatments. These fears were effectively defused through unprecedented levels of involvement by activists and community-based physicians in the design and execution of clinical trials sponsored by the National Institutes of Health. Involvement of community leaders in development of new drugs educated these leaders and fostered the cooperation of their constituencies (primarily urban gay men) in therapeutic research. The reason for systematic, scientific study of promising treatments rather than their immediate widespread distribution was clearer when this process was seen firsthand and was understood. This opening of the therapeutic research process has assured many patients that scientifically based medicine has both the motivation and the ability to help them.

Since 1996, two developments have raised the confidence of many patients receiving conventional medical therapy for HIV. Quantitative assays of HIV in plasma ("viral load") have provided rapid, understandable measures of the need for and effects of antiretroviral drugs (see Chap. 40). Simultaneously, drugs of two new classes, protease inhibitors and nonnucleoside reverse transcriptase inhibitors, were licensed. In combinations with nucleosides, these drugs produce unprecedented CD4 count elevations and clinical benefits (see Chap. 47). The greater potency of current antiretroviral therapy may diminish interest in unconventional approaches for some patients, but many other patients will continue to combine these approaches.

Interest in unconventional therapy may also result from the social marginalization and stigmatization of groups suffering high rates of HIV infection, such as intravenous drug users, homosexuals, and socially disadvantaged urban, ethnic groups (African-Americans and Hispanic-Americans). The experiences of homophobia and racism cause some members of these groups to distrust authority figures, including physicians. A few community leaders have entertained bizarre theories of the origin of HIV in government laboratories. A more rational anxiety was that research and patient care for AIDS would not command adequate resources and priority because AIDS affected marginalized groups.

PSYCHOSOCIAL FACTORS INFLUENCING USE OF UNCONVENTIONAL THERAPY

Before the recent improvements in antiretroviral therapy, diagnosis of HIV infection often promoted a feeling of helplessness in both patients and physicians. Even now, the long-term prognosis remains uncertain, and medical management remains complex, expensive, and demanding. The threat of an early and possibly painful death has provoked understandable confusion and desperation. Under this threat, and knowing that medical science can neither provide a "cure" nor predict the course of HIV infection precisely, patients find alternative approaches attractive for multiple reasons. Unconventional therapy is often promoted as "natural" or "nontoxic," based on "ancient wisdom," effective against many different diseases, and free of side effects. Therapy may address symptoms that have been undertreated by conventional providers (e.g., pain, anxiety, or depression), or it may be less costly, demanding, complex, time consuming, or uncomfortable than conventional treatment. Finally, the therapeutic results may be "guaranteed" or presented with more enthusiasm and assurance than is comfortable for practitioners whose ethical standards demand more realistic assessment and communication.

Another factor is the increasing tendency of patients to challenge medical authority and to demand involvement in decisions affecting them. Suspicion of the motives of pharmaceutical manufacturers, government regulatory agencies, and clinical investigators remains high in the sexual and ethnic minority groups most affected by AIDS. Specifically, the struggle against homophobia by gay Americans and racism by African-Americans and Hispanic-Americans has prepared them to challenge authority and the status quo. Control of personal health decisions and access to unproven or unconventional treatments may be viewed as both a human right and a matter of personal survival.

Finally, interest in "natural" approaches to healing and fear that all antiretroviral drugs are "toxic" make many alternative therapies seem safer. In fact, many antiviral agents have side effects of varying severity that limit their tolerability in some patients and must be weighed in each patient against potential benefits. However, patients may not understand the concepts of individualized and ongoing assessment of drug toxicity and may dismiss all or most drugs as "toxic." To patients conditioned by fear of "pollutants" in the environment and "chemicals" in food and water, the appeal of more "natural and nontoxic" therapy is understandable, but it is often based on misconceptions.

SUMMARY OF COMMONLY USED TREATMENTS

Manipulation

Massage is manual manipulation of the skin, soft tissues, and joints for stimulation, relaxation, pain relief, or healing. It may be combined with or may overlap exercise, acupuncture, hydrotherapy, or other treatments. Many different techniques (e.g., Swedish, Japanese [Shiatsu and Amma], Rolfing, zone, and reflexology) with differing underlying goals and theories are practiced. Because massage is usually administered with bare hands, transmission of herpes simplex or herpes zoster or of HIV from open lesions of HIV-positive patients to the practitioner is a consideration.

Acupuncture is an ancient Chinese system of treatment with slender needles inserted into the skin, subcutaneous tissues, or muscles for 15 to 30 minutes at points along 12 meridians believed to control specific organs. In the United States, its practice and interest both by physicians and the public have increased dramatically. Since the early 1970s, when Western physicians observed acupuncture anesthesia for major surgery in Chinese hospitals, scientific study of acupuncture for relief of chronic pain has increased. Some scientifically acceptable theories of its mechanism have been developed, but they remain speculative hypotheses. The obvious potential risk of transmission of HIV or of hepatitis B or C by blood contamination of these needles can be minimized by appropriate sterilization or use of disposable needles.

Chiropractic is a treatment technique based on the anatomically implausible theory that most pain and disease arise from malalignment of the spine with resulting pressure on spinal nerves. Despite its scientifically unaccepted rationale, chiropractic seems to relieve many musculoskeletal disorders. Rapidly delivered, forceful manual pressure over the paraspinous muscles is said to "adjust" or "realign" the spine. Chiropractors are licensed in nearly all states and have achieved a remarkable level of social, if not scientific, acceptance. Because back pain can arise from the spine, contiguous organs, or systemic disorders that require diagnosis and treatment by a physician, patients should be advised to have a medical evaluation for back pain or other symptoms. No scientific basis for benefits of chiropractic beyond the potentially powerful placebo effect of therapeutic manipulation and the tendency of many pains to resolve over time has been demonstrated.

Altered Mental States

Certain techniques for improving mental and physical health through the induction of specific states of consciousness are popular, and many do not require a provider. Relaxation, hypnosis, meditation, and biofeedback have been useful to persons with life-threatening illness as a means of reducing anxiety or depression or coping with chronic pain. Related, but more specifically therapeutic, methods have been advocated as a treatment for HIV infection. These include *visualization,* to direct destruction of HIV-infected cells mentally, and *positive attitudes,* to promote resistance to HIV. Several popular books that encourage belief in the power of mental approaches to the healing of serious illnesses have been published (16–19). A series on public television, "Healing and the Mind," reviewed this topic in 1993 (20).

The scientific basis for potential influences of mental states on immune function has been explored over the past 30 years. An understanding of the anatomic and chemical connections between the two most complex systems (nervous and immune) in the human body is emerging (21). The popular concept that the course of disease can be powerfully influenced by adverse life experiences, mental attitudes, or alteration of mental states has been studied, with mixed conclusions. Several studies have detected relationships of life stress and mood with changes in markers of progression of HIV infection such as CD4 counts or β_2-microglobulin levels in serum, but other studies have not (22).

The ability of sham treatments (placebos) to improve both objective signs and subjective symptoms of disease is a powerful argument for an influence of psychosocial factors in healing. The placebo effect has been widely studied and provides the primary rationale for blinding both patients and physicians to treatment assignment in controlled clinical trials of therapy (23). However, the underlying conceptual basis and methods for much of this work have been criticized (24).

The concept that patients can influence their disease by mental effort is empowering, but it has the potential for engendering guilt when things do not go well. Although this effect has not been well documented, some critics of the self-healing movement have pointed out the danger of placing so much responsibility on patients with diseases with a high likelihood of progression, such as AIDS or cancer.

Unorthodox Pharmacotherapy

Herbal medicine is almost universally practiced in preindustrial cultures. Much of the herbal medicine practiced in the United States originated in China and India. Plants served as the initial source of various useful and powerful medicines in current use, including digitalis, opiates, quinine, and cocaine. A survey of patients attending the AIDS clinic of the University of California, San Francisco, Medical Center found that 22% (25 of 114) had used medicinal herbs within the past 3 months. A median of 4.5 tablets per day costing a median of $18 per month were consumed. Seven patients reported symptoms possibly caused by one of these herbs (25).

A well-designed placebo-controlled, 12-week pilot study of a mixture of 31 Chinese herbs for treatment of symptomatic HIV-infected patients without AIDS has been reported (26). Trends toward positive changes in "life satisfaction," numbers of symptoms, and severity of symptoms were found in those receiving herbs, but not in the controls. In contrast to subjective end points, more objective measures such as CD4 counts and weight were unchanged. This application of rigorous clinical trials methods to herbal therapy was too small ($n=30$) to achieve adequate power as a phase II efficacy study, but it represents a commendable, pioneering effort. The discussion addresses various methodologic issues such as the lack of traditional Chinese diagnostic methods, individualization of treatment, and other aspects of the "usual therapeutic context" that substantially deviated from clinical practice. Similar limitations often apply to evaluation of orthodox drugs in clinical trials with similar potential impact on assessment of effects.

Two herbally derived drugs for HIV infection have attracted considerable attention: compound Q or trichosantin, an extract of the Chinese cucumber, *Trichosanthes kirilowii,* and hypericin, a polycyclic compound extracted from *Hypericum triquethrifolium* or St. John's wort. Both have in vitro antiviral activity and were used in their herbal form by patients before purification of the active agents. Phase I studies of both trichosantin and hypericin have been reported, and the potential for serious toxicity has been documented with the former (27, 28). Thus, herbal medicines are not free of toxicity, as many patients mistakenly assume.

Homeopathy, a system of herbal treatment invented in the early nineteenth century, is based on the concept that "like cures like." This vague concept arose from the observation that the herbal cure for malaria, cinchona bark (quinine), causes fever in both patients and healthy persons. A second idea central to homeopathy is the need to dilute the active substance to vanishingly small amounts before administering it. Homeopathic physicians may be trained in "allopathic medicine," the name they apply to conventional medicine, and they may use modern diagnostic modalities and laboratory tests, but they generally do not use allopathic medications.

Various *nutritional* and *megavitamin* treatments have been advocated for HIV infection. Deficiencies of zinc or selenium have been postulated to contribute to HIV immune deficiency. The macrocytic anemia of zidovudine therapy and neurologic disease of AIDS have been blamed on vitamin B_{12} or folate deficiency. However, the preventive role of supplemental vitmain B_{12} in zidovudine-induced anemia was tested in a clinical trial and was found not to be helpful (29). Even patients with asymptomatic disease have been found to have decreased levels of multiple nutrients (30). Patients with diarrhea and malabsorption need careful attention to their total nutritional needs, but a role for specific nutrient deficiencies in the pathogenesis of AIDS remains to be proven (31). Likewise, the enthusiasm for high doses of vitamin C as an antiviral agent has been extended from the common cold to AIDS, but this association is unproven (32).

Unproven Drugs and Vaccines

Unproven drugs constitute the most confusing class of "unconventional" therapies because, unlike scientifically unsupportable systems such as chiropractic or homeopathy, each drug, vaccine, or procedure requires evaluation. New candidate drugs and vaccines appear regularly and generate reactions ranging from hopefulness to anger that the drug is not instantly available to all patients to cynicism. A partial list of some of the drugs that have received attention appears in Table 50.2. Most of these agents have not shown enough promise to be carried beyond small phase II trials (33–46). A review of other agents was published along with "an alternative treatment activist manifesto" in early 1994 (47).

ALTERNATIVE MEDICINE AS A MEANS OF PROMOTING EFFECTIVE COMMUNICATIONS WITH PATIENTS

Physicians who value autonomous, communicative, and trusting patients may find it necessary to be nonjudgmental and well informed about unconventional or unproven treatments for AIDS. Impatience or hostility to questions about the latest unproven or unconventional remedy closes discussion, reduces rapport, and may increase the attractiveness of alternative providers. Patients may be less willing to comply with treatments of proven benefit and known risk. At the extreme, they may reject scientific medicine altogether in reaction to their physician's negativity toward their hopes, beliefs, and experiences.

An open attitude does not require a suspension of critical judgment. It provides an opportunity to examine the reasons the patient is seeking help from other providers. Discussion of the patient's underlying information base and beliefs concerning unconventional treatments can be rewarding. Putting the "toxicity" of useful drugs in prospective and explaining the lack of evidence to support extravagant claims by some unconventional providers may prevent patients from making unwise choices. Willingness to be supportive regardless of their choices is crucial. Inviting a discussion of unconventional therapies at multiple times during the patient's course may elicit clinically important information and reassures the patient. Asking about other treatments, providers, or measures the patient is taking to maintain health opens several topics of importance.

First, patients may bring up the need to treat destructive addictions, or they may ask for advice about exercise, nutrition, support groups, or reduction of stress. These nonspecific measures are of uncertain benefit for improving survival or immune function, but for many patients they are empowering and enhance the quality of life.

Second, the physician may discover that their patients have other physicians who are prescribing redundant drugs, a situation that exacerbates the polypharmacy that often characterizes management of AIDS under the best of circumstances.

Third, patients may begin to discuss their fears of pain, disability, and death. This provides an invaluable signal that the patient is ready to deal with these often-neglected issues. Reassurance of support, correction of misinformation, and practical advice about life decisions based on the patient's prognosis can reduce anxiety dramatically. Both physicians

Table 50.2. References for Unorthodox or Unproven Drugs Advocated for the Treatment of AIDS Widely Used in the Early 1990s

Compound	Activity	Phase I Study (reference)	Phase II Study (reference)	Toxicity
AL-721	AV	35	36	Gastrointestinal
Low-dose naltrexone	IE	None	37	None
Disulfiram (Imuthiol)	IE	38	39	Disulfiram (Antabuse) reaction
Trichosanthin	AV	27, 40	41	Coma, dementia, photosensitivity
Hypericin	AV	28, 43	44	Hepatitis
Oral α-interferon (Kemron)	IE	45	46	None
Vitamin C	AV	None	None	Gastrointestinal (diarrhea)
N-acetylcysteine	AV	48	None	None known
Tumeric (curcumin)	AV	49	None	None known
Boxwood extract (SPV-30)	AV	None	None	None known
DNCB	IE	None	50, 51	Contact dermatitis

AV, antiretroviral; IE, immune enhancing.

and patients may avoid facing these issues directly, thus creating a "conspiracy of silence" about the patient's major concerns. Questions about unconventional therapy can be both a symptom of unaddressed concerns and an opening to begin working on them.

KEEPING INFORMED

Unproven drugs of potential scientific merit are reported on regularly in the *AIDS/HIV Treatment Directory*, published by the American Foundation for AIDS Research. Other publications listed in Table 50.1, as well as journals that specialize in educating practitioners such as *AIDS Patient Care* (Mary Ann Leibert, 1651 Third Avenue, New York, NY 10128), provide useful reviews of unproven drugs or relevant unconventional approaches. *The Journal of Alternative and Complementary Medicine*, also published by Mary Anne Liebert, was initiated in January, 1995. Additional references are available in most large biomedical libraries.

Acknowledgment

This effort was funded in part by a grant from the California University-Wide AIDS Research Program to the California Collaborative Treatment Group and the HIV Neurobehavioral Research Center of the University of California, San Diego (NIMH–P50 MH45294). I gratefully acknowledge the help of Emily K. McCutchan, MA, MFCC, and Kim Schulze in the preparation of this chapter.

References

1. Duesberg PH. Inventing the AIDS virus. Washington, DC: Regnery, 1996.
2. Moore J. A Duesberg, Adieu. Nature 1996;380:293–294.
3. Woffendin C, Ranga U, Vang Z, et al. Expression of a protective gene prolongs survival of T cells in human immunodeficiency virus–infected patients. Proc Natl Acad Sci U S A 1996;93:2889–2894.
4. Zwicky JF, Hafner AW, Barrett S, et al. Readers guide to alternative health methods. Chicago: American Medical Associaton, 1993.
5. Eisenberg DM, Kessler RC, Foster C, et al. Unconventional medicine in the United States. N Engl J Med 1993;328:246–252.
6. Maclennan AH, Wilson DH, Taylor AW. Prevalence and cost of alternative medicine in Australia. Lancet 1996;347:569–573.
7. Hand R. Alternative therapies used by patients with AIDS. N Engl J Med 1989;320:672–673.
8. Greenblatt R, Hollander H, McMaster JR, et al. Polypharmacy among patients attending an AIDS clinic: utilization of prescribed, unorthodox, and investigational treatments. J Acquir Immune Defic Syndr 1991;4:136–143.
9. Singh N, Squier C, Sivek C, et al. Determinants of non-traditional therapy use in patients with HIV infection. Arch Intern Med 1996;156: 197–201.
10. Faw C, Ballentine R, Ballentine L, et al. Unproved cancer remedies: a survey of use in pediatric outpatients. JAMA 1977;238:1536–1538.
11. Anderson WH. Patients use and assessment of conventional and alternative therapies for HIV infection and AIDS. AIDS 1993;74: 561–564.
12. Kwitney J. Acceptable risks. New York: Poseidon Press, 1993.
13. Marshall E. Quick release of AIDS drugs. Science 1989;245:345–347.
14. Investigational new drug, antibiotic, and biological drug product regulations: treatment use and sale, final role. Federal Register 1987; 52:19,465–19, 466.
15. Young FE, Norris JA, Levitt JA, Nightingale SL. The FDA's new procedures for use of investigational drugs in treatment. JAMA 1988; 259:2267–2268.
16. Hay L. The AIDS book: creating a positive approach. Santa Monica, CA: Hay House, 1984.
17. Siegal B. Peace, love and healing. New York: Harper Row, 1986.
18. Kubler-Ross E. AIDS: the ultimate challenge. New York: Macmillan, 1987.
19. Coleman D, Gurin J. Mind/body medicine: how to use your mind for better health. Yonkers, NY: Consumer Reports Books, 1993.
20. Moyers B. Healing and the mind. New York: Doubleday, 1993.
21. Ader R, Felten DL, Cohen N. Psychoneuroimmunology. San Diego: Academic Press, 1991.
22. Patterson TL, Shaw WS, Shirley JS, et al. Relationship of psychosocial factors of HIV disease progression. Ann Behav Med 1996;18:30–39.
23. Beecher H. The powerful placebo. JAMA 1955;159:1602–1606.
24. Kienle GS, Kiene H. Placebo effect and placebo concept: a critical methodological and conceptual analysis of reports on the magnitude of the placebo effect. Altern Ther 1996;2:39–54.
25. Kassler WJ, Blanc P, Greenblatt R. The use of medicinal herbs by human immunodeficiency virus–infected patients. Arch Intern Med 1991;151: 2281–2288.
26. Burack JH, Cohen MR, Hahn JA, et al. Pilot randomized controlled trial of chinese herbal treatment for HIV-associated symptoms. J Acquir Immune Defic Syndr Hum Retrovirol 1996;12:386–393.
27. Kahn JO, Kaplan LD, Gambertoglio JG, et al. The safety and pharmacodynamics of GLQ-223 in subjects with AIDS and AIDS-related complex: a phase I study. AIDS 1990;4:1197–1204.
28. Cooper WC, James J. An observational study of the safety and efficacy of hypericin in HIV+ subjects. In: Abstracts of the 6th International Conference on AIDS, San Francisco, 1990.
29. McCutchan JA, Ballard C, Freeman B, et al. Cyanocobalamin (vitamin B_{12}) supplementation does not prevent the hematopoietic toxicity of azidothymidine (AZT) [abstract MBP325]. In: Abstracts of the 5th International Conference on AIDS, Montreal, 1989.
30. Beach RS, Montero-Atienza E, Shor-Posner C, et al. Specific nutrient abnormalities in asymptomatic HIV-1 infection. AIDS 1992;7: 701–708.
31. Cimoch P. Proceedings of the 1992 International Symposium on Nutrition and HIV/AIDS. Nutrition HIV/AIDS 1992;1:3–108.
32. Cathcart R. Vitamin C in the treatment of AIDS. Med Hypotheses 1989;14:3423–3444.
33. Traub A, Margulis SB. Use of dinitrochlorbenzene (DNCB) as an immune modulatory in HIV-positive patients: a pilot study from Brazil. Blood 1995;86:935a.
34. Sarin PS, Gallo RC, Scheer DI, et al. Effects of a novel compound: AL-721 on HTLV III infection in vitro. N Engl J Med 1985;313: 1289–1290.
35. Mildvan D, Armstrong D, Antoniskis D, et al. An open label, dose-ranging trial of AL-721 in PGL and ARC [abstract WPB312]. In: Abstracts of the 5th International Conference on AIDS, Montreal, 1989.
36. Yust I, Vardinon N, Zacut V, et al. Al-721 reduces HIV antigenemia in seropositive asymptomatic subjects [abstract WP2167]. In: Abstracts of the 7th International Conference on AIDS, Florence, Italy, 1991.
37. Bihari B, Drury F, Ragone V, et al. Low dose naltrexone in the treatment of AIDS: long term follow-up results [abstract MCP62]. In: Abstracts of the 5th International Conference on AIDS, Montreal, 1989.
38. Bihari B, Martin J, Seaman D. The use of disulfiram as an immunomodulating agent [abstract 3042]. In: Abstracts of the 4th International Conference on AIDS, Stockholm, 1988.
39. Hersh E, Brewton G, Abrams D, et al. Ditiocarb sodium (diethyldithiocarbamate) therapy in patients with symptomatic HIV infection and AIDS: a randomized, double-blind, placebo controlled study. JAMA 1991;265:1538–1544.
40. McGrath MS, Hwang KM, Caldwell, SE, et al. GLQ-233: an inhibitor of human immunodeficiency virus replication in acutely and chronically infected cells of lymphocytes and mononuclear phagocytic lineage. Proc Natl Acad Sci U S A 1989;86:2844.

41. Byers VS, Levin AS, Waits LA, et al. A phase I-II study of trichosanthin treatment of HIV disease. AIDS 1990;4:1189–1196.
42. Meruelo D, Lavie G, Lavie D. Therapeutic agents with dramatic anti-retroviral activity and little toxicity at effective doses: aromatic polycyclic diones hypericin and pseudohypericin. Proc Natl Acad Sci U S A 1988;85:5232–5234.
43. Cooper WC, James J. An observational study of the safety and efficacy of hypericin in HIV+ subjects [abstract 2063]. In: Abstracts of the 6th International Conference on AIDS, San Francisco, 1990.
44. Furner V, Bek M, Gold J. A phase I/II unblinded dose ranging study of hypericin in HIV-positive subjects [abstract WB2071]. In: Abstracts of the 7th International Conference on AIDS, Florence, Italy, 1991.
45. Koech DK, Obel AO, Minowada J, et al. Low dose oral alpha-interferon for patients seropositive for human immunodeficiency virus type-1. Mol Biother 1990;2:91–95.
46. Kaiser G, Jaeger M, Birkmann J, et al. Oral natural low dose human alpha interferon (HuIFN) in 30 patients with human immunodeficiency virus (HIV-1) infection [abstract WB2140]. In: Abstracts of the 7th International Conference on AIDS, Florence, Italy, 1991.
47. Greenberg J, Burroughs C. An alternative treatment activist manifesto. GMHC Treatment Issues 1994;7:1–4.
48. Walker RE, Lane H, Boenning C, et al. The safety, pharmacokinetics, and antiviral activity of N-acetylcysteine in HIV-infected individuals [abstract MO.B.0022]. In: 8th International Conference on AIDS, Amsterdam, 1992;1:72.
49. Hellinger JA, Cohen CJ, Dugan ME, et al. Phase I/II randomized, open-label study of oral curcumin safety, and antiviral effects on HIV-RT PCR in HIV+ individuals. In: 3rd Conference on Retroviruses and Opportunistic Infections. Washington, DC: American Society of Microbiology, 1996:78.
50. Loveless M, Bradley B, Fields L, et al. Effect of dinitrochlorobenzene (DNCB) cutaneous sensitization on HIV disease progression. In: Infectious Disease Society of America 33rd Annual Meeting, San Francisco, 1995:134.
51. Cohen O, Pantaleo G, Loveless M, et al. Effects of dinitrochlorobenzene therapy on viral load and cytokine expression in lymphoid tissue of HIV-infected individuals. In: Infectious Disease Society of America 33rd Annual Meeting, San Francisco, 1995:135.

51

PSYCHOTHERAPY AND COUNSELING FOR HIV-POSITIVE INDIVIDUALS

George E. Woody, Delinda E. Mercer, and David S. Metzger

Since the first reported case in 1981, the acquired immunodeficiency syndrome (AIDS) and the human immunodeficiency virus (HIV) have become a major challenge to the United States health care system. According to the Centers for Disease Control and Prevention, 548,102 reported cases of AIDS and 343,000 AIDS-related deaths had occurred in the United States as of mid-1996 (1). Investigators estimate that more than 1 million people are infected with HIV in the United States—or 1 in 250 (2), and many more millions are infected worldwide.

In addition to the high-risk groups comprising male homosexuals, bisexuals, and intravenous drug users (IDUs), certain other subpopulations have become infected. These include patients with hemophilia, recipients of blood transfusions, children born to HIV-infected women, and persons from any age or ethnic group who engage in impulsive sexual behavior, especially with many partners. Increased transmission through heterosexual contact is resulting in higher risk among sexually active high school and college students and other young adults, the chronically mentally ill, and abusers of alcohol and nonintravenous drugs. The demographic characteristics of the population becoming newly infected have changed dramatically since the early 1980s, and some authors have asserted that it is no longer appropriate to label people as belonging to particular risk groups (3). However, epidemiologic studies indicate that groups at higher risk continue to emerge. For example, data show a disproportionate impact on minority communities, as reflected in AIDS incidence rates that are six times and three times higher, respectively, among African-Americans and Hispanics/Latinos than among whites (4). Minority women, in particular, are a group now at higher risk mainly because of sexual transmission of the virus from male partners who became infected as a result of substance abuse . African-American and Hispanic/Latino women accounted for 80% of newly reported AIDS cases among women in 1996 (4).

Although physical symptoms of HIV disease may not appear until years after infection, symptoms of emotional distress often begin when a person learns that he or she has become infected. In fact, the need for psychosocial intervention may be substantial at that time. Thus, the need for psychosocial interventions often does not coincide exactly with the need for more intensive medical interventions, and it may extend over a longer period. The recent advances in pharmacotherapy may influence the need for psychosocial interventions, but the direction is unknown. On one hand, treatment advances may magnify the need for psychotherapy or counseling because these advances delay disease progression, or counseling may improve compliance with complex medication schedules. On the other hand, medical advances may reduce the need for psychosocial interventions because the new therapies are resulting in an increasingly positive outcome for those who receive treatment and comply with it.

This chapter provides an overview of individual psychotherapy and counseling for HIV-seropositive individuals. It begins with brief definitions of psychotherapy and counseling, including a few of the most commonly used forms of each. It then reviews research findings on the efficacy of psychotherapy and counseling when they have been used with HIV-infected individuals and with other populations. Although not a focus of this chapter, self-help and support groups are mentioned because of their importance in the management of persons with HIV disease. It also includes an extensive, but by no means exhaustive, discussion of psychological issues that may arise during counseling or psychotherapy and that could serve as a focus for attention. Likely treatment goals and treatment planning issues are discussed, and the chapter concludes with comments about future research. Psychosocial interventions for pediatric AIDS cases and issues surrounding reproductive choices in HIV-positive individuals are not addressed, but they are reviewed elsewhere (5, 6).

DEFINITIONS OF PSYCHOTHERAPY AND COUNSELING

Psychotherapy and counseling, although often discussed as if they are the same thing, have significant differences in orientation, style, content, and the training given to those who deliver them. Psychotherapy is usually performed by doctoral-level persons, typically clinical psychologists or psychiatrists. It is intended to change problematic thoughts, feelings, and behaviors by creating new understandings and then applying them in ways that benefit the patient.

The particular framework used is determined by the orientation of the psychotherapist. For example, cognitive psychotherapy aims to identify and modify false beliefs and attitudes (7, 8); supportive-expressive psychotherapy aims to identify and modify problematic and recurrent relationship themes (9); and interpersonal psychotherapy aims to identify and change current problematic interpersonal relationships (10–12). Thus, cognitive therapists see problems in terms of false beliefs; supportive-expressive therapists see them in terms of problematic relationship "themes," and interpersonal psychotherapists see them in terms of current personal relationships. Therapists practicing any of these techniques always begin by listening to the patient and formulating the problem in terms of their particular orientation. The therapist then works with the patients, using methods specific to their technique, to foster understanding and subsequent affective and behavioral change.

Counseling may be performed by paraprofessionals or professionals, and it is typically done by persons with degrees at the bachelor's or master's level. Counseling focuses on identifying specific, current problems and on delivering concrete services as well as providing structure and support. Its main emphasis is on external problems rather than intrapsychic processes. Examples of counseling are identifying problems that require employment, medical, or legal services and then making referrals to appropriate service providers or crisis intervention in which acute problems such as loss of a place to live, loss of work, or homicidal or suicidal ideation are discussed as a first step for later psychiatric referral, evaluation, and treatment. As in psychotherapy, counselors begin by listening to the patient and then responding with interventions specific to their technique.

In practice, several areas of overlap exist between psychotherapy and counseling and among the various types of psychotherapy, regardless of orientation.

The most important of these include forming a relationship, identifying problems by attentive listening, and providing support. When working with HIV-seropositive patients, most psychotherapists and counselors help the client to obtain accurate information about HIV disease, attempt to bring about reductions in high-risk behavior, and encourage the patient to seek out and comply with medical treatment. The most commonly provided psychosocial intervention in AIDS-related care is pretest and posttest counseling. This intervention is almost always provided for those who are tested for HIV. Pretest counseling explains the test, its limitations, and the implications of a positive test. Pretest counseling also prepares clients for the temporary anxiety that often accompanies the waiting period before results are available. Posttest counseling is provided when results are communicated to the client. Its purpose is to continue education about the meaning of the result, to offer support if necessary, to provide encouragement and advice about how to reduce the risk of viral transmission, and to make referrals to other services if needed.

Another common type of counseling is focused on risk reduction outside the context of HIV testing and is termed simply "risk-reduction counseling." This intervention is offered most often to people who fall into high-risk categories such as drug abusers, gay or bisexual men, women who have sexual relationships with drug abusers, and persons in the sex industry. Often, risk-reduction counseling is provided in the context of a formal treatment program, such as substance abuse treatment, prenatal care, or treatment for the chronically mentally ill.

Risk-reduction counseling is usually brief and informational or psychoeducational and aimed specifically at changing high-risk behavior. It usually provides information on how to reduce the risk associated with sexual and drug using practices, and counselors sometimes distribute condoms and other materials aimed to encourage safer behavior. This type of counseling may also involve assertiveness training that focuses on sexual and drug-using situations, attempts to build self-esteem, and strategies for avoiding high-risk situations. Risk-reduction counseling is usually effective in increasing knowledge about HIV transmission and disease and in reducing high-risk behavior (13–15). As with most psychosocial interventions, it is far from 100% effective, and efforts are constantly under way to improve its efficacy.

Two general approaches to risk-reduction counseling have been used. The informational approach is sometimes referred to as non–theory based. Often, non–theory-based HIV risk-reduction interventions are characterized by a single-session format, and they focus largely on communicating HIV-preventive strategies through individual or group counseling or video presentations. Usually, this type of intervention does not include a skills training component. One limitation of this type of approach is that individuals at high risk are typically knowledgeable about HIV and strategies for prevention (although the information is not always accurate), so it does not appear that lack of information is a primary cause of high-risk behavior.

The second approach is psychoeducational, which often often involves multiple sessions and may be specifically based on psychological theories that appear useful in explaining and predicting change in HIV risk behaviors. One theory often used as the basis for risk-reduction interventions is the social cognitive theory (16), which looks at social, environmental, behavioral, and personal influences on an individual's behavior and assumes that successful behavior change requires skills training, a belief in one's self-efficacy, and access to necessary resources and social support. Another theory is the AIDS risk-reduction model (17), which postulates six mediating variables associated with the process of change to less risky behavior: 1) perceived susceptibility to contracting HIV, 2) anxiety regarding health consequences of HIV, 3) knowledge about HIV transmission, 4) response efficacy involving the belief that effective preventive action can be taken, 5) self-efficacy regarding confidence in one's ability to maintain preventive behaviors, and 6) assertive communication skills. The distinguishing feature of psychoeducational programs is their inclusion of skills training, assertiveness, and strategies to modify perceived peer or partner normative beliefs about risk-taking behavior. Developing and refining these skills usually involve various interactive learning techniques including observing others demonstrate the skills (social modeling) and role play. Generally, psychoeducational approaches are found to be superior to strictly informational approaches (14), and multiple-session interventions are superior to single-session interventions (15, 18).

Particularly important in effective risk-reduction counseling, as well as in other types of psychosocial treatment for persons with HIV disease, are awareness of and sensitivity to issues of race, ethnicity (14, 15, 19), and gender (19). Other cultural factors may be important as well, including the subculture of addiction and, within that, the differences between cocaine and opiate dependence (20), and the norms of workers in the sex industry.

RESEARCH FINDINGS ON PSYCHOTHERAPY AND COUNSELING AND THEIR APPLICATION TO HIV-POSITIVE INDIVIDUALS

Psychotherapy research has made tremendous progress during the last 20 years. Controlled studies have shown that psychotherapy can be helpful in treating many kinds of psychiatric disorders. Among these are major depression, many different anxiety disorders, posttraumatic stress disorder, and probably substance use disorders among those having other psychiatric disorders (i.e., "dual diagnosis patients"). In some studies, psychotherapy has been used alone, and in others it has been used in combination with pharmacotherapy (21–24). Several comprehensive reviews of earlier work supporting the efficacy of psychotherapy are available (25, 26). The gains achieved are usually moderate, but clinically significant.

Fewer studies have compared psychotherapy with counseling, or with a control group wherein support and clinical management (a medically focused intervention that resembles counseling but is briefer) are regularly available. In the few comparative studies that have been done, patients with lower symptom levels or less severe disorders usually showed significant benefits under all treatment conditions (21, 27). In these studies, no differences were noted between counseling or clinical management and psychotherapy. However, patients with more severe forms of the disorder, or with more intense symptoms, did better with psychotherapy than with either counseling or clinical management alone.

Other studies have compared pharmacotherapy, psychotherapy, and counseling in persons with major depression. In some studies, the most severely depressed patients responded better to pharmacotherapy than to cognitive therapy or counseling/clinical management (21), but in others, pharmacotherapy and cognitive therapy did equally well regardless of the severity of the depression (23). The findings from these studies, taken as a whole, suggest that counseling or clinical management and psychotherapy can be helpful, but more severely symptomatic patients have a better chance to improve if given psychotherapy than with counseling or clinical management. These findings also suggest that pharmacotherapy may be needed to supplement either counseling or psychotherapy in persons with the most severe disorders.

As mentioned earlier, a consistent finding from psychotherapy research is that various types of therapies produce approximately equal benefits. Although individual studies have sometimes found one form of therapy better than another, no overall pattern has consistently shown that one type of therapy is superior to others (26, 28). More consistent evidence, however, indicates that psychotherapy produces better results if it is applied according to its specified techniques and if it is administered by a person who forms a good relationship with the patient (29, 30).

Studies also demonstrate that some therapists produce better results than others. This finding is consistent with clinical experience, and it has raised questions regarding whether outcome studies are measuring the effects of *therapy* or of *therapists*. Some more recent studies have adopted methods aimed at addressing this problem. These methods include standardization of treatment techniques by using manuals, consistent training and supervision of therapists, taping therapy sessions for examination of compliance with the specified techniques, and removing therapists from the study protocol who deviate from the technique (31, 32).

Even though both psychotherapy and counseling are regularly used with patients who have HIV disease, few published controlled studies have assessed the outcome of these interventions. One of the few available studies compared four treatment modalities for individual therapy of depressed HIV-positive patients (33). The psychotherapies under study were interpersonal, cognitive-behavioral, supportive, and supportive plus imipramine. The patient population was initially made up of primarily gay and bisexual men with some social and financial resources, but over the years of the study, the patient population changed to reflect the trends in transmission of the virus. In other words, over time, the study had more minority patients with fewer social and financial resources. Drug-addicted clients were not eligible for this study, but drug abuse was sometimes present. Preliminary results (33) examined only the comparison of interpersonal ($n=16$) with supportive therapy ($n=16$), and they suggested that interpersonal psychotherapy produced better outcomes than supportive therapy. More complete outcome data on 101 patients suggest that interpersonal psychotherapy and supportive therapy plus imipramine did better at reducing depression than either supportive therapy alone or cognitive-behavioral therapy (JC Markowitz, unpublished data, 1997). Therapist adherence to treatment condition was monitored by highly reliable raters, and all therapist–patient dyads were rated as adherent to their assigned protocol. This means that any individual therapist effects should be minimized, a finding that implies that differences in outcome are likely to be due to the different treatments.

Another comparative study examined group psychotherapy for HIV-positive patients (34). Thirty-nine asymptomatic HIV-positive gay men were randomly assigned to a 16-week trial of cognitive-behavioral group therapy, existential group therapy, or a wait list control. At the end of the 16-week period, patients in the control group were randomly assigned to either cognitive-behavioral group therapy or existential group therapy. Results showed that participants in either of the active therapies showed significant reduction in psychological distress as compared with the controls. Consistent with most other psychotherapy studies, no significant outcome differences were noted between the two therapies.

The foregoing research suggests that both counseling and psychotherapy (group or individual) can be helpful, including the emotional distress associated with HIV disease. If one were to extrapolate from the existing body of research, one could hypothesize that counseling may be sufficient for most persons with adjustment disorders or for those having more persistent disorders but mild symptoms. In fact, Grant and Anns (35) support this point of view in stating that support and information are enough for most HIV-positive clients, and empathic counseling is often more helpful than probing psychotherapy. Using this same hypothesis, psychotherapy may be useful mainly for patients with more severe disorders or for those whose symptoms are persistent and intense even though they may not meet criteria for a specific disorder. In some cases, pharmacotherapy may be needed in combination with psychotherapy to reduce emotional distress, as discussed earlier (JC Markowitz, unpublished data, 1997).

SELF-HELP GROUPS AND PEER SUPPORT SYSTEMS

Most persons experience a great deal of emotional distress when they learn they are HIV positive. The psychosocial interventions that may be needed at this point, or later, are not limited to psychotherapy or counseling. Institutional social supports, self-help groups, and volunteer services that often serve as "buddies" can be extremely helpful. These services often form the "backbone" of the psychosocial services offered to HIV-positive individuals and, in many cases, are effectively combined with psychotherapy or counseling.

A few studies of the efficacy of these groups have been conducted. One study of HIV-positive individuals found that those who attended support groups had more social contact and lower levels of emotional distress than those who did not (36). Nonattenders had more avoidant coping styles and higher levels of psychological distress. Time since testing positive was an important intervening factor in the level of social isolation. Persons who knew of their serostatus for longer were more likely to participate in a support group than those who had learned that they were HIV seropositive more recently. Even among those who did not attend support groups, longer length of time since testing was associated with less social isolation. However, nonattenders exhibited more emotional distress regardless of how long they had known of their HIV positivity. These findings imply that self-help support groups and other support services such as volunteer "buddies" play an important role in the reduction of psychological distress associated with being HIV positive.

One disadvantage of these social services for HIV-positive individuals is that they are sometimes not available until the person becomes symptomatic with HIV disease. If this type of situation exists, individual psychotherapy or counseling may be the only service available for persons with psychiatric problems who have not yet developed HIV-related medical problems. Another disadvantage is that, given the history of HIV infection in the United States, many support services are strongly oriented toward the gay and bisexual community, and persons who are not members of these social groups may feel uncomfortable or even excluded. Psychotherapy or counseling, because of their focus on the individual, may be more easily adapted to the needs of such persons. Another advantage, at least in theory but not always in practice because of cost, is that psychotherapy and counseling can be given whenever the individual believes that assistance is needed and at any point in the disease progression.

RELATIONSHIP BETWEEN PSYCHOPATHOLOGY AND HIV DISEASE

A few studies have looked at the relationship between psychopathology and HIV infection. The specific areas that have been researched are expressed by the following questions: Is psychopathology a risk factor for HIV infection? Does learning that one is HIV positive cause psychopathology? Do psychiatric disorders such as depression influence the course of HIV disease?

Is psychopathology a risk factor for HIV infection? Perry and colleagues (37) used the Structured Clinical Interview for DSM-III-R (SCID) (38) to arrive at DSM-III-R (39) diagnoses of asymptomatic men and women seeking antibody testing. Persons in this study were an "at-risk" sample including IDUs, sexual partners of those with HIV infection, and homosexual or bisexual men. Results showed higher lifetime and current rates of mood disorders and substance dependence among those seeking testing as compared with a community sample. Although this study examined persons who were at risk of HIV infection, its findings are limited because the subjects were self-selected and may not represent the overall population of those at risk of HIV.

Data from a few studies with drug abusers have consistently found that persons at especially high risk within this population are those with increased levels of psychopathologic features. One study with opioid addicts (40) found that the presence of psychiatric symptoms was associated with risky behavior. In this study, increasing levels of psychiatric symptoms were associated with a stepwise progression of risky behavior. In a later study examining the same cohort but at a later time, increased levels of psychiatric symptoms were associated with not only risky behavior, but also with a higher incidence of HIV infection (41). Another study, also with opioid addicts but conducted by another group of researchers, found that persons with antisocial personality disorder were more likely to engage in risky behavior and to seroconvert than those who were not antisocial (42). In summary, this limited number of studies with drug abusers has consistently found that high levels of psychiatric symptoms, including Axis II psychopathology (i.e., antisocial personality disorder), are associated with risky behavior and subsequent HIV infection.

Most of these studies were conducted in men because most opioid addicts are male. A study of 173 female users of urban health centers in the Baltimore area explored the relationship between depressive symptoms and high-risk behavior (43). These women were not specifically queried about their drug use, but both health centers were located in areas with high levels of intravenous drug use, sexually transmitted diseases, teen pregnancy, unemployment, and poverty. The investigators found that women with higher levels of depressive symptoms were more likely to report high-risk behaviors, including having more than one sexual partner in the past year, having a partner who was an IDU, or having a partner within the last 5 years who was suspected of having a sexually transmitted disease. These results are consistent with the studies described previously (40–42), which focused on male populations.

Given the strength and consistency of the associations found between psychiatric symptoms and risky behavior in this limited number of studies, one could hypothesize that psychiatrically focused therapies, such as psychotherapy or pharmacotherapy, may strengthen risk-reduction interventions among psychiatrically symptomatic individuals. No studies have as yet examined this question, although the available data indicate that this area is worthy of more attention.

Does learning that one is HIV positive cause psychopathologic symptoms? Numerous researchers have examined emotional reactions to learning that one has HIV infection (44, 45). Initial reactions and later responses are usually similar in that patients report heightened levels of anxiety and depression but not necessarily a persistent psychiatric disorder. For example, Dilley and associates (46) and Woo (47) found that adjustment disorder with depressed mood was the most common psychiatric diagnosis for patients hospitalized with HIV disease. This diagnosis is, by definition, transient and consistent with the idea that psychiatric symptoms associated with HIV infection are usually temporary. Similar results were found in another study among persons with substance dependence, in which researchers showed that learning of seropositive status did not result in long-term changes in psychological symptoms (48).

One implication of these studies is that most patients who become HIV positive are initially psychiatrically stable, and learning of HIV-seropositive status does not cause long-term psychiatric disorders. However, this conclusion is limited because much of the research on psychopathology and HIV disease typically lacks detailed information on baseline levels of functioning (49). This finding, if true, would imply that brief counseling and support, rather than psychotherapy, are adequate psychosocial interventions for most persons who become HIV positive.

Do psychiatric symptoms influence the course of HIV disease? Other studies have examined the relationship between psychiatric symptoms and progression of HIV disease (46, 47, 50, 51), on the theory that immunologic function may be negatively influenced by psychopathologic features. Depression has been a special focus of attention because of its common occurrence and because effective treatments, such as psychotherapy and pharmacotherapy, are available (52).

This area has been researched, yielding mostly negative findings (52). For example, Rabkin and colleagues (53) evaluated the extent to which depressive disorders, psychiatric distress, and psychosocial stressors were related to HIV disease and found no relationship between these factors and immune status or disease stage. A meta-analytic review of 21 published studies (54) also found no relationship between depression and decreased immune function or acceleration of HIV disease progression, although depression was associated with more reports of HIV-related symptoms. Thus, the belief that emotional distress is likely to depress immune function, or that a more positive outlook will bolster immune function, is not well supported in the research literature. However, fewer depressive or other psychiatric symptoms may improve one's quality of life and may make HIV-related distress more tolerable.

An area for psychosocial intervention that has received little attention is HIV-related dementia. Patients with dementia often become confused, paranoid, or agitated. Low doses of pharmacotherapeutic agents having distinct antianxiety properties, combined with a supportive psychosocial approach, are generally used to manage such patients. Studies have not yet determined whether cognitive retraining techniques, such as those used with some success in head-injured patients, can be helpful in treating persons with HIV-related dementia.

PSYCHOLOGICAL THEMES ASSOCIATED WITH HIV DISEASE

Psychosocial Issues

Numerous authors have identified psychosocial issues associated with being HIV positive (2, 36). Some of these issues overlap with the stages of death and dying that have been described by Kubler-Ross (55). Issues that arise early include 1) initial response to the diagnosis often involving shock and panic (56); 2) anger and denial; 3) stigma; 4) shame over disclosure of one's HIV status to others; 5) anxiety and depression; 6) problems with self-esteem; 7) loneliness; 8) diminished sexual desire or changes in sexual functioning; 9) changes in health status; 10) difficulty beginning a treatment regimen; 11) choice of a future lifestyle; and 12) problems regarding intimacy and relationships. Later issues often include existential and spiritual concerns, grief over the loss one is facing, and coming to terms with unresolved past issues. Some or all of these issues can become a focus of psychotherapy or counseling.

Existential Issues

As in other situations, such as advanced cancer in which the outcome is expected to be fatal, psychotherapists and counselors treating HIV-positive individuals may be asked to help with existential issues. These issues often deal with finding a purpose in life or creating a meaningful and worthwhile existence before death. They occur in the shadow of premature loss and what it means for one's hopes, dreams, relationships, and health. Many people with HIV may not wish or be able to address these concerns. For others, these concerns are important and may be addressed by psychotherapy or counseling.

Death and Dying

Kubler-Ross' (55) staged model of responses to death and dying is a good starting point to think about some of the emotions experienced by persons who are living with HIV. She identified five progressive phases: denial, anger, bargaining, depression, and acceptance. Several writers have extrapolated from her model to describe emotions reported by persons with HIV disease (56, 57). Nichols (57) suggested that emotional reactions to AIDS often appear more intense and labile than those Kubler-Ross describes.

Alternatively, some clinicians have seen more blunted, even seemingly apathetic, emotional responses to AIDS. These kinds of responses seem more common in clients whose quality of life has already been severely diminished by issues such as drug addiction or chronic mental illness. In these situations, these persons' affective responses appear to have been muted by the painful emotional context of their lives, and further, their ability to recognize and express feelings may be limited. For many of these patients, HIV infection is just one more problem and is not an immediate cause for concern inasmuch as it will probably take years to progress and more pressing problems require an immediate solution, such as food and housing.

Kubler-Ross' staged model has been viewed by some investigators (49) as oversimplified because emotional reactions to terminal illness vary widely. Hoffman (49) also noted no empirical support exists for these stages in HIV-seropositive clients. In response to some of these issues, Kubler-Ross (58) amended her earlier model to acknowledge the variability in people's responses. As with other stage models of development, individuals usually progress at their own pace. They may skip a stage, may be in several at once, or may recycle back to previous stages when new concerns emerge. Thus, although these stages can be helpful guideposts for psychotherapists and counselors, it is inaccurate to think of them as occurring in a rigid progression or as being seen in all persons with HIV disease. Even if these stages are followed, one should also consider other emotional responses that may occur concurrently.

Bartlett and Finkbeiner (59) looked at the association between emotional stress and medical status. They reported that three periods of heightened emotional stress usually occur in persons with HIV disease, each period marked by a change in health status. The first is just after the initial diagnosis. If the initial reaction was marked by intense feelings of anxiety or depression and if the patient had no preexisting psychiatric disorder, these feelings usually diminish over a period of weeks or months as the individual adjusts to the knowledge of being infected. The second period is when the individual has the first bout of illness. At this point, the patient is faced with issues of declining health and vitality, of seeing himself or herself as having an illness and requiring care, and of moving closer to personal mortality and loss. The third period is when the person becomes significantly ill, having experienced two or more AIDS-defining illnesses. Some patients have no change in their attitude or feelings because this point is anticlimactic: they have already defined themselves as having AIDS and have experienced prolonged periods of hopelessness. Others have responded to HIV disease in a more healthful, proactive way and have led full and meaningful lives up to that point. For these patients, becoming ill can be accompanied by a sense of hopelessness and despair, of having "lost the battle."

Changing Dynamics

These medical landmarks have been the traditional ones that serve to precipitate emotional responses that may require intervention. However, the entire emotional landscape is changing with the advent of new therapies and more hope. Studies of emotional responses to these emerging technologies may identify new dynamics that need psychosocial intervention in some individuals. Particularly important will be data on the long-term efficacy of the new treatments, and also on the efficacy of preventive or therapeutic vaccines that may be developed, and the emotional response of persons who are helped by their interventions. Survivor guilt, as occurs in soldiers who survive a battle in which others have died, may emerge is an important theme that could be addressed by psychotherapy or counseling.

THERAPIST QUALITIES

As mentioned earlier, therapist effects have been well documented in earlier studies of psychotherapy and counseling. These effects seem related to the therapist's abilities both to follow the specifications of a particular method and to form a positive relationship with the patient. Therapist qualities are likely to be important factors in the psychosocial treatment of persons with HIV disease as well; however, few data are available to provide information in this important area. In the absence of such data, we describe therapist attributes that are probably important, based on common sense and clinical experience.

Knowledge of HIV Disease

Although one does not need to be an expert, therapists must have basic and up-to-date information on HIV disease. Therapists should know the limitations of their knowledge and should be able to make proper referrals if the patient wishes to obtain more detailed information. Often, the motivated, concerned client aggressively seeks information and may be able to educate the therapist. However, the therapist must also keep in mind that misinformation is prevalent, and thus it is important to be a critical listener and to correct inaccuracies if they arise. Patients with more significant psychiatric or cognitive impairments may not be motivated or able to obtain their own information and may need therapists to provide it at their level and as they are ready to hear it.

Being Comfortable With Sexual Behavior

Psychotherapists and counselors must be comfortable hearing and talking about sexual behavior in detail. It may be necessary to explain what kinds of sexual behaviors are less risky and periodically to use interventions aimed at encouraging the client to limit sexual behavior to these low-risk activities. An example would be dealing with psychological issues that interfere with the use of condoms. Another issue often arises in relation to helping patients deal with shame. Some HIV-seropositive persons may be ashamed of their sexual activities. The therapist must help the patient to eliminate risky behavior, while at the same time being careful to avoid increasing the shame by expressing personal criticism of the patient's lifestyle. Another problem that may emerge, and that can become a focus of therapy, is self-blame over becoming infected. This attitude is likely to be damaging rather than therapeutic, it may be associated with depressive feelings, and it should be reduced or eliminated if possible.

Knowing and Being Comfortable With the Patient's Culture

The therapist should be familiar with the client's culture if it is different from his or her own. The main cultural groups that have typically engaged in high levels of risky behaviors are gay or bisexual males and IDUs. The therapist must be open to hearing about the client's lifestyle and accepting of the client as a valuable person. One should differentiate between high-risk behaviors and high-risk groups, to make it clear that problematic behaviors do not comprise one's entire identity.

This approach is especially meaningful to the person who may feel bad or unworthy because of participation in risky behaviors. Individuals who are members of groups that are often stigmatized by society, such as gay or bisexual men and drug addicts, are encouraged to feel ashamed by cultural attitudes and may even feel that they deserve HIV infection. These feelings can negatively affect the quality of life, they may be associated with increases in risky behavior, and they can be reduced by psychosocial interventions.

Sensitivity to Cultural Differences Extends to Issues of Race and Ethnicity

Therapists and counselors must be aware of this dynamic in attempting to establish a supportive relationship. The therapist should realize that the client will respond to the therapist's perceived similarity or difference to his or her perception of how well the therapist understands the client's cultural experience, and to the therapist's attitude. This issue is particularly important when working with seropositive clients from minority groups in which racial and ethnic differences exist between therapist and patient in important areas such as perception of illness, trust in the medical community, acceptance of homosexuality and bisexuality, sexual behavior, attitudes toward condoms and other contraceptive methods, and drug-using behaviors. Differences may also exist in access to information. People whose command of English is limited, who are less well educated, and who cannot read well may be unable to obtain accurate information without the assistance of a treatment provider.

Social class differences in access to health care can also be an important issue among persons from minority groups. Most important are racial differences in the prevalence of HIV infection, with persons of African-American and Hispanic/Latino descent being disproportionately represented. In fact, about 80% of the cases among women are from these two minority groups (4). In addition, one must take into account the cultural norms, values, expectations, and attitudes of the target group when providing psychotherapy or counseling (15, 19, 60).

Countertransference

The term *countertransference* describes the therapist's emotional reactions to the patient. Just as patients react to therapists, therapists react to patients. These reactions are natural and human. They are studied closely in certain kinds of psychotherapies, such as supportive-expressive therapy, in which the reactions themselves are sometimes used as part of treatment. In other therapies, such as cognitive-behavioral or interpersonal, they are not emphasized. In supportive-expressive therapy, countertransference is often used as a clue to alert the therapist to emotional responses within the patient that require attention.

Countertransference responses can also be harmful if they are associated with negative feelings or attitudes or with otherwise untherapeutic responses. In this regard, all psychotherapists and counselors should have some knowledge of their countertransference. The therapist may err when countertransference is unchecked, whether it is supportive or critical. If the therapist is too empathic and supportive, perhaps because these issues have had a strong impact on the therapist's personal life, the therapist may fail to assist the client in exploring his or her feelings as fully as possible. On the other hand, the patient can be injured if a therapist expresses overt or covert criticism, inattention to important themes, anxiety, or other negative responses. Whatever the origin of these responses, be they fears of HIV, an impulse to create distance from the patient, discomfort with the patient's lifestyle, or other dynamics, they can be harmful, especially if the person is dealing with feelings of shame, guilt, and diminished self-esteem.

In addition to managing these feelings if they occur, therapists must also attempt to understand the limits of their own acceptance of certain behaviors and feelings. For example, a therapist may react negatively to the possibility of a seropositive woman's being pregnant. This situation could create problems if the woman asks for help in deciding whether or not to become pregnant or in deciding whether to continue or terminate a pregnancy. Strong negative emotions may also emerge when working with persons who state that they are not willing to stop sharing needles or have unprotected sex.

In some cases, the intensity of negative or otherwise problematic feelings in the therapist may be reduced by discussing the problem or dilemma with a colleague or supervisor. Occasionally, the therapist may need to refer the patient to another therapist. For these and other reasons, some investigators have suggested that therapy with persons with HIV disease requires a high level of awareness, sensitivity, and skill. In addition to the more "normal" problems associated with managing countertransference, working with persons infected with HIV requires that the therapist assist in dealing with issues surrounding terminal illness and death, and this work can be emotionally demanding.

TREATMENT GOALS

Psychosocial interventions can have many goals, and these must be individualized. Among them are improving compliance with medical treatment, facilitating behavioral change, reducing anxiety, improving self-esteem, decreasing psychiatric symptoms such as anxiety and depression, instilling a sense of hope, reducing guilt and shame, developing realistic life goals, and instilling (or reinstilling) a sense of meaning in the client's life. Therapists may approach these objectives in various ways, depending on their orientation. Specific problems require different approaches, and it is difficult to suggest interventions without knowing the patient or promoting a specific orientation of counseling or psychotherapy. A range of approaches probably can be helpful in addressing the psychosocial needs of persons with HIV disease, and the results achieved by each approach likely will be of approximately equal benefit for patients having similar levels of psychiatric symptoms, as discussed earlier (26, 28, 61).

Facilitating Medical Compliance

A major problem in treating HIV-positive patients is compliance, and this issue is becoming even more important as more effective medication regimens are developed. The incidence of compliance with antiretroviral therapy in HIV-positive patients has been reported to be between 26 and 94% (62–66). In general, patients have difficulty in complying with complicated or burdensome treatment regimens, or those with unpleasant side effects, particularly if the patient does not feel ill or if the illness is chronic.

Medical treatment for HIV has many of the elements that make compliance difficult. One study (67) identified the following reasons gay male, HIV-positive patients gave for rejecting or delaying treatment: 1) difficulty in trusting doctors, 2) feeling that doctors did not look at their condition holistically or see them as individuals, 3) confidentiality, 4) not feeling sick or denial, 5) stress and unpleasant side effects of medical treatment regimens, 6) disinclination to limit the menu of treatment options too early (generally with regard to participation in research protocols), 7) disinclination to risk the chance of a placebo (only in research protocols).

Another study (68), again in an all-male cohort, found that a history of intravenous drug use and African-American race were each associated with noncompliance with antiretroviral therapy. However, these two variables were not independent, so it is difficult to assess the relative strength of the associations. Other research has found that African-American race was associated with noncompliance (65), although this outcome has not been consistently found (69).

Research on service use by HIV-positive women (69) found that, although use of services was high, use of antiretroviral therapy by women with CD4 counts of less than 200 was only 48%, although past or present antiretroviral use was 89%. This finding implies that many women begin treatment regimens but then stop. Race did not predict health care use, but injection drug use did; IDUs were the lowest users of HIV-related health services.

Active drug addiction appears to diminish compliance with medical treatment, probably because addicts are impulsive, give highest priority to using drugs, manage time poorly, and demonstrate impaired judgment. Unfortunately, IDUs make up a significant portion of the population in need of treatment. One study interviewed current and former IDUs with AIDS in New Jersey and New York and found a high level of noncompliance (70). Some of the reasons given for noncompliance with zidovudine (formerly known as azidothymidine or AZT) were the following: some took zidovudine less than prescribed because they believed that combining it with illegal drugs (usually heroin) could cause them to overdose; others stockpiled zidovudine so they could sell it or to give it to a friend who they thought was sicker and needed it more; others wanted to minimize the number of visits to the HIV clinic where they could have to wait a long time; some mentioned being treated rudely; others wished to create a safety margin in case their symptoms worsened or in case insurance coverage was reduced.

Some of these reasons for noncompliance named by participants reflect realistic shortcomings in service provision, whereas others reflect misinformation about appropriate zidovudine use. These latter beliefs could be addressed with psychosocial interventions. Engagement in substance abuse treatment would probably also diminish the effect of these problems because such treatment typically results in a marked reduction in drug use with less impulsive behavior and less time preoccupied with drugs, even in the absence of total cessation of drug use.

One study also found that noncompliant patients demonstrated significantly greater psychological distress, depression, and poor adaptive coping compared with compliant patients (68). In this study, depression was associated with a greater decline in CD4 count and a trend toward accelerated mortality, although this finding has not been supported in other research (52, 53). The authors of this study suggest that their findings may have been due to both the effect of depression on the immune system and the effect of depression on treatment compliance.

Psychosocial treatments may play a central role in fostering treatment compliance. Clearly, compliance with pharmacotherapy for HIV requires prolonged effort because it is complicated, is sometimes associated with unpleasant side effects, and has to be maintained regardless of whether the patient feels ill or not. Many patients require support to comply, and psychosocial interventions including self-help groups and social support services can provide that encouragement and probably increase compliance.

Changing Behavior

A second important reason that psychotherapy, counseling, and social support groups can be important in the presence of HIV disease is to assist seropositive individuals in reducing high-risk behavior. At the most basic level are disseminating information and providing encouragement. Although clients typically have a moderate amount of information about HIV, sometimes the information is incomplete or inaccurate (71). Psychotherapists and counselors, often working in association with other medical personnel, can help the person better to understand the illness and can correct misinformation. The therapist should also know where free condoms are available if the client does not have easy access to these preventive measures. Therapists should be familiar with available drug treatment programs and needle exchanges, if these interventions are appropriate. Social support networks and self-help groups can work alone or in tandem with other interventions to facilitate such change.

Because new developments in pharmacotherapy have increased physical health and may increase life expectancy, assisting patients to change risky behaviors will be necessary for a longer period. From one point of view, an increased life expectancy could mean that HIV-seropositive individuals have more years and more opportunities to transmit the virus. However, the data on this important point are unclear. Because the new therapies often reduce viral load to undetectable levels, they may also reduce transmissibility, at least at some point in time. The answer to this question will probably emerge over the next several years; however, most prudent is to assume that it means that infected persons are morally obligated to sustain responsible behavior throughout their increased life span. Psychotherapy or counseling may have a role in helping individuals to sustain their behavioral change over the extended periods that may be now available to HIV-positive individuals.

Receiving a diagnosis of HIV can be an excellent time to make life changes because the diagnosis often brings the need for meaning and control in one's life to the forefront. For some, at this stressful time it is easier to continue the destructive behavior that contributed to becoming infected. Changing such unhealthy behavior is an essential treatment goal that may be helped by psychosocial interventions. Persons who eliminate unsafe behaviors, initiate a treatment regimen, and choose to maintain a healthy lifestyle often develop a sense of satisfaction and improved sense of well-being.

Studies that have examined the impact of psychosocial interventions on IDUs have examined the relationship between knowledge of avoidance of HIV transmission and reported behaviors. A review by DesJarlais and Friedman (72) found that information is necessary but not sufficient for the elimination of risky behavior. Similarly, increased availability of various means for behavior change, such as condoms and new needles, was necessary but not sufficient. These investigators suggested that changes in needle-sharing behavior are mediated by social learning, and they hypothesized that IDUs will change if they believe that their peer groups are also altering their behavior. This theory implies that subcultural socialization, such as self-help groups, can support reductions in high-risk behaviors, particularly among IDUs.

Problems associated with social support and loneliness are often significant for people coping with HIV. Many individuals believe that they are less able to obtain support from their social network after receiving a diagnosis of HIV because of the associated stigma. Drug addicts with HIV may have trouble developing a drug-free support network because the addiction has destroyed most of their healthy social supports. Members of high-risk groups, most often homosexual or bisexual men, sometimes report difficulty in relying on social supports because many friends have died. Psychotherapists and counselors usually must address issues related to social support and loneliness throughout treatment. This area is one in which participation in HIV-related self-help and support groups can be extremely beneficial.

Reducing Psychiatric Symptoms

Reducing psychopathologic symptoms is a goal in itself, and it also may facilitate behavioral change inasmuch as impulsive behavior and impaired judgment so often accompany anxiety, depression, and other psychiatric symptoms. Data have been reviewed earlier indicating that these symptoms may be associated with risky behavior. Psychotherapy and counseling can be especially helpful in reducing these symptoms and may be maximally useful if these interventions are combined with participation in medical treatment or in support or self-help groups.

The stresses on persons with HIV are numerous and include uncertainty about the future and fears of pain and death, revealing the diagnosis, becoming dependent, expressing sexuality, or being in intimate relationships. These concerns are often associated with anxiety, depression, and anger. A range of interventions can be useful, including encouraging clients simply to express or ventilate their feelings. Therapy or counseling need not be extensive to be helpful. For example, Perry and associates (73) found that a six-session stress-prevention training intervention was helpful in reducing stress in individuals after notification of HIV-positive status.

Participating in risky behaviors often causes a sense that one's life is out of control, with associated feelings of anxiety, depression, and hopelessness. Helping the client to regain a sense of control over such behaviors often reduces these feelings. One strategy that may foster a sense of greater control is to help the client to divide complicated or large problems that seem overwhelming into smaller, more manageable pieces and then to address each one separately.

Many clients have more long-standing, intense, and complex psychiatric symptoms, and they are profoundly depressed about their diagnosis at some point. This depression can be conceptualized as anticipatory grief, which means that one's response to the diagnosis is a rehearsal in preparation for the anticipated death (48, 59). Hopelessness is often a part of this grief and is also a usual response to a diagnosis of HIV infection. Feelings of despair and hopelessness can be explored, and the client can sometimes be helped to reframe them. For example, if unresolved past losses or regrets contribute to the current depression, the person may be helped to work through some of these earlier losses, with subsequent relief of depressive symptoms. This approach can be combined with pharmacotherapy if the symptoms do not resolve with psychosocial interventions alone.

When using psychotherapy or counseling, the therapist must meet the client where he or she is and must be accepting of limitations in the person's willingness to resolve issues and to change unhealthy behaviors. In most cases, it is probably more helpful to support the client in working through any resistance to change than to set ultimatums and to terminate the client from treatment for refusal to comply. However, the therapist must let the client know that even if he or she does not care about health, the therapist does care and so must push the client to take strides toward healthy behavior. This approach includes initiating and participating in treatment for HIV, reducing risky behavior, and participating in drug treatment if necessary.

TREATMENT PLANNING

Initial Assessment

Hoffman (49) elucidated an elaborate model for conceptualizing clients' needs and the provision of treatment to HIV-infected clients. Her psychosocial model focuses on four kinds of variables: special characteristics of HIV seropositivity, social supports, sociomedical situation, and client characteristics.

The first variable, special characteristics of HIV seropositivity, is consistent for all individuals dealing with HIV infection. This variable includes issues related to helping the patient understand the chronic, progressive nature of the illness and the stigma that accompanies it. The second variable, social supports, includes understanding the person's interpersonal network, such as partner or spouse, family, friends, and support groups. It also includes institutional supports that the individual can use, such as community, religious, medical, and psychological services. The third factor is the overall sociomedical situation. This includes the way in which the person became infected, the onset and progression of symptoms, the individual's phase of life (i.e., single, young children, retired), and role changes. The fourth factor involves the patient's characteristics that will be important in administering treatment. These include self-esteem, psychosocial competence, coping style, and general emotional stability. Treatment providers may find it useful to evaluate and address clients' needs within the framework of these four variables.

Later Issues: Loss and Grief

Some additional thoughts on treatment strategies for working with HIV-infected clients come from other work on loss and grief (74) and in working with persons who have other terminal illnesses (75). These issues are important in helping the person come to terms not only with his or her own mortality, but also with the losses that the infected person is likely to have experienced as a result of the death of friends and lovers. Lamb (74) points out that one must identify and reframe the symptoms of grieving to normalize these symptoms or feelings for the client and to facilitate the client's expression of feelings by bringing the "lost object" more directly into the client's experience. Yalom (75) reminds treatment providers of the importance of the client's experience in dealing with loss and the strength the client can gain from the feeling of taking control of his or her life and helping others who are similarly affected.

FUTURE DIRECTIONS

Clients with HIV disease come from many different backgrounds and often have many complex emotional needs. Some of these needs or problems predate HIV infection, and others are a consequence of the infection. Typical issues include feelings of shock and panic, anxiety, denial, anger, fear, depression, guilt, shame, hopelessness, loneliness, grief, and existential issues related to death and dying. Some of these problems are short-lived, whereas others are likely to be more long-lasting.

Psychotherapy, counseling, and participation in self-help and support groups are widely used at all stages in the treatment of persons with HIV disease. These interventions appear to be effective in reducing the distress associated with HIV infection, but little research is available to evaluate their efficacy. The study by Markowitz and colleagues (33) is the first major comparative trial of psychotherapy for persons with HIV in the United States, and thus far, the results suggest that all modalities reduced psychological distress, and further, possibly interpersonal psychotherapy and supportive therapy plus imipramine were more effective at reducing distress than either supportive therapy alone or cognitive-behavioral therapy. Counseling geared toward reducing the distress of being HIV positive (73) and counseling aimed at reducing risky behaviors (13, 15) have generally been found effective relative to no-treatment control groups. Guidelines currently available for assessment and planning of psychosocial treatments for HIV-positive persons derive mainly from psychotherapy research studies in other populations, from work on death and dying, and from some work on counseling and self-help groups in persons who are HIV positive.

Many complex issues present themselves to the psychotherapist or counselor who is treating someone with HIV disease. Among these are the following: a knowledge of the medical consequences and treatments available; sensitivity to the client's identity, including issues of race, ethnicity, gender, sexual orientation, and drug-using patterns; and a knowledge of the availability and location of other services that may be appropriate, including self-help and support groups and drug treatment facilities. The therapist's attitudes toward the patient, either conscious or unconscious, may be important determinants of psychosocial treatment outcome. The social picture and treatment needs of many patients may undergo further change as HIV disease continues to spread into the general population through heterosexual contact.

Because of the large number of persons with HIV disease and longer life expectancy for those who are infected, more research data on the efficacy of both psychotherapy and counseling for persons with HIV disease are needed. Such research could help caregivers better to understand the most useful and cost-effective ways to deliver psychosocial services to this growing population and could reduce HIV-transmitting behaviors, especially among those who have severe psychiatric symptoms.

References

1. Centers for Disease Control and Prevention. HIV/AIDS surveillance report. vol. 8. Atlanta, GA: Centers for Disease Control and Prevention, 1996.
2. O'Brien ME. Living with HIV: experiment in courage. New York: Auburn House, 1992.
3. Strawn JM. The psychosocial consequences of HIV infection. In: Durham JD, Cohen FL, eds. The person with AIDS: nursing perspectives. New York: Springer, 1991:113–134.
4. Centers for Disease Control and Prevention. HIV/AIDS surveillance report. vol. 6. Atlanta, GA: Centers for Disease Control and Prevention, 1994.
5. MacDonald MG, Ginzburg HM, Bolan JC. HIV infection in pregnancy: epidemiology and clinical management. J Acquir Immune Defic Syndr 1991;4:100–108.
6. Mitchell JL. Drug abuse and AIDS in women and their affected off-spring. J Natl Med Assoc 1989;81:841–842.
7. Beck AT, Emery G. Cognitive therapy of substance abuse. Philadelphia: Center for Cognitive Therapy, 1977.
8. Beck AT, Rush J, Shaw B, et al. Cognitive therapy of depression. New York: Guilford Press, 1979.
9. Luborsky L. Principles of psychoanalytic psychotherapy: a manual for supportive-expressive treatment. New York: Basic Books, 1984.
10. Kleber GL, Weissman MM, Rounsaville BJ, et al. Interpersonal psychotherapy of depression. New York: Basic Books, 1984.
11. Rounsaville BJ, Glazer W, Wilber CH, et al. Short-term interpersonal psychotherapy in methadone-maintained opiate addicts. Arch Gen Psychiatry 1983;40:629–636.
12. Markowitz JC, Klerman GL, Perry SW. Interpersonal psychotherapy of depressed HIV-positive outpatients. Hosp Community Psychiatry 1992;43:885–890.
13. Boatler JF, Knight K, Simpson, DD. Assessment of an AIDS intervention program during drug abuse treatment. J Subst Abuse Treat 1994;11:367–372.
14. Malow RM, West JA, Corrigan SA, et. al. Outcome of psychoeducation for HIV risk reduction. AIDS Educ Prev 1994;6:113–125.
15. Peterson JL, Coates TJ, Catania J, et al. Evaluation of an HIV risk reduction intervention among African-American homosexual and bisexual men. AIDS 1996;10:319–325.
16. Bandura A. Social cognitive theory and exercise of control over HIV Infection. In: DiClemente RJ, Peterson J, eds. Preventing AIDS: theories and methods of behavioral interventions. New York: Plenum, 1994:25–29.
17. Gibson DR, Catania J, Peterson JL. Theoretical background. In: Sorensen JL, Wermuth LA, Gibson DR, et al., eds. Preventing AIDS in drug users and their sexual partners. New York: Guilford Press, 1991:99–115.
18. Wingood GM, DiClemente RJ. HIV sexual risk reduction intervention for women: a review. Am J Prev Med 1996;12: 209–217.
19. DiClemente RJ, Wingood GM. A randomized controlled trial of a community-based HIV sexual risk reduction intervention for young adult African-American females. JAMA 1995;274:1271–1276.
20. Cohen E, Navaline H, Metzger D. High-risk behaviors for HIV: a comparison between crack-abusing and opioid-abusing African-American women. J Psychoactive Drugs 1994;26:233–241.
21. Elkin I, Shea T, Watkins J, et al. National Institute of Mental Health treatment of depression collaborative program: general effectiveness. Arch Gen Psychiatry 1989;46:971–982.
22. Kupfer DJ, Frank E, Perel JM, et al. Five-year outcome for maintenance therapies in recurrent depression. Arch Gen Psychiatry 1992;49:769–773.
23. Hollon SD, DeRubeis RJ, Evans MD, et al. Cognitive therapy and pharmacotherapy for depression: singly and in combination. Arch Gen Psychiatry 1992;49:774–781.
24. Frank E, Kupfer DJ, Wagner, et al. Efficacy of interpersonal psychotherapy as a maintenance treatment of recurrent depression: contributing factors. Arch Gen Psychiatry 1991;48:1053–1059.
25. Garfield SL, Bergin AE. Handbook of psychotherapy and behavior change. 3rd ed. New York: John Wiley & Sons, 1986.
26. Smith M, Glass G, Miller T. The benefits of psychotherapy. Baltimore: Johns Hopkins University Press, 1980.
27. Woody GE, McLellan AT, Luborsky L, et al. Severity of psychiatric symptoms as a predictor of benefits from psychotherapy: the Veterans Administration–Penn study. Am J Psychiatry 1984;141:1112–1177.
28. Luborsky L, Singer B, Luborsky L. Comparative studies of psychotherapies: is it true that "everyone has won and all must have prizes"? Arch Gen Psychiatry 1975;32:995–1007.
29. Crits-Christoph P, Beebe KL, Connolly MB. Therapist effects in the treatment of drug dependence: implications for conducting comparative treatment studies. In: Onken LS, Blaine JD, eds. Psychotherapy and counseling in the treatment of drug abuse. National Institute of Drug Abuse research monograph 104. Rockville, MD: US Department of Health and Human Services, 1990:39–48.
30. Luborsky L, McLellan AT, Woody GE, et al. Therapist success and its determinants. Arch Gen Psychiatry 1985;42:602–611.

31. Elkin I, Pilkonis PA, Docherty JP, et al. Conceptual and methodological issues in comparative studies of psychotherapy and pharmacotherapy. I. Active ingredients and mechanisms of change. Am J Psychiatry 1988; 145:909–917.
32. Elkin I, Pilkonis PA, Docherty JP, et al. Conceptual and methodological issues in comparative studies of psychotherapy and pharmacotherapy. II. Nature and timing of treatment effects. Am J Psychiatry 1988;145: 1070–1076.
33. Markowitz JC, Klerman GL, Clougherty KF, et al. Individual psychotherapies for depressed HIV-positive patients. Am J Psychiatry 1995; 152:1504–1509.
34. Mulder CL, Emmelkamp PMG, Antoni MH, et al. Cognitive-behavioral and experiential group psychotherapy for HIV-infected homosexual men: a comparative study. Psychosom Med 1994;56: 423–431.
35. Grant D, Anns M. Counseling AIDS antibody-positive clients: reactions and treatment. Am Psychol 1988;43:72–74.
36. Kalichman SC, Sikkema KJ, Somlai A. People living with HIV who attend and do not attend support groups: a pilot study of needs, characteristics and experiences. AIDS Care 1996;8:589–599.
37. Perry S, Jacobsberg LR, Fishman B, et al. Psychiatric diagnosis before serological testing for the human immunodeficiency virus. Am J Psych 1990;147:89–93.
38. Spitzer RL, Williams JB, Gibbon M, et al. Structured clinical interview for DSM-III R. Washington, DC: American Psychiatric Press, 1990.
39. American Psychiatric Association. Diagnostic and statistical manual of mental disorders. rev. 3rd ed. Washington, DC: American Psychiatric Association, 1987.
40. Metzger DS, Woody GE, DePhillipis D, et al. Risk factors for needle sharing among methadone patients. Am J Psychiatry 1991;148: 636–640.
41. Woody GE, Metzger DS, Navaline H, et al. Psychiatric symptoms, risky behavior and HIV infection. In: Onken L, Blaine J, eds. National Institute of Drug Abuse research monograph. Rockville, MD: US Department of Health and Human Services, 1996.
42. Brooner RK, Schmidt CW, Felch LJ, et al. Antisocial behavior of intravenous drug abusers: implications for diagnosis of antisocial personality disorder. Am J Psychiatry 1992;149:482–487.
43. Orr ST, Celentano DD, Santelli J, et al. Depressive symptoms and risk factors for HIV acquisition among black women attending urban health centers in Baltimore. AIDS Educ Prev 1994;6:230–236.
44. Kaisch K, Anton-Culver H. Psychological and social consequences of HIV exposure: homosexuals in southern California. Psychol Health 1989;3:63–75.
45. Mandel JS. Psychosocial challenges of AIDS and ARC: clinical and research observations. In: McKusick L, ed. What to do about AIDS. Berkeley: University of California Press, 1986:75–86.
46. Dilley JW, Ochitill HN, Perl M, et al. Findings in psychiatric consultations with patients with acquired immune deficiency syndrome. Am J Psychiatry 1985;142:82–86.
47. Woo SK. The psychiatric and neuropsychiatric aspects of HIV disease. J Palliat Care 1988;4:50–53.
48. Davis RF, Metzger DS, Meyers K, et al. Long-term changes in psychological symptomatology associated with HIV serostatus among male injecting drug users. AIDS 1995;9:73–79.
49. Hoffman MA. Counseling the HIV-infected client: a psychosocial model for assessment and intervention. Counsel Psychol 1991;19: 467–542 .
50. Donlou JN, Wolcott D, Gottlieb MS, et al. Psychosocial aspects of AIDS and AIDS-related complex: a pilot study. J Psychosoc Oncol 1985;3:39–55.
51. Hoffman A. Impact of AIDS. Hosp Community Psychiatry 1986;37: 943–944.
52. Stein M, Miller AH, Trestman RL. Depression, the immune system, and health and illness. Arch Gen Psychiatry 1991;48:171–173.
53. Rabkin JG, Williams JB, Remien RH. Depression distress, lymphocyte subsets, and human immunodeficiency virus symptoms on two occasions in HIV-positive homosexual men Arch Gen Psychiatry 1991;48: 111–119.
54. Zorilla EP, McKay JR, Luborsky L, et al. Relation of stressors to clinical progression of viral illness: a meta-analytic review. Am J Psychiatry 1996;153:626–635.
55. Kubler-Ross E. On death and dying. New York, Macmillan, 1969.
56. Barrett RL. Counseling gay men with AIDS: human dimensions. J Counsel Dev 1989;67:573–575.
57. Nichols SE. Psychiatric aspects of AIDS. Psychosomatics 1983;24: 1083–1089.
58. Kubler-Ross E. AIDS: the ultimate challenge. New York: Macmillan 1987.
59. Bartlett JG, Finkbeiner AK. The guide to living with HIV infection. Baltimore: Johns Hopkins University Press, 1991.
60. Peterson JL, Marin G. Issues in the prevention of AIDS among black and Hispanic men. Am Psychol 1988;43:871–877.
61. Woody GE, Luborsky L, MeLellan AT, et al. Psychotherapy for methadone maintained opiate addicts: does it help? Arch Gen Psychiatry 1983;40:639–645.
62. Besch CL, Collins G, Morse E, et al. Cofactors associated with participant compliance in two CPCRA trails [abstract PuB 7040]. In: 8th International Conference on AIDS, Amsterdam, 1992:55.
63. Cortese L, Chung R, Stoute J, et al. Zidovudine usage: patient compliance and factors [abstract PO-33-2233]. In: 9th International Conference on AIDS, Berlin, 1993:507.
64. LoCaputo S, Maggi P, Buccoliero G, et al. Antiretroviral therapy with zidovudine (AZT): evaluation of the compliance in a cohort of HIV positive patients [abstract PO-B26-2124]. In: 9th International Conference on AIDS, Berlin, 1993:489.
65. Muma RD, Ross WW, Parcel G, et al. Zidovudine adherence among individuals with HIV infection. AIDS Care 1995;7:439–448.
66. Wall TL, Sorenson JL, London J, et al. Medication adherence in HIV infected injection drug users [abstract PuB 7581]. In: 8th International Conference on AIDS, Amsterdam, 1992:145.
67. Siegel K, Raveis VH, Krauss BJ. Factors associated with urban gay men's treatment initiation decisions for HIV infection. AIDS Educ Prev 1992;4:135–142.
68. Singh N, Squier C, Sivek C, et al. Determinants of compliance with antiretroviral therapy in patients with human immunodeficiency virus: prospective assessment with implications for enhancing compliance. AIDS Care 1996;8:261–269.
69. Solomon L, Stein M, Flynn CP, et al. Service utilization by HIV-1 infected women from four United States urban centers: the Hers study [abstract]. In: 11th International Conference on AIDS, Vancouver, 1996.
70. Freeman RC, Rodriguez GM, French JF. Compliance with AZT treatment regimen of HIV-seropositive injection drug users: a neglected issue. AIDS Educ Prev 1996;8:58–71.
71. Hanson M, Kramer TH, Gross W, et al. AIDS awareness and risk behaviors among dually disordered adults. AIDS Educ Prev 1992; 4:41–51.
72. DesJarlais DC, Friedman SR. The psychology of preventing AIDS among intravenous drug users. Am Psychol 1988;43:865–870.
73. Perry S, Fishman B, Jacobsberg LB, et al. Effectiveness of psychoeducational interventions in reducing emotional distress after human immunodeficiency virus antibody testing. Arch Gen Psychiatry 1991; 48:143–147.
74. Lamb DH. Loss and grief psychotherapy strategies and interventions. Psychotherapy 1988;25:561–569 .
75. Yalom ID, Greaves C. Group therapy with the terminally ill. Am J Psychiatry 1977;134:396–400.

52

HOSPICE CARE AND SYMPTOM MANAGEMENT

Tom Grothe and Michael Gottlieb

Since the first edition of this textbook, dramatic developments have occurred in the care of the person with acquired immunodeficiency syndrome (AIDS). Combination antiretroviral therapies that include protease inhibitors have contributed to a decline in the number of people dying of AIDS for the first time in the history of the epidemic (1). Additionally, viral load testing is proving to be a valuable tool in ascertaining prognosis (2). These developments in AIDS care have changed the relationship between AIDS and hospice care and palliation. The purpose of this chapter is to review this new relationship and to offer guidelines for physicians to assess when, and for which patients, hospice care and palliation are appropriate. A discussion of hospice philosophy and services is provided, as well as a discussion of the difficulties in accommodating the person with AIDS in a hospice program. Suggestions are made on how and when to make the transition to palliation. We also review symptom management for terminally ill AIDS patients.

In every terminal illness there comes a point when further aggressive, curative care becomes futile and inappropriate. For many patients, AIDS remains a progressive terminal illness. Some AIDS patients are unable to benefit from the new combinations of antiretroviral agents. In many patients infected with human immunodeficiency virus (HIV) who are trying combination therapies, viral load is not reduced below the threshold of detection, and in other patients, viral load responds initially, but then rebounds to high levels. Many patients previously treated with sequential monotherapies carry multiple-drug–resistant viral strains, so the addition of a protease inhibitor has resulted in broad resistances and poor response. Other patients cannot tolerate the side effects of the medications or, for various reasons, are unable to take appropriate doses of the medications. For the present, all these patients are likely to have progressive immunologic decline and eventually to die of opportunistic infections or AIDS-related malignancies. These patients will, at some point, benefit from hospice care and palliation.

HOSPICE CARE

The hospice movement in the United States began in the mid-1970s. It developed in response to the perception that many interventions for dying hospitalized patients were overly aggressive and futile. Advocates of the hospice movement believed that a better way existed to provide care to the dying. In the United States, it is generally agreed that hospice care is appropriate when the physician believes that the patient's prognosis for survival is less than 6 months, and the patient wants no further aggressive, cure-oriented care. The hospice philosophy places the patient in charge of all decisions regarding treatment options. Most hospice care is provided in the home, but some hospices also have residence facilities for patients who cannot stay at home. Hospice workers address problems in three realms: physical, psychosocial, and spiritual; for this reason, every hospice team is multidisciplinary, consisting of a nurse, a social worker, a chaplain, and a physician. Services offered by hospice include expertise in symptom palliation, 24-hour on-call availability of nurses, more intensive case management, team involvement in psychological and social problems, community volunteer involvement, and bereavement care for survivors. In general, home care agencies do not offer this full range of services.

In 1982, United States federal government legislation created a program for reimbursement for hospice services under Medicare (the hospice Medicare benefit). When a dying patient elects "the benefit," the Medicare program provides a capitated daily reimbursement to the hospice providing care. From this daily rate, hospices must pay for all nursing and attendant services, all medications related to the terminal illness, and all medical equipment and supplies used in the home. Short-term hospitalizations for symptom management are reimbursed at a higher rate. These reimbursement rates sustain hospices as long as the patients do not require expensive treatments or services.

The United States government has instituted an intensive retrospective national review of services provided by hospices across the country, by auditing the records of hospice patients receiving the hospice Medicare benefit. If these patients did not die within 6 months of admission to the hospice program, Medicare has claimed that placement or referral was inappropriate and has demanded refund of payment made to the hospice. Because state Medicaid and most private health insurances follow Medicare in insurance policy, this policy could result in more stringent hospice admissions criteria. On a national level, this policy has raised concern at many hospices and has resulted in reluctance to accept patients who do not clearly meet the admission criterion of less than 6 months' prognosis. In the era of improved treatments for HIV, the criterion of less than 6 months' prognosis is more difficult to predict accurately. As a result, hospices could become more reluctant to accept persons with AIDS.

AIDS and Hospice

Hospices have tried to provide care to patients dying of AIDS, with mixed results. Admission of AIDS patients into hospices, and onto the hospice Medicare benefit, will strain hospice budgets if patients are still receiving ongoing treatments such as radiotherapy for neoplasms, antiretroviral drugs, or intravenous treatments for cytomegalovirus (CMV) retinitis. Each hospice will address this problem differently. Therefore, medical professionals need to understand the policies of their local hospice with regard to AIDS admissions and allowable treatments under the hospice Medicare benefit. Many hospices have continued to accept persons with AIDS into their programs, but they do not place them on the hospice benefit to avoid having to pay for expensive palliative treatments. Medical professionals should appreciate the financial constraints placed on hospices and should look for ways to provide palliative care to persons with AIDS within these constraints (Fig. 52.1).

Because hospice developed in response to patients dying of cancer, certain problems from trying to fit AIDS into this model of care. These problems stem from three sources: the disease, the patient, and the agencies.

THE DISEASE

The disease progression of AIDS is not steady, as is that of most cancers, with diagnosis, treatment, treatment failure, and then clear delineation of when to refer to hospice. The course of AIDS is marked by wide swings in the patient's condition. Acute opportunistic infections are followed by recovery and much improved functional status, only to deteriorate with recurrence or additional opportunistic infections. This roller-coaster course makes it difficult to determine when hospice care is appropriate for a person with AIDS. The decision to stop curative treatment and to make the transition to palliation is further confused by the problem that, although many opportunistic infections are curable, the underlying immune suppression is, at this time, not curable. This situation results in varied palliative care treatment plans, sometimes withholding treatments for infections that could

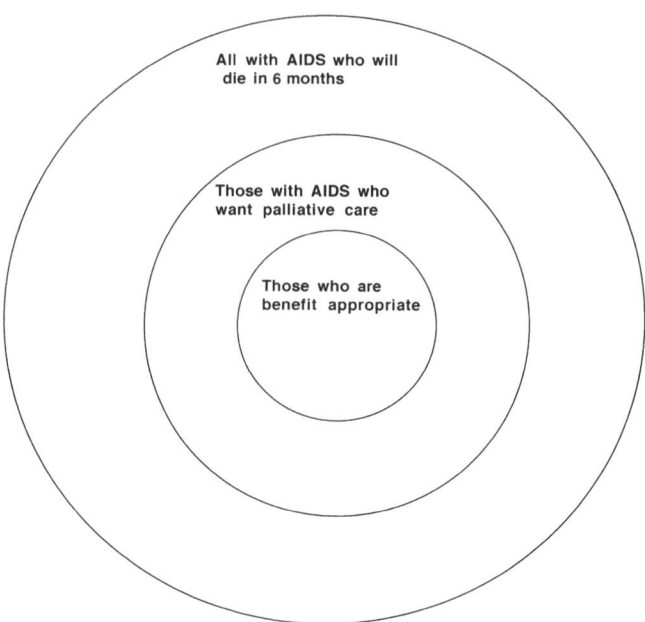

Figure 52.1. Circles within circles. All *circles* indicate AIDS patients with a prognosis of 6 months or less. The *outer circle* consists of those who will die but who do not want palliative care and, as such, are not appropriate candidates for hospice. The *inner circle* is those who will die, who want palliative care, and whose treatments meet the financial constraints of the hospice Medicare benefit. Finally, the *middle circle* consists of those AIDS patients who want palliation, but whose treatments prohibit placement onto the hospice benefit. This *middle circle* is the group of AIDS patients who need creative solutions to provide hospice care. Many hospices have "prehospice" admissions for these patients, in which they are admitted into hospice, but services are billed under the Medicare program, rather than the Medicare hospice benefit.

be cured and at other times providing curative treatments for infection to a dying patient. It is the patient's choice. Finally, responses to treatments and interventions vary, so prognostication cannot be based on responses to therapies. This variability makes the assessment of patients' appropriateness for hospice difficult to determine.

PERSON WITH AIDS

The person with AIDS is not like most other hospice patients. Usually, AIDS patients are younger and are not prepared to confront the dying process. Often, they are from subcultures that are not comfortable in a traditional setting such as a hospice. Some of these subcultures are isolated from the predominant culture, and patients may have conflicts with staff from traditional agencies. Many AIDS patients have histories of substance abuse. Working with active injection drug users can be difficult and requires skills not often found in hospice personnel. Finally, the person with AIDS is often multiply bereaved and experiencing depression, loneliness, and hopelessness as a result of multiple losses. In this regard, hospices are better prepared than other services to provide support and assistance.

Persons with AIDS often cope with their illness by fighting it through activism, protest, and education. It is sometimes difficult for dying AIDS patients psychologically to make the transition to a hospice plan of care when an aggressive posture has worked so well for so long. They sometimes view approaching death as defeat, and they subsequently refuse hospice referral. However, the metaphor of fighting offers little in the way of solace to the AIDS patient who is losing the fight.

HOSPICES AND AIDS SERVICE ORGANIZATIONS

Hospices and AIDS service organizations (ASOs) sometimes have difficulty working together. Boundaries can become confused, and a medical professional can become uncertain about who is in charge. Hospice programs usually want to provide all aspects of care to their patients. However, ASO personnel are often involved for years with AIDS patients before admission to hospice. This situation can result in overlap of services. ASO and hospice staff sometimes have difficulty agreeing on common goals, and this leads to a lack of cooperation between agencies. ASO staff not infrequently regard a patient's admission into a hospice as a failure, and they have a negative perception of hospice professionals. Conversely, hospice staff sometimes perceive ASO personnel to be fostering unrealistic hopes and focusing on futile goals.

Some hospice programs have had limited experience with AIDS patients. Their staff members are sometimes fearful of contagion and uncertain of, what is to them, a new disease and a new patient population. Sometimes, personal or religious beliefs regarding lifestyle can impair the quality of care provided. Additionally, the increased technical skill required to care for a person with AIDS, such as phlebotomy and intravenous infusions, can challenge hospice professionals.

Earlier in the epidemic, hospices in several large cities throughout the United States provided specialized care to persons with AIDS. With the improved prognosis from AIDS, as a result of combination antiretroviral drugs, less demand has been placed on these agencies. In some cases, this improvement in treatment has resulted in the closure of inpatient facilities devoted to care of the dying AIDS patient or in the cutback of specialized service teams for persons with AIDS. This situation may further affect the quality of care provided to persons with AIDS who are merged into traditional hospice and home care teams. However, hospice exists to provide high-quality palliation to dying patients, regardless of disease. The hospice movement contains many caring, skilled practitioners who have much to offer dying AIDS patients.

Transition to Hospice

Hospice is at the end of a spectrum of care, and it should be available to all AIDS patients. Hospice and palliative care are appropriate when therapy offers no prospects for the further improvement of quantity or quality of life. This point is usually not reached at one moment, but is often the result of a series of smaller decisions made during the progression of disease (3). In our opinion, discussion of criteria for palliation and solicitation of the patient's long-term goals should take place shortly after the diagnosis of HIV infection and at regular intervals thereafter. This is especially difficult for health care providers to do in the current era of optimism fostered by the successes of combination antiretroviral regimens, antimicrobial prophylaxis, and improved treatment of opportunistic infections. Open, early discussion of a patient's views on palliative treatment does not mean that the health care provider is giving up on aggressive, life-prolonging treatment. In our view, the two are consistent and constitute optimal patient care. Palliative care needs to be included in the spectrum of care, and, when appropriate, it should be readily available to patients. Discussion needs to take place regarding when palliation will become appropriate before a crisis intervenes and makes it a pressing, imminent option for patients and families.

Palliation is defined by the goal of the therapeutic interventions. Transitions to palliation may take place in a series of small decisions, but once there, the goal of intervention is always comfort. If the goal of a treatment is to sustain or to extend life, then it is curative. Distinguishing between palliative and curative is difficult in AIDS care. When considering which interventions are curative and which are palliative, it is useful to ask: what is the goal of the intervention? AIDS treatments that are clearly palliative include pain and symptom management, wound care, and psychosocial support. AIDS treatments that are probably palliative include suppressive therapies for CMV retinitis and routine *Pneumocystis* and *Mycobacterium avium* complex (MAC) prophylaxis, provided the side effects are minimal. Therapies that are not palliative, based on the goal of the intervention, include total parenteral nutrition, treatments to increase lean body mass, and combination antiretroviral therapies.

New advances in the treatment of AIDS must be continuously evaluated for appropriateness in hospice programs. If the objective of therapy is to provide comfort and to alleviate disturbing symptoms, then it is most likely appropriate for hospice care. Treatments such as retinal implants or laser surgeries could, in some instances, be considered palliative. The more difficult question is how to provide these services within the budgetary constraints of hospice care. Medical doctors, health policy makers, and hospices will need to continue to work together creatively to meet the needs of AIDS patients who are in hospice programs.

Combination antiviral drugs that include protease inhibitors are significantly extending life. For the first time, the possibility exists that HIV infection will be a chronic illness, instead of an inexorably progressive one. Therefore, all patients with HIV infection should exhaust antiretroviral therapy options before making the transition to palliative care. The goal of combination antiretroviral therapy is to extend life; as such, these treatments are not palliative. In the past, hospices provided antiretroviral drugs to dying AIDS patients because of uncertainty about the effects and the goals of these treatments. Many hospices across the United States currently still provide antiretroviral therapy to AIDS patients in their programs. Some hospices claim that the goal of antiretroviral therapy in this circumstance is comfort rather than prolongation of survival. More research is required to determine the value of combination antiretroviral therapies in reducing or stabilizing viral burden and providing relief from constitutional symptoms related to HIV viremia. At this time, we believe that the goal of combination antiretroviral therapy is primarily curative and, as such, should not be part of a hospice plan of care. Continuing antiretroviral therapy while in hospice sends confusing messages to the patient and family regarding prognosis and the goals of therapy. This confusion can impede hospice work.

New advances in reliable measurement of responses to antiretroviral drugs (assays for viral load measurement) have improved delineation of patients who are benefiting from antiretroviral therapy and those who are not. High viral load with multiple opportunistic infections should be a cue for the health care provider that transition to palliation may be appropriate. Viral load testing is a recent measure. Its predictive value with respect to life expectancy is still undetermined. Probably, improved understanding of this parameter will dramatically improve the accuracy of prognostication and will facilitate decisions by patients and their providers to elect hospice care.

Referral to Hospice

When to refer a patient with AIDS to a hospice program has been a difficult decision for many medical providers. In the past, clinicians were uncertain about when it was appropriate to make the transition to palliation. The first criterion for hospice referral is that the patient desires palliative care. Frequently, the option of palliative care has not been discussed, or it is only offered at the last minute in the midst of a crisis, when patients are overwhelmed and are unable to think clearly. A patient's rejection of palliation when it is first discussed does not mean that it should never be considered or brought up again. Palliation needs to remain a discussed option throughout the course of an illness.

Physicians are often reluctant to discuss hospice with patients for fear of being perceived as giving up or of not fighting hard enough. However, hospice only means surrender if the patient and medical doctor have cultivated the metaphor of a battle to cope with HIV. Honest discussion of a patient's condition often results in the choice by the patient and family of less aggressive interventions (4). Hospice has much to offer dying patients. In hospice, patients have an opportunity to reflect on their lives, to achieve closure on unresolved issues and conflicts, and to heal relationships with families and friends. The pain and fear encountered when confronting inevitable death can often be offset by the opportunity to say goodbye and to resolve life issues.

The possibility that a hospice referral is premature is a great concern to physicians, hospices, and patients. In reality, referral to a hospice for patients dying of AIDS often happens too late. Unfortunately, patients are often referred in the last days of life, so symptom management and resolution of unresolved issues become rushed and pressured. To obtain maximum benefit from the services hospices have to offer, a 2-month period for the patient to work with the hospice team is ideal.

Confronted with a patient whose condition is continuing to decline, a physician must ask some difficult questions: What is the purpose of continued aggressive intervention? Am I continuing to treat the patient actively for his or her needs or for my own needs? Is the patient more prepared to accept the terminal nature of the disease than family members, the significant other, or myself? Often, medical providers continue to treat the individual complications (e.g., new-onset lymphoma) without considering the whole condition of the patient. They are so focused on the individual tree that they forget to look at the forest. Although each opportunistic infection may be treatable, the treatment may burden the patient with additional medications, or it may have noxious side effects that impair the quality of remaining life. In considering options for continued aggressive care, the physician should ask the following questions: Has the general condition of the patient deteriorated to a point in which it is inadvisable to treat a new or relapsed infectious or neoplastic complication? Which is more debilitating, further treatment or disease progression?

Palliation Flow Chart

The lack of clarity regarding prognostic markers in AIDS is a large obstacle preventing referral to hospice. In the past, clinicians relied on diagnosed opportunistic infections, general physical condition, and current CD4 count to estimate a patient's prognosis. Advances in assessment of the viral burden may enhance prognostic efforts. Viral load measured in conjunction with CD4 count gives a better approximation of the likelihood of disease progression and prognosis than sole consideration of opportunistic infections.

Figure 52.2 demonstrates possible application of this newer knowledge to improve appropriate hospice referrals. We emphasize that it has not been tested prospectively. This flow chart is developed as a guide to focus physicians on when discussion of, and referral to, hospice may be appropriate. Its design is based on a retrospective review of the literature, but the concept of a flow chart to guide admission to a hospice program is new. We propose that the primary prognostic markers guiding transition to hospice be when the CD4 count is below 50 cells/mm^3 and the viral load is "unresponsive" to antiretroviral therapies. Perhaps the single most important indicator for hospice referral is failure of antiretroviral therapy. It is up to the physician and patient to determine the definition of unresponsive. We believe that antiretroviral treatment failure consists of exhaustion of all available antiretroviral combinations with little, or short-term, decrease in viral load or the patient's inability to tolerate antiretroviral therapies despite aggressive attempts at symptom management.

Exceptions to this flow chart will exist, for example, the patient whose CD4 count is above 50 cells/mm^3 but for whom hospice care is appropriate because of declining physical condition and diagnosed opportunistic infections. However, we believe that this flow chart will significantly clarify who is, and who is not, a hospice candidate (see Fig. 52.2). Past efforts at predicting this focused on unreliable markers such as opportunistic disease progression and declining, but fluctuating, functional status. Although these parameters are important, they do not, by themselves, reliably predict prognosis. A CD4 count that is consistently under 50 cells/mm^3 and a viral load that is not responsive to antiretroviral therapy have a greater predictive value for limited prognosis. In addition, the presence of certain opportunistic infections and neoplasms, some specific demographic variables, and certain clinical manifestations strongly support the notion that hospice care is appropriate for the patient. Table 52.1 lists these criteria, as well as other,

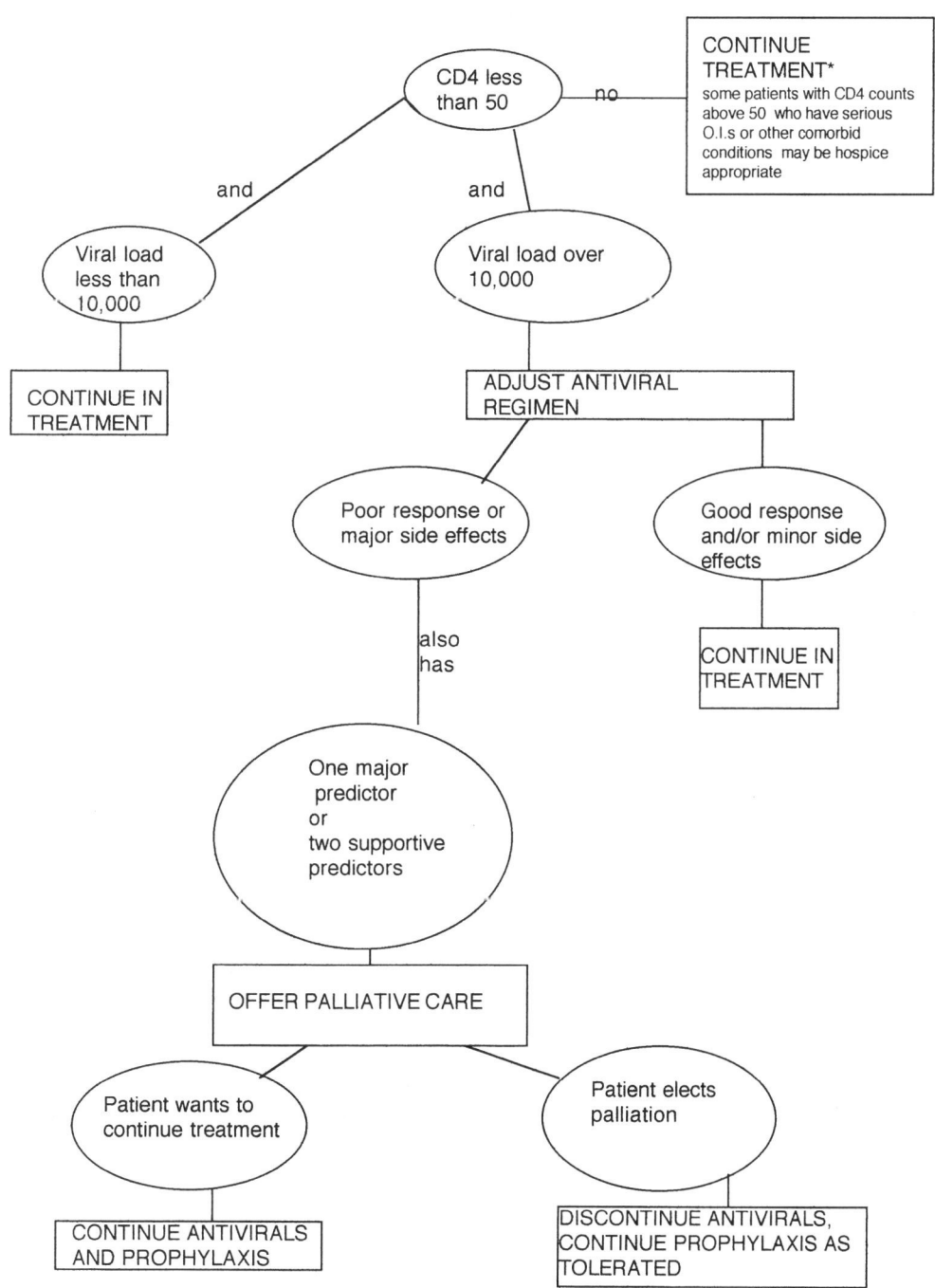

Figure 52.2. Palliative care decision tree. To be appropriate for referral to palliative care, a patient must have a CD4 count below 50 cells/mm^3 and a viral load above 10,000 copies/mL, and the patients must be unresponsive to antiretroviral therapy. In addition, patients should have one major predictor or two supportive predictors (see Table 52.1). Those who do not meet these criteria may be appropriate for palliation based on the medical provider's assessment and the patient's desire.

Table 52.1. Palliative Care Criteria[a]

Major Predictors for Palliation (Reference)	Supportive Predictors for Palliation (Reference)
Central nervous system lymphoma (5)	Karnofsky scale below 70 (8)
Progressive multifocal leukoencephalopathy (5)	Stages 3 or 4 of the Global ADL Scale (9)
Cryptosporidiosis (6)	Loss of 33% lean body mass (6, 10)
Renal failure, with dialysis refused or failed (7)	Persistent serum albumin below 2.5 g/dL (11)
	Visceral Kaposi's sarcoma, unresponsive to treatment and leading to respiratory or gastrointestinal compromise (5)
	Other invasive neoplasias
	End-stage AIDS dementia complex (6)
	Toxoplasmosis, with failed therapy (6)
	Cytomegalovirus, with failed therapy (12)
	Mycobacterium avium complex, disseminated and unresponsive to treatment (13)
	Age over 50 years (14)
	Congestive heart failure (15)

[a] Assumes CD4 count lower than 50 cells/mm^3, viral load higher than 10,000 copies/mL and unresponsive to antiretroviral therapy.

supportive indicators (two or more clearly indicate limited prognosis, in the presence of CD4 count under 50 cells/mm^3 and viral load higher than 10,000 copies/mL that has failed to respond to treatment) (5–15).

The organization of criteria into major (requires one) or supportive (requires two) predictors was a decision based on experience (see Fig. 52.2 and Table 52.1). As newer therapies improve the prognosis of specific conditions on this list, the chart will require modification. The flow chart is designed to ensure that persons with AIDS receive aggressive, interventive care as long as it is valuable, and palliative, comfort-oriented care when appropriate. By following this flow chart, the probability will increase that hospice admissions will be timely and appropriate (i.e., patients will survive between 2 and 6 months).

Case Examples

The following are some examples of appropriate and inappropriate hospice referrals:

CASE EXAMPLE 1

A 45-year-old man with a history of two episodes of *Pneumocystis carinii* pneumonia (PCP) has newly diagnosed cutaneous Kaposi's sarcoma (KS). The CD4 count is 175 cells/mm^3, and the viral load is 24,600 copies/mL. The patient has been on his current antiviral regimen of zidovudine and lamivudine for 2 years. His partner died last year. He requests no further treatment and desires transfer to the hospice home care team.

This patient requires intervention for his depression and support during adjustment to his new KS diagnosis. His antiviral regimen should be adjusted, and KS treatment options should be presented. He would benefit from continued antiviral therapy and prophylaxis. Hospice referral would be inappropriate.

CASE EXAMPLE 2

A 36-year-old woman has long history of multiple opportunistic infections. She has been diagnosed with brain toxoplasmosis, cervical dysplasia, and disseminated *Mycobacterium avium intracellulare* with bacteremia, with weight loss of more than 40 lb in the past 6 months. The patient is now bedridden and wheelchair-bound. She is increasingly unable to tolerate medications because of nausea and vomiting. Her current CD4 count is 11 cells/mm^3, and her viral load is 250,000 copies/mL despite a well-conceived antiretroviral regimen.

This patient is appropriate for hospice referral. Her CD4 count is less than 50 cells/mm^3, and the viral load is unresponsive to treatment. Her prognosis is limited based on multiple opportunistic infections, loss of lean body mass, and functional ability. She has been given an adequate trial of antiviral therapy. Transition to hospice care will assist the patient and her family in preparing for death. Continued treatment would impair her quality of life secondary to side effects and would hinder the patient's acceptance of death.

CASE EXAMPLE 3

A 57-year-old man has had AIDS for 7 years, with three episodes of PCP with residual pulmonary fibrosis and exertional dyspnea, disseminated MAC, peripheral neuropathy, and early cognitive–motor deficit. The patient is bed-bound and incontinent. All antiviral regimens have failed. The patient refuses prophylaxis and most medications. His CD4 count has been under 10 cells/mm^3 for more than 3 years, and the viral load is sustained above 500,000 copies/mL. The patient is now spiking a temperature of 104°F with delirium and rigors.

This patient should have been referred to hospice months ago. Acute symptoms receive palliative attention in hospice, but the decision to transfer to hospice should not be made during a crisis. When the patient failed to respond to antiviral therapies and his condition declined, it would have been appropriate to discuss transition to hospice. Hospices do an excellent job in crisis management, but to benefit from the multidisciplinary approach and holistic view to symptom management that hospices practice, it is best to refer patients to hospice programs when patients have a prognosis of at least 2 months.

SYMPTOM MANAGEMENT OF AIDS

Treatments in Hospice

When a patient is receiving palliative care, the focus is on maintaining comfort at all costs. Each problem is considered in a multifaceted manner to include the physical, emotional, and spiritual aspects of the issues. Under the direction of the physician, the hospice team will intervene to provide symptom relief. This section identifies common palliative symptom management issues and their treatments.

Before discussing symptom management, mention should be made of controversies in treatment in palliation of AIDS. Prophylaxis and suppressive therapies are generally considered palliative because they prevent uncomfortable symptoms in the last months of life. However, if the medications taken to suppress or prevent symptoms are difficult to tolerate, and if they cause prominent side effects, they should be reevaluated, and the physician should consider discontinuing them. For example, discontinuing prophylaxis for PCP may be reasonable if it improves the quality of the few days or weeks left to a patient. The common perception is that dying of PCP is uncomfortable. In fact, the symptoms of dyspnea and air hunger from PCP are readily controlled with skilled palliative interventions.

The goal of combination antiretroviral therapy is life extension and, as such, is not palliative. However, keeping viral load stable could possibly maintain a feeling of well-being, even if the reduced viral load does not affect length of life. More research is required to validate the worth of continuing antiretroviral agents in the face of limited prognosis.

Palliation of Symptoms

When a patient makes the transition to palliative care and hospice, it does not mean that medical care ends. Sometimes, the management of symptoms associated with decline and death is among the most difficult medical treatments in the course of an illness. Most patients with advanced AIDS suffer from multiple symptoms from opportunistic infections that cannot be eradicated. Care givers must become skilled at providing aggressive symptom relief when treatment or cure is no longer possible.

Pain Management in the Hospice Setting

Pain is an underappreciated, underrecognized, and undertreated problem in AIDS. Pain, which is nearly ubiquitous in HIV disease, is present at least 80% of the time in patients with far-advanced AIDS. Despite the results of research (16), pain is still inadequately addressed by AIDS practitioners, for the following reasons:

- Physicians' traditional construct holds that diagnosing and treating the underlying cause of pain will lead to its elimination. Unfortunately, the reality is that, in advanced AIDS, many underlying conditions cannot be treated.
- Physicians who treat AIDS come from various backgrounds and, unlike oncologists, may not have received any specific training in pain management.
- Many physicians continue to hold a largely unfounded bias against opioids and thus believe that these drugs are dangerous and create dependency.

As with terminal cancer, the goal of palliative care in AIDS must be optimal pain and symptom control to improve the patient's quality of life for as long as possible. In the case of late-stage AIDS-related pain, opioids often are the only analgesics that achieve pain control.

EVALUATION OF PAIN

Pain is highly subjective. No chemical or physiologic test can confirm whether, or how much, a person hurts. The best indicator of pain is the patient's own report of that pain (17, 18). In evaluating a patient's pain, it may be helpful to use the Verbal Numerical Scale, used to rate pain from 0 (no pain) to 10 (the worst pain one can imagine). Some physicians have also used pain diagrams, but both this method and the Verbal Numerical Scale can be unreliable in patients with dementia. In such patients, interview by the care giver or the Verbal Numerical Scale may be used to assess the location and intensity of pain (19).

MANAGEMENT OF PAIN

In a 1990 study conducted at the AIDS Home Care and Hospice Program of San Francisco, 53 of 100 patients surveyed had complaints of pain. Their pain fell into 8 general categories, in descending order of frequency: peripheral neuropathy; abdominal pain; headache; skin pain from to KS, pressure sores, or herpes; oropharyngeal pain; chest pain; and diffuse and unrelated pains (20).

One must distinguish between chronic and acute pain. Acute pain is the result of an injury or trauma that will heal. Chronic pain, in AIDS patients, is unrelenting pain that is usually the result of tumor growth, peripheral neuropathy, or severe cachexia; it will not heal. AIDS patients can have both types of pain. Acute pain needs aggressive, rapid intervention with short courses of powerful pain medication. Chronic pain requires long-term use of around-the-clock medication. In chronic pain, the minimal required strength of medication to alleviate pain is preferable because it will almost certainly have to be given around the clock. Poorly controlled pain is one of the reasons chronically ill patients ask for physician-assisted suicide (21).

Peripheral Neuropathy

Neuropathy is most commonly due to HIV infection or to complications of the nucleoside analogs didanosine, dideoxycytidine, and stavudine. Patients often describe a burning sensation in addition to the painful paresthesias usual with most other neuropathies. Neuropathic pain does not respond well to opioids alone. Amitriptyline (Elavil), started at 10 to 25 mg at bedtime, has been helpful. The dose may be increased to 50 to 150 mg as needed. Nortriptyline or desipramine may be useful if amitriptyline leads to excess sedation or other side effects (e.g., dry mouth). Dosages are increased at 10-mg increments until either pain relief occurs or significant side effects appear. If neuropathic pain continues, or if patients are unable to tolerate neuroleptic agents, carbamazepine (Tegretol), 200 mg twice a day, or mexiletine, 200 mg every 8 hours, or gabapentin (Neurontin), 300 mg two or three times a day, may be helpful. Patients taking carbamazepine, mexiletine, and gabapentin need to have laboratory values assessed regularly to assess for toxicity. Although this complication is difficult to manage, most patients have some favorable response to one or more of these agents.

Headache

Chronic headache is a common complaint. Patients may have muscle tension or vascular headache or headache due to chronic sinusitis. Headache may be a side effect of medications including zidovudine, cimetidine, nonsteroidal antiinflammatory drugs (NSAIDs), and even opioids. The physician may start with acetaminophen or an NSAID. If ineffective, ketorolac or tramadol can be used before prescription of orally administered opioids. Newer regimens for chronic intractable headache include such medications as divalproex sodium, carbamazepine, gabapentin, and β-blockers in combination with tricyclic antidepressants.

Abdominal Pain

Abdominal pain is associated with various complications of AIDS; CMV colitis, esophageal gastric ulcers, and duodenal ulcers are typically painful. Disseminated MAC can result in pain because of infiltration of the liver and spleen. Some patients with MAC and hepatosplenomegaly with a homogeneous pattern on a computed tomography scan complain of chronic upper abdominal bloating and discomfort. This effect is presumably due to compression of the gastrointestinal tract by organomegaly. Some patients with known MAC and splenomegaly may experience acute episodes of severe, sharp, or stabbing left upper quadrant, flank, or back pain. Opioids are usually required for relief.

Skin Disorders

Various skin conditions have been noted to cause pain in AIDS patients. KS lesions can obstruct lymphatics and may cause lower extremity edema and pain. Such obstructive pain can initially be treated with a distal compression wrap, but eventually edema progresses and analgesics become necessary (20).

Herpes zoster lesions are painful in the acute phase, and patients with AIDS often suffer from chronic postherpetic neuralgia. In the acute phase, treatment can include acyclovir, amitriptyline, opioids, and occasionally neuroleptics for postherpetic neuralgia.

Decubitus ulcers are common in late stage AIDS because patients are bedridden, weak, and emaciated. Urine or stool incontinence further compounds the risk of developing nonhealing decubitus ulcers. Regular positioning and turning are vital to prevent bedsores.

Oropharyngeal Pain

Oropharyngeal pain has many causes. Oral candidiasis or herpes simplex infection may be painful and is best treated with specific antiviral or antifungal treatments. KS involving the mouth and pharynx may be painful. Odynophagia may be due to oral or esophageal candidiasis, herpes or CMV esophagitis, or aphthous ulcers of the mouth or esophagus. Thalidomide may be effective for treating aphthous ulcers. Amphotericin B lozenges, nystatin pastilles, itraconazole oral suspension, or intermittent infusions of amphotericin B may help to control odynophagia in patients with resistant candidiasis. Esophageal spasm with pain, dysphagia, or vomiting may respond to metoclopramide. Antiulcer agents, especially omeprazole and sucralfate, can be effective in treating pain resulting from upper gastrointestinal ulcerations, thus making it possible for the patient to eat.

Chest Pain

Chest pain occurs in several AIDS-related illnesses. Typical pleuritic pain should suggest a diagnosis of bacterial pneumonia in the patient with fever, productive cough, and pulmonary infiltrate. Acute pneumothorax is a well-recognized complication in late stage AIDS patients, probably resulting from subpleural PCP. Hospice patients experiencing pneumothorax should be managed with opioids.

APPROPRIATE ANALGESIA WITH OPIOIDS

An important rule for control of pain in AIDS is to anticipate the symptoms and not to wait for intense pain to take hold before taking action. The symptom should be treated with appropriate medication and regular dosing to prevent recurrence (19).

The stepladder pain control format used with cancer patients is also effective with AIDS-related pain in hospice, with some important exceptions (20). For example, supplementary management for constipation necessary in cancer patients receiving opioids may not be necessary in the AIDS hospice patient, simply because diarrhea is such a prevalent symptom.

For the most part, pain in advanced AIDS is best suppressed with opioids. Many reservations of the medical community about prescribing opioids simply do not apply to late stage AIDS. Several narcotic agents are effective for managing pain in these patients, among which are morphine, codeine, hydromorphine, and methadone. Most pain specialists agree that morphine is the most effective of these agents (22). One reason for this recommendation is flexibility in route of administration of morphine, from oral to subcutaneous to intravenous by bolus, drip, or patient-controlled analgesia.

Physicians should use the same problem-solving approach they bring to a diagnostic dilemma when deriving the best dose and means of delivery for opioids. Table 52.2 illustrates the correct use of morphine. The following steps are essential for maintaining adequate pain control:

1. Oral morphine should be given every 4 hours, rather than on a PRN ("as needed") basis (20).
2. Prescribe "rescue" doses (usually 25 to 50% of the regular dosage) for breakthrough pain that occurs between the

regularly scheduled doses. More frequent requests for rescue doses provide a signpost to the physician to titrate the 4-hour dosages upward.

Method of Delivery

The type and duration of pain determine the initial route of delivery for the opioid. Practitioners and the American Pain Society agree that oral administration is the preferred route. For severe pain, oral morphine solution offers advantages in titration and provides excellent pain control in most circumstances. Time-release narcotics make around-the-clock dosing easier, but some patients with impaired gut absorption, or motility, do not seem to benefit from this form of delivery. Narcotic suppositories can be prescribed, but this route is often a problem because of chronic diarrhea and perianal lesions in the AIDS hospice patient. Some late stage AIDS patients have nausea, vomiting, or difficulty in swallowing that prevents oral dosing of pain medication. For these patients, transdermal, rectal, subcutaneous, or intravenous delivery of narcotic should be considered. It is best to provide pain medication in the least invasive, and most effective, delivery system. Too often, medical providers graduate to intravenous pain medication infusions before easier, less invasive dosing has been tried. Transdermal fentanyl has significantly decreased the need for intravenous infusions or even subcutaneous lines while providing good pain control. The long-acting nature of the fentanyl patch means that optimum pain relief is not obtained for up to 17 hours after application of the patch. Medical providers need to monitor patients for the amount of pain control provided by the patch, as well as observe for signs of oversedation and respiratory depression. Long-acting narcotics should not be the first narcotic prescribed. Instead, the appropriate dose of narcotic should be determined using short-acting narcotics, such as oral morphine; then the 24-hour dose of required narcotic is converted to the long-acting form. Patients taking long-acting or time-release narcotics (either transdermally or orally) should be prescribed a short-acting narcotic for breakthrough pain.

For severe, acute pain that needs immediate relief, intravenous or intramuscular administration is preferable. When analgesia is reached, the medical provider should consider prescribing a transition to an oral form of the drug. Subcutaneous injections are often preferable in wasted patients whose lack of muscle mass makes intramuscular injections difficult.

Equianalgesic charts are useful in calculating equivalent dosages when switching a patient from one opioid to another or from one method of delivery to another. The equianalgesic chart can also be consulted to prescribe decreasing doses of injectable drug while increasing the oral dosage.

Unwarranted Fears about Opioids

Physicians inexperienced in pain management may underprescribe opioids because of fears of causing respiratory depression or tolerance to the drug. Respiratory depression resulting from opioid analgesics is less of a concern in hospice settings than in patients for whom recovery is anticipated. However, even in hospice, the greatest danger of respiratory depression occurs soon after administration of the first dose; the longer the patient is receiving opioids, the less likely respiratory depression is to occur.

The issue of substance abuse is relevant because many AIDS patients are past or present drug abusers. Control of pain must be the priority. Concern about addiction and dependence are unwarranted in dying patients who are in pain. Patient-controlled analgesia pumps with defined rates and bolus options may be a preferred method of delivery when drug addiction is or has been an ongoing problem.

Physicians should not be afraid to prescribe sufficient opioids to relieve discomfort. Benzodiazepines should not be prescribed as substitutes for analgesics. They are, of course, useful in managing anxiety and for sleep, but given over a long period, barbiturates and benzodiazepines increase the likelihood of depression, thus negatively affecting the patient's quality of life.

Fever

Antipyretics should be prescribed to promote comfort. Acetaminophen (around the clock), NSAIDs such as naproxen (Naprosyn, 250 to 500 mg every 12 hours), and slow-release indomethacin (Indocin SR, 75 mg every 12 hours), may be useful in suppressing hectic fevers associated with uncontrolled infections or lymphoma. For patients who are unable to swallow tablets, choline magnesium salicylate (Trilisate, 1 g) comes in liquid and is given twice a day to prevent recurrent fevers. Rigors, most frequently because of disseminated MAC or disseminated fungal infections, can be lessened by intravenous injections of small doses of morphine. Meperidine should be avoided because of the potential for increasing confusion and restlessness.

Diarrhea

Diarrhea is a common problem in patients with AIDS. It can be caused by the direct effect of HIV on the intestinal tract, or it may be from infection with *Cryptosporidium*, microsporidia, *Isospora belli*, MAC, or CMV. The diarrhea can be severe and debilitating. Diphenoxylate or loperamide

Table 52.2. Correct Use of Morphine[a]

- Administer by mouth (give every 4 h, not PRN)
- Review dose every 24 h
- Titrate dose against the pain (2.5, 5, 10, 15, 20, 30, 45, 80, 90, 120, 180 mg)
- Use a breakthrough dose of 10–25% of 4-h dose
- Use 3:1 dose ratio (mg) when transferring from PO to IV/IM/SC
- Use 1:1 dose ratio (mg) when transferring from oral liquid (every 4 h) morphine to oral sustained release tablets (every 12 h)
- Titrate dose down when morphine no longer needed

[a] From Walsh TD: Prevention of opioid side-effects, J Pain Symptom Manage 1990;5:362–367.

may help, especially if given around the clock, rather than on an as-needed basis. Usually, this diarrhea requires aggressive treatment with around-the-clock constipating narcotics such as codeine, morphine, or tincture of opium. Prophylactic and suppressive antibiotics, or antiretrovirals, suspected of causing or worsening the diarrhea should be discontinued in the hospice setting. In the hospice patient with severe diarrhea, it is of little value to encourage increasing oral intake because this intake only exacerbates the diarrhea. Concerns regarding rehydration are usually unfounded in the hospice patient. Dehydration is a natural process during the end stage of illness that causes little discomfort. If a patient complains of being thirsty, then rehydration may be appropriate.

Nausea and Vomiting

Nausea and vomiting are also common in the AIDS patient. Many of the same opportunistic infections that cause diarrhea can also cause nausea with vomiting. The usual antiemetics are commonly used, with fair results. Some AIDS patients who have used marijuana in the past benefit from smoking marijuana or from taking oral dronabinol to control nausea. Most inpatient hospices do not allow patients to smoke marijuana. Agencies caring for patients in their home have varying policies regarding working with someone who uses substances prohibited by law.

Dyspnea

Shortness of breath often develops in the hospice AIDS patient. Causes can be pneumothorax, KS in the lung, congestive heart failure, severe anemia or pneumonias caused by PCP, CMV, or bacterial infection. Sometimes, the underlying cause can be treated; however, many hospice patients either cannot tolerate the treatments or want no further life-prolonging interventions. Then the practitioner must provide symptom relief from shortness of breath. Oxygen delivered through nasal prongs or a mask may be comforting. Opioid analgesics are essential for suppression of the sensation of shortness of breath. A continuously worsening shortness of breath resulting from untreated pneumonia requires around-the-clock opioids, usually in increasing doses, to stay ahead of the worsening symptom. Continuous subcutaneous narcotic infusions and even intravenous infusion are the best approaches for calming the patient with severe air hunger. In patients with severe shortness of breath, this palliative approach usually results in sedation and may accelerate the patient's death. However, patients requiring this level of intervention are always actively dying and deserve extreme efforts to make their final moments peaceful.

End-Stage Dementia

Not all dying patients manifest dementia; however, the longer patients live with cognitive–motor deficit, the greater is the likelihood of advanced dementia at the time of death. The whole range of cognitive–motor deficit (dementia) is observed in the hospice AIDS patient.

The early symptoms of dementia, such as forgetfulness and confusion, are disturbing to many patients with AIDS. Anxiety can be a presenting symptom of dementia, as well as an appropriate response to the diagnosis of HIV infection. Physicians sometimes mistakenly medicate early dementia with benzodiazepines to calm the patient. In the patient with dementia, benzodiazepines often produce confounding effects, with increased anxiety and breakthrough withdrawal. Additionally, benzodiazepines often increase the disinhibition common in early dementia. For these reasons, these agents should be avoided in hospice AIDS patients. In the actively dying patient, benzodiazepines may be useful in ensuring relaxation and comfort.

Patients with AIDS dementia complex should be considered brain damaged. The family should be assisted in creating a safe environment for the patient. Medications that can be helpful in containing overstimulation are antipsychotics such as perphenazine, chlorpromazine, thioridazine, haloperidol, and resperdal. Practitioners need to be vigilant and regularly assess these patients for extrapyramidal syndromes because these disorders are more common in AIDS-demented patients. Benztropine can be prescribed concomitantly to reduce the likelihood of extrapyramidal symptoms.

Terminal Restlessness

Sometimes, during the dying process, AIDS patients can become agitated and restless to the point of discomfort for patient or family. Under these circumstances, it is not only appropriate, but also necessary, to provide relief by conscious sedation. This goal can be accomplished in several ways. Usually, one should intervene in the most noninvasive manner possible. Around-the-clock oral morphine administration can be increased to cause sedation. Lorazepam may be added to every other 4-hour dose of morphine to sedate the patient further and to create a sense of well-being. Pentobarbital suppositories are an effective means of sedation that requires little intervention or complex care. Dosing of pentobarbital for this purpose is 30 to 60 mg every 6 to 12 hours, increased as needed to obtain relief. Patients who remain restless despite these interventions can be started on a midazolam intravenous drip until death (23). Attempts at conscious sedation are only appropriate in the final week of life.

Family Issues

It is not unusual for a patient to enter a hospice program against the wishes of his or her family (family being defined as those loved ones who are important in the patient's life). The patient may feel resolved regarding palliation, but the significant other or family members may still want the patient to fight for life. Conflicts between patient and family can be difficult. Often, patients decline hospice care even when they are ready because family members are encouraging them to continue to fight. The primary care physician must continuously assess, and advocate for, the patient's wishes.

The patient who has lived in a body that is tired and declining is often aware when it is time to stop active interventions. Family members are not always aware of the internal suffering and fatigue endured by the person with AIDS. They often view their role as that of cheerleaders and motivators, and they feel responsible for supporting and cajoling the patient through treatment. In many cases, the role of care provider supplants the former role of mother, or lover, or friend, and it causes a family member to become consumed by the care giver role. Health care providers' attempts to make the transition from treatment to palliation can be perceived as an assault on their loved one and an assault on their own role in life. Family members may personalize the dying of their relative or spouse or lover as their own failure to love enough. For these reasons, it becomes vital to identify, and then include, important family members in ongoing discussions regarding treatment options. Each office visit should include family; if that is not possible, then physicians can offer updates on the telephone about the patient's condition. As mentioned earlier, discussions of palliation need to begin shortly after HIV diagnosis and at frequent intervals through the course of disease progression. During these discussions, important family members should be present and allowed to ask questions and resolve issues. By regular, ongoing discussion, including the patient's sharing his or her feelings regarding treatment and when to stop, family members have the opportunity to process feelings and to understand the wishes of their loved one, before a crisis develops. Additionally, family members have a chance to work through their feelings in the presence of the physician and patient.

Psychosocial Aspects

AIDS is a disease that causes as much emotional as physical turmoil. As a patient moves toward death, some of these issues can cause real conflict and pain. Many AIDS patients are estranged from their biologic family, sometimes because of sexual orientation and sometimes because of intravenous drug use. Regardless of the cause, this estrangement can become a problem. Some patients want assistance in mending these broken ties; however, others want protection from their biologic family, who could reappear in the last weeks of life and attempt to assume control of finances or health care decisions. One must assess the patient's wishes and respect them. Encouraging early election of the durable power of attorney and making a will can help to guarantee that the patient's wishes are followed.

Depression and withdrawal are not uncommon in the dying patient with AIDS. Sometimes, as a patient moves toward death, he or she becomes more introspective and quiet. This change is natural and does not require medical intervention. However, sometimes patients feel hopeless and depressed. Asking patients how they are feeling and prescribing antidepressant agents with more rapid onset are useful. Sometimes, referral to hospice improves depression because of the increased services available to the patient and the subsequent increased interaction with staff and volunteers.

One must consider the psychological impact on the person dying of AIDS of the deaths of friends, lovers, spouses, and children. The person with AIDS has likely experienced multiple losses from the disease and may be in a state of grief. Manifestations of this unending loss can be depression, anxiety, withdrawal, substance use or abuse, destructive behavior, or thoughts of suicide (24). Sometimes, these feelings are beyond the scope of the patient's ability to process. Interventions can then be focused on maintaining a patient's ability to cope. In some instances, hospices should involve their bereavement programs to provide psychotherapy to the dying patient.

Aid in dying is becoming an accepted fact within the West Coast AIDS communities of the United States (25). The scope of this chapter does not permit an in-depth review, or a moral analysis, of this phenomenon. Physicians should be aware that if they care for persons with AIDS, they will receive requests for aid in dying. Regardless of which action is taken, physicians need to have a clear, morally defensible response to a patient's request for assistance. Timely, appropriate referrals to hospice can change the minds of some persons wishing to die, whereas others remain determined to choose the time of their death.

Spiritual Issues

As a person declines toward death, he or she often contemplates issues beyond the body. Many patients return to childhood beliefs and religions that explain life after death. For some, reconsidering religion is painful because the religion may contain teachings that proclaim that the dying person is sinful. The anxiety and fear that medical care providers sometimes see at the end of their patients' lives often have much to do with these issues. Offering gentle acceptance and support can assist patients in issues of self-worth and acceptance. Referral to a nonjudgmental chaplain can also provide a measure of solace and forgiveness.

Many patients and some physicians are reluctant to refer patients to hospice because they perceive that hospice means giving up hope. However, is false expectation honestly hope? Do we really help patients by supporting their unrealistic hopes of recovery and cure? Can one be hopeful while dying? We believe that hope is more than an expectation, it is a state of being that enriches the moment through a belief in the transcendent. Hope is always present when life is meaningful, regardless of the assigned meaning (26). Each person has different meanings to their life, but if there is meaning, there is hope. Physicians and care providers should listen for what gives meaning to a patient's life and then support and foster that meaning as a way of maintaining hope. One patient may reveal his deep belief in Christ and redemption, another may

Table 52.3. Byock's Milestones or Tasks

1. Sense of completion with world affairs
2. Sense of completion in relation to community
3. Sense of meaning about ones' individual life
4. Love of self
5. Love of others
6. Sense of completion in relationships with family and friends
7. Acceptance of the finality of life—of one's existence as an individual
8. Sense of a new self (personhood) beyond personal loss
9. Sense of meaning about life in general
10. Surrender to the transcendent, to the unknown—letting go

(From Byock I. Beyond symptom management: growth at the end of life. In: National Hospice Organization's Palliative Care Conference, San Francisco, 1994;3:27–32.)

talk of her love of friends and staying sober. Supporting a patient's belief system can sustain a patient's hope, even in the face of death.

Too often, medical health professionals soften the truth based on their belief that patients cannot withstand another disappointment. However, the truth allows patients to make truly informed decisions. Grappling with the hard realities of living can result in increased purpose and meaning in life. Sometimes, this struggle to make meaning of disaster actually strengthens individuals and better prepares them to cope with the future.

Just because someone is dying does not mean that every conversation must be intense. Helping patients to focus on uplifting emotions by asking them what gives them joy now, or what has been an inspiration in their life, will allow patients to refocus on happier times. Happiness can bring just as much meaning to life as contemplative reflection (27).

To provide complete symptom management to the dying AIDS patient, physicians need to consider all aspects of the individual. Providing relief from pain and other physical symptoms is a good beginning, but it is not enough. Often, the dying patient is focused beyond the body. Dr. Ira Byock is a hospice physician who has developed a useful list of milestones, or tasks, that he believes a person who is dying is trying to accomplish (28) (Table 52.3). Providing assistance in working through these milestones may have greater value to some patients and their families than the management of some physical problems.

In conclusion, the dramatic success of combination antiretroviral therapy, including protease inhibitors, one hopes will continue to decrease the numbers of persons with AIDS referred to a hospice for palliative care. However, some patients with AIDS will continue to die, and these patients deserve the option of palliation. Timely referrals allow the palliative care team to work with appropriate patients and their families around symptom management and preparation for death. The goal of therapy at the end of life must be to alleviate suffering while providing an opportunity for the patient to prepare for death. By listening to the patient, working with a palliative care team, and relieving the patient's symptoms, the physician can ease this passage.

References

1. Centers for Disease Control and Prevention.
2. Mellors JW, Rinaldo C, Gupta P, et al. Prognosis in HIV-1 infection predicted by the quantity of virus in plasma. Science 1996;272:55–59.
3. Faber-Langendoen K, Bartels DM. Process of foregoing life-sustaining treatment in a university hospital: an empirical study. Crit Care Med 1992;20:570–577.
4. Cella DF. Measuring quality of life in palliative care. Semin Oncol 1995;22:S73–S81.
5. Neaton JD, Wentworth DN, Rhame F, et al. Considerations in choice of a clinical endpoint for AIDS clinical trials. Stat Med 1994;13: 2107–2125
6. Moore RD. Natural history of opportunistic disease in an HIV-infected urban clinical cohort. Ann Intern Med 1996;124:633–642.
7. Rao TK. Outcome of severe acute renal failure in patients with acquired immunodeficiency syndrome. Am J Kidney Dis 1995;25:390–398.
8. O'Dell MW, Lubeck DP, O'Driscoll P, et al. Validity of the Karnofsky performance status in an HIV-infected sample. J Acquir Immune Defic Syndr Hum Retrovirol 1995;10:350–357.
9. Justice AC, Aiken L H, Smith HL, et al. The role of functional status in predicting in-patient mortality with AIDS: a comparison with current predictors. J Clin Epidemiol 1995;49:193–201.
10. Palenicek JP, Graham NM, He YD, et al. Weight loss prior to clinical AIDS as a predictor of survival. J Acquir Immune Defic Syndr Hum Retrovirol 1995;10:366–370.
11. Herrmann FR. Serum albumin level on admission as a predictor of death, length of stay and readmission. Arch Intern Med 1992;152: 125–130.
12. Lifson AR, Olson R, Roberts SG, et al. Severe opportunistic infections in AIDS patients with late-stage disease. J Am Fam Pract 1994;7: 288–291.
13. Lundgren JD, Pedersen C, Bentsen KD, et al. Survival after the diagnosis of AIDS: study group for HIV infection. Ugeskr Laeger 1995;157:1352–1356.
14. Martin JN, Colford JM, Ngo L, et al. Effects of older age on survival in human immunodeficiency virus (HIV) disease. Am J Epidemiol 1995; 142:1221–1230.
15. Currie PF. Heart muscle disease related to HIV infection: prognostic implications. BMJ 1994;309:1605–1607.
16. Beitbart
17. McCaffery M, Paser CL. Pain ratings: the fifth vital sign. Am J Nurs 1997;97:15–16.
18. McCaffery M, Ferrel BR. Nurses' assessment of pain intensity and choice of analgesic dose. Contemp Nurse 1994;3:68–74
19. Walsh TD. An overview of palliative care in cancer and AIDS. Oncology 1991;5:7–11.
20. Schofferman J, Brody R. Pain in far advanced AIDS. In: Foley KM, Bonica JJ, Ventafridda V, et al., eds. Advances in pain research and therapy. New York: Raven Press, 1990;16:379–386.
21. Abrams DI. Physician-assisted suicide and patients with human immunodeficiency virus disease. N Engl J Med 1997;336:417–421.
22. Levy MH. Pain management in advanced cancer. Semin Oncol 1985; 12:394–410.
23. Burke AL, Diamond PL, Hulbert J, et al. Terminal restlessness: its management and the role of midazolam. Med J Aust 1991;155:485–487.
24. Grothe TM, McKusick L. Coping with multiple loss. Focus 1992; 7:5–6.
25. Batten M. Going early, going late: the rationality of decisions about suicide in AIDS. J Med Philos 1994;19:571–594.
26. Grothe T. Hope in hospice. National Hospice Organization Symposium, Washington, DC, 1994.
27. Kast V. Joy, inspiration, and hope. College Station, TX: Texas A&M University Press, 1991.
28. Byock I. Beyond symptom management: growth at the end of life. In: National Hospice Organization's Palliative Care Conference, San Francisco, 1994;3:27–32.

53

HIV Transmission in the Health Care Environment

David K. Henderson

Few issues created as much anxiety for health care providers as did the introduction of human immunodeficiency virus (HIV) and acquired immunodeficiency syndrome (AIDS) into the health care environment. Early in the HIV epidemic, the risk of occupational HIV infection of health care workers became apparent (1). Even before the first occupational infections were identified, the United States Centers for Disease Control (CDC, now known as the Centers for Disease Control and Prevention) identified the theoretic risk of transmission of the etiologic agent of AIDS and issued guidelines intended to reduce occupational risks for health care workers (2, 3). As more was learned about the risks and routes of nosocomial occupational transmission of HIV, both the United States Public Health Service (USPHS) (4–9) and others (10–11) issued modified guidelines to address the continually accruing information.

In some respects, health care workers' initial, almost visceral, responses to AIDS and HIV infection in the health care workplace were harbingers of society's response to this remarkable infectious disease. Almost from the beginning of the epidemic, health care institutions were faced with practitioners who wanted "zero risk" for occupational HIV infection. Nearly 20 years into the epidemic, health care workers have become more knowledgeable about occupational risks, and, simultaneously, health care institutions and regulatory agencies have developed reasonable strategies to manage patients infected with bloodborne pathogens.

The presence of HIV in the health care workplace has attracted the attention of regulators, as well. The United States Department of Labor's Occupational Safety and Health Administration (OSHA) began inspecting health care workplaces, initially under its "general duty" clause and later for compliance with the notice of proposed rule making issued jointly by the Departments of Labor and Health and Human Services (12). Ultimately, OSHA issued the final standard on bloodborne pathogens (13). Guidelines, process controls, and standards that previously had been applied to industrial settings were, perhaps for the first time, applied to clinical medicine. The broad application of these guidelines has been problematic, particularly for smaller institutions in areas of low prevalence of these bloodborne infections. In addition, the principles endorsed in the final rule have not been uniformly embraced, either in the United States or around the world.

Finally, the occurrence of the initial case cluster of provider-to-patient transmission of HIV (14–18) attracted substantial publicity and public interest, ultimately resulting in remarkable public anxiety about the risk of acquiring HIV infection from an infected health care practitioner. The USPHS issued guidelines for practitioners infected with bloodborne pathogens (19), and, in response to this almost unprecedented anxiety, the United States Congress passed a statute requiring that states implement the July, 1991 CDC guidelines (or guidelines certified as equivalent to the CDC guidelines) for managing HIV-infected or hepatitis B (HBV)-infected providers. Some aspects of the CDC guidelines (e.g., the requirement that infected practitioners who plan to perform "exposure-prone" invasive procedures must notify patients prospectively of the practitioner's infection status) were initially (and remain) controversial and have not been uniformly adopted by the states. A second cluster of HIV infections was linked to an infected provider in 1997. Whereas the details of this case have not yet been published in the refereed medical literature, the case, which involves an HIV-infected orthopedic surgeon, has been described both in the press (20) and at a national meeting (21). Such cases are, in great measure, both rare and inevitable (22–24).

With the exception of a discussion of isolation and management techniques for patients infected with bloodborne pathogens, general infection control issues, such as disinfection, sterilization, and waste disposal are dealt with elsewhere in this text (see Chap. 54). Instead, this chapter focuses on some of the unique issues raised by the introduction of HIV into the health care environment. This chapter discusses the following: 1) the epidemiology of HIV infection in the health care setting; 2) strategies for managing the risk of occupational exposure to, and infection with, bloodborne pathogens in the health care workplace; 3) the management of occupational exposures to HIV, focusing on the safety and efficacy of antiretroviral agents administered as postexposure chemoprophylaxis; and 4) strategies for the administrative management of HIV-infected health care providers in the health care setting.

EPIDEMIOLOGY

Documented Occupational Infections

To date, 52 occupational infections have been documented among health care workers in the United States (25). Each of these cases is a documented seroconversion; that is, the exposed health care worker was known to be HIV seronegative at the time of the exposure, the worker was exposed to blood from a patient known to harbor HIV infection, and, in temporal association with the exposure, the health care worker developed serologic signs of HIV infection. These cases form the nucleus of our knowledge of occupational HIV infection. Several of these cases have been studied in detail (26, 27).

Although definitive data regarding factors influencing the risk of occupational infection are not yet available, evaluation of the 52 cases for which epidemiologic data are available provides some insight into the factors that are likely to influence the risk of transmission of HIV in the health care setting associated with various occupational exposure events (Table 53.1). Further, a retrospective case-control study conducted by public health authorities in the United States, France, and the United Kingdom has provided additional insight into the factors associated with an increased level of risk of occupational infection with HIV (28), as discussed in more detail later in this chapter.

Table 53.1. Factors Possibly Influencing Risks of Occupational or Nosocomial Transmission of HIV-1

- Concentration of circulating virus in source
  Numbers and concentration of cells expressing HIV antigens in the peripheral circulation of the "source" patient[a]
  Presence (and extent) of circulating "free" (as compared with cell-associated) virus
  Strain variation (i.e., strains that rapidly induce syncytia may be more aggressive; differing strains may better adapted to certain routes of exposure)
  Concomitant antiretroviral therapy
- Exposure-specific factors
  Type of exposure (i.e., parenteral, mucosal, or cutaneous)
  Inoculum (extent of exposure[a], type of device [e.g., hollow-bore versus surgical needlestick], body fluid involved, extent to which the device was contaminated with blood[a], whether or not the device had been in the source patient's vascular channel[a])
  Immediacy of the exposure (i.e., time elapsed since the needle or sharp object was contaminated with material from an infected source patient)
- Health care worker–related factors
  Application (and type) of first aid
  For mucosal and cutaneous exposures: status of skin and mucous membranes at the site of exposure (e.g., broken, chapped, inflamed)
- Exposure management-related factors
  Administration of antiretroviral chemoprophylaxis[a]

[a]Identified as significant risk factors for occupational HIV infection in the Center for Disease Control and Prevention's retrospective case-control study (28).

HIV Infections in Health Care Workers Not Documented by Seroconversion

In addition to the 52 documented seroconversions, certain other instances of probable or possible occupational HIV infections have been reported in the medical literature, to local, state, or federal public health authorities, or in the lay press (26, 29). Through December, 1996, 111 such cases had been reported to the CDC in the United States (25). These cases range from individuals who reported occupational exposures to HIV, but who did not have baseline serologic examinations to demonstrate seronegativity at the time of the exposure and were found to be infected weeks or months after the reported exposure, to individuals who have AIDS and who deny community-based risk behaviors and note that they have worked in a health care environment at some time since 1977 (26, 29, 30). A few of these cases almost certainly are community acquired. Based on epidemiologic data from these additional cases, the likelihood that these cases represent true occupational infections (as opposed to situations in which community-based risk behaviors are confounding these data) varies by the type of case report (26), with documented seroconversions representing the most reliable data, and the "no identifiable risk" AIDS cases the most likely to be confounded by community-related risks of HIV infection.

Underreporting of Occupational Infections

Health care workers are, unfortunately, notorious for failing to report occupational exposures to pathogens in the workplace. Some estimates have suggested that as few as one-third of parenteral occupational exposures are reported to employee health services (31–37). Reasons for such underreporting are complex and include, for example, lack of awareness on the part of health care workers of the risks associated with occupational exposures, restriction of health care workers' access (e.g., in terms of location or time) to reporting mechanisms, and trivialization or denial by health care workers of the risks inherent in such exposures. In addition, the problem of occupational infection with HIV or HBV is now complicated by career jeopardy. In light of the federal statute requiring that states implement the July, 1991 USPHS guidelines, health care workers may be increasingly reluctant to reveal either occupationally acquired or community-acquired HIV or HBV infections.

Factors Influencing the Risk of Occupational HIV Infection

Because of the small number of documented seroconversions that have been studied in detail, information about factors contributing to the risk of occupational infection is limited (see Table 53.1) (9, 27, 28, 38). Whereas previous assessments of risk factors for occupational infection were speculative (39), scientific data now available to address this question, in great measure, support earlier speculation.

Perhaps the best available risk factor data come from the case-control study published jointly by public health authorities from the United States, France, and the United Kingdom (28). This study found that the risk of HIV transmission was significantly increased in the following circumstances: 1) when the injury or occupational exposure was "deep," as opposed to superficial; 2) when blood was visible on the device causing the injury; 3) when the injuring device had been placed in the source patient's vein or artery; 4) if the source patient died within 60 days of the exposure (presumably a surrogate marker for viral burden or for circulating "free" virus); and 5) if the exposed health care worker did not take zidovudine as postexposure chemoprophylaxis (28).

The precise mechanics of the seroconversion event are, as yet, poorly understood, nor is the role of host defense in protection against occupational infection clear. Clerici and colleagues demonstrated that health care workers exposed to blood from HIV-infected patients develop HIV-specific T-helper activity (40). Another study from the same laboratory showed that a substantial fraction (i.e., 35%) of a population of health care workers who had sustained occupational exposure to blood from HIV-infected patients developed cytotoxic lymphocyte responses to HIV-related envelope antigens, whereas none of health care workers who had sustained occupational exposures to blood from patients not infected with HIV exhibited such responses (41).

Of the documented cases of occupationally related seroconversions for which epidemiologic data about the exposures resulting in infection are available, most of the "source patients" met surveillance case-definition criteria for AIDS, and many were near the ends of their lives. These data may be confounded by the fact that patients late in the course of HIV infection may be more likely to be hospitalized, to require medical intervention, and to undergo invasive or emergency procedures.

Transfusion of a unit of blood from an infected donor is associated with a nearly 100% risk of HIV infection (42); thus, the extent of exposure (type of wound, depth of injury, extent of contamination with blood, type of instrument) likely influences the risk of infection. Most occupational infections reported in the United States are due to parenteral exposures. Of the infections associated with needlestick exposures to blood, to date, all have been injuries with hollow-bore (i.e., injection) needles; none of these infections have resulted from exposure to a surgical needle. This difference either may be due to an inoculum effect or, at least in part, may reflect the likelihood that exposures caused by surgical needles will not be reported to employee health authorities appropriately.

Finally, the material (i.e., the bodily substance) to which the health care worker is exposed is likely (again, perhaps because of an inoculum effect) to influence the risk of infection. Of the occupational infections studied in detail to date, all have been exposures either to blood (or grossly bloody fluid) or to concentrated viral preparations in laboratories where HIV serologic test kits are manufactured. In the clinical setting, all the reported exposures except one,

Table 53.2. Factors Influencing Nosocomial Risks of Occupational Exposure to HIV-1

- Prevalence of HIV infection among patients served
- Types of medical or surgical procedures performed
- Frequencies with which invasive or risk-associated procedures are performed
- Types of medical or surgical devices used (and the likelihood that these devices could produce parenteral or mucous membrane exposure)
- Circumstances under which procedures are performed
- Technical expertise of the practitioner
- Extent to which the practioner adheres to accepted infection-control practices, procedures, and exposure-prevention strategies

which was an exposure to bloody pleural fluid, have been to blood from a patient known to be HIV infected (27).

The risk of occupational exposure to HIV in the health care workplace is the product of several independent and interdependent factors. Table 53.2 lists several factors that likely contribute to this risk. A major contributor to the risk for exposure and infection is the prevalence of HIV infection among the population of patients served. Risk is clearly higher in the inner city than in rural areas. The characteristics of an individual practitioner's practice also contribute to the risk of occupational exposure. The types and frequencies of procedures performed and the characteristics of the devices used to perform these procedures probably contribute to this risk. Procedures performed with sharp objects that must be handled in other than direct vision are likely to be associated with an increased level of risk. Elective procedures performed under controlled circumstances, such as in an operating room, are likely to be associated with less risk of exposure than are emergency procedures or those performed in less controlled settings. Finally, the technical expertise, personal habits, and attention to detail of the practitioner probably also contribute to the risk. Practitioners who adhere to accepted infection-control practices and who take fewer short-cuts are likely to have a substantially lower risk of occupational exposures.

During the first 16 years' experience with HIV infection in the health care setting, a substantial body of information has been amassed to estimate the single-hit risk of occupational infection with HIV after parenteral exposure to blood from a patient known to be infected with HIV (27, 43–71). More than 25 longitudinal studies evaluated approximately 7000 parenteral exposures to blood from source patients known to be HIV infected. In these studies, 23 infections occurred, for an overall risk estimate of approximately 0.3% per exposure (27, 71). This estimate assumes that all exposures, all "recipients," and all donors are associated with equal risk, an assumption that almost certainly is incorrect. Nonetheless, despite these obvious limitations, this estimate provides perspective, a backdrop for health care workers to consider the overall magnitude of occupational risk of HIV infection in the health care workplace. For example, the 1 in 325 risk can be compared with the approximately 100 in 325 risk of

HBV associated with parenteral occupational exposure to blood from a patient known to carry hepatitis B e antigen. The risk estimate for occupational infection with HIV after parenteral exposure to blood from an HIV-infected patient has actually remained stable (the estimate has consistently ranged from 0.2 to 0.4%) during the past 10 years.

Other routes of exposure have been associated with many fewer occupational infections; for example, to my knowledge, only five occupational infections associated with exposures other than parenteral have been reported anecdotally worldwide. Only one of these cases is reported in a prospective study (62). These other routes of exposure (e.g., cutaneous, mucous membrane) are presumably associated with substantially lower "per-event" occupational infection risks, because such exposures presumably occur much more frequently than do parenteral exposures.

STRATEGIES FOR REDUCING OCCUPATIONAL RISK OF HIV TRANSMISSION

When the risk of occupational infection with HBV first became apparent, the CDC issued guidelines designed to reduce these risks and to assist occupational medical services in the postexposure management of health care workers who sustained occupational exposures to HBV. Even though this recognized risk has been both present and prevalent in the health care environment for decades, health care workers have been remarkably cavalier about it; the estimated 8000 to 12,000 cases of occupational HBV infections (and the 150 to 200 HBV-related deaths) that occur annually among health care workers in the United States stand, unfortunately, as a clear testimonial to the persistence of this largely preventable risk (72).

When the theoretic risk of transmission of the agent or agents responsible for AIDS was first identified, the CDC again issued both clinical and laboratory guidelines for managing this problem. Over the past several years, the CDC has made a special effort to keep these recommendations current. The AIDS and HIV recommendations were, in many regards, identical to the recommendations made earlier for managing patients with bloodborne hepatitis. The USPHS guidelines emphasize that exposure to blood is associated with occupational risk and that health care workers should take "universal" or "standard" precautions when handling blood or other potentially infectious body fluids (7, 9, 73). Rather than "universal" precautions, Lynch and coworkers developed and advocated the use of "body substance isolation" (11). Although in many aspects similar to universal precautions, their approach is broader in scope with respect to overall hospital isolation procedures (11). Both systems require the use of appropriate barriers whenever contact with potentially infectious bodily fluids is anticipated. The CDC issued newer guidelines incorporating many of the aspects of both universal precautions and body substance isolation into what are now called "standard precautions" (73). With the publication of the OSHA bloodborne pathogen standard (13), every health care institution in the in the

Table 53.3. Strategies to Reduce Risks of Occupational Exposures to HIV

- Strict adherence to infection-control guidelines designed to minimize the risk of exposure to blood or other potentially infectious body fluids, such as universal precautions (7), body substance isolation (11), OSHA bloodborne pathogen standard (13), "standard" precautions (73)
- Use of engineered controls (e.g., new devices) or barriers (e.g., "double gloving") (89) demonstrated to reduce the risk of parenteral exposures or the risk of blood exposures of any type
- Appropriate training of staff to understand the epidemiology pathogenesis, and risks of occupational infection with the variety of bloodborne pathogens prevalent in the health care environment
- Consistent evaluation of procedures associated with risks of parenteral, mucous membrane, or cutaneous exposure to blood, with the intent of modifying these procedures to reduce the risks of these types of exposure
- Evaluating occupational exposures to blood that occur in individual health care institutions, again with the intent of intervening to prevent these exposures
- Developing "user-friendly" employee health programs that encourage prompt reporting and appropriate management of occupational exposure to bloodborne pathogens

United States was required to implement these strategies to protect health care workers. These systems of precautions are expensive to implement (74, 75), primarily because of their extensive reliance on the use of barriers to avoid cutaneous contact with blood and bloody materials, and some investigators have questioned whether they may be cost-effective in certain settings (76).

A major barrier to success for any of these strategies is compliance. Each of the systems requires occupational behavior modification. Several studies have demonstrated poor compliance with these recommendations (45, 77, 78). At the Warren G. Magnuson Clinical Center of the National Institutes of Health in Bethesda, MD, implementation of universal precautions was temporally associated with a 50% reduction in health care workers' self-reported cutaneous exposures to blood. Although my colleagues and I found these results encouraging, the reduction was only 50%, and even after implementation of universal precautions, our staff reported an average of nearly 20 cutaneous exposures to blood annually (77).

Based on the first decade of experience in managing HIV-infected patients in the health care setting, my colleagues and I now believe that several interventions may reduce the individual health care worker's risk of occupational HIV infection with bloodborne pathogens (Table 53.3). In our institution, implementation of universal precautions was temporally associated with reductions in cutaneous and mucous membrane exposures to blood, as well as a clear reduction in rates of some types of parenteral exposures (79, 80). Other institutions have reported similar findings (78).

Despite my own experience, the efficacy of universal precautions in preventing occupational exposures remains controversial. Because these precautions involve the extensive use of gloves and other barriers, they are both labor intensive and costly. Concern has been expressed that these expensive precautions may actually increase risk of transmission of some nosocomial infections, because they may foster the inappropriate use of gloves and because they may result in decreased reliance on traditional (clearly effective) infection-control strategies, such as handwashing. Another criticism of universal precautions has been that these precautions do not have a substantial impact on the occurrence of parenteral exposures, the major route of occupational transmission of bloodborne pathogens. Gerberding and her coworkers have demonstrated that gloves may reduce the blood inoculum associated with a needlestick injury by as much as 50% (81–83). In addition, the universal precautions guidelines underscore the careful and appropriate use and handling of sharp objects in the health care setting and emphasize, for example, that needles should not be recapped except when other options are impractical. Although approximately one-third of parenteral occupational exposures have historically been associated with recapping (53), some authorities have argued that many recapping exposures may not be truly preventable, because in some settings recapping of needles may be the best available alternative (84–87). This last argument presents a compelling case for the need for safer medical devices, but it should not deemphasize the importance of discouraging behaviors associated with occupational risks, such as recapping of needles.

In response to some of the complex problems raised by the necessity of managing HIV-infected patients in the health care setting, manufacturers have responded by developing various new and modified devices that may ultimately reduce risks of occupational exposures and, therefore, of occupational infections. Jagger and her coworkers have been perhaps the most eloquent proponents of the importance of instrument and device design in the prevention of adverse parenteral exposures (84–87). Each candidate device should be carefully evaluated in clinical trials to demonstrate safety, efficacy, and risk-reduction benefit. Those devices passing scientific scrutiny should be aggressively implemented, especially in settings serving populations of patients with high prevalences of bloodborne infections. Whether such devices should routinely be used in low-risk settings remains controversial. At the Warren G. Magnuson Clinical Center of the National Institutes of Health, use of several engineering controls (e.g., relatively impervious needle disposal containers, "needleless" intravenous administration sets) has contributed to a persistent decline in needlestick injuries and occupational exposures (88). Ultimately, investigators may be able to make some assessment of the costs and benefits of these devices in the lower-risk environments.

Education is likely to be one of the most effective strategies to reduce the occupational risk of infection with bloodborne pathogens. One reason that health care workers have been cavalier about the occupational risks of HBV infection may be that, although health care workers may have been aware of the epidemiology, pathogenesis, and even the risk of occupational HBV infection, they may have been unaware both of the magnitude of this problem and of the frequency of severe sequelae among those acquiring occupational HBV infections. Making certain that staff members are aware of the risks of infection with bloodborne pathogens, the routes of infection, the severity of the sequelae associated with these occupational infections, and strategies that have been shown to reduce the risks of infection with these organisms is an integral part of any prevention program. Individuals charged with managing these risks in the health care workplace must also remain attuned both to their own unique institutional environments and to individual practitioners in their institutions. Those responsible should evaluate their environments continually to determine factors influencing the risks of occupational exposures to blood or other potentially infectious body fluids. Recurring risk-assessment programs facilitate the identification of procedures and local circumstances that may be modified to reduce risks for staff members.

Individuals who are charged with institutional responsibility for managing occupational risks of exposure to bloodborne pathogens must also be specifically attuned to the unique problems faced by their own institution as well as to the varied microenvironments in their own institutions. For example, the emergency room and the operating suite represent environments that have special requirements that may eclipse basic universal precautions protections. A study from San Francisco General Hospital clearly demonstrates the efficacy of double gloving in reducing the risk of cutaneous exposures to blood in the operating room (89). Various strategies also have been suggested, and some have been at least partially successful, to reduce risks of exposure in the emergency room setting. Thus, this type of virtually continuous risk assessment, with sensible interventions designed to address specifically identified problems, is integral to the management of these occupational risks.

Finally, the role of the institutional occupational medicine team cannot be overemphasized. Efficient, "user-friendly," institutionwide occupational medicine programs that encourage prompt reporting and appropriate management of occupational exposure to bloodborne pathogens must be developed and implemented. Staff members must be made aware of the program's existence. Any such occupational medicine program must take special precautions to protect the medical privacy and confidentiality of health care workers participating in the program.

MANAGEMENT OF OCCUPATIONAL EXPOSURES TO HIV

Because the risk of occupational infection with bloodborne pathogens will likely remain prevalent in the health care environment for some time, institutions should develop and implement a systematic approach to the management of occupational exposures when they occur. Essential components of a program designed to manage occupational exposures to HIV are listed in Table 53.4. Whereas these points are self-explanatory, several deserve additional emphasis. First and foremost, these programs must provide confidential

Table 53.4. Management of Occupational Exposures to HIV in the Health Care Workplace

- Programs designed to manage occupational exposures to bloodborne pathogens must maintain the medical privacy and confidentiality of both the source patient and the exposed employee.
- Each program must develop strategies for stratifying occupational exposures requiring varying types or levels of intensity of follow-up; an algorithm or flow chart for differing types of exposure has been used effectively in some settings.
- Employees must be made aware of both the existence and the mechanics of the postexposure management program; optimally, information about the program should be readily available throughout the institution, even during nontraditional hours.
- Employees must be taught about the appropriate and immediate management of occupational exposures and must be provided ready access to supplies and equipment for adequate "first aid" for occupational exposures of all types.
- Programs must provide appropriate and accurate serologic testing of both the source or donor patient (after informed consent has been obtained, where appropriate) and the exposed employee; as part of the serologic testing program, both the source patient and the employee should be provided with counseling related to the meaning of, and risk associated with, these serologic tests; in addition, the exposed employee should be counseled about the risk of infection after occupational exposure, as well as about strategies suggested to prevent secondary transmission; adequate time should be given to allow the employee to ask questions about these risks, and, optimally, the employee should have the opportunity to return, if necessary, to have additional questions answered.
- The program must provide, and in fact must encourage, clinical and serologic follow-up for the exposed health care worker at specified, periodic intervals; the employee should be instructed to return at these intervals and at any time when the employee develops symptoms consistent with the acute retroviral syndrome often characteristic of acute HIV infection.
- If the institution elects to follow the US Public Health Service Guidelines (105), postexposure chemoprophylaxis is recommended for some types of exposures and may be offered for others (see Table 53.5). The exposed employee should be counseled about the potential risks and benefits of the agent or agents offered; the employee should be made aware of available data relevant to the use of the agents administered as postexposure chemoprophylaxis.

evaluation and follow-up. If one employee's confidentiality is breached, the program is doomed to failure. As is the case for all occupational medicine programs, maintenance of worker privacy and prompt entry into the program are essential elements. Employee education about the program is imperative. Health care workers have to be aware not only of the existence of the program, but also when, where, and how to enroll. The program should be designed such that enrollment and follow-up are as "hassle-free" as possible. Virtually any impediment may be enough to dissuade participation for anxious health care workers who may prefer to "deny" the exposure. Many institutions have used a 24-hour "hotline" approach with success. A trained health care worker is available around the clock to discuss possible exposures and to advise health care workers on appropriate interventions. The role of "first aid" is less clear. Advocating the use of what could be considered routine first aid, such as rinsing the wound with a sterile solution, seems entirely reasonable. In some institutions, workers sustaining occupational exposures are advised to soak the wound in a disinfectant solution, such as an iodophor or chlorhexidine. The efficacy of these solutions in this setting is unknown, but their use is not unreasonable. Counseling the employee about the risks of infection and prevention of secondary transmission is often both time-consuming and anxiety-provoking. Counselors should be prepared to go over the same data on several occasions, if necessary, and should be prepared for the employee to return on several occasions with additional questions. Patience is a key part of this process.

The use of antiretroviral agents as postexposure chemoprophylaxis for occupational exposures is less controversial now than it was at the time this chapter was written for the first edition of this text (39). Whereas sentient arguments can be made for either offering or electing not to offer postexposure chemoprophylaxis with one or a combination of these agents (56, 90–107), the character of these arguments has changed substantially in the past 3 years. Given the 0.3% per exposure risk estimate for infection, because of sample-size requirements, questions of chemoprophylaxis efficacy may never be well addressed in a prospective, placebo-controlled trial. The retrospective case-control study conducted by public health agencies in the United States, France, and the United Kingdom estimated that zidovudine postexposure chemoprophylaxis reduced the risk of HIV infection associated with parenteral exposure to blood from HIV-infected patients by approximately 80% (28). This study has substantial limitations, however. Among them are the following: 1) a retrospective case-control study is clearly not the best study design to address efficacy; efficacy would be optimally determined in a blinded, prospective placebo-controlled prospective clinical trial; 2) most of the "cases" in the study were identified anecdotally; controls were chosen from prospective studies and therefore may not be truly comparable; 3) antiviral regimens varied widely among controls; and 4) the power of the study is limited by population size, because only 33 cases and 679 controls were available for analysis. Nonetheless, the CDC case-control study provided the first clear suggestion of the chemoprophylactic efficacy of antiretroviral agents in health care workers. Other studies have provided similarly encouraging data. For example, the study evaluating the efficacy of zidovudine in preventing maternal–fetal transmission of HIV jointly sponsored by the National Institute of Allergy and Infectious Diseases and the National Institute for Child Health and Human Development demonstrated a 67% reduction in transmission (108). In addition, whereas the early animal studies of chemoprophylaxis produced discouraging results (109–114), subsequent studies have demonstrated true efficacy of antiretrovirals administered as postinfection "prophylaxis" (103, 107, 115, 116). On the strength of this evidence, the USPHS issued new recommendations concerning the use of antiretrovirals as chemoprophylaxis for occupational exposures to HIV, for the first time recommending that chemoprophylaxis be administered to health care workers sustaining certain types of occupational exposures (105). These recommendations are summarized in Table 53.5. Current recommendations advocate the use of zidovudine, lamivudine, and indinavir in combination for a severe occupational exposure, although fewer agents are advocated for less severe exposures (see Table 53.5). Although the data do not prove the efficacy of antiretrovirals used for chemoprophylaxis, taken together, these new studies provide much more compelling rationale for offering these agents in the setting of a documented occupational exposure to HIV.

Some aspects of postexposure management remain problematic. Instances in which the source patient is either unknown or of unknown HIV serologic status occur, especially in some settings, such as the emergency room. Institutional policies should be developed to provide a systematic approach to such issues. Institutions must pay particular heed to local and state laws when developing and implementing policies regarding HIV serologic testing.

PATIENTS' RISKS OF HIV INFECTION FROM INFECTED HEALTH CARE PROVIDERS

Even though the issue of provider-to-patient HIV transmission prompted legislation by the United States Congress, the risk of transmission from an infected provider to a patient is so small that it may never be accurately measured. Most authorities agree that routine patient care activities conducted by an HIV-infected health care worker pose no measurable risk of virus transmission. Practices that involve what has been termed "exposure-prone" invasive procedures (those associated with risk for exposure of a patient's blood to blood or body fluids from a health care worker) have been the focus of the CDC's July, 1991 guidelines (19) and the subsequent congressional legislation. Using data generated from studies of the risk of transmission of HIV from infected patients to health care providers, several modeled estimates of the patient's single-procedure risk have been summarized in the literature (23). Estimates range from a high of 1 infection for every 41,600 "exposure-prone" procedures to 1 infection for every 26,000,000 dental procedures, with most estimates placing the risk at 1 in 100,000 or less (117–120).

Some authorities have argued that even these estimates may be excessively high, because most of the exposure data from the health care setting are based on exposure to hollow-bore needles, whereas the most likely exposure for patients would be to a surgical needle. The CDC risk estimate (117) attempted to take this difference into account by including a factor of 10 multiplier for the presumed differences in HIV transmission risk between hollow-bore and solid-needle occupational exposures. The actual difference in magnitude of risk for these categories of exposure is not known, but it may be substantially higher than the 10-fold difference factored into the CDC model.

From a population-based perspective, a patient's risk assessment will be similar to that constructed previously for

Table 53.5. United States Public Health Service Recommendations for Chemoprophylaxis after Occupational Exposures to HIV

Source Material[a]	Antiretroviral Prophylaxis[b]	Antiretroviral Regimen[c]
Percutaneous Exposures		
Blood		
Highest Risk[d]	Recommend[b]	ZDV plus LMV plus IND
Increased risk[d]	Recommend[b]	ZDV plus LMV, ± IND
No increased risk[d]	Offer[b]	ZDV plus LMV
Fluid containing visible blood, other potentially infectious fluid[e], or tissue	Offer[b]	ZDV plus LMV
Other body fluid (e.g., urine)	Not offer[b]	
"High" or "Increased Risk" Skin Exposures[f]		
Blood	Offer[g]	ZDV plus LMV, ± IND
Fluid containing visible blood, other potentially infectious fluid[e], or tissue	Offer[g]	ZDV ± LMV
Other body fluid (e.g., urine)	Not offer[g]	
Mucous Membrane Exposures		
Blood	Offer[h]	ZDV plus LMV, ± IND
Fluid containing visible blood, other potentially infectious fluid[e], or tissue	Offer[h]	ZDV ± LMV
Other body fluid (e.g., urine)	Not offer[h]	

[a]Any exposure to concentrated HIV (e.g., in a research laboratory or production facility) is treated as percutaneous exposure to blood with highest risk.
[b]Recommend: Postexposure prophylaxis (PEP) should be recommended to the exposed worker with counseling. Offer: PEP should be offered to the exposed worker with counseling. Not offer: PEP should not be offered because these are not occupational exposures to HIV.
[c]Regimens: zidovudine (ZDV) 200 mg TID; lamivudine (LMV) 150 mg BID; indinavir (IND) 800 mg TID (If IND is not available, saquinavir may be used 600 mg TID); prophylaxis is given for 4 weeks. For full prescribing information, see package inserts.
[d]Risk definitions for percutaneous blood exposure: Highest risk: Larger volume of blood (e.g., deep injury with large diameter hollow needle previously in source patient's vein or artery, especially involving an injection of source-patient's blood) AND blood containing high titer of HIV (e.g., source with acute retroviral illness or end-stage AIDS; viral load measurement may be considered, but its use in relation to PEP has not been evaluated). Increased risk: EITHER exposure to larger volume of blood OR blood with high titer of HIV. No increased risk: NEITHER exposure to larger volume of blood NOR blood with high titer of HIV (e.g., solid suture needle injury from source patient with asymptomatic HIV infection. Possible toxicity associated with additional drug(s) may not be warranted.
[e]Includes semen; vaginal excretions; cerebrospinal, synovial, pleural, peritoneal, pericardial, and amniotic fluids.
[f]For skin, risk is increased for exposures involving high titer of HIV, prolonged cutaneous contact with infectious material, contact with an extensive area of skin or contact with an area in which skin integrity is visibly compromised. For skin exposures without increased risk, the risk of drug toxicity may outweigh the benefit of PEP.
[g]Offer: PEP should be offered to the exposed worker with counseling. Not offer: PEP should not be offered because these are not occupational exposures to HIV.
[h]Recommend: PEP should be recommended to the exposed worker with counseling. Offer: PEP should be offered to the exposed worker with counseling. Not offer: PEP should not be offered as these are not occupational exposures to HIV.
(Modified from Centers for Disease Control and Prevention. Update: Provisional Public Health Service recommendations and chemoprophylaxis after occupational exposure to HIV. MMWR 1996;45:468–480.)

transmission in the opposite direction; that is, the various components of the risk determination will include an assessment of the prevalence of HIV infections among health care workers, the procedure contemplated, the risk of exposure associated with that procedure, the types of devices used in that procedure, the technical expertise of the provider, and the extent to which the provider follows appropriate infection-control policies and procedures. Irrespective of the risk-assessment model used, such a calculation will yield an extremely low risk estimate. From a practical perspective, most of this information is not available to the individual patient. For this reason, management strategies have often relied on the worst possible situations.

To date, only two providers have been implicated in transmitting HIV infection to patients: a dentist in Florida (14–18) and an orthopedic surgeon in France (20, 21). The events resulting in transmission of HIV infection in both practices are obscure; nonetheless, both case clusters violate many of the principles laid out in the risk-assessment model described previously. Only half the patients in the dentist's practice have had HIV serologic examinations, and 0.6% (6 of the approximately 1000 who had serologic studies) were found to be infected with a strain of HIV that is genetically almost identical to that of the dentist (16, 18). Similarly, although the details of the case cluster in France are not available, the attack rate is much higher than would be predicted by the risk-assessment model. Precisely what transpired in these two instances to result in this higher rate of iatrogenic transmission of HIV than would be predicted is likely to be impossible to determine with precision. Both case clusters are consistent with what has been observed in clusters of provider-to-patient transmission of HBV (17, 121).

Although several plausible explanations for the high rate of transmission in these practices have been proffered, none will likely ever be established as definitive because of the current inadequacy of information about the epidemiology of occupational infection and because substantial pieces of important data for each cluster are not available for analysis. Nonetheless, one iatrogenic HIV infection, let alone five in the same practice, would be enough to galvanize the anxieties of a populace.

Another approach to estimating patients' risk of HIV infection from infected health care providers has been to conduct so-called "look-back" or retrospective studies of the patients of practitioners who are identified as infected (122–127). To date, thousands of patients have been evaluated, at substantial cost to the investigators and the public (127), without additional instances of iatrogenic infection being identified; these results must not be considered unlikely given the published risk estimates for provider-to-patient transmission.

Public policy simply cannot be driven by unique numerators without considering the relevant denominators. Although public health authorities must make every effort to investigate, and ultimately explain, such case clusters when they occur, sentient policy must be grounded firmly in science. Problems arise when the scientific data seem to conflict with prevailing public sentiment. Twenty years from now, a retrospective analysis of how our society has managed this risk may be both interesting and instructive. In the interim, we must continue to collect additional data and carefully modify policy whenever the scientific evidence warrants a change in policy. Restricting the practices of health care providers infected with bloodborne pathogens will undoubtedly have substantial impact on the lives of the infected practitioners, on the institutions that employ them, and, perhaps, on the delivery of health care, particularly in areas of the country that have high HIV seroprevalences (22–24). Clearly, implementation of any policy that requires serologic testing of health care workers will be extraordinarily expensive (128, 129).

Determining an acceptable level of societal risk for provider-to-patient transmission of HIV seems sensible on first evaluation; however, for this infectious disease (at least in the current societal climate), such a determination may be difficult at best. For various scientific and "nonscience" reasons (22), our society has been, and will likely (at least for the short run) continue to be, reluctant to tolerate any level of risk of provider-to-patient HIV transmission. The lack of societal perspective on this issue is perhaps the most substantive obstacle to the construction of science-based guidelines for the management of HIV-infected health care workers. Although some professional organizations (130, 131), as well as individuals working in the field (24, 70, 130, 132, 133), have published position papers advocating less restrictive postures, the CDC's July, 1991 recommendations (19), although widely ignored, remain the "law of the land."

References

1. Anonymous. Needlestick transmission of HTLV-III from a patient infected in Africa. Lancet 1984;2:1376–1377.
2. Centers for Disease Control. Acquired immune deficiency syndrome: precautions for clinical and laboratory staffs. MMWR Morb Mortal Wkly Rep 1982;31:577–580.
3. Centers for Disease Control. Acquired immunodeficiency syndrome (AIDS): precautions for health-care workers and allied professionals. MMWR Morb Mortal Wkly Rep 1983;32:450–451.
4. Centers for Disease Control. Recommendations for preventing possible transmission of human T-lymphotropic virus type III/lymphadenopathy-associated virus from tears. MMWR Morb Mortal Wkly Rep 1985;34:533–534.
5. Centers for Disease Control. Update: human immunodeficiency virus infections in health-care workers exposed to blood of infected patients. MMWR Morb Mortal Wkly Rep 1987;36:285–289.
6. Centers for Disease Control. Recommendations for preventing transmission of infection with human T-lymphotropic virus type III/lymphadenopathy-associated virus during invasive procedures. MMWR Morb Mortal Wkly Rep 1986;35:221–223.
7. Centers for Disease Control. Recommendations for prevention of HIV transmission in health-care settings. MMWR Morb Mortal Wkly Rep 1987;36(Suppl 2S):1S–19S.
8. Centers for Disease Control. Agent summary statement for human immunodeficiency viruses (HIVs), including HTLV-III, LAV, HIV-1, and HIV-2. MMWR Morb Mortal Wkly Rep 1988;37 Suppl 4:1–17.
9. Centers for Disease Control. Update: universal precautions for prevention of transmission of human immunodeficiency virus, hepatitis B virus, and other bloodborne pathogens in health-care settings. MMWR Morb Mortal Wkly Rep 1988;37:377–382, 387–388.

10. Conte JE Jr, Hadley WK, Sande M. Infection-control guidelines for patients with the acquired immunodeficiency syndrome. N Engl J Med 1983;309:740–744.
11. Lynch P, Jackson MM, Cummings MJ, et al. Rethinking the role of isolation practices in the prevention of nosocomial infection. Ann Intern Med 1986;107:243–246.
12. Department of Labor, Department of Health and Human Services. Joint advisory notice: protection against occupational exposure to hepatitis B virus (HBV) and human immunodeficiency virus (HIV). Fed Register 1987;52:41,818–41,824.
13. Department of Labor OSHA. Occupational exposure to bloodborne pathogens: final rule. Fed Register 1991;56:64,175–64,182.
14. Ou CY, Ciesielski CA, Myers G, et al. Molecular epidemiology of HIV transmission in a dental practice. Science 1992;256:1165–1171.
15. Centers for Disease Control. Possible transmission of human immunodeficiency virus to a patient during an invasive dental procedure. MMWR Morb Mortal Wkly Rep 1990;39:489–493.
16. Centers for Disease Control. Update: transmission of HIV infection during an invasive dental procedure—Florida. MMWR Morb Mortal Wkly Rep 1991;40:21–33.
17. Mishu B, Schaffner W. HIV-Infected surgeons and dentists: looking back and looking forward. JAMA 1993;269:1843–1844.
18. Ciesielski C, Marianos D, Ou C-Y, et al. Transmission of human immunodeficiency virus in a dental practice. Ann Intern Med 1992; 116:798–805.
19. Centers for Disease Control. Recommendations for preventing transmission of human immunodeficiency virus and hepatitis B virus to patients during exposure-prone invasive procedures. MMWR Morb Mortal Wkly Rep 1991;40:1–9.
20. National Public Health Network of France (Réseau National de Santé Publique). HIV transmission from an orthopedic surgeon to a patient. Press release, 1997.
21. Lot FL, National Public Health Network of France (Réseau National de Santé Publique). HIV transmission from an orthopedic surgeon to a patient in France. In: 7th annual meeting of the Society for Health Care Epidemiology of America, St Louis. Thorofare, NJ: Slack, 1997:7.
22. Henderson DK. The HIV- or HBV-infected health care provider and society's perception of risk: science, nonscience, and nonsense. Ann Allergy 1992;68:197–199.
23. Henderson DK. Human immunodeficiency virus infection in patients and providers. In: Wenzel R, ed. Prevention and control of nosocomial infections. 2nd ed. Baltimore: Williams & Wilkins; 1992:42–57.
24. Henderson DK. Management of health-care workers who are infected with the human immunodeficiency virus or other bloodborne pathogens. In: DeVita V, Hellman S, Rosenberg S, eds. AIDS: etiology, diagnosis, treatment, and prevention. 3rd ed. Philadelphia: JB Lippincott, 1993.
25. Centers for Disease Control and Prevention. US HIV and AIDS cases reported through December 1996. HIV/AIDS Surveill Rep 1996;8:21.
26. Beekmann SE, Fahey BJ, Gerberding JL, et al. Risky business: using necessarily imprecise casualty counts to estimate occupational risks for HIV-1 infection. Infect Control Hosp Epidemiol 1990;11:371–379.
27. Henderson DK. Human immunodeficiency virus in the health-care setting. In: Mandell G, Dolin R, Bennett J, eds. Principles and practice of infectious diseases. 4th ed. New York: Churchill Livingstone, 1995:2632–2656.
28. Centers for Disease Control and Prevention. Case-control study of HIV seroconversion in health-care workers after percutaneous exposure to HIV-infected blood: France, United Kingdom, and United States, January 1988–August 1994. MMWR Morb Mortal Wkly Rep 1995;44:929–933.
29. Centers for Disease Control and Prevention. Health-care workers with documented and possible occupationally acquired AIDS/HIV infection, by occupation, reported through September 1993, United States. HIV/AIDS Surveill Rep 1993;5:13.
30. Chamberland ME, Conley LJ, Bush TJ, et al. Health care workers with AIDS: national surveillance update. JAMA 1991;266:3459–3462.
31. Hamory BH. Underreporting of needlestick injuries in a university hospital. Am J Infect Control 1983;11:174–177.
32. Heald AE, Ransohoff DF. Needlestick injuries among resident physicians. J Gen Intern Med 1990;5:389–393.
33. Mangione CM, Gerberding JL, Cummings SR. Occupational exposure to HIV: frequency and rates of underreporting of percutaneous and mucocutaneous exposures by medical housestaff. Am J Med 1991;90:85–90.
34. Bell DM, Shapiro CN, Holmberg SD. Occupational exposure to HIV: frequency and rates of underreporting of percutaneous and mucocutaneous exposures by medical housestaff. Am J Med 1991;90:85–90.
35. Henry K, Campbell S. Needlestick/sharps injuries and HIV exposure among health care workers: national estimates based on a survey of US hospitals. Minn Med 1995;78:41–44.
36. MacDonald MA, Elford J, Kaldor JM. Reporting of occupational exposures to blood-borne pathogens in Australian teaching hospitals. Med J Aust 1995;163:121–123.
37. Campbell S, Cardo D. Reporting of needlestick injuries among health care workers. In: 7th annual meeting of the Society for Health Care Epidemiology of America, St Louis. Thorofare, NJ: Slack, 1997:21.
38. Centers for Disease Control. Pneumocystis pneumonia. MMWR Morb Mortal Wkly Rep 1981;30:250–252.
39. Henderson DK. HIV transmission in the health care environment. In: Broder S, Merigan TC, Bolognesi D, eds. Textbook of AIDS Medicine. Baltimore: Williams & Wilkins, 1994:831–839.
40. Clerici M, Levin JM, Kessler HA, et al. HIV-specific T-helper activity in seronegative health care workers exposed to contaminated blood. JAMA 1994;271:42–46.
41. Pinto LA, Sullivan J, Berzofsky JA, et al. ENV-specific cytotoxic T lymphocyte responses in HIV seronegative health care workers occupationally exposed to HIV-contaminated body fluids. J Clin Invest 1995;96:867–876.
42. Ward JW, Deppe DA, Samson S, et al. Human immunodeficiency virus infection from blood donors who later developed the acquired immunodeficiency syndrome. Ann Intern Med 1987;106:61–62.
43. McCray E, Cooperative Needlestick Surveillance Group. Occupational risk of the acquired immunodeficiency syndrome among health care workers. N Engl J Med 1986;314:1127–1132.
44. Henderson DK, Saah AJ, Zak BJ, et al. Risk of nosocomial infection with human T-cell lymphotropic virus type III/lymphadenopathy-associated virus in a large cohort of intensively exposed health care workers. Ann Intern Med 1986;104:644–647.
45. Gerberding JL, Bryant-LeBlanc C, Nelson K, et al. Risk of transmitting the human immunodeficiency virus, cytomegalovirus, and hepatitis B virus to health care workers exposed to patients with AIDS and AIDS-related conditions. J Infect Dis 1987;156:1–8.
46. Kuhls TL, Viker S, Parris NB, et al. Occupational risk of HIV, HBV, and HSV-2 infections in health care personnel caring for AIDS patients. Am J Public Health 1987;77:1306–1309.
47. McEvoy M, Porter K, Mortimer P, et al. Prospective study of clinical, laboratory, and ancillary staff with accidental exposures to blood or body fluids from patients infected with HIV. BMJ 1987;294:1595–1597.
48. Elmslie K, O'Shaughnessy JV. National surveillance program on occupational exposure to HIV among health-care workers in Canada. Can Dis Wkly Rep 1987;13:163–166.
49. Elmslie K, Mulligan L, O'Shaughnessy M. National surveillance program: occupational exposure to human immunodeficiency virus infection in Canada [abstract Th.A.P. 46]. In: 5th International Conference on AIDS, Montreal, 1989.
50. Ramsey KM, Smith EN, Reinarz JA. Prospective evaluation of 44 health care workers exposed to human immunodeficiency virus-1, with one seroconversion [abstract]. Clin Res 1988;36:22A.
51. Wormser GP, Joline C, Sivak S, et al. Human immunodeficiency virus infections: considerations for health care workers. Bull N Y Acad Med 1988;64:203–215.

52. Marcus R, Cooperative Needlestick Surveillance Group. CDC's health-care workers surveillance project: an update [abstract 9015]. In: 4th International Conference on AIDS, Stockholm, 1988.
53. Marcus R, Cooperative Needlestick Surveillance Group. Surveillance of health care workers exposed to blood from patients infected with the human immunodeficiency virus. N Engl J Med 1988;319:1118–1123.
54. Pizzocolo R, Stellini R, Cadeo GP, et al. Risk of HIV and HBV infection after accidental needlestick [abstract 9012]. In: 4th International Conference on AIDS, Stockholm, 1988.
55. Hernandez E, Gatell JM, Puyuelo T, et al. Risk of transmitting the HIV to health care workers (HCW) exposed to HIV infected body fluids [abstract 9003]. In: 4th International Conference on AIDS, Stockholm, 1988.
56. Henderson DK. Postexposure prophylaxis for occupational exposures to hepatitis B, hepatitis C, and human immunodeficiency virus. Surg Clin North Am 1995;75:1175–1187.
57. Henderson DK. Risks for exposures to and infection with HIV among health care providers in the emergency department. Emerg Med Clin North Am 1995;13:199–211.
58. Rastrelli M, Ferrazzi D, Vigo B, et al. Risk of HIV transmission to health care workers and comparison with the viral hepatitidies [abstract A 503]. In: 5th International Conference on AIDS, Montreal, 1989.
59. Jorbeck H, Marland M, Steinkeller E. Accidental exposures to HIV-positive blood among health-care workers in 2 Swedish hospitals [abstract A 517]. In: 5th International Conference on AIDS, Montreal, 1989.
60. Francavilla E, Cadrobbi P, Scaggiante R, et al. Surveillance on occupational exposure to HIV among health-care workers in Italy [abstract]. In: 5th International Conference on AIDS, Montreal, 1989:795.
61. Ippolito G, Cadrobbi P, Carosi G, et al. Risk of HIV transmission among health care workers: a multicentre study. The Italian Collaborative Study Group on HIV Occupational Risk. Scand J Infect Dis 1990;22:245–246.
62. Ippolito G. HIV infection in health care workers: the European experience. Physicians Assoc AIDS Care Notes 1990;2:273–275, 307.
63. Ippolito G, Puro P, De Carli G, et al. The risk of occupational human immunodeficiency virus infection in health care workers: Italian Multicenter Study. Arch Intern Med 1993;153:1451–1458.
64. Ippolito G, Puro V, De Carli G, et al. Rates of HIV seroconversion by type of exposure: an update of the Italian multicentre study [abstract PO-C18-3021]. In: 9th International Conference on AIDS, Berlin, 1993.
65. Bell DM. Health care worker–to-patient and patient-to-patient transmission of bloodborne infections. In: 5th annual meeting of the Society of Health Care Epidemiology, San Diego. Thorofare, NJ: Slack, 1995:6.
66. Chamberland ME, Ciesielski CA, Howard RJ, et al. Occupational risk of infection with human immunodeficiency virus. Surg Clin North Am 1995;75:1057–1070.
67. Bell DM. Human immunodeficiency virus infection and needle stick injuries. Pediatr Infect Dis J 1996;15:277–278.
68. Deschamps L, Archibald C. National Surveillance of Occupational Exposure to the Human Immunodeficiency Virus. Can Commun Dis Rep 1996;22:52–54.
69. Resnic FS, Noerdlinger MA. Occupational exposure among medical students and house staff at a New York City medical center. Arch Intern Med 1995;155:75–80.
70. Weiss SH. Risks and issues for the health care worker in the human immunodeficiency virus era. Med Clin North Am 1997;81:555–575.
71. Koziol DE, Henderson DK. Nosocomial viral hepatitis in health-care workers. In: Mayhall C, ed. Hospital epidemiology and infection control. Baltimore: Williams & Wilkins; 1994.
72. Centers for Disease Control. Protection against viral hepatitis: recommendations of the Immunization Practices Advisory Committee (ACIP). MMWR Morb Mortal Wkly Rep 1990;39:1–26.
73. Garner JS. Guideline for isolation precautions in hospitals: the Hospital Infection Control Practices Advisory Committee. Infect Control Hosp Epidemiol 1996;17:53–80.
74. Wong ES, Stotka JL, Mayhall CG, et al. Cost-efficacy of hospital infection control before and after the implementation of universal precautions [abstract 786]. In: 29th Interscience Conference on Antimicrobial Agents and Chemotherapy, Houston, TX. Washington, DC: American Society for Microbiology, 1989:233.
75. Doebbeling BN, Wenzel RP. The direct costs of universal precautions in a teaching hospital. JAMA 1990;264:2083–2087.
76. Stock SR, Gafni A, Bloch RF. Universal precautions to prevent HIV transmission to health care workers: an economic analysis. Can Med Assoc J 1990;142:937–946.
77. Fahey BJ, Koziol DE, Banks SM, et al. Frequency of nonparenteral occupational exposures to blood and body fluids before and after universal precautions training. Am J Med 1991;90:145–153.
78. Wong ES, Stotka JL, Chinchilli VM, et al. Are universal precautions effective in reducing the number of occupational exposures among health care workers? A prospective study of physicians on a medical service. JAMA 1991;265:1123–1128.
79. Beekmann SE, Vlahov D, Koziol DE, et al. Temporal association between implementation of universal precautions and a sustained, progressive decrease in percutaneous exposures to blood. Clin Infect Dis 1994;18:562–569.
80. Haiduven DJ, DeMaio TM, Stevens DA. A five-year study of needlestick injuries: significant reduction associated with communication, education, and convenient placement of sharps containers. Infect Control Hosp Epidemiol 1992;13:265–271.
81. Woolwine J, Mast S, Gerberding JL. Factors influencing needlestick infectivity and decontamination efficacy: an ex vivo model [abstract 1188]. In: 32nd Interscience Conference on Antimicrobial Agents and Chemotherapy, Anaheim, CA. Washington, DC: American Society for Microbiology, 1992.
82. Mast S, Gerberding JL. Factors predicting infectivity following needlestick exposure to HIV: an in vitro model. Clin Res 1991;39:58A.
83. Mast S, Woolwine J, Gerberding JL. Efficacy of gloves in reducing blood volumes transferred during simulated needlestick injury. J Infect Dis 1993;168:1589–1592.
84. Jagger J, Hunt EH, Brand-Elnaggar J, et al. Rates of needle-stick injury caused by various devices in a university hospital. N Engl J Med 1988;319:284–288.
85. Jagger J, Hunt EH, Pearson RD. Sharp object injuries in the hospital: causes and strategies for prevention. Am J Infect Control 1990;18:227–231.
86. Jagger J, Pearson RD. Universal precautions: still missing the point on needlesticks. Infect Control Hosp Epidemiol 1991;12:211–213.
87. Jagger J, Hunt EH, Pearson RD. Estimated cost of needlestick injuries for six major needled devices. Infect Control Hosp Epidemiol 1990;11:584–588.
88. Fahey B, Taylor J, Gatt D, et al. Decrease in percutaneous injuries in temporal association with percutaneous-injury-reducing strategies. In: 7th annual meeting of the Society for Health Care Epidemiology of America, St Louis. Thorofare, NJ: Slack; 1997:42.
89. Gerberding JL, Littell C, Tarkington A, et al. Risk of exposure of surgical personnel to patients' blood during surgery at San Francisco General Hospital. N Engl J Med 1990;322:1788–1793.
90. Henderson DK, Gerberding JL. Prophylactic zidovudine after occupational exposure to the human immunodeficiency virus: an interim analysis. J Infect Dis 1989;160:321–327.
91. Henderson DK, Beekmann SE, Gerberding JL. Post-exposure antiviral chemoprophylaxis following occupational exposure to the human immunodeficiency virus. AIDS Updates 1990;3:1–8.
92. Henderson DK. Zeroing in on the appropriate management of occupational exposures to HIV-1. Infect Control Hosp Epidemiol 1990;11:175–177.
93. Henderson DK. Post-exposure chemoprophylaxis for occupational exposure to HIV-1: current status and prospects for the future. Am J Med 1991;91(Suppl 3B):312S–319S.

94. Henderson DK. Prophylaxis for bloodborne infections. In: 31st annual meeting of the Infectious Diseases Society of America, New Orleans, LA, 1993:9.
95. Gerberding JL. Prophylaxis for occupational exposure to HIV. Ann Intern Med 1996;125:497–501.
96. Gerberding JL. Management of occupational exposures to bloodborne viruses. N Engl J Med 1995;332:444–451.
97. Gerberding JL. Prevention of human immunodeficiency virus infection among hospital personnel. Curr Clin Top Infect Dis 1994;14:220–227.
98. Gerberding JL. Is antiretroviral treatment after percutaneous HIV exposure justified? Ann Intern Med 1993;118:979–980.
99. Gerberding JL, Henderson DK. Management of occupational exposures to bloodborne pathogens: hepatitis B virus, hepatitis C virus, and human immunodeficiency virus. Clin Infect Dis 1992;14:1179–1185.
100. Robinson EN Jr. Arguments against the chemoprophylactic use of zidovudine following occupational exposure to the human immunodeficiency virus. Clin Infect Dis 1993;16:357–360.
101. Para MF. Use of zidovudine following occupational exposure to human immunodeficiency virus. Clin Infect Dis 1992;15:884–885.
102. Schmitz SH, Scheding S, Voliotis D, et al. Side effects of AZT prophylaxis after occupational exposure to HIV-infected blood. Ann Hematol 1994;69:135–138.
103. Ruprecht RM, Bronson R. Chemoprevention of retroviral infection: success is determined by virus inoculum strength and cellular immunity. DNA Cell Biol 1994;13:59–66.
104. Beekmann SE, Fahrner R, Koziol DE, et al. Safety of zidovudine (AZT) administered as postexposure chemoprophylaxis to health care workers (HCW) sustaining occupational exposures (OE) to HIV [abstract 1121]. In: 33rd Interscience Conference on Antimicrobial Agents and Chemotherapy, New Orleans, LA. Washington, DC: American Society for Microbiology, 1993.
105. Centers for Disease Control and Prevention. Update: provisional Public Health Service recommendations for chemoprophylaxis after occupational exposure to HIV. MMWR Morb Mortal Wkly Rep. 1996;45:468–480.
106. Malcolm JA, Dobson PM, Sutherland DC. Combination chemoprophylaxis after needlestick injury. Lancet 1993;341:112–113.
107. Van Rompay KK, Marthas ML, Ramos RA, et al. Simian immunodeficiency virus (SIV) infection of infant rhesus macaques as a model to test antiretroviral drug prophylaxis and therapy: oral 3'-azido-3'-deoxythymidine prevents SIV infection. Antimicrob Agents Chemother 1992;36:2381–2386.
108. Connor E, Sperling R, Gelber R, et al. Reduction of maternal–infant transmission of human immunodeficiency virus type 1 with zidovudine treatment. N Engl J Med 1994;331:1173–1180.
109. Gerberding JL, Marx P, Gould R, et al. Simian model of retrovirus chemoprophylaxis with constant infusion zidovudine plus or minus interferon alpha [abstract]. In: 31st Interscience Conference on Antimicrobial Agents and Chemotherapy. Washington, DC: American Society for Microbiology, 1991.
110. Martin LN, Murphey CM, Soike KF, et al. Effects of initiation of 3'-azido,3'-deoxythymidine (zidovudine) treatment at different times after infection of rhesus monkeys with simian immunodeficiency virus. J Infect Dis 1993;168:825–835.
111. McClure HM, Anderson DC, Fultz P, et al. Prophylactic effects of AZT following exposure of macaques to an acutely lethal variant of SIV (SIV/SMM/PBj-14) [abstract]. In: 5th International Conference on AIDS, Montreal, 1989.
112. McCune JM, Namikawa R, Shih CC, et al. Suppression of HIV infection in AZT-treated SCID-hu mice. Science 1990;247:564–566.
113. Ruprecht RM, O'Brien LG, Rossoni LD, et al. Suppression of mouse viraemia and retroviral disease by 3'-azido-3'deoxythymidine. Nature 1986;323:467–469.
114. Tavares L, Roneker C, Johnston K, et al. 3'-Azido-3'deoxythymidine in feline leukemia virus-infected cats: a model for therapy and prophylaxis of AIDS. Cancer Res 1987;47:3190–3194.
115. Tsai CC, Follis KE, Sabo A, et al. Prevention of SIV infection in macaques by (R)-9-(2-phosphonylmethoxypropyl)adenine. Science 1995;270:1197–1199.
116. Tsai C-C, Follis KE, Sabo A, et al. Preexposure prophylaxis with 9-(2-phosphonylmethoxyethyl)adenine against simian immunodeficiency virus infection in macaques. J Infect Dis 1994;169:260–266.
117. Bell DM, Shapiro CN, Culver DH, et al. Risk of hepatitis B and human immunodeficiency virus transmission to a patient from an infected surgeon due to percutaneous injury during an invasive procedure: estimates based on a model. Infect Agents Dis 1992;1:263–269.
118. Gostin L. HIV-infected physicians and the practice of seriously invasive procedures. Hastings Cent Rep 1989;19:32–39.
119. Lowenfels AB, Wormser G. Risk of transmission of HIV from surgeon to patient. N Engl J Med 1991;325:888–889.
120. Rhame FS. The HIV-infected surgeon. JAMA 1990;264:507–508.
121. Schaffner W. Surgeons with HIV infection: the risk to patients. J Hosp Infect 1991;18(Suppl A):191–196.
122. Mishu B, Schaffner W, Horan JM, et al. A surgeon with AIDS: lack of evidence of transmission to patients. JAMA 1990;264:467–470.
123. Porter JD, Cruickshank JG, Gentle PH, et al. Management of patients treated by surgeon with HIV infection. Lancet 1990;335:113–114.
124. Sacks JJ. More on AIDS in a surgeon. N Engl J Med 1986;314:1190.
125. Sacks JJ. AIDS in a surgeon. N Engl J Med 1985;313:1017–1018.
126. Armstrong FP, Miner JC, Wolfe WH. Investigation of a health care worker with symptomatic human immunodeficiency virus infection: an epidemiological approach. Milit Med 1987;152:414–418.
127. Danila RN, MacDonald KL, Rhame FS, et al. A look-back investigation of patients of an HIV-infected physician. N Engl J Med 1991;325:1406–1411.
128. Gerberding JL. Expected costs of implementing a mandatory human immunodeficiency virus and hepatitis B virus testing and restriction program for health-care workers performing invasive procedures. Infect Control Hosp Epidemiol 1991;12:443–447.
129. Russo G, LaCroix S. A second look at the cost of mandatory human immunodeficiency virus and hepatitis B virus testing for health-care workers performing invasive procedures. Infect Control Hosp Epidemiol 1992;13:107–110.
130. Henderson DK, AIDS/Tuberculosis Subcommittee of the Society for Healthcare Epidemiology of America. Position paper (revised): management of health care workers who are infected with HBV, HCV, HIV, and other bloodborne pathogens. Infect Control Hosp Epidemiol 1997;18:349–363.
131. Rhame FS, Pitt H, Tapper ML, et al. Position paper: The HIV-infected health care worker. Infect Control Hosp Epidemiol 1990;11:647–656.
132. Hansen ME, McIntire DD. HIV transmission during invasive radiologic procedures: estimate based on computer modeling. AJR Am J Roentgenol 1996;166:263–267.
133. Rhodes RS. Human immunodeficiency virus transmission and surgeons: update. South Med J 1995;88:251–255.

54

MANAGING OCCUPATIONAL EXPOSURES TO HIV

Julie Louise Gerberding

Occupational exposure to the human immunodeficiency virus (HIV) among health care personnel is not a rare event. More than 50,000 occupational exposures to HIV are believed to have occurred in the United States since the epidemic of acquired immune deficiency syndrome (AIDS) was recognized (1). Although the statistical probability of acquiring infection by this mode of transmission is lower than that associated with many bloodborne infections, the subjective impact on exposed persons is significant. Moreover, at least 150 health care providers have become infected with HIV on the job (1, 2).

Preventing occupational exposure to HIV is a challenge faced in virtually every medical setting and is now also an issue in many other work environments. However, even with scrupulous attention to infection-control practices and implementation of the best current safety devices, health care providers remain at some risk of exposure to HIV. Developing sensible strategies to manage exposed persons is therefore an important priority. Postexposure care must encompass three main goals: 1) to prevent, to the extent possible, HIV infection among those sustaining exposure; 2) to provide information and support during the follow-up interval until infection is diagnosed or excluded with certainty; and 3) to document the relation of occupational exposure to infection adequately among the unfortunate few who do become infected, to implement appropriate antiviral treatment, and to minimize the potential for transmission to their contacts.

POSTOPERATIVE INTERVENTIONS TO DECREASE INFECTION RISK

Immediate postexposure care should emphasize the importance of decontaminating the exposure site as soon as patient safety permits (3, 4). When the exposure involves a needle puncture or similar cutaneous injury, the wound should be washed with soap and water. If the injury is severe enough to warrant suturing, care should be taken to irrigate the site thoroughly before closure. Excision or incision of the exposure site is not recommended. Although use of antiseptics is not contraindicated, no data suggest that their application affects the probability of HIV transmission, and decontamination should not be delayed to obtain these compounds. Most exposed persons attempt to induce bleeding from the wound in the hope that this will enhance decontamination, but again, this approach is of no proven benefit and need not be encouraged.

Exposed mucous membranes of the mouth and nose should be flushed with clean water. Ocular tissue should be irrigated with sterile saline, with eye washes formulated for this purpose, or with clean water. Bite wounds should also be cleaned with soap and water. Antibiotic prophylaxis may be indicated, especially if the bite involves the hand or other tissue vulnerable to bacterial infection.

In 1997, the United States Public Health Service (USPHS) promulgated new guidelines that recommend antiretroviral treatment to prevent infection after occupational exposures to HIV (5). As a consequence, access to postexposure prophylaxis is now a standard of care for occupational exposures that impose a significant risk of HIV transmission. The guidelines were based on data from various sources that strongly suggest that postexposure antiviral treatment may be an efficacious prophylactic strategy.

The pathogenesis of mucosal retroviral infection has been studied in a simian model of transvaginal infection (6). In this model, simian immunodeficiency virus (SIV) remains localized to the antigen-presenting cells in the lamina propria for the first 24 hours after inoculation of the vaginal surface, and little if any local virus replication is apparent. By 24 to 48 hours, SIV appears in the germinal centers of iliac lymph nodes, and active replication is evident. SIV dissemination through the peripheral blood is first detectable within 5 days after inoculation, in both cell-free and cell-associated forms. This model strengthens the hypothesis of a "window of opportunity" after exposure in which antiviral treatment may act to prevent or at least attenuate replication and may allow the host defense system to clear the initial inoculum. The generalizability of this model to transcutaneous HIV exposure has not been established. However, data suggest that dermal dendritic cells, Langerhans' cells, or similar antigen-presenting cells may serve as the initial target cells in the skin, and a similar mechanism of infection is biologically plausible

(7). To date, the effect of antiviral treatment on the histopathogenesis and outcome of SIV infection has not been studied in this simian model.

Newer primate studies postexposure prophylaxis have demonstrated that some antiretroviral drugs can completely prevent infection even when administered after intravenous inoculation (8, 9). Together, these studies suggest that several factors are relevant to the exposure outcome: 1) the titer of virus used for inoculation; 2) the length of the delay before treatment is initiated; 3) the duration of treatment; and 4) the specific antiviral regimen studied. It is premature to extrapolate directly from these models to occupational exposure treatment guidelines, but they do provide additional evidence that immediate antiviral treatment after low-inocula occupational exposures is likely to be efficacious.

Treatment with zidovudine of infected women in the second and third trimesters of pregnancy and of their neonates reduced the risk of perinatal infection by 67% in a randomized placebo-controlled clinical trial (10). The treatment effect was not entirely attributable to a reduction in maternal viral load, and it provides indirect evidence that preexposure or postexposure prophylaxis in the neonate may contribute to the lowered infection risk (11). Ideally, the efficacy of postexposure prophylaxis for preventing occupational infections should be evaluated in a similar controlled clinical trial. However, such a trial is not feasible, given the low frequency of infections after exposure.

The Centers for Disease Control and Prevention (CDC) conducted a retrospective case-control study of risk factors for occupational HIV transmission among health care workers (12). In this study, use of zidovudine after exposure was associated with a 79% reduction in the odds of infection. This effect was independent of exposure characteristics likely to affect transmission risk These data had a major impact on the USPHS decision to create guidelines advocating provision of postexposure drug treatment after risky occupational exposures (5). Taken together, the experiments in animal models, the successful prophylaxis of perinatal infection with zidovudine, and the CDC's case-control study provide strong support for treating workers exposed to HIV with antiretroviral drugs to prevent infection. Nevertheless, proof of efficacy is still lacking, and the decision to treat must consider both the putative benefit as well as the possible risks of exposure to these drugs in otherwise healthy individuals.

Overall, exposure route remains the most important factor predictive of occupational infection. Percutaneous injuries caused by needles or other sharp objects account for more than 95% of occupational infections (1, 2). Transmission through mucous membranes and nonintact skin has occurred, but only in a few cases. The CDC case-control study data have helped to refine the estimate of percutaneous exposure risk and the decision to offer prophylaxis. Deep injuries, visible blood contamination of the implicated sharp object, injury caused by a needle previously inserted into an artery or vein, and preterminal source patient status (defined as a patient who died within 2 months after the exposure) were independent predictors of exposure risk in this study (12). These predictor variables may be surrogates of exposure inoculum (volume, titer), but this concept is not proven. Other determinants of transmission may include the host's immune response, the genotypic or phenotypic characteristics of the HIV strains in the inoculum, and the presence of other viruses in the source patient.

The protection afforded by postexposure prophylaxis is not complete. To date, 11 reports of zidovudine treatment failure among exposed health care workers have been published (13). In all but 1 report, treatment was started within 24 hours of the exposure. The dose of zidovudine used was at least as high as that recommended in the current guidelines, although in some cases treatment was stopped before 28 days because of drug intolerance or the onset of acute seroconversion illness. Zidovudine resistance may have been a factor in some of the treatment failures, because many of the source patients were taking the drug when the occupational exposure occurred. No evidence of delayed seroconversion was seen, but follow-up is not sufficient to determine whether treatment had any effect on the natural history of HIV infection in these patients.

Choosing a prophylactic drug regimen is now complicated by the increased prevalence of antiviral treatment among source patients and the emergence of drug resistance (14–17). The combination of zidovudine and lamivudine is currently recommended for initial treatment after most exposures warranting prophylaxis (5). This decision is based on several relevant facts: 1) zidovudine is the only antiretroviral drug with clinical evidence of prophylactic benefit; 2) primary infection with zidovudine-resistant virus has been demonstrated; 3) the combination of these two drugs may be effective against some strains of zidovudine-resistant HIV; 4) the adverse drug effects associated with lamivudine in combination with zidovudine are the same as those observed with zidovudine alone; and 5) short-term zidovudine treatment is rarely associated with serious objective toxicity (5, 14, 15, 18–20). However, in some circumstances, the source patient harbors circulating strains of HIV that are resistant to both these drugs. This situation is especially likely when the source patient is currently taking this regimen but is nonadherent, fails to respond, or has a high viral load for some other reason. In such cases, alternate drug regimens are usually recommended. The most conservative approach would be to choose an antiviral treatment regimen that includes two drugs the source patient is not currently taking, unless data are available to demonstrate that drug resistance is unlikely (undetectable viral load, laboratory data documenting absence of codon mutations commonly associated with resistance or in vitro susceptibility) (16, 21, 22). In practice, such detailed clinical data are rarely available at the time the exposure is reported and treatment is initiated.

For empiric treatment of exposures occurring when the HIV status of the source patient is not known, when the source patient is not receiving antiviral drugs, when the source patient is known to have a complete response to treatment, or when the source patient is taking other drugs, two-drug therapy with zidovudine and lamivudine is a reasonable choice for prophylaxis of exposed health care workers (5). In other cases, alternate regimens should be considered. One approach is to add a protease inhibitor such as indinavir or nelfinavir to the standard regimen (5, 21, 22). Didanosine and stavudine or stavudine and lamivudine have also been used in some cases. Clinicians who are not familiar with antiretroviral drugs (cross-resistance, toxicity, and drug–drug interactions) are encouraged to seek input from other experts for complicated cases. The National Clinicians' Postexposure Prophylaxis Hotline (PEPLine), at 1-888-HIV-4911, a service funded by the Health Resources and Services Administration and the CDC, also provides free exposure management consultation 24 hours a day, 7 days a week.

Drug toxicity is an important consideration when selecting antiviral drugs. Although data from three large studies indicate that serious objective toxicity is rarely associated with short-term zidovudine prophylaxis among health care workers, long-term follow-up is incomplete (23). No data are yet available to predict the safety of combination regimens (18–20). Subjective drug intolerance is common with zidovudine and most other regimens and may necessitate dose reduction or drug discontinuation. Rarely, symptoms are so severe that treated individuals are unable to work. Symptomatic treatment of common side effects is now encouraged and can improve tolerance and adherence.

Choosing a treatment regimen for pregnant or breast-feeding women exposed to HIV is challenging (23). Although the antiretroviral drugs licensed for HIV are not known to have teratogenic effects in humans, none are classified by the United States Food and Drug Administration as category A (proven to be safe) (24). For serious exposures, zidovudine treatment (with or without lamivudine) is probably safe. Close collaboration with the exposed woman, her obstetrician, and experts in perinatal HIV is important to ensure that the risks and benefits of treatment are clearly articulated and are considered in the decision. All available antiviral drugs for HIV are either proven or suspected to be excreted in breast milk. Women are usually advised to discontinue breast-feeding when HIV prophylaxis is initiated.

In summary, chemoprophylaxis remains a promising but still unproven strategy for preventing occupational infections with HIV. Treatment can be justified only when health care workers are fully informed of the uncertain efficacy and potential toxicities associated with therapy, when monitoring for complications is included in the treatment protocol, and when treatment can be carefully supervised by clinicians with expertise in the use of retrovirus inhibitors (4, 5).

FOLLOW-UP CARE FOR EXPOSED PERSONS

The initial evaluation of a health care worker who is exposed to blood or other potentially infectious material should include an assessment of the exposure's severity and the probability of HIV transmission (3–5). Important aspects of the history include the route of exposure, the volume of material involved, and the timing and adequacy of decontamination. When the exposure involves a needle puncture or similar precutaneous injury, the characteristics associated with increased infection risk in the CDC case-control study (depth, visible blood contamination, use in an artery or vein) should be elicited (12). When the source patient is known to be infected with HIV, the stage of clinical illness, the viral load, and the retroviral treatment history should be ascertained. Viral load can help to predict drug resistance and can aid in selection of the drug regimen. The relationship between viral load (plasma cell-free virus) and transmission risk is not established. Although exposures involving higher viral loads probably would be riskier, the converse is not necessarily true; occupational transmission from a source patient with undetectable viral load has been documented. When the HIV status of the source is not known, a clinical and epidemiologic evaluation should be performed, and unless HIV is deemed unlikely, HIV testing of the source should be encouraged.

A baseline HIV test antibody should be offered to the exposed health care worker when the exposure imparts a risk of HIV transmission (3–5). The baseline test is valuable in excluding prior infection and is necessary to demonstrate that the exposure was temporally related to infection in the few workers who acquire HIV occupationally. Acceptance of HIV testing is enhanced when documentation of test requests and of test results is confidential. Workers who decline baseline testing should be encouraged to have a serum sample stored so testing can be performed later, if needed.

Periodic follow-up antibody testing is recommended at regular intervals (e.g., at 6 weeks, 3 months, and 6 months after exposure) to identify seroconversion (3–5, 25). Although seroconversion after 6 months is possible, it is rare (26). Most experts agree that the adverse psychological consequences of testing beyond the 6-month time point and the low probability of delayed seroconversion contraindicate this practice for most exposures. Supplemental tests, including antigen testing, viral load measurements, and virus cultures, have no role in the routine management of exposed persons. Most persons with documented occupational infection have experienced a febrile illness associated with pharyngitis, lymphadenopathy, fatigue, and other mononucleosis-like symptoms and signs at the time of seroconversion (1, 13). Patients should be advised to report for evaluation if such a syndrome develops. HIV antibody tests may be negative at the onset of seroconversion illness. Testing for HIV p24 or viral load can allow earlier diagnosis of HIV infection and is recommended in this setting. If these special tests are not available, repeating the antibody test in 2 to 4 weeks usually establishes the diagnosis.

Experiencing an occupational exposure to HIV is usually a stressful event for health care providers. Coping styles vary widely and include denial, anger, depression, displacement, anxiety, agitation, and even suicide ideation. Moreover, fears are not readily allayed by provision of statistical information about the "low" risk of infection. Clinicians caring for these patients should evaluate the stress response and should provide access to supportive counseling during the follow-up interval (27, 28). Sometimes, referral to mental health professionals for crisis intervention is needed in the first few weeks after occupational exposure to HIV. Counseling should also include information about sexual practices and other behavior changes to reduce the risk of transmitting HIV to contacts until infection is excluded. It is often helpful to extend counseling services to others, including sexual partners and household members, who may be alarmed about the implications of the exposure event. Coworkers or superiors who learn of the exposure may also require information and support.

Developing an efficient reporting system and providing comprehensive care to the exposed person in a setting in which confidentiality is protected enhance the motivation to report occupational exposures. The reporting process provides an important opportunity to identify causal factors amenable to intervention. Obtaining accurate information from exposed health care providers is critical to this process because these individuals often recognize problems and creative solutions that are not readily apparent to those who are not on the front lines of patient care. A concerted effort should be made to avoid "blaming the victim" during this assessment.

Collated information about reported exposures provides a useful surveillance tool for identifying important aspects of exposure epidemiology and targets for intervention (22). Moreover, the efficacy of prevention strategies can be monitored over time. Ultimately, this approach may lead to improved safety in the health care workplace and reassure the community of health care providers that the benefits of providing care to HIV-infected patients outweigh the risk.

References

1. Bell DM. Occupational risk of human immunodeficiency virus infection in health care workers: an overview. Am J Med 1997;102:9–15.
2. Heptonstall J, Porter KP, Gill ON. Occupational transmission of HIV: summary of published reports to July 1995. London: Public Health Laboratory Service, 1995.
3. Gerberding JL. Management of occupation exposures to blood-borne viruses. N Engl J Med 1995;332:444–451.
4. Gerberding JL. Prophylaxis for occupational exposures to HIV. Ann Intern Med 1996;125:497–501.
5. Centers for Disease Control and Prevention. Update: provisional Public Health Service recommendations for chemoprophylaxis after occupational exposure to HIV. MMWR Morb Mortal Wkly Rep 1998;45:468–472.
6. Spiro Spira AI, Marx PA, Patterson BK, et al. Cellular targets of infection and route of viral dissemination after an intravaginal inoculation of simian immunodeficiency virus into rhesus macaques. J Exp Med 1996;183:215–225.
7. Blauvelt A. The role of dendritic cells in the initiation of human immunodeficiency virus infection. Am J Med 1997;102:16–20.
8. Black RJ. Animal studies of prophylaxis. Am J Med 1997;102:39–44.
9. Tsai CC, Follis KE, Sabo A, et al. Prevention of SIV infection in macaques by (R)-9-(2-phosphonylmethooxypropyl)adenine. Science 1995;270:1197–1199.
10. Connor EM, Sperling RS, Gelber R, et al. Reduction of maternal–infant transmission of human immunodeficiency virus type 1 with zidovudine treatment. N Engl J Med 1994;331:1173–1178.
11. Sperling RS, Shapiro DE, Coombs RW, et al. Maternal viral load, zidovudine teratment, and the risk of human immunodeficiency virus type 1 transmission from mother to infant. N Engl J Med 1996;335:1621–1629.
12. Centers for Disease Control and Prevention. Case-control study of HIV seroconversion in health-care workers after percutaneous exposure to HIV-infected blood: France, United Kingdom, and United States, January 1988–August 1994. MMWR Morb Mortal Wkly Rep 1995;44:929–933.
13. Jochimsen EM. Failures of zidovudine postexposure prophylaxis. Am J Med 1997;102:52–55.
14. Mayers DL. Prevalence and incidence of resistance to zidovudine and other antiretroviral drugs. Am J Med 1997:102:70–75.
15. Richman DD. Resistance of clinical isolates of HIV to antiretroviral agents. Antimicrob Agents Chemother 1993;27:1207–1213.
16. Manion DJ, Hirsch MS. Combination chemotherapy for human immunodeficiency virus type 1. Am J Med 1997;102:76–80.
17. Saag MS. Candidate antiretroviral agents for use in postexposure prophylaxis. Am J Med 1997;102:25–31.
18. Ippolito G, Puro V, Italian Registry of Antiretroviral Prophylaxis. Zidovudine toxicity in uninfected healthcare workers. Am J Med 1997;102:58–62.
19. Tokars JL, Marcus R, Culver DH, et al. Surveillance of HIV infection and zidovudine use among health care workers after occupational exposures to HIV. Ann Intern Med 1993;118:913–919.
20. Beekmann SE, Fahrner R, Henderson DK, et al. Zidovudine safety and tolerance among uninfected health care workers: a brief update. Am J Med 1997;102:63–64.
21. Carpenter CJ, Fischl MA, Hammer S, et al. Antiretroviral therapy for HIV infection in 1996: recommendations of an international panel. JAMA 1996;276:146–154.
22. Gerberding JL. Postexposure prophylaxis for human immunodeficiency virus at San Francisco General Hospital. Am J Med 1997;102:85–89.
23. Struble KA, Pratt RD, Gitterman SR. Toxicity of antiretroviral agents. Am J Med 1997;102:65–67.
24. White A, Andrews E, Eldridge R, et al. Birth outcomes following zidovudine therapy in pregnant women. MMWR Morb Mortal Wkly Rep 1994;43:409,415–416.
25. Ciesielski CA, Metler RP. Duration of time between exposure and seroconversion in healthcare workers with occupationally acquired infection with human immunodeficiency virus. Am J Med 1997;102:115–116.
26. Busch MP, Satten GA. Time course of viremia and antibody seroconversion following human immunodeficiency virus exposure. Am J Med 1997;102:117–124.
27. Dilley JW. Counseling health care workers after accidental exposures. Focus 1990;5:3–4.
28. Tannenbaum J, Anastasoff J. The role of psychosocial assessment and support in occupational exposure management. AIDS Educ Prev 1997;9:275–284.

55
AIDS AND ETHICS: CLINICAL, SOCIAL, AND GLOBAL

John C. Fletcher, Michelle N. Meyer, and Brian Wispelwey

Our chapter has three main sections. The introduction describes the content of each section and identifies the topics discussed in the first and second sections. A transition—on human immunodeficiency virus/acquired immune deficiency syndrome (HIV/AIDS), ethics, and power—leads to the first section. We use HIV/AIDS to encompass issues that arise from a period of vulnerability to HIV infection, to seroconversion, and to the development of the symptoms and sequelae of AIDS.

The first section is about HIV/AIDS and issues in clinical ethics. Specific norms structure the physician–patient relationship in this culture. Whether a patient's medical problems are simple or complex, ethical issues are embedded in every case. For example, each clinical encounter poses issues of confidentiality and privacy, truth telling, informed consent, and determining the capacity of one's patient to participate in decisions. These issues face clinicians (all professionals who interact with the patient, family members, or surrogates such as physicians, nurses, clinical social workers, mental health professionals), adolescent and adult patients, and other decision makers. Moreover, depending on the circumstances, other ethical problems may arise in a case, such as reproductive choices, refusal of treatment, forgoing life-sustaining treatment, requests for assisted suicide or euthanasia, or allocation of scarce resources. A single case may pose several ethical problems that vary in magnitude and complexity. Some ethical problems are preventable by timely planning in the care of patients. Advance directives for end-of-life treatment choices are a good preventive measure, assuming that clinicians respect them. The strengths and weaknesses of these instruments are discussed in the first section. We do not discuss ethical problems in research and treatment of children and young adolescents with HIV/AIDS, because these topics are covered in elsewhere in the literature (1).

HIV/AIDS and clinical ethics, a daunting topic in itself, is followed by a second section about what living with AIDS (2, 3) requires ethically of this and similar societies. This section on social ethics and AIDS addresses regulatory, public policy, and legal issues that have an impact on the clinical situation.

A third section poses hard choices facing world leaders and health policy makers, namely, the ethical considerations of confronting AIDS in the world (4, 5), of conducting HIV/AIDS research with human subjects in developing nations, and of addressing underlying causes that render some nations much more vulnerable to HIV/AIDS than others. HIV/AIDS cases have now been officially reported by 197 countries and territories. HIV infection has been documented in virtually all countries (5). AIDS continues to be a pandemic "relentlessly expanding" (5). An international authority predicts that "if current epidemic trends persist through the end of the century, it is most likely that 60–70 million adults will have been infected with HIV by the end of the year 2000" (5). Forecasts of the total devastation of AIDS in terms of lives that will be lost vary from about 8% (6) to one-quarter (7) of the world population.

HIV/AIDS challenges the discipline of ethics just as severely as it challenges every other discipline. AIDS provokes raw emotions and moralism (8). Those at greatest risk of infection are mostly young, apt to be in turmoil in terms of their own personal and moral development, and AIDS is a lethal disease. AIDS is global, cutting across boundaries of culture, religion, and traditions of morality. The challenge to ethics is for effective tools and resources to meet the individual, social, and global demands to subdue HIV/AIDS within the parameters of clinical, social, and research ethics.

Before moving to the next section and an overview of our ethical perspective for this discussion, the reader is directed to Table 55.1, which identifies and ranks 10 major ethical issues and problems in clinical care and research involving persons with HIV/AIDS. The array of issues and problems shown in Table 55.1 is selective and not complete, as a result of space limitations.

ETHICS, POWER, AND HIV/AIDS

Ethics is concerned with normative questions in the deliberative process that ought to follow the identification of

Table 55.1. HIV/AIDS: Ethical Issues and Problems by Magnitude and Incidence in the Literature

1. Primary prevention and universal access to primary health care[a]
2. Confidentiality and privacy[b]
3. Screening (populations)[a]
4. Obligation to treat persons with HIV infection or AIDS[b]
5. Counseling, testing, and informed consent[b]
6. Counseling HIV-positive women about reproductive choices[b]
7. Notification of partners and at-risk individuals[a]
8. Screening health care workers; their status if HIV positive[a]
9. Drug testing and other research practices[a]
10. Death and dying; forgoing treatment, euthanasia, aiding suicide[b]

[a]Issues of regulation, law, and public policy are discussed in the section of this chapter on social ethics: living with AIDS.
[b]Issues discussed as matters for which clinicians need a reliable approach are addressed in the section of this chapter on HIV/AIDS and clinical ethics.

ethical problems, such as the following: What ought to be done, how, by whom, and why? What causes biomedical ethical problems that confront individuals, groups, and societies? Contrary to popular views, advances in technology are not the primary cause of biomedical ethical problems. Moreover, the unfortunate persons who contract HIV/AIDS are not in themselves an ethical problem, despite a pervasive moralistic tendency to make them so. Rather, such problems are caused by conflicts of widely accepted moral beliefs, ethical principles, and values embedded in the institutions and medical practices of society. Efforts to research, prevent, diagnose, and treat HIV/AIDS are thus merely *occasions* for many dramatic ethical problems, but the causative factors lie deeper.

Ethical problems also threaten valued relationships. In this culture, the physician–patient relationship (9–13) is structured by moral principles of patient-centered beneficence, avoidance of harm, and practices of physician self-regulation aimed to inform and maintain professional integrity and loyalty to patients. Physicians are expected to have character traits that protect patient confidentiality and encourage honesty. Ethical problems in the clinical setting threaten this core relationship as well as others. At such times, the choice of metaphors to understand the physician–patient relationship (14) or AIDS itself (15) has great symbolic power and influence on the action chosen to resolve ethical problems. For example, military metaphors that depict an approach to HIV/AIDS as "war" or the body as a "battlefield" carry high ethical risks of relaxing familiar ethical norms, as is customary in wartime.

Considerations of ethics and forms of power must be mutually informative but not confused one with the other. Brody (12) studied forms of power to illuminate ethical considerations of the physician–patient relationship. In reality, ethical problems always occur in a historical and political context. What ought to be done ethically cannot be answered apart from what can be done practically. Thus, the "ought" depends in part on the "can," but what can be done must not dictate what ought to be done. If it were otherwise, a technologic imperative would totally dominate the relations between science and society. The main point here is that moral agency depends in part on the power and resources to act. Ethical problems are embedded in a matrix of competing social, political, and economic forces. Competition for power, resources, and influence is part of the context for ethics. The actual approaches to ethical problems in any age and culture, including the approaches to HIV/AIDS, cannot be adequately understood apart from issues of power.

In this vein, Bayer's analysis (16–19) of ethical problems in HIV/AIDS in the United States especially succeeds because he takes pains to clarify the social and political matrix of these problems. His work underlines two prominent features of the topic of ethics and AIDS: a high intensity factor and sharp conflict between public health goals and concern for privacy rights of individuals. The bioethics literature that began in the 1960s shows that the ethical problems of HIV infection and AIDS are not new. However, heated debate and political activism indelibly imprinted these problems. Bayer notes: ". . . what is new is the intensity of the discussion, the broad participatory nature of the debate, the political forces called into play, the demands they have made, and the solutions they have sought to fashion" (19).

On the intensity factor, we note the harm done to efforts to cope with HIV/AIDS by conspiracy theories of a "manmade" HIV virus genocidally aimed at blacks or gays by the white power structure. This theory is often linked (20) to the Tuskegee study of untreated syphilis. Jones' peerless history (21) of this experiment now includes a section on its tragic legacy in the age of HIV/AIDS. Wherever possible, the transmission of conspiracy theories must be confronted with the state of knowledge about the origins and history of AIDS (22). Conspiracy theories, born in the bitterness of poverty and discrimination, tear at relationships in settings in which trust is crucial to primary prevention and education.

A second mark of HIV/AIDS ethical issues has been the sharp conflict between societal and individual interests and the claim by those defending individual interests that AIDS is "special." Bayer frames the history of the socioethical debate about HIV/AIDS in terms of competing imperatives between traditional public health goals and methods and guarding the well-being of particular individuals. He depicts the approach shaped in the 1980s to the ethical issues of AIDS as one of "HIV exceptionalism." Bayer (17) defines this position as one that regarded HIV infection as different in kind from other threats to public health. HIV/AIDS is the first epidemic occurring in an era of significant progress in civil rights, gay rights, and heightened concern for the rights of individual patients. The AIDS epidemic and the choices that confronted public health officials and gay men, who were first most severely affected by the epidemic, must be seen against a background of older ethical traditions in public health that justified practices of mandatory screening and reporting, breaching confidentiality, and imposing treatment and quarantine. Bayer notes that in the 1980s, "an alliance of gay leaders, civil libertarians, physicians, and public health officials began to shape a policy for dealing with AIDS that reflected the exceptionalist perspective" (17). He argues that this era is passing, largely because of advances in treatment (16) and other shifts in power, resources, and influence. He also sees other factors for change, such as reduced fears that HIV infection could spread broadly in the population (16), overestimation of the level of infection, and greater influence of black and Hispanic leaders of those affected by HIV/AIDS as compared with the influence of gay spokespersons.

Debate about whether HIV/AIDS is special or deserving of exceptions to traditional ways of fighting epidemics appears destined to continue. Where one stands in the debate depends, in no small part, on one's ethical perspective. We develop this point further in the third section. One can also view the impact of AIDS from either a national or a global perspective. Sharp contrasts emerge from these perspectives. Such a contrast is evident in the tones of a National Research Council report (23) on the social impact of AIDS in the United States and reports on AIDS in the world (4, 5). The Council report assumes that patterns of infection will be contained and mainly will affect the most disadvantaged groups (23) in American society along with a negative impact on public health institutions. The report sees a major danger of the "disappearance" of the majority from concern and action about the epidemic because of the social invisibility of the most severely affected groups. The global report portrays another view, within a perspective of the universal claims of human rights, on the grim policy choices facing nations largely in terms of the devastating global impact of AIDS. On a global scale, the greatest impact of AIDS will be still beyond the year 2000, as stated earlier. More than 31 million persons in the world have been infected with HIV (5), and this number will increase dramatically, especially in Southeast Asia. The tension between the claims of these two views will remain and ought to be balanced in the ways that governments and societies respond to the pandemic.

We also note the steadily rising threat of HIV/AIDS among women and children. The early epidemic largely affected men. The increasing risk and incidence of HIV/AIDS among women in the United States was documented in the late 1980s by a committee of the National Research Council (24) and in 1991 by the Centers for Disease Control and Prevention (CDC) (25). Globally, as of 1996, roughly 15 million women had HIV and or AIDS, compared with 20 million men (5); 5.5 million children had HIV and or AIDS (5). We believe that ethical perspectives open to women's voices will be influential for policy making into the new century.

Advances in therapy and the search for a vaccine do influence the moral evolution of approaches to the ethical problems of HIV/AIDS in clinical and larger social settings. We share Bayer's (16–19) and Grady's (26) historical and evolutionary outlooks on the ways that such progress influences ethics toward increasing personal responsibility and societal accountability for primary prevention of AIDS. This chapter argues a position that ethically justifiable measures can be carried out in primary prevention, screening and testing, reporting of names of those with HIV infection, notification of partners, and limiting the liberty of those who persist in endangering the health of others. A major theme of this chapter is that gaining more control over the epidemic—in the United States and globally—can be done in ethically justifiable ways. A companion theme is that some gains of the past decade in added protection for the rights of HIV-infected persons and of access to services of health care professionals must be enlarged, guarded, and secured.

ETHICS AND BIOMEDICAL ETHICS

As a field, ethics involves critical study of the approaches taken by philosophic and religious traditions to normative questions in every generation. A relatively recent interdisciplinary branch of the field of ethics, biomedical ethics, involves the systematic study of ethical problems in biomedical research and clinical practice. In the middle to late 1960s, the debate about research ethics and protection of human subjects was an impetus for the emergence of biomedical ethics (27). Biomedical ethics also linked older ethical traditions to new problems such as organ transplantation and applied human genetics. Despite the growth of biomedical ethics, some founders (28) and critics (29, 30) criticized its literature as too abstract and distant from clinical realities. More recent work in clinical ethics (31, 32) attempts to enrich biomedical ethics with understanding of the unique factors in each clinical situation and of the clinician's art of caring for patients.

CLINICAL ETHICS

The aims of clinical ethics are to 1) identify and prevent ethical problems in the care of particular patients, 2) analyze these problems in a dialogue open to competing ethical claims and perspectives, and 3) attempt to resolve such problems by shared decision making with the patient or others with moral standing in the case. For these tasks, clinical ethics draws on four general and three specific resources, shown in Table 55.2.

With such resources, clinicians, patients, and other decision makers may cooperate to resolve ethical problems in the care of persons with HIV/AIDS. Timeliness in these efforts

Table 55.2. General and Specific Resources of Clinical Ethics

1. Knowledge of disease processes and approaches to diagnosis and treatment
2. Knowledge of general ethics, biomedical ethics, and different cultural and religious approaches to ethical problems in health care
3. Knowledge of health care law bearing on the clinical encounter
4. Knowledge and skills in interpersonal relations
5. Knowledge of paradigmatic "teaching cases" of clinicians and patients facing ethical problems
6. A method informed by items 1 to 5 to analyze ethical problems that also draws on collective ethical guidance for clinicians, weighs competing ethical perspectives, and aims for the best outcome in the case under study
7. Institutional resources for consultation for ethical problems, when efforts of clinicians, patient, and family reach an impasse

can reduce or avoid harms to patients, particularly the harm of unjustifiable coercion (33). Without such efforts, ethical problems easily become power struggles or unnecessary lawsuits.

No single ethical perspective dominates in a culturally pluralistic society. Herein lies a major source of conflict. Instead of individuals and groups discussing issues from shared moral premises, these parties approach ethical discourse in the United States from different, even "warring" (34), sources of moral authority. This problem is clearly depicted in the current abortion debate and often leads to cynicism about finding common moral ground. Views of sexuality and death and dying are other examples of debates in which opposing groups often talk past each other.

In any event, individuals and groups must both be aware of competing ethical perspectives and must choose among them. We recommend a composite perspective with three major elements: 1) a set of ethical principles based on moral beliefs that are widely held in this and other cultures; 2) commitment to care for patients and their most significant relationships; and 3) a case-based method of moral problem solving that depends on caring professionals, is attentive to ethical principles, and is pragmatic in its primary aim, by which we mean that it aims to guide the development, implementation, and evaluation of action by means of a collaborative method of problem solving involving all those concerned with the case.

A set of five ethical principles is shown in Table 55.3 (28, 35), comprising primary sources of guidance for clinical practice and research. Our recommendations in each section respond to the claims of one or more of these principles. Ethical principles are not absolute. They are tools to weigh and balance judgments about competing claims. "Principlism" (28) has been a major conceptual resource in biomedical ethics, especially for ethical questions of "What ought to be done and why?" Most ethical traditions have a place for basic principles, although views of their force and relevance may vary. Such considerations, on a broad canvas, can provide language and understandings of ethics that can be shared across religious and cultural boundaries in an open, liberal society.

However, when clinicians interact with ethical problems posed within the life histories and needs of patients and families, ethical principles are incomplete guides to action. Principles help to orient to general judgments, but they are often too general to clarify questions of "How?" and "By whom?"—ethical problems that ought to be addressed. The language of principlism tends to focus on issues of individual rights and duties rather than on issues in families and collectivities. Several feminist writers (36–38) argue that principlism is inadequate to the complex, human dimensions of many biomedical dilemmas.

An ethics of "care" (39, 40) is grounded in a responsibility to care for persons and their most significant relationships. To care is to identify with other persons, each of whom is unique, aiming to nurture the web of relationships they share or can share. This perspective provides a personal dimension that is

Table 55.3. Ethical Principles for Practice and Research

Respect for persons: the duty to respect the self-determination and choices of autonomous persons, as well as to protect persons with diminished autonomy (e.g., young children, mentally retarded persons, and those with other mental impairments)

Beneficence: the obligation to secure the well-being of persons by acting positively on their behalf and, moreover, to maximize the benefits that can be attained

Nonmaleficence: the obligation to minimize harm to persons and, wherever possible, to remove the causes of harm altogether

Proportionality: the duty, when taking actions involving risks of harm, to so balance risks and benefits that actions have greatest chance to result in the least harm and the most benefit to persons directly involved

Justice: the obligation to distribute benefits and burdens fairly, to treat equals equally, and to give reasons for differential treatment based on widely accepted criteria for just ways to distribute benefits and burdens

(Adapted from Beauchamp TL, Childress JC. Principles of biomedical ethics. 4th ed. New York: Oxford University Press, 1995; and National Commission for the Protection of Human Subjects of Biomedical and Behavioral Research. The Belmont report, April 18, 1979. Washington, DC: US Government Printing Office, 1986;181–296:41,238.)

a corrective for principlism. It is especially relevant to clinical care of persons with HIV/AIDS, many of whom have been subjected to discrimination and dehumanizing experiences. Caring emphasizes the role of emotions and character traits in ethics and the inseparability of emotions from moral reasoning. In a clinical setting, to care for a patient means to identify with him or her within a plan of care that also considers the patient's relationships in families and with significant others. Instead of seeing individuals in conflict and competing for space, a care-based perspective views patients and clinicians interacting in relationships that have new possibilities. In the following discussion, we propose an integrated perspective, drawing on principlism and caring, in response to ethical problems in HIV/AIDS.

HIV/AIDS and Clinical Ethics

The following is a discussion of approaches to ethical issues and problems in the care of patients with HIV/AIDS. The first step in ethical analysis of an area of practice or in a particular case is to identify ethical issues and problems accurately and to assess their magnitude. What ethical problems in HIV/AIDS are seen most frequently by clinicians, and what is the magnitude of each, that is, which problems pose the greatest risk of harm to the largest number of persons? Because no empiric studies of the magnitude issue have been conducted, this question requires an imaginative approach, with two criteria to limit bias: 1) estimates of numbers of persons adversely affected by the problem; and 2) incidence in the literature. The medical literature is not sufficient to assess magnitude, inasmuch as it has selection bias. For example, the informed consent (to testing) has been the most frequently discussed issue in the AIDS and ethics literature. A search of articles from 1989 to 1997 in English on *Bioethicsline* under the key words of AIDS and ethics produced 2551 items. In addition to items on assorted topics, these were the most frequent topics: informed consent, 979; notification of partners, 465; testing and counseling, 432; prevention, 418; HIV/AIDS and pregnancy, 352; privacy and confidentiality, 36; duty to treat persons with AIDS, 28; drug testing, 22; screening and testing, 9, and death and dying, 2. The problems have been rearranged in this section for the sake of logic of discussion; for example, the obligation to treat comes before the obligation to maintain a valid process of informed consent and to protect privacy and confidentiality. However, poor access to primary health care, complicated by unfair insurance practices, surely has primary place in terms of magnitude. Societal and individual failures in the obligation to treat persons with AIDS are the problems of greatest magnitude, especially on a global basis. When therapy is available to prolong life, many more persons with HIV/AIDS are adversely affected by poor access than are harmed by breaches of informed consent or confidentiality and privacy. Table 55.1 represents our best estimate of the rank and magnitude of ethical problems in HIV/AIDS as a whole. Table 55.4 shows the ethical issues and problems most frequently faced by clinicians and their patients.

OBLIGATION TO TREAT PERSONS WITH HIV/AIDS

Among some physicians, significant reluctance and even open refusal to treat persons with HIV/AIDS was one of the earliest ethical problems in the epidemic. Zuger (41) reviewed and documented the extent of the problem in the 1980s to the best of her knowledge. In the United States, the degree of physicians' resistance to treat persons with HIV/AIDS has probably not lessened (42) in the 1990s, despite a stronger policy position by the American Medical Association (AMA). To explore attitudinal and structural barriers to primary care, in 1990 Gerbert and associates (43) conducted a population-based random sample of 2004 general internists, family physicians, and general practitioners (response rate, 59%). Most physicians (75%) had treated one or more patients with HIV. A majority (68%) believed they had a duty to do so, but half (50%) would not have done so if given a choice. More than 80% believed that they lacked information about AIDS. Negative attitudes (35%) about homosexuals and intravenous drug users (55%) in their practice were evident. Barriers to primary care of persons with HIV/AIDS do exist.

The history of AMA statements about epidemics and AIDS also illustrates the ambivalence of the behavior of physicians in the United States. The original code of ethics of the AMA adopted in 1847 endorsed a position that treating patients in an epidemic was a strong and exceptionless duty (44). This section in the code was removed in 1957 in the belief that massive dangers from infectious diseases had been conquered by medical science. In 1986, the AMA Committee on Ethical and Judicial Affairs made an exception to the obligation to treat based on "emotional inability" to care for patients with AIDS and a duty to transfer the patient (45). Under severe and justified criticism, the Council in 1987 changed positions and asserted that ". . . a physician may not ethically refuse to treat a patient whose condition is within the physician's current realm of competence solely because the patient is seropositive" (46).

Historical studies of previous epidemics and physicians' behavior until the nineteenth century show a consistently mixed, ambivalent response by physicians that was voluntaristic rather than duty oriented (47). In medieval Europe, community leaders negotiated with some physicians for contracts to take extraordinary risks in exposing themselves to bubonic plague. In the nineteenth century, medical ethics in the context of epidemics changed. Zuger and Miles (48) showed that access to physicians was not restricted or difficult in the epidemics of cholera, yellow fever, influenza, or poliomyelitis. Today, organized medicine and the bioethics literature strongly support a duty-based approach to the issue of an obligation to treat patients with HIV/AIDS. This position is not exceptionless, but exceptions are drawn narrowly. Major articles by Arras (49) and Jonsen (50) mark out a situational rather than a categoric approach to the exceptions. These authors stress the record of physicians' courage in exposure to infectious disease and regard treatment of HIV/AIDS patients as normative for the profession rather than an act of supererogation, defined as an act that is beyond the call of duty but not necessarily to the extent of heroism or sainthood. Many authors in biomedical ethics support this position (51–56). No literature exists with an ethical argument defending a right of refusal to treat. Some do argue that surgeons may postpone treatment and mandatorily test prospective patients for HIV infection because of higher occupational risks (57, 58). These pleas reveal the extent to which many physicians still misunderstand the risks of patient-to-physician transmission of HIV. Moreover, in terms of the physician–patient relationship, the ongoing issue reveals how many physicians in the United States view themselves as solo entrepreneurs rather than as members of a profession whose members expect to take special risks for the sake of healing and health.

Is the exception to the obligation to treat based on the "current realm of competence" in the AMA's previously quoted statement ethically acceptable? In the previous edition of this textbook, we argued that experience with the clinical spectrum of HIV/AIDS had been sufficient to establish the standard of care in community practice. Multiple guidelines for management of patients with HIV/AIDS had been published by 1993 (59–63), and it was argued that primary care physicians could no longer conscientiously claim "lack of expertise" as the basis to refuse to treat patients with HIV infection. However, in the intervening 4 years,

Table 55.4. Ethical Issues and Problems in Clinical Care

Obligation to treat persons with HIV infection or AIDS
Confidentiality and privacy
Counseling, testing, and informed consent
Counseling HIV-positive women about reproductive choices
Death and dying; forgoing treatment, euthanasia, aiding suicide

dramatic changes have occurred in our understanding of this disease associated with new and more complex methods to monitor and treat it. Investigators have shown that survival is improved when patients with AIDS are hospitalized in facilities that have more experience with AIDS (64, 65), but the effect of the physician's experience on outcome has only recently been evaluated.

Kitahata and colleagues (66) found a direct relationship between the physician's level of experience in caring for patients with HIV infection and the survival rate of these patients. Patients cared for by the most experienced providers had a mortality rate that was 43% lower than that of a comparable group of patients cared for by less experienced providers. Although it can still be argued that a physician would violate a strong ethical consensus by avoiding or turning away HIV/AIDS patients strictly based on their diagnosis, patients with HIV also have "the right to expect care that is fully informed by the most recent advances in the field" (67). Although new management guidelines continue to be published (68), much of what is now considered accepted practice is complex and still evolving, making it extremely difficult for most physicians to remain optimally informed, particularly if their base of HIV-infected patients is small. Accordingly, the state of Maryland requires that a physician has had experience caring for at least 50 persons with HIV infection to be certified to care for HIV patients receiving Medicaid (J Bartlett, unpublished data). Minimally, less experienced providers will need to work in close consultation with more experienced providers, or, when practical, models of HIV care based on the care of oncology patients should be considered to achieve the goal of optimizing both quality and accessibility of care for persons with HIV/AIDS.

CONFIDENTIALITY AND PRIVACY

Schoeman's (69) extensive review of privacy and AIDS shows how this issue pervades diagnosis, treatment, epidemiology, and reporting of HIV infection, as well as the patient's duty to disclose seropositivity to sexual partners, physician, employer, or insurance provider. In clinical care, from the initial encounter through each stage of the relationship, confidentiality and privacy are vital ethical concerns that jointly face the clinician and the patient. Persons with HIV/AIDS are especially vulnerable to prejudice (70), and thus to violations of confidentiality and privacy, and are at high risk of losing jobs, education, housing, and insurance. Breaches of confidentiality occur when information given "in confidence" to health care professionals is carelessly unprotected or disclosed to others in an unauthorized manner. Privacy is violated when either personal information that would be harmful or disadvantageous to the individual or access to a person's body or body parts is obtained without prior knowledge or consent. Two examples follow.

In 1987, William H. Behringer, an otolaryngologist and plastic surgeon, tested positive for HIV in the context of hospital treatment for *Pneumocystis carinii* pneumonia. He was a patient in the Medical Center of Princeton, New Jersey, where he had privileges to practice. Within hours of his discharge the next day, he received numerous phone calls from friends concerned about his well-being who were also aware of his illness. He also received similar calls from patients. His surgical privileges were suspended within weeks, and he performed no more surgery. His practice declined, and he suffered emotionally and financially until his death in 1989. Dr. Behringer sued the hospital and the treating physician for breaches of confidentiality and for violating the antidiscrimination law of New Jersey. The court agreed with the first complaint and awarded damages (71), but it set aside the second on grounds that the hospital was justified in restricting him because of probability of harm to patients.

Another privacy issue, arguably less egregious, occurred in 1986, when reporters Jack Anderson and Dale Van Atta obtained documents, probably nursing notes, detailing Roy Cohn's diagnosis and treatment for AIDS. They published this information before the patient's death (28). They defended their actions by arguing that the patient was a public figure who had publicly denied that he had AIDS. Their position that the public had "a right to the truth" was criticized by other journalists (72). This situation raises the issue of whether a public figure has privacy rights that transcend the public's right to know. Moreover, does a public denial by a public figure, in effect, change the rules of privacy?

As these cases clearly show, confidentiality and privacy are difficult to protect in the open setting of a modern hospital or even in the physician's office. Many professionals and students see the patient's chart and know the diagnosis and prognosis. For these reasons, Siegler (73) described confidentiality as a "decrepit" concept. However, strong ethical arguments exist to renew and secure the practice. First, protecting confidentiality and privacy is a sign of caring, a virtue indispensable to health care for those with HIV/AIDS and other disorders. Second, persons in greatest need of help, such as those with psychiatric disorders or possibly those who are HIV infected, probably would not seek medical help without an assurance of confidentiality. Studies of psychiatric patients (74, 75) show that they give great weight to the value of confidentiality. Comparable studies are sorely needed with HIV/AIDS patients. Beauchamp and Childress (28) showed that the practice of confidentiality can be defended both in terms of the consequences it produces and by the ethical principle of respect for persons' autonomy and fidelity, which undergirds the keeping of promises.

Gunderson, Mayo, and Rhame (76) examined the arguments by philosophers giving the reasons that privacy is a fundamental human value: 1) privacy is necessary for the development of autonomous individuals and a genuine democracy; 2) privacy is necessary for many projects we value, such as in courtship or in work, or for those with political and economic goals; and 3) privacy protects us from the intolerance, prejudice, ignorance, and malice of others.

Many commentators (77–83) agree that a reasonable probability of infection to unsuspecting others, such as spouses and other sex partners, is a sufficient reason to permit ethically justifiable infringements on patients' confidentiality and privacy. However, wide disagreements exist in the literature on how and by whom infringements may ethically be performed. The most significant division of views exists on the physician's duty to warn unsuspecting third parties when the HIV-infected patient refuses to do so. Marshall (80) argues that physicians have a duty to warn third parties of HIV-infected patients that is grounded in obligations to the larger community. Gunderson and associates (76) give far less weight to the harm principle and pose four criteria for warning. The physician must know "with a high degree of certainty" that 1) the infected patient will have unsafe sexual relations with a partner, 2) the patient will not warn the partner, 3) the potential partner is unaware of the risk, and 4) warning the partner will not so destroy the trust of other patients that more harm than good will result.

In practice, the "high degree of certainty" requirement would effectively nullify action. The criteria cannot be fulfilled by practicing physicians who are not full-time public health officers. If physicians are unwilling to warn third parties who are at significant risk, it is their duty to delegate this task to public health officials, who may carry it out without naming the infected individual.

TESTING, REPORTING, COUNSELING, AND INFORMED CONSENT

Testing and Reporting

The history of testing for antibodies to HIV clearly depicts the dominant themes struck by Bayer in the evolution of ethical issues of HIV/AIDS. In the early to middle 1980s, sharp controversies arose between gay leaders and public health officials on the process of excluding high-risk donors of blood and testing the blood supply for human T-cell lymphotrophic virus type III (HTLV-III) once an antibody test had been licensed by the Food and Drug Administration (FDA). Bayer (16) chronicled the troubling events of this period. He also accurately recorded the acrimony in the ethical debate and resistance to testing, especially among gay men and some of their physicians, when the enzyme-linked immunosorbent assay (ELISA) test was introduced beyond the context of blood donation (16). Gradually, attitudes toward HIV testing among individuals and groups at high or low risk evolved to a new stage. Skepticism or neutrality about the benefits of testing has been effectively succeeded by widespread support for a more assertive but measured approach to testing (84). Ethical debate has shifted to proposals for "routine voluntary testing" for the majority of hospital patients (85, 86), especially those seen in emergency departments (87), and pregnant women either universally or in regions of highest incidence of HIV infection (88–90). Advances in early treatment (91) of opportunistic infections (e.g., see Chaps. 14 and 23) and the role of zidovudine (ZDV, formerly known as azidothymidine or AZT) (92) and other promising drugs in extending the lives of HIV-infected persons (see Chaps. 45 and 47) are clearly important factors in this change of climate. Moreover, progress in protecting persons with HIV/AIDS from discrimination or mistreatment must not be discounted. As a result, publicly funded HIV testing in the United States increased (93) from approximately 79,000 tests in 1985 to nearly 2,091,000 in 1991. Despite these gains, up to 75% or more of persons who are seropositive probably are unaware of their infection (94).

More recently, home test kits have become available that alter the usual paradigm of face-to-face, pretest, and posttest counseling. An additional concern regarding this method of testing is whether it will only increase the testing of those historically at low risk. Data on which to answer this question are at present incomplete.

A topic directly tied to testing for HIV is that of reporting of positive test results to various groups or agencies. Reporting of patients with AIDS by name has been a standard national practice since the earliest phases of the epidemic. Only 26 states require HIV cases to be reported. Investigators now argue that universal AIDS reporting is no longer adequate to monitor epidemic trends (95). AIDS incidence and mortality have recently declined (96), although this decline this may only reflect the effect of improved therapies of HIV and associated infections.

A national HIV surveillance system, as outlined by Gostin and colleagues (95), would likely 1) improve our understanding of the epidemiology of the epidemic, 2) prevent infections by targeting scarce resources for testing, counseling, education, and partner notification, 3) benefit persons with HIV or AIDS by providing an earlier link to medical resources and other services, and 4) promote more equitable allocation of government funding.

Counseling

Counseling before and after HIV testing has also evolved as an ethical requirement for practice in centers, hospitals, and offices. This requirement is global in scope (97), although counseling takes various forms in different societies. In some developing nations, the term *counseling* had not been in the language previously. There counseling mainly means education for prevention and psychosocial support (4). In some African nations, training of community-based workers as counselors with these goals has been effective.

Counseling in the context of HIV testing is done in the United States mainly by nurses, physicians, social workers, and allied health professionals who have been trained for their tasks. Valenti's (94) comprehensive review of the goals and tasks of counseling summarizes standards for practice. Counseling is guided by several ethically relevant goals: to provide education and informed consent before HIV testing and to further primary prevention and effective referral to care in the posttest period.

Two main reasons support an ethical guideline that HIV antibody testing be preceded and followed by competent counseling. The first is the well-documented psychosocial impact of HIV infection (98–101). Evaluative studies of counseling (102, 103) show that it provides reassurance, motivation for change to prevent infection, and reduction of anxiety and depression. The second reason is that HIV antibody testing may be easy to perform, in contrast to other tests (104), but it is not easy to explain to those being tested. Saag's expert discussions of this matter (105) continue in Chapter 4. Knowledge of the natural history of the disease is vital for the most informed approach to counseling after a positive test. Moreover, complex issues affect the specificity and positive and negative predictive values of the ELISA and Western blot approaches to testing for antibodies to HIV. False-positive results in low-prevalence populations have been a problem (106), although not uniformly (107). Positive results require repeated tests and care in explanation to prevent psychological harm or suicide. Counseling persons deemed to be at a lower risk of infection can be difficult after a positive result. For this reasons, persons who conduct counseling must be thoroughly familiar with test performance, laboratory methods, and the particularities of the tests used in their centers (108).

Informed Consent

In the United States, a consensus arose in the mid-1980s (17) that informed consent before HIV testing was an ethical requirement. The consensus was largely shaped in recognition of the negative psychosocial impact of positive results of an antibody test (70). Consequently, the practice of informed consent in HIV testing has probably raised the standard of consent in all clinical tests in adults (17). Several states have passed laws requiring informed consent in this context. Practitioners must be familiar with the law in their states, because some states permit testing without consent (109). In our view, even if it is legal to forego consent, the practice of informed consent in HIV testing is ethically indicated. The reasons for this position are several. First, seeking consent shows respect and caring for persons and their autonomous choices. However, flexibility about the stringency of the requirement for informed consent in treatment and research in cultures in which individualism is not as prevalent has been increasingly supported in the literature (110, 111). Second, when understanding is achieved, it promotes current and future cooperation of patients with professionals in treatment and prevention. Third, communication of a diagnosis of HIV infection is a life-changing event. It should not come as a surprise or be coercive. Even testing patients after exposure of health care workers (HCWs) to their blood or body fluids should be done with prior notification, although consent is not required. Geller and Kass (111) discuss the ethical reasons to seek informed consent from pregnant women in HIV testing, which is relevant to the issues in the next section.

Counseling HIV-Infected Women About Reproductive Choices

Current policy in the United States is to inform all women, especially pregnant women, about HIV testing and to offer the test on a voluntary basis, with appropriate counseling. The features of the policy and supporting arguments are given by Faden and associates (112), who report on a national project sponsored by the American Foundation for AIDS Research. Current practice guidelines for obstetricians and gynecologists (113, 114) reflect this policy. Rising numbers of infected women, infants, and children (24, 25) and the uncertainties regarding vertical transmission of HIV in pregnancy (115) create the occasion for one of the sharpest ethical conflicts in the clinical arena: how ought professionals to counsel HIV-infected women about reproductive choices? Significant harm could be prevented by directive counseling and by advocating abortion as prevention. Kass (116) expertly reviews the debate and literature on this question. She finally advocates a nondirective approach to attempting to influence the woman's moral choice. In our view, this position should prevail in practice, but probably it does not.

In the mid-1980s, before risk data were available from prospective studies on vertical transmission, advice on counseling by governmental and medical statements took a position close to directiveness. The CDC urged that infected women "should be advised to consider delaying pregnancy..." (117), and the American College of Obstetrics and Gynecology stated that such women "should be strongly encouraged not to become pregnant" (118). Arras (119) advocated directive counseling in this period, although he moderated his view in a subsequent publication (120) as accurate risk information was clarified. Prospective studies (121–124) showed a perinatal infection rate of 25 to 35%. Another report (125) found a 13% infection rate. Moreover, preliminary data (126) suggested that the rate of perinatal transmission may be higher if the HIV-infected woman's CD4 cell count is lower than 400 mm^3 and if she is in the later stages of illness (126). The success of ZDV administration during pregnancy in reducing perinatal HIV transmission (127) and the possibility that newer agents could be even more effective also need to be discussed. The issue is complicated by the finding that what is considered optimal therapy for the mother has been inadequately tested for safety and efficacy in the setting of pregnancy.

Informing HIV-infected women who need reproductive advice about relative risks of transmission is current practice (118). However, giving information is not equivalent to "directive" counseling, which involves a moral judgment that "If I were you, I would not have a child." We suspect that, in actual practice, directive counseling of this type occurs often. Bayer (128) documents some of this practice of directiveness and attributes it, among other sources, to a "broad based challenge to the ideological hegemony of individualism in American society." He also identifies eugenic motives at work in the practice. Our recommendation is that clinicians restrain directiveness at this point, with regard to restraint of undue influence or control of women's reproductive choices, including women who are HIV infected. The decision to consent to pregnancy or to continue an unplanned pregnancy is not without ethical and legal challenge, as the ongoing abortion debate shows (129). However, in clinical practice, this decision ethically and legally (130) should remain a choice of the women involved.

The moral acceptability of risk taking in pregnancy varies widely with cultural, educational, and family history. In any ethical theory, it is immoral to cause harm to others that is unjustifiable. With some differences noted later, it is instructive to compare choices in reproduction in HIV/AIDS with the context of human genetics. Shaw (131), an attorney-geneticist, argued that to inflict higher genetic risks on offspring knowingly is morally blameworthy and should carry legal penalties. This view, however, has little effect in the practice of clinical genetics, wherein the conscience of the woman involved, in consultation with the father, is the major guide in many nations (132). Are the risks of HIV/AIDS in children excessive compared with the burdens of heredity?

In terms of overall burden of harm, society tolerates far more harm from heredity that it does from HIV-infected children. Significant birth defects occur in 3 to 4 of each 100 births. Between 25 and 30% of all admissions to pediatric units in developed nations are due to burdens of heredity (133). However, no nation, with the exception of China (134), has coercive policies of pregnancy screening.

A major difference exists between the contexts of genetics and of HIV/AIDS. Children with genetic disorders are usually wanted by their parents, who can, with some exceptions, care for them in their lifetimes. Although about 70 to 90% of infants of HIV-infected mothers are not HIV infected, depending on maternal therapy, each has a 100% chance of being orphaned. The United States will probably have 80,000 AIDS orphans by the year 2000 (135). The social, economic, and personal impacts of this situation are immense (136). AIDS orphans are not highly desirable adoption candidates. AIDS orphans are at higher risk of becoming infected (136). It often requires 3 months or longer to know with a high degree of certainty whether the child is not infected. Those children who acquire HIV infection despite maternal antiretroviral therapy, may live for several years on current therapy, but at great expense and with an uncertain future.

The natural histories of a few genetic disorders are comparable. However, far more therapeutic opportunities are available for many children with genetic disorders. Neither genetic disease nor HIV infection is desirable. However, despite the burdens on society of orphaned children or children slowly dying of AIDS, tolerance for reproductive choice is a better public policy, in principle and in terms of consequences, than the extreme options of mandating preventive abortions or outlawing any abortions. If society were less accepting of reproductive freedom in human genetics, in which even greater risks of harm are routinely taken by parents without requiring a precommitment to preventive abortion, it could logically follow that it should be less tolerant toward the risks of HIV infection for offspring. Further ethical arguments in support of this policy are that it 1) shows respect and caring for the woman and her autonomy, 2) increases chances that she will remain within the health care system to seek help for herself and her child, and 3) respects the influence of cultural differences on moral practices.

If an HIV-infected woman desires to become pregnant, we advocate counseling for her with regard to 1) risks of transmission, 2) treatments available for her and her child, and 3) issues related to who could care for her orphaned child or children (135).

Death and Dying

No effective cure or vaccine exists for AIDS. The complications of AIDS inevitably kill patients, unless either suicide or physician-assisted death (by euthanasia or physician-assisted suicide) is the immediate cause of death.

Having AIDS is a significant risk factor for suicide. Persons with AIDS have a higher risk of suicide (137, 138) than those with other chronic diseases. However, the incidence of deaths from completed suicide among all deaths of AIDS patients has not been ascertained (139).

Since the first edition of this text, a heated ethical and legal debate has focused on physician-assisted death. This issue is, understandably, of significant interest to persons with HIV/AIDS in Europe and the United States. In these nations, suicide has long been decriminalized, but physician-assisted suicide remains clearly a crime, except as modified in the Netherlands. In Dutch law, euthanasia and physician-assisted suicide are technically crimes, but an amendment to that nation's Burial Act provides that physicians will not be prosecuted if they comply with certain conditions and reporting methods (140). The practice of physician-assisted death in the Netherlands occurs frequently in the context of AIDS. For example, a study (141) of 131 homosexual men with AIDS in Amsterdam showed a significant incidence of physician-assisted death. A total of 29 (22%) died by euthanasia or physician-assisted suicide, as compared with 5% of patients with cancer and 2% of the general population.

Persons with HIV/AIDS in the United States are also interested in physician-assisted death. In New York City, a survey (142) published in 1996 of 378 ambulatory HIV-infected patients showed that 63% favored policies permitting physician-assisted suicide, and 55% acknowledged considering this option for themselves. The ethical debate and legal status of physician-assisted death in the United States are reviewed later.

The least morally controversial practices in the medical care of those who die with AIDS are found in hospice care (see Chap. 52) and use of advance directives to refuse all but palliative care. One United States study published in 1991 (143) showed hospice care to be preferred by patients with AIDS, but such a study has not been done recently. Experts on hospice care of patients dying of AIDS describe its four features (144):

1. A unit of care for patient and family (inclusive of closest companions)
2. An interdisciplinary team to assess needs and to develop a plan of care
3. A focus on palliation, pain control, and treatment of symptoms
4. Bereavement services to family and significant others

An advance directive is a statement made by a person during a period of decisional capacity, intended to communicate treatment preferences in the event of a future episode of decisional incapacity. The different types of advance directives are informal (oral) and formal (living will, durable power of attorney for health care, or medical directive) (145).

With a durable power of attorney for health care, now authorized by every state in the United States except Alabama (146), any competent adult may appoint a surrogate decision maker to implement his or her desires in case of incapacity. This type of directive is relevant to persons with HIV/AIDS, inasmuch as about two-thirds of patients with definitive AIDS develop neuropsychiatric symptoms or progressive dementia (147). Grant and colleagues (148) dispute whether an "AIDS dementia complex" exists and prefer the term "AIDS-associated organic mental disorder" to describe a more complex and possibly reversible process. Another directive, the "living will," permits persons to state their preferences to forgo or sustain life-sustaining treatment when terminally ill and if cognitively impaired. Living wills are criticized (149, 150) for unrealistic expectations, because the exact circumstances in which the patient will be dying are beyond prediction. In practice, a durable power of attorney for health care is probably more reassuring for decision makers facing end-stage questions than a living will alone.

Are advance directives effective and helpful tools in the clinical setting? This question has not been specifically studied in the context of cases of end-of-life decision making about patients with AIDS. However, one study showed that advance directives had little effect on discussions of specific treatments (151), and a large controlled trial involving critically ill patients with various diagnoses, including AIDS, showed that advance directives resulted in no difference in outcomes, such as total resources used, do-not-resuscitate orders, or recorded discussions about treatment (152). More research and reflection are needed on physician-assisted "advance care planning" to address these disappointing results (145).

A review is appropriate of the controversy in the United States about physician-assisted death and the Supreme Court's decision regarding the question of a constitutional right to physician-assisted death. Views were sharply divided on this issue. For example, a leader in the disabilities movement favored legalization of physician-assisted death (153), and a leading figure in combating AIDS discrimination (154) viewed the subject itself as motivated by an economic solution for AIDS.

CONTEXTUAL FACTORS AND PUBLIC POLICY

Death in the United States has evolved from a natural event to "death by decision," largely because 61% of Americans now die in hospitals and 17% die in nursing homes (155). The remainder die at home or at the scene of accidents. Sites of dying vary among specific states, for example, Oregon (156): acute care hospitals (32%), nursing homes (32%), and home (31%). A strong ethical and legal consensus has developed (157, 158) that decisions to withhold or withdraw life-sustaining treatments, when the patient lacks capacity to participate, should mainly be based on two factors: 1) an assessment that burdens of particular treatments outweigh the benefits to the patient; and 2) respect for the contemporary or past oral or written directives of the patient to refuse such treatments.

Legal progress toward this consensus began in the Karen Ann Quinlan case in 1976 (159) and prevailed in the United States Supreme Court Cruzan decision in 1991 (160). Variations among the legal requirements of states are important in caring for the dying. However, ethically and legally, "negotiated dying" or "letting die" is the prevailing norm (28). Meanwhile, a renewed debate about legalizing assisted suicide and euthanasia, called "aid in dying" by its proponents and strongly opposed by many authorities in ethics and law, raged in public and in the literature in the early to middle 1990s.

DEBATE ABOUT LEGALIZING PHYSICIAN-ASSISTED DEATH

The euthanasia debate in the twentieth century long predates the AIDS epidemic (161–167). Emanuel (168) provides a thorough historical review of the debate in the United States and Britain. We identify several factors that propelled the debate and the reason the Supreme Court decided to rule on the constitutionality of physician-assisted death. In our view, at least seven factors were involved:

1. Varying assessments of the Netherlands' permissive practice of voluntary euthanasia for competent and terminally ill adults began in the mid-1980s (140, 169–171).
2. Public referenda were held in Washington (172) and California (173), where proposals to legalize aid in dying were narrowly defeated; two referenda were conducted in Oregon, where physician-assisted suicide was approved by the voters (174, 175).
3. Several respected physicians argued that assisted suicide (176–179) or euthanasia (180, 181) would be ethically acceptable provided strong safeguards against abuses are in place (182). These physicians found a vital missing option in the continuum of care for the dying.
4. Strong opposition to legalizing physician-assisted death came from respected bioethicists (183), legal authorities (184), a state bioethics task force (185), and organized medicine (186). These objections were based on the moral line between killing and allowing to die, on the ease of abuse of involuntary euthanasia, and on expectations of the erosion of trust of physicians by patients and family members.
5. Surveys showed that Michigan physicians were largely in favor of liberalization of laws against assisted suicide (187), a small percentage of Washington State residents who had requested suicide (156 reported requests, 38 received prescriptions) from physicians had received assistance (188), and, in San Francisco, the majority of 228

Table 55.5. Public Opinion and Legalizing Euthanasia, 1947 to 1993

When a person has a disease that cannot be cured, do you think that doctors should be allowed by law to end the patient's life by some painless means if the patient and (his) family request it?

Year	Organization	Results
1947	Gallup	37% yes, 54% no, 9% no opinion
1950	Gallup	36% yes, 64% no or no opinion
1973	Gallup	53% yes, 40% no, 7% no opinion
1982	National Opinion Research Center	61% yes, 34% no, 5% don't know
1982	Louis Harris	53% yes, 38% no, 8% not sure
1986	National Opinion Research Center	66% yes, 31% no, 4% don't know
1987	Louis Harris	62% yes, 34% no, 4% not sure
1991	Associated Press	60% yes, 24% no, 8% don't know
1991	Krc Communications	63% yes, 28% no, 9% don't know
1991	National Opinion Research Center	70% yes, 25% no, 5% don't know
1993	Louis Harris	73% yes, 22% no, 5% don't know

(From Roper Center for Public Opinion Research, University of Connecticut, 1994.)

physician respondents caring for persons dying of AIDS stated that they had granted a request for assisted suicide at least once (189).

6. Public opinion increasingly favored the legalization of euthanasia. We reviewed some 85 polls from 1947 to 1993 that asked a question about legalization of euthanasia (190). The results are shown in Table 55.5.
7. Decisions by two federal appellate courts declared unconstitutional state statutes in Washington (191) and New York (192) that banned assisted suicide.

The Ninth Circuit Court of Appeals ruled that the Washington State law was unconstitutional because it violated a person's fundamental liberty right protected by the due process clause of the Fourteenth Amendment to determine the time and manner of her or his death. This court equated the protection of liberty in assisted suicide with protection of liberty in abortion cases. The Second Circuit Court of Appeals found that dying patients in New York State who were not connected to life-support systems were not given equal protection required by the Fourteenth Amendment, because if they were so connected, they could legally refuse treatment and hasten their deaths. This court argued that the right of patients to refuse treatment and to be disconnected and die was, "nothing more nor less than assisting suicide." In its view, patients who were not on respirators and who were refused assistance with suicide were being treated unequally. This court challenged the logic and rationality of a distinction between withholding or withdrawing life-sustaining treatment and assisted suicide.

On June 26, 1997, the United States Supreme Court issued two unanimous rulings on the constitutional issues posed by the lower courts (193, 194). On the first issue, which was posed by the Ninth Circuit's decision, the Supreme Court ruled that no constitutional right to assisted suicide could be found in the nation's history or in the concept of liberty protected by the constitution. The Court also rejected the lower court's appeal to its abortion decisions. On the second issue, which was posed by the Second Circuit's decision, the Supreme Court ruled that a valid distinction exists between refusing unwanted life-sustaining treatment and assisted suicide that has long been respected by the medical profession, and that states having laws based on this distinction were following a long-standing and rational tradition. Annas (195) broadly discussed the Court's decision. Expert commentary on the Court's decision reflects the continuing ethical disagreement on the fundamental issues. Burt (196) saw no justification for a protected right to assisted suicide but interpreted some of the justices' opinions to support a constitutional right to palliative care, thus "requiring states to remove the barriers that their laws and policies imposed on the availability of palliative care." Orentlicher (197) saw the Court's acceptance of arguments from hospice providers and other medical professionals that terminal sedation for intractable pain and suffering was a viable option and thus an argument against assisted suicide was in effect to perform euthanasia, because the sedated patient dies from physician-administered drugs and the physician's withdrawal of feeding and hydration, and not from the disease itself.

Ethics and the Task Ahead: Palliative Care the Standard of Care

The Supreme Court has ruled against the constitutionality of the arguments advanced by the lower courts. Attempts to alter state laws through the court system will not be effective. State voter referenda and actions of state legislatures are possible sources of legal change. Oregon's Death with Dignity Act may be the first state provision for physician-assisted suicide, if it survives legal tests and is not rescinded. Meanwhile, the major task for health care professionals and medical or nursing organizations is to face the issues of death and dying and to learn to provide adequate palliative care for the dying as the standard of care.

Each of us strongly supports the hospice approach (144) to terminal illness, but we have divergent views on physician-assisted death. Wispelwey strongly opposes legalization of this practice because of 1) a potential for abuse of patients who are vulnerable to suggestion, 2) a basically unstable societal context with respect to health care reform and rationing of services, and 3) confidence that improvement of hospice care and preparation for dying will remedy many existing problems. On this view, widening access to hospice care and improving its quality for persons in the end-stage of AIDS comprise the better strategy (198). However, persons with AIDS can be suspicious of hospice care; in large cities, hospice programs designed for AIDS alone are effective and reduce suspicion (23). Three factors led Fletcher to change a position advocating legalization of physician-assisted death (182, 199). Meyer also shares this view. The first factor was the failure in 1993 of a national approach to universal primary health care with a guarantee of palliative care for the terminally ill. It is incoherent to ensure a right to be helped to die without the reality of a right to primary health care and palliative care, which does exist in the Netherlands and many other nations. To pursue legalization of physician-assisted death with so many unrighted wrongs and inequalities in the health care system would also be to court many moral dangers. A second influence was Arras' (200) persuasive arguments about predictable negative social consequences. A third factor involves an appraisal of the current culture of medicine in the United States. Could physicians in the United States really be expected to practice careful self-regulation in the event of legalization of physician-assisted death? The historical and contemporary record of physician self-regulation is not exemplary (13). Moreover, upheavals in medicine and consequent anger among United States physicians about practices and conflicts of interest in managed health care have created instability and mistrust that could negatively affect decision making about death and dying (201). Despite our affirmation that acts to help autonomous and suffering patients to die can be justified morally in specific cases, Fletcher and Meyer conclude that the necessary and sufficient conditions are not yet present in the United States health care system or in organized medicine to justify a public policy of physician-assisted death. When these conditions are realized, then legalization with social controls of physician-assisted death, as a last resort in the face of failure of or a valid refusal of palliative care, could ethically follow.

Given these outcomes of the debate, steps are needed now to improve the situation. Aspects of patients' quality of life and symptom relief (202) need greater emphasis in future studies (203) and not just quantitative issues or T4 count. Greater attention to restructuring hospital care for dying patients (204) is an appropriate response to a clear need and opportunity. More emphasis can be placed on allowing the patient greater control and dignity at the time of death, as well as time to prepare and plan ahead. These considerations pose a strong argument for having primary care physicians treat patients with HIV/AIDS, because trust can only be developed in a consistent relationship over time. However, many AIDS clinics are staffed differently, with infectious disease specialists (23).

The clinical ethics of care for those who die of AIDS depends on the social ethics of how and when to die, as well as who should have control over the circumstances of dying. Many factors in the next section on social ethics have an impact on the clinical care of patients.

SOCIAL ETHICS: LIVING WITH AIDS

The issues shown in Table 55.6 are briefly described and discussed in the next section. In living with AIDS (2, 3), what kind of society and what kind of persons should we be?

Primary Prevention and Universal Access to Primary Health Care

Living with AIDS requires a rebirth of social justice. Specifically, to achieve two interdependent goals requires a cultural and economic revolution in health care. These goals are to establish primary prevention of HIV infection and universal access to primary health care. Walters (205) struck these themes in the social ethics debate in the mid-1980s. Additionally, he called for targeted education programs, expansion of drug treatment programs, exchange of sterile needles and syringes for intravenous drug users, controlled access to intravenous drugs, legalization of prostitution, and decriminalization and antidiscrimination efforts on behalf of homosexuals. Francis (206), a senior CDC official, convincingly made the case for a comprehensive HIV prevention program in his recent retirement address. He documented the slow and moralistic response of United States leaders in the 1980s to HIV/AIDS, which delayed informed warnings and education and increased vulnerability to HIV. Francis described the national response to date as "public health malpractice" (206).

Vulnerability to HIV, a concept used by the Global AIDS Policy Coalition (4), begins on the individual level. Definitions of individual vulnerability to HIV/AIDS are shown in Table 55.7.

Because the private behavior of individuals is the greatest source of risks for HIV/AIDS, primary prevention must focus on individuals, their values, and their education. Empowerment of individuals relates to the preceding discussion of ethics and power. However, the thrust of prevention must also be on communities, key cultural groups, and religious movements, as well as on the nation as a whole. Francis advocated a five-point program for the United States shown in Table 55.8.

An examination of issues facing individuals with HIV infection in the United States provides insight into the reforms needed to achieve universal access to health care. In fact, the HIV epidemic serves to identify the shortcomings in the current "patchwork" system. Although research and development are vital, preventive, regulatory, and economic actions are needed to succeed in living with AIDS.

Health care reform remains one of the most vital domestic policy questions facing the United States (207–211). Reform of health care, as important as it is, must not be separated from the task of addressing economic issues that put individuals at risk of HIV infection. Economic issues are a fulcrum of any effective health care reform. Homelessness, prostitution, drugs, unwed teenage motherhood, and sexual violence are current facets of inner city and rural settings that

Table 55.6. Social and Ethical Issues and HIV/AIDS

Primary prevention and universal access to primary health care
Screening (populations)
Notification of partners and at-risk individuals
Screening health care workers; their status if HIV positive

Table 55.7. Definitions of Individual Vulnerability to HIV/AIDS

In absolute terms: unprotected
In relative terms: exposed to a higher than average risk
In epidemiologic terms: exposed to a higher risk of HIV infection
In medical terms: unable to avail the optimal level and quality of medical care
In operational terms: requiring a higher degree of protection and care
In human rights terms: exposed to the risk of discrimination or unfair treatment challenging basic principles of equity and human dignity
In social terms: deprived of some or all social rights or services
In economic terms: because of financial constraints, unable to offset the risk of infection or to access the optimal level and quality of care
In political terms: unable to achieve full representation or lacking political power

(From Mann J, Tarantola DJM, Netter TW, eds. AIDS in the world. Cambridge, MA: Harvard University Press, 1992:578.)

jeopardize any coherent attempt at health maintenance. HIV is not the only problem generated in these settings: sexually transmitted diseases (STDs), substance abuse, malnutrition, and related maladies may all be traced to economic instability. The most elaborate medical facilities and therapeutics are of little use if children born to children, to destitute women, and to drug addicts are unable to receive the basics of good health, which consist of a nurturing environment in which to thrive, with adequate food and parental attention. These children, as adolescents and young adults, are faced with the frightening array of risk factors mentioned earlier. Prenatal and postnatal care, parental leave, access to the health care system for all levels, incentives to encourage indigent parents to seek routine medical care for their children, job and shelter security, and reasonable wages are cofactors that will contribute to the success of any health care reform.

A focus on primary prevention through education also represents money well spent. In HIV/AIDS, it is apparent that with no current cure, teaching individuals how to avoid contracting infection is a vital focus. Moreover, preventive education works. A CDC report (212) indicated that concurrent to an increase in the amount of HIV instruction received in school and home was a significant decline in the number of high school students who reported having sexual intercourse or who had multiple partners. This finding is an encouraging sign that education does contribute to reducing risk factors to HIV and, by extension, could prevent other sexually transmitted diseases.

Reform of the health insurance industry is needed to live with AIDS and other catastrophic illnesses. Many persons lose their employment because of HIV infection and thus lose health insurance benefits. On the other hand, government assistance is often not available until the individual is completely impoverished or disabled. Although new therapies for HIV have been shown to prolong life and to delay progression of disease, these treatments are often unavailable to the "working poor" who make too much money to qualify for support and too little to afford these beneficial therapies. For people living with HIV/AIDS who lack private insurance coverage, Medicaid and the Health Resources and Services Administration's HIV AIDS programs (funded under the Ryan White Care Act) are both critical components of a safety net. Investigators have estimated that Medicaid pays for the care of half the adults living with AIDS and more than 90% of children living with AIDS. By the end of 1998, half of all people enrolled in Medicaid programs are expected to be in managed care. As discussed by Bartlett, "The financial stakes are high for the movement to managed care, and they are exceptionally high for HIV-care programs" (213). Reimbursement would be shifted from fee-for-service to capitated rates based on an average historical payment. These payments are usually based on the total Medicaid population and range from $37 to $400 per member per month. In Maryland, Medicaid payments for patients with AIDS averaged $2300 per month in 1995. Such a discrepancy in reimbursement would rapidly bankrupt any HIV care program.

A potential solution to this problem includes risk-adjusted rates based on historical payments for the disease in question. However, this approach could be cumbersome if it is applied to diseases other than HIV/AIDS. Newer therapies would need to be initially excluded from these rates because their cost is not reflected in historical payment data. Nonetheless, experts believe that most patients with AIDS will be in managed care systems in 2 to 3 years. The overarching challenge is to ensure that such health plans are well constructed, fairly implemented, and appropriately regulated for patient protection (214).

Facing social rejection, inadequate health care coverage, debilitation, and certain death, HIV/AIDS patients traverse the gauntlet of the current health care system inadequacies. Close examination of the problems encountered by these patients shows the road that must be traveled to bring about the health care reform the United States so badly needs.

Screening Populations

Many diverse proposals for screening populations for HIV were debated or implemented in the 1980s. With some prominent exceptions mainly related to federal and some state policies, a voluntary rather than a mandatory policy of screening exists in the United States. HIV testing is mandatory for all applicants for military service and the Job Corps, for persons wishing to immigrate into the United States, and for many prisoners. Illinois (215) and Louisiana (216) passed

Table 55.8. A Comprehensive HIV Prevention Program

Recognize at the highest levels of government the extreme danger of HIV and make the decision to launch prevention programs equal to the danger.
Establish a categoric financing program to pay for the health care needs of HIV-infected individuals.
Establish a consistent and logical policy regarding drugs and drug addiction.
Increase incentives for the private sector to make vaccines.
Establish clear chains of responsibility.

(Adapted from Francis DP. Toward a comprehensive prevention program for the CDC and the nation. JAMA 1992;268:1444–1447.)

laws requiring premarital screening and then rescinded them because of high costs and ineffectiveness. President Reagan's domestic policy advisor, Gary L. Bauer (217), had earlier advocated universal mandatory premarital screening. His proposals were criticized (218) and not enacted. Gostin's excellent article (219) comprehensively reviews all state and federal mandatory screening practices. Other than these federal and state-based exceptions, voluntariness is a mark of newer proposals for more vigorous screening to detect new cases, to derive the benefits of informing persons about infection, and to refer them to more effective treatment for HIV/AIDS.

In this regard, Rhame and Maki (220) advised vigorous "routine" (but with consent) screening of "all U.S. adults under the age of sixty regardless of their risk history" and universal prenatal testing. By contrast, Weiss and Thier (221) believed that screening be done only before blood and tissue donation. Selective voluntary screening was recommended by three official bodies for persons in high-risk categories (222–224).

Other than the mandatory screening practices named earlier, the practice of voluntary "routine" screening is confined to only some contexts (prenatal care, emergency departments in regions of high HIV prevalence, and STD clinics). "Routine" screening means that it is offered assertively to everyone in that context.

A voluntaristic approach to screening demarcates HIV screening dramatically from earlier public health policies and methods. In this context, an anonymous study by Janssen and associates (225) of blood samples in hospitals has led to new recommendations for routine (but voluntary) screening of all persons between the ages of 15 and 54 years who are admitted to a hospital. Seroprevalence in these hospitals totaled 4.7% and ranged from 0.2 to 14.2%. Like previous studies, that of Janssen and coworkers found that nearly two-thirds of HIV-positive patients came into the hospital with problems apparently unrelated to HIV infection. If these standards were put into effect, Janssen and colleagues claim that screening within these age groups would detect 68% of all HIV-positive patients with conditions other than AIDS. In light of new therapeutic advances in treating AIDS and of the advantages to the individual of knowledge of infection, Quinn (86) advocates expanding the scope of voluntary screening in hospitals to take advantage of the opportunity for counseling, referral, and therapy. We support this recommendation and urge its adoption in all hospitals, especially those in areas of high HIV prevalence. The following is a discussion of Angell's (226) position that such testing in hospitals be done on admission, presumably without consent.

In this period, literature on the ethics of HIV population screening grew rapidly and argued that voluntariness in screening practices was the dominant norm. Many authors were critical of the mandatory practices described earlier. These discussions by Bayer and associates (227), by Gostin (228), and by Lo and colleagues (229) strongly supported voluntary screening practices focused on groups with the highest risk behaviors and exposed the poor cost-to-benefit ratios in mandatory practices. In a later article, Lo (230) cited studies to show that a voluntary testing policy combined with strong methods to protect confidentiality increased the numbers of high-risk persons who accepted testing and decreased the numbers in states with mandatory reporting.

Table 55.9. Justificatory Conditions for Mandatory Screening Policies

Effectiveness: policy probably realizing the goal of protecting the public health
Proportionality: probable benefits of a policy outweighing both the moral rules infringed and any negative consequences
Necessity: policy being one of last resort, with no feasible alternative
Least infringement: policy having to have the least infringement necessary to realize the end sought
Explanation and justification to the persons protected by the rules

(Adapted from Childress JF. Mandatory HIV screening and testing. In: Reamer FG, ed. AIDS and ethics. New York: Columbia University Press, 1991:53–55.)

In a comprehensive review article, Childress (231) analyzed the ethics of large-scale HIV screening using premises widely held in a liberal society. He noted that the most ethically relevant features of these proposals were the extent of screening (universal or selective) and the degree of voluntariness (compulsory or consensual). He argued that the principle of respect for persons (see Table 55.3) was the major source of guidance for screening programs from which rules of liberty, privacy, and confidentiality were derived. As a background test for any screening program that would infringe on these rules or principles, Childress posed five "justificatory conditions," which are shown in Table 55.9.

Angell (226) argued for mandatory screening of all patients on admission to hospitals, of all HCWs who perform invasive procedures, and of all pregnant women and newborns. She did not mention informed consent. One must assume that she would at least rely on some type of notification process. The analysis of this chapter is confined only to patient screening on hospital admission. For the sake of argument, we assume that state laws had been amended to permit Angell's recommendation (219), although such a process would be costly and would create social conflict. Would the conflict be justified in terms of the benefits gained?

How well does Angell's proposal succeed in the light of Childress' tests? First, it would, in fact, contribute to public health. Some 25 million patients would be screened, and about 163,000 new HIV-positive cases (225) would be detected. If these persons received counseling and therapy, benefits would follow. However, what negative consequences are involved? The financial resources needed to test 25 million persons in the hospital (at $50 per test) would total $1.250 billion. Would not this expenditure cut deeply into efforts at research, primary prevention, and education (232)? The entire United States national expenditure on AIDS research in 1991 was only $1.282 billion (4). Is it conceivable that the nation would spend almost as much on testing hospital patients as it does in AIDS research? The cost of HIV and AIDS care in the United States in 1991 was estimated at $5.8 billion (4). The United States spent $736 million on its national AIDS program for prevention and education (4). That national per capita funding of prevention ($2.70) on an annual basis "amounts to less than a month's supply of vitamins" (4). Yet, added to Canadian funding for prevention, the amount exceeds the total amount for the rest of the world. Is it ethically justifiable to spend more annually on HIV testing of hospital patients than on primary prevention and education?

Angell's proposal is not the "last resort." An alternative, proposed by Janssen and associates (225), is more effective than universal screening of hospital patients. Assertively offering tests to all patients between the ages of 15 and 54 years would detect about 143,000 new cases or some 87.7% of all HIV-positive patients in United States hospitals in a total population of 13.7 million patients tested. The cost of annual testing would be between $500 million and $685 million, depending on how many patients accepted testing. If one limited testing in this age range only to hospitals in which the AIDS diagnosis rate is 1.0 or more per 1000 discharges, screening would detect as many as 110,000 new cases (225), and costs of approximately $250 million would be significantly lower. Alternatives, in short, pose less infringement than Angell's and are economically fairer and more feasible.

Finally, to implement Angell's plan, one would be morally obligated to notify all patients and surrogates that screening on admission had occurred. Moreover, disclosure of positive findings would necessarily occur after testing. Much learned about the beneficial relationship of pretest and posttest counseling and informed consent (97) would be sacrificed. After a decade of experience with a practice of informed consent to HIV testing, we doubt that an ethical consensus could be found for universal patient testing with notification. However, it is reasonable to expect support for routine voluntary testing in a patient population likely to result in a high detection rate.

In our view, the preferred strategy is to screen hospital patients between the ages of 15 and 54 years in high-prevalence areas. Rhame and Maki (220) describe the approach to "routine" screening. They expect that patients' responses would fall into three groups:

1. The largest group would deny any risk history and would accept testing with a brief period for counseling.
2. A second group would acknowledge risk histories and would be eligible for lengthy counseling before testing.
3. A smaller group would refuse testing without acknowledging risk behaviors. The latter group could be referred to public health sites offering anonymous testing.

In the 1990s, debate has arisen in earnest on screening pregnant women with HIV infection. The antiretroviral drug ZDV administered to HIV-positive pregnant women in the United States and France has been shown to reduce neonatal HIV infection by two-thirds (127). The results of this randomized controlled trial lends further support to a policy of increased HIV testing of pregnant women, leading some to call for mandatory testing. In New York State, strong efforts were made to introduce mandatory testing, including unblinding serum samples already taken from newborns (233, 234). These proposals generated scrutiny by bioethics committees of the state's medical society (235) and the American Academy of Pediatrics (236). These considerations all favored offering HIV tests and ZDV therapy to pregnant women in voluntary programs. We believe, as Bayer contended at the outset of the debate (237), that mandatory testing remains problematic both ethically and practically, given that mandatory treatment of competent adults is not acceptable. The purpose of prenatal testing is foremost to enable women to make informed choices regarding their health care and their child's health care. Routine voluntary testing meets this goal. If the goal is changed to one focusing on public health, then mandatory testing would seem rational to guarantee the least number of infected infants. A minimum requirement of such a mandatory program would be guaranteed access to potential preventive therapy if the test result was positive.

Notification of Partners and At-Risk Individuals

A social tragedy of great proportions is unfolding, in no small part because, as noted by Quinn (86), most HIV-infected persons are unaware that they are infected and are thus a risk to others. One clear remedy for this situation is a process of contact tracing, notification of sex or needle-sharing partners, and subsequent testing or counseling. The two main approaches to partner notification are by the identified HIV-infected person (patient referral) or by provider referral. Mann and associates (4) reviewed partner notification practices in several nations.

Ethical problems that arise in the notification process include the question of a "right not to know," potential for stigmatization, and whether special duties are created for infected persons that do not apply to uninfected persons (69, 238). In the United States, some literature in ethics and law in the mid-1980s (239) and even later (240) tended to discourage statutory partner notification in public health measures against AIDS. The reasons invoked were lack of a therapeutic option for AIDS and the potential for self-incrimination. However, many benefits clearly flowed from partner notification, such as learning HIV status, decreasing the risks of spread, and increasing information about treatment. This experience with contact tracing and its benefits convinced many, including policy makers, that it should be a major element in the public health response to AIDS. In the United States, partner notification by some method has been required since 1988 to receive federal funds for prevention (4). All publicly funded counseling and testing sites offer patient referral, and provider referral is offered by all states (241). The policy of states is to emphasize provider referral for persons who accept confidential HIV testing at clinics treating STDs (4). Thus, the trend clearly favors provider referral to patient referral. A study in North Carolina (242) comparing the two approaches showed far better results from provider referral. This study illustrates the depth of the unfolding tragedy. Of 162 eligible subjects, 74 agreed to participate: 39 were randomized to provider referral (where 78 of 157 partners were successfully notified), as compared with 35 to patient referral (where only 10 of 153 were successfully notified). Of those notified by providers, 94% were unaware they had been exposed to HIV. Now that drugs exist to ameliorate the harms of HIV/AIDS and to extend the life span, stronger reasons exist to support vigorous measures of provider-initiated and provider-assisted partner notification.

Screening Health Care Workers: Their Status If HIV Positive

In the first decade of HIV/AIDS, a major priority in the health care setting was to define the risk of patient-to-HCW transmission of HIV. In early 1991, the tables were turned. The CDC announced that a dentist in South Florida was a potential source of HIV transmission to one of his patients. Subsequently, it was reported that four other patients of this dentist may have acquired HIV in a similar fashion (243). In the months that followed, a stark confrontation occurred among the medical profession, the public, and politicians. Should all HCWs be routinely tested for HIV, or only subsets of them? Should an HIV-infected HCW allowed to continue to work in the health care setting, or should only certain activities be curtailed?

Scientific data on which to base answers to the foregoing questions are lacking. Although the risk of transmitting HIV in the health care setting can be argued to be real, the magnitude of this risk remains to be defined. However, HCWs have a fiduciary responsibility to their patients, and patient confidence in the health care system is essential; therefore, some investigators believe (244) that any risk to the patient is unacceptable.

At present, only 6 probable cases of transmission of HIV in the setting of a dental practice have been reported. No further cases of documented HCW-to-patient transmission could be found in a retrospective evaluation of more than 15,000 patients of HIV-infected HCWs (mostly dentists and surgeons) (245). The CDC has estimated (246) that the maximal rate of transmission from an HIV-infected surgeon may be in the range of 1 in 41,000 major surgical procedures. Therefore, a retrospective analysis of 15,000 patients may not be adequate to detect additional transmissions. Other investigators (247) have calculated the risk of contracting HIV infection from a surgeon of unknown HIV status as 1 in 21 million per hour of surgery and 1 in 83,000 if the surgeon is HIV positive, a finding that further supports the degree of uncertainty that currently surrounds this issue.

French health officials (248) announced in January, 1997 that an orthopedic surgeon diagnosed with AIDS in 1994 apparently transmitted HIV to a patient during a surgical procedure in 1992. A follow-up investigation has identified 3004 patients who underwent at least 1 invasive procedure by the surgeon. Of 2458 patients who were successfully contacted, 968 had been tested, and no additional infections had been documented thus far. This new case supports the relative rarity of transmission from surgeon to patient, but it also supports the concern that the risk is, however, real.

Despite the rarity of the risks and the uncertainty at the time, the CDC developed controversial guidelines (243), supported by the United States Congress, to address these perceived risks. HCWs who perform exposure-prone procedures are advised to know their HIV status, and if HIV positive, they are required to refrain from performing exposure-prone procedures. Many groups of health professionals including the American College of Surgeons, the American Dental Association, and the Infectious Disease Society of America opposed these guidelines and argued that a list of procedures defined as exposure-prone could not be developed, given the state of available information. The result of this debate was that the CDC authorized each state to decide what constitutes an exposure-prone procedure (249), taking into consideration not only the specific procedure, but also the skill, techniques, and possible impairment of the infected HCW.

This decision leaves open the possibility that each state will have its own set of rules and regulations with regard to HIV-infected HCWs. Examples of this option have already emerged. Some states have begun to develop or already have passed respective laws requiring physicians to disclose their HIV infection. If they do not disclose this information, the penalty is that they will be barred from "medical work" (244). A ruling from the Pennsylvania superior court stated that "disclosure of information regarding the condition of a physician with AIDS is necessary to prevent the spread of AIDS" (244). In this climate, several HCWs have already lost their jobs.

We argue that, although the risk of HIV transmission from an infected HCW to a patient is real, the likelihood is extremely small, supported by the lack of documented cases other than those previously described over a 16-year period. The means of transmission in the six reported cases may have been poor infection-control practices rather than direct transmission from the dentist to each patient. This concern reinforces the principle that implementation and strict enforcement of current infection-control practices comprise an effective strategy for protecting patients and physicians from nosocomial HIV transmission.

To apply a threshold of acceptable risk of HIV transmission in the health care setting at zero, as was done in the case of *Behringer v. Medical Center* (244), is unacceptable and unrealistic because this standard is not applied to any other clinical contact. Therefore, the mandatory removal of an HIV-infected HCW from the health care setting is not ethically defensible. Additionally, mandatory testing of HCWs or only those involved in invasive procedures cannot be recommended. If testing were to be required, how often should it be repeated? Would an HCW need to stop performing invasive procedures for successive months after each potential exposure to HIV? An analysis of a model testing program in Maryland (246) suggests that the cost per case prevented is estimated at $440 million to $4.4 billion. Although every life is important, we believe that reasonable persons would see this option as a patently disproportionate and unjust use of societal resources in living with AIDS.

A requirement that a patient has a right to know whether his or her physician is HIV infected is equally misguided. The risks to which patients are exposed in the course of routine care exceed the risks presented by an HIV-infected physician. One cannot single out HIV infection under the rubric of a patient's "right to know" and ignore the other theoretic or real risks such as potential hepatitis B transmission, the surgeon's complication or infection rates, a history of physician substance abuse, or even how much sleep the surgeon may have had the night before surgery.

Further study is clearly necessary, but at present we favor a program similar to that proposed by the New York Department of Health as a way to maximize patient safety without unnecessary discrimination against HCWs. The first and most important principle is that "HIV infection alone is not sufficient justification to limit professional duties of health care professionals unless specific factors compromise a worker's ability to meet infection-control standards or to provide quality patient care" (244). Each health care facility would be responsible for establishing a panel to evaluate the progress of HIV-infected HCWs in conjunction with their personal physicians. Inherent in this policy would be a requirement for the HIV-infected HCW to report his or her status to the panel. In summary, the strategy emphasizes effective infection-control practices, rather than the infection status of the HCW.

Despite these arguments, according to Larry Gostin (219), the courts have been reluctant to defend health care professionals with HIV under the Americans for Disabilities Act. A review of available cases suggests that the courts have not been convinced by epidemiologic data supporting a low risk of transmission and appear to take a "common sense" approach to health care–related cases suggesting that HIV is bloodborne and therefore can be transmitted in a profession that deals in blood. This debate will continue, and new guidelines are to be anticipated.

Drug Testing and Other Research Practices

Safe and effective drugs to treat AIDS and HIV infection are urgently needed. Limiting the access of HIV-infected individuals to unproven medications has been one of most hotly debated aspects of the epidemic. A turning point in the history of drug regulation in the United States occurred in 1962, coinciding with the link of thalidomide with multiple birth defects (251). The drug approval procedures of the FDA were changed from premarket notification to premarket approval. The regulatory control over the use of human subjects for research purposes followed a parallel course with the subsequent development of the concept of peer review and the establishment of institutional review boards to evaluate the ethical aspects of all investigational protocols. Therefore, the process of developing and approving new drugs in the United States, although arguably safer than in most nations, is frequently long, laborious, costly, and at times frustrating to physicians and patients alike.

The American College of Physicians Ethics Manual (252) summarizes the purposes and ground rules for appropriate clinical investigation as follows: Advances in the diagnosis and treatment of disease are based on well-designed, carefully controlled, and ethically conducted clinical studies. The medical profession must assume the responsibility for ensuring that the experiment is worth doing. Subjects must be instructed concerning the nature of the research; consent must truly be informed and given freely; research must be planned thoughtfully, so that it has a high probability of yielding significant results; risks to the patients must be minimized; and the risk-to-benefit ratio must be sufficiently low to justify the research effort (252).

Does this statement adequately address the concerns of patients with fatal illnesses for which no effective therapy exists? Many individuals in the AIDS activist community (253–255) believe that it does not always apply to drug investigation in the setting of HIV infection. Inherent in this debate are several questions. Does a patient have the right to waive his or her rights as a human subject in an investigational trial? Is the randomized clinical trial the exclusive method for obtaining knowledge concerning the efficacy and safety of a given drug? Should drug testing always include placebo controls, even when the disease under investigation is currently incurable or perhaps fatal? Investigators have argued that a "new context of increased advocacy and empowerment of potential subjects requires a reappraisal of the ethical balance between protecting the rights and welfare of subjects and expanding their options for access to possibly beneficial but still unproven drugs" (254).

Some of these issues are emphasized in debates regarding HIV vaccine trials. A group of physicians from the International Associations for Physicians in AIDS Care announced in late 1997 that they were willing to volunteer to receive a newly developed live-attenuated HIV vaccine. Do they have the right to waive their rights as human subjects and to receive a vaccine that is not yet adequately tested for safety or efficacy and, at least theoretically, could induce a disease similar to AIDS?

Activists have argued that the Kefauver amendment of 1962 requiring the FDA to measure drug efficacy be repealed. Regarding drug regulations, an editorial in the Wall Street Journal stated: ". . . it has become a battle between people who have all the time in the world and people who have little time left in their lives" (253).

In response to these and many other concerns, the FDA has softened some long-held positions. It recognizes that it must balance the risk of introducing a potentially dangerous drug to the public against the costs of delaying the availability of a potentially beneficial drug. In 1987, the FDA issued regulations that allow widespread distribution of investigational drugs for therapeutic purposes provided the disease is serious or life-threatening. Relaxation of these standards, however, has led to some inconsistencies regarding the definition of terms that are becoming part of the language of these new standards. Terms such as a *life-threatening* or *serious* disease can be interpreted in many ways. A disease for which no satisfactory alternative therapy exists leaves open for discussion the broad meaning of "satisfactory."

The result has been the release of drugs before approval for full marketing. Enough data must be available to make a reasonable judgment that the drug is effective and not unduly dangerous. Herein lies another point of controversy. How do we know a drug is effective in the treatment of HIV infection given the prolonged natural history of the disease? Admissible evidence that efficacy has also been relaxed allows the evaluation of surrogate markers of disease progression such as changes in T4 lymphocyte count and more recently viral loading. This allowance is a major concession, given the variability that can be encountered regarding this test at different stages of the disease. Moreover, in 1988, the FDA allowed any desperately ill person to import for their personal use small quantities of an unapproved drug. These drugs must not be for commercial sale, and the patient must supply the name of a physician who will monitor this treatment. The FDA approval merely legitimized the significant use of alternative therapies already occurring in HIV-infected individuals (255). Buyers' clubs began appearing around the United States to increase the availability of unapproved products. This proliferation has led to concern (256) that these clubs have gone beyond the original intention of the 1988 regulation.

The most recent change in drug trial regulation occurred with the development of the parallel track program. In some ways, this program may be viewed as an attempt to step back from the previous liberalization in policy. This program technically limits broader access to investigational drugs to only those patients who are unable to take standard therapy, in whom such therapy is no longer effective, and who cannot participate in the relevant clinical trials. Therefore, the parallel track reestablishes the clinical trial as the first priority for access to new agents. Nonetheless, the overall result of those new regulations has been a steady loosening in the regulatory standards surrounding the drug investigation process. Has the process gone far enough or perhaps too far?

As detailed by other investigators (254), who discuss these complex issues more thoroughly, a new consensus is possible regarding the approach to clinical investigation in the setting of AIDS. The essential factors must still, in our view, include an emphasis on the randomized controlled clinical trial. However, maximal scientific validity must be balanced with individual beneficence. Although no question exists that placebo controls most often yield the best or most valid comparison, this strategy may not always be in a person's best interest in a given trial. We do not intend to imply that placebos are unethical in the setting of AIDS (253), but when the end point of a given study is death, the use of historical controls may be a necessary compromise. Moreover, community consultation should now be a part of the design of any study, if for no other reason than to bring trust back to the investigator–subject relationship. These consultants should include potential subjects or their designated representatives. All groups affected by the research should be eligible for a given protocol whenever possible. Specific exclusion or lack of easy access to trials has been a major criticism of previous investigations. Recent observations suggest that this issue remains a major concern. In a study in Boston, being a person of color or having acquired HIV by injection drug use was independently associated with nonparticipation in clinical trials. In an unadjusted analysis (257), women with HIV were also less likely to enroll in trials.

Despite the appropriate emphasis on controlled clinical trials, there can be no turning back from a policy of increased availability of unproven medications for those with HIV infection. The parallel track program is the best current compromise for medications currently tested or soon to be tested, especially when geography is the main reason for lack of access to a given study. However, this program does not address the numerous unproven therapies that may never be evaluated in a controlled setting. Therefore, expanded access to unproven therapies may be appropriate, but it is not without problems. Risks of such a policy include potential interference with ongoing clinical studies if patients are taking unproven therapies with potential efficacy or confounding toxicities, uncertain risks of toxicity or death, and a significant financial risk for themselves or their families without certainty of benefit. Many individuals with AIDS and other chronic or life-threatening illnesses are significant targets for unscrupulous distributors of expensive bogus remedies. Physicians need to discuss alternative therapies openly and nonjudgmentally with their patients, because immediate condemnation may lead the patient to seek care elsewhere. In the end, one can argue that, after the final calculation of risks and benefits, those living with AIDS should decide what risk to take with regard to therapy.

AIDS IN THE WORLD

At the global level, HIV/AIDS is a tragedy of human suffering from which almost no country and no culture escapes. Some nations, however, continue to be more vulnerable to HIV/AIDS than others, for reasons explored in this section. In their initial study of the pandemic, Mann and colleagues (5) developed a concept of "national vulnerability" to AIDS (ranked as high, medium, and low) using a two-dimensional matrix composed of scores on the AIDS programs of nations and an index of social vulnerability. The index contained several ethically relevant factors, including the overall condition of women (a measure of protection of several freedoms), the ratio of military to health and education spending, and a human development index that combined annual per capita income, life expectancy, adult literacy, and mean years of schooling (5). The conclusion of that study was dire and pessimistic; it reported a basic "dichotomy" in the response to the global crisis, one marked by "relative success at individual and community levels coupled with collective failure at national and international levels" (5). Unfortunately, the message 6 years later is no better. In our view, an adequate global response to this pandemic involves nothing short of a massive worldwide mobilization of resources and commitment that attends to the contextual realities of the pandemic as it affects particular nations and groups of people. The destinies of whole nations are at stake.

Stopping the Spread of the Pandemic: The Gender Gap

The economic and sociocultural conditions of a country often underlie its increased vulnerability to the HIV/AIDS pandemic. A clear correlation, for instance, exists between a country's increased vulnerability to HIV/AIDS and the low status it affords its women citizens. Gupta, Weiss, and Whelan (5), in *AIDS in the World II*, report that "women are increasingly affected in direct, indirect, and complex ways by the HIV/AIDS pandemic" and that "research, prevention, and care activities for women have been slow to develop."

This gender gap results, in part, from the assumptions that underlie the recommendations of most programs aimed at stopping the sexual transmission of HIV. These recommendations are usually the following: 1) abstain from sexual intercourse; 2) practice mutual monogamy; 3) use condoms consistently and correctly; and 4) access appropriate treatment for other STDs (5). Although these recommendations may be appropriate in industrialized nations in which women have greater status and power, they are almost useless in developing countries in which women by and large cannot control these aspects of their lives. Thus, HIV/AIDS prevalence among women in the developing world is 37 times that of the prevalence among relatively more powerful and independent women of industrialized countries. The prevalence of HIV/AIDS in men in developing nations, who have much power relative to their female counterparts despite their status as members of a developing nation, is only 9 times that of the prevalence of men in industrialized nations (5). Gupta, Weiss, and Whelan (5) call for nothing short of new recommendations informed by a new set of assumptions that takes "account of the economic and socio-cultural context within which many women live and the realities of their interactions with men."

Economic and sociocultural factors that are facts of life for women living in developing nations must be considered and made a part of any effective program to combat the spread of HIV in these areas. Women in developing countries have great difficulty in gaining access to education, salaried or wage-earning jobs, credit, training, and support for agricultural work. This already limited economic situation was greatly worsened by the worldwide recession of the 1980s, which affected developing nations especially strongly (5). Thus, women in these countries are in unusually dire straits, especially young, poor, widowed, divorced, and abandoned women and girls. As a result of these economic hardships, women in developing countries often resort to prostitution, either to earn money or other goods or merely to ensure their physical safety. The necessity to survive in the short term through sex with multiple partners, however, endangers the lives of these women in the long term because of their increasing risk of being infected with HIV.

In addition to sexual networking, more women in developing countries are actually put at increased risk of HIV infection by the nonmonogamous sexual activity of their sole male partners. Again, the inaccessibility to economic independence leads these women to view *leaving* the high-risk relationship as more immediately hazardous to them than remaining in the relationship. The option of attempting to change the high-risk behavior of their partners is also not feasible, because addressing the issue of infidelity is likely either to disrupt the financially necessary relationship or to endanger the woman's physical safety. Similarly, many women in these countries believe that if they initiated discussion about condom use during sex, their partners would assume that they were unfaithful and would react violently. Conversely, studies have shown that financially independent women, both in ethnic areas of the United States and in some African countries, are able to wield significant power in their relationships by withholding sex when their partner either refuses to use a condom or has an STD (5).

In addition to economic factors, several sociocultural factors place women living in developing countries at increased risk of HIV infection. These sociocultural factors are both more widespread and complex than the relevant economic factors just discussed and are also more difficult to eradicate. First, many feminine ideals held by cultures in the developing world place women who strive for these ideals at increased risk of HIV infection. According to these ideals, women are to be essentially ignorant of sexual matters and reproductive physiology; ignorance of these matters suggests purity and high virginal value, whereas knowledge suggests promiscuity and decreased value. Thus, most of these women know little about their bodies, contraception (including the correct use of condoms), pregnancy, and STDs (including HIV/AIDS). Men in these cultures, on the other hand, are seen as the teachers in sexual matters, and so their increased knowledge is considered appropriate. When these women do marry, they are expected to surrender their virginity so they may be mothers many times over. Thus, regular sexual activity is integrally tied to women's feminine roles, despite the unparalleled infidelity of their husbands that puts them at risk.

Obviously, this significant lack of information and understanding, as well as the enormous sociocultural pressure to reproduce, ensures that women cannot make informed, voluntary decisions regarding their sexual behavior and reproductive health. For instance, women in these cultures often accept the symptoms of STDs as part of their lives as women, rather than as a disease for which they could seek treatment. Similarly, some women have reported that they abstain from condom use because they fear either that the condom will be lost inside their body, possibly traveling to their throat, or that it will become lodged in the vagina and will bring the woman's reproductive organs with it when it is removed. Unmarried women often engage in anal sex and other sexual activities that safeguard against pregnancy and allow them to remain virgins technically but that, unknown to them, still put them at risk for STDs, including HIV/AIDS (5).

The corresponding masculine ideals in these cultures also place women at risk for HIV infection and other dangers. Although women are condemned for infidelity, men are permitted, and even expected, to have multiple sexual partners, a practice that often begins as early as adolescence, that men believe is necessary for a sense of importance and popularity in the community and that is seen by both men and women as a male biologic imperative (5). A second masculine ideal emphasizes the man's pleasure and control in the sexual relationship. Women, who are socialized to please and to obey men, especially in sexual relationships, believe they must do all they can to make sexual activity more pleasurable for men. They thus acquiesce to male demands not to use condoms and to engage in anal sex. Many women in Africa also insert drying agents made of roots, herbs, and scouring powder into their vagina. They believe that drying the vagina in this matter increases friction, and thus pleasure, for the man, and also that the drying agents will absorb their natural vaginal secretions, which they fear will be construed as a symptom of an STD that they contracted through extramarital sex. Finally, rape, the most extreme expression of male dominance and control, is a reality that women both within and outside of consensual relationships must face. Clearly, in these cases, many of the preventive measures recommended to women, such as condom use and partner control, are not options.

Providing women with HIV prevention methods that contradict both the economic realities and the entrenched sociocultural norms of their societies is to provide no options at all for the 75% of the world's women who live in developing countries (5). A suggestive study conducted by Whelan (5) shows that "the higher the level of women's status or gender equality, the lower the HIV seroprevalence among pregnant women." Any effective plan to halt the spread of HIV/AIDS in most of the world's female population will thus have two components. First, some strategy to improve the status of women in these nations is needed to empower them to take control over their sexual and reproductive health. However, giving women this control would require potentially unrealizable goals, particularly in the short term, such as an enormous overhaul in these countries' systems of financial distribution and their sociocultural concepts of masculinity and femininity. Second, an effective prevention program for these women must also be informed by the realities of their lives. Alternative prevention methods that do not contradict their countries' economic and social realities must be developed and educationally disseminated among women.

Gupta, Weiss, and Whelan (5) offered several specific suggestions to this effect: 1) structural changes are needed to increase women's access to education, credit, training, and employment; 2) resources should be directed toward biomedical research to find a female-controlled method of STD protection that cannot be detected by the woman's partner; 3) the social stigma of seeking STD services should be removed, by integrating these services with family planning and maternal health services; 4) girls and women should be educated about their bodies and about such things as the proper way to use condoms and to negotiate safe sexual behaviors with their male partners; 5) boys and men should be eductaed about the consequences of multiple-partner sex and other high-risk sexual activities, to reduce not only their own HIV risk, but also that of their female partners; and 6) research that continues to explore the economic and sociocultural underpinnings of increasing HIV risk among women should be funded, to enable designers of prevention programs to attend to the realities of women's lives (5).

We have been using women, one of the fastest growing populations of newly HIV-infected people in the world today, as an example of a vulnerable population. We could have chosen other vulnerable, high-risk populations such as children (5). Our discussion, however, is meant to suggest that *all* prevention and treatment programs must attend to the contextual factors in which these programs are intended to be effective. There is no other way to achieve success in combating the spread of this disease. Failure to recognize these contextual realities will ensure the deaths of millions.

Research Ethics on the International Scene

Programs of prevention and treatment of HIV/AIDS, however, must take place within the boundaries of clinical, social, and research ethics. The project to combat the spread of AIDS within ethical boundaries has been challenged with the start of several HIV/AIDS trials sponsored by Western countries in non–Western host countries. In 1994, a double-blind, placebo-controlled study called Protocol 076 revealed that intensive treatment of HIV-infected women and their newborn babies with ZDV (a drug that had been first created and then shelved by Burroughs Wellcome after it failed to be effective in treating cancer) significantly reduced the rate of transmission of the virus from mother to child by two-thirds (258). Since the study, the regimen of ZDV involved in Protocol 076 (ZDV given to the pregnant woman during the last weeks of her pregnancy, intravenously during labor, and to her baby for the first weeks of its life) has become the standard of care in the United States and in other industrialized nations (259). The intense prenatal, obstetric, and postpartum care required by the protocol, however, has a price tag—more than $1000 per pregnancy (260). Unfortunately, this is a cost that most undeveloped nations cannot afford. As a result, some 18 trials involving more than 17,000 women were begun to find more affordable ways for developing countries to reduce the rate of HIV transmission between mother and child. Some of the trials involved lower doses of ZDV for less time; others involved antiseptic vaginal washes, treating the woman with anti-HIV immunoglobulin, and treating either the woman or her baby with various vitamins (261). Of the various trials, many believe that those involving brief treatments of low-dose ZDV are the most promising. In all likelihood, the Protocol 076 regimen involves more ZDV than is actually needed. However, researchers do not yet know which part of that protocol is effective in reducing the HIV transmission rate. In part, answering this question is the goal of the trials in developing countries. If the answer could be found, effective ZDV treatments could cost a mere $50 per pregnancy (260), a cost that most nations may well be able to afford.

These trials have been controversial. First, whereas the sponsoring, "research" countries are wealthy, the host, "subject" countries are not. To many, the image of privileged people conducting research on relatively uneducated, poor Africans understandably raises the specter of the US Public Health Service Syphilis Study (better, if somewhat inappropriately, known as Tuskegee), a 40-year, federally funded study of untreated syphilis in black men in Macon County, Alabama. In this spirit, Angell notes that many trials done in developing countries could not be done in the sponsoring countries: "Clinical trials have become a big business, with many of the same imperatives. To survive, it is necessary to get the work done as quickly as possible, with a minimum of obstacles. When these considerations prevail, it seems as if we have not come very far from Tuskegee after all" (262).

A second point of controversy has centered on the finding that because Protocol 076 proved ZDV to be effective in reducing the chances of transmission of HIV from American women to their children, the women in the African trials receiving the placebos would be denied the best known preventive treatment against perinatal HIV transmission. Such codes as the World Medical Association's (WMA) Declaration of Helsinki, The Nuremberg Code, and the International Ethical Guidelines for Biomedical Research Involving Human Subjects, developed jointly by the Council for International Organizations of Medical Sciences (CIOMS) and the World Health Organization (WHO), stress the importance of putting the welfare of human research subjects above the good of society or scientific inquiry. According to the Helsinki Code: "In any medical study, every patient—including those of a control group, if any—should be assured of the best proven diagnostic and therapeutic method" (263). Thus, a traditional justification of both randomized clinical trials and placebo trials is that they satisfy the principle of clinical equipoise, in which researchers are either indifferent to or torn about which of two treatment options (including, possibly, a no-treatment option) is more effective (264). Moreover, "Every biomedical research project involving human subjects should be preceded by careful assessment of predictable risks in comparison with foreseeable benefits to the subject or to others. Concern for the interests of the subject must always prevail over the interests of science and society" (263).

In the eyes of critics, these principles of human subject research are absolutely necessary to ethical research in any context. Satisfying the elements of informed consent and receiving approval from an institutional review board, albeit also necessary, are seen as insufficient, because of the unequal balance of knowledge and power between researchers and subjects and the variation in institutional review board protection of patients' interests when those interests conflict with the goals of science (262). Universal ethical principles of the type that comprise the Helsinki Code are meant to protect against bias, because they are intentionally applied in a manner that is blind to the particular context of the research. According to critics, the African trials do not meet these essential ethical requirements of guaranteeing the best known treatment and of putting the welfare of all the subjects ahead of society.

We respond, with others (260, 265, 266), as follows. First, the analogy to Tuskegee is misapplied, to say the least. Angell notes that some of the ethical violations that make the Tuskegee study a negative paradigm for human subject research are 1) that the men studied did not give informed consent, and were, in fact, lied to; and 2) that they were denied effective treatment after it became available, and were, in fact, prevented in various extreme ways from receiving treatment when they sought it. In the case of the African trials, however, subjects give fully informed consent, and they are not being denied effective treatment available in their country. The placebo group is, of course, being denied the simplified regimen of ZDV, but ZDV, whether in simplified form or not, has not been shown to be effective in this particular population. Although the full Protocol 076 regimen of ZDV is effective in the United States, it may also prove to be ineffective or even dangerous in African women; additionally, this regimen is simply unavailable in the host countries. Certainly, that wealthy countries can afford medical treatment that poor countries cannot is unjust. However, to fail to conduct research that would potentially help poor populations benefit from that medicine, but within their budgets, is to make the perfect the enemy of the good.

To the charge that the trials violate essential ethical principles such as clinical equipoise, we have two replies. First, it is not clear that clinical equipoise is really being violated. The trials are intended to answer two questions: 1) Are simplified drug regimens of ZDV better than nothing (which is what African women are currently receiving)? and 2) Is ZDV safe for pregnant women and their fetuses, as it so far appears to be in the United States? With respect to these questions, there is not clinical equipoise. Critics of the controlled trials advocate instead equivalency trials, in which simplified regimens of ZDV are tested against the full Protocol 076. For several reasons, researchers collaborating in both the sponsoring and host countries decided that a control trial was necessary. The fastest and most accurate answers to these questions can come only with controlled trials. If all subjects were given ZDV, and some or all of them experienced morbidity or mortality, researchers would not know whether ZDV was dangerous to this population or whether the illness and death were due to an external cause. Similarly, if the simplified regimens proved to be less effective than the full regimen, little benefit could be gained by anyone from these results. Researchers still would not know whether the limited regimens were better than nothing—the current "treatment," and the subjects and their fellow citizens would still not be able to afford the full regimen.

A recent report (267) of preliminary findings from one of the trials in Thailand, presented at the 4th International Conference on AIDS in Asia and the Pacific, demonstrates the importance of placebo-controlled trials. In the Thai study, one group of HIV-positive pregnant women was given a 2-week course of ZDV at 600 mg per day, whereas the control group received a placebo. The transmission rate for the ZDV group was 14.9%; the rate for the control group was slightly (but statistically insignificantly) higher at 16.3% (KE Nelson, unpublished data). Angell argues that "[s]ometimes there may be relevant differences between populations, but that cannot be assumed" (262). Because the rate of perinatal HIV transmission in both groups of women was, for clinical and statistical purposes, the same, the trial results demonstrate that we cannot assume that what we believe to be a protective dose and duration of ZDV will actually protect the particular fetuses in question.

Moreover, a previous study of perinatal HIV transmission in Bangkok, according to Nelson (KE Nelson, unpublished data), found the rate to be 25%. Investigators who support the placebo trials in Thailand and in other developing nations thus noted that had the placebo-controlled group not existed, it would have been assumed that the trial ZDV dose was responsible for reducing the transmission rate from 25 to 14.9%, when in fact, the placebo group's transmission rate of 16.3% shows that the trial dosage of ZDV was ineffective in reducing HIV transmission altogether. The result of this assumption would likely have been a new standard of care in Thailand of a 10- to 14-day course of ZDV, but this care would really have been a waste of ZDV. These investigators concluded that "[c]learly more controlled studies need to be done to establish which dose and duration of AZT that is feasible in a developing country is also effective" (KE Nelson, unpublished data).

This trial is, of course, not perfect. One problem is the low membership in each group (90 subjects receiving ZDV, 92 control subjects receiving a placebo), which renders the results statistically weak (j), a point critics of placebo-controlled trials such as Wolfe, Lurie, and Angell have been quick to note.

Our second, related, response to the charge that the trials fail to meet universal ethical standards is that, although codes such as those of Nuremberg and Helsinki are important sources of ethical guidance in many ways, we argue that they should be viewed as just that—*guidance*—rather than absolute, universal rules that lack flexibility and an appreciation for context. As in our discussion of the design of prevention programs for the spread of HIV/AIDS, research designs, too, must take into account the particular contexts in which that research is being done if we wish to achieve accurate and beneficial results.

References

1. Pizzo PA, Wilfert CM. Pediatric AIDS: the challenge of HIV infection in infants, children, and adolescents. 2nd ed. Baltimore: Williams & Wilkins, 1994.
2. National Commission on AIDS. America living with AIDS: transforming anger, fear, and indifference into action. Washington, DC: National Commission on AIDS, 1991.
3. Graubard S. Living with AIDS. Daedalus 1987;118(2: Special issue):1–201; and 1989;118(3: Special issue):1–254.
4. Mann J, Tarantola DJM, Netter TW, eds. AIDS in the world. Cambridge, MA: Harvard University Press, 1992.
5. Mann J, Tarantola DJM, eds. AIDS in the world II. New York: Oxford University Press, 1996.
6. Johnston WB, Hopkins KR. The catastrophe ahead. New York: Praeger, 1990:148.
7. Gould SJ. The terrifying normalcy of AIDS. New York Times Magazine, April 19, 1987.
8. Jonsen AR. American moralism and the origin of bioethics in the United States. J Med Philos 1991;16:113–130.
9. Katz J. Silent world of doctor and patient. New York: Free Press, 1984.
10. Pellegrino ED, Thomasma D. For the patient's good. New York: Oxford University Press, 1988.
11. Cassell E. The nature of suffering and the goals of medicine. New York: Oxford University Press, 1991.
12. Brody H. The healer's power. New Haven: Yale University Press, 1992.
13. Buchanan AE. Is there a medical profession in the house? In: Spece RG, Shimm DS, Buchanan AE, eds. Conflicts of interest in clinical practice and research. New York: Oxford University Press, 1996:105–136.
14. Childress JF, Siegler M. Metaphors and models of doctor–patient relationships: their implications for autonomy. Theor Med 1984;5:17–30.
15. Sontag S. AIDS and its metaphors. New York: Farrar, Straus, & Giroux, 1989.
16. Bayer R. Private acts, social consequence: AIDS and the politics of public health. New York: Free Press, 1989.
17. Bayer R. Public health policy and the AIDS epidemic: an end to HIV exceptionalism? N Engl J Med 1991;324:1500–1504.
18. Bayer R. As the second decade of AIDS begins: an international perspective on the ethics of the epidemic. AIDS 1992;6:527–532.
19. Bayer R. AIDS and ethics. In: Veatch RM, ed. Medical ethics. 2nd ed. Sudbury, MA: Jones & Bartlett, 1997;395–413.
20. Thomas SB, Quinn SC. The Tuskegee syphilis study, 1932 to 1972: implications for HIV education and AIDS risk education programs in the black community. Am J Public Health 1991;81:1498–1505.
21. Jones JH. Bad blood: the Tuskegee syphilis experiment. 2nd ed. New York: Free Press, 1993.
22. Grmek MD. History of AIDS: emergence and origin of a modern pandemic. Princeton, NJ: Princeton University Press, 1990.
23. National Research Council. The social impact of AIDS in the United States. Washington, DC: National Academy Press, 1993.
24. National Research Council. Committee on AIDS Research and the Behavioral, Social, and Statistical Sciences. AIDS: the second decade. Washington, DC: National Academy Press, 1990:48.
25. Centers for Disease Control and Prevention. The HIV/AIDS epidemic: the first 10 years. MMWR Morb Mortal Wkly Rep 1991;40:359.
26. Grady C. The search for an AIDS vaccine. Bloomington, IN: Indiana University Press, 1995.
27. Rothman D. Strangers at the bedside. New York: Basic Books, 1991.
28. Beauchamp TL, Childress JC. Principles of biomedical ethics. 4th ed. New York: Oxford University Press, 1995.
29. Sider R, Clements CD. The new medical ethics: a second opinion. Arch Intern Med 1985;145:2169–2173.
30. Clauser KD, Gert B. A critique of principlism. J Med Philos 1990;15:219–236.
31. Jonsen AR, Siegler M, Winslade W. Clinical ethics. 4th ed. New York, McGraw-Hill, 1998.
32. Fletcher JC, Miller FG, Lombardo PA, et al. Introduction to clinical ethics. 2nd ed. Frederick, MD: University Publishing Group, 1997.

33. Engelhardt HT. Foundations of bioethics. 2nd ed. New York: Oxford University Press, 1996:16.
34. Hunter JD. Culture wars: the struggle to define America. New York: Basic Books, 1991.
35. National Commission for the Protection of Human Subjects of Biomedical and Behavioral Research. The Belmont report, April 18, 1979. Washington, DC: US Government Printing Office, 1986:181–296:41238.
36. Gilligan C. In a different voice: psychological theory and women's development. Cambridge, MA: Harvard University Press, 1982.
37. Sherwin S. No longer patient. Philadelphia: Temple University Press, 1992.
38. Wolf SM. Introduction: gender and feminism in bioethics. In: Wolf SM, ed. Feminism and bioethics: beyond reproduction. New York: Oxford University Press, 1996:14–16.
39. Baier A. What do women want in a moral theory? Nous 1985;19:53–64.
40. Noddings N. Caring: a feminine approach to ethics and moral education. Berkeley, CA: University of California Press, 1984.
41. Zuger A. AIDS and the obligations of health care professionals. In: Reamer FG, ed. AIDs and ethics. New York: Columbia University Press, 1991:215–218.
42. Wenrich MD, Ramsey PG. Patterns of primary care of patients infected with human immunodeficiency virus. West J Med 1991; 155:380–383.
43. Gerbert B, Maguire BT, Bleecker T, et al. Primary care physicians and AIDS. JAMA 1991;266:2837–2842.
44. Proceedings of the National Medical Convention 1846–1847. In: Reiser SJ, Dyck AJ, Curran WJ, eds. Ethics in medicine: historical perspectives and contemporary concerns. Cambridge: MIT Press, 1977:29–34.
45. American Medical Association, Council on Ethical and Judicial Affairs. Statement on AIDS: proceedings of the 40th interim meeting, Las Vegas, NE, December 7–10, 1986.
46. American Medical Association, Council on Ethical and Judicial Affairs. Ethical issues involved in the growing AIDS crises. JAMA 1988;259: 1360–1361.
47. Fox DM. The politics of physicians' responsibility in epidemics: a note on history. In: Fox E, Fox DM, eds. AIDS: the burdens of history. Berkeley, CA: University of California Press, 1988:86–96.
48. Zuger A, Miles S. Physicians, AIDS, and occupational risks: historical traditions and ethical obligations. JAMA 1987;258:1924–1928.
49. Arras JD. The fragile web of responsibility: AIDS and the duty to treat. Hastings Cent Rep 1988;18:10–20.
50. Jonsen AR. The duty to treat patients with AIDS and HIV infection. In: Gostin LO, ed. AIDS and the healthcare system. New Haven, CT: Yale University Press, 1990:155–168.
51. Pellegrino ED. Altruism, self-interest, and medical ethics. JAMA 1987;258:1939–1940.
52. Loewy E. AIDS and the physician's fear of contagion. Chest 1986; 89:325–326.
53. Emmanuel EJ. Do physicians have an obligation to treat patients with AIDS? N Engl J Med 1988;318:1686–1690.
54. Levine RJ. AIDS and the physician-patient relationship. In: Reamer FG, ed. AIDS and ethics. New York: Columbia University Press, 1991:188–214.
55. Daniels N. Duty to treat or right to refuse? Hastings Cent Rep 1991;21:36–46.
56. Smolkin D. HIV infection, risk taking, and the duty to treat. J Med Philos 1997;22:55–74.
57. Sims AJW, Dudley AJF. Surgeons and HIV. Br Med J 1988;296:80.
58. Gerberding JL, Littell C, Tarkington A, et al. Risk of exposure of surgical personnel to patients' blood during surgery at San Francisco General Hospital. N Engl J Med 1988;322:1788–1793.
59. AMA Physician Guidelines. HIV early care. Chicago: American Medical Association, 1991.
60. White DA, Gold JWM, eds. Medical management of AIDS patients. Med Clin North Am 1992;76(1):19–44.
61. Carey L, ed. AIDS: problems and prospects. New York: Norton Medical Books, 1993.
62. American College of Obstetricians and Gynecologists (ACOG). Human immunodeficiency virus infection. Washington, DC: ACOG technical bulletin no. 162, 1992:1–11.
63. AIDS Care Program. Recommendations for the medical care of persons with HIV infection. 2nd ed. Baltimore: Johns Hopkins Medical Institute, 1992.
64. Bennett CL, Garfinkle JB, Greenfield S, et al. The relation between hospital experience and in-hospital mortality for patients with AIDS-related PCP. JAMA 1989;261:2975–2979.
65. Stone VE, Seage GR III, Hertz T, et al. The relation between hospital experience and mortality for patients with AIDS. JAMA 1992;268: 2655–2661.
66. Kitahata MM, Koepsell TD, Deyo RA, et al. Physicians' experience with the acquired immunodeficiency syndrome as a factor in patients' survival. N Engl J Med 1996;334:701–706.
67. Volberding PA. Improving the outcomes of care for patients with human immunodeficiency virus infection. N Engl J Med 1996;334: 729–731.
68. Carpenter CCJ, Fischl MA, Hammer BA, et al. Antiretroviral therapy for HIV infection in 1997: updated recommendations of the International AIDS Society–USA panel. JAMA 1997;277:1962–1969.
69. Schoeman F. AIDS and privacy. In: Reamer FG, ed. AIDS and ethics. New York: Columbia University Press, 1991:240–276.
70. Blendon R, Donelon K. Discrimination against people with AIDS. N Engl J Med 1988;319:1022–1026.
71. Behringer v. Medical Center at Princeton, 249 N.J. Super. 597 (1991).
72. Alter J, McKillop P. AIDS and the right to know: a question of privacy. Newsweek, August 18, 1986:46–47.
73. Siegler M. Confidentiality in medicine: a decrepit concept. N Engl J Med 1982;307:1518–1521.
74. Schmid D, Appelbaum PS, Roth LS, et al. Confidentiality in psychiatry: a study of the patient's view. Hosp Commun Psychiatry 1983;34: 353–355.
75. Appelbaum PS, Kapeu G, Walters B, et al. Confidentiality: an empirical test of the utilitarian perspective. Bull Am Acad Psychiatry Law 1984;12:109–116.
76. Gunderson M, Mayo DJ, Rhame FS. AIDS: testing and privacy. Salt Lake City, UT: University of Utah Press, 1989:59–73.
77. Smith JW, Allen R. Privacy, medical confidentiality, and AIDS. In: Smith JW, ed. AIDS, philosophy and beyond: philosophical dilemmas of a modern pandemic. Brookfield, VT: Avebury, 1991:195–236.
78. Freedman B. Violating confidentiality to warn of a risk of HIV infection: ethical work in progress. Theor Med 1991;12:309–323.
79. Macklin R. HIV-infected psychiatric patients: beyond confidentiality. Ethics Behav 1991;1:3–20.
80. Marshall S. Doctors' rights and patients' obligations. Bioethics 1990; 292–310.
81. Winston ME. AIDS, confidentiality, and the right to know. Public Affairs Q 1988;2:91–104.
82. Gillett G. AIDS and confidentiality. J Appl Philos 1987;12:7–53.
83. Gillon R. AIDS and medical confidentiality. BMJ 1987;294:1675–1677.
84. HIV counseling in the 1990s [editorial]. Lancet 1991;337:950.
85. Jansen RS, St Louis ME, Satten GA, et al. HIV infection among patients in U.S. acute care hospitals: strategies for the counseling and testing of hospital patients. N Engl J Med 1992;327:445–452.
86. Quinn TC. Screening for HIV infection: benefits and costs. N Engl J Med 1992;327:486–488.
87. Kelen GD, DiGiovanna T, Bisson L, et al. Human immunodeficiency virus infection in emergency department patients: epidemiology, clinical presentations, and risk to health care workers. The Johns Hopkins experience. JAMA 1989;262:516–522.
88. Krasinski K, Borkowsky W, Bebenroth D, et al. Failure of voluntary testing for HIV to identify infected parturient women in a high risk population. N Engl J Med 1988;318:185–189.

89. Gevisser M. Women and children first. Village Voice, October 18, 1989:18.
90. Faden RR, Geller G, Powers M, et al. HIV infection, pregnant women, and newborns: a policy proposal for information and testing. In: Faden RR, Geller G, Powers M, eds. AIDS, women, and the next generation. New York: Oxford University Press, 1991:331–358.
91. Fischl M, Dickinson G, La Vioe L. Safety and efficacy of sulfamethoxazole and trimethoprim chemoprophylaxis for *Pneumocystis carinii* pnuemonia in AIDS. JAMA 1988;259:1185–1189.
92. Volberding P, Lagakos S, Koch M, et al. Zidovudine in asymptomatic human immunodeficiency virus infection: a controlled trial in persons with fewer than 500 CD4 positive cells per cubic millimeter. N Engl J Med 1990;322:941–949.
93. Centers for Disease Control and Prevention. Publicly funded HIV counseling and testing: United States, 1991. MMWR Morb Mortal Wkly Rep 1992;41:613–617.
94. Valenti W. HIV testing and counseling. In: Valenti W, ed. Early intervention in the management of HIV: a handbook for the managed healthcare professional. Rochester, NY: Community Health Network, 1992:13.
95. Gostin LO, Ward JW, Baker AC. National HIV case reporting for the United States: a defining moment in the history of the epidemic. N Engl J Med 1997;337:1162–1167.
96. Centers for Disease Control and Prevention. Update: trends in AIDS incidence, deaths, and prevalence: United States, 1996. MMWR Morb Mortal Wkly Rep 1997;46;165-173.
97. World Health Organization (WHO). Guidelines for counseling about HIV infection and disease. Geneva: WHO, 1990.
98. Strawn JM. The psychosocial consequences of HIV infection. In: Durham JD, Cohen L, eds. The person with AIDS: nursing perspectives. 2nd ed. New York: Springer, 1991:113–134.
99. Ostrow DG. Psychiatric aspects of AIDS: an overview. In: Ostrow DG, ed. Behavioral aspects of AIDS. New York: Plenum, 1990:9–18.
100. Schaffner B. Reactions of medical personnel and intimates to persons with AIDS. In: Ostrow DG, ed. Behavioral aspects of AIDS. New York: Plenum, 1990:341–354.
101. Marzuk PM, Tierney H, Tardiff K, et al. Increased risk of suicide in persons with AIDS. JAMA 1988;260:1333–1337.
102. Cates W, Handsfield HH. HIV counseling and testing: does it work? Am J Public Health 1988;78:1533–1534.
103. Ebright JR, Crane L. Psychological impact of screening for human immunodeficiency virus. AIDS Patient Care 1991;5:29–33.
104. Sloand EM, Pitt E, Chiarello RJ, et al. HIV testing: state of the art. JAMA 1991;266:2861–2865.
105. Saag MS. AIDS testing. Now and in the future. In: Sande MA, Volberding PA, eds. The medical management of AIDS. 3rd ed. Philadelphia: WB Saunders, 1992:47.
106. Meyer KB, Pauker SG. Screening for HIV: can we afford the false positive rate? N Engl J Med 1987;317:239–341.
107. Burke DS, Brundage JF, Redfield RR, et al. Measurement of the false positive rate in a screening program for human immunodeficiency virus infections. N Engl J Med 1988;319:961–964.
108. VanDevanter NL. HIV testing and counseling. In: Durham JD, Cohen L, eds. The person with AIDS: nursing perspectives. 2nd ed. New York: Springer, 1991:81.
109. Gostin L. Ethical principles for the conduct of human subject research: population-based research and ethics. Law Med Health Care 1991;19:191–201.
110. Levine RJ. Informed consent: some challenges to the universal validity of the western model. Law Med Health Care 1991;19:207–213.
111. Geller G, Kass NE. Informed consent in the context of prenatal HIV screening. In: Faden RR, Geller G, Powers M, eds. AIDS, women, and the next generation. New York: Oxford University Press, 1991:288–307.
112. Faden RR, Geller G, Powers M, et al. HIV infection, pregnant women, and newborns: a policy proposal for information and testing. In: Faden RR, Geller G, Powers M, eds. AIDS, women, and the next generation. New York: Oxford University Press, 1991: 331–358.
113. Committee on Obstetrics, Maternal and Fetal Medicine, American College of Obstetricians and Gynecologists (ACOG). Voluntary testing for human immunodeficiency virus. Washington, DC: ACOG opinion no. 97, 1991.
114. Committee on Technical Bulletins, American College of Obstetricians and Gynecologists (ACOG). Human immunodeficiency virus infections. Washington, DC: ACOG technical bulletin no. 169, 1992:7–8.
115. Douglas GC, King BF. Maternal–fetal transmission of human immunodeficiency virus: a review of possible routes and cellular mechanisms of infection. Clin Infect Dis 1992;15:678–691.
116. Kass NE. Reproductive decision making in the context of HIV: the case for nondirective counseling. In: Faden RR, Geller G, Powers M, eds. AIDS, women, and the next generation. New York: Oxford University Press, 1991:308–327.
117. Centers for Disease Control. Recommendations for assisting in the prevention of the perinatal transmission HTLV-III/LAV and acquired immunodeficiency syndrome. MMWR Morb Mortal Wkly Rep 1985;34:721–731.
118. American College of Obstetricians and Gynecologists (ACOG). Prevention of human immune deficiency virus infection and acquired immune deficiency syndrome. Washington, DC: ACOG committee statement no. 53, 1987:1–4.
119. Arras J. HIV infection and reproductive decisions: an ethical analysis [abstract]. In: 5th International Conference on AIDS, Montreal, 1989.
120. Arras J. HIV and childbearing: AIDS and reproductive decisions. Having children in fear and trembling. Milbank Q 1990; 68:353–382.
121. European Collaborative Study. Mother-to-child transmission of HIV infection. Lancet 1988;2:1039–1042.
122. Italian Multicentre Study. Epidemiology, clinical features, and prognostic factors of paediatric HIV infection. Lancet 1988;2:1043–1046.
123. Cowan MJ, Walter C, Culver K, et al. Maternally transmitted HIV infection in children. AIDS 1988;2:437–441.
124. Blanche S, Rouzioux C, Moscato ML, et al. A prospective study of infants born to women seropositive for human immunodeficiency virus type 1: HIV infection in newborns. French Collaborative Study Group. N Engl J Med 1989;320:1643–1648.
125. European Collaborative Study. Children born to women with HIV-1 infection: natural history and risk of transmission. Lancet 1991;337:253–260.
126. Minkoff HL. Duerr A, Schwarz RH. AIDS in obstetrics and gynecology. Washington, DC: ACOG update no. 18, 1992:4.
127. Connor E, Sperling R, Gelber R, et al. Reduction of maternal-infant transmission of human immunodeficiency virus type 1 with zivovudine treatment. N Engl J Med 1994;331:1173-1178.
128. Bayer R. AIDS and the future of reproductive freedom. Milbank Q 1990;68(Suppl 2):178–204.
129. Tribe LH. Abortion. The clash of absolutes. New York: WW Norton, 1990.
130. Planned Parenthood of Southeastern Pennsylvania v. Casey, 112 S. Ct. 2791 (1992).
131. Shaw M. Preconception and prenatal torts. In: Milunsky A, Annas GJ, eds. Genetics and the law. II. New York: Plenum, 1980:225–232.
132. Wertz DC, Mulvihill JJ, Fletcher JC. Medical geneticists confront ethical dilemmas: cross-cultural comparisons among 18 nations. Am J Hum Genet 1990;46:1200–1213.
133. Brent RL. The magnitude of the problem of congenital malformations. In: Brent RL, ed. Prevention of physical and mental congenital defects. A. The scope of the problem. New York: Alan R. Liss, 1985:55.
134. Sun N. Bioethics in medical genetics in China. Presented at the meeting of the Japan Society for Human Genetics, Fukui, Japan, 1990.
135. Michaels D, Levine C. Estimates of the number of motherless youth orphaned by AIDS in the United States. JAMA 1992;268:345–346.
136. Nicholas SW, Abrams EJ. The "silent" legacy of AIDS: children who survive their parents and siblings. JAMA 1992;268:3478–3479.
137. Marzuk PM, Tierney H, Tardiff K, et al. Increased risk of suicide in persons with AIDS. JAMA 1988;259:1333–1337.

138. Kizer KW, Green M, Perkins CI, et al. AIDS and suicide in California. JAMA 1988;260:1881.
139. Starace F. Epidemiology of suicide among persons with AIDS. AIDS Care 1995;7(Suppl 2):S123–128.
140. van der Maas PJ, van der Wal G, Haverkate I, et al. Euthanasia, physician-assisted suicide, and other medical practices involving the end of life in the Netherlands, 1990–1995. N Engl J Med 1996;335: 1699–1705.
141. Bindels PJE, Krol A, van Ameijden E, et al. Euthanasia and physician-assisted suicide in homosexual men with AIDS. Lancet 1996;347: 499–504.
142. Breitbart W, Rosenfeld BD, Passik SD. Interest in physician-assisted suicide among ambulatory HIV-infected patients. Am J Psychiat 1996;153:238–242.
143. McCormick WC, Inui TS, Deyo RA, et al. Long-term care preferences of hospitalized persons with AIDS. J Gen Intern Med 1991;6:524–528.
144. Martin JP. Sustaining care of persons with AIDS. In: Durham JD, Cohen L, eds. The person with AIDS: nursing perspectives. 2nd ed. New York: Springer, 1991:276–299.
145. Emanuel LL, Emanuel EJ. The medical directive: a new comprehensive advance care document. JAMA 1989;261:3288–3293.
146. Meisel A. The right to die. vol. 2. 2nd ed. New York: John Wiley & Sons, 1995:11–13, 133, 211–213.
147. Price RW, Brew BJ. The AIDS dementia complex. J Infect Dis 1988;158:1079–1083.
148. Grant I, Hesselink JR, Kennedy CJ, et al. HIV disease: brain–behavior relationships. In: Ostrow DG, ed. Behavioral aspects of AIDS. New York: Plenum, 1990:247–266.
149. Brett AS. Limitations of listing specific medical interventions in advance directives. JAMA 1991;266:825–828.
150. Menikoff JA, Sachs GA, Siegler M. Beyond advance directives: health care surrogate laws. N Engl J Med 1992;327:1165–1169.
151. Virmani J, Schneiderman LJ, Kaplan RM. Relationship of advance directives to physician–patient communication. Arch Intern Med 1994;154:909–913.
152. Teno J, Lynn J, Phillips RS, et al. Do formal advance directives affect resuscitation decisions and the use of resources for seriously ill patients? J Clin Ethics 1994;5:23–30.
153. Batavia AI. Disability and physician-assisted suicide. N Engl J Med 1997;336:1671–1673.
154. Schulman DI. AIDS discrimination: its nature, meaning, and function. In: McKenzie NF, ed. The AIDS reader. New York: Meridian (Penguin Books), 1991:463–490.
155. National Center for Health Statistics. Mortality. part A, section 1. In: Vital statistics of the United States, 1991. DHHS publication no. (PHS) 96-1101:380–381. Washington, DC: US Government Printing Office, 1996. DHHS publication no. (PHS) 96-1101:380–381.
156. Susan Tolle, MD. Personal communication, 1996, citing Oregon Health Division Vital Statistics, 1995.
157. President's Commission for the Study of Ethical Problems in Medicine and Biomedical and Behavioral Research. Decisions to forego life-sustaining treatment. Washington, DC: US Government Printing Office, 1983:17–18.
158. Weir RF, Gostin L. Decisions to abate life-sustaining treatment for nonautonomous patients. JAMA 1990;264:1846–1853.
159. In re Quinlan, 70 NJ 10, 355 A 2d 647 (1976).
160. Cruzan v. Director, Missouri Dept. of Health, 110 S. Ct. 2841 (1990).
161. Davidson HA. Should we legalize mercy killing? Med Econom 1950;8:64–66.
162. Kamisar Y. Some non-religious views against proposed mercy killing legislation. Minn Law Rev 1958;42:16–36.
163. Fletcher JF. Morals and medicine. Princeton, NJ: Princeton University Press, 1954:
164. St John-Stevas N. Life, death and the law. Cleveland: World Publishing Company (Meridian Book), 1964.
165. Kohl M, ed. Beneficent euthanasia. Buffalo: Prometheus Books, 1975.
166. Russell OR. Freedom to die. New York: Human Sciences Press, 1975.
167. Rachels J. Active and passive euthanasia. In: Baird R, Rosenbaum S, eds. Euthanasia. Buffalo: Prometheus Books, 1989:49–63.
168. Emanuel EJ. The history of euthanasia debates in the United States and Britain. Ann Intern Med 1994;121:793–802.
169. Battin M. Voluntary euthanasia and the risks of abuse: can we learn anything from the Netherlands? Law Med Health Care 1992; 20: 133–143.
170. Gomez C. Regulating death. New York: Free Press, 1991.
171. Van der Mass PJ, van Delden JJM, Pijenborg L, et al. Euthanasia and other medical decisions concerning the end of life. Lancet 1991;338: 669–674.
172. Jonsen AR. Initiative 119: what is at stake? Commonweal 1991; 24(Suppl):2–4.
173. Capron AM, Michel V. California Proposition 161: what is at stake. Commonweal 1992;25(Suppl):2–5.
174. Lee M, Tolle SW. Oregon's assisted suicide vote: the silver lining. Ann Intern Med 1996;124:267-269.
175. Suicide law withstands a challenge. New York Times February 28, 1997:A20.
176. Wanzer SH, Federman DD, Adelstein SJ, et al. The physician's response toward hopelessly ill patients: a second look. N Engl J Med 1989;320:844–849.
177. Quill TE. Death and dignity: a case of individualized decision making. N Engl J Med 1991;324:691–694.
178. Quill TE, Cassel CK, Meier DE. Care of the hopelessly ill: proposed clinical criteria for physician-assisted suicide. N Engl J Med 1992;327: 1380–1384.
179. Brody H. Assisted death: a compassionate response to a medical failure. N Engl J Med 1992;327:1384–1388.
180. Benrubi GI. Euthanasia: the need for procedural safeguards. N Engl J Med 1992;326:197–199.
181. Misbin RI. Physicians' aid in dying. N Engl J Med 1991;325:1307–1311.
182. Miller FG, Quill TE, Brody H, et al. Regulating physician-assisted death. N Engl J Med 1994;331:119–123.
183. Callahan D. The troubled dream of life: living with mortality. New York: Simon & Schuster, 1993.
184. Kamisar Y. Against assisted suicide: even in a very limited form. U Detroit Mercy Law Rev 1995;72:739–753.
185. New York State Task Force on Life and the Law. When death is sought: assisted suicide and euthanasia in the medical context. New York: New York State Task Force on Life and the Law, 1994.
186. American Medical Association. Report B of the Council on Ethical and Judicial Affairs (Richard J. McMurray, MD, Chairperson): decisions near the end of life. Chicago: American Medical Association, 1991.
187. Bachman JG, Alcser KH, Doukas DJ, et al. Attitudes of Michigan physicians and the public toward legalizing physician-assisted suicide and voluntary euthanasia. N Engl J Med 1996;334:303–309.
188. Back AI, Wallace JI, Starks HE, et al. Physician-assisted suicide and euthanasia in Washington state: patient requests and physician responses. JAMA 1996;275:919–925.
189. Slome LR, Mitchell TF, Charlebois E, et al. Physician-assisted suicide and patients with human immunodeficiency virus disease. N Engl J Med 1997;336:417–421.
190. Roper Center for Public Opinion Research at the University of Connecticut, Storrs, CT, 1993.
191. Compassion in Dying v. Washington, 79 F.3d 790 (9th Cir. 1996).
192. Quill v. Vacco, 80 F3d 716 (2d Cir. 1996).
193. Washington v. Glucksberg, 117 S. Ct. 2302 (1997).
194. Vacco v. Quill. 117 S. Ct. 2293 (1997).
195. Annas GJ. The bell tolls for a constitutional right to physician-assisted suicide. N Engl J Med 1997;337:1098–1103.
196. Burt RA. The Supreme Court speaks: not assisted suicide but a constitutional right to palliative care. N Engl J Med 1997;337: 1234–1236.
197. Orentlicher D. The Supreme Court and physician-assisted suicide: rejecting assisted suicide but embracing euthanasia. N Engl J Med 1997;337:1236–1239.

198. Miller RJ. Hospice care as an alternative to euthanasia. Law Med Health Care 1992;20:127–132.
199. Miller FG, Fletcher JC. The case for legalized euthanasia. Perspect Biol Med 1992;36:159–176.
200. Arras JD. Physician-assisted suicide: a tragic view. J Contemp Health Law Policy 1997;13:361–389.
201. Spece RG, Shimm DS, Buchanan AE, eds. Conflicts of interest in clinical practice and research. New York: Oxford University Press, 1996.
202. Foley KM. Pain, physician-assisted suicide, and euthanasia. Pain Forum 1995;4:163–178.
203. Wachtel T, Piette J, Mor V, et al. Quality of life in persons with human immunodeficiency virus infection: measurement by the medical outcomes study instrument. Ann Intern Med 1992;116:129–137.
204. Miller FG, Fins JJ. A proposal to restructure hospital care for dying patients. N Engl J Med 1996;334:1740–1742.
205. Walters L. Ethical issues in the prevention and treatment of HIV infection and AIDS. Science 1988;239:597–603.
206. Francis DP. Toward a comprehensive prevention program for the CDC and the nation. JAMA 1992;268:1444–1447.
207. Himmelstein DU, Woolhandler S, Writing Committee of the Working Group on Program Design. A national health program for the United States: a physicians' proposal. N Engl J Med 1989;320:102–106.
208. President's Commission for the Study of Ethical Problems in Medicine and Biomedical and Behavioral Research. Securing access to health care. Washington, DC: US Government Printing Office, 1985.
209. Engelhardt HT, Rie MA. Morality for the medical-industrial complex: a code of ethics for the mass marketing of health care. N Engl J Med 1988;319:1086–1089.
210. Daniels N. Just health care. New York: Cambridge University Press, 1985.
211. Callahan D. Setting limits: medical goals in an aging society. New York: Simon & Schuster, 1987.
212. Centers for Disease Control. HIV instruction and selected HIV-risk behaviors among high school students: United States, 1989–1991. MMWR Morb Mortal Wkly Rep 1992;41:866–868.
213. Bartlett JG. Human immunodeficiency virus/AIDS Medicaid managed care network. Clin Infect Dis 1997;25(4):803–804.
214. Ashman DJ, et al. In: Conviser R, ed. HIV capitation risk adjustment: conference report. Chicago: Health Research Network, 1997.
215. Turnock BJ, Kelly CJ. Mandatory premarital testing for human immunodeficiency virus. JAMA 1989;261:3415–3418.
216. Petersen LR, White CR, Premarital Screening Study Group. Premarital screening for antibodies to human immunodeficiency virus type 1 in the United States. Am J Public Health 1990;80:1087–1090.
217. Bauer GL. AIDS testing. AIDS Public Pol J 1987;2:1–2.
218. Fletcher JC. AIDS screening: a response to Gary Bauer. AIDS Public Pol J 1987;2:5–7.
219. Gostin LO. Public health strategies for confronting AIDS: legislative and regulatory policy in the United States. JAMA 1989;261:1621–1630.
220. Rhame FS, Maki DG. The case for wider use of testing for HIV infection. N Engl J Med 1989;320:1248–1253.
221. Weiss R, Thier SO. HIV testing is the answer: what's the question? N Engl J Med 1988;319:1010–1012.
222. Institute of Medicine, National Academy of Sciences. Confronting AIDS: update 1988. Washington, DC: National Academy Press, 1988.
223. Report of the Presidential Commission on the Human Immunodeficiency Virus Epidemic, June 24, 1988. GPO publication no. O-214-701:QL3. Washington, DC: US Government Printing Office, 1988. GPO publication no. O-214-701:QL3.
224. Centers for Disease Control. Public Health Service guidelines for counseling and antibody testing to prevent HIV infection and AIDS. MMWR Morb Mortal Wkly Rep 1987;36:509–515.
225. Janssen RS, Michael ESL, Satten GA, et al. HIV infection among patients in U.S. acute care hospitals. N Engl J Med 1992;327:445–452.
226. Angell M. A dual approach to the AIDS epidemic. N Engl J Med 1991;324:1991.
227. Bayer R, Levine C, Wolf SM. HIV antibody screening: an ethical framework for evaluating proposed programs. JAMA 1986;256:1768–1774.
228. Gostin LO. Screening for AIDS: efficacy, cost, and consequences. AIDS Public Pol J 1987;2:14–24.
229. Lo B, Steinbrook RL, Cooke M, et al. Voluntary screening for human immunodeficiency virus (HIV) infection: weighing the benefits and harms. Ann Intern Med 1989;110:727–733.
230. Lo B. Ethical dilemmas in HIV infection: what have we learned? Law Med Health Care 1992;20:98.
231. Childress JF. Mandatory HIV screening and testing. In: Reamer FG, ed. AIDS and ethics. New York: Columbia University Press, 1991:50–76.
232. Rogers DE, Osborn JE. Another approach to the AIDS epidemic. N Engl J Med 1991;325:808.
233. Navarro M. New York AIDS panel encourages doctors to test pregnant women. New York Times, February 25 1994:B4.
234. Kolata G. Discovery that AIDS can be prevented in babies raises debate on mandatory testing. New York Times, November 3 1994:B1439.
235. Berger JT, Rosner F, Farnsworth P. The ethics of mandatory HIV testing in newborns. J Clin Ethics 1996;7:77–84.
236. Scott GB, Beck DT, Fleischman AR, et al. Perinatal human immunodeficience virus testing. Pediatrics 1995;303–307.
237. Bayer R. Ethical challenges posed by zidovudine treatment to reduce vertical transmission of HIV. N Engl J Med 1994;331:1223–1125.
238. Giesecke J, Ramstedt K, Granath F, et al. Efficacy of partner notification for HIV infection. Lancet 1991;338:1096–1100.
239. Gostin LO, Curran W. Limits of compulsion in controlling AIDS. Hastings Cent Rep 1986;16:24–29.
240. Brandt A. Sexually transmitted disease: shadow on the land, revisited. Ann Intern Med 1990;112:481–483.
241. Toomey KE, Cates W. Partner notification for the prevention of HIV infection. AIDS 1989;3(Suppl 1):S57–62.
242. Landis SE, Schoenbach VJ, Weber DJ, et al. Results of a randomized trial of partner notification in cases of HIV infection in North Carolina. N Engl J Med 1992;326:101–106.
243. Centers for Disease Control. Recommendations for preventing transmission of human immunodeficiency virus and hepatitis B virus to patients during exposure prone invasive procedures. MMWR Morb Mortal Wkly Rep 1991;40:1–9.
244. Shuster E. A surgeon with acquired immunodeficiency syndrome: a threat to patient safety? The case of William H. Behringer. Am J Med 1993;94:93–99.
245. Centers for Disease Control. Update: investigation of patients who have been treated by HIV-infected health care workers. MMWR Morb Mortal Wkly Rep 1992;41:344–348.
246. Bartlett JG. AIDS and health care workers. Infect Dis Clin Pract 1992;1:11–20.
247. Lowenfels AB, Wormser G. Risk of transmission of HIV from surgeon to patient. N Engl J Med 1991;325:888–889.
248. Joseph P, ed. CDC: French HIV surgical case will not affect U.S. policy on infected providers. In: Hospital infection control. Am Health Consult Newslett 1997;24:33–36.
249. Bland A. CDC not publishing revised guidelines on infected workers. AIDS Alert 1992;7:113–118.
250. Joseph P, ed. HIV-infected OR nurse sues hospital after dismissal. In: Hospital infection control. Am Health Consult Newslett 1997;24:38.
251. Rothman DJ, Edgar H. AIDS, activism and ethics. Hosp Pract 1991;26:87–94.
252. Anonymous. American College of Physicians ethics manual. II. The physician and society; research; life-sustaining treatment: other issues. Ann Intern Med 1989;111:327–335.
253. Freedman B. Suspended judgment: AIDS and the ethics of clinical trials. Control Clin Trials 1992;13:1–5.

254. Levine C, Dubler NN, Levine R. Building a new consensus: ethical principles and policies for clinical research on HIV/AIDS. IRB Rev Hum Subjects Res 1991;13:1–17.
255. Greenblatt RM, Hollander H, McMaster JR, et al. Polypharmacy among patients attending an AIDS clinic: utilization of prescribed, unorthodox, and investigational treatments. J Acquir Immune Defic Syndr 1991;4:136–143.
256. Mirken B. Buyers' clubs and the FDA. PAACNOTES 1992;4:61–64.
257. Stone VE, Mauch MY, Steger K, et al. Race, gender, drug use and participation in AIDS clinical trials: lessons from a municipal hospital cohort. J Gen Intern Med 1997;12:150–157.
258. Sperling RS, Shapiro DE, Coombs RW, et al. Maternal viral load, zidovudine treatment, and the risk of transmission of human immunodeficiency virus type 1 from mother to infant. N Engl J Med 1996;335:1621–1629.
259. Recommendations of the U.S. Public Health Service Task Force on the use of zidovudine to reduce perinatal transmission of human immunodeficiency virus. MMWR Morb Mortal Wkly Rep 1994;43:1–20.
260. Zimmerman, D. Public Citizen's seriously flawed charges may delay vital research. Probe 1997;June:4–9.
261. Lurie P, Wolfe SM. Unethical trials of interventions to reduce perinatal transmission of the human immunodeficiency virus in developing countries. N Engl J Med 1997;337:853–856.
262. Angell M. The ethics of clinical research in the third world. N Engl J Med 1997;337:847–849.
263. Vanderpool HY, ed. The ethics of research involving human subjects. Frederick, MD: University Publishing Group, 1996.
264. Freedman B. Equipoise and the ethics of clinical research. N Engl J Med 1987;317:141–145.
265. Varmus H, Satcher D. Ethical complexities of conducting research in developing countries. N Engl J Med 1997;337:1003–1005.
266. Bagenda D, Musoke-Mudido P. We're trying to help our sickest people, not exploit them. Washington Post September 28, 1997:C3.
267. Kaiser J. Bangkok study adds fuel to AIDS ethics debate. Science 1997;278:1553.

56
LEGAL MANIFESTATIONS OF AIDS

Mark S. Senak

As with any medical development, the acquired immunodeficiency syndrome/human immunodeficiency virus (AIDS/HIV) epidemic brought with it myriad legal, ethical, and policy issues second in number only to the medical issues it presented. Consider that in the earliest years of the epidemic, when the first health care worker failed to feed a patient out of fear of contagion, the first AIDS ethical and legal crisis was born. Was it an act of discrimination? Did an occupational hazard exist?

AIDS/HIV represents a combination of taboos—sex, death, and drugs, with affected populations traditionally disenfranchised by society socially and, in growing number, economically. It stands to reason under those circumstances that the laws pertaining to the disease would far outnumber laws written about any other single disease in history and that span an enormous spectrum of settings and circumstances.

Initially, a person diagnosed with AIDS faced a host of medical maladies, as well as a new frontier in legal issues, issues that related to him or her as an individual. Consequently, those individual issues began to overflow and directly to affect institutions in contact with the person with AIDS. As a direct result of these changes, society also began to grapple with its own legal and policy concerns pertaining to the epidemic, many of which are still unresolved or, as the epidemic evolves, are faced for the first time. Therefore, this chapter has three sections: legal issues faced by individuals, legal concerns of institutions, and the legal and policy issues of society.

THE INDIVIDUAL

Initially, for the person with AIDS, legal issues appeared in the most immediate sense and were multiple. At the same time they were dying, their partner often was left out of decisions and could not inherit the estate. These patients had trouble obtaining benefits simply because benefits workers were afraid to handle the application; one such worker actually set her dress on fire after an encounter with a person with AIDS. Typically, these patients had considerable problems with their insurance companies, while at the same time, they may have lost their jobs because of discrimination. In terms of legal issues, AIDS was the personal equivalent of world war.

Estate Planning

With depleted immune systems and subject to a host of opportunistic infections, AIDS patients had extremely high mortality in the earliest days of the epidemic, and the length of time between diagnosis with AIDS and death was comparatively short. Given that the epidemic was first recognized among gay men, who were often young and involved in partnering relationships that were unrecognized by the law for purposes of intestate inheritance, wills and estate planning emerged as an early need, usually on an emergency basis.

The laws of intestacy vary by state, but they commonly allow for inheritance to occur without a will to the next of kin, recognized as spouse and children, parents, siblings, grandparents, and perhaps aunts and uncles. If the law finds no living relative, the estate is taken by the state in which the deceased had lived. However, for gay men, this generally meant that the patient's parents stood to inherit an estate that had been shared with a same-sex partner, who had little protection in the eyes of the law. A will was the only way to protect the interests of the persons with AIDS and his or her partner. In addition, a will bestows another advantage. A person writing the will, the testator, always designates an executor, who acts over the estate to ensure that it is executed in a timely and responsible manner. The executor may also be a beneficiary or even the sole beneficiary. In this way, a same-sex partner could inherit the estate and even gain standing to sue a third party on behalf of the decedent, thus giving the relationship a status recognized by law. As such, even with the decreased mortality of today, a person with a life-threatening condition such HIV infection is best advised to consider these matters, and often the physician advises the patient in that capacity.

Powers of Attorney and Directives of Care

A mechanism to delegate one's authority to another individual is called a power of attorney. It allows another to act in your own place and stead as if they were you. A power of attorney may be drawn broadly or narrowly, for several purposes or only for one. For example, a power of attorney can be drawn up that gives another person the authority to sign checks and carry on the affairs of one's business, or it can be drawn so narrowly to allow only action in one capacity and to a limited degree. For example, A allows B to write only one check in an amount of no more than $1000.

Traditionally, powers of attorney have been drawn up for financial or business dealings. However, people began to assign powers of attorney to other individuals for the purpose of making medical decisions. For a time, New York considered this too intimate an authority to delegate; however, many physicians found these documents acceptable, given that many of their patients had no one else to make medical decisions other than the nonfamily power of attorney. However, without color of law, if a conflict arose between the holder of the power of attorney and a family member, the family member was likely to prevail, even if the family's medical directions were in direct conflict with those expressed by the patient before incapacity. This situation led some states, particularly those with large HIV-infected populations, to enact statutes that specifically allowed for one person to designate another as a medical decision maker. In California, the statute is highly enforceable, and any dispute between a designated power of attorney and a family member sees the designated individual prevail.

Not everyone has a partner or significant other to whom one can delegate such authority. However, persons with AIDS have a compelling need to express the limitations on medical procedures that could be performed to save their lives. Although this issue has always been a question for patients, particularly geriatric patients, people with AIDS brought this issue attention in an unprecedented way, partly because this group has arguably been more activist about their disease than any other disease-specific group in history. In New York in the early epidemic years, physicians were presented with "living wills" that, like the power of attorney, did not have the support of law but did provide an indication to the physician of the patient's wishes. Although these documents were not enforceable, they were often followed.

Consequently, many states enacted statutes that allow patients to express wishes on the extent of their medical care in the face of dire or life-threatening circumstances, and the instrument is called by different names in various jurisdictions. Attending physicians or staff members of institutions in which care is administered should not act as formal witnesses to the execution of such instruments. Whether or not the instrument is legal in the jurisdiction, a physician may use it as a guide to the patient's wishes, although following those directives could place the physician in legal jeopardy if family members press for a different level of care and the instrument is without legal support in the state in which care is being delivered.

Discrimination

STATE LAW

When the HIV/AIDS epidemic began in the early 1980s, most states had laws that prohibited discrimination against a person with a handicap or disability in areas of employment and usually in housing or public accommodation. Some states also specifically prohibited discrimination against a person who was perceived to have a disability for one reason or another. However, no disease-specific statutes dealt with AIDS, and whether existing statutes recognized AIDS as a disability was unclear. When discrimination cases first surfaced, there was no such thing as being "HIV-positive" because no test for HIV antibodies existed until 1985. Therefore, the cases brought were cases of AIDS discrimination, not of HIV (then still called HTLV-III) discrimination.

Early cases argued that AIDS was a true disability and that the state statutes protected people with the disease. The earliest cases were successful. Early discrimination was centered primarily on fear of contagion, and as such, persons suspected of having AIDS also often suffered discrimination even though they did not have the disease. It followed that many jurisdictions recognized their statutes to cover the perception of a disability as well as the actual disability itself.

Later, as the population became more knowing about transmission issues and AIDS, discrimination was born less out of fear of contagion than out of economic circumstances. It was expensive for an employer with a small group plan of employees to hire or maintain an employee with the disease. The cost of premiums could become much higher, and days lost to illness would also incur a cost to the employer.

FEDERAL LAW

State statutes did not cover every situation of employment. For example, a federal employee was not covered by any state statute, and some state statutes did not provide a strong enough remedy. This situation caused some to seek the comfort of federal law through the Federal Vocational Rehabilitation Act of 1973, which prohibited discrimination against a person with a handicap in a federal setting. This law meant that any employer with a federal nexus, that is, federal funding of any kind, could fall subject to the jurisdiction of the statute. This group included hospitals that accepted Medicaid or Medicare, as well as schools.

A landmark case occurred in 1987, a year after the United States Department of Justice issued a memorandum stating that, although it was illegal to discriminate against a person with AIDS in the workplace under federal law, if an employer could make a case for genuine fear of contagion in the workplace, then possibly it was not discriminatory. The Arline case involved a Florida school teacher with tuberculosis who sued under the federal statute for discrimination because she lost her job as a result of the tuberculosis. The issue at hand was whether or not a communicable disease could be considered a handicap for federal purposes. Many briefs submitted to the court talked about HIV and AIDS, both for and against the position of the plaintiff. In a decisive 7–2 decision, the court stated that tuberculosis could be considered a handicap for purposes of the federal statute. The court did not address the issue of AIDS or HIV, but the precedent was set that a communicable disease could be considered a handicap for federal purposes.

AMERICANS WITH DISABILITIES ACT

In 1990, President George Bush signed into law the Americans with Disabilities Act, which broke new ground in discrimination protections for people with disabilities. It outlined specific exceptions to the law that made it illegal for people to be discriminated against by reason of a handicap in employment or public accommodation. Included specifically as a disability in this law is HIV.

Insurance

One of the most difficult problems for persons with AIDS early in the epidemic was the area of insurance—health, disability and life.

HEALTH

Many health plans attempted to drop AIDS patients because of the high expense of their care incurred by repeated infections and hospitalizations. For patients who obtained their insurance through individual plans, this denial of coverage often took the form of declaring that the patient had made a material misrepresentation on the application for insurance. Such a claim can generally only be made within 2 years of the issuance of the policy. Patients should be instructed to fill out such applications honestly because an insurance company probably will find any discrepancy if a patient presents claims involving catastrophic illness within the 2-year period of contestability.

For patients in group plans, many insurers attempted to avoid payment in various ways. When the patient was diagnosed with AIDS, some insurers attempted to claim that the disease was a "preexisting condition" within the terms of the contract, meaning that at the time of joining the plan, the insured either knew or should have known that he or she had the illness for which claims were now being presented.

Another method of limiting financial exposure was to "cap" the policy payments for the disease condition. This situation meant that the insured person was notified after the diagnosis that the insurance contract had been revised to state that payments made for AIDS were limited to a dramatically lower amount of money than had been allowed before the change. This cap was specific to AIDS, meaning that if a coworker developed cancer, the payments continued to the original cap. The practice of disease-specific caps went before the courts involving both insured plans and self-insured groups. In these cases, the insured persons sued to state that the disease-specific cap was a violation of the Americans with Disabilities Act, and these cases met with varying responses.

Disability insurance policies also attempted to limit financial exposure by use of material misrepresentation clauses and by testing people for HIV antibodies before issuing a policy. Likewise, life insurers began HIV antibody testing as a condition of granting a policy to an applicant. This is the way in which Magic Johnson reported that he discovered his HIV antibody status.

INSTITUTIONS

Confidentiality

The public health strategy engaged in battling the epidemic relied on people who perceived themselves at risk of HIV to come forward for antibody testing. Because of the extreme nature of various types of discrimination and the finding that such people were subject to loss of employment, insurance, financial well-being, and even family, laws were enacted to bolster the public health strategy and to require confidentiality regarding the HIV status of people infected.

Early confidentiality statutes were deemed overzealous in their efforts to protect patients, sometimes inhibiting the communication of necessary information among treating health care professionals. That stringence has been largely eroded in the statutes, which focus on a middle ground that allows necessary medical personnel to know about the HIV status of a patient being treated.

Informing third parties of test results can be difficult, at best. Although physicians are bound to confidentiality by statute, they are also bound by case law to ensure that harm does not come to third parties when it can be prevented. Confidentiality statutes, in increasing number, permit, but do not necessarily require, a physician to inform a third party that he or she has been exposed to HIV.

An example is when a patient infected with HIV informs the examining physician of an unwillingness to practice safe needle sharing or sexual practices with a known, identifiable third party. In such a case, statutes often allow the physician the option of 1) informing the third party of the exposure without identifying the responsible party; 2) notifying health officers, who, in turn, will notify the third party, again without disclosure; or 3) doing nothing.

The complicating factor in a physician's choice not to inform third parties is the Tarasoff case. This well-known case involved a psychiatrist whose patient stated an intention to murder a known third party. The psychiatrist did not intervene because of the nature of the physician–patient relationship. Sued by the survivors of the known third party after her murder by the patient, the psychiatrist was found liable for not averting the harm. Therefore, it is possible that while satisfying the statutory outline for informing a third party, a physician who elects to do nothing arguably could have some liability.

Whether or not intransigent persons who present a danger to unknown third parties may have their confidentiality breached to protect the public at large is worthy of debate. Although such proposals sound good initially, in fact, they are largely ineffectual, given that no practical way exists to alert the public at large regarding an individual's HIV status and his or her propensity for unsafe sex or needle sharing.

Testing

Testing in almost all jurisdictions requires the consent of the person being tested. Exceptions exist whereby, under some circumstances, a deceased person may be tested without the consent of the next of kin, although the results may need to remain confidential to authorities.

The use of HIV testing as a diagnostic tool took on greater proportions however, when the fear of AIDS reached new heights coincident to a large degree by the alleged transmission of HIV from dentist to patient Kimberly Bergalis in 1990. Before that, many physicians and dentists who were performing invasive procedures wanted to test patients for HIV. Routine screening at the outset of every invasive procedure was deemed ill advised by the Centers for Disease Control. However, with the advent of the Bergalis dental case, new calls were made for the testing of physicians, causing a near standoff in the doctor–patient relationship, with each wanting the other to be tested.

The basis for patients' fears was recognized to some degree by the courts, when patients sued medical practices in which, after patients' treatment, an attending health care worker was discovered to be suffering from HIV or AIDS. Some courts lent credence to the notion by stating that the fear of contagion was enough to evoke a course of action, even if it were found that no HIV transmission occurred between doctor and patient.

SOCIETY: END OF LIFE

As the HIV/AIDS epidemic matured, legal and ethical issues rose from the individual status to the institutional to involve society as a whole. The issue of end-of-life decision making is not new, but it has certainly been brought to the fore by the epidemic, particularly given that the population most affected is young and more activist about their condition than any other disease-specific group. People with AIDS ask society legal and ethical questions that have long been asked of the health care system, but that have reached a new pitch given that it is an epidemic.

What most people know about this subject is gleaned from news reports about the most sensational cases. What is not generally understood is the physician's spectrum of activity, which involves the physician, to various degrees, in the death of the patient. The four identifiable activities during end-of-life decision making range from least involvement to total involvement of the physician.

The option with the least physician involvement is when the patient voluntarily stops eating and drinking, by definition, when a patient decides that he or she will no longer take nourishment, despite the capability to do so. A competent patient has this right because he or she is merely refusing life-prolonging interventions that would include forced feeding. Although this option does not actively involve the physician, it is a long-lasting and miserable effort on the part of the patient.

The next option, which does involve some degree of active participation from the physician, is terminal sedation. This approach involves the administration of pain medication to overcome unrelieved pain for the patient who reaches a point of unconsciousness and is unable to take nourishment when the course of treatment would be legal if done to relieve the patient of pain and if the patient had made the competent decision to forego life-prolonging interventions.

Physician-assisted suicide occurs when the physician makes available the means for a patient to end his or her life, usually by providing drugs that, in large doses, will prove fatal to the patient. That the administration of the drugs is entirely in the patient's hands is advantageous to some degree, but it can result in incomplete suicides that leave the patient in a dire and unintended position. Although this option is illegal, no one has been criminally prosecuted for it with success, although the question exists of the possibility of civil action taken by next of kin.

Finally, voluntary active euthanasia completes the spectrum involving the physician in the active administration of life-ending means, that is, injecting the patient with a lethal drug mixture after receiving informed and competent consent. This practice is invariably illegal.

Section VI
Diseases Associated with Other Retroviruses

57

Human Immunodeficiency Virus Type 2 (HIV-2)

Myron Essex and Phyllis J. Kanki

Human immunodeficiency virus type 2 (HIV-2) is closely related to HIV-1. However, it is more closely related to several of the simian immunodeficiency viruses (SIVs). Most HIV-2 isolates are essentially indistinguishable from the SIVs of such species as mangabeys and macaques, a finding that leads one to conclude that some SIVs and most strains of HIV-2 are essentially the same virus (1, 2). In vivo, this relationship is illustrated by the ability of HIV-2 strains to grow in monkeys (3, 4). HIV-1 does not replicate well in monkeys, but it does readily infect chimpanzees and gibbon apes (5–8).

HIV-2, like the SIVs, was initially detected on the basis of serologic cross-reactivity (9–11). When sera from West African female sex workers were screened for antibodies to HIV-1 antigens, they revealed extensive cross-reactivity for the virus core antigens but weaker or minimal antibody binding reactivity for the HIV-1 envelope (2, 9). Yet when the same West African human sera were assayed on SIV antigens, they reacted strongly with the envelope proteins as well as with the core antigens (Table 57.1).

HIV-2 strains appear to have many similarities to HIV-1 strains. They are transmitted by the same routes, they infect the same cells, and they exhibit considerable diversity in the outer envelope. Although at least some HIV-2 strains are less efficiently transmitted than HIV-1 strains (12), they also establish persistent irreversible infections in people. The disease caused by HIV-2 is apparently also similar, but more strains of HIV-2 may be considerably less virulent than most strains of HIV-1 (13, 14). Because HIV-2 strains have so many characteristics in common with HIV-1, information that applies equally to both viruses is usually not repeated in this chapter. Emphasis is given to information about HIV-2 strains that appears likely to influence differences in distribution, virulence, and clinical outcome. Because research with HIV-2 strains has been much less extensive than for HIV-1 strains, this information is of necessity less complete.

RELATIONSHIP BETWEEN HIV-2 AND OTHER LENTIVIRUSES

Like HIV-1, HIV-2 is a lentiretrovirus with a transactivator gene that regulates expression of the regulatory and structural genes. The entire genome of HIV-2 is about 40 to 45% related to HIV-1 at the nucleotide sequence level. It has been estimated that the HIV-1 and HIV-2/SIV groups of viruses might have diverged from each other as recently as 50 to 60 years ago (15, 16). The SIVs of mangabeys and macaques are the closest relatives of HIV-2 strains (1, 2, 17) (Fig. 57.1). As a group, the SIVs apparently vary more among different species and subspecies of monkeys than different HIV-1 strains vary from each other or than different HIV-2 strains vary from each other (2, 17–19). Because HIV-2 strains appear to be largely limited to West Africa, it is not surprising that they are most closely related to SIVs originating from monkeys in that region (1, 2, 17). The only exception may be the macaque SIV, which is also closely related to both HIV-2 and mangabey SIV. Because SIVs have not been observed in wild Asian monkeys such as macaques, it appears likely that infection of this species occurred accidentally in captivity from African monkeys or human tissues originating from West Africa (2).

HIV-2 GENETIC VARIABILITY

The highest prevalence for infection with HIV-2 strains appears to be in the westernmost regions of Africa, around Guinea-Bissau (20, 21). This suggests that strains of virus identified in that area are more likely to represent the oldest human strains (22). Various HIV-2 strains have been isolated and characterized from about 20 individuals representing such countries as Senegal, Mali, Guinea-Bissau, Ivory Coast, Ghana, and Gambia (22–35).

As with HIV-1, the polymerase activity of HIV-2 is error prone, and as a result extensive variation occurs among isolates (36). This variation is primarily exhibited in the envelope gene against which much of the selective pressure of the immune system is exerted. This results in differences in *env* of as much as 1% per year for evolutionary selection (37, 38). Similar to the genetic variation described for HIV-1, sequence analysis of a limited number of HIV-2 viruses has demonstrated five subtypes, A to E (39). Studies of HIV-2–infected people in Senegal, and Guinea-Bissau have only identified the HIV-2 subtype A (40–43). Thus far, the

Table 57.1. Efficiency for Detection of Antibodies to Major HIV-2 Antigens Using Sera from HIV-2-Infected Persons

Class	Gene	Antigen	Relative Immunogenicity	Cross-reactivity with HIV-1 Antigens
Structural				
	gag	p55 precursor	High	High
		p24 capsid	High	High
		p17 matrix	Moderate	High
	env	gp160 precursor	Very high	Low
		gp120 surface	Very high	Low
		gp41 transmembrane	Very high	Low
	pol	p66/51 polymerase	High	Moderate
		p34 endonuclease	High	Moderate
	vpx	p12	Moderate	Not applicable
	vpr	p13	Moderate	Low
Regulatory				
	tat	p14	Very low	Unknown
	rev	p19	Moderate	Unknown
Accessory				
	nef	p27	Low	High
	vif	p23	Low	Unknown

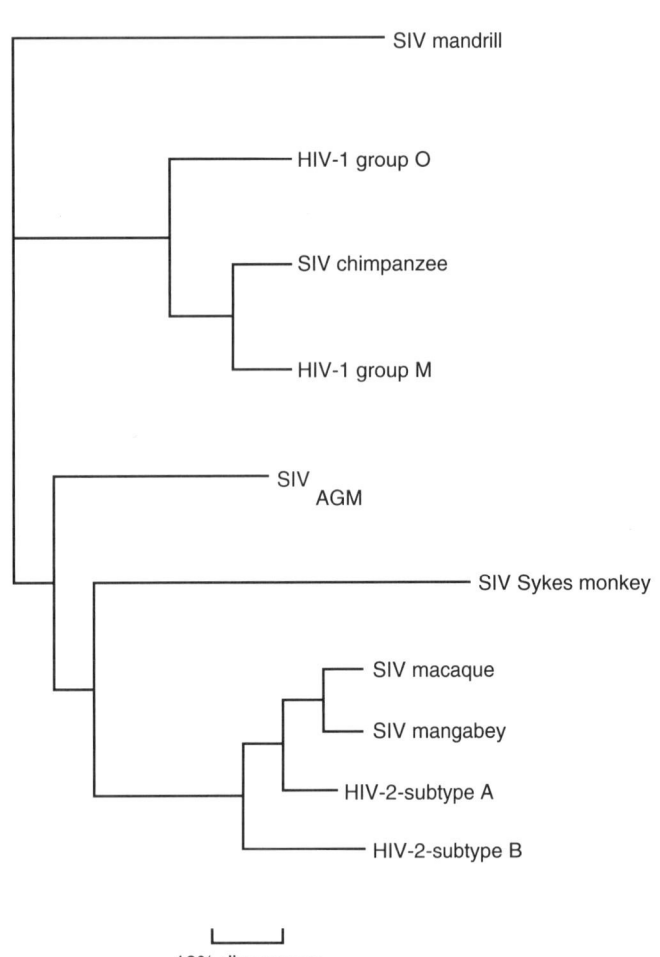

Figure 57.1. Relative genetic relatedness of primate lentiviruses.

Ghanaian isolates, subtype B (31, 32) are believed to be most distant from the prototype HIV-2/mangabey/macaque virus (2). Since the initial description of HIV-2 subtypes, no additional viral sequences have been described for subtypes C through E, which appear to be rare and originally based on one or two viral isolates. Similar to HIV-1, the biologic phenotype of HIV-2, characterized by "slow-low" versus "rapid-high" isolates, appears to correlate with the higher net charge of amino acids in the V3 loop region (44).

Limited studies on the interpatient variability of HIV-2 have shown that the range of variability in the envelope V3 sequence is similar to the interpatient variability of HIV-1 (30, 40). A tissue-specific quasispecies has been identified in HIV-1 infection in vivo, and this has also been demonstrated in the analysis of blood and brain viral sequences from an HIV-2–infected individual (40, 41). Evaluation of intrapatient variation in the V3 envelope region of HIV-2 in asymptomatic and symptomatic persons followed over time has shown a lower variation when compared with HIV-1 (42) This lower intrapatient variation appears to be a distinct feature of HIV-2 infection that may result from decreased viral burden and may also contribute to lower rates of transmission and disease development.

EPIDEMIOLOGY

Rates of HIV-2 infection are highest in sexually active populations such as commercial sex workers, a finding indicating that this virus, like HIV-1, is transmitted sexually (12, 20, 45–47). Rates are also higher in adults with sexually transmitted diseases, in prisoners, and in people hospitalized with infectious diseases (20, 45–48). Such risk groups usually have seroprevalence rates that are 5- to 10-fold higher than those of the general population (Table 57.2).

The prevalence rates appear highest in West Africa, particularly in the region of Guinea-Bissau (20, 21, 47, 49). In this region, which includes southern Senegal, seroprevalence rates in female prostitutes may be 10 to 50% or higher (see Table 57.2). In countries such as Guinea-Bissau, the Gambia, Cape Verde, and Senegal, the prevalence of HIV-2 infection exceeds that of infection with HIV-1, but HIV-1 infection appears to be increasing and in some cases may soon overtake infection with HIV-2. Evidence from cross-sectional prevalence studies has been presented from Guinea-Bissau (49), the Ivory Coast (48, 50), and Senegal (12, 20, 48, 51), where a disproportionate increase in HIV-1 prevalence compared with HIV-2 infection has been described.

In most other countries of West Africa—Burkina Faso, Ghana, the Ivory Coast, Nigeria, and Mali, infection with HIV-1 is more prevalent than with HIV-2, ranging from a 3-fold to a 24-fold rate ratio (HIV-1 versus HIV-2) (45, 52–57). The rapid spread of HIV-1 in West Africa has been documented, and prevalence and incidence trends indicate that HIV-1 will become the predominant HIV type in much of the region (51, 57). The existence of significant rates of HIV-1 and HIV-2 in many of these countries begs the question of what outcome will result after these viruses interact at a population level.

Geographically, the distribution of HIV-2 seems to be totally independent from the distribution of HIV-1 (45, 58). Countries in central or eastern Africa appear to be relatively free of HIV-2, as are most regions of Europe and North America. In these low-risk regions, almost all the rare infections observed are either in West African immigrants or in persons who had contact with West Africans. Countries such as Angola, Mozambique, Spain, and Portugal appear to have low but stable rates of HIV-2 in the population (45, 59, 60). These countries share a common language and trade with Guinea-Bissau. HIV-2 has also been detected in the large cities of southwestern India (61), perhaps because of exchange with the former Portuguese colonies of Africa. Goa, a former Portuguese colony, situated south of Bombay on the western coast, has reported a 4.9% rate of HIV-2 infection and a 9.8% rate of HIV-1 infection in patients with sexually transmitted diseases (62). Significant HIV-2 infection has not been reported in other parts of Asia to date.

France was one of the first countries to institute HIV-2 testing in blood donors, and several HIV-2 cases were identified (63). Of 75 HIV-2–infected persons studied in Paris, 58 were of African origin, 12 were European, and 5 were Caribbean (64). To a lesser degree, other European countries have reported sporadic cases of HIV-2 infection in large serosurveys, usually with a link to West Africa (45, 65, 66). It is interesting to speculate that the relatively high rates of HIV-2 infection reported in France (67) may be due to significant ties with former colonies in French West Africa, and perhaps they may reflect some bias in the populations surveyed.

Although HIV-2 is transmitted by sex and blood, as is HIV-1, the rate of infection in West Africa appears more stable than that of HIV-1. In the Ivory Coast, for example, HIV-1 appears to be introduced more recently than HIV-2, but it is already present at higher rates (20, 48, 68, 69). In Senegal, during an 8-year period of follow-up, a 26-fold increase in HIV-1 infection occurred, whereas HIV-2 infection rates remained relatively constant (51, 70). This finding implies that HIV-2 may have been in the human population in Africa at least as long as HIV-1, and in West Africa HIV-2 has apparently been present considerably longer. The relative lack of significant HIV-2 prevalence in Europe, North America, and Asia in the face of HIV-1 expansion also supports the general observation that HIV-2 is spread less efficiently than HIV-1 (58, 66, 71–80).

Case reports of HIV-2 transmitted by blood and blood products have been published; however, widespread HIV testing in blood bank settings has limited the risk of this mode of transmission (81, 82). The most common modes of HIV transmission in HIV-2–endemic areas are perinatal and heterosexual transmission; because most West African countries have been afflicted with both HIV-1 and HIV-2 infections, direct comparison of transmission rates between the two viruses has been possible. In Senegalese female commercial sex workers followed over an 11-year period, the annual incidence of HIV-1 dramatically increased, with a 1.18-fold increased risk per year and a 13-fold increase in risk over the entire study period. The incidence of HIV-2 remained stable, despite higher HIV-2 prevalence (51, 83). In this high-risk group, heterosexual transmission of HIV-2 was significantly slower than that of HIV-1, a finding that strongly suggests differences in the infectivity potential of these two related immunodeficiency viruses (51, 83). Using mathematic modeling techniques, the efficiency of heterosexual transmission of HIV-2 has been estimated to range from 5 to 9 times less than that of HIV-1 per sexual act with an infected partner (70). Based on the differences in transmission and disease-causing potential of HIV-2 compared with HIV-1, Anderson and May (80) postulated that pathogenicity of the virus is associated with reproductive success of

Table 57.2. Estimates of Prevalence Rates of HIV-2 in Different Geographic Areas

Location	Seroprevalence (%) General Population[a]	High-Risk Groups[b]	References
Highest rates			
Burkina Faso	1–2	15–20	45, 52
Cape Verde	0–1	10–20	46, 52, 65
The Gambia	1–2	20–30	84, 85, 87
Guinea-Bissau	5–10	20–50	20, 21, 47, 49
The Ivory Coast	1–5	20–50	48, 50, 57, 69
Mali	1–5	10–40	56
Senegal	1–2	10–40	12, 45, 46, 51, 52
Low but stable rates			
Angola	0–1	5–10	59
Ghana	0–1	3–5	53
India	0–1	1–5	61, 62
Mozambique	0–1	5–10	45, 52
Portugal	0–1	5–10	60
Extremely low rates			
Brazil	<.01	<.01	71
Burundi	<.01	<.01	58
Denmark	<.01	<.01	72
Greece	<.01	<.01	73
Italy	<.01	<.01	74
Kenya	<.01	<.01	58
Spain	<.01	<.01	75, 76
Uganda	<.01	<.01	77
United States	<.01	<.01	78–79
Zaire	<.01	<.01	58

[a]Blood donors, pregnant women, and hospital workers.
[b]Female commercial sex workers, sexually transmitted disease patients, hospitalized infectious disease, and prisoners.

the infectious disease organism. Mathematic models applied to the existing epidemiology data of HIV-1 and HIV-2 suggest that HIV-1 will competitively displace HIV-2 in the longer term, in areas where both viruses are transmitted within the same sexually active populations (80).

The sexual transmission of HIV-2, like that of HIV-1, appears to be enhanced by the presence of other sexually transmitted diseases such as chancroid or syphilis (84). Enhanced risk of infection with HIV-2 was also associated with an increase in years of sexual activity and with non-Senegalese nationality, and HIV-2–infected women tend to be older than HIV-1–infected women (12). In a cross-sectional discordant-couple study of HIV-2 transmission, older women were more likely to have a seropositive spouse than younger women (85).

Maternal or neonatal transmission of HIV-2 also occurs (86), but it appears to be less efficient than of HIV-1 (68, 87, 88). Prospective studies of HIV-2 perinatal transmission have been conducted in Guinea-Bissau, the Ivory Coast, France, and Senegal, all demonstrating extremely low rates of perinatal transmission of HIV-2 (0 to 3.7% transmission), in contrast to that of HIV-1 (15 to 45% transmission) (89–93). In studies that measured perinatal transmission of both viruses, the rate of HIV-1 transmission was 10- to 20-fold higher than that of HIV-2. No information is available concerning HIV-2 transmission by breast milk. Because all available data have shown HIV-2 infection to be uncommon in children, transmission of HIV-2 by breast milk must be extremely rare.

MORPHOLOGIC AND GENETIC STRUCTURE

HIV-2 strains are morphologically similar to HIV-1 strains. They are spheric, 100 to 120 nm. All have a conical electron-dense core with a surrounding lucent space, all enclosed within an envelope (94–96). The matrix protein at the small end of the core is probably attached to the inner surface of the transmembrane protein through the carboxy terminus of the latter (97, 98).

HIV-2 strains morphologically appear slightly different from HIV-1 but are probably indistinguishable from the mangabey/macaque group of SIVs (1, 10, 99). Protruding envelope projections are often apparent on HIV-2 or SIV, but not on mature HIV-1, a finding suggesting that the gp120 projections are more tightly bound (96, 100, 101). The electron-lucent paranucleoid space is also a distinguishing characteristic. In the case of HIV-2, this space is usually limited to an open ring around the triangular core, whereas in HIV-1, the entire space between the core and the envelope appears lucent, except for diffuse lateral paranuclear bodies peripheral to the long sides of the triangular core. HIV-2 may also be more uniform in size and shape than HIV-1. HIV-2 and HIV-1 both bud from the cell surface in the same manner. The major core and envelope proteins are situated in the same positions in budding and extracellular virions (Fig. 57.2). Vpx, the only protein unique to HIV-2, appears to be situated just below the envelope (102).

The replication cycle of HIV-2 includes 1) adsorption to CD4 and fusion with the cell surface, 2) penetration and uncoating, 3) reverse transcription, 4) transport of viral DNA to nucleus, 5) chromosomal integration, 6) transcription of viral mRNA and splicing, 7) translation of regulatory and structural proteins, 8) transport of structural proteins to cytoplasmic membrane and virus assembly, and 9) budding, maturation, and release through CD4 sites. The length of the entire genome of HIV-2 is about 10 kb, as it is for HIV-1. The open-reading frames of HIV-2 are also similar to those of HIV-1. For different HIV-1, HIV-2, and SIV strains, the genes may be in different reading frames, but the level of conservation within each gene is still high. The regulatory gene sequences appear to vary more among HIV-2 strains when compared with HIV-1 strains (24, 103, 104). The *gag* and *pol* messages are unspliced, the *env* is singly spliced, and the major regulatory genes are doubly spliced and made from multiple messages. HIV-1 has one gene, *vpu*, which is not found in HIV-2 (105–107). However, the function of the HIV-1 *vpu*, the ability to increase viral particle release, may be provided by the HIV-2 envelope (108). HIV-2 has one gene, *vpx*, which is not found in HIV-1 (25, 109–111). Although Vpx is distantly related to the *vpr* gene found in both HIV-1 and HIV-2, *vpu* and *vpx* are totally unrelated to each other (112, 113).

CELL ATTACHMENT

HIV-2 apparently infects the same range of cells as HIV-1: T4 helper lymphocytes, monocytes, macrophages, and microglia cells in the central nervous system. Although HIV-2 infects through the same CD4 receptor, it apparently does so with a 10- to 100-fold greater affinity than HIV-1 (114–116). Although the HIV-2 glycoprotein appears to be slightly less glycosylated than HIV-1, this property does not appear to account for their differences in binding efficiency (116). Investigators believe that infection by HIV-2 is inhibited more efficiently by soluble CD4 than is HIV-1 (117). This is probably because HIV-2 has more stable gp120 at its surface (97, 100, 101).

Different strains of HIV-2 show different abilities to bind to CD4, as well as varying degrees of infectivity and syncytia-inducing ability (118, 119). The possibility that HIV-2 may use a receptor in addition to CD4 has been raised, because some cell lines transfected with the CD4 receptor show different sensitivity to HIV-2 compared with HIV-1 (120). However, HIV-2 can cross-interfere with HIV-1 in vitro (121, 122). In fact, HIV-2 strains appear to interfere well with HIV-1 strains, whereas HIV-1 strains only partially interfere with HIV-2 strains (121).

Several members of the chemokine receptor family have been shown to function in association with CD4 to permit HIV-1 entry and infection in various types of cells (117, 120, 123). Like HIV-1, certain HIV-2 strains have been shown to use fusin/CXCR4 as both a coreceptor (in the presence of CD4) and an alternative receptor, in the absence of CD4 (123, 124). Studies with the related SIV have demonstrated

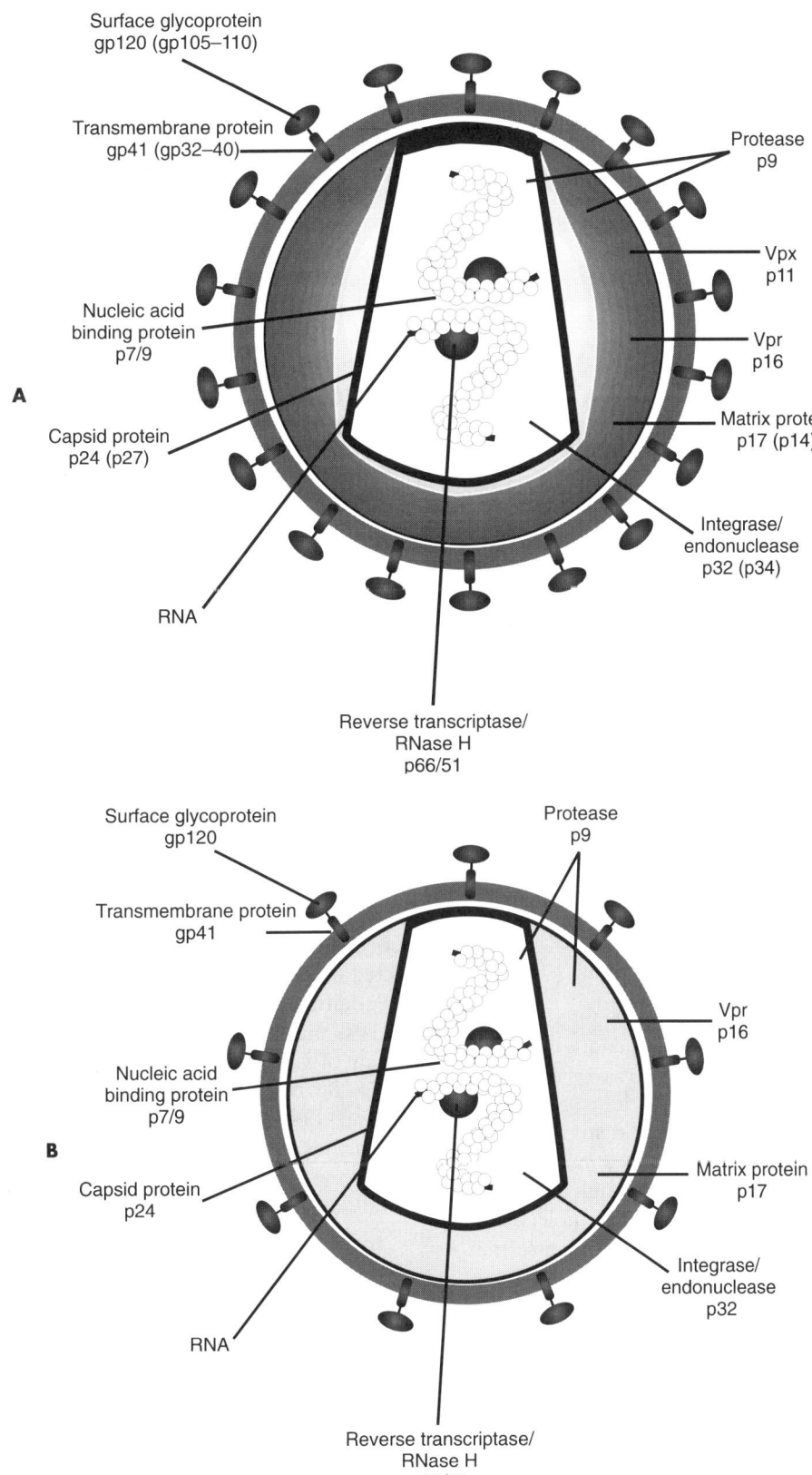

Figure 57.2. Schematic illustration of HIV-2 and HIV-1 virions. A. HIV-2 virion. **B.** HIV-1 virion. *Numbers in parentheses* for HIV-2 indicate reported protein size designations that may be different for those of HIV-1. For consistency in **A** and in the text, the more commonly used generic terms based on HIV-1 protein size designations are listed first.

that, unlike in HIV-1, CCR5 is used by both macrophage-tropic and T-cell–tropic SIVs, and that receptor use may be important in viral tropism (125). This expanding area of research is rapidly identifying and characterizing the various coreceptors involved in this process, and a better appreciation of HIV tropism will likely emerge in the near future.

REVERSE TRANSCRIPTION AND INTEGRATION

The *pol* gene encodes three proteins: protease, reverse transcriptase, which also has RNase H activity, and endonuclease/integrase. The protease of HIV-2 is assumed to be similar to HIV-1 protease, which apparently functions as a dimer (126). The HIV-2 protease, as expressed in yeast, was also shown to be efficient at hydrolyzing HIV-1 peptide junctions (127). This finding suggests that the substrate specificities of both viral proteins are analogous.

The reverse transcriptase/RNase H molecule of HIV-2 is similar in size to the HIV-1 reverse transcriptase and is serologically cross-reactive with human antibodies (128). The HIV-2 polymerase appears to be equally error prone to that of HIV-1 (36). Both are more error prone than other retroviral polymerase enzymes. Functional mutants of HIV-2 polymerase were found to have the same likelihood for loss of RNA-dependent DNA polymerase activity as the HIV-1 polymerase, a finding suggesting a high degree of overlap between their respective catalytic domains (129). No such relationship was found between the HIV-1 and HIV-2 enzymes for their efficiency to demonstrate DNA-dependent DNA polymerase activity (129). As for other retroviral reverse transcriptases, the DNA polymerase is associated with the amino terminus of the molecule, and RNase H is associated with the carboxy terminus (130). However, the specific RNase H activity of HIV-2 appears to be about 10-fold lower than the comparable activity of the HIV-1 enzyme (131).

The integrase/endonuclease protein functions by nicking linear viral DNA at a specific site to remove two or three bases at each end (132). The integrase appears to have only one site for catalysis cutting of the donor DNA and strand transfer (133). The DNA then integrates apparently at random. The protease molecule is small, about 9 kd, although it is usually functional as a dimer (134). Antibodies to this molecule are not readily detectable in infected people. The reverse transcriptase/RNase H molecule of HIV-1 exists as a heterodimer described as p66/p51. The HIV-2 pol products, except the protease, are highly immunogenic in infected people, and the antibodies are cross-reactive between HIV-1 and HIV-2 (9, 128). The same is true for the endonuclease/integrase p34 molecule of HIV-2 (128, 135). These observations confirm the high degree of conservation at the protein level between the major pol gene products of HIV-1 and HIV-2.

REGULATORY GENE FUNCTIONS

The long terminal repeat (LTR) regions at the ends of the viral genome contain sequences necessary for activation of transcription and for termination of the transcripts, but an important element of control for these viruses occurs through RNA processing or splicing. One of the most important characteristics of HIVs that makes them different from other retroviruses is their ability to regulate their own expression (37). The 5′ LTR is the initiation region for transcription, which terminates at the 3′ LTR (136).

The expression of HIVs can be activated by cellular transcription factors such as NF-κB and T-cell mitogens, which bind to the LTR (137). The LTR of HIV-1 may be more responsive to cellular activation signals than the HIV-2 LTR, a finding indicating that the HIV-2 has different response elements (138, 139). Whereas HIV-1 has two NF-κB enhancer binding sites, only one can be identified for HIV-2 or most SIVs (140). This finding may have biologic significance, because studies of two different strains of SIV with dramatic difference in virulence in vivo have demonstrated duplication of the NF-κB binding sites in the virulent strain (141).

For HIV-1, the NF-κB transcription factor may be sufficient for inducible transcriptional activation (142). For HIV-2, additional factors are used (138, 139, 143–145). One that appears to bind to purine-rich motifs in the HIV-2 enhancer is Elf-1, a transcription factor related to the *ets* cellular oncogene, and a novel peri-ets (pets) site (146). Some studies suggest that activation of the HIV-2 enhancer may require four or more *cis*-acting elements, most of which are not in HIV-1 (147). Such differences in sensitivity to cellular transcription factors may also help to explain potential differences in virus load and cell tropism at the host level. Combined with the lower CD4 affinity seen with HIV-2 gp120, this finding may help to explain why HIV-2–infected persons apparently have lower levels of virus than persons infected with HIV-1.

In addition to the cell factors and the regulatory proteins of HIVs, the LTRs are also responsive to the regulatory proteins of various other viruses such as cytomegalovirus, hepatitis B virus, and the human T-cell leukemia virus type 1 (HTLV-I) (145, 148, 149). However, except for HTLV-I, these viruses ordinarily do not infect the same cells as the HIVs in the intact host.

The *tat* and *rev* products, both made from doubly spliced messages, are the most important viral regulators of transcription (136). Tat is a 16-kd protein that is active early in the viral infection to enhance additional production of regulatory gene messages. *Rev* expression occurs later and acts to enhance expression of structural gene messages. Tat binds to a Tat response element (TAR) in viral RNA. It can activate mRNA expression and protein synthesis by more than 100-fold (138, 139). Studies have demonstrated that RNA polymerase II is the cellular target for Tat resulting in Tat-mediated increase in transcriptional elongation from the HIV LTR (150).

For HIV-2, *tat* gene transactivation may be more complex than for HIV-1. HIV-2 appears to have two stem-loop TAR structures, whereas HIV-1 has one (151, 152). The *tat* gene of HIV-1 *(tat-1)* has a high degree of homology with the tat

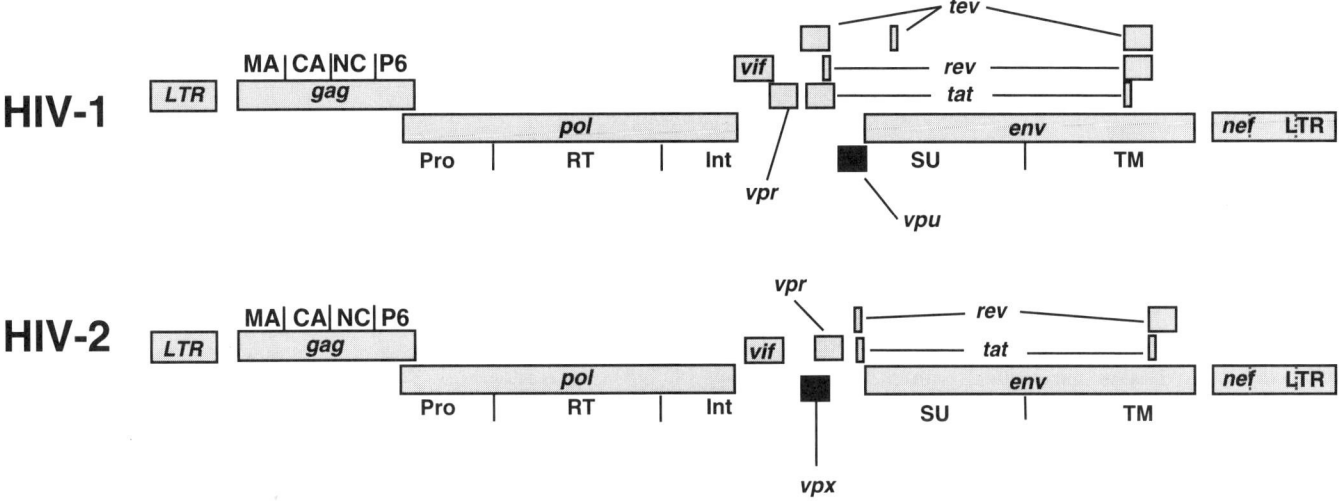

Figure 57.3. Schematic illustration of HIV-1 and HIV-2 genomes.

gene of HIV-2 *(tat-2)*. Yet, *tat-1* activates the LTRs of HIV-1 TAR (TAR-1) and HIV-2 (TAR-2) equally, and *tat-2* activates TAR-1 poorly (153).

Rev is a 19-kd protein that acts to increase transcription of RNA for the *gag, pol, env, vif,* and *vpr* genes and to transport the messages for these genes out of the nucleus (154–156). It has a negative effect on expression of *rev, tat,* and *nef* messages. HIV-2 rev appears to act similarly, although it appears to be less phosphorylated (157). Rev acts through a rev response element (RRE) stem-loop structure in the envelope open-reading frame (154, 158). Although HIV-1 *rev* functions on both the HIV-1 RRE and the HIV-2 RRE, HIV-2 *rev* functions only on RRE of HIV-2 (159, 160). Investigators have hypothesized that the low level of HIV-2 *rev* function on HIV-1 RRE may be because the HIV-2 *rev* is inhibited from polymerization after binding the HIV-1 RRE (161).

ACCESSORY GENES AND GENE PRODUCTS

Tat and *rev* appear to be the only regulatory genes essential for virus replication. Several others have some lesser effect on virus replication rate, but the effect appears to be variable according to the virus strain and cell type. In this context, the other genes are categorized as accessory.

Open-reading frames for *nef* overlap the 3′ LTR (Fig. 57.3). The nef product is a 27-kd myristoylated protein that is highly cross-reactive between HIV-1 and HIV-2 (162, 163). In some studies, *nef* was believed to downregulate virus replication in cell cultures (164–166). In another study with the *nef* of SIV$_{mac}$, a close relative of HIV-2, *nef* appeared to enhance the replication capacity of the virus (167). The HIV-2 *nef* is proteolytically cleaved by the HIV-2 encoded protease, independent of Nef myristoylation (168). The full-length *nef* of HIV-2 and the core domain are part of the HIV-2 particles, analogous to the situation reported for HIV-1.

The *vif* gene encodes a 23-kd protein (169). It was initially assumed to enhance the spread of free virus (170–172), but current studies suggest that it may be more important as a determinant of cell tropism (173). The *vpu* gene is not present on HIV-2 strains or SIVs, only in HIV-1 strains.

The two remaining genes, *vpr* and *vpx*, are related to each other (112, 113). Although *vpx* is only in HIV-2 strains and most SIVs, *vpr* is present in HIV-1 strains as well as HIV-2 strains and SIVs (111). Studies show that *vpr* encodes a protein of about 13 kd (174–176), and *vpx* encodes a protein of about 12 kd (25, 109, 110). Both these proteins are packaged in virus particles (109, 110, 174–176). The observation that the Vpx protein is packaged in amounts equimolar to *gag* has been used to argue that it is essential (110); studies have found 2000 to 3000 copies of the Vpx per particle with a half-life of 36 hours (177, 178). Vpx appears to be dispensable, with negligible effects in established T-cell lines (172, 179–181). However, when fresh lymphocytes are used, Vpx mutants grow poorly, with a reduction of 10-fold or more in early DNA synthesis (179, 182, 183). Vpx in the SIV system has been shown to be both necessary and sufficient for the nuclear import of the viral reverse transcription complex (184). Vpr is thought to enhance growth of HIV-2 in macrophages (185) and to inhibit the progression of infected cells from the G2 to the M phase of the cell cycle (184). An infectious molecular clone of HIV-2 (UC2) has been described with a defective *vpr*, yet it is still capable of limited replication in baboons (186).

A significant proportion of HIV-2–infected persons make antibodies to Vpx (97). When present, such antibodies can be used to establish infection with HIV-2 as opposed to HIV-1. A few infected people also make antibodies to the Vpr product (176). Data suggest that Vpr may function as a regulator of cellular permissiveness to HIV-1 replication. Like HIV-1 Vpr, the Vpr of HIV-2 causes cells to accumulate in G$_2$ of the cell cycle, although this effect is attenuated in HIV-2 relative to HIV-1 (178). The distant genetic relatedness of Vpr to Vpx has suggested that the Vpx in HIV-2/SIV results from a ancient duplication of the Vpr gene (112), The relevance of this observation to the function of these genes in HIV-2 is still not known.

STRUCTURAL GENES: *GAG* AND *ENV*

The *gag* gene products are essentially the same for HIV-1 and HIV-2 (187) and are highly conserved. A 55-kd precursor is myristoylated and cleaved by the viral protease to form p17 (MA), p24 (CA), p2, p7 (NC), p1, and p6. The matrix protein (MA) p17 is at the amino terminus, and in its cleaved form it surrounds the nucleocapsid. The capsid (CA) p24 is slightly larger for HIV-2 or SIV and is sometimes described as p27 (9, 188). It provides the structure for the core that contains the genome and the polymerase and integrase enzymes (136). Workers have identified NC p7-8 as a nucleic acid binding protein (189), and both zinc finger motifs are involved with the specificity of packaging the genomic viral RNA into the virions (190).

The envelope glycoprotein precursor is slightly smaller for HIV-2, as are the external glycoprotein and the transmembrane protein. Although usually described using the terminology for HIV-1 (gp160, gp120, gp41, respectively), the HIV-2 glycoproteins are sometimes designated with lower sizes (e.g., gp140B145, gp105B110, gp32B40). By analysis of the primary amino acid sequence for N-linked glycosylation sites, the HIV-2 and SIV gp120s have significantly fewer conserved sites. This feature could presumably account for the lower molecular weight of the HIV-2 gp120, because carbohydrates make up 50% or more of the HIV-1 gp120 (191–193). The HIV-2 has at least one glycosylation site near the carboxy terminus that seems important for CD4 binding and infectivity (194). For HIV-1, all the N-linked glycosylation sites that are important for infectivity appear to be on the amino terminus side (191).

HIV-2 envelope sequences vary to approximately the same degree as HIV-1 sequences (23–30). Although the V3 regions correspond in both virus types, HIV-2 strains do not have the conserved GPGR amino acid sequence at the tip of the V3 loop (25, 30).

In general, however, sites on the external glycoprotein appear to be conserved between HIV-1 and HIV-2. This is true for CD4 binding (104, 195), precursor processing (196), fusion (196, 197), principal neutralizing domain at V3 (30, 197, 198), cytolytic T-cell activity (199), and perhaps for antibody-dependent cell cytotoxicity (198, 200, 201). With HIV-1, much of the envelope glycoprotein appears to generate binding antibodies. Binding activity as assayed, using antibodies from people infected with HIV-2, appears to be more concentrated to specific areas in the middle of gp120, including the V3 loop (202, 203). Another area for antibody binding activity is at the amino terminus of the transmembrane protein (202, 204). Another region, at the carboxy terminus of gp120, may be slightly less immu-

Table 57.3. Functional Activities of Envelope Gene Mapped to Specific Epitopes of HIV-2

Function	Amino Acid Position	References
Antibody binding for diagnosis		
Greatest immunogenicity	224–230, 524–763	202, 203
Type specificity	307–327, 479–511, 537–707	204, 216, 223
Virus neutralization		
Principal neutralizing domain	311–337	30, 197, 198
Other neutralization domains	119–137, 472–509, 595–614, 714–729	198
Antibody-dependent cell cytotoxicity	291–311, 446–461	198
Cytolytic T-cell function	265–279	199
Cleavage	501–511	276, 208
Fusion/syncytia induction	308–340, 506–521	276, 197, 277
Glycosylation site for infectivity	331–445	115, 116, 278
CD4 binding	331–445	115, 116, 278
Cytoplasmic domain	700–850	208

nogenic, but it appears to be the most cross-reactive (204). The various sites for activity on the envelope proteins are summarized in Table 57.3.

The most type-specific region of HIV-2 g120, the V3 loop region, is also the principal neutralizing domain, as it is for HIV-1 (30, 197, 198). However, other neutralizing regions of lower activity have been described, including a linear epitope in V2 and one conformational epitope outside V1, V2, and V3 (198, 205), and some investigators have described cross-neutralization between HIV-1 and HIV-2 with human antibodies (206, 207). Although the reactions are usually weak in both directions, they appear stronger for serum from HIV-2–infected people for neutralization of HIV-1 (206, 207). Although the fusion domains for syncytia induction have been mapped to the hydrophobic amino terminus of the transmembrane protein, loss of syncytia-inducing ability does not appear to have much of an effect on the infectivity of HIV-2 (196).

Both HIV-1 and HIV-2 have a long cytoplasmic domain on the transmembrane protein. This domain often becomes truncated, at least on culturing the virus in T-cell lines. Even small truncations of this sort appear to enhance fusion activity (208, 209). Whether this has any importance in vivo is unclear.

SEROLOGIC TESTING

The same procedures for antibody blood testing and clinical diagnosis that were developed for HIV-1 are used for HIV-2. Because most of the tests were developed for HIV-1 using HIV-1 antigens, the degree of cross-reactivity and specificity for HIV-2 is variable. Most of the first-generation tests used whole-virus antigens, in which core antigens such as p24 and pol p66/p51 are well represented. These antigens are more strongly cross-reactive than envelope antigens, especially gp120 (9, 20, 210–212). Similarly, enzyme-linked immunosorbent assays using core antigens or whole HIV-1 virus are likely to be more sensitive for HIV-2 antibodies than Western blot (WB), which may rely more on a profile of antigens that includes envelope activity. Radioimmunoprecipitation (RIPA) may be more sensitive than WB because it allows more conformational cross-reactivity for the larger envelope molecules (10, 20, 210–212). Competition assays are generally much less sensitive when using HIV-1 antigens to detect HIV-2 antibodies. In general, a trade-off occurs between sensitivity and specificity. The HIV-1–based tests that are best to detect HIV-2 are likely to be highest in general sensitivity but lowest in specificity, whether for HIV-1 or HIV-2. Although much less common, cross-reactivity between gp120s of HIV-1 and HIV-2 can be seen, perhaps best by RIPA (213). HIV-2–infected persons tend to have envelope cross-reactive antibodies for HIV-1 antigens more often than do HIV-1–infected persons for HIV-2 antigens (213, 214). This situation is fortunate, because most reference tests are made with HIV-1 antigens.

Even when confirmatory tests are made with HIV-2 whole-virus antigen, a problem with HIV-2 WB and RIPA assays may be the tendency of the transmembrane protein to form trimers of about the same size as the gp120 (215). This is particularly important when the criteria of "two envelope reactivities" are used, resulting in potential false-positive confirmation.

Various investigations have focused on identifying type-specific antigens to allow confirmatory tests that will distinguish between HIV-1 and HIV-2. Most have been made as synthetic peptides (216–221), but some were larger, bacterially expressed peptides (222, 223) (see Table 57.3). These peptides have varied in sensitivity and specificity. Because most were selected for specificity, one may expect that sensitivity could be compromised. Thus, although they are appropriate for type-specific confirmation, they may not be as useful as larger HIV-2–specific antigens for initial screening.

When human serum samples are screened in such places as the Ivory Coast, Senegal, and Burkina Faso, a disproportionately large fraction of the samples often test as "dual positive" because they appear reactive on both HIV-1 and HIV-2 confirmatory tests (20, 48, 223). These sites have increasing numbers of HIV-1–infected persons on a population background with significant levels of HIV-2 infection. Whether the true fraction of dual positives is higher than one should expect by chance is unclear. Most of the dual reactives fall out when polymerase chain reaction (PCR) tests are done that are specific for HIV-1 or HIV-2, and an even larger number fails to yield both types of virus after cultivation (224–227). One can also use Vpu antibody tests that are specific for HIV-1 and Vpx antibody tests that are specific for HIV-2 (105, 109). Unfortunately, significant numbers of infected persons fail to make detectable antibodies to these antigens.

The HIV dual antibody profile is characterized by antibodies with strong reactivity to the env antigens of both HIV-1 and HIV-2 by immunoblot and RIPA (211, 228, 229). Several possible biologic explanations for this phenomenon can be entertained, including extensive cross-reactivity by either of the HIVs, dual infection, and infection with an intermediate virus such as a recombinant. Isolation of both HIV-1 and HIV-2 has been reported from selected HIV-dual cases, and PCR evidence of both viruses has ranged from 30 to 80%, in serologically defined dual reactives reported from similar populations (225–227). Whether the low and variable rate of concordance between serologic studies and PCR is due to extensive HIV-1 cross-reactivity as suggested, misclassification of samples based on serodiagnosis, or insensitivity of the PCR assays is unclear. Recent refinement of PCR assays with Southern blot detection of the amplified product has maximized the sensitivity and specificity for HIV-2 provirus detection (230). The further development of such assays is critical to studies that seek to characterize HIV-2 biology and its interaction with HIV-1 in vivo.

PATHOGENESIS

Few studies have evaluated deterioration of the immune system or alternatives in the virus load over time in HIV-2–infected people. To our knowledge, the only long-term follow-up cohort of healthy HIV-2–infected people is in Senegal (12). The number of acquired immunodeficiency syndrome (AIDS) cases that have developed in that cohort remains low (see later). Most early changes in HIV-1–infected people have been studied most readily after infection through blood transfusion or intravenous drug use. HIV-2–infected individuals with known infection times have rarely been available in West Africa, thus making it difficult to establish parameters such as the interval between infection and disease, or the possible presence of an early flu-like syndrome. Much is now becoming known about sites of replication, cell tropism, and genetic variation of HIV-1 during the course of infection, but this information is almost completely lacking for HIV-2. The possibility also exists that some strains of HIV-2 may be more virulent, but this possibility has not been established.

In cross-sectional studies, T4 lymphocyte counts and T4:T8 ratios appear reduced in HIV-2–infected healthy carriers, but less dramatically than for HIV-1–infected carriers (14, 231–235). Alterations in T-cell subsets evaluated prospectively have shown similar results, in which immunosuppression in HIV-2–infected people was significantly slower than HIV-1 and could not be demonstrated in all followed subjects (236, 237). Similarly, neopterin and β_2-microgloloulin levels are elevated in HIV-2–infected individuals, but less so than in persons infected with HIV-1 (234, 235). Skin test anergy to various antigens is also less pronounced in HIV-2 infection (14, 231, 235).

Investigators have established that new genotypes of HIV-1 evolve over time in the same individual after infection. The earliest isolates generally grow in macrophages as well as lymphocytes. They do not cause syncytia in established T-cell lines and are associated with a "slow-low" phase in which the load of virus in blood and blood cells is low. As disease develops, HIV-1 strains that have changes in the envelope V3 loop evolve. These viruses are often associated with higher virus loads in blood and syncytia induction in T-cell lines and are called "rapid-high" viruses (238–242).

The ability of HIV-2 strains to induce syncytia may be lower than for HIV-1 strains (243). HIV-2 is more difficult to isolate from asymptomatic persons than is HIV-1, but when it is isolated, it appears to show the "slow-low" pattern (244, 245). Similarly, the "rapid-high" isolates are more likely to be from HIV-2–infected people with disease. The determinants of cell tropism and replication capacity for HIV-2 have not yet been mapped. However, a correlation among the number of charged residues in the V3 loop, the nature of the residues at positions 18 and 19 of the V3 loop, and the phenotype of HIV-2 isolates has been described (44). Evidence of a lower viral burden in HIV-2–infected persons has been reported from both virus isolation and PCR studies (246–248). The isolation rate of HIV-2 from peripheral blood mononuclear cells or plasma of asymptomatic HIV-2–infected persons was lower than the isolation rate for HIV-1 (246). At lower CD4+ lymphocyte counts, virus isolation was equally efficient in both infections. Studies in the Gambia and Senegal suggest that proviral HIV-2 copies increase with disease development and with the decrease in CD4+ lymphocytes (247, 249). The methods for measurement of HIV-1 plasma RNA have provided researchers with an important and predictive marker of HIV-1 pathogenesis. These assays are currently being developed for HIV-2 and will provide an important measurement of viral burden to characterize HIV-2 pathogenesis and compare it with that of HIV-1.

CLINICAL OUTCOME

HIV-2 appears to be less virulent than HIV-1, but it still is associated with AIDS development. Along with lower rates of transmission, less dramatic immune alterations, and lower virus loads, HIV-2–infected persons with disease appear to progress less rapidly (14, 232, 234, 250–252). HIV-2 infection is also more frequent in older women than is HIV-1 infection (12, 250), a finding suggesting that progression to disease is either slower or less frequent, or both (231, 250, 252).

Early surveys included various case reports of AIDS in HIV-2–infected persons (46, 253, 254). The disease characteristics, including tuberculosis, chronic diarrhea, and *Candida* infections, seemed similar to those seen in HIV-1–associated AIDS (46, 232, 255). Central nervous system involvement was also occasionally seen in HIV-2–infected persons (256, 257). However, classic African AIDS-associated diseases such as tuberculosis often had only a weak epidemiologic association with HIV-2, even in HIV-2–endemic areas (13, 14, 20, 258).

In one prospective study, HIV-2 infection was associated with subsequent disease development 5- to 10-fold less frequently than HIV-1 infection in the same cohort (14, 231). Because transmission rates for HIV-2 were 3- to 4-fold lower than for HIV-1 in the same cohort, this finding also suggests that HIV-2–infected persons were usually infected longer than those infected with HIV-1 (14, 231). Whether all HIV-2 strains may be slightly less aggressive or some strains and isolates in certain geographic areas may be less virulent or even nonvirulent remains to be determined. In the female sex worker cohort study in Dakar, Senegal, an update of their cohort study showed a 20-fold difference in the incidence rate of AIDS, comparing seroincident women with HIV-1 versus HIV-2 infection (259, 260). Although the rate of long-term nonprogression for HIV-1 varies between 2 and 20% according to the definition used, 16 of 21 HIV-2–infected women (76%) followed for longer than 8 years fit a common definition of long-term nonprogressors (237).

Studies of HIV-2 humoral immunity have now been extended to evaluate the highly related mucosal immune response. Evaluation of HIV-2 antibody responses in the cervicovaginal secretions showed that only one-third of infected women generate IgA responses to HIV-2 envelope antigens in this compartment, a finding suggesting lower levels of viral replication compared with HIV-1. The cross-reactivity by IgG and IgA to heterologous envelope antigens was more frequent with HIV-2 infection (261).

VACCINATION AND THERAPY

Drugs that have efficacy against HIV-1 are generally assumed to be effective against HIV-2. However, with a few exceptions of in vitro analysis (262–265), most drugs effective against HIV-1 have not been tested for activity against HIV-2. A case can therefore be made that HIV-2 infection in monkeys also provides a valuable in vivo model for drug testing that is not readily available for HIV-1 (266). Antiretroviral therapy has been infrequently reported in HIV-2 infection. A recent report of two HIV-2 AIDS cases undergoing zidovudine treatment in the Netherlands demonstrated mutations in the RT genes similar to those associated with zidovudine resistance in HIV-1 (267).

Studies from the Dakar, Senegal cohort showed that HIV-2–positive women were at lower risk of HIV-1 infection than were HIV-negative women; the original report of 70% protection was based on 9 years of observation (268). Demonstrated differences in the infectivity and disease potential of HIV-2 compared with HIV-1 support the notion that the mechanism for such protection may be analogous to the attenuated virus vaccine model. An update of the study with 11 years of observation indicates that HIV-2 protection ranges from 64 to 74%, depending on the method of analysis (268, 269). Further studies of this viral interaction are critical to confirming and defining the protective mechanism. In vitro studies of HIV-2 and HIV-1 suggest that viral determinants may be responsible for the inhibition of HIV-1 (270).

HIV-2 is primarily found in West Africa, where it infects an estimated 1 to 2 million people. It is also spread less efficiently than HIV-1, thus making projections for future infections much lower than for HIV-1. For these reasons, development of an HIV-2 vaccine has not been a high research priority. However, HIV-2 infects monkeys, whereas HIV-1 does not, and the SIV vaccine model uses viruses that are closer to HIV-2 than to HIV-1. The development and testing of an HIV-2 vaccine could therefore be simpler than the development of an HIV-1 vaccine. A few reports of HIV-2 have described experimental studies with limited vaccine protection (271, 272); immune correlates of protection have not been identified (273–275). Data from human studies suggesting that HIV-2 may afford protection from HIV-1 indicate that a candidate vaccine based on HIV-2 possibly could provide necessary cross-immunity for HIV-1 protection.

References

1. Gao F, Yue L, White A, et al. Human infection by genetically diverse SIVSM-related HIV-2 in West Africa. Nature 1992;358:495–499.
2. Essex M, Kanki P. The origins of the AIDS virus. Sci Am 1988;259:64–71.
3. Stahl Hennig C, Herchenroder O, Nick S, et al. Experimental infection of macaques with HIV-2ben, a novel HIV-2 isolate. AIDS 1990;4:611–617.
4. Castro BA, Nepomuceno M, Lerche NW, et al. Persistent infection of baboons and rhesus monkeys with different strains of HIV-2. Virology 1991;184:219–226.
5. Alter HJ, Eichberg JW, Masur H, et al. Transmission of HTLV-III from human plasma to chimpanzees: an animal model for AIDS. Science 1984;226:549–552.
6. Francis DP, Feorino PM, Broderson JR, et al. Infection of chimpanzees with lymphadenopathy-associated virus. Lancet 1984;2:1276–1277.
7. Gajdusek DC, Amyx HL, Gibbs CJJ, et al. Infection of chimpanzees by human T-lymphotropic retroviruses in brain and other tissues from AIDS patients. Lancet 1985;1:55–56.
8. Fultz PN, McClure HM, Swenson RB, et al. Persistent infection of chimpanzees with human T-lymphotropic virus type III/lymphadenopathy–associated virus: a potential model for acquired immunodeficiency syndrome. J Virol 1986;58:116–124.
9. Barin F, M'Boup S, Denis F, et al. Serological evidence for virus related to simian T-lymphotropic retrovirus III in residents of West Africa. Lancet 1985;2:1387–1390.
10. Kanki P, McLane MF, King NWJ, et al. Serologic identification and characterization of a macaque T-lymphotropic retrovirus closely related to HTLV-III. Science 1985;228:1199–1201.
11. Kanki P, Kurth R, Becker W, et al. Antibodies to simian T-lymphotropic retrovirus type III in African green monkeys and recognition of STLV III viral proteins by AIDS and related sera. Lancet 1985;1:1330–1332.
12. Kanki P, M'Boup S, Marlink R, et al. Prevalence and risk determinants of human immunodeficiency virus type 2 (HIV-2) and human immunodeficiency virus type 1 (HIV-1) in West African female prostitutes. Am J Epidemiol 1992;136:895–907.
13. Marlink RG, Ricard D, M'Boup S, et al. Clinical, hematologic, and immunologic cross-sectional evaluation of individuals exposed to human immunodeficiency virus type 2 (HIV-2). AIDS Res Hum Retroviruses 1988;4:137–148.
14. Marlink R. The biology and epidemiology of HIV-2. In: Essex M, M'Boup S, Kanki PJ, et al., eds. AIDS in Africa. New York: Raven Press, 1994:47–65.
15. Smith TF, Srinivasan A, Schochetman G, et al. The phylogenetic history of immunodeficiency viruses. Nature 1988;333:573–575.
16. Myers G, MacInnes K, Korber B. The emergence of simian/human immunodeficiency viruses. AIDS Res Hum Retroviruses 1992;8:373–386.
17. Marx P, Li Y, Lerche N, et al. Isolation of a simian immunodeficiency virus related to human immunodeficiency virus type 2 from a West African pet sooty mangebey. J Virol 1991;65:4480–4485.
18. Emau P, McClure HM, Isahakia M, et al. Isolation from African Sykes' monkeys (*Cercopithecus mitis*) of a lentivirus related to human and simian immunodeficiency viruses. J Virol 1991;65:2135–2140.
19. Allan JS, Kanda P, Kennedy RC, et al. Isolation and characterization of simian immunodeficiency viruses from two subspecies of African green monkeys. AIDS Res Hum Retroviruses 1990;6:275–285.
20. Kanki P, M'Boup S, Ricard D, et al. Human T-lymphotropic virus type 4 and the human immunodeficiency virus in West Africa. Science 1987;236:827–831.
21. Harrison LH, José da Silva AP, Gayle HD, et al. Risk factors for HIV-2 infection in Guinea-Bissau. J Acquir Immune Defic Syndr 1991;4:1155–1160.
22. Tristem M, Hill F, Karpas A. Nucleotide sequence of a Guinea-Bissau–derived human immunodeficiency virus type 2 proviral clone (HIV-2CAM2). J Gen Virol 1991;72:721–724.
23. Guyader M, Emerman M, Sonigo P, et al. Genome organization and transactivation of the human immunodeficiency virus type 2. Nature 1987;326:662–669.
24. Zagury JF, Franchini G, Reitz M, et al. Genetic variability between isolates of human immunodeficiency virus (HIV) type 2 is comparable to the variability among HIV type 1. Proc Natl Acad Sci U S A 1988;85:5941–5945.
25. Franchini G, Fargnoli KA, Giombini F, et al. Molecular and biological characterization of a replication competent human immunodeficiency type 2 (HIV-2) proviral clone. Proc Natl Acad Sci U S A 1989;86:2433–2437.
26. Kuhnel H, von Briesen H, Dietrich U, et al. Molecular cloning of two West African human immunodeficiency virus type 2 isolates that replicate well in macrophages: a Gambian isolate, from a patient with neurologic acquired immunodeficiency syndrome, and a highly divergent Ghanian isolate. Proc Natl Acad Sci U S A 1989;86:2383–2387.
27. Hasegawa A, Tsujimoto H, Maki N, et al. Genomic divergence of HIV-2 from Ghana. AIDS Res Hum Retroviruses 1989;5:593–604.
28. Kumar P, Hui HX, Kappes JC, et al. Molecular characterization of an attenuated human immunodeficiency virus type 2 isolate. J Virol 1990;64:890–901.
29. Klemm E, Schneweis KE, Horn R, et al. HIV-II infection with initial neurological manifestation. J Neurol 1988;235:304–307.
30. Boeri E, Giri A, Lillo F, et al. In vivo genetic variability of the human immunodeficiency virus type 2 V3 region. J Virol 1992;66:4546–4550.
31. Dietrich U, Adamski M, Kreutz R, et al. A highly divergent HIV-2–related isolate. Nature 1989;342:948–950.
32. Kawamura M, Katahira J, Fukasawa M, et al. Isolation and characterization of a highly divergent HIV-2[GH-2]: generation of an infectious molecular clone and functional analysis of its rev-responsive element in response to primate retrovirus transactivators (Rev and Rex). Virology 1992;188:850–853.
33. Miura T, Sakuragi J, Kawamura M, et al. Establishment of a phylogenetic survey system for AIDS-related lentiviruses and demonstration of a new HIV-2 subgroup. AIDS 1990;4:1257–1261.
34. Kuhnel H, von Briesen H, Dietrich U, et al. Molecular cloning of two West African HIV2 isolates that replicate well in macrophages. Res Virol 1990;141:233–237.
35. Castro B, Barnett S, Evans L, et al. Biologic heterogeneity of human immunodeficiency virus type 2 (HIV-2) strains. Virology 1990;178:527–534.
36. Bakhanashvili M, Hizi A. Fidelity of the RNA-dependent DNA synthesis exhibited by the reverse transcriptases of human immunodeficiency virus types 1 and 2 and of murine leukemia virus: mispair extension frequencies. Biochemistry 1992;31:9393–9398.
37. Myers G, Pavlakis GN. Evolutionary potential of complex retroviruses. In: Levy JA, ed. The Retroviridae. New York: Plenum Press, 1992:1–37.
38. Luke W, Fendrich C, Schreiner D, et al. Structural comparison of the external glycoproteins of human and simian immunodeficiency virus. Intervirology 1991;32:198–203.

39. Gao F, Yue L, Robertson DL, et al. Genetic diversity of human immunodeficiency virus type 2: evidence for distinct sequence subtypes with differences in virus biology. J Virol 1994;68:7433–7447.
40. Sankalé JL, De La Tour RS, Marlink RG, et al. Distinct quasi-species in the blood and the brain of an HIV-2–infected individual. Virology 1996;226:418–423.
41. Sankalé JL, M'Boup S, Marlink R, et al. HIV-2 and HIV-1 quasispecies in cervical secretions and blood. AIDS Res Hum Retroviruses (in press).
42. Sankalé JL, Sallier de la Tour R, Renjifo B, et al. Intra-patient variability of the human immunodeficiency virus type-2 (HIV-2) envelope V3 loop. AIDS Res Hum Retroviruses 1995;11:617–623.
43. Norrgren H, Leithner T, Aaby P, et al. Comparison of CD4 counts, viral load and genetic variation in HIV-2 infection: AIDS cases, old non-progressors and young asymptomatic subjects in Guinea-Bissau. In: 9th International AIDS in Africa Conference, Kampala, Uganda, 1995.
44. Albert J, Stalhandske P, Marquina S, et al. Biological phenotype of HIV type 2 isolates correlates with V3 genotype. AIDS Res Hum Retroviruses 1996;12:821–828.
45. Kanki P, Marlink R, Siby T, et al. Biology of HIV-2 infection in West Africa. In: Papas TS, ed. Gene regulation and AIDS. Houston: Portfolio Publishing Company of Texas, 1990:255–271.
46. Romieu I, Marlink R, Kanki P, et al. HIV-2 link to AIDS in West Africa. J Acquir Immune Defic Syndr 1990;3:220–230.
47. Naucler A, Andreasson PA, Costa CM, et al. HIV-2-associated AIDS and HIV-2 seroprevalence in Bissau, Guinea-Bissau. J Acquir Immune Defic Syndr 1989;2:88–93.
48. Denis F, Barin F, Gershy-Damet G, et al. Prevalence of human T-lymphotropic retroviruses type III (HIV) and type IV in Ivory Coast. Lancet 1987;1:408–411.
49. Naucler A, Anderson B, Norrgren H, et al. Prevalence and incidence of HIV-1, HIV-2, HTLV, and *Treponema pallidum* infections among police officers in Guinea Bissau. In: 8th International Conference on AIDS in Africa, Yaounde, 1993.
50. De Cock K, Odehouri K, Moreau J, et al. Rapid emergence of AIDS in Abidjan, Ivory Coast. Lancet 1989;2:408–410.
51. Kanki P, Travers K, Hernandez-Avila M, et al. Slower heterosexual spread of HIV-2 compared with HIV-1. Lancet 1994;343:943–946.
52. Kanki P, DeCock KM. Epidemiology and natural history of HIV-2. AIDS 1994;8(Suppl):S1–S9.
53. Ankrah T, Roberts M, Antwi P, et al. The African AIDS case definition and HIV serology in medical in-patients at Komfo Anokye Teaching Hospital, Kumasi, Ghana. West Afr J Med 1994;13:98.
54. Olaleye O, Bernstein L, Ekweozor C, et al. Prevalence of human immunodeficiency virus types 1 and 2 infections in Nigeria. J Infect Dis 1993;167:710.
55. Kline R, Dada A, Blattner W, et al. Diagnosis and differentiation of HIV-1 and HIV-2 infection by two rapid assays in Nigeria. J Acquir Immune Defic Syndr Hum Retrovirol 1994;7:623.
56. Maiga Y, Sissoko Z, Maiga M. Étude de la séroprévalence de l'infection à VIH dans les 7 régions économiques du Mali. In: 8th International Conference on AIDS in Africa/8th African Conference on Sexually Transmitted Diseases, Marrakech, 1993.
57. Koffi K, Gershy-Damet G, Peeters M, et al. Rapid spread of HIV infections in Abidjan, Ivory Coast, 1987–1990. Eur J Clin Microbiol Infect Dis 1992;11:271.
58. Kanki P, Allan J, Barin F, et al. Absence of antibodies to HIV-2/HTLV-4 in six Central African Nations. AIDS Res Hum Retroviruses 1987;3:317–322.
59. Santos-Ferreira M, Cohen T, Lourenco M, et al. A study of seroprevalence of HIV-1 and HIV-2 in six provinces of People's Republic of Angola: clues to the spread of HIV infection. J Acquir Immune Defic Syndr 1990;3:780.
60. Victorino RMM, Guerreiro D, Lourenço MH, et al. Prevalence of HIV-2 infection in a family planning clinic in Libson. Int J STD AIDS 1992;3:281–284.
61. Rubsamen-Waigmann H, Briesen H, Maniar J, et al. Spread of HIV-2 in India. Lancet 1991;337:550–551.
62. Rubsamen-Waigmann H, Maniar J, Gerte S, et al. High proportion of HIV-2 and HIV-1/2 double-reactive sera in two Indian states, Maharashtra and Goa: first appearance of an HIV-2 epidemic along with an HIV-1 epidemic outside of Africa. Int J Med Microbiol Virol Parasitol Infect Dis 1994;280:398.
63. Courouce AM, Barin F, Baudelot J, et al. HIV-2 infection among blood donors and other subjects in France. Transfusion 1989;29:368.
64. Matheron S, Simon F, Sassi G, et al. Infection HIV-2 chez l'adulte: étude de cohorte, Paris, 1986–1993. In: 8th International Conference on AIDS in Africa and 8th African Conference on Sexually Transmitted Diseases, Marrakech, 1993.
65. De Cock K, Brun-Vezinet F. Epidemiology of HIV-2 Infection. AIDS 1989;3(Suppl 1):S89–S95.
66. Smallman-Raynor M, Cliff A. The spread of human immunodeficiency virus type 2 into Europe: a geographical analysis. Int J Epidemiol 1991;20:480.
67. Mazeron M, Cerboni J, Alain S, et al. Prevalence of HIV infections among patients attending a Parisian anonymous testing center between 1988 and 1993. Pathol Biol (Paris) 1994;42:520.
68. Gayle H, Gnaore E, Adjorlolo G, et al. HIV-1 and HIV-2 infection in children in Abidjan, Cote D'Ivoire. J Acquir Immune Defic Syndr 1992;5:513.
69. Gershy-Damet G, Koffi K, Soro B, et al. Seroepidemiological survey of HIV-1 and HIV-2 infections in the five regions of Ivory Coast. AIDS 1991;5:462–463.
70. Donnelly C, Leisening W, Sandberg S, et al. Comparison of transmission rates of HIV-1 and HIV-2 in a cohort of prostitutes in Senegal. Bull Math Biol 1993;55:731–741.
71. Hendry R, Parks D, Campos Mello D, et al. Lack of evidence for HIV-2 infection among at-risk individuals in Brazil. J Acquir Immune Defic Syndr 1991;4:623.
72. Kvinesdal BB, Worm AM, Lindhardt BO, et al. HIV-2 infection in Denmark. Scand J Infect Dis 1992;24:419–421.
73. Georgoulias V, Agelakis A, Fountouli P, et al. Seroprevalence of HIV-2 infection in Greece (Crete). J Acquir Immune Defic Syndr 1990;3:1188–1192.
74. Costigliola P, Ricchi E, Manfredi R, et al. No evidence of HIV-2 infection amongst HIV-1 Ab positive people in the largest cities of north-eastern Italy. Eur J Epidemiol 1992;8:140–141.
75. Soriano V, Aguado I, Fernandez JL, et al. Multicenter study of the prevalence of type 2 human immunodeficiency virus infection in Spain (1990). Med Clin 1992;98:771–774.
76. Estebanez P, Sarasqueta C, Rua-Figueroa M, et al. Absence of HIV-2 in Spanish groups at risk for HIV-1 infection. AIDS Res Hum Retroviruses 1992;8:423–424.
77. Downing RG, Biryahwaho B. No evidence for HIV-2 infection in Uganda. Lancet 1990;336:1514–1515.
78. O'Brien TR, George JR, Epstein JS, et al. Testing for antibodies to human immunodeficiency virus type 2 in the United States. MMWR Morb Mortal Wkly Rep 1992;41:1–9.
79. Myers RA, Patel JD, Joseph JM. Identifying HIV-2-seropositive individuals by reevaluating HIV-1 indeterminate sera. J Acquir Immune Defic Syndr 1992;5:417–423.
80. Anderson RM, May RM. The population biology of the interaction between HIV-1 and HIV-2: coexistence or competitive exclusion? AIDS 1996;10:1663–1673.
81. Parkman PD. Recommendations for the prevention of human immunodeficiency virus (HIV) transmission by blood and blood products. Bethesda, MD: Food and Drug Administration, Center for Biologics Evaluation and Research, 1990.
82. Dufoort G, Courouce A, Ancelle-Park R, et al. No clinical signs 14 years after HIV-2 transmission via blood transfusion. Lancet 1988;2:510.
83. Kanki PJ, Hamel D, Sankalé J-L, et al. HIV-1 subtypes differ in disease progression. Bethesda, MD: National Conference Development AIDS Vaccine Groups, 1997.

84. Pepin J, Quigley M, Todd J, et al. Association between HIV-2 infection and genital ulcer diseases among male sexually transmitted disease patients in the Gambia. AIDS 1992;6:489–493.
85. Aaby P, Ariyoshi K, Buckner M, et al. Age of wife as a major determinant of male-to-female transmission of HIV-2 infection: a community study from rural West Africa. AIDS 1996;10:1585–1590.
86. Morgan G, Wilkins HA, Pepin J, et al. AIDS following mother-to-child transmission of HIV-2. AIDS 1990;4:879–882.
87. Del Mistro A, Chotard J, Mali A, et al. HIV-1 and HIV-2 seroprevalence rates in mother-child pairs living in the Gambia, West Africa. J Acquir Immune Defic Syndr 1992;5:19.
88. Poulsen AG, Kvinesdal BB, Aaby P, et al. Lack of evidence of vertical transmission of human immunodeficiency virus type 2 in a sample of the general population in Bissau. J Acquir Immune Defic Syndr 1992;5:25–30.
89. Andreasson P, Dias F, Naucler A, et al. A prospective study of vertical transmission of HIV-2 in Bissau, Guinea-Bissau. AIDS 1993;7:989.
90. Adjorlolo-Johnson G, DeCock K, Ekpini E, et al. Prospective comparison of mother-to-child transmission of HIV-1 and HIV-2 in Abidjan, Ivory Coast. JAMA 1994;272:462.
91. Anonymous. Comparison of vertical human immunodeficiency virus type 2 and human immunodeficiency virus type 1 transmission in the French prospective cohort: the HIV Infection in Newborns French Collaborative Study Group. Pediatr Infect Dis J 1994;13:502.
92. Ngagne M, Diouf A, Kebe F, et al. Histoire naturelle de la transmission verticale VIH1 et VIH 2 à Dakar. In: 9th International Conference on AIDS and Associated Cancers in Africa, Kampala, Uganda, 1995.
93. Abbott RC, Ndour-Sarr A, Diouf A, et al. Risk determinants for HIV infection and adverse obstetrical outcomes in pregnant women in Dakar, Senegal. J Acquir Immune Defic Syndr Hum Retrovirol 1994;7:711–717.
94. Gonda MA, Wong-Staal F, Gallo RC, et al. Sequence homology and morphologic similarity of HTLV-III and visna virus, a pathogenic lentivirus. Science 1985;227:173–177.
95. Palmer E, Sporborg C, Harrison A, et al. Morphology and immuno-electron microscopy of AIDS virus. Arch Virol 1985;85:189–196.
96. Palmer E, Martin ML, Goldsmith C, et al. Ultrastructure of human immunodeficiency virus type 2. J Gen Virol 1988;69:1425–1429.
97. Yu X, Yuan X, Matsuda Z, et al. The matrix protein of human immunodeficiency virus type 1 is required for incorporation of viral envelope protein into mature virions. J Virol 1992;66:4966–4971.
98. Yu X, Yuan X, McLane MF, et al. Mutations in the cytoplasmic domain of human immunodeficiency virus type 1 transmembrane protein impair the incorporation of Env proteins into mature virions. J Virol 1993;67:213–221.
99. Daniel MD, Letvin NL, King NW, et al. Isolation of T-cell tropic HTLV-III-like retrovirus from macaques. Science 1985;228:1201–1204.
100. Hockley DJ, Wood RD, Jacobs JP, et al. Electron microscopy of human immunodeficiency virus. J Gen Virol 1988;69:2455–2469.
101. Yu Q-C, Matzuda Z, Yu X-F, et al. An electron-lucent region within the virion distinguishes human immunodeficiency virus (HIV) type 1 from HIV-2 and simian immunodeficiency virus. AIDS Res Hum Retroviruses 1994;10:745–749.
102. Yu X, Matsuda Z, Yu QC, et al. Vpx of simian immunodeficiency virus is localized primarily outside the virus core in mature virions. J Virol 1993;67:4386–4390.
103. Tristem M, Mansinho K, Champalimaud JL, et al. Six new isolates of human immunodeficiency virus type 2 (HIV-2) and the molecular characterization of one (HIV-2CAM2). J Gen Virol 1989;70:479–484.
104. Kirchhoff F, Jentsch KD, Bachmann B, et al. A novel proviral clone of HIV-2: biological and phylogenetic relationship to other primate immunodeficiency viruses. Virology 1990;177:305–311.
105. Matsuda Z, Chou MJ, Matsuda M, et al. Human immunodeficiency virus type 1 has an additional coding sequence in the central region of the genome. Proc Natl Acad Sci U S A 1988;85:6968–6972.
106. Strebel K, Klimkait T, Maldarelli F, et al. Molecular and biochemical analyses of human immunodeficiency virus type 1 vpu protein. J Virol 1989;63:3784–3791.
107. Cohen EA, Terwilliger EF, Sodroski JG, et al. Identification of a protein encoded by the vpu gene of HIV-1. Nature 1988;334:532–534.
108. Bour S, Strebel K. The human immunodeficiency virus (HIV) type 2 envelope protein is a functional complement to HIV type 1 Vpu that enhances particle release of heterologous retroviruses. J Virol 1996;70:8285–300.
109. Yu XF, Ito S, Essex M, et al. A naturally immunogenic virion-associated protein specific for HIV-2 and SIV. Nature 1988;335:262–265.
110. Henderson L, Sowder R, Copeland T, et al. Isolation and characterization of a novel protein (X-ORF product) from SIV and HIV-2. Science 1988;241:199–201.
111. Kappes J, Morrow C, Lee S, et al. Identification of a novel retroviral gene unique to human immunodeficiency virus type 2 and simian immunodeficiency virus SIVMAC. J Virol 1988;62:3501–3505.
112. Tristem M, Marshall C, Karpas A, et al. Origin of vpx in lentiviruses. Nature 1990;347:341–342.
113. Tristem M, Marshall C, Karpas A, et al. Evolution of the primate lentiviruses: evidence from vpx and vpr. EMBO J 1992;11:3405–3412.
114. Moore JP. Simple methods for monitoring HIV-1 and HIV-2 gp120 binding to soluble CD4 by enzyme-linked immunosorbent assay: HIV-2 has a 25-fold lower affinity than HIV-1 for soluble CD4. AIDS 1990;4:297–305.
115. Morikawa Y, Moore JP, Fenouillet E, et al. Complementation of human immunodeficiency virus glycoprotein mutations in trans. J Gen Virol 1992;73:1907–1913.
116. Bahraoui E, Benjouad A, Guetard D, et al. Study of the interaction of HIV-1 and HIV-2 envelope glycoproteins with the CD4 receptor and role of N-glycans. AIDS Res Hum Retroviruses 1992;8:565–573.
117. Looney DJ, Hayashi S, Nicklas M, et al. Differences in the interaction of HIV-1 and HIV-2 with CD4. J Acquir Immune Defic Syndr 1990;3:649–657.
118. Hoxie JA, Brass LF, Pletcher CH, et al. Cytopathic variants of an attenuated isolate of human immunodeficiency virus type 2 exhibit increased affinity for CD4. J Virol 1991;65:5096–5101.
119. Mulligan MJ, Ritter GD, Chaikin MA, et al. Human immunodeficiency virus type 2 envelope glycoprotein: differential CD4 interactions of soluble gp120 versus the assembled envelope complex. Virology 1992;187:233–241.
120. Clapham P, McKnight A, Weiss RA. Human immunodeficiency virus type 2 infection and fusion of CD4-negative human cell lines: induction and enhancement by soluble CD4. J Virol 1992;66:3531–3537.
121. Hart AR, Cloyd MW. Interference patterns of human immunodeficiency viruses HIV-1 and HIV-2. Virology 1990;177:1–10.
122. Le Guern M, Levy JA. Human immunodeficiency virus (HIV) type 1 can superinfect HIV-2–infected cells: pseudotype virions produced with expanded cellular host range. Proc Natl Acad Sci U S A 1992;89:363–367.
123. Feng Y, Broder C, Kennedy P, et al. HIV-1 entry cofactor: functional cDNA cloning of a seven-transmembrane, G protein-coupled receptor. Science 1996;272:872–877.
124. Endres MJ, Clapham PR, Marsh M, et al. CD4-independent infection by HIV-2 is mediated by fusin/CXCR4. Cell 1996;87:745–756.
125. Edinger AL, Amedee A, Miller K, et al. Differential utilization of CCR5 by macrophage and T cell tropic simian immunodeficiency virus strains. Proc Natl Acad Sci U S A 1997;94:4005–4010.
126. Oroszlan S, Luftig RB. Retroviral proteinases. Curr Top Microbiol Immunol 1990;157:153–185.
127. Pichuantes S, Babe LM, Barr PJ, et al. Recombinant HIV2 protease processes HIV1 Pr53gag and analogous junction peptides in vitro. J Biol Chem 1990;265:13,890–13,898.
128. Allan JS, Coligan JE, Lee TH, et al. Immunogenic nature of a *pol* gene product of HTLV-III/LAV. Blood 1987;69:331–333.

129. Shaharabany M, Hizi A. The DNA-dependent and RNA-dependent DNA polymerase activities of the reverse transcriptases of human immunodeficiency viruses types 1 and 2. AIDS Res Hum Retroviruses 1991;7:883–888.
130. Hizi A, Tal R, Hughes SH. Mutational analysis of the DNA polymerase and ribonuclease H activities of human immunodeficiency virus types 2 reverse transcriptase expressed in *Escherichia coli*. Virology 1991;180:339–346.
131. Hizi A, Tal R, Shaharabany M, et al. Catalytic properties of the reverse transcriptase of human immunodeficiency viruses type 1 and type 2. J Biol Chem 1991;266:6230–6239.
132. Whitcomb JM, Hughes SH. The sequence of human immunodeficiency virus type 2 circle junction suggests that integration protein cleaves the ends of linear DNA asymmetrically. J Virol 1991;65:3906–3910.
133. van Gent DC, Groeneger AA, Plasterk RH. Mutational analysis of the integrase protein of human immunodeficiency virus type 2. Proc Natl Acad Sci U S A 1992;89:9598–602.
134. Navia MA, Fitzgerald PM, McKeever BM, et al. Three-dimensional structure of aspartyl protease from human immunodeficiency virus HIV-1. Nature 1989;337:615–620.
135. Vinga-Martins C, Schneider T, Werno A, et al. Mapping of immunodominant epitopes of the HIV-1 and HIV-2 integrase proteins by recombinant proteins and synthetic peptides. AIDS Res Hum Retroviruses 1992;8:1301–1310.
136. Haseltine WA. The molecular biology of HIV-1. In: DeVita VT Jr, Hellman S, Rosenberg SA, et al., eds. AIDS, etiology, diagnosis, treatment and prevention. 3rd ed. Philadelphia: JB Lippincott, 1992:39–59.
137. Cullen BR. Human immunodeficiency virus as a prototypic complex retrovirus. J Virol 1991;65:1053–1056.
138. Tong-Starksen S, Welsh T, Peterlin M. Differences in transcriptional enhancers of HIV-1 and HIV-2 response to T-cell activation signals. J Immunol 1990;145:4348–4354.
139. Markovitz DM, Hannibal M, Perez VL, et al. Differential regulation of human immunodeficiency viruses (HIVs): a specific regulatory element in HIV-2 responds to stimulation of the T-cell antigen receptor. Proc Natl Acad Sci U S A 1990;87:9098–9102.
140. Arya S, Gallo C. Human immunodeficiency virus type 2 long terminal repeat: analysis of regulatory elements. AIDS 1988;85:9753–9757.
141. Courgnaud V, Laure F, Fultz PN, et al. Genetic differences accounting for evolution and pathogencity of simian immunodeficiency virus from a sooty mangabey after cross-species transmission to a pig-tailed macaque. J Virol 1992;66:414–419.
142. Nabel G, Baltimore D. An inducible transcription factor activates expression of human immunodeficiency virus in T cells. Nature 1987;326:711–713.
143. Arya SK. Human immunodeficiency virus type 2 (HIV-2) gene expression: downmodulation by sequence elements downstream of the transcriptional initiation site. AIDS Res Hum Retroviruses 1991;7:1007–1014.
144. Arya SK. Human immunodeficiency virus type-2 gene expression: two enhancers and their activation by T-cell activators. New Biologist 1990;2:57–65.
145. Arya SK, Sethi A. Stimulation of the human immunodeficiency virus type 2 (HIV-2) gene expression by the cytomegalovirus and HIV-2 transactivator gene. AIDS Res Hum Retroviruses 1990;6:649–658.
146. Fu GK, Markovitz DM. Purification of the pets factor: a nuclear protein that binds to the inducible TG-rich element of the human immunodeficiency virus type 2 enhancer. J Biol Chem 1996;271:19,599–19,605.
147. Markovitz DM, Smith MJ, Hilfinger J, et al. Activation of the human immunodeficiency virus type 2 enhancer is dependent on purine box and kappa B regulatory elements. J Virol 1992;66:5479–5484.
148. Seto E, Yen TS, Peterlin BM, et al. Trans-activation of the human immunodeficiency virus long terminal repeat by the hepatitis B virus X protein. Proc Natl Acad Sci U S A 1988;85:8286–8290.
149. Rimsky L, Hauber J, Dukovich M, et al. Functional replacement of the HIV-1 rev protein by the HTLV-1 rex protein. Nature 1988;335:738–740.
150. Mavankal G, Ignatius Ou SH, Oliver H, et al. Human immunodeficiency virus type 1 and 2 Tat proteins specifically interact with RNA polymerase II. Proc Natl Acad Sci U S A 1996;93:2089–2094.
151. Arya SK. Human and simian immunodeficiency retroviruses: activation and differential transactivation of gene expression. AIDS Res Hum Retroviruses 1988;4:175–186.
152. Berkhout B, Gatignol A, Silver J, et al. Efficient trans-activation by the HIV-2 Tat protein requires a duplicated TAR RNA structure. Nucleic Acids Res 1990;18:1839–1846.
153. Chang Y, Jeang KT. The basic RNA-binding domain of HIV-2 Tat contributes to preferential trans-activation of a TAR2-containing LTR. Nucleic Acids Res 1992;20:5465–5472.
154. Malim MH, Hauber J, Le SY, et al. The HIV-1 rev trans-activator acts through a structured target sequence to activate nuclear export of unspliced viral mRNA. Nature 1989;338:254–257.
155. Hammarskjold ML, Heimer J, Hammarskjold B, et al. Regulation of human immunodeficiency virus env expression by the rev gene product. J Virol 1989;63:1959–1966.
156. Emerman M, Vazeux R, Peden K. The rev gene product of the human immunodeficiency virus affects envelope-specific RNA localization. Cell 1989;57:1155–1165.
157. Dillon P, Nelbock P, Perkins A, et al. Structural and functional analysis of the human immunodeficiency virus type 2 *rev* protein. J Virol 1991;65:445–449.
158. Dayton AI, Terwilliger EF, Potz J, et al. *Cis*-acting sequences responsive to the rev gene product of the human immunodeficiency virus. J Acquir Immune Defic Syndr 1988;1:441–452.
159. Sakai H, Siomi H, Shida H, et al. Functional comparison of transactivation by human retrovirus rev and rex genes. J Virol 1990;64:5833–5839.
160. Dillon PJ, Nelbock P, Perkins A, et al. Function of the human immunodeficiency virus types 1 and 2 Rev proteins is dependent on their ability to interact with a structured region present in env gene mRNA. J Virol 1990;64:4428–4437.
161. Garrett ED, Cullen BR. Comparative analysis of Rev function in human immunodeficiency virus types 1 and 2. J Virol 1992;66:4288–4294.
162. Allan J, Coligan J, Lee TH, et al. A new HTLV-III/LAV encoded antigen detected by antibodies from AIDS patients. Science 1985;230:810–813.
163. Arya SK, Gallo RC. Three novel genes of human T-lymphotropic virus type III: immune reactivity of their products with sera from acquired immune deficiency syndrome patients. Proc Natl Acad Sci U S A 1986;83:2209–2213.
164. Terwilliger E, Sodroski JG, Rosen CA, et al. Effects of mutations within the 3′ orf open reading frame region of human T-cell lymphotropic virus type-III (HTLV/LAV) on replication and cytopathology. J Virol 1986;60:754–760.
165. Luciw PA, Cheng-Mayer C, Levy JA. Mutational analysis of the human immunodeficiency virus: the orf-B region down-regulates virus replication. Proc Natl Acad Sci U S A 1987;84:1434–1438.
166. Cheng Mayer C, Iannello P, Shaw K, et al. Differential effects of nef on HIV replication: implications for viral pathogenesis in the host. Science 1989;246:1629–1632.
167. Kestler HWD, Ringler DJ, Mori K, et al. Importance of the nef gene for maintenance of high virus loads and for development of AIDS. Cell 1991;65:651–662.
168. Schorr J, Kellner R, Fackler O, et al. Specific cleavage sites of Nef proteins from human immunodeficiency virus types 1 and 2 for the viral proteases. J Virol 1996;70:9051–9054.
169. Lee TH, Coligan J, Allan J, et al. A new HTLV-III/LAV protein encoded by a gene found in cytopathic retroviruses. Science 1986;231:1546–1549.
170. Strebel K, Daugherty D, Clouse K, et al. The HIV 'A' (sor) gene product is essential for virus infectivity. Nature 1987;328:728–730.

171. Fisher AG, Ensoli B, Ivanoff L, et al. The sor gene of HIV-1 is required for efficient virus transmission in vitro. Science 1987;237:888–893.
172. Shibata R, Miura T, Hayami M, et al. Mutational analysis of the human immunodeficiency virus type 2 (HIV-2) genome in relation to HIV-1 and simian immunodeficiency virus SIVagm. J Virol 1990;64:742–747.
173. Gabuzda D, Lawrence K, Langhoff E, et al. Role of vif in replication of human immunodeficiency virus type 1 in CD4+ T lymphocytes. J Virol 1992;66:6489–6495.
174. Yuan X, Matsuda Z, Matsuda M, et al. Human immunodeficiency virus vpr gene encodes a virion-associated protein. AIDS Res Hum Retroviruses 1990;6:1265–1271.
175. Cohen EA, Dehni G, Sodroski JG, et al. Human immunodeficiency virus vpr product is a virion-associated regulatory protein. J Virol 1990;64:3097–3099.
176. Yu X-F, Matsuda M, Essex M, et al. Open reading frame vpr of simian immunodeficiency virus encodes a virion-associated protein. J Virol 1990;64:5688–5693.
177. Kewalramani VN, Emerman M. Vpx association with mature core structures of HIV-2. Virology 1996;218:159–168.
178. Kewalramani VN, Park CS, Gallombardo PA, et al. Protein stability influences human immunodeficiency virus type 2 Vpr virion incorporation and cell cycle effect. Virology 1996;218:326–334.
179. Marcon L, Michaels F, Hattori N, et al. Dispensable role of the human immunodeficiency virus type 2 Vpx protein in viral replication. J Virol 1991;65:3938–3942.
180. Hu W, Vander Heyden N, Ratner L. Analysis of the function of viral protein X (VPX) of HIV-2. Virology 1989;173:624–630.
181. Dedera D, Hu W, Vander Heyden N, et al. Viral protein R of human immunodeficiency virus types 1 and 2 is dispensable for replication and cytopathogenicity in lymphoid cells. J Virol 1989;63:3205–3208.
182. Kappes J, Conway J, Lee S, et al. Human immunodeficiency virus type 2 vpx protein augments viral infectivity. Virology 1991;184:197–209.
183. Yu XF, Yu QC, Essex M, et al. The vpx gene of simian immunodeficiency virus facilitates efficient viral replication in fresh lymphocytes and macrophage. J Virol 1991;65:5088–5091.
184. Fletcher TM, Brichacek B, Sharova N, et al. Nuclear import and cell cycle arrest functions of the HIV-1 Vpr protein are encoded by two separate genes in HIV-2/SIV(SM). EMBO J 1996;15:6155–165.
185. Hattori N, Michaels F, Fargnoli K, et al. The human immunodeficiency virus type 2 vpr gene is essential for productive infection of human macrophages. Proc Natl Acad Sci U S A 1990;87:8080–8084.
186. Barnett SW, Legg HS, Sun Y, et al. Molecular cloning of the human immunodeficiency virus subtype 2 strain HIV-2UC2. Virology 1996;222:257–261.
187. Voss G, Kirchhoff F, Nick S, et al. Morphogenesis of recombinant HIV-2 gag core particles. Virus Res 1992;24:197–210.
188. Henderson L, Sowder R, Copeland T, et al. Gag precursors of HIV and SIV are cleaved into six proteins found in the mature virions. J Med Primatol 1990;19:411–419.
189. Gorelick RJ, Nigida SM Jr, Bess JW Jr, et al. Noninfectious human immunodeficiency virus type 1 mutants deficient in genomic RNA. J Virol 1990;64:3207–3211.
190. Komatsu H, Tsukahara T, Tozawa H. Viral RNA binding properties of human immunodeficiency virus type-2 (HIV-2) nucleocapsid protein-derived synthetic peptides. Biochem Mol Biol Intern 1996;38:1143–1154.
191. Lee WR, Syu WJ, Du B, et al. Nonrandom distribution of gp120 N-linked glycosylation sites important for infectivity of human immunodeficiency virus type 1. Proc Natl Acad Sci U S A 1992;89:2213–2217.
192. Lee WR, Yu XF, Syu WJ, et al. Mutational analysis of conserved N-linked glycosylation sites of human immunodeficiency virus type 1 gp41. J Virol 1992;66:1799–1803.
193. Leonard CK, Spellman MW, Riddle L, et al. Assignment of intrachain disulfide bonds and characterization of potential glycosylation sites of the type 1 recombinant human immunodeficiency virus envelope glycoprotein (gp120) expressed in Chinese hamster ovary cells. J Biol Chem 1990;265:10,373–10,382.
194. Hoxie JA. Hypothetical assignment of intrachain disulfide bonds for HIV-2 and SIV envelope glycoproteins. AIDS Res Hum Retroviruses 1991;7:495–499.
195. Franchini G, Gurgo C, Guo HG, et al. Sequence of simian immunodeficiency virus and its relationship to the human immunodeficiency viruses. Nature 1987;328:539–543.
196. Steffy K, Kraus G, Looney D, et al. Role of the fusogenic peptide sequence in syncytium induction and infectivity of human immunodeficiency virus type 2. J Virol 1992;66:4532–4535.
197. Robert-Guroff M, Aldrich K, Muldoon R, et al. Cross-neutralization of human immunodeficiency virus type 1 and 2 and simian immunodeficiency virus isolates. J Virol 1992;66:3602–3608.
198. Bjorling E, Broliden K, Bernardi D, et al. Hyperimmune antisera against synthetic peptides representing the glycoprotein of human immunodeficiency virus type 2 can mediate neutralization and antibody-dependent cytotoxic activity. Proc Natl Acad Sci U S A 1991;88:6082–6086.
199. Nixon DF, Huet S, Rothbard J, et al. An HIV-1 and HIV-2 cross-reactive cytotoxic T-cell epitope. AIDS 1990;4:841–845.
200. Norley SG, Mikschy U, Werner A, et al. Demonstration of cross-reactive antibodies able to elicit lysis of both HIV-1– and HIV-2– infected cells. J Immunol 1990;145:1700–1705.
201. Ljunggren K, Chiodi F, Biberfeld G, et al. Lack of cross-reaction in antibody-dependent cellular cytotoxicity between human immunodeficiency virus (HIV) and HIV-related West African strains. J Immunol 1988;140:602–605.
202. Huang M, Essex M, Lee TH. Localization of immunogenic domains in the human immunodeficiency virus type 2 envelope. J Virol 1991;65:5073–5079.
203. Mannervik M, Putkonen P, Ruden U, et al. Identification of B-cell antigenic sites on HIV-2 gp125. J Acquir Immune Defic Syndr 1992;5:177–187.
204. Norrby E, Putkonen P, Bottiger B, et al. Comparison of linear antigenic sites in the envelope proteins of human immunodeficiency virus (HIV) type 2 and type 1. AIDS Res Hum Retroviruses 1991;7:279–285.
205. McKnight A, Shotton C, Cordell J, et al. Location, exposure, and conservation of neutralizing and nonneutralizing epitopes on human immunodeficiency virus type 2 SU glycoprotein. J Virol 1996;70:4598–4606.
206. Weiss RA, Clapham PR, Weber JN, et al. HIV-2 antisera cross-neutralize HIV-1. AIDS 1988;2:95–100.
207. Bottiger B, Karlsson A, Andreasson PA, et al. Cross-neutralizing antibodies against HIV-1 (HTLV-IIIB and HTLV-IIIRF) and HIV-2 (SBL-6669 and a new isolate SBL-K135). AIDS Res Hum Retroviruses 1989;5:525–533.
208. Mulligan MJ, Yamshchikov GV, Ritter GD Jr, et al. Cytoplasmic domain truncation enhances fusion activity by the exterior glycoprotein complex of human immunodeficiency virus type 2 in selected cell types. J Virol 1992;66:3971–3975.
209. Kong L, Lee S, Kappes J, et al. West African HIV-2-related human retrovirus with attenuated cytopathicity. Science 1988;240:1525–1529.
210. Bottiger B, Karlsson A, Andreasson PA, et al. Envelope cross-reactivity between human immunodeficiency virus types 1 and 2 detected by different serological methods: correlation between cross-neutralization and reactivity against the main neutralizing site. J Virol 1990;64:3492–3499.
211. Holzer T, Allen R, Heynen C, et al. Discrimination of HIV-2 infection from HIV-1 infection by Western blot and radioimmuno-precipitation analysis. AIDS Res Hum Retroviruses 1990;6:515–524.
212. De Cock KM, Porter A, Kouadio J, et al. Cross-reactivity on Western blots in HIV-1 and HIV-2 infections. AIDS 1991;5:859–863.
213. Syu WJ, Du B, Essex M, et al. Association between cross-reactive HIV-2 gp120 antibody and disease progression in HIV-1 infection.

In: Lerner R, ed. Vaccines 1990. Cold Spring Harbor, NY: Cold Spring Harbor Press, 1990:373–377.
214. Espejo RT, Uribe P. Immunoprecipitation of human immunodeficiency virus type 2 glycoproteins by sera positive for human immunodeficiency virus type 1. J Clin Microbiol 1990;28:2107–2110.
215. Parekh BS, Pau CP, Granade TC, et al. Oligomeric nature of transmembrane glycoproteins of HIV-2: procedures for their efficient dissociation and preparation of Western blots for diagnosis. AIDS 1991;5:1009–1013.
216. Baillou A, Janvier B, Mayer R, et al. Site-directed serology using synthetic oligopeptides representing the C-terminus of the external glycoproteins of HIV-1, HIV-2, or SIV_{mac} may distinguish subtypes among primate lentiviruses. AIDS Res Hum Retroviruses 1991;7:767–772.
217. De Cock KM, Porter A, Kouadio J, et al. Rapid and specific diagnosis of HIV-1 and HIV-2 infections: an evaluation of testing strategies. AIDS 1990;4:875–878.
218. Ayres L, Avillez F, Garcia Benito A, et al. Multicenter evaluation of a new recombinant enzyme immunoassay for the combined detection of antibody to HIV-1 and HIV-2. AIDS 1990;4:131–138.
219. Baillou A, Barin F, Leonard G, et al. Competitive enzyme-immunoassays using native viral antigens to discriminate between HIV-1 and HIV-2 infections. J Virol Methods 1990;29:81–89.
220. Baillou A, Janvier B, Leonard G, et al. Fine serotyping of human immunodeficiency virus serotype 1 (HIV-1) and HIV-2 infections by using synthetic oligopeptides representing an immunodominant domain of HIV-1 and HIV-2/simian immunodeficiency virus. J Clin Microbiol 1991;29:1387–1391.
221. Broliden PA, Ruden U, Ouattara AS, et al. Specific synthetic peptides for detection of and discrimination between HIV-1 and HIV-2 infection. J Acquir Immune Defic Syndr 1991;4:952–958.
222. Gueye-Ndiaye A, Clark R, Samuel K, et al. Cost-effective diagnosis of HIV-1 and HIV-2 by recombinant-expressed env peptide (566/966) dot blot analysis. AIDS 1993;7:481–495.
223. Zuber M, Samuel KP, Lautenberger JA, et al. Bacterially produced HIV-2 env polypeptides specific for distinguishing HIV-2 from HIV-1 infections. AIDS Res Hum Retroviruses 1990;6:525–534.
224. Pieniazek D, Peralta JM, Ferreira JA, et al. Identification of mixed HIV-1/HIV-2 infections in Brazil by polymerase chain reaction. AIDS 1991;5:1293–1299.
225. Evans L, Moreau J, Odehouri K, et al. Simultaneous isolation of HIV-1 and HIV-2 from an AIDS patient. Lancet 1988;2:1389–1391.
226. Rayfield M, De Cock K, Heyward W, et al. Mixed human immunodeficiency virus (HIV) infection in an individual: demonstration of both HIV type 1 and type 2 proviral sequences by using polymerase chain reaction. J Infect Dis 1988;158:1170–1176.
227. Peeters M, Gershy-Damet GM, Fransen K, et al. Virological and polymerase chain reaction studies of HIV-1/HIV-2 dual infection in Cote d'Ivoire. Lancet 1992;340:339–340.
228. Tedder R, O'Connor T, Hughs A, et al. Envelope cross-reactivity in Western blot for HIV-1 and HIV-2 may not indicate dual infection. Lancet 1988;2:927–930.
229. Kanki PJ, Barin F, Essex M. Antibody reactivity to multiple HIV-2 isolate. In: 4th International Conference on AIDS, Stockholm, 1988.
230. Dieng-Sarr A, Hamel DG, Travers KU, et al. HIV-1 and HIV-2 dual infection: lack of HIV-2 proviral correlates with low CD4+ lymphocyte counts. AIDS 1998;12:131–137.
231. Kanki P. Virologic and biologic features of HIV-2. In: Wormser GP, ed. AIDS and other manifestations of HIV infection. 2nd ed. New York: Raven Press, 1992:85–93.
232. De Cock K, Odehouri K, Colebunders R, et al. A comparison of HIV-1 and HIV-2 infections in hospitalized patients in Abidjan, Cote d'Ivoire. AIDS 1990;4:443.
233. Lisse IM, Poulsen A-G, Aaby P, et al. Immunodeficiency in HIV-2 infection: a community study from Guinea-Bissau. AIDS 1990;4:1263–1266.
234. Kestens L, Brattegard K, Adjorlolo G, et al. Immunological comparison of HIV-1, HIV-2 and dually-reactive women delivering in Abidjan, Cote d'Ivoire. AIDS 1992;6:803–807.
235. Pepin J, Morgan G, Dunn D, et al. HIV-2-induced immunosuppression among asymptomatic West African prostitutes: evidence that HIV-2 is pathogenic, but less so than HIV-1. AIDS 1991;5:1165–1172.
236. Lisse IM, Poulsen AG, Aaby P, et al. Serial CD4 and CD8 T-lymphocyte counts and associated mortality in an HIV-2–infected population in Guinea-Bissau. J Acquir Immune Defic Syndr Hum Retrovirol 1996;13:355–362.
237. Traore I, Marlink R, Thior I, et al. HIV-2 as a model for long term non-progression. In: 11th International Conference on AIDS, Vancouver, 1996.
238. Cheng-Mayer C, Seto D, Tateno M, et al. Biologic features of HIV-1 that correlate with virulence in the host. Science 1988;240:80–82.
239. Asjo B, Albert J, Karlsson A, et al. Replicative capacity of human immunodeficiency virus from patients with varying severity of HIV infection. Lancet 1986;2:660–662.
240. Fenyo E, Albert J, Asjo B. Replicative capacity, cytopathic effect and cell tropism of HIV. AIDS 1989;3(Suppl 1):S5–S12.
241. Tersmette M, De Goede R, Al B, et al. Differential syncytium-inducing capacity of human immunodeficiency virus isolates: frequent detection of syncytium-inducing isolates in patients with acquired immunodeficiency syndrome (AIDS) and AIDS-related complex. J Virol 1988;62:2026–2032.
242. Schuitemaker H, Koot M, Kootstra NA, et al. Biological phenotype of human immunodeficiency virus type 1 clones at different stages of infection: progression of disease is associated with a shift from monocytotropic to T-cell-tropic virus population. J Virol 1992;66:1354–1360.
243. Mulligan MJ, Kumar P, Hui HX, et al. The env protein of an infectious noncytopathic HIV-2 is deficient in syncytium formation. AIDS Res Hum Retroviruses 1990;6:707–720.
244. Albert J, Naucler A, Bottiger B, et al. Replicative capacity of HIV-2, like HIV-1, correlates with severity of immunodeficiency. AIDS 1990;4:291–295.
245. Schulz T, Whitby D, Hoad J, et al. Biological and molecular variability of human immunodeficiency virus type 2 isolates from The Gambia. J Virol 1990;64:5177–5182.
246. Simon F, Matheron S, Tamalet C, et al. Cellular and plasma viral load in patients infected with HIV-2. AIDS 1993;7:1411–1417.
247. Berry N, Ariyoshi K, Jobe O, et al. HIV type 2 proviral load measured by quantitative polymerase chain reaction correlates with CD4+ lymphopenia in HIV type 2–infected individuals. AIDS Res Hum Retroviruses 1994;10:1031–1037.
248. Korber B, Kanki P, M'Boup S, et al. PCR Analysis of HIV-2 viral isolates and peripheral blood lymphocytes from HIV-1 and HIV-2 seropositive West Africans. In: Chermann JC, Barré-Sinoussi F, eds. 4th International Conference on AIDS and Associated Cancers in Africa. Paris: SO-FRAMACOM, 1989.
249. Korber B, Kanki P, Barin F, et al. Genetic and antigenic variability in different HIV-2 viral isolates. In: Chermann JC, Barré-Sinoussi F, eds. 4th International Conference on AIDS and Associated Cancers in Africa. Paris: SO-FRAMACOM, 1989:170.
250. Gody M, Ouattara SA, de The G. Clinical experience in relation to HIV-1 and HIV-2 infection in rural hospital in Ivory Coast, West Africa. AIDS 1988;2:433–436.
251. Saimot AG, Matheron S, Brun-Vezinet F. Manifestations cliniques de l'infection HIV-2. Med Mal Infect 1988;S:707–S712.
252. Ancelle R, Bletry O, Baglin AC, et al. Long incubation period for HIV-2 infection. Lancet 1987;1:688–689.
253. Clavel F, Guetard D, Brun-Vezinet F, et al. Isolation of a new human retrovirus from West African patients with AIDS. Science 1986;233:343–346.
254. Saimot AG, Coulaud JP, Mechali D, et al. HIV-2/LAV-2 in Portuguese man with AIDS (Paris, 1978) who had served in Angola in 1968–74. Lancet 1987;1:688.
255. Le Guenno BM, Barabe P, Griffet PA, et al. HIV-2 and HIV-1 AIDS cases in Senegal: clinical patterns and immunological perturbations. J Acquir Immune Defic Syndr 1991;4:421–427.

256. Schneider J, Luke W, Kirchhoff F, et al. Isolation and characterization of HIV-2 obtained from a patient with predominantly neurological defects. AIDS 1990;4:455.
257. Dwyer D, Matheron S, Bakchine S, et al. Detection of human immunodeficiency virus type 2 in brain tissue. J Infect Dis 1992;166:888.
258. De Cock KM, Gnaore E, Adjorlolo G, et al. Risk of tuberculosis in patients with HIV-I and HIV-II infections in Abidjan, Ivory Coast. Br Med J 1991;302:496–499.
259. Marlink R, Kanki P, Thior I, et al. Reduced virulence of HIV-2 compared to HIV-1. Science 1994;265:1587–1590.
260. Marlink R, Kanki P, Thior I, et al. Reduced rate of disease development with HIV-2 compared to HIV-1. Science 1994;265:1587–1590.
261. Belec L, Tevi-Benissan C, Dupre T, et al. Comparison of cervicovaginal humoral immunity in clinically asymptomatic (CDC A1 and A2 category) patients with HIV-1 and HIV-2 infection. J Clin Immunol 1996;16:12–20.
262. Mohan P, Singh R, Baba M. Potential anti-AIDS agents: synthesis and antiviral activity of naphthalenesulfonic acid derivatives against HIV-1 and HIV-2. J Med Chem 1991;34:212–217.
263. De Clercq E, Yamamoto N, Pauwels R, et al. Potent and selective inhibition of human immunodeficiency virus (HIV)-1 and HIV-2 replication by a class of bicyclams interacting with a viral uncoating event. Proc Natl Acad Sci U S A 1992;89:5286–5290.
264. Mohan P, Schols D, Baba M, et al. Sulfonic acid polymers as a new class of human immunodeficiency virus inhibitors. Antiviral Res 1992,18. 139–150.
265. Nakashima H, Masuda M, Murakami T, et al. Anti-human immunodeficiency virus activity of a novel synthetic peptide, T22 ([Tyr-5,12, Lys-7]polyphemusin II): a possible inhibitor of virus-cell fusion. Antimicrob Agents Chemother 1992;36:1249–1255.
266. Bottiger D, Putkonen P, Oberg B. Prevention of HIV-2 and SIV infections in cynomolgus macaques by prophylactic treatment with 3′-fluorothymidine. AIDS Res Hum Retroviruses 1992;8:1235–1238.
267. van der Ende ME, Schutten M, Ly TD, et al. HIV-2 infection in 12 European residents: virus characteristics and disease progression. AIDS 1996;10:1649–1655.
268. Travers K, M'Boup S, Marlink R, et al. Natural protection against HIV-1 infection provided by HIV-2. Science 1995;268:1612–1615.
269. Kanki P, Eisen G, Travers KU, et al. HIV-2 and natural protection against HIV-1 infection [technical comment]. Science 1996;272:1959–1960.
270. Arya S, Gallo RC. Human immunodeficiency virus (HIV) type 2 mediated inhibition of HIV type 1: a new approach to gene therapy of HIV infection. Proc Natl Acad Sci U S A 1996;93:4486–4491.
271. Putkonen P, Thorstensson R, Albert J, et al. Infection of cynomolgus monkeys with HIV-2 protects against pathogenic consequences of a subsequent simian immunodeficiency virus infection. AIDS 1990;4:783–789.
272. Putkonen P, Thorstensson R, Walther L, et al. Vaccine protection against HIV-2 infection in cynomolgus monkeys. AIDS Res Hum Retroviruses 1991;7:271–277.
273. Andersson S, Makitalo B, Thorstensson R, et al. Immunogenicity and protective efficacy of a human immunodeficiency virus type 2 recombinant canarypox (ALVAC) vaccine candidate in cynomolgus monkeys. J Infect Dis 1996;174:977–985.
274. Biberfeld G, Thorstensson R, Putkonen P. Protection against human immunodeficiency virus type 2 and simian immunodeficiency virus in macaques vaccinated against human immunodeficiency virus type 2. AIDS Res Hum Retroviruses 1996;12:443–446.
275. Myagkikh M, Alipanah S, Markham PD, et al. Multiple immunizations with attenuated poxvirus HIV type 2 recombinants and subunit boosts required for protection of rhesus macaques. AIDS Res Hum Retroviruses 1996;12:985–992.
276. Freed E, Myers DJ. Identification and characterization of fusion and processing domains of the human immunodeficiency virus type 2 envelope glycoprotein. J Virol 1992;66:5472–5478.
277. Bosch ML, Earl PL, Fargnoli K, et al. Identification of the fusion peptide of primate immunodeficiency viruses. Science 1989;244:694–697.
278. Morikawa Y, Moore JP, Wilkinson AJ, et al. Reduction in CD4 binding affinity associated with removal of a single glycosylation site in the external glycoprotein of HIV-2. Virology 1991;180:853–856.

58

HUMAN T-LYMPHOTROPIC VIRUSES: HTLV-I AND HTLV-II

William A. Blattner and Maria S. Pombo de Oliveira

The worldwide pandemic of acquired immunodeficiency syndrome (AIDS) has focused attention on the role of retroviruses as etiologic agents in human disease. The discovery that the cause of AIDS is a retrovirus, human immunodeficiency virus type 1 (HIV-1), was made possible by pioneering basic research stimulated by the search for a human leukemia virus. First described by Rous in 1911 as filterable agents capable of inducing sarcomas in chickens (1), retroviruses (initially called RNA tumor viruses) are among the earliest known viruses. In the 1950s and 1960s, these agents were found to cause various mammalian cancers and leukemias and were shown to be RNA viruses. The discovery in the early 1970s of reverse transcriptase, a virally encoded enzyme that promotes the synthesis of a proviral DNA from an RNA template, facilitated development of a sensitive assay capable of detecting low-level retrovirus expression (2, 3). The discovery of the first human retrovirus, human T-lymphotropic virus type I (HTLV-I), depended on the development of culture techniques that would permit the long-term growth of target hematopoietic cells through the use of a growth factor now known as interleukin-2 (IL-2) (4). This first human retrovirus, HTLV-I, identified in 1979 by Gallo, Poiesz, and coworkers, proved the existence of human retroviruses (5). Its T-cell tropism provided the intellectual framework that implied a related virus as the cause of AIDS (6). The tools and techniques developed in the search for HTLV-I were adapted to detect and grow HIV-1 successfully (7, 8) (see Chap. 3).

These discoveries in the early 1980s ushered in a new age of medical virology. These initial breakthroughs were followed by the molecular characterization of both the human oncorna- (HTLV) and lenti- (HIV) retroviruses (9–11), establishing their associations with various diseases. The challenge for the beginning of the next millennium is to translate insights from pathogenesis to the development of effective treatment of associated diseases and to apply these insights to broadening therapies of related cancers, neurologic disorders, and other diseases. This chapter focuses on the HTLV family of viruses: their biology, virology, occurrence in humans, and associated diseases.

VIRUS AND HOST INTERACTIONS

HTLV-I, initially isolated in 1979, is the first known human retrovirus (5). It has been linked to certain human diseases, its epidemiology, virology, and pathophysiology are well described. HTLV-II, isolated in 1982 (12), demonstrated a close relationship with HTLV-I, with a molecular homology of approximately 60%. Although much is known about the molecular biology and virology of HTLV-II, its epidemiology and disease associations are less well understood.

HTLV-I and HIV are morphologically and molecularly distinctive, and they differ in cell biology and pathogenesis. For example, HTLV-I causes cell transformation in tissue culture and stimulates target cell proliferation by activating growth-promoting cellular lymphokines and cytokines. HIV also disrupts the normal lymphokine and cytokine pathway, but it induces cytopathic or cytolytic effects and immune paralysis that result in ablation of immune cell functions (13). HIV-1 primarily induces immunodeficiency; HTLV-I does it rarely. Both viruses cause lymphoproliferative malignancies. HIV induces immunodeficiency-associated B-cell tumor and Kaposi's sarcoma; HTLV-I causes T-cell malignancies. HIV-1 induces various neurologic syndromes such as encephalopathy, progressive multiple leukoencephalopathy, and peripheral neuropathies; HTLV-I is strongly linked to a chronic demyelinating neurologic syndrome.

HTLV-I and HTLV-II, like all retroviruses, are single-stranded RNA viruses containing a diploid genome that replicates through a DNA intermediate (14). This unique life cycle is made possible by the presence of a virally encoded enzyme, reverse transcriptase, which converts a single-stranded viral RNA into a double-stranded DNA provirus copy. Proviral DNA can be integrated into the host genome by a recombination mechanism using a viral protein, integrase (14). This capacity for genomic integration is important to the ability of retroviruses to cause lifelong infection, to evade immune clearance, and to produce diseases in the host that may take years to decades to develop.

Morphologically, the HTLV viruses were first classified as type C, but subsequently they were assigned to their own morphologic group. HTLV has a diameter of approximately 100 nm and a thin, electron-dense outer envelope and an electron-dense, roughly spheric core (Fig. 58.1). Surface projections of the lipid envelope are formed by viral envelope glycoproteins. During budding of the mature virion from the cell surface, a portion of the cell membrane is incorporated in the viral envelope. The core protein encloses the ribonucleoprotein complex of genomic RNA with viral reverse transcriptase and other internal structural proteins.

Molecularly, the 5′ and 3′ ends of the HTLV genome and those of all other retroviruses contain repeated sequences called long terminal repeats (LTRs) (6) (Fig. 58.2). These sequences are necessary for efficient replication and contain various regulatory elements (see Chap. 3), which may be required for integration of viral DNA into the host genome. The genomic structure of HTLV contains coding regions common to all retroviruses: gag (group-specific antigen), pol (polymerase), and env (envelope), arranged in 5′ to 3′ order, with LTR at each end. The *gag* gene encodes the protein products p15, p19, p24 (intermediate breakdown product), p28, and (precursor) p53 observed on HTLV-I Western blot (WB). The *pol* gene codes for reverse transcriptase, protease, endonuclease, and integrase. The *env* gene encodes the major components of the viral coat, the surface and transmembrane glycoproteins gp46, gp21, and (precursor) gp61/68. Retroviral genes generally code for large overlapping polyproteins that are later processed into functional peptide products by the virally encoded protease (14).

The HTLV viruses, like HIV, have additional genes mapped to the pX region of the genome 3′ to the viral envelope with various regulatory functions (15) (see Fig. 58.2). One gene, *tax* (transactivator), encodes a protein responsible for enhanced transcription of viral and cellular gene products by a transactivating mechanism. The second gene, called *rex* (regulator of expression of virion proteins), acts to modulate *tax* gene-mediated transactivation (16, 17). The tax protein has been postulated to play a critical role in leukemogenesis (18–22). The additional regulatory element of HIV-1 are not found in the HTLV-I genome.

The life cycle of HTLV involves an infection phase (including viral attachment, entry, reverse transcription, and proviral integration) and an expression phase (including transcription, translation, assembly, and budding of the virion) (14). HTLV-I appears to be tropic for the CD4 positive lymphocyte; for HTLV-II, CD8 cells are the primary target (23). Analogous to HIV-1, which enters its target cell through the CD4 molecule, HTLV probably also binds by a similar mechanism, although clearly the CD4 molecule alone is not the target for viral attachment for HTLV-I. Sommerfelt and colleagues (24) suggested that a gene, possibly a T-cell activation marker, on chromosome 17 is necessary for HTLV-I infection. Studies from Guyot, Newbound, and Lairmore (25) suggest that the viral tropism be largely determined by *tat* gene sequences, which promote effective growth in CD4 cells. Furthermore, the expression of mediated cell adhesion molecules and lymphocyte activation receptors have been also suggested as important elements in promote viral replication and homing of the virally infected cells (25). CD2 overexpression and additional stimulation of the T-cell receptor CD3 complex leads to upregulation of the infected cell receptors such as CD28, CD69, and CD25 (22). Further details of the life cycle of human retroviruses are discussed in Chapter 2.

The integration of HTLV into the host cell is a critical event in the pathogenesis of HTLV-associated diseases because, in all cases of HTLV-I–associated adult T-cell leukemia/lymphoma (ATL), the virus is monoclonally integrated, but not at a specific site (26). This suggestion that the process of leukemogenesis results from the clonal expansion of an HTLV-I–infected cell is supported by the observation that tumor cells have clonal rearrangements of the TCR-β gene (26–28). Clonal expansion of HTLV-I–infected cells in vivo is associated with mutations of the suppressor genes p53, p16, and p21 and clonal integration patterns of HTLV-I provirus (21). Recent analyses of infected cells in different individuals (asymptomatic persons and patients with HTLV-I–associated diseases) have demonstrated that the pattern of

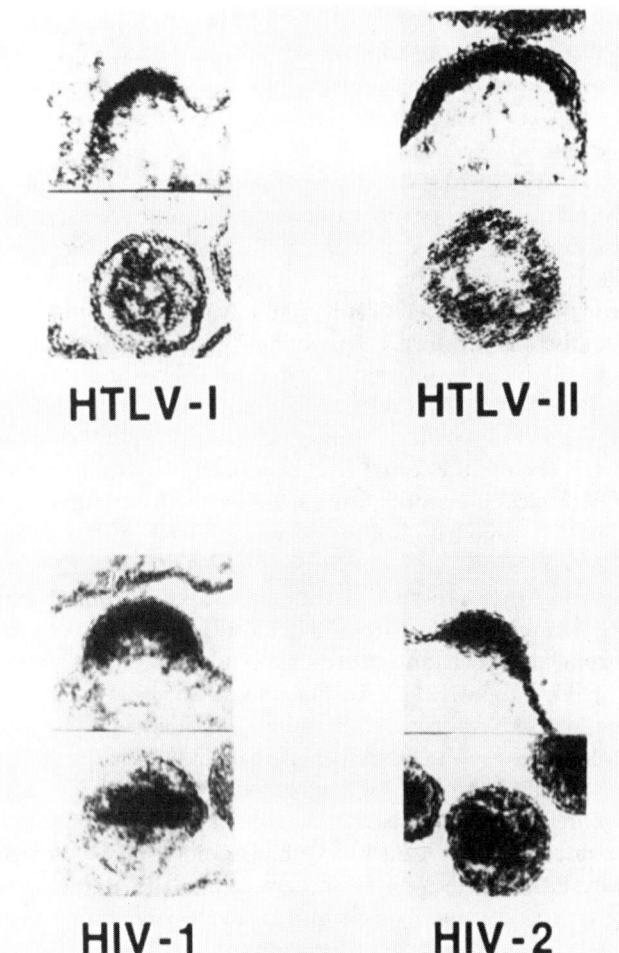

Figure 58.1. Thin-section electron micrographs of the four known human retroviruses. Mature virion are shown in the *lower panel*, and budding particles are shown in the *upper panel* for each virus. (From Blattner WA. Retroviruses. In: Evans AS, ed. Viral infections of humans: epidemiology and control. 3rd ed. New York: Plenum Medical Book, 1988:545–592.)

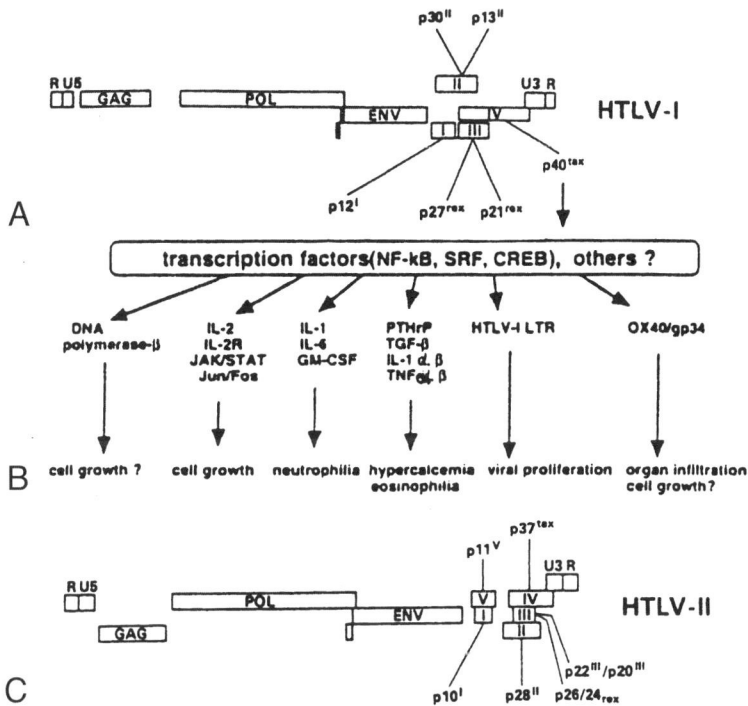

Figure 58.2. Schematic representation of the genomic structure of HTLV-I and HTLV-II. The overall genetic structure is similar to all other mammalian retroviruses that contain repeated sequences (LTR) located at the 5' and 3' ends of the viral genome, gag, pol, and env regions. The pX region in the 3' end codes for the regulatory protein isoforms, Tax and Rex. The regulatory proteins are Rex, a posttranscriptioal regulator of viral expression, and Tax, the viral transactivator of transcription; Tax gene product mediates certain transcriptional factors (see text for details). **A.** Structure of coding region for HTLV-I. **B.** The transcriptional pathways of tax mediation through all their effects. **C.** The genomic structure of HTLV-II (see text for details.)

integration of HTLV-I provirus can show different HTLV-I sequences as multiple, complete, and defective types. In the defective types, deletion occurs in gag, pol, or env regions, but the pX region is always conserved (29, 30). For HTLV-I–associated myelopathy and other syndromes involving presumptive mechanisms of HTLV-I–induced immunologic perturbation, integration is almost always oligoclonal or polyclonal (27, 31).

Unlike HIV, the rate of mutational change in the HTLV-I virus is negligible, so the issue of latency is pathogenically important (28). HTLV-I expression requires activation of host cell mechanisms for transcription, translation, and processing of viral components. HTLV-I has developed sophisticated strategies for subverting cellular function, particularly by means of the tax viral regulatory element that can activate cellular cytokine pathways to promote cell growth (17). The lack of substantial diversity for HTLV-I suggests that the virus uses novel strategies for remaining invisible to the host immune system (28). For example, the high frequency of defective virus found in ATL cells can be explained by the hypotheses that cells harboring these defective viruses escaped killing by cytotoxic T-lymphocytes (CTLs) and immunosurveillance (30). The strategies used by this relatively stable virus to evade immune surveillance are not yet fully characterized. They may involve a lower level of virus proliferation, altered immune response due to viral effects on immune recognition, or more frequent cell-to-cell transmission (31–33). Data reported by Bangham and colleagues suggest that selective mutation of *tat* gene sequence may contribute to disease pathogenesis (unpublished data presented at 8th International Conference on Human Retrovirology, 1997). On the other hand, certain autoimmune-type diseases associated with HTLV-I appear to result from a loss of control of viral expression inasmuch as virus load is high in persons with some of these diseases, and levels of antibody are markedly elevated in response to presumed elevations in viral expression.

Factors that control viral replication, especially *tax* and cellular genes, are emerging as important cofactors in disease pathogenesis. For instance, after infection of CD4+ T cells by HTLV-I, an initial phase of IL-2–dependent cell growth occurs. Over time, the cells became IL-2 independent (34, 35). This phenomenon may be associated with the dysregulation of the T-cell growth cycle (36, 37). The *tax* gene is responsible for the transactivation of virus transcription by a *tax*-responsive element of 21 bp containing a cAMP. Tax binds directly to several members of nuclear factor κB (NF-κB) proteins and thus leads to activation of the cellular genes for IL-2 and IL-2 receptor and the transactivation of cellular suppressor genes (18, 21, 35). Mutations in suppressor gene p53 (an important cell-cycle regulator) and the activation of tyrosine kinase family may represent important intermediates in the transformation of T cells infected by HTLV-I to malignant leukemic cells (36, 37).

DETECTION OF HTLV

The original isolation of HTLV-I and HTLV-II used complex techniques of tissue culture involving exogenous growth factors, detection of reverse transcriptase, and electron microscopic examination (5). The establishment of permanent cell lines allowed for the viral antigens to be characterized and for serologic tests to be developed. Originally, antigen-specific assays for the gag p24 and p19 assays were used to prove specificity, but these assays lacked sensitivity. Whole-virus assays improved sensitivity but in some populations lost specificity (38). The latest generation of serologic assays use a combination of whole-virus and recombinantly produced peptides to detect virus infection with a high degree of sensitivity and specificity (39–42). Because of the high frequency of HTLV-II positive results in blood donors, a newly licensed screening assay includes lysate of both virus types simultaneously with improved sensitivity and specificity (43). For HTLV-I and HTLV-II, a combination of enzyme-linked immunoassay (ELISA) confirmed by WB is the standard approach, although alternative strategies using immunofluorescent assays and agglutination approaches are also used by some investigators (44–46). The criteria for WB blot positivity is the presence of reactivity to both a *gag* and *env* gene product, and in the case of *env*, this usually entails a recombinantly produced antigen because of the paucity of HTLV envelope antigens in whole-virus preparations. To date, no confirmatory essay has been licensed (47).

Early epidemiologic studies of HTLV-I were complicated by the cross-reactivity of HTLV-I and HTLV-II because their standard serologic assays were unable to differentiate between HTLV-I and HTLV-II reactivity. However, the most recent screening assay with lysate of both virus and WB technology, which includes the addition of synthetic peptides both to confirm positively and to distinguish virus type, have enhanced such studies (45–48). A modified WB has been developed that contains both group-specific conserved motifs from the transmembrane protein and type-specific motifs from the external glycoproteins (rgp46) of HTLV-I (MTA1) and HTLV-II (K55). These have been coated on the strips to allow simultaneous confirmation and differentiation of both HTLV-I and HTLV-II in 98% of cases (49) (Fig. 58.3).

The epidemiology of HTLV-I and HTLV-II has been largely defined through the use of antibody testing. The use of the polymerase chain reaction (PCR) technique has also been useful for facilitating epidemiologic studies by providing a precise tool for distinguishing virus type and for quantifying viral presence (50, 51). For example, because virus-positive antibody-negative individuals could be missed by antibody tests, the true prevalence of virus may be underestimated. In fact, several surveys using PCR have not detected large numbers of virus-positive antibody-negative individuals, although some instances have been reported (52–54). On the other hand, in tropical countries, especially in Africa, repeatable ELISA reactive samples exhibit a high frequency of indeterminate WB. The interpretation of WB results such as reactivities to gag-encoded proteins (p19, p24 or p53) without reactivity to env-encoded glycoproteins

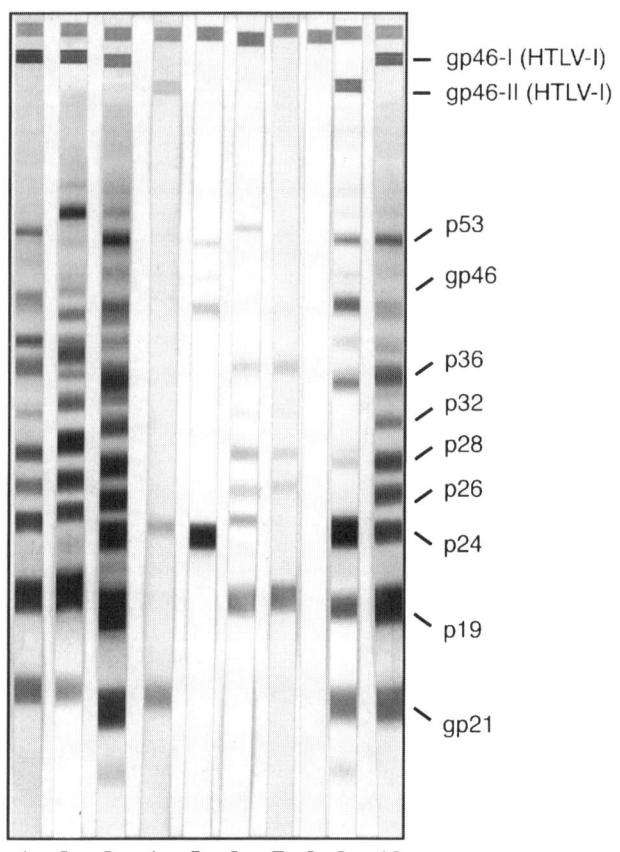

Figure 58.3. Western blots using type specific motifs from the external glycoproteins (rgp46) of HTLV-I and HTLV-II; reactivity to HTLV-I and HTLV-II sera as indicated. *1, 2,* and *3,* HTLV-I positive: reactivity to gag (p19 or p24), and env (gp46 or rgp46-I) and rgp21 bands; *4,* HTLV-II positive: reactivity to gag (p24), and env (rgp46-II) and rgp21 bands; *5, 6,* and *7,* indeterminate pattern, viral bands p19 or p24 present, but pattern does not meet the criteria for HTLV-I positive or HTLV-II positive; *8,* negative control; *9* and *10,* HTLV-I–and HTLV-II–positive controls (From Lipka JJ, Miyoshi I, Madlock KG, et al. Segregation of human T cell lymphotropic virus type I and II infections by antibody reactivity to unique viral epitopes. J Infect Dis 1992;165:268–272; Horal P, Hall WW, Svennerholm B, et al. Identification of type-specific linear epitopes in the glycoproteins gp46 and gp21 of human T-cell leukemia viruses type I and type II using synthetic peptides. Proc Natl Acad Sci U S A 1991;88:5754–5758.)

(gp21, gp46) is still a question that needs to be resolved to avoid overestimating the rate of HTLV-I/II seroprevalence in these regions (55–57). PCR is a useful technique for distinguishing virus type but in large scale is not suitable for epidemiologic work.

EPIDEMIOLOGY AND MODES OF TRANSMISSION OF HUMAN RETROVIRUSES

Origin of HTLV-I and Molecular Epidemiology

Retroviruses related to HTLV-I, called simian T-lymphotropic virus, have been isolated from African and other Old World primate species (58–60). These viruses share significant homology to human HTLV-I; this observation suggests the possibility of enzootic transmission of HTLV-I to humans at some point (61). How HTLV-I spread among various human populations is controversial, particularly given the unusual distribution of the virus worldwide. So far, five major molecular subtypes of HTLV-I have been identified: the Cosmopolitan (C, widespread all over the world), Japanese (J), West African (WA) subtype, Central African (CA), and Melanesian (Papua New Guinea, Melanesia, and Australian aborigine). Among the major types (e.g., Cosmopolitan versus Melanesian), one can note up to an 8 to 10% difference (62, 63).

An African origin of HTLV-I is supported by the occurrence of HTLV-I clusters in Africa (56, 64, 65) and among persons of African descent residing in the Caribbean, but not among other migrant populations residing in the region (66). On the other hand, clusters of HTLV-I in southern Japan and northeastern Iran and the isolation of a closely related virus in aboriginal peoples of Papua New Guinea, Northern Australia, and the Solomon Islands make the origin of this class of virus more difficult to discern (67–70). Molecular analysis of these isolates indicates little genetic variation; the opposite is true of the HIV family of viruses, which are prone to significant genetic alteration. Speculation exists regarding the spread of HTLV-I, possibly through the African slave trade; for example, a high degree of homology (less than 1%) is present between viruses isolated from west Africa and those from the Caribbean (63). The difference between Japanese and Caribbean isolates varies by as much as 2%, indicating a close homology but distinctive origin (9, 71), whereas a variant African strain was isolated from Zaire that differs from the West African strain by about 3 to 4% (72–74). However, the most significant variant HTLV-I viruses have been isolated from seropositive persons in various parts of Melanesia (75). The original isolate was obtained from an unacculturated hunter gatherer tribe, the Hagahai, residing in the highlands of Papua New Guinea. Their only contact with the outside world had occurred within weeks of the original blood sample collection. These viruses differ by as much as 9 to 10% from the prototype Japanese strain and by as much as 4 to 6% from the viruses isolated in Australia and the Solomon Islands (69, 75, 76). In some cases, these strains have been isolated from persons with ATL and HTLV-associated myelopathy, suggesting that despite genetic differences, the virus has pathogenic potential (73, 77, 78). A large study of the LTR by restriction fragment length polymorphisms covering the major HTLV-I endemic area and including new specimens has demonstrated that variations are more closely linked to the geographic origin of the infected individuals than to the patient's clinical status (63, 78–81).

Molecular Epidemiology of HTLV-II

The origin of HTLV-II is less certain. HTLV-II is documented in intravenous drug users (IVDUs) in the United States and Italy (82–87). A natural reservoir has been detected among various Amer-Indian populations residing in the United States and Central and South America (88–98). Virus isolates from these populations have revealed two basic families of HTLV-II that differ molecularly by approximately 2 to 4% (99, 100). These two major HTLV-II subtypes, A and B, occur throughout the Americas, and reports exist of African strains related to the B subtype as well as a report of subtype A in the Cameroon (99, 100). The hypothesis that HTLV-II is a New World virus that diverged from a common ancestor of HTLV-I has been challenged by a report of an HTLV-II virus in pygmies residing in northwest Zaire (101). Furthermore, new phylogenetic analyses performed in strains of diverse geographic origin suggest that the current known HTLV-I subtypes probably have originated from geographically distinct interspecies transmission events (102, 103).

Although much remains to be learned about the origins of the HTLV viruses, the current data support the hypotheses that these viruses are either extremely old, dating back to early humans, or that they evolved in nonhuman primates and penetrated humans through enzootic exposure (61). In any event, their apparently slow rate of evolution could make them a useful marker for tracking the migrations of these early peoples. For example, the differences between the Melanesian and Japanese prototype are consistent with a rate of evolution that corresponds with the separation of the Melanesian subpopulation from other human populations (75).

An unanswered puzzle is the evolution of HTLV-II. In view of what is known about the slow rate of evolution of these viruses, it would seem impossible for HTLV-II to have evolved independently from a common prototype HTLV in the time since humans first migrated to the New World. This consideration has led to speculation that a primate intermediary could have been a host to this strain and passed it into humans. Primate viruses do transfer to other species. HTLV-I and HTLV-II could have been transferred to humans sufficiently long ago to permit adaptation to occur, resulting in a relatively low rate of disease occurrence (62).

The introduction of the HIV pathogen in humans is a recent event, possibly the result of an enzootic exposure (104). The mutable nature of the virus, coupled with insufficient time for adaptation, has resulted in serious clinical consequences, with HIV causing a devastating array of diseases in a large proportion of those infected.

DESCRIPTIVE EPIDEMIOLOGY

HTLV-I

HTLV-I infections occur worldwide; HTLV-II infections have been confirmed by culture or sequencing PCR and newer serologic technique clusters in the Americas and Africa. The distribution of antibody positivity for both viruses varies by geographic region and by racial, ethnic, or risk-group subpopulation (105). Geographic clustering of HTLV-I is exemplified by endemic foci of HTLV-I in southern Japan (Kyushu, Shikoku, and the islands of the Ryukyu chain including Okinawa) (106–110). Nationwide surveys document small pockets of seropositivity in some isolated villages in Honshu and the most northern island of Hokkaido among aboriginal Ainu populations, but most positive results detected in northern Japan are among persons who migrated there from viral endemic areas in the south (111, 112). Surveys within HTLV-I–endemic areas of Japan have documented marked variations in seroprevalence. A survey of Miyazaki prefecture documented a gradient toward higher seropositivity in the more southern districts, with highest rates in coastal and more rural areas (113). In other surveys of isolated populations living on some of the many small islands off the coast of Kyushu, this tendency for microclustering was also documented, with each village having a distinctive pattern of prevalence (114, 115). The highest rates of seropositivity are found in Okinawa and surrounding districts (106).

Surveys of mainland China, Taiwan, Korea, Thailand, India, and Vietnam are largely negative (105). However, in view of the propensity of HTLV-I to cluster geographically, additional systematic surveys in Taiwan and Vietnam documented a significantly higher prevalence in prostitutes and drug abusers than in the general population (79, 105, 116).

Surveys in Melanesia have documented unexpectedly high seroprevalence rates, particularly in Papua New Guinea (67, 117, 118). As noted earlier, molecular epidemiologic studies have shown that these infections are caused by closely related but distinctive variants of HTLV-I that are associated with HTLV clinical outcomes. An isolate from an Australian aborigine and one from a Solomon Islander are molecularly as different from each other as they are from prototype strains (69). Detailed seroepidemiologic studies have not been conducted, but high rates of positivity including unusually high rates of infection in children have been reported, a finding suggesting a distinctive epidemiologic pattern (117).

A major endemic focus of HTLV-I infection occurs in the Caribbean. The first clues leading to this discovery came from the observation that a cluster of cases of ATL cases detected in the United States and the United Kingdom occurred among migrants from this region (119–123). Subsequent broad serosurveys have documented significant rates of positivity in Jamaica, Trinidad and Tobago, Martinique, Barbados, St. Lucia, Haiti, and the Dominican Republic (66, 105, 124–126). In addition, the adjacent areas of South America, including Venezuela, Guyana, and Surinam and some areas of Central America, Panama, and Honduras have been shown to harbor foci of seropositivity (90, 105, 127).

In Trinidad and Tobago, seropositivity is restricted almost exclusively to persons of African descent, even though persons of Indo-Asian ethnic background have shared a common environment for more than 100 years (66). In one study, rates of positivity were reported to be higher in Tobago, but a follow-up study has shown this was an artifact of sampling (125). A large-scale survey of the Jamaican population documented varying rates of seropositivity in different regions, but not the type of microepidemiologic clustering reported in Japan (124). In Jamaica, the highest rates of positivity are observed in the lowland, high-rainfall areas (128). Other ecologic correlates appear to reflect the finding that HTLV-I is most prevalent among persons of the lowest socioeconomic class (129). This prevalence is mirrored in a survey of pregnant women in which the highest rates were observed in women attending the hospital serving the indigent population (130). Men and women attending clinics to treat sexually transmitted diseases have the highest rate of seropositivity (131); the rate is lower in blood donors (132).

Some countries in South and Central America are HTLV-I–endemic areas, but the distribution of HTLV-I infection varies markedly. In Colombia, HTLV-I clusters along the Pacific Coast in an area with an unusually high rate of the associated neurologic syndrome compared with the presence of ATL (133–134). Persons of African descent predominate in this isolated area. Rates are significantly higher in this low-altitude area compared with rates at higher-altitude areas, controlling for race. Controlling for altitude, rates are higher in persons of African descent than in persons of Mestizo background (135). Other areas of South America with documented foci of HTLV-I include Brazil, Venezuela, Surinam, and Guyana (105, 127, 136–140). Most positive results occur in persons of African descent. However, one survey in Chile identified pockets of HTLV-I in persons of non-African descent and raised the possibility of a trans-Pacific introduction of the virus (74, 141).

In the United States, large-scale screening of the blood supply has documented rates of HTLV-I/II of 0.43 per 1000, with approximately half the positive cases being HTLV-II (142, 143). In a significant proportion of HTLV-I–positive cases, donors have backgrounds linking them to a viral endemic area or behaviors such as drug abuse linked to transmission (142). Smaller regional surveys and studies of military populations show a similar pattern, with persons of African ancestry having elevated rates of seropositivity. Migrant populations often acquire infection early in life and carry their viral infection to nonendemic areas, where disease may appear years later. Migrant populations from Okinawa to Hawaii and from the Caribbean to the United States and the United Kingdom constitute risk groups for HTLV positivity, as are Americans who experience exposure through sexual contact or transfusion in viral endemic areas (121–123, 143, 144).

Results of surveys conducted on the African continent (Ivory Coast, Ghana, Nigeria, Zaire, Kenya, Tanzania) show that rates of HTLV-I seropositivity are similar to those in the Caribbean region (56, 65, 105, 146–148). Systematic surveys have not been performed to document the exact pattern of viral occurrence. One of the difficulties in conducting surveys in African populations has been the presumably false-positive, nonspecific reactivity on standard serologic screening assays. Furthermore, confirmatory WB assays often have an array of detectable banding patterns that may resemble weak positive reactions (54, 55, 147). In other cases the pattern of reactivity is identical to that seen in Japan and the Caribbean; WB reactivity has a classic banding profile. In one survey in Zaire with clearly positive reactivity, an area of microgeographic clustering was detected in the northern equatorial region by studying rates among female prostitutes from different provinces residing in the capital, Kinshasa (64). This region was also found to be a focus of the virally associated neurologic disease (148). Further study is needed to define more precisely the microgeographic pattern of viral occurrence.

Studies in Europe and in the Middle East are largely negative, save for occasional positive cases among migrants from viral endemic areas (105, 121, 149). However, a focus of HTLV-I was found among Iranian Jews from northeastern Iran residing in Israel and New York (70). Follow-up studies in Iran have confirmed a focus of viral endemicity among persons residing in Mashad (150, 151, 81). The origin of this cluster is unclear, but this area historically was a crossroads for travel from the Far East to Europe and could represent the residual of historic exposure of some migrant population with the high frequency of intermarriage acting to amplify viral endemicity. Surveys in southern India, where an HTLV-like neurologic disease has been reported, are largely negative for HTLV-I (152). The Seychelles in the Indian Ocean are an endemic hot spot for HTLV-I (154, 155).

HTLV-II

Much less is known about the epidemiology of HTLV-II, largely because it is difficult to distinguish this type from HTLV-I by conventional serologic techniques. Recently, the application of a reliable WB algorithm (see earlier), the development of sensitive recombinant peptide assays, and the newly licensed dual screening test have enhanced the study of this virus (147). The first HTLV-II–specific studies relied on complex competitive binding assays. These studies documented the high prevalence of this virus type among IVDUs in Italy and East Coast United States sites (87, 156). This finding was subsequently confirmed by the use of PCR in a group of IVDUs in New Orleans (83). Virtually every population of IVDUs in the United States has evidence of HTLV-II infection, with rates ranging up to as high as 10 to 15% and more (87). Retrospective surveys documented the presence of HTLV-II in this risk group as early as the late 1960s (85). Studies of Italian IVDUs who may have had contact with IVDUs in the United States had significantly elevated rates of HTLV-II (153).

Amer-Indians residing in North, Central, and South America have varying rates of positivity for HTLV-II; this observation has created an opportunity to evaluate the natural history of this virus in a non-IVDU population. In a manner that resembles the geographic clustering of HTLV-I, HTLV-II is distributed in clustering patterns as well (90). In North America, pockets of positivity are encountered among the Seminoles in south Florida (91) and the Pueblo and Navajo in New Mexico (92), but not among various tribes in Alaska (157). In Central America, the major studies have been conducted in Panama, where a pocket of positivity was identified in the Guaymi Indians residing in northeastern Panama near the border of Costa Rica (89, 158); similarly high rates were not observed in other Guaymi enclaves in southwest Panama or among various other tribes in other parts of Panama (90). In Colombia, occasional pockets of HTLV-I have been observed in some Amer-Indian populations, but HTLV-II is rare (98, 141). A large survey of sera from numerous tribes collected years ago as part of anthropologic studies identified two remote tribes in the interior of Brazil infected with HTLV-II (93). A survey of HTLV-II infection in Indian communities in the Amazon region of Brazil demonstrated an overall seroprevalence rate of greater than 30% (94). This previous study was confirmed by others with the demonstration that HTLV-II is widespread in the Brazilian Amazon region, and in urban areas HTLV-II has been documented mainly in IVDUs (95). Further, Argentinian and Paraguayan Indians were also identified as clusters of HTLV-II infections (96, 97). These hunter–gatherer tribes who share a common linguistic group are separated by hundreds of miles from each other; they had extremely high rates of seropositivity of as much as 20% and more in older age groups. The seroprevalence rates tended to increase with age, a finding supporting the importance of sexual transmission of the virus; vertical transmission was also demonstrated in family studies (93, 158).

The evidence of HTLV-II antibodies and later characterization of isolates (subtypes A and B) from persons living in large West and Central African cities strongly suggested that HTLV-II is also prevalent in Africa. The discovery of HTLV-II subtype B virus in pygmies living in Zaire, and further and further isolated and characterized within a family in Gabon for three generations, confirms the hypothesis of an ancient presence of this HTLV-II subtype B on the African continent (101, 159–163).

DEMOGRAPHIC PATTERNS

A characteristic age-dependent rise in HTLV-I seroprevalence is observed in diverse geographic areas. For example, as shown in Figure 58.4, the patterns of infection in Jamaica and Okinawa, Japan, are similar. In both locales, one sees a parallel rise in male and female rates that begins in adolescence but plateaus in men around age 40 years but continues to rise in women into their 60s. In Jamaica, this rise is steeper for women compared with men, and overall the rates in Okinawa are higher than in Jamaica (106, 125, 164). The explanation for this age-dependent rise in HTLV-I seroprevalence is not fully understood. Three hypotheses have been put forth to explain the pattern: 1) reactivation of latent infection throughout life; 2) ongoing infections throughout life with more efficient male-to-female transmission; or 3) a "cohort effect" representing declining rates of infection in younger birth cohorts (145, 165). The issue of "immunosilent" HTLV-I infection is as controversial in the HTLV field as it is in the field of HIV study. One group in Japan reported a high prevalence of PCR-positive and antibody-negative individuals (52), most likely the result of laboratory contamination, whereas others in similarly exposed cohorts have been unable to document this phenomenon, including exposed blood bank recipients and the children of antibody-positive women who have breast-fed their children and have had at least one child with HTLV-I infection (53, 166). Other investigators have reported isolated instances of patients with

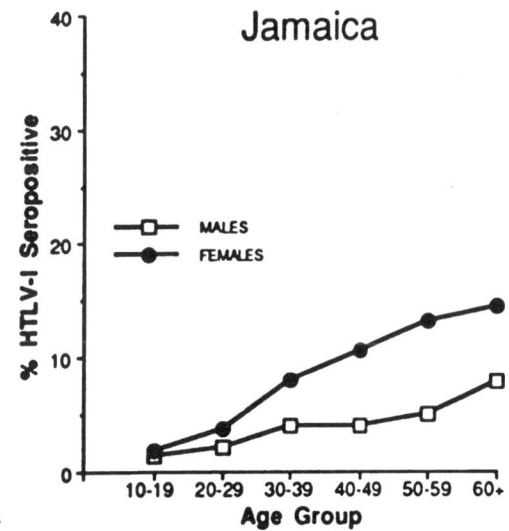
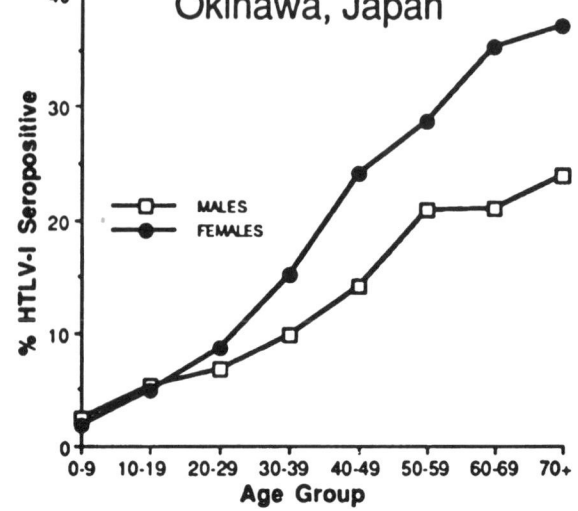

Figure 58.4. **Age-specific seroprevalence of HTLV-I.** Age-specific seroprevalence in Jamaica (**A**) and Okinawa (**B**) showing the similarity of shape of curve but with higher rates in Okinawa. The possible explanations for these patterns are discussed in the text. (**A**. From Murphy EL, Figueroa JP, Gibbs WN, et al. Human T-lymphotropic virus type I (HTLV-I) seroprevalence in Jamaica. I. Demographic determinants. Am J Epidemiol 1991;133: 1114–1124. **B**. From Kajiyama W, Kashiwagi S, Norura H, et al. Seroepidemiologic study of antibody to adult T-cell leukemia virus in Okinawa, Japan. Am J Epidemiol 1985;123:41–47.)

HTLV-associated diseases and PCR positively, usually with defective viruses (29, 167). In these instances, the virus was able to infect a host cell but was unable to be expressed at a level high enough to elicit an antibody reaction. Given the magnitude of the rise in seroprevalence and the marked male-to-female difference, this phenomenon alone would not account for most unexplained infections. Considerable evidence documents the incidence of new infections, but rates of new infection in younger birth cohorts do not appear sufficient to account for the higher rates in older groups, at least in Japan. This finding has led to the conclusion that, for unexplained reasons, rates of infection appear to be declining in younger birth cohorts (107). Possible explanations include changes in standard of living, such as improved nutrition, changes in breast-feeding patterns, elimination of environmental cofactors that facilitate transmission, and declines in other sexually transmitted diseases that enhance transmission. In a study of migrants from viral endemic areas of Japan to Hawaii, rates of HTLV-I were highest in those born in Okinawa, lower in first-generation Hawaiian born, and lowest in the grandchildren of migrants (144). The likely factors explaining this pattern of declining prevalence include changes in environment and improvement in socioeconomic status (145, 168–170).

For HTLV-II, a characteristic age-dependent rise in seroprevalence also occurs (93). However, data from studies of endemic populations of Amer-Indians document that, although the shape of the curve resembles that for HTLV-I, no differences between male and female patients occur at any age (158, 171). In IVDUs, unusually high rates of seropositivity in older age groups have been linked to the sharing of primitive "eyedropper" injection equipment, thus raising the possibility of a "cohort effect" resulting from changes in injection techniques (156). No evidence exists for the frequent occurrence of a virus-positive antibody-negative state.

MODES OF TRANSMISSION

Summarized in Table 58.1 are the routes, modes, and cofactors associated with HTLV-I and HTLV-II transmission. Many similarities exist between the modes of transmission of HTLV-I and those of HIV-1. Factors associated with transmission of HTLV-II are less well defined.

Mother-to-Child Transmission

A major route of transmission is from mother to child (172). Both HTLV-I and HTLV-II virus have been detected in breast milk (130, 172), and, in the case of HTLV-I, the virus has been successfully transmitted through breast milk in nonhuman primate and rabbit animal models (173). In studies from Japan, breast-feeding has been documented to be more efficient in transmitting the virus than perinatal transmission (172–176). For example, although 20% of breast-fed infants seroconvert to HTLV-I, 1 to 2% of bottle-fed infants of HTLV-I–positive mothers become infected. This finding contrasts with studies of perinatal HIV-1 transmission, wherein up to 30% of offspring of positive mothers acquire infection by the transplacental or perinatal route (177–179). In prospective studies from Jamaica, a similar rate of transmission has been documented (130). During the first 6 months of life, maternal antibodies are present; and in serial WBs, all bands often disappear before new bands appear as a result of neonatal infection (130). In some cases, breast-feeding had ceased up to several months before seroconversion, but study of cells from exposed but nonseroconverting children identified none with latent HTLV-I viral infection. The major predictor of maternal-to-child transmission is the viral load of the mother, as measured by antibody titer and viral antigen level on short-term culture. The presence of antibody to the tax or env antigen has also been associated with transmission of the virus (180–183).

In studies from Jamaica and Japan, antibodies to envelope glycoprotein (gp46) epitope were associated with enhanced transmission, thus raising the possibility that maternal antibodies may contribute to transmission of the virus (180, 181). Furthermore, in a prospective cohort study conducted in Jamaica, timing of breast-fed was strongly associated with the efficiency of transmission (182). Among children born from HTLV-I–positive mothers in follow-up for more than 2 years, 32% of children breast-fed for 12 months or longer were HTLV-I seropositive, compared with 9% of those breast-fed for less than 12 months (182) (Fig. 58.5). These data strongly suggest that limiting the duration of breast-feeding to less than 12 months could reduce significantly the mother-to-child transmission of HTLV-I. Based on population studies, investigators estimate that approximately 2 to 5% of HTLV-I infections result from maternal-to-child transmission in the first few years of life; this infection in early life may have considerable significance for subsequent risk of disease, particularly ATL (184, 185).

HTLV-II transmission from mother to child is still controversial, because prospective surveys are still under investigation (162). For instance, in studies of IVDU mothers who are HTLV-II positive, none transmitted the virus to their bottle-fed infants, whereas among Indians of the Gran Chaco (Argentina) and Kayapo (Brazil), a high rate (30% and 46% respectively) of mother-to-child transmission was observed (186; Poiez et al., Novoa, Hall et al., unpublished data presented at the 8th International Conference on Human Retrovirology, Rio de Janeiro, 1997). In Panama, the Guayami Indians have a 1 to 2% prevalence among preadolescent children (158). This finding is consistent with infection in early life and an excess of seropositive children when the mother is seropositive compared with the virtual absence of seropositive children when the mother is seronegative (187, 188). HTLV-II has been detected in the breast milk of HTLV-II–positive women (189).

Table 58.1. Transmission of HTLV-I

	Modes of Transmission	
	HTLV-I	HTLV-II
Mother to infant		
Transplacental	Yes	Unknown
Breast milk	Yes	Yes
Sexual		
Male to female	Yes	Yes
Female to male	Yes	Yes
Male to male	Yes	Possible
Parenteral		
Blood transfusion	Yes	Yes
Intravenous drug use	Yes	Yes
Cofactors		
Elevated virus load		
Mother to infant	Yes	Yes
Heterosexual	Yes	Yes
Ulcerative genital lesions	Yes	Possible
Cellular transfusion products	Yes	Yes
Sharing of "works"	Yes	Yes

Kataoka R, Takehara N, Iwahara Y, et al. Transmission of HTLV-I by blood transfusion and its prevention by passive immunization in rabbits. Blood 1990;76:1657–1661.

Sexual Transmission

Evidence of sexual transmission of HTLV-I has come primarily from cross-sectional studies of married couples or from surveys of sexually active risk groups, but also from prospective studies. Sexual transmission of HTLV-I from male to female and from female to male as well as from male to male has been suggested from these data (190). HIV-1

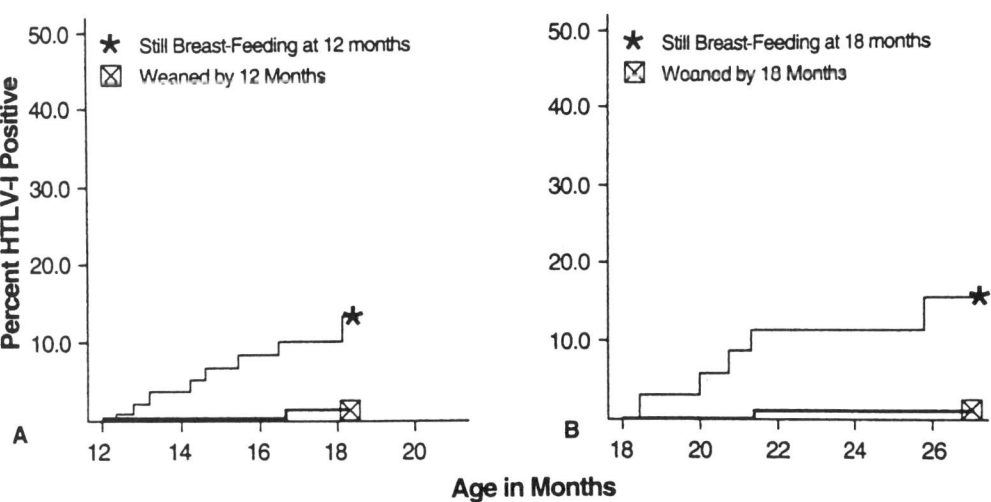

Figure 58.5. Incidence of HTLV-I infection among children who were still HTLV-I negative (A) at 12 months and (B) at 18 months. The values are stratified according to whether a child had been weaned at 12 months ($n = 84$) or at 18 months ($n = 88$) or was still being breast-fed (*) beyond that age ($n = 64$ in **A**; $n = 37$ in **B**). (From Wiktor SZ, Pate EJ, Rosenberg PS, et al. Mother-to-child transmission of human T lymphotropic virus type I associated with prolonged breast-feeding. J Hum Virol 1977;1:37–44.)

shares these routes of infection, but it appears to be an order of magnitude more infectious than HTLV-I. This discrepancy may reflect differences in virus load or the finding that HTLV-I is highly cell associated, whereas HIV-1 is both cell associated and cell free (191–193). Numerous studies of married or steady heterosexual couples have documented a significant excess of couples concordant for HTLV-I infection (168). In general, discordant couples more often have a seropositive woman and seronegative man than vice versa. However, younger discordant couples have a more equal prevalence in which either the man or the woman is seropositive. This pattern is consistent with the hypothesis that male-to-female transmission is more efficient than female-to-male transmission (146, 168). This conclusion is supported by prospective studies with a small number of seroconversion events that have documented a higher occurrence of male-to-female than female-to-male HTLV-I transmissions.

Several markers of sexual activity are associated with HTLV-I transmission. In one study of a sexually transmitted disease clinic in Jamaica, seropositivity in women was associated with a large number of sexual partners; no such association was observed among men (131, 191). In a study of homosexual men in Trinidad, however, the number of lifetime partners was positively associated (192). Another cofactor for sexual transmission of HTLV-I in these and other studies is the coincidence of other sexually transmitted diseases, particularly ulcerative genital lesions such as occur in syphilis (131, 193, 194). A current diagnosis of syphilis was also associated with HTLV-I positivity in the study of the sexually transmitted disease clinic in Jamaica (193). Similar associations of the occurrence of ulcerative genital lesions and the risk of HIV-1 infection have been reported from Africa and elsewhere (195). These data suggest that the difference in HTLV-I prevalence between men and women may result from the low efficiency of female-to-male transmission and a potential role for cofactors that interrupt normal mucosal barriers and promote transmission. However, female-to-male transmission can occur in the absence of detectable cofactors, as observed among a group of Marine Corps veterans married to seropositive Okinawan women (196). Duration of a steady sexual relationship with a seropositive partner is also associated with seroconversion (113). This finding may be related to increases in virus load, which occur over time in relation to changes in immune status, so as a person carrying the virus ages, the HTLV-I virus load increases. This hypothesis may explain the late seroconversion of some sexual partners with long-standing sexual relationships with a seropositive partner. For HTLV-I, elevated antibody titer appears to correlate with virus load (197, 198). In the case of HTLV-I, this relationship of elevated titer and heterosexual transmission has been shown in one prospective cohort study in Japan (111). Recently, this relation has been more directly shown by quantitative PCR (197). In addition, the presence of anti-tax antibody has been shown to be associated with heightened transmission, possibly related to a state of virus proliferation induced by tax and measured indirectly by anti-tax antibody (198).

Sexual transmission of HTLV-II has been difficult to study because of the frequent coincidence of intravenous drug abuse in the study populations. In virtually all studies of female prostitutes, intravenous drug abuse was the major risk factor for seropositivity (199, 200). Preliminary analyses of the Guaymi in Panama and Amer-Indians residing in New Mexico report an excess concordance for seropositivity among married couples; this pattern is consistent with that observed in cross-sectional studies of HTLV-I suggesting seroconversion (201). In a recent serosurvey of Guaymi Indians, both univariate and multivariate analysis demonstrated that, among women, early age at first intercourse (less than 13 years of age), number of lifetime sexual partners, and number of long-term sexual relationships were significantly associated with HTLV-II positivity (Armien, Giusti et al., unpublished data presented at the 8th International Conference on Human Retrovirology, Rio de Janeiro, 1997).

Parenteral Transmission

A third major route of transmission is parenteral, either by blood transfusion or intravenous drug abuse. In the case of transfusion transmission, cellular components are associated with transmission of HTLV-I; approximately 50% of recipients of HTLV-I–positive blood seroconvert (202–205). Seroconversion has not been associated with plasma or cryoprecipitate; donor units of whole blood or packed cells are less likely to be associated with viral transmission the longer they are stored in the blood bank, presumably because of the loss of white blood cell viability (206). No characteristic of the donor such as elevated antibody titer is associated with increased risk of viral transmission. Among transfusion recipients, the use of immunosuppressive drugs such as corticosteroids is associated with heightened susceptibility to infection, possibly because of a blunting of the immune response to HTLV-I in the recipient (207).

The only documented illness linked to HTLV-I transfusion transmission is the HTLV-associated demyelinating neurologic syndrome described later (207). Among blood donors in the United States who are confirmed HTLV positive, approximately half are infected with HTLV-I and the other half with HTLV-II. The major risk factors are drug abuse, birthplace in a virally endemic area, or sexual contact with a person with this profile. Viral load, as measured by proviral DNA level on lymphocytes, seems to be related to seroconvertion after exposure to contaminated blood transfusion. Proviral DNA among seroconverters has a profile with an initially increased load and then stabilizes over time; increase of DNA is also observed before the onset of symptoms of HTLV-I–related disease progression (Manns et al., unpublished data presented at the 8th International Conference on Human Retrovirology, Rio de Janeiro, 1997).

The benefit of blood donor screening in preventing transfusion transmission has been documented in Japan, and a decrease of incidence rate of ATL has been observed by the T- and B-cell Malignancy Study Group (208; K Tajima, unpublished data).

HTLV-I transfusion transmission has been documented in retrospective surveys of recipients of known positive units of blood, with approximately half the recipients seroconverting. Longer shelf life of blood is also associated with diminished transmission (206, 209). Parenteral drug abuse has also been associated with transmission of HTLV-I and HTLV-II. Most HTLV-positive IVDUs are infected with HTLV-II and not with HTLV-I, a finding that suggests a biologic difference in the efficiency of transmission of these viruses in the drug abuse setting (84, 205). Risk factors for seroconversion include sharing of drug abuse "works," particularly a history of using an eyedropper in place of a syringe, which was a common apparatus before the wide availability of disposable syringes (205). This historical circumstance may help to explain the exceptionally high rates of seropositivity in older IVDUs because this method was associated with a larger exchange of blood during the sharing of equipment. Transmission involving "casual contact" does not appear to occur. Health care and laboratory workers who experience a needle-stick or skin or mucous membrane exposure in the absence of protective barriers have not been documented to have acquired HTLV-I or HTLV-II infection (210).

A single Japanese health care worker who experienced a "microtransfusion" when a loaded syringe punctured his foot was documented to have seroconverted to HTLV-I. The issue of insect-borne transmission has been raised from several ecologic studies. In one study in Trinidad, this hypothesis was raised by the correlation of HTLV-I positivity among study subjects who lived near water courses where mosquitoes could breed (129). In Jamaica, however, no correlation was found between antibodies to HTLV-I and arthropod-born vector diseases (211). The correlation of HTLV-I positivity with low altitude in Jamaica and Colombia has also been invoked to suggest a vector-borne phenomenon (128, 133). However, such associations may correlate with circumstances of immune activation that may enhance HTLV-I transmission. However, given the relatively inefficient transmission of HTLV-I, vector transmission appears most unlikely.

CLINICAL MANIFESTATIONS OF HTLV-I AND HTLV-II INFECTION

The list of HTLV-I–associated diseases has grown since ATL was first etiologically linked to HTLV-I (Table 58.2). The two main categories of HTLV-I–associated diseases are those resulting from the direct effects of the virus in transforming the leukemia cell, such as for ATL, and those resulting from the immunologic perturbation induced by the virus, such as postulated for HTLV-I–associated myelopathy (212).

HTLV-I–Associated Malignancies

ATL was first recognized by Takatsuki and colleagues in 1977 (213, 214), before the discovery of HTLV-I, as an aggressive leukemia/lymphoma of mature T lymphocytes

Table 58.2. HTLV-Associated Diseases

	HTLV-I	HTLV-II
Childhood		
Infective dermatitis	++++	No
Persistent lymphadenopathy	++	No
Infant death	+	Unknown
Glomerular nephritis	Unknown	++
Adult T-cell leukemia/lymphoma	+++	No
HTLV-associated myelopathy	++++	Unknown
Adulthood		
Adult T-cell leukemia/lymphoma	++++	No
Large granular lymphocyte leukemia	No	Possible
HTLV-associated myelopathy	++++	++
Infective dermatitis	+++	Eczema, herpes
Polymyositis	++	Unknown
Uveitis	+++	Unknown
HTLV-associated arthritis	+++	Possible
Pulmonary infiltrative pneumonitis	++	Bronchitis
Small cell carcinoma of lung	+	Unknown
Invasive cervical cancer	+	Unknown

++++, proven association; +++, probable association; ++ likely association; +, suspected association.

with varied clinical manifestations: generalized lymphadenopathy, visceral involvement, hypercalcemia, cutaneous skin involvement, lytic bone lesions, and peripheral blood involvement with cells manifesting pleotropic features (so-called "flower cells") in a large number of cases.

Although these original cases were diagnosed in Kyoto, most of these patients were born in the southern islands of Kyushu, Shikoku, and the Ryuku archipelago, including Okinawa. Systematic case findings organized by the T-cell and B-cell leukemia/lymphoma group confirmed this clinical impression, and descriptive epidemiologic surveys suggested a role for a transmissible agent to explain this clustering (111). This etiologic agent is HTLV-I, which was originally isolated from a patient thought to have a variant of mycosis fungoides (5). Subsequently, a second cluster of ATL was identified among patients of West Indian ancestry who were diagnosed with ATL in Great Britain and the United States (120, 121). The prevalence of these HTLV-I–associated leukemia/lymphomas worldwide is unknown; the incidence in any population depends on the prevalence of viral infection (215, 216). Cases have been identified in North and South America, Africa, Europe (among migrants from viral endemic areas), the Middle East, Australia (among aboriginal people who harbor the HTLV-I Melanesian variant), the Caribbean basin, and Japan (134, 217–226). In endemic areas such as southern Japan and the Caribbean islands, the annual incidence of virus-associated leukemia is approximately 3 in 100,000 and may account for half of all adult lymphoid malignancies in HTLV-I–endemic areas (114, 216). The chance of an infected individual's developing ATL over a lifetime is 1 to 5%, with early-life exposure associated with the greatest risk of subsequent disease. The male-to-female ratio is approximately 1, and the peak occurrence is in the 40-year-old range in the West Indies and the 50-year-old range in Japan (111, 215). In Jamaica and Trinidad and

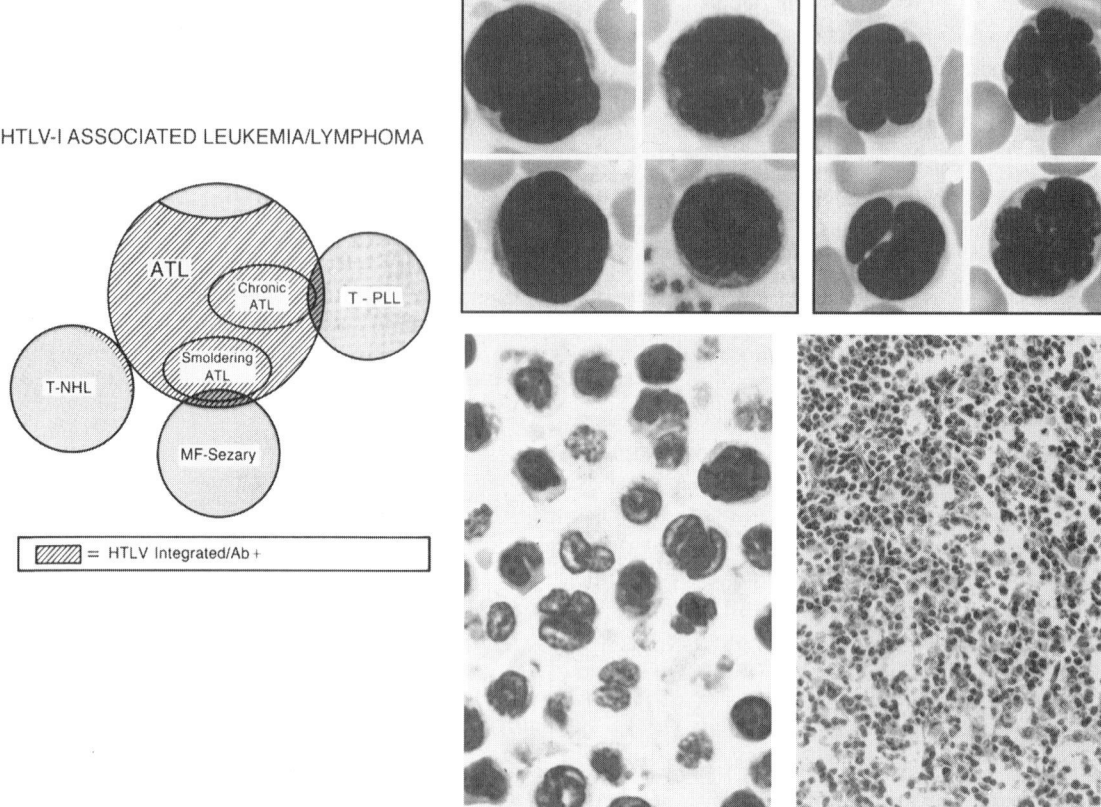

Figure 58.6. Spectrum of T-cell lymphoproliferative diseases entities associated with HTLV-I. *ATL*, adult T-cell leukemia/lymphoma, especially the acute type and the variants, chronic and smoldering originally described in Japan; *T-PLL*, T-cell prolymphocytic leukemia; *T-NHL*, T-cell non–Hodgkin's lymphoma; *MF-Sezary*, mycosis fungoides and Sézary syndrome, both examples of cutaneous T-cell lymphomas. (See color section.)

Tobago, a case-control analysis performed over 3 years demonstrated that patients with non–Hodgkin's lymphoma (NHL) were 10 times more likely to be HTLV-I positive than were controls, and the relative risk of HTLV-I infection was much higher at a younger age and declined after the age of 50 years. Furthermore, taking advantage of the data generated from the two regions, a study was performed to evaluate the age-specific incidence rates of NHL among HTLV-I–positive and HTLV-I–negative individuals. In this study, the incidence of NHL increased with age and was higher in males than in females. The incidence of T-cell NHL was higher in patients infected with HTLV-I early in life (227, 228).

The attributable risk of HTLV-I as a cause of leukemia/lymphoma peaks in the 40- and 50-year ranges and thereafter declines, a finding supporting the concept that exposure early in life with a long latent period from exposure to disease accounts for the observed pattern. Before the age of 50 years, HTLV-I is the major single cause of lymphoma in virally endemic areas (227–228). In some instances, ATL occurs in the pediatric age group, with cases as young as 2 and 10 years reported, but these instances are rare (111, 229, 230). Initially, confusion was considerable about the relation of HTLV-I to mycosis fungoides/Sézary syndrome (231, 232, 218). As more experience with ATL has been gained in virally endemic areas, the breadth of clinical variants has become more evident (233–237) (Fig. 58.6).

The Lymphoma Study Group in Japan classified ATL into four clinical subtypes based on clinicopathologic features: acute, chronic, smoldering, and lymphoma types (236). The acute form of ATL is characterized by an aggressive, mature T-cell lymphoma whose clinical course is often associated with a high white cell count with pleomorphic morphology, hypercalcemia, and cutaneous involvement. Other cases resemble T-prolymphocytic leukemia (237, 238) and are termed chronic ATL subtype; the white blood cells are often elevated, and the abnormal lymphocytes have a characteristic cleaved morphology and are called "buttock cells." Some patients manifest mild lymphadenopathy, hepatosplenomegaly, and elevated serum lactate dehydrogenase. Smoldering subtype ATL may clinically resemble mycosis fungoides/Sézary syndrome, with cutaneous involvement presenting as erythema or as infiltrative plaques or tumors. Pautrier's microabscesses may be observed, as in the first patient from whom the virus was isolated. Sometimes a long prodrome of symptoms or signs, usually in the context of chronic or smoldering ATL, is noted before transformation to acute ATL, which is rapidly fatal. Sometimes ATL presents as a T-cell NHL with no other clinical features of ATL except for monoclonal integration of HTLV-I in proviral DNA in the tumor cells. These cases are classified as adult T-cell leukemia, lymphoma type and are indistinguishable from peripheral T-cell lymphomas (233). Most patients with acute ATL die within 6 months of diagnosis, particularly if they have hypercalcemia (226, 239). The cause of death is usually an explosive growth of tumor cells, hypercalcemia, bacterial sepsis, and various opportunistic infections including *Pneumocystis carinii* pneumonia and other infections observed in patients with immunodeficiency.

The diagnosis of ATL should be considered in adults with mature T-cell lymphoma and hypercalcemia or cutaneous involvement, particularly if the individual is from a known risk group or endemic region. The diagnosis is established by testing serum for HTLV-I antibodies and finding leukemic cells with the provirus in the blood or in biopsy specimens. In some patients with ATL who are from virally endemic areas, as well as in patients without this profile, antibody is absent (215, 218). In some cases, evidence indicates HTLV-I integrated in the tumor tissue, often representing a defective virus or portions of the virus that include critical genes of the virus thought to be essential for transformation such as *tax* (21–30, 240–242). Especially perplexing are sporadic reports of patients with mycosis fungoides with evidence of HTLV-I genes integrated in the absence of antibodies in patients without identifiable risk factors (243–246). It appears that these cases are exceedingly rare, and considerable potential for misclassification exists, given the spectrum of ATL variants observed in Japan and elsewhere. Retroviral particles observed by electron microscopy have been reported from some patients with mycosis fungoides in HTLV-nonendemic areas in Europe (247, 248). Some unambiguous cases of Sézary syndrome associated with the presence of unusual retroviral infection markers were described. The blood smear showed typical Sézary cells and atypical lymphocytes with convoluted nuclei as flower cells. Although the patient did not have any clinical or biologic manifestations of ATL, and HTLV-I serologic studies were consistently negative, his peripheral blood lymphocytes in medium-term culture produced typical type C retrovirus–like particles with budding forms strongly resembling HTLV virions. The producer cells did not express HTLV-I–specific antigens, but Southern blotting submitted to digestion with the restriction enzymes and hybridized with a full genomic HTLV-I probe showed the presence of specific homologous sequences (247). However, these HTLV-I–like sequences presented a restriction enzyme pattern distinct from that of the HTLV-I prototype genome and of other HTLV-I proviruses studied up to now.

Molecular and virologic studies have provided much information about the pathogenesis of HTLV-I–associated ATL. Investigators believe that, early in infection, HTLV-I infects only a few T cells and perhaps monocyte/macrophages. As shown in Figure 58.7, activated T cells are postulated to represent a particularly suitable target for HTLV-I infection. This concept is supported from several perspectives. First, chromosome 17 has been identified as essential for viral infection, perhaps involving a T-cell activation marker on this chromosome (24). Second, HTLV-I induces spontaneous lymphocyte proliferation when cells from HTLV-I–infected persons are placed in tissue culture in the absence of mitogens and antigens (246, 250). The finding that normal Jamaicans in the absence of HTLV-I infection have significantly higher spontaneous lymphocyte proliferation levels than blood bank controls in the United States supports the concept that an activated T cell is the prime target for HTLV-I infection. Figure 58.7 outlines the initial events of HTLV-I infection, requiring that HTLV-I bind to

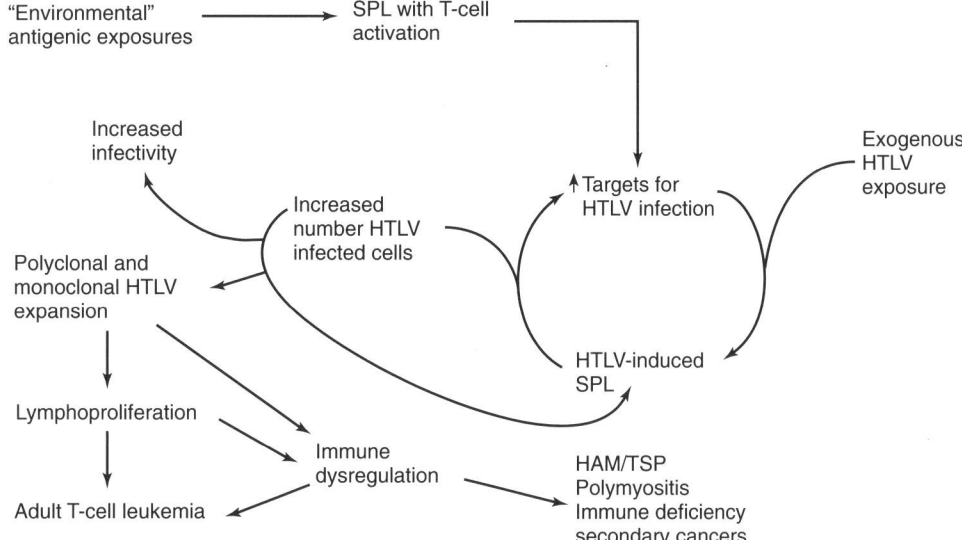

Figure 58.7. Interaction of HTLV-I and spontaneous proliferating lymphocytes *(SPL)* could amplify the risk of HTLV-I infection, thus explaining some aspects of the peculiar geographic distribution of HTLV-I. Furthermore, this ongoing property of HTLV-I–induced proliferation may contribute to the pathogenesis of both the leukemia and the neurologic and related conditions. (Courtesy of W.A. Blattner and S.Z. Wiktor.)

an as yet undefined receptor with subsequent uncoating, reverse transcription, and production of a DNA provirus. The DNA provirus randomly integrates into the DNA of infected cells. Although HTLV-I may exist as a latent virus, the genes of the virus promote cell proliferation by direct and indirect mechanisms, including various lymphokine pathways and in the process may promote the expression of additional activated target cells for amplification of virus spread (251) (see Fig. 58.7). Clearly, host immune responses to the virus are activated, resulting in development of viral antibodies and CTLs targeted at viral antigens (250). The finding that blood bank recipients who are taking exogenous immunosuppressive medications are more susceptible to infection is best explained by a situation wherein the host immune response is blunted and clearance of virus infection is impaired (178). Investigators have observed that some persons develop polyclonal and oligoclonal populations that resemble transformed, but not malignant, cells (197, 240). Such polyclonal, oligoclonal, and monoclonal expansions have been noted to appear and sometimes disappear spontaneously. After a long latent period (years to several decades), a monoclonal malignancy may develop, presumably involving additional oncogenic mutations (29, 240).

Studies have suggested that some genes of the virus may modify the clearance of the p53 and other suppressors gene by different pathways (252–257). Studies in vitro have demonstrated that binding of viral tax to a receptor on NF-κB or other latent cytoplasmic proteins such as signal transducers and activators of transcription (STATs) can induce a dysregulated T-cell transformation (18, 36, 256). Immunosuppressive events may also play a role inasmuch as tumor necrosis factor β is turned on in ATL (258, 259).

Why only a few infected individuals develop malignancy (1 to 3% lifetime risk), why the latency from infection to disease appears so long, and why CD4 cells are selectively transformed (although CD8 cells can also be infected) remain unknown. In ATL, the HTLV-I provirus is found integrated in the DNA of the leukemic cells in a clonal fashion, with one or multiple copies of the provirus integrated in the same chromosomal location in each cell. Two different cases of ATL in which parts of the HTLV-I virus are deleted have been described. One deleted case retains some LTR sequences but lacks viral structural sequences, whereas the other case has a deleted 5'-LTR plus the structural and regulatory sequences (9, 29, 30, 167). Although this finding is still controversial, the deleted type integration pattern seems to be associated with a particularly aggressive form of ATL (258). Besides, deletions of cell-cycle genes such as p15, p16, or p21 have been also described as predictors of different clinical subtypes and prognosis (258, 259).

ATL is a tumor derived from a single transformed cell that expanded from a virus infection before transformation and clonal expansion, rather than later as a passenger virus; tumors from different patients have proviral integration in different locations and monoclonal TCR-β gene rearrangements (21, 28). Unlike some animal models, leukemogenesis does not result from a *cis*-activation of a nearby cellular gene by the LTR of the virus (6, 9). Growing evidence suggests that transformation at some stage involves the expression of the Tax protein encoded by the pX gene of HTLV-I (21, 22, 260). Because the Tax protein induces expression of cellular genes critical for T-cell proliferation, including IL-2 and its receptor (IL-2R), an autocrine mechanism may be involved, particularly in the first steps of leukemogenesis. For the development of malignancy, additional genetic changes are postulated because leukemia cells become independent of IL-2 requirements for growth (21). Nonetheless, several investigators have observed that *tax* gene expression is detectable in tumor samples, even in some cases of antibody-negative ATL (19, 166). ATL cells also secrete many kinds of cytokines vivo such as IL-1α, IL-1β, LD78 (macrophage-inflammatory protein-α or MIP-1α), tumor necrosis factor-α, interferon-γ, and granulocyte–macrophage colony-stimulating factor (GM-CSF), but not secreting IL-1α, IL-1β, IL-1 receptor antagonist (IL-1 Ra), IL-4, interferon-α, and G-CSF, irrespective of the stimulatory agents (260, 261). In a recent study, elevated IL-10 levels were observed in fresh leukemic cells of 33 of 45 patients with ATL, as well as HTLV-I–infected T-cell lines MT-2, SLB-1, and C10/MJ (262, 263).

The most frequent chromosomal abnormalities reported in ATL are the breakpoints at 6p15 and 6q21. Multiple chromosome and complex karyotype are also observed. The nature of additional genetic changes is unknown, but it may involve chromosomal alterations that are frequent but not at a specific locus in ATL (264, 265).

Two cases of B-cell chronic lymphocytic leukemia with a possible HTLV-I association involving an indirect mechanism were reported from Jamaica, but no statistical excess of such cases has been seen among prospectively ascertained incident cases over several years (266). No viral sequences are found in the tumor, but the immunoglobulins of the tumor cell react to HTLV-I–specific antigens. Investigators hypothesized for these cases that chronic stimulation of B-cell proliferation by viral antigens, coupled with virus-induced impairment of CD4 cell function, resulted in malignant transformation and B-cell chronic lymphocytic leukemia.

HTLV-I has also been associated with isolated cases of other malignancies (139, 267, 268). In one case of small cell cancer of the lung, viral sequences were monoclonally integrated into the tumor cells (268). A statistically increased prevalence of HTLV-I antibodies is seen in patients with invasive carcinoma of the cervix, but this could result from shared sexual risk factors rather than from a direct effect of HTLV-I in carcinogenesis (269). Surveys of hospitalized patients in Japan with various malignant diseases have elevated rates of HTLV-I compared with "normal populations," but ascertainment biases could have influenced this association.

HTLV-I–Associated Neurologic Disease

HTLV-I has been linked to a neurologic syndrome called tropical spastic paraparesis/HTLV-I–associated myelopathy

(TSP/HAM) (270, 271). TSP/HAM is a chronic neurologic syndrome associated with demyelination of the long motor neurons of the spinal cord. Symptoms often begin with a stiff gait, progressing (usually slowly) to increasing spasticity and lower extremity weakness, back pain, urinary incontinence, and impotence in men developing later during the course of the illness (272–274). Sometimes ataxia develops. On nuclear magnetic resonance scan, isolated lesions of the central nervous system are detected in some cases (273). The syndrome differs from classic multiple sclerosis because of the generally slow, progressive course and absence of waxing and waning of symptomatology and changes in affect (275). Some cases are acutely progressive. Dramatic examples of such rapidly progressive cases are sometimes associated with the transfusion of HTLV-I from a positive blood donor (207, 276). Studies from Japan have documented a significant excess of blood transfusion in TSP/HAM cases compared with ATL and in normal donors (276, 278). At present, about 2000 cases of TSP/HAM have been reported in HTLV-I–endemic cases including Japan, the Caribbean, Brazil, Colombia, Chile and Africa (141, 273, 279, 280). The incidence of disease has been measured in Japan to be approximately half that of ATL, although the prevalence of disease is much higher inasmuch as the syndrome is rarely fatal but chronically disabling (279). The annualized incidence of TSP/HAM per 100,000 inhabitants in Jamaica and Trinidad is 2.8 and 1.9, respectively. These rates are inversely related to the rates of ATL in these countries, with ATL rates falling in age strata where TSP/HAM rates are rising. These data, coupled with the much higher and rising rate of TSP/HAM with age and female sex, suggest that adult acquired infection is a major source of exposure related to this disease complex. In fact, based on transfusion experience, in which the highest incidence of TSP/HAM is observed within a few months to years after exposure, it is likely that, in contrast to ATL, in which years to decades transpire between exposure and ATL development, the latency between exposure and TSP/HAM development is likely to be much shorter (Maloney et al., unpublished data). Death results from complicating infections of the lung or urinary tract. Women are approximately twofold more likely to be infected, and in one analysis, markers of sexual transmission were observed, especially in female cases (273, 279). Cases tend to peak in the 30- to 50-year age group, but pediatric cases have been reported in children as young as 3 years of age (279). The pattern of occurrence, links with blood transfusion, and markers of sexual transmission suggest that perinatally acquired, postnatally acquired, and adult-acquired infection are linked to disease. A shorter latency between infection and disease occurrence is likely. Genetic susceptibility factors have been postulated, based on associations of certain antigens of the major histocompatibility complex and TSP/HAM risk (32). In southern Japan, a significantly higher frequency of HLA A-26 and B61 was found in patients with ATL, whereas HLA-B7 and DrB1 *0101 was seen in patients with TSP/HAM. These results suggest that a genetic segregation of HTLV-I immune response may occur with HLA haplotypes of ATL and TSP/HAM (Sonoda et al, unpublished data from HLA and HLTV: 12th International Histocompatibility Workshop Study). Cases combining ATL and TSP/HAM have been reported; in a series of 186 ATL cases described in Brazil, 12 patients had TSP/HAM. In 6 cases, the patients had suffered from myelopathy more than 4 years before the diagnosis of ATL, and 2 patients were brother and sister. In the remaining 6 cases, the diagnosis of both diseases was made during admission for ATL treatment (Pombo-de-Oliveira, Blattner, et al., unpublished data).

Persons with TSP/HAM have high levels of spontaneous lymphocyte proliferation, and carriers of the associated genetic phenotype also strongly react to the virus in the proliferation assay (31, 33, 242, 281, 282). These data suggest that persons affected with TSP/HAM are prone to aberrant reactions to the virus, and virus loads in excess of those seen in ATL have been reported in TSP/HAM cases from Japan (32). Proviral load can differ more than 100 times among infected individuals; Bangham and collegues (283, 284) proposed a model for the dynamics of immune responses to persistent viruses based on variation of CTL responsiveness and viral load. They analyzed the interaction between virus replication and CTL responses measured by a simple mathematic model (Fig.58.8). Individuals differ in their CTL responsiveness to HTLV-I according to diversity of variable epitopes. However, strong and weak responders may differ in virus load but can maintain the same levels of CTL responses (283, 284).

An indirect mechanism of pathogenesis has been postulated (285, 286). As shown in Figure 58.7, perturbation in immune function caused by HTLV-I has been suggested, although direct viral infection of nervous system tissue has not been excluded. As seen in multiple sclerosis, oligoclonal immunoglobulin bands are present in the cerebrospinal fluid, but with reactivity for HTLV-I–specific bands (242, 286). The demyelinating lesions from these cases involve infiltration with CD8 cells, and only rarely is an HTLV-I–positive cell observed based on in situ hybridization analysis (246). Possibly, HTLV-I induces an autoimmune type of mechanism either through a molecular mimicry process or by indirect effects on immune function (212). The high virus loads suggest a deficiency in the ability of the host to control viral proliferation. The diagnosis is suspected in unexplained central nervous system disease with loss of pyramidal tract functions and is confirmed by testing sera for HTLV-I antibodies.

Other HTLV-I–Associated Diseases

Polymyositis of skeletal muscle is frequently associated with HTLV-I seropositivity in viral endemic areas. These cases are indistinguishable from polymyositis seen in HTLV-I–nonendemic areas. Large-joint polyarthropathy has been reported in Japan among elderly patients (287, 288). A distinguishing feature of these cases is the presence of HTLV-I–producing cells in the synovial infiltrate. A unique

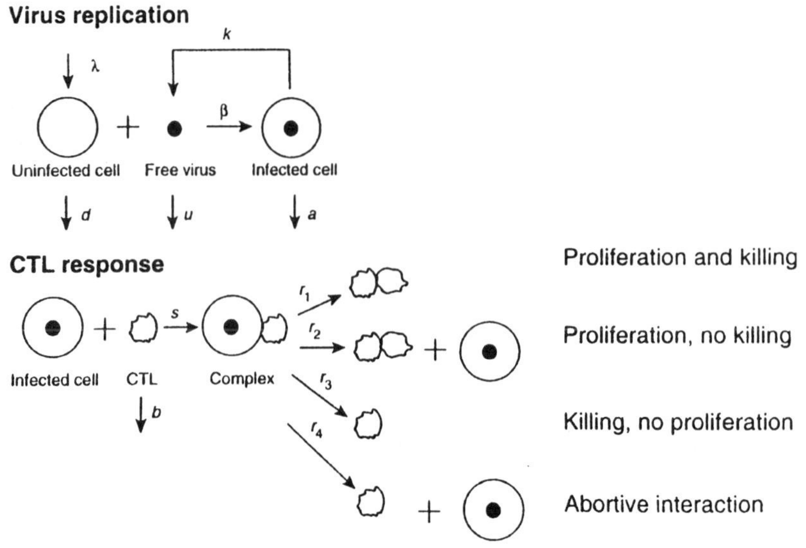

Figure 58.8. A model for virus cytotoxic lymphocyte (CTL) interaction. In virus replication, free virus particles, uninfected cells, and infected cells are population dynamics with different rates of productions (λ, κ, β) and declinations (u, a, d). This complex dissociated in four pathways: target cells can be killed CTL stimulated to be divided; CTLs can be divided without killing the target cells; the target cell may be killed, but the CTLs may not divide; and there may be killing but no proliferation. (From Nowak AM, Bangham CRM. Population dynamics of immune responses to persistent viruses. Science 1996;272:74–79.)

form of uveitis has been observed in HTLV-I–positive individuals. These cases account for about 30 to 40% of idiopathic uveitis in HTLV-I–endemic areas (289). The first evidence of an association of HTLV-I infection with uveitis was reported in Japan by Ohba and colleagues (290), who detected ocular involvement in patients with ATL, TSP/HAM, and asymptomatic carriers. The ocular manifestation were then classified in three groups: 1) opportunistic infections and tumor infiltration in ATL patients; 2) ocular alterations in TSP/HAM patients including Sjögren's syndrome, retinal pigmentary degeneration, optic atrophy, vitreous opacities, cotton-wool spots and retinal vasculitis; 3) HTLV-I uveitis in asymptomatic carriers. Proviral DNA of HTLV-I was identified in 60% of T cells from intraocular fluid of these patients (290, 292). HTLV-I–associated infiltrative pneumonitis has also been reported in some individuals in Japan (293, 294).

HTLV-I appears to be immunosuppressive based on clinical and laboratory observations. AIDS-like illnesses associated with HTLV-I (in the absence of underlying malignancy) have been reported in Japan (295). The association of HTLV-I with parasitic infestations (e.g., strongyloidosis) refractory to treatment has also been interpreted to suggest that HTLV-I may have immunosuppressive effects (296–298). Decreased skin test response to recall antigens has also been reported among HTLV-I–infected older individuals (299). Various subclinical perturbations in hematologic markers such as depressed hemoglobin and lymphopenia have been reported in healthy HTLV-I carriers (300). The infective dermatitis syndrome was first shown to be associated with HTLV-I in Jamaica (301). It appears to represent the first childhood HTLV-I syndrome. Patients are born of HTLV-I–positive mothers and experience a syndrome of "failure to thrive." They are prone to refractory generalized eczema and infection with saprophytic *Staphylococcus* and *Streptococcus* bacteria that are suppressed by long-term antibiotic therapy and recur when the therapy is stopped. This syndrome usually emerges early in life, in the first few years after birth, and in cases followed for many years it persists into adulthood. Anecdotal cases emerging in adolescence suggest that some may result from infection at older age. Investigators have postulated that infective dermatitis is an immunodeficiency syndrome induced by HTLV-I. Some patients go on to develop ATL and TSP/HAM (302, 303). Further study of the pathogenesis of this syndrome should provide valuable insights into the pathogenesis of HTLV-I–associated diseases.

Other possible pediatric consequences of HTLV-I infection include the persistent lymphadenopathy syndrome, which has been identified among offspring of HTLV-I-positive women (130). Its relation to HTLV-I is unclear inasmuch as the virus has not been detected in many children with this syndrome. Possibly it represents an immunologic response to the virus because some children with the syndrome have seroconverted later than most children exposed through breast-feeding. Others are persistently virus antibody negative but with modest elevations in CD8 cells. Some studies have also suggested that infant mortality is higher in women who are HTLV-I seropositive (315). It is possible that this association results from the higher infant mortality of women of lower socioeconomic status, who are at higher risk of HTLV-I infection, rather than from a direct effect of HTLV-I on the infant.

Coinfection with HTLV-I and HIV-1 seems to result in a faster progression to AIDS (304). A direct effect of viral gene interactions has been postulated by some investigators, based on molecular interactions of the two viruses that infect the same target cell (17, 35). Alternatively, the cell proliferative effects of HTLV-I may amplify the cytopathic effects of HIV-1 on infected T cells (305-307). Additional data from prospectively followed cohorts are needed to clarify this association. HTLV-I infection has been associated with *Strongyloides*.

HTLV-II DISEASE ASSOCIATIONS

HTLV-II remains an orphan virus with no clearly established disease link, although a growing body of case reports is starting to suggest some possible associations. The original isolations of HTLV-II came from patients reported to have hairy cell leukemia (HCL); however, surveys of HCL cases have identified only sporadic examples of HTLV-II positivity (12, 308, 309). One of these cases had tumor cells involving B cells and the HTLV-II virus in the T cells, a finding suggesting an indirect mechanism (210). Subsequently, several cases of large granular lymphocyte (LGL) leukemia, a T-cell malignancy with a natural killer (NK) cell phenotype, have been reported (310). However, several surveys of LGL cases did not documented a clear excess of HTLV-I antibodies or molecular sequences of HTLV-II genome (218, 238, 315, 311, 312).

New Mexico, which has a large Amer-Indian population, has no detectable perturbation in the incidence of HTLV-II–suspect lymphoproliferative diseases such as HCL, suspected to be HTLV-II associated, but the power of this approach to detect a true association is weakened by the inability to measure HTLV-II status directly in the registered cases (313). One case of HTLV-II–associated mycosis fungoides has been reported based on detection of virus positivity in the absence of antibody (246). A syndrome of severe skin disease, eosinophilia, and dermatopathic lymphadenopathy has been reported among some IVDUs coinfected with HTLV-II and HIV-1 (244). Pathogenically, HTLV-II, like HTLV-I, induces spontaneous lymphocyte proliferation in vitro but at a lower level than HTLV-I (210).

A growing number of TSP/HAM cases associated with HTLV-II is being reported (314, 315). In one prospective transfusion cohort with a small number of clinical events, HTLV-I–associated TSP/HAM appeared more frequently than detected in the small number of HTLV-II recipients. Some of the case reports noted features reminiscent of the ataxic form of TSP/HAM reported from Jamaica. Patients have oligoclonal bands in the cerebrospinal fluid reminiscent of that observed in HTLV-I-positive patients with specific reactivity for viral-specific antigens.

Other possible conditions identified in medical surveys of the Guaymi Indians, IVDU, and transfusion cohorts that are being evaluated in association with HTLV-II are adult polyarthritis, eczema of the skin, and asthma. In one prospective study of IVDUs, HTLV-II–positive subjects had an excess of medical deaths including elevated asthma-related deaths. In the Guaymi survey glomerular nephritis appeared significantly elevated in children. Given the streptococcal association in HTLV-I–associated infective dermatitis, this intriguing association needs additional follow-up. Bronchitis, bladder or kidney infection, and oral herpes are the most frequent infectious diseases associated with HTLV-II observed in a cross-sectional study of infected IVDUs and blood donors, all HIV negative (E Murphy, et al., unpublished data). Nonetheless, at this time, HTLV-II remains a true orphan virus without a clear disease association.

TREATMENT

HTLV-I–associated diseases have a poor prognosis because effective therapies have not yet been developed. ATL is refractory to most conventional and experimental chemotherapeutic regimens; however, some cases do respond with prolonged remission to multidrug regimens developed for treating high-grade T-cell NHL (316, 317). Prognosis varies by subtype. Among the 50 to 60% of patients with ATL who have acute-type ATL and the 25 to 30% with lymphoma type, survival is short, whereas among the 10 to 15% with chronic and smoldering types, long-term prognosis is good, although some patients progress to a more aggressive type. Most patients with acute and lymphoma-type ATL die within 6 to 10 months of diagnosis (Fig. 58.9). Patients with chronic and smoldering ATL are treated with either no therapy or with prednisone with or without cyclophosphamide. Patients with these more indolent forms of ATL when treated with aggressive therapy have a high rate of complicating infections resulting from the intrinsic immunodeficiency of ATL as well as the cytoreductive effects of therapy. The acute and lymphoma-type ATL are aggressive high-grade lymphomas with a generally poor prognosis, although some patients do respond with prolonged remission to multidrug regimens. For example, in Japan, large trials of VEPA (vincristine, cyclophosphamide, prednisolone, and doxorubicin) or VEPA-M (adding methotrexate) as well as more complex 9- and 10-drug regimens have shown some success, but with poor long-term survival (225). Although initial response rates, even for the poorest risk categories, are higher than 50% and complete remissions are achieved in 20%, these responses can be short lived, with relapses occuring with weeks to months (318). An intensive combination chemotherapy regimen supported by G-CSF was evaluated in patients with ATL in a multi-institutional cooperative study in Japan and yielded a better response rate and longer survival compared with previous reports (320, 321). Significant prognostic factors include poor performance status at diagnosis, age older than 40 years, extensive disease, hypercalcemia, and high serum lactate dehydrogenase level. Approximately 13 to 15% of patients with such aggressive cases experience long-term survival (more than 2 years) that, in one study, was associated with several factors: complete remission, longer time to remission, and total doxorubicin dose. Relapses in these long-term survivors often occurred in the central nervous system and proved refractory to subsequent therapy (18). Other studies employing combinations of doxorubicin and etoposide have resulted in complete remission rates of

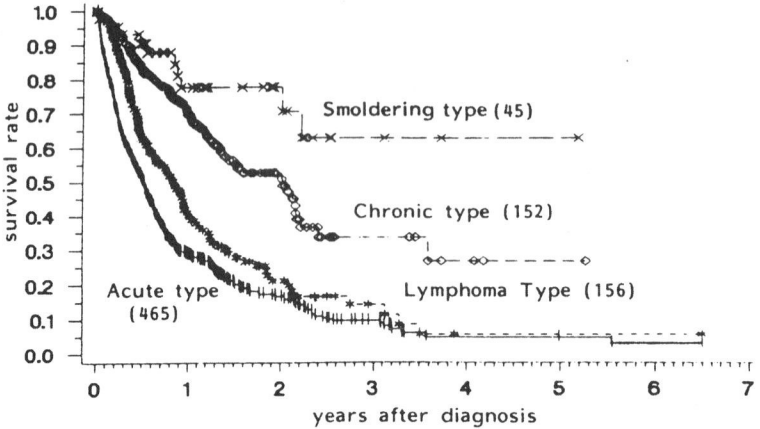

Figure 58.9. Survival patterns of adult T-cell leukemia/lymphoma (ATL) in different subtypes after treatment with polychemotherapy. Acute and lymphoma-type ATL have the poorest prognosis after chemotherapy. (From Tsukasaki K, Ikeda S, Murata K, et al. Characteristics of chemotherapy induced clinical remission in long survivors with aggressive adult T-cell leukemia/lymphoma. Leuk Res 1993;17:157–163.)

40%, but they have not improved survival. Phase I trials with topoisomerase inhibitors and dioxopiperazine inhibitors have shown some promise (321). Deoxycoformycin was thought to offer some benefit in early trials, but it has proven to be ineffectual in aggressive disease (322–324). Ubenimex has been tried and was shown to be antedodally beneficial in chronic ATL (325). Experimental approaches that use humanized monoclonal antibodies to the IL-2 receptor that can be linked with cell toxins selectively targeted to the leukemic cells are being tested, with some evidence of at least partial responses (326). This approach, in turn, may lead to a more rational approach to targeting therapies, perhaps with implications for treating other forms of T-cell lymphoproliferative disease. The complicating hypercalcemia of ATL often responds to standard therapeutic approaches, but in a significant proportion may be refractory. Bacterial sepsis and opportunistic infections are frequent and should be treated with appropriate antimicrobial agents; however, despite therapy, these infections are frequently the cause of death. An intriguing advance in the treatment of ATL was reported in two independent studies with the combination of an antiretroviral agent (zidovudine) and interferon-α (327–329). Complete remission rate was observed in 75% of the untreated patients in acute and lymphoma type ATL. Despite the good initial response and mild toxicity of the treatment, relapses occurred after a median follow up of 1 year. The success of this antiretroviral approach in the treatment of ATL would suggest that the postulated oncogenic effect of HTLV-I can be controllable or reversible. A postremission treatment needs to be developed to consolidate the long-term benefit of this treatment approach.

Treatment of TSP/HAM is equally challenging. Oral corticosteroids have beneficial effects in some patients with TSP/HAM, particularly those with rapidly progressive disease (274). Intrathecal hydrocortisone, intravenous methylprednisolone, interferon-α, azathioprine, danazol, and intermittent high-dose vitamin C also have been suggested as beneficial to patients with TSP/HAM. However, none of these treatment has been systematically studied to evaluate the remission and prolongation of survival of these patients (273). Treatment with androgenic steroids, such as danazol, has resulted in improvement in urinary and fecal incontinence but not in the underlying neurologic condition (330, 331). Intermittent high-dose vitamin C has been beneficial in the mobility, but it had no effect in the urinary symptoms (J Edwards, unpublished data presented at the 8th International Conference on Human Retrovirology, Rio de Janeiro, 1997). Based on the association between the IL-2 complex and the immune activation in TSP/HAM, a humanized anti-Tac (anti-interkeukin-2 receptor antibody) has been safety used in seven patients in different clinical stages of TSP/HAM. The efficiency of this approach was measured by the reduction of viral load confirmed by PCR. No clinical progression of disease was noted in all patients, and one patient had some improvement in neurologic symptoms.

PREVENTION

Guidelines for prevention and counseling have been developed for HTLV-I and HTLV-II by a Centers for Disease Control and Prevention (CDC) Working Group (332). Standard prevention approaches are similar for both viruses. In the blood bank, blood should be screened before transfusion, and if a donor is identified as positive, the CDC recommends that positive donors not give blood. Such blood bank screening has been recommended since 1987 in Japan, since 1988 in the United States and in Brazil, since 1993 (47, 280). Unfortunately, in many virally endemic areas of the developing world, HTLV-I blood bank screening is not feasible because of budgetary constraints and competing public health priorities. HTLV-I/II–positive mothers should be discouraged from breast-feeding when practicable to prevent mother-to-infant transmission. In tropical settings in which diarrheal disease has a high mortality in non–breast-fed infants, breast-feeding is recommended. However, based on emerging data, it may be possible to recommend breast-feeding in the critical first few months of life when maternal antibodies may offer some protection with safe introduction of bottle feeding where feasible (182). This issue is far from settled and will require additional study before precise recommendations can be made. Use of condoms is recommended for couples discordant for HTLV-I/II serostatus; given the relatively low frequency of sexual transmission per sexual encounter, couples who desire pregnancy could time their unprotected sexual times to coincide with periods of maximal fertility. Such decisions require careful discussion between physician and patient, and no absolute guidelines exist in this particular area. Counseling seropositive persons should be based on knowledge of virus type with clear discussion of the distinction between the HTLV viruses and the HIV viruses. In addition, virus type should be defined by serologic methods, and the distinctions in disease associations of the two virus types as outlined previously should be emphasized.

Vaccines containing whole virus and recombinant HTLV-I envelope antigens have successfully prevented HTLV-I infection in monkeys and rabbits, and maternal antibodies appear to protect newborns in the first 6 months of life (323–335). Unlike HIV-1, which varies considerably in its envelope, HTLV-I is constant and appears to protect even major variant strains (336). Using rabbit antisera to portions of the HTLV-I envelope, Japanese investigations have neutralized both American and Japanese HTLV-I isolates in vitro (333, 337). In one primate challenge study, HTLV-I–infected cells were used as the challenge vehicle. Protection correlated with the presence of neutralizing antibodies, a finding indicating that humoral immunity can be an effective barrier against infection (335). Because human or animal antisera to Japanese and American HTLV-I envelope will cross-neutralize, it is likely that the envelope antigens of HTLV-I represent a single serotype worldwide. Thus, unlike the isolate-specific neutralizing epitopes of HIV, a synthetic vaccine against one HTLV-I isolate should protect against other HTLV-I isolates (338, 339). Whether a vaccine for HTLV-I or HTLV-II will ever be implemented in human populations is the subject of ongoing debate. In Japan, epidemiologic data suggest that the rate of new infections is declining spontaneously, presumably as a result of changing socioeconomic conditions and lifestyle. In the Caribbean, the incidence of HTLV-I infections in a sexually transmitted disease clinic is as high as 1 to 1.5% per year. In other parts of the world, HTLV-I and HTLV-II infections continue to occur, but rates are poorly defined. Whether the disease burden associated with these viruses warrants a vaccine is also a matter of discussion. The incidence of disease is not dissimilar to the estimated incidence of hepatocellular carcinoma in hepatitis B antigen carriers, but without the acute morbidity associated with acute hepatitis. Final decisions on this issue will require additional definition of the cost and benefits of such an intervention.

In conclusion, the study of HTLV-I and HTLV-II represents an important chapter in the history of contemporary medicine. In the 10 years since the discovery of the first human leukemia virus, significant progress has been made in the understanding of the epidemiology and modes of transmission of the HTLVs. Their mechanisms for transmission similar to those of HIV but less efficient. This inefficiency of viral transmission may explain the low rates of transmission from mother to non–breast-fed infant and from females to males sexually, and it also may explain why only half of the recipients of HTLV-positive blood seroconvert. We have also discovered that increased viral load or replication may be an important factor in the transmission of HTLV-I from mother to infant as well as in sexual contact cases, and genital ulcer disease may enhance sexual transmission of the virus. Risk factors for transmission are becoming more clearly defined, as are the opportunities for making specific suggestions and recommendations for the prevention of these HTLV-associated infections.

Knowledge of HTLV-associated diseases has expanded since the discovery of the relationship between HTLV-I/ATL and HTLV-I/TSP/HAM and includes a growing array of syndromes of altered immunity and malignant potential. Based on current knowledge, mortality resulting directly from the effects of the virus is probably between 5 and 10% among carriers during their lifetime, and morbidity may be twice as high. In the near future, the disease associations of HTLV-II should be clarified.

HTLV viruses offer new avenues for expanding knowledge of disease causation, and they provide a conceptual model for exploring disease pathogenesis. Additional examples of viruses of this class with shared properties of long latency, low-level replication, with cellular tropism to other tissues are candidate agents for unexplained autoimmune, immunodeficiency, and neurologic diseases and for some human malignancies. Critical to this process will be the development of techniques for detecting and growing these putative viruses.

References

1. Rous P. A sarcoma of the fowl transmissible by an agent separable from the tumor cells. J Exp Med 1911;13:397.
2. Baltimore D. RNA dependent DNA polymerase in virions of RNA tumor viruses. Nature 1970;226:1209–1211.
3. Temin TM, Mitzutani S. RNA-directed DNA polymerase in virions of Rous sarcoma virus. Nature 1970;226:1211.
4. Morgan DA, Ruscetti FW, Gallo RC. Selective in vitro growth of T-lymphocytes from normal human bone marrow. Science 1976;193:1007–1008.
5. Poiesz BJ, Ruscetti FW, Gazdar AF, et al. Detection and isolation of type-C retrovirus particles from fresh and cultured lymphocytes of a patient with cutaneous T-cell lymphoma. Proc Natl Acad Sci U S A 1980;77:7415–7419.
6. Gallo R, Wong-Staal F, Montagnier L, et al. HIV/HTLV gene nomenclature. Nature 1988;333:504.
7. Barre-Sinoussi F, Chermann JC, Rey F, et al. Isolation of a T-lymphotropic retrovirus from a patient at risk for acquired immune deficiency syndrome (AIDS). Science 1983;220:868–871.
8. Popovic M, Sarngadharan MG, Read E, et al. Detection, isolation, and continuous production of cytopathic retroviruses (HTLV-III) from patients with AIDS and pre-AIDs. Science 1984;224:497–500.
9. Seiki M, Hattori S, Hirayama Y, et al. Human adult T-cell leukemia virus: complete nucleotide sequence of the provirus genome inte-

grated in leukemia cell DNA. Proc Natl Acad Sci U S A 1983;80: 3618–3622.
10. Shimotohno K, Takahashi Y, Shimizu N, et al. Complete nucleotide sequence of an infectious clone of human T-cell leukemia virus type II: an open reading frame for the protease gene. Proc Natl Acad Sci U S A 1985;82:3101–3105.
11. Ratner L, Haseltine W, Patarca R, et al. Complete nucleotide sequence of the AIDS virus, HTLV-III. Nature 1985;313:277–284.
12. Kalyanaraman VS, Sarngadharan MG, Robert-Guroff M, et al. A new subtype of human T-cell leukemia virus (HTLV-II) associated with a T-cell variant of hairy cell leukemia. Science 1982;218:571–573.
13. Gallo RC. Mechanism of disease induction by HIV. J Acquir Immune Defic Syndr 1990;3:380–389.
14. Varmus H. Retroviruses. Science 1988;240:1427–1435.
15. Wong-Staal F, Gallo RC. Human T-lymphotropic retroviruses. Nature 1985;317:395–403.
16. Rosenblatt JD, Cann AJ, Slamon DJ, et al. HTLV-II transactivation is regulated by the overlapping *tax/rex* nonstructural genes. Science 1988;240:916–919.
17. Siekevitz M, Josephs SF, Dukovich M, et al. Activation of the HIV-1 LTR by T cell mitogens and the trans-activator protein of HTLV-I. Science 1987;238:1575–1578.
18. Hirai H, Fujisawa J, Suzuki T, et al. Transcriptional activator tax of HTLV-I binds to the NF-kB precursor p105. Oncogene 1992;7: 1737–1742.
19. Okayama A, Chen YA, Tachibana N, et al. High incidence of antibodies to HTLV-I tax in blood relatives of adult T cell leukemia patients. J Infect Dis 1991;163:47–52.
20. Berneman A, Gartenhaus RB, Reitz MS Jr, et al. Expression of alternatively spliced human T-lyphotropic virus type I pX mRNA in infected cell lines and in primary uncultured cells from patients with adult T-cell leukemia/lymphoma and healthy carriers. Proc Natl Acad Sci U S A 1992;89:3005–3009.
21. Franchini G. Molecular mechanisms of human T-cell leukemia/ lymphotropic virus type I infection. Blood 1995;86:3619–3639.
22. Chlichlia K, Moldenhauer G, Daniel PT, et al. Immediate effects of reversible HTLV-1 *tax* function: T-cell activation and apoptosis. Oncogene 1995;10:269–227.
23. Igichi S, Ramundo MB, Takahashi H, et al. In vivo cellular tropisms of human T-cell leukemia virus type II (HTLV-II). J Exp Med 1992; 176:293–296.
24. Sommerfelt MA, Williams BP, Clapham PR, et al. Human T cell leukemia viruses use a receptor determined by human chromosome 17. Science 1988;242:1557–1559.
25. Guyot DJ, Newbound GC, Lairmore MD. Signaling via the CD2 receptor enhances HTLV-1 replication in T lymphocytes. Virology 1997;234:123–129.
26. Yoshida M, Seiki M, Yamaguchi K, et al. Monoclonal integration of human T-cell leukemia provirus in all primary tumors of adult T-cell leukemia suggests causative role of human T-cell leukemia virus in the disease. Proc Natl Acad Sci U S A 1984;81:2534–2537.
27. Cavrois M, Wain-Hobson S, Gessain A, et al. Adult T-cell leukemia/ lymphoma on a background of clonally expanding human T-cell leukemia virus type-1-positive cells. Blood 1996;88: 4646–4650.
28. Okamoto T, Mori S, Ohno Y, et al. Stochastic analysis of the carcinogenesis of adult T-cell leukemia-lymphoma. In: Blattner W, ed. Human retrovirology: HTLV. New York: Raven Press, 1990:307–313.
29. Tsukasaki K, Tsushima H, Yamamura M, et al. Integration patterns of HTLV-I provirus in relation to the clinical course of ATL: frequent clonal change at crisis from indolent disease. Blood 1997;89:948–956.
30. Tamiya S, Matsuoka M, Etoh K, et al. Two types of defective human T-lymphotropic virus type I provirus in adult T-cell leukemia. Blood 1996;88:3065–3073.
31. Jacobson S, Gupta A, Mattson D, et al. Immunologic studies in tropical spastic paraparesis. Ann Neurol 1990;27:149–156.
32. Usuku K, Sonoda S, Osame M, et al. HLA haplotype-linked high immune responsiveness against HTLV-I in HTLV-I-associated myelopathy: comparison with adult T-cell leukemia/lymphoma. Ann Neurol 1988;23:S143–S150.
33. Daenke S, Kermode AG, Hall SE, et al. High activated and memory cytotoxic T-cell responses to HTLV-I in healthy carriers and patients with tropical spastic paraparesis. Virology 1996;217:139–146.
34. Gallo RC. Human retroviruses: a decade of discovery and link with human disease. J Infect Dis 1991;164:235–243.
35. Gallo RC. Human retroviruses in the second decade: a personal perspective. Nature Med 1995;8:753–759.
36. Migone T-S, Lin JX, Cereseto A, et al. Constitutively activated Jak-STAT pathway in T cells transformed with HTLV-I. Science 1995;269:79–81.
37. Xu X, Heidenrich O, Nerenberg M. Role of kinases in HTLV-I transformation. J Invest Med 1996;44:113–123.
38. Robert-Guroff M, Nakao Y, Notake K, et al. Natural antibodies to human retrovirus HTLV in a cluster of Japanese patients with adult T-cell leukemia. Science 1982;215:975–978.
39. Chen YMA, Lee TH, Wiktor SZ, et al. Type-specific antigens for serological discrimination of HTLV-I and HTLV-II infection. Lancet 1990;336:1153–1155.
40. Lillehoj EP, Alexander SS, Dubrule CJ, et al. Development and evaluation of a human T-cell leukemia virus type-I serologic confirmatory assay incorporating a recombinant envelope polypeptide. J Clin Microbiol 1990;28:2653–2658.
41. Hartley TM, Malone GE, Khabbaz RF, et al. Evaluation of a recombinant human T-cell lymphotropic virus type I (HTLV-I) p21E antibody detection enzyme immunoassay as a supplementary test in HTLV-I/II antibody testing algorithms. J Clin Microbiol 1991;29: 1125–1127.
42. Lal RB, Heneine W, Rudolph DL, et al. Synthetic peptide-based immunoassays for distinguishing between human T-cell lymphotropic virus type I and II infections in seropositive individuals. J Clin Microbiol 1991;29:2253–2258.
43. Lipka JJ, Miyoshi I, Madlock KG, et al. Segregation of human T cell lymphotropic virus type I and II infections by antibody reactivity to unique viral epitopes. J Infect Dis 1992;165:268–272.
44. Roberts BD, Foung SK, Lipka JJ, et al. Evaluation of an immunoblot assay for serologic confirmation and differentiation of human T-cell lymphotropic virus types I and II. J Clin Microbiol 1993;31:260–264.
45. Kleinman SK, Kaplan JE, Khabbaz RF, et al. Evaluation of a p21e spiked Western blot (immunoblot) in confirming human T-cell lymphotropic virus type I and II infection in volunteer blood donors: the Retrovirus Epidemiology Donor Study Group. J Clin Microbiol 1994;32:602–607.
46. Lipka JJ, Santiago P, Chan L, et al. Modified Western blot assay for confirmation and differentiation of human T-cell lymphotopic virus types I and II. J Infect Dis 1991;164:400–403.
47. Licensure of screening tests for antibody to human T-lymphotropic virus type I. MMWR Morb Mortal Wkly Rep 1988;37:736–747.
48. Blomberg J, Robert-Guroff M, Blattner W, et al. Type- and group-specific continuous antigenic determinants of HTLV: use of synthetic peptides for serotyping of HTLV-I and -II infection. J Acquir Immune Defic Syndr 1992;5:294–302.
49. Horal P, Hall WW, Svennerholm B, et al. Identification of type-specific linear epitopes in the glycoproteins gp46 and gp21 of human T-cell leukemia viruses type I and type II using synthetic peptides. Proc Natl Acad Sci U S A 1991;88:5754–5758.
50. Heneine W, Khabbaz RF, Lal RB, et al. Sensitive and specific polymerase chain reaction assays for diagnosis of human T-cell lymphotropic virus type I (HTLV-I) and HTLV-II infections in HTLV-I/II-seropositive individuals. J Clin Microbiol 1992;30: 1605–1607.
51. Deffer C, Coste J, Descamps F, et al. Contribution of polymerase chain reaction and radioimmunoprecipitation assay in the confirmation of human T-lymphotropic virus infection in French blood donors. Transfusion 1995;35:596–600.

52. Saito S, Ando Y, Furuki K, et al. Detection of HTLV-I genome in seronegative infants born to HTLV-I seropositive mothers by polymerase chain reaction. Jpn J Cancer Res 1989;80:808–812.
53. Pate EJ, Wiktor SZ, Shaw GM, et al. Lack of viral latency of human T-lymphotropic virus type-I (HTLV-I). N Engl J Med 1991;325:284.
54. Rios M, Khabbaz RF, Kaplan JE, et al. Transmission of human T-cell lymphotropic virus (HTLV) type II by transfusion of HTLV-I screened blood products. J Infect Dis 1994;170:206–210.
55. Gallo D, Diggs JL, Hanson CV. Evaluation of two commercial human T-cell lmphotropic virus Western blot (immunoblot) kits with problem specimens. J Clin Microbiol 1994;32:2046–2049.
56. Garin B, Gosselin S, de Thé G, et al. HTLV-I/II infection in a high viral endemic area of Zaire, Central Africa: a comparative evaluation of serology, PCR and significance of indeterminate Western blot pattern. J Med Virol 1994;44:104–109.
57. Gessain A, Mahieux R, de Thé G. HTLV-I indeterminate Western blot patterns observed in sera from tropical regions: the situation revisited. J Acquir Immune Defic Syndr Hum Retrovirol 1995;9:316–319.
58. Miyoshi I, Yoshimoto S, Fujishita M, et al. Natural adult T-cell leukaemia virus infection in Japanese monkeys. Lancet 1982;2:658.
59. Guo H, Wong-Staal F, Gallo RC. Novel viral sequences related to human T-cell leukemia virus in T-cells of a seropositive baboon. Science 1984;223:1195–1197.
60. Kanki P, Essex M. Simian T-lymphotropic viruses and related human viruses. Vet Microbiol 1988;17:309–314.
61. Benveniste RE. The contributions of retroviruses to the study of mammalian evolution. In: MacIntyre RJ, ed. Molecular evolutionary genetics. New York: Plenum, 1985:359–417.
62. Gessain A, Gallo RC, Franchini G. Low degree of human T-cell leukemia/lymphoma virus type I genetic drift in vivo as a means of monitoring viral transmission and movement of ancient human populations. J Virol 1992;66:2285–2295.
63. Vidal AU, Gessain A, Yoshida M, et al. Phylogenetic classification of human T cell leukaemia/lymphoma virus type I genotypes in five major molecular and geographical subtypes J Gen Virol 1994;75:3655–3666.
64. Wiktor SZ, Piot P, Mann JM, et al. Human T-cell lymphotropic virus type I (HTLV-I) among female prostitutes in Kinshasa, Zaire. J Infect Dis 1990;161:1073–1077.
65. Delaporte E, Dupont A, Peeters M, et al. Epidemiology of HTLV-I in Gabon (Western Equatorial Africa). Int J Cancer 1988;42:687–689.
66. Bartholomew C, Charles W, Saxinger C, et al. Racial and other characteristics of human T cell leukemia/lymphoma (HTLV-I) and AIDS (HTLV-III) in Trinidad. Br Med J 1985;290:1243–1246.
67. Yanagihara R, Jenkins CL, Alexander SS, et al. Human T lymphotropic virus type I infection in Papua New Guinea: high prevalence among the Hagahai confirmed by Western blot analysis. J Infect Dis 1990;162:649–654.
68. Yanagihara R, Ajdukiewicz AB, Garruto RM, et al. Human T-lymphotropic virus type I infection in the Solomon Islands. Am J Trop Med Hyg 1991;44:122–130.
69. May J, Stent G, Schnagl R. Antibody to human T-cell lymphotropic virus type I in Australian aborigines. Med J Aust 1988;149:104.
70. Meytes D, Schochat B, Lee H, et al. Serological and molecular survey for HTLV-I infection in a high-risk Middle Eastern group. Lancet 1990;336:1533–1535.
71. Schulz TF, Calabro ML, Hoad JG. HTLV-I envelope sequences from Brazil, the Caribbean, and Romania: clustering of sequences according to geographic origin and variability in an antibody epitope. Virology 1991;184:483–491.
72. Cartier L, Araya F, Castillo JL, et al. Southernmost carriers of HTLV-I/II in the world. Jpn J Cancer Res 1993;84:1–3.
73. Hahn BH, Shaw GM, Popovic M, et al. Molecular cloning and analysis of a new variant of human T-cell leukemia virus (HTLV-Ib) from an African patient with adult T-cell leukemia-lymphoma. Int J Cancer 1984;34:613–618.
74. Gessain A, Yanagihara R, Franchini G, et al. Highly divergent molecular variants of human T-lymphotropic virus type I from isolated populations in Papua New Guinea and the Solomon Islands. Proc Natl Acad Sci U S A 1991;88:7694–7698.
75. Sherman MP, Saksena NK, Dube DK, et al. Evolutionary insights on the origin of human T-cell lymphoma/leukemia virus type I (HTLV-I) derived from sequence analysis of a new HTLV-I variant from Papua New Guinea. J Virol 1992;66:2556–2563.
76. Bastian I, Gardner J, Webb D, et al. Isolation of a human T-lymphotropic virus type-I strain from Australian aboriginals. J Virol 1993;67:843–851.
77. Ajdukiewicz AB, Yanagihara R, Garruto RM, et al. HTLV-I myeloneuropathy in the Solomon Islands. N Engl J Med 1989;321:615–616.
78. Song K-J, Nerurkar VR, Cortez AJP, et al. Sequence and phylogenetic analysis of human T cell lymphotropic virus type I from a Brazilian woman with adult T cell leukemia: comparison with virus strains from South America and Caribbean basin. Am J Trop Med Hyg 1995;52:101–108.
79. Yang Y-C, Hsu T-Y, Liiu M-Y, et al. Molecular subtyping of T-lymphotropic virus type I (HTLV-I) by a nested polymerase chain reaction-restriction fragment polymorphism analysis of the envelope gene: two distinct lineages of HTLV-I in Taiwan. J Med Virol 1997;51:25–31.
80. Voevodin A, Al-Mufti S, Farah S, et al. Molecular characterization of human T-lymphotropic virus type I (HTLV-I) found in Kuwait: close similarity with HTLV-I isolates originating from Mashhad, Iran. AIDS Res Hum Retroviruses 1995:1255–1259.
81. Yamashita M, Achiron A, Miura T, et al. HTLV-I from Iranian Mashhadi Jews in Israel is phylogenetically related to that of Japan, India, and South America rather than that of Africa and Melanesia. Virus Genes 1995;10:85–90.
82. Robert-Guroff M, Weiss SH, Giron JA, et al. Prevalence of antibodies to HTLV-I, -II, and -III in intravenous drug abusers from an AIDS endemic region. JAMA 1986;255:3133–3137.
83. Lee H, Swanson P, Shorty VS, et al. High rate of HTLV-II infection in seropositive IV drug abusers in New Orleans. Science 1989;244:471–475.
84. Cantor KP, Weiss SH, Goedert JJ, et al. HTLV-I/II seroprevalence and HIV/HTLV coinfection among U.S. intravenous drug users. J Acquir Immune Defic Syndr 1991;4:460–467.
85. Khabbaz RF, Hartel D, Lairmore M, et al. Human T lymphotropic virus type II (HTLV-II) infection in a cohort of New York intravenous drug users: an old infection? J Infect Dis 1991;163:252–256.
86. Calabro ML, Luparello M, Grottola A, et al. Detection of human T-lymphotropic virus type IIb in human immunodeficiency virus type I coinfected persons in southeastern Italy. J Infect Dis 1993;168:1273–1277.
87. Biggar RJ, Buskell-Bales Z, Yakshe PN, et al. Antibody to human retroviruses among drug users in three East Coast American cities, 1972–1976. J Infect Dis 1991;163:57–63.
88. Lairmore MD, Jacobson S, Gracia F, et al. Isolation of human T-cell lymphotropic virus type 2 from Guaymi Indians in Panama. Proc Natl Acad Sci U S A 1990;87:8840–8844.
89. Heneine W, Kaplan JE, Gracia F, et al. HTLV-II endemicity among Guaymi Indians in Panama. N Engl J Med 1991;324:565.
90. Reeves WC, Levine P, Cuevas M, et al. Seroepidemiology of human T-cell lymphotropic virus type-I in the Republic of Panama. Am J Trop Med Hyg 1990;42:374–379.
91. Levine PH, Jacobson S, Elliott R, et al. HTLV-II infection in Florida Indians. AIDS Res Hum Retroviruses 1993;9:123–127.
92. Hjelle B, Scalf R, Swenson S. High frequency of human T-cell leukemia-lymphoma virus type II infection in New Mexico blood donors: determination by sequence-specific oligonucleotide hybridization. Blood 1990;76:450–454.
93. Maloney EM, Biggar RJ, Neel JV, et al. Endemic human T cell lymphotropic virus type II infection among isolated Brazilian Amerindians. J Infect Dis 1992;166:100–107.

94. Ishak R, Harrington WJ, Azevedo VN, et al. Identification of human T cell lymphotropic virus type IIa infection in the Kayapo, an indigenous population of Brazil. AIDS Res Hum Retroviruses 1995; 11:813–821.
95. Eiraku N, Novoa P, Ferreira MC, et al. Identification and characterization of a new and distinct molecular subtype of human T-cell lymphotropic virus type 2. J Virol 1996;70:1481–1492.
96. Ferrer JF, Esteban E, Dube S, et al. Endemic infection with human T cell leukemia/lymphoma virus type IIB in Argentinian and Paraguayan Indians: epidemiology and molecular characterization. J Infect Dis 1996;174:944–953.
97. Ferrer JF, del Pino N, Esteban E, et al. High rate of infection with human T-cell leukemia retrovirus type II in four Indian population of Argentina. Virology 1993;1997:576–584.
98. Ijichi S, Zaninovic V, Leon FE, et al. Identification of human T cell leukemia virus type IIb infection in the Wayu, an aboriginal population of Colombia. Jpn J Cancer Res 1993;84:1215–1218.
99. Hall W, Takahashi H, Liu C, et al. Multiple isolates and characteristics of human T-cell leukemia virus type II. J Virol 1992;66:2456–2463.
100. KuboT, Zhu SW, Ijichi S, et al. Molecular characterization of human T-cell leukemia virus type II (HTLV-II). AIDS Res Hum Retroviruses 1994;10:465–471.
101. Goubau P, Desmyter J, Ghesquiere J, et al. HTLV-II among pygmies. Nature 1992;359:201.
102. Liu H-F, Goubau P, Van Brussel M, et al. The three human T-cell leukemia virus type I subtypes arose from three geographically distinct simian reservoirs. J Gen Virol 1996;77:359–368.
103. Vandamme A-M, Liu H-F, Van Brussel M, et al. The presence of a divergent T-lymphotropic virus in a wild-caught pygmy chimpanzee (Pan paniscus) support an African origin for the human T-lymphotropic/simian T-lymphotropic group of viruses. J Gen Virol 1996;77: 1089–1099.
104. Schulz TF. Origin of AIDS. Lancet 1992;339:867.
105. Blattner W. Retroviruses. In: Evans AS, ed. Viral infections of human epidemiology and control. 3rd ed. New York: Plenum, 1989:545–592.
106. Kajiyama W, Kashiwagi S, Norura H, et al. Seroepidemiologic study of antibody to adult T-cell leukemia virus in Okinawa, Japan. Am J Epidemiol 1985;123:41–47.
107. Mueller N, Tachibana N, Stuver SO, et al. Epidemiologic perspectives of HTLV-I. In: Blattner W, ed. Human retrovirology: HTLV. New York: Raven Press, 1990:281–294.
108. Hinuma Y, Komoda H, Chosa T, et al. Antibodies to adult T-cell leukemia virus-associated antigen (ATLA) in sera from patients with ATL and controls in Japan: a nation-wide sero-epidemiologic study. Int J Cancer 1982;29:631–635.
109. Clark JW, Robert-Guroff M, Ikehara O, et al. Human T-cell leukemia-lymphoma virus type 1 and adult T-cell leukemia-lymphoma in Okinawa. Cancer Res 1985;45:2849–2852.
110. Kashiwagi S, Ikematsu H, Hayashi J, et al. Seroepidemiologic study of adult T-cell leukemia virus (HTLV) and hepatitis B virus infection in Okinawa, Japan. Microbiol Immunol 1988;32:917–923.
111. Tajima K, T- and B-Cell Malignancy Study Group, et al. The 4th nation-wide study of adult T-cell leukemia/lymphoma (ATL) in Japan: estimates of risk of ATL and its geographical and clinical features. Int J Cancer 1990;45:237–243.
112. Hinuma Y. Seroepidemiology of adult T-cell leukemia virus (HTLV-I/ATLV): origin of virus carriers in Japan. AIDS Res Hum Retroviruses 1986;2(Suppl. 1):S17–S22.
113. Stuver SO, Tachibana N, Okayama A, et al. Determinants of HTLV-I seroprevalence in Miyazaki prefecture, Japan: a cross-sectional study. J Acquir Immune Defic Syndr 1992;5:12–18.
114. Tajima K, Kamura S, Ito S, et al. Epidemiological features of HTLV-I carriers and incidence of ATL in an ATL-endemic island: a report of the community-based co-operative study in Tsushima, Japan. Int J Cancer 1987;40:741–746.
115. Yamaguchi K. Human T-lymphotropic virus type I in Japan. Lancet 1994;343:213–216.
116. Zhuo J, Yang T, Zeng Y, et al. Epidemiology of anti-human T-cell leukemia virus type I antibody and characteristics of adult T-cell leukemia in China. Chin Med J (Engl) 1995;108:902–906.
117. Kazura JW, Saxinger WC, Wenger J, et al. Epidemiology of human T-cell leukemia virus type I infection in East Sepik province, Papua New Guinea. J Infect Dis 1987;155:1100–1107.
118. Currie B, Hinuma Y, Imai J, et al. HTLV-I antibodies in Papua New Guinea. Lancet 1989;2:1137.
119. Blattner W, Kalyanaraman VS, Robert-Guroff M, et al. The human type-C retrovirus, HTLV, in blacks from the Caribbean region, and relationship to adult T-cell leukemia/lymphoma. Int J Cancer 1982; 30:257–264.
120. Catovsky D, Greaves MF, Rose M, et al. Adult T-cell lymphoma-leukaemia in blacks from the West Indies. Lancet 1982;1:639–643.
121. Greaves MF, Verbi W, Tilley R, et al. Human T-cell leukemia virus in immigrants to the United Kingdom. In: Gallo RC, Essex ME, Gross L, eds. Human T-cell leukemia/lymphoma viruses. New York: Cold Spring Harbor Laboratory, 1984:297–306.
122. Dosik H, Goldstein MF, Poiesz BJ, et al. Seroprevalence of human T-cell lymphotropic virus in blacks from a selected central Brooklyn population. Cancer Invest 1994;12:289–295.
123. Cruickshank JK. HTLV-I infection in Britain. BMJ 1990;301:442.
124. Murphy EL, Figueroa JP, Gibbs WN, et al. Human T-lymphotropic virus type I (HTLV-I) seroprevalence in Jamaica. I. Demographic determinants. Am J Epidemiol 1991;133:1114–1124.
125. Blattner W, Saxinger C, Riedel D, et al. A study of HTLV-I and its associated risk factors in Trinidad and Tobago. J Acquir Immune Defic Syndr 1990;3:1102–1108.
126. Riedel DA, Evans AS, Saxinger C, et al. A historical study of human T lymphotropic virus type I transmission in Barbados. J Infect Dis 1989;159:603–609.
127. Merino F, Robert-Guroff M, Clark J, et al. Natural antibodies to human T-cell leukemia/lymphoma virus in healthy Venezuelan populations. Int J Cancer 1984;34:501–506.
128. Maloney EM, Murphy EL, Figueroa JP, et al. Human T-lymphotropic virus type I (HTLV-I) seroprevalence in Jamaica. II. Geographic and ecologic determinants. Am J Epidemiol 1991;133:1125–1134.
129. Miller GJ, Pegram SM, Kirkwood BR, et al. Ethnic composition, age and sex, together with location and standard of housing as determinants of HTLV-I infection in an urban Trinidian community. Int J Cancer 1986;38:801–808.
130. Wiktor SZ, Pate E, Murphy EL, et al. Maternal infant transmission of HTLV-I in Jamaica [abstract]. AIDS 1990;6:136.
131. Murphy EL, Figueroa JP, Gibbs WN, et al. Sexual transmission of human T-lymphotropic virus type I (HTLV-I). Ann Intern Med 1989;111:555–560.
132. Manns A, Wilks RJ, Murphy EL, et al. A prospective study of transmission by transfusion of HTLV-I and risk factors associated with seroconversion. Int J Cancer 1992;51:886–891.
133. Maloney EM, Ramirez HC, Levin A, et al. A survey of the human T-cell lymphotropic virus type I (HTLV-I) in south-western Colombia. Int J Cancer 1989;44:419–423.
134. Blank A, Yamaguchi K, Blank M, et al. Colombian patients with adult T-cell leukemia/lymphoma. Leuk Lymphoma 1993;9:407–412.
135. Lillo F, Varnier OE, Sabbatani S, et al. Detection of HTLV-I and not HTLV-II infection in Guinea Bissau (West Africa). J Acquir Immune Defic Syndr 1991;4:541–542.
136. Andrada-Serpa M, Tosswill J, Schor D, et al. Seroepidemiologic survey for antibodies to human retroviruses in human and non-human primates in Brazil. Int J Cancer 1989;44:389–393.
137. Cortes E, Detels R, Aboulafia D, et al. HIV-1, HIV-2, and HTLV-I infection in high-risk groups in Brazil. N Engl J Med 1990;320: 953–958.
138. Gabbai AA, Bordin JO, Viera-Filho JPB, et al. Selectivity of human T lymphotropic virus type I (HTLV-I) and HTLV-II infection among different population in Brazil. Am J Trop Med Hyg 1993; 49:664–671.

139. Carvalho SMF, Pombo de Oliveira MS, Thuler LCS, et al. HTLV-I and HTLV-II infections in hematologic disorder patients, cancer patients, and healthy individuals from Rio de Janeiro, Brazil. J Acquir Immune Defic Syndr Hum Retrovirol 1997;15:238–242.
140. Galvão-Castro B, Lourrres L, Rodriques LGM, et al. Distribution of human T-lymphotropic virus type I among blood donors: a nationwide Brazilian study. Transfusion 1997;37:242–243.
141. Zamora T, Zaninovic V, Kajiwara M, et al. Antibody to HTLV-I in indigenous inhabitants of the Andes and Amazon regions in Colombia. Jpn J Cancer Res 1990;81:715–71.
142. Williams AE, Fang CT, Slamon DJ, et al. Seroprevalence and epidemiological correlates of HTLV-I infection in US blood donors. Science 1988;240:643–646.
143. Lee HH, Swanson P, Rosenblatt JD, et al. Relative prevalence and risk factors of HTLV-I and HTLV-II infection in US blood donors. Lancet 1991;337:1435–1439.
144. Blattner W, Nomura A, Clark JW, et al. Modes of transmission and evidence for viral latency from studies of HTLV-I in Japanese migrant populations in Hawaii. Proc Natl Acad Sci U S A 1986;83:4895–4898.
145. Ho GY, Nomura A, Nelson K, et al. Declining seroprevalence and transmission of HTLV-I in Japanese families who immigrated to Hawaii. Am J Epidemiol 1991;134:981–987.
146. Verdier M, Denis F, Sangare A, et al. Prevalence of antibody to human T cell leukemia virus type I (HTLV-I) in populations of Ivory Coast, West Africa. J Infect Dis 1989;160:363–370.
147. Madeleine MM, Wiktor SZ, Goedert JJ, et al. HTLV-I and HTLV-II worldwide distribution: reanalysis of 4,832 immunoblot results. Int J Cancer 1993;54:255–260.
148. Kayembe K, Goubau P, Desmyter J, et al. A cluster of HTLV-I associated tropical spastic paraparesis in Equateur (Zaire): ethnic and familial distribution. J Neurol Neurosurg Psychiatry 1990;53:4–10.
149. Soriano V, Gutierrez M, Vallejo A, et al. HTLV-I associated illnesses in Spain. Vox Sang 1995;69:261–262.
150. Kitze B, Turner RW, Burchardt M, et al. Differential diagnosis of HTLV-I associated myelopathy and multiple sclerosis in Iranian patients. Clin Invest 1992;70:1013–1018.
151. Achiron A, Pinhas-Hauriel O, Doll L, et al. Spastic paraparesis associated with human T-lymphotropic virus type I: a clinical, serological and genomic study in Iranian born Mashad Jews. Ann Neurol 1993;34:670–675.
152. Richardson JH, Newell AL, Newman PK, et al. HTLV-I and neurological disease in south India. Lancet 1989;1:1079–1080.
153. Zella D, Mori L, Sala M. HTLV-II infection in Italian drug abusers. Lancet 1990;336:575–576.
154. Roman GC, Spencer PS, Schoenberg BS, et al. Tropical spastic paraparesis in the Seychelles Islands: a clinical and case-control neuroepidemiologic study. Neurology 1987;37:1323–1328.
155. Lavanchy D, Bovet P, Hollanda J, et al. High seroprevalence of HTLV-I in the Seychelles. Lancet 1991;337:248–249.
156. Lee HH, Weiss SH, Brown LS, et al. Patterns of HIV-1 and HTLV-I/II in intravenous drug abusers from the Middle Atlantic and Central regions of the USA. J Infect Dis 1990;162:347–352.
157. Davidson M, Kaplan JE, Hartley TM, et al. Prevalence of HTLV-I in Alaska natives. J Infect Dis 1990;161:359–360.
158. Vitek CR, Gracia FJ, Giusti R, et al. Evidence for sexual and mother-to-child transmission of human T-lymphotropic virus type II among Guaymi Indians, Panama. J Infect Dis 1995;171:1022–1026.
159. Gessain A, Mauclere P, Froment A, et al. Isolation and characterization of a human T-cell lymphotropic virus type II (HTLV-II), subtype B from a healthy pygmy living in a remote area of Cameroon: an ancient origin for HTLV-II in Africa. Proc Natl Acad Sci U S A 1992;92:4041–4045.
160. Gessain A, de Thé G. What is the situation of human T cell lymphotropic virus type II (HTLV-II) in Africa? Origin and dissemination of genomic subtypes. J Acq Immune Def Syn Hum Retrovir 1996;13(Suppl 1):S228–S235.
161. Tuppin P, Gessain A, Kazanji M, et al. Evidence in Gabon for an intrafamilial clustering with mother-to-child and sexual transmission of a new molecular variant of human T-lymphotropic virus type-II subtype B. J Med Virol 1996;48:22–32.
162. Andersson S, Dias F, Mendez PJ, et al. HTLV-I and -II infections in a nationwide survey of pregnant women in Guinea-Bissau, West Africa. J Acquir Immune Defic Syndr Hum Retrovirol 1997;15:320–322.
163. Goubau P, Liu HF, De Lange GG, et al. HTLV-II seroprevalence in pygmies across Africa since 1970. AIDS Res Hum Retroviruses 1993;9:709–713.
164. Takezaki T, Tajima K, Komoda H, et al. Incidence of human T-lymphotropic virus type I seroconversion after age 40 among Japanese residents in an area where the virus is endemic. J Infect Dis 1995;171:559–565.
165. Morofuji-Hirata M, Kajiyama W, Nakashima K, et al. Prevalence of antibody to human T-cell lymphotropic virus type I in Okinawa, Japan, after an interval of 9 years. Am J Epidemiol 1993;137:43–48.
166. Nakashima M, Itagaki A, Yamada O, et al. Evidence against a seronegative HTLV-I carrier rate among children. AIDS Res Hum Retroviruses 1990;6:1057–1058.
167. Korber B, Okayama A, Donnelly R, et al. Polymerase chain reaction analysis of defective human T-cell leukemia virus type I proviral genomes in leukemic cells of patients with adult T-cell leukemia. J Virol 1991;65:5471–5476.
168. Kajiyama W, Kashiwagi S, Ikematsu H, et al. Intrafamilial transmission of adult T cell leukemia virus. J Infect Dis 1986;154:851–857.
169. Hall WW, Liu CR, Scheenwind O, et al. Deleted HTLV-I provirus in blood and cutaneous lesions of patients with mycosis fungoides. Science 1991;253:317–320.
170. Ueda K, Kusuhara K, Tokugawa K, et al. Cohort effect on HTLV-I seroprevalence in southern Japan. Lancet 1989;2:979.
171. Proletti F, Vlahov D, Alexander S, et al. Correlates of HTLV-II/HIV-1 seroprevalence and incidence of HTLV-II infection among intravenous drug users [abstract C310]. In: 8th International Conference on AIDS, Amsterdam, 1992.
172. Hino S, Yamaguchi K, Katamine S, et al. Mother-to-child transmission of human T-cell leukemia virus type-I. Jpn J Cancer Res 1985;76:474–480.
173. Kinoshita K, Yamanouchi K, Ikeda S, et al. Oral infection of a common marmoset with human T-cell leukemia virus type-I (HTLV-I) by inoculating fresh human milk of HTLV-I carrier mothers. Jpn J Cancer Res 1985;76:1147–1153.
174. Hino S, Kubota K, Doi H, et al. Preliminary follow-up of survey of children born to HTLV-I carrier mothers who refrained from breast feeding [abstract]. Proc Annu Meet Jpn Cancer Assoc 1990;49:118.
175. Kinoshita K, Amagasaki T, Hino S, et al. Milk-borne transmission of HTLV-I from carrier mothers to their children. Jpn J Cancer Res 1987;78:674–680.
176. Kinoshita K, Hino S, Amagasaki T, et al. Demonstration of adult T-cell leukemia virus antigen in milk from three sero-positive mothers. Gann 1984;75:103–105.
177. Goedert JJ, Mendez H, Drummond JE, et al. Mother-to-infant transmission of human immunodeficiency virus type 1: association with prematurity or low anti-gp120. Lancet 1989;2:1351–1354.
178. Cohen ND, Munoz A, Reitz BA, et al. Transmission of retroviruses by transfusion of screened blood in patients undergoing cardiac surgery. N Engl J Med 1989;320:1172–1176.
179. Hino S, Doi H, Yoshikuni H, et al. HTLV-I carrier mothers with high-titer antibody are at risk as a source of infection. Jpn J Cancer Res 1987;78:1156–1158.
180. Hino S, Katamine S, Miyamoto T, et al. Association between maternal antibodies to the external envelope glycoprotein and vertical transmission of HTLV-I: maternal anti-env antibodies correlate with protection in non–breast-fed children. J Clin Invest, 1995;95:2920–2925.
181. Wiktor SZ, Pate EJ, Murphy EL, et al. Mother-to-child transmission of human T-cell lymphocytic virus type I (HTLV-I) in Jamaica: association with antibodies to envelope glycoprotein (gp46) epitopes. J Acquir Immune Defic Syndr 1993;6:1162–1167.

182. Wiktor SZ, Pate EJ, Rosenberg PS, et al. Mother-to-child transmission of human T lymphotropic virus type I associated with prolonged breast-feeding. J Hum Virol 1977;1:37–44.
183. Yoshinaga M, Yashiki S, Oki T, et al. A maternal risk factor for mother-to-child HTLV-I transmission: viral antigen-producing capacities in culture of peripheral blood and breast milk cells. Jpn J Cancer Res 1995;86: 649–654.
184. Sugiyama H, Doi H, Yamaguchi K, et al. Significance of postnatal mother-to-child transmission of human T-lymphotropic virus type-I on the development of adult T-cell leukemia/lymphoma. J Med Virol 1986;20:253–260.
185. Murphy EL. The epidemiology of HTLV-I: modes of transmission and their relation to patterns of seroprevalence. In: Blattner W, ed. Human retrovirology: HTLV. New York: Raven Press, 1990: 295–306.
186. Black F, Biggar RJ, Maloney E, et al. Endemic transmission of HTLV type II among Kayapo Indians of Brazil. AIDS Res Hum Retroviruses 1994;10:1165–1171.
187. Wilks R, Hanchard B, Morgan O, et al. Patterns of HTLV-I infection among family members of patients with adult T-cell leukemia/lymphoma and HTLV-I associated myelopathy/tropical spastic paraparesis [letter]. Int J Cancer 1996;65:272–273.
188. Nyambi PN, Ville Y, Louwagie J, et al. Mother-to-child transmission of human T-cell lymphotropic virus type I and II (HTLV-I/II) in Gabon: a prospective follow-up of 4 years. J Acquir Immune Defic Syndr Hum Retrovirol 1996;12:187–192.
189. Heneine W, Woods T, Greene D, et al. Detection of human T-lymphotropic virus type II in breast milk of HTLV-II infected mothers by using the polymerase chain reaction [abstract]. Lancet 1992;340:1157–1158.
190. Sullivan MT, Williams CT, Fang EP, et al. Human T-lymphotropic virus (HTLV) types I and II infection in sexual contacts and family members of blood donors who are seropositive for HTLV) types I or II. Transfusion 1993;33:585–590.
191. Bulterys M, Landesman S, Burns DN, et al. Sexual behavior and injection drug use during pregnancy and vertical transmission of HIV-1. J Acquir Immune Defic Syndr Hum Retrovirol 1997;15:76–82.
192. Bartholomew C, Saxinger WC, Clark JW, et al. Transmission of HTLV-I and HIV among homosexual men in Trinidad. JAMA 1987;257:2604–2608.
193. Figueroa JP, Ward E, Morris J, et al. Incidence of HIV and HTLV-I infection among sexually transmitted disease clinic attendees in Jamaica. J Acquir Immune Defic Syndr Hum Retrovirol 1997;15: 232–237.
194. Kleinman S, Fitzpatrick L, Lee H. Transmission of HTLV-I/II from blood donors to their sexual partners [abstract]. In: Program and Abstracts, International Society of Blood Transfusion/American Association of Blood Banks, Joint Congress Meetings, Los Angeles, 1990.
195. Simonsen JN, Plummer FA, Ngugi EN, et al. HIV infection among lower socioeconomic strata prostitutes in Nairobi. AIDS 1990;4: 139–144.
196. Brodine SK, Oldfield EC, III, Corwin AL, et al. HTLV-I among US marines stationed in a hyperendemic area: evidence for female-to-male sexual transmission. J Acquir Immune Defic Syndr 1992;5:158–162.
197. Tachibana N, Okayama A, Ishihara S, et al. High HTLV-I proviral DNA level associated with abnormal lymphocytes in peripheral blood from asymptomatic carriers. Int J Cancer 1992;51:593–595.
198. Chen YMA, Okayama A, Lee TH, et al. Sexual transmission of human T-cell leukemia virus type I associated with the presence of anti-tax antibody. Ann Intern Med 1991;88:1182–1186.
199. Khabbaz RF, Onorato IM, Cannon RO, et al. Seroprevalence of HTLV-I and HTLV-II among intravenous drug users and persons in clinics for sexually transmitted diseases. N Engl J Med 1992; 326:375–380.
200. Kaplan JE, Khabbaz Rf, Murphy EL, et al. Male-to-female transmission of HTLV-I and II: association with viral load. J Acquir Immune Defic Syndr Hum Retrovirol 1996;12:193–201.
201. Hjelle B, Cyrus S, Swenson SG. Evidence for sexual transmission of human T lymphotropic virus type II. Ann Intern Med 1992;116: 90–91.
202. Okochi K, Sato H, Hinuma Y. A retrospective study on transmission of adult T cell leukemia virus by blood transfusion: seroconversion in recipients. Vox Sang 1984;46:245–253.
203. Kleinman S, Swanson P, Allain JP, et al. Transfusion transmission of human T-lymphotropic virus types I and II: serologic and polymerase chain reaction results in recipients identified through look-back investigations. Transfusion 1993;31:14–18.
204. Sullivan MT, Williams AE, Fang CT, et al. Transmission of human T-lymphotropic virus types I and II by blood transfusion. Arch Intern Med 1991;151:2043–2048.
205. Vlahov D, Khabbaz R, Cohn, et al. Risk factors for HTLV-II seroconversion among injecting drug users in Baltimore. AIDS Res Hum Retroviruses 1994;10:448–454.
206. Donegan E. Comparison of HTLV-I/II with HIV-1 transmission by component type and shelf storage before administration [abstract]. Transfusion 1989;29:38S.
207. Gout O, Baulac M, Gessain A, et al. Rapid development of myelopathy after HTLV-I infection acquired by transfusion during cardiac transplantation. N Engl J Med 1990;322:383–388.
208. Kamihira, Nakasima S, Oyakawa Y, et al. Transmission of human T-cell lymphotropic virus type I by blood transfusion before and after mass screening of sera from seropositive donors. Vox Sang 1987;52:43–44.
209. Donegan E, Busch MP, Galleshaw JA, et al. Transfusion of blood components from a donor with human T-lymphotropic virus type II (HTLV-II) infection. Ann Intern Med 1990;113:555–556.
210. Wiktor SZ, Jacobson S, Weiss SH, et al. Spontaneous lymphocyte proliferation in HTLV-II infection. Lancet 1991;337:327–328.
211. Murphy EL, Calisher CH, Figueroa JP, et al. HTLV-I infection and arthropod vectors. N Engl J Med 1989;320:1146–1140.
212. Kramer A, Blattner W. The HTLV-I model and chronic demyelinating neurologic diseases. In: Notkins AL, Oldstone MBA, eds. Concepts in viral pathogenesis. New York: Springer-Verlag, 1989:204–214.
213. Takatsuki K, Uchiyama T, Sagawa K, et al. Adult T cell leukemia in Japan [abstract]. In: Seno S, Takaku F, Irino S, eds. Topics in hematology. No. 1825. Amsterdam: Excerpta Medica, 1976:73–78.
214. Uchiyama T, Yodoi J, Sagawa K, et al. Adult T-cell leukemia: clinical and hematologic features of 16 cases. Blood 1977;50:481–492.
215. Tajima K, Kuroishi T. Estimation of rate of incidence of ATL among ATLV (HTLV-I) carriers in Kyushu, Japan. Jpn J Clin Oncol 1985; 15:423–430.
216. Murphy EL, Hanchard B, Figueroa JP, et al. Modelling the risk of adult T-cell leukemia/lymphoma in persons infected with human T-lymphotropic virus type I. Int J Cancer 1989;43:250–252.
217. Levine PH, Manns A, Jaffe ES, et al. The effect of ethnic differences on the pattern of HTLV-I associated T-cell leukemia/lymphoma (HATL) in the United States. Int J Cancer 1994;56:177–181.
218. Pombo de Oliveira MS, Matutes E, Schulz T, et al. T-cell malignancies in Brazil. clinico-pathological and molecular studies of HTLV-I positive and negative cases. Int J Cancer 1995;60:823–827.
219. Cabrera ME, Labra S, Catovsky D, et al. HTLV-I positive adult T-cell leukemia/lymphoma (ATLL) in Chile. Leukemia, 1994;8: 1763–1767.
220. Gerard Y, Lepere J-F, Pradinaud R, et al. Clustering and clinical diversity of adult T-cell leukemia/lymphoma associated with HTLV-I in a remote black population of French Guiana. Int J Cancer 1995;60:773–776.
221. Delaporte E, Peeters M, Martin-Prevel Y, et al. Non–Hodgkin lymphoma in Gabon and its relation to HTLV-I. Int J Cancer 1993;53:48–50.
222. Veelken H, Kohler G, Schneider J, et al. HTLV-I associated adult T-cell leukemia/lymphoma in two patients from Bucarest, Romania. Leukemia 1996;10:1366–1369.
223. Sidi Y, Meytes D, Shohat B, et al. Adult T-cell lymphoma in Israeli patients of Iranian origin. Cancer 1990;65:590–593.

224. Gibbs WN, Lofters WS, Campbell M, et al. Non-Hodgkin's lymphoma in Jamaica and its relation to adult T-cell/lymphoma. Ann Intern Med 1987;106:361–368.
225. Takatsuki K, Matsuoka M, Yamaguchi K. Adult T-cell leukemia/lymphoma in Japan. J Acquir Immune Defic Syndr Hum Retrovirol 1996;13(Suppl 1):S15–S19.
226. Hanchard B. Adult T-cell leukemia/lymphoma in Jamaica: 1986–1995. J Acquir Immune Defic Syndr Hum Retrovirol 1996;13(Suppl 1):S20–S25.
227. Manns A, Cleghorn FR, Falk RT, et al. Role of HTLV-I in development of non–Hodgkin lymphoma in Jamaica and Trinidad and Tobago. Lancet 1993;342:1448–1450.
228. Cleghorn F, Manns A, Falk R, et al. Effect of human T-lymphotropic virus type I infection on non–Hodgkin's lymphoma incidence. J Natl Cancer Inst 1995;87:1009–1014.
229. Ikai K, Uchiyama T, Maeda M, et al. Sézary-like syndrome in a 10-year old girl with serologic evidence of human T-cell lymphotropic virus type I infection. Arch Dermatol 1987;123:1351–1355.
230. Pombo de Oliveira MS, Matutes E, Famadas LC, et al. Adult T-cell leukaemia/lymphoma in Brazil and its relation to HTLV-I. Lancet 1990;336:987–990.
231. Kawano F, Tsuda H, Yamaguchi K, et al. Unusual clinical courses of adult T-cell leukemia in siblings. Cancer 1984;54:131–134.
232. Blayney DW, Blattner W, Robert Guroff M, et al. The human T cell leukemia/lymphoma virus (HTLV) in the southeastern United States. JAMA 1983;250:1048–1052.
233. Jaffe ES, Blattner W, Blayney DW, et al. The pathologic spectrum of HTLV-associated leukemia/lymphoma in the United States. Am J Surg Pathol 1984;8:263–275.
234. Broder S, Bunn PA, Jaffe ES, et al. T-cell lymphoproliferative syndrome associated with human T-cell leukemia/lymphoma virus. Ann Intern Med 1984;100:543–557.
235. Kawano F, Yamaguchi K, Nishimura H, et al. Variation in the clinical courses of adult T-cell leukemia. Cancer 1985;55:851–856.
236. Shimoyama M. Diagnostic criteria and classification of clinical subtypes of adult T-cell leukemia lymphoma: a report from the Lymphoma Study Group (1984–78). Br J Haematol 1991;79:428–437.
237. Catovsky D, Matutes E. Leukemias of mature T cells. In: Knowles DH, ed. Neoplastic hematopathology. Baltimore: Williams & Wilkins, 1992:1267–1279.
238. Pawson R, Schulz TF, Matutes E, et al. The human T-cell lymphotropic viruses types I/II are not involved in T-prolymphocytic leukemia and large granular lymphocytic leukemia. Leukemia 1997;11:1305–1311.
239. Yamaguchi K, Kiyokawa T, Futami G, et al. Pathogenesis of adult T-cell leukemia from clinical pathologic features. In: Blattner W, ed. Human retrovirology: HTLV. New York: Raven Press, 1990:163–171.
240. Yamaguchi K, Seiki M, Yoshida M, et al. The detection of human T cell leukemia virus proviral DNA and its application for classification and diagnosis of T cell malignancy. Blood 1984;63:1235–1240.
241. Yamaguchi K, Matsuoka M, Takemoto S, et al. DNA diagnosis of HTLV-I. Intervirology 1996;39:158–164.
242. Furukawa Y, Fujisawa J, Osame M, et al. Frequent clonal proliferation of human T-cell leukemia virus type I (HTLV-I)–infected T cells in HTLV-I–associated myelopathy (HAM-TSP). Blood 1992;80:1012–1016.
243. Kubota T, Ikezoe T, Hakoda E, et al. HTLV-I seronegative, genoma-positive adult T-cell leukemia: report of a case. Am J Hematol 1996;53:133–136.
244. Kaplan MH, Hall WW, Susin M, et al. Syndrome of severe skin disease, eosinophilia and dermatopathic lymphadenopathy in patients with HTLV-II complicating human immunodeficiency virus infection. Am J Med 1991;91:300–309.
245. Vahlne A. Deleted HTLV-I provirus in blood and cutaneous lesions of patients with mycosis fungoides. Science 1991;253:317–320.
246. Zucker-Franklin D, Hooper WC, Evatt BL. Human lymphotropic retroviruses associated with mycosis fungoides: evidence that human T-cell lymphotropic virus type II (HTLV-II) as well as HTLV-I may play a role in the disease. Blood 1992;80:1537–1545.
247. van der Loo EM, van Muijen GNP, van Vloten WA, et al. C type virus-like particles specifically localized in Langerhans' cells and related cells of skin and lymph nodes of patients with mycosis fungoides and Sézary's syndrome. Virchows Arch B Cell Pathol 1979;31:193–203.
248. Bazarbachi A, Saal F. Laroche L, et al. HTLV-1–like particles and HTLV-1–related DNA sequences in an unambiguous case of Sézary syndrome. Leukemia 1994;8:201–207.
249. Kramer A, Jacobson S, Reuben JS, et al. Spontaneous lymphocyte proliferation is elevated in asymptomatic HTLV-I–positive Jamaicans. In: Blattner W, ed. Human retrovirology: HTLV. New York: Raven Press, 1990:79–85.
250. Jacobson S, Shida H, McFarlin DE, et al. Circulating CD8+ cytotoxic T lymphocytes specific for HTLV-I pX in patients with HTLV-I–associated neurological disease. Nature 1990;348:245–248.
251. Greenberg SJ, Tendler CL, Manns A, et al. Altered cellular expression in human retroviral-associated leukemogenesis. In: Blattner W, ed. Human retrovirology: HLTV. New York: Raven Press, 1990:87–104.
252. Sakashita A, Hattori T, Miller C, et al. Mutations of the p53 gene in adult T-cell leukemia. Blood 1992;79:477–480.
253. Yamato K, Oka T, Hiroi M, et al. Aberrant expression of the p53 tumor suppressor gene in adult T-cell leukemia and HTLV-I–infected cells. Jpn J Cancer Res 1993;84:4–8.
254. Reid R, Lindholm P, Mireskandari A, et al. Stabilization of wild-type p53 in human T-lymphocytes transformed by HTLV-I. Oncogene 1993;8:3029–3036.
255. Nagai H, Kinoshita T, Imamura J, et al. Genetic alteration of p53 in some patients with adult T-cell leukemia. Jpn J Cancer Res 1991;82:1421–1427.
256. Cereseto A, Diella F, Mulloy JC, et al. p53 functional impairment and high p21$^{waf1/cip1}$ expression in human T-cell lymphotropic/leukemia virus type I–transformed T cells. Blood 1996;88:1551–1560.
257. Hatta Y, Yamada Y, Tomonaga M, et al. Extensive analysis of the retinoblastoma gene in adult T cell leukemia/lymphoma (ATL). Leukemia 1997;11:984–989.
258. Shimamoto Y, Kobayashi M, Miyamoto Y. Clinical implication of the integration patterns of human T-cell lymphotropic virus type I proviral DNA in adult T-cell leukemia/lymphoma. Leuk Lymphoma 1996;20:207–215.
259. Yamada Y, Hatta Y, Murata K, et al. Deletions of p15 and/or p16 genes as a poor-prognosis factor in adult T-cell leukemia. J Clin Oncol 1997;15:1778–1785.
260. Weiss RA, Schulz TF. Transforming properties of the HTLV-I tax gene. Cancer Cells 1990;2:281–283.
261. Tendler CL, Greenberg SJ, Burton JD, et al. Cytokine induction in HTLV-I associated myelopathy and adult T-cell leukemia: alternate molecular mechanisms underlying retroviral pathogenesis. J Cell Biochem 1991;46:302–311.
262. Yamada Y, Ohmoto Y, Hata T, et al. Features of the cytokines secreted by adult T cell leukemia (ATL) cells. Leuk Lymphoma 1996;21:443–447.
263. Mori N, Gill PS, Mougdil T, et al. Interleukin-10 gene expression in adult T-cell leukemia. Blood 1996;88:1035–1045.
264. Fujita K, Yamasaki Y, Sawada H, et al. Cytogenetic studies on the adult T-cell leukemia in Japan. Leuk Res 1989;13:535–543.
265. Kamada N, Sakurai M, Miyamoto K, et al. Chromosome abnormalities in adult T-cell leukemia/lymphoma: a karyotype review committee report. Cancer Res 1992;52:1481–1493.
266. Mann DL, Desantis P, Mark G, et al. HTLV-I-associated B-cell CLL: indirect role for retrovirus in leukemogenesis. Science 1987;236:1103–1106.
267. Asou N, Kumagai T, Uekihara S, et al. HTLV-I seroprevalence in patients with malignancy. Cancer 1986;58:903–907.
268. Matsuzaki H, Asou N, Kawaguchi Y, et al. Human T-cell leukemia virus type I associated with small cell lung cancer. Cancer 1990;66:1763–1768.

269. Strickler HD, Rattray C, Escoffery C, et al. Human T-cell lymphotropic virus type I and severe neoplasia of the cervix in Jamaica. Int J Cancer 1995;61:23–26.
270. Gessain A, Barin F, Vernant JC, et al. Antibodies to human T-lymphotropic virus type-I in patients with tropical spastic paraparesis. Lancet 1985;2:407–410.
271. Gessain A, Caudie C, Gout O, et al. Intrathecal synthesis of antibodies to human T lymphotropic virus type I and the presence of IgG oligoclonal bands in the cerebrospinal fluid of patients with endemic tropical spastic paraparesis. J Infect Dis 1988;157:1226–1234.
272. Osame M, Matsumoto M, Usuku K, et al. Chronic progressive myelopathy associated with elevated antibodies to human T-lymphotropic virus type I and adult T-cell leukemia like cells. Ann Neurol 1987;21:117–122.
273. Ijichi S, Osame M. Human T lymphotropic virus type I (HTLV-I) associated myelopathy/tropical spastic paraparesis (HAM/TSP): recent perspectives. Intern Med 1995;34:713–721.
274. Osame M, Igata A, Matsumoto M, et al. HTLV-I associated myelopathy (HAM): treatment trials, retrospective survey and clinical and laboratory findings. Hematol Rev 1990;3:271–274.
275. Ehrlich GD, Glaser JB, Bryz-Gornia V, et al. Multiple sclerosis, retroviruses, and PCR: the HTLV-MS Working Group. Neurology 1991;41:335–343.
276. Osame M, Izumo S, Igata A, et al. Blood transfusion and HTLV-I associated myelopathy. Lancet 1986;2:104–105.
277. McFarlin DE, Blattner W. Non-AIDS retroviral infections in humans. Annu Rev Med 1991;42:97–105.
278. Osame M, Janssen R, Kubota H, et al. Nationwide survey of HTLV-I associated myelopathy in Japan: association with blood transfusion. Ann Neurol 1990:28:50–56.
279. Kaplan JE, Osame M, Kubota H, et al. The risk of development of HTLV-I-associated myelopathy/tropical spastic paraparesis among persons infected with HTLV-I. J Acquir Immune Defic Syndr 1990; 3:1096–1101.
280. Matutes E, Schulz T, Serpa MJA, et al. Report of the Second International Symposium on HTLV-I in Brazil. Leukemia 1994;8:1092–1094.
281. Jacobson S, Zaninovic V, Mora C, et al. Immunological findings in neurological diseases associated with antibodies to HTLV-I: activated lymphocytes in tropical spastic paraparesis. Ann Neurol 1988;23(Suppl):S196–S200.
282. Gessain A, Saal F, Giron ML, et al. Cell surface phenotype and human T lymphotropic virus type I antigen expression in 12 T cell lines derived from peripheral blood and cerebrospinal fluid of West Indian, Guyanese and African patients with tropical spastic paraparesis. J Gen Virol 1990;71:333–341.
283. Nowak AM, Bangham CRM. Population dynamics of immune responses to persistent viruses. Science 1996;272:74–79.
284. Bangham CRM, Kermode AG, Hall SE, et al. The cytotoxic T-lymphocytes response to HTLV-I: the main determinant of disease? Semin Virol 1996;7:41–48.
285. Hollsberg P, Hafler DA. Pathogenesis of diseases induced by human lymphotropic virus type 1 infection. Beth Israel 1993;328:1173–1182.
286. Jacobson S, McFarlin DE, Koenig S. Demonstration of HTLV-I specific CTL in the CSF of patients with HAM/TSP [abstract]. Nature 1990;245.
287. Morgan OS, Rodgers-Johnson P, Mora C, et al. HTLV-I and polymyositis in Jamaica. Lancet 1989;1184–1187.
288. Nishioka K, Maruyama I, Sato K, et al. Chronic inflammatory arthropathy associated with HTLV-I. Lancet 1989;1:441.
289. Mochizuki M, Watanabe T, Yamaguchi K, et al. HTLV-I uveitis: a distinct clinical entity caused by HTLV-I. Jpn J Cancer Res 1992;83:236–239.
290. Ohba N, Matsumoto M, Sameshima Y, et al. Ocular manifestations in patients with human T-lymphotropic virus type I. Jpn J Ophthalmol 1989;33:1–12.
291. Mochizuki M, Tajima K, Watanabe T, et al. Human T lymphotropic virus type-I uveitis. Br J Ophthalmol 1994;78:149–154.
292. Sagawa K, Mochizuki M, Masuoka K, et al. Immunopathological mechanisms of human T lymphotropic virus type I (HTLV-I) uveitis: detection of HTLV-I infected T cells in the eye and their constitutive cytokine production. J Clin Invest 1995;95:852–858.
293. Sugimoto M, Nakashima H, Kawano O, et al. Bronchoalveolar T-lymphocytosis in HTLV-I-associated myelopathy. Chest 1989;95:708.
294. Mita S, Sugimoto M, Nakamura M, et al. Increased human T lymphotropic virus type I (HTLV-I) proviral DNA in peripheral blood mononuclear cells and bronchoalveolar lavage cells from Japanese patients with HTLV-I–associated myelopathy. Am J Trop Med Hyg 1993;48:170–177.
295. Miyoshi I, Kobayashi M, Yoshimoto S, et al. ATLV in Japanese patient with AIDS [letter]. Lancet 1983;2:275.
296. Robinson RD, Lindo JF, Neva FA, et al. Immunoepidemiologic studies of *Strongyloides stercoralis* and human T lymphotropic virus type I infections in Jamaica. J Infect Dis 1994;169: 692–696.
297. Nakada K, Kohakura M, Komoda H, et al. High incidence of HTLV antibody in carriers of *Strongyloides stercoralis* [letter]. Lancet 1984;1:633.
298. Nakada K, Yamaguchi K, Furugen S, et al. Myoclonal integration of HTLV-I proviral DNA in patients with strongyloidiasis. Int J Cancer 1987;40:145–148.
299. Tachibana N, Okayama A, Ishizaki J, et al. Suppression of tuberculin skin reaction in healthy HTLV-I carriers from Japan. Int J Cancer 1988;42:829–831.
300. Ho GYF, Nelson K, Nomura AMY, et al. Markers of health status in an HTLV-I-positive cohort. Am J Epidemiol 1992;136:1349–1357.
301. LaGrenade L, Hanchard B, Fletcher V, et al. Infective dermatitis of Jamaican children: a marker for HTLV-I infection. Lancet 1990;336:1345–1347.
302. Tsukasaki K, Yamada Y, Ikeda S, et al. Infective dermatitis among patients with ATL in Japan. Int J Cancer 1994;57:293.
303. Hanchard B, LaGrenade L, Canberry C, et al. Childhood infective dermatitis evolving into adult T-cell leukaemia after 17 years [letter]. Lancet 1991;338:1593–1594.
304. Bartholomew C, Blattner W, Cleghorn F. Progression to AIDS in homosexual men co-infected with HIV and HTLV-I in Trinidad [letter]. Lancet 1987;2:1469.
305. Zack JA, Cann AJ, Lugo JP, et al. HIV-I production from infected peripheral blood T-cells after HTLV-I induced mitogenic stimulation. Science 1988;240:1026–1029.
306. Kobayashi M, Yoshimoto S, Fujishita M, et al. HTLV-positive T-cell lymphoma/leukaemia in an AIDS patient [letter]. Lancet 1984;1:1361–1362.
307. Schechter M, Lee HH, Halsey NA, et al. Coinfection with human T-cell lymphotropic virus type I and HIV in Brazil: impact on markers of HIV disease progression. JAMA, 1994;271:353–357.
308. Rosenblatt JD, Golde DW, Wachsman W, et al. A second isolate of HTLV-II associated with atypical hairy cell leukemia. N Engl J Med 1986;315:372–377.
309. Rosenblatt JD, Gasson JC, Glaspy J, et al. Relationship between human T-cell leukemia virus-II and atypical hairy cell leukemia: serologic study of hairy cell leukemia patients. Leukemia 1987;1397–401.
310. Fouchard N, Flageul B, Bagot M, et al. Lack of evidence of HTLV-I/II infection in T-CD8 malignant or reactive lymphoproliferative disorders in France: a serological and/or molecular study of 169 cases. Leukemia, 1995;9:2087–2092.
311. Loughran TP, Sherman MP, Ruscetti FW, et al. Prototypical HTLV-I/II infection is rare in patients with large granular lymphocyte leukemia. Leukemia Res 1994;18:423–429.
312. Loughran TP, Coyle T, Sherman MP, et al. Detection of human T-cell leukemia/lymphoma virus, type II, in patient with large granular lymphocyte leukemia. Blood 1992;80:1116–1119.
313. Hjelle B, Mills R, Swenson S, et al. Incidence of hairy cell leukemia, mycosis fungoides, and chronic lymphocytic leukemia in a first known HTLV-II-endemic population. J Infect Dis 1991;163:435–440.

314. Hjelle B, Appenzeller O, Mills R, et al. Chronic neurodegenerative disease associated with HTLV-II infection. Lancet 1992;339:645–646.
315. Jacobson S, Lehky T, Nishimura M, et al. Isolation of HTLV-II from a patient with chronic, progressive neurological disease clinically indistinguishable from HTLV-I–associated myelopathy/tropical spastic paraparesis. Am Neurol Assoc 1993;14:392–396.
316. Bunn PA, Schechter GP, Jaffe E, et al. Clinical course of retrovirus-associated adult T-cell lymphoma in the United States. N Engl J Med 1983;309:257–264.
317. Shimoyama M, Ota K, Kikuchi M, et al. Major prognostic factors of adult patients with advanced T-cell lymphoma/leukemia. J Clin Oncol 1988;6:1088–1093.
318. Tsukasaki K, Ikeda S, Murata K, et al. Characteristics of chemotherapy induced clinical remission in long survivors with aggressive adult T-cell leukemia/lymphoma. Leuk Res 1993;17:157–163.
319. Taguchi H. An intensive chemotherapy of adult T-cell leukemia/lymphoma. Rinsho Ketsueki 1996;37:654–660.
320. Taguchi H, Kinoshita KC, Takatsuki K, et al. An intensive chemotherapy of adult T-cell leukemia/lymphoma: CHOP followed by etoposide, vincristine, ranimustine and mitoxantrone with granulocyte colony-stimulating factor support. J Acquir Immune Defic Syndr Hum Retrovirol 1996;12:182–186.
321. Ohno R, Masaoka T, Shirakawa S, et al. Treatment of adult T-cell leukemia/lymphoma with a new oral anti-tumor drug and a derivative of bis(2,6 dioxopiperazine). Cancer 1993;71:2217–2221.
322. Ishihashi T, Kiyoi H, Fukutani H, et al. Effective treatment of adult T-cell with a novel oral anti-tumor agent, MST-16. Oncology 1992;49:333–337.
323. Dearden C, Matutes E, Catovsky D, et al. Deoxycoformicin in treatment of mature T-cell leukemias. Br J Cancer 1991;65:903–907.
324. Tobinai K, Shimoyama M, Inoue S, et al. Phase I study of YK-176 (2′-deoxycoformicin) in patients with adult T-cell leukemia/lymphoma. Jpn J Clin Oncol 1992;22:164–169.
325. Okamura T, Shibuya T, Harada M, et al. Successful treatment of chronic adult-cell leukemia with ubenimex. Acta Haematol 1992;87:94–98.
326. Waldmann TA. Adult T-cell leukemia: prospects for immunotherapy. In: The human retroviruses. New York: Academic Press, 1991:319–334.
327. Bernard S, Gill P, Rosen P, et al. A phase I trial of alpha-interferon in combination with pentostatin in hematologic malignancies. Med Pediatr Oncol 1991;19:276–282.
328. Gill PS, Harrington W, Kaplan MH, et al. Treatment of adult T-cell leukemia-lymphoma with a combination of interferon alfa and zidovudine. N Engl J Med 1995;332:1744–1748.
329. Bazarbachi A. Hermine O. Treatment with a combination of zidovudine and alpha-interferon in naive and pretreated adult T-cell leukemia/lymphoma patients. J Acquir Immune Defic Syndr Hum Retrovirol 1996;13(Suppl 1):S186–190.
330. Harrington W, Sheramata W, Cabral L, et al. Tropical spastic paraparesis/HTLV-I- associated myelopathy (TSP/HAM): treatment with an anabolic steroid danazol. AIDS Res Hum Retroviruses 1991;7:1031–1036.
331. Bartholomew C, Edwards J, Maharaj M. A trial of danazol in TSP patients in Trinidad [abstract 1:14B]. In: Proceedings of the Conference on HTLV, Kumamoto, 1992.
332. Centers for Disease Control. Guidelines for counseling persons infected with human T-lymphotropic virus type I (HTLV-I) and type II (HTLV-II). Ann Intern Med 1993;118:448–454.
333. Cockerell GL, Lairmore M De B, Rovnak J, et al. Persistent infection of rabbits with HTLV-I patterns of anti-viral antibody reactivity and detection of virus by gene amplification. Int J Cancer 1990;45:127–130.
334. Kotani S, Yoshimoto S, Yamato K, et al. Serial transmission of human T-cell leukemia virus type I by blood transfusion in rabbits and its prevention by use of X-irradiated stored blood. Int J Cancer 1986;37:843–847.
335. Dezzutti CS, Frazier DE, Huff LY, et al. Subunit vaccine protects *Macaca nemestrina* (pig-tailed macaque) against simian T-cell lymphotropic virus type-I challenge. Cancer Res 1990;50(Suppl):5687–5691S.
336. Ibuki K, Funahashi S-I, Yamamoto H, et al. Long-term persistence of protective immunity in cynomolgus monkeys immunized with a recombinant vaccinia virus expressing the human T cell leukemia virus type I envelope gene. J Gen Virol 1997;78:147–152.
337. Takahashi K, Takezaki T, Oki T, et al. Inhibitory effect of maternal antibody on mother-to-child transmission of human T-lymphotropic virus type 1. Int J Cancer 1991;49:673–677.
338. Miyoshi I, Sawada T, Iwara Y, et al. Immunoprophylaxis against milk-borne transmission of HTLV-I in rabbits [abstract]. In: Proceedings of the 5th Conference on HTLV, Kumamoto, Japan, 1992.
339. Kataoka R, Takehara N, Iwahara Y, et al. Transmission of HTLV-I by blood transfusion and its prevention by passive immunization in rabbits. Blood 1990;76:1657–1661.

INDEX

Page numbers in *italics* denote figures; those followed by "t" denote tables.

A-77003, 760, 768
Abacavir (1592U89), 149, 751, 757–758, 788–789, 863
 for children, 172
 clinical trial of, 788
 combined with other drugs, 878
 penetration of blood-brain barrier by, 489
 pharmacology of, 757–758, *833*, 833–834
 structure and antiviral activity of, *753*
 viral resistance to, 788, 875t, 895
Abdominal masses, 558
Abdominal pain, 930
Abortion, 958–959
Abscesses
 in children, 169
 cutaneous, 504
 intraperitoneal, 558
 pancreatic, 557
 renal and perirenal, 596
ABT-378, 796
ABT-538. *See* Ritonavir
Acalculous cholecystitis, 333, 553, 556, 578
Access to care, 882
 for travelers, 320
 for unconventional therapies, 904–905
 for women, 153
Acetaminophen, 931
N-Acetylcysteine, 770, 907t
Achromycin-V. *See* Tetracycline
Acid-base disorders, 585–586
ACTG. *See* AIDS Clinical Trials Group
ACTH. *See* Corticotropin
Actinic dermatitis, 512
Actinomyces esophagitis, 539
Activator protein (AP-1), 406
Acupuncture, 903, 905
Acute infections, 87–90
 immune responses during, 87–89
 recovery from, 89–90, 90t
Acute renal failure (ARF), 586–588
 definition of, 586
 etiology of, 586–587, 586t
  acute intrarenal or extrarenal obstruction, 587
  acute tubulointerstitial nephritis, 587
  myoglobinuria, 587
  prerenal azotemia and acute tubular necrosis, 586–587
  prevalence of, 586
  rapidly progressive immune-complex glomerulonephritis, 587
  thrombotic thrombocytopenic purpura and hemolytic-uremic syndrome, 587

 in HIV vs. non-HIV patients, 588t
 management of, 588, 588t
 outcome of, 587–588, 588t
Acute retroviral seroconversion syndrome, 53–54, 54t, 62, 139. *See also* Primary HIV infection
Acute tubular necrosis, 586–587
Acute tubulointerstitial nephritis, 587
Acyclic nucleoside phosphonates (ANPs), 819, *838*, 838–839
Acyclovir, 144, 770
 for cytomegalovirus infections, 384
 for herpesvirus infections, 501, 572
  efficacy in immunosuppressed patients, 394
  esophageal, 541
  gastrointestinal, 547
  genital, 393
  herpes simplex virus, 393–394
  long-term suppressive therapy, 393
  oral, 503
  postexposure prophylaxis, 500
  varicella-zoster virus, 397, 465, 468
 lack of effect on Kaposi's sarcoma, 431–432
 myelosuppression induced by, 615
 for oral hairy leukoplakia, 501, 527
 in pregnancy, 158
 renal toxicity of, 586
 resistance to, 394–395, 398, 501
 therapeutic ratio for, 393
Adaptive immunity, 88–89
ADC. *See* AIDS dementia complex
ADCC. *See* Antibody-dependent cellular cytotoxicity
Addison's disease, 585, 630, 631
ADE. *See* Antibody-dependent enhancement
Adefovir dipivoxil (GS 840), 757, 788, 875t
Adefovir (PMEA), 751, 757, *838*, 838–839
 for cytomegalovirus infection, 385
 for Kaposi's sarcoma, 432
 structure and antiviral activity of, *753*
Adenine arabinoside (ARA-A; vidarabine)
 effects in progressive multifocal leukoencephalopathy, 414, 415
 for herpes simplex virus infection, 392, 394–395
 for varicella-zoster virus infection, 398
Adenine phosphoribosyl transferase (APRT), 818
Adenosine diphosphate (ADP), 815, *816*, 818
Adenosine monophosphate (AMP), 815, *816*, 818, *818*
Adenosine triphosphate (ATP), 815, *816*, 818
Adenovirus infection, 544, 550, 572
ADP. *See* Adenosine diphosphate
Adrenal disorders, 585, 629–632
 adrenocortical secretion in AIDS, 630–631
 clinical approach to, 631

 cytomegalovirus adrenalitis, 376, 629
 evaluation of adrenal glucocorticoid secretion, 629–630
 evaluation of adrenal mineralocorticoid secretion, 631–632
 pathologic processes, 629
Adult T-cell leukemia/lymphoma (ATL), 1013–1016, *1014*, *1015*
 prognosis for, 1019, *1020*
 treatment of, 1019–1020
Advance directives, 960, 979–980
Advanced HIV disease, 56, 64, 148
 clinical manifestations of, 148
 management of, 148
 neurologic complications of, 480–491
Advances in knowledge, 3–8
 basic science, 3–5
 clinical care, 5–7
 prevention and vaccine development, 7–8
Africa, 111–113, *112–113*, 112t, 118, *119*, 693, 725. *See also* Developing countries
 HIV-2 infection in, 113, 986–987, 987t
AG-1343. *See* Nelfinavir
Agitation, 932
AGM-1470, for microsporidiosis, 344
Aid in dying, 933, 960–961, 961t, 982
AIDS case definition, 49, 50t, 55, 123, 146
AIDS Clinical Trials Group (ACTG), 166, 174
 ACTG 019, 783
 ACTG 076, 155–156, 746, 783
 ACTG 114, 786
 ACTG 116, 865
 ACTG 117, 865
 ACTG 119, 786
 ACTG 143, 888
 ACTG 152, 680
 ACTG 155, 786
 ACTG 164, 789
 ACTG 175, 783–785, 786
 ACTG 214, 743
 ACTG 229, 792
 ACTG 241, 789
 ACTG 261, 790
 ACTG 290, 784
 ACTG 328, 747
 ACTG 334, 747
 ACTG 343, 880
 ACTG 372A, 880
AIDS dementia complex (ADC), 413, 485–489
 alternative terms for, 486
 clinical features of, 485–486
 definition of, 485
 imaging of, 487, *487*
 laboratory studies in, 487
 neuropsychological testing in, 487
 palliative care for, 932
 pathology and pathogenesis of, 487–489

1031

AIDS dementia complex (ADC)—*Continued*
  staging of, 486, 486t
  treatment of, 489
AIDS enteropathy, 538, 546–547, 649
AIDS vaccine development, 7–8, 89, 95–96, 106–107, 689–714, 728–739, 743–744
  animal models for, 706–709
    baboons, 706
    chimpanzees, 706
    immunization and challenge studies, 707–709, 708t
    macaques, 706–707
    nonprimate models, 707
  antigen targets and immunologic effector mechanisms, 694–697
    antigenic diversity, 694, 729–730
    cell-mediated immune responses, 695–696
    humoral responses, 694–695
    mucosal immunity, 696, *697*
    potential disease-inducing antigens, 696–697
  approaches to vaccine formulation, 697–705, 698t–701t
    DNA vaccines, 699t, 730
    live attenuated vaccines, 704–705, 730, 735
    live recombinant vectors, 702–703
    nucleic acid vaccination, *703*, 703–704
    recombinant protein subunits, 697–698
    strategies for vaccine adjuvants and delivery systems, 705–706
    synthetic peptides, 698–702
    virus-like particle vaccines, 702
    whole inactivated HIV-1 vaccines, 704
  challenges in, 91, 95, 728, 728t
  clinical trials in developing countries, 728–739
    addressing skepticism, mistrust, and political commitment, 731
    benefits of, 730–731, 731t
    building infrastructure for, 732
    community preparedness for, 732
    counseling and, 734
    data collection, management, and analysis for, 733–734
    ethics of, 736
    health services and service referrals for, 734
    human resources and economic costs of, 731–732
    institutional review boards and informed consent for, 733
    logistical challenges in, 730
    logistical challenges of, 730
    participant recruitment for, 732–733, 733t
    participant retention in, 734
    specimen handling and laboratory facilities for, 733
    trained researchers and staff for, 732
    vaccine administration and clinical monitoring for, 734
  clinical trials of safety and immunogenicity, 8, 709–713
    breakthrough infections, 710
    conduct of, 709–710
    live recombinant vectors and nucleic acid vaccines, 712
    peptide vaccines, 711
    recombinant envelope protein subunit vaccines, 710–711
    safety, 710
    summary of immunogenicity data from, *712–713*, 713
  current status of, 713–714, 738, 738t
  design of vaccine efficacy trials, 735–736, 735t
  durability of protection provided by vaccines, 728
  ethics of, 736–738
    building structures for ethical research, 737–738
    in developing countries, 736
    informed consent and independent, non-coerced participation, 737
    just distribution of risk and benefit, 736—737
    maximizing benefits and minimizing risks, 737
  factors affecting vaccine utility, 728
  features of vaccines for other viruses, 689–691
    successful viral vaccines, 689–690, 726t, 727t
    unsuccessful vaccine efforts, 690–691
  goal of, 728
  for HIV-2 infection, 994–995
  ideal properties of HIV vaccine, 728
  International AIDS Vaccine Initiative (IAVI), 739
  natural immunity against HIV-1 as potential guide for, 693–694, *694*
  novel approaches for acceleration of, 738–739
  partially protective vaccines, 728
  pathogenesis of HIV-1 infection relevant to immune intervention, 691–693
    chronic persistence and progression to clinical disease, 693
    early events, 691–693
  selecting sites for vaccine efficacy trials, 734
  therapeutic use of HIV vaccines, 743–744
AIDS Vaccine Evaluation Group (AVEG), 709
AIDS-related complex (ARC), 49, 55
AL-721, 907t
Albendazole, 344, 548, 552
Aldosterone, 631–632
Allergic drug reactions, 513–514
Allopathic medicine, 906–907
Alopecia, 514
Alternative therapies. *See* Unconventional therapies
ALX40-4C, 762
AMD3100, 21, 761–762
Amebiasis, 316, 546, 550
Amenorrhea, 636
Americans with Disabilities Act, 967, 981
Amikacin, 291–292, 291t, 548
Aminoglycosides, 312, 787
Aminooxypentane (AOP)-RANTES, 21
8-Aminoquinolines, 208
Aminosidine, 337, 547
Amitriptyline, 929
Amoxicillin, 317

AMP. *See* Adenosine monophosphate
Amphotericin B
  adverse effects of
    endocrine, 632t
    hepatic, 552
    renal, 585, 586
  alternative formulations of, 363
  for aspergillosis, 366
  for blastomycosis, 366
  for candidiasis, 359, 359t, 540
  for coccidioidomycosis, 365
  for cryptococcosis, 362–363, 362t, 467
  for hepatic fungi, 573
  for histoplasmosis, 364
  interaction with zalcitabine, 787
  for penicilliosis, 318, 366
  in pregnancy, 157–158
  for sporotrichosis, 366
Ampicillin, 317
Amprenavir (141W94; Vx-478), 149, *755*, 761, 795–796, 875t, 878t
Amyloidosis, 592
Anabolic therapies
  for thrombocytopenia, 614
  for wasting, 652–653
Anal carcinoma, 148, 432
Anal intercourse, 104, 115, 117, 151, 537
Analgesics, opioid, 930–931, 931t. *See also* Pain management
  interaction with ritonavir, 793
  method of delivery of, 931
  unwarranted fears about, 931
Ananthamebiasis, 507
Anemia, 54, 140, 612–613
  cause of, 612
  correlation with disease progression, 612
  in thrombotic thrombocytopenic purpura/hemolytic-uremic syndrome, 587
  vitamin B_{12} deficiency and, 612–613
  zidovudine-induced, 822, 864
Angioedema, 512
Angiotensin-converting enzyme (ACE) inhibitors, 593–594
Angular cheilitis, 358, 524
Animal models in vaccine development, 706–709, 708t
Anogenital complications, 144, 438t
  carcinoma, 148, 432
  perianal condylomata acuminata, 502
Anorexia, 146, 148, 315, 644, 647. *See also* Wasting syndrome
ANPs. *See* Acyclic nucleoside phosphonates
Antacids, 541, 786, 790
Antibodies, neutralizing, 20, 64, 91–92, 691–692, 695, 744–745
  AIDS vaccine development and, 697–698
  in long-term nonprogressors, 67
  in rapid progressors, 68
  role in perinatal HIV transmission, 166
Antibody response, 53, 89, 139–140
  strategies for enhancement of, 745–746
    monoclonal antibody, 746
    polyclonal antisera, 745–746
Antibody testing. *See also* Laboratory testing
  for *Bartonella* infection, 303, 304, 307
  for herpes simplex virus infection, 392
  for HIV-1 infection, 53, 140, 662–663
    (*See also* Diagnosis of HIV infection)

counseling before and after, 912, 957–958
ethical issues related to, 957–958
informed consent for, 958
after occupational exposures, 949
to qualify for insurance coverage, 981
reporting results of, 957
for HIV-2 infection, 985, 986t, 992–993
for HTLV-I and HTLV-II infection, 1006, *1006*
for syphilis, 300
for toxoplasmosis, 235–236, 481
Antibody-dependent cellular cytotoxicity (ADCC), 63, 72–73, 89, 139, 695
Antibody-dependent enhancement (ADE), 696–697
Anticonvulsants, 248, 485, 793
Anti-D (anti-Rh) antibody, 614
Antidepressants, 929
Antidiarrheal agents, 338, 548, 793, 931–932
Antidiscrimination legislation, 980–981
Antiemetics, 793, 932
Antifungal therapy, 56. *See also* specific drugs
for aspergillosis, 366
for blastomycosis, 366
for candidiasis, 358–359, 359t, 524–525, 540
for coccidioidomycosis, 365
for cryptococcosis, 361–363, 362t
for disseminated infections, 509
hepatic effects of, 552, 576
for hepatic infections, 573
for histoplasmosis, 364–365
for penicilliosis, 318, 366
in pregnancy, 157–158
for sporotrichosis, 366
Antigenic diversity of HIV-1, 117, 694
Antigenic drift, 87
Antigenic properties of viral proteins, 90–92
determinants recognized by T cells, 92
epitopes recognized by B cells, 90–91, *91*
neutralization of field strains of HIV-1 by antibody, 91–92
Antigenic shift, 87
Antigen-presenting cells (APCs), 88, 93, 692
Antigens
Epstein-Barr virus, 441–442, 446
potential disease-inducing, 696–697
Toxoplasma, 236–237
Antihistamines
for eosinophilic folliculitis, 511
interaction with ritonavir, 793
for scabies, 507
Antimalarial therapy, 320, 320t
Antimicrobial therapy
for bacillary angiomatosis, 311–312, 505
for *Campylobacter*, 317
for cholangiopathy, 578
for *Clostridium difficile* infection, 317, 548
for cryptosporidiosis, 336–338, 547
hepatic effects of, 576
interaction with ritonavir, 794
for isosporiasis, 317, 650
for microsporidiosis, 317, 344, 548
for nontuberculous mycobacterial infection, 290–294, 291t, 293t, 548
for *Pneumocystis carinii* pneumonia, 200–208, 201t
for pyogenic cutaneous infections, 505
for salmonellosis, 317

for shigellosis, 317
for syphilis, 300–301
topical microbicides to prevent sexually transmitted diseases, 726–728
for toxoplasmosis, 241–244, 246–248, 247t
retinochoroiditis, 466
for traveler's diarrhea, 320, 322
for tuberculosis, 271–272, 271t
Antiphospholipid antibodies, 620–621
Antipyretics, 931
Antiretroviral drug development, 5, 149, 751–771, 780–798. *See also* Clinical trials; Investigational drugs
bringing anti-HIV drugs into the clinic, 754–756
combination therapy, 769–771
to combat viral resistance, 770–771
rationale for, 769–770, 770t
drug testing in vitro, 751–753, 756t
drugs acting at early stages of HIV replication, 761–762
inhibitors by chemokine-related or chemokine receptor-related strategy, 761–762
inhibitors of virus adsorption to target cells, 761
drugs acting at late stages of HIV replication, 762–765
inhibitors of budding, 764–765
inhibitors of integrase, 762
inhibitors of nuclear migration, 762
inhibitors of viral transcription and translation, 762–763
viral assembly and maturation, 763–764
capsid and matrix proteins, 764
nucleocapsid p7 protein, 764
ethics of drug testing, 967–968
rational drug design, 753–754
stages in HIV replication cycle that may be targets for therapeutic intervention, 751, 756t, 780, 781t
targeting reverse transcriptase, 756–759 (*See also* Reverse transcriptase inhibitors)
nonnucleoside reverse transcriptase inhibitors, *758*, 758–759
nucleoside reverse transcriptase inhibitors, 757–758
structure of reverse transcriptase, 756–757, *757*
targeting viral protease, 759–761 (*See also* Protease inhibitors)
design of symmetry-based inhibitors, 760
pharmacokinetics, 760–761
protease structure and substrate-based inhibitors, *759*, 759–760
structure-based inhibitors, 760–761
Antiretroviral drug resistance, 6, 678, 743, 765–769, 841, 869, 874, 875t, 887–888, 891–898, 923
assays of drug susceptibility, 897–898
genotypic assays, 898
phenotypic assays, 897–898
in children, 680–681
combination therapy to overcome, 770–771, 874, 887–888
drug-resistance testing in patient management, 881, 898, 898t

genotypes associated with, 678, 680–681, 853–855, 891
to nonnucleoside reverse transcriptase inhibitors, 756, 759, 766–767, 841, 874, 875t, 891, 892, 895–896, *896*
delavirdine, 790, 867
nevirapine, 766–767, 789, 841, 867, 891
to nucleoside reverse transcriptase inhibitors, 765–766, 782, 874, 875t, 892–893, 892–895, 894t
abacavir, 788, 895
didanosine, 782, 894
lamivudine, 788, 866, 891, 892, 895
multiple nucleoside resistance, 895
zalcitabine, 786–787, 894–895
zidovudine, 765–766, 864, 891–894, *892–893*, 894t
plasma HIV-1 RNA level and, 678, 892
to protease inhibitors, *760*, 761, 767–769, 790–791, 848, 853–857, 874, 875t, 891, 897, 897t
A-77003, 768
active site mutants, 767–768
cleavage site mutants, 769
cross-resistance, 768, 855–857, *856*
emergence of, 767, 791
genetic basis of, 853–855
indinavir, 794, 851, 853–854, 868
nelfinavir, 795, 855
nonactive site mutants, 768
ritonavir, 793, 850, 854
saquinavir, 792, 854–855, 867–868
resistance interactions of reverse transcriptase mutations, 896–897
viral mutations associated with, 678, 765–769, 782, 874, 875t, 891–898
Antiretroviral therapy, 5–7, 148–149, 437, 601, 780–798, 815–857, 861–888, 863t, 874t, 905. *See also* Pharmacology; Protease inhibitors; Reverse transcriptase inhibitors; specific drugs
access to treatment with, 320, 882
for acute exanthem of HIV disease, 499
for acute primary infection, 53, 140
adverse effects of, 863t
diarrhea, 543
hepatotoxicity, 552–553, 552t, 576
myelosuppression, 615
neuropathies, 147, 490
pancreatitis, 543
risk of lymphoma, 439
for AIDS dementia complex, 489
for children, 172–174
considerations for, 173–174
guidelines for, 173
improvement in neurologic disease after, 169
initiation in newborns and infants less than 1 year of age, 173
initiation in older children, 173
making changes in, 173
combination therapy, 769–771, 780, 798, 869, 872–882, 885–888 (*See also* Combination antiretroviral therapy)
dosages of, 863t
drug interactions with (*See* Drug interactions)
effect on hepatitis B virus coinfection, 570

Antiretroviral therapy—*Continued*
effect on infectiousness and HIV transmission, 103–104
ethics of drug testing, 967–968
evaluating response to, 874–876
failure of, 149, 881
future considerations for, 798, 870, 880–882
for glomerulosclerosis, 592–593
goal of, 797, 873, 885
highly active (HAART), 3, 4, 6, 8, 537, 538
history of, 780
for HIV-2 infection, 994
initiation of, 6, 149, 796–797, 869, 873
in asymptomatic infection, 675–676
based on plasma viral RNA level, 675–677, 679–680
in children, 679–680
in primary infection, 676–677, 869
in symptomatic infection, 676
making changes in, 149, 797, 869, 878–879, 879t
other treatment modalities and, 881
patient monitoring during, 869, 881–882
penetration of blood-brain barrier by, 489
pharmacology of, 815–857, 881
for postexposure prophylaxis, 869–870, 940–941, 941t, 947–949
during pregnancy, 155–156, 157t, 166, 174–175, 948, 970–971
protease inhibitors, 148–149, 751, 759–761, 790–796, 848–857, 867–869
provided by hospice programs, 925–926
reverse transcriptase inhibitors, 148–149, 751, 756–759, 781–790, 815–842, 863–867
stages in HIV replication cycle that may be targets for, 751, 756t, 780, 781t
attachment, 863–867
protein processing, 867–868
staging HIV infection in era of, 56–57
strategic approaches for, 6, 796–798, 869–870, 879–880, 879t
current standard, 879
eradication, 880
induction and maintenance, 879–880
intensification, 880
trade names and drug manufacturers, 863t
viral load monitoring and, 51, 673–682
(*See also* Plasma HIV-1 RNA)
for women, 154
Antituberculosis therapy, 270–273
drug interactions with, 272–273, 273t
delavirdine, 790
indinavir, 794
ritonavir, 794
hepatic effects of, 576
in pregnancy, 157
Antiviral therapy
for cytomegalovirus retinitis, 461–463
for herpes simplex virus infection, 392–395
for herpes zoster ophthalmicus, 468
for Kaposi's sarcoma, 431–432
for varicella-zoster virus retinitis, 465
AP-1. *See* Activator protein
Aphthous ulcers, 144
esophageal, 539, *539*
recurrent, 529, *529*
thalidomide for, 529, 539, 541

Apoptosis, 73–74, 539
Appetite loss, 146, 148, 315, 644, 647
Appetite stimulants, 148, 651
APRT. *See* Adenine phosphoribosyl transferase
ARA-A. *See* Adenine arabinoside
ARA-C. *See* Cytosine arabinoside
ARC. *See* AIDS-related complex
Arginine vasopressin, 633, *633*
Arprinocid, 244
Arthritis
cryptosporidiosis and, 333
psoriatic, 509
Reiter's syndrome, 510
Aryloxyphosphoramidate prodrugs, *834, 835–836, 837*
Ascites, 558–559
Ascorbate, 614
Asia, *112,* 112t, 114–115, *115. See also* Developing countries
Aspergillosis, 366
central nervous system, 484
clinical features of, 366
cutaneous, 366, 509
diagnosis of, 366
hepatic, 550, 572–573
oral, 525
orbital, 470
thyroid, 634
treatment of, 366
Astemizole interactions with protease inhibitors, 792, 795, 852
Asymptomatic HIV infection, 140–143
of nervous system, 479
plasma viral RNA level to determine suitability of initiating antiretroviral therapy in, 675–676
children, 679–680
Ataxia, 411
ATL. *See* Adult T-cell leukemia/lymphoma
Atopic dermatitis, 511–512
Atovaquone
adverse effects of, 244
for cryptosporidiosis, 338
for microsporidiosis, 344
for *Pneumocystis carinii* pneumonia, 201t, 203t, 207
in pregnancy, 157
prophylactic, 146, 211
for toxoplasmosis, 244, 247t
retinochoroiditis, 466
ATP. *See* Adenosine triphosphate
Australia, *112,* 112t
Austrian's syndrome, 602
Autoimmune mechanisms, 73
AVEG. *See* AIDS Vaccine Evaluation Group
Avian leukosis virus, 23
Azathioprine, 1020
3'-Azido-2',3'-dideoxythymidine (AzddThd, AZT). *See* Zidovudine
3'-Azido-2',3'-dideoxyuridine (AzddUrd), 824, *824–825*
Azithromycin
for bacillary angiomatosis, 311, 505
for cryptosporidiosis, 337, 547
hepatotoxicity of, 552
for *Mycobacterium avium* complex infection, 290, 291t, 548
prophylaxis, 146, 292

in pregnancy, 158
for toxoplasmosis, 243, 247t
Azotemia, 585, 586

B cells, 407
dysfunctions of, 75
in children, 169
epitopes recognized by, 90–91, *91*
migration into nonlymphoid tissues, 407–408
Bacillary angiomatosis, 143t, 303–312
clinical manifestations of, 309–311
bone marrow, 310
central nervous system, 311
cutaneous, 309, *309,* 505
esophageal, 539
fever and bacteremia, 310–311
hepatosplenic, 310, 575
HIV-associated dementia, 311
mucous membrane, 309–310
musculoskeletal, 309
pulmonary, 310
diagnosis of, 305–307
differential diagnosis of, 308, 309, 505
epidemiology of, 304–305
etiology of, 303, 304
histopathology of, 307–308, *307–308,* 505
historical recognition of, 303–304
link between cats and, 305, 312
microbiology of, 305–306, 505
pathogenesis of, 308
prevention of, 312
treatment of, 311–312, 505
Bacillary peliosis hepatis, 304, 310, 549, *550,* 576
Bacille Calmette-Guérin (BCG) vaccine, 275, 321
Bacitracin, 505
Back pain, 906
Bacteremia
bacillary angiomatosis and, 311
Campylobacter jejuni, 317
in children, 169
Mycobacterium avium complex, 289, 290, 291t, 292
Salmonella, 317
Bacterial infections. *See also* specific bacteria
in children, 169
cutaneous, 504–506
diarrhea due to, 546, 548
esophageal, 539, 541
oral, 528–529
Bactrim. *See* Trimethoprim-sulfamethoxazole
Bartonella henselae and *B. quintana,* 303–307, 304t, 505. *See also* Bacillary angiomatosis
Basal cell carcinoma, 514, 515, 523
Basal ganglia calcifications, 169
Baseline clinical and laboratory evaluation, 873–874
Basic fibroblast growth factor, in Kaposi's sarcoma, 424–425
B-cell stimulatory factor-1. *See* Interleukin-4
B-cell stimulatory factor-2. *See* Interleukin-6
BCG. *See* Bacille Calmette-Guérin vaccine
bcl-2 gene, 441, 442
bcl-6 gene, 441
Beau's lines, 514

Behavioral risk factors, 101, 104, 116t, 117, 117t, 919
Bell's palsy, 491
Bereavement, 920
Bicyclams, 728
BILA-2011, 760
Biliary tract disease, 553, 576–578
 acalculous cholecystitis, 553, 578
 in bacillary angiomatosis, 310
 cholangiopathy, 553, 576–578, 577–578
 cryptosporidiosis, 332–333, 377, 576, 578
 cytomegalovirus, 376–377
 treatment of, 556
Biofeedback, 903, 906
Biologic variables affecting spread of HIV, 117
BI-RG-587. See Nevirapine
Birth control pills, 101, 104, 151
Bis(isopropyloxycarbonyloxymethyl) prodrugs, 834, 835, 836
Bis(pivaloyloxymethyl) prodrugs, 751, 834–835, 834–835
Bis(S-acryl-2-thioethyl) prodrugs, 834, 835, 836
BIV. See Bovine immunodeficiency virus
BK virus, 403, 404
Blastocystis hominis infection, 546
Blastomycosis, 147, 366, 508–509
Bleach distribution programs, 182–184, 186
Bleomycin, 453, 453t, 516
Blinded studies, 809
Blindness, 470. See also Ocular sequelae
Blood supply protection, 125–126, 130, 134, 661
Blood transfusion
 effects on disease progression, 617
 erythropoietin administration as alternative to, 617
 HIV-1 transmission by, 116, 125–126, 151, 937
 HIV-2 transmission by, 987
 HTLV-I and HTLV-II transmission by, 1012–1013
Blood-brain barrier, 489
Blood-retina barrier, 471
BOB/GPR-15, 14, 15t
Body composition in disease, 643–644
Bone and mineral homeostasis, 638, 638–639
Bone marrow abnormalities, 614–615, 614t
 bacillary angiomatosis, 310
 drug-induced myelosuppression, 615
 HIV infection, 61
 morphologic changes, 614–615
Bone marrow microenvironment, 620
Bone marrow progenitor cells, 618–619
BONZO/STRL-33, 14, 15t
Botryomycosis, 504
Bovine dialyzable leukocyte extract (DLE), 338
Bovine immunodeficiency virus (BIV), 25
Bowenoid papulosis, 501, 502, 503, 514–515
Boxwood extract, 907t
Brachial plexopathy, 479
Brain abscesses, 230–232, 231
Brain biopsy, 238, 245
Breast-feeding
 HIV transmission by, 116, 127, 153, 165–166

HTLV-I and HTLV-II transmission by, 1010–1011, 1011
 postexposure prophylaxis during, 949
Bronchoalveolar lavage (BAL), 198–199
Bronchopulmonary fistula, 195
Buffergel, 727
Burkitt's lymphoma, 440
BW 1592, 5
BW 348U87, 395

CA. See Capsid protein
Cachectin. See Tumor necrosis factor-α
Cachexia, 148, 643–645. See also Wasting syndrome
CAEV. See Caprine arthritis/encephalitis virus
Calciphylaxis, 586
Calcium, 638–639
 hypercalcemia, 586, 637
 hypocalcemia, 586, 637–638
 nephrocalcinosis, 596
Calcium channel blocker interactions with antiretroviral agents, 790, 792
Caloric intake, 644, 651–652
Campylobacter infection, 315, 546
 acalculous cholecystitis and, 578
 antimicrobial therapy for, 317
 traveler's diarrhea, 316–317
Candidiasis, 357–360
 brain, 484
 bronchopulmonary, 358
 cardiac, 601, 602
 in children, 168–170
 clinical features of, 358
 diagnosis of, 358
 epidemiology of, 357–358
 esophageal, 55, 139, 147, 358, 523, 538, 540
 hepatic, 572
 host defense mechanisms against, 357
 intraocular, 467
 microbiology of, 357
 oral, 139, 144, 147, 195, 357–358, 508, 521, 523–525
  angular cheilitis, 524
  diagnosis of, 523–524
  erythematous, 524, 524
  pathogenesis of, 524
  prevalence of, 522
  pseudomembranous, 524, 525
  relapses of, 525
  risk factors for, 523
 prophylaxis for, 360
 relation to CD4+ cell count, 360
 systemic, 358
 treatment of, 154, 358–359, 359t, 524–525, 540
 vaginal, 152, 154, 357, 358
Canker sores, 529, 529
Caprine arthritis/encephalitis virus (CAEV), 25, 32
Capsid (CA) protein, 24, 29–30, 764, 989
Captopril, 593
Carbamazepine, 485
 hepatotoxicity of, 553
 interaction with protease inhibitors, 485, 792, 852
 for neuropathic pain, 930
Carbovir, 753, 757, 833, 833–834

Cardiac involvement, 601–607
 cardiomyopathy, 604–607
  cytokines and, 605–606
  drug-induced, 606
  due to immune system impairment, 605
  frequency of, 606–607
  HIV myocarditis leading to, 604–605
  nutritional, 606
  opportunistic infections and, 605
 incidental, 601–602
  toxoplasmosis, 232, 234
 myocarditis, 603–604
 neoplasms, 602
 pericarditis, 602–603
 pulmonary hypertension, 603
 types of, 601
 valvular, 602
Cardiovascular surgery in AIDS patients, 607
Caregivers, 932–933
Caribbean nations, 112, 112t, 113–114. See also Developing countries
Case definition
 for AIDS, 49, 50t, 55, 123, 146, 391
 for pediatric HIV infection, 163, 164t
Castanospermine, 20
Castleman's disease, 444
CAT. See Chloramphenicol acetyl transferase
Catabolism
 fat cell, 644–645
 protein, 647
Cat-scratch disease, 304, 307
CCR1, 761
CCR2-V64I, 17
CCR2b, 14, 15t, 761
CCR3, 14–15, 15t, 761
CCR5, 4, 14–15, 15t, 28–29, 60, 60, 611, 691, 695, 781, 861
 development of drugs aimed at, 21, 761–762, 798
 discovery of, 761
 disease progression and heterozygosity for, 52, 67
 HIV-2 and, 990
 Langerhans cell expression of, 19
 role in HIV transmission, 18–19, 102
 role in natural resistance to HIV entry, 4, 17–19, 691
CCR8, 14, 15t
CD4+ cells, 59, 71–75, 91, 611
 AIDS case definition based on count of, 49, 50t, 146
 in children, 163, 164t
 autologous infusion of expanded cells, 745
 characteristics of, 88t
 daily turnover rate of, 612
 depletion and dysfunction of, 4–5, 71–75, 72t, 140–141, 320–321, 612, 862
  antibody-dependent cellular cytotoxicity, 72–73
  apoptosis, 73–74
  autoimmune mechanisms, 73
  discordant with plasma viral RNA level, 678
  HIV-mediated direct cytopathicity, 72
  HIV-mediated syncytia formation, 72
  HIV-specific cytotoxic T lymphocytes, 72, 696
  lymphocyte regeneration, 74

CD4+ cells—*Continued*
  depletion and dysfunction of—*Continued*
    nature of T-cell dysfunction in HIV infection, 73–74, 74t
    superantigen-mediated perturbation of T-cell subsets, 73
  disease progression and count of, 49–50, *50, 52*
    advanced disease, 56, 64
    early disease, 55
    late disease, 55
    latent period, 64
    middle stage disease, 55
    primary infection, 54, 62, 139
  diseases related to depletion of, 103
    candidiasis, 357
    coccidioidomycosis, 365
    cryptococcosis, 360
    cryptosporidiosis, 332
    lymphomas, 437
    Mycobacterium avium complex, 286, 288, 294
    Pneumocystis carinii pneumonia, 191, 194, 197
    in splenectomized patients, 614
    toxoplasmosis, 227, 229, 229t, 237–238, 249
    tuberculosis, 261–263
  HIV attachment to, 4, 15–16, *15–16*, 59, 611, 861
    CD4-gp120 interactions, 13, 15, 695
    chemokine inhibition of, 71
    HIV-2, 988
    infection of, 60
  initiation of antiretroviral therapy based on count of, 675, 874
  interleukin-2 effects on level of, 68
  intracellular complex between CD4 molecules and gp160, 26
  natural function of, 13
  Nef-mediated downregulation of, 36
  perinatal transmission rate related to maternal count of, 166
  during pregnancy, 155
  sexual HIV transmission related to count of, 102
  Th1 and Th2, 71, 88, 88t
  thymocytes, 61
CD8+ cells, 73
  in advanced disease, 64
  autologous infusion of expanded cells for Kaposi's sarcoma, 745
  characteristics of, 88t
  in long-term nonprogressors, 67, 612
  during primary infection, 54, 62–63, 139
  in rapid progressors, 68
  role in host resistance to *Toxoplasma gondii*, 227
  thymocytes, 61
  Vβ families of, 62–63, 73
CD34+ cells, 61, 62, 618
CD38+ cells, 68
Ceftriaxone, 301
Cell adhesion molecules, 72
Cell-mediated immunity, 88, 611, 695–696, 744–745. *See also* Cytotoxic T lymphocytes

Cellular targets
  of HIV-1, 13–21, 14t, 59, 611–612, 691–692, 861
    fusion of viral and cell membranes, 861
    therapeutic strategies and, 20–21
    viral tropism, 18, *18*, 102, 691–692
  of HIV-2, 988
  of HTLV-I and HTLV-II, 1004
Centers for Disease Control and Prevention (CDC), 123, 146, 163, 911
Central nervous system involvement. *See* Neurologic complications
Cephalexin, 505
Cerebral atrophy, 169
Cerebral hemorrhage, 233
Cerebrospinal fluid (CSF)
  in AIDS dementia complex, 487
  in cytomegalovirus infection, 377
  HIV in, 407
    in children, 169
  in neuropathies, 479
  in progressive multifocal leukoencephalopathy, 413
  in syphilis, 299, 299t, 301
  in toxoplasmosis, 238
Cervical dysplasia/cancer, 143, 148, 152, 154
Cervical ectopy, 104
Chancroid, 319, 319t, 506
Chemokine receptors, 15, 101, 102, 861. *See also* CCR2, CCR3, CCR5, CCR8
  modification for therapeutic use, 761
Chemokines, 4, 14–15
  α- and β- types of, 14–15
  definition of, 14
  inhibition of HIV entry by β-chemokines, 71, 91, 437, 695
  macrophage-derived, 4
  modification for therapeutic use, 21, 761–762
  specificity of, 15
Chemoprophylaxis, 7, 56, 145–146
  for candidiasis, 360
  for cryptococcosis, 363–364
  for cytomegalovirus, 146, 384, 464
  for herpesvirus infections, 500
  for malaria, 320, 320t
  for *Mycobacterium avium* complex, 146, 292–293
    in children, 170
  after occupational HIV exposure, 869–870, 940–941, 941t, 947–949
    choice of drugs for, 869–870, 941t, 948–949
    drug toxicity and, 949
    evidence in support of, 948
    follow-up care and, 949–950
    National Clinicians' Postexposure Prophylaxis Hotline, 949
    for pregnant or lactating women, 949
    primate studies of, 947–948
    protection afforded by, 948
    window of opportunity for, 947
  for *Pneumocystis carinii*, 145–146, 209–211
    in children, 170, 170t, 171
  for toxoplasmosis, 146, 228, 248–249, 249t
  for traveler's diarrhea, 320
  for tuberculosis, 146, 273–275

Chemotherapy
  for adult T-cell leukemia/lymphoma, 1019
  for cloacogenic carcinoma, 432
  for Kaposi's sarcoma, 429–430, 454
    intralesional, 428
  for lymphomas, 445, 445t, 453–454, 453t, 516
Chest pain, 930
Chest radiography, 146t
  aspergillosis on, 366
  coccidioidomycosis on, 365
  histoplasmosis on, 364
  penicilliosis on, 318, 366
  Pneumocystis carinii pneumonia on, 197–198, *198*
  toxoplasmosis on, 241
  in tuberculosis, 267, *267*, 268
Chickenpox, 396, 397, 500, 525. *See also* Varicella-zoster virus infection
Childhood HIV infection. *See* Pediatric HIV infection
Children orphaned by AIDS, 119, *119*
Chinese herbs, 906
Chiropractic, 905–906
Chlamydia trachomatis infection, 319t, 726, 727
Chloramphenicol acetyl transferase (CAT), 404
Chlorhexidine, 505, 529, 727
Chloroquine, 320, 320t
Cholangiopathy, 552, 576–578
  diagnosis of, 577–578, *577–578*
  microbiology of, 576–578
  treatment of, 556, 578
Cholecystitis, acalculous, 333, 553, 556, 578
Cholestyramine, 548
Choroidal infections. *See also* Ocular sequelae
  fungal, 466–467
  metastatic bacterial infections, 466
  pneumocystosis, 196, 375, 467
  toxoplasmic retinochoroiditis, 232, 234, 375, 457, *465*, 465–466
  tuberculosis, 467
Chronic infections, 87
Cidofovir
  for acyclovir-resistant herpesvirus infections, 395, 398–399
  adverse effects of, 379t, 382, 462–463
    renal, 382, 586
    uveitis, 457, 470
  for cytomegalovirus infection, 382–383
    cutaneous, 501
    retinitis, 378t, 382–383, 461–463
      intravitreal injection, 383, 463
    probenecid administered with, 463
  for progressive multifocal leukoencephalopathy, 484
Ciliary neurotropic factor, 645
Cimetidine, 786
Ciprofloxacin
  for bacillary angiomatosis, 311, 505
  for *Campylobacter*, 317
  for drug-resistant tuberculosis, 272
  for *Mycobacterium avium* complex infection, 291, 291t, 548
  for pyogenic cutaneous infections, 505
  renal toxicity of, 587
  for traveler's diarrhea, 320, 322
Circumcision, 103

Cisapride interactions with antiretroviral agents, 790, 795, 852
Clarithromycin
  for cryptosporidiosis, 337
  interaction with ritonavir, 794
  for *Mycobacterium avium* complex infection, 290–291, 291t, 548
    prophylaxis, 146, 292
  in pregnancy, 158
  for toxoplasmosis, 243, 247t
Clindamycin
  adverse effects of, 242
  interaction with saquinavir, 792
  for *Pneumocystis carinii* pneumonia, 201t, 204–207, 206t
  in pregnancy, 158
  for toxoplasmic retinochoroiditis, 466
Clinical course of HIV disease, 49–57, 62–64, 63, 92, 92–93, 612, 673–675
  acute retroviral seroconversion syndrome, 53–54, 54t, 62, 139
  advanced disease, 56, 64, 148
  in children, 167–169, 678–679
  clinical latency, 64, 92–93, 612
  disease staging, 52, 56–57
  early disease, 54–55, 54t, 143–146
  HIV-2 infection, 994
  host factors affecting, 52–53
  indicators of disease progression, 49–52
  late disease, 54t, 55, 146–148
  long-term nonprogression, 52, 66–67, 93, 691, 694
  middle stage disease, 54t, 55
  neurologic complications and, 478
  pathogenesis and, 693
  primary infection, 62–64, 92, 139–140
  rapid disease progression, 52, 67–68
  time course to progression to AIDS, 62, 67
  transfusion effects on, 617
  treatment effects on, 49
  variability of, 49
  viral load, CD4 counts, and clinical staging, 49–52, 50–52, 50t
Clinical manifestations of HIV disease, 139–148, 140t, 142t
  bacillary angiomatosis, 303–312
  cardiac, 601–607
  in children, 163–175
  cryptosporidiosis, 327–339
  cutaneous, 499–516
  cytomegalovirus, 373–385
  endocrine, 629–638
  fungi, 357–366
  gastrointestinal, 537–559
  hematologic, 611–621
  hepatobiliary, 567–578
  herpes simplex and varicella-zoster virus infections, 391–402
  Kaposi's sarcoma and cloacogenic carcinoma, 421–432
  lymphomas, 437–447, 451–454
  microsporidiosis, 339–344
  neurologic, 477–491
  nontuberculous mycobacterial infections, 285–294
  ocular, 457–472
  oral, 521–530
  Pneumocystis carinii pneumonia, 191–211
  progressive multifocal leukoencephalopathy, 403–415
  renal, 585–596
  by stage of disease, 139–148
    advanced disease, 56, 148
    asymptomatic infection, 140–143
    early symptomatic disease, 54–55, 143–146
    late symptomatic disease, 55, 146–148
    middle stage disease, 55
    primary infection, 53–54, 54t, 62–64, 92, 139–140
  syphilis, 297–302
  toxoplasmosis, 225–249
  tropical diseases, 315–322
  tuberculosis, 261–275
  wasting syndrome, 643–654
  in women, 151–159
Clinical trials, 807–813. See also Antiretroviral drug development; Investigational drugs
  access to, 904–905
    for women, 153
  AIDS Clinical Trials Group (ACTG), 166, 174 (See also AIDS Clinical Trials Group for specific trials)
  of AIDS vaccines, 8, 699t–701t, 728–739, 738t, 745–749 (See also AIDS vaccine development)
  analyzing and interpreting data from, 811–813
    effects of noncompliance, 812
    intent to treat analyses, 811–812
    losses to follow-up, 812
    surrogate markers, 812–813
  of antiretroviral therapy effects on plasma viral RNA level, 675
  in children, 679
  definition of, 807
  design of, 807–811
    determining how many data to collect, 811
    overall research strategy, 807–809, 808, 808t
    randomization and ethical issues, 809–810, 809t
    selecting end points, 809
    selecting treatments and blinding, 809
    statistical power, 810
  evaluating literature on, 813, 813t
  "induction trials," 809
  interim monitoring of, 811
    assessing definitions, logic, and data quality, 811
    safety and efficacy assessment, 811
  Pediatric AIDS Clinical Trials Group (PACTG), 172, 174
  phases I–III, 807–808
  placebo-controlled trials, 971–972
  research ethics of, 967–968
    internationally, 970–972
  short- vs. long-term, 808–809
Cloacogenic carcinoma, 432
Clofazimine, 291, 291t
Clostridium difficile infection, 147, 546, 547
  traveler's diarrhea, 317
  treatment of, 317, 548
Clotrimazole, 359t, 524
CMV. See Cytomegalovirus infection
CNI-H0294, 762
Coagulation disorders, 620–621
Cocaine, 606
Coccidioidomycosis, 147, 365
  clinical features of, 365
  cutaneous manifestations of, 507–508
  diagnosis of, 365
  epidemiology of, 365
  hepatic, 550, 572
  meningitis, 365, 490
  microbiology of, 365
  in travelers, 318
  treatment of, 365
Codes of ethics, 971. See also Ethical issues
Cognitive impairment
  AIDS dementia complex, 485–489
  cotton-wool spots and, 459
  in progressive multifocal leukoencephalopathy, 411, 412t
Colitis, 146, 541–548. See also Diarrhea
Colonoscopy, 542
Colony-stimulating factors (CSFs), 540, 616–618
  erythropoietin, 617
  granulocyte colony stimulating factor, 617
  granulocyte-monocyte colony-stimulating factor, 617
  interleukin-3, 618
  pharmacokinetics of exogenous administration of, 617
  production in HIV infection, 616
  sources of, 616
  stem cell factor, 617
Colostral immunoglobulin concentrates, 338
Combination antiretroviral therapy, 769–771, 780, 798, 863–864, 869, 872–882, 885–888
  antiretoviral resistance and, 770–771, 874, 875t, 878–879, 887–888 (See also Antiretroviral drug resistance)
  baseline clinical and laboratory evaluation before, 873–874
  evaluating response to, 874–876
  factors involved in selecting drugs for, 872, 873t
  goal of, 873
  in vitro, 885–886, 886t
  initial approaches for, 876–878
    nonnucleoside reverse transcriptase inhibitor plus two nucleoside analog reverse transcriptase inhibitors, 877
    protease inhibitor plus nonnucleoside reverse transcriptase inhibitor plus nucleoside analog reverse transcriptase inhibitor, 878
    protease inhibitor plus two nucleoside analog reverse transcriptase inhibitors, 876–877
    three nucleoside analog reverse transcriptase inhibitors, 878
    two nucleoside analog reverse transcriptase inhibitors, 877
    two protease inhibitors, 877–878, 878t
  initiation of, 873
  level of patient commitment required for, 873
  managing failure or toxicity of initial regimen for, 878–879, 879t

Combination antiretroviral therapy—*Continued*
  optimism about, 872
  pharmacokinetics and, 881, 886–887, 886t
  for postexposure prophylaxis, 870, 948–949
  potential advantages of, 885
  in pregnancy, 156
  rationale for, 769–770, 770t
  strategic approaches for, 879–880, 879t
    current standard, 879
    eradication, 880
    induction and maintenance, 879–880
    intensification, 880
    triple therapy, 873
Communicating with patients, 907–908
Compazine. *See* Prochlorperazine
Complement system, 17, 88
Compliance with treatment, 918–919
  combination therapy, 873
  effect on clinical trial results, 812
  psychosocial interventions for improvement of, 918–919
  reasons for lack of, 918
Compound Q, 906
Computed tomography (CT)
  in cryptosporidiosis, 332, 333
  hepatic, 555
  pancreatic, 557
  in *Pneumocystis carinii* pneumonia, 198
  in progressive multifocal leukoencephalopathy, 412, *413*
  in toxoplasmosis, 238, *239*, 481, *482*
  in tuberculosis, 267, *268*
Condoms, 101, 104–106, 128–129
  effectiveness for blocking HIV transmission, 104
  female, 105, 129
  use by injecting drug users, 187–188
Condylomata acuminata, 501–503
Confidentiality issues, 956–957, 981
Congestive heart failure, 606
Conjunctival microvasculopathy, 458, 458t
Conscious sedation, 932
Constitutional symptoms, 143–144, 146
Contact lenses, 471
Contact tracing, 131–132, 965–966
Continuum of care options, 132
Conus medullaris syndrome, 233
Coombs test, positive, 613
Coreceptors, 4, 13–16, 15t, 59–60, *60*, 91, 691, 781, 861
  development of drugs aimed at, 21
  evidence for, 13–14
  for HIV-2, 988–990
  triggering of HIV entry by, 15–16, *15–16*
Corneal transplantation, 471
Corneal ulcers, 468, 470
Corticosteroids
  for aphthous ulcers, 144
  for chronic actinic dermatitis, 512
  for glomerulosclerosis, 593
  for herpes zoster, 398
  inhibition of proinflammatory cytokines by, 747
  for *Pneumocystis carinii* pneumonia, 200, 201t, 202–204, 205t, 206–208
  for postscabetic id reactions, 507
  for recurrent aphthous ulcers, 529
  for seborrheic dermatitis, 509
  for thrombocytopenia, 614
  for toxoplasmosis, 248
  for tropical spastic paraparesis/HTLV-I-associated myelopathy, 1020
Corticotropin (ACTH), 629–630
Corticotropin-releasing hormone (CRH), 629–630
Cortisol, 629–630, 648
Cost of care, 132, 965
Cotrimoxazole, 576, 585
Cotton-wool spots, 55, 375, 457–459, *458*
Counseling. *See* Psychosocial interventions
Countertransference issues, 917–918
"Crack" cocaine, 126
Cranial neuropathies, 479
C-reactive protein, 88
CRH. *See* Corticotropin-releasing hormone
Crixivan. *See* Indinavir
Cryotherapy
  for basal cell carcinoma, 515
  for human papillomavirus lesions, 503
  for Kaposi's sarcoma, 428
  for molluscum contagiosum, 504
  for squamous cell carcinoma, 515
Cryptococcosis, 147, 360–364
  adrenal, 629
  bone marrow failure and, 615
  cardiac, 602
  clinical features of, 360–361
  cutaneous, 361, 507–508
  diagnosis of, 361
  epidemiology of, 360
  hepatic, 550, *550*, 572
  intraocular, 466–467
  meningitis, 360, 361, 363, 470, 484
  microbiology of, 360
  oral, 525
  pancreatic, 556
  prognostic factors in, 361
  prophylaxis against, 363–364
  pulmonary, 360–361
  relapses of, 363
  relation to CD4+ cell count, 360
  suppressive therapy for, 363
  thyroid, 634
  treatment of, 361–363, 362t, 467
    in pregnancy, 157–158
Cryptosporidial infection, 55, 147, 148, 316, 327–339, 545
  asymptomatic, 332
  CD4+ cell count and, 332
  clinical manifestations of, 332–333
  diagnosis of, 335–336
  differential diagnosis of, 332
  disinfection and, 331
  esophageal, 539
  geographic distribution of, 329
  historical recognition of, 327
  immune response to, 334–335
  incubation period for, 332
  joint involvement in, 333
  liver, gallbladder, or biliary tract, 332–333, 377
    acalculous cholecystitis, 578
    cholangiopathy, 576, 578
  Milwaukee outbreak of, 327, 330–331
  molecular epidemiology of, 331
  other infections concurrent with, 333
    pancreatic, 333, 556
    parasite causing, 327–328
      life cycle of, *328*, 328–329
    pathology and pathogenesis of, 333–334, *334*
    in pregnancy, 331
    prevalence of, 329–330
    prevention of, 339
    pulmonary, 333
    recurrent, 332
    spectrum of clinical illness from, 331–332
    susceptibility to, 331
    transmission of, 330–331
    traveler's diarrhea, 316
    treatment of, 333, 336–338, 547
      antiretroviral therapy, 338
      benzeneacetonitrile derivatives, 338
      immunomodulatory agents, 338
      macrolides, 336–337
      nitazoxanide, 337–338
      other antiprotozoan agents, 338
      paromomycin, 337
      supportive therapy, 338
CSFs. *See* Colony-stimulating factors
CTLs. *See* Cytotoxic T lymphocytes
CTP. *See* Cytidine triphosphate
Cultural sensitivity, 917
Curcumin, 907t
Cutaneous manifestations, 54, 143t, 144, 499–516
  bacterial infections, 504–506
    bacillary angiomatosis, 309, *309*, 505
    folliculitis, abscesses, furuncles, impetigo, and related infections, *504*, 504–505
    mycobacterial infections, 505–506
    syphilis, 297, 506
  in children, 169
  fungal infections, *507*, 507–509
    aspergillosis, 366, 509
    blastomycosis, 508–509
    cryptococcosis, 361, 508
    histoplasmosis, 508, *508*
    other fungi, 509
    penicilliosis, 366, 509
    sporotrichosis, 366, 508
  managing pain of, 930
  neoplastic disorders, 514–516
    lymphoreticular malignancies, *515*, 515–516
    primary cutaneous neoplasms, 514–515
      basal cell carcinoma, 514
      Bowenoid papulosis, *502*, 514–515
      epidermodysplasia verruciformis, 514–515
      melanoma, 515
      squamous cell carcinoma, 515
  noninfectious disorders, 509–514
    atopic dermatitis, 511–512
    chronic actinic dermatitis, 512
    drug eruptions, 513–514
    eosinophilic folliculitis, 511, *511*
    hair and nail abnormalities, 514
    papular pruritic disorders, 510
    papular urticaria, 512
    porphyria cutanea tarda, 512–513
    prurigo nocularis, 510
    psoriasis, 509–510
    Reiter's syndrome, 510

seborrheic dermatitis, 509, *509*
xerotic dermatitis, 512, *512*
parasitic infections and ectoparasitic infestations, 506–507
acanthamebiasis, 507
pneumocystosis, 195, 507
scabies, 506–507
strongyloidiasis, 507
toxoplasmosis, 234–235
viral infections, 499–504
acute exanthem, 499
cytomegalovirus, *500*, 501
herpesvirus infections, 499–501, *500*
human papillomavirus infections, 501–503, *502*
molluscum contagiosum, *502*, 503–504
oral hairy leukoplakia (Epstein-Barr virus), 501
CXCR4 (fusin), 4, 14–15, 15t, 17–18, 28–29, 59–60, *60*, 611, 691, 781, 861
development of drugs aimed at, 21, 761–762
discovery of, 761
HIV-2 and, 988
in rapid progressors, 52, 67
role in HIV transmission, 19, 102
Cyclophilin A, 30, 763–764
Cyclophosphamide
for adult T-cell leukemia/lymphoma, 1019
for lymphomas, 453, 453t, 516
Cyclosaligenyl prodrugs, *834*, 836–837, *837*
Cyclospora infection, 538, 546, 576
Cyclosporine, 593, 747
Cytarabine (ARA-C), 414, 415
Cytidine triphosphate (CTP), 815, *817*
Cytokines, 7, 68–71, 88, 611–612. *See also* specific cytokines
effects on hematopoiesis, 70–71, 616–620
enhancement of immune response by, 747
HIV effects on production of, 68
induction of HIV expression by, 68–69, *70*
lymphomagenesis and, 443–444
role in cardiomyopathy, 605–606
role in Kaposi's sarcoma, 422–425
role in metabolic disturbances and wasting, 644, 648
effect of anticytokine therapy, 653–654
fat cell catabolism, 644–645
hypertriglyceridemia, 646
in vivo lipid metabolism, 645
role in progressive multifocal leukoencephalopathy, 407–408
role in toxoplasmosis, 227–228
secretion by Th1 and Th2 cells, 5, 71, 88, 88t
strategies to inhibit proinflammatory cytokines, 746–747
suppression of HIV expression by, 69–70, *70*
for toxoplasmosis therapy, 244–245
Cytomegalovirus (CMV) infection, 148, 373–385
adrenalitis, 376, 629
clinical presentations of, 373
coagulation disorders and, 621
colitis, 376, 378, 381, 543–544, *544–545*
cutaneous, *500*, 501
diagnosis of, 374
epidemiology of, 373–374
esophagitis, 376, 538, *539*
gastrointestinal, 648

hematologic abnormalities and, 616
hepatobiliary, 376–377, 549–550, 572, 577, *577*
histopathology of, 374, *374*
HIV disease and, 373–374
neurologic complications of, 377, 470, 485, 489, 490
oral, 526
pancreatic, 556
pituitary, 633
pneumonitis, 376
prevalence in HIV infection, 373, 385
prevention of, 384
prophylaxis for, 146, 384, 464
renal, 596
retinitis, 234, 373–376, 375, 457, 459–464, *460*
autopsy studies of, 463
bilateral, 375
choroidal pneumocystosis and, 467
diagnosis of, 374, *374–375*, 375, 384, 460
differential diagnosis of, 375, 464
natural history of, 461
in pregnancy, 158
prevalence of, 460
rhematogenous retinal detachment and, 464
strains with UL97 mutations, 378, 462, 463
visual loss due to, 375, 460–461
risk related to CD4+ cell count, 373, 374, 460
screening for, 384
testicular, 635
of thyroid, 634
Cytomegalovirus (CMV) treatment, 377–384, 378t
cidofovir, 382–383
for colitis, 378, 547
contribution to mortality of CMV in persons with AIDS, 383–384
for esophagitis, 378
foscarnet, 380–382
future of, 385
ganciclovir, 377–380
for pneumonitis, 378
in pregnancy, 158
for retinitis, 378t, 461–464
combination therapy, 383, 462
development of antiviral resistance, 462
ganciclovir intraocular device, 379–380, 463
intravitreal injections, 379, 382, 463
long-term efficacy, 462–464
salvage therapy, 383
systemic antiviral therapy, 461–463
toxicities of drugs for, 379t
Cytomegalovirus Retinitis Retreatment Trial, 462
Cytosine arabinoside (ARA-C), 414, 415
Cytotoxic T lymphocytes (CTLs), 63, 64, 73, 88, 92–94, 139, 690, 695–696, 744–745
AIDS vaccine development and, 698, 729–730
autologous infusion of expanded cells, 745
CD4+ cells, 73, 696

CD8+ cells, 73, 93–94, 695
disease progression and, 693
long-term nonprogressors, 67, 93, 745
rapid progressors, 67
role of Nef, 37–38
role in control of viral infections, 90, 90t, 92, 695
in tropical spastic paraparesis/HTLV-I-associated myelopathy, 1017, *1018*
Cytovene. *See* Ganciclovir

Danazol, 1020
Dapsone
interaction with didanosine, 786
interaction with saquinavir, 792
for *Pneumocystis carinii* pneumonia, 207
plus trimethoprim, 201t, 206, 206t, 467
in pregnancy, 157
prophylactic, 146, 210–211
for psoriasis, 510
for thrombocytopenia, 614
for toxoplasmosis, 243, 247t
Data collection in clinical trials, 811
Daunorubicin, liposomal, for Kaposi's sarcoma, 429–430
DCs. *See* Dendritic cells
ddAdo. *See* 2′,3′-Dideoxyadenosine
ddC. *See* Zalcitabine
ddI, ddIno. *See* Didanosine
"Dealer's works," 181
Death and dying, 959–961, 982. *See also* Mortality from AIDS
advance directives and powers of attorney, 960, 979–980
aid in dying, 933, 960–961, 961t, 982
estate planning, 979
hospice care, 923–929, 959
palliative care, 929–932, 961–962
staged model of, 916
suicide, 959
tasks of dying patient, 934, 934t
Decubitus ulcers, 930
Dehydroepiandrosterone (DHEA), 631
Delavirdine, 5, 149, 751, 789–790, 839, 863t, 867, 875t
adverse effects of, 784t, 790, 863t, 867
antiretroviral activity of, 790
chemical structure of, *754*, 840
for children, 172
clinical experience with, 790, 867
dosage of, 790, 863t, 867
drug interactions with, 273t, 790, 867
metabolism of, 790
in pregnancy, 157t
viral resistance to, 790, 867
Dementia, 56, 147, 148, 485–489. *See also* AIDS dementia complex
bacillary angiomatosis and, 311
management of, 932
Demographic impact of AIDS epidemic, 118, *118–119*
Demographic variables affecting spread of HIV, 117–118
Demyelination
in AIDS dementia complex, 413
in cytomegalovirus, 413
in progressive multifocal leukoencephalopathy, 403, 410, *410*

Dendritic cells (DCs), 62–66
  dysfunctions of, 76
  follicular (FDCs), 18, 64–66, 89, 94, 693
  functions of, 62
  HIV tropism for, 18, 692
  infection of, 62
  in lymphoid organs, 65
  role in viral persistence, 693
  types of, 62
Dengue fever, 318
Deoxycoformycin, 1020
Deoxycorticosterone, 630
Deoxynojirimycin, 20
17-Deoxysteroids, 630–631
2′-Deoxy-3′-thiacytidine (3TC). *See* Lamivudine
2′-Deoxyuridine, 824, *824*
Depression, 933
Dermatitis. *See also* Cutaneous manifestations
  atopic, 511–512
  chronic actinic, 512
  infective, 1018
  seborrheic, 509, *509*
  xerotic, 512, *512*
Desciclovir, 527
Desipramine, 793, 929
Developing countries, 101, 111–119, 134
  Africa, 101, 111–113, *112–113*, 112t, 118, *119*
  Asia, 114–115, *115*
  benefits of clinical research to, 730–731, 731t
  factors affecting dynamics of HIV spread in, 116–118
    behavioral, 117, 117t
    biologic, 117
    demographic, 117–118
    economic and political, 118
  gender gap in stopping spread of pandemic in, 969–970
  HIV vaccine trials in, 728–739 (*See also* AIDS vaccine development)
  impact of AIDS/HIV epidemic in, 118–119
    accompanying tuberculosis epidemic and, 119
    on demographics, 118, *118–119*
    economic and social, 119, *119*
    on health sector, 118–119
  Latin America, 101, 113–114, *114*
  logistical challenges of conducting clinical trials in, 730
  modes of HIV transmission in, 115–116, 116t
  sexually transmitted diseases in, 725–726
  traditional healing practices in, 903
Development of drugs. *See* Antiretroviral drug development
Dexamethasone
  interaction with protease inhibitors, 792, 852
  for lymphomas, 453, 453t
Dextrin sulfate, 727
DHEA. *See* Dehydroepiandrosterone
Diabetes, drug-induced, 637, 852
Diabetes insipidus, 634, 873
  toxoplasmosis and, 233, 234
Diagnosis of HIV infection, 53, 661–669
  in blood specimens from adults, 661–664
    antibody testing, 53, 140, 662–663
    defining window of seroconversion, 661–662, *662*
    testing algorithms, 664, 664t
    testing for p24 antigen and HIV RNA, 663–664, 673–682
    Western blot for confirmation of reactivity, 663
  in developing countries, 733
  in donated blood, 661
  ethical issues related to HIV testing, 957–958
  HIV-2, 985, 986t, 992–993
  HIV-1 variability and, 668–669
    emerging variants, 669
    HIV clades, 668
    testing HIV variants, 668–669
  home testing systems for, 668, 957
  in infants and children, 167, 171, 664–667
    considerations in infants, 664–665, 665t
    peripheral blood mononuclear cell culture, 665–666
    plasma HIV-1 RNA detection, 666
    qualitative DNA polymerase chain reaction, 666
    specificity of, 665
    testing algorithm, 666–667
  late in infection, 661
  after occupational exposures, 949
  in oral fluids, 667
  rapid assays for, 667–668
  in urine specimens, 667
  in women, 153–154, 158–159
Dialysis, 587, 588, 588t, 594
Diarrhea, 144, 146, 147, 538, 541–548
  adenovirus, 544
  AIDS enteropathy, 546–547, 649
  approach to patient with, 542, *543*
  bacterial, 546, 548
  Clostridium difficile, 546, *547*
  cryptosporidiosis, 327–339, 545, 547
  cytomegalovirus, 376, 378, 543–544, *544–545*, 547
  diagnostic evaluation of, 538, 542
  drug-induced, 543
  empiric therapy for, 542
  etiology of, 542–547, 544t
  fungal, 545
  herpes simplex virus, 545, 547
  microsporidiosis, 339–344, 545–546, 548
  mycobacterial infection, 292, 546
  prevalence of, 541
  prognostic significance of, 542
  protozoa, 545–546
  traveler's, 315–317, 320, 322
  treatment of, 547–548, 931–932
  wasting syndrome and, 648–649
Diclazuril sodium, 338
Dicloxacillin, 505
Didanosine (ddI, ddIno), 5, 149, 601, 728, 751, 780, 785–786, 863t, 864–865
  adverse effects of, 784t, 785–786, 863t, 865t
    hepatic, 552, 576
    neuropathy, 490, 865
    pancreatitis, 543, 557, 865
    renal, 585
  antiretroviral activity of, 785
  chemical structure of, *753, 830*
  for children, 172–173
    atrophy of peripheral retinal pigment epithelium and, 470
  clinical trials of, 785, 865
  combined with other drugs, 876–878 (*See also* Combination antiretroviral therapy)
    interferon-α, 765
    zidovudine, 783–785
  dosage of, 782t, 785, 863t, 865t
  drug interactions with, 786
    antituberculosis drugs, 273t
    ganciclovir, 379
    indinavir, 795
  formulations of, 785
  metabolism of, 785, 830–832, *831*
  pharmacology of, 785, 830–832, 864–865
  for postexposure prophylaxis, 949
  during pregnancy, 156, 157t, 785
  viral resistance to, 782, 875t, 894
2′,3′-Didehydro-2′,3′-dideoxythymidine (d4T). *See* Stavudine
2′,3′-Dideoxyadenosine (ddAdo), 753, *830–831*, 830–832
2′,3′-Dideoxycytosine (ddC). *See* Zalcitabine
2′,3′-Dideoxy-2′-fluoro-9-β-D-arabinofuranosyadenine (2′-FddaraA), 832, *832*
−2′,3′-Dideoxy-5-fluoro-3′-thiacytidine (FTC), 828–829, 828–830
2′,3′-Dideoxyinosine. *See* Didanosine
2′,3′-Dideoxynucleosides, 752, *752*, 819–833, 819–834. *See also* Reverse transcriptase inhibitors
−2′,3′-Dideoxy-3′-thiacytidine (3TC). *See* Lamivudine
Diet, 148
  hyperalimentation, 644, 650–651
  lactose-free, low-fat, 542
α-Difluoromethylornithine, 338
DiGeorge syndrome, 168
1,25-Dihydroxy vitamin D level, 637–638
Dilantin. *See* Phenytoin
Diphenoxylate, 931
Diphtheria vaccine, 171, 321, 322
Direct cytopathicity, HIV-mediated, 72
Directives of care, 960, 979–980
Disability insurance, 981
Discrimination, 132–133, 980–981
  federal law and, 967, 980–981
  state law and, 980
Distal sensory polyneuropathy (DSPN), 490
Disulfiram, 907t
DLE. *See* Bovine dialyzable leukocyte extract
DMP-266, 149, 840, *840*
  combined with indinavir, 851
  viral resistance to, 875t
DMP-450, *755*, 760
DNCB, 907t
N-Docosonal, 727
Doxepin cream, 507, 511
Doxorubicin
  for adult T-cell leukemia/lymphoma, 1019
  cardiotoxicity of, 606
  liposomal, for Kaposi's sarcoma, 429–430
  for lymphomas, 453, 453t, 516
Doxycycline
  for bacillary angiomatosis, 311, 505
  for *Campylobacter*, 317

for malaria, 320, 320t
pill esophagitis due to, 539–540
for toxoplasmosis, 244
for traveler's diarrhea, 322
DPM 266. *See* Efavirenz
Dronabinol, 651, 932
Drug abuse. *See* Injecting drug users
Drug interactions
among antiretroviral agents, 885–887
in vitro, 885–886, 886t
pharmacokinetic, 886–887, 886t
with antituberculous agents, 272–273, 273t
with delavirdine, 790
with didanosine, 786
with fluconazole, 525
with foscarnet, 382
with ganciclovir, 379
with protease inhibitors, 850–852, 850t, 867–868
with zalcitabine, 786, 787
with zidovudine, 785
Drug-induced disorders. *See also* adverse effects listed under specific drugs
acid-base and electrolyte disorders, 585–586, 586t
cardiomyopathy, 606
cutaneous eruptions, 143t, 513–514
diarrhea, 543
endocrine abnormalities, 631, 632t, 637, 852
gonadal dysfunction, 636
hepatotoxicity, 552–553, 552t, 575–576
hypocalcemia, 637–638
myelosuppression, 615
ocular, 457, 470
pancreatitis, 543, 556–557, 637, 865, 866
pill esophagitis, 539–540
Drug-resistant infections
cytomegalovirus, 378–379, 462
herpesviruses, 501
HIV (*See* Antiretroviral drug resistance)
in patients with hematologic abnormalities, 612
tuberculosis, 265–266, 266t
DSPN. *See* Distal sensory polyneuropathy
d4T. *See* Stavudine
Duffy antigen, 15
Durable power of attorney, 960, 979–980
Duty to treat persons with HIV/AIDS, 955–956
Duty to warn persons at risk of HIV, 981
Dying patient. *See* Death and dying
Dyspepsia, 541
Dysphagia, 147, 358, 538, 650
Dyspnea, 932

Early intervention, 53, 130–131
Early symptomatic disease, 54–55, 143–146
diarrhea, 144
fatigue, 144
fever and night sweats, 144
headache, 143–144
laboratory abnormalities in, 145
management of, 145
mucocutaneous conditions, 143t, 144
oral complications, 143t, 144, 521
preventing opportunistic infections, 145–146

EBV. *See* Epstein-Barr virus
Economic impact of HIV/AIDS, 119
"Ecstasy," 576
Eczema craquele, 512
Edema, peripheral, 592
Educational programs for prevention, 128, 963
Efavirenz, 149, 840, *840*
combined with indinavir, 851
viral resistance to, 875t
Efudex. *See* 5-Fluorouracil
EIAV. *See* Equine infectious anemia virus
Elavil. *See* Amitriptyline
Electroencephalography (EEG), 413
Electrolyte disorders, 585–586, 586t
ELISA. *See* Enzyme-linked immunosorbent assay
Emotional distress, 911, 933. *See also* Psychosocial interventions
E-mycin. *See* Erythromycin
Encephalitis, 479
cytomegalovirus, 377, 470, 485, 489
herpes simplex, 485
toxoplasmic, 225, 230–234, *231*, 233t, 245
Encephalitozoon infection. *See* Microsporidiosis
Encephalopathy
bacillary angiomatosis and, 311
in children, 169, 486
progressive multifocal leukoencephalopathy, 403–415
Endocarditis, 311, 602
Endocrine abnormalities, 629–638
adrenal gland, 629–632
bone and mineral homeostasis, 637–638
drug-induced, 631, 632t
gonadal function, 635–636
hypothalamic-pituitary axis, 632–634
pancreas, 636–637
thyroid, 634–635
in toxoplasmosis, 233, 234
wasting syndrome and, 648
End-of-life decision making, 933, 960–961, 961t, 982
Endophthalmitis, fungal, 457
Endoscopic retrograde cholangiopancreatography (ERCP), 555, 577
Endoscopy, diagnostic, 542
Endothelin-1, 458
Endotoxin, 645, 653
Energy balance, 644, 646–649. *See also* Wasting syndrome
Entamoeba histolytica infection, 316, 546, 550
Enteral nutrition, 650–651
Enterocytozoon bieneusi infection. *See* Microsporidiosis
Enteropathy, 649
env gene, 23–24, *32*, 59, 90, 611, 696
of HIV-2, 985, 988
of HTLV-I and HTLV-II, 1004, *1005*
Envelope glycoproteins, 26–28, 59, 611, 618, 694–695
AIDS vaccine development and, 697–698, 699t, 701t
of HIV-2, 992
Enzyme-linked immunosorbent assay (ELISA), 140, 167, 698
Eosinophilic folliculitis, 143t, 511, *511*
Eosinophils, 88

Epidemiology of HIV infection, 3, 911
among injecting drug users, 180
among women, 151–152
in children, 112t, 116, 163
in developing world, 111–119 (*See also* Developing countries)
future of AIDS epidemic, 8–9
global nature of pandemic, 111, *112*, 112t, 134, 968–969
HIV-2 infection, 986–988, 987t
incidence of HIV/AIDS, 611
public health issues, 123–134
sexual transmission, 101–107 (*See also* Sexual transmission of HIV)
variables influencing dynamics of spread, 116–118, 116t
behavioral, 117, 117t
biologic, 117
demographic, 117–118
economic and political, 118
Epidemiology of HTLV-I and HTLV-II infections, 1007–1010
Epidermodysplasia verruciformis, 501, 503, 514–515
Epitopes recognized by B cells, 90–91, *91*
Epivir. *See* Lamivudine
Epstein-Barr virus (EBV) infection, 75, 144, 501, 526–527, *527*
hepatic, 572
oral hairy leukoplakia, 144, 501, 526–527, *527*
role in lymphomagenesis, 440–442, 452
oral lymphomas, 523
as therapeutic target, 446
Equine infectious anemia virus (EIAV), 25, *32*
ERCP. *See* Endoscopic retrograde cholangiopancreatography
Ergot derivative interactions with protease inhibitors, 852
Ery-Tab. *See* Erythromycin
Erythema multiforme, 513–514
Erythromycin
for bacillary angiomatosis, 311, 505, 575
for *Campylobacter*, 317
hepatotoxicity of, 552
Erythropoiesis, 70
Erythropoietin, 70, 617
Escherichia coli infection, 316, 546, 587
Esophageal disease, 147, 538–541
approach to patient with, *540*
bacterial, 539, 541
candidal, 55, 139, 147, 523, 538
in children, 170
diagnosis of, 540
treatment of, 170, 540
cytomegaloviral, 376, 538, *539*
diagnosis of, 540
foscarnet for, 381, 540–541
ganciclovir for, 378, 540–541
diagnosis of, 540
etiology of, 538–540, 539t
fungal, 538
malignant, 539
pill esophagitis, 539–540
prevalence of, 538
symptoms of, 538
treatment of, 540–541

Esophageal disease—*Continued*
  ulcers, 539, *539*, 541
  viral, 538–539
Estate planning, 979
Estradiol, 635
Ethambutol
  for *Mycobacterium avium* complex infection, 291, 291t, 548
  in pregnancy, 158
  renal toxicity of, 585
  for tuberculosis, 271–272, 271t
Ethical issues, 951–972, 952t
  biomedical ethics, 953
  clinical ethics, 953–962
    aims of, 953
    competing ethical perspectives, 954
    confidentiality and privacy, 956–957
    counseling before and after testing, 957–958
    counseling HIV-infected women about reproductive choices, 958–959
    death and dying, 959–961, 961t
    ethical principles, 954, 954t
    HIV testing and reporting, 957
    HIV/AIDS and, 954–955, 955t
    informed consent for testing, 958
    obligation to treat persons with HIV/AIDS, 955–956
    palliative care as standard of care, 961–962
    resources of, 953t
  ethics, power, and HIV/AIDS, 951–953
  at global level, 968–972
    international research ethics, 970–972
    stopping spread of pandemic: gender gap, 969–970
  HIV vaccine research, 736–738
    building structures for ethical research, 737–738
    in developing countries, 733, 736
    informed consent and independent, non-coerced participation, 737
    just distribution of risk and benefit, 736–737
    maximizing benefits and minimizing risks, 737
  physician-patient relationship, 952
  randomized trials, 810
  social ethics, 962–968, 962t
    drug testing and other research practices, 967–968
    notification of partners and at-risk persons, 131–132, 965–966
    population screening, 129–131, 963–965, 964t
    primary prevention and universal access to primary health care, 962–963, 963t
    screening health care workers and their status if HIV positive, 966–967
Ethionamide, 552
Etoposide, 453, 453t
Etretinate, 510
Europe, *112*, 112t
European Collaborative Study, 166, 167
Euthanasia, 933, 960–961, 961t, 982
Euthyroid sick syndrome, 634, 648
Exanthem of HIV disease, 499

Exercise, 652
Existential issues, 916
Experimental design, 807–811. *See also* Clinical trials
Experimental drugs. *See* Antiretroviral drug development; Investigational drugs
Eye Bank Association of America, 471
Eye disease. *See* Ocular sequelae

Facial palsy, 491
Failure to thrive, 633
Famciclovir
  effects on hepatitis B virus coinfection, 570
  for herpesvirus infections, 393–394, 501
    herpes zoster, 397–398
    postexposure prophylaxis, 500
Family issues, 932–933
Fansidar. *See* Pyrimethamine-sulfadoxine
Fat, body, 643–644, 651
Fat cell catabolism, 644–645
Fatigue, 144, 146, 651–652
Fatty acid synthesis, 645
Fc receptors, 17, 611
FDA. *See* U.S. Food and Drug Administration
FDCs. *See* Dendritic cells, follicular
FddA. *See* 2′-β-Fluoro-2′,3′-dideoxyadenosine
2′-FddaraA. *See* 2′,3′-Dideoxy-2′-fluoro-9-β-D-arabinofluranosyadenine
Federal Vocational Rehabilitation Act of 1973, 980
Feline immunodeficiency virus (FIV), 25, 32
Female condom, 105, 129
Fentanyl transdermal patch, 931
Ferritin serum levels, 612
Fever, 144, 146, 148
  bacillary angiomatosis and, 310–311
  differential diagnosis in HIV-infected travelers, 315, 317–319, 318t
  management of, 931
Fialuridine, 553
Fibrinolytic defects, 621
Fibroblasts, 611
Fifapentine, 244
Filariasis, 318
Filgrastim. *See* Granulocyte colony-stimulating factor
Fish oil, 653
Fistula, bronchopulmonary, 195
FIV. *See* Feline immunodeficiency virus
Flagyl. *See* Metronidazole
FLT. *See* 3′-Fluoro-2′,3′-dideoxythymidine
Fluconazole
  for candidiasis, 154, 359, 359t, 525, 540
    prophylactic, 360
  for coccidioidomycosis, 365
  for cryptococcosis, 362–363, 362t
    prophylactic, 363–364
    for suppression, 363
  for disseminated infections, 509
  drug interactions with, 525
  for hepatic fungi, 573
  for histoplasmosis, 364–365
  in pregnancy, 157–158
Flucytosine, 362–363, 467
Fludrocortisone, 632
2′-β-Fluoro-2′,3′-dideoxyadenosine (FddA), 751, *753*, 757, 788

3′-Fluoro-2′,3′-dideoxythymidine (FLT), *752*, 824–825, *825–826*
5-Fluorouracil
  for Bowenoid papulosis, 515
  for cloacogenic carcinoma, 432
  for toxoplasmosis, 244
  for verruca plana and filiform verrucae, 503
Focal epithelial hyperplasia, 527, *528*
Follicle-stimulating hormone (FSH), 635, 636
Follicular dendritic cells (FDCs), 64–66, 89, 94
Folliculitis, 143t, *504*, 504–505
  eosinophilic, 511, *511*
Follow-up
  of clinical trial subjects, 812
  after occupational HIV exposure, 949–950
Fomivirsen, 385, 470
Fortovase. *See* Saquinavir
Foscarnet
  for acyclovir-resistant herpesvirus infections, 395, 398, 501, 541
  adverse effects of, 379t, 381–382, 395, 541
    cutaneous ulcerations, 513–514
    endocrine, 632t
    hypocalcemia, 586, 637–638
    renal, 541, 585–587
  for cytomegalovirus infection, 380–382
    colitis, 378, 381, 547
    cutaneous, 501
    esophageal, 381, 540–541
    retinitis, 378t, 380–381, 461–463
      intravitreal injection, 382, 463
  drug interactions with, 382, 787
  for Kaposi's sarcoma, 431–432
  mechanism of action of, 380
  in pregnancy, 158
  for varicella-zoster virus retinitis, 465
Foscarnet-Ganciclovir CMV Retinitis Trial, 461
Fosinopril, 593
French Collaborative Study, 166
FSH. *See* Follicle-stimulating hormone
FTC. *See* −2′,3′-Dideoxy-5-fluoro-3′-thiacytidine
Fumagillin, 344
Funding
  for AIDS vaccine research, 731–732
  for HIV prevention and treatment, 101–102
Fungal infections, 357–366. *See also* specific fungi
  aspergillosis, 366, 509
  blastomycosis, 366
  bone marrow failure and, 615–616
  candidiasis, 357–360
  in children, 169
  coccidioidomycosis, 318, 365
  corneal ulcers, 468
  cryptococcosis, 360–364, 508
  cutaneous, *507*, 507–509
  diarrhea due to, 545
  endocarditis, 602
  endophthalmitis, 457
  esophageal, 538
  hepatic, 550, *550*, 572–573, *573*
  histoplasmosis, 318, 364–365, 508, *508*
  management in pregnancy, 157–158
  mucormycosis, 366
  of nails, 514
  oral, 523–525, *524–525*
  penicilliosis, 318, 365–366, 509

of retina and choroid, 466–467
sporotrichosis, 366, 508
in travelers, 318
Fungizone. *See* Amphotericin B
fur gene, 441
Furunculosis, 504, *504*
Fusarium infection, 467
Fusin (CXCR4), 4, 14–15, 15t, 17–18, 28–29, 59–60, *60*, 611, 691, 781, 861
development of drugs aimed at, 21, 761–762
discovery of, 761
HIV-2 and, 988
in rapid progressors, 52, 67
role in HIV transmission, 19, 102
Fusobacterium infection, 575
Futile care, 923
Future considerations
AIDS epidemic, 8–9
antiretroviral therapy, 798, 870, 880–882
cytomegalovirus therapy, 385
psychosocial interventions, 920–921

Gabapentin, 930
gag gene, 23–24, 611, 702, 759
of HIV-2, 988, 992
of HTLV-I and HTLV-II, 1004, *1005*
gag gene products, 24, 29–31, 90
capsid protein, 24, 29–30, 764, *989*
matrix protein, 24, 30, 764, *989*
NC protein, 30
p6, 30–31
gag/pol polyprotein, 31, 790
Galactocerebroside, 16, 692
Galactosylceramide, 611
Gallbladder disease. *See* Biliary tract disease
Ganciclovir
adverse effects of, 379, 379t, 462
hepatotoxicity, 552
myelosuppression, 540, 615
for cytomegalovirus infection, 377–380
colitis, 547
cutaneous, 501
development of resistance to, 378–379, 383, 462
esophageal, 540–541
retinitis, 377–378, 378t, 461–464
intraocular device, 379–380, 383, 463
intravitreal injection, 379, 463
prophylaxis, 464
drug interactions with, 379
for Kaposi's sarcoma, 431–432
leukocyte growth factors used with, 462
oral formulation of, 377, 541
for oral hairy leukoplakia, 527
oral vs. intravenous formulations of, 377, 462
pharmacokinetics of, 377
in pregnancy, 158
valine ester prodrug of, 385
for varicella-zoster virus retinitis, 465
Gastrointestinal manifestations, 147, 537–559
AIDS enteropathy, 538, 649
bacillary angiomatosis, 309–310
clinical significance of, 537
cryptosporidiosis, 327–339
cytomegalovirus colitis, 376
enterocolitis and diarrhea, 541–548
esophageal disease, 538–541

gastric disease, 541
general approach to patient with, 537–538, 538t
hepatobiliary disease, 548–553, 567–578
microsporidiosis, 327, 339–344
pancreatic disease, 556–558, 636–637
peritoneal and mesenteric disease, 558–559
prevalence of, 537
toxoplasmosis, 232, 234
treatment of, 650
wasting syndrome and, 648–649
G-CSF. *See* Granulocyte colony-stimulating factor
GDP. *See* Guanine diphosphate
Gene products, viral, 23–41, 862
accessory, 23, 36–41
effects on virus life cycle, 37, *38*
of HIV-2, 991–992
Nef protein, 36–38
Vif protein, 38–39
Vpr/Vpx proteins, 39–41
Vpu protein, 39
envelope and virus-mediated cytopathicity, 28–29
envelope glycoproteins, 26–28
gag gene products, 29–31
of HIV-2, *991*, 991–992
interaction with cellular ligands, 23
long terminal repeat, 24, *32*, 35, 568
pol gene products, 31–35, *32–34*
Tat and Rev proteins, 24–25, 35–36
Gene therapy, 21
Genetics
accessory genes, 25
genes involved in disease progression, 67
genetic variability of HIV-1, 3–4, 117, 668–669, 694, 765, 891
genetic variability of HIV-2, 985–986
genomic organization of HTLV-I and HTLV-II, 1004, *1005*
genomic organization of lentiviruses, 3, 23–26, *24–25*, *32*, 611
genotypes associated with natural resistance to HIV entry, 17
molecular genetics of AIDS-related lymphomas, 440–441
mutations associated with drug resistance, 678, 765–769, 782, 874, 875t, 891–898 (*See also* Antiretroviral drug resistance)
risk of sexual HIV transmission and, 102–103
role in Kaposi's sarcoma, 422
Genital warts, 501–503
Gentamicin
for bacillary angiomatosis, 311, 505
for *Mycobacterium avium* complex infection, 291–292, 291t
Geotrichosis, oral, 525
Germinal center hyperplasia, 65, *65*
G31G, 727
GGP64222, 763
GH. *See* Growth hormone
Giardia lamblia infection, 316, 546
Gingivitis, 528
Glial cells, 611
neurotropism of JC virus for, 404
in progressive multifocal leukoencephalopathy, 403, 410, *410*

Glial specific factor (GF1), 405–406
Global HIV/AIDS pandemic, 111, *112*, 112t, 134, 968–969. *See also* Epidemiology of HIV infection
γ-Globulin preparations, 126, 614
for children, 169–170, 172
Glomerulonephritis, immune-complex, 595–596
rapidly progressive, 587
Glomerulopathies, chronic, 588, 589t
Glomerulosclerosis, 588–594
clinical course of, 592
demography and epidemiology of, 588–589
dialysis for, 594
medical treatment of, 592–594
pathogenesis of, 590–591, 590t
pathology of, 589–590, 589t
prevalence of, 589
renal transplantation for, 594
Glucocorticoid resistance, 631
Glucocorticoid secretion, 629–632
abnormalities in HIV infection, 630–631
medication effects on, 631, 632t
Glucose-6-phosphate dehydrogenase (G6PD) deficiency, 322
Glutathione, 770
Glycosylation, 26
GM-CSF. *See* Granulocyte-macrophage colony-stimulating factor
GMP. *See* Guanine monophosphate
GnRH. *See* Gonadotropin-releasing hormone
Gonadal function, 635–636
Gonadotropin-releasing hormone (GnRH), 635–636
Gonorrhea, 319–320, 506, 726, 727
gp41 (TM), 13, 20, 26, 59, 73, 90, 694–695, 730–731, 781, 861, *989*
fusogenic activity of, 15, *16*, 28
gp120 (SU), 20, 26–28, 59, *60*, 68, 72, 90, 611, 618, 695, 780–781, 861, *989*
binding to CD4, 13, 15, *16*, 695
in HIV vaccine research, 697–698, 743
viral tropism and, 18
gp160, 26, 59, 618, 695, 861
in HIV vaccine research, 697–698, 744
Granulocyte colony-stimulating factor (G-CSF), 573, 617, 864
administered with ganciclovir, 462
exogenous administration of, 617
for lymphomas, 453
production in HIV infection, 616
Granulocyte-macrophage colony-stimulating factor (GM-CSF), 68, 193, 617
administered with ganciclovir, 462
administered with zidovudine, 617
induction of HIV expression by, 69
for lymphomas, 453
production in HIV infection, 616
regulatory influence on early T-cell development, 70
Granulocytopenia, 613
Granuloma inguinale, 319, 319t, 506
Grief counseling, 920. *See also* Psychosocial interventions
Growth hormone (GH), 633, 652
GS 840 (adefovir dipivoxil), 757, 788, 875t
GTP. *See* Guanine triphosphate
Guanine diphosphate (GDP), 815, *816*, 818

Guanine monophosphate (GMP), 815, *816*, 818, *818*
Guanine triphosphate (GTP), 815, *816*, 818
Guillain-Barré syndrome, 479
Gut-associated lymphoid tissue, 537
Gynecologic complications, 152. *See also* Women and HIV infection
 cervical dysplasia/cancer, 143, 148, 152, 154
 management of, 154
 menstrual cycle, 152, 636
 pelvic inflammatory disease, 152, 154
 vaginal candidiasis, 152, 154, 357, 358

H_2 blockers, 541, 786
HAART. *See* Antiretroviral therapy, highly active
Haemophilus ducreyi infection, 319, 319t, 506
Haemophilus influenzae infection, 55, 169
 endocarditis, 602
 of head and neck, 504
Haemophilus influenzae vaccine, 169, 171, 322
 during pregnancy, 155
Hair abnormalities, 514
Hairy cell leukemia (HCL), 1019
Hairy leukoplakia (HL), 144, 501, 521, 526–527, *526–527*
 differentiation from candidiasis, 358
 Epstein-Barr virus and, 144, 501, 526–527, *527*
 histology of, 526–527, *527*
 prevalence of, 522
 prognostic significance of, 526
 treatment of, 501, 527
Harm reduction, 188, 912–913
HAV. *See* Hepatitis A virus infection
HBV. *See* Hepatitis B virus infection
HBY-097, 839, *840*, 875t
HCL. *See* Hairy cell leukemia
HCV. *See* Hepatitis C virus infection
HD. *See* Hodgkin's disease
HDV. *See* Hepatitis delta virus infection
Headache, 143–144, 479, 489–490, 930
Health care environment and HIV transmission, 127, 152, 935–942, 947–950
 during cardiovascular surgery, 607
 documented occupational infections, 936, 947
 guidelines for providers infected with blood-borne pathogens, 935
 HIV infections in health care workers not documented by seroconversion, 936
 managing occupational exposures, 869–870, 939–941, 940t–941t, 947–950 (*See also* Postexposure prophylaxis)
  follow-up care for exposed persons, 949–950
  postoperative interventions to decrease infection risk, 947–949
 OSHA standard on bloodborne pathogens, 935
 patients' risks of infection from HIV-infected health care workers, 941–942, 966–967
 related to ocular infections and procedures, 471–472
 reporting occupational infections, 936, 950
 risk factors for occupational transmission, 936–938, 936t–937t, 948
 screening health care workers, 966–967, 982
 strategies for reducing occupational risk, 938–939, 938t, 947
 stress response to occupational exposure, 949–950
Health care reform, 962–963
Health insurance, 963, 981
Heart. *See* Cardiac involvement
Heck's disease, 527, *528*
Helicobacter pylori infection, 541
Helper T lymphocytes, 59
Helplessness, 905
Helsinki Code, 971
Hematologic abnormalities, 61, 140, 611–621
 anemia, 612–613
 bone marrow abnormalities, 614–615, 614t
 causes of, 612t, 615–620
  altered hematopoiesis from tumor, infection, or medications, 60–61, 615–616
  cytomegalovirus, 616
  parvovirus B19, 616
  zidovudine, 615, 784, 822, 864
 bone marrow progenitor cells, 618–619
 colony-stimulating factors, 616–618
  erythropoietin, 617
  granulocyte colony-stimulating factor, 617
  granulocyte-monocyte colony-stimulating factor, 617
  interleukin-3, 618
  stem cell factor, 617
 hematopoietic microenvironment, 620
 other cytokines and interleukins, 70–71, 619–620
  interferons, 619
  interleukin-1, 619
  interleukin-2, 619
  interleukin-6, 619
  transforming growth factor-β, 620
  tumor necrosis factor, 619–620
 coagulation disorders, 620–621
 effect of reducing or interrupting therapy due to, 612
 neutropenia, 613
 thrombocytopenia, 613–614, 614t
Hemolysis, immune, 613
Hemolytic-uremic syndrome (HUS), 587
Heparin cofactor II deficiency, 621
Hepatic fatty acid synthesis, 645
Hepatitis, 139–141, 550–551, 567–572. *See also* Liver disease
Hepatitis A virus (HAV) infection, 318, 567
Hepatitis B virus (HBV) infection, 319t, 550–551, 567–571, *568*
 among injecting drug users, 185
 bone marrow suppression and, 616
 clinical course in HIV-infected persons, 568–569, 569t
 guidelines for health care providers infected with, 935
 hepatitis delta and, 571–572
 immunization against, 322
  for children, 171
  effects of HIV infection on response to, 551, 570
  for pregnant women, 155
 molecular interactions with HIV, 568
 prevalence in HIV-infected persons, 550, 567
 therapeutic implications of HIV coinfection, 569–571
  famciclovir, 570
  interferon-α, 555, 569–570
  lamivudine, 570
  protease inhibitors, 570
  reactivation of hepatitis B viral replication, 570–571
  reduced response to hepatitis B vaccine, 570
  zidovudine, 570
 transmission of, 550, 567
 in travelers, 318
Hepatitis C virus (HCV) infection, 458, 551, 571
 among injecting drug users, 185, 571
 bone marrow suppression and, 616
 clinical course in HIV-infected persons, 551, 571
 diagnosis of, 551
 therapeutic implications of HIV coinfection, 571
  interferon-α, 555, 571
  ribavirin, 571
  zidovudine, 571
 transmission of, 551, 571
Hepatitis delta virus (HDV) infection, 571–572
 hepatitis B and, 571–572
 transmission of, 571
Hepatitis E virus (HEV) infection, 572
Hepatitis G virus (HGV) infection, 572
Hepatocytes, 551
Hepatomegaly, 553, 567
Hepatotoxic drugs, 552–553, 552t, 575–576
Herbal medicine, 906
Herpes simplex virus (HSV) infection, 391–396, 499–501, *500*
 acyclovir-resistant, 394–395
 clinical features of, 391–392
 coagulation disorders and, 621
 complications of, 392
 diagnosis of, 392
 diarrhea due to, 545
 encephalitis, 485
 epidemiology of, 391
 esophageal, 541
 genital, 319t, 391–393
 hepatic, 550, 572
 histopathology of, 500
 mucocutaneous, 143t, 144, 391
 oral, 525, *526*
 pathogenesis of, 391
 retinitis, 465
 treatment of, 392–395, 501, 547
 vaccines for prevention of, 395–396, 690, 691
Herpes zoster, 143t, 144, 396–397, 499–501, *500*
 clinical features of, 396
 neurologic complications of, 397
 ophthalmicus, 397, 468

orofacial, 525–526
  pain of, 930
  postherpetic neuralgia and, 397, 500, 526
  treatment of, 397–398, 930
Heterosexual HIV transmission, 104, 115, 151
HEV. *See* Hepatitis E virus infection
HGPRT. *See* Hypoxanthine/guanine phosphoribosyl transferase
HGV. *See* Hepatitis G virus infection
HHV8. *See* Human herpesvirus-8
"Hiccups," 538
Histamine-2 blockers, 541, 786
Histiocytic erythrophagocytosis, 615
Histopathology
  acute exanthem of HIV disease, 499
  of AIDS dementia complex, 487–489
  bacillary angiomatosis, 307–308, *307–308*, 505
  bacillary peliosis hepatis, 549, *550*
  chronic actinic dermatitis, 512
  condylomata acuminata, 503
  cryptosporidiosis, 333–334, *334*
  cutaneous cytomegalovirus, 501
  cutaneous lymphoma, 515–516
  cutaneous syphilis, 506
  cytomegalovirus, 374, *374*
  glomerulosclerosis, 589–590, 589t
  herpesvirus infections, 500
  impetigo, 505
  Kaposi's sarcoma, 425, *425*
  lymphomas, 439, 451–452
  molluscum contagiosum, 503–504
  morbilliform drug eruptions, 513
  mycobacterial infections
    cutaneous, 506
    Mycobacterium avium complex, 287–288
    tuberculosis, 268, *268*
  nonspecific liver lesions, 576
  oral hairy leukoplakia, 501, 526–527, *527*
  Pneumocystis carinii pneumonia, 194–195
  porphyria cutanea tarda, 513
  progressive multifocal leukoencephalopathy, 403, *404*, 410, *410–411*
  psoriasis, 510
  seborrheic dermatitis, 509
  toxoplasmosis, 230–232, *231*, 237
Histoplasmosis, 147, 364–365
  bone marrow failure and, 615
  clinical features of, 364
  cutaneous manifestations of, 507–508, *508*
  diagnosis of, 364
  epidemiology of, 364
  gastrointestinal, 545
  hepatic, 550, 572–573, *573*
  intraocular, 467
  meningitis, 364, 490
  microbiology of, 364
  myocardial, 601
  oral, 525, *525*
  prophylaxis against, 365
  renal, 596
  in travelers, 318
  treatment of, 364–365
History of early epidemic, 124
Hivid. *See* Zalcitabine
HIVIG. *See* Hyperimmune anti-HIV immunoglobulin
HIVNET, 731

HLAs. *See* Human leukocyte antigens
HMG I(Y), 33
Hodgkin's disease (HD), 148, 439–440, 451–452. *See also* Lymphomas
  cutaneous, 515
  hepatic, 551, 575
  prognostic indicators for, 453
  treatment of, 453
Home HIV testing systems, 668, 957
Homelessness, 132
Homeopathy, 906–907
Homophobia, 905
Homosexual HIV transmission, 188, 537
Hormones. *See* Endocrine abnormalities
Hospice care, 923–929. *See also* Palliative care
  admission of AIDS patients into, 924–925
  AIDS services organizations and, 925
  antiretroviral therapy in, 925–926
  family issues, 932–933
  indications for, 923
  Medicare reimbursement for, 923–924
  multidisciplinary team for, 923
  psychosocial issues, 933
  referral to, 926
    case examples of, 928
    palliation flow chart for, 926–928, *927*
  settings for, 923
  spiritual issues, 933–934
  symptom management, 929–932
  tasks of dying patient, 934, 934t
  transition to, 925–926
  treatments in, 928–929
Host cell receptors, 4, 13–21, 59–60, *60*, 91, 691, 861
  CD4+ cells, 4, 13, 59, 91
  coreceptors, 4, 13–16, *15–16*, 15t, 59–60, *60*, 91, 691
  other, 16–17, 16t
  therapeutic strategies related to, 20–21
  viral evolution and, 17–18
  viral tropism and, 18, *18*
Housing, 132
HPV. *See* Human papillomavirus infection
HSV. *See* Herpes simplex virus infection
HTLV-I and HTLV-II. *See* Human T-lymphotropic viruses
Human foamy virus, 25
Human herpesvirus-6, 616
Human herpesvirus-8 (HHV-8), 4, 423–424, 442–443, 447, 521–522
Human immunodeficiency virus type 1 (HIV-1), 13–21, 611–612
  antigenic properties of viral proteins, 90–92
    determinants recognized by T cells, 92
    epitopes recognized by B cells, 90–91, *91*
    neutralization of field strains of HIV-1 by antibody, 91–92
  cellular targets for, 13–21, 14t, 59, 611–612, 691–692, 861
  drug resistant, 765–769, 891–898 (*See also* Antiretroviral drug resistance)
  evolution of, 17–18
  genetic variability of, 3–4, 117, 668–669, 694, 765, 891
    clades, 3–4, 668
    emerging variants, 9, 669
    group M strains, 3, 60

group O strains, 3, 668–669
  mutations associated with drug resistance, 678, 765–769, 782, 874, 875t, 891–898
  testing for, 668–669
  vaccine development and, 729–730
genomic organization of, 3, 23–26, *32*, 611
host cell receptors for, 4, 13–21, 59–60, *60*, 92 (*See also* Host cell receptors)
initial identification of, 59
interactions with hepatitis B virus, 568
life cycle of, 861–862 (*See also* Viral replication)
natural resistance to, 4, 17, 52, 693–694
neutralization of, 20 (*See also* Antibodies, neutralizing)
plasma HIV-1 RNA level, 51, 139–141, 140t, 148, 673–682, 862–863, 876 (*See also* Plasma HIV-1 RNA level)
reservoir for, 148
routes of infection by, 94–95
sanctuary sites for, 94, 876, 885
structure of, 90, *989*
tropism of, *18*, 18–19, 102, 691–692
Human immunodeficiency virus type 2 (HIV-2), 985–995
  accessory genes and gene products of, *991*, 991–992
  cell attachment of, 988–990
  cellular targets of, 988
  clinical outcome of infection with, 994
  compared with HIV-1, 985
  epidemiology of, 113, 986–988, 987t
  genetic variability of, 985–986
  morphologic and genetic structure of, 23–26, *32*, 985, 988, *989*
  pathogenesis of infection with, 993–994
  regulatory gene functions and, 990–991
  relationship with other lentiviruses, 23, *24*, 985, *986*
  replication cycle of, 988
  reverse transcription and integration of, 990
  serologic testing for, 985, 986t, 992–993
  structural genes of (*gag* and *env*), 992, 992t
  transmission of, 987–988
  vaccination and drug therapy against, 994–995
Human immunodeficiency virus type 1 (HIV-1) infection
  among injecting drug users, 179–188
  asymptomatic, 140–143
  in children, 163–175 (*See also* Pediatric HIV infection)
  classification of, 49, 50t
  clinical course of, 49–57, 62–64, *63*, 92, 92–93, 612, 673–675 (*See also* Clinical course of HIV disease)
  clinical manifestations of, 139–148 (*See also* Clinical manifestations of HIV disease)
  cytotoxic T lymphocytes and, 63, 64, 73, 88, 92–94, 139, 690, 695–696, 744–745
  diagnosis of, 53, 661–669 (*See also* Diagnosis of HIV infection)
  education about, 128
  history of early epidemic, 124

Human immunodeficiency virus type 1 (HIV-1) infection—*Continued*
  immunopathogenesis of, 3–5, 59–76, 611–612, 780–781, 862–863 (*See also* Immunopathogenesis of HIV infection)
  incidence of, 611 (*See also* Epidemiology)
  incubation period for, 139, 661–662, *662*
  role in pathogenesis of Kaposi's sarcoma, 422–423
  transmission of, 94–95, 124–127 (*See also* Transmission of HIV infection)
  in women, 123, 151–159 (*See also* Women and HIV infection)
Human leukocyte antigens (HLAs), 101, 102, 422
Human papillomavirus (HPV) infection, 319, 319t, 501–503, *502*, 521
  cervical dysplasia and, 152
  clinical lesions associated with, 501
  differential diagnosis of, 503
  histology of, 503
  oral lesions of, 527–528, *528*
  treatment of, 503
Human spuma retrovirus, 25
Human subject research, 967–968, 970–972
Human T-lymphotropic viruses (HTLV-I and HTLV-II), 25, 29, 751, 1003–1021
  clinical manifestations of, 1013–1019, 1013t
    HTLV-I, 1013–1019
      in children, 1018
      co-infection with HIV-1, 1018–1019
      malignancies, 1013–1016, *1014, 1015*
      neurologic disease, 1016–1017, *1018*
      other disease, 1017–1019
    HTLV-II, 1019
  compared with HIV-1, 1003
  cutaneous, 515
  descriptive epidemiology of, 1007–1010
    demographic patterns, 1009–1010, *1010*
    HTLV-I, 1007–1009
    HTLV-II, 1009
  genomic organization of, 1004, *1005*
  laboratory testing for, 1006, *1006*
  life cycle of, 1004
  morphology of, 1003–1004, *1004*
  mutations of, 1005
  origin and molecular epidemiology of, 1006–1007
    HTLV-I, 1006–1007
    HTLV-II, 1007
  pathogenesis of infection with, 1005–1006
  preventing infection with, 1020–1021
    vaccines, 1021
  prognosis for patients with, 1019, *1020*
  replication of, 1003, 1005–1006
  transmission of, 1010–1013, 1011t
    mother-to-child, 1010–1011, *1011*
    parenteral, 1012–1013
    sexual, 1011–1012, 1021
  treating infection with, 1019–1020
  virus-host interactions, 1003–1005
Humoral responses, 694–695
HUS. *See* Hemolytic-uremic syndrome
Hydrocortisone, 632, 1020

Hydroxychloroquine, 512, 513
18-hydroxy-deoxycorticosterone, 630
17-Hydroxysteroids, 629, 630
Hydroxyurea, 6
Hyperalimentation, 644, 650–651
Hyperamylasemia, 556–557
Hypercalcemia, 586, 637
  adult T-cell leukemia/lymphoma and, 1019–1020
Hypericin, 906, 907t
Hyperimmune anti-HIV immunoglobulin (HIVIG), 174, 728, 746
Hyperimmune egg yolks, 338
Hyperkalemia, 201, 585, 586, 632
Hypermetabolism, 643, 644, 646–647
Hypernatremia, 585
Hyperpigmentation, oral, 530
Hypertriglyceridemia, 644–646
Hyperuricemia, 586
Hypervolemia, 585
Hypnosis, 906
Hypoalbuminemia, 621
Hypocalcemia, 586, 637–638
  foscarnet-induced, 382
  nephrocalcinosis and, 596
Hypochlorhydria, 541
Hypoglycemia, pentamidine-induced, 201–202, 637
Hypokalemia, 585
Hypomagnesemia, 586, 638
Hyponatremia, 585, *633*, 633–634
Hypopituitarism, 233, 234, 633
Hyporeninemic hypoaldosteronism, 585, 632
Hypotension, pentamidine-induced, 201
Hypothalamic-pituitary axis abnormalities, 632–634
Hypouricemia, 586
Hypovolemia, 585
Hypoxanthine/guanine phosphoribosyl transferase (HGPRT), 818
Hypoxemia, 196

IAVI. *See* International AIDS Vaccine Initiative
ICAM-1. *See* Intracellular adhesion molecule-1
Idoxuridine, 414, 415
IDUs. *See* Injecting drug users
IDV. *See* Indinavir
IFN. *See* Interferon
IGF-1. *See* Insulin-like growth factor-1
IL. *See* Interleukin
Illicit drug use. *See* Injecting drug users
Ilosone. *See* Erythromycin
Imaging. *See also* specific imaging modalities
  in AIDS dementia complex, 487, *487*
  in central nervous system lymphoma, 452
  in cryptosporidiosis, 332, 333
  in *Pneumocystis carinii* pneumonia, 197–198, *198*
  in progressive multifocal leukoencephalopathy, 412–413, *413–414*, 483–484, *484*
  in toxoplasmosis, 238–241, *239–241*, 481–482, *482*
  in tuberculosis, 267, *267–269*
Imiquimod, 503
Immigration restrictions, 133–134
Immune plasma, 745–746

Immune response, 5, 694–696
  during acute viral infection, 87–89
    adaptive immunity, 88–89
    innate immunity, 87–88
  cell-mediated, 88, 611, 695–696, 744–745
  in children, 679
  to cryptosporidial infection, 334–335
  humoral, 694–695
  to microsporidiosis, 342–343
  mucosal, 696
  to *Mycobacterium avium* complex, 287–288
  to *Mycobacterium tuberculosis*, 261
  risk for *Pneumocystis carinii* pneumonia and, 193–194
  roles of, 89–90
    limitation of viral replication, 89
    prevention of infection, 89
    recovery from infection, 89–90, 90t
    therapies to enhance HIV-specific response, 743
Immune thrombocytopenic purpura, 530
Immune-based therapies, 7, 743–748
  for cryptosporidiosis, 338
  to enhance HIV-specific immune response, 743
  enhancement of antibody response, 745–746
    transfer of monoclonal antibody, 746
    trials of polyclonal antisera, 745–746
  general immune enhancement, 746–748
    by cytokines and lymphokines, 747–748
    inhibition of proinflammatory cytokines, 746–747
  HIV-1 pathogenesis and, 691–693
  HIV vaccines, 689–714, 743–744 (*See also* AIDS vaccine development)
  HIV-specific cytotoxic T-cell responses, 744–745
    transfer of HIV-specific cell populations, 745
  for lymphomas, 445–446, 454
  strategies of, 743, 744t
  for toxoplasmosis, 244–245
Immune-complex glomerulonephritis, 595–596
  rapidly progressive, 587
Immunizations for HIV-infected persons
  contraindications to, 322t
  efficacy of, 320–321
  recommendations for children, 171–172, 172t
  recommendations for pregnant women, 155
  recommendations for travelers, 321–322, 322t
  safety of, 321, 322t
Immunoglobulin A, 89, 696
  IGA nephropathy, 595–596
Immunologic memory, 89
Immunopathogenesis of HIV infection, 3–5, 59–76, 611–612, 780–781, 862–863
  AIDS dementia complex, 487–489
  B-cell dysfunctions, 75
  cellular activation and endogenous cytokines, 68–71
    cytokine induction of HIV expression, 68–69, *70*
    cytokine suppression of HIV expression, 69–70, *70*
    cytokines and hematopoietic cells, 70–71
    HIV effects on cytokine production, 68

inhibition of HIV entry by chemokines, 71, 91
Th1/Th2 cytokine patterns, 71
chronic persistence and progression to clinical disease, 693
clinical course and, 62–64, *63*
dendritic cell dysfunctions, 76
early events, 691–693
HIV-2, 993–994
host cell receptors, 13–21, 59–60, 611–612 (*See also* Host cell receptors)
infection of lymphoid cells, 60–61
CD4+ cells, 60
hematopoietic cells, 60–61
infection of nonlymphoid cells, 61–62
dendritic cells, 62
monocyte/macrophages, 61–62, 611–612, 692
long-term nonprogression, 52, 66–67, 93, 691
lymphoid organs and HIV, 64–66, *65*
mechanisms of depletion and dysfunction of CD4+ cells, 71–75, 72t
antibody-dependent cellular cytotoxicity, 72–73
apoptosis, 73–74
autoimmune mechanisms, 73
HIV-mediated direct cytopathicity, 72
HIV-mediated syncytia formation, 72
HIV-specific cytotoxic T lymphocytes, 72, 744–745 (*See also* Cytotoxic T lymphocytes)
lymphocyte regeneration, 74
nature of T-cell dysfunction in HIV infection, 74–74, 74t
superantigen-mediated perturbation of T-cell subsets, 73
monocyte/macrophage dysfunctions, 75–76
natural killer cell dysfunctions, 75, 75t
natural resistance to HIV, 17, 52, 693–694
plasma viral RNA and, 673–675
portals of entry, 691
rapid disease progression, 52, 67–68
in children, 168
relevance to immune intervention, 691–693
therapeutic strategies and, 20–21
viral tropism and, 19, 691–692
IMP. *See* Inosine monophosphate
Impetigo, 504–505
α and β Importins, 30
Impotence, 635–636
IN. *See* Integrase
In vitro drug interactions among antiretroviral agents, 885–886, 886t
In vitro drug testing, 751–753, 756t
Incidence of HIV/AIDS, 611. *See also* Epidemiology of HIV infection
Incubation period, 139, 661–662, *662*
Indinavir (IDV; MK-639), 5, 149, 601, 751, 761, 780, 794–795, 850t, 851, 863t, 868
adverse effects of, 552, 587, 794, 850t, 851, 863t, 868
antiviral activity of, 851
chemical structure of, *755*, 791, *849*
clinical experience with, 794, 868

combined with other drugs, 794, 851, 853, 868, 876–878, 878t (*See also* Combination antiretroviral therapy)
dosage of, 795, 850t, 851, 863t, 868
drug interactions with, 794–795, 850t
antituberculosis drugs, 273t
delavirdine, 790
penetration of blood-brain barrier by, 489
pharmacokinetics of, 794
for postexposure prophylaxis, 949
in pregnancy, 157t
use in hepatic disease, 794
viral resistance to, 794, 851, 853–854, 868, 875t
Indomethacin (Indocin), 931
"Induction trials," 809
Infection control guidelines, 938–939, 938t
to prevent tuberculosis, 275
Infective dermatitis, 1018
Infective endocarditis, 311, 602
Inflammatory bowel disease, 538
Influenza, 87, 89, 318
Influenza vaccine, 321
for children, 172
for pregnant women, 155
for travelers, 322
Informed consent
for HIV testing, 958
for vaccine efficacy trials, 733, 737
Ini1. *See* Integrase interactor 1
Injecting drug users (IDUs), 126, 179–188
epidemic numbers of, 179–180
glomerulosclerosis in, 588
harm reduction for, 188
HIV infection among, 180–182
in developing countries, 116
outcomes of, 180
rapid transmission of, 180–182, *181*
in women, 151
HIV prevention programs for, 129, 182–188
bleach distribution programs, 182–184, 186
early studies of, 182
in high-seroprevalence areas, 187
insufficiency of, 188
integrating multiple programs, 186
methadone maintenance therapy, 185–186, 185t
modifying sexual behavior, 187–188
problematic issues in, 187
providing services, 188
standards for assessment of, 186–187
street outreach, 182–184, 183t
syringe exchange, 126, 129, 184–185, 184t
impact of psychosocial interventions for, 919
infective endocarditis in, 602
lymphomas in, 439
parenteral HTLV-I and HTLV-II transmission, 1012–1013
potential for transmission of infectious pathogens, 116, 179
"shooting galleries" and "dealer's works" used by, 181
Injections for medical reasons, 116, 126
"Innocent bystander mechanism," 605
Inosine monophosphate (IMP), 815, *816*, 818, *818*

Insect bite reactions, 143t
Insect-borne infections, 318
Institutional review boards, 733
Insulin, 637, 648
Insulin-like growth factor-1 (IGF-1), 633, 652
Insurance coverage, 963, 981
Integrase (IN), 29, 762, 781, *989*
of HIV-2, 990
inhibitors of, 762
structure of, 762
Integrase interactor 1 (Ini1), 762
Intensive care for *Pneumocystis carinii* pneumonia, 208–209
"Intent to treat" analyses, 811–812
Interferon-α (IFN-α), 88, 619, 907t
for adult T-cell leukemia/lymphoma, 1020
adverse effects of, 555, 606
antiviral activity of, 764–765
combination therapy with, 765
for condylomata acuminata, 503
effects on hematopoiesis, 619
for hepatitis B virus infection, 555, 568–570, 764
for hepatitis C virus infection, 555, 571, 764
for hepatitis delta virus infection, 572
for Kaposi's sarcoma, 431, 764
for progressive multifocal leukoencephalopathy, 415
regulatory influence on early T-cell development, 70, 764
role in wasting, 648
fat cell catabolism, 645
hypertriglyceridemia, 645, 646
suppression of HIV expression by, 69, 568, 747
for thrombocytopenia, 614, 747
trichomegaly of eyelashes induced by, 514
for tropical spastic paraparesis/HTLV-I-associated myelopathy, 1020
Interferon-β (IFN-β), 88, 619
fat cell catabolism and, 645
for progressive multifocal leukoencephalopathy, 415
regulatory influence on early T-cell development, 70
suppression of HIV expression by, 69
for toxoplasmosis, 244
Interferon-γ (IFN-γ), 66, 88, 407, 616, 619
effects on HIV production, 69
for *Pneumocystis carinii* pneumonia, 208
regulatory influence on early T-cell development, 70
role in host resistance to *Toxoplasma gondii*, 227
role in wasting, 648
fat cell catabolism, 645
for toxoplasmosis, 244–245
Interim monitoring of clinical trials, 811
Interleukin-1 (IL-1), 193, 407–408, 616, 619
effects on adrenal glucocorticoid secretion, 629
effects on hematopoiesis, 619, 620
IL-1β
HIV effects on production of, 68
induction of HIV expression by, 69
role in Kaposi's sarcoma, 422–424
regulatory influence on early T-cell development, 70

Interleukin-1 (IL-1)—*Continued*
  role in wasting, 648
    fat cell catabolism, 645
    hypertriglyceridemia, 645
  for toxoplasmosis, 244
Interleukin-2 (IL-2), 7, 619, 697, 1003
  cardiotoxicity of, 606
  effects on hematopoiesis, 619, 620
  induction of HIV expression by, 68
  therapy with, 68, 747
    combined with interferon-α, 765
    for lymphomas, 446
Interleukin-3 (IL-3), 68, 69, 618
Interleukin-4 (IL-4), 88, 407–408
  effects on HIV expression, 69
  immunotherapy for lymphomas, 445–446
  reciprocal relationship with interleukin-6, 445
  regulatory influence on early T-cell development, 70
  role in host resistance to *Toxoplasma gondii*, 227
Interleukin-6 (IL-6), 66, 193, 407–408, 619
  effects on adrenal glucocorticoid secretion, 629
  effects on hematopoiesis, 619
  HIV effects on production of, 68, 616, 619
  induction of HIV expression by, 69, 619
  reciprocal relationship with interleukin-4, 445
  regulatory influence on early T-cell development, 70
  role in host resistance to *Toxoplasma gondii*, 227
  role in Kaposi's sarcoma, 422–425
  role in lymphomagenesis, 440, 443–444
    therapy targeted to, 445
  role in wasting, 648
    fat cell catabolism, 645
    hypertriglyceridemia, 645
Interleukin-8 (IL-8), 193
  role in Kaposi's sarcoma, 422–424
  role in *Pneumocystis carinii* pneumonia, 193
Interleukin-10 (IL-10), 66
  effects on HIV expression, 69–70
  role in lymphomagenesis, 444
  in toxoplasmosis, 228
Interleukin-12 (IL-12), 88
  induction of HIV expression by, 68
  role in host resistance to *Toxoplasma gondii*, 228
  therapeutic uses of, 744, 747
  for toxoplasmosis, 244, 245
Interleukin-13 (IL-13), 70
International AIDS Vaccine Initiative (IAVI), 739
International travel. *See* Travel-related diseases
Intestinal parasites, 327–344, 545–546
  cryptosporidiosis, 327–339, 545
  microsporidiosis, 339–344, 545
Intracellular adhesion molecule-1 (ICAM-1), 408
Intracranial hypertension, 363
Investigational drugs, 5, 20–21, 149, 807–808, 874t. *See also* Antiretroviral drug development; Clinical trials
  access to, 904–905
  clinical trials of, 807–813
  nucleoside reverse transcriptase inhibitors, 788–789

process for approval of, 807
  protease inhibitors, 795–796
  for toxoplasmosis, 242–244
Invirase. *See* Saquinavir
Iridocyclitis, 457
Iritis, cidofovir-induced, 382
Iron overload, 576
Iron stores, 612
Isoniazid
  for bacillary angiomatosis, 311
  hepatotoxicity of, 552
  in pregnancy, 158
  for tuberculosis, 271, 271t
Isosporiasis, 55, 147, 315, 317, 546
  acalculous cholecystitis and, 578
  antimicrobial therapy for, 317, 650
Isotretinoin
  for eosinophilic folliculitis, 511
  for oral hairy leukoplakia, 501
  for verruca plana and filiform verrucae, 503
"Itchy red bump disease," 510
Itraconazole
  for aspergillosis, 366
  for blastomycosis, 366
  for candidiasis, 359, 359t, 540
  for coccidioidomycosis, 365
  for cryptococcosis, 362, 362t
  for disseminated infections, 509
  for eosinophilic folliculitis, 511
  for histoplasmosis, 364
    prophylactic, 365
  interaction with saquinavir, 792
  for microsporidiosis, 344
  for penicilliosis, 318, 366
  for sporotrichosis, 366
Ivermectin, 507

Jarisch-Herxheimer-like reactions, 311
JC virus, 403–407, 483
  biology of, 404, *404–405*
  chronic meningoencephalitis due to, 408
  molecular control of gene expression for, 404–406
  molecular interactions with HIV-1, 406
  prevalence of antibodies to, *408*, 408–409
  role in progressive multifocal leukoencephalopathy, 403, 406–408
  types of cells infected with, 406
JM3100 (AMD3100), 21, 761–762
c-jun gene, 406

Kala-azar, 319
Kaposi's sarcoma herpesvirus/human herpesvirus-8 (KSHV/HHV-8), 4, 423–424, 442–443, 447, 522
Kaposi's sarcoma (KS), 55, 143t, 147–148, 421–432, 437, 615
  clinical course of, 426
  clinical manifestations of, 425–426
  diagnosis of, 426
  differential diagnosis of, 426–427
  epidemiology of, 421–422
  etiology and pathogenesis of, 422–425, 438t
    cytokines, 422–425
    genetic factors, 422
    HIV, 422–423

human herpesvirus-8, 4, 423–424, 442–443, 447, 522
    sexual practices, 422
  histopathology of, 425, *425*
  history of, 421
  prognosis for, 426
  risk factors for, 421
  sites of, 421, *422–424*, 425
    adrenal, 629
    esophageal, 539
    hepatic, 552, 575, *575*
    myocardial and pericardial, 602
    ophthalmic, 426, 458t, 469, *469*
    oral, *423*, 522–523, *523*
    pulmonary, 426
    renal, 596
    testicular, 635
    thyroid, 634
  staging of, 427
  treatment of, 427–432
    antiherpes medications, 431–432
    chemotherapy, 429–430, 454
    cryotherapy, 428
    expanded CD8 cells, 745
    interferons, 430–431, 764
    intralesional therapy, 428
    investigational agents, 432
    laser therapy, 428
    pain management, 930
    principles of, 427–428
    radiation therapy, 428
Keratinocyte growth factor, 645
Keratoconjunctivitis, microsporidial, 342
Ketoconazole
  for candidiasis, 359, 359t, 525, 540
  drug interactions with
    didanosine, 786
    indinavir, 794
    saquinavir, 792
  endocrine effects of, 632t
    adrenal, 630, 631
    bone and mineral homeostasis, 638
    testicular, 636
  hyperkalemia induced by, 586
Ketotifen, 653
Kidney disease. *See* Renal disease
kit ligand (stem cell factor), 70, 617
KNI-272, *755*, 760, 767–769
KS. *See* Kaposi's sarcoma
KSHV/HHV-8. *See* Kaposi's sarcoma herpesvirus/human herpesvirus-8
Kupffer cells, 551, 567, 576

L-697,661, 758, 839, *840*
L-735,524. *See* Indinavir
Labor and delivery management, 153, 156, 166–167, 166t
Laboratory testing, 141, 141t
  baseline, before initiating antiretroviral therapy, 873–874
  for candidiasis, 358, 524
  for cervical dysplasia/cancer, 154
  for cervical intraepithelial neoplasia, 143
  for coccidioidomycosis, 365
  for cryptococcosis, 361
  for cryptosporidial infection, 335–336
  for hepatitis, 141, 551
  for herpes simplex virus infection, 392

for histoplasmosis, 364
for HIV-1 infection, 53, 124, 661–669
(*See also* Diagnosis of HIV infection)
in children, 167, 171
in developing countries, 733
findings during acute primary infection, 54, 139
findings during asymptomatic infection, 140
findings during early symptomatic infection, 145
as preventive strategy, 129–130
in women, 153–154, 158–159
for HIV-2 infection, 985, 986t, 992–993
for HTLV-I and HTLV-II infection, 1006, *1006*
for human papillomavirus infection, 503
for microsporidiosis, 343
for *Mycobacterium avium* complex, 289–290
for syphilis, 141, 300
for toxoplasmosis, 141–142, 235–238, 235t
for tuberculosis, 141, 269–270, 269t
for varicella-zoster virus infection, 397
Lactate dehydrogenase (LDH), 197
Lactic acidosis, 585
Lactobacillus suppositories, 727
Lamivudine (3TC), 5, 149, 728, 780, 787–788, 863t, 866
adverse effects of, 784t, 788, 863t, 866
antiretroviral activity of, 752, 787
chemical structure of, *752, 828*
for children, 172
clinical experience with, 866
combined with other drugs, 866, 876–878
(*See also* Combination antiretroviral therapy)
indinavir, 851
nelfinavir, 852
zidovudine, 784, 788
dosage of, 782t, 788, 863t
for hepatitis B virus infection, 555–556, 570
for hepatitis delta virus infection, 572
metabolism of, 787, 828–830, *829*
penetration of blood-brain barrier by, 489
pharmacology of, 787–788, 828–830, 866
for postexposure prophylaxis, 948–949
in pregnancy, 157t
viral resistance to, 788, 866, 875t, 891, 892, 895
Langerhans cells (LCs), 19, 62
expression of CCR5 on, 19
HIV tropism for, 18, 19, 692
Laparotomy, 559
Laser therapy for Kaposi's sarcoma, 428
Late symptomatic disease, 55, 146–148
gastrointestinal disease, 147
malignancies, 147–148
management of, 148
neurologic disease, 147
pulmonary disease, 146–147
Latent phase of HIV infection, 14, 64, 92–93, 612, 862
nervous system during, 479–480
Latin America, *112,* 112t, 113–114, *114.* *See also* Developing countries
LCs. *See* Langerhans cells
LDH. *See* Lactate dehydrogenase

Legal concerns, 979–982
of individuals with HIV, 979–981
discrimination, 132–133, 980–981
estate planning, 979
insurance, 981
powers of attorney and directives of care, 960, 979–980
of institutions, 981–982
confidentiality, 981
HIV testing, 981–982
of society, 982
aid in dying, 933, 960–961, 961t, 982
Leishmaniasis
esophageal, 539
hepatic, 550, 574, *574*
in travelers, 315, 319
visceral, 319
Lentiviruses, 13, 23, 611
genomic organization of, 23–26, *32*
HIV-1, 13–21, 611–612
HIV-2, 985–995
phylogenetic relationships among, 23, *24,* 985, *986*
replication of, 13, *14,* 611
postintegration events in, 26, *27*
preintegration events in, 24, *25*
viral gene products, 23, 26–41 (*See also* Gene products, viral)
virion composition, 26
Leptin, 648
Lethargy, 651–652
Letrazuril, 338
Leucovorin, 247t
Leukemia
adult T-cell leukemia/lymphoma, 1013–1016, *1014, 1015,* 1019–1020, *1020*
hairy cell, 1019
Leukemia-inhibiting factor (LIF), 70, 645, 648
Leukocyte functional antigen 1 (LFA-1), 17, 72, 692
Leukocytosis, 139
Leukopenia, 139, 140
Levofloxacin
for drug-resistant tuberculosis, 272
for *Mycobacterium avium* complex infection, 291, 291t
for toxoplasmosis, 244
LFA-1. *See* Leukocyte functional antigen 1
LGV. *See* Lymphogranuloma venereum
LH. *See* Luteinizing hormone
LIF. *See* Leukemia-inhibiting factor
Life cycle of HIV, 861–862. *See also* Viral replication
attachment, 13–21, 14t, 59, 611–612, 691–692, 861
CD4+ cells, 4, 15–16, *15–16,* 59, 611, 861
coreceptors, 4, 13–16, 15t, 59–60, *60,* 91, 691, 781, 861
fusion of viral and cell membranes, 861
genome activation, 862
integration, 862
possible targets for antiretroviral therapy in, 751, 756t, 761–765, 780, 781t
(*See also* Antiretroviral drug development)
attachment, 863–867
protein processing, 867–869

protein processing, *759,* 759–760, 790, 862
reverse transcription, 29, 31, *34,* 861–862
viral assembly and budding, 862
viral gene product translation, 23–41, 862
Life insurance, 981
Lindane, 507
Linear gingival erythema, 528
LIP. *See* Lymphoid interstitial pneumonitis
Lipid metabolism, 645–646
Lipoprotein lipase, 646
Listeriosis, 575
Literature evaluation, 813, 813t
Liver biopsy, 538, 548, 552, 554–555, 567
Liver disease, 548–553, 567–578
adenovirus, 550, 572
bacillary angiomatosis, 310, 575
bacillary peliosis hepatis, 304, 310, 549, *550,* 576
cytomegalovirus, 376–377, 549–550, 572
diagnosis of, 553–555, *554*
drug-induced, 552–553, 552t, 575–576
Epstein-Barr virus, 550, 572
etiologies of, 549, 549t
fungal infections, 550, *550,* 572–573, *573*
hepatitis A, 567
hepatitis B, 550–551, 567–571, *568*
hepatitis C, 551, 571
hepatitis delta, 571–572
hepatitis E, 572
hepatitis G, 572
herpes simplex virus, 550, 572
HIV infection, 551, 567
Kaposi's sarcoma, 552, 575, *575*
leishmaniasis, 574, *574*
listeriosis, 575
lymphomas, 551–552, *552,* 575, *575*
mycobacterial infection, 407, 549, 567, 574, *574*
nonspecific lesions, 576
other bacteria, 575
Pneumocystis carinii, 550, *573,* 573–574
symptoms of, 548
toxoplasmosis, 550, 574
treatment of, 555–556
varicella-zoster virus, 550, 572
veno-occlusive disease, 576
Living will, 960
Lobucavir
for cytomegalovirus infection, 385
for Kaposi's sarcoma, 432
Long terminal repeat (LTR) regions
of HIV-1, 24, *32,* 35, 568, 984, *991*
of HIV-2, 990, *991*
of HTLV-I and HTLV-II, 1004
Long-term nonprogressors (LTNPs), 52, 66–67, 93, 691, 694
CD8+ cells in, 67, 612
cytotoxic T lymphocyte activity in, 67, 93, 745
role of *nef* in, 36–38, 66–67
Loperamide, 548, 931
Lorazepam, 932
Loviride, *754,* 839, *840,* 875t
LTNPs. *See* Long-term nonprogressors
LTR. *See* Long terminal repeat regions
Lumbar puncture, 301, 361
Luminal agents, 548
Lupus anticoagulant, 620–621

Luteinizing hormone (LH), 635, 636
LY-300046, 754, 839, 840
Lymphadenitis, streptococcal axillary, 504, 504
Lymphadenopathy, 54, 65, 139, 140, 143
　HTLV-I-associated persistent lymphadenopathy syndrome, 1018
　mediastinal, 147
　Pneumocystis carinii pneumonia and, 195, 196
　in tuberculosis, 266–267, 267–268
Lymphocyte regeneration, 74
Lymphogranuloma venereum (LGV), 319, 319t, 469, 506
Lymphoid cells, 60–61, 537
Lymphoid interstitial pneumonitis (LIP), 163–164, 169
Lymphoid organs and HIV, 59, 64–66, 65
Lymphokine-activated killer (LAK) cells, 227, 228
Lymphokines, 747
Lymphomas, 55, 75, 143, 147, 437–447, 451–454
　adrenal, 629
　adult T-cell leukemia/lymphoma, 1013–1016, 1014, 1015, 1019–1020, 1020
　affecting bone marrow, 615
　Burkitt's, 440
　clinical manifestations of, 438–439, 451
　cutaneous, 515, 515–516
　diagnosis of, 451
　epidemiology of, 438
　esophageal, 539
　hepatic, 551–552, 552, 575, 575
　histology of, 439, 451–452
　Hodgkin's disease, 439–440, 451–452
　immunodeficiency and, 437
　intraocular and orbital, 375, 458t, 470
　myocardial and pericardial, 602, 603
　oral, 523, 523
　pathogenesis of, 437–444, 438t
　　cytokines, 443–444
　　Epstein-Barr virus, 440–442, 452
　　Kaposi's sarcoma herpesvirus/human herpesvirus-8, 442–443
　　molecular genetics, 440–441
　　primary central nervous system, 438–439, 452, 482–483, 483
　　differentiation from toxoplasmosis, 238–240, 452, 482
　　treatment of, 453–454, 482–483
　prognostic indicators for, 452–453
　relation to CD4+ cell depletion, 437
　remission of, 439, 445
　renal, 596
　risk in patients receiving antiretroviral therapy, 439
　staging of, 451
　strategies for prevention of, 446–447
　T-cell, 441
　treatment of, 444–446, 445t, 453–454, 453t, 516
Lymphopenia, 54, 139, 140

MA. *See* Matrix protein
MAC. *See* Mycobacterial infections, nontuberculous, *M. avium* complex

Macroamylasemia, 557
Macrophage colony-stimulating factor (M-CSF), 616
Macrophage inflammatory protein-1α (MIP-1α), 4, 14, 60, 60, 67, 70, 91, 93, 691, 761
Macrophage inflammatory protein-1β (MIP-1β), 4, 14, 60, 60, 67, 91, 761
Macrophages. *See* Monocytes/macrophages
Magnetic resonance imaging (MRI)
　in AIDS dementia complex, 487, 487
　in progressive multifocal leukoencephalopathy, 412–413, 413–414, 483, 484
　in toxoplasmosis, 238, 240–241, 481
　in tuberculosis, 269
Magnetic resonance spectroscopy, 413
Major histocompatibility complex (MHC), 13, 88, 695–696
Malabsorption, 148, 332, 648–649
Malaria, 318, 320, 320t
Malignancies
　HIV-associated, 55, 59, 147–148
　　bone marrow, 615
　　cardiac, 602
　　cloacogenic carcinoma, 432
　　cutaneous, 514–516
　　esophageal, 539
　　hepatic, 551–552, 552, 575, 575
　　Kaposi's sarcoma, 147–148, 421–432
　　lymphomas, 147, 437–447, 451–454
　　ocular, 458t, 468–470, 469
　　pathogenesis of, 437–438, 438t
　　renal, 596
　HTLV-I associated, 1013–1016, 1014, 1015
Managed care, 963
Management of HIV disease, 5–7
　advanced disease, 148
　antiretroviral therapy, 148–149, 780–798, 815–857, 861–888
　　combination therapy, 769–771, 780, 798, 863–864, 869, 872–882, 885–888
　appetite stimulants, 148
　based on viral load monitoring, 673–682
　chemoprophylaxis for opportunistic infections, 145–146
　in children, 171–174
　early symptomatic disease, 145
　ethical issues in, 951–972, 952t
　evolving standard of care, 873
　future considerations for, 880–882
　goal of, 797, 873, 885
　hospice care, 923–929
　late symptomatic disease, 148
　pain management, 929–931
　palliative care, 923, 929–932, 961–962
Manipulation, 903, 905–906
Mantoux test, 141
Manufacturers of antiretroviral drugs, 863t
Marantic endocarditis, 602
Marijuana, 932
Massage, 905
Mast cells, 88
Matrix (MA) protein, 24, 30, 764, 989
MD 266, 5
Measles, 318–319
Measles vaccine, 171–172, 318–319, 321, 322
　for pregnant women, 155

Mechanical ventilation, 208–209
Medicaid and Medicare, 963, 980
Medical directives, 960, 979–980
Meditation, 906
Mefloquine, 320, 320t
Megakaryocytes, 613, 615
Megestrol acetate, 651
　endocrine effects of, 632t
　　adrenal, 631
　　diabetes mellitus, 637
　　testicular, 636
Melanoma, 515
Membranoproliferative glomerulonephritis, 595
Membranous glomerulonephritis, 595
Meningismus, 479
Meningitis, 139, 147, 489–490. *See also* Neurologic complications
　aseptic, 489–490
　in children, 169
　Coccidioides immitis, 365, 490
　cryptococcal, 360, 361, 363, 470, 484, 489
　Histoplasma, 364, 490
　other causes of, 490
Meningococcal vaccine, 322
Menstrual cycle, 152, 636
Mental state alterations, 906. *See also* Cognitive impairment
Mesangial hyperplasia, 594–595
Mesangial proliferative glomerulonephritis, 595
Mesenteric disease, 558–559, 558t
Metapyrone stimulation test, 629–631
Methadone maintenance treatment, 185–186, 185t
Methotrexate
　for adult T-cell leukemia/lymphoma, 1019
　interaction with trimethoprim, 510
　for lymphomas, 453, 453t, 516
　for psoriasis, 510
Methylprednisolone, 1020
Metronidazole
　for acanthamebiasis, 507
　for *Clostridium difficile* infection, 317
　for eosinophilic folliculitis, 511
　hepatotoxicity of, 552
　interaction with ritonavir, 794
　for microsporidiosis, 317, 344
Mexiletine, 930
MHC. *See* Major histocompatibility complex
Microbicides, topical, 105, 726–728
　broad-spectrum, 727
　HIV-specific, 727–728
　ideal properties of, 726–727
　rationale for use of, 726
Microcephaly, 169
Microsporidiosis, 147, 317, 327, 339–344, 538
　acalculous cholecystitis and, 578
　antimicrobial therapy for, 317
　cholangiopathy and, 576–578
　clinical features of, 341–342
　corneal, 468
　diagnosis of, 343
　epidemiology of, 341
　hepatic, 550
　immune response to, 342–343
　parasite causing, 339–341, 339t, 340
　renal, 596
　transmission of, 341
　treatment of, 317, 344, 548

Microsporum canis infection, 509
Midazolam interactions with protease inhibitors, 795, 852
Migrant workers, 117–118
Mineralocorticoids
　deficiency of, 585
　secretion of, 631–632
Minimal-change disease, 594–595
Minocycline, 244
MIP-1α. *See* Macrophage inflammatory protein-1α
MIP-1β. *See* Macrophage inflammatory protein-1β
Mitomycin C, 432
Mitral valve prolapse, 602
MK-639. *See* Indinavir
MKC-442, *840*, 875t
MLV. *See* Murine leukemia virus
Molluscum contagiosum, 143t, *502*, 503–504
　of eyelids, 468–469
Monoclonal antibodies
　for adult T-cell leukemia/lymphoma, 1020
　for lymphomas, 446
　to prevent HIV infection, 727, 728
　transfer of HIV-specific antibodies, 746
　for tropical spastic paraparesis/HTLV-I-associated myelopathy, 1020
Monocytes/macrophages, 14, 59, 88, 611–612
　dysfunctions of, 75–76
　HIV tropism for, 18, 692
　infection of, 61–62
　role in host resistance to *Toxoplasma gondii*, 227, 228
Mononeuritis multiplex, 490–491
Morphine, 930–931, 931t
Mortality from AIDS, 537. *See also* Death and dying
　in developing countries, 118
　wasting as predictor of, 643, 644
Mother-to-child transmission. *See also* Pediatric HIV infection
　of HIV-1, 164–167, 174–175
　of HIV-2, 988
　of HTLV-I and HTLV-II, 1010–1011, *1011*
Mucocutaneous conditions, 143t, 144
Mucormycosis, 366
　rhino-orbitocerebral, 470
Mucosal immunity, 696, *697*
Muehrcke's nails, 514
Multicenter AIDS Cohort Study, 51, 104, 431, 676
Multiple sclerosis-like disease, 479
Mumps vaccine for pregnant women, 155
Mupirocin, 505
Murine leukemia virus (MLV), 23, *32*
c-*myc* gene, 440, 442
Mycelex. *See* Clotrimazole
Mycobacterial infections, nontuberculous, 285–294
　classification of, 285, 286t
　clinical disease associated with, 285, 286t
　cutaneous, 505–506
　drug susceptibilities of, 293t
　M. avium complex (MAC), 56, 147, 148, 285–293, 316–317, 505
　　adrenal, 629
　　bacteremia, 289, 290, 291t, 292
　　bone marrow failure and, 615

　　in children, 170
　　clinical features of, 288–289, 288t
　　course of, 289
　　decision to treat, 290
　　diagnosis of, 289–290
　　esophageal, 539
　　gastrointestinal, 546, 648–650
　　hepatobiliary, 377, 549, 567, 574
　　immune response and pathogenesis of, 287–288
　　incidence and epidemiology of, 285–287, 286t, *287*
　　nephrocalcinosis and, 596
　　pathology of, 288
　　pericardial, 603
　　in pregnancy, 158
　　prevention of, 56, 146, 292–293
　　prognosis for, 289, 293
　　testicular, 635
　　thyroid, 634
　　treatment of, 290–292, 291t, 294, 548
　M. bovis, 506
　M. fortuitum, 293
　M. chelonae, 293
　M. genovense, 294
　M. gordonae, 293
　M. haemophilum, 293, 505
　M. kansasii, 293
　M. malmoenseum, 293
　route of acquisition of, 287
　in tropical countries, 315
Mycobacterium tuberculosis. *See* Tuberculosis
Mycophenolate mofetil, 208
Mycostatin, 524
Myelodysplasia, 615
Myelopathy, 147, 479
　cytomegalovirus-induced spastic, 377
　toxoplasmosis and, 233
　tropical spastic paraparesis/HTLV-I-associated myelopathy, 1016–1017, *1018*, 1019–1020
　vacuolar, 147
Myelopoiesis, 70, 613
Myelosuppressive drugs, 615
Myocarditis, 603–604
　toxoplasmic, 232, 234, 601–602
Myopathies, 491, 587

N-9. *See* Nonoxynol 9
NADR/ATOM. *See* National AIDS Demonstration Research/AIDS Targeted Outreach Model
Nail abnormalities, 513, 514
Naltrexone, 907t
Naproxen (Naprosyn), 931
Narcotic analgesics, 930–931, 931t. *See also* Pain management
　interaction with ritonavir, 793
　method of delivery of, 931
　unwarranted fears about, 931
National AIDS Demonstration Research/AIDS Targeted Outreach Model (NADR/ATOM), 182–184, 183t
National Clinicians' Postexposure Prophylaxis Hotline, 949
National HIV-1 Surveillance of HIV-1 Seropositivity Among Childbearing Women Project, 163

"Natural" healing approaches, 905
Natural history. *See* Clinical course of HIV disease
Natural killer (NK) cells, 88
　dysfunctions of, 75, 75t
　role in host resistance to *Toxoplasma gondii*, 227, 228
Natural resistance to HIV, 4, 17, 52, 693–694
Nausea and vomiting, 146, 541
　management of, 932
　zidovudine-induced, 864
NBC. *See* Normal bovine colostrum
NC protein, 30
Necrotizing ulcerative periodontitis, 528, *528*
Needle exchange programs, 126, 129, 184–186, 184t
Needle sharing. *See* Injecting drug users
Needlestick injuries, 127, 869, 947. *See also* Health care environment and HIV transmission
nef gene, 3, *32*, 90, 695
　of HIV-2, 991
　role in long-term nonprogression, 36–38, 66–67
Nef protein, 36–38, 616
　CD4 downregulation mediated by, 36
　enhancement of viral infectivity by, 37, *38*
　interaction with cellular kinases, 36–37
　lymphocyte activation and, 37
　major histocompatibility complex class I downregulation and, 37–38
　properties of, 36
Neisseria gonorrhoeae infection, 319–320, 506, 726, 727
Nelfinavir (NFV; AG-1343), 5, 149, 751, 761, 780, 795, 850t, 852, 863t, 868–869
　adverse effects of, 552, 795, 850t, 852, 863t, 869
　antiviral activity of, 795, 852
　chemical structure of, *755*, *791*, *849*
　clinical experience with, 795, 868–869
　combined with other drugs, 795, 852, 853, 868–869, 876–878, 878t (*See also* Combination antiretroviral therapy)
　dosage of, 850t, 852, 863t, 868
　drug interactions with, 273t, 795, 850t
　pharmacokinetics of, 795
　for postexposure prophylaxis, 949
　in pregnancy, 157t
　viral resistance to, 795, 855, 875t
Neonatal HIV infection, 126–127, 153, 164–167. *See also* Pediatric HIV infection
Nephrocalcinosis, 596
Nephrotic syndrome, 592
Nerve growth factor, 645
Neuroleukin, 697
Neurologic complications, 55–56, 147, 477–491, 478t
　asymptomatic HIV-1 infection of nervous system, 479
　bacillary angiomatosis, 311
　in children, 169, 486
　clinical presentation of, 477–478
　cytomegalovirus, 377, 470, 485
　diagnostic evaluation of, 478–479
　of herpes zoster infection, 397
　HIV encephalopathy, 486

Neurologic complications—*Continued*
    HIV stage-specific, 478
        acute infection, 479
        advanced disease, 480–491
        clinically latent infection, 479–480
    meningitis, 489–490
        aseptic, 489–490
        in children, 169
        Coccidioides immitis, 365, 490
        cryptococcal, 360, 361, 363, 470, 484, 489
        Histoplasma, 364, 490
        tuberculous, 490
    multiple sclerosis-like disease, 479
    myopathies, 491
    neuro-ophthalmic disorders, 411, 458t, 470
    neuropathies, 479–480
    neurosyphilis, 147, 298–302, 490
    nonfocal, 485–490
    opportunistic infections, 478t
    other diseases, 484–485
    peripheral neuropathy, 147, 479–480, 490–491, 929–930
    predominantly focal, *480,* 480–485, 481t
    primary central nervous system lymphoma, 238–240, 438–439, 452–454, 482–483
    progressive multifocal leukoencephalopathy, 403–415, 483–484
    seizures, 485
    stroke, 485
    temporal profile of evolution of, 477–478
    toxoplasmosis, 225–249, 480–482
    tuberculosis, 267
Neurontin. *See* Gabapentin
Neuropathic pain, 929–930
Neuropsychological testing, 487
Neurotropism, 488–489
Neutropenia, 140, 613, 864
    drug-induced, 573
        foscarnet, 381
        ganciclovir, 379, 540
        zidovudine, 864
    due to invasive aspergillosis, 572–573
Neutrophils, 88
Nevirapine (BI-RG-587), 5, 149, 751, 758, 789, 839, 863t, 867
    adverse effects of, 784t, 789, 863t, 867
    chemical structure of, *754, 840*
    for children, 172–173
    clinical experience with, 867
    combined with other drugs, 789, 867
    dosage of, 789, 863t
    interaction with antituberculosis drugs, 273t
    penetration of blood-brain barrier by, 489
    pharmacokinetics of, 789
    during pregnancy, 156, 157t
    viral resistance to, 766–767, 789, 841, 867, 875t, 891
New Zealand, *112,* 112t
NF-1. *See* Nuclear factor-1
NFV. *See* Nelfinavir
Night sweats, 144
Nitazoxanide, 337–338
Nitrogen balance, 644, 645, 652
NK. *See* Natural killer cells
NNRTIs. *See* Nonnucleoside reverse transcriptase inhibitors

Nocardiosis
    esophageal, 539
    retinal, 466
Noncompliance, 918–919
    effect on clinical trial results, 812
    psychosocial interventions for, 918–919
    reasons for, 918
Non-Hodgkin's lymphomas. *See* Lymphomas
Nonnucleoside reverse transcriptase inhibitors (NNRTIs), 149, 751, 756, 758–759, 789–790, 839–842, 863t, 866–867. *See also* specific drugs
    binding of, 758, *758,* 766–767
    chemical structures of, *754, 840*
    combination therapy with, 872–882 (*See also* Combination antiretroviral therapy)
    delavirdine, 789–790, 863t, 867
    development of, 758–759
    interaction with protease inhibitors, 852
    mechanism of action of, 758–759, 840–841, 867
    nevirapine, 789, 863t, 867
    penetration of blood-brain barrier by, 489
    strategies for use of, 867
    treatment with high concentrations of, 842
    viral resistance to, 756, 759, 766–767, 841, 867, 875t, 891, 892, 895–896, *896*
Nonoxynol-9 (N-9), 727
Nonprimate models in vaccine development, 707
Nonsyncytium-inducing (NSI) viruses, 28, 60, 91
Norfloxacin
    for bacillary angiomatosis, 505
    for traveler's diarrhea, 320, 322
Normal bovine colostrum (NBC), 338
North America, *112,* 112t
Nortriptyline, 929
Norvir. *See* Ritonavir
Nosema infection. *See* Microsporidiosis
Nosocomial tuberculosis, 275
NSI viruses. *See* Nonsyncytium-inducing viruses
Nuclear factor-1 (NF-1), 405–406
Nuclear migration inhibitors, 762
Nucleoside analogs. *See* Reverse transcriptase inhibitors
Nucleotide biosynthesis, 815, *816–818*
Null hypothesis, 810
Nuremberg Code, 971
Nutrition, patient's refusal of, 982
Nutritional cardiomyopathy, 606
Nutritional status and HIV transmission, 104–105
Nutritional support, 548, 644, 650–651, 907
Nydrazid. *See* Isoniazid
Nystatin, 359t

O-9. *See* Octoxynol-9
Obligation to treat persons with HIV/AIDS, 955–956
Obstetric management, 153, 156, 166–167, 166t
Obstructive nephropathy, 587
Occupational exposures to HIV. *See* Health care environment and HIV transmission
Octoxynol-9 (O-9), 727

Octreotide, 548
    for cryptosporidiosis, 338
    for microsporidiosis, 344
    pancreatitis due to, 557
Ocular sequelae, 375, 457–472, 458t
    diagnosis of, 457
    drug-induced, 470
    HIV transmission related to, 471–472
    neoplasms, 458t, 469–470
        Kaposi's sarcoma, 426, 469, *469*
        lymphomas, 470
        squamous cell carcinoma, 469–470
    neuro-ophthalmic disorders, 458t, 470
    ocular HIV infection, 457
    opportunistic infections, 459–469, 459t
        of ocular surface and adnexa, 468–469
            corneal microsporidiosis, 468
            fungal and bacterial corneal ulcers, 468
            herpes simplex epithelial keratitis, 468
            herpes zoster keratitis, 397, 468
            herpes zoster ophthalmicus, 397, 468
            molluscum contagiosum lesions of eyelids, 468–469
            ocular lymphogranuloma venereum, 469
        of retina and choroid, 459–467
            choroidal pneumocystosis, 196, 467
            cytomegalovirus, 234, *374–375,* 375, 459–464, *460*
            fungi, 466–467
            herpes simplex virus, 465
            metastatic bacterial infections, 466
            syphilis, 466
            toxoplasmosis, 232, 234, 457, *465,* 465–466
            tuberculosis, 467
            varicella-zoster, *464,* 464–465
    other disorders, 470–471
    vasculopathy, 457–459, *458,* 458t
Odynophagia, 147, 358, 538
Ofloxacin, 272
Oncogenes in AIDS-related lymphomas, 440
1592U89. *See* Abacavir
141W94 (amprenavir; Vx-478), 149, *755,* 761, 795–796, 875t
1263W94, 385
Onychomycosis, 54
Open lung biopsy, 199
Open-reading frames, 23–24
Ophthalmic disorders. *See* Ocular sequelae
Opioid analgesics, 930–931, 931t. *See also* Pain management
    interaction with ritonavir, 793
    method of delivery of, 931
    unwarranted fears about, 931
Opportunistic infections, 55, 59, 145–146
    cardiomyopathy and, 605
    chemoprophylaxis for, 7, 145–146
    in children, 169–170
    impact on course of HIV disease, 770
    management in pregnancy, 157–158
    mortality from, 145, *145*
    neurologic, 478t
    ocular, 459–469, 459t
    renal, 596
Optic neuropathy, 470
    due to varicella-zoster virus infection, 464
    ischemic, 458

Oral contraceptives, 101, 104, 151
Oral fluid testing for HIV infection, 667
Oral manifestations, 143t, 144, 521–530
    bacterial infections, 528–529
        periodontal diseases, 528, 528–529
    in children, 530
    classification of, 522, 522t
    fungal lesions, 523–525
        candidiasis, 139, 144, 147, 195, 357–358, 508, 521, 523–525, 524–525
        histoplasmosis, 525, 525
        other fungi, 525
    idiopathic/autoimmune lesions, 529–530
        abnormal pigmentation, 530
        immune thrombocytopenic purpura, 530
        recurrent aphthous ulcers, 529, 529
        salivary gland disease, 529, 529–530
    neoplasms, 522–523
        Kaposi's sarcoma, 423, 522–523, 523
        lymphoma, 523, 523
        oral cancer, 523
    other problems, 530
    prevalence and incidence of, 521–522
    significance of, 521
    viral lesions, 525–528
        cytomegalovirus, 526
        hairy leukoplakia, 54, 144, 501, 526–527, 526–527
        herpes simplex virus, 525, 526
        human papillomavirus, 527–528, 528
        varicella/herpes zoster virus, 525–526
Oropharyngeal pain, 930
Osteomyelitis, 169
Ovarian function, 636

p6, 30–31
p7, 90, 764, 989
p9, 90, 989
p17, 3, 90, 764, 989
p24, 90, 139, 611, 764, 989
    antigen testing, 663–664
    in infants, 665, 665t
p41, 611
p55, 90
p53 gene, 440
P values, 810, 813
Paclitaxel, 429, 430
PACTG. *See* Pediatric AIDS Clinical Trials Group
Pain management, 929–931
    for abdominal pain, 930
    for acute vs. chronic pain, 929
    for chest pain, 930
    evaluation of pain, 929
    for headache, 930
    opioid analgesics for, 930–931, 931t
        method of delivery of, 931
        unwarranted fears about, 931
    for oropharyngeal pain, 930
    for peripheral neuropathy, 929–930
    for skin disorders, 930
Palliative care, 923, 929–932, 961–962. *See also* Hospice care
    criteria for, 928t
    for diarrhea, 931–932
    for dyspnea, 932
    for end-stage dementia, 932
    for fever, 931
    flow chart for, 926–928, 927
    goal of, 925
    for nausea and vomiting, 932
    for pain, 929–931
    for terminal restlessness, 932
    transition to, 925–926
Pan American Health Organization definition of AIDS, 521
Pancreatic biopsy, 557–558
Pancreatic disease, 556–558, 636–637
    approach to patient with, 557
    cryptosporidial, 333
    diagnosis of, 557
    drug-induced, 543, 556–557, 637, 865, 866
    etiologies of, 556, 556t
    infectious mass lesions, 557
    pancreatitis, 556
    prevalence of, 556
    treatment of, 558
PAP. *See* Pulmonary alveolar proteinosis
Papanicolaou smear, 143, 154
Paracentesis, 558
Paraproteinemia, 613
Parasitic infections
    cutaneous, 506–507
    HTLV-I–associated, 1018
    intestinal, 327–344
Parathyroid hormone (PTH), 637, 637
Paromomycin, 337, 547
Parotid gland enlargement, 530
Partner notification, 131–132, 965–966
Parvovirus B19 infection, 616
Pathogenesis. *See* Immunopathogenesis of HIV infection
Pathology. *See* Histopathology
PBMCs. *See* Peripheral blood mononuclear cells
PC213, 727
PCR. *See* Polymerase chain reaction
Peau d'orange appearance, 512
Pediatric AIDS Clinical Trials Group (PACTG), 172, 174
Pediatric HIV infection, 163–175
    case definition and classification of, 163, 164t–166t
    clinical stages of, 163–164, 165t
    diagnosis of, 167, 171, 664–667, 665t
    epidemiology of, 112t, 116, 163
    ethics and, 953
    growth hormone deficiency and, 633
    infections in, 169–170
        bacterial, 169
        esophageal candidiasis, 170
        fungal, 169
        Mycobacterium avium-intracellulare, 170
        Pneumocystis carinii pneumonia, 170, 170t
        prophylaxis for, 169–170
        toxoplasmosis, 235
    management of infant at risk for, 170–171, 171
    natural history of, 167–168, 678–679
        rapid progressors, 168, 679
    oral complications of, 530
    organ system diseases in, 169
        central nervous system, 169, 486
        lymphoid interstitial pneumonitis, 169
    perinatally (vertically) acquired, 126–127, 153, 164–167
        by breast-feeding, 116, 127, 153, 165–166
        detection at birth, 164
        in developing countries, 116
        discordant outcomes in twins, 164
        HIV-2 infection, 988
        intrapartum transmission, 153, 164–165
        intrauterine infection, 164
        maternal factors related to, 166, 166t
        obstetric factors related to, 153, 156, 166–167, 166t
        prevention of, 116, 155–156, 174–175, 746
            hyperimmune anti-HIV immunoglobulin, 746
            zidovudine, 155–156, 157t, 166, 174, 728, 746, 948, 970–971
        rates of, 166
        time from birth to development of AIDS, 167, 168
    plasma virus levels in, 168
    prognosis for, 168–169
        age at diagnosis and, 168
        by race/ethnicity, 163
    reporting of, 163
    "transient," 665
    treatment and management of, 171–174
        antiretroviral therapy, 172–174
        immunization recommendations, 171–172, 172t
        laboratory assessments, 171
Peer support systems, 914
Peliosis hepatis, 304, 310, 549, 550, 576
Pelvic inflammatory disease (PID), 152, 154
Penciclovir, 431–432
Penicillin, 300–301, 506, 552
Penicilliosis, 365–366
    clinical features of, 318, 366
    cutaneous manifestations of, 366, 509
    diagnosis of, 318, 366
    epidemiology of, 365–366
    hepatic, 572
    microbiology of, 365
    mortality from, 318
    oral, 525
    in travelers, 315, 318
    treatment of, 318, 366
Penicillium marneffei infection, 509
Pentamidine
    adverse effects of, 201–202, 209
        endocrine, 632, 632t
        hepatotoxicity, 552
        hyperkalemia, 586
        hypocalcemia and hypomagnesemia, 638
        myelosuppression, 615
        pancreatitis, 543, 556–557, 637
        renal, 585–587
    interaction with didanosine, 786
    interaction with foscarnet, 382
    for *Pneumocystis carinii* pneumonia, 201t, 203t
        aerosolized, 207, 467
        choroidal pneumocystosis, 467
        cutaneous pneumocystosis, 507
        parenteral, 201–202
        in pregnancy, 157

Pentamidine—*Continued*
  prophylactic, 146, 196, 209
  for toxoplasmosis, 244
Pentamidine analogs, 208
Pentobarbital, 932
Pentoxifylline, 653, 746–747, 770, 798
Peptic ulcer disease, 538, 541
Peptide T, 697
Pericardial effusion, 603
Pericardiocentesis, 603
Pericarditis, 602–603
Peridex. *See* Chlorhexidine mouth rinse
Perinatal infection. *See also* Pediatric HIV infection
  HIV-1, 126–127, 153, 164–167
  HIV-2, 988
  HTLV-I and HTLV-II, 1010–1011, *1011*
Periodontal disease, 528–529
  etiology of, 529
  gingivitis/linear gingival erythema, 528
  periodontitis, 528, *528*
  treatment of, 529
Peripheral blood mononuclear cells (PBMCs)
  antiviral activity of dideoxynucleosides in, 770t
  culture of, 665–666, 673
Peripheral edema, 592
Peripheral neuropathy, 147, 479–480, 490–491, 865, 929–930
Peritoneal disease, 558–559, 558t
Permethrin cream, 507
Pertussis vaccine, 171, 321
PET. *See* Positron emission tomography
Pharmacology, 815–857. *See also* Protease inhibitors; Reverse transcriptase inhibitors
  combination drug therapy and, 881, 886–887, 886t
  protease inhibitors, 148–149, 790–796, 848–857, 867–868
  reverse transcriptase inhibitors, 148–149, 815–842
    acyclic nucleoside phosphonates, *838*, 838–839
    2′,3′-dideoxynucleosides, 819–834
      3′-azido-2′,3′-dideoxyuridine, 824, *824–825*
      carbovir and 1592U89, *833*, 833–834
      2′,3′-dideoxyadenosine and didanosine, 785, 830–832, *830–832*, 864–865
      3′-fluoro-2′,3′-dideoxythymidine, 824–825, *825–826*
      lamivudine and (-)-2′,3′-dideoxy-5-fluoro-3′-thiacytidine, 787–788, *828–829*, 828–830, 866
      stavudine, 787, 822–823, *822–824*, 866
      zalcitabine, 786, 826–828, *827*, 865
      zidovudine, 783, *819–821*, 819–822, 864
    nonnucleoside, 789–790, 839–842, *840*, 866–867
    prodrugs of nucleotide analogs that deliver nucleoside-5′-monophosphates directly into intact cells, 834–837, *834–837*
      aryloxyphosphoramidate approach, 835–836
      bis(isopropyloxycarbonyloxymethyl) approach, 835
      bis(pivaloyloxymethyl) approach, 834–835
      bis(S-acryl-2-thioethyl) approach, 835
      cyclosaligenyl approach, 836–837
    purine nucleotide metabolism, *816, 818*, 818–819
    pyrimidine 2′-deoxyribonucleotide metabolism, 815–818, *817*
Phenobarbital interactions with protease inhibitors, 792, 852
Phenytoin, 485
  hepatotoxicity of, 552
  interaction with protease inhibitors, 485, 792, 852
9-(2-Phosphonylmethoxyethyl)adenine (PMEA), 751, 757, *838*, 838–839
  for cytomegalovirus infection, 385
  for Kaposi's sarcoma, 432
  oral prodrug form of, 757, 788
  structure and antiviral activity of, *753*
9-(2-Phosphonylmethoxypropyl)adenine (PMPA), 728, 751, *753*, *838*, 838–839
5-Phosphoribosyl-1-pyrophosphate (PRPP), 818
Photophobia, 479
Photosensitivity, 143t
Physician-assisted death, 933, 960–961, 961t, 982
Physician-patient relationship, 907–908, 952
Physicians' obligation to treat persons with HIV/AIDS, 955–956
PID. *See* Pelvic inflammatory disease
Pill esophagitis, 539–540
Piritrexim
  for *Pneumocystis carinii* pneumonia, 208
  for toxoplasmosis, 243
Pituitary function, *633*, 633–634
Pituitary pathology, 632–633
Placebo effect, 906
Placebo trials, 971–972
Placental HIV transmission, 153
Placental membrane binding protein (PMBP), 16–17
Plantar warts, 502, 503
Plaquenil. *See* Hydroxychloroquine
Plasma HIV-1 RNA level, 51, 139–141, 140t, 148, 673–682, 862–863
  adequacy in explaining clinical response to therapy, 681–682
  in AIDS dementia complex, 487
  assays for detection of, 663–664, 666, 673, 674t
  roles in therapeutic management of adults, 673–678
    to define virologic failure, 677–678, 876
      discordant viral RNA and CD4 cell responses, 678
      viral resistance, 678, 892
    to initiate therapy, 675–677, 874
      in asymptomatic infection, 675–676
      in primary infection, 676–677
      in symptomatic infection, 676
    to monitor therapy, 677, 881
    pregnant women, 678
    for prognosis, 673–675
      clinical trials, 675
      natural history, 673–675
  roles in therapeutic management of children, 678–681
    to initiate therapy, 679–680
      in asymptomatic infection, 679–680
      in symptomatic infection, 680
    to monitor therapy and describe treatment failure, 680–681
      viral resistance, 680–681
    for prognosis, 678–679
      clinical trials, 679
      natural history, 678–679
  steady state, 674
  suppression below level of quantification, 873
  uncertainty in measurement of, 681, 681t
Plasmapheresis, 587
Plasmodium infection, 318, 320, 320t
Platelets, 613–614
Pleistophora infection. *See* Microsporidiosis
Pleural effusions, tuberculous, 267, *267*
PMBP. *See* Placental membrane binding protein
PMEA. *See* 9-(2-Phosphonylmethoxyethyl)adenine
PML. *See* Progressive multifocal leukoencephalopathy
PMPA. *See* 9-(2-Phosphonylmethoxypropyl)adenine
Pneumococcal vaccine, 143
  for children, 172
  for pregnant women, 155
  for travelers, 322
Pneumocystis carinii pneumonia (PCP), 55, 147, 191–211
  ascites and, 559
  on chest radiography, 197–198, *198*
  in children, 170–171
  clinical manifestations of, 195–196
    extrapulmonary, 196
      choroidal, 196, 375, 467
      cutaneous, 195, 507
      diarrhea, 538
      esophageal, 539
      hepatic, 550, *573*, 573–574
      pituitary, 633
      SIADH, 633–634
      thyroid, 634
    lung cavitation and spontaneous pneumothorax, 195–196
    signs and symptoms, 191, 195
  diagnosis of, 191, 198–200
    bronchoalveolar lavage, 198–199
    cyst wall stains, 199
    immunochemical stains, 199
    molecular identification, 199–200
    noncyst wall stains, 199
    open lung biopsy, 199
    sputum induction, 198
    transbronchial biopsy, 199
  epidemiology of, 192, 315
  histopathology of, 194–195
  immunoresponse and risk for, 193–194
    humoral response, 194
    T-cell-mediated response, 193–194

incidence of, 191
laboratory abnormalities associated with, 196–197
   CD4+ cell count, 191, 194, 197
   lactate dehydrogenase, 197
   pulmonary function tests, 196–197
mortality from, 191, 200
organism causing, 191–192
outcome predictors for, 208
pathogenesis and pathophysiology of, 193, 197
transmission of, 192
Pneumocystis carinii pneumonia (PCP) treatment, 200–208, 201t
for choroidal pneumocystosis, 467
cost of, 191
experimental agents, 208
   pentamidine analogs and 8-aminoquinolines, 208
   piritrexim, 208
initial therapy, 200
mechanical ventilation and ICU care, 208–209
for mild episodes, 206–208, 206t
   aerosolized pentamidine, 207
   atovaquone, 207
   clindamycin-primaquine, 206–207
   corticosteroids, 207–208
   dapsone alone, 207
   trimethoprim-dapsone, 206
in pregnancy, 157
prophylaxis, 145–146, 191, 209–211
   aerosolized pentamidine, 209
   atovaquone, 211
   in children, 170, 170t, 171
   dapsone, 210–211
   pyrimethamine-sulfadoxine, 211
   recommendations for, 211
   trimethoprim-sulfamethoxazole, 209–210
salvage therapy, 204–206
   clindamycin-primaquine, 204–206
   corticosteroids, 206
   trimetrexate, 204
for severe episodes, 200–204
   corticosteroids, 202–204, 205t
   parenteral pentamidine, 201–202
   trimethoprim-sulfamethoxazole, 200–201, 202t–203t
   trimetrexate, 202
supportive care, 208
Pneumonitis
   cytomegalovirus, 376, 378
   lymphoid interstitial, 163–164, 169
Pneumothorax, spontaneous, 195–196
PNPase. *See* Purine nucleoside phosphorylase
Podophyllin resin
   for condylomata acuminata, 503
   for oral hairy leukoplakia, 501, 527
pol gene, 90, 611, 759, 897
   drug resistance and mutations of, 782
   of HIV-2, 988, 992
   of HTLV-I and HTLV-II, 1004, *1005*
pol gene products, 31–35, *32–34*
Poliomyelitis, 689–690, 691t
Poliovirus vaccine, 171, 321, 689
   for pregnant women, 155
Polyclonal antisera, 745–746

Polymerase chain reaction (PCR), 61, 140, 163, 167, 407, 673
   in central nervous system lymphoma, 452
   in cryptosporidiosis, 336
   in cytomegalovirus, 374, 384, 489
   to detect *Bartonella* species, 306
   to detect HIV infection in infants, 665, 666
   in herpes simplex virus infection, 392
   in *Pneumocystis carinii*, 192, 199–200
   in progressive multifocal leukoencephalopathy, 403, 413, 484
   in toxoplasmosis, 237, 481
Polymyositis, HTLV-I-associated, 1017
Polymyxin B, 505
Polyneuropathies, 479–480, 490
Polyomaviruses, 403, 404
Polyradiculopathy, cytomegalovirus, 377, 490
Population screening, 129–131, 963–965, 964t
Porphyria cutanea tarda, 512–513
Positron emission tomography (PET), 452, 482
Postexposure prophylaxis, 869–870, 940–941, 941t, 947–949
   choice of drugs for, 869–870, 941t, 948–949
   drug toxicity and, 949
   evidence in support of, 948
   follow-up care and, 949–950
   National Clinicians' Postexposure Prophylaxis Hotline, 949
   for pregnant or lactating women, 949
   primate studies of, 947–948
   protection afforded by, 948
   window of opportunity for, 947
Postherpetic neuralgia, 397, 500, 526
Potassium
   hyperkalemia, 586, 632
   hypokalemia, 585
   pill esophagitis due to, 539–540
Poverty, 118
Powers of attorney, 960, 979–980
Prednisone
   for adult T-cell leukemia/lymphoma, 1019
   effects in progressive multifocal leukoencephalopathy, 414, 415
   for glomerulosclerosis, 593
   for lymphomas, 516
Pregnancy and HIV infection, 7, 152, 154–158. *See also* Women and HIV infection
   in Africa, 113, *113*
   antiretroviral therapy, 155–156, 157t, 166, 174–175, 948, 970–971
      ACTG 076 trial, 155–156, 746
      carcinogenicity of zidovudine, 156
      current principles, 156
      drug combinations, 156
   CD4+ cell count and viral load monitoring, 155, 678
   counseling HIV-infected women about reproductive choices, 958–959
   immunization recommendations, 155
   labor and delivery management, 156
   mandatory HIV testing, 130, 965
   opportunistic infections, 157–158
      cryptosporidiosis, 331
      fungal infections, 157–158
      mycobacterial infections, 158
      Pneumocystis carinii pneumonia, 157

      toxoplasmosis, 158, 228, 235, 249
      viral infections, 158
   postexposure prophylaxis, 949
Prevention of HIV transmission, 7–8, 89, 101–102, 102t, 127–130, 537, 725–739
   among injecting drug users, 129, 182–188
   among women, 64t, 105–106, 158
      gender gap in developing countries, 969–970
   blood supply protection, 125–126, 130, 134
   education for, 128, 963
   ethical issues related to, 962–963, 963t
   lack of priority given to, 101–102, 102t
   microbicides, 105, 726–728
   modalities for, 725, 726t
   from mother to child, 155–156, 157t, 174–175, 746, 948, 970–971
   need for, 725
   postexposure prophylaxis, 869–870, 940–941, 941t, 947–949
   sexual transmission, 101, 104–106, 128–129
   strategies for reducing occupational risk, 938–939, 938t
   testing and screening for, 129–130, 957–958
      screening health care workers, 966–967
   treatment of sexually transmitted diseases, 105–106, 725–726
   vaccine development, 89, 95–96, 106–107, 689–714, 728–739, 728t (*See also* AIDS vaccine development)
Primaquine
   for malaria, 320, 320t
   plus clindamycin for *Pneumocystis carinii* pneumonia, 201t, 204–207, 206t
   in pregnancy, 157
Primary HIV infection, 53–54, 62–64, 139–140, *140*
   definition of, 62
   diagnosis of, 53, 661–664
   immune response to, 62–64
   incubation period for, 139, 661–662, *662*
   laboratory findings in, 54, 139
   neurology of, 479
   signs and symptoms of, 53–54, 54t, 62, 139
   viral replication and plasma viremia during, 62
      initiation of antiretroviral therapy based on, 676–677
Primate models in vaccine development, 706–709, 708t
Prison health care, 133
Privacy issues, 956–957
PRO2000, 727
Probenecid, 300, 463, 785
Prochlorperazine, 553
Progenitor cells, 618–619
Progesterone, 635
Programmed cell death, 73–74, 539
Progression of disease. *See* Clinical course of HIV disease
Progressive multifocal leukoencephalopathy (PML), 148, 403–415, 470, 483–484
   association with AIDS, 403, 407–408
   cerebrospinal fluid and other studies in, 413, 484
   clinical features of, 410–411, 412t, 483
   definition of, 403

Progressive multifocal leukoencephalopathy (PML)—Continued
  epidemiology of, 403, *408*, 408–409
  etiology and pathogenesis of, 403–407, 483
    biology of JC virus, 404, *404–405*
    molecular control of JC virus gene expression, 404–406
    molecular interactions between JC virus and HIV-1, 406
    molecular pathogenesis, 406–407
  histopathology of, 403, *404*, 410, *410–411*
  historical descriptions of, 403, 409
  host factors and underlying diseases associated with, 403, 409
  neuroimaging in, 412–413, *413–414*, 483–484, *484*
  prognosis for, 411–412
  treatment of, 414–415, 414t, 484
Progressive outer retinal necrosis syndrome, 375, 397, *464*, 464–465
Prophylaxis. *See* Chemoprophylaxis
Proptosis, 470
Proquanil, 320, 320t
Protease, *759*, 759–760, 790, 862, *989*
  of HIV-2, 990
Protease inhibitors, 5, 140, 148–149, 537, 601, 751, 759–761, 790–796, 848–857, 863t, 867–869. *See also* specific drugs
  adverse effects of, 791, 791t, 850t, 863t
    endocrine, 632t, 637
    hepatic, 552
    rare, 852
  characteristics of, 850t
  chemical structures of, *755*, *791*, *849*
  for children, 172
  combination therapy with, 852–853, 872–882 (*See also* Combination antiretroviral therapy)
  for cryptosporidiosis, 338
  for cytomegalovirus retinitis, 461–462
  development of, 759–761
  drug interactions with, 793t, 850t, 852
    anticonvulsants, 485, 792, 852
    antituberculosis drugs, 272, 273t
    delavirdine, 790
  for hepatitis B, 570
  history of, 780, 790
  indinavir, 794–795, 851, 863t, 868
  investigational, 795–796
  mechanism of action of, 848, 862
  nelfinavir, 795, 852, 863t, 868–869
  penetration of blood-brain barrier by, 489
  pharmacokinetics of, 761
  for postexposure prophylaxis, 949
  during pregnancy, 156, 157t
  ritonavir, 792–794, 849–851, 863t, 868
  saquinavir, 791–792, 848–849, 863t, 867–868
  structure-based, 760–761
  substrate-based, 759–760
  symmetry-based, 760
  treatment compliance with, 761
  viral resistance to, 760, 761, 767–769, 790–791, 848, 853–857, 874, 875t, 897–898
    active site mutants, 767–768
    cleavage site mutants, 769
    cross-resistance, 768, 855–857, *856*
    emergence of, 767, 791
    genetic basis of, 853–855
    nonactive site mutants, 768
Protein C, 621
Protein S deficiency, 621
Protein wasting, 647
Proteins, retroviral, *759*, 759–760, 790, 862
Proteinuria, 585, 592
Protocol 076, 970–971
Pruritus, 54, 510
Pseudallescheria boydii infection, 509
Pseudomembranous colitis, 546, *547*
Pseudomonas infections, 55, 504, 505
Psoriasis, 143t, 509–510
Psychopathology
  interventions for reduction of, 919–920
  relationship between HIV disease and, 914–915
  in toxoplasmosis, 233
Psychosocial interventions, 130–131, 911–921
  in conjunction with HIV vaccine efficacy trials, 734
  counseling before and after HIV testing, 912, 957–958
  counseling HIV-infected women about reproductive choices, 958–959
  definitions of counseling and psychotherapy, 911–913
  future directions for, 920–921
  goals of, 918–920
    changing behavior, 919
    facilitating medical compliance, 918–920
    reducing psychiatric symptoms, 919–920
  initial assessment for, 920
  persons performing, 911–912
  psychological themes associated with HIV disease, 915–916
    changing dynamics, 916
    death and dying, 916
    existential issues, 916
    psychosocial issues, 915–916
  related to loss and grief, 920
  relationship between psychopathology and HIV disease, 914–915
  research findings on outcome of, 913–914
  risk-reduction counseling, 912–913
  self-help groups and peer support systems, 914
  therapist qualities, 916–918
    being comfortable with sexual behavior, 917
    countertransference, 917–918
    cultural sensitivity, 917
    knowing and being comfortable with patient's culture, 917
    knowledge of HIV disease, 917
PTH. *See* Parathyroid hormone
Public health issues, 123–134
  AIDS in developing world, 134
  case definition for AIDS, 49, 50t, 55, 123, 146, 391
  early features of epidemic as determinant of subsequent public perception, 124
  early intervention and care, 130–132
    continuum of care options, 132
    partner notification, 131–132
    screening, counseling, and testing, 130–131
  HIV/AIDS as sexually transmitted disease, 115, 133
  immigration and travel restrictions, 133–134
  modes of transmission, 124–127 (*See also* Transmission of HIV infection)
  patients' risks of infection from HIV-infected health care workers, 941–942
  prevention, 127–130 (*See also* Prevention of HIV transmission)
  related to demographic features of epidemic, 132–133
    discrimination, 132–133
    housing, 132
    prison health care, 133
    rural health care, 133
Pulmonary alveolar proteinosis (PAP), 195
Pulmonary disease, 146–147
  aspergillosis, 366
  bacillary angiomatosis, 310
  chest radiographic findings of, 146t
  coccidioidomycosis, 365
  cryptococcosis, 360–361
  cryptosporidiosis, 333
  cytomegalovirus pneumonitis, 376
  histoplasmosis, 364
  Kaposi's sarcoma, 426
  lymphoid interstitial pneumonitis, in children, 163–164, 169
  Mycobacterium avium complex infection, 288
  penicilliosis, 366
  Pneumocystis carinii pneumonia, 147, 191–211
  toxoplasmosis, 232, 234, 241
  tuberculosis, 261–275
Pulmonary function tests, 196–197
Pulmonary hypertension, 603
Pulse oximetry, 196
Purified protein derivative (PPD) test, 141
Purine nucleoside phosphorylase (PNPase), 819
Purine nucleotide metabolism, 815, *816*, *818*, 818–819
Pyelonephritis, 596
Pyrazinamide
  hepatotoxicity of, 552
  in pregnancy, 158
  renal toxicity of, 585
  for tuberculosis, 271–272, 271t
Pyridinone, *840*
Pyrimethamine
  adverse effects of, 210, 242
    myelosuppression, 615
  in pregnancy, 158
  prophylactic, 146
    plus dapsone for *Pneumocystis carinii* pneumonia, 210–211
    plus sulfadoxine for *Pneumocystis carinii* pneumonia, 211
  for toxoplasmosis, 248, 249t
  for toxoplasmic retinochoroiditis, 466
Pyrimethamine-sulfadoxine
  prophylaxis for isosporiasis, 317
  prophylaxis for toxoplasmosis, 248, 249t

Stevens-Johnson syndrome induced by, 320
therapy for toxoplasmosis, 243, 247t
Pyrimidine 2'-deoxyribonucleotide metabolism, 815–818, *817*

Qinghaosu, 244
Quasispecies of RNA virus, 891
Quinidine, 792
Quinine, 320, 320t

R-82150, *754*
R-82913, 839
R-86183, 839
R-89439. *See* Loviride
Race/ethnicity
  of children with HIV infection, 163
  therapist sensitivity to issues of, 917
Radiation therapy
  for cloacogenic carcinoma, 432
  for Kaposi's sarcoma, 428
  for lymphomas, 453–454, 482–483
Randomized trials, 809–810, 809t
Ranitidine, 786
RANTES. *See* Regulated-on-activation normal T-cell expressed and secreted
Rapid disease progression, 52, 67–68
  in children, 168, 679
ras gene, 440
Rash. *See* Cutaneous manifestations
Receptors. *See* Host cell receptors
Reed-Sternberg cells, 440, 444, 516
Regulated-on-activation normal T-cell expressed and secreted (RANTES), 4, 14, 60, *60*, 67, 91, 93, 691, 761–762
  modification for therapeutic use, 21
Rehydration therapy, 932
Reiter's syndrome, 143t, 333, 510
Relaxation, 906
Renal disease, 585–596
  acute renal failure, 586–588, 586t, 588t
  chronic glomerulopathies, 588–596, 589t
    focal or global glomerulosclerosis, 588–594
    immune-complex glomerulonephritis, 595–596
    minimal-change disease and mesangial hyperplasia, 594–595
  drug use in patients with, 586
    trimethoprim-sulfamethoxazole, 201, 202t
  drug-induced, 585–586, 586t
    cidofovir, 382
    foscarnet, 541
    pentamidine, 201
  electrolyte and acid-base disorders, 585–586, 586t
  neoplasms, 596
  nephrocalcinosis, 596
  opportunistic infections, 596
  renal cell carcinoma, 596
Renal transplantation, 594
Renin-angiotensin system, 632
Reporting HIV test results, 957
Rescriptor. *See* Delavirdine
Research design, 807–811. *See also* Clinical trials

Research ethics, 967–968, 970–972. *See also* Ethical issues
Resistance to antiretroviral agents. *See* Antiretroviral drug resistance
Respiratory syncytial virus (RSV), 690–691, 691t
Respiratory tract infections, 318. *See also* Pulmonary disease
Resting energy expenditure, 647, 651
Restlessness, terminal, 932
Restriction fragment length polymorphisms (RFLP), 264, *265*
Retin-A. *See* Isotretinoin
Retinal biopsy, 457
Retinal disease, 55, 457. *See also* Ocular sequelae
  cytomegalovirus retinitis, 234, *374–375*, 375, 457, 459–464, *460*
  fungal infections, 466–467
  herpes simplex virus retinitis, 465
  metastatic bacterial infections, 466
  microvasculopathy, 457–459, 458t
  retinal vein occlusions, 458
  syphilitic, 466
  toxoplasmic retinochoroiditis, 232, 234, 375, 465, 465–466
  varicella-zoster virus retinitis (progressive outer retinal necrosis syndrome), 375, 397, *464*, 464–465
Retrovir. *See* Zidovudine
Retroviruses, 13, 611, 1003. *See also* Lentiviruses
  HIV-1, 13–21, 611–612
  HIV-2, 985–995
  HTLV-I and HTLV-II, 1003–1021
  proteins of, *759*, 759–760, 790, 862
rev gene, 14, *32*, 90, 763, 781
  of HIV-2, 990–991
  as target for therapeutic intervention, 763
Rev protein, 24–25, 35–36, 763, 990
Reverse T_3 (rT_3), 634–635, 635t
Reverse transcriptase (RT), 13, 29, 31, 611, 781, *989*, 1003
  of HIV-2, 990
  structure of, 31, *33*, 756–757, *757*
Reverse transcriptase inhibitors, 5, 140, 148–149, 751, 757–759, 781–790, 815–842, 863–867. *See also* specific drugs
  acyclic nucleoside phosphonates, 819, *838*, 838–839
  adverse effects of, 784t, 863t
  categories of, 756
  for children, 172
  combination therapy with, 149, 769–771, 780, 863–864, 872–882 (*See also* Combination antiretroviral therapy)
  2',3'-dideoxynucleosides, 757–758, 781–789, 782t, 819–834
    3'-azido-2',3'-dideoxyuridine, 824, *824–825*
    carbovir and abacavir, 757–758, *833*, 833–834
    comparison of, 865t
    development of, 757–758, 781
    2',3'-dideoxyadenosine and didanosine, 785–786, 830–832, *830–832*, 864–865

3'-fluoro-2',3'-dideoxythymidine, 824–825, *825–826*
lamivudine and −2',3'-dideoxy-5-fluoro-3'-thiacytidine, 787–788, *828–829*, 828–830, 866
stavudine, 787, *822–823*, 822–824, 866
zalcitabine, 786–787, 826–828, *827*, 865–866
zidovudine, 783–785, *819–821*, 819–822, 864
dosages of, 782t, 863t, 865t
history of, 780
investigational, 788–789
nonnucleoside, 149, 751, 756, 758–759, 789–790, 839–842, 863t, 866–867
  binding of, 758, *758*, 766–767
  chemical structures of, *754*, *840*
  delavirdine, 789–790, 867
  development of, 758–759
  interaction with protease inhibitors, 852
  mechanism of action of, 758–759, 840–841
  nevirapine, 789, 867
  treatment with high concentrations of, 842
  viral resistance to, 756, 759, 766–767, 841, 874, 875t, 891, 892, 895–896, *896*
nucleoside analogs, 149, 863–864
nucleotide biosynthesis pathways, 815, *816–818*
for patients with tuberculosis, 272–273
penetration of blood-brain barrier by, 489
for postexposure prophylaxis, 870, 948–949
during pregnancy, 156, 157t
prodrugs of nucleotide analogs that deliver nucleoside-5'-monophosphates directly into intact cells, 834–837, *834–837*
  aryloxyphosphoramidate approach, 835–836
  bis(isopropyloxycarbonyloxymethyl) approach, 835
  bis(pivaloyloxymethyl) approach, 834–835
  bis(S-acyl-2-thioethyl) approach, 835
  cyclosaligenyl approach, 836–837
purine nucleotide metabolism, *816*, *818*, 818–819
pyrimidine 2'-deoxyribonucleotide metabolism, 815–818, *817*
strategies for use of, 863–864
structures and antiviral activity of, 752–754
viral resistance to, 765–766, 782, 874, 875t, 892–895 (*See also* Antiretroviral drug resistance)
Reverse transcription, 29, 31, *34*, 861–862
Rev-responsive element (RRE), 36
Rhabdomyolysis, 479
Rhodococcus equi infection, 466
Ribavirin, 785
Ribonuclease H, 781
Rickettsioses, 318
Rifabutin
  drug interactions with, 272–273, 273t, 852
    delavirdine, 790
    indinavir, 794
    macrolide antibiotics, 470
    nelfinavir, 795
    ritonavir, 794

Rifabutin—Continued
    for *Mycobacterium avium* complex infection, 291, 291t, 548
        prophylaxis, 146, 292
    for toxoplasmosis, 244
    uveitis induced by, 457, 470
Rifadin. *See* Rifampin
Rifampicin
    for bacillary angiomatosis, 311, 505
    effects on bone and mineral homeostasis, 638
Rifampin
    adverse effects of
        adrenal, 630, 631
        endocrine, 632t
        hepatic, 552
        renal, 585, 587
        thyroid, 635
    drug interactions with, 272–273, 273t, 852
        delavirdine, 790
        fluconazole, 525
        indinavir, 794
        nelfinavir, 795
        ritonavir, 794
    for *Mycobacterium avium* complex infection, 291, 291t, 548
    in pregnancy, 158
    for tuberculosis, 271, 271t
Rimactane. *See* Rifampin
Risk-reduction counseling, 188, 912–913
Ritonavir (RTV; ABT-538), 5, 149, 601, 760, 780, 792–794, 849–851, 850t, 863t, 868
    adverse effects of, 552, 793, 850t, 851, 863t, 868
    antiretroviral activity of, 792, 849–850
    chemical structure of, 755, 791, 849
    clinical experience with, 849–850, 868
    combined with other drugs, 792, 793, 849–850, 852–853, 868, 876–878, 878t (*See also* Combination antiretroviral therapy)
    dosage of, 792, 849, 850t, 863t, 868
    drug interactions with, 273t, 793–794, 793t, 850t, 851, 868
    formulations of, 792
    pharmacokinetics of, 792–793, 850–851
    in pregnancy, 157t
    viral resistance to, 793, 850, 854, 875t
RNA. *See* Plasma HIV-1 RNA
Ro 5-3335, 763
Ro 24-7429, 763
Ro 31-8959. *See* Saquinavir
Rolipram, 798
Roseola, 616
Rous sarcoma virus, 23, 1003
Roxithromycin, 243, 248, 505
RRE. *See* Rev-responsive element
RSV. *See* Respiratory syncytial virus
RT. *See* Reverse transcriptase
rT_3. *See* Reverse T_3
RTV. *See* Ritonavir
Rubella vaccine, for pregnant women, 155
Rural health care, 133
Ryan White Care Act, 963

Sabin-Feldman dye test, 227
Safer sex practices, 187–188
Saliva testing for HIV infection, 667
Salivary gland disease, 529, 529–530, 557
Salmonellosis, 55, 315, 546
    acalculous cholecystitis and, 578
    antimicrobial therapy for, 317
    traveler's diarrhea, 316–317
Sanctuary sites for HIV, 94, 876, 885
Sandostatin. *See* Octreotide
Saquinavir (SQV; Ro 31-8959), 5, 149, 601, 751, 760, 780, 848–849, 850t, 863t, 867–868
    administration of, 849
    adverse effects of, 792, 849, 850t, 863t, 868
    antiretroviral activity of, 792, 848–849
        Invirase vs. Fortovase formulations, 849
    chemical structure of, 755, 791, 849
    clinical experience with, 867–868
    combined with other drugs, 792, 848–849, 852–853, 868, 876–878, 878t (*See also* Combination antiretroviral therapy)
    dosage of, 791–792, 848, 849, 850t, 863t, 867
    drug interactions with, 792, 850t
        delavirdine, 790
    formulations of, 791, 849
    pharmacokinetics of, 791
    in pregnancy, 157t
    viral resistance to, 792, 854–855, 867–868, 875t
Sargramostim. *See* Granulocyte-macrophage colony-stimulating factor
Scabies, 506–507
    causative organism in, 506
    clinical features of, 506–507
    postscabetic id reactions, 507
    treatment of, 507
Scalded skin syndrome, 514
Scedosporium inflatum infection, 509
Schistosomiasis, 550
SCID-hu mice, 61, 91, 93, 193–194, 342–343, 441–442, 446, 752–753
Sclerosing cholangitis, 577, 577
Screening, 129–131, 963–965, 964t
    estimated cost of, 964
    of health care workers, 966–967, 982
    justification for mandatory screening, 964, 964t
    premarital, 964
    prenatal, 130, 965
    voluntaristic approach to, 964
S-CSF. *See* Stem cell factor
SDF-1. *See* Stromal cell-derived growth factor-1
SDZ-NIM-811, 763
Seborrheic dermatitis, 143t, 509, 509
Secretory immunoglobulin A, 89
Sedation, conscious, 932
Sedative-hypnotic interactions with antiretroviral agents, 790, 793
Seizures, 485
    anticonvulsants for, 485
    foscarnet-induced, 381
    in toxoplasmosis, 233, 248
Self-help groups, 914
Sensory deficits, 411, 412t
Sensory neuropathies, 490
Septic arthritis, 169
Septra. *See* Trimethoprim-sulfamethoxazole

Seroconversion
    acute retroviral seroconversion syndrome, 53–54, 54t, 62, 139
    defining window of, 661–662, 662
Seven-transmembrane (7TM) family of receptors, 14, 18, 59–60
Severe combined immunodeficient (SCID)-hu mice, 61, 91, 93, 193–194, 342–343, 441–442, 446, 752–753
Sex hormone-binding globulin, 636
Sex steroids, 635
Sexual abuse, 163
Sexual transmission of HIV, 101–107, 115, 125, 187–188
    by anal intercourse, 104, 115, 117, 151, 537
    behavioral risk factors and, 101, 104, 115, 116t, 117, 117t
    circumcision and, 103
    coinfection, genital ecology and, 103
    in developing countries, 101, 115
    effects of antiretroviral therapy on infectiousness, 103–104
    genetics and risk of, 102–103
    genital anatomic variations and, 103
    heterosexual, 104, 115, 151
    HIV-2, 987–988
    Kaposi's sarcoma occurrence related to sexual behavior, 422
    prevention of, 101, 104t–105t, 105–107
        condoms and barrier methods, 101, 104–106, 128–129
        sexually transmitted disease control, 105–106
        for women, 105–106, 106t
    related to sexual norms of society, 118
    risk factors for high susceptibility, 104
    sexually transmitted diseases and, 101, 103, 105–106, 117, 151
    viral factors in infectiousness, 102
Sexual transmission of HTLV-I and HTLV-II, 1011–1012
Sexually transmitted diseases (STDs), 128, 144, 506
    chancroid, 319, 319t, 506
    Chlamydia trachomatis infection, 319t, 726, 727
    clinical course in HIV infection, 319, 319t
    in developing countries, 725–726
    gonorrhea, 319–320, 506, 726, 727
    herpes simplex virus, 319t, 391–393
    HIV transmission and, 101, 103, 105–106, 117, 151, 725–726
    HIV/AIDS as, 115, 133
    human papillomavirus, 319, 319t, 501–503, 502, 521
    incidence of, 725
    syphilis, 141, 297–302
    in travelers, 319–320, 319t
    treatment of, 725–726
    Trichomonas vaginalis infection, 319t, 726, 727
"Sharps" accidents, 127, 869, 947. *See also* Health care environment and HIV transmission
Shigellosis, 315–317, 546
Shingles. *See* Herpes zoster
"Shooting galleries," 181
SI viruses. *See* Syncytium-inducing viruses

SIADH. *See* Syndrome of inappropriate secretion of antidiuretic hormone
Sigmoidoscopy, 542
Simian immunodeficiency virus (SIV), 63, 90, 692, 696, 985, *986*
   genomic organization of, 23, *24*, 26, *32*
   Nef protein and, 36–37
   pathogenesis of infection with, 947–948
Simple Use Diagnostic System (SUDS), 667–668
Single-photon emission computed tomography (SPECT), 452, 482
SIV. *See* Simian immunodeficiency virus
Skin disease. *See* Cutaneous manifestations
"Slim disease," 315, 537, 643
Social ethics, 962–968, 962t
   drug testing and other research practices, 967–968
   notification of partners and at-risk persons, 131–132, 965–966
   population screening, 129–131, 963–965, 964t
   primary prevention and universal access to primary health care, 962–963, 963t
   screening health care workers and their status if HIV positive, 966–967, 982
Social impact of HIV/AIDS, 119, 905
Sodium balance
   hypernatremia, 585
   hyponatremia, 585, *633*, 633–634
SP-303, 395
Sparfloxacin, 291, 291t
SPECT. *See* Single-photon emission computed tomography
Spermatogenesis, 635
Spermicides, 105, 727
Spinal cord involvement in toxoplasmosis, 232, 233, 238
Spiramycin, 336–337
Spiritual issues, 933–934
Spleen
   bacillary angiomatosis involving, 310
   irradiation of, 614
   splenectomy for thrombocytopenia, 614
Sporotrichosis, 366
   cutaneous, 366, 508
   hepatic, 550
   intraocular, 467
Sputum induction, 198
SPV-30, 907t
Squamous cell carcinoma, 515
   Bowenoid papulosis and, 501, *502*, 503, 514–515
   of conjunctiva and eyelid, 469–470
   oral, 523
   treatment of, 515
SQV. *See* Saquinavir
St. John's wort, 906
Staging
   of AIDS dementia complex, 486, 486t
   of HIV infection, 49, 52, 56–57
   of Kaposi's sarcoma, 427
   of lymphomas, 451
Standard of care, 873
Staphylococcal infections
   blepharitis, 471
   in children, 169
   cutaneous, 504, *504*
   endocarditis, 602
   folliculitis, 143t
   pericarditis, 603
   S. aureus, 55, 169
   scalded skin syndrome, 514
Statistical power of clinical trials, 810
Stavudine (d4T), 5, 149, 780, 787, 863t, 866
   adverse effects of, 490, 784t, 787, 863t, 866
   antiretroviral activity of, *752*, 787
   chemical structure of, *752*, *822*
   for children, 172
   clinical trials of, 787, 866
   combined with other drugs, 787, 866, 876–877 (*See also* Combination antiretroviral therapy)
      indinavir, 851
      zidovudine, 784
   dosage of, 782t, 787, 863t
   penetration of blood-brain barrier by, 489
   pharmacology of, 787, 822–824, *823*, 866
   for postexposure prophylaxis, 949
   in pregnancy, 157t
   use in renal disease, 787
STDs. *See* Sexually transmitted diseases
Stem cell factor (S-CSF; kit ligand), 70, 617
"Sterilizing immunity," 89
Stevens-Johnson syndrome, 320, 513
Stigmatization, 905, 965
Stomach disease, 541, *541*
Street outreach programs for injecting drug users, 182–184, 183t
Streptococcal infections
   axillary lymphadenitis, 504, *504*
   endocarditis, 602
   pericarditis, 603
   pneumonia, 55, 143
      in children, 169
      immunization against, 143, 155, 172, 322
Streptomycin
   for *Mycobacterium avium* complex infection, 291, 291t
   for tuberculosis, 271–272, 271t
Stroke, 485
Stromal cell-derived growth factor-1 (SDF-1), 14, 60, *60*
Strongyloidiasis, 507
Studies of the Ocular Complications of AIDS, 378, 461
Sucralfate, 541
Suicide, 959. *See also* Death and dying
   physician-assisted death, 933, 960–961, 961t, 982
Sulfadiazine
   adverse effects of, 242, 587
   in pregnancy, 158
   for toxoplasmosis, 242, 247t
Sulfadoxine
   for malaria, 320t
   for *Pneumocystis carinii* prophylaxis, 211
Sulfamerazine, 242
Sulfamethazine, 242
Sulfonamides, 615, 632t
Superantigens, 73
Support groups, 914
Suramin, 761
Surfactant, 193
Sustiva. *See* Efavirenz

SV 40, 403
Symptom management, 928–934
   diarrhea, 931–932
   dyspnea, 932
   end-stage dementia, 932
   fever, 931
   nausea and vomiting, 932
   pain, 929–931
   terminal restlessness, 932
   treatments in hospice, 928–929
Syncytium formation, 28, 72
Syncytium-inducing (SI) viruses, 4, 28, 59, 91
Syndrome of inappropriate secretion of antidiuretic hormone (SIADH), 585, 633–634
   toxoplasmosis and, 233, 234
Syphilis, 141, 297–302
   animal models of, 297
   cerebrospinal fluid examination in, 301
   cutaneous manifestations of, 297, 506
   disseminated, 297
   follow-up care for, 301–302
   HIV infection and, 298, 319, 319t
   latent, 297
   natural history of, 297–298
   neurosyphilis, 147, 298–302, 298t, 299t, 319, 490
   primary, 297
   retinal, 466
   secondary, 297
   serologic tests for, 141, 300
   tertiary, 298
   topical microbicides for prevention of, 727
   treatment of, 300–301, 506, 726
   Tuskegee study of, 971
Syringe exchange programs, 126, 129, 184–186, 184t
Systemic lupus erythematosus, 595

T_3. *See* Triiodothyronine
T_4. *See* Thyroxine
T22, 762
TAR. *See* Tat-response element
tat gene, 3, 14, *32*, 90, 762, 781
   of HIV-2, 990–991
   role in Kaposi's sarcoma, 423
   as target for therapeutic intervention, 762–763
Tat protein, 24–25, 35, 68, 762–763, 990
Tat-response element (TAR), 24, 763, 990
tax gene, 1004, 1005
TBG. *See* Thyroid-binding globulin
3TC. *See* Lamivudine
T-cell line-adapted (TCLA) viruses, 695
T-cell receptor (TCR), 88
TCLA. *See* T-cell line-adapted viruses
Tegretol. *See* Carbamazepine
Terfenadine interactions with protease inhibitors, 795, 852
Terry's nails, 514
Testis, 635–636
   function of, 635–636, *636*
   involvement in toxoplasmosis, 232, 234
   pathology in, 635
Testosterone, 635–636, *636*, 651–653
Tetracycline, 244, 466, 552
TGF-β. *See* Transforming growth factor-β

Thalidomide, 798
  for aphthous ulcers, 529, 539, 541
  to induce weight gain, 653
  inhibition of TNF-α by, 747
  for microsporidiosis, 344
Therapeutic failure defined by plasma viral RNA level, 677–678
  in children, 680–681
Thiabendazole, 507
Thrombocytopenia, 54, 140, 613–614
  causes of, 613
  ganciclovir-induced, 379, 540
  prevalence of, 613
  spontaneous remission of, 613
  treatment of, 613–614, 614t, 747
Thromboembolic events, 621
Thrombopoietin, 70
Thrombotic thrombocytopenic purpura (TTP), 587
Thrush. *See* Candidiasis, oral
Thymidine kinase inhibitors, 500, 501
Thymidine triphosphate, 40, 815, *817*
Thymosin α, 697
Thymus
  CD4+ thymocytes, 61
  double-positive (DP) thymocytes, 61
  HIV infection of, 61
  T-cell development in, 61
    cytokine influences on, 70
Thyroid disorders, 634–635, *635*, 635t, 648
Thyroid-binding globulin (TBG), 634, 635t
Thyroid-stimulating hormone (TSH), 634, *635*, 635t
Thyrotropin-releasing hormone (TRH), 633, 634
Thyroxine (T_4), 634, 635t, 648
Tilorone, 415
Tivirapine, *840*
TNF-α. *See* Tumor necrosis factor-α
TNF-β. *See* Tumor necrosis factor-β
TNP-470, for microsporidiosis, 344
Topotecan, 484
Total parenteral nutrition (TPN), 650–651
Toxic axonal neuropathy, 490
Toxic epidermal necrolysis, 513–514
Toxoplasma gondii, 225–227
  biotypes of, 225
  forms of, 225–226
    oocyst, 225
    tachyzoite, 225–226
    tissue cyst, 226
  host-parasite relationship, 227
  hosts of, 225
  life cycle of, *226*, 226–227
  strains of, 227
Toxoplasmosis, 55, 141–142, 225–249, 480–482
  ascites and, 559
  clinical manifestations of, 225, 232–235
    cardiac, 234, 601–602
    extracerebral, 230, 230t
    hepatic, 550, 574
    neurologic, 233–234, 233t
    other organ involvement, 234–235
    pancreatic, 556
    pulmonary, 234
    retinochoroiditis, 234, 375, 457, *465*, 465–466
  congenital, 235
  diagnosis of, 141–142, 235–241, 235t, 481
    antibody tests, 235–236, 481
    antigen detection, 236–237
    brain biopsy, 238, 245
    cerebrospinal fluid analysis, 238, 481
    histology, 237
    imaging, 238–241, *239–241*, 481–482, *482*
    isolation of *Toxoplasma*, 237
    other laboratory abnormalities, 237–238
    polymerase chain reaction, 237, 481
  differentiation from central nervous system lymphoma, 238–240, 452, 482
  epidemiology and incidence of, 228–229, 229t, 481
  etiology of, 225–228
    causative organism, 225–227
    nonspecific effector cells, 228
    role of cytokines, 227–228
    specific immunity, 227
  histopathology of, 230–232
    adrenal, 629
    central nervous system, 230–232, *231*
    eye, 232
    heart, 232
    intestinal tract, 232
    liver, 574
    lungs, 232
    other organ involvement, 232
    pituitary, 633
    skeletal muscle, 232
    testicular, 635
    testis, 232
  historical recognition of, 225
  outcome of, 248
  pathophysiology of, 229–230
  in pregnancy, 228, 235, 249
  prevention of, 229, 229t, 248–249
    newly acquired infection, 229, 249
    primary prophylaxis, 146, 228, 248–249, 249t
  transmission of, 228, 249
  vertical, 228, 235
Toxoplasmosis treatment, 241–245
  antimicrobial therapy, 241–244
    clindamycin, 242
    combination therapy, 244
    experimental/investigational, 242–244
      atovaquone, 244
      dapsone, 243
      macrolides-azalides and ketolides, 243–244
      other drugs, 244
      Piritrexim, 243
      pyrimethamine-sulfadoxine, 243
      tetracyclines, 244
      trimethoprim and trimethoprim-sulfamethoxazole, 243
      trimetrexate, 243
    pyrimethamine, 241–242
    sulfonamides, 242
  immunotherapy, 244–245
  for patient with suspected disease, 245–248, *246*
    anticonvulsants, 248
    antimicrobial therapy, 246–248, 247t
    corticosteroids, 248
    encephalitis, 245
    extraneural disease, 245–246
  in pregnancy, 158
TPN. *See* Total parenteral nutrition
Trachipleistophora hominis infection. *See* Microsporidiosis
Transbronchial biopsy, 199
Transfer of HIV-specific cell populations, 745
Transforming growth factor-β (TGF-β), 408, 620
  effects on hematopoiesis, 620
  HIV effects on production of, 68, 616
  regulatory influence on early T-cell development, 70
  role in wasting, 648
  in toxoplasmosis, 228
Transient ischemic attacks, 55
Transmission of HIV infection, 94–95, 124–127
  by blood transfusion, 116, 125–126, 151, 937
  in developing countries, 101, 115–116, 116t, 725
  in health care environment, 127, 152, 935–942, 947–950 (*See also* Health care environment and HIV transmission)
  historical recognition of, 124
  HIV-2, 987–988
  inefficiency of casual contact, 125
  injection for medical reasons, 116, 126
  injection of illicit drugs, 116, 126, 179–188
  mother-to-child, 116, 153, 164–167, 174–175 (*See also* Pediatric HIV infection)
    by birth to infected mother, 126–127, 164–167
    by breast-feeding, 116, 127, 153, 165–166
    HIV-2 infection, 116
    uninfected infants of infected mothers, 694
  prevention of, 127–130, 725–739 (*See also* Prevention of HIV transmission)
  sexual, 101–107, 115, 116t, 125, 151, 187–188 (*See also* Sexual transmission of HIV)
  statistics on, 101
  viral factors in infectiousness, 102
  viral tropism and, 18–19, 102
  to women, 151–152
Travel restrictions, 133–134
Travel-related diseases, 315–322
  clinical course of, 316t
  diarrhea, 315–317
  differential diagnosis of febrile illness, 317–319, 318t
  rare clinical problems, 317t
  risk of exposure to, 315, 316t
  sexually transmitted diseases, 319–320, 319t
  special problems for HIV-infected travelers, 320, 320t
  treatment and vaccination issues, 320–322
    access to medications, 320
    malaria prophylaxis and treatment, 320, 320t
    during pregnancy, 155
    vaccination recommendations, 321–322, 322t

vaccine efficacy, 320–321
vaccine safety, 321
tuberculosis, 262, 265, 315, 319
Trecator. *See* Ethionamide
Treponema pallidum infection. *See* Syphilis
TRH. *See* Thyrotropin-releasing hormone
Triacsin C, 764
Triamcinolone, 507, 510
Triazolam interactions with protease inhibitors, 792, 795, 852
Trichomegaly of eyelashes, 514
Trichomonas vaginalis infection, 319t, 726, 727
Trichosanthin, 906, 907t
Trifluridine, 395
Triglycerides, 644–646
Triiodothyronine (T_3), 634, 635t, 648
Trimethoprim
    adverse effects of, 615, 632, 632t
    interaction with methotrexate, 510
    for *Pneumocystis carinii* pneumonia, 201t, 206, 206t, 467
    for toxoplasmosis, 243
Trimethoprim-sulfamethoxazole (TMP-SMX)
    adverse effects of, 201, 320, 322
        cutaneous, 513, 514
        hepatic, 552–553
        hyperkalemia, 586
        pancreatitis, 543
        renal, 587
    for bacillary angiomatosis, 311, 505
    for isosporiasis, 317, 650
    managing intolerance to, 210, 514
    for microsporidiosis, 344
    for *Pneumocystis carinii* pneumonia, 200–201, 201t–203t, 206t, 574
        choroidal pneumocystosis, 467
        interferon-γ and, 208
        in pregnancy, 157
        prophylactic, 146
            for children, 170, 171
            for isosporiasis, 317
            for *Pneumocystis carinii* pneumonia, 196, 209–211
            for toxoplasmosis, 146, 228, 248, 249t
        ramped dosing with, 210
    for salmonellosis, 317
    for shigellosis, 317
    for toxoplasmosis, 243, 247t
Trimetrexate
    for *Pneumocystis carinii* pneumonia, 201t, 202, 203t, 204
    in pregnancy, 157
    for toxoplasmosis, 243
Trisodium phosphonoformate hexahydrate. *See* Foscarnet
Tropical spastic paraparesis/HTLV-I-associated myelopathy (TSP/HAM), 1016–1017, *1018*
    HTLV-II-associated, 1019
    treatment of, 1020
Trovafloxacin, 244
Troviridine (LY-300046), 754, 839, *840*
TSH. *See* Thyroid-stimulating hormone
TSP/HAM. *See* Tropical spastic paraparesis/HTLV-I-associated myelopathy
TTP. *See* Thrombotic thrombocytopenic purpura

Tuberculosis, 55, 131, 141, 146–147, 261–275
    ascites and, 559
    bone marrow failure and, 615
    clinical features of, 266, 268
    diagnosis of, 268–270, *269*, 269t
        radiographic findings, 267, *267–268*
        sensitivity of tuberculin skin testing in HIV-infected patients, 267–269, 274, 274t
    epidemiology of, 261, *262*, 264–265, *264–265*, 315
        in children, 264–265
        coinfection with HIV, 119, 261–264, 262t, 263t
        outside United States, *119*, *262*, 265, 315
        transmission, 261, 264–265, *265*
    histopathology of, 268, *268*
    impact on course of HIV infection, 263–264
    microbiology of, 270
    mortality from, 261
    multidrug-resistant, 265–266, 266t, 271–272
    nosocomial, 275
    pathogenesis of, 261–264
        development of active disease, 262–263, 263t
        immunologic response, 261
        infectiousness, 263
        Mycobacterium tuberculosis infection, 261
    prevention of, 146, 273–275
        BCG vaccine, 275
        infection control guidelines, 275
        preventive therapy, 273–275
    research and public health priorities related to, 275
    sites of, 266–267, 269
        adrenal, 629
        brain, 484–485
        esophageal, 539
        hepatic, 549, 574, *574*
        ocular, 467
        pericardium, 603
        testicular, 635
    in travelers, 315, 319
    treatment of, 270–273
        in developing countries, 273
        drug toxicity and interactions related to, 272–273, 273t
        effectiveness in HIV-infected persons, 270–271
        nonadherence and directly observed therapy, 272
        in pregnancy, 158
        recommendations for, 271–272, 271t
    wasting syndrome and, 649
Tubulointerstitial nephritis, 587
Tumor necrosis factor-α (TNF-α; cachectin), 66, 193, 407–408, 616, 619–620
    effects on cortisol secretion, 629
    effects on hematopoiesis, 619–620
    HIV effects on production of, 68, 619
    induction of HIV expression by, 68–69, 568
    in microsporidiosis, 344
    in *Pneumocystis carinii* pneumonia, 193
    regulatory influence on early T-cell development, 70
    role in cardiomyopathy, 605–606

    role in host resistance to *Toxoplasma gondii*, 227
    role in Kaposi's sarcoma, 422–424
    role in wasting, 644–645, 648
        effects of TNF-inhibiting drugs, 653
        hypertriglyceridemia, 645, 646
    strategies for inhibition of, 746–747, 770, 798
        thalidomide, 539, 747
    for toxoplasmosis, 244
Tumor necrosis factor-β (TNF-β), 68
Tuskegee syphilis study, 971
Typhoid fever, 318
Typhoid fever vaccine, 321
Tzanck smear, 392

U-90152. *See* Delavirdine
U-96988, 755, 761
Ubenimex, 1020
UDG. *See* Uracil DNA glycosylase
UDP. *See* Uridine diphosphate
U-87201E, 839
Ulcers
    aphthous, 144
        esophageal, 539, *539*
        recurrent, 529, *529*
        thalidomide for, 529, 539, 541
    corneal, 468, 470
    decubitus, 930
    foscarnet-induced cutaneous, 513–514
    necrotizing ulcerative periodontitis, 528, *528*
    peptic, 538, 541
Ultrasound
    in cryptosporidiosis, 333
    hepatic, 555
    pancreatic, 557
Ultraviolet irradiation
    for eosinophilic folliculitis, 511
    for scabies, 507
    for seborrheic dermatitis, 509
UMP. *See* Uridine monophosphate
Unconventional therapies, 903–908
    definition of, 903
    as means of promoting effective communications with patients, 907–908
    media announcements of, 903
    patterns of use of, 903–904
    psychosocial factors influencing use of, 905
    social factors influencing attitudes about and access to, 904–905
    sources of information about, 904t, 908
    types of, 903, 905–907
        altered mental states, 906
        manipulation, 905–906
        unorthodox pharmacotherapy, 906–907
        unproven drugs and vaccines, 907, 907t
    use by patients with HIV infection, 904
Universal precautions, 938–939
Uracil DNA glycosylase (UDG), 40
Urbanization, 117
Uridine diphosphate (UDP), 815, *817*
Uridine monophosphate (UMP), 815, *817*
Uridine triphosphate (UTP), 40, 815, *817*
Urine testing for HIV infection, 667
Urticaria, papular, 512
U.S. Food and Drug Administration (FDA), 807
UTP. *See* Uridine triphosphate

Uveitis
　drug-induced, 457, 470
　HTLV-I-associated, 1018

Vaccine research. *See* AIDS vaccine development
Vaccines for HIV-infected persons
　　contraindications to, 322t
　　efficacy of, 320–321
　　recommendations for children, 171–172, 172t
　　recommendations for pregnant women, 155
　　recommendations for travelers, 321–322, 322t
　　safety of, 321, 322t
Vaginal candidiasis, 152, 154, 357, 358
Vaginal spermicides, 105, 727
Valacyclovir, 393–394, 501
　for herpes zoster, 397–398
　for postexposure prophylaxis, 500
Valvular heart disease, 602
Van der Waals contacts, *758*, 766
Vancomycin
　for bacillary angiomatosis, 311
　for *Clostridium difficile* infection, 317
Varicella-zoster immune globulin (VZIG), 399, 500
Varicella-zoster vaccine, 172, 399, 500
Varicella-zoster virus (VZV) infection, 396–399, 499–501
　acyclovir-resistant, 398–399
　clinical features of, 396–397
　of corneal epithelium, 468
　epidemiology of, 396
　hepatic, 572
　histopathology of, 500
　immunity to, 399
　laboratory diagnosis of, 397
　neurologic, 485
　oral, 525–526
　pathogenesis of, 396
　prevention of, 172, 399, 500
　retinitis, 375, 397, *464*, 464–465
　treatment of, 397–399
Vascular disorders
　hepatic veno-occlusive disease, 576
　ocular, 457–459
Vascular endothelial cell growth factor (VEGF), 424–425
Vasoactive polypeptide, 697
VEGF. *See* Vascular endothelial cell growth factor
Ventilatory support, 208–209
Ventricular enlargement, 169
Verrucae vulgares, 502, *502*
Verrucous carcinoma, *502*, 503, 515
Vertical transmission. *See also* Pediatric HIV infection
　of HIV-1, 164–167, 174–175
　of HIV-2, 988
　of HTLV-I and HTLV-II, 1010–1011, *1011*
Very low density lipoprotein (VLDL), 645
Vidarabine
　effects in progressive multifocal leukoencephalopathy, 414, 415
　for herpes simplex virus infection, 392, 394–395
　for varicella-zoster virus infection, 398

Videx. *See* Didanosine
vif gene, 25–26, *32*, 38, 90
　of HIV-2, 991
Vif protein, 38, 38–39
Villous atrophy, 649
Vinblastine, for Kaposi's sarcoma, 428
Vincristine
　for adult T-cell leukemia/lymphoma, 1019
　for Kaposi's sarcoma, 428
　for lymphomas, 453, 453t, 516
　for thrombocytopenia, 614
Viracept. *See* Nelfinavir
Viral budding, 862
　inhibitors of, 764–765
Viral infections. *See also* specific infections
　cutaneous, 499–504
　cytomegalovirus, 148, 373–385
　esophageal, 538–539, *539*
　features of successful vaccines for, 689–690, 690t, 691t
　hepatitis, 139–141, 550–551, 567–572
　herpes simplex virus, 391–396, 499–501, *500*
　herpes zoster, 143t, 144, 396–397, 499–501, *500*
　immune responses during, 87–89
　management in pregnancy, 158
　oral, 525–528, *526–528*
　during pregnancy, 158
　varicella-zoster virus, 396–399, 499–501
Viral load, 50–51, *50–52*, 612, 862–863, 905. *See also* Plasma HIV-1 RNA level
　AIDS dementia complex and, 487
　daily production of HIV virions, 891
　"induction trials" for reduction of, 809
　methods for assessment of, 673
　monitoring during pregnancy, 155, 678
　prognostic significance of, 673–675
　sexual HIV transmission and, 102
　suppression below level of quantification, 873
　therapeutic management based on, 51, 673–682
　　in adults, 673–678
　　in children, 678–681
Viral replication, 13, *14*, 59, 611–612, 673, 780–781, 848
　during advanced disease, 64
　antiretroviral therapy for suppression of, 148–149
　during clinical latency, 64
　cytokine induction of, 68–69, *70*
　cytokine suppression of, 69–70, *70*
　effect on lymphoid architecture, 66
　of HIV-2, 988–992
　HIV-1 life cycle, 861–862
　immune responses for limitation of, 89
　during initial infection, 62–64
　interleukin-2 effects on, 68
　opportunistic infections and, 146
　role of cytotoxic T lymphocytes in, 63, 64
　site of, 59
　stages that may be targets for therapeutic intervention, 751, 756t, 780, 781t
　viral "set-point" and, 674
Viral tropism, 18, *18*
　HIV transmission and, 18–19, 102
　pathogenesis and, 19, 691–692

Viramune. *See* Nevirapine
Virologic failure, 677–678, 876
Virologic set-point, 62, 64
Visual disturbances, 457. *See also* Ocular sequelae
Visualization, 906
Vitamin A deficiency, 101, 104–105
Vitamin B_{12} deficiency, 612–613, 649
Vitamin C, for tropical spastic paraparesis/HTLV-I-associated myelopathy, 1020
Vitamin treatments, 907
Vitreous humor biopsies, 457
Vittaforma corneae infection. *See* Microsporidiosis
VLDL. *See* Very low density lipoprotein
von Willebrand factor, 621
vpr gene, 3, 26, *32*, 39, 90, 988, *989*
　of HIV-2, 991
Vpr protein, 39–41
　cell-cycle arrest by, 40
　interaction with uracil DNA glycosylase, 40
　nuclear transport and, 40–41
vpu gene, 26, *32*, 90, 988
Vpu protein, 39
vpx gene, 26, 988, *989*, 991–992
Vpx protein, 39–41
Vx-478 (amprenavir; 141W94), 149, *755*, 761, 795–796, 875t
VZIG. *See* Varicella-zoster immune globulin
VZV. *See* Varicella-zoster virus infections

Wasting syndrome, 56, 148, 643–654
　body composition in disease, 643–644
　clinical approach to, 649–654
　　anabolic therapies, 652–653
　　anticytokine therapy, 653–654
　　appetite stimulants, 651
　　documenting weight trends, 649–650
　　hyperalimentation, 650–651
　　nutritional status improvement related to treatment for infection, 650
　　role of such symptoms as lethargy and fatigue, 651–652
　　treating gastrointestinal disease, 650
　energy balance and, 646–649
　　gastrointestinal disease, 648–649
　　hypermetabolism, 646–647
　　malabsorption, 148, 649
　　protein wasting, 647
　　role of cytokines, 648
　　role of secondary infection and anorexia, 647
　mechanisms and mediators of, 644–646
　　cytokines and hypertriglyceridemia, 646
　　cytokines and in vivo lipid metabolism, 645
　　disturbances in triglyceride metabolism, 646
　　energy balance and weight loss, 644
　　fat cell catabolism and cachectin hypothesis, 644–645
　　role of cytokines in metabolic disturbances and wasting, 644
　　TNF-induced changes in lipid metabolism, 645
　mortality related to, 643, 644
　nutritional cardiomyopathy, 606

valvular heart disease and, 602
weight loss, 146, 315, 643
 in women, 644
Western blot assay, 140, 167, 663
 for HTLV-I and HTLV-II, 1006, *1006*
Wills, 979
Women and HIV infection, 123, 151–159
 counseling HIV-infected women about reproductive choices, 958–959
 epidemiology of, 151–152
 ethics and, 953
 gynecologic complications, 152
  cervical dysplasia/cancer, 143, 148, 152, 154
  management of, 154
  menstrual cycle, 152, 636
  pelvic inflammatory disease, 152, 154
  vaginal candidiasis, 152, 154, 357, 358
 impact on women's health care, 153
 injection drug use and, 151
 management in nonpregnant women, 153–154
  antiviral therapy, 154
  initial assessment, 153
  laboratory testing and monitoring, 153–154
  opportunistic infections, 154
 management in pregnancy, 152, 154–158 (*See also* Pregnancy and HIV infection)
 mother-to-child HIV transmission, 116, 153, 164–167, 174–175 (*See also* Pediatric HIV infection)
 natural history of, 152
 prevention of, 158
  gender gap in developing countries, 969–970
  sexual transmission, 105–106, 106t
  testing women at risk for, 158–159
 wasting syndrome, 644
World Health Organization (WHO)
 Global Programme on AIDS, 124
 Multi-Centre Study, 182
Wound decontamination after HIV exposure, 947
WR-6026, 208

Xanthosine monophosphate, 818, *818*
Xerosis, 512, *512*
Xerostomia, 529

Yellow fever, 318, 321, 322

Zalcitabine (ddC), 5, 149, 601, 751, 780, 786–787, 863t
 adverse effects of, 784t, 787, 863t, 865t, 866
  pancreatitis, 543, 557
  peripheral neuropathy, 490, 866
  pill esophagitis, 539–540
 antiviral activity of, *752*, 786
 chemical structure of, *752*, 786, *827*
 for children, 172–173
 clinical trials of, 786, 866
 combined with other drugs, 866, 876–878 (*See also* Combination antiretroviral therapy)
  ritonavir, 849
  saquinavir, 849
  zidovudine, 783–784, 786
 dosage of, 782t, 786, 863t, 865t
 drug interactions with, 786, 787
 metabolism of, 786, *827*, 828–830
 pharmacology of, 786, 826–828, 865
 in pregnancy, 157t
 use in renal disease, 786
 viral resistance to, 786–787, 875t, 894–895
ZDV. *See* Zidovudine
Zerit. *See* Stavudine
Zidovudine (ZDV), 5, 149, 601, 751, 780, 783–785, 863t, 864
 for acute exanthem of HIV disease, 499
 for adult T-cell leukemia/lymphoma and, 1020
 adverse effects of, 784–785, 784t, 822, 863t, 864, 865t
  carcinogenicity, 156
  cardiac, 606
  central nervous system symptoms, 864
  cutaneous, 513
  hematopoietic, 615, 784, 822, 864
  hepatic, 552, 576
  management of, 864
  myopathy, 491, 587
  nausea, 864
  pill esophagitis, 539–540

antiretroviral activity of, *752*, 783
chemical structure of, *752*, *819*
for children, 172–173
 improvement of neurologic disease after, 169
 infants at risk for HIV infection, 170–171
clinical trials of, 783–784, 864
combined with other drugs, 769, 783–784, 864, 876–878 (*See also* Combination antiretroviral therapy)
 didanosine, 783–785
 indinavir, 851
 lamivudine, 784, 788
 nelfinavir, 852
 ritonavir, 849
 saquinavir, 792, 849
 zalcitabine, 783–784, 786
for cryptosporidiosis, 338
for cytomegalovirus retinitis, 461
development of, 783
dosage of, 782t, 784, 863t, 865t
drug interactions with, 785
 antituberculosis drugs, 273t
 ganciclovir, 379
formulations of, 784
for glomerulosclerosis, 592–593
GM-CSF administered with, 617
for hepatitis B virus infection, 570
for hepatitis C virus infection, 571
mechanism of cell penetration by, 819
metabolism of, 783, 819–822, *820–821*
for oral hairy leukoplakia, 527
penetration of blood-brain barrier by, 489
pharmacology of, 783, 819–822, 864
for postexposure prophylaxis, 870, 948–949
in pregnancy to prevent vertical HIV transmission, 155–156, 157t, 166, 174, 728, 746, 948, 970–971
for progressive multifocal leukoencephalopathy, 415
for psoriasis, 510
for thrombocytopenia, 614
use in renal or hepatic disease, 783, 785
viral resistance to, 765–766, 864, 875t, 891–894, *892–893*, 894t
Zinc fingers, 764, 798
Zithromax. *See* Azithromycin
Zonalon. *See* Doxepin cream